Principles
and
Practice of Pediatric Oncology

Principles
and
Practice of

Pediatric
Oncology

edited by

Philip A. Pizzo, M.D.

Chief of Pediatrics
Head, Infectious Diseases
National Cancer Institute
Bethesda, Maryland

David G. Poplack, M.D.

Head, Leukemia Section
Pediatric Branch
National Cancer Institute
Bethesda, Maryland

with 107 contributors

**J. B. Lippincott
Company
Philadelphia**
London · Mexico City · New York · St. Louis · São Paulo · Sydney

Sponsoring Editor: Delois Patterson
Coordinating Editor: Leslie E. Hoeltzel
Indexer: Barbara Littlewood
Senior Designer: Anita Curry
Designer/Cover Designer: Anthony Frizano
Production Manager: Kathleen P. Dunn
Production Coordinator: Fred Wood/Charlene C. Squibb
Compositor: Tapsco
Printer/Binder: Halliday Lithograph

6   5   4   3   2   1

Library of Congress Cataloging-in-Publication Data

Principles and practice of pediatric oncology.

Includes bibliographies and index.
1. Tumors in children.   I. Pizzo, Philip A.
II. Poplack, David G. [DNLM: 1. Neoplasms—in infancy
and childhood. QZ 200 P957]
RC281.C4P65 1988   618.92'994   87-35353
ISBN 0-397-50821-2

The authors and publisher have exerted every effort to
ensure that drug selection and dosage set forth in this text
are in accord with current recommendations and practice
at the time of publication. However, in view of ongoing
research, changes in government regulations, and the
constant flow of information relating to drug therapy and
drug reactions, the reader is urged to check the package
insert for each drug for any change in indications and
dosage and for added warnings and precautions. This is
particularly important when the recommended agent is a
new or infrequently employed drug.

To Ted. Friend and teacher in matters of life and death

c o n t r i b u t o r s

associate editors

Surgery
Daniel M. Hays, M.D.

Radiation Therapy
Laurence E. Kun, M.D.

Genetics and Immunology
John J. Mulvihill, M.D.

Pathology
Timothy J. Triche, M.D.

Arthur Ablin, M.D.
Clinical Professor of Pediatrics
Chief, Pediatric Clinical Oncology
University of California at San Francisco
Children's Hospital Medical Center
San Francisco, California

Saresh Advani, M.D.
Head, Department of Medical Oncology
Tata Memorial Hospital
Parel, Bombay, India

Leland A. Albright, M.D.
Associate Professor of Neurosurgery
University of Pittsburgh
Attending Neurosurgeon
Children's Hospital
Pittsburgh, Pennsylvania

Arnold J. Altman, M.D.
Professor of Pediatrics
Head, Division of Hematology/Oncology
University of Connecticut Health Center
Farmington, Connecticut

Frank M. Balis, M.D.
Senior Staff Fellow
Pediatric Branch
National Cancer Institute
Bethesda, Maryland

J. B. Beckwith, M.D.
Professor of Pathology
Clinical Professor of Pediatrics
University of Colorado
Chairman, Department of Pathology
The Children's Hospital
Denver, Colorado

Luis Becu, M.D.
Professor and Chairman, Department of
Pathology
Children's Hospital of Buenos Aires
Oncology Unit
Buenos Aires, Argentina

Helga Binder, M.D.
Associate Professor, Child Health and
Development
George Washington University Medical
School
Associate Physiatrist
Children's Hospital National Medical
Center
Washington, District of Columbia

Julie Blatt, M.D.
Associate Professor, Division of Hema-
tology-Oncology
Department of Pediatrics
University of Pittsburgh School of Medi-
cine
Children's Hospital of Pittsburgh
Pittsburgh, Pennsylvania

W. Archie Bleyer, M.D.
American Cancer Society
Professor of Clinical Oncology
University of Washington School of
Medicine
Children's Hospital and Medical Center
Fred Hutchinson Cancer Research
Center
Seattle, Washington

Shirley Bonnem
Vice President, Public Relations and
Development
The Children's Hospital of Philadelphia
Philadelphia, Pennsylvania

N. Breslow, Ph.D.
Professor and Chairman
Department of Biostatistics
University of Washington
Seattle, Washington

George R. Buchanan, M.D.
Professor of Pediatrics
University of Texas–Southwestern Medi-
cal Center
Director, Hematology-Oncology
Children's Medical Center of Dallas
Dallas, Texas

Beatriz de Camargo, M.D.
Pediatric Oncologist
São Paulo, Brazil

Andrea O. Cavazzana, M.D.
Institute of Anatomic Pathology
Padova, Italy

George P. Chrousos, M.D.
Clinical Professor of Pediatrics
Georgetown University Medical Center
Senior Investigator
National Institute of Child Health and
  Human Development
Bethesda, Maryland

Harvey J. Cohen, M.D., Ph.D.
Professor of Pediatrics
Chief, Division of Pediatric Hematol-
  ogy/Oncology
University of Rochester School of Medi-
  cine
Rochester, New York

Jeffrey Cossman, M.D.
Senior Investigator
Laboratory of Pathology
National Cancer Institute
National Institutes of Health
Bethesda, Maryland

Carol M. Cronin, M.S.
Associate Director
Clinical Research
The Purdue Frederick Company
Norwalk, Connecticut

Giulio J. D'Angio, M.D.
Professor of Radiation Therapy, Pediat-
  ric Oncology, and Radiology
School of Medicine, University of Penn-
  sylvania
Director, Children's Cancer Research
  Center
The Children's Hospital of Philadelphia
Philadelphia, Pennsylvania

Patricia Deasy–Spinetta, M.A., M.S.
School Psychologist
San Diego Unified School District
San Diego, California

Blanca Diez, M.D.
Pediatric Oncologist
Children's Hospital of Buenos Aires
Oncology Unit
Buenos Aires, Argentina

Sarah S. Donaldson, M.D.
Associate Professor of Radiology
Division of Radiation Therapy
Stanford University Medical Center
Stanford, California

Lorah D. Dorn, R.N., M.S.N.
Department of Individual and Family
  Studies
The Pennsylvania State University
University Park, Pennsylvania
National Institute of Mental Health
Bethesda, Maryland

Edwin C. Douglass, M.D.
Department of Hematology/Oncology
Associate Member, St. Jude Children's
  Research Hospital
Assistant Professor of Pediatrics
University of Tennessee
Memphis, Tennessee

Janie Eddy, R.N., M.S.N., P.N.P.
Pediatric Branch, National Cancer Insti-
  tute
Bethesda, Maryland

Peter R. Egbert, M.D.
Department of Ophthalmology
Stanford University Medical Center
Stanford, California

Frederick Eilber, M.D.
Professor of Surgery
Division of Surgical Oncology
UCLA School of Medicine
Los Angeles, California

Susan S. Ellenberg, Ph.D.
Biometric Research Branch
Cancer Therapy Evaluation Program
Division of Cancer Treatment
National Cancer Institute
Bethesda, Maryland

Judith Falloon, M.D.
Medical Officer, AIDS Section
Critical Care Medicine Department
Clinical Center
National Institutes of Health
Bethesda, Maryland

Robert M. Filler, M.D., F.R.C.S.(C)
Professor of Surgery
The University of Toronto
Surgeon-in-Chief
The Hospital for Sick Children
Toronto, Ontario, Canada

J. Finklestein, M.D.
Adjunct Professor of Pediatrics
UCLA School of Medicine
Director of Pediatric Hematology/On-
  cology
Jonathan Jaques Children's Cancer
  Center
Los Angeles, California

John C. Fletcher, Ph.D.
Chief, Bioethics Program
The Clinical Center
The National Institutes of Health
Bethesda, Maryland

**Carolyn R. Freeman, M.B., B.S.,
  F.R.C.P.(C)**
Professor and Chairman
Department of Radiation Oncology
McGill University
Montreal, Quebec, Canada

Nazli Gad-el-Mawla, M.D.
Professor and Head, Department of
  Medical Oncology
National Cancer Institute
Fom-el-Khalig
Cairo, Egypt

Lynn H. Gerber, M.D.
Adjunct Associate Professor
George Washington University
Chief, Department of Rehabilitation
  Medicine
Warren Grant Magnuson Clinical Center
National Institutes of Health
Bethesda, Maryland

D. M. Green, M.D.
Associate Professor of Pediatrics
State University of New York, Buffalo
Cancer Research Pediatrician
Roswell Park Memorial Institute
Buffalo, New York

**Mark Greenberg, M.B.Ch.B.,
  F.R.C.P. (C)**
Associate Professor of Pediatrics
University of Toronto
Senior Oncologist
Hospital for Sick Children
Toronto, Ontario, Canada

Holcombe E. Grier, M.D.
Assistant Professor of Pediatrics
Harvard Medical School
Dana-Farber Cancer Institute
The Children's Hospital
Boston, Massachusetts

James W. Hathorn, M.D.
Assistant Professor of Medicine
Divisions of Hematology/Oncology and
  Infectious Diseases
Department of Medicine
Duke University School of Medicine
Durham, North Carolina

Frances Ann Hayes, M.D., F.R.C.P.(C)
Professor, Department of Pediatrics
University of Tennessee, Memphis
Member, Department of Hematology-
  Oncology
St. Jude Children's Research Hospital
Memphis, Tennessee

Daniel M. Hays, M.D.
Professor of Surgery and Pediatrics
University of Southern California School
  of Medicine
Section Head, Hematology/Oncology
Children's Hospital of Los Angeles
Los Angeles, California

Richard L. Heideman, M.D.
Pediatric Branch
National Cancer Institute
Bethesda, Maryland

Stephen P. Hersh, M.D., F.A.P.A.
Clinical Professor of Psychiatry and
    Child Health and Human Develop-
    ment
George Washington University School
    of Medicine
Washington, District of Columbia
Consultant, Pediatric Branch
National Cancer Institute
Bethesda, Maryland

John S. Holcenberg, M.D.
Professor of Pediatrics and Biochemistry
University of Southern California
Los Angeles, California

Doris A. Howell, M.D.
Professor of Pediatrics
Department of Pediatrics
University of California at San Diego
School of Medicine
San Diego, California

Hart Isaacs, Jr., M.D.
Assistant Professor of Pathology
University of Southern California
School of Medicine
Attending Pathologist
Department of Pathology
Children's Hospital of Los Angeles
Los Angeles, California

Mark A. Israel, M.D.
Head, Molecular Genetics Section
Pediatric Branch
National Cancer Institute
Attending Physician, Clinical Center
Bethesda, Maryland

Elaine S. Jaffe, M.D.
Laboratory of Pathology
National Cancer Institute
Bethesda, Maryland

P. Kelalis, M.D.
Chairman, Department of Urology
Mayo Clinic
Professor of Pediatric Urology
Mayo Medical School
Rochester, Minnesota

Timothy Kinsella, M.D.
Professor and Chairman
Department of Human Oncology
University of Wisconsin Medical School
Madison, Wisconsin

Laurence E. Kun, M.D.
Chairman, Department of Radiologic
    Oncology
St. Jude Children's Research Hospital
Memphis, Tennessee

Stephan Ladisch, M.D.
Associate Professor of Pediatrics
Department of Pediatrics
Division of Hematology/Oncology
UCLA School of Medicine and Medical
    Center
Los Angeles, California

Beverly Lange, M.D.
Associate Professor of Pediatrics
School of Medicine, University of Penn-
    sylvania
Director, Oncology Ambulatory Services
Children's Hospital of Philadelphia
Philadelphia, Pennsylvania

Shirley B. Lansky, M.D.
Professor of Psychiatry
University of Illinois
President and Director, Illinois Cancer
    Council
Chicago, Illinois

Brigid G. Leventhal, M.D.
Associate Professor of Pediatrics and
    Oncology
Johns Hopkins Hospital
Baltimore, Maryland

Frederick P. Li, M.D.
Head, Clinical Studies Section
Clinical Epidemiology Branch
National Cancer Institute
Bethesda, Maryland

Hai Peng Lin, M.D.
Associate Professor of Paediatrics
Department of Medicine
Faculty of Medicine
University of Malaysia
Lembah Pantai, Kuala Lumpur

Michael P. Link, M.D.
Associate Professor of Pediatrics
Stanford University School of Medicine
Staff Hematologist/Oncologist
Children's Hospital at Stanford
Palo Alto, California

Marcy A. List, Ph.D.
Instructor of Psychology
Department of Psychiatry
University of Illinois at Chicago
Chicago, Illinois

**Ian T. Magrath, M.B.B.S., F.R.C.P.,
    F.R.C.Path.**
Head, Lymphoma Biology Section
Pediatric Branch
National Cancer Institute
Bethesda, Maryland

Ida M. Martinson, R.N., Ph.D.
Professor and Chair
Department of Family Health Care
School of Nursing
University of California, San Francisco
San Francisco, California

June L. McCalla, R.N., M.S.N., C.P.N.P.
Clinical Nurse Specialist/Practitioner
Cancer Nursing Service
Clinical Center
National Institutes of Health
Bethesda, Maryland

Robert W. Miller, M.D.
Chief, Clinical Epidemiology Branch
Division of Cancer Etiology
National Cancer Institute
Bethesda, Maryland

Angela W. Miser, M.B.B.S.
Special Project Associate
Mayo Clinic
Rochester, Minnesota

James S. Miser, M.D.
Senior Investigator
Pediatric Branch
National Cancer Institutes
Bethesda, Maryland

Grace Powers Monaco, J.D.
Chair, Board of Directors, The Candle-
    lighters Childhood Cancer Foundation
Washington, District of Columbia

John E. Moulder, Ph.D.
Department of Radiation Oncology
The Medical College of Wisconsin
Milwaukee, Wisconsin

John J. Mulvihill, M.D.
Head, Clinical Genetics Section
National Cancer Institute
Bethesda, Maryland

Mark E. Nesbit, Jr., M.D.
Professor of Pediatrics
Department of Pediatrics
Health Science Center
The University of Minnesota
Minneapolis, Minnesota

Jeffrey A. Norton, M.D.
Head, Surgical Metabolism Section
Surgery Branch
National Cancer Institute
Bethesda, Maryland

James A. O'Neill, Jr., M.D.
Professor of Pediatric Surgery
School of Medicine, University of Penn-
    sylvania
Surgeon-in-Chief
The Children's Hospital of Philadelphia
Philadelphia, Pennsylvania

Jorge A. Ortega, M.D.
Section Head for Oncology
Division of Hematology-Oncology
Children's Hospital of Los Angeles
Professor of Pediatrics
University of Southern California
School of Medicine
Los Angeles, California

Roger J. Packer, M.D.
Associate Professor of Neurology and
    Pediatrics
School of Medicine, University of Penn-
    sylvania
Associate Attending of Neurology and
    Pediatrics
Director of Neuro-Oncology Program
The Children's Hospital of Philadelphia
Philadelphia, Pennsylvania

Bruce R. Parker, M.D.
Professor of Clinical Radiology and
    Clinical Pediatrics
Division of Diagnostic Radiology
Stanford University Medical Center
Stanford, California

Robertson Parkman, M.D.
Director, Bone Marrow Transplant Ser-
    vice
Children's Hospital of Los Angeles
Los Angeles, California

Jane Peter, B.S., R.D.
Clinical Research Dietician
Clinical Center
National Institutes of Health
Bethesda, Maryland

Antonio Sergio Petrilli, M.D.
Assistant, Pediatric Oncology Depart-
    ment
Fundacao Antonio Prudente
Instituto Central
Hospital A.C. Camargo
Chief, Pediatric Oncology
Paulista Medical School
São Paulo, Brazil

Sherry L. Phillips, M.P.A., O.T.R.
Therapist Officer
United States Public Health Service
Food and Drug Administration
Rochester, New York

Philip A. Pizzo, M.D.
Chief of Pediatrics
Head, Infectious Diseases
National Cancer Institute
Bethesda, Maryland

David G. Poplack, M.D.
Head, Leukemia Section
Pediatric Branch
National Cancer Institute
Bethesda, Maryland

Charles B. Pratt, M.D.
Professor of Pediatrics
Department of Pediatrics
University of Tennessee, Memphis
Member, Hematology-Oncology
St. Jude Children's Research Hospital
Memphis, Tennessee

Douglas J. Pritchard, M.D.
Professor of Orthopedic Surgery
Mayo Clinic
Rochester, Minnesota

Norma K. C. Ramsay, M.D.
Professor, Department of Pediatrics
University of Minnesota
Minneapolis, Minnesota

R. Beverly Raney, Jr., M.D.
Professor of Pediatrics
University of Virginia School of Medicine
Chief, Division of Pediatric Hematol-
    ogy/Oncology
University of Virginia Hospital
Charlottesville, Virginia

Gregory H. Reaman, M.D.
Associate Professor of Pediatrics
George Washington University School
    of Medicine
Department of Pediatrics
Children's Hospital National Medical
    Center
Washington, District of Columbia

Chris Ritter–Sterr, M.S., R.N.
Nurse Specialist
Department of Psychiatry
University of Illinois at Chicago
Chicago, Illinois

Maryann Roper, M.D.
Senior Investigator
Biologics Evaluation Section
Investigatonal Drug Branch
Cancer Therapy Evaluation Program
National Cancer Institute
Bethesda, Maryland

Lucy B. Rorke, M.D.
Professor of Pathology and Neurology
University of Pennsylvania
Neuropathologist
Children's Hospital of Philadelphia
Philadelphia, Pennsylvania

Arthur J. Ross III, M.D.
Assistant Professor of Pediatric Surgery
School of Medicine, University of Penn-
    sylvania
Attending Surgeon
The Children's Hospital of Philadelphia
Philadelphia, Pennsylvania

Judith Ross, M.S.W., A.C.S.W.
Coordinator, Oncology Social Services
The Children's Hospital of Philadelphia
Philadelphia, Pennsylvania

Stephen E. Sallan, M.D.
Associate Professor of Pediatrics
Harvard Medical School
Clinical Director of Pediatric Oncology
Dana-Farber Cancer Institute
The Childrens Hospital
Boston, Massachusetts

**Sheila Judge Santacroce, R.N.,
    M.S.N., C.P.N.P., C.N.A.**
Head Nurse, Pediatric Oncology
Cancer Nursing Service
Warren Grant Magnuson Clinical Center
National Institutes of Health
Bethesda, Maryland

Cindy L. Schwartz, M.D.
Division of Hematology/Oncology
Department of Pediatrics
The Cancer Center
University of Rochester Medical Center
Rochester, New York

Nita L. Seibel, M.D.
Assistant Professor of Child Health and
    Development
George Washington University School
    of Medicine and Health Sciences
Attending, Hematology/Oncology
Children's Hospital National Medical
    Center
Washington, District of Columbia

V. Shanta, M.D.
Director and Scientific Director
Cancer Institute (W.I.A.)
Madras, India

Stuart E. Siegel, M.D.
Professor of Pediatrics
Chief, Division of Hematology/Oncol-
    ogy
Children's Hospital of Los Angeles
Los Angeles, California

Edwin Ide Smith, M.D.
Professor of Surgery
University of Oklahoma
College of Medicine
Pediatric Surgeon
Oklahoma Children's Memorial Hospital
Oklahoma City, Oklahoma

John J. Spinetta, Ph.D.
Professor of Psychology
Department of Psychology
San Diego State University
San Diego, California

Melvin Tefft, M.D., F.A.C.R.
Director and Chairman, Department of
    Radiation Therapy
Rhode Island Hospital
Professor of Radiation Medicine
Brown University
Providence, Rhode Island

Timothy J. Triche, M.D., Ph.D.
Chief, Ultrastructural Pathology Section
Laboratory of Pathology
National Cancer Institute
Bethesda, Maryland

Richard S. Ungerleider, M.D.
Head, Pediatrics Section
Clinical Investigations Branch
Cancer Therapy Evaluation Program
National Cancer Institute
Bethesda, Maryland

Jan van Eys, Ph.D., M.D.
Mosbacker Professor of Pediatrics
Head, Division of Pediatrics
University of Texas System Cancer
    Center
M. D. Anderson Hospital and Tumor In-
    stitute
Houston, Texas

Kenneth I. Weinberg, M.D.
Division of Research Immunology/Bone
    Marrow Transplantation
Children's Hospital of Los Angeles
Assistant Professor of Pediatrics
University of Southern California School
    of Medicine
Los Angeles, California

Howard J. Weinstein, M.D.
Associate Professor of Pediatrics
Department of Pediatric Hematology/
    Oncology
Dana-Farber Cancer Institute
Boston, Massachusetts

Lori S. Wiener, Ph.D.
Clinical Social Worker
Department of Social Work
National Institutes of Health
Bethesda, Maryland

Christopher Williams
Consultant Hematologist/Oncologist
Hamad General Hospital
Doha, Qatar

foreword

Being up-to-date on the clinical and scientific base of pediatric oncology is invaluable for all of us who practice cancer medicine. Pediatric malignancies have been a wellspring of information regarding all cancers. *Principles and Practice of Pediatric Oncology* promises to continue that tradition. Most of the current generation of medical oncologists, for example, began their education with the study of pediatric tumors. It was there that they learned the lessons of the need for, and the value of, systemic therapy, and the relation between tumor volume and outcome. The most important lesson of all, as it turned out, was applicable to all cancer specialists: the need for a combined-modality approach, to integrate regional and systemic treatments. This approach has now evolved in both pediatric and adult cancer medicine to more than just adding one therapy to another; it involves a carefully crafted matching of the right amounts of the different modalities to effect maximum benefit and minimize side-effects. In adults, this approach in breast cancer, sarcomas, and lymphomas—to name just a few tumors for which the benefits of combined modality treatment are apparent—came from lessons learned in childhood leukemia, Wilms' tumor, and rhabdomyosarcomas. We have also learned from pediatric oncologists that advances can be rapidly translated into practice. To the credit of pediatricians, it is an unusual child with cancer who is not part of a program that both standardizes the delivery of optimum treatment and collects information vital to the next generation of protocols, all the while preserving the practice of pediatric cancer medicine. Sadly, medical, surgical, and radiation oncologists have yet to learn this valuable lesson of constancy from our pediatric colleagues.

As we close in on cancer at the molecular level, we can continue to learn by focusing on the clinical differences and similarities between pediatric and adult tumors. In the flurry of new information available to us concomitant with the biologic revolution, for example, the puzzle of the histologic differences between pediatric and adult malignancies is yielding to our curiosity. In experimental animals, carcinogens that induce, say, breast cancer in an exposed adult can produce neuroblastoma and other types of tumors characteristic of the pediatric population, if exposure takes place during embryogenesis when more genetic programs are apparently vulnerable to damage. We now have, I believe, an understanding of what the cancer cell is trying to do: it is trying to create a whole human being. In this somewhat animated view of the cancer process, exposure to carcinogenic influences very likely triggers highly conserved genetic programs, under the influence of what we now know as oncogenes, that are essential to embryologic growth and development—hence the different phenotypes in pediatric and adult malignancies, vis-à-vis time of exposure. Most of the programs required to create a whole human being are, of course, not available in adults, although teratomas with hair and teeth tell us how frighteningly close the cancer cell can come to its goals. The most lethal of these developmental programs is the capacity for rapid cellular expansion and the ability to migrate, the malignant counterparts being unrestricted growth and lethal metastases.

All these lessons, learned and unlearned, are in *Principles and Practice of Pediatric Oncology* in their modern-day version. This is the most comprehensive textbook of pediatric oncology yet assembled. The first section is sufficiently broad on the basics of the new biology and genetics to bring the physician up-to-date in the science behind the management of pediatric cancers. The remainder of the book covers every aspect of childhood cancers, including the most important aspects of managing the fruits of the success in this field, the complications of long survival.

Those of us concerned with cancer medicine in adults can, I suppose, never really catch up with the pediatric oncologists. Long survivors of combined modality treatment from the pediatric population will always be the benchmark for observing the consequences of successful treatment. The need to continue to share our experiences is even greater today. These long survivors of combined modality therapy are now becoming adults, and, in addition to giving us the vital information we need on the consequences of successful treatment in the patients themselves, the normal children of these patients are now just beginning to provide us some assurance that the genetic consequences of our treatments in offspring appear to be minimal.

Given the fluid nature of the practice of cancer medicine these days and the maturity of pediatric oncology as a specialty, it is an unusual oncologist or general physician who does not or will not have the occasion to deal with problems related to pediatric oncology in his or her practice. *Principles and Practice of Pediatric Oncology,* at long last, gives the physician the long-needed single, up-to-date reference source missing for so many years.

Vincent T. DeVita, Jr., M.D.

preface

The education of the pediatric oncologist and all who engage in the care of children with cancer must be comprehensive and complete. The range of knowledge that must be acquired needs to include the principles of epidemiology, cell biology, molecular genetics, and immunology as well as the fundamentals of pharmacology, surgery, and radiation therapy. Moreover, because cancer impacts on the *total child and family,* every caregiver must also be knowledgeable about the physical and psychosocial care and rehabilitation of the patient and his or her family. The scope of the pediatric oncologist also includes an in-depth understanding of the long-term sequelae of cancer and its treatment, including its impact on the education and occupation of cancer survivors. *Principles and Practice of Pediatric Oncology* has been structured to provide a comprehensive review of the multiple disciplines that make up the care and research agendas for children with cancer.

Pediatric oncology serves as a unique model for the study, treatment, and, possibly, prevention of cancer. The successful use of combination chemotherapy and multimodal regimens for acute lymphoblastic leukemia (Chapter 16) and a variety of solid tumors (Chapters 24–34) represents a cornerstone of modern oncology. With effective therapies, however, the complexity and the heterogeneity of cancer in children have become more apparent (Chapter 6), and it is increasingly common for clinical and biological prognostic factors to be included in the design of treatment regimens. Accordingly, just as immunophenotyping and cytogenetics provided evidence of tumor diversity (Chapter 2 and 4) in the 1970s, gene rearrangements, oncogene profiles, and other techniques of modern molecular biology are being employed in the 1980s to evaluate tumor tissue (Chapter 3), provide biological markers (Chapter 8), and guide management. Indeed, the boundaries between pathology, immunology, cell biology, and molecular biology are becoming increasingly blurred and coalesced in pediatric oncology.

Because cancer is a rare entity in children, the pediatrician must be able to differentiate its signs and symptoms from other more common clinical entities. Knowing when a child requires more intensive and invasive investigation is a critical component of the diagnostic process (Chapters 1 and 5). Understanding which tests to perform, in what sequence, and what their advantages and limitations are requires special expertise in relation to the pediatric patient (Chapter 7).

Because cancer in children interrupts normal growth and development, unique care must be taken in defining the dose, route, and schedule of chemotherapy and radiation therapy (Chapters 9 and 11) as well as in the choice of the surgical procedures that may be required for diagnosis or for achieving local tumor control (Chapter 10). These issues are particularly critical in the management of the infant with cancer (Chapter 12), further emphasizing that any physician involved in the care of children with cancer must be cognizant of the principles that ensure the optimal safety and quality of treatment.

Skill in the supportive care of the child or adolescent undergoing cancer treatment is also an essential element of successful treatment. This must include a detailed knowledge of the metabolic and mechanical emergencies that may ensue from cancer or its treatment (Chapter 37), including the diagnosis, management, and prevention of infectious complications (Chapter 39) as well as the management of nausea and vomiting (Chapter 45), pain (Chapter 44), and hematologic (Chapter 38) and nutritional supportive care (Chapter 40). An awareness and understanding of the impact of cancer and its treatment on the psychological health of the patient and family are also necessary prerequisites for appropriate intervention (Chapters 41, 42, and 46).

The impact of cancer in the child reaches beyond medical and emotional health issues. The financial cost of care can be considerable, and awareness of the direct and out-of-pocket expenses and resources for reimbursement is critical (Chapter 43). A number of important ethical, legal, and advocacy issues may also arise in the treatment of the child or adolescent with cancer, revolving about such issues as compliance, consequences of therapy, and experimental regimens (Chapters 15 and 53).

The pediatric oncologist must also be knowledgeable in the design, execution, analysis, and interpretation of clinical trials (Chapter 13). This is underscored by the relative rarity of childhood tumors, which makes it important that clinical studies be designed to address critical questions and provide meaningful answers in an efficient manner. Limited numbers of patients also requires close cooperation among investigators. The development of cooperative trials in pediatric oncology thus serves as a highly successful model for medical oncology.

Today, more than 50% of children with cancer will survive. Attention to the long-term rehabilitation (Chapter 47), educational needs (Chapter 51), and vocational and occupational needs (Chapter 52) of cancer survivors has therefore become increasingly important. The long-term complications of cancer (Chapter 50) and its treatment require close monitoring. New

and unanticipated diseases, such as AIDS (Chapter 36), can also impact on the child with cancer and the practice of the pediatric oncologist.

Despite the available therapy and current advances, many children who are diagnosed with cancer will not survive. Helping these children and their families to face terminal illness and death, whether it occurs in the hospital, at home, or in a hospice, becomes an important consideration for all caregivers (Chapters 46 and 49).

The success of pediatric oncology in the western world is unprecedented. Although malnutrition and infectious diseases are numerically more important, children in developing countries still develop cancer. Understanding the epidemiologic and biological aspects of childhood cancer around the world and developing and modifying methods for intervention are important considerations (Chapters 1 and 54).

In *Principles and Practice of Pediatric Oncology* we have attempted to deal with a broad range of important topics in conceptual and practical detail. We acknowledge the efforts, care, and patience of the contributors to *Principles and Practice of Pediatric Oncology*. To develop a textbook that presents a current and unified approach required considerable integration and organization. The process, although demanding, was a stimulating and exciting venture, and it is our hope that the final product reflects well on the cooperation and enthusiasm of all who have been involved.

Finally, we acknowledge the help and assistance of the J. B. Lippincott Company, especially Stuart Freeman, Sanford Robinson, Delois Patterson, and Leslie Hoeltzel. We particularly appreciate the wisdom of our co-workers and fellows at the National Cancer Institute and the continued motivation to advance our knowledge that we receive from caring for children with cancer. We especially hope that the words contained in these pages will help to improve the care and treatment of children with cancer everywhere.

Philip A. Pizzo, M.D.
David G. Poplack, M.D.
Bethesda, Maryland

contents

Basic Issues
in Pediatric
Oncology

part

o n e

one

Frequency and Environmental Epidemiology of Childhood Cancer

Robert W. Miller

Epidemiologic studies have provided important new information on the causes and end-results of childhood cancer. Studies of peculiarities in the occurrence of specific cancers with respect to age, sex, race, and clustering of cases may be helpful in determining etiology. Population-based data, for example, at the state or national level, are usually required. Death certificates are a ready source for this purpose when they list the causes of death, as in the United States, but as therapy increasingly diminishes mortality, the value of death-certificate data for etiologic studies is reduced. In this circumstance, data on incidence must be used instead. Incidence can be determined through the use of data from population-based cancer registries. End-results can be determined if the registries collect information on treatment and outcome.

At the bedside, peculiarities of occurrence can be observed in individual or series of cases. Clinical and epidemiologic delineation of syndromes has led to laboratory research that has revealed previously unknown mechanisms of carcinogenesis: deletion or inactivation of genes that regulate normal development (Wilms' tumor and retinoblastoma, as well as cancers that occur excessively as bilateral primary tumors); DNA repair defects that move the age distribution of skin cancer from late adulthood to childhood (in xeroderma pigmentosum); immunodeficiency disorders that greatly raise the risk of lymphoma and, to a lesser extent, certain other cancers; and preexistent chromosomal abnormalities that are associated with an increased risk of leukemia.[1]

Environmental influences have also been first recognized by clinicians who have observed clusters of cases and traced them to their causes. The latent period must be relatively short for the exposure to induce cancer during childhood. It is more likely that, because of long latent periods, exposures during childhood will lead to cancers in adulthood, but diethylstilbestrol, ionizing radiation, ultraviolet light, and chemotherapy may have short enough latent periods for exposures and carcinogenic effects to occur in childhood (see Chap. 55).

In this chapter key aspects of the epidemiology of childhood cancer will illustrate the methods involved. These methods include retrospective studies in which the histories of patients and controls are examined for clues to etiology; prospective studies in which a cohort of persons with an exposure or other characteristic puts them at high risk of cancer are followed to determine how the subsequent cancer experience compares with that of a control group; and special disease registries through which risks and detailed relationships can be defined.

CANCER INCIDENCE

The cancer incidence rate is the number of new cases in a time-interval divided by the population at risk. The data generally must be derived from a population-based registry. Rates will differ geographically and by ethnic group. In the United States about 12% of all new cases have been ascertained since 1973 through the

Surveillance, Epidemiology and End Results (SEER) Program of the National Cancer Institute.[2] The data on incidence, collected from hospitals and other medical facilities in five states, four metropolitan areas, and Puerto Rico, show patterns of occurrence that provide clues to the etiology of cancer. In addition to incidence, data on mortality are collected from death certificates and data on survival from medical records. About 90% of diagnoses are based on histologic findings. The resource provides excellent data on all three measures of the impact of cancer on the population. In addition, it provides starting points for epidemiologic studies of etiology and the progression of site-specific cancers. Data from the SEER Program are especially useful for studies of the distribution of cancer by age, sex, ethnic group, and geography (clusters) over time.

In the United States, about 6550 new cases of cancer are diagnosed annually in children under the age of 15 years, and about 2175 deaths occur (Table 1-1). Some childhood cancer deaths do not occur until after 15 years of age, especially those cancers with high rates in adolescence. Only a small number of patients die after 15 years of age from cancers with peak incidence rates early in life, for example, leukemia, kidney cancer, and retinoblastoma. The data in Table 1-1 show that among children with leukemia 42.5% die of the disease, as compared with 18% of children with kidney cancer and 10% of those with retinoblastoma.

The cancer rate for black children is only 80% that for white children (Table 1-2). This difference is largely due to lower rates among blacks for acute lymphocytic leukemia (53% lower), lymphomas (41%), Ewing's sarcoma (89%), melanomas (85%), and thyroid cancer (50%). Lesser deficiencies occur in brain tumors and neuroblastoma. Incidence rates are slightly higher in blacks than in whites for kidney tumors, retinoblastoma, and osteosarcoma. Ethnic differences in the occurrence of childhood cancer are discussed more fully below.

The incidence rates for the most frequent cancers among white children in the United States by 5-year age groups for each sex are shown in Table 1-3. As is well known, the distribution by type of cancer is very different among the three age groups. Several cancers have peaks in rates soon after birth, suggesting prenatal origins of these tumors. The frequencies of lymphoma and bone cancer increase with age, suggesting that postnatal events are responsible. Cancers that occur predominantly in males are leukemia, lymphoma, and, to a lesser extent, brain tumors. The only similar predominance in females involve cancers of "other sites" at 10 to 14 years, largely due to thyroid cancer.

From the histologic classifications of SEER data it has been shown that nonepithelial cancers account for 92% of all cancer in children under 15 years of age.[4] A steep rise in the rates for epithelial cancers causes a crossover (equal frequency) to occur at 15 to 19 years of age; in middle and late life 80% to 88% of all cancer is epithelial. These relative frequencies are deceptive, however, for they do not reveal that, beginning in mid-childhood, the rates for both types of cancer increase throughout life but at a much higher level for epithelial than for nonepithelial cancers (Fig. 1-1).

MORTALITY

When information about cancer occurrence is not available from incidence data, mortality data are used. To detect changes in cancer rates of childhood cancer by single years of age, one must turn to past mortality data because incidence data are not numerous enough for this purpose. Thus it has been found that mortality from leukemia among white children in the United States varied markedly by single years of age (Fig. 1-2A). Data grouped by 5-year intervals of time show that the huge peak at 4 years of age began to shrink in 1965–1969 and barely showed any elevation by 1975–1979.

Changes over time as portrayed by mortality data also show survival rates today compared with those a few years ago. With regard to leukemia, the number of deaths per year began to decline from the expected number in 1964 and has moved steadily downward since (Fig. 1-2B). There were 8000 fewer deaths than expected from 1964 through 1980. The decrement by 5-year birth cohorts is shown in Figure 1-2C. The greatest benefit has been for children under 5 years of age, whose leukemia is usually of the acute lymphocytic type.

Among other main categories of childhood cancers, long-term steep declines have occurred in mortality from kidney cancers, Hodgkin's disease, bone sarcoma, and only recently in non-Hodgkin's lymphoma (Fig. 1-3). For cancers other than leukemia, there were about 9300 fewer deaths than expected during the interval 1964–1980.

ETHNIC DIFFERENCES

Leukemia

Court-Brown and Doll[5] found that a peak in mortality from acute lymphocytic leukemia (see Chap. 16) at 2 to 3 years of age emerged in England and Wales in 1920–1930, in whites in the United States about 15 years later, and not at all in blacks or Japanese (Table 1-4). Later, in the 1960s, a peak began to emerge among the Japanese.[6] It is not known why these international differences occurred or why blacks have not developed the peak (Fig. 1-4).

A peculiar cluster of acute monomyelogenous leukemia (AMML) in Ankara, Turkey, was reported by Cavdar and colleagues in 1971.[7] Chloroma of the eye was a common feature. The frequency of all forms of childhood leukemia in Ankara was similar to that elsewhere in Europe and in the United States, but the proportion attributable to AMML, 34%, was far above the usual 4%. The excess is at the expense of acute myelocytic leukemia (AML) (see Chap. 17), which made up only 4% of the cases. The reason for this shift in cell type was

Table 1-1
*Estimated Number of New Cancers and Cancer Deaths
in Children Under 15 Years of Age in the United States, 1985*

Site	Number of New Cases	Number of Deaths
All sites	6550	2175
Leukemias	2000	850
Brain and nervous system	1230	550
Lymphomas	780	160
Sympathetic nervous system	525	250
Soft tissues	420	110
Kidney	410	75
Bone	320	85
Retinoblastoma	200	20
Other sites	665	75

(Modified from Young JL Jr, Ries LG, Silverberg E et al: Cancer incidence, survival, and mortality for children younger than age 15 years. Cancer 58:598–602, 1986)

Table 1-2
Annual Cancer Incidence by Type for Children Under 15 Years of Age by Race (SEER, 1973–1982)

Diagnosis	White Children		Black Children	
	Number	Rate	Number	Rate
Leukemia	1583	40.0	140	24.1
Acute lymphocytic	1166	29.4	80	13.7
Acute granulocytic	189	4.8	27	4.6
Other and unspecified	228	5.8	33	5.8
Brain and nervous system	971	24.5	124	21.3
Glioma	634	15.9	81	13.9
Medulloblastoma	218	5.5	28	4.8
Ependymoma	86	2.2	12	2.1
Other and unspecified	33	0.9	3	0.5
Lymphomas	649	16.4	57	9.8
Hodgkin's	290	7.3	30	5.2
Non-Hodgkin's lymphoma	359	9.1	27	4.6
Sympathetic nervous system	416	10.5	51	8.8
Neuroblastoma	344	8.7	43	7.4
Other	72	1.8	8	1.4
Kidney	308	7.8	64	11.0
Wilms' tumor	305	7.7	58	10.0
Other	3	0.1	6	1.1
Retinoblastoma	129	3.3	25	4.3
Bone	248	6.3	28	4.8
Osteosarcoma	116	2.9	23	4.0
Ewing's sarcoma	110	2.8	2	0.3
Chondrosarcoma	12	0.3	1	0.2
Other and unspecified	10	0.3	2	0.3
Soft tissue sarcomas	315	8.0	45	7.7
Rhabdomyosarcoma	172	4.3	19	3.3
Fibrosarcoma	48	1.2	11	1.9
Embryonal sarcoma	20	0.5	4	0.7
Other and unspecified	75	1.9	11	1.9
Gonadal and germ cell	95	2.4	14	2.4
Ovary	53	1.3	9	1.5
Testis	42	1.1	5	0.9
Nongonadal germ cell	62	1.6	9	1.5
Teratomas	25	0.3	1	0.2
Embryonal carcinoma	23	0.6	3	0.5
Germinomas	13	0.6	5	0.9
Liver	58	1.5	6	1.0
Hepatoblastoma	35	0.5	1	0.2
Hepatoma	20	0.9	4	0.7
Other and unspecified	3	0.1	1	0.2
Melanomas	51	1.3	1	0.2
Skin	44	1.1	1	0.2
Eye	6	0.2	—	—
Other	1	0.0	—	—
Miscellaneous	244	6.2	42	7.2
Thyroid	68	1.8	5	0.9
Reticuloendothelial	36	0.9	5	0.9
Carcinoid	19	0.5	4	0.5
Nerve sheath tumors	16	0.4	6	1.0
Blood vessel tumors	11	0.3	—	—
Adrenal cortical	10	0.3	1	0.2
Other and unspecified	84	2.1	21	3.5
Total	5129	129.5	606	104.1

(Modified from Young JL Jr, Ries LG, Silverberg E et al: Cancer incidence, survival, and mortality for children younger than age 15 years. Cancer 58:598–602, 1986)

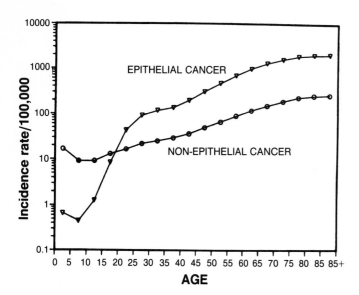

FIGURE 1-1. Age distributions of patients with epithelial as compared with nonepithelial cancers. (Miller RW, Myers MH: Lancet 2:1250, 1983)

not revealed by cytogenetic, immunologic, or virologic studies.[8] AMML is also the only form of leukemia for which patients with Fanconi's anemia are at high risk,[9] and it is the most common form of leukemia induced by alkylating agents used as treatment for cancer.[10] Thus clusters of AMML have been geographic, genetic, or drug-induced. Apparently development of this form of leukemia has something to do with alteration in host response.

Lymphoma

Denis P. Burkitt, a surgeon, observed in 1958 that a previously undescribed form of lymphoma (see Chap. 20) clustered in tropical Africa.[11] This finding provided a powerful stimulus to research in cancer epidemiology and virology. Other forms of lymphoma also show peculiarities in geographic distribution.

Hodgkin's disease had two age peaks in all except one country studied by MacMahon in 1966.[12] The exception was Japan, where cases early in life are rare and the first age peak is absent. The scarcity has also been observed among Japanese migrants to Hawaii[13]; thus an inherent resistance appears to be responsible.

The distribution of Hodgkin's disease by subtype varies geographically: The more aggressive forms predominate in underdeveloped countries.[14] Subtypes of non-Hodgkin's lymphoma (NHL) have many geographic and ethnic dissimilarities.[15] For example, B-cell lymphomas are less frequent in Japan than in Western countries.[16] The Japanese also have a seemingly reciprocal excess of certain autoimmune disorders, for example, systemic lupus erythematosus, Hashimoto's thyroiditis, and Takayasu's aortitis.[16] As compared with whites, Japanese appear to be protected against B-cell lymphomas but predisposed to autoimmune disease.

Persons at high risk of lymphomas characteristically have immunosuppression, which may be inborn, as in Wiskott–Aldrich syndrome, ataxia-telangiectasia, or the X-linked lymphoproliferative syndrome; acquired, as from drugs given to organ-transplant patients, or from a virus, such as HIV (see also Chaps. 4 and 22). One can expect geographic clusters of lymphoma whenever severe immunosuppression occurs as a result of viruses or chemicals.

Neuroblastoma

A study of consecutive cases of childhood cancer in various countries conducted by the Union Internationale Contre le Cancer (UICC) revealed a near-absence of neuroblastoma (see Chap. 28) in Tanzania, 1959–1966, and in the several countries covered by the Kenya Regional Cancer Registry, 1968–1969.[17] Rates could not be calculated; thus data were compared with those from the Manchester (England) Children's Tumour Registry through the use of a ratio of neuroblastoma to Wilms' tumor. In Manchester the ratio was 1.35, whereas the lowest frequency in Africa had a ratio of 0.09. In Uganda, Ibadan, and the Dakar Regional Registry, the ratios were 0.25 to 0.45. Ratios below 0.5 were observed in Puerto Rico, Bombay, and Cali, Colombia. The pathologists involved were highly skilled; thus

Table 1-3
Annual Incidence per Million of Cancer by Type, Age Groups, and Sex Among White Children Under 15 Years of Age in the United States, SEER Program, 1973–1982

Type of Cancer	Age of Males			Age of Females		
	0–4	*5–9*	*10–14*	*0–4*	*5–9*	*10–14*
All sites	190.3	114.6	114.4	172.2	90.1	104.6
Leukemia	72.5	35.6	27.9	61.3	32.5	16.8
Lymphoma	10.1	22.5	28.3	5.2	6.4	22.1
Brain and central nervous system	27.3	28.1	23.3	25.0	22.5	21.4
Sympathetic nervous system	28.3	4.3	1.3	28.5	2.9	1.8
Kidney	16.1	4.7	1.1	19.8	6.7	1.1
Retinoblastoma	9.1	0.6	—	10.9	0.5	—
Bone	1.4	3.8	12.2	1.7	4.5	12.0
Soft tissues	8.6	8.2	7.4	9.0	6.7	7.9
Other	16.8	6.7	12.9	10.7	7.6	21.5

(Modified from Young JL Jr, Ries LG, Silverberg E et al: Cancer incidence, survival, and mortality for children younger than age 15 years. Cancer 58:598–602, 1986)

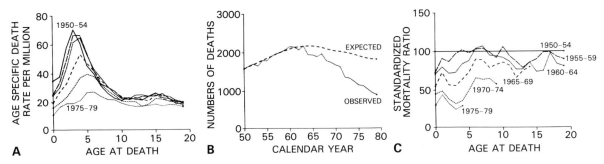

FIGURE 1-2. Mortality from leukemia in patients under 20 years of age in the United States, 1950–1979. **A.** Rates by single year of age. **B.** Number of deaths per year, observed versus expected at 1950 rates. **C.** Standardized mortality ratios by 5-year birth cohorts, 1950–1954 through 1975–1979. (Miller RW, McKay FW: JAMA 251:1567–1570, 1984)

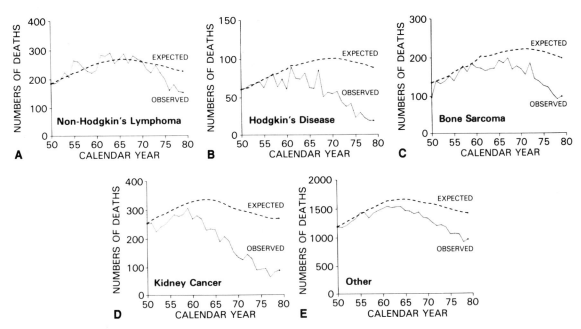

FIGURE 1-3. Annual numbers of deaths in patients under 20 years of age in the United States, observed versus expected at the 1950 rate (1951 for bone sarcoma). **A.** Non-Hodgkin's lymphoma. **B.** Hodgkin's disease. **C.** Bone sarcoma. **D.** Kidney cancer. **E.** All other cancers (Miller RW, McKay FW: JAMA 251:1567–1570, 1984)

it is unlikely that neuroblastoma went unrecognized. A possible explanation is that, in these parts of the world, some inhibiting factor transmitted from the mother to the fetus or newborn infant enhances regression of neuroblastoma *in situ,* thus removing this potential precursor for clinical neuroblastoma.

Retinoblastoma

In Manchester and in the United States, the frequency of neuroblastoma and of Wilms' tumor was higher than that for retinoblastoma, but in Israel, where diagnosis and reporting of cases is presumably similar, retinoblastoma was more frequent than the other two tumors. Similar high frequencies of retinoblastoma were reported in Sudan, Uganda, Ibadan, Bombay, and Karachi. Retinoblastoma was thus more frequent in certain parts of the Indian subcontinent and Africa than elsewhere. Other studies show no excess of bilateral (hereditary) cases.

Thus the high frequency may be due to an environmental influence (see Chap. 25).

Wilms' Tumor

Wilms' tumor (see Chap. 27) was thought to have a constant rate worldwide,[18] but the All-Japan Children's Cancer Registry consistently shows the frequency there to be about half that elsewhere.[19] The possibility thus arises that the gene locus on the short arm of chromosome 11 may be less mutable in the Japanese than in other ethnic groups.

Bone Cancer

In coding death certificates for bone cancer, the same numbers are used for all types. Hence, from coded data, Ewing's sarcoma (see Chap. 31) cannot be distinguished from osteosar-

Table 1-4
Examples of Ethnic and Geographic Differences in the Rates of Childhood Cancer

Cancer	Childhood Group	Rate Low	High	Comments
Leukemia	Blacks	+		No peak in ALL*
	Ankara, Turkey		+	High AMML instead of ALL
NHL	Central Africa		+	Due to Burkitt's lymphoma
	Japan	+		B-cell lymphoma
	Developing areas	+	+	Shift from less to more aggressive subtypes
Hodgkin's disease	Japan	+		No early age-peak
	Developing areas	+	+	Shift from less to more aggressive subtypes
Neuroblastoma	Central Africa	+		Nearly absent
Retinoblastoma	Indian subcontinent		+	Very high rates
	Israel		+	1.7 times the U.S. rate
Wilms' tumor	Japan	+		Half the rates elsewhere
Ewing's sarcoma	Japan, Korea, China and blacks	+		Very low rates
Skin cancer	North Africa		+	Due to XP
Testicular cancer	Blacks, Japan	+		No adolescent age-peak
Pineal (germ cell)	Japan		+	12 times the U.S. rate

* ALL = acute lymphocytic leukemia; AMML = acute monomyelogenous leukemia; NHL = non-Hodgkin's lymphoma; XP = xeroderma pigmentosum.

FIGURE 1-4. Mortality from leukemia by single year of age, U.S. whites compared with nonwhites, 1960–1969.

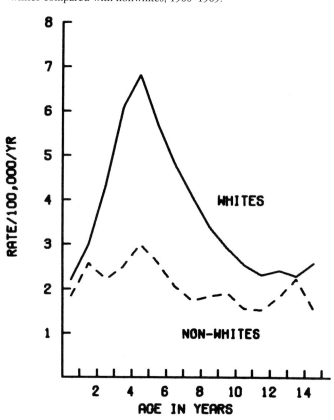

coma (see Chap. 32). By recoding death-certificate diagnoses of bone cancer according to cell type for all children in the United States who died of cancer during the 1960s, it was found that blacks rarely develop Ewing's sarcoma.[20] The UICC study showed that Ewing's sarcoma is also rare among blacks in Africa and among the Chinese and Japanese. Data collected for the Atlas of Cancer Mortality in the People's Republic of China show this deficiency,[21] as do those from the Bone Cancer Registry maintained by orthopedic surgeons in Japan.[22] Apparently whites are much more susceptible than other races to this form of bone cancer. No such difference exists with regard to osteosarcoma.

Testicular Cancer

The frequency of testicular cancer (see Chaps. 33 and 35) in whites in the United States begins to rise at 15 to 19 years of age to a tremendous peak at 25 to 29 years. There is no corresponding peak among blacks[23] (Fig. 1-5) or Japanese.[24] These differences indicate that whites are especially susceptible to various types of testicular cancer in adolescence and early adulthood. Small peaks in the frequency of embryonal cancer of the testis occur soon after birth in whites in the United States and among the Japanese but not among blacks in the United States.[24]

Skin Cancer

The UICC study revealed that at the Institut Salah Azaiz in Tunis, 14% of all cancer in children 15 years of age or younger was skin cancer.[17] This high frequency, equal to that for Wilms'

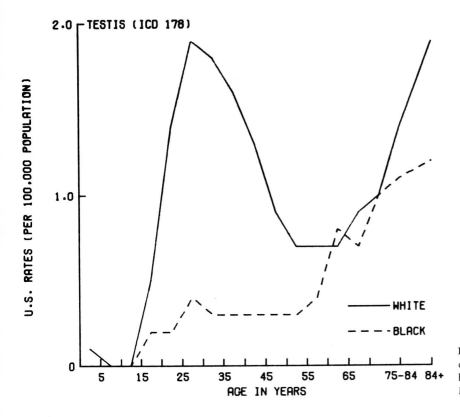

FIGURE 1-5. Age distribution of mortality from cancer of the testis, U.S. whites compared with blacks, 1950–1967. (Burbank F: Natl Cancer Inst Monogr 33:316, 1971)

tumor plus neuroblastoma in Europe and the United States, occurs throughout North Africa but has barely been mentioned in the medical literature.[25] The great excess of xeroderma pigmentosum (XP) in North Africa was evident from the hundreds of cases that had been quickly assembled for laboratory research on the DNA repair defect in this disease, and this genetic defect is closely associated with skin cancer. Ideally, protection from sunlight can prevent skin cancers so highly lethal among children in this part of the world (see Chap. 55).

Brain Tumors

Geographic or ethnic peculiarities in the occurrence of brain tumors (see Chap. 24) are not easy to recognize because ascertainment and pathologic classification are so variable from place to place. A noteworthy exception is pineal neoplasia of the teratomatous type, including germinomas, which are about 12 times more common in Japan than elsewhere.[26] In a small series of patients with pineal tumors in Hawaii, a disproportionate number were Japanese,[27] a finding that suggests an inherent high risk that is not modified by the environment upon migration.

Nasopharyngeal Carcinoma

The rates for nasopharyngeal carcinoma are inordinately high in southern China and among people who have migrated from that area to other parts of the world (see Chap. 35).[28] This ethnic propensity is related to the histocompatibility antigens HLA-A2 and HLA BW26 linked with DRW9 and to Epstein–Barr virus infection.[29,30]

CANCER CLUSTERS

Interest in clusters of childhood cancer first developed in 1963 when a concentration of cases of childhood leukemia was observed in a single parish in Niles, Illinois, in conjunction with a cluster of a rheumatic-like illness.[31] Virologists, persuaded that the sort of viruses found in animal studies would be found in humans, took this episode as evidence for their belief. A large number of childhood leukemia clusters were studied in the next 15 years by the Centers for Disease Control, but none revealed a cause for the cluster.[32] Interest in the viral etiology of leukemia diminished, but clusters gained renewed interest in 1978 when an aggregation of cases occurred among children in Rutherford, New Jersey. A chemical cause was suspected because factories there have caused heavy chemical pollution, but no cause was proved.[33]

An even more perplexing cluster of leukemia occurred in Woburn, Massachusetts. In 1979, 12 cases were noted in a small geographic area. Investigation by the CDC revealed no identifiable cause, but 8 more cases developed over the next 6 years. A group of statisticians at Harvard[34] published data that were thought to implicate water pollution from factories in the area, but other investigators strongly disagreed with the analysis and interpretation of findings.[35] This is the only cluster that has persisted after the initial investigation, and it is receiving the research attention it deserves.

To show how easy it is to find clusters, Glass and associates made scatter maps of the geographic distribution of deaths resulting from leukemia in children under age 15 years in Los Angeles County, 1960–1964.[36] By drawing boundaries as tightly as possible around groups of deaths, they found at least nine clusters as large or larger than that in Niles, Illinois.

The other side of this story is that virtually all known human carcinogens were first recognized by alert clinicians who observed clusters of cancer and traced them to their causes. Examples include vaginal or cervical adenocarcinoma from diethylstilbestrol, mesothelioma from asbestos exposure, lung cancer from the manufacture of mustard gas, and liver neoplasia from oral contraceptives.[37] Confirmation of clinical observations has come from special disease registries or cancer registries. In theory, cancer clusters caused by environmental agents should be detectable from data in registries, but the unavoidable lag in registration and difficulties in sensing unusual aggregates from tables of numbers are handicaps. The new epidemic of Kaposi's sarcoma due to AIDS is detectable in the SEER data but was noted much earlier by clinicians. The increase in the frequency of DES-induced clear cell adenocarcinoma of the cervix or vagina among young women occurred before the SEER Program was initiated, and, in fact, no change in rates can be detected in the SEER data. The increase of one to eight cases annually over two organ-sites would not have attracted notice. Under the circumstances, recognition of the change in rates was more readily made by clinicians than by cancer registries.

ENVIRONMENTAL CARCINOGENS

Thirty chemicals or industrial processes are known to cause human cancer.[38] Some, with short latent periods, cause cancer in childhood. Other cancers occur in adults as the result of childhood exposures (see Chap. 55). The carcinogenicity of environmental agents may be enhanced or diminished by interaction with one another or with genetic influences (see Chap. 2).

Physical Agents

Solar Radiation

A substantial proportion of all cancers in humans affect the skin and are induced by ultraviolet light. Because of the long latent period, skin cancers rarely occur in childhood except when there is markedly heightened sensitivity, as in XP, in which there is a DNA repair defect, or in albinism, in which there is no pigment in the skin to protect against the effects of ultraviolet light. In the general population, the darker the complexion, the lower is the frequency of skin cancer. The role of exposure to solar radiation in producing skin cancer is evidenced by maps of cancer mortality which show that in the southern United States, mortality from malignant melanoma is significantly higher than that in the northern United States.[39]

Ionizing Radiation

LEUKEMIA. Exposure to ionizing radiation from the atomic bombs in Japan caused an increase in the frequency of the usual acute leukemias of childhood and of chronic myelogenous leukemia (CML).[40] The peak in radiogenic leukemia occurred 5 years after exposure, and, with such a short latent period, the leukemogenic effect could easily be seen during childhood (Fig. 1-6).

Children are more susceptible than adults to radiation-induced leukemia, the relative risk being two to three times greater when exposure to the atomic bomb occurred before the age of 10 years than when it occurred later.[41] By the 15th year after exposure, CML no longer occurred excessively, and the increase in acute myelogenous leukemia disappeared soon thereafter.[40]

The exposures to the atomic bomb and fallout involved whole-body radiation. Partial-body exposures are also leukemogenic, as demonstrated in British men given radiotherapy for ankylosing spondylitis[42] and more recently in survivors of childhood cancer, especially Hodgkin's disease treated with x-irradiation.[43]

A study of leukemia mortality among children in Utah showed an excess of leukemia and a deficiency of other forms of cancer after weapons tests in Nevada in the early 1950s. Subsequent studies have given conflicting results.[44] The doses were far below the leukemogenic doses in studies elsewhere.

Twenty-five years ago radiation was widely used for shoe-fitting, for fluoroscopic examinations done routinely in pediatric office practice, and for therapy of benign diseases, such as "enlarged" thymus. In 1956 expert committees in the United States (National Academy of Sciences) and Great Britain (Medical Research Council) issued widely publicized reports warning against potential adverse effects from such indiscriminate use of ionizing radiation.[45,46] Subsequently, these exposures were sharply curtailed or eliminated, and radiation protection in general became much more stringent. Either as a result or coincidentally, leukemia mortality rates in children under five years of age dropped substantially.[47] From 1960 to 1966 about 1000 fewer children died of leukemia than

FIGURE 1-6. Schematic diagram of the excess risk of leukemia among atomic-bomb survivors, by age at the time of the bomb (ATB), the number of years since then (latent period), and city (Hiroshima, dark shading; Nagasaki, light shading). (Ichimaru M, Ohkita T, Ishimaru T: Gann Monogr Cancer Res 32:113–127, 1986)

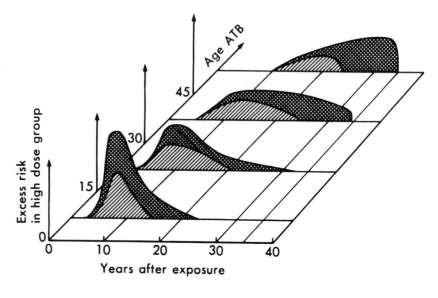

were expected at the rates for 1950 to 1959. At that time, chemotherapy was not increasing survival as it is today.

Beginning in 1956, Bithell and Stewart published a series of papers on the increased frequency of leukemia and all other forms of childhood cancer after exposure of the mother's abdomen during pregnancy to diagnostic irradiation. Much of the evidence supports a causal relationship.[48] Questions have been raised, however, about the biological plausibility of a radiation-induced increase of the same magnitude (relative risk = 1.5) for leukemia, lymphosarcoma, cerebral tumors, neuroblastoma, Wilms' tumor, and all other childhood cancer—each of which has dissimilar epidemiologic characteristics that suggest dissimilar etiologies.[49] Also, other investigators have claimed that maternal or paternal irradiation before conception increases the frequency of childhood leukemia,[50] a finding that is of questionable biological plausibility. Studies of atomic-bomb survivors have not confirmed the increased risk of leukemia after low-dose intrauterine or preconception irradiation.[51,52] MacMahon, who has labored long over this question, has concluded that it is unlikely that the association between fetal irradiation and childhood cancer will ever be resolved.[53] Possibly the hospital-based studies that showed such an increase reflected subtle abnormalities of maternal physiology or "lifestyle" associated with diagnostic radiation during pregnancy and, independently, an increased rate for cancer in the offspring.

THYROID TUMORS. In 1950 Duffy and Fitzgerald noted that 10 of 28 patients with carcinoma of the thyroid (see Chap. 34) had a history of radiotherapy for thymic enlargement.[54] Soon after, Hempelmann began a prospective study of nearly 3000 persons treated with radiotherapy for enlargement of the thymus, as compared with about 5000 nonirradiated siblings. The most recent report by this group, which concerned subjects up to 50 years of age or older, revealed thyroid carcinoma in 30 in the exposed group as compared with 1 in the control group, and benign thyroid tumors in 59 as compared with 8 in the control group.[55] Within the radiation field, benign tumors of bone were observed in 18 versus 2.26 expected, of breast in 13 versus 9.65 expected, and of other sites (mostly in peripheral nerves) in 38 versus 20.46 expected.[56] Malignant thyroid tumors tended to develop earlier in life than benign ones, and females were affected 1.9 times more often than males. The shortest latent period for development of carcinoma of the thyroid was 6 years and the longest, more than 35 years. The risk of thyroid cancer was proportional to the dose, with an estimated three to four cases developing per million people per cGy per year.[55]

In Israel an increase in the frequency of thyroid neoplasia was noted after radiotherapy for ringworm of the scalp; the average dose to the thyroid was less than 9 cGy.[57] Other studies in the United States have revealed an increased frequency of benign or malignant neoplasms of the thyroid 30 to 45 years after radiotherapy for benign disorders of the head or neck, including tonsillar and adenoidal hyperplasia and acne.[58] The latent period in these instances usually extended well beyond pediatric age span. Among the survivors of the atomic bombs in Japan, a substantial increase in thyroid carcinoma was observed, especially among females, with no heightened susceptibility during childhood.[59]

Thyroid-seeking radioisotopes of iodine have been a special problem to the children of the Marshall Islands, accidentally caught in the fallout from a nuclear weapons test at Bikini in 1954.[60,61] Among those on the most heavily exposed island, Rongelap, 2 who were younger than 1 year of age at the time suffered ablation of the thyroid. Among the other 17 Rongelap islanders exposed under the age of 10 years, 15 have developed thyroid nodules, including 1 with carcinoma. Of 4 children exposed *in utero,* 1 developed a thyroid nodule in 1974. Other islanders, who received lower doses, developed nodules—3 of them carcinomatous, after an extended latent period. The estimated dose to the thyroid glands of the Rongelap children was 335 to 1150 cGy.

OTHER CANCERS. Girls who were younger than age 10 at the time of exposure to the atomic bomb in Japan have now reached middle age and are showing an increased rate of breast cancer, higher than that of older cohorts.[62] The capacity of ionizing radiation to induce cancer of the salivary glands has also been observed in Japan.[59] Studies of children who received radiotherapy for tinea capitis in Israel or New York City have revealed an excess of brain tumors, especially meningioma,[63] which has not been observed among Japanese atomic-bomb survivors.

Radiotherapy for cancers in children has induced second neoplasms of connective tissue, bone, and skin.[64] In some genetic disorders, such as familial (usually bilateral) retinoblastoma, there may be greater susceptibility to radiogenic oncogenesis.[65]

In Germany, among 218 persons under 20 years of age experimentally given intravenous ^{224}Ra (radium) primarily for tuberculosis of bone, 1944–1951, 35 have developed bone sarcoma. The latent period ranged from 4 to 21 years. Twenty patients developed benign bone tumors, 18 of which were osteomas.[66]

Thorotrast, used as a radiopaque dye for cerebral angiography, among other purposes, contains radioisotopes that can induce liver cancer, especially hemangioendothelioma, leukemia, and occasionally osteosarcoma.[67] Thorotrast was used primarily in adults, but even among the small number of children exposed some have developed neoplasia.

The threat of accidental releases of radiation from nuclear reactors was largely theoretical until 1979. Then, in Pennsylvania at Three Mile Island (TMI), a failure of highly fallible equipment occurred in the hands of people insufficiently trained to deal with it. The equipment failures were predictable, and in fact were predicted, for everything that went wrong at TMI had gone wrong elsewhere, but not in combination or with the plant functioning at 97% capacity.[68,69] The doses received by the general population nearby were too small for detectable increases in cancer rates, mutations, or teratogenic effects.[70] The main effect was psychological, caused by the experience itself augmented by stories in the news media that greatly alarmed the people of the area.

In 1986 a partial meltdown at a nuclear reactor in Chernobyl, USSR, occurred because of operator error. Substantial amounts of radioactive isotopes were released into the atmosphere. Fallout occurred especially in the Ukraine and Byelorussia, in neighboring countries, and, to a lesser extent, throughout the world. Twenty-nine workers at the reactor who were heavily exposed died. Near the plant 135,000 people were evacuated. Twenty-five thousand people who lived 3 to 15 km from the plant were estimated to have received 350 to 550 mSv (35–55 rem) from external irradiation.[71] This is 7 to 11 times the annual dose limit for radiation workers. The dose is in the range of the lowest exposure at which a leukemogenic effect was observed in Japanese atomic-bomb survivors.[72] Over all of European Russia the cumulative dose from external radiation in the next 50 years is estimated to be only three times greater than background.[71] Additional exposures occurred from the ingestion of radioisotopes which, as fallout, contaminated food and water.

Another new radiation problem is caused by ^{222}Rn (radon, a decay product of radium) in the soil in certain areas of the

United States. Studies of uranium miners in the United States and Europe years ago revealed an excess of lung cancer among them.[73] Extrapolation downward from those doses reveals that lung cancer may occur from the levels of exposure found in some homes.[74] In eastern Pennsylvania, 55% of homes had radon levels in air that exceeded the upper limit suggested by the Environmental Protection Agency for homes built on tailings from uranium mines in Colorado. No study has yet demonstrated an excess of lung cancer in relation to long-time residence in these homes. Several studies are in progress. Up to 10,000 cases of lung cancer per year in the United States may be due to radon exposures in the home, according to some estimates. It has been recommended that remedial action be taken if children are exposed to radon levels at home of more than 3 pCi/liter.[75] There may be an interaction with cigarette smoke in the induction of lung cancer. Measurements in the home can be made with radon detectors, which are readily available commercially.

Asbestos

Solar and ionizing radiation are not the only physical agents known to be oncogenic. The chemical agent asbestos is apparently carcinogenic because of the physical properties of its fibers (thin diameter and length of 5 μm or greater). Glass fibers of the appropriate dimension produce analogous neoplasms in rats.[76]

The discovery that asbestos induces mesothelioma of the pleura was made with the help of an alert clinician in South Africa, who observed a cluster of 33 adults with this rare neoplasm. The affected persons were in diverse occupations; only a small proportion had worked with asbestos. As children, however, most had lived near open pits where asbestos was mined, and some had often played on the dumps.[77] Elsewhere asbestos has been carried home on the father's workclothes and has caused mesothelioma in the wife or child three or four decades later.[78] Mesotheliomas in persons under 20 years of age are apparently not due to asbestos and are histologically unlike those produced by this agent.[79]

Asbestos also greatly multiplies the capacity of cigarette smoking to induce lung cancer, the frequency being up to 53 times greater than that in people who do not smoke and who are not occupationally exposed to asbestos.[80] Ceilings of an estimated 9000 schools built in the United States between 1950 and 1973 were sprayed with asbestos.[81] Some have deteriorated with abuse so that the fibers float free and may be inhaled by the students, possibly raising the risk of mesothelioma or, among future smokers, bronchogenic carcinoma. Asbestos should be removed or contained by barriers to prevent the occurrence of these cancers.

CHEMICALS

Diethylstilbestrol

In 1971 a simple retrospective study revealed that a cluster of a rare vaginal cancer in adolescent and young adult females was attributable to maternal use of diethylstibestrol (DES) during pregnancy.[82] Among 262 white women with such cancers, 1948–1965, the youngest was 7 years old. Generally those affected were 15 to 22 years of age, with a peak at ages 17 to 22. The risk that clear-cell adenocarcinoma of the vagina or cervix will develop after intrauterine exposure to DES through 34 years of age is 1 case per 1000.[83] (The low rate among exposed

women was taken to signify that DES is an incomplete carcinogen and that another factor is involved in this carcinogenic process.) The drug was given to pregnant women with diabetes or threatened abortion. No delayed effects were anticipated, and the carcinogenic effect of the drug was detected only because the tumor was so rare that clusters were noticed. It is not known whether other neoplasms will occur for the daughters or sons of the DES-treated women. In both sexes there are malformations of the genital tract—minor anomalies of the vagina or cervix (ridging, vaginal adenosis) and cysts of the epididymis.[84,85] The reproductive performance of DES daughters is below normal because of a high frequency of adverse outcomes (ectopic pregnancy, miscarriage, and prematurity).[86] Presumably these outcomes are due to an abnormality in uterine contour, which is T shaped on hysterosalpingogram.[87]

The excess of this rare cancer is detectable in the data of the SEER Program, 1973–1984, during which time 42 cases of clear-cell adenocarcinoma of the vagina or cervix were reported in females ranging from 15 to 29 years of age (Kim and Miller: Unpublished data). In 1984 new cases were still being diagnosed. The most recent year of birth was 1968.

Any known human carcinogen that can cross the placenta may in theory induce cancer in the offspring, perhaps after a latent period of several decades. Phenytoin seems a good candidate for transplacental carcinogenicity because it occasionally causes a hypersensitivity reaction resembling Hodgkin's disease, which may be fatal or may regress if the drug is withdrawn in time.[88] In the fetal hydantoin syndrome, however, instead of lymphoma, four cases with neuroblastoma have been reported in the United States.[89,90]

Chemotherapy

Of the several categories of cancer chemotherapy, only alkylating agents have caused an increased frequency of second primary cancers in humans.[10] The effect was most pronounced after treatment for Hodgkin's disease. Fifteen years after therapy, among 1036 patients with this neoplasm, 12 (4.2%) had developed leukemia as compared with 0.14 expected. Among 8134 children with primary cancers other than Hodgkin's disease, 10 developed leukemia (4 after Wilms' tumor treated only with radiation) as compared with 1.48 expected.[91] The risk of leukemia was related to the dose of the alkylating agents rather than to duration of treatment. A study in adults has indicated that melphalan is a more potent carcinogen than cyclophosphamide.[92]

An excess of bone cancer has also occurred after therapy for childhood cancer. Most is attributable to radiotherapy, given in very high doses, but alkylating agents have also been implicated.[93]

Anabolic Androgenic Steroids

A small number of patients have reportedly developed liver cancer after treatment of their aplastic anemia with anabolic androgenic steroids.[94] Patients with Fanconi's anemia may have been especially prone to this effect. Occasionally the neoplasm regressed when the drug was withdrawn.[95] A small number of cases occurred in patients treated for disorders other than aplastic anemia.[96] There has been concern that athletes, who take the drug to build their musculature, might develop liver cancer. Only a few such cases are known to have occurred.[97]

Immunosuppressants

Patients on immunosuppressive therapy after renal transplantation have a marked propensity—150 times greater than normal—to immunoblastic lymphoma, which often first affects the brain, an unusual site for this neoplasm (see Chap. 4 and 22). The latent period may be as short as 2 weeks. An excess of other cancers, principally hepatobiliary, begins 2 years after transplantation.[98] The risk for lymphoma and for other cancers seems to be greatest in patients under 20 years of age. In one series, 7 developed lymphoma compared with 0.161 expected, and 6 developed other cancers compared with 0.649 expected.[98]

Lymphoma of the brain may also occur in Wiskott–Aldrich syndrome, which is characterized by genetically determined immunosuppression. Cerebral lymphoma has been reported occasionally in nonsurgical patients taking immunosuppressive drugs.[99]

Tobacco

In the past few years attention has turned to the risk to nonsmokers from passive exposure to tobacco smoke. An expert panel of the National Research Council has concluded that, overall, studies on the health effects of passive smoking indicate an increase in the frequency of lung cancer, which is biologically plausible given the known carcinogens in tobacco smoke.[100] The Surgeon General's report on this subject concludes with the statement that involuntary smoking can cause disease, including lung cancer, in healthy nonsmokers.[101] These reports have generated federal and statewide bans on smoking in public places. The risk of respiratory cancer after exposure in childhood to passive smoking is not known, but it may well be increased, given that early exposure to other agents, such as ionizing radiation, can cause certain cancers later in life (see Chap. 55).

When maps of cancer mortality in the United States by county were published in 1975, an excess of oral cancer among women in the South was noted. A case-control study revealed that dipping snuff (placing it between the gum and buccal mucosa) was responsible.[102] At about the same time individual cases of oral cancer in young adults who had used chewing tobacco came to national attention. The habit was popularized among high school students by professional athletes. A Consensus Development Panel of the National Institutes of Health estimated that at least 10 million persons in the United States had used smokeless tobacco in 1985 and concluded that there is strong evidence that it causes cancer of the mouth.[103] The Council on Scientific Affairs of the American Medical Association concurred and urged that the restrictions that apply to advertising cigarettes be applied to the advertising of snuff and chewing tobacco.[104] Pediatricians have an opportunity and responsibility to prevent tobacco-related cancers by educating their patients.

Endogenous Chemicals

When one excludes cancers caused by sunlight or cigarette smoking, only a small fraction of the remainder are known to be due to other environmental agents. A hypothesis, recently in favor, is that most cancers are induced by chemicals that form within the body through metabolic activation, sometimes dependent on the effects of intestinal bacteria. For example, it is believed that nitrate in the diet is endogenously reduced to nitrite by bacteria and, as a result, mutagenic/carcinogenic N-nitroso compounds are formed.[105] Among foods that have produced mutagens after nitrosation experimentally are beans, fermented soy products, and certain moldy foods. Internal body fluids, such as gastric juice or bile, may reveal differences in levels of N-nitroso compounds in high-risk as compared with normal populations. Studies of this type, which combine chemical carcinogenesis and epidemiology, have recently been called metabolic epidemiology. Identifying metabolic carcinogens may be aided by applying bacterial mutagenicity tests and other screening procedures to body fluids, such as urine or bile.

Diet

Laboratory studies suggest that a variety of chemicals in food may be carcinogenic in humans. Among them are aflatoxins, cycasin, and bracken fern carcinogens (natural constituents) as well as protein pyrolysates produced when certain foods are cooked.[106] Some food constituents protect against cancer in experimental animals. Among these anticarcinogens are carotenoids and dietary fiber.

It has been difficult to derive strong evidence that individual components of the diet are carcinogenic in humans because of the long latent periods involved, the role of metabolic conversion, and possibly interactions that may be potentiating or inhibiting.

Willett and MacMahon have made a comprehensive analytical review of the literature on the diet as a cause of cancer.[107] They noted that laboratory experimentation and human correlation studies suggest that overnutrition contributes to cancer of the endometrium, and fats in particular contribute to cancer to the breast or colon. The composition of the diet is thought to affect the bacterial flora of the intestines, which in turn produce carcinogenic metabolites through degradation of bile acids and cholesterol. In addition, high fiber content is thought to diminish the frequency of colon cancer by speeding transit time and thus diminishing the contact between dietary carcinogens and intestinal mucosa. Recent studies have failed to confirm this hypothesis.[107]

From their review of the literature, Willett and MacMahon[107] concluded that, although individual ingredients may predispose to cancer or protect against it, the available data were generally inconsistent or incomplete. They believe that the data from epidemiologic studies, clinical observations, and animal experimentation are insufficient for strong recommendations to be made about specific dietary factors but that no harm would be done and other health benefits might be derived from following the recommendations that several medical organizations have issued concerning diet and cancer. The main recommendations are to reduce fat consumption from 40% to 30% of calories (in the United States); to include in the daily diet whole grain cereals, citrus fruits, and green or yellow vegetables; to limit consumption of salt-cured and smoke-cured foods and alcoholic beverages; and to maintain optimal body weight.[108]

The potential human carcinogenicity of certain food additives (e.g., saccharin, Red Dye 2) has been highly controversial and is based on animal experimentation and bacterial mutagenicity tests.[109] Diabetics have not experienced increased cancer of the urinary bladder in the somewhat limited time that these sugar substitutes have been used.[110] On the basis of animal tests, Red Dye 2 has been banned in the United States but not elsewhere.[111]

Chemical Contaminants

Chemical contaminants are another category of potential carcinogens, exposure to which is usually at low levels. Among the suspects are pesticides, polychlorinated biphenyls (PCBs), polybrominated biphenyls (PBBs), dioxin, and kepone, each of which has polluted land areas and waterways.[112] At the Love Canal in Niagara Falls, New York, a mixture of 82 chemicals buried in a large abandoned trench covering 16 acres contaminated a school and the surrounding neighborhood.[113] No carcinogenic effect in humans has yet been demonstrated. Dioxin, which produces a variety of noncancerous effects in animals, including congenital malformations, has to date caused only chloracne after heavy exposure of children or adults.[114]

Some of these chemicals are deposited in adipose tissues and are removed from the body primarily in the fat of breast milk.[115] This circumstance raises the possibility that in rare instances, when the mother has been heavily exposed to one of these agents, breast-feeding may transmit the chemicals to the infant at a time when susceptibility is high and life expectancy is long, allowing ample time for development of cancers with latent periods of 50 years or more.

Practitioners are usually the first to encounter medical problems attributed to heavy pollution. A plan is needed to deal with the health effects or fear of them. Public health authorities should take steps to limit and define the exposure and its effects. Characterizing the exposure may be difficult, for the agent may disappear before it can be measured, or effects may be due to impurities in trace amounts. Prompt identification of the contaminant will help diminish the emotional reactions that arise from uncertainty. The literature must be searched for clues to the effects, based on animal experimentation and previous observations in humans. If possible, specimens of tissues, body fluids, and contaminated objects should be obtained for current or future study. The situation should be dealt with locally, with advice from state health authorities first, who can call on national experts if necessary.

Other Environmental Influences

Three lines of evidence implicate as yet ill-defined environmental influences on human carcinogenesis. First, studies of people who migrate from one country to another have revealed that certain cancer rates of the old country persist among the first generation in the new country, even when migration occurred relatively early in life.[116] The rates of the new country are usually observed in the children of the immigrants. Second, maps of cancer mortality by county in the United States, 1950–1969, show distinctive patterns of excessive mortality from specific forms of cancer, indicative of environmental exposures. Some clues to the nature of the exposures have emerged from studies of mortality with respect to specific industries within high-risk counties, for example, the high rate of lung cancer among counties having smelters for lead, copper, or zinc, which emit arsenic, a known pulmonary carcinogen.[117] Third, there are differences in cancer risk within a given country related to lifestyle, as in Seventh Day Adventists in the United States, whose total cancer mortality rates are 50% to 70% of those for the general population for most sites, unrelated to the carcinogenic effects of smoking or drinking.[118] In the aggregate, these studies indicate that exogenous agents encountered early in life influence various cancer rates for many years to come. The experience with DES reveals that carcinogenic exposures may begin during intrauterine life.[83]

VIRUSES

Leukemia

In the 1960s there was great anticipation on the basis of laboratory research that viruses would soon be proved to be causes of human cancer. Murine leukemia and feline leukemia/lymphoma, which are so induced, were thought to be counterparts of human leukemia. A wide variety of hypotheses have been tested concerning the vertical or horizontal transmission of childhood leukemia, but none has been proved. Clusters of leukemia attracted great publicity and led to the development by statisticians of ingenious procedures to test dispassionately for excessive clusters of rare events.[119] As discussed previously, the results showed that leukemia clusters occur no more often than is expected by chance.

Well after interest in the viral etiology of leukemia faded, clusters of adult T-cell leukemia in Kyushu, Japan, and in islands of the Caribbean were independently found to be due to the retrovirus HTLV-I.[120] Soon after, clusters of Kaposi's sarcoma, a rare lymphoma, occurred in New York and San Francisco among homosexual males with acquired immune deficiency syndrome (AIDS)[121] due to another retrovirus, HTLV-III, which has since been designated as HIV (see Chap. 36). At about the same time the cause of hairy cell leukemia was found to be another retrovirus, HTLV-II. These neoplasms rarely, if ever, occur in children, although children may harbor the virus because of vertical transmission.

X-Linked Lymphoproliferative Syndrome

In 1975 families were first recognized in which more than one boy developed B-cell lymphoproliferative disorders: lymphoma, chronic or fatal infectious mononucleosis, or acquired agammaglobulinemia.[122] These disorders are believed to occur in this syndrome because of overwhelming infection with EBV due to an X-linked genetic susceptibility to the virus (see Chap. 22).

Cancers Associated with Human Papilloma Virus

Epidemiologic patterns suggest that carcinoma of the uterine cervix is venereally transmitted, apparently by human papilloma virus (HPV) types 16 and 18. The recent marked increase in sexual activity of teenagers should result in an increase in the frequency of cancer of the uterine cervix.[123] Juvenile laryngeal papillomatosis, in which the neoplasms are usually benign, is associated with HPV types 6 and 11.[123] Treatment with radiotherapy or bleomycin has caused malignant transformation of the neoplasm.[124] The peak age at onset is 2 years, reflecting probable infection of the infant passing through the birth canal.[125]

Another disorder attributed to HPV type 5 in particular is epidermodysplasia verruciformis, a familial skin disorder, which may develop early in life and may later undergo malignant transformation, especially in sun-exposed skin.[126]

Hodgkin's Disease

In Albany, New York, a cluster of Hodgkin's disease (see Chap. 21) was observed among children and young adults who either knew one another (case–case transmission) or knew an unaffected person in close contact with other cases (case–carrier–case transmission). In effect, these observations generated a hypothesis which at first seemed to be supported when tested elsewhere by the original investigator[127] but not when tested later by other investigators.[128] A group at Harvard, however, has found an excess of Hodgkin's disease in like-sex young sibpairs, a finding that suggests horizontal transmission of the disease early in life may come from close sharing of activities and sleeping quarters.[129]

Burkitt's Lymphoma

In Africa, Burkitt's lymphoma (see Chap. 20) is apparently related to infection with EBV[130] and exhibits temporal and geographic changes in occurrence that reflect environmental influences. It is thought that holoendemic malaria causes a continuous intense antigenic stimulus that alters susceptibility to EBV so that it gives rise to African lymphoma. In North America there is no malaria, and the rare occurrence of Burkitt's lymphoma is usually unrelated to EBV.[131] In both geographic areas, however, the patients typically have one of three chromosomal translocations: t(8;14), t(8;22), and t(2;8), which are independent of infection with EBV.[132]

Hepatocellular Carcinoma

In Africa and Asia high rates of hepatocellular carcinoma occur that are believed to result from chronic infection with hepatitis B-virus (HBV) (see Chap. 26). In these areas perinatal infection is common: 70% to 90% of infants are affected if the mother is positive for both hepatitis surface antigen (HBsAg) and hepatitis B e antigen. Almost all of these infants become chronic carriers who, decades hence, will be at high risk of cirrhosis and primary cancer of the liver.[133] The virus crosses the placenta, but HBsAg is seldom found in the fetus. It is detectable soon after birth. Two hypotheses have been proposed to explain these peculiarities of occurrence: [a] maternal antibodies provide passive immunity while the child is *in utero,* or [b] maturation of the liver is required before the virus can replicate.[134] Vaccination on the first day of life is important to protect the infant from the lethal sequelae of the carrier state.[135] Thus a preventive measure at birth can protect against cancer and cirrhosis in the adult.

SOME EPIDEMIOLOGIC GUIDELINES

What to Do When Clusters Are Observed

In pediatric oncology units or in office practice the clinician can make novel observations concerning environmental or inherent causes of type-specific childhood cancers. Clusters occur often by chance and occasionally because of environmental carcinogens, as revealed usually by retrospective studies; that is, the histories of the affected persons revealed a large exposure in common, usually a drug or occupational chemical. Sometimes a single case draws attention to the suspected carcinogen, as in respiratory cancers induced by war-time exposure to mustard gas during its manufacture in Japan, or liver neoplasia due to oral contraceptives in Michigan.[37]

When a cluster is suspected, the clinician should determine whether the cancers are of the same or related subtypes (*e.g.,* B-cell leukemias rather than a mixture of B-cell and other leukemias). The date of onset should be compared with the date of the arrival of each child at the location of the cluster. Cases should be excluded if the latent period is too short or if the neoplasm was present before the child took up residence, attended school, or was otherwise exposed in the area. If the exclusions do not dispel the concern of a cluster, the occurrence should be reported to the state epidemiologist. This official, after evaluating the data, may request assistance from the Epidemiologic Intelligence Service of the Centers for Disease Control in Atlanta, Georgia.

When two rare events are observed in the same child, such as the fetal hydantoin syndrome and neuroblastoma, a general rule is that if three of these concurrences have been observed nationally within a few years, the relationship between the two disorders is unlikely to be due to chance.

A second step, when an association has been made, is to establish a special disease registry, as exemplified by those for DES-induced clear cell adenocarcinoma of the cervix or vagina, or for liver neoplasia attributed to the use of oral contraceptives. Data from special disease registries improve estimates of risk, as well as information about the latent period, age of susceptibility to the carcinogen, age of onset of the cancer, definition of the clinical manifestations, outcome of therapy, and distribution over time, especially useful when a decrease in the number of new cases occurs as the cause is controlled.

Another approach, more costly and technically difficult, involves prospective studies of cohorts of persons exposed to the carcinogen, as compared with similar persons who were not exposed. Cohort studies, as used, for example, in the follow-up of Japanese atomic-bomb survivors, allow a wide variety of health effects to be evaluated over time in relation to the dose of radiation received. In this way differences in cancer rates in the heavily exposed as compared with the lightly or unexposed groups of survivors reveal which neoplasms were radiation induced. (Radiogenic cancers are indistinguishable from those that occur in nonexposed persons, except for the difference in rates.)

Causal Associations

The association between two events need not be causal. The establishment of causality is enhanced by showing [a] a logical time-sequence, that is, the presumed causal event precedes the effect; [b] specificity of the effect, that is, one rather than multiple cancers caused by a given exposure; [c] a dose-response relationship; [d] biologic plausibility, that is, the new information is consonant with previous knowledge; [e] consistency with other observations on cause and effect, for example, determining whether the relationship of fat consumption to colon cancer rates is the same throughout the world; [f] the exclusion of concomitant variables (alternative explanations) in the analysis, for example, referral bias; and [g] disappearance of the effect when the cause is removed. Not all of these elements can be evaluated or will be true for even the most fully studied effects of an environmental exposure. Ionizing radiation, for example, induces various but not all forms of cancer.

Incidence or Prevalence?

The word *incidence* is commonly misused in the medical literature. Its meaning is narrow: the number of new cases in a specific interval of time. *Point prevalence* is the number of cases, new or old, at a point in time. When more general words are needed, *frequency* or *occurrence* should be used.

SEARCHING FOR CLUES TO CANCER ETIOLOGY

In searching for clues to cancer etiology a few questions can produce a high yield of new information. The family history ranks first. Ideally each medical record for patients with cancer should include a recent pedigree showing illnesses in each first-degree relative (parents, siblings, and children of the index case), as well as information about other relatives with cancer or other potentially related diseases, such as immunologic disorders, blood dyscrasias, or congenital malformations. Second, physicians should inquire about the mother's occupational and other exposures during pregnancy and about the child's exposures to chemicals, radiation, and unusual infections. The following findings may be etiologically important: coexistent disease, such as multiple congenital malformations; multifocal or bilateral cancer in paired organs (a possible clue to hereditary transmission); cancer of an unusual histologic type; cancer at an unusual age (*e.g.*, adult-type cancers in childhood); cancer at an unusual site; or marked overreaction to conventional cancer therapy (*e.g.*, acute reaction to radiotherapy for lymphoma in ataxia-telangiectasia). From such occurrences, new understanding of the origins of childhood cancer may be derived in the future, as in the past.

REFERENCES

1. Miller RW: Genes, syndromes, and cancer. Pediatr Rev 8:153–158, 1986
2. Young JL Jr, Percy CL, Asire AJ et al: Cancer incidence and mortality in the United States, 1973–77. Natl Cancer Inst Monogr 57:1–9, 1981
3. Young JL Jr, Ries LG, Silverberg E et al: Cancer incidence, survival, and mortality for children younger than 15 years. Cancer 58:598–602, 1986
4. Miller RW, Myers MH: Age distribution of epithelial cancers. Lancet 2:1250, 1983
5. Court–Brown WM, Doll R: Leukaemia in childhood and young adult life. Trends in relation to aetiology. Br Med J 1:981–988, 1961
6. Miller RW: Childhood cancer mortality in USA and Japan. Tohoku J Exp Med 91:103–107, 1967
7. Cavdar AO, Arcasoy A, Gozdasoglu S et al: Chloroma-like ocular manifestations in Turkish children with acute myelomonocytic leukemia. Lancet 1:680–682, 1971
8. Cavdar AO, Arcasoy A, Babacan E et al: Ocular granulocytic sarcoma (chloroma) with acute myelomonocytic leukemia in Turkish children. Cancer 41:1606–1609, 1978
9. O'Gorman Hughes DW: Aplastic anaemia in childhood: III. Constitutional aplastic anaemia and related cytopenias. Med J Aust 1:519–526, 1974
10. Greene MH: Epidemiologic studies of therapy-related acute leukemia. In Castellani A (ed): Epidemiology and Quantitation of Environmental Risks in Humans from Radiation and Other Agents—Potential and Limitations, pp. 499–514. New York, Plenum Press, 1985
11. Burkitt DP: A sarcoma involving the jaws of African children. Br J Surg 46:218–223, 1958
12. MacMahon B: Epidemiology of Hodgkin's disease. Cancer Res 26:1189–1200, 1966
13. Mason TJ, Fraumeni JF Jr: Hodgkin's disease among Japanese Americans. Lancet 1:215, 1974
14. Motawy MS, Omar YT: Hodgkin's disease in children of Kuwait. Cancer 57:2255–2259, 1986
15. Magrath I, O'Conor GT, Ramot B (eds): Pathogenesis of Leukemias and Lymphomas: Environmental Influences. New York, Raven Press, 1984
16. Kadin ME, Berard CW, Nanba K et al: Lymphoproliferative diseases in Japan and western countries. Hum Pathol 14:745–772, 1983
17. Miller RW: Ethnic differences in cancer occurrence: Genetic and environmental influences with particular reference to neuroblastoma. In Mulvihill JJ, Miller RW, Fraumeni JF Jr (eds): Genetics of Human Cancer, pp 1–14. New York, Raven Press, 1977
18. Innis MD: Nephroblastoma: Possible index cancer of childhood. Med J Aust 1:18–20, 1972
19. Hirayama T: Descriptive and analytical epidemiology of childhood malignancy in Japan. In Kobayashi N (ed): Recent Advances in Management of Children with Cancer, pp 27–43. Tokyo, The Children's Cancer Association of Japan, 1980
20. Miller RW: Contrasting epidemiology of childhood osteosarcoma, Ewing's tumor, and rhabdomyosarcoma. Natl Cancer Inst Monogr 56:9–14, 1981
21. Li FP, Tu J, Liu F et al: Rarity of Ewing's sarcoma in China. Lancet 1:1255, 1980
22. Bone Tumor Committee of Japanese Orthopedic Association: Bone Tumor Registry in Japan: The Incidence of Bone Tumors in Japan, pp 122–123. Tokyo, National Cancer Center, 1982
23. McKay FW, Hanson MR, Miller RW: Cancer mortality in the United States: 1950–1977. Natl Cancer Inst Monogr 59:1–197, April 1982
24. Miller RW, Sugano H: Report on a U.S.–Japan Cooperative Cancer Research Program workshop on adult-type cancer under age 30. Gann Monogr Cancer Res: 33:193–204, 1987
25. Marshall J: Skin Diseases in Africa, p 91. Cape Town, Maske W. Miller, 1964
26. Koide O, Watanabe Y, Sato K: A pathological survey of intracranial germinoma and pinealoma in Japan. Cancer 45:2119–2130, 1980
27. Miller RW: Relation between cancer and congenital malformations. The value of small series, with a note on pineal tumors in native and migrant Japanese. Isr J Med Sci 7:1461–1464, 1971
28. Cammoun M, Horener GV, Mourali N: Tumors of the nasopharynx in Tunisa. An anatomic and clinical study of 143 cases. Cancer 33:184–192, 1974
29. Chan SH, Day NE, Kunaratham N et al: HLA and nasopharyngeal carcinoma in Chinese—A further study. Inst J Cancer 32:171–176, 1983
30. de-Thé G: Role of the Epstein–Barr virus in human diseases: Infectious mononucleosis, Burkitt's lymphoma, and nasopharyngeal carcinoma. In Klein G (ed): Viral Oncology, pp 769–797. New York, Raven Press, 1985
31. Heath CW Jr, Hasterlik RJ: Leukemia among children in a suburban community. Am J Med 34:796–812, 1963
32. Caldwell GG, Heath CW Jr: Case clustering in cancer. South Med J 69:1598–1602, 1976
33. Halperin W, Altman R, Stemhagen A et al: Epidemiologic investigation of clusters of leukemia and Hodgkin's disease in Rutherford, New Jersey. J Med Soc NJ 77:267–273, 1980
34. Lagakos SW, Wessen BJ, Zelen M: An analysis of contaminated well water and health effects in Woburn, Massachusetts. J Am Stat Assoc 81:583–596, 1986
35. MacMahon B: Comment. J Am Stat Assoc 81:597–599, 1986
36. Glass AG, Hill JA, Miller RW: Significance of leukemia clusters. J Pediatr 73:101–107, 1968
37. Miller RW: The discovery of human teratogens, carcinogens and mutagens. Lessons for the future. In Holländer A, de Serres FJ (eds): Chemical Mutagens: Principles and Methods for Their Detection, vol 5, pp 101–126. New York, Plenum Press, 1978
38. IARC Monographs on the Evaluation of the Carcinogenic Risk of Chemicals to Humans. Chemicals, Industrial Processes and Industries Associated with Cancer in Humans. IARC Monographs 1-29, Supplement 4, pp 14–16. Lyon, France, International Agency for Research on Cancer, October 1982
39. Pickle LW, Mason TJ, Howard N et al: Atlas of Cancer Mortality Among U.S. Whites, 1950–1980, pp 102–105. DHHS Publ. No. (NIH) 87-2900. Bethesda, MD, Natl Institutes of Health, 1987
40. Ichimaru M, Ohkita T, Ishimaru T: Leukemia, multiple myeloma and malignant lymphoma. Gann Monogr Cancer Res 32:113–127, 1986
41. Miller RW, Boice JD Jr: Radiogenic cancer after prenatal or childhood exposure. In Upton AC, Albert RE, Burns FJ et al (eds): Radiation Carcinogenesis, pp 379–386. New York, Elsevier, 1986
42. Darby SC, Nakashima E, Kato H: A parallel analysis of cancer mortality among atomic bomb survivors and patients with ankylosing spondylitis given X-ray therapy. J Natl Cancer Inst 75:1–21, 1985
43. Tucker MA, Meadows AT, Boice JD Jr et al: Cancer risk following treatment of childhood cancer. In Boice JD Jr, Fraumeni JF Jr (eds): Radiation Carcinogenesis: Epidemiology and Biological Significance, pp 211–224. New York, Raven Press, 1984
44. Machado SG, Land CE, McKay FW: Cancer mortality and radioactive fallout in southwestern Utah. Am J Epidemiol 125:44–61, 1987
45. Summary Reports of the Committees on the Biological Effects of Atomic Radiation, p 108. Washington, DC, National Academy of Sciences–National Research Council, 1956
46. Medical Research Council: Hazards to Man of Nuclear and Allied Radiations. London, Her Majesty's Stationery Office, 1956

47. Miller RW: Decline in U.S. childhood leukemia mortality. Lancet 2:1189–1190, 1969

48. Bithell JF, Stewart AM: Pre-natal irradiation and childhood malignancy: A review of British data from the Oxford survey. Br J Cancer 31:271–287, 1975

49. Miller RW: Delayed radiation effects in atomic-bomb survivors. Science 166:569–574, 1969

50. Graham S, Levin ML, Lilienfeld AM et al: Preconception, intauterine, and postnatal irradiation as related to leukemia. Natl Cancer Inst Monogr 19:347–371, 1966

51. Jablon S, Kato H: Childhood cancer in relation to prenatal exposure to atomic-bomb radiation. Lancet 2:1000–1003, 1970

52. Kato H, Schull WJ, Neel JV: A cohort-type study of survival in the children of parents exposed to the atomic bombings. Am J Hum Genet 18:339–373, 1966

53. MacMahon B: Prenatal x-ray exposure and twins. N Engl J Med 312:576–577, 1985

54. Duffy BJ, Fitzgerald P: Cancer of the thyroid in children: A report of 28 cases. J Clin Endocrinol Metab 10:1296–1308, 1950

55. Shore RE, Woodward E, Hildreth N et al: Thyroid tumors following thymus irradiation. J Natl Cancer Inst 74:1177–1184, 1985

56. Hempelmann LH, Hall WJ, Phillips M et al: Neoplasms in persons treated with x-rays in infancy: Fourth survey in 20 years. J Natl Cancer Inst 55:519–530, 1975

57. Ron E, Modan B: Thyroid and other neoplasms following childhood scalp irradiation. In Boice JD Jr, Fraumeni JF Jr (eds): Radiation Carcinogenesis: Epidemiology and Biological Significance, pp 139–151. New York, Raven Press, 1984

58. Shore RE, Woodward ED, Hempelmann LH: Radiation-induced thyroid cancer. In Boice JD Jr, Fraumeni JF Jr (eds): Radiation Carcinogenesis: Epidemiology and Biological Significance, pp 131–138. New York, Raven Press, 1984

59. Ezaki H, Ishimaru T, Hayashi Y et al: Cancer of the thyroid and salivary glands. Gann Monogr Cancer Res 32:129–142, 1986

60. Conard RA: Late radiation effects in Marshall Islanders exposed to fallout 28 years ago. In Boice JD Jr, Fraumeni JF Jr (eds): Radiation Carcinogenesis: Epidemiology and Biological Significance, pp 57–71. New York, Raven Press, 1984

61. Conard RA et al: Review of Medical Findings in a Marshallese Population Twenty-six Years after Accidental Exposure to Radioactive Fallout, pp 1–138. Upton, NY, Brookhaven National Laboratory, 1980

62. Land CE, Boice JD Jr, Shore RE et al: Breast cancer risk from low-dose exposure to ionizing radiation: Results of parallel analysis of three exposed populations of women. J Natl Cancer Inst 65:353–376, 1980

63. Shore RE, Albert RE, Pasternack BS: Follow up study of patients treated by x-ray epilation for tinea capitis: Resurvey of post-treatment illness and mortality experience. Arch Environ Health 31:21–26, 1976

64. Sagerman RH, Cassady JB, Tretter P et al: Radiation induced neoplasia following external beam therapy for children with retinoblastoma. Am J Roentgenol 105:529–535, 1969

65. Strong LC: Theories of pathogenesis: Mutation and cancer. In Mulvihill JJ, Miller RW, Fraumeni JF Jr (eds): Genetics of Human Cancer, pp 401–416. New York, Raven Press, 1977

66. Mays CW, Spiess H: Bone sarcomas in patients given Radium-224. In Boice JD Jr, Fraumeni JF Jr (eds): Radiation Carcinogenesis: Epidemiology and Biological Significance, pp 241–252. New York, Raven Press, 1984

67. da Motta LC, da Silva Horta J, Tavares MH: Prospective epidemiological study of thorotrast-exposed patients in Portugal. Environ Res 18:152–172, 1979

68. Ford DF: Three Mile Island. Thirty Minutes to Meltdown. New York, Penguin, 1982

69. Behling UH, Hildebrand JE: Radiation and Health Effects. A Report of the TMI-2 Accident and Related Health Effects, pp 48–69. Issued by the GPU Nuclear Corporation, Middletown, PA 17057, June 1986

70. Fabrikant JI: Health effects of the nuclear accident at Three Mile Island. Health Physics 40:151–161, 1981

71. Editorial: Living with radiation—after Chernobyl. Lancet 2:609–610, 1986

72. Ishimaru T, Hoshino T, Ichimaru M et al: Leukemia in atomic bomb survivors, Hiroshima and Nagasaki, 1 October 1950–30 September 1966. Radiation Res 45:216–233, 1971

73. Lorenz E: Radioactivity and lung cancer, a critical review in miners of Schneeberg and Joachimstahl. J Natl Cancer Inst 5:1–15, 1944

74. Nero AV, Schwer MB, Nazaroff WW et al: Distribution of airborne radon-222 concentrations in U.S. homes. Science 234:992–997, 1986

75. Environmental Protection Agency and the Department of Health and Human Services: Citizen's Guide to Radon, pp 1–14. Washington, DC, Superintendent of Documents, OPA 86-004, 1986

76. Wagner JC: Mesothelioma and mineral fibers. Cancer 57:1905–1911, 1986

77. Wagner JC, Sleggs CA, Marchand P: Diffuse pleural mesothelioma and asbestos exposure in the North Western Cape Province. Br J Indust Med 17:260–271, 1960

78. Anderson HA, Lilis R, Baum SM et al: Household-contact asbestos. Neoplastic risk. Ann NY Acad Sci 271:311–323, 1976

79. Grundy GW, Miller RW: Malignant mesothelioma in childhood. Report of 13 cases. Cancer 30:1216–1218, 1972

80. Fraumeni JF Jr, Blot WJ: Lung and pleura. In Schottenfeld D, Fraumeni JF Jr (eds): Cancer Epidemiology and Prevention, pp 564–582. Philadelphia, WB Saunders, 1982

81. Committee on Environmental Hazards, American Academy of Pediatrics: Asbestos exposure in schools. Pediatrics 79:301–305, 1987

82. Herbst AL, Ulfelder H, Poskanzer DC: Adenocarcinoma of the vagina. N Engl J Med 284:878–881, 1971

83. Melnick S, Cole P, Anderson D et al: Rates and risks of diethylstilbestrol related clear-cell adenocarcinoma of the vagina and cervix: An update. N Engl J Med 316:514–516, 1987

84. Robboy SJ, Noller KL, O'Brien P et al: Increased incidence of cervical and vaginal dysplasia in 3,980 diethylstilbestrol-exposed young women. JAMA 252:2979–2983, 1984

85. Leary FJ, Resseguie LJ, Kurland LT et al: Males exposed in utero to diethylstilbestrol. JAMA 252:2984–2989, 1984

86. Barnes AB, Colton T, Gundersen J et al: Fertility and outcome of pregnancy in women exposed in utero to diethylstilbestrol. N Engl J Med 302:609–613, 1980

87. Kaufman RH, Binder GL, Grey PM Jr et al: Upper genital tract changes associated with exposure in utero to diethylstilbestrol. Am J Obstet Gynecol 128:51–59, 1977

88. Anthony JJ: Malignant lymphoma associated with hydantoin drugs. Arch Neurol 22:450–454, 1970

89. Allen RW, Ogden B, Bently FL et al: Fetal hydantoin syndrome, neuroblastoma, and hemorrhagic disease in a neonate. JAMA 244:1464–1465, 1980

90. Miller RW: Transplacental carcinogenesis. Cancer Bull 38:300–302, 1986

91. Tucker MA, Meadows AT, Boice JD Jr et al: Leukemia after therapy with alkylating agents for childhood cancer. J Natl Cancer Inst 78:459–464, 1987

92. Greene MH, Harris EL, Gershenson DM et al: Melphalan may be a more potent leukemogen than cyclophosphamide. Ann Intern Med 105:360–367, 1986

93. Tucker MA, D'Angio GJ, Boice JD Jr et al: Bone sarcomas linked to radiotherapy and chemotherapy in children. N Engl J Med 317:588–593, 1987

94. Johnson FL, Feagler JR, Lerner KG et al: Association of androgenic-anabolic steroid therapy with development of hepatocellular carcinoma. Lancet 2:1273–1276, 1972

95. McCaughan GW, Bilous MJ, Gallagher ND: Long-term survival with tumor regression in androgen-induced liver tumors. Cancer 56:2622–2626, 1985

96. Carrasco D, Prieto M, Pallardo L et al: Multiple hepatic adenomas after long-term therapy with testosterone enanthate. Review of the literature. J Hepatol 1:573–578, 1985

97. Haupt HA, Rovere GD: Anabolic steroids: A review of the literature. Am J Sports Med 12:469–484, 1984

98. Hoover R: Effects of drugs—Immunosuppression. In Hiatt HH, Watson JD, Winstein JA (eds): Origins of Human Cancer, pp 369–379. Cold Spring Harbor, NY, Cold Spring Harbor Laboratory, 1977

99. Uhl GS, Williams, JE, Arnett FC Jr: Intracerebral lymphoma in a patient with central nervous system lupus on cyclophosphamide. J Rheumatol 1:282–286, 1974

100. Committee on Passive Smoking, Board on Environmental Studies and Toxicology, National Research Council: Environmental Tobacco Smoke. Measuring Exposures and Assessing Health Effects, p 337. Washington, DC, National Academy Press, 1986

101. A Report of the Surgeon General: The Health Consequences of Involuntary

Smoking. Rockville, MD, U.S. Public Health Service Office on Smoking and Health, 1987

102. Winn DM, Blot WJ, Shy CM et al: Snuff dipping and oral cancer among women in the southern United States. N Engl J Med 304:745–749, 1981

103. Consensus Development Panel, National Institutes of Health: Health applications of smokeless tobacco use. JAMA 255:1045–1048, 1986

104. Council on Scientific Affairs, American Medical Association: Health effects of smokeless tobacco. JAMA 255:1038–1044, 1986

105. Tannenbaum SR: Diet and exposure to N-nitroso compounds. Int Symp Princess Takamatsu Cancer Res Fund 16:67–75, 1985

106. Wogan GN: Diet and nutrition as risk factors for cancer. Int Symp Princess Takamatsu Cancer Res Fund 16:3–10, 1985

107. Willett WC, MacMahon B: Diet and cancer—an overview. N Engl J Med 310:633–638, 697–703, 1984

108. Committee on Diet, Nutrition and Cancer, National Research Council: Diet, Nutrition and Cancer. Washington, DC, National Academy Press, 1982

109. Tomatis L, Breslow NE, Bartch H: Experimental studies in the assessment of human risk. In Schottenfeld D and Fraumeni JF Jr (eds): Cancer Epidemiology and Prevention, pp 44–73. Philadelphia, WB Saunders, 1982

110. Hoover R, Strasser PH: Artificial sweeteners and human bladder cancer. Lancet 1:837–840, 1980

111. Boffey PM: Color additives: Botched experiment leads to banning of Red Dye No. 2. Science 191:450, 1976

112. Miller RW: Areawide chemical contamination. Lessons from case histories. JAMA 245:1548–1551, 1981

113. Levine AG: Love Canal: Science, Politics, and People, pp 1–263. Lexington, MA, Lexington Books, 1982

114. Gough T: Dioxin, Agent Orange, The Facts, pp 1–289. New York, Plenum, 1986

115. Rogan WJ, Gladen BC, McKinney JD et al: Polychlorinated bipenyls (PCBs) and dichlorodiphenyl dichloroethene (DDE) in human milk: Effects of maternal factors and previous lactation. Am J Public Health 2:172–177, 1986

116. Haenszel W: Migrant studies. In Schottenfeld D, Fraumeni JF Jr (eds): Cancer Epidemiology and Prevention, pp 194–207. Philadelphia, WB Saunders, 1982

117. Blot WJ, Fraumeni JF Jr: Arsenical air pollution and lung cancer. Lancet 2:142–144, 1975

118. Phillips RL: Role of lifestyle and dietary habits in risk of cancer among Seventh Day Adventists. Cancer Res 35:3513–3522, 1975

119. Smith PG: Spatial and temporal clustering: In Schottenfeld D, Fraumeni JF Jr (eds): Cancer Epidemiology and Prevention, pp 391–407. Philadelphia, WB Saunders, 1982

120. Gallo RC, Wong–Staal F: Human T-lymphotropic retroviruses. Nature 317:395–403, 1985

121. Centers for Disease Control: Kaposi's sarcoma and pneumocystis pneumonia among homosexual men. New York City and California. MMWR 30:305–308, 1981

122. Purtilo DT, Sakamoto K, Barnabei V et al: Epstein–Barr virus-induced diseases in boys with the X-linked lymphoproliferative syndrome (XLP). Update on studies of the registry. Am J Med 73:48–56, 1982

123. McCance DJ: Human papillomaviruses and cancer. Biochim Biophys Acta 823:195–205, 1986

124. Schouten TJ, van den Broek P, Cremers CW et al: Interferons and bronchogenic carcinoma in juvenile laryngeal papillomatosis. Arch Otolaryngol 109:289–291, 1983

125. Freij BL, Sever JL: Congenital susceptibility to papillomavirus infection. In Buyse ML (eds): Birth Defects Encyclopedia. New York, National Foundation March of Dimes and Alan R. Liss (in press)

126. Lutzner MA: Papillomaviruses and neoplasia in man. Monogr Pathol 27:126–170, 1986

127. Vianna NJ, Polan AK: Epidemiologic evidence for transmission of Hodgkin's disease. N Engl J Med 289:499–502, 1973

128. Smith PG, Pike MC, Kinlen LJ et al: Contacts between young patients with Hodgkin's disease. Lancet 2:59, 1977

129. Grufferman S, Cole P, Smith PG et al: Hodgkin's disease in siblings. N Engl J Med 296:248–250, 1977

130. Morrow RH Jr: Burkitt's lymphoma. In Schottenfeld D, Fraumeni JF Jr: Cancer Epidemiology and Prevention, pp 779–794. Philadelphia, WB Saunders, 1982

131. Magrath IT, Sariban E: Clinical features of Burkitt's lymphoma in the USA. In Lenoir GM, O'Conor GT, Olweny CLM (eds): Burkitt's Lymphoma: A Human Cancer Model, pp 119–127. Lyon, IARC Publ. No. 60, 1985

132. Berger R, Bernheim A: Cytogenetics of Burkitt's lymphoma-leukemia. A review. In Lenoir GM, O'Connor GT, Olweny CLM (eds): Burkitt's Lymphoma: A Human Cancer Model, pp 65–80. Lyon, IARC Publ. No. 60, 1985

133. Wright J, Rosa F: Perinatal hepatitis B infection. In Buyse ML (eds): Birth Defects Encyclopedia. New York, National Foundation March of Dimes and Alan R. Liss (in press)

134. London WT, O'Connell AP: Transplacental transmission of hepatitis B virus. Lancet 1:1037–1038, 1986

135. Stevens CE, Taylor PE, Tong MY et al: Yeast-recombinant hepatitis B immune globulin in prevention of prenatal heptitis B virus transmission. JAMA 257:2612–2616, 1987

two

Clinical Genetics of Pediatric Cancer

John J. Mulvihill

Knowledge *Versus* Opinion

Why a child has cancer is usually unknown. In the only such study to date,[1] parents of 175 Australian children with acute lymphoblastic leukemia were asked, "What do you feel caused your child's illness?" (Fig. 2-1). Only 9% had no idea. Half believed that environmental factors could be implicated; almost a third knew another child in the same area with the same malignancy. Radiation fallout was mentioned by 14%. Other reasons given were exposure to insecticides, "always sick" in the past, and cancer in other family members.

The parents' perceptions echo popular scientific beliefs that 80% of cancers are due to the environment, including factors grouped as lifestyle, such as diet.[2] However, this notion, developed in relation to adult tumors, does not withstand critical examination when applied to the 1% to 2% of malignancies that occur before 20 years of age. The generalization was founded on the rapid changes in cancer mortality rates in recent decades, on observations of cancer in migrant populations, and on a few well-documented cancers arising after certain occupational and radiation exposures and following use of some drugs.[3] However impressive this evidence may be for adult tumors, it is nearly absent with regard to childhood cancer.

On the other hand, cancer biologists know that, at the level of the cell, cancer is always a genetic disease. Clinicians recognize many genetic, congenital, or familial determinants of childhood cancer, as seen when parents of 503 children were interviewed and medical records reviewed for clues to etiology.[4]

This chapter tries to reconcile these apparently opposing views and is based on two premises. First, despite slow, steady progress in understanding the origins of childhood and adolescent cancer, it must be admitted that, for many tumor types in general and certainly for most individual patients, we cannot with much confidence point to a single cause. Second, to avoid the polarizing simplification of considering environmental and genetic determinants as mutually exclusive, it seems reasonable to think that, in each child, cancer arises from a complex interaction of diverse environmental factors with genetic variations, a notion embraced by the term "ecogenetics."[5]

After a brief explanation of the terms and techniques of genetics and cytogenetics as they relate to the etiology of cancer of the young, the prototype disorder of ataxia-telangiectasia (AT) will be discussed as an example of a disorder predisposing to cancer. Other human gene traits that predispose to cancer upon exposure to specific environmental agents are explained in detail. The chromosomal abnormalities associated with childhood malignancies are then enumerated, whether they are constitutional (present in every normal cell) or acquired (seen just in the cancer cells). Even when the chromosomes may be normal, certain birth defects are associated with an excess risk of childhood cancer, and investigation of them provides opportunities for prevention, screening, and early detection and at the same time sheds light on the mechanisms of teratogenesis and carcinogenesis. Oncologists and pediatricians know that the occurrence of

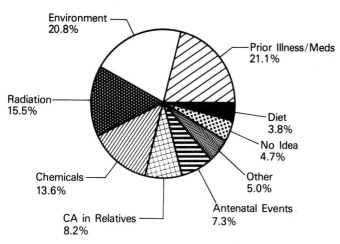

FIGURE 2-1. Parents' thoughts about why their child developed acute lymphoblastic leukemia. (Derived from Reference 1)

cancer in a child is inevitably a family affair, and the special situation of several cancers in a family deserves consideration. Finally, clinical recommendations are given to guide busy cancer therapists in identifying the patient who deserves special etiologic attention and counseling.

Terms and Techniques

The discipline of human genetics studies inborn variations of normal characteristics and of disease.[6–10] All major areas within human genetics have to address the problem of human cancer through their special approaches and perspectives, which often involve specialized terms and techniques.

Population genetics considers variations in disease by ethnic and racial groups and by kindred. For example, pinealoblastoma occurs to excess in Japanese children,[11] whereas Ewing's sarcoma is rare among blacks both in the United States and in Africa.[12] The samples of subjects for study may be groups of families or entire populations. Special areas of mathematical genetics have developed techniques to dissect genetic and environmental determinants of cancers within large families, including the interaction of single major genes (mendelian traits) with shared environment.

Clinical genetics, as practiced in the United States, addresses diseases in individual patients and their relatives that appear to be genetic, congenital, or familial. (*Genetic* refers to genes or chromosomes, the DNA of the cell. *Congenital* means present at birth for environmental, genetic, or unknown reasons. *Familial* refers to aggregation within a kindred for genetic, environmental, or unknown reasons; although family members share many genes, they usually also have a common environment. All three terms can appropriately describe many disorders.) The subjects for study are individual patients and their relatives. The special area of malformations is handled clinically by dysmorphologists and experimentally by developmental geneticists. By recognizing the occasional patient with a birth defect that carries a high risk of cancer, the clinician hopes to detect cancer early and prevent serious morbidity and the researcher hopes to understand the related phenomena of carcinogenesis and teratogenesis by standing at their interface. The clinical geneticist recognizes some 200 single-gene traits that predispose to or are complicated by neoplasia; these 200 represent some 5% of the 4000 recognized genetic traits of humans, who seem to have enough DNA for 50,000 genes.

Such classic mendelian traits include about half that have autosomal dominant inheritance (passed from one generation to the next with 50% probability, including sometimes from father to son), one-third with autosomal recessive inheritance (occurring only when the mutant gene is present in two copies, presumably one from each carrier parent), and one-sixth with X-linked recessive inheritance (such as hemophilia and Duchenne's muscular dystrophy).

Cytogenetics and cell genetics are closely related tools for the clinician and researcher alike. Every technical improvement in distinguishing the 46 chromosomes in every human somatic cell has supported Theodor Boveri's 1914 hypothesis that, with sufficiently refined methods, every cancer cell will prove to have abnormal chromosomes.[13] The sample for analysis is a living cell: blood lymphocytes, fresh tumor cells obtained by bone-marrow aspiration, or tissue from a biopsy specimen (for tumor cells or fibroblasts). Laboratory techniques approach an art, but all involve arresting growing cells in metaphase or in prophase for long chromosomes and staining the mitotic figures with colored or fluorescent dyes so that each chromosome may be distinguished from all others, usually by its unique pattern of alternately light and dark bands. Sometimes, the karyotypic abnormalities are constitutional (present in every body cell from conception) and may account for birth defects associated with a risk of cancer. More often, a child with a normal constitutional karyotype has a cancer the cells of which have chromosomes in the wrong number (aneuploidy) or with the wrong structure (translocation, inversion, breaks, homogeneously staining regions), or both (double minutes).

Molecular genetics brings the focus to the gene—the segment of DNA, with its precise sequence of the four nucleotide bases, that seems to have a discrete function. The techniques of the molecular geneticist in a sense reveal cancer genes directly in the form of activated oncogenes, transposed elements, single-base changes, and so forth, as explained in Chapter 3.

ECOGENETICS

Considering cancer as *either* genetic *or* environmental in origin is a polarizing oversimplification. A single tumor type—even a single cancer in one child—is likely to have many determinants; hence, the appropriate conceptualization for the origins of all cancers may be "ecogenetics."[14] By analogy to *pharmacogenetics* (the study of genetic variations in response to drugs), ecogenetics means the study of genetic variations in response to any environmental agent.[15,16] Although examples of ecogenetics in childhood cancer are few (Table 2-1),[17] they provide the models for understanding all human cancer through intense study of just a small number of patients. These traits will be emphasized here and in other comprehensive reviews[5,18–22]; exclusively environmental determinants are explained in detail in Chapters 1 and 55.

Ataxia-Telangiectasia (AT): Ecogenetic Prototype

In 1963, Miller identified five pairs of sibs who had died of childhood leukemia years before.[23] He suggested recall of one family to look for genetic traits recognized to predispose to leukemia, such as Down's syndrome, Fanconi's pancytopenia, and Bloom's syndrome.[24] Specifically, he suggested the diagnosis of AT because the records showed that the leukemic sibs and a brother had a neurologic problem. Patients with AT, an autosomal recessive trait, have dilated scleral blood vessels, progressive cerebellar dysfunction, immunodeficiency, and a

Table 2-1
Genetic–Environmental Interactions (Ecogenetics) in Tumors of the Young

Environmental Agent	Genetic Trait	Tumor or Outcome
Ionizing radiation	Ataxia-telangiectasia with lymphoma	Radiation toxicity
	Retinoblastoma	Sarcoma
	Nevoid basal-cell carcinoma syndrome	Basal cell carcinoma
Ultraviolet radiation	Xeroderma pigmentosum	Skin cancer, melanoma
	Cutaneous albinism	Skin cancer
	Hereditary dysplastic nevus syndrome	Melanoma
Stilbestrol	XO Turner's syndrome	Adenosquamous endometrial carcinoma
Androgen	Fanconi's pancytopenia	Hepatoma
Iron	Hemochromatosis	Hepatocellular carcinoma
Tyrosine	Tyrosinemia	Hepatocellular carcinoma
Monosaccharides	Glycogen storage disease type 1	Hepatic adenoma
? Epstein–Barr virus	Purtilo X-linked lymphoproliferative syndrome	Burkitt's and other lymphomas
Papillomavirus type 5	Epidermodysplasia verruciformis	Skin cancer

(Adapted from Reference 14)

risk of leukemia and lymphoma (also see Chap. 4).[25–29] AT was indeed diagnosed in the brother in Oregon.[30]

Similar etiologic observations are amassed slowly because therapists must pursue diagnosis and therapy rather than the origins of a disease like cancer. But such a tactic continues to work, even in AT. For example, Hecht and colleagues studied chromosomes in the surviving sib and found a minor clone of lymphocytes with abnormal chromosomes.[31] Over time, the minor clone became a major one, as if this were the cell line that would become frankly malignant. This boy died of intercurrent lung disease, but patients who did indeed go on to have leukemia have since been described. Also, markers have been documented to involve regions of chromosome 14.[32]

Hecht and others further confirmed the place of AT among the chromosomal breakage syndromes popularized by German.[33] The three classic syndromes—AT, Fanconi's pancytopenia, and Bloom's syndrome—are autosomal recessive traits with an excess of broken chromosomes *in vitro* and a high risk of malignancy, mostly leukemia.

An additional insight into AT came from Birmingham, England, where an AT patient developed lymphoma.[34] After the usual radiotherapy, he suffered acute radiation toxicity. Two similarly radiosensitive AT patients had previously been reported.[35,36] What was different in Birmingham was the presence of the radiobiological laboratory of D. G. Harnden, who could assay radiosensitivity *in vitro*. The assay involves growing fibroblasts to confluence in a laboratory dish, exposing them to several doses of ionizing radiation, and evaluating the fraction of cells that survive to establish new colonies after further incubation. Harnden found the cells to be unduly sensitive to gamma radiation.[34] Although the exact molecular defects of AT remain unclear, they may prove to relate to carcinogenesis in general, even in the absence of AT.[28,29]

AT is rare, seen perhaps in 1 in 100,000 Americans,[37] yet the Hardy–Weinberg principle of gene frequencies in populations implies that AT could have public health consequences, since carriers occur at a frequency of 1 in 70. Such heterozygotes (*e.g.,* parents of affected children) are clinically normal except for a possible excess of cancer (suggested by two independent but controversial studies from one team.[38,39]) It is conceivable that the gene, which clearly predisposes to cancer in the double dose, may also predispose in a single dose. In support of this notion, some laboratories report that fibroblasts from heterozygotes have a degree of radiosensitivity *in vitro* that is intermediate between those of normal and AT persons.[34,40]

In summary, a few patients studied intensively by alert clinicians and collaborating scientists provided insight into the interrelations of gamma radiation, cancer, and the molecular mechanisms of carcinogenesis. Such interactions would be hard to study otherwise, since appropriate animal models have not been found.

Ionizing Radiation

No human carcinogen is better understood than ionizing radiation.[41–44] Besides clinical observations as early as 1902,[45] large epidemiologic studies document the carcinogenicity of radiation in children.[46] Data come from retrospective cohort studies of survivors of the atomic bombs in Japan,[47] survivors of other nuclear explosions,[48] and patients given radiation for malignancy,[49] tinea capitis, or an enlarged thymus and as contrast media (radioisotopic agents) (see Chaps. 1 and 55).[50,51] Such studies rarely address the possibility that the effect seen in a large population could be accounted for by unusual host sensitivity of a segment of the group.[52] Radiation is not associated with an excess of all types of cancer in adults and certainly not in children. Even though radiation may be received during childhood, most tumors do not appear until later in life. Although not seen by pediatricians, their occurrence serves as a general warning that adult tumors certainly may have their origins in childhood, including in medical practices and personal habits. Details of radiation carcinogenesis in children vary with the site and type of exposure, age at exposure, and the type of tumor.

Postnatal Exposure

Because of the long latency for most radiogenic cancers, few tumors appearing in childhood can be attributed to radiation.[46] One exception is leukemia: excessive acute and chronic myelogenous leukemia and acute lymphoblastic leukemia were seen 3 to 10 years after the atomic bombs in Japan. Children are generally more susceptible than adults to radiogenic tumors, including benign and malignant thyroid and salivary gland tumors, bone and other sarcomas, and brain tumors. In contrast, lung and colon cancers have not (yet) been associated with radiation exposure in those younger than 20 years. The male breast seems spared, as does the prepubertal female breast; on the other hand, the adolescent female breast appears highly sensitive to radiation. X-rays are unlikely to contribute to the origins of embryonal tumors, Hodgkin's disease, and testicular cancer.

In the past, malignancy has been recognized repeatedly as a late complication of enthusiastic application of radiation for nonmalignant diseases, such as tinea capitis,[53] and of new radioisotopes, such as ^{131}I for diagnostic thyroid studies, thorium dioxide (Thorotrast) in contrast media, and ^{224}Ra for treating disseminated tuberculosis.[44,50] Such experiences mandate critical evaluation of new uses of radioactive agents. Controversy continues concerning the alleged excesses of childhood leukemia in Utah due to fallout from nuclear testing[46,54,55] or in English districts with nuclear power plants.[56] Prudent use of dental radiation is highly unlikely to cause harm.[57]

Prenatal Exposure

In England, prenatal exposure to medical radiation, usually for routine pelvimetry in the third trimester four decades ago, was associated with a 60% excess of all types of malignancy during the first decade of life, with a linear response to dose (inferred from the number of films).[58] In Boston, a 50% excess of all cancer was confined to the first 7 years.[59] The Tristate Leukemia Survey showed an excess of leukemia, the only malignancy studied, especially in children with some immune dysfunction, including allergies, (which may have been the indication for maternal radiography).[60] Superficially concordant, these studies were not sufficiently similar in design and results to support a causal relation. The association was not seen among children *in utero* at the time of the Japanese atomic bombs.[61] There is no confirmatory animal model, and one agent is not likely to increase the frequency of all types of childhood cancer.

Although the controversy seems irresolvable,[62] it is prudent to restate that only essential radiation exposure should be permitted during pregnancy, since fetal exposure to as few as 10 to 19 cGy of neutrons apparently caused small head size among the Hiroshima bomb survivors.[63]

With Susceptible Genotype

RETINOBLASTOMA. AT is not an isolated example of radiation interacting with a sensitive host. Another example is retinoblastoma, the embryonal tumor of the eye, which continues to serve as an example of a cancer gene (see Chap. 25).[64-66] The gene has been isolated and its base sequence determined,[67] and prenatal diagnosis has been accomplished.[68] Like all children given radiotherapy, retinoblastoma patients have an excess risk of second tumors arising in the field of radiation.[69-71] They also manifest other pleiotropic effects of the retinoblastoma gene: an excess of osteosarcoma outside the radiation port[72] and of pinealoblastoma ("trilateral retinoblastoma").[73] Radiogenic tumors seem to occur earlier in retinoblastoma patients than in those with other types of cancer that are not considered to be hereditary.[74] Further, children with hereditary retinoblastoma seem to get radiogenic tumors more often than do patients with sporadic retinoblastoma. (Of course, they receive radiotherapy more often because of their bilateral tumors.) In any case, an *in vitro* manifestation of this clinical radiosensitivity has been reported by one laboratory.[75,76] Unusual sensitivity to gamma radiation was found in fibroblasts from infants with bilateral (hereditary) retinoblastoma but not those with unilateral (sporadic) tumor or retinoblastoma associated with a specific chromosomal anomaly, 13q. Other laboratories failed to confirm the initial observation, although some reported other abnormalities (and some none) involving irradiated cells from retinoblastoma patients.[77,78]

NEVOID BASAL-CELL CARCINOMA SYNDROME. An autosomal dominant disease, Nevoid basal-cell carcinoma syndrome—also called Gorlin's syndrome—is characterized by craniofacial anomalies such as synophrys (fused eyebrows), telecanthus (lateral displacement of the lacrimal duct punctum), and broad nasal bridge; palmar and plantar pits; and multiple basal-cell carcinomas of the skin (Fig. 2-2).[79,80] How one mutant gene causes such diverse effects remains unknown. Two clinical observations suggest that radiation contributes to the development of skin cancers. First, the basal cell carcinomas seem to appear first on sun-exposed areas. Second, in children given radiotherapy for medulloblastoma (a feature of the syndrome), crops of basal cell carcinomas arise first around the margins of the radiation port before they occur elsewhere on the skin.[74] The peculiar distribution and short latency period suggest an unusual clinical response to gamma radiation. However, in assays using colony survival (described above), *in vitro* radiosensitivity was not detected.[81]

Ultraviolet Radiation

Sunlight is the most common cause of cancer in adults.[82] The incidence and the mortality rate of skin cancers other than malignant melanoma correlate well with latitude in both the Northern and the Southern Hemispheres: skin cancer rate decreases as distance from the equator increases. These observations are in whites only. Blacks in the United States have a skin cancer rate about 10% that of whites, a difference best explained by genetically determined skin color; that is, the amount of melanin granules in the epidermis. Skin cancer is virtually absent in children without a genetic predisposition; however, as in many other adult tumors, the risk for skin cancer begins in childhood, when habits of sun exposure are often determined.

With Susceptible Genotypes

XERODERMA PIGMENTOSUM. Although skin cancer rarely occurs in children, in Tunisia it accounts for 14% of all childhood cancers.[12] The apparent explanation is the intense solar radiation at that latitude plus the frequency of autosomal recessive xeroderma pigmentosum in a highly inbred community. In the 1960s, radiobiologist J. Cleaver investigated ultraviolet radiosensitivity *in vitro* when he heard of the San Francisco "moon people," so called because they knew they had to avoid sunlight to prevent recurrent skin tumors. The discovery of a defect in the repair of ultraviolet-induced damage to the genetic material brought clinical relevance to

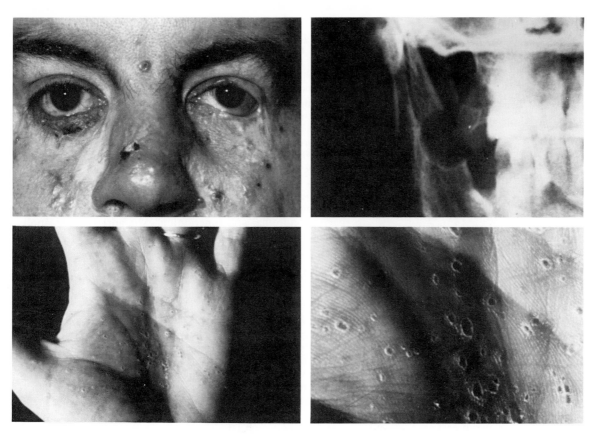

FIGURE 2-2. Nevoid basal cell carcinoma syndrome with palmar pits, mandibular cysts, and multiple basal cell carcinomas of the skin, even in childhood. (Courtesy of A. E. Bale, National Cancer Institute)

years of fundamental research in microbes, demonstrating the interaction of radiation, mutagenesis, and carcinogenesis.[83]

DYSPLASTIC NEVUS SYNDROME. Everyone has some moles, properly called pigmented nevi. Nevi with histopathologically dysplastic melanocytes are called dysplastic nevi and, in contrast to ordinary moles, are numerous; are variable in size, shape, and color; and continue to appear past childhood (see Chap. 35).[84-86] Most importantly, they carry a high risk of cutaneous malignant melanoma, about 400 times the risk of the general population. An interaction of the trait with ultraviolet radiation is suggested by two observations: dysplastic nevi predominate in sun-exposed areas, and fibroblasts and lymphocytes from affected persons are unusually sensitive to ultraviolet light and chemicals that mimic its action.[87] The dysplastic nevus syndrome may be sporadic but is often hereditary, appearing in families as an autosomal dominant trait. In children, dysplastic nevi have been seen in the scalp, an unusual site for normal nevi. When the syndrome is diagnosed early, an educational and surveillance program can be launched so that any melanoma can be removed simply at its earliest stage.

ALBINISM. The various hereditary forms of cutaneous albinism are less well studied but probably more common than xeroderma pigmentosum. In Africa, blacks with albinism have a high frequency of skin cancer even in childhood.[88] Search for DNA repair defects in albinotic cells seems desirable, although the lack of pigment to protect the DNA from mutagenic ultraviolet light is probably a sufficient explanation for the increased risk of skin cancer.

Chemicals, Including Drugs

Human exposure to chemicals is immense and often beneficial to health. The numbers, amounts, and exact types of chemicals are changing rapidly. To the extent that chemistry is the physical foundation of life, all cancers can be considered chemically mediated.

The fetus and child have special sensitivities to chemical pollutants.[89] In rare situations, intense exposure to drugs is firmly associated with subsequent neoplasia, either as a result of interaction with a genetic disorder or by action on the fetus; that is, transplacentally.[90,91]

Estrogens in Turner's Syndrome

Affected individuals with this condition are phenotypic females with short stature, primary amenorrhea, and minor dysmorphic features. They often receive estrogen replacement for many years to improve their secondary sex characteristics, since their streak gonads produce insufficient hormones. In some such patients, a rare type of cancer, adenosquamous carcinoma of the endometrium, occurs in the rudimentary uterus before age 30 years.[92] An absence of case reports suggests that the tumor has not been seen in Turner's syndrome without estrogen replacement. Although estrogen use has been associated with endometrial cancer in the general population,[93] the usual cell type is adenocarcinoma, and it occurs at a later age than in patients with Turner's syndrome.

Androgens in Fanconi's Pancytopenia

Long-term use of androgens, especially the steroid oxymetholone, has been associated with hepatomas in patients with this autosomal recessive disease (pancytopenia, radial dysplasia, microcephaly, and renal anomalies).[94] Although metastasizing hepatocellular carcinoma has occurred, the tumors are more often benign hepatic cell adenomas, the same type associated with long-term use of the oral contraceptive pill. Patients with pancytopenia may, in fact, not be uniquely susceptible, because similar tumors have been reported in patients receiving androgens for infertility and non-Fanconi aplastic anemia.[95] Still, a possible ecogenetic interaction can be seen *in vitro:* fibroblasts from patients with Fanconi's pancytopenia are unduly sensitive to the chromosome-breaking effects of the alkylating agent diepoxybutane.[96] This assay has permitted prenatal diagnosis of an affected fetus and can help identify carriers of just one mutant gene, that is, heterozygotes.

Iatrogenic Cancer

Cancer therapy has proved to be a two-edged sword. Substantial improvements in survival have been achieved,[97] but chemotherapy and radiotherapy have proved to be powerful carcinogens. Children who survive 5 years after a diagnosis of cancer have 20 times more cancer than expected in those without a cancer history.[98] On average, 6 per 1000 children who have survived cancer develop a second malignancy in each year of follow-up. Of 36 such children with double cancers, 28 second tumors were attributed to radiotherapy given for the first: 12 sarcomas, four acute leukemias, four thyroid carcinomas, two skin cancers, two breast cancers, and one case each of hepatoma, renal cell carcinoma, mesenchymoma, and oligodendroglioma. In two of the remaining eight patients, host susceptibility was likely, since one had had bilateral retinoblastoma and malignant melanoma and the other had two sibs with a total of three other cancers.

Thirteen pediatric oncology centers in North America and Europe assembled 222 patients with multiple primary cancers, some of whom were included in the list above.[49,71] Among 9170 2-year survivors, the frequency of a second malignancy was 12% by 25 years, an average rate of three extra cancers per 1000 persons per year. The rate of second cancers fails to level off (Fig. 2-3), in contrast to observations on radiogenic leukemia[41] and malignancy following radiotherapy and chemotherapy for Hodgkin's disease.[99] Some patients with second

cancers had them in radiation fields with no known genetic preneoplastic disease; others had predisposing genetic disorders, such as hereditary retinoblastoma, neurofibromatosis, nevoid basal-cell carcinoma syndrome, and xeroderma pigmentosum. Whereas the one series demonstrated no effect attributable to chemotherapy alone,[98] the collaborative series showed a 14-fold excess of leukemia, mostly attributable to alkylating-agent therapy.[100] In short, host and environmental factors are determinants of second malignant neoplasms in children; hence, there is an obvious need to devise less-toxic treatments while maintaining or bettering the survival rates.

Even without carcinogenic treatments, multiple neoplasms, not all malignant, occur to excess in certain families[101] with mendelian traits such as neurofibromatosis and the newly delineated triad of gastric epithelioid leiomyosarcoma, pulmonary chondroma, and functioning extra-adrenal paraganglioma, especially in young women (Carney triad).[102]

Transplacental Carcinogenesis

Diethylstilbestrol

By the early 1970s, the world's literature contained about a dozen cases of clear-cell adenocarcinoma of the vagina in women younger than 30 years of age. Then, Herbst and Scully encountered six in a few years at one Boston hospital.[103] The retrospective search for etiologic clues included, at a mother's suggestion, questions on *in utero* exposure to diethylstilbestrol (DES), which was given to perhaps a million women in the 1940s and 1950s to prevent miscarriages. (Reanalysis of a study that launched such DES treatment showed no benefit for this indication and an excess of malformations.[104])

With 519 cases now assembled,[105] it is clear that (1) exposure to DES in any trimester can be carcinogenic; (2) the lowest dose associated with abnormalities seems to be 1.5 mg daily or 135 mg total; (3) most of the cancers are diagnosed between ages 15 and 27 years; (4) vaginal ridges and adenosis are precursor lesions detectable in early childhood[106]; and (5) the cancer may arise in the cervix as well as the vagina (see Chaps. 1, 35, 55). Cancer is still a rare complication: 1 per 100 exposed women through age 34 years. Hence, DES is an incomplete carcinogen, and other factors must operate. Cancer has not been reported in male offspring who, nonetheless, may have oligospermia, epididymal cyst, hypoplastic testes, and microphallus as teratogenic manifestations.[107]

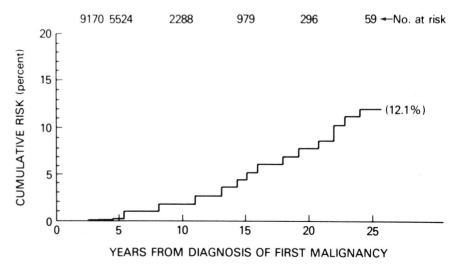

FIGURE 2-3. Cumulative frequency of second malignant neoplasms in 9170 persons who survived at least 2 years after the diagnosis of an initial childhood cancer.

YEARS FROM DIAGNOSIS OF FIRST MALIGNANCY

The association of the maternal use of DES with malformations and cancer in offspring has refocused attention on the overlap of carcinogenesis and teratogenesis. The principle has emerged that any agent suspected of causing human malformations may be suspected of causing cancer, and *vice versa;* however, the mechanisms of action may well be different.[108] For example, *in utero* radiation may cause small head size and mental retardation in the fetus by killing brain cells,[63] whereas it may cause cancer in a child or adult by inducing mutation in still-viable cells.

Phenytoin (Diphenylhydantoin; Dilantin)

A rare complication of chronic use of phenytoin for epilepsy is lymph node hyperplasia that often regresses when the drug is withdrawn but which can progress malignantly.[109] Phenytoin use in pregnancy has been associated with a syndrome of growth, mental retardation, and hypoplasia of the midface and nails.[110] Of some 100 cases of fetal hydantoin syndrome reported since 1976, 7 had neoplasia: 4 neuroblastomas and 1 each of ganglioneuroblastoma, extrarenal Wilms' tumor, and melanotic ectodermal tumor.[111-114]

One action of phenytoin is suppression of T-cell function. Because inborn immunodeficiencies are associated with a high risk of childhood cancer,[115,116] it is reasonable to speculate that the neoplasia, and perhaps the malformations, associated with phenytoin might relate to its immunosuppression.[117]

Arsenic

A brief report suggested that basal cell carcinomas in a teenager were related to his mother's use of Fowler's solution, also associated with similar tumors in the mother.[118] Since the nevoid basal-cell carcinoma syndrome was not thought to be present, transplacental carcinogenesis by arsenic was a possible, albeit unlikely, explanation.

Other

The point remains that cancer in childhood and adolescence may arise following *in utero* exposures to various agents. A comprehensive case–control study of 11,169 children with cancer found maternal epilepsy and pulmonary tuberculosis in excess, although no association with a specific drug was detected.[119] A controversial study incriminated maternal use of barbiturates in childhood brain tumors.[120] Rarely, maternal cancer metastasizes to the placenta and fetus.[121]

Diet

The role of dietary factors in the origins of adult cancer is controversial.[122] For childhood cancers, there is no evidence apart from three ecogenetic traits. Children with autosomal recessive tyrosinemia benefit from a diet low in tyrosine and phenylalanine; otherwise, and sometimes nonetheless, hepatic cirrhosis may worsen and be complicated by malignant hepatoma as early as 15 years of age.[123] Presumably, if the diet were free of the precursors of tyrosine, the metabolites would not accumulate to toxic, carcinogenic levels. Similar reasoning applies to the postcirrhotic hepatoma complicating hereditary hemochromatosis and perhaps to hepatic adenoma arising in the majority of children with glycogen storage disease, type 1.[124]

Pediatricians should be concerned about the trend toward manipulating children's diets in the hope of preventing adult cancers, given current plans to establish "cancer-prevention" diets during the critical childhood and adolescent years. One concern arises because some recommended foods are not popular among the young, such as cruciferous vegetables (cabbage, broccoli, and cauliflower). Although the crucial elements in these foods have not been identified, well-meaning caretakers might substitute vitamin and mineral pills, perhaps in large doses ("If a little is good, a lot is better"). Pediatricians might start to see liver toxicity or fetal malformation syndrome caused by, for example, poisoning by vitamin A.[125]

Viruses

As with diet, few viruses have been implicated in childhood and adolescent cancer, but prenatal and childhood exposure to viruses has been associated with cancers later in life. Examples include perinatal infection with hepatitis B virus and hepatocellular carcinoma; Epstein–Barr virus (EBV) infection and Burkitt's lymphoma or nasopharyngeal carcinoma (see Chaps. 20 and 35); and papilloma viruses and laryngeal papillomatosis or cervical carcinoma.[126-128]

Despite many murine models, few human neoplasias have been suspected of arising from the interaction of a possibly oncogenic virus with a susceptible genome. The chief candidate is the lymphoproliferative syndrome of Purtilo.[129] Inherited as an X-linked trait, so mostly males are affected, the features include fulminating, sometimes fatal, infectious mononucleosis; Burkitt's lymphoma; Hodgkin's disease; and bone-marrow aplasia. Other studies have etiologically associated all of these disorders with EBV. With only a half-dozen reported families, much clinical and laboratory investigation remains to be done, and a registry has been established at the University of Nebraska to expedite studies. The trait should be considered whenever a male presents with an EBV-associated disorder, so that special efforts can be made to place the family under surveillance to improve understanding of the proposed virus–gene interaction.

Similar interactions are postulated in EBV-associated nasopharyngeal carcinoma, which seems to occur to excess in Chinese with HLA-A Singapore 2. There is suspicion that some families may be especially susceptible to hepatitis infection, and such host susceptibility could explain ethnic and familial aggregations of the hepatocellular carcinoma.[131] Papillomavirus type 5 may well interact with a susceptible genotype to produce warts with unusually high rates of malignant degeneration in epidermodysplasia verruciformis, generally thought to be an autosomal recessive skin disorder.[132]

GENETIC FACTORS

Even in the absence of known ecogenetic interactions, a multitude of genetic and congenital disorders predispose to childhood and adolescent cancer.[5,133] Such genetic factors may be considered in three groups:

1. *Chromosomal:* entire lengths of genetic material are translocated, absent, or present in excess either in every body cell (constitutional) or just in the malignant tissue (acquired).
2. *Single locus:* disease arising from a mutation in either one allelic member as a dominant trait or in a double dose, as in a recessive trait.
3. *Polygenic or multifactorial:* many genes interact, perhaps with environmental factors, to cause disease, with no one factor or gene playing a predominant role.

Twin and Epidemiologic Observations

A classic resource for delineating genetic factors is twins. For cancer, however, study of twins has been minimally informative. The one exception is an identical twin who develops leukemia in infancy; the risk of leukemia in the other twin then is nearly 100%.[23] The risk decreases after 1 year of age and approaches the risk of any family member by 6 years. This age-dependent difference in risk has been attributed to one twin developing leukemia *in utero* and passing leukemic cells to the other through placental vascular anastomoses. This phenomenon was especially well demonstrated by karyotyping of leukemic cells in one report of childhood leukemia in twins.[134]

Epidemiologic surveys have provided some evidence of hereditary determinants in childhood cancer. The early age at diagnosis of retinoblastoma, Wilms' tumor, and several other embryonal cell tumors[135] suggests their prenatal origin and, with other observations, supports Knudson's mutational hypothesis described below. Racial differences, which in theory may be either environmental or genetic, are often unexplained. The worldwide absence of Ewing's sarcoma in blacks could be genetic.[12] Childhood pineal tumors occur much more frequently in Japan than elsewhere in the world.[11] The strongest evidence of genetic factors comes from the study of small numbers of patients with associated congenital defects, laboratory evidence of genetic abnormalities, and positive family histories. Retinoblastoma is an enduring example.

Retinoblastoma: Prototype of a Cancer Gene

In 1922, the Galton Laboratory in London, the originator of modern medical genetics, published a monograph on glioma retinae, as retinoblastoma was then known, concluding that the disease was "of great interest to the clinician but has been of no very great interest from the point of view of the student of heredity."[64] In fact, the tumor continues to serve as a model of progress made in understanding the origins of childhood cancer through genetics. In addition to the ecogenetic interaction of the gene with ionizing radiation (above), five developments in the last two decades illustrate how insights from clinical observations can lead to laboratory discoveries that have wide application.

Recognition of Hereditary Subgroups

Studies of large groups of patients with retinoblastoma resolved the confusion about the many cases that did not seem to be familial even though the trait was the best known example of a cancer gene. It is now obvious that bilateral retinoblastoma is much more likely to be familial than is unilateral retinoblastoma (see also Chap. 25). A further characteristic of hereditary retinoblastoma is early age of onset: 50% of cases are identified by 1 year of age for bilateral tumors or 3 years for unilateral tumors.[136,137]

FIGURE 2-4. Four pleiotropic effects of the retinoblastoma gene on chromosome 13q14.

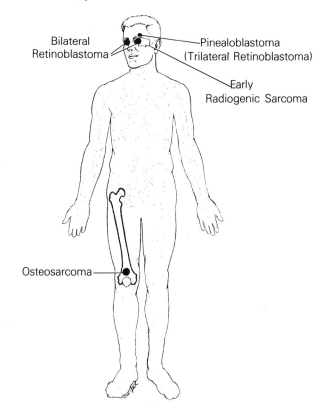

FIGURE 2-5. Abbreviated family tree of a man (*arrow*) who carried the retinoblastoma gene and manifested it as an osteosarcoma at age 37 years, never having had retinoblastoma. (Modified from Reference 138)

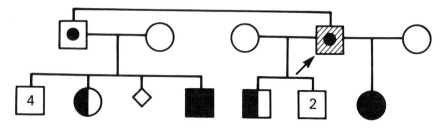

Pleiotropic Effects

The usual therapy for bilateral retinoblastoma is enucleation of the more involved eye and radiotherapy to the other eye. Survivors of such therapy have an excess of bony and soft-tissue sarcomas.[69-72] Some of these sarcomas arise in the field of radiation, perhaps earlier than in patients given similar radiotherapy for nonhereditary tumors.[74] Other second primary tumors occur far from the radiation field, such as in the distal femur, the usual site for osteosarcoma. The risk for such tumors is about 50 times normal and seems confined to patients with hereditary, bilateral retinoblastoma. This is the pleiotropic effect of the retinoblastoma gene; namely, it is expressed not only in the eye but also in other tissues that have the mutant gene from conception (Fig. 2-4). Additional evidence that sarcoma is a manifestation of the retinoblastoma gene comes from pedigrees that include individuals who must have the gene (because they transmitted it) but who had sarcoma, not retinoblastoma (Fig. 2-5).[138] Pinealoblastoma, the embryonic tumor of the "third eye" in lower vertebrates, seems to be an additional pleiotropic effect of the gene, giving rise to the term "trilateral retinoblastoma."[73]

Two-Mutation Hypothesis

Knudson melded these clinical and epidemiologic observations into a credible mutational model that resurrected previous multiple-hit theories of carcinogenesis (Fig. 2-6).[137] He theorized that all retinoblastomas arise from at least two mutations. The second mutation always occurs after conception; that is, postzygotically, as a result of an environmental or an unknown agent. The first mutation may be postzygotic, as in sporadic cases, or prezygotic, as in hereditary cases. In other words, the first mutation, leading to an instability, may come from a rare somatic mutation or from a hereditary or germinal mutation that would be present in all body cells. Some pathologists believe there is a benign retinal tumor, a retinoma, that could represent a penultimate step in carcinogenesis in line with the Knudson model except that the precursor cell is a mature retinoblast, not an immature one that could lead to retinoblastoma.[139]

Associated Birth Defects

In some patients with retinoblastoma but without a family history of retinoblastoma, a syndrome of birth defects, including mental retardation, was observed in association with a deletion in the long arm of chromosome 13 (13q−).[27,124] These few patients were in fact the clue to the location of the retinoblastoma gene. Improved cytogenetic techniques revealed a few patients with retinoblastoma but no congenital defects and

with a deletion of a specific band, 13q14 (read as "band four of region one of the long arm of chromosome 13") (see Chap. 3).[140] Then, a similar deletion was seen in most tumor cells, even in patients with normal constitutional (lymphocytic) karyotypes.

FIGURE 2-6. Knudson's two-mutation hypothesis. In all tumors, the same cell must undergo at least two mutations in order to become malignant, and the second mutation always occurs after conception. In sporadic nonhereditary tumor (**right**), the first hit also occurs after conception. In hereditary tumor (**left**), the first mutation is in a germ cell, such that all body cells in the offspring have the first mutation. (Reprinted from Miller RW: Genetics and familial predisposition. In Calabresi P, Shein PS, Rosenberg SA (eds): Medical Oncology: Basic Principles and Clinical Management of Cancer, p 130. New York, Macmillan, 1985)

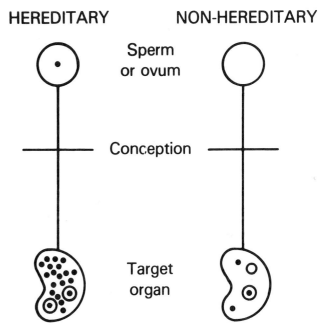

HEREDITARY   NON-HEREDITARY

Sperm or ovum

Conception

Target organ

- • First mutation (pre- or post-conception)
- ○ Second mutation (post-conception only)

Table 2-2
Two Classes of Oncogenes

Feature	Oncogene	Antioncogene
Example	*myc, ras, met*	*Rb-1,* Wilms' tumor, renal cell carcinoma, meningioma
Normal action	Growth factor, ?embryogenesis	Represses cancer
Carcinogenic action	When activated (*e.g.,* by translocation or point mutation)	When lost (*e.g.,* by deletion, recombination)
Mode of carcinogenic action	Dominant	Recessive
Inheritance of active gene	Not inherited	Inherited and not inherited
Tissue specificity	Broad	Narrow

Loss of Genetic Heterozygosity

These clinical observations on double primary cancers, pleiotropic effects, Knudson's two-hit model, and a chromosome abnormality demanded a unifying hypothesis. Molecular dissection was expedited by the discovery of the linkage of the retinoblastoma locus to a polymorphic protein.[27] In certain tumors and patients without visible chromosomal deletions, the nearby locus, esterase D, served as a marker of the retinoblastoma locus and was found to be deleted.[23] The fascinating story then emerged that launched a fresh generalization concerning childhood carcinogenesis and a new term, "antioncogene" (Table 2-2).[141] To summarize, although retinoblastoma acts as a dominant trait at the level of the person, it acts as a recessive trait at the cellular level, since it is not manifested until two alleles at the locus are lost or otherwise changed. By various genetic mechanisms, the end-result is loss of heterozygosity (gain of homozygosity or hemizygosity) at the retinoblastoma locus on chromosome 13q14 (see Chaps. 3 and 25). The normal allele at the locus acts to suppress cancer development when present in two copies (as in normal persons) or even as one copy, for example, in persons with one mutant retinoblastoma gene or a constitutional deletion of the normal allele—hence the term antioncogene. A retinoblastoma can

Table 2-3
Childhood and Adolescent Neoplasia Associated with Acquired Nonrandom Cytogenetic Abnormalities

Chromosome	Abnormality	Neoplasm
1	Deletion p32p36	Neuroblastoma
1	Deletion q25–q41	Various lymphoproliferative disorders
2	Translocation 2p11–13;8q24	Burkitt's lymphoma
2	Translocation 2q37;13q14	Alveolar rhabdomyosarcoma
3	Translocation 3p25;8q21	Mixed salivary gland tumor
5	Monosomy	Environmental myeloid leukemia
5	Deletion q21–qter	Lymphoproliferative neoplasia
6	Translocation 6p21–23;9q33–34	Myeloid leukemia (M2) with basophilia
6	Deletion q21–qter	Lymphoproliferative neoplasia
7	Monosomy	Environmental myeloid leukemia (M2)
8	*cf.* chromosomes 2, 3, 14	
8	Trisomy; translocation 8q22;21q11	Acute myelogenous leukemia (M2)
8	Translocation 8q24;22q11 or 2p13 or 14q32.3	Burkitt's lymphoma
9	*cf.* chromosome 6	
9	Translocation 11q24;22q11 (Philadelphia)	Chronic myelogenous leukemia
11	Translocation 11q24;22q12	Ewing's sarcoma, Askin tumor, peripheral neuroepithelioma, esthesioneuroblastoma
11	Deletion p13	Miller's syndrome of sporadic aniridia ± Wilms' tumor
12	Isochromosome 12p	Germ cell tumors
12	Translocation 12q13;16q11	Myxoid liposarcoma
13	*cf.* chromosome 2	
13	Deletion q14	Retinoblastoma
14	Translocation 14q12;14q32	Lymphoproliferative in ataxia-telangiectasia
14	*cf.* chromosomes 2, 6, 8	
14	Translocations from 8, 11	Lymphocyte B-cell neoplasia, including Burkitt's and other lymphomas and acute lymphatic leukemia
15	Translocation 15q22;17q21	Acute myelomonocytic leukemia
16	*cf.* chromosome 12	
16	Inversion p13;q22	Acute myelomonocytic leukemia with eosinophilia
17	*cf.* chromosome 15	
20	Deletion q11–qter	Preleukemia, including polycythemia vera
21	*cf.* chromosome 8	
22	*cf.* chromosome 8, 9, 11	
22	Monosomy, deletion q	Meningioma
X	Translocation Xp11.2; 11q11.2	Synovial sarcoma

(Compiled from References 147 and 148)

appear clinically only when both copies of the antioncogene are lost, for example, through point mutation or mitotic recombination. Because osteosarcoma is an occasional feature of the presence of the retinoblastoma gene, it is satisfying to find that some osteosarcomas have cytogenetic and molecular evidence of involvement of 13q14.[142] Indeed, evidence is mounting for the similar action of recessive mutant genes in the pathogenesis of Wilms' tumor (see Chap. 27), hepatoblastoma (see Chap. 26), rhabdomyosarcoma (see Chap. 30), and, in adults, small cell carcinoma of the lung, renal cell carcinoma, meningioma, and, in neurofibromatosis type 2 (bilateral acoustic neurofibromatosis), acoustic neuroma and neurofibroma.[143–146]

Cytogenetics of Cancer in the Young

Boveri's hypothesis in 1914 that malignancy is caused by chromosomal imbalance has been increasingly substantiated as techniques improve for studying chromosomes.[13] Quantum advances include successful *in vitro* culture techniques for lymphocytes, differential staining techniques to distinguish one chromosome from all others, assays for sister chromatid exchange, and prophase staining to improve resolution of chromosome structure and function. Excellent reviews of cancer cytogenetics are available that encompass all age groups, with an emphasis on acquired cytogenetic defects; that is, those seen only in the neoplastic tissue, closely related tissue, or tumor cell lines (Table 2-3).[18,148–152] Therefore, what follows deals with constitutional chromosomal syndromes that predispose to childhood and adolescent cancer (Table 2-4).

Wilms' Tumor

Many of the observations associating retinoblastoma with birth defects, chromosomal and gene marker deletions, and loss of genetic heterozygosity within the tumor have parallel findings in Wilms' tumor, which could, likewise, be attributed to an antioncogene.[144] When Miller's syndrome of aniridia, urogenital abnormalities, and Wilms' tumor was clinically delineated,[153] available techniques of karyotyping failed to identify the small chromosomal deletion (see also Chap. 27).[154] Technical advances since have permitted the recognition of a small chromosomal deletion, 11p13,[155] and a linked protein marker, catalase, that support loss of heterozygosity as a plausible mechanism for development of Wilms' tumor. It is of interest,

although of uncertain significance, that in all five Wilms' tumors studied for parental origin of the lost allele, it was the mothers' alleles that were missing and the fathers' that were retained.[156]

It may be expected that, as techniques improve, additional chromosomal syndromes will be recognized. In any case, the association of cancer with various birth defects remains of clinical and research importance.[157]

Wilms' tumor itself occurs excessively in three other syndromes, each with urogenital malformations but without cytogenetic anomalies: (1) pseudohermaphroditism and a congenital nephron disorder (Drash syndrome),[97] (2) hemihypertrophy, which may affect just one extremity or the tongue and may be contralateral to the tumor,[133,153] and (3) the visceral cytomegaly syndrome of Wiedemann and Beckwith consisting of large tongue, omphalocele, and large viscera, resulting from cells that are both large and excessive in number.[144,158] When any one of these defects is recognized, Wilms' tumor should be looked for in the hope of improving the prognosis through early detection. A reasonable surveillance program would include abdominal examination, perhaps urinalysis, and renal ultrasound, probably after a baseline intravenous urogram. This program could be repeated every other month until age 2 years, then three or four times a year to age 6 years. Additional tumors seen with hemihypertrophy and Wiedemann–Beckwith syndrome are hepatoblastoma and adrenocortical carcinoma.

Other Birth Defects Predisposing to Cancer

Sacrococcygeal Teratomas

Sacrococcygeal teratomas may be associated with major malformations of the lower spine, and perhaps duplication of the lower intestinal and urogenital region but not of other areas.[159]

Cryptorchidism

The risk of malignancy, about 35 times normal, is a chief reason for repairing cryptorchidism.[160] The risk increases with the degree of maldescent, being four times greater in abdominal than in inguinal testes. Neoplasia can occur in normally descended testes of patients with unilateral cryptorchidism. Orchiopexy has been recommended at age 12 to 18 months in the hope of decreasing the risk of malignancy and preserving fertil-

(*Text continues on p. 32*)

Table 2-4
Childhood and Adolescent Neoplasms in Constitutional Cytogenetic Disorders

Chromosome	Abnormality	Neoplasms
8	Trisomy	Preleukemia
11	Deletion q13	Miller's syndrome of sporadic aniridia with and without Wilms' tumor
13	Deletion q14	Sporadic retinoblastoma with and without birth defects; osteosarcoma; early radiogenic sarcomas; pinealoblastoma
21	Trisomy	Acute leukemia in Down's syndrome
X	Monosomy	Endometrial adenosquamous carcinoma in estrogen-treated Turner's syndrome; possibly neural tumors
X	Extra	Breast carcinoma; extragonadal germ-cell tumors in Klinefelter's syndrome
Y	Present	Gonadoblastoma in gonadal dysgenesis syndromes

Table 2-5
Selected Single-Gene Traits Associated with Childhood and Adolescent Neoplasia

Gene Trait, Neoplasm, or Disorder	Inheritance Chromosome* (if known)	Associated Neoplasms
Phakomatoses		
von Recklinghausen's neurofibromatosis	AD† 17q	Sarcoma, neuroma, schwannoma, meningioma, optic glioma, pheochromocytoma, leukemia
Tuberous sclerosis	AD† 9q	Adenoma sebaceum, periungual fibroma, glial tumors, rhabdomyoma of heart, renal tumor, lung cysts
von Hippel–Lindau syndrome	AD†	Retinal angioma, cerebellar hemangioblastoma, other hemangiomas, pheochromocytoma, hypernephroma, cysts
Sturge–Weber syndrome	AD	Angioma of numerous organs
Nervous System		
Retinoblastoma	AD†;13q;14	Sarcoma, pinealoblastoma
Acoustic neuromas, bilateral	AD†;22	
Neuroblastoma	AR AD	
Macroencephaly	AD†	Ganglioneuroblastoma
Endocrine		
Multiple endocrine neoplasia 1 (Werner's syndrome; MEN-1)	AD† 11q	Adenomas of islet cells, parathyroid, pituitary, and adrenal glands; malignant schwannoma; nonappendiceal carcinoid
Multiple endocrine neoplasia 2 (Sipple's syndrome; MEN-2)	10p	Medullary carcinoma of thyroid, parathyroid adenoma, pheochromocytoma
Multiple mucosal neuroma syndrome	AD†	Pheochromocytoma, medullary carcinoma of the thyroid, neurofibroma, submucosal neuromas of tongue, lips, eyelids
Paraganglioma (chemodectoma)	AD†	
Pheochromocytoma	AD†	Parathyroid adenoma, chief cell hyperplasia
Thyroid goiter and dyshormonogenesis, including Pendred's syndrome	AD	Benign goiter
Mesoderm (Soft Tissue)		
Nevoid basal cell carcinoma syndrome (Gorlin's syndrome)	AD†	Basal cell carcinoma, ovarian fibroma
Leopard syndrome	AD†	Multiple lentigines
Gingival fibromatosis ± hypertrichosis or other anomalies	AD†	
Juvenile fibromatosis	AR†	Multiple subcutaneous
Familial cutaneous collagenoma	AR	Multiple skin nodules
Multiple lipomatosis, sometimes site specific, neck or conjunctiva	AD†	Skin cancer
Goldenhar's syndrome	AR	Lipodermoid of conjunctiva, hemangioma
Macrosomia adiposa congenita	AR	Obese soon after birth, eosinophilia, adrenocortical adenoma
Alimentary Tract		
Familial polyposis coli	AD†;5p	Intestinal carcinoma of colon
Gardner's syndrome	AD†;5p	Intestinal polyps, osteomas, fibromas, sebaceous cysts, carcinoma of colon, ampulla of Vater, pancreas, thyroid, and adrenal
Peutz–Jeghers syndrome	AD†	Intestinal polyps, ovarian (granulosa cell) tumor
Turcot syndrome	AR	Brain tumor, intestinal polyposis
Hereditary pancreatitis	AD†	Carcinoma of pancreas
Tylosis with esophageal cancer	AD†	Carcinoma of esophagus
Familial, juvenile, and neonatal cirrhosis	AD AR†	Hepatocellular carcinoma
Hemochromatosis	AD† AR†;6p	Hepatocellular carcinoma

(Modified from Reference 166)
* AD = autosomal dominant; AR = autosomal recessive; XD = X-linked dominant; XR = X-linked recessive.
† Mode of inheritance considered proved.

Table 2-5 *(continued)*

Gene Trait, Neoplasm, or Disorder	Inheritance Chromosome* (if known)	Associated Neoplasms
Urogenital		
Gonadal dysgenesis,	AR†	Gonadoblastoma, dysgerminoma
hermaphroditism,	AR	
Reifenstein's syndrome,	XR†	
testicular feminization		
Wilms' tumor	AD†;11p13	
Nephroblastomatosis		
Vascular		
Multiple glomus tumors	AD†	
Hereditary hemorrhagic telangiectasia of Rendu–Osler–Weber	AD†	Angioma
Lymphedema with distichiasis	AD†	Lymphangiosarcoma of edematous limb
Skeletal		
Multiple exostosis	AD†	Osteosarcoma, chondrosarcoma
Cherubism	AD†	Fibrous dysplasia of jaws, giant cell tumor
Fibro-osseous dysplasia	AD	Osteosarcoma, medullary fibrosarcoma
Paget's disease of bone	AD	Osteosarcoma
Enchondromatosis (Ollier's syndrome)	AD	Bone tumors, hemangioma (Maffucci's syndrome)
Lymphatic and Hematopoietic		
Histiocytic reticulosis	AR†	
generalized or neural only	AR	
(Letterer–Siwe disease)	XR†	
Familial lipochrome histiocytosis	AR†	
Kostmann infantile genetic agranulocytosis	AR†	Acute monocytic leukemia (chromosomal breaks)
Polycythemia rubra vera	AR	Acute myelogenous leukemia
Glutathione reductase deficiency	AR†	Leukemia (chromosomal breaks)
Leukemia	AD	
Other lymphoproliferative disorders	AD	
Immunodeficiency		
Burton agammaglobulinemia	XR†	Leukemia, lymphoreticular
Wiskott–Aldrich syndrome	XR†	Lymphoreticular
Ataxia-telangiectasia	AR†	Lymphoreticular, leukemia, carcinoma of stomach, brain tumors (chromosomal breaks)
Chediak–Higashi syndrome	XR†	Pseudolymphoma
Multiple System		
Bloom's syndrome	AR†	Leukemia, intestinal cancer (chromosomal breaks)
Fanconi's pancytopenia	AR†	Acute monomyelogenous leukemia, squamous cell carcinoma of mucocutaneous junctions, hepatic carcinoma and adenoma (chromosomal breaks)
Dyskeratosis congenita	XR†	Leukoplakia with squamous cell carcinoma, including of cervix
Zinsser–Cole–Engman syndrome	AD	
Beckwith–Wiedemann syndrome	AR†	Visceromegaly, cytomegaly, macroglossia, adrenocortical neoplasia, Wilms' tumor, hepatoma
Rothmund–Thomson syndrome	AR†	Squamous cell carcinoma
Werner's syndrome	AR†	Sarcoma
Osteopoikilosis	AD†	Nevi
Noonan's syndrome	AD†	Schwannoma
Focal dermal hypoplasia (Goltz's syndrome)	XD†	Mucocutaneous papillomas

(continued)

(Modified from Reference 166)
* AD = autosomal dominant; AR = autosomal recessive; XD = X-linked dominant; XR = X-linked recessive.
† Mode of inheritance considered proved.

Table 2-5 (continued)

Gene Trait, Neoplasm, or Disorder	Inheritance Chromosome* (if known)	Associated Neoplasms
Inborn Errors of Metabolism		
Angiokeratoma diffusa (Fabry's syndrome)	XR†	
Tyrosinemia, hypermethioninemia, galactosemia, Wilson's disease, glycogen storage disease IV	AR† AR	Postcirrhotic hepatoma
Alpha-1-antitrypsin deficiency	Codominant	Hepatoma
Vitamin-D-resistant rickets	XR†	Parathyroid adenoma

(Modified from Reference 166)
* AD = autosomal dominant; AR = autosomal recessive; XD = X-linked dominant; XR = X-linked recessive.
† Mode of inheritance considered proved.

ity; in any case, a scrotal testis seems cosmetically desirable and is easier to monitor for tumor. Testicular dysgenesis often occurs in the non-neoplastic tissue surrounding testicular cancers; biopsies taken at orchiopexy show diminished or no spermatogonia. To sort out these relations, future large studies will have to consider also the heterogeneity of the etiology of cryptorchidism.

Neoplasia in Other Anomalous Tissue

Heterotopic or persisting fetal rest tissues predispose to malignancy. Examples include craniopharyngioma in vestiges of Rathke's pouch, chordoma in notochordal remnants within the nucleus pulposus, clear-cell adenocarcinoma of the genital tract in mesonephric remnants (vaginal adenosis), and various carcinomas in brachial cleft cysts, thyroglossal duct cysts, gut duplications, and biliary tract defects.[159]

Candidate Syndromes of Cancer and Malformations

Suspected associations that await additional case reports and innovative explanations that might be explored in the laboratory are acute leukemia in Rubenstein–Taybi syndrome,[161] Poland anomaly (absent pectoralis major and ipsilateral syndactyly),[162] Schwachman's syndrome (exocrine pancreatic insufficiency and neutropenia),[163] familial ataxia with monosomy C,[130] and various childhood cancers occurring with Sotos' syndrome of cerebral gigantism.[164]

Single-Gene Defects

The seventh edition of McKusick's *Mendelian Inheritance in Man* enumerates 1906 certain single-gene traits and 2001 others with suggestive but inconclusive evidence of mendelian behavior.[165] Elsewhere, a table is presented of McKusick's 200 conditions (and several additional ones) that have neoplastic tendencies as a sole feature, a frequent concomitant, or a rare complication in childhood or adult life.[166] The inference can be drawn that a small percentage of the known human genome influences the expression or suppression of neoplasia. Many of the traits were selected for inclusion in Table 2-5 because they are certainly mendelian and should be recognized by the pedi-

atrician because the tumor or other significant complication arises in childhood.

Familial Aggregation

Sometimes, childhood cancer occurs more than once in a family. Occasionally, such clusters will occur by chance or be explained by chromosomal (Tables 2-3 and 2-4) or mendelian (Table 2-5) traits or, rarely, by environmental carcinogenic exposure. Often, however, no etiology is evident, and such families represent opportunities for etiologic research.[167,168]

Epidemiologic Surveys

Empirical recurrence risks are similar when derived from national cancer registries in the United States and the United Kingdom.[23,169] When cancer occurs in one sib, the relative risk of cancer in the remaining sibs is three times the expected risk based on population rates. In both studies, specific types of malignancies were seen in excess, suggesting that the familial association is not a random or chance occurrence. In the United States the significant excess neoplasms of sib pairs included brain–brain, brain–sarcoma, and sarcoma–sarcoma.[23] In the United Kingdom the same combinations were seen, as was lymphoma–lymphoma.[169]

Individual families are known that verify these national data, which are minimum estimates. Reports suggest that some families may have tumors all of one cell type, whereas others may have diverse cell types. Each family is an important challenge, both as a clinical problem and as an opportunity to learn more about the origins of the tumors in the general population.[170] In the clinic, family members should be examined for subtle signs of known hereditary diseases, such as neurofibromatosis or the multiple neoplasia syndromes, that could explain tumors and provide a basis for counseling the family and offering surveillance.

Toward a Definition

The notion of "cancer family" remains poorly defined. Because one in four Americans develops a cancer in a lifetime (about 1 in 300 by age 15 years), everyone probably will have relatives with cancer, even in childhood; simply by chance some will have many affected family members. An excessive aggregation within a family can be suspected when it occurs

- in more than two generations;
- in a high percentage of siblings;
- at an unusual age for the tumor type;
- in an atypical gender; or
- in association with other cancers, genetic disorders, or birth defects in the same individual.

A Specific Syndrome

One pattern of cancer family that features childhood cancer is the Li–Fraumeni cancer family syndrome[171] or the SBLA syndrome[172] after the tumor types seen to excess: sarcoma; breast, bone, or brain cancer; lung and laryngeal cancer; and adrenocortical neoplasms. The excess of tumors in the Li–Fraumeni syndrome has been rigorously validated by 13 years of follow-up of the original four families: 16 cancers occurred in 10 of 31 relatives, compared with 0.5 that would be expected from general population rates.[171] The pattern is frequent enough to account for a high frequency of breast cancer in the young mothers of children with sarcomas.[173] The pediatrician caring for a child with a sarcoma perhaps should alert the patient's mother to her higher risk of breast cancer, which is about three times normal. Familial cancer, starting with childhood sarcoma, seems to behave as an autosomal dominant trait,[174] but no biological marker or gene localization has been identified.

Research Opportunities

In research centers, a comprehensive clinical–laboratory investigation could shed light on pathogenesis.[157] For example, when three of six sibs developed acute myelogenous leukemia, a new assay for *in vitro* transformation of fibroblasts on exposure to simian virus 40[175] and for survival of fibroblast colonies following increasing doses of ionizing radiation[176] was applied to available family members. Normal results were obtained in the father and the two brothers who had no malignancy; abnormal results were seen in the mother, who had distant relatives with cancer and a personal history of cervical cancer; in the leukemic proband; and in one sib who was normal at the time of testing but developed acute myelogenous leukemia 6 years later.[177]

CONCLUSION

Why a young person develops cancer is usually unexplained. As detailed here and elsewhere in *Principles and Practice of Pediatric Oncology,* known factors include a few environmental and therapeutic agents and prenatal exposures; some congenital and genetic disorders, such as chromosomal and mendelian traits and birth defects of unknown origins; and interacting environmental and host factors (ecogenetics). Progress in etiology occurs most rapidly when clinical and laboratory investigations can be made on peculiar occurrences of cancer. Health professionals caring for young patients with cancer may initiate such research by being alert to etiologic opportunities. Clinicians must know enough of the demographic features of a tumor, such as patterns by age, gender, and race, and the patient's medical and family history to recognize the unusual patient who could shed light on cancer etiology in general.

CLINICAL RECOMMENDATIONS

Many genetic and congenital conditions increase the risk of childhood cancer enormously. Individually they are rare, but in the aggregate they may be numerous. How can clinicians identify patients who might benefit from referral to specialists knowledgeable about cancer genetics? Tentative guidelines that should be integral to the practice of pediatric oncology were developed at a National Institutes of Health Workshop on Strategies for Controlling Cancer Through Genetics.[178] The suggestions address two situations: *individuals* and *families.*

Identifying Individuals for Genetic Evaluation

The occurrence of cancer in an individual under any of the following circumstances may indicate an increased susceptibility to malignancy as a result of predisposing host factors:

1. Cancer occurring in both of paired organs that is thought not to be the result of metastases (*e.g.,* cancer in both adrenal glands or in both kidneys).
2. More than one focus of cancer in a single organ (multicentric tumors) (*e.g.,* multiple retinoblastomas in one eye, multiple foci of Wilms' tumor in one kidney).
3. Two or more distinct cancers (multiple primary malignancies) (*e.g.,* sarcoma after a brain tumor, colon cancer after Wilms' tumor).
4. Cancer that has occurred at an atypical age (*e.g.,* breast or ovarian cancer in young women, an embryonal tumor in an adolescent or young adult), at an atypical site (*e.g.,* osteosarcoma in the midhumerus), or in the less usually affected gender (*e.g.,* breast cancer in a young man).
5. Cancer associated with birth defects (*e.g.,* Wilms' tumor in a patient with sporadic aniridia, urogenital malformations, mental retardation, and growth abnormalities); one of many single-gene disorders known to be complicated by neoplasia (Table 2-5) (*e.g.,* neurofibrosarcoma or optic nerve glioma in a person with neurofibromatosis, hepatocellular carcinoma in a person with tyrosinemia, or basal cell carcinomas or medulloblastoma in a person with the nevoid basal-cell carcinoma syndrome); precursor lesions (*e.g.,* malignant melanoma in a person with dysplastic nevi or atypical moles, colon cancer in a person with multiple adenomatous polyps); or other diseases (*e.g.,* lymphoma or other cancers in a person with an existing autoimmune disorder or immunodeficiency).
6. Unusual or rare cancers (*e.g.,* pheochromocytoma).

To aid in identifying such patients, who deserve referral to an "etiologist," a few questions about medical history should be routinely asked: Does the patient have a history of cancer, tumors, or unusual growths? A relevant clinical examination, especially seeking minor dysmorphic features, should also be done: does the patient exhibit any birth defects, genetic disease, or precursor lesions? Other information that is often relevant includes the gross pathology and histopathology of the primary malignant neoplasm.

Identifying Families for Genetic Evaluation

A child may be predisposed to cancer because of his or her family history. A family history of cancer may also be significant in evaluating a patient with cancer who does not meet any of the criteria just listed. Therefore, two additional guidelines incorporate knowledge of the family history:

1. One first-degree relative (*e.g.*, brother, sister, or parent) who has cancer and meets any of the above criteria.
2. Two first-degree relatives (one of whom may be the patient) with any cancer. However, if sibships in the family are large and the tumor types common for both the ages at diagnosis and the patients' genders, then further evaluation is not necessary.

A family history adequate for this purpose can be collected by asking patients who among their blood relatives has or had a cancer, tumor, or an unusual growth? If the solicited family history appears significant by either of the above criteria, then all persons with cancer—and their blood relatives—merit evaluation.

Interpreting a family history is problematic. As noted earlier, no firm definition of a "cancer family" is available. A working definition depends on the type and site of cancers, the ages at diagnosis, the patients' genders, the number of tumors, and the absolute numbers of affected and unaffected relatives. Guidance concerning the significance of a particular family history can be provided by a consultant with experience in evaluating families with cancer.

REFERENCES

1. McWhirter WR, Kirk D: What causes childhood leukaemia? Some beliefs of parents of affected children. Med J Austral 145:314–316, 1986
2. Higginson J, Muir CS: Environmental carcinogenesis: Misconceptions and limitations to cancer control. JNCI 63:1291–1298, 1979
3. Doll R, Peto R: The causes of cancer: Quantitative estimates of avoidable risks of cancer in the United States today. JNCI 66:1191–1308, 1981
4. Li FP, Jamison DS, Meadows AT: Questionnaire study of cancer etiology in 503 children. JNCI 76:31–36, 1986
5. Mulvihill JJ: Ecogenetic origins of cancer in the young: Environmental and genetic determinants. In Levine AS (ed): Cancer in the Young, pp 13–27. New York, Masson, 1982
6. Camerini–Otero D, Mulvihill JJ, Schechter AN: Medical Genetics: 1987. Bethesda, Foundation for Advanced Education in the Sciences, 1987
7. Emery AEH, Rimoin DL: Principles and Practice of Medical Genetics. Edinburgh, Churchill Livingstone, 1983
8. Fraser Roberts JA, Pembrey ME: An Introduction to Medical Genetics, 8th Edition. Oxford, Oxford University Press, 1985
9. McKusick VA: Human Genetics, 2nd Edition. Englewood Cliffs, NJ, Prentice–Hall, 1969
10. Thompson JS, Thompson MW: Genetics in Medicine, 4th Edition. Philadelphia, WB Saunders, 1986
11. Miller RW: Relation between cancer and congenital malformations: The value of small series, with a note on pineal tumors in native and migrant Japanese. Isr J Med Sci 7:1461–1464, 1971
12. Miller RW: Ethnic differences in cancer occurrence: Genetic and environmental influences with particular reference to neuroblastoma. In Mulvihill JJ, Miller RW, Fraumeni JF Jr (eds): Genetics of Human Cancer, pp 1–14. New York, Raven Press, 1977
13. Boveri T: Zur Frage der Entstehung maligner Tumoren. Jena, Gustav Fischer, 1914
14. Mulvihill JJ: Clinical observations of ecogenetics in human cancer. Ann Intern Med 92:809–813, 1980
15. Brewer GJ: Human ecology, an expanding role for the human geneticist. Am J Hum Genet 23:92–94, 1971
16. Omenn GS, Motulsky AG: "Eco-genetics": Genetic variation in susceptibility to environmental agents. In Cohen BH, Lilienfeld AM, Huang PC (eds): Genetic Issues in Public Health and Medicine, pp 83–111. Springfield, IL, Charles C Thomas, 1978
17. Li FP, Bader J: Epidemiology of cancer in childhood. In Oski F, Nathan DG (eds): Hematology of Infancy and Childhood, 3rd ed, pp 918–941. Philadelphia, WB Saunders, 1987
18. Chaganti RSK, German J: Genetics in Clinical Oncology. New York, Oxford University Press, 1985
19. Greenberg RS, Shuster JL Jr: Epidemiology of cancer in children. Epidemiol Rev 7:22–48, 1985
20. Li FP: Cancers in children. In Schottenfeld D, Fraumeni JF Jr (eds): Cancer Epidemiology and Prevention, pp 1012–1024. Philadelphia, WB Saunders, 1982
21. Miller RW: Etiology of childhood cancer. In Sutow WW, Vietti TJ, Fernbach DJ (eds): Clinical Pediatric Oncology, 2nd Edition, pp 33–45. St Louis, CV Mosby, 1977
22. Miller RW: Environmental causes of cancer in childhood. Adv Pediatr 25:97–119, 1978
23. Miller RW: Deaths from childhood leukemia and solid tumors among twins and other sibs in the United States, 1960–67. J Natl Cancer Inst 46:203–209, 1971
24. Miller RW: Persons with exceptionally high risk of leukemia. Cancer Res 27:2420–2423, 1967
25. Boder E: Ataxia-telangiectasia: Some historic, clinical and pathologic observations. Birth Defects 11:255–270, 1975
26. Bridges BA, Harnden DG (eds): Ataxia-Telangiectasia: A Cellular and Molecular Link between Cancer, Neuropathology, and Immune Deficiency. Chichester, John Wiley & Sons, 1982
27. Cavenee WK, Dryja TP, Phillips RA, Benedict WF, Godbout R, Gallie BL, Murphree AL, Strong LC, White RL: Expression of recessive alleles by chromosomal mechanisms in retinoblastoma. Nature 305:779–784, 1983
28. Gatti RA, Swift M (eds): Ataxia-Telangiectasia: Genetics, Neuropathology, and Immunology of a Degenerative Disease of Childhood. New York, Alan R Liss, 1985
29. Waldmann TA, Misiti J, Nelson DL, Kraemer KH: Ataxia-telangiectasia: A multisystem hereditary disease with immunodeficiency, impaired organ maturation, x-ray hypersensitivity, and a high incidence of neoplasia. Ann Intern Med 99:367–379, 1983
30. Hecht F, Koler RD, Rigas DA, Dahnke GS, Case MP, Tisdale V, Miller RW: Leukaemia and lymphocytes in ataxia-telangiectasia. Lancet 2:1193, 1966
31. Hecht F, McCaw BK, Koler RD: Ataxia-telangiectasia—clonal growth of translocation lymphocytes. N Engl J Med 289:286–291, 1973
32. McCaw BK, Hecht F, Harnden DG, Teplitz RL: Somatic rearrangement of chromosome 14 in human lymphocytes. Proc Natl Acad Sci USA 72:2071–2075, 1975
33. German J: Genes which increase chromosomal instability in somatic cells and predispose to cancer. Prog Med Genet 8:61–101, 1972
34. Taylor AMR, Harnden DG, Arlett CF, Harcourt SA, Lehmann AR, Stevens S, Bridges BA: Ataxia-telangiectasia: A human mutation with abnormal radiation sensitivity. Nature 258:427–429, 1975
35. Gotoff SP, Amirmokri E, Liebner EJ: Ataxia-telangiectasia: Neoplasia, untoward response to x-irradiation, and tuberous sclerosis. Am J Dis Child 114:617–625, 1967
36. Morgan JL, Holcomb TM, Morrissey RW: Radiation reaction in ataxia telangiectasia. Am J Dis Child 116:557–558, 1968
37. Swift M, Morrell D, Cromartie E, Chamberlin AR, Skolnick MH, Bishop DT: The incidence and gene frequency of ataxia-telangiectasia in the United States. Am J Hum Genet 39:573–583, 1986
38. Swift M, Sholman L, Perry M, Chase C: Malignant neoplasms in the families of patients with ataxia-telangiectasia. Cancer Res 36:209–215, 1976
39. Swift M, Reitnauer PJ, Morrell D, Chase CL: Breast and other cancers in families with ataxia-telangiectasia. N Engl J Med 316:1289–1294, 1987
40. Paterson MC, Smith BP, Lohman PHM, Anderson AK, Fishman L: Defective excision repair of γ-ray-damaged DNA in human (ataxia-telangiectasia) fibroblasts. Nature 260:444–447, 1976
41. Boice JD Jr, Fraumeni JF Jr: Radiation Carcinogenesis: Epidemiology and Biological Significance. New York, Raven Press, 1984
42. National Research Council Committee on the Biological Effects of Ionizing Radiations: The Effects on Populations of Exposure to Low Levels of Ionizing Radiation. Washington, DC, National Academy of Sciences–National Research Council, 1980
43. United Nations Scientific Committee on the Effects of Atomic Radiation: Sources and Effects of Ionizing Radiation: Report to the General Assembly. New York, United Nations, 1977
44. Upton AC, Albert RE, Burns FJ, Shore RE (eds): Radiation Carcinogenesis. New York, Elsevier, 1986
45. Frieben A: Demonstration lines Cancroids des rechten Handruckens, das sich nach langdauernder Einwirkung von Röntgenstrahlen entwickelt hatte. Fortschr Geb Röntgenstr 6:106, 1902
46. Miller RW, Boice JD Jr: Radiogenic cancer after prenatal or childhood exposure. In Upton AC, Albert RE, Burns FJ, Shore RE (eds): Radiation Carcinogenesis, pp 379–386. New York, Elsevier, 1986
47. Beebe GW: Reflections on the work of the Atomic Bomb Casualty Commission in Japan. Epidemiol Rev 1:184–210, 1979
48. Conard RA: Summary of thyroid findings in Marshallese 22 years after

exposure to radioactive fallout. In DeGroot LJ, Frohman LA, Kaplan EL, Refetoff S (eds): Radiation-Associated Thyroid Carcinoma, pp 241–257. New York, Grune & Stratton, 1977

49. Miké V, Meadows AT, D'Angio GJ: Incidence of second malignant neoplasms in children: Results of an international study. Lancet 2:1326–1331, 1982

50. Boice JD Jr, Land CE: Ionizing radiation. In Schottenfeld D, Fraumeni JF Jr (eds): Cancer Epidemiology and Prevention, pp 231–253. Philadelphia, WB Saunders, 1982

51. Mays CW (ed): Biological effects of ^{224}Ra and Thorotrast. Health Phys 35:1–174, 1978

52. Baum JW: Population heterogeneity hypothesis on radiation induced cancer. Health Phys 25:97–104, 1973

53. Modan B, Ron E, Werner A: Thyroid cancer following scalp irradiation. Radiology 123:741–744, 1977

54. Land CE: The hazards of fallout or of epidemiologic research? N Engl J Med 300:431–432, 1979

55. Lyon JL, Klauber MR, Gardner JW, Udall KS: Childhood leukemias associated with fallout from nuclear testing. N Engl J Med 300:397–402, 1979

56. Black D: New evidence on childhood leukaemia and nuclear establishments. Br Med J 294:591–592, 1987

57. Wall BF, Fisher ES, Paynter A, Hudson A, Bird PD: Doses to patients from pantomographic and conventional dental radiography. Br J Radiol 52:727–734, 1979

58. Stewart A, Webb J, Giles D, Hewitt D: Malignant disease in childhood and diagnostic radiation *in utero.* Lancet 2:447, 1956

59. MacMahon B: Prenatal x-ray exposure and childhood cancer. J Natl Cancer Inst 28:1173–1191, 1962

60. Graham S, Levin ML, Lilienfeld AM, Schuman LM, Gibson R, Dowd JE, Hempelmann L: Preconception, intrauterine, and postnatal irradiation as related to leukemia. Natl Cancer Inst Monogr 19:347–371, 1966

61. Jablon S, Kato H: Childhood cancer in relation to prenatal exposure to atomic-bomb radiation. Lancet 2:1000–1003, 1970

62. MacMahon B: Prenatal x-ray exposure and twins. N Engl J Med 312:576–577, 1985

63. Miller RW, Mulvihill JJ: Small head size after atomic irradiation. Teratology 14:355–357, 1976

64. Bell J: Glioma retinae. Eugenics Laboratory Memoirs, Series 21: The Treasury of Human Inheritance: Anomalies and Diseases of the Eye, vol. 2, pp 112–123. London, Cambridge University Press, 1922

65. Francois J, DeBie S, Matton–Van Leuven MT: Genesis and genetics of retinoblastoma. J Pediatr Ophthalmol Strabismus 16:85–100, 1979

66. Vogel F: Genetics of retinoblastoma. Hum Genet 52:1–54, 1979

67. Lee W-H, Bookstein R, Hong F, Young L-J, Shew J-Y, Lee EY-HP: Human retinoblastoma susceptibility gene: Cloning, identification, and sequence. Science 235:1394–1399, 1987

68. Cavenee WK, Murphree AL, Shull MM, Benedict WF, Sparkes RS, Kock E, Nordenskjold M: Prediction of familial predisposition to retinoblastoma. N Engl J Med 314:1201–1207, 1986

69. Abramson DH, Ellsworth RM, Kitchin FD, Tung G: Second nonocular tumors in retinoblastoma survivors: Are they radiation-induced? Ophthalmology 91:1351–1355, 1984

70. Draper GJ, Sanders BM, Kingston JE: Second primary neoplasms in patients with retinoblastoma. Br J Cancer 53:661–671, 1986

71. Tucker MA, Meadows AT, Boice JD Jr, Hoover RN, Fraumeni JF Jr: Cancer risk following treatment of childhood cancer. In Boice JD Jr, Fraumeni JF Jr (eds): Radiation Carcinogenesis: Epidemiology and Biological Significance, pp 211–224. New York, Raven Press, 1984

72. Kitchin FD, Ellsworth RM: Pleiotropic effects of the gene for retinoblastoma. J Med Genet 11:244–246, 1974

73. Bader JL, Meadows AT, Zimmerman LE, Rorke LB, Voute PA, Champion LA, Miller RW: Bilateral retinoblastoma with intracranial retinoblastoma: Trilateral retinoblastoma. Cancer Genet Cytogenet 5:203–213, 1982

74. Strong LC: Theories of pathogenesis: Mutation and cancer. In Mulvihill JJ, Miller RW, Fraumeni JF Jr (eds): Genetics of Human Cancer, pp 401–414. New York, Raven Press, 1977

75. Nove J, Nichols WW, Weichselbaum RR, Little JB: Abnormalities of human chromosome 13 and in vitro radiosensitivity: A study of 19 fibroblast strains. Mutat Res 84:157–167, 1981

76. Weichselbaum RR, Little JB: Familial retinoblastoma and ataxia telangiectasia: Human models for the study of DNA damage and repair. Cancer 45:775–779, 1980

77. Ejima Y, Sasaki MS, Utsumi H, Kaneko A, Tanooka H: Radiosensitivity of fibroblasts from patients with retinoblastoma and chromosome 13 anomalies. Mutat Res 103:177–184, 1982

78. Morten JEN, Harnden DG, Taylor AMR: Chromosome damage in G_0 x-irradiated lymphocytes from patients with hereditary retinoblastoma. Cancer Res 41:3635–3638, 1981

79. Gorlin RJ: Nevoid basal cell carcinoma syndrome. Medicine 66:98–113, 1987

80. Southwick GJ, Schwartz RA: The basal cell nevus syndrome: Disasters occurring among a series of 36 patients. Cancer 44:2294–2305, 1979

81. Featherstone T, Taylor AMR, Harnden DG: Studies on the radiosensitivity of cells from patients with basal cell naevus syndrome. Am J Hum Genet 35:58–66, 1983

82. Scotto J, Fraumeni JF Jr: Skin (other than melanoma). In Schottenfeld D, Fraumeni JF Jr (eds): Cancer Epidemiology and Prevention, pp 996–1011. Philadelphia, WB Saunders, 1982

83. Cleaver JE: Defective repair replication of DNA in xeroderma pigmentosum. Nature 218:652–656, 1968

84. Elder DE, Greene MH, Bondi EE, Clark WH Jr: Acquired melanocytic nevi and melanoma: The dysplastic nevus syndrome. In Ackerman AB (ed): Pathology of Malignant Melanoma. New York, Masson, 1981

85. Greene MH: The dysplastic nevus syndrome: Precursors of hereditary and nonfamilial cutaneous melanoma. In DeVita VT Jr, Hellman S, Rosenberg SA (eds): Important Advances in Oncology 1986, pp 173–192. Philadelphia, JB Lippincott, 1986

86. Kraemer KH, Greene MH, Tarone R, Elder DE, Clark WH Jr, Guerry D IV: Dysplastic naevi and cutaneous melanoma risk. Lancet 2:1076–1077, 1983

87. Perera MIR, Um KI, Greene MH, Waters HL, Bredberg A, Kraemer KH: Hereditary dysplastic nevus syndrome: Lymphoid cell ultraviolet hypermutability in association with increased melanoma susceptibility. Cancer Res 46:1005–1009, 1986

88. Okoro AN: Albinism in Nigeria: A clinical and social study. Br J Dermatol 92:485–492, 1975

89. Miller RW: Susceptibility of the fetus and child to chemical pollutants. Science 184:812–814, 1974

90. Fraumeni JF Jr, Miller RW: Drug-induced cancer (and addendum). Natl Cancer Inst Monogr 52:67–73, 1979

91. Stolley PD, Hibberd PL: Drugs. In Schottenfeld D, Fraumeni JF Jr (eds): Cancer Epidemiology and Prevention, pp 304–317. Philadelphia, WB Saunders, 1982

92. McCarty KS Jr, Barton TK, Peete CH Jr, Creasman WT: Gonadal dysgenesis with adenocarcinoma of the endometrium: An electron microscopic and steroid receptor analysis with a review of the literature. Cancer 42:512–520, 1978

93. Marrett LD, Meigs JW, Flannery JT: Trends in the incidence of cancer of the corpus uteri in Connecticut, 1964–1979, in relation to consumption of exogenous estrogens. Am J Epidemiol 116:57–67, 1982

94. Mulvihill JJ, Ridolfi RL, Schultz FR, Borzy MS, Haughton PBT: Hepatic adenoma in Fanconi anemia treated with oxymetholone. J Pediatr 87:122–124, 1975

95. Ziegenfuss J, Carabasi R: Androgens and hepatocellular carcinoma. Lancet 1:262, 1973

96. Auerbach AD, Adler B, Chaganti RSK: Prenatal and postnatal diagnosis and carrier detection of Fanconi anemia by a cytogenetic method. Pediatrics 67:128–135, 1981

97. Miller RW, McKay FW: Decline in US childhood cancer mortality, 1950–1980. JAMA 251:1567–1570, 1984

98. Li FP, Myers MH, Heise HW, Jaffe N: The course of five-year survivors of cancer in childhood. J Pediatr 93:185–187, 1978

99. Blayney DW, Longo DL, Young RC, Greene MH, Hubbard SM, Postal MG, Duffey PL, DeVita VT Jr: Decreasing risk of leukemia with prolonged follow-up after chemotherapy and radiotherapy for Hodgkin's disease. N Engl J Med 316:710–714, 1987

100. Tucker MA, Meadows AT, Boice JD Jr, Stovall M, Oberlin O, Stone BJ, Birch J, Voute PA, Hoover RN, Fraumeni JF Jr: Leukemia after therapy with alkylating agents for childhood cancer. JNCI 78:459–464, 1987

101. Mulvihill JJ, McKeen EA: Discussion: Genetics of multiple primary tumors: A clinical etiologic approach illustrated by three patients. Cancer 40:1867–1871, 1977

102. Carney JA: The triad of gastric epithelioid leiomyosarcoma, pulmonary chondroma, and functioning extra-adrenal paraganglioma: A five-year review. Medicine 62:159–169, 1983

103. Herbst AL, Scully RE: Adenocarcinoma of the vagina in adolescence: A report of 7 cases including 6 clear-cell carcinomas (so-called mesonephromas). Cancer 25:745–757, 1970

104. Brackhill Y, Berendes HW: Dangers of diethylstilboestrol: Review of a 1953 paper. Lancet 2:520, 1978

105. Melnick S, Cole P, Anderson D, Herbst A: Rates and risks of diethylstilbestrol-related clear-cell adenocarcinoma of the vagina and cervix: An update. N Engl J Med 316:514–516, 1987

106. O'Brien PC, Noller KL, Robboy SJ, Barner AB, Kaufman RH, Tilley BC, Townsend DE: Vaginal epithelial changes in young women enrolled in the National Cooperative Diethylstilbestrol Adenosis (DESAD) Project. Obstet Gynecol 53:300–308, 1979

107. Gill WB, Schumacher GFB, Bibbo M, Straus FH II, Schoenberg HW: Association of diethylstilbestrol exposure in utero with cryptorchidism, testicular hypoplasia and semen abnormalities. J Urol 122:36–39, 1979

108. Miller RW: Relationship between human teratogens and carcinogens (and addendum). Natl Cancer Inst Monogr 52:59–63, 1979

109. Li FP, Willard DR, Goodman R, Vawter G: Malignant lymphoma after diphenylhydantoin (Dilantin) therapy. Cancer 36:1359–1362, 1975

110. Hanson JW: Fetal hydantoin effects. In Sever JL, Brent RL (eds): Teratogen Update: Environmentally Induced Birth Defects Risks, pp 29–33. New York, Alan R Liss, 1986

111. Lipson A, Bale P: Ependymoblastoma associated with prenatal exposure to diphenylhydantoin and methylphenobarbitone. Cancer 55:1859–1862, 1985

112. Pendergrass TW, Hanson JW: Fetal hydantoin syndrome and neuroblastoma. Lancet 2:150, 1976

113. Seeler RA, Israel JN, Royal JE, Kaye CI, Rao S, Abulaban M: Ganglioneuroblastoma and fetal hydantoin–alcohol syndromes. Pediatrics 63:524–527, 1979

114. Sherman S, Roizen N: Fetal hydantoin syndrome and neuroblastoma. Lancet 2:517, 1976

115. Fraumeni JF Jr, Hoover RN: Immunosurveillance of cancer: Epidemiologic observations. Natl Cancer Inst Monogr 47:121–126, 1977

116. Kinlen LJ, Sheil AGR, Peto J, Doll R: Collaborative United Kingdom–Australasian study of cancer in patients treated with immunosuppressive drugs. Br Med J 2:1461–1466, 1979

117. MacKinney AA, Booker HE: Diphenylhydantoin effects on human lymphocytes in vitro and in vivo: An hypothesis to explain some drug reactions. Arch Intern Med 129:988–992, 1972

118. Aldick HJ, Fabry H: Multiple Basaliome durch Arseneinwirkung in der Fetalperiode. Hautarzt 24:496, 1973

119. Sanders BM, Draper GJ: Childhood cancer and drugs in pregnancy. Br Med J 1:717–718, 1979

120. Gold E, Gordis L, Tonascia J, Szklo M: Risk factors for brain tumors in children. Am J Epidemiol 109:309–319, 1979

121. Potter JF, Schoeneman M: Metastasis of maternal cancer to the placenta and fetus. Cancer 25:380–387, 1970

122. Willett WC, MacMahon B: Diet and cancer: An overview. N Engl J Med 310:633–638 and 697–701, 1984

123. Weinberg AG, Mize CE, Worthen HG: The occurrence of hepatoma in the chronic form of hereditary tyrosinemia. J Pediatr 88:434–438, 1976

124. Lele KP, Penrose LS, Stallard HB: Chromosome deletion in a case of retinoblastoma. Ann Hum Genet 27:171–174, 1963

125. Hall JG: Vitamin A: A newly recognized human teratogen: Harbinger of things to come? J Pediatr 105:583–584, 1984

126. Evan AS: Viruses. In Schottenfeld D, Fraumeni JF Jr (eds): Cancer Epidemiology and Prevention, pp 364–390. Philadelphia, WB Saunders, 1982

127. Jose DG: Virus-associated malignant diseases in animals and man. Aust NZ J Med 8:195–214, 1978

128. de-Thé G: The epidemiology of Burkitt's lymphoma: Evidence for a causal association with Epstein–Barr virus. Epidemiol Rev 1:32–54, 1979

129. Purtilo DT: Epstein–Barr-virus-induced oncogenesis in immune-deficient individuals. Lancet 1:300–303, 1980

130. Li FP, Potter NU, Buchanan GR, Vawter G, Whang–Peng J, Rosen RB: A family with acute leukemia, hypoplastic anemia and cerebellar ataxia. Am J Med 65:933–940, 1978

131. Ohbayashi A: Genetic and familial aspects of liver cirrhosis and hepatocellular carcinoma. In Okuda K, Peters RL (eds): Hepatocellular Carcinoma, pp 43–57. New York, John Wiley, 1976

132. Orth G, Jablonska S, Jarzabek–Chorzelska M, Obalek S, Rzesa G, Favre M, Croissant O: Characteristics of the lesions and risk of malignant conversion associated with the type of human papillomavirus involved in epidermodysplasia verruciformis. Cancer Res 39:1074–1082, 1979

133. Mulvihill JJ: Congenital and genetic diseases. In Fraumeni JF Jr (ed): Persons at High Risk of Cancer: An Approach to Cancer Etiology and Control, pp 3–37. New York, Academic Press, 1975

134. Chaganti RSK, Miller DR, Meyers PA, German J: Cytogenetic evidence of the intrauterine origin of acute leukemia in monozygotic twins. N Engl J Med 300:1032–1034, 1979

135. Hanson MR, Mulvihill JJ: Epidemiology of cancer in the young. In Levine AS (ed): Cancer in the Young, pp 3–12. New York, Masson, 1982

136. Hethcote HW, Knudson AG Jr: Model for the incidence of embryonal cancers: Application to retinoblastoma. Proc Natl Acad Sci USA 75:2453–2457, 1978

137. Knudson AG Jr: Mutation and cancer: Statistical study of retinoblastoma. Proc Natl Acad Sci USA 68:820–823, 1971

138. Gordon H: Family studies in retinoblastoma. Birth Defects 10(10):185–190, 1974

139. Gallie BL, Ellsworth RM, Abramson DH, Phillips RA: Retinoma: Spontaneous regression of retinoblastoma or benign manifestation of the mutation? Br J Cancer 45:513–521, 1982

140. Johnson MP, Ramsay N, Cervenka J, Wang N: Retinoblastoma and its association with a deletion in chromosome #13: A survey using high-resolution chromosome techniques. Cancer Genet Cytogenet 6:29–37, 1982

141. Knudson AG Jr: Hereditary cancers of man. Cancer Invest 1:187–193, 1983

142. Dryja TP, Rapaport JM, Epstein J, Goorin AM, Weichselbaum R, Koufos A, Cavenee WK: Chromosome 13 homozygosity in osteosarcoma without retinoblastoma. Am J Hum Genet 38:59–66, 1986

143. Casalone R, Granata P, Simi P, Tarantino E, Butti G, Buonaguidi R, Faggionato F, Knerich R, Solero L: Recessive cancer genes in meningiomas? An analysis of 31 cases. Cancer Genet Cytogenet 27:145–159, 1987

144. Koufos A, Hansen MF, Copeland NG, Jenkins NA, Lampkin BC, Cavenee WK: Loss of heterozygosity in three embryonal tumours suggests a common pathogenetic mechanism. Nature 316:330–334, 1985

145. Seizinger BR, Rouleau G, Ozelius LJ, Lane AH, St George–Hyslop P, Huson S, Gusella JF, Martuza RL: Common pathogenetic mechanism for three tumor types in bilateral acoustic neurofibromatosis. Science 236:317–319, 1987

146. Zbar B, Brauch H, Talmadge C, Linehan M: Loss of alleles of loci on the short arm of chromosome 3 in renal cell carcinoma. Nature 327:721–724, 1987

147. Mulvihill JJ, Madigan P: Neoplasia of man (Homo sapiens). In O'Brien SJ (ed): Genetic Maps 1984: A Compilation of Linkage and Restriction Maps of Genetically Studied Organisms, vol 3, Cold Spring Harbor Laboratory, pp 446–449. Cold Spring Harbor, New York, 1984

148. Sandberg AA, Turc–Carel C: The cytogenetics of solid tumors: Relation to diagnosis, classification and pathology. Cancer 59:387–395, 1987

149. Golomb HM, Rowley JD, Bahr GF (eds): Banded chromosomal abnormalities in human malignancy: Basic mechanism and clinical implications. Virchows Arch [Cell Pathol] 29:1–150, 1978

150. Hsu TC: Human and Mammalian Cytogenetics: An Historical Perspective. New York, Springer-Verlag, 1979

151. Sandberg AA: The Chromosomes in Human Cancer and Leukemia. New York, Elsevier/North Holland, 1979

152. Yunis JJ: Chromosomal rearrangements, genes, and fragile sites in cancer: Clinical and biologic implications. In DeVita VT, Hellman S, Rosenberg SA (Eds): Important Advances in Oncology 1986, pp 93–128. Philadelphia, JB Lippincott, 1986

153. Miller RW, Fraumeni JF Jr, Manning MD: Association of Wilms's tumor with aniridia, hemihypertrophy and other congenital malformations. N Engl J Med 270:922–927, 1964

154. Fraumeni JF Jr, Geiser CF, Manning MD: Wilms' tumor and congenital hemihypertrophy: Report of five new cases and review of literature. Pediatrics 40:886–899, 1967

155. Riccardi VM, Sujansky E, Smith AC, Francke U: Chromosomal imbalance in the aniridia–Wilms' tumor association: 11p interstitial deletion. Pediatrics 61:604–610, 1978

156. Schroeder WT, Chao L-Y, Dao DD, Strong LC, Pathak S, Riccardi V, Lewis WH, Saunders GF: Nonrandom loss of maternal chromosome 11 alleles in Wilms' tumors. Am J Human Genet 40:413–420, 1987

157. Mulvihill JJ: Laboratory approach to familial cancer. In Fleisher M (ed): The Clinical Biochemistry of Cancer, pp 90–106. Washington, DC, American Association for Clinical Chemistry, 1979

158. Sotelo–Avila C, Gooch WM III: Neoplasms associated with the Beckwith–Wiedemann syndrome. Perspect Pediatr Pathol 3:255–271, 1976

159. Bolande RP: Developmental pathology. Am J Pathol 94:627–684, 1979

160. Martin DC: Malignancy in the cryptorchid testis. Urol Clin North Am 9:371–376, 1982

161. Jonas DM, Heilbron DC, Ablin AR: Rubinstein–Taybi syndrome and acute leukemia. J Pediatr 92:851–852, 1978

162. Armendares S: Absence of pectoralis major muscle in two sisters associated with leukemia in one of them. J Pediatr 85:436–437, 1974

163. Caselitz J, Kloppel G, Delling G, Gruttner R, Holdhoff U, Stern M:

Schwachman's syndrome and leukemia. Virchows Arch [Pathol Anat] 385:109–116, 1979

164. Sugarman GI, Heuser ET, Reed WB: A case of cerebral gigantism and hepatocarcinoma. Am J Dis Child 131:631–633, 1977

165. McKusick VA: Mendelian Inheritance in Man, 4th Edition. Baltimore, Johns Hopkins University Press, 1978

166. Mulvihill JJ: Genetic repertory of human neoplasia. In Mulvihill JJ, Miller RW, Fraumeni JF Jr (eds): Genetics of Human Cancer, pp 137–143. New York, Raven Press, 1977

167. Fraumeni JF Jr: Clinical patterns of familial cancer. In Mulvihill JJ, Miller RW, Fraumeni JF Jr (eds): Genetics of Human Cancer, pp 223–231. New York, Raven Press, 1977

168. Müller H-J, Weber W: Familial Cancer. Basel, S Karger, 1985

169. Draper GJ, Heaf MM, Kinnier Wilson LM: Occurrence of childhood cancers among sibs and estimation of familial risks. J Med Genet 14:81–90, 1977

170. Mulvihill JJ: Clinical ecogenetics: Cancer in families. N Engl J Med 312:1569–1570, 1985

171. Li FP, Fraumeni JF Jr: Prospective study of a family cancer syndrome. JAMA 247:2692–2694, 1982

172. Lynch HT, Katz DA, Bogard PJ, Lynch JF: The sarcoma, breast cancer, lung cancer, and adrenocortical carcinoma syndrome revisited: Childhood cancer. Am J Dis Child 139:134–136, 1985

173. Hartley AL, Birch JM, Marsden HB, Harris M: Breast cancer risk in mothers of children with osteosarcoma and chondrosarcoma. Br J Cancer 54:819–823, 1986

174. Williams WR, Strong LC: Genetic epidemiology of soft tissue sarcomas in children, pp 151–153. In Müller H-J, Weber W (eds): Familial Cancer. Basel, S Karger, 1985

175. Snyder AL, Li FP, Henderson ES, Todaro GJ: Possible inherited leukaemogenic factors in familial acute myelogenous leukaemia. Lancet 1:586–589, 1970

176. Bech–Hansen NT, Sell BM, Mulvihill JJ, Paterson MC: Association of in vitro radiosensitivity and cancer in a family with acute myelogenous leukemia. Cancer Res 41:2046–2050, 1981

177. McKeen EA, Miller RW, Mulvihill JJ, Blattner WA, Levine AS: Familial leukaemia and SV40 transformation. Lancet 2:310, 1977

178. Parry DM, Berg K, Mulvihill JJ, Carter CL, Miller RW: Strategies for controlling cancer through genetics: Report of a workshop. Am J Hum Genet 41:63–69, 1987

three

Molecular and Cellular Biology of Pediatric Malignancies

Mark A. Israel

Only within the past 40 years has there been widespread recognition that the biologic alterations indicative of malignancy are closely related to events central for the development of complex, multicellular organisms. Coordinated growth regulation, differentiation, tissue invasion, and cell migration are now under intense scrutiny, as are the environmental factors that contribute to the development of malignancy. With great success, it has become possible to identify the chemical and biological agents that can transform normal cells to malignant ones, and to catalogue a broad array of cellular changes that may accompany this transformation. Laboratory investigators have also begun to reveal the biochemical basis for malignant transformation.

The dramatic advances in cellular biology and recombinant DNA technology are particularly noteworthy. They have combined to focus attention on cancer as a genetic disorder and provide a framework within which to reconcile many of the diverse laboratory and clinical observations that have placed cancer among the most enigmatic diseases. This chapter, by highlighting selected topics in genetics, biology, and biochemistry, presents some of the important themes in ongoing cancer research that have begun to influence clinical management and can be expected to lead to novel approaches to the prevention, diagnosis, staging, and treatment of pediatric malignancies. In this regard, the identification of specific genetic alterations that seem to be intimately related to malignancy has been of particular importance and has opened new lines of investigation toward elucidating the biochemical pathways that mediate the development of cancer and its numerous clinical features.

GENETIC ISSUES

Cytogenetics

Pediatric malignancies such as retinoblastoma and Wilms' tumor, which were among the first malignancies to be recognized as occurring in familial clusters, provided important early evidence of a heritable, genetic component of cancer etiology.[1-4] The pursuit of specific genetic alterations that might be associated with these tumors was futile, however, until advanced techniques for the visualization and characterization of chromosomes led to the identification of disease-associated, nonrandom genetic rearrangements in a wide variety of tumors. The most important of such technical advances was the identification of dyes such as quinacrine that could reproducibly and differentially stain chromosomes, thereby enabling the geneticist to identify an unambiguous staining pattern for each of the different chromosomes.[5-7] This pattern appears as a series of dark and light, wide and narrow bands that is unique to any particular region of any particular chromosome and thereby allows the recognition of chromosomal rearrangements (Fig. 3-1). More recently, gene mapping has made it possible to

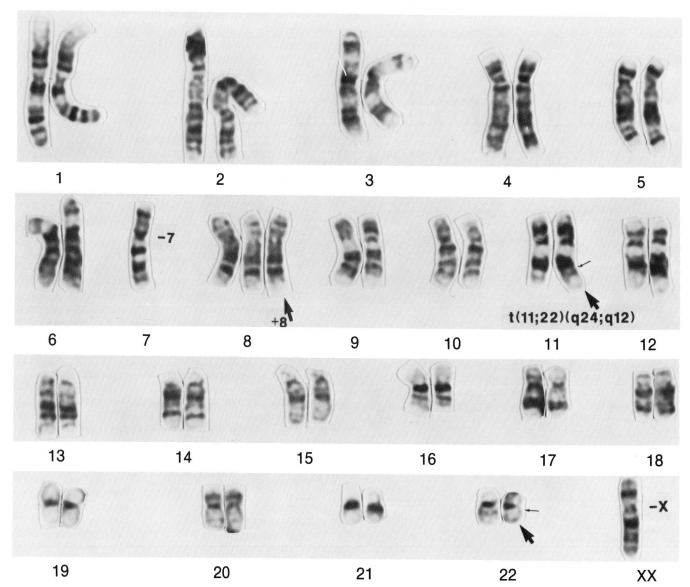

FIGURE 3-1.   Banding pattern of tumor cell chromosomes. Karyotype of a Ewing's sarcoma tumor cell: 44X, −X, −7, +8, t(11;22) (24;q12). This karyotype demonstrates cytogenetic alterations frequently found in Ewing's sarcoma, including supernumerary chromosome 8 and a reciprocal translocation of genetic material between chromosomes 11 and 22.

identify both the precise location and the structural alteration of genes involved in tumor-specific chromosomal rearrangements.[8,9] An ever-increasing number of malignancies have been recognized to be associated with specific genetic alterations (see below), and the importance of genetic rearrangements for the diagnosis and classification of patients with cancer is likely to increase. Table 3-1 describes the common types of rearrangements seen in tumor cells and details the abbreviation system used for describing the cellular chromosomal constitution.

Cytogenetic studies of leukemias and lymphomas have proceeded much more rapidly than similar studies of solid tumors. Although the precise reasons for this are unclear, evaluable chromosomes are more easily prepared from hematopoietic tumors and there seems to be less cell-to-cell variation in chromosomes from these tumors than is observed in many common solid tumors. Many nonrandom genetic rearrangements can now be recognized in different lymphomas and

leukemias (Table 3-2), and a number have been identified in solid tumors (Table 3-3). A listing of such rearrangements emphasizes the apparent specificity of many translocations for different malignancies, but there is still considerable debate about the proportion of any specific tumor type that exhibits a particular cytogenetic rearrangement. In Burkitt's lymphoma, for example, virtually every tumor has a recognizable translocation (see Chap. 20). In other tumor types, the proportion is lower. Because it seems likely that cytogenetically detected chromosomal rearrangements mark sites of alterations in oncogenes and other genes that are of potential etiologic importance[10–12] (see below), many investigators now believe that all tumors have a genetic rearrangement, although some may be too small to be easily recognized by currently available techniques.[47–49]

Occasionally, similar chromosomal changes are found in tumors that appear to be histologically distinct.[49] In some cases this may indicate a common genetic basis for some aspect of the development of these apparently different tumors. For example, the same chromosomal deletion that can occur in retinoblastoma[33] is also found in osteogenic sarcoma tumor cells.[50] The occasional occurrence of both these tumors in the same patient lends credence to the possibility of a common genetic origin (see Chaps. 25 and 32). Other tumors with cytogenetically indistinguishable rearrangements may indicate that there can be considerable variation, histologic or otherwise, among a number of tumors that constitute a singular genetic

and perhaps biological entity. For example, both Ewing's sarcoma and peripheral neuroepithelioma have indistinguishable cytogenetic rearrangements[40,42–45,51] (see Chaps. 29 and 31). Emerging evidence that Ewing's sarcoma (historically known as a tumor of bone) has a number of neuronal features suggests not only that these tumors may arise by a common genetic mechanism, but also that they may share common ontologic and biological features.[52] Recognition of the diversity of tumors associated with specific, nonrandom, clonal chromosomal alterations has provided considerable impetus for geneticists and oncologists to consider seriously the notion that tumors might be better classified by their genetic characteristics than by their histopathologic appearance.[53]

Although we do not yet know the precise mechanisms that mediate tumor-specific chromosomal changes, the very small number of rearrangements that have been studied in detail do bear some common features that provide hints as to what the correct answers to these questions might be. For example, rearrangements in B-cell and T-cell lymphoid disorders all tend to occur in chromosomal sites at which tissue-specific genes expressed at high levels are located.[54] In B-cell malignancies such as Burkitt's lymphoma, rearrangements occur near the immunoglobulin locus.[55–57] In T-cell disorders, breakpoints cluster near the loci encoding subunits of the T-cell receptor.[14,58,59] Perhaps the open chromatin configuration or other structural features common to highly expressed genes predisposes these sites to rearrangement. Another possibility is that these rearrangements result from a malfunctioning of normal developmental processes important for the rearrangement of the gene segments that are required for the formation of functional immunoglobulin and T-cell receptor genes.[60] In this regard, there is an intriguing possibility that cytogenetic changes in tumors of other tissues could identify other gene systems that are not yet recognized to undergo rearrangement as part of their normal developmental process.

Table 3-1
Abbreviations Used in Cytogenetic Descriptions

p	the short arm of a chromosome
q	the long arm of a chromosome
+	trisomy or an extra copy of a chromosome
t	translocation, an exchange of chromosomal material between two chromosomes
dup	duplication of a chromosome band or segment
del	deletion of a chromosome band or segment
i	isochromosome, an abnormal chromosome that has identical short or long arms
DM	double minute chromosome, an extrachromosomal stretch of highly repeated DNA sequences that segregates independently of the chromosomes during mitosis
HSR	homogeneous staining region, a stretch of chromosomal DNA that is amplified producing a repetitious, monotonous staining pattern

(ISCN: An international system for human cytogenetic nomenclature—high resolution banding. Cytogenet Cell Genet 31:1–23, 1981)

Table 3-2
Cytogenetic Rearrangements in Selected Pediatric Hematopoietic Tumors

Tumor Type	Chromosomal Rearrangement	References
Acute lymphoblastic leukemia		
Pre-B-cell leukemia	t(1;19) (q23;p13.3)	11
B-cell leukemia	t(2;8), t(8;14), t(8;22)	12
	t(11;14) (q13;q23)	11
Not defined	t(4;11) (q21;q23)	13
Acute T-cell lymphocytic leukemia	t(11;14) (p13;q13)	14
Acute nonlymphocytic leukemia		
Acute myelogenous leukemia (M2)	t(8;21) (q22;q22)	15
Acute promyelocytic leukemia (M3)	t(15;17) (q25;q22)	16,17
Acute myelomonocytic leukemia (M4)	t(11;21) (q22;q21), 16q	18
Acute monoblastic leukemia (M5)	11q, t(9;11) (p21;q23)	19, 20
Acute nonlymphocytic leukemia with basophils	t(6;9)	21
Acute nonlymphocytic leukemia with eosinophils	inv16(p13q22)	22–24
Chronic myelogenous leukemia	t(9;22) (q34;q11)	25, 26
Non-Hodgkin's lymphoma		
B-cell lymphoma		
Burkitt's lymphoma	t(8;14) (q24;q32)	27, 28
	t(2;8) (p13;q24)	
	t(8;22) (q24;q11)	
Large cell lymphoma	del(6) (q21), +7	
T-cell lymphoma	inv(14) (q11.2;q32.2)	
	t(8;14) (q24;q11.2)	
	t(14;14) (q11.2q32)	29

Table 3-3
Cytogenetic Rearrangements in Pediatric Tumors

Solid Tumors	Cytogenetic Rearrangements	References
Germ cell tumors	i(12p)	30–32
Retinoblastoma	del(13) (q14)	33, 34
Osteogenetic sarcoma	del(13) (q14)	35
Wilm's tumor	del(11) (p13) ;t(3;17)	36, 37
Neuroblastoma	del(1) (p32) (p36), DMs, HSRs	38, 39
Rhabdomyosarcoma	3p, t(2;13) (q37;q14), t(2,11)	40, 41
Ewing's sarcoma	t(11;22) (q24;q12)	40, 42–44
Peripheral neuroepithelioma	t(11;22) (q24;q12)	40, 45
Synovial sarcoma	t(x;18) (q22.1;q11.2)	46

Also not known is the basis for the common phenotypic and clinical features that characterize most tumors bearing any particular genetic rearrangement.[61] Perhaps specific rearrangements orchestrate a specific cellular phenotype. Alternatively, to become manifest as malignancy, different rearrangements may require different cellular machinery that is present only in a limited number of cell types. An intriguing finding of recent cytogenetic studies that should shed light on this question is the identification of genes now thought to be of central importance in the etiology of human tumors (*e.g.,* oncogenes) near or at the site of tumor-specific chromosomal alterations.[62–64] It seems reasonable to expect that alterations in the expression or structure of such genes will play a central role in the expression of malignancy. Research to characterize these genes has expanded greatly since the application of recent advances in recombinant DNA technology to molecular biology and is already making important contributions.

Molecular Biology

An appreciation of the impact that developments in recombinant DNA technology and molecular biology are likely to have on clinical oncology requires a familiarity with this discipline and its experimental approaches (Table 3-4). Remarkably, this entire approach to nucleic acid biochemistry hinges on an understanding of the primary structure of the DNA molecule. DNA is a double-stranded molecule in which only two types of nucleotide base pairing across strands can occur: adenosine with thymidine, and guanosine with cytosine.[65] This complementarity of base pairing is the basis upon which the linear arrangement of nucleotides in one DNA strand specifies with precise fidelity the structure of the opposite strand. This structural characteristic gives DNA its remarkable ability to encode its own replication and, indirectly, to mediate the synthesis of proteins.[66] Similarly, this complementarity provides the biochemical basis for the central techniques of recombinant DNA technology.[67]

Among these techniques, DNA hybridization analysis is of particular importance (Fig. 3-2). Hybridization is the process by which two complementary strands of nucleic acid anneal to form a double-stranded molecule[68–70] and forms the basis for all experiments analyzing DNA or RNA from tumor specimens for any particular gene. For such experiments, a probe consisting of isotopically labeled, single-stranded DNA that corresponds to the gene of interest is prepared. Following treatment to render the nucleic acid specimen being examined single-stranded, a mixture of the probe and experimental sample is incubated under the proper reaction conditions and allowed to

Table 3-4
Glossary of Molecular Biological Terms

DNA Sequence: The precise order of the four nucleotides adenine, guanine, cytosine, and thymidine as they are linked together to form the DNA strand. This DNA sequence encodes the genetic information of the organism.

Genome: All the chromosomal DNA sequences of an organism.

Hybridization: The annealing or base pairing of two single-stranded DNA molecules that are complementary.

Messenger RNA: A modified RNA molecule from which noncoding sequences have been removed and translation signals added. It is a precise copy of the amino acid coding sequences of a gene.

Molecular Cloning: The insertion of a foreign DNA segment into a DNA vector molecule that replicates independently of the host cell chromosome.

Oncogene: A gene that causes the malignant transformation of tissue culture cells or tumor formation in animals.

Probe: Isotopically labeled DNA or RNA that can be base paired with a complementary stretch of RNA or DNA during a hybridization reaction.

Proto-oncogenes: Normal cellular genes that become oncogenes after activation.

Recombinant DNA: A DNA molecule constructed by joining a fragment of DNA to a vector, such as a circular bacterial plasmid.

Restriction Enzymes: Enzymes that cut DNA at specific recognition sites.

Transcription: Synthesis of an RNA molecule by polymerization of nucleotides complementary to a DNA template. This RNA molecule is a precursor of mRNA and represents a precise, complementary copy of the DNA sequence from which it was transcribed.

Translation: Synthesis of proteins by the sequential addition of amino acids as defined by a messenger RNA molecule.

anneal, thus producing double-stranded molecules. Because the probe DNA is complementary to the gene of interest within the tumor cell genome, the characterization of molecules that contain one strand of nucleic acid from the clinical biopsy specimen and one strand of DNA from the probe can reveal both the configuration and the amount of nucleic acid that correspond to the gene of interest in the tumor material. Experimental manipulations yielding double-stranded molecules

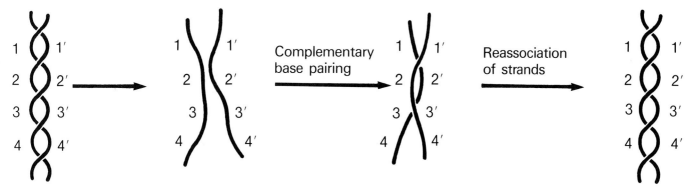

FIGURE 3-2.   Molecular hybridization. Separated complementary strands of either DNA or DNA and RNA can form double-stranded duplex molecules under the proper experimental conditions. The frequency of molecular collisions and the stability of the duplex molecules formed determine the rate of hybridization. Such experiments are usually carried out with one nucleic acid strand which has been isotopically labeled (probe) so that its association with nucleic acid sequences in the experimental sample can be identified.

Table 3-5
Types of DNA Hybridization Analysis Useful in the Evaluation of Human Tumor Specimens

Southern Blotting Analysis: A technique for characterizing DNA. A DNA sample digested with restriction enzymes is fractionated by size in agarose gels, transferred to a nitrocellulose membrane, and hybridized to an isotopically labeled nucleic acid probe.

Northern Blotting Analysis: A technique for evaluating gene expression by characterizing mRNA sequences. RNA is purified from cells, fractionated by size on agarose gels, transferred to a nitrocellulose membrane, and analyzed by hybridization as described for Southern analysis.

In situ *Hybridization to Histologic Tissue Specimens:* Isotopically labeled nucleic acid probes are hybridized to tissue sections mounted for microscopic evaluation. After the reaction has been completed, the tissue is covered with a photographic emulsion in which silver grains mark sites of probe reactivity. With emulsion in place, slides can be stained for routine histologic evaluation.

In situ *Hybridization to Chromosomal Spreads:* Isotopically labeled nucleic acid probes are hybridized to metaphase chromosome preparations on a microscope slide. After the reaction has been completed, the specimen is analyzed and stained for G-banding in a manner analogous to that described above for tissue specimens.

Table 3-6
Selected Restriction Enzyme Cleavage Sites*

Enzyme	Cleavage Site 5′,3′						Microorganism
BamHI	G	G	A	T	C	C	*Bacillus amyloliquefaciens* H
	C	C	T	A	G	G	
EcoRI	G	A	A	T	T	C	*Escherichia coli* RY13
	C	T	T	A	A	G	
Hind III	A	A	G	C	T	T	*Hemophilus influenzae* Rd
	T	T	C	G	A	A	

* Restriction endonuclease are enzymes that recognize specific pallandromic arrangements of DNA. Within these sequences the cleavage sites are always exact and are indicated in this table by arrows. Different restriction enzymes are isolated from different strains of bacterium, each of which has a companion methylase that specifically methylates bases within the restriction sites, thereby protecting each type of bacteria from its own restriction enzyme while it remains sensitive to cleavage by all others.

---

consisting of an isotopically labeled probe and cellular nucleic acid are now routine and form the basis of all hybridization analyses (Table 3-5).

Restriction endonucleases, enzymes that catalyze the cleavage of both strands of DNA at sequence-specific locations,[71,72] play an important role in the hybridization analysis of clinical specimens (Table 3-6). Because the human genome contains more than 100,000 different genes spread over more than a billion total DNA base pairs per cell, preparations of cellular DNA must be enriched for a gene being studied before that gene can be detected. Cleavage of DNA from clinical specimens by restriction endonucleases is the first step in the enrichment procedure.[73] Since every cell contains only one stretch of DNA containing any given gene, and the location of

restriction enzyme recognition sites in DNA flanking any particular gene is identical in the DNA of every cell, the restriction enzyme products resulting from the digestion of cellular DNA include fragments of only one size that contain any particular gene of interest. These fragments can then be separated from most of the other reaction products that are of a different size by gel electrophoresis (Fig. 3-3). In this technique, the collection of restriction fragments to be separated by size is loaded at the top of a porous, gel-like material that is then subjected to an electrical field. The individual DNA fragments migrate in the electrical field at a rate approximately proportional to their size, so that all DNA fragments of a particular size are found in the same location along the migration path. All locations along the gel migration path are therefore greatly enriched in specifically sized fragments of DNA.

After the restriction enzyme-cleaved DNA from a specimen of interest has been size fractionated in a gel, genes of interest can be examined by Southern blot analysis[73] (Fig. 3-3). First, the gel is treated with denaturing reagents that render the DNA single-stranded. The DNA is then transferred out of the gel onto a solid matrix, typically a sheet of nitrocellulose, where it is immobilized such that the matrix binds all DNA fragments at a position that corresponds exactly to their migra-

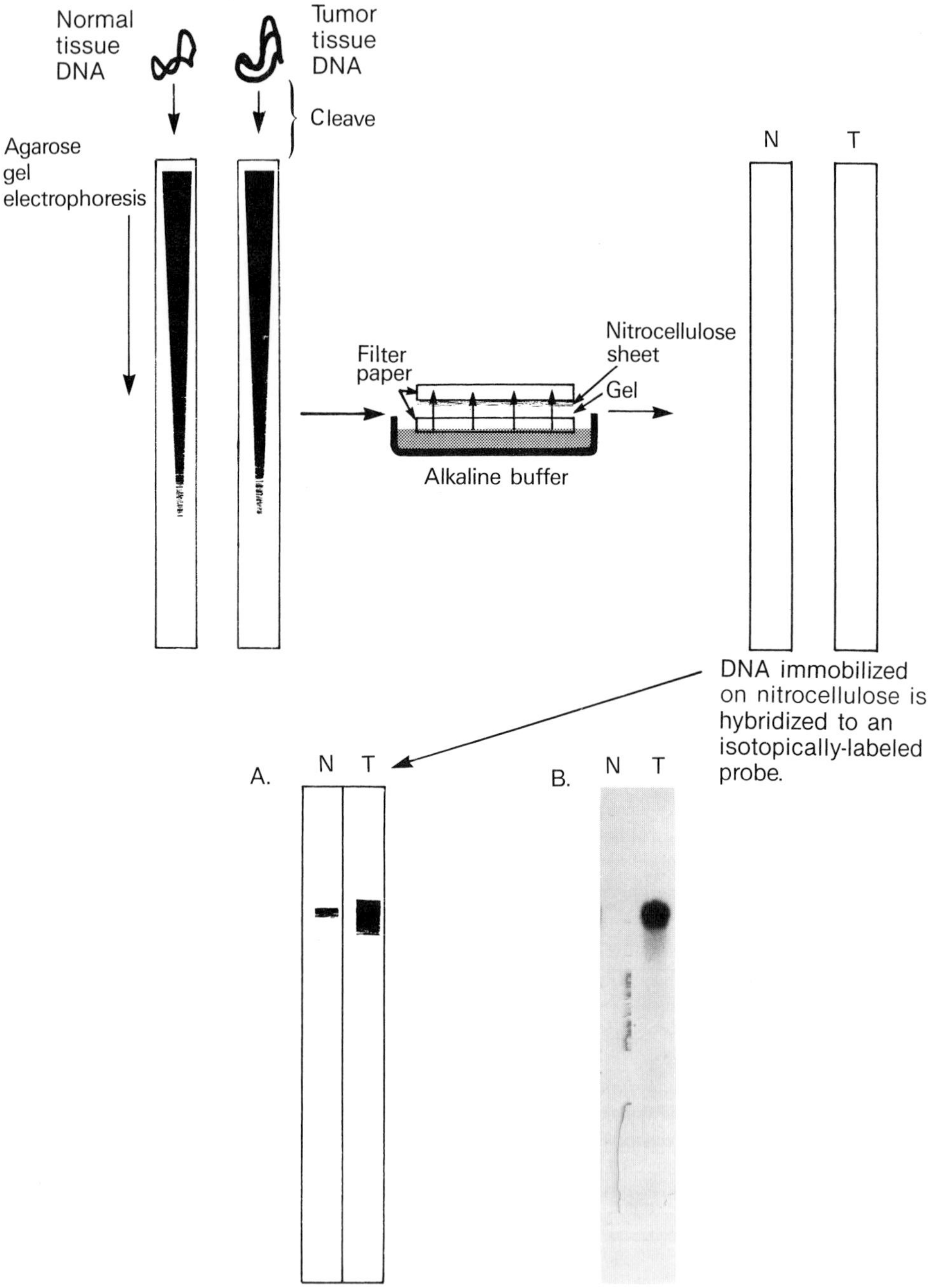

FIGURE 3-3. Southern blot hybridization analysis of tumor cell DNA. **Panel A.** Steps through which one might proceed in the analysis of DNA, which is amplified during the development of a particular malignancy. Cleavage of DNA from both a normal cell and a tumor cell results in innumerable different-sized fragments that can be distributed along a migration path during gel electrophoresis. Denaturation of this DNA, transfer *in situ* to a solid matrix such as nitrocellulose, and hybridization analysis using a radiolabeled molecular probe that corresponds to the amplified gene lead to an increased amount of radioactivity at a location in the gel path where the DNA fragment that contains the gene of interest has migrated. The location and the intensity of this DNA fragment can be identified by autoradiography, revealing both the structure and copy number of DNA fragments that contain the gene of interest. **Panel B.** Actual autoradiogram of experiment depicted in Panel A.

tion position in the gel. The DNA on the solid matrix is then hybridized to isotopically labeled DNA that corresponds to the gene that is being studied. After the matrix has been washed free of all nonhybridizing probe and exposed to x-ray film, hybridization of the labeled probe DNA to the single-stranded DNA on the matrix is detected as a specific "gel band" that was recognized by the probe.

Southern blot analysis can be used to detect several types of genetic rearrangements that are now recognized to occur in malignant cells. Examples of such rearrangements include chromosomal translocations, gene amplifications, deletions, viral insertions, or even single base pair mutations. Each of these alter the DNA structure of tumor cells and can be identified as changes from the Southern hybridization pattern found in DNA of normal tissues. The clinical application of this type of analysis has been most extensively pursued in lymphoid malignancies in which rearrangements of immunoglobulin[74] and T-cell receptor[75] genes are being actively studied. In some cases, the aberrant rearrangement of immunoglobulin genes may play a role in oncogenesis by bringing an oncogene into the vicinity of the DNA regulatory elements responsible for the expression of immunoglobulins[74] (see Chaps. 4, 16, 20). In other lymphoid malignancies, immunoglobulin and T-cell receptor gene rearrangements may have taken place as part of normal development.[75] If such rearrangements have occurred before the oncogenic event, however, they can be used to identify malignant clones and to subclassify leukemias and lymphomas in terms of both their lineage and the developmental stage at which they arise.[76] For example, the cells of most childhood leukemias, including the category previously called "null cell" leukemias, are now recognized to have undergone immunoglobulin gene rearrangement. While this indicates that they originate in B cells, the finding that they have often undergone rearrangement of only one (the heavy-chain gene) of the two types of immunoglobulin genes required for immunoglobulin production suggests that the oncogenic event leading to this type of leukemia must occur at a precise time during development before immunoglobulin light-chain rearrangement.[77] In acute lymphoblastic leukemia occurring during infancy, a significant number of patients show an unrearranged or embryonal pattern for both heavy- and light-chain immunoglobulin genes, suggesting that these tumors correspond to the malignant transformation of a less-differentiated cell type than that in which most acute lymphoblastic leukemias of childhood arise[78] (see Chaps. 12 and 16).

Similar hybridization analyses have also been used to examine RNA and to determine the level of expression of various genes in malignant and normal tissues. If RNA from a clinical specimen is immobilized after gel fractionation by means of a procedure called Northern blot analysis (a technique that is exactly analogous to Southern blot analysis), the amount of a specific RNA corresponding to a particular molecular probe can be determined. In such an evaluation, the location and intensity of the bands again correspond to the structure and amount of RNA being expressed in the tissue of interest. As seen in Figure 3-4, the level of RNA encoding the N-*myc* protein in a neuroblastoma tumor cell line known to contain many copies of the N-*myc* gene is higher than that found in an Epstein–Barr virus-transformed lymphoblastoid cell line from the same patient that contains only a single copy of this gene.

Hybridization of a probe to histologic tissue specimens *in situ* can give information about the particular cell type expressing a gene of interest (also see Chap. 6). For example, the analysis of a tissue homogenate for the structure or expression of specific genes may be confounded by the presence of cellular elements that are not of particular interest to the investigation (*i.e.,* tumor stroma or adjacent, contaminating normal tissue). Hybridization of molecular probes to histologic sections addresses this problem by providing a hybridization signal, namely, silver grains, over each cell in which the gene whose expression is being examined is detected (Fig. 3-5). Similarly, hybridization of such probes to metaphase spreads of chromosomes can identify the specific chromosomal band in which a gene is located.[80,81]

Each of these techniques, of course, relies on the availability of molecular probes for a gene of interest. Such probes are usually stretches of DNA encoding at least enough of a gene to allow its identification in a hybridization analysis. Originally, only a limited number of probes were available so that only a few genes could be evaluated. Recently, a large array of genes have become available through the use of recombinant DNA technology to identify and clone specific stretches of DNA known to encode proteins of particular interest to the oncologist (Table 3-7). Foremost among these are the oncogenes, whose altered expression or function may play a central role in the etiology of specific malignancies; tissue lineage-specific genes, whose highly limited pattern of expression makes them effective indicators of the tissue in which a tumor may arise; and genes that may encode proteins important for the development of metastases, drug resistance, and other clinically important features of malignancy.

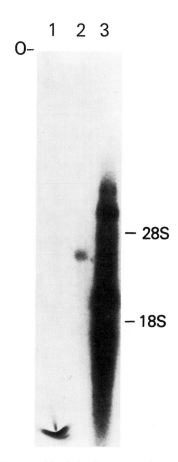

FIGURE 3-4. Northern blot hybridization analysis of cellular RNA. Northern blot analysis of RNA is precisely analogous to Southern blot analysis of DNA as demonstrated in Figure 3-3. The autoradiogram shown here depicts the analysis of five micrograms of poly (A)⁺ RNA isolated from a childhood rhabdomyosarcoma cell line, A204 (lane 1), a human lymphoblastoid cell line, DeF (lane 2), and a simian-sarcoma-virus-infected fibroblast cell line, ssv-3T3 (lane 3) hybridized to a ³²P-radiolabeled v-*sis* DNA probe. The migration of ribosomal RNA as detected by ethidium bromide staining is indicated.

Cancer Genes

Oncogenes

Cellular oncogenes (proto-oncogenes), which are present in the genome of every cell, can be activated and thereby cause a cell to acquire and maintain malignant characteristics.[82,83] Such activated proto-oncogenes are known as oncogenes (Table 3-8). Oncogenes were originally identified as the genetic loci responsible for the ability of retroviruses (RNA tumor viruses) to cause tumors in animals and to initiate and maintain the neoplastic transformation of cells in culture.[84,85] Molecular analyses of these genetic loci revealed that they were not viral genes but copies of cellular genes that, having been taken up into the viral genome (transduced), could be activated and thereby cause the malignant transformation of infected cells.[83,86] Indeed, these genes were originally named by an abbreviation of the virus in which they were first identified (*e.g.,* v-*sis* is the name of the viral tumor-causing gene in simian sarcoma virus; c-*sis* is the cellular proto-oncogene that corresponds to it).

Oncogenes have also been identified by other techniques, the best known of which is based on the ability of some onco-

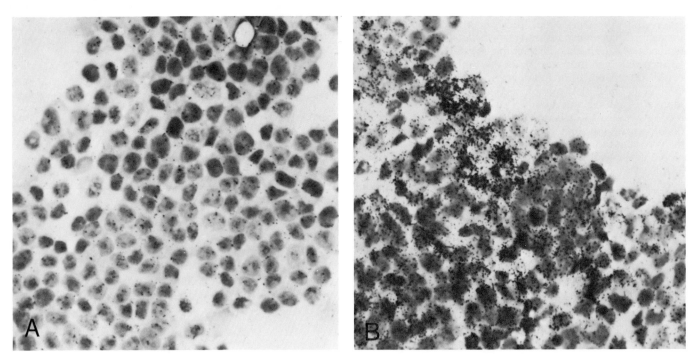

FIGURE 3-5. *In situ* hybridization analysis of tissue specimens. Hybridization of a ^{35}S-methionine *in vitro* labeled N-*myc* DNA probe to a human tumor cell line containing a single copy of the N-*myc* proto-oncogene and no detectable N-*myc* RNA expression (**Panel A**) reveals only background hybridization compared to the very frequently observed silver grains in an autoradiogram of a parallel analysis of an N-*myc* amplified human neuroblastoma tumor cell line in which N-*myc* is known to be very highly expressed (**Panel B**).

Table 3-7
Types of Molecular Probes (Cloned Genes) Available for Tumor Evaluation

Gene Type	Selected Examples
Potential Cancer Genes	
Dominant oncogenes	c-src, N-ras
Recessive cancer genes	"Retinoblastoma gene"
Growth Regulators	
Growth factors	PDGF, TGF-α, NGF, EGF
Growth factor receptors	EGF-receptor, insulin receptor
Cytoplasmic Messenger Protein	
G-proteins	c-ras, G-protein subunit of adenylate cyclase
Cyclic AMP dependent protein kinases	Protein kinase A
Potential Nuclear Regulatory Factors	
Nuclear binding proteins	c-myc, c-fos
Cytoskeletal Proteins	Actins, myosin, tubulin
Extracellular Matrix	
Matrix proteins	Laminin, fibronectin
Matrix receptors	Laminin receptor, fibronectin receptor
Drug Resistance Genes	
Genes related to specific agents	DHFR, aspartate transcarbamylase (CAB)
Multidrug resistance	Mdr, glutathione S-transferase

genes to change the growth characteristics of the murine fibroblast cell line NIH/3T3 (Fig. 3-6).[87–90] These cells normally stop growing once the surface on which they are being propagated has been completely covered by a cellular monolayer. When purified tumor DNA is transfected into these cells, a few may take up and express an oncogene. These cells are no longer growth inhibited by contact with their neighbors and simply overgrow adjacent cells, giving rise to a thick pile of cells known as a focus. Such a focus can be easily recognized and separated from adjacent growth-arrested cells. Human genes in the tumor DNA that are transfected and lead to the altered growth pattern of the murine cells can then be isolated

Table 3-8

Characterization of Selected Viral Oncogenes and Their Human Homologues

Oncogene	Viral Origin	Species of Origin	Animal Tumors Expressing Oncogene	Apparent Subcellular Localization of Cellular Gene Product	Associated Biochemical Activity or Putative Function	Chromosome Location of Human Homologue	Pediatric Tumors in Which Expression Has Been Detected or Activation Prediction
Growth Factor Family							
sis	Simian sarcoma v.	Monkey	Sarcomas	Cytoplasm/ secreted	PDGF-like growth stimulation	22q13.1	Glioblastoma
Protein Kinases							
src	Rous sarcoma v.	Chicken	Sarcoma	Plasma membrane	Tyrosine kinase	20q	Rhabdomyosarcoma, osteogenic sarcoma leukemia, Ewing's sarcoma, neural tumors
abl	Abelson murine leukemia v.	Mouse	Lymphoma	Plasma membrane	Tyrosine kinase	9q34-1	CML, ALL
erb B	Avian erythro- blastosis v.	Chicken	Sarcoma, erythro- leukemia	Plasma membrane	Tyrosine kinase truncated EGF receptor	7pter-q22	Glioblastoma
p21 ras Family							
N-ras	None	Human		Plasma membrane	Binds quanine nucleotides, GTPase activity	1p13	Neuroblastoma, carcinomas, leukemia
H/K-ras	Harvey/Kristen murine sarc. v.	Rat	Sarcomas, erythro- leukemia	Plasma membrane	Binds quanine nucleotides, GTPase activity	11p14–15/ 12p12 12q24	Neuroblastoma, rhabdomyosarcoma, leukemia, carcinoma
Nuclear Protein Family							
c-myb	Avian myelo- blastosis v.	Chicken	Myeloblastic leukemia	Nucleus	DNA binding protein	6q22–24	Neural tumors, leukemia, lymphoma, rhabdomyosarcoma, astrocytoma, neuroblastoma, Wilm's tumor
N-myc	None	Human	—	Nucleus		2p23–24	Neuroblastoma
c-myc	Avian myelo- blastosis v.	Chicken	Carcinoma, sarcoma, myelocytoma	Nucleus	DNA binding protein	8q24	Burkitt's lymphoma, neuroepithelioma
FOB	FBJ murine leukemia v.	Mouse	Sarcoma, leukemia	Nucleus		14q21–q31	Leukemias, neuroblastoma
Miscellaneous							
ets-1	E26 Avian erythro- blastosis v.	Chicken	Leukemia	Cytoplasmic	—	11q23.3–24	Ewing's sarcoma, neuroepithelioma
rel	Avian reticulo- endotheliosis virus	Turkey	Lymphatic leukemia		Homology to protein kinase		Rhabdomyosarcoma

from these foci by molecular cloning techniques and characterized.[87–90]

In a few cases, several different experimental approaches seeking oncogenes have led independently to the identification of the same genes. For example, some oncogenes identified by the NIH transfection assay were independently shown to have been transduced by retroviruses.[87,88,90] This finding, along with the recognition that some oncogenes encode growth-regulatory functions,[57,91–93] has provided important confirmation of a role for these genes in the malignant transformation of cells. Indeed, the finding that purified preparations of some oncogenes and combinations of other such genes can be transfected into freshly cultured normal cells and lead to the expression of a malignant phenotype has provided important evidence for the involvement of these genes in cancer.[94]

No fewer than 30 proto-oncogenes are now thought to be in the genome of every mammalian cell.[83] Although we have little hint of precisely what functions the proteins encoded by most oncogenes may serve, biochemical activities of several oncogene products have been identified (Table 3-8). As noted above, a few of these products have been recognized to correspond to proteins known to play important roles in the regulation of growth. As discussed later, the cellular pathways of growth regulation are now known to include distinct steps that can be experimentally evaluated. Among the important components of these pathways are growth factors, their receptors, cytoplasmic proteins that transfer the growth message through the cytoplasm to the nucleus, and nuclear proteins that somehow induce the changes in gene activity required for the expression of malignancy (Fig. 3-7). Table 3-8 lists the gene products or classes of gene products known to be encoded by

A

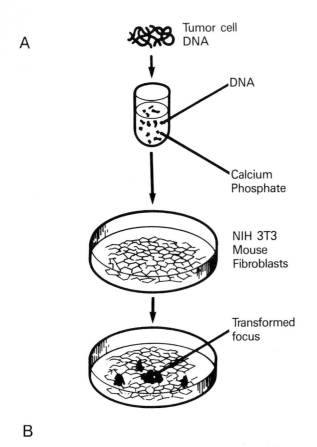

Tumor cell
DNA

DNA

Calcium
Phosphate

NIH 3T3
Mouse
Fibroblasts

Transformed
focus

B

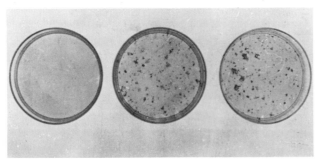

FIGURE 3-6.   Panel A. Fibroblast transfection assay for activated on-cogenes. DNA extracted from human tumors can be coprecipitated with calcium phosphate, which enhances its uptake by NIH-3T3 immortalized mouse fibroblasts. Rare cells that take up and express an activated oncogene become transformed and are recognized by their characteristic morphology and an associated loss of growth control leading to the piling up of these cells into thick foci. After repeated cycles of DNA purification and transfection of sequentially transformed cells, DNA nonspecifically taken up is diluted out, and eventually only a single stretch of human DNA in which the transforming gene must reside can be identified within the genome of the transformed mouse fibroblasts. **Panel B.** The appearance of experimental dishes in which 3T3 cells have been transfected by either mock, control DNA (dish on the *far left*), or DNA encoding an activated oncogene (dishes on the *right*). In this case, the adherent cell sheets have been stained with a vital dye to demonstrate the presence of thickly piled-up foci that correspond to the location of transformed cells in the experimental dishes.

specific oncogenes, emphasizing their potential for involvement in each of these steps in growth regulation. The finding that genes responsible for virus-induced tumors encoded proteins that could be important for the regulation of cell growth has provided impetus for investigators to identify their role in the development of specific malignancies: It seems likely that cancer may occur when one or more genes in these pathways go awry.[83]

ONCOGENE ACTIVATION.   The identification of human proto-oncogenes within or near various chromosomal rearrangements that mark specific human tumors has provided yet another important line of evidence suggesting a role for these genes in human carcinogenesis[62-64] (Table 3-9). Indeed, the conversion of a cellular proto-oncogene to an oncogene occurs by various mechanisms, several of which seem to be closely linked to the chromosomal rearrangements that mark the probable involvement of oncogenes in specific tumor types (Table 3-10). The first such observation, the recognition of the c-*myc* proto-oncogene at the site of each of the three different chromosomal translocations that occur in Burkitt's lymphoma[97] (see Chap. 20), has spearheaded an expanding research effort in this area of investigation detailing the involvement of altered chromosomal structure in activating proto-oncogenes. For example, in chronic myelogenous leukemia, the t(9;22) chromosomal rearrangement is thought to interrupt the structure of the c-*abl* gene and bring the distal portion of the gene encoding the c-*abl* protein into juxtaposition with another gene on chromosome 22 whose precise identity is unknown[98] (see Chap. 18). The resulting hybrid messenger RNA mole-

FIGURE 3-7.   Pathway of stimulated cell proliferation. Cellular proliferation can be modified by extracellular signals such as growth factors that interact with receptors on the surface membrane. These receptors can be transmembrane proteins (see text) that transduce the regulatory signal through the membrane, initiating an intracellular cascade of molecular messages that culminate in the alteration of nuclear proteins regulating the expression of genes important for cellular proliferation and tumorigenesis.

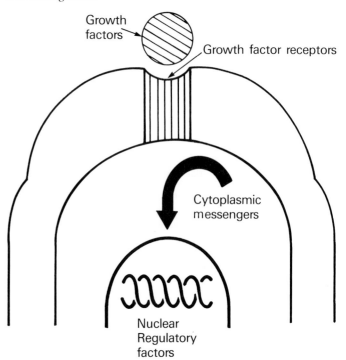

Growth
factors

Growth factor receptors

Cytoplasmic
messengers

Nuclear
Regulatory
factors

cule, which includes a fragment of a gene normally located on chromosome 22 and a portion of the c-*abl* proto-onco-gene,[99-101] encodes a presumably aberrant c-*abl* gene product. Similarly, the amplification of the N-*myc* gene in advanced stage neuroblastoma is thought to alter its expression such that either an abnormal protein is made or the normal protein is present but in inappropriate amounts or at inappropriate times in the cell's life cycle, thereby causing altered regulation of tumor cell growth[102-104] (see Chap. 28). These studies, as well as ongoing studies of other tumors, have lead to the recognition that translocations, amplifications, deletions, and other chromosomal rearrangements might mark not only the involvement of known oncogenes in tumorigenesis but also the location of other genes not previously recognized to be involved in malignant transformation.[105]

Recessive Cancer Genes

Since every gene in a cell is present as two alleles, the ability of structural alterations in even one of the two proto-oncogene alleles to lead to malignancy indicates that these changes are manifested in a manner that is dominant over the activity of the normal allele. As noted above, the altered structure of the c-*abl* locus in chronic myelogenous leukemia is thought to play a central role in the development of this disease. Yet a second c-*abl* gene remains intact on the unrearranged chromosome 9. Although this second locus is not altered in any way, its normal function seems to be overridden by that of the rearranged c-*abl* locus. To date, all known oncogenes have been thought to act in this dominant manner.[106] However, a number of clinical and cytogenetic observations made during the study of inherited forms of retinoblastoma led to the suggestion that recessive genes important for the development of cancer might be profitably sought in this tumor[2,107-109] (see Chap. 25). For example, a loss of genetic material from chromosome 13 is sometimes found in patients with retinoblastoma.[2,108,110] Also, the development of retinoblastoma has been closely associated with the inheritance of an unbalanced chromosome 13 deletion.[111] Finally, some patients with sporadic retinoblastoma have a deletion of chromosome 13 in their tumor tissue.[2] This association of a loss of genetic material with the development of cancer has suggested that the mutation leading to retinoblastoma is in a recessive allele that requires inactivation or deletion of the normal allele before tumor development occurs.[107,112]

Recombinant DNA technology has provided an approach for molecular geneticists to evaluate this hypothesis. Ultimately, such studies require the cloning and characterization of the DNA that encompasses both alleles of the recessive cancer gene, and these efforts are ongoing in the study of retinoblastoma.[113] Before such experiments in other tumors can be undertaken, however, it is necessary to identify the chromosomal regions in which such recessive genes might be located (Table 3-11). The current experimental approach to this problem asks simply whether one of the two alleles at a particular chromosomal site has been lost during the development of a tumor, suggesting the presence of a recessive gene important in the development of that malignancy. The ability to identify the loss of DNA at a particular genetic locus rests on the fact that there is considerable "silent" variation in the actual arrangement of nucleotide bases that make up DNA, and therefore the arrangement of restriction enzyme recognition sites in any one individual's DNA may be different from that in DNA from anyone else. Such differences are recognized as variations in the size of the DNA fragments produced by endonuclease cleavage of cellular DNA from different individuals[116,117] and have been called "*restriction fragment length polymorphisms*" (RFLPs). At many genetic loci, the paired alleles of any particular individual—one on the maternally derived chromosome and one on the paternally derived chromosome—may be different from one another. These RFLP sites can then be recognized by Southern blotting, and the locus in DNA isolated from normal tissue can be compared to that isolated from tumor tissue, revealing whether one of the two alleles has been lost.[116-118]

Exploiting this approach, an investigator can distinguish each of the two chromosomes of an individual who is heterozygous at a particular locus. Using molecular probes to examine the chromosomal region 13q14 in patients with retinoblastoma,[108] 11q13 in patients with Wilm's tumor,[4] and 22q in patients with acoustic neuroma,[114] it is possible to show that tissue derived from these tumors has lost DNA corresponding to one of the two alleles at these loci. Remarkably, this has been possible even in tumors whose karyotype appears normal, suggesting that chromosomal deletions too small to be detected by conventional analysis as well as other less obvious genetic alterations (such as the loss of an entire chromosome and duplication of its homologue) must have occurred in association with tumor formation.[108]

Table 3-9
Oncogenes Located near Structural Genetic Rearrangements in Selected Pediatric Malignancies

Oncogene	Genetic Rearrangement	Tumor
myc	t(8;14)(q24;q32)	Burkitt's lymphoma
abl	t(9;22)(q34;q11)	Chronic myelogenous leukemia
N-myc	DMs, HSRs	Neuroblastoma
rel	t(2;11)(q37;q14)	Rhabdomyosarcoma
ets	t(11;22)(q24;q12)	Ewing's sarcoma, neuroepithelioma

Table 3-10
Mechanisms by Which Proto-oncogenes May Be Activated in Pediatric Tumors

Mechanisms	Example Oncogene	Tumors
Gross structural rearrangement	abl	Chronic myelogenous leukemia
Point mutation	N-ras	Thoracic neuroblastoma
Amplification	N-myc	Neuroblastoma
Regulatory changes	myc	Burkitt's Lymphoma

Table 3-11
Pediatric Malignancies with Recognized Recessive Genetic Alterations

Tumor	Chromosomal Alterations	References
Retinoblastoma	13q14	33
Osteosarcoma	13q14	35
Wilm's tumor	11p13	37
Embryonal tumors of Beckwith–Wiedemann syndrome	11p	4
Acoustic neuroma and meningioma	22	114
Meningioma	22	114, 115

The molecular analysis of DNA from members of families in which the inheritance of a tumor can be associated with specific genetic loci has made it possible to recognize the specific allele associated with tumor development. This approach to the identification of the genotype required for the development of retinoblastoma has been used clinically to predict the risk of individuals in affected families for developing overt disease.[119] As cancer predisposition and the genetic basis of other malignancies is better understood, there can be little doubt that novel approaches to genetic counseling will become an increasingly important aspect of pediatric oncology (also see Chaps. 2 and 25).

CELLULAR ISSUES

Cell Growth

To date, unbridled growth has been the focus of cancer research directed at characterizing the molecular alterations that play a crucial role in the development of malignancies. Most human tissues turn over at perceptible rates, and it is the imbalance between the growth of new cells and the death of senescent cells that results in the growth of a tumor. At present, we have no means to measure efficiently growth rates in individual tumor tissues.[120] In particular, we know little about the mechanisms by which cell loss occurs in tumors, and therefore descriptions of tumor growth at best reflect only the balance between cell growth and cell loss. Nonetheless, some remarkable observations have been made that should influence our thinking about the biological regulation of tumor growth.[121] For one, pathologically indistinguishable tumors grow at dramatically different rates in different individuals.[122,123] Also, metastases seem to grow faster than primary tumors,[124,125] and multiple metastases sometimes appear to grow at very similar rates and sometimes at very disparate rates. Different areas of the same tumor may grow at different rates, and it has sometimes appeared that the surgical removal of a primary tumor mass can lead to more rapid growth of residual primary and metastatic tumor tissue.

Each of these clinical observations suggests that the regulation of tumor growth must be a function not only of the tumor itself but also of its environment. Recently, it has been possible to identify some of these regulatory influences (see below), and emerging knowledge of the molecular mechanisms by which such regulation is mediated has emphasized the importance of the cell cycle as a framework within which to understand these events (Fig. 3-8). The most easily recognized phase of the cell cycle is the M phase, the time during which cellular division occurs.[128] This period begins with nuclear division (mitosis) and ends with cytoplasmic division (cytokinesis).

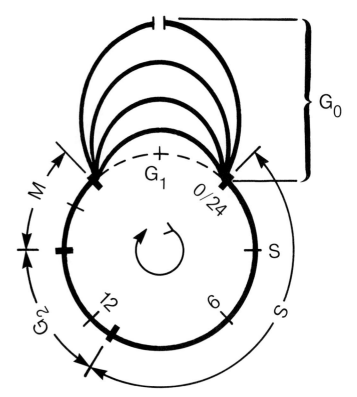

FIGURE 3-8. Cellular growth cycle. Depicted are the phases through which a tumor cell might proceed during growth. These phases are divided in an idealized manner for a cell with a generation time of 24 hours. G_1, G_2, M, and S refer to the phases of the cell cycle as outlined in the text. Restriction points during G_1 are times at which a cell might enter a quiescent interface or move out of the cell cycle into G_0 for an indeterminate period of time.

Nuclear division in the absence of cellular division is a frequent event in some tumors, as evidenced by the finding of hyperdiploidy in many of the tumors that occur during childhood, including leukemias and several solid tumors.[127] When a cell is not dividing, it is said to be in interphase. During interphase the only discrete period that can be recognized is the S phase, when new DNA is synthesized. The gap between the end of DNA synthesis and the beginning of mitosis is called G_2, and the period that follows mitosis before the next round of DNA synthesis is called G_1.[126]

The dramatic differences in cell cycle duration that characterize neoplastic cell types are largely a reflection of variations in the duration of G_1.[128] This is the only portion of the cell cycle in which normal cells may either become quiescent and growth arrested or proceed with proliferation. If cell division is initiated, cells proceed through the cell cycle and divide without any further requirement for external stimulation. Daughter cells then proceed into G_1, where they can again divide or remain arrested at a restriction point at which the cell awaits further signals to proceed with the next round of division.[129,130] Late G_1, where the restriction point has been mapped, seems to be the only position in the cell cycle at which cell division can become physiologically arrested and the time when extracellular signals that regulate cell division are most active (see below).

Normal cells are growth arrested during most of their lifetime. During this long interphase, they carry out the designated functions associated with their particular differentiated phenotype. Although highly differentiated cells may be thought of as arrested for long periods of time at a restriction point in G_1, some investigators find it more accurate to characterize this period as entirely distinct from the cell cycle and therefore designate it G_0.[131] Since the precise physiologic events that mediate the growth arrest of cells are not yet known, laboratory research is currently focused on the cellular proteins that are required for the regulation of DNA synthesis and how these proteins are regulated at the restriction point.[132] An understanding of these molecular events has obvious implications for cancer research because the inability of cancer cells to enter G_0 may be a fundamental feature of their unbridled proliferation.[131] Such issues are also of importance to clinical oncologists in their attempts to improve the effectiveness of chemotherapy and radiation in the management of patients with cancer, since tumor cells that are not traversing the cell cycle are likely to be an important source of treatment failure.[133–137]

In this regard, improved techniques to characterize the cell cycle kinetics of human tumors are needed. In the past, examination of the cell cycle in human tumors was particularly difficult,[124] requiring microscopic examination of biopsied tumor tissue labeled *in vitro* or obtained after the administration of bromodeoxyuridine (BrdU) or isotopically labeled thy-

midine to the patient. The percentage of cells that incorporated radioactive thymidine or immunologically detectable BrdU was designated as the labeling index, a parameter that provided an indirect estimate of the proliferative activity of a tumor.[126,138] The availability of fluorescence-activated cell-sorter (FACS) analysis, however, has opened new avenues for studies of the cell cycle in both experimental systems and biopsy specimens.[139] With this approach, cells are treated with a fluorescent dye that binds to DNA, and the amount of fluorescence associated with each cell in a biopsy specimen is analyzed (Fig. 3-9). This procedure enables the proportion of cells at various stages in the cell cycle, as indicated by varying amounts of fluorescence, to be rapidly, easily, and repeatedly estimated. Although this approach is still limited by the availability of tumor tissue, it greatly enhances the possibility that cell cycle analysis can be used routinely in the management of patients with cancer.

Growth Regulation

With few exceptions, human tissues are characterized by their ability to divide rather than their ability to remain growth arrested. Most human tissues are renewable and proliferate both

FIGURE 3-9. Components of a flow cytometer. In the center a jet stream of cells in suspension are depicted as emerging from a flow cell and into a focused laser beam. The forward angle light scatter is detected by a photodiode, whereas scattered fluorescent light is detected by a photomultiplier after fractionation by a variety of filters, allowing discrimination of varying fluorescent wavelengths. The jet stream that is broken into precise drops by an ultrasonic transducer can be electrically charged and sorted by the use of electronic deflection plates (not shown).

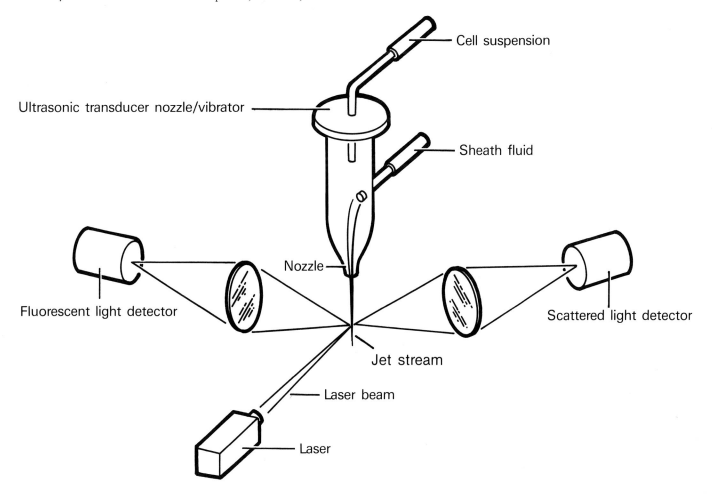

as a normal physiologic feature of tissue maintenance and in response to injury. Some normal cells, such as skin, bone marrow, and mucosa, contain stem cells that have the ability to give rise not only to additional cells that go on to develop predictable features of terminal differentiation but also to other stem cells that have a capacity for unlimited division.[140,141] These tissues tend to turn over at a very rapid rate. In contrast, hepatocytes turn over at an almost imperceptible rate, yet more than half the liver can be regenerated in less than a week in response to the loss of liver tissue.[142] As one might expect from these diverse and tissue-specific features of growth regulation, growth regulatory influences emerge from many different sources (Table 3-12).

Much of our information about the regulation of cellular proliferation comes from studies *in vitro*. In this regard, a most remarkable characteristic of cells from malignant tissue that distinguishes them from cells of normal tissue is their ability to grow indefinitely in culture, that is, to become immortalized and thereby form a cell line.[143] Specialized cells that make up various normal tissues can be maintained in culture for only short periods and eventually cease to divide, age, and die.[144,145] To date, only three sources of immortalized normal cells in culture exist: Epstein–Barr virus lymphoblastoid cell lines,[146] cells experimentally transfected with specific viral genes known to confer the property of unlimited cellular growth,[147,148] and a few cell cultures, usually fibroblasts, that are presumed to have become immortalized because of an as-yet-unrecognizable mutational event.[149]

Several decades of experiments have detailed the cellular features of malignant cells in culture (Table 3-13); however, only a very limited number of these effectively distinguish malignant cells *in vitro* from proliferating normal tissues. To date, all such characteristics are related to differences in growth. Nonmalignant cells in monolayer culture tend to become growth inhibited once they come into contact with a neighboring cell.[150,151] Transformed malignant cells, on the other hand, continue to grow, changing their shape to achieve a higher cell density than that obtained by normal cells. Eventually, transformed cells simply pile up on neighboring cells, sometimes even growing as floating clumps in either liquid or semisolid media containing agar. Most malignant cells exhibit this anchorage-independent growth,[152] whereas normal cells require contact with a surface such as glass before they can thrive *in vitro*. Because growth in semisolid media correlates closely with tumorigenesis in mice that are immunosuppressed[152,153]—the most stringent test of malignant cellular behavior—growth in agar is the most frequently employed labora-

Table 3-12
Potential Sources of Growth Regulatory Influences

Soluble Factors
  Hormones
  Growth factors
  Nutritional elements

Extracellular Factors
  Vascular and supportive tissues
  Stromal matrix
  Cell-to-cell contact/position in a tissue

Cellular Factors
  Plasma membrane
  Cytoplasmic regulatory proteins
  Growth-related gene expression
  Differentiation-related gene expression

Table 3-13
Cellular Features of Transformed Cell Lines

Growth
  Ability to form tumors in immunosuppressed mice
  Diminished requirement for substrate adherence
  High cloning efficiency in semi-solid agar
  Diminished requirement for growth factors in serum
  Rapid doubling time in low concentrations of serum
  High cloning efficiency in liquid media
  High saturation density

Morphology
  Heterogeneous shape
  Thick, convex, refringent cells
  Disoriented growth pattern

Cytoskeleton
  Loss of actin cables and microtubules
  Altered organization of microtubules

Surface Structures
  Enhanced agglutination by lectins
  Altered surface proteins, glycoproteins, and glycolipids
  Decreased collagen production

Biochemical
  Increased rate of glucose transport
  Increased anaerobic glycolysis
  Production of plasminogen activator

tory test of malignant growth and forms the basis of the widely used "clonogenic assay," which measures the efficacy of tumor cell growth in agar before and after exposure to cytotoxic agents.[154–156]

A central requirement for the regulation of normal cell growth is that it be coordinated among the different cells of a tissue. It therefore is of interest that some cellular processes thought to be important for the control of proliferation seem to be mediated through the cell's milieu (see Table 3-12). At present, we understand few details of the processes by which physical constraints,[150,151] positional effects,[157] and cell–cell contacts mediate alterations in cell growth, and their involvement in tumorigenesis has not been demonstrated. Recent advances in our understanding of soluble regulators of cellular proliferation, however, have provided insights into how mediators of growth such as hormones and peptide growth factors influence the development of a number of different tumors[158–160] (Table 3-14). Peptide growth factors both stimulate and inhibit cellular proliferation and may play important physiologic roles in wound healing, bone repair, and other processes involving regulated growth.[161,162] Some growth factors are highly specific in terms of the cell types that they can stimulate; others stimulate a wide variety of cells.[160] For example, epidermal growth factor stimulates most cells of mesenchymal origin that have been evaluated, whereas few of the many factors that stimulate the growth of hematopoietic cells can stimulate other cell types. Some tissues do not seem to have receptors for any known growth factor, whereas other tissues, such as fibroblasts, have receptors for multiple growth factors and seem to require more than one growth factor before they can reach their full proliferative potential.[163]

An important characteristic of growth factors is that their activity is mediated through binding to a specific cell membrane receptor.[51,164,166] Because growth factors are bound at the cell surface and need not be internalized to stimulate cell growth, their activity is not mediated through their direct binding to DNA and subsequent activation or repression of the

Table 3-14
Selected Polypeptide Growth Factors and Receptors of Potential Oncogenic Significance

Growth Factor	Source	Selected Target Tissues	Size (# of Amino Acids)	Receptor Characteristics	Tumors with Evidence of Expressing Growth Factor or Receptor
Insulin-like growth factor I (IGF-I)	Human plasma	Multiple tissue types		Four subunits, receptor-like	
Insulin-like growth factor II (IGF-II)	Human plasma	Multiple tissue types	67aa		Wilm's tumor, rhabdomyosarcoma
Epidermal growth factor (EGF)	Human urine	Epidermal and epithelial cells	53aa	Single polypeptide chain, tyrosine kinase activity	
Type α transforming growth factor (TGF-A)	Placenta, malignant cells	Same as EGF	50	Utilizes EGF receptor	
Type β transforming growth factor (TGF-B)	Placenta, kidney	Fibroblasts and epithelial cells	224	Very large dimeric molecule	
Platelet derived with factor (PDGF)	Platelets, endothelial cells	Smooth muscle, mesenchymal cells	241 + A	Single polypeptide chain, tyrosine kinase activity	Gliomas, osteosarcoma
Colony stimulating factor-1 (CSF-1)	Murine tumor cells	Macrophage progenitors	Unknown	Single polypeptide chain, tyrosine kinase activity	
Interleukin-2 (IL-2)	T-helper cells	Cytotoxic T-cells	169	Heterodimer	

Table 3-15
Plasma Membrane Receptors with Putative Tyrosyl Kinase Activity

Epidermal growth factor receptor
Platelet-derived growth factor receptor
Insulin receptor
Insulin-like growth factor receptor
Colony stimulating factor I receptor

expression of specific genes. Rather, growth factors seem to work by activating their receptor, which is either itself transported intracellularly or transmits across the cell membrane a message that initiates a series of intracellular events, culminating in the altered expression of genes important for cell division.[166–168] Because growth requires the activation of many different cellular activities, the recent recognition that some growth factor receptors have protein kinase activity was particularly interesting[169] (Table 3-15). Protein kinases transfer phosphate molecules from a donor substrate to other enzymes and thereby modulate the enzyme's specific activity. Cascades of enzymatic activity allowing for the precise regulation of complex biochemical systems can be based on kinase-mediated enzyme activation, providing an explanation for the diverse cellular effects of growth factor stimulation.[170]

Among the best studied growth factor receptors of this type is the epidermal growth factor receptor (EGF), a 170-kD glycoprotein that has three functional domains arranged in a transmembrane configuration.[170–173] The extracellular domain binds EGF to the cell surface, transmitting a signal through a hydrophobic transmembrane domain to an intracellular segment that has tyrosine kinase activity. The finding that the protein kinase activity of several growth factor receptors specifically phosphorylated tyrosine adds an important degree of specificity to this enzymatic activity,[174] since serine and threonine are the most commonly phosphorylated amino acids. Phosphotyrosine constitutes less than 0.01% of all the phosphorylated amino acid in cellular proteins,[175] suggesting that only a very limited number of proteins are substrates for these kinases.

We do not yet know the critical cellular proteins that are physiologically phosphorylated and presumably activated after the interaction of a growth factor with its receptor. Nevertheless, an outline of the pathway by which such interactions are likely to stimulate cell growth, and how alterations in these pathways might lead to malignancy, is emerging. Figure 3-7 provides a schematic view of the cellular pathways that might be involved in the conversion of a growth signal to alterations in gene expression. Such a model outlines four broad categories of events that might occur during growth factor stimulated cell proliferation. Recent studies demonstrating that known oncogenes may encode proteins that can function at each of these stages in growth signal transduction (see Table 3-8) suggest strongly that malignancies may arise as a result of pathologic alterations in these pathways. Determining precisely how such alterations are manifested as the spectrum of features that characterize malignant cells remains a major challenge for cancer research. The interaction of oncogene products, however, with such pleiotropic mediators of cellular response as cell membrane lipids and cytoplasmic protein kinase C (see below),[176] suggests that an integrated model for the expression of malignancy may emerge.

Growth factors are distinguished from other extracellular stimulants of proliferation in that they are produced close to their target cell. They reach the target cell by diffusion, a process dubbed paracrine growth regulation (Fig. 3-10). For example, platelets associated with a clot might produce platelet-derived growth factor (PDGF), a stimulant of fibroblast division, and thereby influence wound healing.[177] Although a

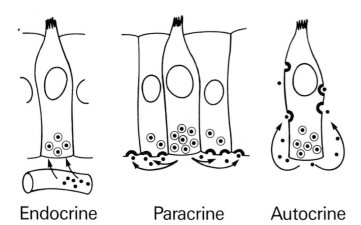

Endocrine   Paracrine   Autocrine

FIGURE 3-10. Autocrine growth regulation. A hypothesis to explain the unregulated proliferation of human tumor cells is that the genetic alterations leading to malignancy effect steps in stimulated growth critical for the production of a growth factor or its receptor. If the same cell that contains receptors for a particular growth factor also makes that growth factor, important steps in the regulation of cellular growth might be bypassed (Sporn MB, Todaro GJ: Autocrine secretion and malignant transformation of cells. N Engl J Med 303:878–880, 1980. Used with permission).

precise role for paracrine-mediated, growth-factor-stimulated proliferation has not yet been defined for malignant cells,[178] one can easily imagine that growth factors produced by cancer cells could be important stimulants of stromal tissue growth, a prerequisite for the development of large tumors. Conversely, stromal cells or subpopulations of tumor cells could produce growth factors that play a regulatory role in either stimulating or limiting tumor growth.

A novel mechanism of growth factor-stimulated proliferation, namely, autocrine growth regulation, has been proposed and demonstrated to be of importance in a number of experimental tumor systems[158,179] (Fig. 3-10). Such a mechanism of growth signal transduction hypothesizes that a cell can respond to the same growth factor that it produces. This mechanism of altered growth regulation in tumor cells is in concert both with the finding that some tumors can be shown to produce growth stimulatory substances[180] (see Table 3-14) and with much earlier cancer research demonstrating a decreased requirement for growth factor-containing serum when growing malignant cells *in vitro*.[181–183] In experimental systems, this line of investigation has been pursued further. For example, in a growth factor-dependent murine cell line the expression of a hematopoietic growth factor results in the autonomous growth of that cell line and confers tumorigenicity upon it,[184] providing direct evidence for the involvement of autocrine growth pathways in tumorigenesis. Other investigators have studied virus-transformed cell lines and identified tumor growth factors (TGFs) not previously recognized in any normal tissues (see Table 3-14). TGFs were originally defined by their ability to stimulate the growth of specific indicator cell lines, and they have assumed increasing importance because of the large number of different types of human tumor cell types in which their expression can be identified. Neither TGF-alpha nor TGF-beta, the most extensively studied human TGFs, have as yet been reported to be expressed in pediatric tumors, however.

A number of experimental approaches have been used to demonstrate and characterize the presence of autocrine growth pathways in human tumors. Among tumors that occur in pediatric patients, only osteogenic sarcoma has been studied in detail (see Chap. 32). To date, it has been possible to show that

the U-2 OS osteogenic sarcoma-derived cell line both contains functional PDGF receptors and synthesizes PDGF.[185,186] While the interaction of some autocrine growth factors and their receptors can be blocked by antisera to either the growth factor or the receptor, the growth of these cells is not inhibited by antiserum to PDGF.[186] Among the explanations for this finding is that the interaction of the growth factor and its receptor may take place within the cell before secretion rather than at the cell surface. Such a possibility has obvious implications for the development of therapeutic strategies directed at interfering with autocrine growth pathways and is an important area of ongoing research.

Differentiation

Pathologists recognized long ago that few malignant tumors expressed the full complement of tissue-specific features that characterize differentiated, mature tissues. For the oncologist, the fully differentiated state might frequently be defined by growth arrest, since it appears that the regulation of growth is intimately related to the development of tissue-specific, differentiated features.[31,32] The precise relationship between differentiation and malignant transformation is, however, unknown, and we do not know why tumors appear immature.[187,188] On the one hand, terminally differentiated cells cannot be transformed *in vitro* and are not thought to give rise to tumors *in vivo*. Perhaps cells giving rise to tumors simply are too immature to express the features that characterize a specific cell type. On the other hand, the loss of tissue specific markers is sometimes progressive over the course of tumor growth.[189] Such a loss can also occur in association with the continued passage of tumor cell lines in culture,[190] suggesting that tumor cells can undergo dedifferentiation in association with their malignant growth.

Remarkably, the tendency of tumors to become progressively less differentiated is not as common in pediatric tumors as in adult tumors. Some tumors, such as neuroblastoma[191] and rhabdomyosarcoma,[192] even undergo differentiation after diagnosis. While this has generally been observed in association with systemic treatment, it does indicate that the loss of differentiated features is not an invariant event associated with the progressive growth of a malignant tumor and that some tumors retain potential for the expression of features associated with their fully differentiated counterpart. Other important evidence suggesting that the absence of differentiated features in tumors of developing tissues does not always indicate dedifferentiation comes from the study of lymphoid malignancies. In lymphocytes, the immunoglobulin and T-cell receptor genes rearrange in a programmed manner marking specific stages in the differentiation of lymphoid tissue (see Chaps. 4, 20). Recent findings characterizing the structure of these genes in various lymphoid malignancies indicate that such tumors have a recognizable pattern of gene rearrangement corresponding to that seen at different stages along the normal pathway of lymphocyte differentiation.[76] These data extend biochemical studies suggesting that these tumors are clonal expansions of cells at different stages along the normal differentiation pathway[193,194] and are of importance because they provide a clinical counterpart for an emerging body of information suggesting that malignancy can arise in close association with arrested differentiation.

When normal tissues differentiate, there is a precisely balanced expansion of cells at various stages along the differentiation pathway. The more mature the cell, the more limited is its growth potential. Although the precise kinetics by which the various stages of a particular tissue expand during differentiation is unknown, a predictable imbalance would occur between the emergence of new cells (indeed, new cells with proliferative capacity) and physiologic cell loss if differentiating cells were unable to proceed along the programmed pathway to terminal differentiation.[195] Experimental evidence in support of cancer arising as a disorder of developmental processes comes from several sources. Among the most provocative of these is the study of murine teratocarcinoma cells, which are malignant but become benign in association with the induction of differentiation.[188,196,197] The apparent reversibility of malignancy in these[198] and other cells[199] suggests that under some circumstances there can be an intimate interplay between the molecular mechanisms that mediate differentiation and those that induce malignancy.

Other evidence for the possibility that tumors arise in association with arrested differentiation comes from laboratory studies utilizing transforming viruses to block cellular differentiation. In such experiments, a virus that carries a temperature-sensitive mutation in its transforming gene is used to transform cells. At the permissive temperature, the transforming gene product is stable and the cells display characteristics of malignant cells. At the nonpermissive temperature the transforming protein is unstable and the cells are normal by all measurable criteria. When cells that can be induced to undergo differentiation culture are infected by such viruses, differentiation is blocked at the permissive temperature.[200] Because it is unlikely that any specific transforming viral gene product would interact directly with the series of structural genes responsible for a particular differentiated phenotype, differentiation probably is blocked by transformation-induced changes in the mechanisms that regulate tissue-specific differentiation. An important implication of these studies is that although cancer may arise as the result of a somatic mutation, alterations of gene expression—epigenetic phenomena—can contribute to the development of malignancy (also see Chap. 2).

Pediatric tumors, including those of solid tissues, are a particularly fruitful area in which to look further for the clinical implications of arrested differentiation during tumorigenesis. Most of the embryonal tumors, such as neuroblastoma, Wilms' tumor, rhabdomyosarcoma, and brain tumors present with varying degrees of differentiation that can be recognized histologically and biochemically. In some cases, for example, in gliomas, the degree of differentiation of the tumor is a strong predictor of clinical behavior (see Chap. 24). If this is a reflection of the origin of such tumors in different cells along the differentiation pathway, it is possible that therapies directed at the modulation of differentiation might be profitably pursued in such tumors. It is even possible to imagine that under such circumstances therapeutic approaches directed at correcting or bypassing the oncogenic lesion might be successful in inducing a fully differentiated, growth arrested cell.

Because there are so few markers that identify different stages along the maturational pathway of most tissues, it is possible that within current histologically defined tumor groups there are distinct subgroups that correspond to different stages in the differentiation of the particular tissue in which they arise. For example, recent data have indicated that among neuroblastomas, those arising outside known sites of sympathetic ganglia are cholinergic[201] and those arising within the sympathetic ganglia are adrenergic.[202] Clearly these are tumors of cells committed to a neuronal lineage but at different stages in differentiation. Further, those that are cholinergic invariably carry a t(11;22) translocation, suggesting that these two different types of neuroblastoma may have different etiologies and require different therapeutic approaches. The finding that a t(2;13) chromosomal arrangement exists in some alveolar rhabdomyosarcomas but not in embryonal rhabdomyosar-

comas[41] suggests that such diversity may also be found among other embryonal tumors of solid tissues (also see Chap. 30). Whether a subclassification of solid tumors based on their corresponding to recognizable stages in the differentiation of the tissue in which they arise (similar to that currently used to describe lymphomas) will be possible is as yet unclear; however, it raises the possibility of new nosologies and perhaps novel approaches to therapy based on a diagnosis that is more specific and reflects more closely the etiologic mechanisms by which embryonal tumors may arise.

BIOCHEMICAL ISSUES

Expression of Malignancy

Historically, efforts to characterize the causes of altered cellular growth regulation and tissue-specific differentiation have sought to describe the biochemical differences between normal and malignant tissues or between immortalized and transformed tissue culture cells. A large number of parameters have been measured, and there are many reports of changes in both the cellular structure[203–205] and the metabolism[206–208] of malignant cells. Foremost among the structural changes are those that occur in the cytoskeleton. The cytoskeleton is a complex network of proteins that plays a key role in the maintenance of cell shape, cell mobility, and the intracellular organization of cytoplasmic organelles and cellular compartments. Microfilaments, also known as actin filaments, and microtubules are two prominent components of the cytoskeleton. In transformed cells the cytoskeleton is invariably disturbed, and the normal arrangement of actin filaments into cables that span the length of the cell is unrecognizable[209] (also see Chap. 6). This phenomenon may explain the altered shape of transformed cells and suggests that cellular functions in which the cytoskeleton takes part may be compromised in the transformed cell. In contrast to the paucity of information detailing the physiologic implications of these structural changes, a number of biochemical changes[206–208] have been recognized providing insight into the molecular mechanisms that may play important roles in tumorigenesis, whereas others have provided opportunities for novel approaches to the management of patients with cancer.

Among the biochemical changes that have been exploited clinically, those that are manifested as altered expression of cell surface markers have been the most important. Monoclonal antibody technology (see Chaps. 4 and 14) has provided the opportunity for investigators to develop antibody preparations directed against a single epitope, thereby increasing greatly the specificity of immunologic reagents to identify precisely defined subgroups of cells. Interestingly, while the search for cell surface markers that are specific for particular malignancies has been largely unsuccessful, the identification of oncofetal antigens (antigens expressed not only in malignancies but also during specific stages of normal differentiation) has been remarkably fruitful. This is best exemplified for lymphoid malignancies[210,211] (see Chap. 16) and selected non-lymphocytic leukemias[212] (see Chap. 17), where surface markers have made possible novel approaches to the identification and classification of these hematopoietic malignancies and have provided insight into the ontologic relationships among the various tumors arising in these tissues (also see Chap. 4). The success of immunologic assays for the characterization of solid tumors has been much more limited, and among pediatric tumors only neuroblastoma has been extensively studied.[213–215] Several monoclonal antibodies with varying degrees of specificity for neuroblastoma have been described, and a role for these in the differential diagnosis of the small blue round cell tumors of childhood has been proposed[216] (see Chaps. 6 and 28). The usefulness of cell surface markers for classifying solid tumors into clinically relevant subgroups, however, has not yet been demonstrated.

Studies are also being pursued that exploit the cell surface changes in tumor cells and explore the usefulness of monoclonal antibodies to target tumor cells for staging studies and therapeutic intervention. One important approach to targeting requires that a radionuclide be covalently bound to a tumor-specific monoclonal antibody without affecting its immunologic specificity. Different radionuclides are used in such studies, depending on whether the goal is to visualize or to treat the tumor (see Chaps. 4, 14). Other approaches to targeting therapy with monoclonal antibodies include the *in vivo* use of monoclonal antibodies bound to toxins or chemotherapeutic agents and the *in vitro* use of such antibodies for treatment and complement-dependent lysis of tumor cells that contaminate autologous bone marrow transplants (see Chap. 48).

Surface membrane changes in malignant cells have also been a focus of studies evaluating the biochemical pathways that mediate tumorigenesis.[217-219] The most revealing of these studies to date are those that have characterized the various mechanisms by which cells receive growth regulatory signals and communicate these signals to the cellular machinery necessary for the expression of malignancy. The preceding section described the role of growth factor receptors with intrinsic protein kinase activity in signal transduction. Receptors for other growth regulatory substances, including some hormones, are distinct from this type of transmembrane receptor in that the molecular activities, which initiate the cellular response culminating in altered growth, are not intrinsic to the receptor molecule.

Plasma membrane receptors that lack intrinsic protein kinase activity are now known to communicate with cytosolic enzyme systems through other proteins, of which the G-proteins are the best characterized.[220,221] G-proteins are a group of guanine-nucleotide-binding proteins with guanosinetriphosphatase (GTPase) activity. They are located on the cytoplasmic side of the plasma membrane, where they are activated in association with the formation of a ligand-surface receptor complex.[222,223] After activation of receptors associated with guanylnucleotide-binding proteins, a complex sequence of reactions is initiated that leads to the stimulation or inhibition of the catalytic activity of various cytoplasmic enzymes thought to take part in the development of malignancy (see below).[224,225] This role of G-proteins in mediating the communication between surface receptors and effector proteins has led to their being dubbed "second messengers." Although a precise role for G-proteins in the development of malignancy has been elusive, a group of oncogenes, the *ras* family, is known to share sequence similarities and functional activities with the G-proteins.[226] *Ras* family oncogenes are known as p21 proteins (because of their molecular size, 21 kD) (see Table 3-8).[227] Although most normal and abnormal cells produce a p21 *ras*-encoded protein, the activated oncogene in *ras*-transformed cells has a single amino acid change that distinguishes this protein from that encoded by the proto-oncogene in normal cells[105,228,229] (Fig. 3-11). Both the normal and the activated p21 *ras* proteins bind guanyl nucleotides; however, the GTPase activity of the oncogenic p21 protein is greatly reduced in comparison to the activity of the normal cellular protein.[230] Although it is not yet known whether the *ras* family proteins belong to a specific receptor pathway, activated *ras* genes very efficiently induce cell transformation *in vitro*[228] and are found to be activated in a broad spectrum of human tumors, including neuroblastoma and rhabdomyosarcoma (see Table 3-8).

One of the most important enzymes whose activity is mod-

ulated by G-proteins after cellular stimulation by various hormones is adenylate cyclase, the rate-limiting enzyme in the synthesis of cyclic adenosine monophosphate (cyclic AMP).[231] Cyclic AMP is itself a "second messenger" and thought to exert all of its effects (Table 3-16) by means of the phosphorylation of specific enzyme substrates. Of particular interest in this regard has been the observation that cyclic AMP metabolism, as measured by the steady-state levels of cyclic AMP and the activity of enzymes important in its synthesis and degradation, seems to be defective in many transformed cells.[232,233] Although it is not known whether such changes are of etiologic significance, modulation of the transformed properties of cell lines from different tumor types by treatment *in vitro* with cyclic AMP provides evidence of its importance in the expression of malignancy.[234,235]

Receptor-mediated transduction of signals from growth factors, hormones, and other biologically active substances is also known to be mediated by the hydrolysis of inositol phospholipids.[236-238] After the initiation of stimulated growth in many different cell types, including tumor cell lines, there is a rapid breakdown of cell membrane components into various phosphatidyl inositol derivatives of which 1,2-diacylglycerol is one of the best characterized[238] (Fig. 3-11). 1,2-Diacylglycerol synthesis is of considerable interest to oncologists because it dramatically increases the activity of protein kinase C,[239-242] an enzyme thought to be the primary target of tumor promotors such as phorbol esters when they complement the activity of tumor initiators in model systems of chemical carcinogenesis.[243-245] It appears that whether activated by a tumor promotor or endogenous lipids, protein kinase C can mediate the pleiotropic effects of membrane stimulation[246] on the post-translational phosphorylation of specific cellular proteins[239,240] (Table 3-17). Phorbol esters can also induce the differentiation *in vitro* of cell lines from such tumors as neuroblastoma, rhabdomyosarcoma, and promyelocytic leukemia.[247-249] If differentiation is physiologically mediated by protein kinase C, as experimental evidence would suggest, it is possible that this regulatory enzyme provides another molecular site at which the relationship between malignancy and altered differentiation might be sought.

The stimulation of surface receptors leading to inositol phospholipid breakdown also causes the mobilization of intracellular calcium ions.[250,251] In addition to enhancing the catalytic activity of protein kinase C itself, calcium ions are known to regulate the activity of cellular enzymes that play important roles in many different cellular functions, including proliferation.[252,253] In this regard, intracellular calcium ions are thought to play a synergistic role with protein kinase C in mediating the intracellular component of growth stimulatory signal transduction.[254,255] Since alterations in calcium ion metabolism are frequently found in malignant cells,[256-258] alterations in the avail-

---

Table 3-16

Selected Cellular Processes Mediated by cAMP

Cellular Process	Proposed Mechanisms
Cellular proliferation	Regulation of cells entering the cell cycle
In vitro differentiation	Altered gene expression
Hormonal stimulation	Second messenger function
Enzyme induction	Enhanced enzymatic activity
Cell motility and migration	Regulator of microfilament function
Membrane transport	Unknown

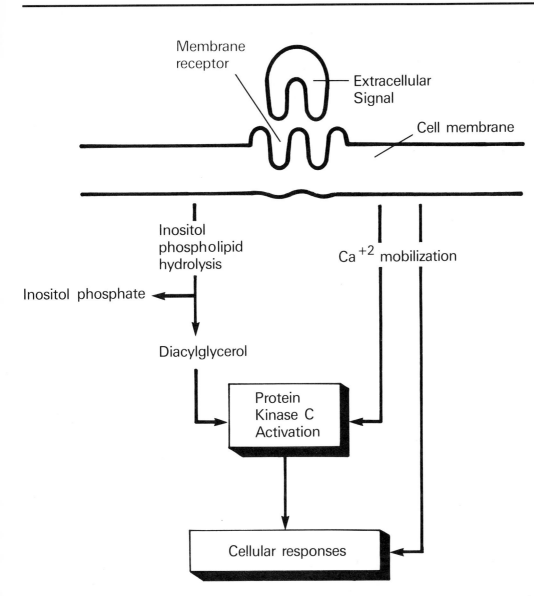

FIGURE 3-11. Signal transduction pathways. The cellular mechanisms by which extracellular signals effect altered cellular behavior are diverse. Important components of these pathways include the products of phospholipid hydrolysis and intracellular calcium. An important intermediary through which the effects of these agents might be mediated is protein kinase C, an enzyme that phosphorylates an increasing number of intracellular proteins that may play important regulatory or structural roles.

ability of intracellular calcium ions may be yet another mechanism by which the function of diverse metabolic pathways is altered in cancer cells.

Tumor Progression

A central feature of clinical and preclinical cancer research is recognition of the progressive changes in tumor growth and behavior that occur during the course of virtually all malignant illnesses that cannot be cured by currently available treatment. It often appears that a tumor becomes more aggressive, more malignant, during its course. This evolution of virulence is called tumor progression. While the morphologic and chemical changes that take place during tumor progression have been the most extensively studied aspect of tumor progression, it is the increased rate of tumor growth, the increased tissue invasiveness, and the development of metastases and drug resistance that are of profound significance in determining a patient's outcome.[259]

An appealing hypothesis to explain these changes characterizes malignancy as the final common phenotype that arises after a series of genetic alterations in a tumor cell during the course of its growth.[260] According to such a model, malignant cells undergo a number of random genetic changes, and, among the emerging, genetically distinguishable clones, those that acquire a growth advantage grow out. Even among tumors that arise from a single malignant cell, it is possible that the repetition of this selection process may be one source of the recognizable heterogeneity that characterizes most tumors. Such a model could explain tumor subpopulations that are inherently more metastatic or drug resistant than others.[261] Since most tumors in which genetic stability has been evaluated have been found to become more unstable over their course, it is possible that continued tumor growth is itself a key mechanistic element in tumor progression.[262]

Metastases and increased tissue invasiveness are among the most prominent clinical features marking recognizable tumor progression. Because early events leading to metastases must include the invasion of tumor cells into the circulatory system, the biologic mechanisms mediating invasiveness must also play a central role in metastases. The migration of cells in the body and the invasion of cells from one tissue into another during embryogenesis are among normal developmental processes. In matured tissues, however, cellular compartments are separated from one another by an extracellular matrix[263] across which cells can migrate only in a limited number of physiologic states (such as inflammation). Two important compo-

Table 3-17
Protein Kinase C Substrates of Oncologic Potential

Receptor proteins
  Epidermal growth factor receptor
  Insulin receptor
  Somatomedin C receptor
  Transferrin receptor
  Interleukin-2 receptor

Neurotransmitter receptors

Other membrane proteins
  Ca^{2+}-transport
  Na^+/K^+ ATPase
  Na^+ channel protein
  Glucose transporter
  GTP-binding protein
  HLA antigens

Cytoskeletal proteins
  Vinculin
  Filamin
  Caldesmon
  Microtubule-associated proteins

Other proteins
  Retinoid-binding proteins
  Vitamin D-binding protein
  Ribosomal S6 protein
  Stress proteins
  Middle T antigen
  pp60[src] protein

(Adapted from Nishizuka Y: Studies and perspectives of protein kinase C. Science 233:305–312, 1986)

nents of the extracellular matrix are the basement membrane, a continuous structure whose components are synthesized by most parenchymal cell types, and the interstitial stroma. The basement membrane is a complex structure consisting of various glycoproteins, such as laminin and type IV collagen.[264] Because the extracellular matrix provides a physical barrier for cellular movement from one tissue compartment to another, and because the cellular membrane adjacent to invasive tumors is often disrupted,[265,266] the ability of tumor cells to pass through basement membranes has been studied as a key element in the invasion process[267,268] (also see Chap. 6). In this regard, specific cell surface structures that recognize components of the extracellular matrix, such as laminin receptors,[269] have recently been recognized and may be important in mediating the attachment of tumor cells to the basement membrane at the initiation of the invasion process. Altered expression of the gene encoding the laminin receptor in various types of carcinomas has also been recognized, raising the possibility that the ability of tumor cells to recognize regulatory signals emerging from the extracellular matrix may also be compromised.[270]

After attachment to the basement membrane, tumor cells must find a way through this structure and the stromal elements of the interstitial space. Although cellular proliferation is not absolutely required for such invasion, proteolysis seems to play a key role.[271] Tumor cell proteases that can dissolve collagens and other structural components of the basement membrane have been identified, and the production of plasminogen-activator substances, which can lead to the generation of plasmin A and thereby the activation of latent proteases, has been extensively studied as an important characteristic of

the transformed phenotype of malignant cells in culture.[271] In some experimental systems, it has been shown that production of tumor cell proteolytic enzymes can be correlated with a tumor's metastatic potential.[272] Other studies have demonstrated that invasive tumor cells produce greater amounts of proteolytic enzymes than do other cells within the tumor.[273] Cells destined to become metastatic must also survive passage through the circulation, emerge in a new location, and initiate autonomous growth. Specific basement membrane receptors and recently identified tumor-produced motility factors[274,275] may be important for the movement of tumor cells both out of the circulation and into new tissue locations, providing further evidence that the invasion of normal tissues is not simply a result of forceful tumor growth.

The survival of cells at sites distant from the primary tumor is an early and key element in the establishment of metastatic disease. Establishment of a metastatic focus has also been recognized to be a function not only of the individual tumor cell but also of its new location.[261,276] To date, no biochemical explanation for the host contribution to organ-specific tumor metastases has emerged, although laboratory model systems have shown that the expression of undefined cell surface antigens on tumor cells correlates with organ-specific patterns of metastatic tumor cell growth.[277] The identification of such markers on metastatic populations of spontaneously arising human tumors might identify potential targets for therapeutic intervention directed at limiting metastatic spread while contributing to other studies aimed at identifying host factors important for the development of metastatic disease.

Because the pathologic events that accompany tumor progression are so complex, it is likely that a very broad spectrum of cellular and genetic alterations, many of which are not yet recognized, contribute to the enhancement of tumor virulence. For example, the role of such factors as blood supply in tumor progression is an area of investigation that may be of considerable clinical relevance.[278–280] Laboratory studies designed to characterize the development of new blood vessels during tumor growth have identified several tumor-produced factors that stimulate endothelial cell division[265] and vessel formation.[281,282] The recent isolation of the gene for one such protein, angiogenin,[283] suggests that it will soon be possible to investigate whether alterations in the regulation of such rarely evaluated features of tumors as their ability to induce a vascular supply are important determinants of clinical virulence and whether the inhibition of such tumor-specific features might have therapeutic potential (also see Chap. 14).

FUTURE CONSIDERATIONS

The recognition of specific genes involved in the malignant growth of tumor tissues has importance even beyond providing starting points for laboratory investigations focused on identifying the actual molecular and regulatory alterations of etiologic significance in cancer. More effective tumor nosologies based on genotype rather than histopathologic appearance might be expected to follow the molecular genetic characterization of tumors. Indeed, much of the heterogeneity that characterizes both the clinical behavior and the therapeutic responsiveness of most tumors may eventually be seen as reflecting the different genetic disorders among currently designated pathologic entities. Some oncogene products may be useful as tumor markers, and it is easy to imagine that beyond simply indicating the presence of tumors, such markers could reflect clinically important tumor characteristics such as virulence, invasiveness, metastatic potential, and therapeutic responsiveness. The analysis of oncogenes may also provide new opportunities for the study of cancer predisposition and thereby herald an era of more effective prenatal counseling and premorbid monitoring of high-risk groups. Preventive measures can be envisioned as a result of accurate and effective environmental screening based on the potential of agents to affect these critical genes. Even novel therapeutic approaches based on the modulation of gene expression to correct specific genetic defects are being considered.

Although the molecular changes leading to unregulated growth are still being defined, and although we are only beginning to investigate clinical features of cancer other than unregulated growth, an unprecedented degree of optimism and enthusiasm pervades cancer research. The cancer researcher currently has available a set of tools and a conceptual framework dramatically different from those available even 10 years ago. Investigators are now challenged to demonstrate how alterations in cell growth and differentiation contribute to the development of cancer and how correcting them might change the course of these life-threatening diseases. Pediatric malignancies have historically been particularly fruitful models for the study of both the basic cellular alterations that give rise to cancer and the therapeutic approaches aimed at curing it. The current era is no exception. It would be inaccurate to think that we understand the pathologic underpinnings of even one tumor type, but it would be equally inaccurate to ignore the surge of basic science that will be applicable to the management of cancer patients. There is no adult tumor for which the amount of relevant molecular pathologic information available rivals what we currently know about childhood leukemias, Burkitt's lymphoma, or neuroblastoma. These are diseases in which the diagnostic and therapeutic implications of current research advances will probably be best pursued, and their investigation should set the pace and the direction of research in other malignancies for exploring the clinical application of currently evolving scientific advances.

REFERENCES

1. Yunis JJ, Ramsay N: Retinoblastoma and subband deletion of chromosome 13. Am J Dis Child 132:161–163, 1978
2. Vogel F: Genetics of retinoblastoma. Hum Genet 52:1–54, 1979
3. Riccardi VM, Hittner HM, Francke U et al: The aniridia-Wilm's tumor association: The critical role of chromosome band 11p13. Cancer Genet Cytogenet 2:131–137, 1980
4. Koufos A, Hansen MF, Copeland NG, Jenkins NA, Lampkin BC, Cavenee WK: Loss of heterogeneity in three embryonal tumors suggests a common pathogenic mechanism. Nature 316:330–334, 1985
5. Casperson T, Zech L, Johansson C, Modest EJ: Identification of human chromosomes by DNA-binding fluorescent agents. Chromosoma 30:215–227, 1970
6. Yunis JJ: Human chromosome methodology. New York, Academic Press, 1974
7. Yunis JJ: High resolution of human chromosomes. Science 191:1268–1270, 1976
8. Croce CM: Chromosome translocations and human cancer. Cancer Res 46:6019–6023, 1986
9. Sandberg AA, Gemmill RM, Hecht BK, Hecht F: The Philadelphia chromosome: A model of cancer and molecular cytogenetics. Cancer Genet Cytogenet 21:129–146, 1986
10. ISCN: An international system for human cytogenetic nomenclature—high resolution banding. Cytogenet Cell Genet 31:1–23, 1981
11. Williams DL, Look AT, Melvin SL, Robertson PK, Dahl G, Flake T, Stass S: New chromosomal translocations correlate with specific immunophenotypes of childhood acute lymphoblastic leukemia. Cell 36:101–109, 1984
12. Rowley JD: Principles of cancer biology: Chromosomal abnormalities. In DeVita VT Jr, Hellman S, Rosenberg SA (eds): Cancer: Principles and Practice of Oncology, pp 67–78. Philadelphia, JB Lippincott, 1982
13. Crist WC, Cleary ML, Grossi CE, Prasthofer EF, Heggie GD, Omura GA, Carroll AJ, Link MP, Slar J: Acute leukemias associated with the 4;11 chromosome translocation have rearranged immunoglobulin heavy chain genes. Blood 66:33–38, 1985
14. Erikson J, Williams DL, Finan J et al: Locus of the alpha-chain of the T-cell receptor is split by chromosome translocation in VT-cell leukemias. Science 229:784–786, 1985
15. Rowley JD: Identification of a translocation with quinacrine fluorescence in a patient with acute leukemia. Ann Genet 16:109–112, 1973
16. Kaneko Y, Sakurai M: 15/17 translocation in acute promyelocytic leukemia. Lancet 1:961, 1977
17. Rowley JD, Golomb HM, Vardman JW, Fukuhara S, Dougherty C, Potter D: Further evidence for non-random chromosomal abnormality in acute promyelocytic leukemia. Int J Cancer 20:869–872, 1977
18. Berger R, Berheim A, Weh JH, Daniel MT, Flandrin G: Cytogenetic studies on acute monocytic leukemia. Leuk Res 4:119–127, 1980
19. Hagemeijer A, Hahlen K, Sizoo W, Abels J: Translocation (9;11)(p21;q23) in three cases of acute monoblastic leukemia. Cancer Genet Cytogenet 5:95–105, 1982
20. Kaneko Y, Rowley JD, Maurer HS, Variakojis D, Moohr JW: Chromosome pattern in childhood acute nonlymphocytic leukemia. Blood 60:389–399, 1982
21. Pearson MG, Vardiman JW, LeBeau MM, Rowley JD, Cohen MM, Prigogina EL: A new cytogenetic subset of acute nonlymphocytic leukemia: t(6;9) associated with bone marrow basophilia (abstr). Blood 62(suppl 1):180a, 1983
22. LeBeau MM, Larson RA, Bitter MA, Vardiman JW, Golomb HM, Rowley JD: Association of an inversion of chromosome 16 with abnormal marrow eosinophils in acute myelomonocytic leukemia: A unique cytogenetic-clinicopathological association. N Engl J Med 309:630–636, 1983
23. Arthur DC, Bloomfield CD: Partial deletion of the long arm of chromosome 16 and bone marrow eosinophilia in acute nonlymphocytic leukemia: A new association. Blood 61:994–998, 1983
24. DelaChapelle A, Lantinen R: Chromosome 16 and bone-marrow eosinophilia. N Engl J Med 309:1394, 1983
25. Nowell PC, Hungerford DA: A minute chromosome in human granulocytic leukemia. Science 132:1497, 1960
26. Rowley JD: A new consistent chromosomal abnormality in chronic myelogenous leukemia. Nature 243:290–293, 1973
27. Zech L, Haglund U, Nilsson K et al: Characteristic chromosomal abnormalities in biopsies and lymphoid-cell lines from patients with Burkitt and non-Burkitt lymphomas. Int J Cancer 17:47–56, 1976
28. Manolov G, Manolova Y: Marker band in one chromosome 14 from Burkitt lymphomas. Nature 237:33–34, 1972
29. Kaiser-McCaw B, Hecht F, Hamden DG, Teplitz L: Somatic rearrangement of chromosome 14 in human lymphocytes. Proc Natl Acad Sci USA 72:2071–2075, 1975
30. Atkin NB, Baker MC: Specific chromosomal change, i(12p), in testicular tumours? Lancet 2:1349, 1982
31. Atkin NB, Baker MC: Specific chromosomal marker in seminoma and malignant teratoma of the testis? Cancer Genet Cytogenet 10:199–204, 1983
32. Gibas Z, Prout GR, Pontes JE, Sandberg AA: Chromosome changes in germ cell tumors of the testis. Cancer Genet Cytogenet 19:245–252, 1986
33. Sparkes RS, Sparkes MC, Wilson MG et al: Regional assignment of genes for human esterase D and retinoblastoma to chromosome 13q14. Science 208:1042–1044, 1980
34. Sparkes RS, Murphree AL, Lingua RW et al: Gene for hereditary retinoblastoma assigned to human chromosome 13 by linkage to esterase D. Science 219:971–973, 1983
35. Dryja TP, Rapaport JM, Epstein J, Goorin AM, Weichselbaum R, Koufos A, Caveñee WK: Chromosome 13 homozygosity in osteosarcoma without retinoblastoma. Am J Hum Genet 38:59–66, 1986
36. Riccardi VM, Sujansky E, Smith AC, Francke U: Chromosomal imbalance in the aniridia-Wilms tumor association: 11 p interstitial deletion. Pediatrics 61:604, 1978
37. Francke U, Holmes LB, Atkins L et al: Aniridia-Wilm's tumor association: Evidence for specific deletion of 11p13. Cytogenet Cell Genet 24:185–192, 1979
38. Biedler JL, Spengler BA: A novel chromosome abnormality in human neuroblastoma and antifolate resistant Chinese hamster cell lines in culture. J Natl Cancer Inst 57:683–695, 1976
39. Brodeur GM, Green AA, Hayes FA: Cytogenetic Studies of Primary Human Neuroblastomas. In Evans AE (eds): Advances in Neuroblastoma Research, p 344. New York, Raven Press, 1980
40. Whang-Peng J, Triche TJ, Knutsen T, Miser J, Kao-Shan S, Tsai S, Israel M: Cytogenetic characterization of selected small round cell tumors of childhood. Cancer Genet Cytogenet 21:185–208, 1986
41. Turc-Carel C, Lizard-Nacol S, Justrabo E, Favrot M, Philip T, Tabone E:

Consistent chromosomal translocation in alveolar rhabdomyosarcoma. Cancer Genet Cytogenet 19:361–362, 1986

42. Aurias A, Rimbaut C, Buffe D, Zucker JM, Mazabraud A: Translocation of band q12 of chromosome 22 in Ewing's sarcoma: A cytogenetic study of four fresh tumors. Cancer Genet Cytogenet 12:21–25, 1984

43. Turc–Carel C, Philip I, Berger MP, Philip T, Lenoir GM: Chromosome study of Ewing's sarcoma (ES) cell lines: Consistency of a reciprocal translocation t(11;22)(q24;q12). Cancer Genet Cytogenet 12:1–19, 1984

44. Aurias A, Rimbaut C, Buffee D, Zucker JM, Mazabraud A: Translocation involving chromosome 22 in Ewing's sarcoma. Cancer Genet Cytogenet 12:21–25, 1984

45. Whang–Peng J, Triche TJ, Knutsen T, Miser J, Douglass EC, Israel MA: Chromosome translocation in peripheral neuroepithelioma. N Engl J Med 311:584–585, 1984

46. Turc–Carel C, Cin PDal, Limon J, Li F, Sandberg AA: Translocation X:18 in synovial sarcoma. Cancer Genet Cytogenet 23:93, 1986

47. Yunis JJ, Bloomfield CD, Ensrud K: All patients with acute non-lymphocytic leukemia may have a chromosomal defect. N Engl J Med 305:135–319, 1981

48. Yunis JJ: The chromosomal basis of human neoplasia. Science 221:227–236, 1983

49. Yunis JJ: Chromosome rearrangements, genes, fragile sites in cancer: Clinical and biologic implications. In DeVita VT Jr, Hellman S, Rosenberg SA (eds): Important Advances in Oncology, pp 93–128. Philadelphia, JB Lippincott, 1986

50. Hansen MF, Koufos A, Gallie BL, Phillips RA, Fodstad O, Brgger A, Gedde–Dahl T, Cavanee WK: Osteosarcoma and retinoblastoma: A shared chromosomal mechanism revealing recessive predisposition. Proc Natl Acad Sci USA 82:6216–6220, 1985

51. Griffin CA, McKeon C, Israel MA, Gegonne A, Ghysdael J, Stehelin D, Douglass EC et al: Comparison of constitutional and tumor-associated 11;22 translocations: Nonidentical breakpoints on chromosomes 11 and 22. Proc Natl Acad Sci USA 83:6122–6126, 1985

52. Lipinski M, Braham K, Philip I, Wiels J, Philip T, Goridis C, Lenoir GM, Tursz T: Neuroectoderm-associated antigens on Ewing's sarcoma cell lines. Cancer Res 47:183–187, 1987

53. Yunis JJ: Chromosomes and cancer: New nomenclature and future directions. Hum Pathol 12:494–503, 1981

54. Kirsch IR, Brown JA, Lawrence J, Korsmeyer SJ, Morton CC: Translocations that highlight chromosomal regions of differentiated activity. Cancer Genet Cytogenet 18:159–171, 1985

55. Klein G: Specific chromosomal translocations and the genesis of B-cell derived tumors in mice and men. Cell 32:311–315, 1983

56. Leder P, Battey J, Lenoir G, Moulding C, Murphy W, Potter H, Stewart T, Taub R: Translocations among antibody genes in human cancer. Science 222:765–771, 1983

57. Croce CM: Chromosomal translocations, oncogenes, and B-cell tumors. Hosp Pract 41–48, 1985

58. Williams DL, Look AT, Melvin SL et al: New chromosomal translocations correlate with specific immunophenotypes of childhood acute lymphoblastic leukemia. Cell 36:101–109, 1984

59. Shima EA, LeBeau MM, McKeithan TW et al: Gene encoding the alpha-chain of the T-cell receptor is moved immediately downstream of c-myc in chromosomal 8;14 translocation in a cell line from a human T-cell leukemia. Proc Natl Acad Sci USA 83:3439–3443, 1986

60. Adesnik M, Darnell JE: Biogenesis and characterization of histone messenger RNA in HeLa cells. J Mol Biol 67:397–406, 1972

61. Kaneka Y, Rowley JD, Variakojis D, Chilcote RR, Check I, Sakurai M: Correlation of karyotype with clinical features in acute lymphoblastic leukemia. Cancer Res 42:2918–2929, 1982

62. Rowley JD: Identification of the chromosome region involved in human hematologic malignant disease. Science 216:749–751, 1982

63. Yunis JJ: Chromosome rearrangements, genes, fragile sites in cancer: Clinical and biologic implications. In DeVita VT Jr, Hellman S, Rosenberg SA (eds): Important Advances in Oncology, pp 93–128. Philadelphia, JB Lippincott, 1986

64. Heim S, Mitelman F: Nineteen of 26 cellular oncogenes precisely localized in the human genome map to one of the 83 bands involved in primary cancer-specific rearrangements. Hum Genet 75(1):70–72, 1987

65. Watson JD, Crick FHC: Molecular structure of nucleic acid: A structure for deoxyribose nucleic acid. Nature 171:737–738, 1953

66. Watson JD: Molecular Biology of the Gene, 3rd ed. Menlo Park, Benjamin/Cummings, 1976

67. Maniatas T, Fritsch EF, Sambrook J: Molecular Cloning: A Laboratory Manual. Cold Spring Harbor, Cold Spring Harbor Laboratory, 1982

68. Bonner TI, Brenner DJ, Beufeld BR et al: Reduction in the rate of DNA reassociation by sequence divergence. J Mol Biol 81:123–135, 1973

69. Casey J, Davidson N: Rates of formation and thermal stabilities of RNA:DNA and DNA:DNA duplexes at high concentrations of formamide. Nucl Acids Res 4:1539–1552, 1977

70. Hutton JR: Renaturation kinetics and thermal stability of DNA in aqueous solutions of formamide and urea. Nucl Acids Res 4:3537–3555, 1977

71. Smith HO, Wilcox KW: A restriction enzyme from Hemophilus influenzae: II. Base sequence of the recognition site. J Mol Biol 51:393–409, 1970

72. Roberts R: Restriction and modification enzymes and their recognition sequences. Nucl Acid Res 10:117–144, 1982

73. Southern EM: Detection of specific sequences among DNA fragments separated by gel electrophoresis. J Mol Biol 98:503–517, 1975

74. Leder P, Battey J, Lenoir G, Moulding C, Murphy W, Potter H, Stewart T, Taub R: Translocations among antibody genes in human cancer. Science 222:765–771, 1983

75. Seidman JG, Leder P: The arrangement and rearrangement of antibody genes. Nature (Lond) 276:790–795, 1978

76. Magrath IT: Lymphocyte differentiation: An essential basis for the comprehension of lymphoid neoplasia. JNCI 67:501–514, 1981

77. Korsmeyer SJ, Arnold A, Bakhshi A et al: Immunoglobulin gene rearrangements and cell surface antigen expression in acute lymphocytic leukemias of T cell and B cell precursor origins. J Clin Invest 71:301, 1983

78. Korsmeyer SJ, Hieter PA, Ravetch JV et al: Developmental hierarchy of immunoglobulin gene rearrangements in human leukemic pre-B cells. Proc Natl Acad Sci USA 78:7096, 1981

79. Alwine JC, Kemp DJ, Stark GR: Method for detection of specific RNAs in agarose gels by transfer to diazobenzyloxy-methyl-paper and hybridization with DNA probes. Proc Natl Acad Sci USA 74:5350–5354, 1977

80. Solomon E, Goodfellow P: Human gene mapping rolls along. Nature 306:223–224, 1983

81. Harper ME, Saunders GF: Localization of single copy DNA sequences of G-banded human chromosomes by in situ hybridization. Proc Natl Acad Sci USA 78:4458–4460, 1981

82. Bishop JM: Viral oncogenes. Cell 42:23–38, 1985

83. Bishop JM: The molecular genetics of cancer. Science 235:305–311, 1987

84. Watson JD, Tooze J: The DNA Story. San Francisco, WH Freeman and Company, 1981

85. Tooze J: The Molecular Biology of Tumor Viruses. Cold Spring Harbor, Cold Spring Harbor Laboratory, 1980

86. Stehelin D, Varmus HE, Bishop JM, Vogt PK: DNA related to the transforming gene(s) of avian sarcoma viruses is present in normal avian DNA. Nature 260:170–173, 1976

87. Shih C, Shilo BZ, Goldfarb MP et al: Passage of phenotypes of chemically transformed cells via transfection of DNA and chromatin. Proc Natl Acad Sci USA 76:5714–5718, 1979

88. Cooper GM, Okenquist S, Silverman L: Transforming activity of DNA of chemically transformed and normal cells. Nature 284:418–421, 1980

89. Murray MJ, Shilo BZ, Shih C et al: Three different human tumor cell lines contain different oncogenes. Cell 25:355–361, 1981

90. Blair DG, Cooper CS, Oskarsson ME et al: New method for detecting cellular transforming genes. Science 218:1122–1125, 1982

91. Robbins KC, Antoniades HN, Devare SG et al: Structural and immunological similarities between simian sarcoma virus gene product(s) and human platelet-derived growth factor. Nature 305:605–608, 1983

92. Downward J, Yarden Y, Mayes E et al: Close similarity of epidermal growth factor receptor and v-erb-B oncogene protein sequences. Nature 307:521–527, 1984

93. Waterfield MD, Scrace GT, Wittle N et al: Platelet-derived growth factor is structurally related to the putative transforming protein p28sis of simian sarcoma virus. Nature 304:35–39, 1983

94. îand H, Parada LF, Weinburg RA: Tumorigenic conversion of primary embryo fibroblasts requires at least two cooperating oncogenes. Nature 304:596–601, 1983

95. Doolittle RF, Hunkapiller MW, Hood LE, Devare SG, Robbins KC, Aaronson SA, Antoniades HN: Simian sarcoma virus onc gene, v-sis is derived from the gene (or genes) encoding a platelet derived growth factor. Science 221:275–277, 1983

96. Macara IG: Oncogenes, ions, and phospholipids. Am J Hum Genet 248:3–11, 1985

97. Dalla–Favera R, Bregni M, Erikson J, Patterson D, Gallo R, Croce CM:

Human c-myc onc gene is located on region of chromosome 8 that is translocated in Burkitt lymphoma cells. Proc Natl Acad Sci USA 79:7824–7827, 1982

98. de Klein A, van Kessel AG, Grosveld G, Bartram CR, Hagemeijev A, Bootsma D, Spurr NK et al: A cellular oncogene is translocated to the Philadelphia chromosome in chronic myelocytic leukemia. Nature 300:765–767, 1982

99. Shtivelman E, Lifshitz B, Gale RP et al: Alternative splicing of RNAs transcribed from the human abl gene and from the bcr-abl fused gene. Cell 47:277–284, 1986

100. Shtivelman E, Lifshitz B, Gale RP, Canaani E: Fused transcript of abl and bcr genes in chronic myelogenous leukemia. Nature 315:550–554, 1985

101. Groffen J, Stephenson JR, Heisterkamp N et al: Philadelphia chromosomal breakpoints are clustered within a limited region, bcr, on chromosome 22. Cell 36:93–99, 1984

102. Schwab M, Alitalo K, Klempnauer K et al: Amplified DNA with limited homology to myc cellular oncogene is shared by human neuroblastoma cell lines and a neuroblastoma tumour. Nature 305:245–248, 1983

103. Michitsch RW, Montgomery KT, Melera PW: Expression of the amplified domain in human neuroblastoma cells. Mol Cell Biol 4:2370–2380, 1984

104. Kohl NE, Gee CE, Alt FW: Activated expression of the N-myc gene in human neuroblastomas and related tumors. Science 226:1335–1337, 1984

105. Tsujimoto Y, Yunis J, Onorato–Showe L, Erikson J, Nowell PC, Croce CM: Molecular cloning of the chromosomal breakpoint of B-cell lymphomas and leukemias with the T(11;14) chromosome translocation. Science 224:1403–1406, 1984

106. Bishop JM: Cellular oncogenes and retroviruses. Annu Rev Biochem 52:301–354, 1983

107. Knudson AG: Mutation and Cancer: Statistical study of retinoblastoma. Proc Natl Acad Sci, USA 68:820–823, 1971

108. Cavenee WK, Dryja TP, Phillips RA et al: Expression of recessive alleles by chromosomal mechanisms in retinoblastoma. Nature 305:779–784, 1983

109. Murphree AL, Benedict WF: Retinoblastoma: Clues to human oncogenesis. Science 223:1028–1033, 1984

110. Cross HE, Hansen RE, Morrow G, Davis JR: Retinoblastoma in a patient with a 13qXp translocation. Am J Hum Genet 84:548–554, 1977

111. Riccardi VM, Hittner HM, Francke U et al: Partial triplication and deletion of 13q: Study of a family presenting with bilateral retinoblastomas. Clin Genet 15:332–345, 1979

112. Knudson AG: Hereditary cancers in man. Cancer Invest 1:187–193, 1983

113. Friend SH, Bernards R, Rogel S, Weinberg RA, Rapaport JN, Albert DM, Dryja TP: A human DNA segment with properties of the gene that predisposes to retinoblastoma and osteosarcoma. Nature 323:643–646, 1986

114. Seizinger BR, Martuza RL, Gusella JF: Loss of genes in tumorigenesis of human acoustic neuroma. Nature 322:644–667, 1986

115. Mark J, Mitelman F, Levan G: On the specificity of the G abnormality in human meningiomas studied by the fluorescence technique. Acta Pathol Microbiol Scand [A] 80:812–820, 1972

116. Bishop DT, Williamson JA, Skolnick MH: A model for restriction fragment length distributions. Am J Hum Genet 35:795, 1983

117. Cavenee W, Leach R, Mohandas T, Pearson P, White R: Isolation and regional localization of DNA segments revealing polymorphic loci from human chromosome 13. Am J Hum Genet 36:10–24, 1984

118. Orkin SA: Reverse genetics and human disease. Cell 47:845–850, 1986

119. Cavenee WK, Murphree AL, Shull MM, Benedict WF, Sparkes RS, Kock E, Nordenskjold M: Prediction of familial predisposition to retinoblastoma. N Engl J Med 314:1201–1207, 1986

120. Foulds L: Neoplastic Development. New York, Academic Press, 1969

121. Collins VP, Loeffler RK, Twey H: Observation on growth rates of human tumours. Am J Roentgenol 76:988–1000, 1956

122. Steel GG: Growth kinetics of tumours. Oxford, Clarendon Press, 1977

123. Malaise F, Chavaudra N, Tubiana M: The relationship between growth rate, labelling index and histological type of tumours. Eur J Cancer 9:305–312, 1973

124. Tubiana M, Malaise EP: Growth rate and cell kinetics in human tumours: Some prognostic and therapeutic implications. In Symington T, Carter RL (eds): Scientific Foundations of Oncology, pp 126–136. Chicago, Year Book Medical Publishers, 1976

125. Charbit A, Malaise E, Tubiana M: Relation between the pathological nature and the growth rate of human tumours. Eur J Cancer 7:307–315, 1971

126. Howard P, Pelc SR: Nuclear incorporation of 32P as demonstrated by autoradiographs. Exp Cell Res 2:178–187, 1951

127. Heim S, Mitelman F: Numerical chromosome aberrations in human neoplasia. Cancer Genet Cytogenet 22(2):99–108, 1986

128. Baserga R: The relationship of the cell cycle to tumor growth and control of cell division. Cancer Res 25:581–595, 1965

129. Pardee AB: A restriction point for control of normal animal cell proliferation. Proc Natl Acad Sci USA 71:1286–1290, 1974

130. Brooks RF, Bennett DC, Smith JA: Mammalian cell cycles need two random transitions. Cell 19:493–504, 1980

131. Baserga R: Multiplication and Division in Mammalian Cells. New York, Marcel Dekker, 1976

132. Pardee AB: Molecules involved in proliferation of normal and cancer cells: Presidential address. Cancer Res 47:1488–1491, 1987

133. DeVita VT: Cell kinetics and the chemotherapy of cancer. Cancer Treat Rep 2:23–33, 1971

134. Schackney SE, McCormack GW, Cuchural GH Jr: Growth rate patterns of solid tumors and their relation to responsiveness to therapy: An analytical review. Ann Intern Med 89:107–121, 1978

135. Steel GG, Lamerton LF: Cell population kinetics and chemotherapy. Natl Cancer Inst Monogr 30:29–50, 1968

136. DeVita VT: Cell kinetics and the chemotherapy of cancer. Cancer Treat Rep 2:23–33, 1971

137. Skipper HE, Simpson–Herren L: Relationship between tumor stem cell heterogeneity and responsiveness to chemotherapy. In DeVita VT Jr, Hellman S, Rosenberg SA (eds): Important advances in Oncology, pp 63–77. Philadelphia, JB Lippincott, 1985

138. Mendelsohn ML: The growth fraction: A new concept applied to tumors. Science 132:1496, 1960

139. Gray JW, Carva JH, George YS et al: Rapid cell cycle analysis by measurement of the radioactivity per cell in a marrow window in 5 phases (RCSi). Cell Tissue Kinet 10:97–104, 1977

140. Mackillop WJ, Buick RN: Cellular heterogeneity in human ovarian carcinoma studies by density gradient fractionation. Stem Cells 1:355–366, 1981

141. Potten CS, Schofield R, Lajtha LG: A comparison of cell replacement in bone marrow, testis and three regions of surface epithelium. Biochim Biophys Acta 560:281–299, 1979

142. Becker FF: The normal hepatocyte in division: Regeneration of the mammalian liver. Prog Liver Dis 3:60–76, 1970

143. Giard DJ, Aaronson SA, Todaro GJ et al: In vitro cultivation of human tumors: Establishment of cell lines derived from a series of solid tumor. J Natl Cancer Inst 51:1417–1423, 1973

144. Clarkson B, Baserga R: Control of Proliferation in Animal Cells. Cold Spring Harbor, Cold Spring Harbor Laboratory, 1976

145. Jakoby WB, Pastan IH: Methods in Enzymology: Cell Culture. New York, Academic Press, 1979

146. Gerber P, Whang–Peng J, Monroe JH: Transformation and chromosome changes induced by Epstein–Barr virus in normal human leukocyte cultures. Proc Natl Acad Sci USA 63:740–747, 1969

147. Rassoulzadegan M, Naghashfar Z, Cowie A, Carr A, Grisoni M, Kamen R, Cuzin F: Expression of the large t protein of polyoma virus promotes the establishment in culture of "normal" rodent fibroblast cell lines. Proc Natl Acad Sci USA 80:4354–4358, 1983

148. Steinberg ML, Defendi V: Transformation and immortalization of human keratinocytes by SV40. J Invest Dermatol 81:131s–136s, 1983

149. Tadaro GJ, Green H: Quantitative studies of the growth of mouse embryo cells in culture and their development into established cell lines. J Cell Biol 17:299–313, 1963

150. Abercrombie M: Contact inhibition and malignancy. Nature 281:259–262, 1979

151. Smets LA: Cell transformation as a model for tumor induction and neoplastic growth. Biochim Biophys Acta 605:93–111, 1980

152. Barrett JC, Crawford BD, Mixter LO, Schechtman LM, Ts'o PO, Pollack R: Correlation of in vitro growth properties and tumorigenicity of syrian hamster cell lines. Cancer Res 39:1504–1510, 1979

153. Smith IE, Courtenay VD, Gordon MY: A colony-forming assay for human tumour xenografts using agar in diffusion chambers. Br J Cancer 34:476–483, 1976

154. Salmon SE, Hamburger AW, Soehnein B, Durie BGM, Alberts DS, Moon TE: Quantitation of differentiation sensitivity of human tumor stem cells to anticancer drugs. N Engl J Med 298:1321–1327, 1978

155. VonHoff DD, Casper J, Bradley E, Jones D, Makuch R: Association between human tumor colony forming assay results and response of an individual patient's tumor to chemotherapy. Am J Med 70:1027–1032, 1981

156. VonHoff DD, Clark GM, Stogdill BJ, Sarosdy MF, O'Brien MT, Casper JT,

Mattox DE et al: Prospective clinical trial of a human tumor cloning system. Cancer Res 43:1926–1931, 1983

157. Watt FM, Green H: Stratification and terminal differentiation of cultured epidermal cells. Nature 295:434–436, 1982

158. Sporn MB, Todaro GJ: Autocrine secretion and malignant transformation of cells. N Engl J Med 303:878–880, 1980

159. James R, Bradshaw RA: Polypeptide growth factors. Annu Rev Biochem 53:259–292, 1984

160. Goustin AS, Leof EB, Shipley GD, Moses HL: Growth factors and cancer. Cancer Res 46:1015, 1986

161. Schultz GS, White M, Mitchell R, Brown G, Lynch J, Twardzik DR, Todaro GJ: Epithelial wound healing enhanced by transforming growth factor-alpha and vaccinia growth factor. Science 235:350–352, 1987

162. Canalis E: Effect of growth factors on bone cell replication and differentiation. Clin Orthop 193:246–263, 1985

163. Leof EB, Wharton W, Wyk JJVan, Piedger WJ: Epidermal growth factor (EGF) and somatomedin C regulate GI progression in competent BALB/c-3T3 cells. Exp Cell Res 141:107–115, 1982

164. Huang JS, Huang SS, Deuel TF: Transforming protein of simian sarcoma virus stimulates autocrine growth of ssv-transformed cells through PDGF cell-surface receptors. Cell 39:79–87, 1984

165. Leal F, Williams LT, Robbins KC, Aaronson SA: Evidence that the v-sis gene product transforms by interaction with the receptor for platelet-derived growth factor. Science 230:327–330, 1985

166. Chinkers MJ, McKanna JA, Cohen S: Rapid induction of morphological changes in human carcinoma cell line A-431 by epidermal growth factor. J Cell Biol 83:260–265, 1979

167. Pastan I, Willingham MC: Journey to the center of the cell: Role of the receptosome. Science 214:504–509, 1981

168. Herman B, Pledger WJ: Platelet-derived growth factor-induced alterations in vinculin and actin distribution in BALB/C-3T3 cells. J Cell Biol 100:1031–1040, 1985

169. Carpenter G, King L, Cohen S: Epidermal growth factor stimulates phosphorylation in membrane preparations in vitro. Nature 276:409–410, 1978

170. Stoscheck CM, King LE Jr: Role of epidermal growth factor in carcinogenesis. Cancer Res 46:1030–1037, 1986

171. Conen S, Ushiro H, Stoscheck C, Chinkers M: A native 170,000 epidermal growth factor receptor-kinase complex from shed membrane vesicles. J Biol Chem 257:1523–1531, 1982

172. Ullrich A, Coussens L, Hayflick JS, Dull TJ, Gray A, Tam A, Lee J et al: Human epidermal growth factor receptor cDNA sequence and aberrant expression on amplified gene in A431 epidermoid carcinoma cells. Nature 309:418–425, 1984

173. Hunter T, Cooper JA: Protein-tyrosine kinases. Annu Rev Biochem 54:897–930, 1985

174. Ushiro H, Cohen SJ: Identification of phosphotyrosine as a product of epidermal growth factor-activated protein kinase in A431 cell membranes. J Biol Chem 255:8363–8365, 1980

175. Sefton BM, Hunter T, Beemon K, Eckhart W: Evidence that phosphorylation of tyrosine is essential for transformation by Rous sarcoma virus. Cell 20:807–816, 1980

176. Macara IG: Oncogenes, ions, and phospholipids. Am J Hum Genet 248:3–11, 1985

177. Ross R, Bowen-Pope DF, Raines EW: Platelet derived growth factor: Its potential roles in wound healing, atherosclerosis, neoplasia, and growth and development. Ciba Found Symp 116:98–112, 1985

178. Gol-Winkler R: Paracrine action of transforming growth factors. Clin Endocrinol Metab 15:99–115, 1986

179. Temim HM: Studies on carcinogenesis by avian sarcoma viruses: VI. The differential effect of serum and polyanions on multiplication of uninfected and converted cells. J Natl Cancer Inst 37:167–175, 1966

180. Kaplan PL, Anderson M, Ozanne B: Transforming growth factor production enables cells to grow in the absence of serum: An autocrine system. Proc Natl Acad Sci USA 79:485–489, 1982

181. Dulbecco R: Topoinhibition and serum requirement of transformed and untransformed cells. Nature 227:802, 1970

182. Paul D, Lipton A, Klinger I: Serum factor requirements of normal and simian virus-40-transformed 3T3 mouse fibroblasts. Proc Natl Acad Sci USA 68:645–648, 1971

183. Holley RW, Kiernan JA: Control of the initiation of DNA synthesis in 3T3 cells: Serum factors. Proc Natl Acad Sci USA 71:2908–2911, 1974

184. Lang RA, Metcalf D, Gough NM, Dunn AR, Gonda TJ: Expression of a hemopoietic growth factor cDNA in a factor-dependent cell line results in autonomous growth and tumorigenicity. Cell 43:531–542, 1985

185. Graves DT, Owen AJ, Barth RK, Tempst P, Winoto A, Fors L, Hood LE: Detection of c-sis transcripts and synthesis of PDGF-like proteins by human osteosarcoma cells. Science 226:972–974, 1984

186. Betsholtz C, Westermark B, Ek B, Heldin CH: Co-expression of a PDGF-like growth factor and PDGF receptors in a human osteosarcoma cell line: Implications for autocrine receptor activation. Cell 39:447–457, 1984

187. Pierce GB, Shikes R, Fink LM: Cancer: A problem of developmental biology. Englewood Cliffs, NJ, Prentice-Hall, 1978

188. Mintz B, Fleischman RA: Teratocarcinomas and other neoplasms as developmental defects in gene expression. Adv Cancer Res 34:211–278, 1981

189. Miner KM, Kawaguihi T, Uba GW, Nicholson GL: Clonal drift of cell surface, melanogenic and experimental metastatic properties of in vivo selected, brain meninges-colonizing murine B16 melanoma. Cancer Res 42:4631–4638, 1982

190. Barrett JC, Ts'o PO: Evidence for the progressive nature of neoplastic transformation in vitro. Proc Natl Acad Sci USA 75:3761–3765, 1978

191. Dyke PC, Mulkey DA: Maturation of ganglioneuroblastoma to ganglioneuroma. Cancer 20:1343–1349, 1967

192. Bale PM, Parsons RE, Stevens MM: Pathology and behavior of juvenile rhabdomyosarcoma. In Finegold M, Bennington JL (eds): Pathology of Neoplasia in Children and Adolescents, pp 196–222. Philadelphia, WB Saunders, 1986

193. Greaves MF: Maturation and differentiation in leukemias. Cancer Surv 1:189–342, 1982

194. McCulloch EA: Stem cells in normal and leukemic hemopoiesis. Blood 62:1–13, 1983

195. Sachs L: Constitutive uncoupling of pathways of gene expression that control growth and differentiation in myeloid leukemia: A model for the origin and progression of malignancy. Proc Natl Acad Sci USA 77:6152–6156, 1980

196. Pierce GB, Dixon FJ: Testicular teratomas: I. The demonstration of teratogenesis by metamorphosis of multipotential cells. Cancer 12:573–583, 1959

197. Pierce GB, Dixon FJ, Verney EL: Teratocarcinogenic and tissue forming potentials of the cell types comprising neoplastic embryoid bodies. Lab Invest 9:583–602, 1960

198. Pierce GB: The cancer cell and its control by the embryo. Rous-Whipple award lecture. Am J Pathol 113:117–124, 1983

199. Sachs L: Control of normal cell differentiation and the phenotypic reversion of malignancy in myeloid leukemia. Nature 274:535–539, 1978

200. Fiszman MY, Fuchs P: Temperature-sensitive expression of differentiation in transformed myoblasts. Nature 254:429–431, 1975

201. McKeon C, Thiele CJ, Ross RA, Kwan M, Triche TJ, Miser JS, Israel MA: Indistinguishable and predictable patterns of proto-oncogene expression in two histopathologically distinct tumors: Ewing's sarcoma and neuroepithelioma. (in press)

202. Ross RA, Biedler JL, Spengler BA, Reis DJ: Neurotransmitter-synthesizing enzymes in 14 human neuroblastoma cell lines. Cell Mol Neurobiol 1:301–311, 1981

203. Emmelot P: Biochemical properties of normal and neoplastic cells surfaces: A review. Eur J Cancer 9:319–333, 1973

204. Tucker RW, Sanford KK, Frankel FR: Tubulin and actin in paired nonneoplastic and spontaneously transformed neoplastic cell lines in vitro. Cell 13:629–642, 1978

205. McClain DA, Edelman GM: Density-dependent stimulation and inhibition of cell growth by agents that disrupt microtubules. Proc Natl Acad Sci USA 77:2748–2752, 1980

206. Hatanaka M: Transport of sugars in tumor cell membranes. Biochim Biophys Acta 355:77–104, 1974

207. Naiditch WP, Cunningham DD: Hexose uptake and control of fibroblast proliferation. J Cell Physiol 92:319–332, 1977

208. Rozengurt E: Early events in growth stimulation. In Hynes RO (ed): Surfaces of Normal and Malignant Cells, pp 323–353. New York, John Wiley & Sons, 1979

209. Pollack R, Osborn M, Weber K: Patterns of organization of actin and myosin in normal and transformed cultured cells. Proc Natl Acad Sci USA 72:994–998, 1975

210. Giraldo AA, Meis JM: The use of immunocytochemical techniques in the diagnosis of lymphoreticular proliferations. Dev Oncol 34:141–173, 1985

211. Warnke RA, Weiss LM: Practical approach to the immunodiagnosis of

lymphomas emphasizing differential diagnosis. Cancer Surv 4:349–358, 1985

212. Thiel E: Cell surface markers in leukemia: Biological and clinical correlations. CRC Crit Rev Oncol Hematol 2:209–260, 1985

213. Miraldi FD, Nelson AD, Kraly C, Ellery S, Landmeier B, Coccia PF, Strandjord SE, Cheung NK: Diagnostic imaging of human neuroblastoma with radiolabeled antibody. Radiology 161:413–418, 1986

214. Reynolds CP, Seeger RC, Vo DD, Black AT, Wells J, Ugelstad J: Model system for removing neuroblastoma cells from bone marrow using monoclonal antibodies and magnetic immunobeads. Cancer Res 46:5882–5886, 1986

215. Darbyshire PJ, Bourne SP, Allan PM, Berry J, Oakhill A, Kemshead JT, Coakham HB: The use of a panel of monoclonal antibodies in pediatric oncology. Cancer 59:726–730, 1987

216. Donner L, Triche TJ, Israel MA, Seeger RC, Reynolds CP: A panel of monoclonal antibodies which discriminate neuroblastoma from Ewing's sarcoma, rhabdomyosarcoma, neuroepithelioma and hematopoietic malignancies. In Evans E, D'Angio G, Seeger RC (eds): Advances in Neuroblastoma Research. New York, Alan R. Liss (in press)

217. Burger MM: Cell surfaces in neoplastic transformation. In Horecker BL, Stadtman ER (eds): Current Topics in Cellular Regulation, pp 135–193. New York, Academic Press, 1971

218. Nicolson GL, Poste G: The cancer cell: Dynamic aspects and modifications in cell-surface organization. N Engl J Med 295:197–203, 1976

219. Hynes RO: Cell surface proteins and malignant transformation. Biochim Biophys Acta 458:73–107, 1976

220. Lefkowitz RJ, Michel T: Plasma membrane receptors. J Clin Invest 72:1185–1189, 1983

221. Gilman AG: G proteins and dual control of adenylate cyclase. Cell 36:577–579, 1984

222. Smigel M, Katada T, Northup JK, Bokoch GM, Ui M, Gilman AG: Mechanisms of guanine nucleotide-mediated regulation of adenylate cyclase activity. Adv Cyclic Nucleotide Protein Phosphorylation Res 17:1–18, 1984

223. Lefkowitz RJ, Caron MG: Adrenergic receptors: Molecular mechanisms of clinically relevant regulation. Clin Res 33:395–406, 1985

224. Birnbaumer L, Codina J, Mattera R, Cerione RA, Hildenbrandt JD, Sunyer T, Rojas FJ et al: Regulation of hormone receptors and adenyl cyclases by guanine nucleotide binding N proteins. Recent Prog Horm Res 41:41–99, 1985

225. Sibley DR, Benovic JL, Caron MG, Lefkowitz RJ: Regulation of transmembrane signaling by receptor phosphorylation. Cell 48:913–922, 1987

226. Hurley JB, Simon MI, Teplow DB: Homologies between signal transducing G proteins and ras gene products. Science 226:860–862, 1984

227. Shih TY, Weeks MO, Young HO, Scolnick EM: Identification of a sarcoma virus-coded phosphoprotein in nonproducer cells transformed by Kirsten or Harvey murine sarcoma virus. Virology 96:64–79, 1979

228. Reddy EP, Reynolds RK, Santos E, Barbacid M: A point mutation is responsible for the acquisition of transforming properties of the T24 human bladder carcinoma oncogene. Nature 300:149–152, 1982

229. Taparowsky E, Suard Y, Fasano O, Shimizu K, Goldfarb MP, Wigler M: Activation of T24 bladder carcinoma transforming gene is linked to a single amino acid change. Nature 300:762–765, 1982

230. McGrath JP, Capon DJ, Goeddel DV, Levinson AD: Comparative biochemical properties of normal and activated human ras p21 protein. Nature 310:644–649, 1984

231. Gilman AG: Guanine nucleotide-binding regulatory proteins and dual control of adenylate cyclase. J Clin Invest 73:1–4, 1984

232. Willingham MC: Cyclic amp and cell behavior in cultured cells. Int Rev Cytol 44:319–363, 1976

233. Hunt NH, Martin TJ: Hormone receptors and cyclic nucleotides: Significance for growth and function of tumors. Mol Aspects Med 3:59–118, 1980

234. Prasad KN, Hsie AW: Morphologic differentiation of mouse neuroblastoma cells induced in vitro by dibutyryl adenosine 3'-5'-cyclic monophosphate. Nature (Lond) 233:141–142, 1971

235. Johnson GS, Friedman RM, Pastan I: Restoration of several morphological characteristics of normal fibroblasts in sarcoma cells treated with adenosine-3':5'-cyclic monophosphate and its derivatives. Proc Natl Acad Sci USA 68:425–429, 1971

236. Nishizuka Y: Turnover of inositol phospholipids and signal transduction. Science 225:1365–1370, 1984

237. Nishizuka Y, Takai Y, Kishimoto A, Kikkawa U, Kaibuchi K: Phospholipid turnover in hormone action. Recent Prog Horm Res 40:301–345, 1984

238. Williamson JR: Role of inositol lipid breakdown in the generation of intracellular signals. State of the art lecture. Hypertension 8:I1140–I1156, 1986

239. Michell RH: Inositol phospholipids and cell surface receptor function. Biochem Biophys Acta 415:81–147, 1975

240. Berridge MJ: Phosphatidylinositol hydrolysis: A multifunctional transducing mechanism. Mol Cell Endocrinol 24:115–140, 1981

241. McCaffrey PG, Rosner MR: Growth state-dependent regulation of protein kinase C in normal and transformed murine cells. Cancer Res 47:1081–1086, 1987

242. Kishimoto A, Takai Y, Mori T, Kikkawa U, Nishizuka Y: Activation of calcium and phospholipid-dependent protein kinase by diacylglycerol, its possible relation to phosphatidylinositol turnover. J Biol Chem 255:2273–2276, 1980

243. Nishizuka Y: Studies and perspectives of protein kinase C. Science 233:305–312, 1986

244. Castagna M, Takai Y, Kaibuchi K, Sano K, Kikkawa U, Nishizuka Y: Direct activation of calcium-activated, phospholipid-dependent protein kinase by tumor-promoting phorbol esters. J Biol Chem 257:7847–7851, 1982

245. Kikkawa U, Takai Y, Tanaka Y, Miyake R, Nishizuka Y: Protein kinase C as a possible receptor protein of tumor-promoting phorbol esters. J Biol Chem 258:4768–4773, 1983

246. Nishizuka Y: The role of protein kinase C in cell surface signal transduction and tumour promotion. Nature 308:693–698, 1984

247. Miao RM, Fieldsteel AH, Fodge DW: Opposing effects of tumour promoters on erythroid differentiation. Nature 274:271–272, 1978

248. Mufson RA, Fisher PB, Weinstein IB: Effect of phorbol ester tumor promoters on the expression of melanogenesis in B-16 melanoma cells. Cancer Res 39:3915–3919, 1979

249. Spinelli W, Sonnenfeld KH, Ishii DN: Effects of phorbol ester tumor promoters and nerve growth factor on neurite outgrowth in cultured human neuroblastoma cells. Cancer Res 42:5067–5073, 1982

250. Michell RH, Kirk CJ, Jones LM, Downes DP, Creba J: The stimulation of inositol lipid metabolism that accompanies calcium mobilization in stimulated cells: Defined characteristics and unanswered questions. Philos Trans R Soc [B] 296:123–137, 1981

251. Exton JH: Mechanisms involved in calcium-mobilizing agonist responses. Adv Cyclic Nucleotide Protein Phosphorylation Res 20:211–262, 1986

252. Takai Y, Kishimoto A, Kawahara Y, Minakuchi R, Sano K, Kikkawa U, Mori T et al: Calcium and phosphatidylinositol turnover as signalling for transmembrane control of protein phosphorylation. Adv Cyclic Nucleotide Res 14:301–313, 1981

253. Takai Y, Kishimoto A, Nishizuka Y: In Cheung WY (ed): Calcium and Cell Function, pp 385–412. New York, Academic Press, 1982

254. Berridge MJ: Phosphatidylinositol hydrolysis and calcium signaling. Adv Cyclic Nucleotide Research 14:289–299, 1981

255. Kaibuchi K, Tsuda T, Kikuchi A, Tanimoto T, Yashita T, Takai Y: Possible involvement of protein kinase C and calcium ion in growth factor-induced expression of c-myc oncogene in Swiss 3t3 fibroblasts. J Biol Chem 261:1187–1192, 1986

256. Tupper JT, Zorgniotti F: Calcium content and distribution as a function of growth and transformation in the mouse 3T3 cell. J Cell Biol 75:12–22, 1977

257. Smith JW, Tupper JT: Intracellular calcium pools and their metabolic dependence in normal versus Simiam virus 40-transformed human fibroblasts. J Cell Physiol 120:309–314, 1984

258. Moss DJ, Burrows SR, Parsons PG: Calcium concentration defines two stages in transformation of lymphocytes by Epstein-Barr virus, 33:587–590, 1984

259. Fidler IJ, Hart IR: Principles of cancer biology: Cancer metastasis. In DeVita VT Jr, Hellman S, Rosenberg SA (eds): Cancer: Principles and Practice of Oncology, pp 113–124, 2nd ed. Philadelphia, JB Lippincott, 1985

260. Nowell PC: Mechanisms of tumor progression. Cancer Res 46:2203–2207, 1986

261. Fidler IJ, Kripke ML: Metastasis results from preexisting variant cells within a malignant tumor. Science 198:893–895, 1977

262. German J (ed): Chromosome mutation and neoplasia. New York, Alan R. Liss, 1983

263. Hay ED: Cell Biology of Extracellular Matrix. New York, Plenum, 1982

264. Vracko R: Basal lamina scaffold—Anatomy and significance for maintenance of orderly tissue structures. Am J Pathol 77:313–346, 1974

265. Burtin P, Chavanel G, Foidart JM, Martin E: Antigens of basement membrane in the peritumoral stroma in human colon adenocarcinomas: An immunofluorescence study. Int J Cancer 30:13–18, 1982

266. Barsky SH, Siegal G, Jannotta F, Liotta LA: Loss of basement membrane components by invasive tumors but not by their benign counterparts. Lab Invest 49:140–148, 1983

267. Liotta LA, Rao CN, Barsky SK: Tumor invasion and the extracellular matrix. Lab Invest 49:636–649, 1983

268. Wewer UM, Albrechtsen R, Rao CN, Liotta LA: The extracellular matrix in malignancy. Rheumatology 10:451–478, 1986

269. Graf J, Iwamoto Y, Sasaki M, Martin GR, Kleinman HK, Robey FA, Yamada Y: Identification of an amino acid sequence in laminin mediating cell attachment, chemotaxis, and receptor binding. Cell 48:989–996, 1987

270. Wewer UM, Liotta LA, Jaye M, Ricca GA, Drohan WN, Claysmith AP, Rao CN, Wirth P, Coligan JE, Albrechtsen R et al: Altered levels of laminin receptor mRNA in various human carcinoma cells that have different abilities to bind laminin. Proc Natl Acad Sci USA 83:7137–7141, 1986

271. Goldfarb RH, Liotta LA: Proteolytic enzymes in cancer invasion and metastasis. Semin Thromb Hemost 12:294–307, 1986

272. Turpeenniemi–Huganen T, Thorgeirsson UP, Hart IR, Grant SS, Liotta LA: Expression of collagenase IV (basement membrane collagenase) activity in murine tumor cell hybrids that differ in metastatic potential. JNCI 74:99–103, 1985

273. Liotta LA, Tryggvason K, Garbisa S, Hart I, Foltz CM, Shafie S: Metastatic potential correlates with enzymatic degradation of basement membrane collagen. Nature (Lond) 284:67–68, 1980

274. Russo RG, Foltz CM, Liotta LA: New Invasion assay using endothelial cells grown on native human basement membrane. Clin Exp Metastasis 1:115–127, 1983

275. Liotta LA, Mandler R, Murano G, Katz DA, Gordon RK, Chiang PK, Schiffmann E: Tumor cell autocrine motility factor. Proc Natl Acad Sci USA 83:3302–3306, 1986

276. Paget J: Lectures on Surgical Pathology, p 580. London, Longman, Brown, Green and Longmans, 1863

277. Shearman PJ, Gallatin WM, Longenecker BM: Detection of a cell-surface antigen correlated with organ-specific metastases. Nature 286:267–269, 1980

278. Tannock IF: The relation between cell proliferation and the vascular system in a transplanted mouse mammary tumour. Br J Cancer 22:258–273, 1968

279. Folkman J, Cotran R: Relation of vascular proliferation to tumor growth. Int Rev Exp Pathol 16:207–248, 1976

280. Gullino PM: Angiogenesis, tumor vascularization, and potential interference with tumor growth. Biol Responses Cancer 4:1–20, 1985

281. Folkman J: Tumor angiogenesis. Adv Cancer Res 43:175–203, 1985

282. Vallee BL, Riordan JF, Lobb RR, Higachi N, Fett JW, Crossley G, Buhler R et al: Tumor-derived angiogenesis factors from rat walker 256 carcinoma: An experimental investigation and review. Experientia 41:1–15, 1985

283. Kurachi K, Davie EW, Strydom DJ, Riordan JF, Vallee BL: Sequence of the cDNA and gene for angiogenin, a human angiogenesis factor. Biochemistry 24:5494–5499, 1985

four

Interface Between Immunodeficiency and Pediatric Cancer

Kenneth I. Weinberg and Robertson Parkman

The proposed role for immunology in neoplastic diseases has continuously changed. Over the past 25 years attempts have been made to define a role for the immune system in the "natural" control of neoplastic disease. Recently attempts were made to "stimulate" the immune system as adjunct therapy in the treatment of cancer. Despite the attractiveness for a role of the immune system in the control of cancer, clear-cut evidence is still lacking. This chapter will review the immunologic response to tumors and neoplastic disease seen in patients with primary and acquired immunodeficiencies.

Although there is controversy regarding a therapeutic role for immunology in oncology, no debate exists concerning a diagnostic role for immunology, especially in characterizing diseases of lymphoid and hematopoietic origin. The use of surface differentiation markers and DNA rearrangements has markedly improved our understanding of the pathophysiology of some diseases. In this chapter we will review the present status of immunologic markers in lymphoid and hematopoietic neoplastic diseases. To understand better the terminology that will be used herein, a glossary is provided in Table 4-1.

IMMUNOLOGIC MARKERS IN NEOPLASTIC DISEASE

Although tumor-specific transplantation antigens (TSTA) have been identified in experimental animal systems, primarily virally induced leukemias and chemically induced carcinomas, TSTA rarely occurs in human neoplastic disease. Human T lymphotrophic virus-1 (HTLV-1) infected T-ALL, Epstein–Barr virus (EBV) infected lymphomas and nasopharyngeal carcinomas, and hepatitis B infected hepatocellular carcinomas may represent the only human analogues of murine virally induced tumors.[1,2] Therefore, the majority of immunologic markers used in diagnosing human leukemia/lymphoma are normal differentiation antigens found in unique and informative clusterings on the neoplastic cells. The normal differentiation antigens are thus tumor-associated transplantation antigens (TATA) rather than being true TSTA. A review of the normal differentiation of lymphoid and myeloid cells is necessary before immunologic marker use in the diagnosis of neoplastic disease can be understood.

Both T and B lymphocytes have specific receptors for antigen. The B-lymphocyte receptor for antigen is analogous to the immunoglobulin (Ig) molecule produced by mature B lymphocytes. T lymphocytes express a surface antigen receptor, the T-cell receptor (TCR), which recognizes antigen in the context of the major histocompatibility complex. Each T or B lymphocyte expresses a single antigenic specificity. The heterogeneity of antigenic specificities found in the lymphocyte repertoire is too great to be explained by a single gene encoding for each specificity. The basis of antigenic diversity was not resolved until recently. Antibody molecules consist of polypeptide chains, regions of which vary significantly in their amino acid composition (variable regions), whereas others are

Table 4-1
Glossary of Immunologic Terms Used in This Chapter

Class I—histocompatibility antigens; HLA-A, -B, -C in humans and H-2 in mice

Cytokine—biologically active proteins produced by leukocytes

Differentiation antigens—cell-associated antigens found only at discrete stages of differentiation

DNA probes—A radiolabeled DNA fragment complementary to fragments of a specific gene which will bind to the gene fragments

EBV—Epstein–Barr virus, the etiologic agent of infectious mononucleosis, is a DNA virus that infects B lymphocytes and nasal epithelial cells. B lymphocytes spontaneously proliferate *in vivo* after EBV infection

Episomal DNA—foreign DNA, for example, from a virus, which is present in a cell in a nonintegrated or extrachromosomal form

FACS—fluorescent activated cell sorter, an electron machine that can characterize (size, fluorescence, light scatter) a population of cells on a single cell basis

Fc Receptor—the receptor on NK cells, macrophage/monocytes, and granulocytes for the Fc portion of the IgG molecule

Germ line—the embryonic form of a gene

Histocompatibility—cell-associated antigens involved in transplantation immunity

LAK—IL-2 stimulated leukocytes that can destroy both histocompatible and nonhistocompatible tumor cells

Monoclonal antibody—antibody produced by the fusion of one B lymphocyte with a myeloma cell; the resultant hybrid cell is expanded and the secreted antibody with a unique specificity purified

Monoclonal/polyclonal—a population of identical cells descended from a single precursor is monoclonal. A population of heterogeneous cells descended from many precursor cells is polyclonal. Most leukemias are monoclonal, whereas the proliferating B lymphocytes in infectious mononucleosis are polyclonal

Oncogene—genes that cause cancer. Oncogenes are altered versions of normal cellular genes (proto-oncogenes), which are involved in the regulation of cellular growth and differentiation

Rearrangement—the genetic recombination of germ-line segments into a complete gene

Restriction endonuclease—bacterial enzymes that break phosphodiester bonds of DNA at specific nucleotide sequences, thus cleaving the DNA at specific sites

Southern blot—a technique developed by E. M. Southern in which DNA that has been cleaved into specific fragments by a restriction endonuclease is separated by molecular weight on an agarose gel and transferred to a nitrocellulose or nylon membrane. Specific DNA fragments can then be hybridized to DNA probes

relatively consistent in their amino acid sequences (constant regions). The germ-line genes for the immunoglobulin molecule consist of a restricted number of gene segments that encode for the variable region and a limited number of gene segments that encode for the constant regions. Each individual cell inherits the genes in an unrearranged configuration, which persists in differentiated nonlymphoid cells. During lymphocyte ontogeny, recombinations occur resulting in unique combinations, which define the lymphocyte's antigenic specificity

(Fig. 4-1). Similar processes occur for both the immunoglobulin heavy- and light-chain genes and the TCR genes. Some combinations produced by the recombinant process result in receptor genes that cannot be transcribed or translated; such nonproductive rearrangements are aborted. The recombination process is regulated so that the recombination of immunoglobulin genes occurs only in B lymphocytes and the recombination of the TCR genes only in T lymphocytes.

The use of monoclonal antibodies to surface differentiation antigens and DNA probes to detect rearrangements of the Ig or the TCR genes, or both, and the expression of messenger RNA for differentiation antigens have permitted the evaluation of the lineage and state of differentiation of neoplastic cells. The routine identification of surface differentiation antigens is possible because of the wide availability of monoclonal antibodies, the specificity of which has been determined in a series of international workshops. A standard nomenclature (cluster determinant [CD]) has been established that replaces the heterogeneous nomenclature previously used (Leu and OKT, among others) (Table 4-2).[3] Most immunologic analysis of surface determinants is done by fluorescence-activated cell sorter (FACS) analysis, in which the fluorescent intensity of cells stained with a fluorescent-labeled monoclonal antibody is compared to cells stained with a fluorescent-labeled immunoglobulin without antibody specificity (Fig. 4-2). From FACS analysis the percentage of antigen-positive cells and their antigenic density can be determined.

Detection of Ig or TCR gene rearrangements is done on DNA after the DNA has been partially digested by appropriate restriction endonucleases (depending on the probe in use) and electrophoresed. Both Ig and TCR genes are found in their unrearranged germ-line form rearrangements in nonlymphoid tissues (*e.g.,* fibroblasts, hepatocytes) and in lymphoid tissues before rearrangements occur. After the Ig and TCR genes have been rearranged, normally no single rearrangement occurs in high enough frequency for a distinct single band pattern to be detected (Fig. 4-3). Thus, a TCR-β probe will detect the germ-line TCR-β gene in normal B lymphocytes but no specific rearrangement in normal T lymphocytes. If, however, clonal T-ALL cells are analyzed, a single rearrangement will be detected. The converse occurs in B-lymphocyte neoplasms. An Ig heavy-chain (IgH) gene probe will reveal germ-line heavy chains in normal and malignant T lymphocytes but no unique rearrangements in normal B lymphocytes. However, monoclonal or polyclonal B-lymphocyte lymphomas/leukemias will give one or more discrete bands depending on the clonality of the disease. Monoclonal diseases demonstrate a single Ig gene rearrangement pattern; polyclonal diseases contain several Ig gene rearrangements, each one corresponding to an individual clone.

Central to the use of differentiation antigens and gene rearrangements to determine the lineage and state of differentiation of neoplastic cells is the assumption that the phenotype of the neoplastic cell is related to the normal cell from which the neoplastic cell has been derived (Fig. 4-4). Although many leukemia/lymphomas exhibit phenotypes present on normal lymphoid/myeloid cells, a proportion of cells exhibit "lineage infidelity," that is, they express a phenotype not easily demonstrated on normal cells. Possible explanations for the "inappropriate" expression of lineage markers are that chromosomal translocations have occurred that have produced cells with unique recombination events, that the neoplastic process permits the "deregulation" of genes normally not expressed, or that the cells exhibit a phenotype found on a small number of normal cells.[4] Evidence points to most cases of lineage infidelity resulting from cells that exhibit a rare phenotype found on a small percentage of normally differentiating cells rather than

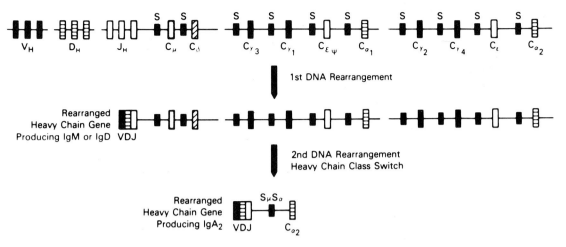

FIGURE 4-1. Schematic representation of DNA rearrangement in the embryonic/germ-line human heavy-chain gene (14q 32). The rearrangement results in the joining of one V_H, D_H, and J_H segment, which then encodes for the antigen-specific variable region of the heavy chain of the antibody molecule.

being a primary consequence of the neoplastic state of the cells.

Leukemia/lymphomas can be divided into three primary phenotypes: B lymphocyte, T lymphocyte, or myeloid lineage.

B-Lymphocyte Lineage

The lymphoid stem cell can differentiate into cells of either B- and T-lymphocyte lineage. The *sine qua non* of the B-lymphocyte lineage is the rearrangement of one or more Ig genes in conjunction with the presence of cytoplasmic or surface immunoglobulin (SIg) or both.[5] Thus, a spectrum of phenotypes exists starting with early pre-B cells that have rearranged IgH genes as the earliest phenotype (Fig. 4-5). After IgH rearrangement, cytoplasmic heavy chains (C_μ) can be detected in pre-B cells. The rearrangement of κ-light chains occurs before λ-light chain rearrangement. If a κ-rearrangement is nonexpressible, then the other κ-allele can be rearranged, and, if that rearrangement is unsuccessful, a λ-rearrangement occurs (Fig. 4-6).[6] Thus, two nonpermissive κ-rearrangements (one for each chromosomal allele) must occur before a λ-rearrangement can occur, explaining the increased incidence of κ as compared to λ expressing malignant cells. The persistence of germ-line λ-chain genes can be detected in cells with κ-chain rearrangements. After immunoglobin light-chain (IgL) gene rearrangement has been completed, light-chain protein is produced, and surface expression of a complete immunoglobulin molecule occurs.

In addition to the sequential changes in Ig expression, parallel changes in the expression of surface differentiation antigens occur. Ia (HLA-Dr) is expressed on pre-B, immature B, and mature B lymphocytes.[7] The differentiation antigens (CD19, CD10, CD20, CD9, and CD21) are then sequentially expressed on the cell surface (see Fig. 4-5).[8] CD19 and CD20 are B-lymphocyte-specific antigens expressed on most B lymphocytes regardless of their state of differentiation. Expression of CD10 (common acute lymphoblastic leukemia antigen [CALLA]) occurs before the detection of cytoplasmic μ-chains. CD10 was originally thought to be uniquely expressed on non-T, non-B leukemia cells; however, some normal bone marrow cells express CD10, as do kidney tubule and bile duct cells.[9] CD9 expression occurs after CD10 expression and persists when CD10 expression is no longer detected.

Most pediatric leukemias exhibit a pre-B or immature B lymphocyte phenotype with the frequency of leukemias with a mature B lymphocyte phenotype being relatively rare (see Chap. 16). B-CLL, a disease of mature B lymphocytes, is rarely found in pediatric patients. Several phenotypes exist in pediatric acute lymphoblastic leukemia. The most frequent is Ia^+, $CD19^+$, $CD10^+$, $CD9^+$, $CD20^-$, SIg^-, with Ia^+, $CD19^+$, $CD10^+$, $CD20^+$, $CD9^-$, SIg^- and Ia^+, $CD19^+$, $CD10^+$, $CD20^+$, $CD9^+$, SIg next in frequency.[7,10,11] Occasional leukemias that express a $CD19^+$ or SIg^+ phenotype have been identified. A correlation exists between the surface phenotype and the response to chemotherapy. The response of leukemia with a pre-B phenotype is better than that with an immature B-lymphocyte (Burkitt leukemia) phenotype. The majority of pediatric B-lymphocyte lymphomas have a mature B-lymphocyte phenotype since the receptor for the third component of complement (C3d, CD21) is also the receptor for EBV and is expressed only in the late pre-B-cell stage, making it biologically impossible for most pre-B lymphocytes to be infected by EBV (see Fig. 4-2), a prerequisite for many pediatric lymphomas.[12] Thus, pediatric non-T-lymphocyte leukemias have a pre-B or immature B lymphocyte phenotype, whereas pediatric non-T lymphomas have an immature or mature B-lymphocyte phenotype (Table 4-3).

A minority of leukemias in addition to B-lymphocyte markers (Ig rearrangements, C_μ) exhibit either myeloid differentiation antigens or evidence of T-lymphocyte lineage (CD2 expression, TCR-γ or β-chain rearrangements).[13] Leukemias with multiple lineage specificities may represent stages of normal differentiation that are abortive, leading to cells that cannot terminally differentiate. However, because of their neoplastic transformation and clonal expansion, neoplastic cells with the unique phenotype can be identified.

T-Lymphocyte Lineage

The earliest definable characteristic of cells of T-lymphocyte lineage is the presence of messenger RNA for the δ- and ϵ-subunits of CD3 (Fig. 4-7).[13] CD3 is an antigen made up of several invariant subunits, which are associated in the cell membrane with the T-lymphocyte receptor for antigen. After CD3 RNA is

Table 4-2
Nomenclature for Standard Cluster Determinants and Expression on Neoplastic Cells

Determinant	Normal Expression	Neoplastic Cells
CD1	Thymocytes	T-ALL; T lymphoma
CD2	All T lymphocytes	T-lymphocyte malignancies
CD3	Mature T lymphocytes	T-CLL; T-ALL; T lymphoma
CD4	Helper T lymphocytes	T-ALL; T-CLL; cutaneous T lymphomas
CD5	Pan T lymphocytes + some B lymphocytes	B-CLL; T-lymphocyte malignancies
CD6	Mature T lymphocytes + some B lymphocytes	T-ALL; T-CLL; B-CLL
CD7	Pan T lymphocytes	T-ALL; T-CLL
CD8	Cytotoxic/suppressor T lymphocytes	T-ALL; T-CLL
CD9	Monocytes	Acute non-T, non-B leukemia; B-CLL
CD10	Pre-B lymphocytes; granulocytes	Acute non-T, non-B lymphoblastic leukemia
CD11a	LFA-1α chain	
CD11b	Monocytes; granulocytes	M4 and M5, ANLL; CML
CD12	Monocytes; granulocytes	M4 and M5, ANLL
CD13	Monocytes; granulocytes	M1, ANLL; CML
CD14	Monocytes	M4 and M5, ANLL
CD15	Granulocytes	M4 and M5, ANLL; CML
CD16	Fc receptor; NK cells; granulocytes	
CD17	Granulocytes; monocytes; platelets	
CD18	LFA-1β chain	
CD19	B lymphocytes	B-lymphocyte malignancies; B lymphomas
CD20	B lymphocytes	B-lymphocyte malignancies
CD21	C3d receptor (EBV receptor)	B-lymphocyte malignancies
CD22	B lymphocytes	B-lymphocyte malignancies
CD23	Some B lymphocytes	
CD24	B lymphocytes, granulocytes	Acute non-T, non-B lymphoblastic leukemia
CD25	IL-2 receptor	HTLV-1-infected T-ALL

produced, immature thymocytes express CD2, the membrane protein that is the receptor for sheep erythrocytes (E). More than 98% of thymocytes and all peripheral T lymphocytes express CD2. As in B lymphocytes, the generation of diverse antigen-specific T lymphocytes is accomplished by rearrangement of sequential genes that encode for the polypeptide chain of the TCR. The γ- and β-chains of the TCR undergo rearrangements prior to the rearrangement of the α-chain genes. During the developmental stages, in which rearrangements are occurring, terminal deoxynucleotidyl transferase (TdT) can be detected in the nucleus.[14] TdT increases genetic diversity of antigen receptors by catalyzing the addition of new nucleotides without a DNA template.[15] After TCR rearrangement has been completed, cytoplasmic TCR can be detected and then surface TCR expression. After the early differentiation events relating to surface expression of CD2 and TCR-β rearrangement, there is the sequential expression in the thymus of a series of cell surface glycoproteins: Stage 1 thymocytes express CD2 and CD9 but no other determinants[16]; Stage 2 thymocytes express CD4, CD8, and CD6; and Stage 3 (mature) thymocytes lose the expression of CD6 concomitantly with the surface expression of CD3 and TCR. Mature thymocytes, S-TCR+, CD3+, and CD4+ or CD8+, migrate from the thymus to the periphery and acquire antigen-specific responsiveness. Most normal T lymphocytes require exogenous interleukin-2 (IL-2) for their *in vivo* proliferation.[17] The effects of IL-2 are

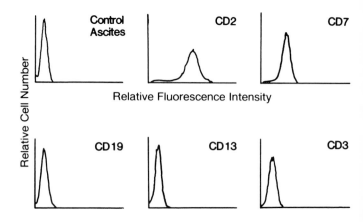

FIGURE 4-2. Fluorescence-activated cell sorter analysis of bone marrow cells from a child with T-acute lymphoblastic leukemia. Intensity of fluorescence after staining with fluorescein-labeled monoclonal antibodies is compared with nonspecific staining of cells with a fluoresceinated mouse myeloma protein (control ascites). Cells stained with antibodies to T-lymphocyte-specific surface antigens (CD2, CD7) but not with the antibodies to the B-lymphocyte-specific antigen (CD19) or the myeloid-specific antigen (CD13). The leukemic cells do not express CD3, surface expression of which occurs only in latest stages of T-lymphocyte differentiation.

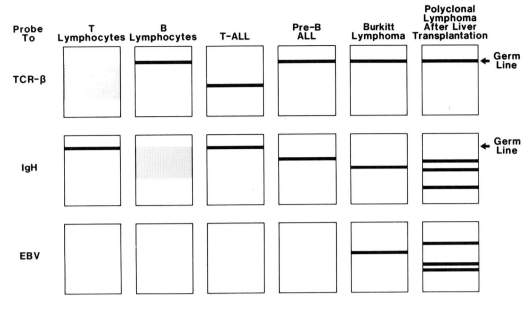

FIGURE 4-3. DNA analysis of leukemia and lymphomas by Southern blot analysis. DNA from neoplastic and normal cells is digested by appropriate enzymes and electrophoresis and probed with TCR-β and IgH-chain cDNA. Persistence of the germ line DNA configuration occurs in differentiated cells of inappropriate lineage (IgH in unrearranged T lymphocytes, TCR-β in unrearranged B lymphocytes). A heterogeneous mixture of rearrangements is seen in normal T and B lymphocytes since no single DNA rearrangement occurs in high frequency. Clonal neoplastic cells display one or more discrete bands depending on whether the disease is monoclonal or polyclonal.

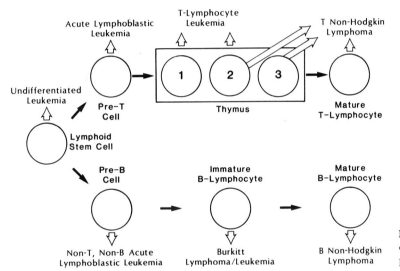

FIGURE 4-4. Schematic representation of normal lymphoid differentiation with potential cells of origin for the common pediatric lymphoid malignancies.

mediated through the IL-2 receptor (CD25), which can be detected on all activated T lymphocytes.[18]

The incidence of malignancies of T-lymphocyte origin in children is significantly less than that of neoplastic disease of T-lymphocyte origin in adults. When T-lymphocyte leukemias/lymphomas occur in the pediatric population, they usually have a phenotype of Stages 1 and 2 thymocytes (CD6+ with or without the expression of CD4 or CD8) (see Chap. 16). T lymphomas usually have rearranged TCR-γ and -β genes but show germ-line TCR-α genes (Fig. 4-7) (see Chap. 20).

The preponderance of lymphoid leukemias among children as compared to adults may be a reflection of the developmental biology of the lymphoid system. The generation of the diversity of Ig and TCR specificities occurs by genetic recombination during lymphocyte ontogeny. Errors in the recombination process are likely to produce lymphocytes uniquely susceptible to the events that result in malignancy. Best characterized of the recombinational events is the translocation of the c-*myc* oncogene and one of the immunoglobulin genes seen in Burkitt's lymphoma. The translocation results in the deregulation of the c-*myc* gene and is a key step in onco-

genesis of Burkitt's lymphoma.[19] The mechanisms of recombination do not differ significantly between B and T lymphocytes, and thus it is not surprising that recombination events similar to those seen in Burkitt's lymphoma have been described in some T-ALL. A translocation between the c-*myc* locus on chromosome 8 and the locus for the TCR-α gene on chromosome 14 results in the deregulation of the c-*myc* gene.[20]

Myeloid Leukemias

Myeloid leukemias are derived from myeloid progenitors that are committed to granulocyte or monocyte differentiation, or both (see Chaps. 17–19). Myeloid leukemias, therefore, share morphologic, enzymatic, and antigenic similarities to normal granulocytes and monocytes. Whereas certain surface glycoproteins (CD11) are found on both mature granulocytes and monocytes, other antigens are found only on cells of monocyte lineage (CD14). Other differentiation antigens (CD13) are found on both immature and mature myeloid cells. Thus, both

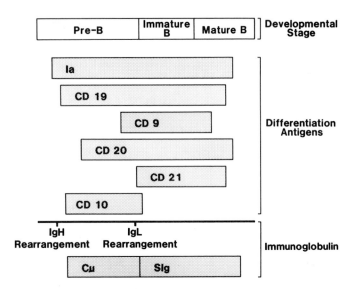

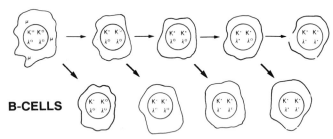

FIGURE 4-5. Schematic representation of normal B-lymphocyte differentiation showing association among the surface expression of differentiation antigens, immunoglobulin rearrangements, and immunoglobulin expression.

PRE B-CELLS

B-CELLS

FIGURE 4-6. A model of light-chain rearrangements within pre-B-cell differentiation. After heavy-chain gene rearrangements and production of cytoplasmic μ, rearrangement of the germ-line light-chain genes (κ^0 and λ^0) begins with the κ genes. Effective rearrangement (κ^+) results in a cell producing κ light chain. λ rearrangements can occur if there are ineffective rearrangements or loss of both κ gene alleles ($\kappa^\times$).

the state of differentiation and the lineage of myeloid leukemias can be determined by the surface expression of their differentiation antigens as well as by their morphology. Most pediatric myeloid leukemias are derived from relatively immature forms of the granulocyte series, although congenital leukemias with a monocytic phenotype and chronic myelogenous leukemia are found. At present, the correlation between antigenic expression and clinical responsiveness to chemotherapy is not as well defined for myeloid leukemias as it is for leukemias of B-lymphocyte origin.

IMMUNOLOGIC RESPONSE TO TUMORS

The primary immunologic response to tumors is cell-mediated immunity with little or no role for antibody. Potential effectors of cell-mediated immunity include cytotoxic T lymphocytes and the family of natural killer/cytotoxic cells (also see Chap. 14). The cytotoxic T lymphocytes require partial histocompati-

bility identity between the cytotoxic T lymphocytes and the target cells, prior antigenic exposure, and a specific TCR-α β-receptor. Natural killer cells do not require histocompatibility identity with their target cells or previous antigenic exposure. Cytotoxic T lymphocytes can destroy human tumor cells expressing TSTA but have minimal reactivity against human tumors expressing only TATA. Natural killer cells have reactivity against some TATA expressing tumor cells as well as virally infected fibroblasts.

As discussed previously, TSTA can be identified in many experimental animal systems but are infrequently found in human tumors; virally induced TSTA can be detected in some human neoplastic disease (HTLV-1 in T-ALL and EBV in some B-lymphocyte lymphoma). Most antigens associated with tumors in humans are related to normal differentiation antigens and therefore are TATA rather than being true TSTA uniquely expressed on tumor cells. The lack of TSTA in humans makes comparisons between experimental tumor systems in animals and human disease difficult. Animal research has demonstrated a role for T lymphocytes in the destruction of virally induced leukemias and chemically induced sarcomas; the cytotoxic destruction is due to the immunologic response directed against the unique TSTA. Analogous events mediated by cytotoxic T lymphocytes rarely occur in human disease. In humans the cellular immunologic responses are directed against tissue antigens that are a normal component of the host repertoire at some time in development (self-antigens). The immunologic response to human tumors, therefore, appears to reside in cell types (natural killer cells, natural suppressor cells, natural cytotoxic cells), the specificity of which is determined not by TSTA but by undefined components of the cell surface present on both neoplastic and virally infected normal cells (Fig. 4-8). These "nonspecific" effector cells appear to have the primary role in the control of human neoplastic disease as opposed to the TSTA-specific cytotoxic T lymphocytes seen in experimental tumor systems.

T Lymphocytes

The antigenic specificity of T lymphocytes is determined by their TCR. Early animal studies with tumors expressing TSTA demonstrated that animals could be innoculated with tumors and that after tumor excision the animals were resistant to subsequent challenge with the same tumor, although they were still susceptible to tumor challenge with antigenically dissimilar tumors of the same type.[21] Besides being tumor specific, the resistance to subsequent tumor challenge was transferrable to nonimmune animals and was eliminated by *in vitro* treatment with antibodies to T lymphocytes. *In vitro* experiments demonstrated that T lymphocytes from immune animals or animals in whom tumors had undergone spontaneous regression were able specifically to lyse the challenging tumor but not appropriate controls. Thus the classic antigenic specificity associated with histocompatibility transplantation antigens was confirmed with TSTA.

However, if animals were transplanted with larger doses of tumors that were not surgically removed, the tumor grew progressively and the animals died. Questions arose as to why, if antigen-specific cytotoxic T lymphocytes could be demonstrated, animals were unable to destroy the tumors. Sequential analysis of animals receiving lethal tumor challenges revealed that cytotoxic T lymphocytes could be detected early after tumor injection (7–10 days); however, later no cytotoxic T-lymphocyte activity could be detected.[22] Transfer experiments using spleen cells from animals with progressively growing tumors mixed with spleen cells from immune animals demon-

Table 4-3
Comparison of Pediatric Lymphoblastic Leukemias and Lymphomas

	Leukemia	*Lymphoma*
T/B lymphocyte origin (%)	30/70	10/90
EBV genome	Absent	Present in B-lymphoid disease
State of differentiation	B: Pre-B cell	B: Immature B lymphocyte
	B: Immature B lymphocyte	B: Mature B lymphocyte
	T: Stage 1 thymocyte	T: Stage 2 thymocyte
	T: Stage 2 thymocyte	T: Stage 3 thymocyte

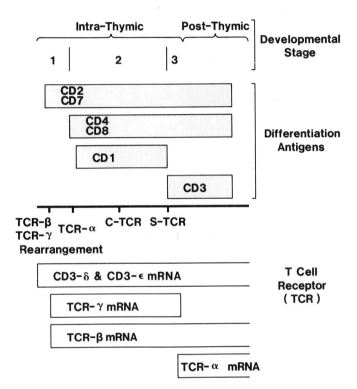

FIGURE 4-7. Schematic representation of normal T-lymphocyte differentiation showing association among developmental stage, surface differentiation antigen expression, and T-cell receptor (TCR) rearrangement and expression.

strated that the spleen cells from animals with progressively growing tumors were able to inhibit the protective effect of the immune spleen cells. Thus, the absence of detectable cytotoxic activity in the spleen cells of animals with progressively growing tumors was due to an active suppressor mechanism rather than the absence of cytotoxic cells. The functional presence of the suppressor cells could further be demonstrated by the use of cyclophosphamide, which has a specific effect on the rapidly proliferating suppressor cells, or antibodies to differentiation antigens uniquely expressed on the suppressor cells (I–J).[23] The administration of cyclophosphamide or anti-I–J antibodies reduced the *in vivo* growth of tumors and in some cases resulted in tumor regression. Thus, the first immunologic response to TSTA was that of cytotoxic T lymphocytes, which might destroy the tumor depending on its antigenicity and proliferative capacity. If, however, the initial cytotoxic response was inadequate, then suppressor T lymphocytes, which blocked the cytotoxic activity of the T lymphocytes, appeared, permitting tumor growth. The underlying mechanisms by which the balance of the immunologic response changes from protective (cytotoxic) to suppressive is not understood and is central to any considerations for using immunotherapy.

Cytotoxic T lymphocytes can recognize TSTA only on cells that express Class I major histocompatibility complex proteins. In animal models, evasion of target recognition by tumor cells has recently been described in which Class I gene and protein expression is inhibited by several oncogene products, including proteins from oncogenic adenoviruses and from the *myc* family of proto-oncogenes. Transfection of the oncogene induces the down-regulation of Class I gene expression and increases the tumorigenicity of the transfectants. Neuroblastoma and small-cell lung carcinomas frequently have low levels of Class I gene (HLA-A, -B, -C) expression and amplification of N-*myc* (see Chaps. 3 and 28).[24] The role of Class I expression in the control of human tumors is uncertain at present.

Although much work has been done attempting to demonstrate cytotoxic T lymphocytes with TSTA specificity in humans, few clear-cut examples exist. Most *in vitro* evaluations of human peripheral blood for T-lymphocyte effectors have focused on the inhibition of tumor growth or the promotion of tumor lysis. In some patients the concomitant presence of cytotoxic and suppressor lymphocytes has been demonstrated.[25] *In vivo* responsiveness to TSTA has been detected by the intradermal injection of tumor cells or solubilized tumor membranes to detect delayed hypersensitivity. Both the *in vivo* and the *in vitro* evaluation of T-lymphocyte responses to human TSTA have been difficult, particularly since most tumor cells have been cultured *in vitro* for prolonged periods and many are contaminated with microorganisms (microplasma, viruses), which induce surface antigens that can be targets for the observed immunologic responses. Relatively few studies have been done with fresh tumor cells. Most human tumor systems appear to be antigenically diverse, with multiple antigens rather than a single dominant antigen being associated with the malignant cells. Some patients receive longitudinal chemotherapy, which may have a significant effect on their immune system, making longitudinal evaluation difficult even if the timing of the chemotherapy is consistent. Studies have shown T-lymphocyte reactivity to various tumor cells (*e.g.,* breast, prostate, intestine, kidney). However, correlation of the T-lymphocyte reactivity with long-term clinical outcome is poor. In summary, cytotoxic T lymphocytes do not have a role in controlling most pediatric tumors.

Primary attempts to stimulate the immune system of patients have included nonspecific stimulation with agents like BCG and specific stimulation with modified autologous or allogeneic tumor cells.[26] Only in rare cases has the use of specific or nonspecific immunotherapy shown improvement in controlled clinical trials over chemotherapy/surgery alone. More recent attempts using IL-2 are reviewed in Chapter 14.

Effector Cell   Target Cell   Outcome

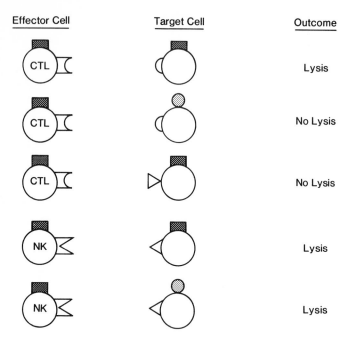

FIGURE 4-8. Comparison of cytotoxic specificity of cytotoxic T lymphocytes (CTL) and natural killer (NK) cells. Histocompatibility antigen (*solid symbols*) identity is a prerequisite for the interaction of CTL effector cells and target cells. Histocompatibility antigen identity is not a prerequisite for the lysis of target cells by NK effector cells. The specificity of the CTL is determined by the TCR, whereas the specificity of the NK cells is determined by unknown recognition structures.

B Lymphocytes

The antigenic specificity of B lymphocytes is determined by the antigen-combining site of the immunoglobulin molecule. In animal experiments antibodies directed against TSTA can either lyse tumor cells or inhibit tumor growth. In most cases the systems studied have been chemically induced sarcomas or virally induced leukemias rather than spontaneous tumors, which are more analogous to human disease. The role of antibody in preventing virally induced leukemia can be seen in cats, in which a feline leukemia vaccine prevents the animals from developing feline leukemia following their natural exposure. Experiments to demonstrate the role of antibodies as compared to the role of cellular immunity in the *in vivo* control of tumor growth are difficult to perform and generally have been uninformative.

In the early 1970s the serum of oncology patients and normal persons was tested for antibodies to tumors by immunofluorescence and complement fixation. Reactivity was detected in the serum of both normal subjects and oncology patients, in part resulting from contamination of the target cells with infectious organisms. Generally it is believed that antibodies do not play a major role in human defenses against neoplastic disease.

Natural Killer Cells

With specific T- or B-lymphocyte immunity having no clear-cut role in human neoplastic disease, the focus of the immunologic response to human tumors has shifted from specific reactivity to general reactivity. During initial attempts to identify

cytotoxic T lymphocytes in the peripheral blood of patients with neoplastic disease, lymphocytes from normal persons, who were not family members of patients, were able to lyse one or more tumor cell lines.[27] Since these people had no previous antigenic exposure to the tumors, the cells responsible for such lysis were termed natural killer (NK) cells. Besides their large granular lymphocyte (LGL) morphology, NK cells have surface antigenic determinants of both lymphoid and myeloid origin (CD2 and CD11) and the presence of Fc receptors (CD16).[28] Thus NK cells may represent a remnant from a time in phylogeny before mononuclear cells diverged into lymphoid and hematopoietic lineages. If such is the case, it might explain the relatively broad specificity demonstrated by NK cells.

The functional activity of NK cells is defined by the capacity of leukocytes from nonimmune persons to lyse susceptible targets (the myeloid leukemia, K562, and herpes simplex virus infected fibroblasts by human NK cells and the leukemia YAC-1 by murine NK cells). Although the physical attachment of NK cells to susceptible targets can be identified microscopically before their destruction, the chemical nature of either the NK receptor or the membrane target components has not been biochemically characterized. At present, much work is directed at the factors released by the cytoplasmic granules (cytolysins), which are responsible for the lysis of susceptible targets.[29] NK lysis has many parallels to that of cytotoxic T lymphocytes in that direct physical contact is needed before target cells are destroyed by cytolysins. Killing occurs by pore-forming proteins (PFP) disrupting the target cell membrane. PFP are serine esterases that are antigenically related to C9, the terminal component of the complement system, and are released by the cytotoxic cell after it has attached to the target.[30]

The role of NK cells in normal immune surveillance is still uncertain. Beige mice, which have a genetic deficiency in NK activity, show no significant increase in tumors throughout their life span.[31] Further, the spectrum of tumors susceptible to NK lysis is limited. Recent work has focused, therefore, not on the role of NK cells in immune surveillance but on their possible therapeutic role. The cytolytic capacity of NK cells is significantly increased by incubation with IL-2. Investigators have demonstrated that *in vivo* infusion of NK cells following their *in vitro* stimulation with IL-2 results in decreased tumor growth in mice.[32] Since IL-2 is produced by T lymphocytes, it is possible that antigen-specific T lymphocytes produce IL-2 *in vivo,* which then locally stimulates NK cells. The success of *in vitro* IL-2-activated murine NK cells is the basis for the clinical investigation of human IL-2-activated leukocytes (LAK cells) in cancer therapy (see Chap. 14).[33]

Cytokines

Cytokines are biologically active proteins produced by lymphocytes, monocytes, and fibroblasts that have immunoregulatory or antiviral and antitumor activities (Table 4-4). They were initially evaluated for their *in vivo* and *in vitro* properties as single agents. Recent evidence has demonstrated significant synergy between cytokines in both the lysis and cytostasis of tumor cells. Because the clinical administration of single cytokines has been associated with clinical toxicity, the future clinical use of cytokines will be based on their synergy, which mimics the normal *in vivo* immunologic response.

The first cytokines identified were the interferons (INF-α, INF-β, and INF-γ). INF-α is produced by leukocytes, INF-β by fibroblasts, and INF-γ by T lymphocytes. INF-α and -β have primarily antiviral activity, although recently INF-α has been

Table 4-4
Cytokines

Name	Source	Effect	Theoretical Role in Cancer Therapy
IL-1	Phagocytic cells	T-lymphocyte activation; fever; fibroblast proliferation	Synergy with other cytokines in tumor cytostasis
IL-2	T lymphocytes	Stimulates T lymphocytes; stimulates LAK cells	Immunotherapy
IL-3 (CSF)	T lymphocytes	Stimulates hematopoietic differentiation and proliferation	↑ rate of hematopoietic recovery after chemotheray
INF-α	Leukocytes	Antiviral	↑ NK activity; immunotherapy
INF-β	Fibroblast	Antiviral	↑ NK activity
INF-γ	T lymphocytes	Immunoregulatory	Synergy with other cytokines in tumor cytostasis
TNF-α	Leukocytes	Cytotoxic	Immunotherapy
TNF-β	Lymphocytes	Cytotoxic	Immunotherapy

shown to be effective in treating hairy cell leukemia.[34] The antiviral activity of INF-α and -β is related to their inhibition of viral protein and nucleic acid synthesis. The mechanism of action of the antitumor activity of INF-α is uncertain but may be a direct antiproliferative effect resulting from reduction of c-*myc* expression.[35] Recently, IFN-γ in conjunction with tumor necrosis factor (TNF-α) has been shown to mediate the cytostatic inhibition of tumor growth *in vitro,* possibly by altering the expression of the proto-oncogene c-*myc*.[35] INF-γ, immune interferon, produced by antigen-specific T lymphocytes has immunoregulatory activities, including the activation of macrophages/monocytes.

Interleukin-1 (IL-1) is produced by monocytes/macrophages after their stimulation with either specific stimuli (antigens) or nonspecific stimuli (*e.g.,* lipopolysaccharide). IL-1 in conjunction with specific antigen can trigger the proliferation of antigen-specific T lymphocytes or the production of cytokines.[36] Without IL-1, no specific lymphocyte activity is detected unless alternative "first signals" are provided. IL-1 has a wide range of biological function, including fever production, stimulation of fibroblast proliferation, and chemotaxis. IL-2 is produced by antigen-specific T lymphocytes and is required for the proliferation of non-IL-2-producing T lymphocytes. IL-2 activity is mediated through the IL-2 receptor (CD25). CD25 can be detected on HTLV-1 T-ALL but not on other T-lymphocyte malignancies. In addition to its immunoregulatory role, IL-2 enhances the cytolytic activity of NK cells and is the basis for the clinical investigational use of IL-2-activated leukocytes (LAK cells).

Tumor necrosis factor (TNF) is a family of proteins that have the capacity to lyse susceptible tumors.[37] TNF-α is produced by macrophages, whereas TNF-β (lymphotoxin, LT) is produced by lymphocytes. TNF can lyse susceptible tumor cells directly, although there is a significant lag period (16 hours) between the addition of the TNF and cell destruction. Recently, synergy between IL-1 and TNF-α and between INF-γ and TNF in the cytostatic inhibition of tumor growth has been reported.[38]

The demonstration of synergy between cytokines represents a more realistic picture of what occurs *in vivo* than do previous experiments with pharmacologic doses of cytokines. The local concentrations of cytokines produced *in situ* will be significantly higher than those achieved with systemically administered cytokines; however, it is impossible to achieve physiologic concentrations at the site of tumors with systemic administration. Therefore, the clinical use of cytokines will have to take advantage of the synergy that exists between cytokines.

Macrophages/Monocytes

Although macrophages/monocytes have a primary role in eliminating antibody-coated bacteria and destroying fungi and other microorganisms (see Chap. 39), their role in controlling neoplastic disease is less certain. *In vitro* experiments have demonstrated that INF-γ-activated macrophages can lyse tumor cells *in vitro.* Further, macrophages/monocytes produce INF-α, which has antitumor activity. However, the clear demonstration of either of these functions in controlling tumors *in vivo* is lacking.

NEOPLASTIC DISEASE IN PRIMARY HUMAN IMMUNODEFICIENCY STATES

Severe Combined Immune Deficiency

Clinical Presentation

Severe combined immune deficiency (SCID) is a clinical phenotype in which affected infants have no T- or B-lymphocyte protection.[39] Affected children are usually well for the first 3 months of life in part because of the presence of transplacentally derived maternal antibody. Affected infants present with a clinical triad of failure to thrive, diarrhea, and recurrent pulmonary infections, especially with *Pneumocystis carinii.* Because of their combined T- and B-lymphocyte defects, they are at increased risk of infection with encapsulated respiratory bacteria, DNA viruses, and fungi. The treatment of choice is bone marrow transplantation with either untreated histocompatible or T-lymphocyte-depleted haploidentical bone marrow. Affected children who are not transplanted usually die by 1 year of age. No other effective form of therapy exists.

Pathophysiology

SCID is caused by a variety of primary defects, including the absence of lymphoid stem cells, the absence of the enzyme adenosine deaminase, the lack of thymic endocrine function, and peripheral defects in terminal T-lymphocyte differentiation and function. Common to all these primary defects is an inability of either T or B lymphocytes to mount a specific immunologic response. The initial cases of SCID were called "the Swiss form of agammaglobulinemia" and were characterized by lymphopenia, probably caused by an absence of lymphoid stem cells. Lymphopenia, however, is a rare finding because most forms of SCID are due to peripheral defects in lymphocyte differentiation and function rather than an absence of lymphoid stem cells. Patients with SCID are heterogeneous with regard to the presence of phenotypic T lymphocytes, B lymphocytes, and NK cells. Most patients (80%) with SCID have no detectable T lymphocytes. A few patients have phenotypic T lymphocytes with or without the ability to proliferate to nonspecific mitogenic stimulation but without *in vitro* blastogenesis following immunization with antigens (tetanus, diphtheria). Whereas most SCID patients have an absence of phenotypic T lymphocytes, almost half have phenotypic (surface Ig positive) B lymphocytes. Without antigen-specific T lymphocytes, specific antibodies are not produced, although some patients can synthesize immunoglobulin without antibody production. The presence of functional NK cells varies between 10% and 50%. A complete review of the pathophysiology of all the primary defects of SCID is beyond the scope of this chapter and has been reviewed.[39]

Neoplastic Disease

The primary neoplastic diseases found in children with SCID involve the lymphoid system, particularly lymphoma and leukemia. The incidence of true neoplastic disease in SCID patients is difficult to ascertain because many patients die at an early age if not diagnosed and treated. The early reports of intestinal lymphomas may have been lymphoid hyperplasia and hyperreactivity rather than true neoplasms. The establishment of the Immunodeficiency Cancer Registry has provided a mechanism for analyzing neoplastic disease attributed to patients with the primary immunodeficiencies.[40] Thirty-one of 42 neoplasms found in SCID patients reported to the Registry were lymphomas and 5 were leukemias.[41] Most lymphomas were non-Hodgkin's lymphomas (NHL) and generally had a B-lymphocyte morphology. The lymphomas were frequently widely distributed at diagnosis, with a median age of onset of 2 years. Thus, the SCID patients who develop a neoplastic disease represent a subset of patients who live beyond the expected age of death. DNA analysis has demonstrated that multiple copies of the EBV genome are frequently found in the NHL tumors, suggesting that the lymphomas are caused by the uncontrolled proliferation of EBV-infected B lymphocytes. Only SCID patients with phenotypic B lymphocytes are theoretically at risk of associated EBV-induced lymphoma. No prospective studies, however, have been done to determine the incidence of NHL in SCID patients with phenotypic B lymphocytes, since most diagnosed patients receive either histocompatible or T-cell-depleted haploidentical bone marrow transplants.

Wiskott–Aldrich Syndrome

Clinical Presentation

The Wiskott–Aldrich syndrome (WAS) is an X-linked disorder in which affected patients suffer from progressive T-lymphocyte immunodeficiency, an inability to make antibodies to carbohydrate antigens, eczema, thrombocytopenia with platelets of reduced size and function, and an increased incidence of lymphomas, particularly of the central nervous system.[42] Although patients clinically may present with thrombocytopenia at birth, the diagnosis of WAS is difficult because eczema clinically is not usually present during the first year of life and normal newborn infants have a decreased capacity to produce anticarbohydrate antibodies. Because of their T-lymphocyte immunodeficiency and inability to make antibodies to the car-

bohydrate antigens of bacterial cell walls, patients suffer from infection with both encapsulated respiratory bacteria and DNA viruses.

Pathophysiology

A unitarian hypothesis to explain both the lymphoid and the hematopoietic components of WAS did not exist until abnormalities were observed in the membrane glycoproteins of both the T lymphocytes and platelets of WAS patients. Defects in 115,000 molecular weight glycoprotein (gpL-115) and abnormalities in platelet glycoprotein Ia-Ib have been demonstrated and suggest that the primary defect in WAS is due to membrane glycoproteins that undergo spontaneous degradation.[43] The abnormal membranes are removed by the *in vivo* action of the spleen, resulting in lymphocytes and platelets of reduced size with morphologic abnormalities that can be identified by scanning electron microscopy.[44] The resultant abnormal lymphocytes and platelets have a shortened *in vivo* survival, resulting in thrombocytopenia and an absence of long-lived T lymphocytes needed for normal immunologic memory and immunoregulation.

Neoplastic Disease

Fifty-nine of the 79 cases of neoplastic disease reported in WAS patients were non-Hodgkin's lymphoma.[41] The most frequent NHL histology was B-cell lymphoma (27%). The central nervous system was the primary site in 33% of patients. The median age of diagnosis was 6.7 years. Whereas NHL had a young age of onset, the age of onset of Hodgkin's disease or immunoblastic sarcoma was older (25 and 17 years, respectively).[40] Copies of the EBV genome have been identified in many of the NHL specimens. Three cases of Hodgkin's disease and 7 cases of leukemia have been reported.

X-Linked Lymphoproliferative Syndrome

Clinical Presentation

The X-linked lymphoproliferative syndrome (XLP) is an X-linked recessive disorder in which affected males develop fatal infectious mononucleosis following infection with EBV; 70% of patients will die of their initial EBV infection, and 15% will have a lymphoproliferative disorder at autopsy.[45,46] Of the 30% who survive, most develop common variable immunodeficiency with recurrent pyogenic infections, and 30% will die of a lymphoproliferative disorder.

Pathophysiology

The primary defects in XLP are an inability to control EBV infection and the proliferation of EBV-infected B lymphocytes. The capacity of T lymphocytes from XLP patients to lyse EBV-infected targets is normal; however, the NK activity of these patients is significantly less than that of normal persons or carriers even after incubation with INF-γ.[47] Both INF-α and -γ production are normal. The hypogammaglobulinemia seen in surviving XLP patients results from the destruction of EBV-infected B lymphocytes by either productive EBV infection or their lysis by cytotoxic T lymphocytes. B lymphocytes that may be nonproductively infected with EBV become transformed, resulting in their uncontrolled proliferation.

Neoplastic Disease

All of the lymphoproliferative disorders identified in patients with XLP have a B-lymphocyte phenotype (Burkitt's lymphoma, NHL, immunoblastic sarcoma). In all cases tested the EBV genome can be detected in the neoplastic cells, demonstrating that the malignant transformation is related to the integration of the EBV genome into the B lymphocytes. Chemotherapy has not been successful in treating any of the B-lymphocyte neoplasms identified in XLP patients.

Ataxia-Telangectasia

Clinical Presentation

Patients with ataxia-telangectasia (AT) have a clinical triad consisting of cerebellar ataxia, ocular telangectasia, and immunodeficiency. Clinical immunodeficiency is characterized by an increased susceptibility to viral infections particularly of the herpes virus group, a decrease in serum IgA, and a predisposition to bronchopulmonary infections with encapsulated respiratory pathogens.[48]

Pathophysiology

The underlying primary defect in patients with AT is an increased susceptibility to DNA damage.[49] Investigations have demonstrated an increased susceptibility of all tissues from AT patients to damage by X-irradiation. It has been proposed that the increased incidence of neoplastic disease seen in these patients is a consequence of their DNA damage and is not due to their immunodeficiency. Recently, translocations of chromosome 7q32-35, the region of the gene for TCR-β gene (7q32); chromosome 14q11, the site of the TCR-α gene; and chromosome 7p15, the site of the TCR-γ gene, have been identified in T-lymphocyte malignancies of AT patients, suggesting that the malignancies are due to the interaction of an oncogene with the translocated TCR genes, resulting in the uncontrolled proliferation of the T lymphocytes.[50] The relationship between increased susceptibility to DNA damage and ataxia and telangectasia is still uncertain.

Neoplastic Disease

Patients with AT have an overall tumor incidence of 12%.[51] Most neoplastic disease in AT patients is lymphoid in origin. About half of the malignancies reported in AT patients are non-Hodgkin's lymphoma (67 of 145), with 31 cases of leukemia and 15 cases of Hodgkin's disease. The presence of the EBV genome has been identified in many NHL tumors. The mean age of diagnosis of NHL is 10 years. The morphologic features of NHL seen in AT patients are similar to those of NHL seen in non-AT children. Analysis of AT patients with and without immunodeficiency has revealed that the incidence of NHL is the same, suggesting that the increased incidence of lymphomas in AT patients is due to their DNA abnormalities rather than their immunodeficiency.

In addition to lymphoid tumors, 21 nonlymphoid tumors, including 7 gastric carcinomas and 3 dysgerminomas of the ovary, have been reported. Five of the 7 gastric cancers occurred in females. Whereas the lymphoid malignancies had their onset before the age of 15, most of the carcinomas had their onset in adult life. An increased frequency of carcinomas is seen in the family members of AT patients and suggests that the genes controlling malignancy may be active in the heterozygote state. Analysis of AT patients indicates that the degree of immunodeficiency, either cell-mediated immunodeficiency or IgA deficiency, does not correlate with the incidence of neoplastic disease, suggesting that increased incidence of malignancy is related to the underlying primary defect (*e.g.,* chromosomal fragility) rather than to the immunodeficiency.

Bloom's Syndrome

Clinical Presentation

Bloom's syndrome is an autosomal recessive disorder in which affected individuals display stunted growth, telangiectatic erythema of the face, and sun sensitivities. Some patients have low immunoglobulin levels and mild anemia.

Pathophysiology

The primary defect in Bloom's syndrome is a deficiency of DNA ligase 1, which is necessary for most DNA repair.[52] Thus, Bloom's syndrome, like AT, is due to a primary defect in DNA repair.

Neoplastic Disease

Of 78 patients followed long-term, 16 patients (21%) developed 18 neoplasms (8 leukemias, 4 lymphomas, and 6 solid tumors).

Selective IgA Deficiency

Clinical Presentation

The absence of serum IgA is the most frequently described human immune deficiency state and occurs in about 1 of 700 individuals. In some cases, however, IgA deficiency is due to an absence of serum IgA 1 (90% of the total IgA) rather than to a total absence of IgA. Surveys differ as to the clinical consequence of IgA deficiency. Most patients with IgA deficiency have no definable sequellae; however, some series report an increased incidence of either autoimmune diseases or sinopulmonary infections. The increased incidence of infections may be due to a concomitant absence of IgG2 and IgG4 in some patients.

Pathophysiology

Patients with IgA deficiency have immature lymphocytes that coexpress IgA and IgM.[53] Thus, the terminal differentiation of IgA-bearing cells does not occur, resulting in either no or partial IgA1 production. In rare cases absence of the joining piece (J chain) has been reported. Acquired IgA deficiency occurs in some cases secondary to drugs such as phenytoin. Drug-induced IgA deficiency may be due to suppressor T lymphocytes, which interfere with the terminal differentiation of B lymphocytes into mature IgA-secreting lymphocytes.

Neoplastic Disease

Whereas lymphoid malignances are the predominant neoplastic disease in patients with defects of T-lymphocyte immunity, carcinomas and sarcomas occur most frequently in patients with IgA deficiency.[41] Of 37 neoplasms reported, 28 are nonlymphoid and 9 are lymphoid. The most frequent neoplastic disease is gastric carcinoma (24 cases), which occurred in patients with selective IgA deficiency and in patients with common variable immunodeficiency and AT who also lack IgA. Questions as to whether the lack of secretory IgA may lead to increased stimulation of gastric cells or the uncontrolled proliferation of DNA viruses within the gastrointestinal tract are a matter of speculation; however, no solid data exist.

Common Variable Immunodeficiency

Clinical Presentation

Patients with common variable immunodeficiency (CVID) have recurring infections with encapsulated respiratory pyrogenic organisms, including pneumonia, meningitis, osteomyelitis, and boils. The age of onset can be during the first year of life if the condition is congenital or later if the condition is acquired.

Pathophysiology

CVID is a heterogeneous group of diseases, all of which are characterized by significant reductions in circulating immunoglobulin levels (IgM, IgG, IgA) and a profound inability to produce specific antibodies. Patients have circulating B lymphocytes although they may be low in number or have a relatively immature phenotype. A variety of primary defects exist in CVID, including an inability to respond to T-lymphocyte signals and an inability to synthesize or secrete immunoglobulin. In addition, some patients have normal B lymphocytes but no helper T lymphocytes or an excess of suppressor T lymphocytes, both of which result in the lack of T-lymphocyte signals required for normal B-lymphocyte activation.[54]

Neoplastic Disease

Malignancies are equally divided between lymphoid and non-lymphoid malignancies, with non-Hodgkin's lymphoma representing the single largest diagnosis (54 of 116 cases).[41] CVID patients with NHL have an age of diagnosis of 36 years compared to greater than 60 years in the general population. The tumors are usually extranodal in origin. Nineteen adenocarcinomas and 26 other tumors have been reported. Some of the gastric carcinomas may be secondary to the absence of IgA.

X-Linked Agammaglobulinemia

Clinical Presentation

Affected male infants develop recurrent infections with encapsulated respiratory pathogens during the second 6 months of life. Patients have decreases in all immunoglobulin classes (IgG, IgA, IgM) once transplacental maternal IgG disappears. The patients can be treated successfully by the routine administration of intramuscular or intravenous gammaglobulin. Some patients are at increased risk of developing infections with ECHO viruses particularly of the central nervous system, presumably owing to the low frequency of protective antibodies in pooled immunoglobulin, whereas others develop autoantibodies.

Pathogenesis

Patients with X-linked agammaglobulinemia (X-AG) have no detectable circulating B lymphocytes, although pre-B lympho-

cytes can be demonstrated in the bone marrow of some patients.[55] Thus, the patient's lack of immunoglobulin production is due to a total absence of mature B lymphocytes.

Neoplastic Disease

Patients with X-AG have no significant increase in tumors compared to normal individuals, in contrast to patients with SCID and CVID in whom an increased incidence of lymphoid neoplasms is seen. The primary difference between patients with X-AG and those with the other immunodeficiencies is the lack of any immature or mature B lymphocytes, indicating that the presence of immature/mature B lymphocytes is a prerequisite for developing B-lymphocyte lymphomas.

T-Lymphocyte-Depleted Bone Marrow Transplants

Clinical Presentation

Whereas graft-versus-host-disease (GVHD) is clinically controllable following histocompatible bone marrow transplantation, the transplantation of histoincompatible bone marrow after the ablative preparation of the recipient uniformly results in fatal GVHD. Based on animal studies, the removal of mature T lymphocytes from the transplantation innoculum allows successful lymphoid and hematopoietic engraftment without clinically significant GVHD. Two principal methods have been used to remove mature T lymphocytes: [1] soybean lectin and E-rosette formation, and [2] lysis with anti-T-lymphocyte monoclonal antibodies and complement.[56,57] Following transplants with monoclonal antibody and complement treatment, there has been about a 30% incidence of B-lymphocyte lymphomas, whereas a lower incidence has been observed in patients receiving soybean and E-rosette-depleted marrow.

Pathophysiology

Evaluation of the B-lymphocyte lymphomas that develop after transplantation has found the neoplastic cells to be of both donor and recipient origin.[58] Analysis for the presence of the EBV genome has demonstrated the presence of EBV in most cases, suggesting that the lymphomas represent either the uncontrolled proliferation of donor B lymphocytes, which already contained the EBV genome before transplantation, or the transmission of the EBV genome from donor B lymphocytes to recipient lymphocytes after transplantation in EBV-negative recipients. The elimination of mature T lymphocytes may remove the lymphocytes that can control the proliferation of EBV-infected B lymphocytes as normally occurs in infectious mononucleosis. EBV virus contains linear double-stranded DNA, whereas EBV DNA in tumor cells is in the form of circularized episomal DNA.[59] The length of the linear termini varies, producing EBV DNA of variable length. The variations in the length allows the determination of episomal clonality and, by implication, of cellular clonality. As a terminal event, however, a clone with the greatest selective advantage may expand, resulting in a monoclonal rather than a polyclonal process.

Neoplastic Diseases

Malignancies other than EBV-induced lymphomas have not been seen in patients receiving T-lymphocyte depleted transplants.

Solid Organ Transplantation

Clinical Presentation

Patients successfully transplanted with renal grafts have routinely received prednisone and azathioprine; the recent introduction of cyclosporine A has permitted the successful transplantation of livers, hearts, and kidneys. An evaluation of neoplastic disease in recipients of solid organ grafts before the introduction of cyclosporine revealed an increased incidence of malignant disease, primarily skin cancers (40%) and lymphomas (12%). The introduction of cyclosporine has markedly increased the proportion of lymphomas (41%) and shortened the time to onset (20 months versus 60 months).[60] Thus the incidence of lymphoma is significantly increased by adding cyclosporine to the post-transplantation immune suppression regimen. In many cases the lymphomas have been sensitive to the reduction or the cessation of cyclosporine therapy. The lymphomas are of B-lymphocyte origin, the EBV genome can be detected in the lymphomas, and the disease is multifocal. The regression of the lymphomas following the reduction or cessation of cyclosporine therapy suggests that the lymphomas can still potentially be regulated by normal host defense mechanisms.[61] If the immunosuppression is not adequately reduced, the disease then progresses to a neoplastic process that is unresponsive to later reductions in immunosuppression. At that time, the disease becomes monoclonal, suggesting that an evolution of the EBV transformed B lymphocytes has occurred. The noncytotoxic suppressor T lymphocytes that have been identified in patients with infectious mononucleosis may be inhibited by cyclosporine, permitting the proliferation of the EBV-infected B lymphocytes.[62] Without such suppressor cells, patients with primary cellular immunodeficiencies or those receiving significant immunosuppression may not be able to suppress the proliferation of EBV-infected B lymphocytes.

CLINICAL OUTCOME OF IMMUNODEFICIENT PATIENTS WITH CANCER

Patients with primary immunodeficiencies develop neoplastic disease at a younger age than do nonimmunodeficient patients who develop the same neoplastic processes.[45] The cure and response rates of immunodeficient patients are significantly less than those of nonimmunodeficient patients. Whereas the survival rate of nonimmunodeficient patients with Hodgkin's disease is 80% at 5 years, fewer than 20% of immunodeficient patients with Hodgkin's disease are alive. The response and cure rates with other tumors are equally poor, suggesting that the absence of normal defense mechanisms results in the decreased effectiveness of normal therapy. The success of chemotherapy in normal persons is, therefore, due to the additive effects of chemotherapy and the normal components of the immune system.

ROLE OF IMMUNE SYSTEM IN CONTROL OF HUMAN MALIGNANT DISEASE

Based on the neoplastic disease seen in patients with primary immunodeficiencies, certain conclusions about the role of the immune system in the control of human neoplastic disease can be made. First, most neoplastic disease in patients with cellular immunodeficiencies consists of lymphomas/leukemias primarily of B-lymphocyte origin (Table 4-5). Further, EBV DNA can be identified in many lymphomas, particularly from patients with WAS, SCID, CVID, and XLP. The singular increase in the frequency of EBV-related B-lymphocyte neoplasms suggests that normal control of EBV-infected B lymphocytes as seen in infectious mononucleosis does not occur in patients with primary cellular immune defects. The EBV-related lymphomas/leukemias are one of the few human tumor systems in which TSTA exist; therefore, it is not surprising that the congenital or acquired deficiency of T lymphocytes would result in the increased frequency of TSTA expressing tumors. The demonstration of the presence of T lymphocytes, which can noncytolytically inhibit EBV-infected B-lymphocyte proliferation, in patients with infectious mononucleosis suggests that the absence of analogous cells in immunodeficient patients is the basis for the increased incidence of B-lymphocyte neoplasms. Synergy between cytokines (TNF and IL-1/TNF and INF-γ) in the inhibition of tumor growth indicates that the cytostatic effect of T lymphocytes may be mediated through such cytokines. The nonrandom translocations of biologically active genes, as in the case of the TCR in AT or Ig in Burkitt's lymphoma, may result in cells with the potential for uncon-

Table 4-5
Neoplastic Disease in Immunodeficient Patients

Disease	Immune Function		Neoplastic Disease
	Cellular	Humoral	
SCID	↓	↓	EBV-associated B lymphocyte lymphoma/leukemia
WAS	↓	↓	EBV-associated B lymphocyte lymphoma (35% CNS)
XLP	↓ (NK)	Normal	EBV-associated B lymphocyte lymphoma
AT	Normal or ↓	↓ IgA	EBV-associated B lymphocyte lymphoma; gastric carcinoma
Bloom's syndrome	Normal	Normal	Leukemia/lymphoma
IgA deficiency	Normal	↓ IgA	Gastric carcinoma
CVID	Normal	↓	Non-Hodgkin lymphoma; gastric carcinoma
X-AG	Normal	↓	None
T-cell-depleted BMT	↓	↓	EBV-associated B lymphocyte lymphoma
Organ transplant			
− cyclosporin	↓	Normal	Skin cancer; EBV-associated B lymphocyte lymphoma
+ cyclosporin	↓	Normal	EBV-associated B lymphocyte lymphoma

trolled proliferation. The increased incidence of gastric carcinoma in female patients with an absence of IgA suggests that at least two factors (sex and IgA deficiency) are involved, since an increased incidence of gastric carcinoma is not seen in male patients with X-linked agammaglobulinemia who also have an absence of IgA. The analysis of both primary and acquired immunodeficiencies shows an increase only in EBV-associated lymphoid neoplasms, gastric carcinomas, and cutaneous carcinomas, with no increase in any other tumor types. Thus, the role that the immune system plays in the control of most tumors is extremely limited.

This work was supported by a grant from the Concern Foundation.

REFERENCES

1. de-The G, Geser A, Day NE et al: Epidemiological evidence for casual relationship between Epstein-Barr virus and Burkitt's lymphoma from Ugandan prospective study. Nature 274:756–761, 1978

2. Poiesz BJ, Ruscetti FW, Gazdar AF et al: Detection and isolation of type C retrovirus particles from fresh and cultured lymphocytes of a patient with cutaneous T-cell lymphoma. Proc Natl Acad Sci USA 77:7415–7419, 1981

3. Shaw S: Characterization of human leukocyte differentiation antigens. Immunol Today 8:1–3, 1987

4. Greaves MF: Differentiation-linked leukemogenesis in lymphocytes. Science 234:697–704, 1986

5. Korsmeyer SJ, Hieter PA, Ravetch JV et al: A developmental hierarchy of immunoglobulin gene rearrangements in human leukemic pre-B-cells. Proc Natl Acad Sci USA 78:7096–7100, 1981

6. Hieter PA, Korsmeyer SJ, Waldman TA et al: Human immunoglobulin kappa light chain genes are deleted or rearranged in lambda producing B-cells. Nature 290:368–372, 1981

7. Melink GB, LaBien TW: Construction of an antigenic map for human B-cell precursors. J Clin Immunol 3:260–267, 1983

8. Nadler LM, Anderson KC, Mouti G et al: B₄, a human B-lymphocyte associated antigen expressed on normal, mitogen-activated, and malignant B-lymphocytes. J Immunol 131:244–250, 1983

9. Metzgar RS, Borowitz MJ, Jones NH et al: Distribution of common acute lymphoblastic leukemia antigen in nonhematopoietic tissues. J Exp Med 154:1249–1254, 1981

10. Nadler LM, Korsmeyer SJ, Anderson KC et al: The B-cell origin of non-T-cell acute lymphoblastic leukemia: A model for discrete stages of neoplastic and normal pre-B-cell differentiation. J Clin Invest 74:332–340, 1984

11. Korsmeyer SJ, Arnold A, Bakhshi A et al: Immunoglobulin gene rearrangement and cell surface antigen expression in acute lymphocytic leukemias of T-cell and B-cell precursor origins. J Clin Invest 71:301–313, 1983

12. Siaw MFE, Nemerow GR, Cooper NR: Biochemical and antigenic analysis of the Epstein Barr virus/C3d receptor (CR2). J Immunol 136:4146–4151, 1986

13. Van Dongen JJM, Quertermous T, Bartram CR: T cell receptor-CD3 complex during early T cell differentiation. Analysis of immature T cell acute lymphoblastic leukemias (T-ALL) at DNA, RNA, and cell membrane level. J Immunol 138:1260–1269, 1987

14. Van Dongen JJM, Hooijkaas H, Comans–Bitter M et al: Human bone marrow cells positive for terminal deoxynucleotidyl transferase (TdT), HLA-DR, and a T cell marker may represent prothymocytes. J Immunol 135:3144–3150, 1985

15. Desiderio SV, Yancopoulos GD, Paskind M et al: Insertion of regions into heavy-chain genes is correlated with expression of terminal deoxytransferase in B cells. Nature 311:752–755, 1984

16. Reinherz EL, Kung PC, Goldstein G: Discrete stages of human intrathymic differentiation: Analysis of normal thymocytes and leukemic lymphoblasts of T cell lineage. Proc Natl Acad Sci USA 77:1588–1592, 1980

17. Smith KA: Interleukin 2. Annu Rev Immunol 2:319–333, 1984

18. Greene WC, Leonard WJ, Depper JM: The human interleukin-2 receptor: Normal and abnormal expression in T cells and in leukemias induced by the human T-lymphotropic retroviruses. Ann Intern Med 105:560–572, 1986

19. Kelly K: The regulation and expression of c-myc in normal and malignant cells. Annu Rev Immunol 4:317–338, 1986

20. Erikson J, Finger L, Sun L: Deregulation of c-myc by translocation of the α-locus of the T-cell receptor in T-cell leukemias. Science 232:884–886, 1986

21. Fujimoto A, Greene M, Sehon AH: Regulation of the immune response to tumor antigens: I. Immunosuppressor T cells in tumor-bearing hosts. J Immunol 116:791–799, 1976

22. Treves AJ, Carnaud C, Trainin N et al: Enhancing T lymphocytes from tumour-bearing mice suppress host resistance to a syngeneic tumour. Eur J Immunol 4:722–727, 1974

23. Greene MI, Dorf ME, Pierres M et al: Reduction of syngeneic tumor growth by an anti-I-J alloantiserum. Proc Natl Acad Sci USA 74:5118–5121, 1977

24. Bernards R, Dessain SK, Weinberg RA: N-myc amplification causes downmodulation of MHC Class I antigen expression in neuroblastoma. Cell 47:667–674, 1986

25. Yu A, Watts H, Jaffe N, Parkman R: Concomitant presence of tumor-specific cytotoxic and inhibitor lymphocytes in patients with osteogenic sarcoma, N Engl J Med 297:121–127, 1977

26. Hersh EM: Current status of active non-specific immunotherapy. In Reif AE, Mitchell MS (ed): Immunity to Cancer, pp 443–451. New York, Academic Press, 1985

27. Herberman RB, Holden HT: Natural cell-mediated immunity. Adv Cancer Res 27:305–377, 1978

28. Ortaldo JR, Sharrow SO, Timonen T: Analysis of surface antigens on highly purified human NK cells by flow cytometry with monoclonal antibodies. J Immunol 127:2401–2414, 1981

29. Herberman RB, Reynolds CW, Ortaldo JR: Mechanism of cytotoxicity by natural killer (NK) cells. Annu Rev Immunol 4:651–680, 1986

30. Young JDE, Cohn ZA, Podack ER: The ninth component of complement and the pore-forming protein (Perforin 1) from cytotoxic T cells: Structural, immunological, and functional similarities. Science 233:184–190, 1986

31. Argov S, Cochran AJ, Karre K: Incidence and type of tumors induced in C57BL b9/b9 mice and +/b9 littermates by oral administration of DMBH. Int J Cancer 28:739–746, 1981

32. Mazumder A, Rosenberg SA: Successful immunotherapy of NK-resistant established pulmonary melanoma metastases by the intravenous adoptive transfer of syngeneic lymphocytes activated in vitro by interleukin-2. J Exp Med 159:495–507, 1984

33. Rosenberg SA, Lotze MT, Muul LM et al: Observations on the systemic administration of autologous lymphokine-activated killer cells and recombinant interleukin-2 to patients with metastatic cancer. N Engl J Med 313:1485–1492, 1985

34. Einat M, Resnitzky D, Kimchi A: Close link between reduction of c-myc expression by interferon and G₀/G₁ arrest. Nature 313:597–600, 1985

35. Yarden A, Kimchi A: Tumor necrosis factor reduces c-myc expression and cooperates with interferon-γ in HeLa cells. Science 234:1419–1421, 1986

36. Durum SK, Schmidt JA, Oppenheim JJ: Interleukin 1: An immunological perspective. Annu Rev Immunol 3:263–287, 1985

37. Beutler B, Cerami A: Cachectin: More than a tumor necrosis factor. N Engl J Med 316:379–385, 1987

38. Ruggiero V, Baglioni C: Synergistic anti-proliferative activity of interleukin 1 and tumor necrosis factor. J Immunol 138:661–663, 1987

39. Parkman R: Treatment of immune deficiency states with organ transplantation. In Schwartz R (ed): Progress in Clinical Immunology, pp 85–102. New York, Grune & Stratton, 1976

40. Filipovich AH, Robison L, Heinitz KJ: Tumors in Patients with Naturally Occurring Immunodeficiency Disorders: Report from the Immunodeficiency Cancer Registry. In Muller HJ, Weber W (eds): Familial Cancer, pp 222–225. Basel, S Karger, 1985

41. Filipovich AH, Heinitz KJ, Robison LL, Frizzera G: The immunodeficiency cancer registry: A research resource. Am J Pediatr Hematol/Oncol (in press)

42. Cooper MD, Chasse HP, Lowman JT et al: Wiskott-Aldrich syndrome: An immunologic deficiency disease involving the afferent limb of immunity. Am J Med 44:499–513, 1968

43. Reisinger D, Parkman R: Molecular heterogeneity of a lymphocyte glycoprotein in immunodeficient patients. J Clin Invest 79:595–599, 1987

44. Kenney DM, Cairns L, Neustein H et al: Morphological abnormalities in the lymphocytes of patients with the Wiskott-Aldrich syndrome. Blood 68:1329–1332, 1986

45. Henle G, Henle W: Observations on childhood infections with the Epstein-Barr virus. J Infect Dis 121:303–310, 1970

46. Tamir D, Benderly A, Levy J et al: Infectious mononucleosis and Epstein-Barr virus in childhood. Pediatrics 53:330–335, 1974

47. Sumaya C: Primary Epstein–Barr virus infections in children, Pediatrics 59:16–21, 1977

48. Boder E, Sedgwick RP: Ataxia telangiectasia. A familiar syndrome of progressive cerebellar ataxia, oculocutaneous telangiectasia and frequent pulmonary infection. Pediatrics 21:526–554, 1958

49. Taylor AM, Harnden DG, Arlett CF et al: Ataxia-telangiectasia: a human mutation with abnormal radiation sensitivity. Nature 258:427–429, 1975

50. Fiorilli M, Carbonari M, Crescenzi M et al: T-cell receptor genes and ataxia telangiectasia, Nature 313:186, 1985

51. Spector BD, Filipovich AH, Perry GS et al: Epidemiology of cancer in ataxia-telangiectasia. In Bridges BA, Harnden DG (eds): Ataxia-teleangiectasia—A Cellular and Molecular Link Between Cancer, Neuropathology, and Immune Deficiency. New York, John Wiley & Sons, 1982

52. Chan JYH, Becker FF, German J et al: Altered DNA ligase I activity in Bloom's syndrome cells, Nature 325:357–359, 1987

53. Conley ME, Cooper MD: Immature IgA B cells in IgA-deficient patients. N Engl J Med 305:495–497, 1981

54. Reinherz EL, Rubinstein AJ, Geha RS et al: Abnormalities of immunoregulatory T cells in disorders of immune function. N Engl J Med 301:1018–1022, 1979

55. Pearl ER, Vogler LB, Okos AJ et al: B lymphocyte precursors in human bone marrow: An analysis of normal individuals and patients with antibody-deficiency states. J Immunol 120:1169–1175, 1978

56. Reisner Y, Kapoor N, Kirkpatrick D et al: Transplantation for severe combined immunodeficiency with HLA-A, B, D, DR incompatible parental marrow cells fractionated by soybean agglutinin and sheep red blood cells. Blood 61:341–348, 1983

57. Reinherz E, Geha R, Rappeport JM et al: Reconstitution after transplantation with T-lymphocyte-depleted HLA haplotype-mismatched bone marrow for severe combined immunodeficiency. Proc Natl Acad Sci USA 79:6047–6051, 1982

58. Shearer WT, Ritz J, Finegold MJ: Epstein-Barr virus-associated B-cell proliferations of diverse clonal origins after bone marrow transplantation in a 12-year-old patient with severe combined immunodeficiency. N Engl J Med 312:1151–1159, 1985

59. Raab–Traub N, Flynn K: The structure of the termini of the Epstein-Barr virus as a marker of clonal cellular proliferation. Cell 47:883–889, 1986

60. Penn I: Cancers following cyclosporine therapy. Transplantation 43:33–35, 1987

61. Starzl TE, Nalesnik MA, Porter KA et al: Reversibility of lymphomas and lymphoproliferative lesions developing under cyclosporine-steroid therapy. Lancet 1:583–587, 1984

62. Wang F, Blaese RM, Zoon KC, Tosato G: Suppressor T cell clones from patients with acute Epstein-Barr virus-induced infectious mononucleosis. J Clin Invest 79:7–14, 1987

Diagnosis and Evaluation of the Child with Cancer

part

two

five

Clinical Assessment and Differential Diagnosis of the Child with Suspected Cancer

Mark E. Nesbit, Jr.

SIGNS AND SYMPTOMS IN THE CHILD WITH CANCER

The diagnosis of cancer in a child starts with the history and physical examination. For a pediatric oncologist the index of suspicion for cancer is of course very high, but for the practicing physician the opposite is true. If anything, there is a general reluctance to consider such a diagnosis, since cancer still carries with it the fear of death. It should be remembered that even though the parents do not say so, they are often worried about whether a fever or lump represents cancer. It is not inappropriate for all concerned that this suspicion of cancer be there when the initial history is taken as long as the fear is not manifest as a delay in the diagnosis.

The history is the first step in the diagnostic process, with the chief complaint being the most important initial clue. What are the chief complaints that should increase the index of suspicion of cancer in a child? Listed in Table 5-1 are the more common ones. Some of the signs and symptoms that the public associates with cancer are in fact very rare in children. These include nose bleed, a nonhealing sore, bleeding from the rectum, a change in bowel habits, and chronic cough. Most of the signs and symptoms of childhood cancer are due either to a mass and its effect on surrounding normal structures or to secretion by the tumor of a substance that disturbs normal function. The former mechanism is by far the more common. However, significant advances have been made recently that identify cellular and extracellular tumor markers that may be responsible for some of the signs and symptoms of a malignancy, and although many of these cellular markers have no direct clinical application, they will in the future provide an important clue to the presence of a cancer (see Chap. 8).

Another important area in the history taking is the family's medical history. The history of the parents and siblings as well as of first cousins should be noted on a family tree or family group record. The minimal data collected should include a list of serious illnesses, family members' ages, and, if dead, the cause of death. The occurrence of any malignancy should be documented with as much demographic data as are available on the diagnosis. Certain familial and genetic diseases such as neurofibromatosis, Down's syndrome, and autoimmune diseases should be documented.

Both environmental and genetic factors have been associated with an increased risk of childhood cancer. Of the known environmental factors, ionizing radiation[1] and alkylating agents[2] are most commonly reported. More important when dealing with most pediatric tumors are genetic factors (Table 5-2). The major categories of disease with an increased risk of cancer are immune deficiency disorders, metabolic disorders, disorders of chromosomal instability, and the phakomatoses. There also are those children who have had one childhood cancer linked with an increased incidence of a second cancer. The association of osteosarcoma and bilateral retinoblastoma[3] and that of acute lymphocytic leukemia and brain tumors[4] are good examples (see Chap. 2).

At least 85% of the pediatric cancers are associated with the signs and symp-

Table 5-1
Common Chief Complaints Given by Parents That Suggest a Pediatric Cancer

Chief Complaints	Suggested Cancer
Chronic drainage from ear	Rhabdomyosarcoma; Langerhans cell histiocytosis
Recurrent fever with bone pain	Ewing's sarcoma; leukemia
Morning headache with vomiting	Brain tumor
Lump in neck that does not respond to antibiotics	Hodgkin's or non-Hodgkin's lymphomas
White dot in eye	Retinoblastoma
Swollen face and neck	Non-Hodgkin's lymphoma; leukemia
Mass in abdomen	Wilms' tumor
	Neuroblastoma; hepatoma
Paleness and fatigue	Leukemia; lymphoma
Limping	Osteosarcoma; other bone tumors
Bone pain	Leukemia; Ewing's sarcoma; neuroblastoma
Bleeding from vagina	Yolk sac tumor; rhabdomyosarcoma
Weight loss	Hodgkin's lymphoma

Table 5-2
Hereditary Diseases Predisposing to Childhood Cancer*

Disorder	Mechanism of Inheritance†	Cancer
"Phakomatoses"		
Neurofibromatosis	AD	Brain tumor, sarcoma, acute leukemia
Tuberous sclerosis	AD	Brain tumor
Nevoid basal-cell carcinoma syndrome	AD	Medulloblastoma Basal cell carcinoma
Metabolic disorders		
Glycogen storage disease IV	AR	Postcirrhotic hepatoma
Hereditary tyrosinemia	AR	Postcirrhotic hepatoma
Galactosemia	AR	Postcirrhotic hepatoma
Hypermethionemia	AR	Postcirrhotic hepatoma
Alpha-1-antitrypsin deficiency	AR	Postcirrhotic hepatoma
Immune deficiency disorders		
Bruton's agammaglobulinemia	SR	Leukemia, lymphoreticular
Severe combined immunodeficiency	SR	Leukemia, lymphoreticular
Wiskott-Aldrich syndrome	SR	Leukemia, lymphoreticular
Common variable immunodeficiency	?	Leukemia, lymphoreticular, brain
IgA deficiency	AD?	Lymphoreticular, gastrointestinal
Disorders of chromosomal stability or DNA repair		
Xeroderma pigmentosum	AR	Skin cancers, melanoma
Ataxia telangiectasia	AR	Lymphoreticular, ovarian, brain, gastrointestinal
Bloom's syndrome	AR	Acute leukemia, gastrointestinal, other
Fanconi's anemia	AR	Acute leukemia, hepatoma

* Reprinted in part with permission from Sutow WW, Fernbach DJ, Vietti JJ (eds): Clinical Pediatric Oncology. St Louis, CV Mosby, 1984.
† AD = autosomal dominant; AR = autosomal recessive; SR = sex-linked recessive.

toms listed in Tables 5-1 and 5-3. It is the other 15% of tumors —those associated with unusual signs and symptoms that make diagnosis more difficult. The most common pediatric tumor to be associated with unusual signs and symptoms is neuroblastoma (Table 5-4). Table 5-5 lists the unusual presentations for the other pediatric tumors.

ESTABLISHING THE DIAGNOSIS

Treatment of a malignancy can begin only after the tumor has been diagnosed. Recent radiologic techniques have dramatically improved the assessment for cancer, and we are now in the era of noninvasive techniques such as computed tomography (CT), diagnostic ultrasound, and magnetic resonance imaging (MRI) (see Chap. 7). It should be remembered, however, that even with these advances, the only sure way to establish the diagnosis of cancer is by pathologic confirmation.

When working up a child for a suspected cancer, it helps to discuss the overall plans with the parents and the child (if of appropriate age). Most parents are frustrated with the length of time that the diagnostic tests will take; for example, processing and examining the tissue specimen usually takes 2 or 3 days. This frustration is heightened when the signs and symptoms have persisted for months. It helps to emphasize to the parents that enough time must be taken to ensure the correct diagnosis and to determine the extent of the tumor accurately. Such care will prevent later errors and the need to repeat examinations and biopsies after treatment has begun.

Pathologic Diagnosis

After the clinical, laboratory, and roentgenographic examination and other tests point to the possibility of a neoplasm, the next decision is selection of the quickest and most reliable method to establish the pathologic diagnosis (see Chap. 6). Prior to obtaining any tissue for pathologic study, the primary physician should confer with both the surgeon and the pathologist and discuss the site to biopsy, the amount of tissue needed, and the specimens to be obtained. It is always better to remove enough material initially so that further biopsies are not necessary.

When it appears that the mass is localized to an organ such as the adrenal gland or the kidney and there is no evidence of metastatic disease, the approach is one of surgical exploration, with total extirpation if possible. Intraoperative frozen-section study is often unnecessary in such cases, since an immediate diagnosis is unlikely to alter the operative management, although review of the surgical margins may help determine the adequacy of the excision (e.g., in cases of a partial hepatectomy for hepatoblastoma or resection of a soft-tissue sarcoma).

Excisional and incisional biopsies are the standard techniques for obtaining tissue for a diagnosis, although recently Aspiration, Biopsy, Cytology (ABC) has been recommended in some clinical situations. An excisional biopsy is preferred by most pathologists because it yields the greatest amount of tissue and fewer artifactual distortions than does the smaller incisional biopsy. However, if an excisional biopsy could compromise future therapy in some fashion, then it should not be performed. The prototypical clinical situation for an excisional biopsy is the suspicious lymph node. Too often, an accessible lymph node is removed in fragments rather than as an intact structure. If a suspicious lesion is smaller than 4 cm and located superficially in the dermis or subcutaneous tissues, an excision would generally be recommended. A larger mass in a deeper location should be approached more cautiously with an incisional biopsy except when a total resection is contemplated.

Frozen-section examination is recommended during an incisional biopsy to be certain the lesion has been sampled. However, if the amount of tissue is small or if the surgeon is reluctant to remove additional tissue because of a difficult approach, a frozen section should not be performed. Disadvantages of the frozen section include artifact, exhaustion of tissue in the block through sectioning, and the loss of the opportunity to perform additional studies such as electron microscopy. On the other hand, frozen section of tissue that is subsequently fixed in Formalin generally does not interfere with the application of most immunohistochemical stains.

Regardless of the particular biopsy procedure, the tissue should be placed in 0.9% saline and immediately transported to the surgical pathology laboratory. This will ensure the most expeditious handling of the tissue for special studies such as cell markers, cytogenetics, freezing for a variety of analyses, preparation of a suspension for flow cytometry, and fixation for electron microscopy. It is desirable for a pathologist to be available to supervise these activities. A gross examination of the tissue is preferred beforehand so that a judgment can be made about the representativeness and adequacy of the specimen.

Aspiration, Biopsy, Cytology has generated a great deal of enthusiasm by virtue of its cost efficiency and reliability in experienced hands, and the procedure has been widely ap-

---

Table 5-3

Presenting Signs and Symptoms of Some Common Pediatric Cancers and Their Differential Diagnosis

Presenting Signs or Symptoms	Common Differential Diagnoses (nonmalignant conditions)	Cancer
Headache, morning vomiting	Migraine, sinusitis	Brain tumor
Lymphadenopathy	Infection	Lymphoma
Bone pain	Infection, trauma	Bone tumor
Abdominal mass	Constipation, kidney cyst, full bladder	Wilms' tumor
Mediastinal mass	Infection, cysts	Lymphoma
Pancytopenia	Infection	Leukemia
Bleeding	Coagulation disorders, platelet disorders	Leukemia

Table 5-4
Unusual Presentations of Childhood Neuroblastoma

Unusual signs and symptoms not related directly to tumor growth
  Chronic diarrhea[5]
  Polymyoclonus–opsoclonus[6]
  Cog-wheel erythrocytes[7]
  Failure to thrive[8]
  Cushing's syndrome[9]
  Pseudomuscular dystrophy*
  Congestive heart failure†
  Ondine's curse†

Unusual signs and symptoms related directly to tumor growth
  Horner's syndrome[10]
  Superior vena caval syndrome[11]
  Hydrocephalus
    Meningeal involvement[12]
    Cavernous or lateral sinus involvement[13]
    Choroid papilloma[14]
  Blindness[15]
  Subcutaneous nodules[16]
  Leukemoid reaction[17]
  Myasthenia gravis[18]
  Heterochromia[19]

* T Silberman, Marshfield (WI) Clinic; personal communication.
† Case records of the University of Minnesota Hospitals and Clinics.

plied in adults for thyroid or breast masses. The method also can be used for the more deeply situated mass, with thin-needle aspirations being guided by CT scan. The skill of the operator and the confidence of the cytopathologist are the critical elements for a reliable diagnosis. An ideal clinical indication for ABC is the child with a previously treated neoplasm who presents with a suspected recurrence.[56] The tumor type will have already been established by an earlier biopsy or excision, so that this is not a consideration unless there is a question of a second primary tumor. Even then, if the histologic types of the two primary tumors are sufficiently divergent, this may be appreciated even in the ABC. The recognition of a recurrent neuroblastoma or rhabdomyosarcoma in an ABC is usually straightforward. As the primary diagnostic procedure, however, the ABC does not yield sufficient material for the myriad special studies that most pediatric oncologists prefer before the institution of therapy for these tumors. It is certainly not practical to perform studies for N-*myc* gene amplification on an ABC of a neuroblastoma.

Electron microscopy, immunohistochemistry, immunophenotyping of suspected lymphomas, cytogenetic DNA analysis through flow cytometry, and oncogene amplification studies are specialized diagnostic procedures that are available in many laboratories (see Chap. 6). Few laboratories will have all of these techniques immediately available. The point cannot be overemphasized that these studies must be prefaced by an accurate pathologic diagnosis or reasonable differential diagnosis (see below). The pathologist is in the best position in most cases to decide the appropriate special studies in consultation with the clinician

Differential Diagnosis

The following section discusses some of the more common signs and symptoms seen with pediatric cancer and suggests a method of work-up for each one. Table 5-3 lists these signs and symptoms and their differential diagnosis.

Headaches

Headache is one of the most common symptoms seen in pediatric practice. Although few of these headaches are caused by an intracranial tumor, it is always important to rule out tumor when dealing with complaints of repeated headaches (see Chap. 24).

The diagnosis of a brain tumor is initially suspected on the basis of a symptom complex that most often depends on the site of the tumor. Because most brain tumors are situated so that they interfere with cerebrospinal fluid circulation, increased intracranial pressure is a common occurrence. An analysis of the early prominent symptoms in a group of children with brain tumors revealed that in supratentorial tumors, vomiting occurred in 46% of cases and headache in 43%, whereas in infratentorial tumors, 59% of patients had coordination difficulties, 76% vomited, and 56% had headache.[57]

Table 5-5
Unusual Presentations of Childhood Cancers Other Than Neuroblastoma

Cancer	Unusual Signs or Symptoms
Acute lymphoblastic leukemia	Hypercalcemia[20]
	Cyclic neutropenia[21]
	Eosinophilia[22]
	Pulmonary nodules[23]
	Lupus erythematosus[24]
	Isolated renal failure*
	Rheumatoid arthritis[25]
	Virus-associated hemophagocytic syndrome[26]
	Bone marrow necrosis[27]
	Skin nodules[28]
	Pericardial effusion[29]
	Aplastic anemia[30]
	Hypoglycemia[31]
Acute nonlymphocytic leukemia	Myelofibrosis[32]
	Mediastinal mass[33]
	Clitorism[34]
	Ovarian mass[35]
	Pericarditis[36]
	Chloroma[37]
Hodgkin's disease	Nephrotic syndrome[38]
	Pruritus[39]
	Acute dysautonomia[40]
	Dermatomyositis[41]
Germ cell tumor	Parinaud's syndrome[42]
Thymoma	Myasthenia gravis[43]
Central nervous system tumor	Diencephalic syndrome[44]
Wilms' tumor	Hypoglycemia[45]
	Uterine mass[46]
	Inferior vena cava thrombosis[47]
	Anemia[48]
Hepatoma/hepatocellular carcinoma	Erythrocytosis[49]
	Thrombocytopenia[50]
	Inferior vena cava thrombosis†
Ewing's sarcoma	Superior vena cava syndrome[51]
	Inflammatory syndrome[52]
Rhabdomyosarcoma	Pericardial effusion[53]
	Pulmonary bronchial cyst[54]
Chronic myelogenous leukemia	Priapism[55]

* WG Woods; case records of the University of Minnesota Hospitals and Clinics.
† Case records of the University of Minnesota Hospitals and Clinics.

With the advent of CT and MRI, noninvasive means are available to rule out a brain tumor (see Chaps. 7 and 24).[63] However, these tests cannot be recommended routinely for all children with headache or vomiting. Honig and Charney have analyzed the history, physical examination findings, and skull radiographs of 72 children with headaches secondary to a brain tumor. Their findings suggest that the best method of screening for tumor in a patient with a headache is a careful neurologic examination, since all but 5% to 6% of children with a headache and a brain tumor had an abnormal neurologic finding on clinical examination.[58]

Obtaining a good clinical history is extremely important. The following variables need to be determined: duration of symptoms, their location, timing, severity, precipitating events, and mode of onset. The study by Honig and Charney has indicated the importance of the following symptoms suggestive of brain tumors: recurrent morning headache, headaches that awaken the child, intense incapacitating headache, and changes in the quality, frequency, and pattern of the headaches.[58] The conditions that suggest the need for further radiologic examination are outlined in Table 5-6. As noted above, these examinations should be combined with a thorough neurologic examination.

Lymphadenopathy

Lymphadenopathy is a common presenting finding in children with both malignant and nonmalignant tumors. A lymph node is considered enlarged if it is more than 10 mm in its greatest diameter; exceptions are epitrochlear nodes, for which 5 mm is considered abnormal, and inguinal nodes, which are not considered abnormal unless they are larger than 15 mm. Most children have palpable small cervical, axillary, and inguinal nodes, but adenopathy in the posterior auricular, epitrochlear, or supraclavicular area is definitely abnormal.

Certainly, a thorough physical examination and history are essential. One of the first determinations to be made is whether the nodal enlargement is isolated or a part of a generalized lymphadenopathy. Most of the malignant diseases such as acute lymphoblastic leukemia and acute nonlymphocytic leukemia present with generalized rather than localized lymphadenopathy. In leukemia, regional lymphadenopathy that predominates in the noncervical areas is more suggestive of a malignancy than is enlargement around the head and neck. Of the other common malignant conditions that present with lymphadenopathy, non-Hodgkin's lymphoma and neuroblas-

toma are usually associated with other evidence of systemic disease such as a chest mass, abdominal mass, or peripheral blood changes.

Usually, there is no problem in categorizing generalized lymphadenopathy fairly quickly after a good history and physical examination and a few radiographic and blood tests. Much more difficult problems relate to localized enlargement, especially in the head and neck area. Infection is the most common cause for acute cervical adenopathy, with *Staphylococcus aureus* and beta-hemolytic *Streptococcus* the most common bacterial pathogens.[59] Other infectious causes are cat-scratch disease, nontuberculous mycobacteria, toxoplasmosis, Epstein–Barr virus, cytomegalovirus, and the Human Immunodeficiency Virus (HIV).

With chronic lymphadenopathy in the head and neck, malignancy becomes a more likely diagnosis. Although it is impossible to generalize, malignant tumors are usually firm, rubbery, and matted; and when seen over several examinations, they will increase in size. The primary malignant tumors that involve the head and neck in children are most often malignant lymphomas. Age is an important determining factor; in children under 6 years of age, the most common cancers are neuroblastoma, non-Hodgkin's lymphoma, rhabdomyosarcoma, and Hodgkin's lymphoma. From ages 7 to 13, Hodgkin's lymphoma and lymphosarcoma are the most common and are seen with equal frequency. Thyroid cancer and then rhabdomyosarcoma follow in frequency.

Lymphadenopathy in the mediastinum presents a diagnostic problem. In a report by Bower and coworkers of 173 cases of mediastinal masses, 41% were malignant neoplasms.[60] At the University of Minnesota, of 68 anterior or middle mediastinal masses, 43% proved to be Hodgkin's lymphoma, 25% non-Hodgkin's lymphoma, and 17% leukemia. Of interest, 9% were histoplasmosis[61] (see discussion of mediastinal masses below).

The diagnostic work-up for lymphadenopathy should include the important clues from the clinical presentation as a guide. In general, if a chronic lymphadenopathy is increasing in size, it should be biopsied. Children with mildly enlarged nodes at the first visit can be followed by serial examinations. Within 2 or 3 weeks, most noncancerous nodes should have returned to normal. In cases of localized cervical adenitis with moderate inflammation and fever, the child can be started on oral antibiotic therapy empirically. The coverage should include both *Streptococcus* and *Staphylococcus,* and anaerobic coverage should be included if a dental source is suspected. A complete blood count and a throat culture are indicated in these situations.

When a child either does not respond to antibiotic therapy or has a fluctuant lymph node or a node larger than 3 cm, a more extensive work-up is necessary. This should include a PPD skin test, chest radiography, complete blood count with a differential and platelet count, and cultures from other sites that may be the source of an infection. Viral, bacterial, and fungal serologies are useful only if indicated by the history and physical examination. A bone-marrow biopsy and aspiration are indicated if the chest film is abnormal or the blood work shows thrombocytopenia or anemia and there is significant hepatosplenomegaly.

The need for lymph node biopsy is suggested by the following signs and symptoms: (1) an enlarging node or nodes that remain enlarged after 2 to 3 weeks; (2) nodes that have not diminished in size after 5 to 6 weeks or that do not reach normal size by 10 to 12 weeks (especially if associated with unexplained fever, weight loss, or hepatosplenomegaly; enlarged supraclavicular or lower neck nodes should be biopsied earlier); and (3) any abnormal chest film finding. At the time of

---

Table 5-6
Conditions Suggesting Need for CT in Children with Headache

Presence or onset of neurologic abnormality
Ocular findings such as papilledema, decreased visual acuity, or loss of vision
Vomiting that is persistent, increasing in frequency, or preceded by recurrent headaches
Change in character of headache, such as increased severity and frequency
Recurrent morning headaches or headaches that repeatedly awaken child from sleep
Short stature or deceleration of linear growth
Diabetes insipidus
Age 3 years or less
Neurofibromatosis
Cured of acute lymphoblastic leukemia with irradiation of central nervous system as part of initial treatment

biopsy, the largest and firmest node should be taken for evaluation (also see Chap. 39). Material should be cultured for aerobic and anerobic bacteria and for mycobacteria. In endemic regions, fungal cultures (*e.g., Histoplasma, Cryptococcus*) should be done. In addition, the node should be examined by light and electron microscopy and portions sent for chromosomal analysis as well as for cell markers. When possible, extra material should be frozen to have available if other tests become necessary.

Bone Pain

Most pain associated with cancer is due to bone, nerve, or hollow viscus involvement (see Chap. 44). The early presentation of childhood cancer rarely includes pain except in cancer of the bone and leukemia. For the two most common malignant bone tumors in children (osteogenic sarcoma and Ewing's sarcoma), bone pain is common; in a series of 229 patients with Ewing's sarcoma, 89% had pain as a presenting symptom (see Chaps. 31 and 32).[62] This pain tends to be intermittent at first and increases in severity with time. A peculiarity of the pain associated with Ewing's sarcoma is that it often disappears spontaneously for weeks or months. A similar incidence of bone pain is seen with osteogenic sarcoma, with pain as a presenting symptom in 79% of the cases.[63] For both Ewing's sarcoma and osteogenic sarcoma, the time between the onset of symptoms and the diagnosis can be as long as 8 to 12 months.

Arthritis may be a prominent feature of acute leukemia, and leukemic arthritis can be mistaken for various rheumatic diseases. The presence of anemia or leukopenia or inconsistent bone scan results in a child with arthritis should prompt the physician to examine the bone marrow. Clinical findings and constitutional complaints do not help to differentiate the causes of bone pain. Bone pain as a presenting complaint of leukemia has been reported in 27% to 33% of cases.[64] Most of the cases are related to acute lymphocytic leukemia rather than to acute nonlymphocytic leukemia. A review of 107 consecutive children presenting with acute lymphoblastic leukemia reported 21% with bone pain and 44% with radiologic bone changes.[65] A significant correlation was found between the severity of the bone pain and the number of bones involved on radiography, but there was no significant correlation between the presence or absence of bone pain and the prognosis.

If a child complains of persistent pain, especially if the pain is associated with swelling, mass, or limitation of motion, a radiograph should be obtained promptly and examined by an experienced observer. Although the films are extremely important in judging the extent of the abnormality and the behavior of the skeletal lesion, they should not be used to make a definitive diagnosis of the cause, since there are no pathognomonic radiologic signs of malignant bone lesions. Biopsy and pathologic study are absolutely necessary to establish the diagnosis.

Abdominal Masses

A palpable abdominal mass is the most common sign that should suggest the diagnosis of a malignant solid tumor, although statistically the mass is most likely to be either benign or a pseudotumor such as feces, the abdominal aorta, a distended bladder, or hydronephrotic kidneys. For example, in a report by Melicow and Uson on 653 palpable abdominal masses seen in children from 1934 to 1956, 293 (45%) had a nonmalignant cause.[66]

The age of the patient is a helpful clue. For an abdominal mass in a newborn infant, a renal cause is most common; if the mass turns out to be malignant, it will most likely be a Wilms' tumor or a neuroblastoma (Table 5-7) (see Chap. 27). In older patients, a mass is more likely to be secondary to leukemia or to lymphomatous involvement of the liver and spleen. Despite the statistics, all suspicious abdominal masses require work-up to ensure that the proper diagnosis is made. Histologic confirmation is always necessary. Although a great deal has been written about the importance of the size, mobility, and consistency of a mass, such information is unrewarding in determining its nature.

In the history, it helps to determine whether there have been symptoms referable to the abdominal mass and, if so, their type and duration. Because of the high incidence of a renal cause for an abdominal mass, a good history relative to the urinary tract is important.

The initial step in working up an abdominal mass is a good abdominal examination. This is frequently not easy. Every attempt should be made to have the child relaxed before palpating the abdomen. Attempting to divert the child's attention is perhaps the best method but does not always work. For a younger child, a bottle or pacifier can be helpful. When examining the abdomen, it is always important to remember that a number of structures are palpable in normal children (liver edge, spleen, kidneys, aorta, sigmoid colon, feces, and spine). If the abdominal mass is suspected of being feces, it may be practical to give an enema and reexamine the patient. Similarly, if the mass is suspected to be the bladder, it may be necessary to catheterize the patient and repeat the examination. A rectal examination is absolutely necessary. Vaginal and pelvic examinations are important in the older adolescent female, but bimanual abdominal and rectal examinations are preferred to vaginal examinations in infants and younger girls. Pelvic examinations should be performed by an experienced physician.

Table 5-7
Relative Incidence of Retroperitoneal Tumors in 442 Cases*

Retroperitoneal Tumors (442 cases)	Number of Patients
Kidney	
Wilms' tumor	202
Other malignant tumors	10
Benign tumors	18
Sympathetic tumors	
Neuroblastomas with metastases at presentation	125
Neuroblastomas without metastases	60
Neuroblastomas (Pepper's syndrome)	15
Ganglioneuromas	5
Adrenocortical tumors	7
Malignant lymphomas	65
Liver	
Benign tumors	9
Malignant tumors	14
Ovary	
Dysgerminomas	4
Teratomas	27
Embryonic sarcomas	22
Other	9

* Data from the Institut Gustave-Roussy as presented in Shweisguth 0 (ed): Solid Tumors in Children. New York, John Wiley & Sons, 1982. Reprinted with permission.

After the physical examination has been completed, the work-up should proceed to radiologic examination: a flat plate of the abdomen with anteroposterior and lateral views, a chest film, and abdominal CT with and without contrast. A urinalysis and stool specimen (examined for guaiac positivity) are helpful. The results will suggest the need for any further tests such as ultrasonography, intravenous urography, tumor marker assays, and bone-marrow examination.

Mediastinal Masses

A number of benign and malignant tumors are found in the thorax, and the mediastinum is the site of most intrathoracic masses in children. The location of the masses in one of the three anatomic regions of the mediastinum suggests important clues to the nature of the mass. (Fig. 5-1). The posterior mediastinum is bounded posteriorly by the anterior surface of the curve of the ribs, anteriorly by the posterior border of the pericardium, and inferiorly by the diaphragm. The anterior mediastinum is bounded by the first rib superiorly, by the posterior surface of the sternum anteriorly, by the anterior border of the upper dorsal vertebra posteriorly, and by a curved line along the cardiac border extending back to the border of the dorsal vertebra. The middle mediastinum occupies the area between the other two regions, with its base on the diaphragm (Fig. 5-1).

The common lesions in the anterior mediastinum are lymphoid tumors, bronchogenic cysts, aneurysms, lipomas, and thyroid tumors. In the middle mediastinum, lymph node le-

sions, angiomas, pericardial cysts, teratomas, bronchogenic cysts, esophageal lesions, and hernias through the foramen of Morgagni are found. In the posterior mediastinum, neurogenic tumors are some of the most common tumors, accounting for approximately 20% of all primary mediastinal tumors and cysts.[67] These lesions arise from the nerve roots and sympathetic ganglia in the paravertebral sulcus. The types seen are neuroblastomas, ganglioneuroblastomas, neurilemomas, neurofibromas, ganglioneuromas, and pheochromocytomas. The other masses seen in the posterior mediastinum are bronchogenic and enterogenous cysts, thoracic meningocele, and malignant tumors such as Ewing's sarcoma, lymphoma, and rhabdomyosarcoma.

Patients with mediastinal tumors may be asymptomatic or may present with symptoms secondary to compression or erosion of the adjacent organs, such as the respiratory tract (cough, stridor, and hemoptysis) (see Chap. 37). Commonly, the mass is discovered during routine chest radiographs. Tomography, barium swallow, fluoroscopy, ultrasound, and CT scans may be helpful in localizing and identifying mediastinal tumors (see Chap. 7). In all cases, however, the definitive diagnosis has to await histologic examination.

After the usual infectious causes of hilar adenopathy or mediastinal masses have been ruled out, it is necessary to perform a CT scan of the chest and more invasive diagnostic procedures. A bone-marrow aspiration and biopsy for evaluation of both tumor and infection are indicated. If marrow and lung tests are negative, then either mediastinotomy or open biopsy is indicated to obtain tissue for histologic study.

One of the common malignant diagnoses made on tissue from the mediastinum is tumors classified as small blue round-cell tumors (see Chap. 6). These include Ewing's sarcoma, soft-tissue Ewing's sarcoma, rhabdomyosarcoma, lymphoma, and a leukemic mass. Electron microscopy, histochemical evaluation, and cell-membrane studies may be necessary to establish a definitive diagnosis. If one is in doubt and a portion of a rib is involved, resection of the rib above and below the lesion as well as resection of the rib and intercostal muscle along with the tumor is justified. This procedure satisfies the criteria for treatment of Ewing's sarcoma, rhabdomyosarcoma, and small blue round-cell tumors of thoracopulmonary origin (see Chaps. 29, 30, and 31).

Pancytopenia and Leukocytosis

PANCYTOPENIA. Anemia, leukopenia, and thrombocytopenia occur alone or in combination as a common presenting sign in acute leukemia of childhood, both lymphocytic and nonlymphocytic (see Chaps. 16 and 17). In 936 newly diagnosed and untreated children with acute lymphoblastic leukemia, 51% presented with hemoglobin less than 7.5 g/dl, 73% presented with platelet counts less than 150,000/mm^3 and 30% presented with a total peripheral white blood cell counts of less than 5,000/mm^3.[68] A similar analysis of 171 children with acute nonlymphocytic leukemia revealed that 82% presented with platelet counts less than 100,000/mm^3 and 39% presented with a total white blood cell count of less than 5,000/mm^3. This pancytopenia is primarily due to replacement of the bone marrow by tumor, although such replacement often does not completely explain the degree of pancytopenia. There are other explanations for anemia associated with malignancy (see Chap. 38). In general, the anemia is characterized as one of chronic disease. Autoimmune hemolytic anemias are reported with lymphoma. Except with marrow involvement, leukopenia is rarely a part of extramedullary malignancies. This is also true of thrombocytopenia except for the rare instance of idiopathic thrombocytopenia purpura

FIGURE 5-1. Principal anatomic regions of mediastinum with most common types of masses.

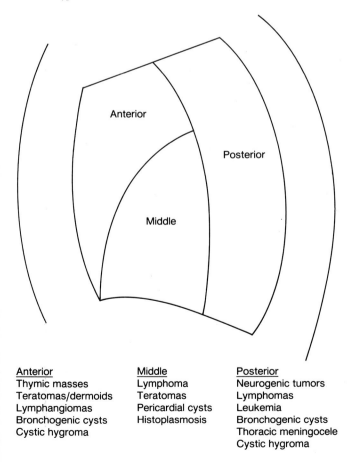

Anterior	Middle	Posterior
Thymic masses	Lymphoma	Neurogenic tumors
Teratomas/dermoids	Teratomas	Lymphomas
Lymphangiomas	Pericardial cysts	Leukemia
Bronchogenic cysts	Histoplasmosis	Bronchogenic cysts
Cystic hygroma		Thoracic meningocele
		Cystic hygroma

associated with Hodgkin's disease or the low platelet counts seen with disseminated intravascular coagulopathy, which may occur with widely disseminated sarcomas such as rhabdomyosarcoma and neuroblastoma.

Any other malignancy that involves the marrow also can produce pancytopenia or depression of only one of the cell lines. The tumors that most often involve the bone marrow are neuroblastoma, lymphomas, and, less commonly, Ewing's sarcoma and rhabdomyosarcoma.

LEUKOCYTOSIS. An elevated white blood cell count (leukocytosis) is commonly seen with acute leukemia of childhood (Chap. 16 and 17). Counts of greater than 10,000/mm³ are reported in 45% of children with acute lymphoblastic leukemia; 10% will have an initial count of greater than 100,000/mm³.[68] Among newly diagnosed cases of acute nonlymphocytic leukemia, 21% of patients will have white blood cell counts of greater than 100,000/mm³.[69] Most nonmalignant cases of leukocytosis are due to infections, especially staphylococcal and pneumococcal infections. Exaggerated elevations (leukemoid reactions) of greater than 50,000/mm³ may occur with septicemia, especially with infections due to *Staphylococcus, Haemophilus influenzae,* meningococcus, and *Salmonella.*[70] Lymphoid leukemoid reactions have been observed in infectious lymphocytosis[71] and mumps,[72] varicella,[73] adenovirus,[74] cytomegalovirus,[75] and pertussis[76] infections. Peripheral white cell counts greater than 100,000/mm³ are almost always due to acute or chronic leukemia. A myeloid leukemoid reaction (100,000/mm³) has been reported in premature infants whose mothers received corticosteroids during pregnancy.[77] Leukocytosis due to exaggerated eosinophilia, with white blood cell counts in the range of 20,000 to 100,000/mm³ with predominantly eosinophils, is often seen with parasitic infections, especially visceral larval migrans.[78] Other nonmalignant causes of eosinophilia include the hypereosinophilic syndrome, periarteritis nodosa, allergy, and hypersensitivity reactions. The

Table 5-8
*Predominant Pediatric Cancers by Age and Site**

Tumors	Newborn (<1 year)	Infancy (1–3 years)	Child (3–11 years)	Adolescent and Young Adult (12–21 years)
Leukemias	Congenital leukemia AML AMMoL CML-juvenile	ALL AML CML-juvenile	ALL AML	AML ALL
Lymphomas	Very rare	Lymphoblastic	Lymphoblastic Undifferentiated	Lymphoblastic Undifferentiated Burkitt's Hodgkin's
Solid CNS tumors	Medulloblastoma Ependymoma Astrocytoma Choroid plexus papilloma	Medulloblastoma Ependymoma Astrocytoma Choroid plexus papilloma	Cerebellar astrocytoma Medulloblastoma Astrocytoma Edendymoma Craniopharyngioma	Cerebellar astrocytoma Astrocytoma Craniopharyngioma Medulloblastoma
Head and neck	Retinoblastoma Rhabdomyosarcoma Neuroblastoma Multiple endocrine neoplasia	Retinoblastoma Rhabdomyosarcoma Neuroblastoma	Rhabdomyosarcoma Lymphoma	Lymphoma Rhabdomyosarcoma
Thoracic	Neuroblastoma Teratoma	Neuroblastoma Teratoma	Lymphoma Neuroblastoma Rhabdomyosarcoma	Lymphoma Ewing's sarcoma Rhabdomyosarcoma
Abdominal	Neuroblastoma Mesoblastic nephroma Hepatoblastoma Wilms' tumor (>6 mon)	Neuroblastoma Wilm's tumor Hepatoblastoma Leukemia	Neuroblastoma Wilm's tumor Lymphoma Hepatoma	Lymphoma Hepatocellular carcinoma Rhabdomyosarcoma

Gonadal	Yolk sac tumor of testis
	  (endodermal sinus
	  tumor)
	Teratoma
	Sarcoma botryoides
	Neuroblastoma
		Rhabdomyosarcoma
		Yolk sac tumor of testis
		Clear-cell sarcoma
		  (kidney)
			Rhabdomyosarcoma	Rhabdomyosarcoma
				Dysgerminoma
				Teratocarcinoma,
				  teratoma
				Embryonal carcinoma of
				  testis
				Embryonal carcinoma
				  and endodermal
				  sinus tumors of
				  ovary

Extremity	Fibrosarcoma	Fibrosarcoma Rhabdomyosarcoma	Rhabdomyosarcoma Ewing's sarcoma	Osteosarcoma Rhabdomyosarcoma Ewing's sarcoma

* Reprinted with permission from Pizzo PA, Miser JS, Casady JR, Fuller RM: Solid tumors of childhood. In DeVita VT Jr, Hellman S, Rosenberg SA (eds): Cancer: Principles and Practice of Oncology, 2nd ed, pp 1511–1589. Philadelphia, JB Lippincott, 1985.

malignant causes are eosinophilic leukemia, Hodgkin's disease, and acute lymphoid leukemia (see Chaps. 16, 17, 19, and 21).

WORK-UP OF PANCYTOPENIA AND LEUKOCYTOSIS.   Careful assessment for infectious causes is of paramount importance in working up a patient with abnormal peripheral blood counts. A bone-marrow study is the most appropriate means to rule out malignant causes. The indications for bone-marrow examination include (1) finding of atypical or blast cells on peripheral blood smears; (2) significant depression of more than one blood cell element; (3) association with unexplained lymphadenopathy or hepatosplenomegaly; and (4) absence of an infectious cause for the blood abnormality. Both aspiration and biopsy are required to determine morphology and marrow cellularity.

Bleeding

Bleeding is an uncommon initial sign in children with cancer. When it does occur, it is usually related to thrombocytopenia and marrow involvement (see Chap. 38). In newly diagnosed acute leukemia, bleeding can also be related to impaired platelet function if the patient has been treated with aspirin or non-steroidal anti-inflammatory drugs for fever or bone pain. Also, high-dose penicillin, carbenicillin, ticarcillin, and moxalactam have been associated with platelet dysfunction and can add to the bleeding tendency of these patients.[79] Although coagulation abnormalities can be associated with disseminated malignancies, they rarely cause signs or symptoms unless disseminated intravascular coagulation occurs. This complication has been reported in acute lymphocytic leukemia (especially T-cell), lymphoma, rhabdomyosarcoma, and the acute nonlymphocytic leukemias.[80] A very high incidence is present in acute promyelocytic leukemia (M3) and to a lesser extent with myelomonocytic leukemia (M4) and acute monoblastic leukemia (M5a) when associated with initial leukocytosis.[81,82]

When significant bleeding is encountered as a presenting sign, acute leukemia must be ruled out. This requires examination of the peripheral blood, with a complete blood count, and a bone-marrow aspiration. Initial work-up of bleeding usually also requires comprehensive screening coagulation studies using a standard panel of tests: one-stage prothrombin time (PT), activated partial thromboplastin time (PTT), thrombin time (TT), fibrinogen level, serum fibrin–fibrinogen degradation (split products), and platelet count. In disseminated intravascular coagulation, the PT is prolonged and the PTT usually prolonged; the TT is slightly prolonged, and fibrinogen is decreased with decreased platelet count and the presence of fibrin degradation products. The presence of fibrin degradation products usually separates disseminated coagulation from other causes of bleeding that are associated with abnormal PT, PTT, and fibrinogen levels. Only rarely will the bleeding associated with malignancy be difficult to detect clinically. Consultation with coagulation experts will assist in selecting more specialized studies.

SUMMARY

Throughout this chapter, there has been an emphasis on the influence of the signs and symptoms on making the diagnosis of cancer in children. As shown in Table 5-8, the impact of age and site is also important and should be considered when working up a sick child. With recent technical advances, the armamentarium of diagnostic tests available to establish the diagnosis of malignant diseases is extensive. Unfortunately, if the possibility of a cancer is never considered by the physician, there is an increased chance of making a mistake or delaying the diagnosis. Although the incidence of malignant disease in children is low, the impact of cancer makes it imperative that all professionals handling children have a high index of suspicion of cancer.

This investigation was supported by Public Health Service grant CA07306 awarded by the National Cancer Institute and by the Children's Cancer Research Fund of the University of Minnesota.

REFERENCES

1. Bithell JF, Steward AM: Prenatal irradiation and childhood malignancy: A review of British data from the Oxford survey. Br J Cancer 31:271–287, 1975
2. Reiner RR, Hoover R, Fraumeni JF Jr et al: Acute leukemia after alkylating-agent therapy of ovarian cancer. N Engl J Med 297:177–181, 1977
3. Farwell J, Flannery JT: Cancer in relatives of children with central nervous system neoplasms. N Engl J Med 311:749–753, 1984
4. Meadows AT, Baum E, Fossati-Bellani F et al: Second malignant neoplasm in children: An update from the Late Effects Study Group. J Clin Oncol 3:532–538, 1985
5. Ilda Y, Nose O, Kai H et al: Watery diarrhea with vasoactive intestinal peptide-producing ganglioneuroblastoma. Arch Dis Childh 55:929–936, 1980
6. Altman AJ, Baehner RL: Favorable prognosis for survival in children with coincidental opsomyoclonus and neuroblastoma. Cancer 37:846–852, 1976
7. Williams TH, House RF, Burgert EO et al: Unusual manifestations of neuroblastoma: Chronic diarrhea, polymyoclonia–opsoclonus and erythrocyte abnormalities. Cancer 29:475–480, 1972
8. Balakrishnan V, Rice MS, Simpson DA: Spinal neuroblastoma: Diagnosis, treatment, and prognosis. J Neurosurg 40:631–638, 1974
9. Cummins GE, Cohen D: Cushing's syndrome secondary to ACTH-secreting Wilms' tumor. J Pediatr Surg 9:535–539, 1974
10. Bukerman BL, Seaver R: Congenital Horner's syndrome and thoracic neuroblastoma. J Pediatr Ophthalmol Strabismus 15:24–25, 1978
11. Familusi TB, Samuel I, Jaiyesimi et al: Superior vena cava occlusion in a 12 year old girl with neuroblastoma. Clin Pediatr 16:1160–1172, 1977
12. Farr GH, Hajdu SI: Exfoliative cytology of metastatic neuroblastoma. Acta Cytol 16:203–206, 1972
13. Mones RJ: Increased intracranial pressure due to metastatic disease of venous sinuses. Neurology 152:1000–1007, 1965
14. Krivit C: Central nervous system presentation of a child with neuroblastoma. Northwest Pediatric Abstract, 1986
15. Donohus JP, Garrett RA, Baehner RL, Thomas MH: The multiple manifestations of neuroblastoma. J Urol 111:260–264, 1974
16. D'Angio GJ, Evans AE, Koop CE: Special pattern of widespread neuroblastoma with a favourable prognosis. Lancet 12:1046–1049, 1971
17. Gaffrey PC, Hausman CF, Fetterman GH: Experience with smears of aspirates from bone marrow in the diagnosis of neuroblastoma. Am J Clin Pathol 31:213–221, 1959
18. Robinson MJ, Howard RN: Neuroblastoma presenting as myasthenia gravis in a child age 3 years. Pediatrics 43:111–113, 1969
19. Albert DM, Rubenstein RA, Scheie HG: Tumor metastasis to the eye. Am J Ophthalmol 63:727–738, 1967
20. Cohn SL, Margon ER, Mallette LE: The spectrum of metabolic bone disease in lymphoblastic leukemia. Cancer 59:346–350, 1987
21. Lensink DB, Barton A, Applebaum FR, Hammond WP: Cyclic neutropenia as a premalignant manifestation of acute lymphoblastic leukemia. Am J Hematol 22:9–16, 1986
22. Troxell ML, Mills GM, Allen RC: The hypereosinophilic syndrome in acute lymphocytic leukemia. Cancer 54:1058–1061, 1984
23. Corbaton J, Munoz A, Modero L, Camarero C: Pulmonary leukemia in a child presenting with infiltrative and nodular lesions. Pediatr Radiol 14:431–432, 1984
24. Saulsbury FT, Sabid H, Conrad D, Kesler RW, Levien G: Acute leukemia with features of systemic lupus erythematosus. J Pediatr 105:57–62, 1984
25. Saulsbury FT, Sabid H: Acute leukemia presenting as arthritis in children. Clin Pediatr 24:625–628, 1985

26. Risdall RJ, McKenna RW, Nesbit M et al: Virus-associated hemophagocytic syndrome. Cancer 44:993–1002, 1979
27. Niebrugge DJ, Benjamin DR: Bone marrow necrosis preceding acute lymphoblastic leukemia in childhood. Cancer 52:2162–2164, 1983
28. Dunn NL, McWilliams NB, Mohanokumer T: Clinical and immunological correlates of leukemia cutis in childhood. Cancer 50:2049–2051, 1982
29. Mancuso L, Marchi S, Giuliano P, Pitrolo F: Cardiac tamponade as first manifestation of acute lymphoblastic leukemia in a patient with echographic evidence of mediastinal lymph nodal enlargement. Am Heart J 110:1303–1304, 1985
30. Alarcon PA, Miller ML, Stuart MJ: Erythroid hypoplasia. Am J Dis Child 132:763–764, 1978
31. Canivet B, Squara P, Elbaze P et al: Consommation de glucose in vitro au cours des grandes hyperleucocytoses. Une cause d'hypoglycemie factice. Pathol Biol 30:843–846, 1982
32. Cairney AG, McKenna R, Arthur DC et al: Acute megakaryoblastic leukaemia in children. Br J Haematol 63:541–554, 1986
33. Baanerjee D, Silva E: Mediastinal mass with acute leukemia. Arch Pathol Lab Med 105:126–129, 1981
34. Williams DL, Bell BA, Ragash AH: Clitorism at presentation of acute non-lymphocytic leukemia. J Pediatr 106:754–757, 1985
35. Morgan ER, Labotka RJ, Gonzalez-Crussi F et al: Ovarian granulocytic sarcoma as the primary manifestation of acute infantile myelomonocytic leukemia. Cancer 48:1819–1824, 1981
36. Chu J, Demello D, O'Connor DM et al: Pericarditis as presenting manifestation of acute non-lymphocytic leukemia in a young child. Cancer 52:322–324, 1983
37. Rajantie J, Tarkkanen A, Rapola J et al: Orbital granulocytic sarcoma as a presenting sign in acute myelogenous leukemia. Opthalmologica 189:158–161, 1984
38. Powderly WG, Cantwell BM, Fennelly JJ èt al: Renal glomerulopathies associated with Hodgkin's disease. Cancer 56:874–875, 1985
39. Higgins FK: Hodgkin's disease. In Molander DW, Pack GT (eds): Hodgkin's Disease. Springfield, IL, Charles C Thomas, 1968
40. Van Lieshout JJ, Wieley W, Van Montfrans GA et al: Acute dysautonomia associated with Hodgkin's disease. J Neurol Neurosurg Psychiatr 49:830–832, 1986
41. Dowsett RJ, Wong RL, Robert NJ, Abeles M: Dermatomyositis and Hodgkin's disease. Am J Med 80:719–723, 1986
42. Barrett A: Germ cell tumors. In Voute PA, Barrett A, Bloom HJG, Lemerle J, Neidhardt MK (eds): Cancer in Children. pp. 185–196. Berlin, Springer-Verlag, 1986
43. Furman WL, Buckley PJ, Green AA, Stokes DC, Chien LT: Thymoma and myasthenia gravis in a 4 year old child. Cancer 56:2703–2706, 1985
44. Nellhaus G: Brain tumors in childhood. Pediatr Ann 2:18–38, 1974
45. Loutfi AH, Mehrez I, Shahbender S et al: Hypoglycemia with Wilms' tumor. Arch Dis Childh 39:197–203, 1964
46. Bittencourt AL, Britto JF, Fonseca LE: Wilms' tumor of the uterus. Cancer 47:2496–2499, 1981
47. Slovis TL, Philppart AI, Cushing B: Evaluation of the inferior vena cava by sonography and venography in children with renal and hepatic tumors. Radiology 140:767–772, 1981
48. Ramsay NKC, Dehner LP, Coccia PF et al: Acute hemorrhage into Wilms' tumor: A cause of rapidly developing abdominal mass with hypertension, anemia and fever. J Pediatr 91:763–765, 1977
49. Jacobson RJ, Lowenthal MN, Kew MC: Erythrocytosis in hepatocellular cancer. S Afr Med J 53:658–660, 1978
50. Nickerson HJ, Silberman T: Hepatoblastoma, thrombocytosis and increased thrombopoietin. Cancer 45:315–317, 1980
51. Dvorak PF, Vorlicky LN, Nesbit ME: Ewing's sarcoma presenting as the superior mediastinal syndrome. Clin Pediatr 10:607–610, 1971
52. Wang CC, Schulz M: Ewing's sarcoma: A study of fifty cases treated at the Massachusetts General Hospital, 1930–1952 inclusive. N Engl J Med 248:571–576, 1953
53. Small EJ, Gordon GJ, Dahms BB: Malignant rhabdoid tumor of the heart in an infant. Cancer 55:2850–2853, 1985
54. Allan BT, Day DL, Dehner LP: Primary pulmonary rhabdomyosarcoma of the lung in children. Cancer 59:1005–1011, 1987
55. Spiers AS: Chronic granulocytic leukemia. Med Clin North Am 68:713–727, 1984
56. Frable WJ: Fine needle aspiration biopsy—a review. Hum Pathol 14:9–28, 1983
57. Bergstrand CG, Bergstedt J, Herrlin KM: Pediatric aspects of brain tumors in infancy and childhood. Acta Paediatr 47:688–705, 1958
58. Honig PJ, Charney EB: Children with brain tumor headaches. Am J Dis Child 136:121–124, 1982
59. Lascari AD: Hematological Manifestations of Childhood Diseases. New York, Thieme-Stratton, 1984
60. Bower RJ, Kiesewetter WB: Mediastinal masses in infants and children. Arch Surg 112:1003–1009, 1977
61. Woods WG, Singher L, Krivit W, Nesbit ME: Histoplasmosis simulating lymphoma in children. J Pediatr Surg 14:423–425, 1979
62. Pritchard DJ, Dahlin DC, Dauphine RT et al: Ewing's sarcoma. J Bone Joint Surg 57A:10–16, 1975
63. McKenna BJ, Schwinn CD, Soong KY et al: Sarcoma of the osteogenic series: Analysis of 552 cases. J Bone Joint Surg 48A:1–26, 1966
64. Hann IM, Guptas, Palmer MK, Morris-Jones PH: The prognostic significance of radiologic and symptomatic bone involvement in childhood acute lymphoblastic leukemia. Med Pediatr Oncol 6:51–55, 1979
65. Rogalsky RJ, Black B, Reed MH: Orthopaedic manifestations of leukemia in children. J Bone Joint Surg 68A:494–501, 1986
66. Melicow MM, Uson AC: Palpable abdominal masses in infants and children: A report based on a review of 653 cases. J Urol 81:705–710, 1959
67. Leonard AS, Alyono D, Fischel RJ et al: Role of the surgeon in the treatment of children's cancer. Surg Clin North Am 65:1387–1422, 1985
68. Robison LL, Sather H, Coccia PF et al: Assessment of the interrelationship of prognostic factors in childhood acute lymphoblastic leukemia. Am J Pediatr Hematol Oncol 2:5–13, 1980
69. Choi S-I, Simone JV: Acute nonlymphocytic leukemia in 171 children. Med Pediatr Oncol 2:119–146, 1976
70. Holland P, Mauer AM: Myeloid leukemoid reactions in children. Am J Dis Child 105:568–575, 1963
71. Barnes GR, Yannet H, Liberman R: A clinical outbreak of infectious lymphocytosis. Am J Med Sci 218:646–654, 1954
72. Garcia R, Rasch CA: Leukemoid reactions to mumps virus. N Engl J Med 271:251–252, 1964
73. Goldman D: Chickenpox with a blood picture simulating that in leukemia. Am J Dis Child 40:1282–1284, 1930
74. Connor JD: Evidence for an etiologic role of adenoviral infections in pertussis syndrome. N Engl J Med 283:390–394, 1970
75. Okum DB, Tanaka KR: Profound leukemoid reaction in cytomegalovirus mononucleosis. JAMA 240:1888–1894, 1978
76. Brooksaler F, Nelson JD: Pertussis: A reappraisal and report of 190 confirmed cases. Am J Dis Child 114:389–396, 1967
77. Bielwaski D, Hiatt IM, Hegyi T: Betamethasone-induced leukaemoid reaction in premature infants (letter). Lancet 1:218, 1978
78. Lukens JN: Eosinophila in children. Pediatr Clin North Am 19:969–979, 1972
79. Brown CH, Bradshaw MW, Natelson EA et al: Defective platelet function following the administration of penicillin compounds. Blood 47:949–956, 1976
80. Hasegawa DK, Bloomfield CD: Thrombotic and hemorrhagic manifestions of malignancy In Yarbo JW, Bornstein R (eds): Oncologic Emergencies, pp. 141–196. New York, Grune and Stratton, 1981
81. Hasegawa DK: Coagulation abnormalities in acute leukemia. Lab Med 17:388–394, 1986
82. Ribeiro RC, Pui C-H: The clinical and biological correlates of coagulopathy in children with acute leukemia. J Clin Oncol 4:1212–1218, 1986

six

Pathology in Pediatric Oncology

Timothy J. Triche and Andrea O. Cavazzana

Historical Perspective

Before the advent of combination therapy, precise diagnoses of childhood cancers were generally neither relevant nor required. Wilms' tumor was Wilms' tumor; no prognostic subtypes were known, particularly since virtually all children with the disease died. With the appearance of chemotherapy and radiation, however, all this changed. The first National Wilms' Tumor Study Group quickly documented certain unfavorable histopathologic groups; patients with localized disease (stage I) whose tumors displayed features of anaplasia proved to have a markedly worse survival (about 5%) than those whose tumors had conventional histologic appearance (survival better than 90%).[1] Thus, for the first time, pathologic analysis was directly related to prognosis within a tumor type. It must be emphasized that this prognostic significance became evident only with effective therapy; those types of tumors that proved resistant to treatment were necessarily all considered "poor prognosis," and histopathologic distinctions remained irrelevant.

As effective treatment regimens were developed for a variety of other childhood tumors, similar prognostic distinctions emerged. Embryonal rhabdomyosarcoma appears to be less aggressive and more amenable to treatment than alveolar rhabdomyosarcoma, for example.[2] Telangiectatic osteosarcoma appears more lethal than conventional forms.[3] Lymphoblastic lymphoma appears more treatment resistant than Burkitt's lymphoma.[4] Even neuroblastoma, for which little effective therapy beyond surgery can be offered, appears to be divisible at least into "better" and "worse" prognostic groups based on features such as the mitosis/karyorrhexis index, presence of foci of primitive neuroblastic cells, and diffuse versus fibrous trabecular pattern.[5]

Beyond the recognition of more- or less-aggressive subtypes of conventional childhood tumors, the widespread development of effective treatment protocols tailored to specific tumor types has necessitated accurate diagnosis of even the most primitive forms of childhood cancer, the so-called small round blue-cell tumors. The response of each tumor is generally best when the patient is treated according to the specific protocol developed for that tumor; disastrous results can be expected in many cases when erroneous diagnoses lead to inappropriate therapy. One need only consider the differential treatment response of Ewing's sarcoma, metastatic neuroblastoma, and primary lymphoma of bone to appreciate the importance of distinguishing one from another.

Age Distribution of Childhood Cancer

Another important consideration in the pathologic evaluation of childhood tumors is their occurrence in adults. Because of the conventional separation of pediatric and adult patient populations, highly artificial separation of certain childhood and adult tumors occurs. Most oncologists and pathologists are unaware, for example, that the third most common solid tumor of childhood (rhabdomyosarcoma) occurs in two major forms with a distinctive bimodal age distribution; the second, ascribable to the alveolar type, actually peaks around 15 to 16 years of age, just at the outside limits of most pediatric populations, and occurs in patients 30 to 40 years of age.[2] Similarly, Ewing's sarcoma, Burkitt's lymphoma, osteosarcoma, acute lymphocytic leukemia, gliomas, and even neuroblastoma and Wilms' tumor have been described in adults. Conversely, hepatocellular carcinoma, renal cell carcinoma, adrenocortical carcinoma, and melanoma are found in children.[6] Thus, it is imperative to approach each tumor with an open mind and an awareness of the possibilities.

The Current Approach to Childhood Tumor Diagnosis

Pathology, like all areas of medicine, has benefited greatly from the enormous increase in biomedical research since World War II. New techniques, equipment, and basic knowledge have irrevocably altered the methods used to arrive at a diagnosis. Before 1945, gross examination and light microscopy in conjunction with clinical information were the only tools available to derive a diagnosis. Since then, histochemistry, electron microscopy, immunocytochemistry, cytogenetics, hybridoma technology, and molecular genetics, to name some of the more important methods, have been developed and applied routinely to the problems of tumor classification. The tools available now to the pathologist have enormously increased the possibility for diagnostic precision and, most importantly, allow far better correlation of tumor characteristics with clinical behavior.

The improved methods of diagnosis are especially relevant in connection with recent observations of oncogene expression in neuroblastoma. Here, a single factor, overexpression of the oncogene N-*myc,* has been associated with unusually aggressive clinical behavior independent of any conventional pathologic features in this disease.[7] Nevertheless, at least one half of the neuroblastomas in patients with ultimately fatal disease do not overexpress this oncogene, once again demonstrating the hazard of over-reliance on any single feature in the evaluation of a tumor. Noteworthy in this regard is the straightforward morphologic analysis of neuroblastomas reported by Shimada and coworkers that appears to have a better than 90% predictive value in identifying poor-prognosis patients.[5] In this scheme, elements such as persistent undifferentiated neuroblasts, paucity of stroma, persistence of nodular areas of tumor growth within abundant stroma, and, especially, a high mitosis and karyorrhexis index are associated with a poor prognosis independent of age, treatment, or other factors. This is superior to the 50% predictive value of N-*myc* amplification. Morphologic analysis is also simple and requires no specialized tissue handling or methodology. The lesson is that it is important not to overlook the conventional in the face of attractive new technology when the former is more useful.

The Interplay of Multiple Diagnostic Techniques in Tumor Diagnosis

The above comments highlight another truism of tumor diagnosis: the most reliable approach to analysis is a multimodality approach, always beginning with conventional light microscopy in the context of the clinical history. The importance of this cannot be overemphasized; examples of overzealous ap-

plication of the latest technology to the exclusion of routine tumor analysis, with resultant misdiagnosis and poor treatment results, only emphasize this axiom. We have seen, for instance, spurious false-positive lymphoid markers in a bone tumor that led to inappropriate treatment on a lymphoma protocol, with disastrous results. Routine morphologic examination, as well as the clinical history, failed to corroborate the marker result, but the "objective" immunologic result unfortunately held sway in the face of "subjective" evaluation. The latter, although more difficult to quantitate and explain, is nonetheless less prone to gross error. Thus, technologic wizardry is no substitute for sound pathologic analysis; it should complement the latter, not supplant it. This combined-modality approach to tumor analysis will be emphasized throughout *Principles and Practice of Pediatric Oncology.*

DIAGNOSIS OF CHILDHOOD TUMORS

The Character of Childhood Cancer

The spectrum of disease encountered in childhood cancer is both more limited than that of adult cancer and more challenging. Adult cancer is overwhelmingly carcinoma; childhood cancer is rarely so.[6] Brain tumors are of overriding concern in childhood cancer by virtue of sheer numbers, yet categorization is perhaps less compelling for these than for other childhood cancers in view of the almost uniformly poor prognosis among brain tumors.[8] The greatest challenge in childhood cancer diagnosis relates to precise identification of sometimes similar appearing tumors and certainly to recognition of subpopulations of tumors within a larger group, such as Wilms' tumor, that possess an innately more aggressive biological behavior.

Thus, although a handful of tumors account for the overwhelming majority of childhood cancers, the variety within a diagnostic group can be extraordinary. Because certain of these subsets possess an extremely good (such as botryoidal rhabdomyosarcoma) or poor (such as rhabdoid tumor of the kidney) prognosis, they must be identified. Unlike treatment of the common tumors in adults, particularly those of the lung and colon, multimodality therapy in pediatric patients is frequently very effective—if appropriate to the tumor, which assumes that the tumor is correctly diagnosed. Such diagnosis is not always possible by routine methods, and the general problem of diagnosis of undifferentiated or primitive tumors is particularly troublesome, especially in view of the possibility of successful therapy. On a percentage basis, more childhood than adult tumors present such problems. In fact, most of the common types of tumors of childhood at one time or another must be considered in the differential diagnosis of a primitive tumor.

Small Round-Cell Tumors of Childhood

A group of difficult-to-diagnose tumors in children have frequently been referred to as "small round-cell tumors of childhood" in deference to their usual appearance. This simple description is somewhat misleading, because the cells are often neither small nor round nor uniformly blue. Nonetheless, as a group, they are primitive or embryonal in appearance, often present in misleading clinical situations (*i.e.,* bone-marrow metastases from an occult primary) and lack any particular morphologic feature that would allow a precise diagnosis. As a result, they have engendered an entire literature.[9–12]

Table 6-1
Small Round-Cell Tumors of Childhood

Traditional	Revised
Ewing's sarcoma	Ewing's sarcoma
Neuroblastoma	Metastatic neuroblastoma
Rhabdomyosarcoma	Extranodal lymphoma
Lymphoma	Metastatic primitive alveolar rhabdomyosarcoma
	Small-cell osteosarcoma
	Mesenchymal chondrosarcoma
	Primitive *neuro*ectodermal *tumor* of bone (PNET)
	"Askin tumor" of bone/soft tissue
	*P*eripheral *n*euroepithelioma (PN; often called peripheral neuroblastoma, adult neuroblastoma)

Table 6-2
Methods in the Diagnosis of Small Round-Cell Tumors

Light microscopy
Electron microscopy
Immunocytochemistry (paraffin sections)
Immunophenotyping (monoclonal antibody; frozen sections)
Imprints for
 Catecholamine fluorescence
 Periodic acid Schiff (PAS) and special stains
 Immunophenotyping (polyclonal and monoclonal antibodies)
 In situ hybridization
Viable tumor tissue for
 Short-term tissue culture
 Cytogenetic studies
 Molecular genetic analysis
Biochemical analysis
 Neurotransmitter enzymes
 Extracellular matrix protein synthesis/degradation
 Whole-cell or tissue electrophoresis
Combined electrophoresis/immunologic analysis ("Western" analysis)

As a consequence of their uniform morphologic appearance, these small blue-cell tumors are especially suited to analysis by the new technology; traditional light microscopy is inadequate for reliable diagnosis. As such, they provide a model system to demonstrate the benefits of a multi-modality approach to tumor diagnosis. These nonmorphologic techniques provide not only diagnoses, but also prognostic information. This may well lead to other clinically useful information such as chemotherapy sensitivity and drug resistance, much as estrogen-receptor analysis of breast carcinoma biopsy specimens identifies patients whose tumors are likely to be responsive (resistant) to hormonal therapy. Thus, an integrated picture of tumor features is emerging that should provide a great deal more information than the current "carcinoma/sarcoma/lymphoma" or "high-grade/low-grade" evaluations common to light microscopic evaluation alone. It is likely that future diagnoses will incorporate information about histogenesis, antigen expression (both tissue-specific and immunologically relevant, such as HLA), oncogene and growth factor/growth factor-receptor expression, cytogenetic

abnormalities, and possibly other measures of biologic behavior, such as drug-resistance-gene amplification and laminin-receptor expression, protease activity, and other indices of malignancy. Thus, pathologic evaluation of most tumors is likely to become far more complex and will likely draw on the experience gained from attempts to better understand and categorize the small blue-cell tumors of childhood.

Members of this informal group of childhood tumors vary with the author, but most would agree that the group includes at least Ewing's sarcoma, lymphoma, rhabdomyosarcoma, and (supposedly) neuroblastoma (Table 6-1). Although historically valid, this rather simplistic scheme completely fails to address new concepts in tumor types and interrelations. A more timely list would include the tumors listed on the right in Table 6-1. These are the tumors that present a real problem in differential diagnosis, based on our experience with patients admitted to the National Cancer Institute (NCI) Ewing's sarcoma protocol. In this revised listing, specific new entities (Askin tumor,[13] small-cell osteosarcoma[14]) and, even more importantly, specific forms of conventional tumors (extranodal lymphoma, metastatic neuroblastoma, and primitive rhabdomyosarcoma) are precisely defined. It is the specific form of the disease that is relevant to the differential diagnosis of small round-cell tumors; no one will mistakenly identify botryoidal rhabdomyosarcoma as a small round-cell tumor!

DIAGNOSTIC METHODOLOGY

The preceding classification introduces several new entities and concepts into diagnosis. This is the direct result of the application of a host of newer diagnostic techniques, which as a group have brought an enormous increase in our understanding of the basic biology of these tumors. Because of the importance of these methods to the diagnosis of the round-cell tumors in particular, and childhood cancer in general, they are discussed in some detail. The basic approach to tumor diagnosis that we employ is outlined in Table 6-2.

Although most tumors would require only a few of the procedures listed, certain individual cases are candidates for all of them. This is especially true of Ewing's sarcoma, the perennial undifferentiated round-cell tumor of childhood (even when it occurs in adults). The specific methodology is discussed below, with some examples of expected results; a more comprehensive discussion of typical results with specific groups of tumors follows.

Specific Methods

Light Microscopy

As normally performed, light microscopy does not even begin to approach its inherent potential, yet it alone provides more information than any other technique and is the standard against which all other methods are compared. This is so not because of any technical consideration but rather in spite of poor technique. The tremendous advantage of light microscopic morphology is that it is a direct link between the specimen and the mind of the observer. Unfortunately, most diagnoses are proffered despite a somewhat tenuous link. Fortunately, the reliability and information content of this technique can be enormously enhanced with a few simple precautions, as summarized in Table 6-3.

Although the above may seem self-evident, it is all too apparent that these simple principles are eschewed by many;

review of any group of cases assembled from material submitted from a variety of laboratories makes this painfully obvious. Because of this single oversight, many of the techniques to follow are often pursued with no chance of success: a poorly fixed tissue block yields little useful immunocytochemical evidence, and a frozen section of a non-tumor-bearing area of a specimen is useless.

When performed properly and with attention to the quality of the final product, light microscopy will provide sufficient evidence for diagnosis in most cases—the better the quality, the less the need for other techniques. There is surprisingly little appreciation of the sophistication inherent in the human mind's analysis of the microscopic appearance of a tumor or of the experience of the observer. One need only consider the disappointment surrounding the progress to date in the application of artificial intelligence to image-analysis problems to appreciate the truth of this. The reader should recognize that the following methods are no substitute for thoughtful inter-

---

Table 6-3

Handling of Specimens for Light and Electron Microscopy and Immunocytochemistry

Optimization of Light Microscopic Analysis of Tumor Tissue
1. Fixation
   a. Tissue should always be fixed promptly in high-quality *buffered* 10% neutral (*p*H 7.4) Formalin (4% formaldehyde) in small pieces no thicker than 3 mm.
   b. Rapidly penetrating fixatives that optimize the light microscopic image, such as B5 or Bouin's, should be used in parallel with Formalin. Because they have certain disadvantages, they should *not* be used alone.
2. Embedding
   a. Tissue should be embedded in a hard paraffin or paraffin/plastic formulation in order that high-quality thin (<5*f*) sections can be cut.
   b. Some specimens will benefit from embedding in methacrylate epoxy resin. This method provides the highest quality light microscopic images but is not suitable for the large volume of routine specimens. For biopsies, especially rebiopsies in the face of an uncertain diagnosis, methacrylate is an extremely desirable addition to routine embedding but should not exclude same. Certain stains and procedures are not possible on methacrylate sections; the value of the method is the high-quality light microscopic morphology.
3. Staining
   a. Attention to the quality of hematoxylin and eosin (H & E) staining is mandatory; all the preceding is otherwise for naught.
   b. Commonly used special stains (PAS with and without diastase digestion, reticulin) should be ordered at the outset if diagnostic problems are anticipated (as in rebiopsy).
   c. Blank sections for immunocytochemistry are beneficially cut in advance pending choice of antibodies upon review of the H & E sections. We cut six sections and dry them at <50°C for this purpose.
4. Relation of Light Microscopy Specimens to Specimens for Special Studies (Some thought to relatedness of specimens should be given at the time routine specimens are taken for light microscopy. A gross photograph (Polaroid), labeled with section or specimen codes, is invaluable in this regard.)
   a. Tissue for electron microscopy or frozen sections should be from the same area as at least one of the routine tissue blocks for comparison.

   b. Tissue fragments used for culture, extraction of nucleic acids or proteins, or archival freezing should be from proven tumor-bearing areas based on a gross examination of the specimen, with frozen section confirmation as indicated.

Optimization of Electron Microscopy Results
1. Tissue should be minced into small pieces (<1 mm in least dimension) while immersed in 2.5% glutaraldehyde in buffer.
2. Fixation should exceed 6 hours but not 24 hours.
3. Specimens should be chosen from more than one site within large specimens.
4. Even the core of tissue and clot from a fine-needle biopsy is adequate.
5. All specimens should be previewed as lf sections for light microscopy to determine whether representative and of adequate technical quality.
6. In no case should a final diagnosis based on ultrastructural findings be tendered in the absence of concurrent evaluation of the light microscopy findings.
7. Electron microscopy is best performed in conjunction with immunocytochemistry.

Optimization of Immunocytochemistry
1. Antibody specificity
   No antibody is specific for a given epitope; binding is always *relatively* more or less to a given epitope.
2. Antigenic epitope distribution in tissues
   The same epitope may occur on several different antigens of vastly different character and tissue distribution.
3. Effect of fixation
   No antibody will bind to poorly fixed or excessively denatured antigens; alcohol-labile antigens such as glycolipids will not reliably survive normal tissue processing.
4. Importance of controls
   Results are meaningless in the absence of relevant positive and negative controls processed exactly in parallel with the specimen. Normal tissue is not always a relevant control for tumor.
5. Optimal control specimens
   Known tumors represent the preferred positive controls for unknown tumors because of the comparably reduced antigenic expression in both relative to normal tissues.

pretation of the light microscopic appearance of a tumor in the context of clinical information and laboratory data; rather, they extend the scope of the analysis.

Electron Microscopy

The first major change in the microscopic analysis of tumors since the last century occurred after World War II, when biological electron microscopy first appeared. At first only a research tool, the methodology was translated into diagnostic applications by the 1950s. The 1960s saw the rapid growth of an information base of normal and tumor ultrastructure. The past decade and a half has been a period of enormous productivity for the field, which is now mature; current papers focus on specific details or, more commonly, document ultrastructural features in conjunction with other findings from additional techniques.[15] Thus, an immense information base exists that can be used to great gain in tumor diagnosis.

The main value of electron microscopy is not that it answers questions of benign versus malignant but rather that it is an accurate determinant of histogenesis.[16] Thus, in the context of primitive round-cell tumors in children and adults, it remains an invaluable diagnostic tool. Neuroblastoma is easily diagnosed when dense core granules are found by electron microscopy; the same is true of rhabdomyosarcoma and myofilaments, or acute megakaryocytic leukemia and platelet granules. To achieve this, however, one must observe certain conditions and requirements of the technique, as listed in Table 6-3.

Surprisingly, these principles are routinely overlooked in our experience. Failure to appreciate these few basic needs of the technique reduces its contributions to the diagnosis. The specter of a patient sent for rebiopsy whose specimen for electron microscopy is received in B5 fixative illustrates the problem, and this exact scenario has occurred repeatedly for lack of awareness of these few points.

A number of new methods of electron microscopic examination of tissues have been introduced subsequent to transmission electron microscopy, including scanning electron microscopy (SEM), scanning transmission electron microscopy (STEM), and hybrid methods such as ultrastructural immunocytochemistry with electron-dense-labeled antibodies. In general, none of these methods has had any appreciable impact on tumor analysis. SEM, although aesthetically pleasing and useful in a research setting, has had no value in tumor diagnosis. STEM is increasingly useful in environmental pathology, as in the pneumoconioses and, especially, certain pulmonary tumors, particularly mesothelioma, where identification of asbestos particles has assumed major medicolegal significance; for childhood tumors, no parallel value exists.

The only new method likely to have significance for tumor analysis is immunocytochemistry. This is, unfortunately, a tedious and difficult technology, but when successful it provides information unobtainable by any other method. The inherent need for a solid substrate (the epoxy resin used in transmission microscopy), that cannot be removed during examination in the electron microscope (since there is no glass supporting substrate for the section, as there is with light microscopic sections) enormously complicates efforts to bind antibodies (or any other biological molecules, for that matter) to tissue antigens. This problem has in part been circumvented by incubation of the tissue with reagents prior to embedding, but, in this case, problems of cell and tissue penetration have proved insurmountable for routine tissue applications. It is likely that until highly porous hydrophilic resins are developed, immunoelectron microscopy will remain predominantly a research tool. Such efforts have thus far been only marginally successful.

Immunocytochemistry

The most visible development in diagnostic pathology in the past decade has been the introduction of light microscopic immunocytochemistry as a routine diagnostic technique.[17] This is a fundamentally different approach to tumor diagnosis: unlike light or electron microscopy, it is a nonmorphologic method intended to detect the tumor-cell content of a marker substance (an antigen) that will react with an antibody presumed specific for that substance. The antigen can be proteinaceous, carbohydrate, or even glycolipid in nature, but it must be stable and retained after tissue processing, including fixation, if it is to be detected. Many substances easily detected by radioimmunoassay or enzyme-linked immunosorbent assay, for example, are not detectable in fixed tissue.

Further, the bound antibody–antigen complexes must be seen in relation to the tumor tissue. Fluorescein was used initially but is not nearly as useful as peroxidase reaction products. The introduction of various methods, especially the Sternberger unlabeled antibody-bridge technique[18] (in which a second antibody binds bivalently to both the tissue-bound first antibody and a complex of peroxidase/antiperoxidase antigen–antibody aggregates), revolutionized the method. More recently, the avidin–biotin method has been introduced[19] (in which biotin-labeled antibody binds avidin–peroxidase complexes with remarkably high affinity (10^{12} M^{-1})). This method is gaining popularity because it appears to be more sensitive and to have lower background than the Sternberger method. Further refinements, such as predigestion of tissue sections with protease, appear to enhance this sensitivity. The basic method is illustrated schematically in Figure 6-1.

Unlike its ultrastructural counterpart, light microscopic immunocytochemistry has made the transition to the diagnostic pathology laboratory. Before 1980, the technique was purely a research tool, but since then it has grown enormously; in our laboratory, the total number of requests for diagnostic immunocytochemistry has doubled each year for 5 consecutive years. Recent improvements in the sensitivity and quality of available antibodies have further enhanced the value of the technique.

Although an extremely valuable tool, immunocytochemistry is not without serious shortcomings.[20] It is no substitute for light microscopy or even for electron microscopy; the methods provide two completely different perspectives on problems of diagnosis. The most serious shortcoming of immunocytochemistry is the failure of its occasional practitioners to appreciate the pitfalls of antibody binding to antigens. The problems can be summarized in a few short axioms, as seen in Table 6-3. Because of neglect of these cautions, huge numbers of specimens are processed inappropriately, with predictably useless results. Moreover, negative results are of limited utility, and positive results are significant only if all controls are appropriately positive and negative, and especially if only tumor cells (and possibly appropriate normal elements) are positive in the tumor section. Under these circumstances, immunocytochemistry can provide invaluable evidence of a tumor's origins, degree of differentiation, and possibly even malignancy. For the careful practitioner, immunocytochemistry has vastly increased the power of the pathologist to document a tumor diagnosis objectively; the combination of electron microscopy and immunocytochemistry is even more potent.

Unfortunately, in the minds of some, immunocytochemistry is rapidly assuming the role once played by electron microscopy: it is becoming the first alternative to traditional light microscopy in the surgical pathologist's mind.[21] This is unfortunate in that the relation between electron microscopy and immunocytochemistry is synergistic: each provides informa-

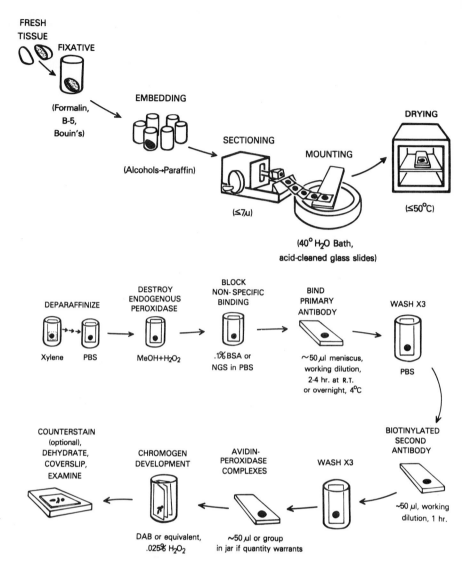

FIGURE 6-1. Schematic diagram of immunocytochemistry technique. The basic methodology of one standard immunoperoxidase method is illustrated; many variations exist (see text).

tion not provided by the other. For example, electron microscopy can readily document the presence of cytoplasmic filaments but cannot distinguish vimentin from desmin or neurofilament triplet protein. Immunocytochemistry, on the other hand, can easily distinguish the three (or others) if they are present and if the tissue is antigenically intact and the antibodies active. A negative result in no way excludes a finding; it is not uncommon to see obvious intermediate filaments in a tumor that was nonreactive with any intermediate-filament-specific antibody. The reasons are rarely obvious, but electron microscopy then assumes a primary role in such cases.

A detailed discussion of the immunocytochemical results expected from every antibody and every tumor is obviously beyond the scope of this chapter. However, an overview of the expected results in the context of small round-cell tumor diagnosis is quite appropriate.

Experience over the past several years has increasingly focused on certain families or clusters of antibodies useful in the analysis of routinely fixed and embedded tumors. Three of those groups are especially relevant to childhood tumor diagnosis: a group of neural markers, the cytoskeletal or intermediate-filament proteins, and hematopoietic markers. A tabular summary of the specificity of each antibody and of the results typically obtained with these antibodies in any given tumor is presented in Tables 6-4 and 6-5. The details are discussed below.

The most important point concerning the data listed in Tables 6-4 and 6-5 is that they are only a guide to the expected results; they are not individually reliable, and anomalous results are the rule, not the exception.[20] The more antibodies used in a given case, the greater is the probability of an untoward result. Thus, we interpret the results of immunocytochemistry only in the context of light and electron microscopic findings, and inappropriate results are viewed with skepticism.

NEURAL MARKERS. Neuron-Specific Enolase (NSE). Among neural markers useful in paraffin-embedded tissue, NSE is the most sensitive[22] but also the most prone to spurious but valid positive results on non-neural tissues due to the low content of neuron-specific γ enolase subunit in many, if not all, cells and tissues.[23] The alpha and beta subunits are ubiquitous in most tissues and are nonspecific. For some time, possible heterodimers ($\alpha\gamma$ or $\beta\gamma$) were thought to be the source of the problem, but recent studies have demonstrated that all tissues studied contain detectable levels of $\gamma\gamma$ enolase or NSE.[23] Despite these problems, the levels in neural tissues and tumors are far

Table 6-4
Antibodies Useful in the Diagnosis of Small Round-Cell Tumors of Childhood

Antibody	Specificity
Neuron-specific enolase (NSE)	Gamma subunit of enolase, ubiquitous in brain and neural tissue and found in virtually all neuroepithelial-derived tumors. Also present in muscle and, at low levels (normally undetectable in tissue sections, in all tissues
Leu7 (human natural killer cell)	Epitope on T lymphoid cells with "killer" (*i.e.,* cytotoxic) ability. Same epitope found in nerve (on myelin-associated glycoprotein; MAGP) and in other neural tumors (on a complex glycoconjugate)
Neurofilament triplet protein (NFTP)	Actually a family of three distinct proteins (68, 160, and 200 kD) that compose the intermediate filaments of neural tissue. Any given antibody usually is specific for only one of the subunits
Desmin	The intermediate filament of myogenous tissues; reliable but may be present in myofibroblasts also. Not specific for skeletal muscle *per se*
Vimentin	Ubiquitous intermediate-filament protein of all mesenchymal tissue, sarcomas, and lymphoid malignancies. Also present in neural tissue, pleural effusions of carcinoma, and renal and hepatic carcinoma. Most useful in childhood tumors as a technique control; if negative, all results are potentially meaningless
Keratin	The intermediate-filament protein of epithelia, benign or malignant. Negative among childhood tumors except carcinomas, germ cell tumors, and synoviosarcoma, epithelioid sarcoma, and neurofibrosarcoma with glandular differentiation

beyond those found in normal tissues and non-neural tumors, and appropriately titered antibody used with positive and negative controls yields reliable results.

Leu7 (HNK.1; Myelin-Associated Glycoprotein-Binding Antibody). Leu7, a monoclonal antibody developed as part of a series of hematopoietic monoclonals and found specific for human natural killer cells (thus the designation HNK),[24] was subsequently found to bind nerves and neurons,[25] owing to its ability to bind myelin-associated glycoprotein.[26] Despite this apparent exquisite specificity for a neural-tissue marker, the antibody has proved less reliable than expected, since other epitopes, often glycolipid or complex carbohydrate (and therefore easily removed or degraded in routinely fixed and processed tissues), have been documented in other neural and non-neural tissues.[27] This is particularly problematic since only these determinants, and no myelin-associated glycoprotein,

have been identified in non-neuroblastomatous neural tumors of childhood.[28]

Neural Filament Triplet Protein (NFTP). A third neural marker is NFTP. This marker is in fact a member of the next group to be discussed but is at the same time a highly specific neural marker. NFTP forms intermediate filaments in neural but not neural supportive tissues and is actually a triad of three discrete subunits: 68-, 160-, and 200-kD proteins. Each is immunologically distinct, but they are all derived from the same primordial gene and share significant amino acid sequence homology (as do all the intermediate filaments to be discussed).[29] For this reason, there is a real possibility of immunologic overlap; we have documented this at a research level and suspect it in clinical specimens as well. Antibodies against each of the subunits, as well as pan-NFTP antibodies, have been produced. The latter is not unexpected, in view of the partial homology. Fortunately, all seem to be highly specific except for as-yet-unexplained nuclear staining that may be due to cross reactivity with nuclear lamins A, B, and C, which are filamentous proteins localized to the inner surface of the nuclear envelope that appear to be primordial cytoskeletal proteins.[30] In any event, anti-NFTP antibodies are quite reliable but unlikely to bind to primitive neural tumors, and they are less useful than NSE in identifying a given tumor as neural or not.[31] When positive, the results are unassailable, but negativity does not preclude a neural histogenesis.

CYTOSKELETAL PROTEINS. Desmin (Myogenous Tumors and Tissues). Desmin is another cytoskeletal protein of diagnostic value in childhood tumors. It occurs only in myogenous tissues, including smooth and skeletal muscle and, probably, myofibroblasts. In the context of childhood tumors, this reactivity reduces to rhabdomyosarcoma.[32] Leiomyosarcoma, a not-uncommon soft-tissue sarcoma in adults, is virtually unreported in children; a recent article documented only 12 cases over a 40-year period at the Boston Children's Hospital.[33] Thus, myogenous tumors in children are overwhelmingly of skeletal-muscle origin or at least differentiation. Although primary rhabdomyosarcoma of bone is rare,[34] metastatic bone involvement is not, and antibodies to desmin can be extremely useful in the differential diagnosis of metastatic tumor in bone.

Ideally, antibodies to desmin should be teamed with antibodies to another myogenous marker, especially a skeletal muscle-specific marker such as myoglobin (present in high concentrations in skeletal muscle tissue and tumors) or the creatine kinase MM isozyme (CK-MM), which is specific for skeletal or cardiac muscle.[35] Positivity for two or more of these markers is irrefutable evidence of rhabdomyosarcoma in the NCI experience.[36] This is important because NSE reactivity is often positive in rhabdomyosarcoma.[22] Again, this should be no surprise, since normal skeletal and smooth muscle stains with antibodies to this enzyme; neoplastic counterparts would be expected to express the same antigens, as they often do. The actual incidence is difficult to quantitate, but there is no question that it is high enough to necessitate a confirmation of a diagnosis of neural tumor other than NSE alone. We routinely use either the group of neural-associated antibodies discussed above or the muscle-associated antibodies noted here.[37]

Vimentin (Mesenchymal Tissues). Another widely used cytoskeletal protein, vimentin, is not particularly useful in differential diagnosis, as should be apparent from Table 6-3. This protein is ubiquitous among eukaryotic cells, and its detection serves more as a positive technique control than as a discriminant of histogenesis. Only its absence in *most* carcinomas

Table 6-5
Typical Immunocytochemistry Results in Small Round-Cell Tumors of Childhood

Tumor	Antibody						
	NSE	*Leu7*	*NFTP*	*Desmin*	*Vimentin*	*Keratin*	*LCA**
Ewing's sarcoma	−	−	−	−	+	−	−
Neuroblastoma	+	+	+	−	+	−	−
Askin tumor	+	−	±	−	+	−	−
PNET of bone	+	−	±	−	+	−	−
Small-cell osteosarcoma	−	−	−	−	+	−	−
Mesenchymal chondrosarcoma	−	−	−	−	+	−	−
Rhabdomyosarcoma	±	−	−	+	+	−	−
Synoviosarcoma	−	−	−	−	+	+	−
Lymphoma	−	∓	−	−	∓	−	+

* Leukocyte common antigen.

makes it useful in the differential diagnosis of anaplastic tumors of adults; in small round-cell tumors of childhood, it is of little utility.

Keratin (Epithelial Tissues and Malignancies). Keratin is widely used in adult tumor diagnosis because of its widespread presence in carcinomas. However, at least 19 isotypes of keratin have been described,[38] and no pankeratin antibody has been made available. Thus, "cocktails" such as AE1/AE3 mixed monoclonal antibody have been marketed[39] that largely alleviate the problem, although unexpected negativity among epithelial tissues and tumors continues. A large number of polyspecific keratin antibodies have been offered to address this problem, but, as of this writing, no single antibody appears to offer a clear advantage.

Most salient for pediatric tumors is the virtual absence of epithelial malignancies, except for Wilms' tumor, germ cell tumors, and teratomas, none of which is of concern in identifying round-cell tumors. Thus, although of potential value in this specific instance, in reality keratin antibodies are of little practical value in childhood tumor diagnosis. We have had isolated cases, such as a tumor of the superior pole of the kidney with a differential diagnosis of monomorphic Wilms' tumor versus undifferentiated neuroblastoma; keratin antibodies were weakly positive, but the electron microscopic appearance was unequivocal, showing desmosomes and keratin filament bundles but no neural differentiation. Among adolescents, rare examples of poorly differentiated extragonadal germ cell tumors can be studied usefully with keratin antibodies. We have even encountered an "epithelial" malignancy in pelvic soft tissue that was negative for keratin antibodies but positive for glial fibrillary acidic protein, another cytoskeletal filamentous protein limited to the glia of the central nervous system; in this case, the results confirmed the suspicion of a singular example of a medulloepithelioma outside the central nervous system.

HEMATOPOIETIC MARKERS. The final marker listed in Table 6-5, LCA, is a generic marker for hematopoietic cells and their tumors. Several such antibodies have been popularized, such as the anti-T200 antigen of Battifora and Trowbridge,[40] but fail to work reliably on paraffin-embedded, formaldehyde-fixed tissues. Anti-LCA, as marketed by DAKO, among others, is a

mixture of monoclonals and works well on paraffin-embedded tissues.[41] We have never encountered a false-positive result to our knowledge, and only one or two cases have been nonreactive among dozens of childhood lymphomas.

The particular value of this antibody, as well as of those already discussed, is that they work reliably on ordinary tissue sections and do not require any special specimen handling. This is of greatest significance to pathologists in referral centers, where the patient often has been biopsied elsewhere and only sections and paraffin blocks are available to establish a diagnosis short of a rebiopsy of the tumor, which is impossible if the original procedure was an excisional biopsy. Thus, this fairly limited panel of antibodies has been of enormous practical value, not because it is the best or most comprehensive, but because it works. Predictably, failures do occur, and anomalous results occasionally force a more extended diagnostic evaluation. In such cases, the procedures to follow become extremely important.

IMMUNOPHENOTYPING. Many of the problems of nonspecific binding or nonreactivity noted in connection with conventional immunocytochemistry are readily redressed by using monoclonal antibodies on frozen sections or tumor imprints (see Chap. 4). This approach circumvents antigenic degradation by covalent fixation with formaldehyde. Further, the heat denaturation that results from drying of conventional sections is avoided. The cumulative effect is enormously improved immunoreactivity, a necessary consequence of the use of monoclonal antibodies. This alone warrants the special handling (*i.e.,* freezing, preferably in OCT or similar cyroprotectant/ mordant) necessary for tissue-section immunophenotyping with monoclonal antibodies.

This is not to say that monoclonal antibodies have not been used successfully on alcohol-fixed paraffin-embedded tissues; they have.[42] Of necessity, though, even this method fails to address all the unique requirements of monoclonal antibodies and of certain classes of antigens. On the one hand, alcohol extracts lipids, glycolipids, and any antigens attached thereto and not otherwise cell bound. Also, the subsequent heat denaturation that results from paraffin embedding (at least 45°C) and, especially, subsequent drying (often 60°C or more) are deleterious. The advantage, however, is optimal morphologic preservation, on a par with that of conventional fixation and paraffin embedding. Thus, this method is preferable if the antigens to be sought are known to be nonlipid and stable.

The results with Leu7 (HNK.1) epitomize this problem: although this antibody binds myelin-associated glycoprotein in nerves and neuroblastoma, the equivocal and nonreproducible results obtained with other neural tumors such as PNET can now be ascribed to the alcohol-labile glycolipid determinant "seen" by the antibody in these tumors. No myelin-associated glycoprotein is present in these tumors,[28] and only variable and scant amounts of unextracted glycolipid antigen remain to be detected in conventionally or alcohol-fixed and processed tissues. Thus, when in doubt, air-dried frozen sections or tumor imprints are the preferred specimen despite their inferior morphology compared to conventionally processed or alcohol-fixed specimens.

Although highly specific for the particular epitope recognized by the hybridoma clone, monoclonal antibodies lack the multipoint attachment of polyclonal antibodies. If the epitope is fixation sensitive or is labile during processing, as many are, the reactivity is lost. This was the case with most of the first monoclonal antibodies; more recent offerings have been evaluated with this problem in mind and sometimes circumvent it. Nonetheless, the vast majority of the targets of the most useful monoclonals are exquisitely sensitive to normal tissue fixation and processing, and the antibodies are reactive only on alcohol- or acetone-fixed specimens. Some, as noted in connection with Leu7, are only reactive on air-dried, unfixed specimens.

For all of the above reasons, it is extremely useful to augment conventional immunocytochemistry with a panel of monoclonal antibodies of known specificity. In some cases, these are the same antibodies used on paraffin sections (such as LCA), but the results are far more impressive and unequivocal.

We have beneficially used a relatively limited panel of such antibodies in connection with the small round-cell tumors of childhood (Table 6-6).[43] Using just three antibodies, we have distinguished neuroblastoma, Ewing's sarcoma, peripheral neural tumors (peripheral neuroepithelioma, Askin tumor, PNET of bone and soft tissue), and lymphoma of bone. This panel does not distinguish each of the peripheral neural tumors (peripheral neuroepithelioma, Askin tumor, and PNET of bone), which was one early piece of evidence for a relation between these tumors. It was also the earliest piece of information strongly indicating that metastatic neuroblastoma, which is easily identified by the monoclonal antibody HSAN 1.2, is only rarely an issue among neural tumors of bone. Rather, almost all have fit the phenotype of the non-neuroblas-

toma neural tumors (HSAN 1.2 weakly positive, W6/32 [HLA-A, B, C, or class I] positive). Neuroblastoma, in contrast, is uniformly HLA-I negative and strongly HSAN 1.2 positive.

The limited panel listed in Table 6-6 also fails to distinguish Ewing's sarcoma readily from the non-neuroblastoma neural tumors. Ewing's sarcoma is HLA-I positive but negative or weakly positive for HSAN 1.2. In reality, the positivity among the peripheral neural tumors ranges from strong to weak; tumors with the latter result are indistinguishable from Ewing's sarcoma (see Fig. 6-6). These data also support the concept that Ewing's sarcoma is at least immunophenotypically similar to peripheral neural tumors and markedly dissimilar from neuroblastoma.

The antibody panel discussed here represents the pragmatic application of a few monoclonals to diagnosis of a limited spectrum of tumors. Although literally hundreds of such antibodies are available, and at least a dozen "neuroblastoma-specific" monoclonals, very few monoclonals bind only one antigen in one tissue type. Most bind such a small, precisely define epitope that the probability of its occurrence in several tissues is high. Caution is therefore in order when using a new or uncharacterized monoclonal antibody with presumed single-epitope specificity. Only the exceptional monoclonal will prove to be so specific, and extensive evaluation is mandatory before relying on such antibodies for tumor diagnosis.

Tumor-Cell Imprints ("Touch Preparations")

Although imprints are hardly a high-technology procedure, new life has been breathed into this old method by virtue of its unique potential to provide optimal cytology with intact antigenicity and cell content. Thus, a variety of procedures impossible on routine formaldehyde-fixed, alcohol-dehydrated, and paraffin-embedded tissue are readily consummated on imprints. Typical procedures include the following:

1. Catecholamine fluorescence assays of suspected neural crest tumors
2. Special stains of labile substances, such as PAS stains for glycogen
3. Immunocytochemistry with both polyclonal and monoclonal antibodies, especially for cell-surface and labile determinants
4. *In situ* hybridization using DNA or RNA probes.

This potential of tumor imprints for use in multiple assays is particularly valuable when only a small amount of material is available. Currently, the most common example of this is fine-needle aspiration; such specimens usually provide more than adequate material for evaluation as imprints.

CATECHOLAMINE FLUORESCENCE. Tumor imprints, cytospins, smears, and similar preparations offer the unique opportunity to detect tumor-cell contents otherwise beyond the scope of more routine methods. In particular, these preparations readily allow the detection of catecholamines in even single neuroblastoma cells using fluorescence, either by glyoxylic acid[44] or by paraformaldehyde vapor-induced "autofluorescence."[45] Differential diagnosis is rarely a problem in older patients, but bone-marrow involvement in young patients with neuroblastoma (in whom neuroblasts may be exceedingly difficult to distinguish from normal blastic marrow elements) is not an uncommon problem.[46]

SPECIAL STAINS. Another major value of imprints is as specimens for special stains such as PAS (periodic acid oxidation of glycosylated compounds, with Schiff's base reduction

---

Table 6-6
Monoclonal Antibody Reactivity of Small Round-Cell Tumors

| Tumor | Antibody | | |
	HSAN 1.2	W6/32	LCA
Neuroblastoma	+++	−	−
Ewing's sarcoma	∓	+	−
Peripheral neural tumors*	±	+	−
Lymphoma	−	+	+
Osteosarcoma; rhabdomyosarcoma	−	+	−

* Askin tumor, PNET of bone, peripheral neuroepithelioma.

and color development). This stain is generally used both with and without diastase digestion to distinguish glycogen which is diastase labile, from glycoprotein and other glycosubstances that are diastase resistant.

IMMUNOPHENOTYPING. Imprints are an ideal source of tumor cells for immunocytochemistry with any antibody, polyclonal or monoclonal, and these air-dried specimens are easily prepared. They thus offer a simple and inexpensive alternative to frozen sections. Not surprisingly, similar preparations are of increasing value in cytology, where immunoanalysis augments cytologic evaluation.

***IN SITU* HYBRIDIZATION WITH DNA OR RNA PROBES.** This technology is discussed in detail elsewhere (see Chap. 3), but a short note here is appropriate. Although most attention has focused on the application of probe technology to chromosomes[47] or tissue sections (Fig. 6-2),[48] one should not overlook the usefulness of tumor imprints for this same method. Specimens are exceedingly easy to prepare, they are a single cell thick, the backgrounds are low due to low nonspecific binding (which often is not true of frozen sections), and photographic emulsions (for radiolabeled probes) are easily and uniformly applied, again rarely true of tumor sections. For this reason, imprints may yet become a preferred method of tumor preparation for such studies. This is analogous to the situation with peripheral-blood and bone-marrow smears; they, too, are a single cell thick and provide ideal conditions for single-cell hybridizations with probes. The results are often spectacular.

Viable Tumor Tissue

Once a surgical specimen has been obtained for other studies, it is rather simple to continue the analysis *in vitro,* at least for short-term culture. The potential benefits of this approach are unique; virtually all cultured tumors are amenable to cytogenetic analysis,[49] and in many cases a stable long-term culture may be established. Most tumors cultured in our laboratory over the past several years have yielded at least short-term growth;[50] from this, cytogenetic analysis is readily obtained. Culture also represents a renewable resource of pure tumor cells for diverse studies, from molecular genetics to *in vitro* chemotherapy- and radiation therapy-sensitivity testing. Thus, the added burden of the difficult technique is more than com-

pensated for by the immense variety of potential diagnostic information. Culture is obviously not a first-line technique for all tumors, but unusual tumors, such as the round-cell tumors of childhood, stand to benefit from such analysis.

SHORT-TERM CULTURE. Short-term culture itself can be quite useful in diagnosis. Neural tumors in general (neuroblastoma and, to a lesser extent, peripheral neural tumors) frequently undergo spontaneous differentiation *in vitro.*[46] Osteosarcoma, chondrosarcoma, lymphoma, and metastatic soft-tissue sarcomas all fail to undergo such differentiation but show decidedly different morphology.[12]

In addition to light microscopic morphology, electron microscopy of cultured tumors can be diagnostic, even when ultrastructural study of the uncultured, surgically excised tumor is not, simply because cellular and subcellular differentiation that remains undetectable by light microscopy can readily be seen by electron microscopy. Further, reversible cell injury incurred during the relative hypoxia surrounding intraoperative devascularization and excision can be reversed under the relatively rich culture conditions, resulting in viable, normal-appearing cells, unlike the swollen, artifactually distorted cells common in many biopsies. Only the frequent overgrowth of tumor cells by fibroblasts prevents short-term culture from being utterly reliable; these undesired cells are readily recognized, but tumor cells may be completely lost with time.

CYTOGENETICS. Perhaps the greatest potential utility of short-term culture is its direct application to a particularly promising new area of tumor characterization, cytogenetics. Although not new *per se,* tumor cytogenetics has found new relevance to oncology with the description of characteristic chromosomal abnormalities in certain tumors.[51-53] This analysis is appropriate to the round-cell tumors of bone and to Ewing's sarcoma in particular. Ewing's sarcoma, which lacks any specific feature or marker that allows a positive identification by any other technique, possesses a highly characteristic reciprocal translocation of the long arms of chromosomes 11 and 22 (see Chaps. 2 and 3). This change, first reported by Turc–Carel[54] and Aurias[55] and their coworkers, has subsequently been confirmed by others[56,57] and appears to be nearly constant in Ewing's sarcoma. Rather unexpectedly, this same abnormality has been found in peripheral neural tumors such

FIGURE 6-2. Schematic diagram of *in situ* hybridization of tissue sections; radiolabeled *in situ* hybridization of typical frozen sections is illustrated. Newer methods under development are expected to replace radioactive probes as their sensitivity approaches that of present techniques.

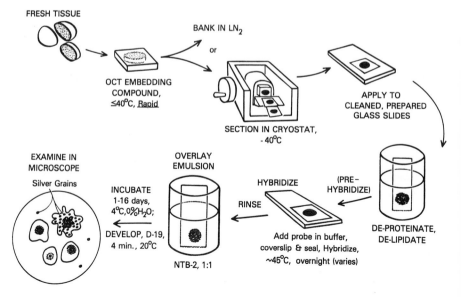

as the Askin tumor of the chest wall,[56,58] peripheral neuroepithelioma, and one of two extraosseous Ewing's sarcomas.[56,60] This concordance has been the single most compelling datum so far of a common histogenesis for this group of tumors. It also fails to support any close histogenetic relation to neuroblastoma, which has never been reported to possess this translocation but which routinely displays abnormalities of chromosome 1, along with homogeneously staining regions (HSRs) and double minutes (DMs) or fragments of extrachromosomal DNA.[61,62] Thus, at least two distinct families of tumors can be identified by cytogenetic analysis alone. Further, a recent report has documented other cytogenetic abnormalities (*i.e.*, 1q+ in all of five PNETs and monosomy 13 in two of five).[63]

Although it is far less advanced, cytogenetic analysis of other childhood tumors has been illuminating. Alveolar rhabdomyosarcoma has been reported to possess a chromosome 2;13 translocation,[64] and a chromosome 15X translocation has been identified in synovial sarcoma (see Chaps. 30 and 31).[65] No characteristic cytogenetic abnormality of small-cell osteosarcoma or mesenchymal chondrosarcoma has been reported, which is not surprising in view of the small number of cases in the literature. Lymphoma is a heterogeneous group of tumors, certain of which have a high frequency of one or more abnormalities; Burkitt's lymphoma is likely to show translocations of chromosome 8 and either 2, 14, or 22.[66,67]

Thus, tumor cytogenetics alone has the potential to distinguish between different diagnostic possibilities in certain cases. The situation is likely to become more precise with the advent of probes that allow mapping of chromosome fine structure. This possibility is best exemplified by the recent description of a reproducible gene or gene-cluster deletion in retinoblastoma that is responsible for the development of the disease and which is only sometimes visible as a chromosome 13q rbl-locus deletion.[68–71] Often, the deleted portions are too small to be detected by conventional chromosome studies, and newer methods of mapping will be required to detect such deletions, rearrangements, and translocations. This molecular cytogenetic analysis of tumors will most probably revolutionize cytogenetics and appears likely to unmask a host of consistent abnormalities in human tumors that are currently undetectable. Recent studies of the Philadelphia chromosome abnormality in chronic myelogenous leukemia[72] and a similar abnormality in acute lymphoblastic leukemia[73] have revealed subtle differences in the gene rearrangement leading to c-*abl* activation, which correlates with the different clinical presentation of the two diseases. Observations such as this virtually mandate allocation of portions of appropriate biopsy specimens to molecular and cytogenetic studies; the latter studies require viable tumor placed in at least short-term culture.

MOLECULAR GENETIC ANALYSIS. Although this subject is discussed in detail in Chapter 3, it is worth noting here that cultures provide an inexhaustible source of tumor DNA and RNA for molecular genetic analysis. Fresh, rapidly frozen tumor and corresponding normal tissue are the mainstays of this powerful new technology, yet adequate tissue samples are often unavailable in this era of limited biopsy procedures. Without adequate tumor tissue, no molecular genetic studies are possible. For this reason, short-term culture can provide another crucial resource: both cytogenetics and molecular genetic analysis of tumors become possible when such cultures are available.

It is difficult to estimate at this time the ramifications of this new method for tumor diagnosis and, perhaps even more importantly, for predictions of tumor "malignancy" or likely clinical behavior. Recent work on the *neu/erbB* oncogene in breast cancer[74] and on the even more relevant role of N-*myc* in childhood neuroblastoma[75–77] clearly indicates the need to evaluate such factors in tumors. Which tumors and which oncogenes or other genes have not yet been determined, but it is safe to say that this approach will grow in frequency and importance. It is also safe to say that paraffin-embedded specimens will *not* be adequate for these studies, and viable tumor tissue, at least frozen promptly at $-80°C$ (or better, $-190°C$) and preferably kept viable for a period of time in culture, will become increasingly important.

Biochemical Analysis

A far less precisely defined area of tumor analysis, also made possible by maintenance of viable tumor cells *in vitro*, is the study of tumor cell products. This approach has many possible manifestations, from the study of extracellular matrix constituents synthesized and secreted by tumor cells to the study of cell-specific synthesis of biologically active substances such as hormones and enzymes. The latter possibility has proved particularly useful in the study of neural tumors, which as a group secrete neurotransmitter enzymes unique to neural tissues.

NEUROTRANSMITTER ENZYME ANALYSIS. The best-described neurotransmitter enzymes in neuroblastoma are dopamine beta hydroxylase (DBH) and tyrosine hydroxylase (TH), which together form the common adrenergic (epinephrine and norepinepherine) neurotransmitter enzymes, and choline acetyl transferase (CAT), the common enzyme for cholinergic neurotransmission.[78,79] Neuroblastoma usually expresses both in the patient (whence positivity for catechols in urine or serum) and *in vitro*, where these enzymes have been readily identified in conditioned culture medium and in tumor cells themselves.[79] This expression is also the basis of the positive assay for catecholamine fluorescence described earlier. Thus, bioassay for these enzymes, or immunologic detection of their presence with appropriate antibodies, constitutes reliable evidence for a diagnosis of metastatic neuroblastoma among the round-cell tumors of bone.

Interestingly, only neuroblastoma among the tumors being discussed herein expresses adrenergic neurotransmitter enzymes (Ross RA, Triche TJ: Unpublished data). The other neural tumors noted previously do not secrete catecholamines *in vivo*, and the tumor cells do not express detectable levels of the necessary enzymes. Conversely, these tumors are routinely positive for CAT, the most ubiquitous of the cholinergic enzymes. Likewise, antibodies against another cholinergic enzyme, acetylcholinesterase, give positive reactions in those cases in which they have been used (Cavazzana AO, Triche TJ: Unpublished data).[80] Both neuroblastoma and other neural tumors are positive for cholinergic enzymes; the presence of adrenergic neurotransmitter enzymes distinguishes neuroblastoma from all other neural tumors, which are exclusively cholinergic.

EXTRACELLULAR MATRIX SYNTHESIS AND DEGRADATION. The extracellular matrix (ECM) produced by normal tissues is usually duplicated by their tumorous counterparts.[81] The ECM-degradative capabilities of tumor cells provide yet another insight into the relative "malignancy" of a given tumor, since invasion of the tumor or vascular basement membrane (composed of the ECM proteins laminin, basal lamina proteoglycan, and type IV collagen) is the required first step in invasion and metastasis, the hallmark of malignant tumors.[82] For these reasons, numerous studies over the past decade have attempted to relate either synthesis or degradation to tumor behavior.

Extracellular Matrix Synthesis.   At least in a developmental biology setting, ECM synthesis studies have been illuminating. At a simplistic level, certain generalizations can be made:[83]

Hematopoietic cells and lymphoma synthesize no ECM proteins, consonant with their mobility within the body.

Sarcomas in general synthesize stromal, as opposed to basal lamina, ECM proteins, particularly types I, II, III, V, and other collagens, plus fibronectin or other high-molecular-weight "binding" glycoproteins (osteonectin, chondronectin).

Neural tumors synthesize scant amounts of basal lamina and stromal ECM; with neural differentiation of the tumor cells, ECM synthesis virtually ceases except for scant amounts of fibronectin.

Ewing's "sarcoma," like neural tumors, synthesizes small amounts of both basal lamina and stromal ECM.

Although these studies have shed light on relative tumor histogenesis, they are not readily applied to tumor diagnosis because of the cumbersome biosynthetic methods used to date. Immunocytochemistry with antibodies against these ECM constituents[84] has sometimes led to erroneous results due to its inability to distinguish host from tumor stroma.[85] These problems may well be circumvented with the development of simple methods of *in situ* hybridization, whence DNA probes for each of the ECM proteins could be applied to tumor sections. For the time being, this is not feasible other than in a research setting, where it has been successful (DeClerk YA: Personal communication).

Extracellular Matrix Degradation.   The other major area of interest with regard to ECM is its degradation by tumor cells. Whereas benign neoplasms can degrade ECM, malignant tumors all do. This fundamental difference can be evaluated by a number of methods and provides an index of malignancy, and presumably therefore of prognosis. This relatively novel approach to tumor evaluation is well established in the research laboratory but is not yet a practical diagnostic tool. The most likely development will be antibodies or probes to biologically relevant proteins. On one hand, collagenases appear to be an important part of early invasion and metastasis; antibodies to such proteins have been developed and are reactive with collagenases within tumor cells.[86] Further, membrane receptors for substances such as laminin appear to play a major role in tumor-cell attachment to ECM, perhaps the earliest event in tumor invasion and metastasis.[87] Both antibodies to the receptor and cloned fragments of its DNA have been publicized.[88] Widespread availability of such antibodies or DNA probes could prove extremely useful in evaluating the degree of malignancy manifest by a given tumor. This, in conjunction with other techniques designed to determine tumor histogenesis reliably, could provide a truly comprehensive evaluation of a tumor's origins and clinical behavior. Such developments are expected in the near future.

ELECTROPHORESIS OF WHOLE-CELL AND TISSUE EXTRACTS. Another general approach to tumor analysis, which unfortunately has seen little application in conventional pathologic analysis, is the biochemical analysis of tumor-cell products or tumor extracts by gel electrophoresis. Although immunocytochemistry and biological assays (as with enzymatic techniques) offer straightforward methodology and seemingly clear-cut results, the reality is that false-positive immunoassays are common, and proof of identity is not forthcoming by immunocytochemistry alone. How, then, to identify a putative substance positively?

Fortunately, biochemical analysis of proteins by gel electrophoresis has become routine with highly reproducible results. Highly automated equipment has been introduced (as the Phastpage by Pharmacia) that makes such analysis routine. It seems likely such analytic methods for tumor-product characterization will prove necessary to verify other, less reliable, methods such as immunocytochemistry. What sort of substance might one wish to identify in a given tumor?

The possibilities for tumor characterization are virtually limitless. With little imagination, one can easily anticipate verification of, say, seeming skeletal-muscle myosin in a tumor by simple tissue extraction into detergent buffer (sodium dodecyl sulfate [SDS]/Tris) and electrophoresis; myosin is characterized by the presence of a 200-kD band (myosin heavy chain) and a family of lower-molecular-weight proteins, about 15 to 20 kD (myosin light chains) on SDS/polyacrylamide gel electrophoresis (SDS/PAGE).[89]

Although exquisitely precise in its ability to identify substances of interest in a tumor, simple whole-tissue extract SDS/PAGE is nonetheless hampered by the often extremely low level of a given protein in an extract. Although innumerable purification methods are available, they subvert the speed and ease of analysis that are essential for practical tumor diagnosis. However, recent improvements and modifications in this technology have largely solved this problem.

Electrophoresis/Immunoblot Analysis ("Western" Analysis)

The universal use of the Southern method of DNA gel electrophoresis followed by blotting to nitrocellulose membranes and detection with DNA probes inevitably spawned a similar technique for RNA analysis ("Northern" analysis) and protein analysis ("Western" analysis). The great virtue of all three methods is their ability to pick out a single entity separated on the basis of size even when it is present in extraordinarily small amounts. In Western analysis, proteins are separated by size by SDS/PAGE, electrophoretically transferred to a nitrocellulose or similar membrane, and incubated with an antibody to the substance of interest. It is possible not only to detect minute amounts of material, but also to verify that identification, since the relative molecular weight of the substance is generally known, and this is easily determined by the migration in the gel. Thus, the power of Western analysis stems from extraordinary sensitivity plus a positive identification. The only loss is information regarding cell or tissue localization; this is readily obtained from concordant immunocytochemical analysis. In our opinion, immunocytochemistry is never absolute evidence in the absence of Western analysis with the same antibody on extracts from the same tissue.

CONTROVERSIES IN PEDIATRIC PATHOLOGY

The preceding discussion of diagnostic methods and corresponding findings has obvious implications for the appropriate categorization or diagnosis of a number of the tumors under discussion here. In particular, the effect on our understanding of Ewing's sarcoma, undifferentiated neuroblastoma, neuroepithelioma, extraosseous Ewing's sarcoma, primitive rhabdomyosarcoma, monophasic synoviosarcoma, fibrosarcoma, and lymphoma will be discussed.

What Is the Origin of Ewing's Sarcoma?

The controversy surrounding the origin of Ewing's sarcoma and its relation, if any, to other childhood tumors, especially neuroblastoma, is a well-known issue in pathology.[90] The long-standing assertion by Rupert Willis that Ewing's tumor was only metastatic neuroblastoma[91] is especially interesting in view of the data discussed above. Willis was both right and wrong; Ewing's sarcoma is not metastatic neuroblastoma, but it is almost certainly neural. The body of ultrastructural, immunologic, cytogenetic, molecular genetic, and biochemical data discussed herein overwhelmingly supports such a histogenesis for the tumor, yet the problem remains: is Ewing's sarcoma just a misdiagnosed PNET, or is it somehow different?

Before addressing that question, it is useful to consider the following observations:

1. Ewing's sarcoma is widely regarded as a tumor devoid of any evidence of neural differentiation by light or electron microscopy.
2. The original description of the Askin tumor noted suggestive evidence of neural differentiation in three cases in which ultrastructural information was available.
3. The original description of PNET of bone noted that all cases were referred as being Ewing's sarcoma, but further study, especially in culture, revealed obvious neural characteristics.
4. Peripheral neuroepithelioma (or the same tumor by many other names, including peripheral neuroblastoma, most adult neuroblastoma, and most PNETs) is a primitive neural tumor lacking ganglion cell differentiation and frank neuropil but possessing rosettes by light microscopy and obvious neurites and dense core granules by electron microscopy.

These points lead to a logical conclusion: there is an overlapping spectrum of neural differentiation among these tumors, such that absolute distinction between, say, Ewing's sarcoma and the Askin tumor in each and every case is impossible (see Chaps. 29 and 31). What of the published accounts of NSE positivity in Askin[92] tumor but not Ewing's sarcoma?[22] Recent work from this laboratory has demonstrated that, although typical cases of Ewing's sarcoma are indeed negative for NSE by conventional Sternberger peroxidase–antiperoxidase methods, they are positive if the more-sensitive avidin–biotin complex method is used, especially following protease

FIGURE 6-3. Typical light microscopic appearance of Ewing's-class tumors. **A.** Ewing's sarcoma. **B.** Askin tumor (malignant small-cell tumor of thoracopulmonary region). **C.** Primitive neuroectodermal tumor of bone. **D.** Peripheral neuroepithelioma.

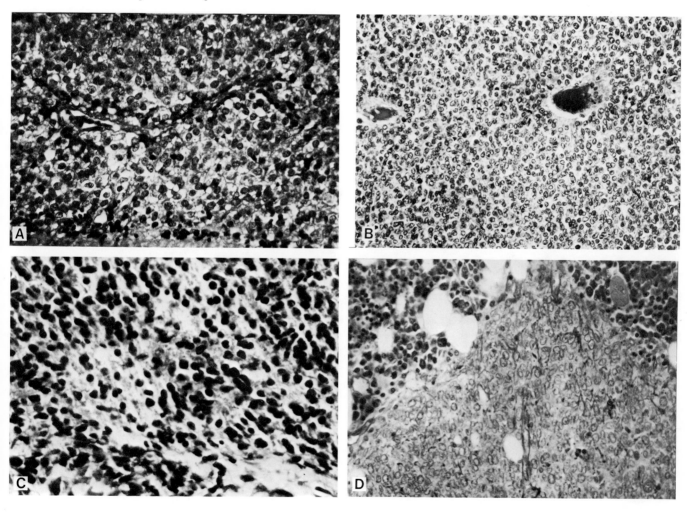

digestion.[93] Further, others have published reports of NSE positivity in apparently typical Ewing's sarcoma,[94] and Leu7 (HNK.1) positivity, typical of neural tissue, has also been documented in some cases of Ewing's sarcoma.[27]

The obvious conclusion from data such as these is that there is no single, simple distinction between these tumors other than at the extremes of the spectrum. No one would confuse a peripheral neuroepithelioma having rosettes, cell processes, and dense core granules with Ewing's sarcoma devoid of all these neural features, yet, by analogy, we accept totally undifferentiated neuroblasts as a possible neuroblastoma. Given the wide-ranging body of data tying Ewing's sarcoma, Askin tumor, the PNET of bone, and peripheral neuroepithelioma together, it should not be difficult to accept the concept of a range of peripheral neural tumors of presumed common histogenesis, with Ewing's sarcoma as the extreme undifferentiated member of the group, overt peripheral neuroepithelioma as the most differentiated (and the only one readily confused with neuroblastoma), and the Askin tumor and PNET of bone intermediate between these extremes.[80] Typical examples of these tumors are illustrated by light microscopy in Figure 6-3 and by electron microscopy in Figure 6-4. This concept of an overlapping spectrum of peripheral neural tumors is diagrammed in Figure 6-5.

Although the concept of a tumor family is well substantiated, a corollary to this is the issue of whether any of these family members should be distinguished from one another. What is the point of separating Ewing's sarcoma from peripheral neuroepithelioma if they are basically the same tumor? Pathologic findings aside for the moment, the most justifiable reason for making any such distinction is to convey clinically useful information with treatment implications. In this regard, evidence from two separate studies suggests that neural differentiation in this group of tumors is associated with a lesser response to treatment and ultimately poorer prognosis.[95,96] This point was also made in the original paper describing the Askin tumor.[13] For this reason, we continue to distinguish between tumors with no detectable neural differentiation by conventional pathologic techniques (Ewing's sarcoma), those with atypical features but no absolute evidence of neural histogenesis (atypical Ewing's sarcoma), and those with obvious neural differentiation (PN or PNET, including the Askin tumor). The criteria we use to make these distinctions are illustrated in Figure 6-6 and depicted in tabular form in Table 6-7.

The important point regarding these criteria is that, as noted previously, they are not absolute; exceptions do occur, and it is often impossible to assign a given tumor confidently to one or another category. Further, what does one do if only H&E slides are available? If the histologic appearance is typically bland, diffuse, and uniform, we categorize the tumor as Ewing's sarcoma pending availability of additional tissue for

FIGURE 6-4. Typical ultrastructural appearance of the same tumors as shown in Figure 6-3. **A.** Ewing's sarcoma. **B.** Askin tumor. **C.** PNET of bone. **D.** Peripheral neuroepithelioma.

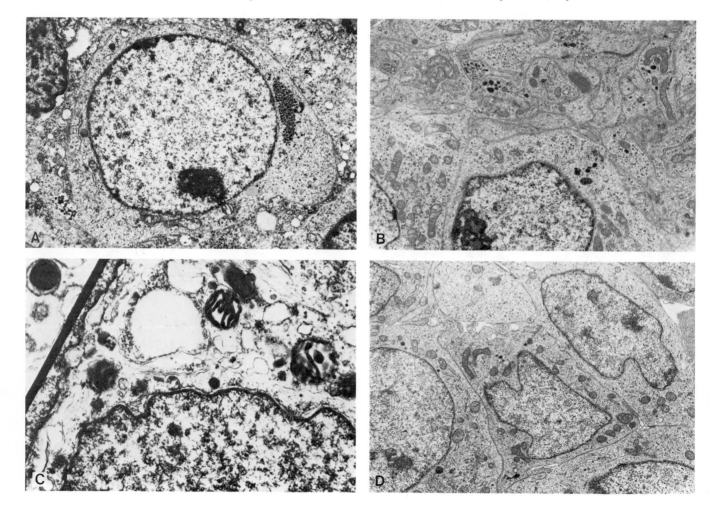

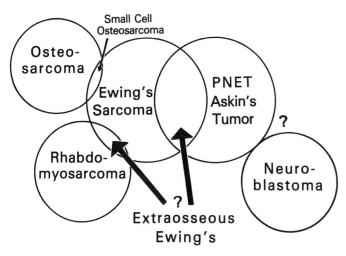

FIGURE 6-5. Diagram of the relationship of Ewing's sarcoma, Askin tumor, PNET of bone, peripheral neuroepithelioma, and neuroblastoma.

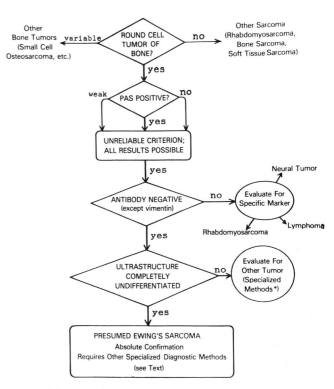

FIGURE 6-6. Flow diagram for the differential diagnosis of Ewing's sarcoma and related tumors by conventional pathologic methods.

further study. If features such as a lobular pattern, obvious stroma, suggestive rosettes, or PAS negativity are present, we categorize the tumor as atypical pending further study. If obvious rosettes are present, and especially if the PAS stain is either weakly positive or negative, we tentatively categorize the tumor as peripheral neuroepithelioma or PNET pending the outcome of electron microscopy and immunocytochemistry if available. If not, we do not make an absolute diagnosis of peripheral neuroepithelioma. On the one hand, the tumor may lack true neural differentiation; on the other, it rarely represents metastatic neuroblastoma. For the latter, ultrastructural characteristics can suggest the diagnosis (as opposed to PN/PNET), since the latter rarely, if ever, displays the regular, small dense core granules and long, regular, slender neurites typical of neuroblastoma. In such cases, the methods discussed in detail previously become imperative for precise diagnosis. In their absence, one simply cannot be sure of the diagnosis.

Another point that should be made regarding this group of tumors is that a bone versus soft-tissue origin is frequently impossible to discern. The Askin tumor has been thought to arise from soft tissue,[13] yet rib involvement is almost universal. The PNET of bone, as indicated by its name, is purely a bone tumor,[97] yet peripheral neuroepithelioma or PNET of soft tissue with no obvious bone involvement appears identical by all the measures discussed above and may involve multiple bones, presumably secondarily. Under these circumstances, and re-

membering that even straightforward Ewing's sarcoma may present as a soft-tissue sarcoma with no overt bone origin (until detected on further clinical evaluation, including bone biopsy), it is wise to consider bone and soft-tissue lesions in the differential diagnosis of these round-cell tumors.

A further complication, in light of the above, is categorization of extraosseous Ewing's sarcoma. Although at this point too little information is available to be certain, such data as exist indicate that this is a heterogeneous group of tumors, probably with two major constituents. On the one hand, definite progression to rhabdomyosarcoma has been reported[98] and seen in our laboratory, whereas cytogenetic analysis has both confirmed and refuted the presence of the Ewing's-associated rcp(11:22) chromosomal translocation.[56,60] Further, a recent study of more than 80 cases from the Intergroup Rhabdomyosarcoma Study (IRS), which had categorized such tumors originally as special types I and II and more recently as

Table 6-7
Criteria for Distinction Between Ewing's Sarcoma, Atypical Ewing's Sarcoma, and Peripheral Neural Tumors

Tumor	Light Microscopy	Electron Microscopy	Immunocytochemistry
Ewing's	Diffuse sheets of undifferentiated round cells	No neural differentiation	Negative NSE and Leu7 (Sternberger technique)
Atypical Ewing's	PAS negative, rosettes, stroma, pleomorphic	Cell processes, no dense core granules	Negative or weak-positive NSE; negative EM
PN/PNET	Lobular pattern, rosettes	Neurites and dense core granules	Definitely NSE positive, possibly Leu7 Positive

extraosseous Ewing's, has detected clear-cut neural differentiation by immunocytochemistry with NSE and S100 antibodies in about half the tumors studied.[99] Thus, no simple yes or no answer is possible: some are almost certainly peripheral neural tumors, others are certainly primitive rhabdomyosarcomas, and some may well be other soft-tissue sarcomas such as synoviosarcoma. Further study will be needed to know for sure. For now, such tumors should be considered as candidates and evaluated as detailed earlier in this chapter.

From the preceding discussion, it should be clear that although certainties are scarce in this group of tumors, the overall relation of Ewing's sarcoma to peripheral neural tumors, including the Askin tumor, neuroepithelioma, and PNET of bone, is fairly straightforward.[80,100] The problem is appropriate categorization of individual tumors, and this is possible only with extended study by the techniques discussed in detail previously.

What Other Ewing's-like Sarcomas Occur in Bone?

Missing from the discussion thus far is a consideration of well-described tumors such as small-cell osteosarcoma and mesenchymal chondrosarcoma and their relation to Ewing's sarcoma. Very little is known about these tumors other than their light[101-103] and, to some degree, electron[104,105] microscopic appearance. The extensive analysis performed on Ewing's sarcoma and other peripheral neural tumors has not been possible on these bone sarcomas for lack of cases and established tumor cell lines. Nonetheless, certain observations have been made that suggest little direct relation to Ewing's sarcoma on morphologic grounds.

The first and most obvious point to be made, particularly in connection with mesenchymal chondrosarcoma (Fig. 6-7A), which some believe to be only another presentation of small-cell osteosarcoma[103,106] (Fig. 6-7B), is that the tumor cells look different from Ewing's sarcoma by electron microscopy. Specifically, Ewing's sarcoma cells lack the specialized organelles for synthesis and secretion of extracellular matrix constituents (extensive rough endoplasmic reticulum [RER], prominent Golgi apparatus, and numerous mitochondria), a well-developed cytoskeleton, and any evidence of extracellular matrix (collagen fibers) (Fig. 4A)[107,108] In contrast, mesenchymal chondrosarcoma cells possess all these and more:[105] RER con-

taining flocculent electron-dense secretory product (unpolymerized collagen or proteoglycan), prominent cytoskeleton, and obvious extracellular matrix, including proteoglycan granules and fine fibrillar collagen, are all present at least focally (Fig. 6-8A).

To date, there are no published reports of the ultrastructural appearance of small-cell osteosarcoma, although two cases were reported in abstract form at the International Association of Pathologists in 1982,[104] and we have observed two additional cases (unpublished observations). Both groups of observers noted the presence of typical osteoblast features in these tumors, especially abundant RER and at least focal well-developed collagen fibers (Fig. 6-8B). Both features clearly set these tumors apart from ordinary Ewing's sarcoma.

Although ultrastructural criteria allow reasonably reliable evidence in conjunction with the requisite light-microscopic evidence of bone or cartilage formation of a difference between these two tumors and Ewing's sarcoma, this does not necessarily preclude commonality of histogenesis. The light and electron microscopic appearance of Ewing's sarcoma and peripheral neuroepithelioma/PNET is vastly different, as discussed previously, yet these tumors appear to be closely related. Could small-cell osteosarcoma and mesenchymal chondrosarcoma be related to them as well? This intriguing possibility remains unsubstantiated at present for lack of data derived from cytogenetics, immunocytochemistry, and biochemical studies but would be especially intriguing for the following reason: simple neural lineage is a reasonable idea but combined neural and mesenchymal differentiation or lineage is a far less familiar concept. Rare tumors such as malignant ectomesenchymoma,[109,110] and even the less rare nerve-sheath tumor with neural crest derivatives (Schwann cells, ?melanocytes) and sarcomatous elements (cartilage, muscle), confirm the possibility of coexistent mesenchymal and neuroepithelial differentiation.[111] Clearly, such a possibility exists in this context as well, but *in vitro* studies, or at least analysis of fresh tumor tissue from mesenchymal chondrosarcoma and small-cell osteosarcoma, will be needed to confirm any such suspicion.

Some obvious bone sarcomas lack any evidence of bone, cartilage, or any other differentiation. The proper conceptual and nosologic placement of such tumors is unknown. Even a universally acceptable diagnostic term has thus far not been put forward. We use the term "primitive sarcoma of bone" to

FIGURE 6-7. Bone-matrix-forming round-cell tumors of bone (light microscopy). **A.** Mesenchymal chondrosarcoma. **B.** Small-cell osteosarcoma.

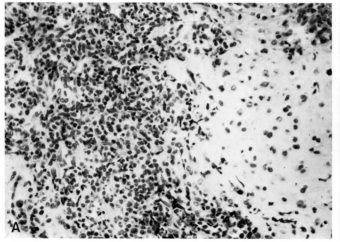
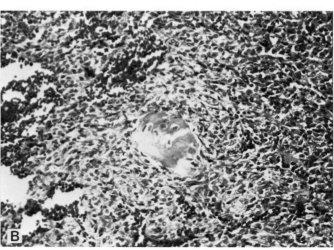

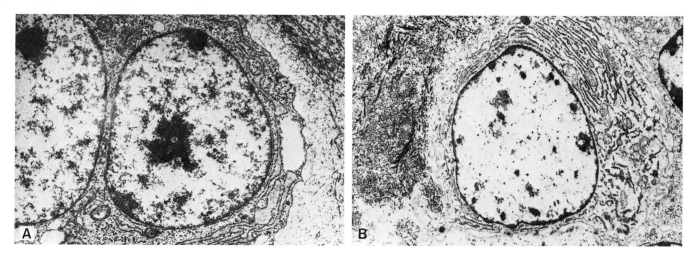

FIGURE 6-8. Ultrastructural appearance of tumors illustrated in Figure 6-7. **A.** Mesenchymal chondrosarcoma. **B.** Small-cell osteosarcoma.

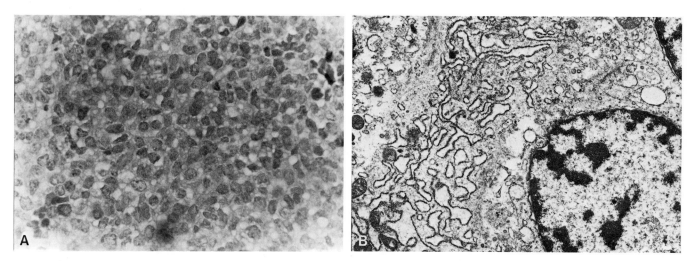

FIGURE 6-9. Light- and electron-microscopic appearance of nonmatrix-forming round-cell sarcoma of bone. **A.** Primitive sarcoma of bone by light microscopy; the tumor is virtually indistinguishable from Ewing's sarcoma. **B.** Same tumor by electron microscopy. Organelles associated with osteoblasts and chondroblasts (rough endoplasmic reticulum, Golgi apparatus) and collagenous stroma, none of which are found in Ewing's sarcoma, are evident.

identify such tumors, at the same time avoiding any presumption of a histogenesis. Others, such as Llombart–Bosch, and coworkers,[112] prefer the term "blastemic mesenchymal sarcoma of bone." Many such tumors are simply called Ewing's sarcoma, but careful review of the light microscopy findings invariably reveals a spindle-cell tumor (Fig. 6-9A) at least focally, which precludes a diagnosis of Ewing's sarcoma. Because selection among the treatment possibilities turns on whether these tumors are more similar to osteosarcoma or a related tumor or to Ewing's sarcoma, this is a practical as well as conceptual question. Ultrastructural studies would support the former view (Fig. 6-9B) but in no way exclude a specific histogenesis. There are only subtle differences between this tumor and Ewing's sarcoma by light microscopy but rather striking differences by electron microscopy. Too few of these tumors have been studied by electron microscopy to generalize, but certain cases have demonstrated neural markers by immunocytochemistry (Llombart–Bosch: Personal communi-

cation), an observation that has suggested that they represent another facet of the PNET of bone. Until sufficient numbers of these cases have been studied, it is unwise to emphatically rule in or out any specific relationship, especially with osteosarcoma and Ewing's sarcoma.

Can Soft-Tissue Sarcomas Arise in Bone, or Are Such Bone Lesions Always Metastatic?

In addition to these usual bone tumors, there are scattered reports in the literature of presumed soft-tissue sarcomas arising within bone. Both rhabdomyosarcoma[113] and synoviosarcoma[114] have been seen, although the latter often presents in such contiguity with bone that direct extension cannot be excluded. Always, however, the possibility of metastasis from an occult primary tumor must be considered in such cases. The primary importance of such entities, however, is the possible confusion of these tumors with "true" bone sarcomas. This becomes particularly relevant when the tumor is exceedingly primitive and rather "round cell" in character; both synovio-sarcoma and rhabdomyosarcoma, despite their usual images as spindle-cell sarcomas, can present a somewhat round-cell appearance (see below), with the obvious potential for confusion with the more common members of this group.

What Are the Common *Bona Fide* Metastatic Tumors of Bone?

The final issue to contend with in the differential diagnosis of round-cell tumors of bone is the problem of metastatic bone tumors. This problem is generally confined to neuroblastoma and rhabdomyosarcoma among childhood round-cell bone tumors but becomes vastly more complex in adults, in whom all manner of metastatic tumors, especially carcinomas such as small-cell carcinoma of lung, becomes the dominant issue. Although Ewing's sarcoma has been reported in patients in their fifth decade,[115] such cases more commonly prove to be metastatic tumor, especially small-cell carcinoma of lung. Rarely, primary brain tumors, including gliomas and medullo-blastomas, present as primary bone tumors, but careful clinical evaluation in this era of magnetic resonance imaging and computed tomography scans should readily clarify the issue. If not, such cases are readily diagnosed by careful histologic evaluation augmented by immunocytochemistry and electron microscopy, if necessary.

Are All Undifferentiated Neural Tumors in Bone Metastatic Neuroblastoma?

Most pathologists, if asked for a differential diagnosis of round-cell tumors of bone, would probably mention first Ewing's sarcoma (because it is the standard against which all others are measured) followed by metastatic neuroblastoma, to name only two. In fact, metastatic neuroblastoma is almost never the culprit. Most cases of "metastatic neuroblastoma with regressed primary" are really primary tumors. Despite this, rare cases of true metastatic neuroblastoma do occur as apparent primary bone or soft-tissue tumors.[116] This is distinct from the common presentation of a nearly leukemic picture of diffuse bone-marrow involvement. These latter patients have no radiologic evidence of an apparent single focus of tumor but instead have diffuse marrow involvement with few, if any, radiologic changes. These cases almost invariably follow a known primary somewhere in the autonomic nervous system. The challenge arises when there is no known sympathetic nervous system primary but there is seemingly a primary bone tumor. We have seen rare cases of this syndrome but more often have found no evidence of a regressed or inapparent primary tumor elsewhere. It is precisely in this situation that the diagnostic methods discussed above become invaluable.

The light microscopic appearance of undifferentiated neuroblastoma is not particularly enlightening (Fig. 6-10A). The usual rosettes and neuropil so characteristic of neuroblastoma are generally not evident. The ultrastructural appearance, in contrast, is generally strikingly neural in character (Fig. 6-10B). Tumor cells with regular nuclei, "salt-and-pepper" chromatin, cytoplasmic dense core granules of regular size and shape and, frequently, quite regular cell processes or neurites are often present even in seemingly undifferentiated cases. This degree of neural differentiation, incidentally, is almost exclusively the realm of neuroblastoma; the other neural tumors of childhood usually have obvious neural features but look like poorly wrought caricatures of real neuroblastomas when compared point by point. This fact is not readily appreciated from the literature. Nonetheless, there is sufficient overlap of ultrastructural features that most cases cause at least some degree of diagnostic uncertainty. For these, even more precise methods are available.

A simple method of detecting and characterizing tumor cells in marrow is catecholamine fluorescence.[117,118] Air-dried imprints or smears are adequate specimens. Simple exposure to paraformaldehyde vapor at 80°C for 1 hour is sufficient to condense the catechols into ring compounds that fluoresce bright green to yellow when illuminated by fluorescein-specific light sources.[119] Alternatively, a fresh solution of glyoxylic acid can be used to immerse the smears or imprints, with similar final results and no inconvenience or toxic vapor.[120,121]

FIGURE 6-10. Metastatic neuroblastoma mimicking Ewing's sarcoma. **A.** Light microscopic appearance of apparently undifferentiated neuroblastoma in bone. (H&E) **B.** Electron microscopic appearance of same tumor. Unequivocal neurites and dense core granules firmly establish the diagnosis of neural tumor, and quality of the differentiation (which is classic) establishes this as neuroblastoma.

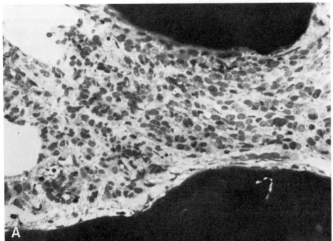

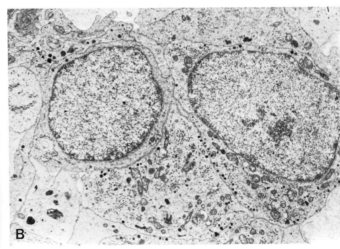

Either way, the tumor cells are easily detected, even as single cells in a field of hundreds of normal cells (Fig. 6-11).

Catecholamine fluorescence has been popularized as a method of positively identifying neuroblastoma, but even simpler methods are now available. Most are not technically as simple to perform as catecholamine fluorescence but have nonetheless largely supplanted this method, perhaps due to their reproducibility. Most pathologists are comfortable with immunocytochemical methods, for example, but less comfortable with a method they use only rarely that is totally divorced from other diagnostic methods. Presumably for this reason, NSE antibodies have become the method of choice for identifying neuroblastoma cells.[122] Unfortunately, NSE does not discriminate between real neuroblastoma and a host of other neural or neural crest-derived tumors of childhood. Catecholamine fluorescence is apparently specific for adrenergic tumors (such as almost all neuroblastomas), although melanoma is reportedly also positive despite absence of catechols.[123] The reason for this is unclear, but the fact is of little consequence in the diagnosis of neuroblastoma. In any event,

NSE staining is generally preferred, and the results are often striking (Fig. 6-12).

When imprints or frozen sections of tumor are available, neuroblastoma-"specific" monoclonal antibodies can be employed to verify the neural origin of the specimen. This test is particularly useful when paired with an HLA class I-specific antibody, as discussed above.[43] Neuroblastoma is positive for the former but not the latter; other neural tumors are positive for both or only the latter. An example of a true neuroblastoma is seen in Figure 6-13. The result with the neuroblastoma antibody HSAN 1.2 is strongly positive (Fig. 6-13A); the result with the HLA class I-specific antibody W6/32 is negative (Fig. 6-13B).

Neuroblastoma was apparently the first childhood tumor to be grown *in vitro,* by Murray and Stout in 1948.[124] As a rule, these tumors spontaneously produce characteristic neurites

FIGURE 6-12. Neuroblastoma; NSE staining. Conventional immunocytochemical staining of virtually all neuroblastomas with antisera to NSE yields results similar to these; the greater the differentiation, the more intense is the staining.

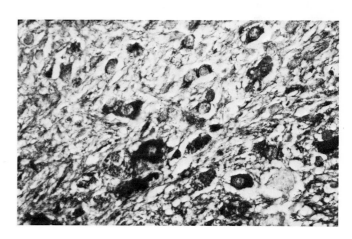

FIGURE 6-11. Neuroblastoma; catecholamine fluorescence. Treatment of tumor imprints or frozen sections with formaldehyde vapor at 80°C for 1 hour and examination by fluorescence microscopy typically results in images such as this.

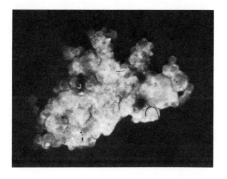

FIGURE 6-13. Neuroblastoma; monoclonal antibody staining. **A.** HSAN 1.2, an antibody raised against neuroblastoma, stains all neuroblastomas intensely (*left*) and most other peripheral neural tumors to a lesser extent (*right*). **B.** W6/32 (HLA class-I-specific monoclonal) does not stain neuroblastoma (*left*) but stains all other neuroectodermal tumors (*right*) tested to date. Beta-2-microglobulin antibody yields similar results.

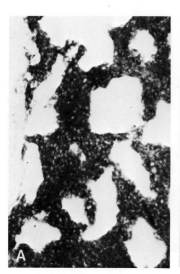
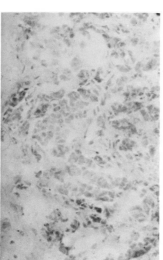
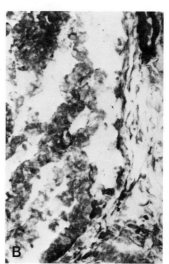
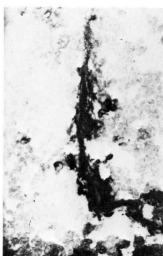

within days, especially in medium with a low serum concentration (Fig. 6-14). Perhaps even more intriguing is the apparent adverse prognostic significance of successful growth and establishment of a stable tumor cell line: patients whose tumors grow in culture do not survive.[125] The explanation for this has recently become apparent: virtually all such neuroblastoma lines overexpress the N-*myc* oncogene,[126] and this has been strongly correlated with advanced-stage disease and ultimate death.[76,77] Conversely, single-copy-N-*myc* neuroblastoma apparently does not grow indefinitely in culture, at least not without eventually overexpressing N-*myc*.

As discussed elsewhere, molecular genetic analysis of

FIGURE 6-14. Spontaneous differentiation of neuroblastoma *in vitro* (phase contrast microscopy). Short-term culture generally results in colony formation and neurite extension within days of explant. No agents are required to induce this differentiation in even the most primitive neuroblastomas, although low serum concentrations enhance the change.

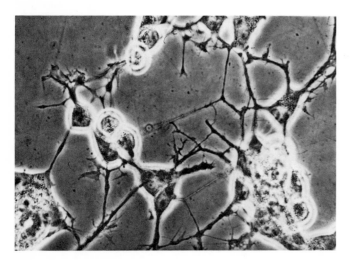

neuroblastoma for N-*myc* amplification and expression can provide prognostically useful information. A recent development that may further simplify this analysis is the availability of highly specific antibody for the N-*myc* oncogene product.[127,128] These antibodies readily and specifically detect the N-*myc* protein product in tumor cell nuclei when the cells overexpress mRNA for the protein. The cellular protein levels are correspondingly elevated in such cases (as determined by Western analysis),[129,130] and this is easily detected immunocytochemically as illustrated in Figure 6-15. Figure 6-15A shows a neuroblastoma in which N-*myc* is overexpressed and Figure 6-15B another neuroblastoma in which N-*myc* is not overexpressed. The first case shows amplification and overexpression of the oncogene; the second has only a single copy of the oncogene, and no mRNA for N-*myc* was detected by Northern analysis. Thus, this method is easily applied in the course of pathologic analysis of the tumors and should soon become routine in the evaluation of new cases.

A number of extremely promising neural-associated antibodies have become available in the past few years. These differ from general markers such as NSE and also from the usual monoclonal antibody, which detects cell-surface determinants. In contrast, these antibodies were developed to detect normal constituents of neural tissue. Two examples are chromogranin and synaptophysin. The former seems to be specific for the adrenergic granules of neuroblastoma and other tumors such as pheochromocytoma and islet-cell tumors[131] and shows striking sequence homology with pancreastatin,[132] which has suggested a possible hormonal activity for chromogranin although none has been demonstrated to date. In any case, in our experience, this protein is routinely expressed by neuroblastoma but not by any other childhood tumor, including the other neural tumors.[133] This observation has been confirmed by Western analysis (Fig. 6-16). This may become an increasingly important antibody for diagnostic use, especially since it works on paraffin-embedded tissues.

Synaptophysin is thought to be localized in the clear neurosecretory granules of the cholinergic neurons.[134] This antibody is less well characterized but shows promise for distin-

FIGURE 6-15. Immunocytochemistry of N-*myc* protein in neuroblastoma. **A.** N-*myc*-amplified neuroblastoma with increased N-*myc* mRNA. Rather intense staining of tumor cell nuclei is evident due to excessive accumulation of the 64-kD N-*myc* protein. **B.** Single-copy N-*myc* tumor with no expression of the oncogene. No nuclear staining is evident because no N-*myc* protein has accumulated in such cases. (Avidin–biotin–peroxidase method with nuclear fast green counterstain)

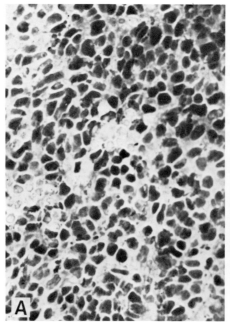

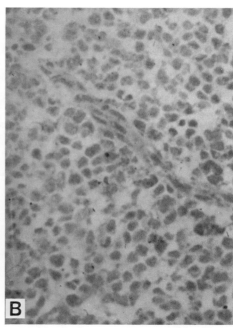

guishing between the two; immunofluorescence readily detects punctate fluorescence, suggesting localization to neurosecretory granules (Fig. 6-17).

Clearly, many methods can be applied to the diagnosis of neuroblastoma. Fortunately, few are actually needed in most cases because the histology is generally characteristic. Probably the greatest value of these methods is in distinguishing *bona fide* neuroblastoma from the many other childhood neural tumors.

FIGURE 6-16. Western analysis of chromogranin expression in childhood tumors; a panel of typical childhood tumors, including neuroblastoma, is illustrated. Note that only neuroblastoma shows evidence of chromogranin expression, as detected by antichromogranin-antibody staining of cell extracts.

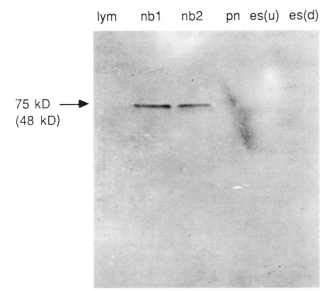

lym   nb1   nb2   pn   es(u)   es(d)

75 kD →
(48 kD)

How Do You Define Primitive Peripheral Neuroectodermal Tumors of Bone?

It is probably safe to assume that we have a great deal to learn about this complex and diverse group of tumors. It also is safe to say that they are only distantly related to neuroblastoma, despite their similar morphologic appearance. The clinical differences are striking, as discussed above and in other chapters. The routine pathology picture is generally rather primitive and usually reminiscent only of a neural lineage (Fig. 6-18). The tumors seem to be rather similar by all available criteria whether they arise in bone or soft tissue; in fact, the

FIGURE 6-17. Immunofluorescence of synaptophysin in cholinergic neural tumor. Synaptophysin antibody stains cholinergic neural tumors, as here, unlike chromogranin antibody. This new antibody is currently under investigation to determine specificity, and early reports are favorable.

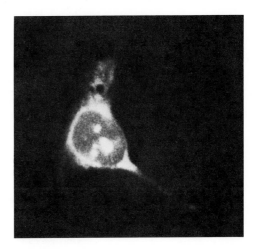

FIGURE 6-18. Light microscopic appearance of peripheral neuroepithelioma; a lobular pattern with suggestion of rosettees is seen. Neuropil, convincing rosettes, and ganglion cells are not normally seen in this group of tumors.

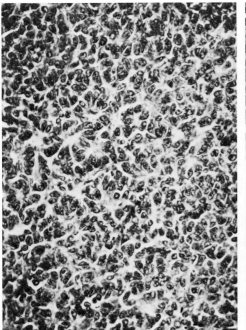
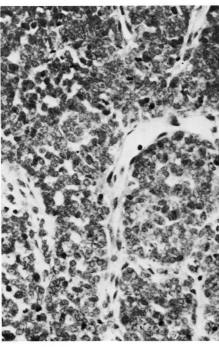

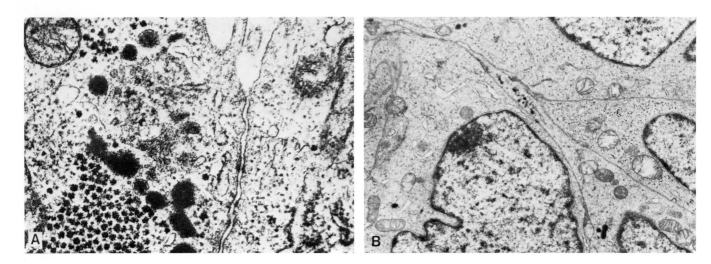

FIGURE 6-19. Ultrastructure of peripheral neuroepithelioma. **A.** Pleomorphic dense core granules are the rule, as here. Occasionally, classic neuroblastoma-type granules are found but are uncommon. **B.** Neurite formation is typically poor or infrequent in these tumors, as least in *ex vivo* specimens.

Table 6-8
Neuroblastoma and Other Neural Tumors of Childhood Compared

Parameter	Neuroblastoma	Peripheral Neural Tumors
Age of patient	Usually <5 years	Usually adolescence
Race	All	Rare in blacks, Asians
Catecholamine secretion	>95% cases	Never, or close to it
Cytogenetics	1p+, HSR, DMs	rcp (11:22) trans
Neurotransmitter enzymes	Adrenergic and cholinergic	Cholinergic only
Immunophenotype		
HSAN 1.2	Strongly positive	Weakly positive or negative
W6/32 (HLA I)	Negative	Positive
Oncogenes		
N-*myc*	Positive (50%)	Always negative
c-*myc*	Always negative	Always positive
Response to treatment	Very poor; survival <1 year	50% long-term survival (est.)

distinction is more often blurred and an osseous versus an extraosseous origin impossible to determine with certainty.

Because these tumors as a group (which includes at least obvious neural tumors, often called PNET, the PNET of bone, the Askin tumor of the chest wall, and the tumor we call peripheral neuroepithelioma) are readily and successfully treated, unlike stage IV neuroblastoma with which they would otherwise be confused—as they historically were in most cases—it is important to distinguish the two. The past 5 years have witnessed a remarkable growth in the availability of the necessary tools. Several of these have already been touched on in connection with neuroblastoma (catecholamine fluorescence, monoclonal antibodies, N-*myc* expression), but a unified discussion of how to make a positive diagnosis has yet to be provided.

After light microscopy, the first piece of objective evidence for a neural histogenesis is usually obtained by electron microscopy. Figure 6-19 is a typical example of this class of tumor; obvious dense core granules are present (Fig. 6-19A) but are quite different from those seen in Figure 6-10B. In peripheral neural tumors as a class, the quality of neural differentiation is markedly inferior to that routinely found in true

neuroblastoma. This is also true of neurites, which typically contain few neurotubules and neurofilaments, unlike neuroblastoma, in which they are a dominant part of the overall picture (Fig. 6-19B versus Fig. 6-10B).

If doubt still remains especially in distinguishing peripheral neuroepithelioma and related tumors from neuroblastoma, there are numerous methods of doing so. (Here we refer to all the non-neuroblastoma neural tumors as PNETs but not necessarily to indicate that they are all the same; we do not know that at this time.) Sufficient studies have not been performed on all members to make subtle distinctions. The methods to follow are in fact the means of doing so.

Some of the most compelling data to distinguish these tumors as a group from neuroblastoma come from cytogenetic, biochemical, immunologic, and molecular genetic analysis, as discussed above and in Chapter 3 (Table 6-8). In aggregate, there is a striking dissimilarity between neuroblastoma and all other neural tumors, which as a group show remarkable homogeneity. A note of caution is in order, however; the tumors studied to date were all readily confused with Ewing's sarcoma by light microscopy. Morphologically widely divergent neural tumors were not included in this study, nor have they been studied by these techniques. They, too, would qualify as PNETs in the broad sense of the word, but their relation, if any, to the tumors discussed here is unclear.

As Table 6-8 makes clear, many of the diagnostic procedures successfully employed for the diagnosis of neuroblastoma are also exceedingly useful for the diagnosis of these neural tumors. Although subtle morphologic differences exist between the two groups of tumors, real objective evidence of their differences becomes manifest only when the additional techniques discussed in connection with neuroblastoma and listed in Table 6-8 are employed. The expected results with these techniques are listed in that table.

The more interesting challenge in the diagnosis of these other neural tumors is discerning evidence of a neural histogenesis in the first place. This same issue was discussed in connection with Ewing's sarcoma, where a number of techniques to unmask the neural character of Ewing's were considered in some detail.[80] The same methods have convincingly

demonstrated neural differentiation in even the most primitive PNETs. The difference from Ewing's, as was discussed, is that PNETs undergo these changes spontaneously, whereas they must be induced in Ewing's sarcoma with *in vitro* differentiating agents and do not occur in the patient even after multiple tumor recurrences and treatment. The light and electron microscopic appearances of the PNETs have already been illustrated (see Figs. 6-3 and 6-4). Additional evidence of a diagnosis of PNET frequently arises from spontaneous neural differentiation in even short-term culture (Fig. 6-20). The appearance in short-term culture of the PNET of bone (illustrated in Figures 6-3C and 6-4C) is characterized by very nice neurites with bulbous swellings ("varicosities"). Using electron microscopy of the cultured cells, convincing evidence of neural differentiation is often readily apparent (Fig. 6-21).

Because the granules are often pleomorphic and the neurites abortive (unlike the case in Fig. 6-21), many other techniques have been used to verify the neural character of these features. One new method is illustrated in Figure 6-22. Here, short-term cultured cells that have undergone differentiation have been treated with uranium salts under conditions that allow specific binding of the heavy-metal salts to neurosecretory granules (regardless of shape, size, or number); this "uraniffin" reaction[135] is simple and reliable and yields convincing results, confirming the impression of neural differentiation.

The judicious application of a select few of the many techniques discussed thus far generally leads to an unequivocal diagnosis of peripheral neural tumor in even the most primitive cases. In fact, the number of techniques employed is usually a direct reflection of the diagnostic uncertainty surrounding the case: the more methods, the less the overt differentiation. Fortunately, the methods exist, and the diagnosis will eventually become clear.

Are Extraosseous Ewing's Sarcomas Simply Soft-Tissue PNETs?

A clear-cut statement distinguishing PNET of bone from peripheral neuroepithelioma of soft tissue has not been presented here because they are frequently impossible to distin-

FIGURE 6-20. Spontaneous differentiation of PNET of bone in short-term culture. Like neuroblastoma and unlike Ewing's sarcoma, PNET of bone undergoes spontaneous neural differentiation, producing neurites and even varicosities, when placed in culture.

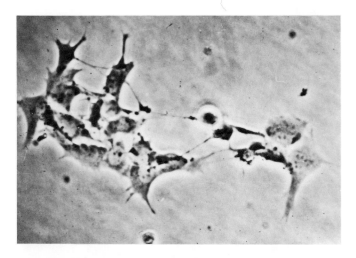

FIGURE 6-21. Peripheral neuroepithelioma *in vivo* and *in vitro*. **A.** Patient biopsy material; no convincing neural differentiation is seen, although the ultrastructure is suggestive of neural tumor. **B.** After 3 days of growth *in vitro*, the tumors cells have spontaneously developed conspicuous neurites with dense core granules.

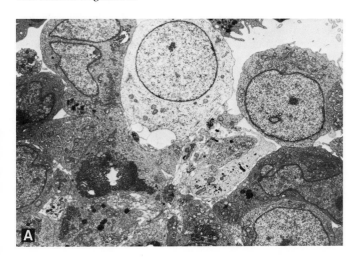
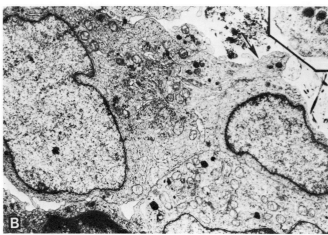

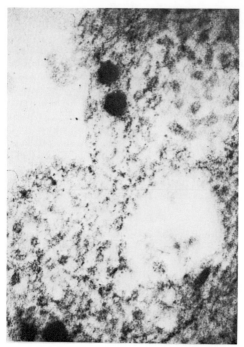 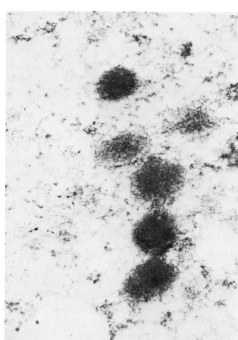

FIGURE 6-22. Uraniffin reaction of peripheral neuroepithelioma. Confirmation of the neural nature of the often-pleomorphic granules found in primitive neurotectodermal tumors is easily obtained by uranyl salt staining of the tissue, as here. Only neurosecretory granules show an affinity for uranium under the conditions of the uraniffin reaction.

guish. Figure 6-23 illustrates such an example. The CT scan clearly demonstrates a large soft-tissue mass and at least two bone lesions. Is it a bone tumor involving soft tissue, or a soft-tissue tumor involving bone? This particular patient was referred with a diagnosis of Ewing's sarcoma of bone, yet at surgery the soft-tissue mass was encapsulated and appeared to involve bone secondarily in two separate sites. This, then, would appear to be extraosseous Ewing's sarcoma. Other cases have no osseous involvement and are simple to distinguish from osseous Ewing's; some cases are certainly only massive soft-tissue involvement from an inconspicuous osseous primary. This suspicion has been substantiated by cytogenetic analyses, as discussed above. At least one tumor has been reported to possess the characteristic rcp(11:22) chromosomal translocation[60]; a second lacks the translocation.[56]

These results are perhaps not surprising in a tumor as ill defined as extraosseous Ewing's sarcoma. The entity was not described as such prior to 1975,[136] although one or two papers described the entity by other names.[137] What, then, is extraosseous Ewing's? The light and electron microscopic appearances are generally indistinguishable from those of osseous Ewing's sarcoma[138] (Fig. 6-24). However, sufficient numbers of cases have now been studied by various methods to suggest that, as might be suspected, the "tumor" is almost certainly a group of tumors, from primitive rhabdomyosarcoma to peripheral neuroepithelioma, with others in between. Recently, more than 80 cases were analyzed from the IRS, and half were found to express neural markers such as NSE and S100.[99]

Results such as this would certainly suggest a close relation between peripheral neuroepithelioma of bone and soft-tissue and extraosseous Ewing's sarcoma. The analogous situation exists with the Askin tumor of the chest wall. This tumor, now recognized as a peripheral neuroectodermal tumor,[92] has been described as a soft-tissue tumor, but rib is almost always involved. It now appears that the Askin tumor is a clinicopathologic entity; the same tumor almost certainly occurs in virtually any location. The data from the IRS would substantiate this. Although half of the cases from that series of extraosseous Ewing's showed evidence of a neural histogenesis, half did

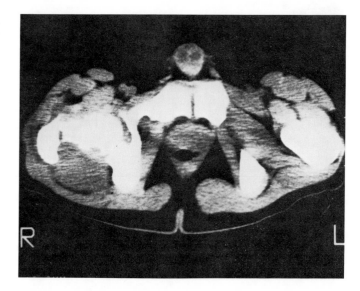

FIGURE 6-23. Computed tomography scan of peripheral neuroepithelioma; a dominant soft-tissue mass is seen in the posterior thigh, but at least two foci of osseous involvement are evident as well. Bone versus soft-tissue origin for this tumor is impossible to determine with certainty, although the latter seems more likely.

not.[99] The origin of these tumors remains speculative, but certain studies have strongly suggested that some, if not most, are related to rhabdomyosarcoma.

Are the Other Extraosseous Ewing's Sarcomas Simply Primitive Rhabdomyosarcoma?

The entire issue of diagnosis in rhabdomyosarcoma is currently under scrutiny; much of this debate is reviewed in Chapter 30. The special problem of tumors with virtually no

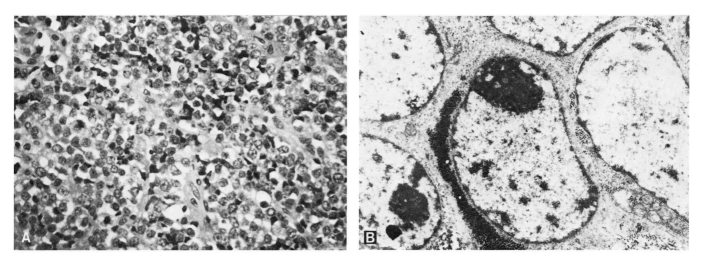

FIGURE 6-24. Extraosseous Ewing's sarcoma. **A.** Light microscopic appearance of this Ewing's sarcoma look-alike. **B.** Ultrastructure of this tumor is generally indistinguishable from that of osseous Ewing's sarcoma. If not, it is not considered extraosseous Ewing's (see text).

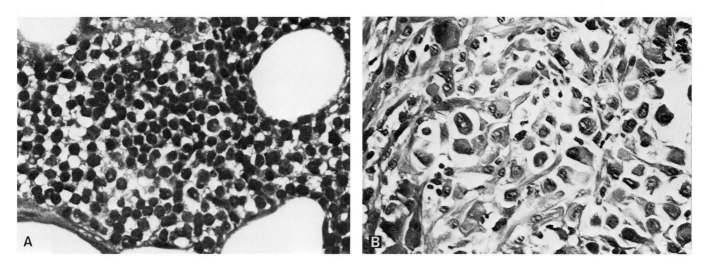

FIGURE 6-25. Primitive rhabdomyosarcoma simulating extraosseous Ewing's sarcoma. **A.** Initial biopsy in this patient revealed cutaneous infiltrate and bone-marrow involvement indistinguishable from Ewing's sarcoma. **B.** Repeat bone biospy some months later after treatment revealed this obvious highly differentiated rhabdomyosarcoma.

evidence of myogenous differentiation is addressed here as a continuation of the above discussion.

As suggested above, fragmentary evidence indicates that certain Ewing's-like soft-tissue tumors are really very primitive rhabdomyosarcomas. Figure 6-25 illustrates such a case; the skin lesion in this patient was indistinguishable from Ewing's sarcoma, but no bone primary tumor was found (Fig. 6-25A). The tumor was interpreted as extraosseous Ewing's sarcoma and, because of a positive NSE stain, as most likely neural in character. Several months later, the patient developed bone-marrow metastases; these were very obviously myogenic (Fig. 6-25B). Thus, the case was certainly a rhabdomyosarcoma from the beginning. It is safe to say that light microscopy is not a sufficient method for making such diagnoses.

A well-documented example of this phenomenon has been published, along with extensive supportive studies. This tumor showed no evidence of myogenesis in the patient or for months in culture;[139] only after the patient had died with metastases having areas of alveolar rhabdomyosarcoma was the diagnosis clear.[98]

The examples noted above are not isolated instances; 10 to 17% of the cases entered in the IRS are candidates for the misdiagnosis. As noted for peripheral neural tumors, perhaps half of these cases appear to be covert neural tumors; the other half in large part may represent additional cases of this tumor. When all were regrouped under the category of "undifferentiated," they had the worst prognosis of any form of rhabdomyosarcoma. In our opinion, every effort should be made to ferret out cases of this highly aggressive form of rhabdomyosarcoma.[2,140]

The methods to detect primitive rhabdomyosarcoma are as yet unsophisticated compared to those for the neural tumors discussed above. No consistent cytogenetic, enzymatic, or monoclonal antibody marker has been identified. At this point, the most useful tools are electron microscopy and immunocytochemistry with muscle markers (desmin, myoglobin, CK-MM, skeletal muscle myosin)[141,142] (Table 6-9). An example of the electron microscopy and immunocytochemistry results with desmin is illustrated in Figure 6-26.

Several studies are in progress to evaluate the reliability and sensitivity of various markers and immunocytochemistry techniques in detecting myogenesis in a putative rhabdomyosarcoma. It appears that no matter how sensitive the methodology, some cases will not have any evidence of myogenesis at the outset yet will develop such differentiation with treatment, as discussed above.[142,143] Are such cases rhabdomyosarcoma, and how does one diagnose them? This is a problem because true extraosseous Ewing's sarcoma seems to respond well to a moderate-dose Ewing's regimen,[144] whereas primitive rhabdo-

myosarcoma appears to be an unusually aggressive tumor poorly responsive to the same type of regimen.[2,140] There is obviously a need for other indices of impending or nascent myogenesis. Future efforts in immunophenotyping and molecular genetics may resolve this dilemma.

What Other Soft-Tissue Sarcomas Should Be Considered in the Diagnosis?

Although most primitive round-cell sarcomas of soft tissue probably fall into one of two categories—peripheral neuroepithelioma or rhabdomyosarcoma—some, and certainly the majority of undifferentiated spindle-cell sarcomas, do not. The spectrum of soft-tissue sarcomas in childhood is limited, and, for the reasons discussed above, many of the apparently undif-

Table 6-9
Primitive Rhabdomyosarcoma Versus Extraosseous Ewing's Sarcoma

Marker	Rhabdomyosarcoma	Extraosseous Ewing's
Electron microscopy		
Cytoplasmic filaments	Abundant	Scant or absent
Dense plaques (Z bands)	Often present	Always absent
Glycogen	Always present*	Always abundant*
Basal lamina	Often present	Never present
Fibrillar collagen stroma	Usually present	Never between tumor cells
Pleomorphic nuclei	Routine	Rare
Marginated dense chromatin	The rule	The exception
Immunocytochemistry		
Desmin	Positive, >90%	Negative
Myoglobin	Positive, >90%	Negative
CK-MM	Positive, majority	Negative
Skeletal muscle myosin	Positive, ~50%	Negative
Vimentin	Always positive	Always positive
Actin (fibroblast)	Always positive	Always positive
Actin (muscle)	Positive	Negative

* "Always" = >95% estimated.

FIGURE 6-26. Primitive rhabdomyosarcoma. **A.** Ultrastructure of this tumor is readily distinguishable from Ewing's sarcoma by abundance of cytoplasmic intermediate filaments, among other things, but is not otherwise diagnostic. **B.** Same tumor, stained with antibodies to desmin; positive reaction in single myoblastic cells appears to identify these filaments as desmin, and therefore to identify the tumor as rhabdomyosarcoma.

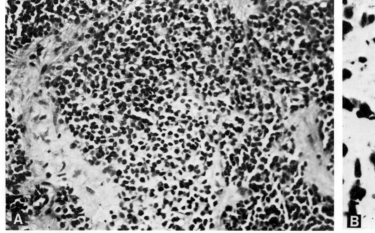

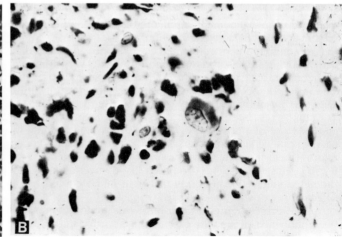

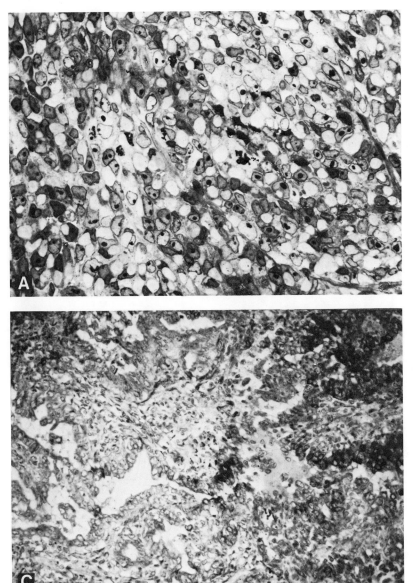

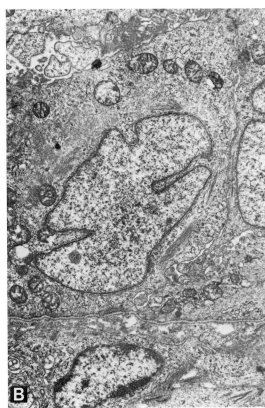

FIGURE 6-27. Monophasic synoviosarcoma. **A.** Light microscopic appearance is not diagnostic of synoviosarcoma. In this case, it was even misleading, with extensive pink cytoplasmic inclusions suggesting a rhabdoid tumor. **B.** By electron microscopy, tumor displayed unequivocal features of synoviosarcoma, including basal lamina, epithelial cell differentiation, microvilli, and lumen formation. **C.** Antikeratin antibodies confirm keratinous nature of cytoplasmic filaments noted in *B.*

ferentiated sarcomas probably would be categorized as rhabdomyosarcoma or peripheral neural tumor if sufficiently sensitive markers and extensive diagnostic evaluation were available (see Chap. 31).

Despite these caveats, there are some tumors that are not "closet" rhabdomyosarcoma or PNET. One of the two likely candidates is synoviosarcoma, not the conventional form with both a spindle stromal-cell and an epithelioid glandular component, but rather the "monophasic synoviosarcoma." This type lacks any clear-cut distinction between the two components and appears undifferentiated by routine light microscopic examination (Fig. 6-27A); both electron microscopy (Fig. 6-27B) and immunocytochemistry with antibodies to either keratin (Fig. 6-27C) or epithelial membrane antigen have been useful in identifying this tumor.[146] The advent of these tools has enormously improved the chances of identifying this tumor, which was heretofore undiagnosed, especially if primitive.

The existence of predominantly stromal or epithelial monophasic synoviosarcoma has been documented, but the stromal cell-predominant form presents certain problems in interpretation. How can one make a diagnosis of synoviosarcoma, whose unique characteristic is the development of epithelial differentiation manifest as glands, in the absence of epithelial cells? In most cases, elements of epithelial differentiation, such as keratin filament bundles or basal lamina or elaborate cell-to-cell junctions, are present in otherwise sarcomatous cells (*i.e.,* with features of fibroblastic cells, including elaborate RER, actin cables, and prominent Golgi apparatus). These cases can be reasonably diagnosed by ultrastructural features alone. Without such features, a diagnosis of monophasic synoviosarcoma cannot be substantiated, and overlap with fibrosarcoma and related lesions, especially neurofibrosarcoma and fibromatosis, is inevitable.

What Is the Relation, If Any, of Fibrosarcoma to Neurofibrosarcoma?

Childhood fibrosarcoma should be a straightforward diagnosis but is not because of its overlap with undifferentiated rhabdomyosarcoma on the one hand (the undifferentiated spindle

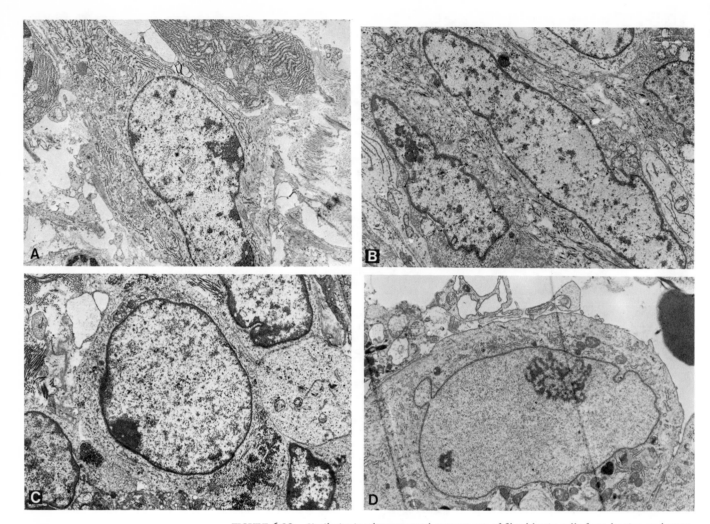

FIGURE 6-28.   Similarity in ultrastructural appearance of fibroblastic cells from benign and sarcomatous conditions. **A.** Reactive fibroblast. **B.** Fibrosarcoma cell. **C.** Embryonal rhabdomyosarcoma; undifferentiated cell. **D.** Neurofibrosarcoma cell.

cells in even "garden variety" embryonal rhabdomyosarcoma look like fibroblasts) and monophasic synoviosarcoma on the other. Further, the distinction between benign (*i.e.,* fibromatosis) and malignant (fibrosarcoma) is often not possible by pathologic examination alone; the clinical history and presentation are crucial to such a distinction.[111] Even if the tumor is malignant, the distinction between high-grade (neurofibrosarcoma) and low- (fibrosarcoma in patients younger than 5 years) to moderate-grade (older children with histologically identical fibrosarcoma) can be extraordinarily difficult.

Once again, both electron microscopy and immunocytochemistry have become critical in the evaluation of these tumors. Fibrosarcoma is rather typical in its ultrastructural features; it is composed of cells very similar in appearance to activated normal fibroblasts, as in healing wounds (Fig. 6-28A, B). Unfortunately, as noted, undifferentiated rhabdomyosarcoma cells can be identical in appearance (Fig. 6-28C). Neurofibrosarcoma cells are superficially the same, but careful search will usually reveal elements of normal nerve-sheath development, especially extensive but fragmented basal lamina (typical of Schwann cells) and a peculiar tendency for a caricature of unmyelinated nerve-sheath formation (called pseudome-

saxon formation) (Fig. 6-28D). When present, these features allow easy distinction of neurofibrosarcoma from the others.

Although neurofibrosarcoma can be distinguished by electron microscopy, it cannot be distinguished reliably. This has become apparent with the advent of immunocytochemistry and correlation with ultrastructural data. Immunocytochemistry is capable of surveying vastly greater amounts of tumor than is electron microscopy, and this seeming nerve-sheath differentiation is often focal. As such, a marker for Schwann cells is usually employed—S100 protein antibody. When this is done, most neurofibrosarcomas will show at least focal positivity[147] (Fig. 6-29). The practical consequences of this finding are potentially devastating: fibrosarcoma is generally regarded as a low-grade malignancy not beneficially treated by aggressive chemotherapy and radical surgery; neurofibrosarcoma is just the opposite. What, then, should one do with a positive S100 result and no other evidence of malignant nerve-sheath tumor? There is no good answer at this point, but, as always, judgment and interpretation in the context of clinical and routine pathologic examination are mandatory. There is no body of evidence yet to support dogmatic assertions. Our feeling is simply that immunocytochemistry results alone should not precipitate a significant change in treatment without support by other clinical or pathologic data. The tumor illustrated in Figure 6-29, in fact, was present at birth, diagnosed as fibrosarcoma, and surgically excised yet later recurred locally with evidence of well-developed nerve-sheath differentiation (Fig. 6-30). The patient is alive and well at 3 years' follow-up, with no evidence of recurrence after only reexcision and local radiation therapy. This is hardly the usual evolution of high-grade neurofibrosarcoma.

Lymphoma in Unusual Locations

The last tumor to be considered in this chapter is lymphoma. Of all the round-cell tumors, lymphoma is the truest candidate yet an uncommon problem in the differential diagnosis. When it occurs, however, misdiagnosis can be devastating.

FIGURE 6-29. S100 antibody staining of neurofibrosarcoma. Despite light microscopic similarity to fibrosarcomatous lesions, neurofibrosarcoma is generally easily distinguishable therefrom by virtue of its S100 protein content as detected by routine immunocytochemistry.

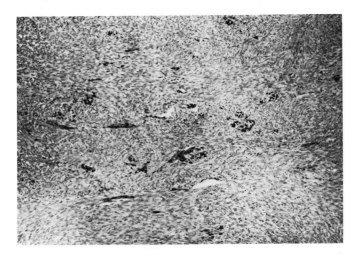

Lymphoma in lymph nodes is usually a straightforward histologic diagnosis.[148] Any uncertainty can be alleviated with any of a number of studies, from monoclonal antibodies to immunoglobulin or T-cell receptor gene rearrangement analyses, but none of these will help if there is no index of suspicion. This is unfortunately the case when this most common extracranial solid tumor of childhood presents in an unusual site such as bone or extranodal soft tissue or with unusual clinical features such as multiple lytic bone lesions that simulate metastatic tumor. Here, the challenge is to *consider* lymphoma in the differential diagnosis, not to decide whether the tumor mass in question is lymphoid hyperplasia or lymphoma. In these cases, the diagnosis of malignancy is manifest; it is the histogenesis that is not. It is for these cases that the discussion which follows is presented.

Although diffuse large-cell lymphoma is the more common problem in adults, children have an unusual predisposition to lymphoblastic lymphoma in general[148] and a correspondingly frequent incidence of a bony presentation of lymphoblastic lymphoma.[149] The radiographic appearance can simulate that of Ewing's sarcoma, but any doubt can be readily allayed by immunocytochemistry with LCA antibodies (Fig. 6-31A). The ultrastructural appearance is characteristic as well (Fig. 6-31B). The distinction from marrow involvement by acute lymphoblastic leukemia is conceptually more difficult than the reality; lytic bone lesions are characteristic of the presentation of primary lymphoma of bone even if multifocal, whereas diffuse, radiologically inapparent involvement is the more common situation with acute lymphoblastic leukemia.

CONCLUSION

The preceding discussion will appear to many readers to be arcane, academic, and of little practical value, with expensive implications. To others, it will appear interesting but too superficial to be of any personal value. For a few (plagued with the same diagnostic problems as the authors), it will perhaps offer a number of possibilities for other approaches when no diagnosis is evident after a conventional pathologic evaluation. We would be pleased if this chapter offers a starting point for physicians involved in the diagnosis and treatment of children

FIGURE 6-30. Recurrent neurofibrosarcoma previously identifiable only as fibrosarcoma. **A.** Light microscopy demonstrates vague neural appearance, with fascicles of tumor cells. **B.** By electron microscopy, absolute evidence of far-advanced nerve-sheath differentiation is evident. Even neurites were identified, suggesting tumor more hamartomatous than the usual neurofibrosarcoma.

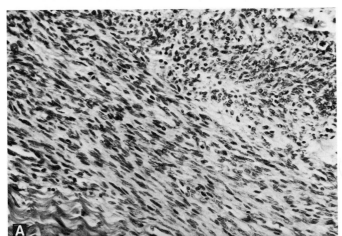
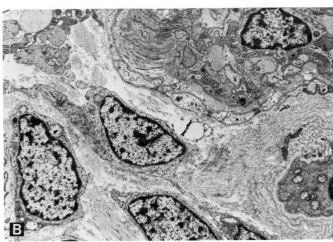

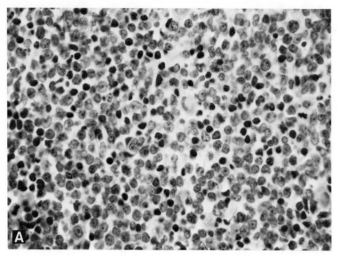
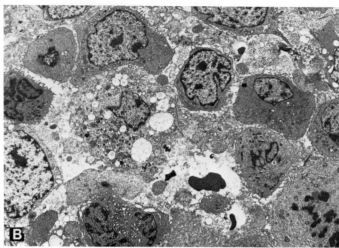

FIGURE 6-31. Extranodal, extraosseous lymphoma of soft tissue. **A.** Immunocytochemistry with LCA monoclonal antibodies, even on paraffin sections, provides unequivocal evidence of hematopoietic differentiation. **B.** Ultrastructural appearance of the same tumor confirmed not only its hematopoietic nature (which could include granulocytic sarcoma) but also its lymphoid character.

with cancer, but we are more concerned with those who might ignore this information out of hand. We would consider this unwise, for the following reasons:

1. Ewing's sarcoma treated as lymphoma of bone is unlikely to have a good outcome in our experience.
2. Primitive rhabdomyosarcoma had the worst prognosis of any form of rhabdomyosarcoma in a recent review, yet this is precisely the tumor most likely to be called either embryonal rhabdomyosarcoma or not even rhabdomyosarcoma, and treated accordingly, with often-disastrous results.
3. The prognosis for advanced-stage neuroblastoma patients remains bleak, except perhaps for bone-marrow transplantation. In contrast, most tumors historically diagnosed as metastatic neuroblastoma in patients older than 5 years are peripheral neural tumors that have responded well to an aggressive regimen of vincristine, Adriamycin, and cyclophosphamide with 400 Gy of local radiation.
4. No new tumors or well-described tumors with aberrant clinical behavior will be identified unless these methods are used prospectively to segregate tumor types into groups with differing biological behavior. This is the necessary first step in the design of therapeutic regimens that neither overtreat nor undertreat the patient.

Despite these profound differences in biology, origin, response to treatment, and clinical evolution (to death in most untreated or ill-treated cases), these tumors can be virtually indistinguishable to even the most practiced eye using only light microscopy. Correct diagnosis and thus treatment demand the best possible diagnostic evaluation. The methods described in this chapter, whether established or new, can provide the means of doing so. For the patient's sake, they should be utilized as needed.

REFERENCES

1. Beckwith JB, Palmer NF: Histopathology and prognosis of Wilms' tumor: Results from the First National Wilms' Tumor Study. Cancer 41:1937–1978
2. Newton WA, Soule EH, Hamoudi AB, Reiman HM, Shimada H, Beltangady M, Maurer HM: Histopathology of childhood sarcomas, Intergroup Rhabdomyosarcoma Studies I and II: Clinicopathologic correlation. J Clin Oncol (in press)
3. Spjut HJ, Ayala AG: Skeletal tumors in childhood and adolescence. Major Probl Pathol 18:256–281, 1986
4. Magrath IT, Janus C, Edwards BK et al: An effective therapy for both undifferentiated (including Burkitt's) lymphomas and lymphoblastic lymphomas in children and young adults. Blood 63:1102–1111, 1984
5. Shimada H, Chatten J, Newton WA et al: Histopathologic prognostic factors in neuroblastic tumors: Definition of subtypes of ganglioneuroblastoma and an age-linked classification of neuroblastomas. JNCI 73:405, 1984
6. Marsden HB, Steward JK: Epithelial and other rare tumours. In Recent Results in Cancer Research: Tumors in Children, pp 403–444. New York, Springer-Verlag, 1976
7. Seeger RC, Brodeur GM, Sather H et al: Association of multiple copies of the N-myc oncogene with rapid progression of neuroblastomas. N Engl J Med 313:1111, 1985
8. Sutow WW: General aspects of childhood cancer. In Sutow WW, Fernbach DJ, Vietti TJ (eds): Clinical Pediatric Oncology, pp 1–13 St Louis, CV Mosby, 1984
9. Dehner LP: Soft tissue sarcomas of childhood: The differential diagnostic dilemma of the small blue cell. Natl Cancer Inst Monogr 56:43–59, 1981
10. Triche TJ, Askin FB: Neuroblastoma and the differential diagnosis of small-, round-, and blue-cell tumors. Hum Pathol 14:569–595, 1983
11. Variend S: Small cell tumours in childhood: A review. J Pathol 145:1–25, 1985
12. Triche TJ, Askin FB, Kissane JM: Neuroblastoma, Ewing's sarcoma, and the differential diagnosis of small-, round-, and blue-cell tumors. In Finegold M (ed): Pathology of Neoplasia in Children and Adolescents, pp 145–195. Philadelphia, WB Saunders, 1986
13. Askin FB, Rosai J, Sibley RK, Dehner LP, McAlister WH: Malignant small cell tumor of the thoracopulmonary region in childhood: A distinctive clinicopathologic entity of uncertain histogenesis. Cancer 43:2438–2451, 1979
14. Sim FH, Unni KK, Beabout JW et al: Osteosarcoma with small cells simulating Ewing's tumor. J Bone Joint Surg [Am] 61:207, 1979
15. Ghadially FN: Diagnostic Electron Microscopy of Tumours. London, Butterworths, 1985
16. Triche TJ: Morphologic tumor markers. Semin Oncol 14:139–172, 1987
17. DeLellis RA, Sternberger LA, Mann RB, Banks PM, Nakane PK: Immunoperoxidase technics in diagnostic pathology: Report of a workshop sponsored by the National Cancer Institute. Am J Clin Pathol 71:483–488, 1979
18. Sternberger LA: Immunocytochemistry. Englewood Cliffs, Prentice Hall, 1974
19. Hsu SH, Raine L, Fanger H: Use of avidin–biotin–peroxidase techniques: A comparison between ABC and unlabeled antibody (PAP) procedures. J Histochem Cytochem 29:577–580, 1981

20. Erlandson RA: Diagnostic immunohistochemistry of human tumors. Am J Surg Pathol 8:615–624, 1984

21. Hammar SP: Is electron microscopy dying? (editorial). Ultrastruct Pathol 10:iii–v, 1986

22. Tsokos M, Linnoila RI, Chandra RS, Triche TJ: Neuron-specific enolase in the diagnosis of neuroblastoma and other small, round-cell tumors in children. Hum Pathol 15:575–584, 1984

23. Schmechel DE: b-Subunit of the glycolytic enzyme enolase: Nonspecific or neuron specific? (editorial). Lab Invest 52:239–242, 1985

24. Abo T, Balck CM: A differentiation antigen of human NK and K cells identified by a monoclonal antibody (HNK-1). J Immunol 127:1024–1029, 1981

25. Kruse J, Mailhammer R, Wernecke H, Faissner A, Sommer I, Goridis C, Schachner M: Neural cell adhesion molecules and myelin-associated glycoprotein share a common carbohydrate moiety recognized by monoclonal antibodies L2 and HNK-1. Nature 311:153–155, 1984

26. McGarry KH, Ilyas AA, Quarles RH, Roder JC: Recognition of myelin-associated glycoprotein by the monoclonal antibody HNK-1. Nature 306:376–378, 1983

27. Lipinski M, Braham K, Philip I et al: Neuroectoderm-associated antigens on Ewing's sarcoma cell lines. Cancer Res 47:183–187, 1986

28. Chou KH, Ilyas AA, Evans JE, Quarles RH, Jungalwala FB: Structure of a glycolipid reacting with monoclonal IgM in neuropathy and with HNK-1. Biochem Biophys Res Commun 128:383–388, 1985

29. Osborn M, Weber K: Tumor diagnosis by intermediate filament typing: A novel tool for surgical pathology. Lab Invest 48:372–394, 1983

30. Fisher DZ, Chaudhary N, Blobel G: cDNA sequencing of nuclear laminins A and C reveals primary and secondary structural homology to intermediate filament proteins. Proc Natl Acad Sci USA 83:6450–6454, 1986

31. Osborn M, Dirk T, Kaser H et al: Immunohistochemical localization of neurofilaments and neuron-specific enolase in 29 cases of neuroblastoma. Am J Pathol 122:433–442, 1986

32. Altmannsberger M, Osborn M, Treuner J et al: Diagnosis of human childhood rhabdomyosarcoma by antibodies to desmin, the structural protein of muscle specific intermediate filaments. Virchows Arch [B] 39:203–215, 1982

33. Lack EE: Leiomyosarcomas in childhood: A clinical and pathologic study of 10 cases. Pediatr Pathol 6:181–197, 1986

34. Hsueh S, Hsih SN, Kuo TT: Primary rhabdomyosarcoma of long bone: A case report. Orthopedics 9:705–707, 1986

35. Tsokos M: The role of immunocytochemistry in the diagnosis of rhabdomyosarcoma. Arch Pathol Lab Med 110:776–778, 1986

36. Tsokos M, Howard R, Costa J: Immunohistochemical study of alveolar and embryonal rhabdomyosarcoma. Lab Invest 48:148–155, 1983

37. Triche TJ, Tsokos M, Miser JS, Reynolds CP, Israel MA, Donner L: Peripheral neuroepithelioma: A bone or soft tissue tumor resembling Ewing's sarcoma and distinct from neuroblastoma. Proceedings of the XVII Meeting of SIOP, Venice, Italy, September 30–October 4, 1985

38. Moll R, Franke WW, Schiller DL, Geiger B, Krepler R: The catalog of human cytokeratins: Patterns of expression in normal epithelia, tumors and cultured cells. Cell 31:11–24, 1982

39. Sun T-T, Eichner R, Schermer A, Cooper D, Nelson WG, Weiss RA: Classification, expression and possible mechanisms of evolution of mammalian epithelial keratins: A unifying model. In: Levine A, Topp W, Vande Woude G, Watson JD (eds): The Cancer Cell, Vol 1: The Transformed Phenotype, pp 169–176. New York, Cold Spring Harbor Laboratory, 1984

40. Battifora H, Trowbridge IS: A monoclonal antibody useful for the differential diagnosis between malignant lymphoma and non-hematopoietic neoplasms. Cancer 51:816, 1983

41. Kurtin PJ, Pinkus GS: Leukocyte common antigen. A diagnostic discriminant between hematopoietic and nonhematopoietic neoplasms in paraffin sections using monoclonal antibodies: Correlation with immunologic studies and ultrastructural localization. Hum Pathol 16:353–365, 1985

42. Stein H, Gatter K, Asbahr H, Mason DY: Methods in laboratory investigation: Use of freeze-dried paraffin-embedded sections for immunohistologic staining with monoclonal antibodies. Lab Invest 52:676–683, 1985

43. Donner L, Triche TJ, Israel MA, Seeger RC, Reynolds CP: A panel of monoclonal antibodies which discriminate neuroblastoma from Ewing's sarcoma, rhabdomyosarcoma, neuroepithelioma and hematopoietic malignancies. Progr Clin Biol Res 175:347–366, 1985

44. Lindvall O, Bjorklund A: The glyoxylic acid fluorescence histochemical method: A detailed account of the methodology for the visualization of central catecholamine neurons. Histochemistry 39:97, 1974

45. Falck B, Hillarp N-A, Thieme G et al: Fluorescence of catecholamines and related compounds condensed with formaldehyde. J Histochem Cytochem 10:348–354, 1962

46. Reynolds CP, Smith RG, Frenkel EP: The diagnostic dilemma of the "small round cell neoplasm": Catecholamine fluorescence and tissue culture morphology as markers for neuroblastoma. Cancer 48:2088–2094, 1981

47. Harper ME, Saunder GF: Localization of single copy DNA sequences on G-banded chromosomes by in situ hybridization. Chromosoma 83:431–439, 1981

48. Obara T, Conti CJ, Baba M, Resau JH, Trifillis AL, Trump BF, Klein–Szanto AJP: Rapid detection of xenotransplanted human tissues using in situ hybridization. Am J Pathol 122:386–391, 1986

49. Yunis JJ: The chromosomal basis of neoplasia. Science 221:227–235, 1983

50. Cavazzana AO, Navarro S, Navarro R, Mims S, Triche TJ: Short term tissue culture in the differential diagnosis of small round cell tumors of childhood. Presented at the International Academy of Pathology, Chicago, March 8–13, 1987

51. Sandberg AA: The chromosomes in human cancer and leukemia. New York, Elsevier North Holland, 1980

52. Gilbert F: Chromosomes, genes, and cancer: A classification of chromosome changes in cancer. JNCI 71:1107–1114, 1983

53. Mitelman F: Catalogue of chromosome aberrations in cancer. Cytogenet Cell Genet 36:1–515, 1983

54. Turc–Carel C, Philip T, Berger M-P et al: Chromosome study of Ewing's sarcoma (ES) cell lines: Consistency of a reciprocal translocation t(11;22) (q24;q12). Cancer Genet Cytogenet 12:1, 1984

55. Aurias A, Rimbaut C, Buffe D et al: Translocation involving chromosome 22 in Ewing's sarcoma: A cytogenetic study of four fresh tumors. Cancer Genet Cytogenet 12:21, 1984

56. Whang–Peng J, Triche TJ, Knutsen T, Miser J, Kao-Shan S, Tsai S, Israel MA: Cytogenetic characterization of selected small round cell tumors of childhood. Cancer Genet Cytogenet 21:185–208, 1986

57. Prieto F, Baudia L, Montalar J, Massuti B: Translocation (11;22) in Ewing's sarcoma. Cancer Genet Cytogenet 17:87–89, 1985

58. de Chadarevian JP, Vekemans M, Seemayer TA: Reciprocal translocation in small-cell sarcomas (lett). N Engl J Med 311:1702–1703, 1984

59. Whang–Peng J, Triche TJ, Knutsen T, Miser J, Douglass EC, Israel MA: Chromosome translocation in peripheral neuroepithelioma. N Engl J Med 311:584–585, 1984

60. Becroft DMO, Pearson A, Shaw RL, Swi LJ: Chromosome translocation in extraskeletal Ewing's tumour. Lancet 2:400, 1984

61. Gilbert F, Balaban G, Moorhead P, Bianchi D, Schlesinger H: Abnormalities of chromosome 1p in human neuroblastoma tumors and cell lines. Cancer Genet Cytogenet 7:33–42, 1982

62. Gilbert F, Feder M, Balaban G et al: Human neuroblastomas and abnormalities of chromosomes 1 and 17. Cancer Res 44:5444–5449, 1984

63. Potluri VR, Gilbert F, Helsen C, Helson L: Primitive neuroectodermal tumor cell lines: Chromosomal analysis of five cases. Cancer Genet Cytogenet 24:75–86, 1987

64. Turc–Carel C, Philip T: Consistent chromosomal translocation t(2;13) (q37C4) in alveolar rhabdomyosarcoma. Proceedings of the XVII Meeting of SIOP, Venice, September 30–October 4, 1985

65. Turc–Carel C, Cin PD, Limon J, Li F, Sandberg AA: Translocation X;18 in synovial sarcoma (lett). Cancer Genet Cytogenet 23:93, 1986

66. Croce CM, Thierfelder W, Erikson J, Nishikure K, Finan J, Lenoir GM, Nowell PC: Transcriptional activation of an unrearranged and untranslocated c-myc oncogene by translocation of a C lambda locus in Burkitt lymphoma cells. Proc Natl Acad Sci USA 80:6922–6926, 1983

67. Magrath IT, Erikson J, Whang–Peng J et al: Synthesis of kappa light chains by cell lines containing an 8;22 chromosomal translocation derived from a male homosexual with Burkitt's lymphoma. Science 222:1094–1098, 1983

68. Yunis JJ, Ramsay N: Retinoblastoma and subband deletion of chromosome 13. Am J Dis Child 132:161–163, 1978

69. Balaban G, Gilbert F, Nichols W, Meadows A, Shields J: Abnormalities of chromosome 13 in retinoblastomas from individuals with normal constitutional karyotypes. Cancer Genet Cytogenet 6:213–221, 1983

70. Benedict WF, Banerjee A, Mark C, Murphree AL: Nonrandom chromosomal changes in untreated retinoblastomas. Cancer Genet Cytogenet 10:311–333, 1983

71. Friend SH, Bernareds R, Rogelj S, Weinberg RA, Rapaport JM, Albert DM, Dryja TP: A human DNA segment with properties of the gene that predisposes to retinoblastoma and osteosarcoma. Nature 323:643–646, 1986

72. Shtivelman E, Lifshitz B, Gale RP, Canaani E: Fused transcript of abl and bcr genes in chronic myelogenous leukemia. Nature 315:550–554, 1985

73. Kurzrock R, Shtalrid M, Romero P et al: A novel c-abl protein product in Philadelphia-positive acute lymphoblastic leukaemia. Nature 325:631–635, 1987

74. Slamon DJ, Clark GM, Wong SG, Levin WJ, Ullrich A, McGuire WL: Human breast cancer: Correlation of relapse and survival with amplification of the HER-2/neu oncogene. Science 235:177–182, 1987

75. Schwab M, Alitalo K, Klempnauer KH et al: Amplified DNA with limited homology to myc cellular oncogene is shared by human neuroblstoma cell lines and a neuroblastoma tumour. Nature 305:245, 1983

76. Brodeur GM, Seeger RC, Schwab M et al: Amplification of N-myc in untreated neuroblastomas correlates with advanced disease stage. Science 224:1121–1124, 1984

77. Seeger RC, Brodeur GM, Sather H et al: Association of multiple copies of the N-myc oncogene with rapid progression of neuroblastomas. N Engl J Med 313:1111–1116, 1985

78. Brewster MA, Berry DA: Serial studies of serum dopamine beta hydroxylase and urinary vanillylmandelic and homovanillic acids in neuroblastoma. Med Pediatr Oncol 6:93–99, 1979

79. Ross A, Tong HJ, Reis DJ et al: Neurotransmitter-synthesizing enzymes in human neuroblastoma cells: Relationship to morphological diversity. In Advances in Neuroblastoma Research, p 151. New York, Raven Press, 1980

80. Cavazzana AO, Miser JS, Jefferson J, Triche TJ: Experimental evidence for a neural origin of Ewing's sarcoma of bone. Am J Pathol 127:507–518, 1987

81. Alitalo K, Vaheri A: Pericellular matrix in malignant transformation. Adv Cancer Res 37:111–158, 1982

82. Liotta LA, Rao CN, Barsky SH: Tumor invasion and the extracellular matrix. Lab Invest 49:636–649, 1983

83. Scarpa S, Modesti A, Triche TJ: Extracellular matrix synthesis by undifferentiated childhood neoplasia. Am J Pathol (in press)

84. Barsky SH, Rao CN, Grotendorst GR, Liotta LA: Increased content of type V collagen in desmoplasia of human breast carcinoma. Am J Pathol 108:276–283, 1982

85. Harvey W, Squier MV, Duance VC, Pritchard J: A biochemical and immunohistological study of collagen synthesis in Ewing's tumour. Br J Cancer 46:848–855, 1982

86. Grigioni WF, Biagini G, Errico AD, Milani M: Behaviour of basement membrane antigens in gastric and colorectal cancer. Acta Pathol Jpn 36:173–184, 1986

87. Liotta LA: Tumor invasion and metastases—Role of the extracellular matrix: Rhoads Memorial Award Lecture. Cancer Res 46:1–7, 1986

88. Wewer UM, Liotta LA, Jaye M et al: Altered levels of laminin receptor mRNA in various human carcinoma cells that have different abilities to bind laminin. Proc Natl Acad Sci USA 83:7137–7141, 1986

89. Adelstein RS, Conti MA, Daniel JL, Anderson W Jr: The interaction of platelet actin, myosin and myosin light chain kinase. In Biochemistry and Pharmacology of Platelets (Ciba Foundation Symposium 35), 1975

90. Yunis EJ: Ewing's sarcoma and related small round cell neoplasms in children. Am J Surg Pathol 10(suppl 1):54–62, 1986

91. Willis RA: Metastatic neuroblastoma in bone presenting the Ewing's syndrome, with a discussion of "Ewing's sarcoma." Am J Pathol 16:317–331, 1940

92. Linnoila RI, Tsokos M, Triche TJ, Marangos PJ, Chandra RS: Evidence for neural origin and PAS positive variants of the malignant small cell tumor of thoracopulmonary region ("Askin tumor"). Am J Surg Pathol 10:124–133, 1986

93. Cavazzana AO, Navarro S, Triche TJ: Ewing's sarcoma and peripheral neuroepithelioma compared. Presented at the International Academy of Pathology, Chicago, March 8–13, 1987

94. Kawaguchi K, Koike M: Neuron-specific enolase and Leu-7 immunoreactive small round-cell neoplasm: The relationship to Ewing's sarcoma in bone and soft tissue. Am J Clin Pathol 86:79–83, 1986

95. Hartman KR, Triche TJ, Kinsella TJ, Miser JS: Histopathology—A significant prognostic factor in Ewing's sarcoma: A review of 56 cases of distal extremity primary tumors. Cancer (submitted)

96. Hashimoto H, Kiryu H, Enjoji M, Daimaru Y, Nakajima T: Malignant neuroepithelioma (peripheral neuroblastoma). Am J Surg Pathol 7:309–318, 1983

97. Jaffe R, Santamaria M, Yunis EJ et al: The neuroectodermal tumor of bone. Am J Surg Pathol 8:885–898, 1984

98. Garvin AJ, Stanley WS, Bennett DD, Sullivan JL, Sens DA: In vitro growth, heterotransplantation, and differentiation of a human rhabdomyosarcoma cell line. Am J Pathol 125:208–217, 1986

99. Shimada H, Newton WA, Soule EH et al: Pathological features of extraosseous Ewing's sarcoma: A report from the Intergroup Rhabdomyosarcoma Study. Hum Pathol (in press)

100. Thiele CJ, McKeon C, Triche TJ, Ross RA, Reynolds CP, Israel MA: Differential proto-oncogene expression characterizes histopathologically indistinguishable tumors of the peripheral nervous system. Cancer (submitted)

101. Sim FH, Unni KK, Beabout JW et al: Osteosarcoma with small cells simulating Ewing's tumor. J Bone Joint Surg [Am] 61:207, 1979

102. Martin SE, Dwyer A, Kissane JM et al: Small-cell osteosarcoma. Cancer 50:990, 1982

103. Dabska M, Huvos AG: Mesenchymal chondrosarcoma in the young: A clinicopathologic study of 19 patients with explanation of histogenesis. Virchows Arch [A] 399:89, 1983

104. Ringus JC, Riddell RH: Small cell osteosarcoma: Ultrastructural description and differentiation from atypical Ewing's sarcoma (abstrt). Lab Invest 44:55A, 1981

105. Martinez–Tello FJ, Navas–Palacios JJ: Ultrastructural study of conventional chondrosarcomas and xyoid- and mesenchymal-chondrosarcomas. Virchows Arch [A] 396:197–211, 1982

106. Hutter RVP, Foote FW, Francis KC et al: Primitive multipotential primary sarcoma of bone. Cancer 19:1, 1965

107. Mahoney JP, Alexander RW: Ewing's sarcoma: A light- and electron-microscopic study of 21 cases. Am J Surg Pathol 2:283–298, 1978

108. Dickman PS, Triche TJ: Extraosseous Ewing's sarcoma versus primitive rhabdomyosarcoma: Diagnostic criteria and clinical correlation. Hum Pathol 17:881–893, 1986

109. Schmidt D, Mackay B, Osborne BM et al: Recurring congenital lesion of the cheek. Ultrastruct Pathol 3:85, 1982

110. Karciogulu Z, Someren A, Mathes SJ: Ectomesenchymoma: A malignant tumor of migratory neural crest (ectomesenchyme) remnants showing ganglionic, Schwannian, melanocytic, and rhabdomyoblastic differentiation. Cancer 39:2486–2496, 1977

111. Coffin CM, Dehner LP: Soft tissue neoplasms in childhood: A clinicopathologic overview. Major Probl Pathol 18:223–255, 1986

112. Llombart–Bosch A, Contesso G, Henry–Amar M, Lacombe JJ et al: Histopathological predictive factors in Ewing's sarcoma of bone and clinicopathological correlations: A retrospective study of 261 cases. Virchows Arch [A] 409:627–640, 1986

113. Chasin WD: Rhabdomyosarcoma of the temporal bone. Ann Otol Rhinol Laryngol 112:71–73, 1984

114. Spjut HA: Case presentation. Presented at the International Association of Pathologists Bone Specialty Conference, New Orleans, March, 1986

115. Kissane J, Askin F, Foulkes M et al: Ewing's sarcoma of bone: Clinicopathologic aspects of 303 cases from the Intergroup Ewing's Sarcoma Study. Hum Pathol 14:773–779, 1983

116. Triche TJ, Ross WE: Glycogen-containing neuroblastoma with clinical and histopathologic features of Ewing's sarcoma. Cancer 41:1425–1432, 1978

117. Reynolds CP, Smith RG, Frenkel EP: The diagnostic dilemma of the "small round cell neoplasm": Catecholamine fluorescence and tissue culture morphology as markers for neuroblastoma. Cancer 48:2088, 1981

118. Reynolds CP, German CD, Weinberg AG et al: Catecholamine fluorescence and tissue culture morphology: Techniques in the diagnosis of neuroblastoma. Am J Clin Pathol 75:275, 1981

119. Falck B, Hillarp N-A, Thieme G et al: Fluorescence of catecholamines and related compounds condensed with formaldehyde. J Histochem Cytochem 10:348, 1962

120. Lindvall O, Bjorklund A: The glyoxylic acid fluorescence histochemical method: A detailed account of the methodology for the visualization of central catecholamine neurons. Histochemistry 39:97, 1974

121. De La Torre JC, Surgeon JW: A methodological approach to rapid and sensitive monoamine histofluorescence using a modified glyoxylic acid technique: The SPG method. Histochemistry 49:81, 1976

122. Triche TJ, Tsokos M, Linnoila RI, Marangos PJ, Chandra R: NSE in neuroblastoma and other round cell tumors of childhood. Progr Clin Biol Res 175:295–317, 1985

123. Inoshita T, Youngberg GA: Fluorescence of melanoma cells. Am J Clin Pathol 78:311–315, 1982

124. Murray MR, Stout AP: Distinctive characteristics of the sympathicoblastoma cultivated in vitro: A method for prompt diagnosis. Am J Pathol 23:429, 1947

125. Reynolds CP, Frenkel EP, Smith RG: Growth characteristics of neuroblastoma in vitro correlate with patient survival. Trans Assoc Am Physicians 43:203–211, 1980

126. Rosen N, Reynolds CP, Thiele CJ, Biedler JL, Israel MA: Increased N-myc expression following progressive growth of human neuroblastoma. Cancer Res 46:4139–4142, 1986

127. Slamon DJ, Boone TC, Seeger RC et al: Identification and characterization of the protein encoded by the human N-myc oncogene. Science 232:768–772, 1986

128. Ikegaki N, Bukovsky J, Kennett RH: Identification and characterization of the NMYC gene product in human neuroblastoma cells by monoclonal antibodies with defined specificities. Proc Natl Acad Sci USA 83:5929–5933, 1986

129. Seeger RC, Moss TJ, Bjork RL et al: Expression of N-myc by neuroblastomas with one or multiple copies of the oncogene. Fourth Symposium on Advances in Neuroblastoma Research, Philadelphia, May 1987 (in press)

130. Triche TJ, Cavazzana AO, Navarro S, Reynolds CP, Slamon DJ, Seeger RC: NMYC protein expression in small round cell tumors. Fourth Symposium on Advances in Neuroblastoma Research, Philadelphia, May 1987 (in press)

131. Eiden LE: Is chromogranin a prohormone? Nature 325:301, 1987

132. Huttner WB, Benedum UM: Chromogranin A and pancreastatin (lett). Nature 325:305, 1987

133. Cavazzana AO, Magnani JL, Miser JS, Triche TJ: Ewing's sarcoma in an undifferentiated neuroectodermal tumor. Fourth Symposium on Advances in Neuroblastoma Research, Philadelphia, May 1987 (in press)

134. Gould VE, Wiedenmann B, Lee I et al: Synaptophysin expression in neuroendocrine neoplasms as determined by immunocytochemistry. Am J Pathol 126:243–257, 1987

135. Payne CM, Nagle RB, Borduin V: An ultrastructural cytochemical stain specific for neuroendocrine neoplasms. Lab Invest 51:350–365, 1984

136. Angervall L, Enzinger FM: Extraskeletal neoplasm resembling Ewing's sarcoma. Cancer 36:240, 1975

137. Tefft M, Vawter GF, Mitus A: Paravertebral "round cell" tumors in children. Radiology 92:1501, 1969

138. Wigger HJ, Salazar GH, Blanc WA: Extraskeletal Ewing's sarcoma: An ultrastructural study. Arch Pathol Lab Med 101:446, 1977

139. Garvin AJ, Stanley WS, Bennett DD, Sullivan JL, Sens DA: In vitro growth, heterotransplantation, and differentiation of a human rhabdomyosarcoma cell line. Am J Pathol 125:208–217, 1986

140. Tsokos M, Miser A, Pizzo P, Triche TJ: Histologic and cytologic characteristics of poor prognosis childhood rhabdomyosarcoma (abstr). Lab Invest 50:61A, 1984

141. Tsokos M, Howard R, Costa J: Immunohistochemical study of alveolar and embryonal rhabdomyosarcoma. Lab Invest 48:148, 1983

142. Tsokos M, Miser A, Wesley R et al: Solid variant alveolar rhabdomyosarcoma: A primitive rhabdomyosarcoma with poor prognosis and distinct histology. Presented at the XVII Meeting of SIOP, Venice, September 30–October 4, 1985

143. Dickman PS, Triche TJ: A comparative analysis of immunocytochemistry and electron microscopy in the diagnosis of primitive rhabdomyosarcoma. (In preparation)

144. Kinsella TJ, Triche TJ, Dickman PS, Costa J, Tepper JE, Glaubiger D: Extraskeletal Ewing's sarcoma: Results of combined modality treatment. J Clin Oncol 1:489–495, 1983

145. Krall RA, Kostianovsky M, Patchefsky AS: Synovial sarcoma: A clinical, pathological, and ultrastructural study of 26 cases supporting the recognition of the monophasic variant. Am J Surg Pathol 5:137–151, 1981

146. Miettinen M, Lehto V-P, Virtanen I: Monophasic synovial sarcoma of spindle cell type. Virchows Arch [B] 44:187, 1983

147. Weiss WW, Langloss JM, Enzinger FM: Value of S-100 protein in the diagnosis of soft tissue tumors with particular reference to benign and malignant Schwann cell tumors. Lab Invest 49:299–308, 1983

148. Kjeldsberg CR, Wilson JF: Malignant lymphoma in children. Major Probl Pathol 18:87–125, 1986

149. Smith RG: Parosteal lymphoblastic lymphoma: A human counterpart of Abelson virus-induced lymphosarcoma of mice. Cancer 54:471–476, 1984

seven

Imaging Studies in the Diagnosis of Pediatric Malignancies

Bruce R. Parker

The past two decades have seen not only a remarkable improvement in the survival rate of children with malignant disorders, but also a technologic explosion in the field of diagnostic imaging that has made accurate assessment of tumor size and spread more precise than ever before possible. These advances in imaging technology, however, require increased knowledge and sophistication on the part of the imaging specialist, increase the cost of equipment, and increase the difficulty in choosing the appropriate modality for the quickest, most accurate, and least expensive patient evaluation.

This chapter will deal with the relative merits of the imaging procedures available to us and make recommendations concerning general problems in pediatric oncology. The imaging characteristics and the imaging evaluation of patients with specific tumors are dealt with in the appropriate specific chapters.

RELATIVE MERITS OF IMAGING PROCEDURES

Plain Film Radiography

At a time when we are seeing remarkable advances in sophisticated imaging modalities, the plain film radiograph continues to play a central role in the diagnosis, evaluation, and follow-up of children with malignant disease (Table 7-1). Although less sensitive than computed tomography (CT) (see below), plain film chest radiography continues to be the examination of choice for short-interval evaluation of pulmonary metastases. The examination is fast, technologically easy, and relatively inexpensive; requires no anesthesia or sedation; and delivers minimal radiation to the bone marrow and gonads. The chest film also continues to be the procedure of choice for evaluating such complications of therapy as drug reactions and pulmonary infections in the immunologically altered host.

Plain films of the abdomen, however, have been superseded by more technologically advanced procedures for evaluation of masses and other problems found in pediatric oncologic patients. Nevertheless, enough information can be gleaned from the abdominal plain film that it should precede more sophisticated procedures. Although not as sensitive as CT for finding calcification within tumors, the plain film still permits most calcifications to be identified. On rare occasions, a specific diagnosis can be made, but further diagnostic imaging studies are rarely obviated. Finally, the plain film still represents the best simple evaluation of the abdominal gas pattern and of the presence or absence of intestinal obstruction or free intraperitoneal air. For these reasons, plain film abdominal radiography should always be performed prior to, or concomitant with, ultrasound, CT, or magnetic resonance imaging (MRI) in evaluating abdominal abnormalities.

Abdominal contrast studies, on the other hand, are used with much less frequency since the advent of the newer imaging modalities. In particular, ex-

Table 7-1
*Comparative Value of Imaging Procedures on a Scale of 1 to 5**

	Plain Film	Isotope Scan	US	CT	MRI
CNS–Intracranial					
Sensitivity	1	3	0	5	5
Anatomic delineation	0	1	0	4	5
Potential complications	0	0	0	1	0
Cost	1	2	2	4	4
CNS–Intraspinal					
Sensitivity	1	0	0	4	5
Anatomic delineation	0	0	0	4	5
Potential complications	0	0	0	1	0
Cost	1	2	2	4	4
Thoracic					
Sensitivity	3	0	0	4	3–4
Anatomic delineation	3	0	0	5	4
Potential complications	0	0	0	1	0
Cost	1	2	2	4	5
Abdominal					
Sensitivity	2	4†	4	5	4
Anatomic delineation	1	3†	3	5	4–5
Potential complications	0	0	0	2	0
Cost	1	2	2	4	5
Skeletal					
Sensitivity	4	5	0	5	5
Anatomic delineation	2	3	0	4	5
Potential complications	0	0	0	0	0
Cost	1	2	2	3	5

* On a scale of 1 to 5, 5 is the highest value.
† Liver and spleen.

cretory urography has little role in the evaluation of the patient with oncologic disease. Retroperitoneal disease, whether intrinsic or extrinsic to the genitourinary system, is studied with a higher degree of accuracy by various combinations of ultrasound, CT, and MRI. Even complications of therapy, such as renal infection in the altered host, are better defined by a combination of ultrasound and radionuclide imaging than by excretory urography.[1]

Barium studies are a simple and sensitive means of evaluating gastrointestinal lesions (Fig. 7-1). Except in lymphoma, however, primary neoplastic involvement of the gastrointestinal tract is rare in children. CT offers the advantage of being able to evaluate the mesentery and the mesenteric lymph nodes (Fig. 7-2), as well as the solid abdominal viscera. Mucosal lesions of the gastrointestinal tract, however, still are better seen with traditional barium studies; esophagitis, duodenal ulcer, drug-induced colitis, and radiation enterocolitis are al best identified in this way (Fig. 7-3). However, contrast enemas must be used with extreme caution, and are generally contraindicated, in neutropenic patients because of the bacteremia that invariably occurs during the procedure. Studies performed after ingestion of contrast agents are safe even in immunocompromised children.

Skeletal radiographs are sensitive in detecting abnormalities, although most neoplastic and infectious processes will be apparent on radionuclide bone scan before they are obvious on plain films.[2] Nevertheless, by the time most patients with primary bone tumors are symptomatic, the plain film is abnormal

and so should be the first screening modality in the symptomatic patient (Fig. 7-4A). CT has proved better than either plain films or radionuclide studies in determining the extent of disease[3] (Fig. 7-4B) but has now been superseded by MRI for this purpose[4] (Fig. 7-4C). Except in histiocytosis X and, possibly, neuroblastoma, bone scanning is more sensitive to the presence of early metastatic disease than is plain film radiography (see below).

Skull radiography, in the era of CT and MRI, is rarely useful.[5] A skull film should always be included as part of a radiographic survey to detect calvarial metastases, but virtually any other abnormality is better seen on CT or MRI. Even destructive lesions of the sella turcica, sphenoid wings, or other cranial bones are seen better using a bone window setting on CT. CT is also the method of choice for imaging the base of the skull.[6] Evaluation of the intracranial structures has been revolutionized by MRI. Even as a screening mechanism, plain skull radiography adds nothing but cost to the evaluation of the patient and can always be obtained following the CT or MRI scan if there is reason to think it might add useful information. MRI is unable to detect small intracranial calcifications, but CT is superior to skull films for this purpose.[7]

Spinal radiographs are valuable as a screening examination for metastatic disease and for compression fractures secondary to disease-induced or drug-induced osteoporosis. However, radioisotope bone scanning is more sensitive for the early detection of metastatic disease or occult bone tumor, and CT will give better definition of spinal lesions.

The need for routine myelography has been virtually obviated first by CT with intrathecal contrast injection and now by MRI of the spinal canal and its contents. MRI has already shown itself to be the modality of choice for evaluation of lesions of the spinal cord and its coverings.[8] Not only are the images more diagnostic, but they are obtained without intrathecal contrast material and are thus better tolerated by patients. Of particular importance in children is that MRI is extremely sensitive in detecting encroachment of paraspinous tumors through the neural foramina into the spinal canal[9] (Fig. 7-5).

Angiography and Lymphangiography

The use of angiography has diminished dramatically since the advent of the newer imaging modalities. Inferior vena cavography has been replaced by lymphangiography and CT for evaluation of retroperitoneal lymphadenopathy and by ultrasound and CT for evaluation of the intravascular spread of a malignancy such as in Wilms' tumor.[10] Arteriography was commonly used in the past for evaluation of tumor volume but has been superseded by CT and MRI for this purpose.

Abdominal arteriography is occasionally indicated when the surgeon needs information about the blood supply to a particular tumor or when preoperative tumor embolization is to be performed. Hepatic arteriography is important in the evaluation of both benign and malignant disease of the liver because CT, even with intravenous contrast material, does not always give sufficient information, especially when partial hepatectomy is contemplated (see Chap. 26).[11] However, preliminary studies with MRI suggest that not only is the tumor volume well defined by this procedure but also that there may be sufficient differences in the appearance of the liver and the hepatic vessels to differentiate the common tumors that may involve the liver.[12]

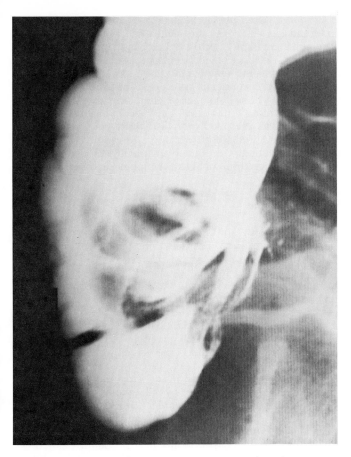

FIGURE 7-1. *Burkitt's lymphoma* presenting as ileocolic intussusception in 4-year-old boy. Barium enema demonstrates typical "coiled-spring" appearance of intussusception.

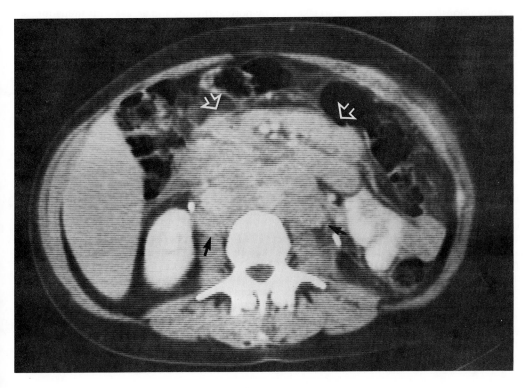

FIGURE 7-2. *Non-Hodgkin's lymphoma* in 17-year-old girl. CT demonstrates mesenteric lymphadenopathy (*open arrows*) as well as retroperitoneal lymphadenopathy (*closed arrows*).

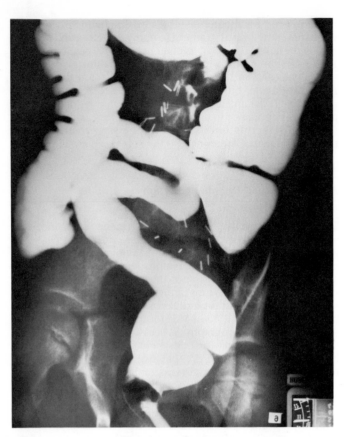

FIGURE 7-3. *Radiation colitis* in 6-year-old boy presenting 2 years after therapy for pelvic rhabdomyosarcoma. Barium enema shows rigiity, narrowing, and mucosal effacement of sigmoid colon.

CT and MRI have obviated extremity arteriography both in primary bone tumors and in soft-tissue sarcomas. Some surgeons continue to request arteriography prior to limb salvage procedures in order to define the relations of the tumor to major arteries, but other surgeons are content with the excellent delineation of soft-tissue tumor extent on MRI studies and believe they gain no necessary further information from arteriograms (see Chap. 32).

Neuroangiography has been superseded by CT and MRI, although arteriography is still the best way of evaluating intravascular disease in the vessels supplying the central nervous system. Such abnormalities are uncommon in children, but they occur rarely as a complication of antitumor therapy.

Lymphangiography remains controversial in the diagnostic evaluation of patients with lymphoma[13] (Table 7-2) (see Chaps. 20 and 21). The procedure is technically difficult in inexperienced hands, invasive, and expensive; has a definite although small incidence of complications; and usually requires heavy sedation or general anesthesia in preadolescent children. On the other hand, it is the only imaging procedure that allows evaluation of intrinsic lymph node architecture (Fig. 7-6). Lymphangiography can be successful in children as young as 14 months when performed by experienced personnel.[14] Body CT, when performed with exquisite attention to technical detail and appropriate use of intravenous and oral contrast agents, is capable of identifying lymph nodes greater than 1 cm in diameter. However, CT is not able to determine whether a lymph node is enlarged because of tumor or because of reactive hyperplasia. Because reactive hyperplasia is present

in 12% of children under the age of 16 and 19% of children under the age of 11,[15] the specificity of CT is low. The accuracy of lymphangiography, on the other hand, approaches 95%.[16] However, CT evaluation of the retroperitoneal lymph nodes is gradually replacing lymphangiography in some institutions where the lymphangiogram is reserved for patients with negative CT scans who will not receive chemotherapy. MRI can also demonstrate retroperitoneal lymph node involvement but cannot differentiate reactive hyperplasia from malignant disease. However, measurement of relaxation times, in vivo MR spectroscopy, or both may eventually enable this procedure to differentiate benign from malignant lymph node disease.

Nuclear Medicine

Nuclear medicine studies, especially when performed by imaging specialists with a particular interest in and experience with pediatric diseases, can be an effective diagnostic tool. Bone scanning is of less value than either CT or MRI in the evaluation of the extent of involvement by primary bone tumors[4] but continues to be the most sensitive and easily performed modality for the early identification of skeletal metastases.[2] Except in neuroblastoma and histiocytosis X, for reasons discussed below, bone scanning is more sensitive than radiographic skeletal surveys and is the screening examination of choice. Positive bone scans can result from abnormalities other than metastases, however, and any area that is positive on bone scan should be studied further by radiography.

Even with the best of equipment, liver scans are generally not as sensitive as ultrasound or CT for metastatic disease in patients with solid tumors.[17] However, infiltrating diseases such as leukemia and lymphoma may be better defined on radioisotope liver scans than with the other imaging modalities.

There is some controversy about the utility of gallium scans. In some centers, they are used in the evaluation of Hodgkin's disease and non-Hodgkin's lymphoma, especially in the search for recurrences.[18] However, the radionuclide is also taken up by normal thymus and areas of inflammation, so its overall usefulness is diminished. Nevertheless, in some experienced hands, gallium scanning does seem to provide useful information in patients with lymphoma.

As a further aid to the detection of focal infectious processes in the immunocompromised patient, white cell scans using ^{111}In have been shown to identify involved organs (Fig. 7-7). In children, an accuracy of 86% has been reported.[19] Although as many as one third of patients with occult infections may show false-negative results, the absence of false-positive results makes a positive scan a reliable indication of a focal infectious process (see Chap. 39).[20] It may be necessary to follow a white-cell scan with ultrasound, CT, or MRI to define a lesion better, but the white-cell scan offers the advantage of finding focal infections in a shorter period of time and at less cost than are required for total body imaging with other modalities.

The use of ^{131}I-meta-iodobenzylguanidine (MIBG) as a specific radioisotope marker in neuroblastoma is being explored (see Chap. 28).[21] MIBG has been used for the detection of pheochromocytomas, but, because it is associated with the cytoplasmic portion of the adrenal medulla, which contains neurosecretory granules,[22] it also can locate neuroblastomas. Initial interest in the method has been for localization purposes, but the potential for specifically directed treatment with a therapeutic dose of a radiopharmaceutical is exciting.[23]

Recent advances in nuclear medicine imaging based on

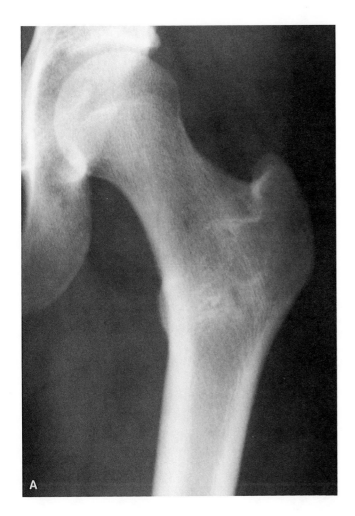

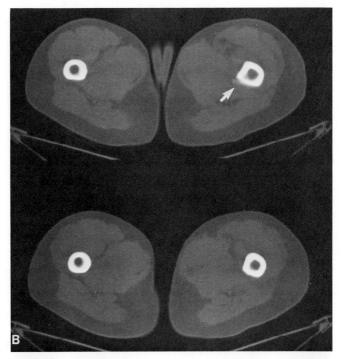

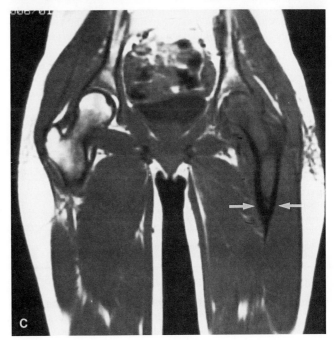

FIGURE 7-4. *Ewing's sarcoma* in a 16-year-old girl. **A.** Anteroposterior film of left femur demonstrates vague mottled lucent and sclerotic abnormalities in region of greater trochanter. **B.** Axial CT scans of subtrochanteric region demonstrate apparent inferior extent of tumor in the immediate subtrochanteric region (*upper scan*), with normal medullary cavity bilaterally 1 cm below this level (*lower scan*). **C.** Coronal MRI scan demonstrates intramedullary extent of tumor to be 4 to 5 cm below level of trochanter.

computer-aided technology are becoming available for clinical practice. Single-photon emission computed tomography (SPECT) utilizes essentially the same technology as CT scanning (see below). In the case of SPECT, however, the energy input is from gamma-emitting radioactive isotopes rather than from x-rays as in CT. The same isotopes now used in clinical practice are used with SPECT. Positron-emission tomography (PET) utilizes positron-emitting isotopes and has significant potential for evaluation of physiological and metabolic activity rather than just anatomic structure. Labeling of antitumor agents may permit localization of neoplastic tissue. The necessity for a nearby cyclotron to produce the positron-emitting isotopes limits the availability of the technique.

Ultrasound

Although high-frequency sound was first used for diagnostic purposes more than 30 years ago, its real value has been realized only in the past decade with the rapid development of advanced technology.[24] The procedure utilizes sound waves in the range of 2 to 10 million cycles per second (2–10 megahertz

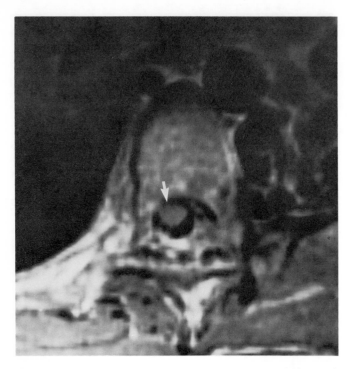

FIGURE 7-5. *Extraosseous Ewing's sarcoma* in 15-year-old boy. Left paraspinous primary is seen to extend through neural foramen to displace spinal cord (*arrow*) to the right on this axial MRI scan.

Table 7-2
*Retroperitoneal Lymphadenopathy: Comparison of Utility of Imaging Procedures on a Scale of 1 to 4**

	LAG†	CT	US	MRI
Accuracy	4	3	2	2–3
Technical skill required	4	1	3	1
Invasiveness	4	1	0	0
Potential complications	3	1	0	0
Cost	4	3	2	3

* On a scale of 1 to 4, 4 is the highest value.
† Lymphangiography.

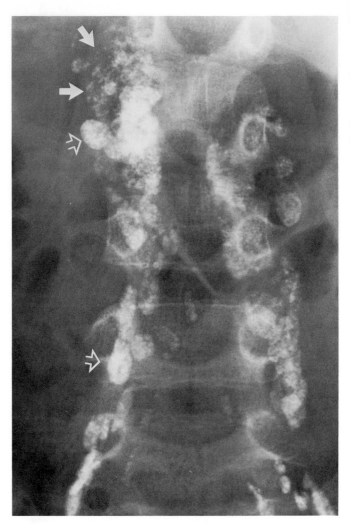

FIGURE 7-6. *Hodgkin's disease.* Bipedal lymphangiogram in 11-year-old boy demonstrates areas of tumor involvement (*closed arrows*) and reactive hyperplasia (*open arrows*) documented at staging laparotomy. Note that nontumorous nodes are at least as large as the involved nodes, making differentiation by CT, ultrasound, or MRI difficult.

[MHz]), well above the 20,000 Hz that is the upper limit of aural perception by humans. The sound waves are generated by a hand-held transducer that contains a piezoelectric crystal. This crystal vibrates when an electric current is passed through it, and sound waves at a specific frequency are thereby propagated. The sound can be directed toward a particular body part and can be focused to greater or lesser degrees, depending on technologic factors. The transducer's crystal also acts as a receiver for sound waves reflected back from internal structures. The vibration generated in the crystal by these echos produces an electrical signal, which can be digitized, processed, and displayed, usually in real time, on a television monitor.

The number and strength of the echos depends on tissue interfaces. Because there are no interfaces in a fluid-filled cyst, for instance, no echos are seen within it, and the structure is known as sonolucent or anechoic. However, tissue interfaces, such as those found in solid tumors, produce echos of various numbers and intensities. The resulting image is described as echogenic. Interfaces between air and soft tissue produce such strong echos that diagnostic anatomic detail often is not possible. Also, interfaces between bone and soft tissues attenuate the sound wave to such a degree that acoustic shadows are produced that interfere with image quality. Thus, bowel gas, air in the lungs, and bones all interfere with the production of satisfactory images and limit the anatomic areas that are susceptible to accurate diagnostic ultrasound evaluation.

Ultrasound examination, particularly when performed with the newest computerized equipment, is an excellent tool in the evaluation of the abdomen, pelvis, and scrotal contents of children. Its utility in other areas of the body depends on the amount of bone or gas present in or near the structure to be imaged. Because ultrasound examinations are relatively quick, relatively inexpensive, use no ionizing radiation, have no known complications or side effects, and do not require sedation or anesthesia, they are the ideal screening examination for the abdomen following plain film examination. Technically successful ultrasound examinations are easier to perform in children than in adults and in younger children than in older children because of the relative paucity of abdominal fat. Ul-

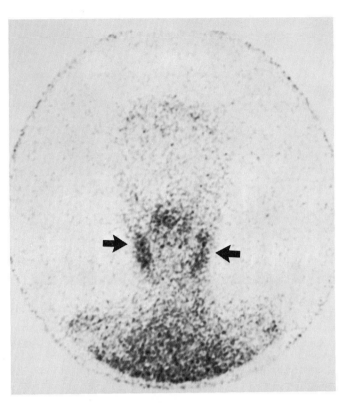

FIGURE 7-7. *Cervical lymphadenitis* in 4-year-old boy undergoing chemotherapy for rhabdomyosarcoma. Indium-111 white cell scan demonstrates increased uptake in both sides of neck (*arrows*). (Courtesy of IR McDougall, Division of Nuclear Medicine, Stanford Medical Center)

trasound is particularly useful in the evaluation of the retroperitoneum, the liver, the spleen, and the pelvic organs. In children, the pancreas and the aorta and inferior vena cava can usually be identified. Retroperitoneal lymphadenopathy can frequently be identified, although not as routinely as with CT. Intraperitoneal abnormalities may be difficult to image, especially if small, because of the presence of intestinal gas. Ultrasound is able to differentiate solid from fluid-filled masses easily and quickly and usually, although not always, can distinguish the organ of origin of an abdominal mass (Fig. 7-8). The principal disadvantages of ultrasound are that the resolution is poor when compared with CT or MRI; the examination is highly dependent on the skill, experience, and expertise of the sonographer; and the presence of bone or gas interferes with image production, limiting its utility in many anatomic areas.

Computed Tomography

A CT image represents a display of a thin section of anatomy. However, rather than being produced by radiation from a stationary x-ray tube striking a piece of film after passing through the patient, as plain films are, the CT image comes from a fan-shaped x-ray beam produced by a tube that rotates around the body part being examined. Instead of film, the x-rays strike a series of small crystal detectors, which convert the energy into electrical signals. These thousands of signals are fed into a computer that analyzes them based on its software program and constructs an image that can be displayed on the computer console. By changing various settings on the console, the radi-

ologist can manipulate the image to bring out those features of particular interest. The image can be photographed and displayed on radiographic film for ease of evaluation and permanent storage. If desired, the computer-generated information can also be stored on tape or disk.

The patient is placed on a movable table, and the body part to be examined is then placed into the gantry of the CT unit, which looks like an elongated doughnut. Because the geometry of satisfactory image production necessitates a relatively small diameter for the gantry, patients other than the smallest infants can be imaged only in cross section, producing axial slices through the body. These slices characteristically are perpendicular to the long axis of the body part being examined.

For reasons described below, more diagnostic information is frequently obtained when the images are enhanced by the use of the same intravenous contrast material that is used for excretory urography. Scans performed without the use of contrast material are referred to as unenhanced scans.

The advantages of CT in the evaluation of the cranial contents were apparent immediately following its introduction in 1972. Pneumoencephalography has disappeared from the armamentarium of the neuroradiologist, and intracranial arteriography is rarely used for pediatric patients with tumors. As the CT equipment has become technologically more sophisticated over the past 15 years, resolution has improved dramatically, allowing identification of tumor masses, even small calcifications, hydrocephalus, and cerebral and cerebellar complications of anticancer therapy.

Although unenhanced cranial CT scanning frequently is sufficient to identify a tumor, the use of intravenous iodinated contrast material often aids in the differentiation of neoplastic from normal brain tissue and helps differentiate the tumor mass from edema that may occur in the area of a tumor. Although there is a small but definite incidence of morbid, even fatal, reactions to contrast material in adults, the incidence is so low in children that contrast material can be used with safety.[25] Even patients with a previous history of contrast reaction can be studied with intravenous contrast material if proper premedication is given and appropriate equipment and trained personnel are available in the event of an untoward incident. The primary concern in the use of intravenous contrast material in children is potential compromise of renal function, and this can be obviated by having patients well hydrated prior to the procedure and by maintaining the total intravenous dose of iodinated contrast material at no more than 3 ml per kilogram of body weight. Iodinated contrast material is contraindicated in patients with significantly elevated uric acid concentrations and should be used with appropriate caution in patients with markedly impaired renal function, although it is usually safe even in this group.

Until recently, one of the disadvantages of CT was its ability to scan patients only in axial projection. However, recent advances in computer technology have enabled neuroradiologists to produce computer-reconstructed images in coronal and sagittal planes (Fig. 7-9). Many institutions also have the necessary software for three-dimensional reconstruction of CT images, but this method is not commonly used in the evaluation of oncologic patients.

Over the past decade, the increasing technologic sophistication of CT has permitted excellent axial images of the thorax, abdomen, spine and its contents, and extremities to be obtained. Intravenous contrast material is often useful in the thorax to differentiate vascular from nonvascular structures; in the abdomen better to define hepatic, splenic, renal, and adrenal masses; and to differentiate retroperitoneal and mediastinal vessels from masses (Fig. 7-10). Appropriate use of oral contrast material is necessary to differentiate intestinal loops from

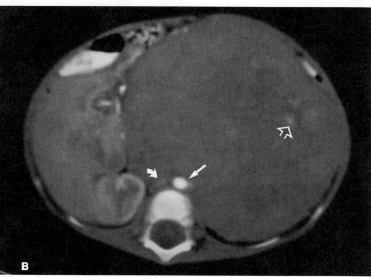

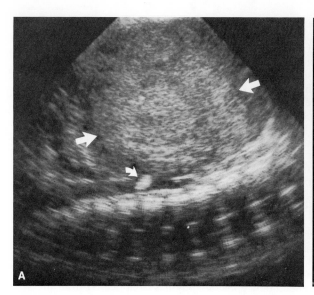

FIGURE 7-8. *Wilms' tumor* in a 1-year-old girl presenting as huge left-sided mass replacing kidney and extending across the midline. **A.** Longitudinal ultrasound scan of right side demonstrates large echogenic mass (*straight arrows*) with bright echogenic focus in inferior vena cava (*curved arrow*), suggesting tumor or thrombus. **B.** Enhanced CT scan demonstrates contrast in aorta (*straight arrow*), extrinsic compression of inferior vena cava (*curved arrow*), and calcification in the tumor (*open arrow*). No tumor thrombus was seen either on CT or at surgery. Echogenic focus was secondary to flow phenomena in the compressed inferior vena cava.

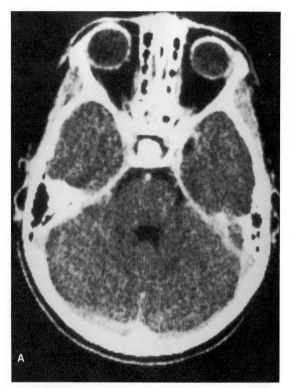

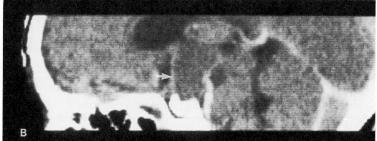

FIGURE 7-9. *Craniopharyngioma* in 13-year-old boy. **A.** Contrast-enhanced axial cut demonstrates intrasellar portion of tumor. **B.** Computer reconstruction in sagittal plane demonstrates cystic suprasellar component (*arrow*). (Courtesy of Charles Griffin, Advanced Imaging Center, Stanford Medical School)

intra-abdominal masses. In children, because of the lack of the retroperitoneal and mesenteric fat found in adults, judicious use of gastrointestinal contrast material is particularly important in the production of diagnostically adequate examinations (Fig. 7-11).

Lesions of the spine and other bones are usually well-defined without the use of contrast material. Soft-tissue masses, however, are best studied with intravenous infusion of contrast. Computer reconstruction in sagittal and coronal planes of body CT studies can be performed when needed.

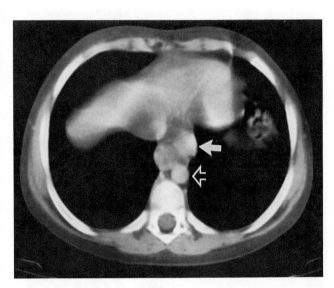

FIGURE 7-10. *Prespinous mass* in 7-year-old boy is easily distinguished from esophagus (*closed arrow*) and aorta (*open arrow*), both of which contain contrast material.

Modern CT equipment offers excellent resolution for body studies and, until the advent of MRI, was the modality of choice for most solid tumors. Its principal disadvantages for pediatric cancer patients are its cost, the need for heavy sedation or general anesthesia in the young patient, and the necessary reliance on axial studies. Nevertheless, these disadvantages are slight when compared with the information to be gleaned from these studies, and CT continues to be the foremost imaging tool in the diagnosis and staging of patients with solid tumors and lymphomas.

Magnetic Resonance Imaging

Magnetic resonance imaging is based on the concept of nuclear magnetic resonance first described by Bloch[26] and Purcell and associates[27] 40 years ago. The machine looks much like a CT unit, but the gantry is surrounded by a large magnet rather than x-ray generating equipment and receivers. Several different types of magnets are used, depending on the type of equipment and manufacturer, but all produce a static field many times the strength of the earth's magnetic field. Certain nuclei in the body with a nonzero magnetic moment will rotate with a wobbling motion (precess) around the direction of the magnetic field. Energy in the form of radio waves can be applied to these precessing nuclei, causing them to change the axis of their spin by absorption of some of the energy of the radio waves. Each of the nuclei thus affected will absorb energy only at a specific radio frequency, known as the resonance frequency. The radio frequency (RF) is generated through a coil placed on or around the patient that also acts as a receiver for the returning signals. When the radio transmission is stopped, the nuclei return to their original spinning position, giving up their energy in the form of an RF signal that is received by the coil. This return of the nuclei to their baseline state in the magnetic field is known as relaxation. Two different parameters of relaxation can be measured: T1 and T2. The operator can select for T1 or T2 imaging by altering the RF pulses generated by the coil. The RF signal returning from the nuclei to the coil is converted into an electrical signal, which is then treated by a computer in the way previously described for CT. Images are generated on the computer console, and photographic images can be produced.

Hydrogen is by far the most common charged nucleus in the body, and virtually all clinically useful MRI studies to date have involved hydrogen nuclei, although research involving other nuclei is being pursued in many institutions. Depending on the parameters selected, the areas having the largest number of free hydrogen nuclei will produce the greatest signal intensity, whereas those having the least number will give lowest signal intensity. Thus, on T1-weighted images, fat gives a very bright signal, whereas bone gives no signal at all.

MRI has proved to be as revolutionary in the 1980s as CT was in the 1970s. It has already proved itself superior to CT in most instances of intracranial tumors, especially those in the posterior fossa (Fig. 7-12). The spinal contents are better studied with MRI than with CT, and the need for myelography has diminished since the advent of MRI[28,29] (see Fig. 7-5). The principal advantage of MRI is its spectacular level of resolution, even with first-generation machines. Its other major advantage is its ability to provide direct coronal and sagittal images as well as axial images. If indicated, any variation of obliquity can also be obtained. Because there is signal dropout from calcified structures, MRI is not useful in detecting intracranial calcification or in evaluating the cranial bones. However, these areas are easily studied with plain film radiography or CT, which can be used as a worthwhile adjunct to MRI scanning.

Application of MRI to extracranial structures occurred even more rapidly than was the case with CT. Some early studies have shown MRI to be the equal of CT in the anatomic definition of many mediastinal[30,31] and intra-abdominal tumors,[32,33] but its principal advantage so far has been its ability to scan directly in coronal and sagittal planes. Carefully designed clinical protocols to evaluate the relative merits of CT and MRI in the thorax and abdomen are necessary before the full utility of MRI in these areas is established.

FIGURE 7-11. *Non-Hodgkin's lymphoma* presenting as posterior intraperitoneal mass in 5-year-old boy. Mass (*arrows*) is well demarcated from bowel by contrast material and air in the colon. Retroperitoneal lymphadenopathy (*open arrow*) is present, as is benign parapelvic cyst in right kidney and extrarenal pelvis in left kidney.

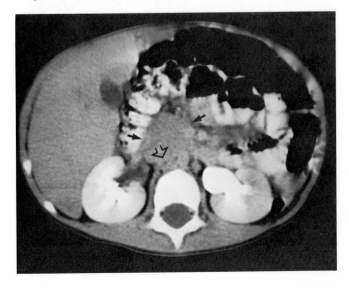

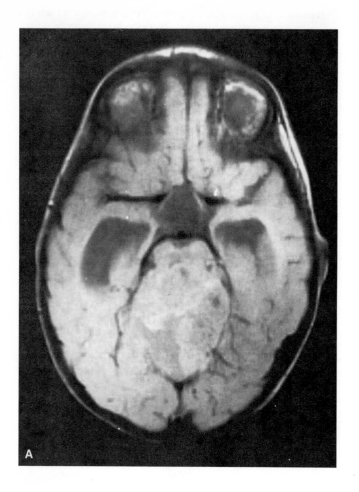

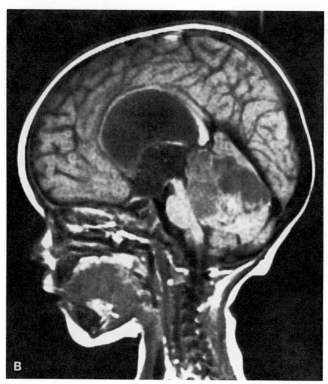

FIGURE 7-12. *Medulloblastoma.* T1-weighted axial (**A**) and sagittal (**B**) MRI scans demonstrate large midline mass in posterior fossa involving fourth ventricle and cerebellar vermis.

For bone and extremity tumors, however, it is already obvious that MRI offers distinct advantages over CT[3] (see Fig. 7-4). Both the soft-tissue and the intramedullary extent of primary bone tumors are better evaluated with MRI than with CT (see Chaps. 31 and 32). This is particularly important when primary radiation therapy or other limb salvage procedures are being considered. MRI cannot always differentiate between edema and tumor in the soft tissue surrounding a bone primary, but this is frequently true of CT as well.

A striking advantage of MRI has been shown in childhood leukemia. For the first time, an imaging modality appears to be able to differentiate normal bone marrow from marrow infiltrated by tumor cells.[34,35] Moore and coworkers found that a statistically significant prolongation of T1 relaxation times in the bone marrow correctly differentiated eight children with newly diagnosed acute lymphocytic leukemia (ALL) and four children will ALL in relapse from five children with ALL in remission and eleven age-matched controls.[36] Although more clinical research studies need to be done, it already seems possible that routine MRI imaging may rival the success of routine bone-marrow aspiration when looking for recurrent leukemia. It is also possible that MRI may be able to identify leukemia at presentation, again obviating bone-marrow aspiration for screening symptomatic patients, although not for cell-specific diagnosis.

The value of the calculation of T1 and T2 relaxation times, which has such potential utility in leukemia, is also being studied in the evaluation of solid tumors. The possibility that this method may lead to a way of differentiating neoplastic and non-neoplastic tissue is being explored, but insufficient data are at present available to determine its ultimate utility. In vivo MR spectroscopy is also being explored in a number of clinical research centers and may be even more useful for differentiating neoplastic from non-neoplastic tissue. It also has the potential, as yet largely unexplored, of differentiating one form of malignant tumor from another. Although great excitement has been generated by this possibility, thorough animal experiments and clinical trials will be necessary before reasonable conclusions can be reached.

The principal disadvantages of MRI include its cost, the necessity for sedation or anesthesia in the young child, and the length of time required by the procedure. A new generation of machines is already on the horizon that may permit faster scanning, which will have the advantage of decreasing both examination time and cost, since patient throughput will be increased. MRI already is the imaging study of choice for central nervous system tumors[37] and primary bone tumors.[4] It is probably the imaging study of choice for extremity soft-tissue tumors,[3,38] and technologic advances may soon make it the primary modality for intrathoracic and intra-abdominal disease as well.

There are few risks involved in MRI. Radio waves can cause heat in animal tissues, but there is no proof that this happens to a dangerous extent with the frequencies used for medical imaging. Although the magnetic fields are very strong, no deleterious effects have been described even in patients and animals exposed for long periods or repeatedly.

The only contraindication to the procedure is the presence of ferrous metallic objects in the body. Foreign bodies, especially in the eye; surgical clips, especially on blood vessels; and orthopedic devices may undergo torsion in a strong magnetic field, with resultant damage. A careful history should be taken and radiographs obtained if there is a question of a ferrous metallic foreign body.

Interventional Radiology

Interventional procedures by diagnostic radiologists have played an increasing role in both diagnosis and therapy during the past decade. Needle biopsies of various organs under fluoroscopic control have been done for some years, but the development of ultrasound and CT guidance methods for needle biopsy has greatly increased the utility of this procedure. Lesions in the lungs, liver, retroperitoneum, abdomen, and bone are readily accessible to biopsy with appropriate imaging guidance (see Chaps. 5 and 6). Diagnostic accuracy of 95% has been reported.[39,40] In experienced hands, the procedures are accurate and safe and do not typically require anesthesia, although sedation may be necessary for young children. Small-bore needles are frequently used, yielding cytologic specimens that usually are adequate to determine whether a biopsied lesion is benign or malignant, although they may not be sufficient to differentiate various types of malignancies. Thus, thin-needle biopsies have been more useful for determination of recurrent disease than for making a specific primary diagnosis. If a specific histologic diagnosis is needed, larger needles or cutting needles can be used. However, their use entails a higher risk of complications, especially bleeding. Patients undergoing such procedures must therefore have a thorough screen of bleeding times and clotting factors. The procedure should be performed only by an experienced interventional radiologist capable of treating potential complications.

Interventional radiologists also perform intravascular catheterization for infusion of chemotherapeutic agents. This procedure is less widely used in pediatric oncology than it is in adult oncology but may play a role particularly in tumors of the liver. Interventionalists have also been active in the treatment of complications of tumor or therapy. For example, percutaneous biliary drainage can readily be performed when the biliary system becomes obstructed. Similarly, percutaneous nephrostomies can relieve hydronephrosis produced by obstruction to urinary flow.

GENERAL CONCEPTS IN PEDIATRIC TUMOR IMAGING

Diagnosis

Although the approach to the diagnostic imaging of specific tumors is dealt with in appropriate chapters elsewhere in this book, an understanding of a logical imaging approach to the common presenting problems of children with tumors can make the initial evaluation more rapid and more efficient (Table 7-3).

Central Nervous System Tumors

Although cranial CT is an excellent tool for the evaluation of the central nervous system (CNS) in children with neurologic symptoms, MRI has clearly become the study of choice in institutions where it is available. One of the particular problems with cranial CT in children has been adequate evaluation of the posterior fossa because of bone artifacts produced on CT. Since most CNS tumors in childhood are located in the posterior

fossa, MRI should be utilized because of its superior imaging capabilities for subtentorial lesions (Fig. 7-12). Although no imaging study can replace histologic diagnosis in tumors of the CNS, the characteristic location and the imaging patterns of many brain tumors in children allow reliable presurgical evaluation.

MRI has also become the modality of choice for identifying lesions of the spinal cord and other abnormalities of the spinal contents.[41,42] The need for plain film myelography and for spinal CT with intrathecal contrast material has been substantially reduced by MRI.

A thorough discussion of imaging studies in the evaluation of CNS tumors can be found in Chapter 24.

Thoracic Tumors

Primary tumors of the bronchi and lungs are extremely rare in children. Most malignancies involving the pulmonary parenchyma are metastatic and are discussed below.

Primary tumors of the mediastinum are best defined by the compartment in which they arise. Tumors arising in the posterior mediastinum are largely of neurogenic origin. Neuroblastoma is the most common malignant tumor in this area (see Chap. 28). Erosion of ribs, widening of spinal neural foramina, and calcification of the mass are plain film signs that suggest the correct diagnosis (Fig. 7-13). Although the range of possible diagnoses is large, the common benign lesions have radiographic features that usually differentiate them from neuroblastoma, ganglioneuroma, and ganglioneuroblastoma. For example, neurenteric cysts are always associated with congenital anomalies of the thoracic spine. Neurofibromas frequently are associated with acute-angle scoliosis and multiple small paraspinous masses at several levels along the spine. Calcifications are not present in these two benign entities.

CT is essential in the evaluation of posterior mediastinal masses and is typically performed in association with myelography using water-soluble contrast material to evaluate the spinal canal for extension of the neurogenic tumor. CT also helps in pointing to the specific diagnosis, since 90% of neuroblastomas are calcified on CT whereas only 50% are calcified on plain film radiography.[43] MRI, with its ability to evaluate the spinal canal without intrathecal contrast material, may supplant CT in the evaluation of posterior mediastinal masses.[9,44] However, its inability to detect the small punctate calcifications of neuroblastoma is a potential disadvantage. Further studies are necessary to determine the relative efficacy of CT and MRI in evaluation of these masses.

The middle mediastinum may be involved by lymphadenopathy secondary to leukemia or lymphoma, but this rarely occurs in the absence of anterior mediastinal lymphadenopathy or thymic infiltration (see Chaps. 16, 20, 21, 35, and 37). Acute myelogenous leukemia and chronic lymphocytic leukemia may be exceptions. Plexiform neurofibromatosis and juvenile fibromatosis may involve the middle mediastinum as a large infiltrating mass rather than the multiple paraspinous masses typical in neurofibromatosis. Although histologically benign, plexiform neurofibromatosis and juvenile fibromatosis are potentially fatal because of involvement of the tracheobronchial tree or the great vessels. CT is the method of choice for evaluation of the middle mediastinum.[44] As in any evaluation of the mediastinum, intravenous contrast material should always be used in an attempt to differentiate cardiovascular structures from abnormal masses. Again, MRI has potential utility in evaluation of this area, but further study is necessary to determine its proper role.

Evaluation of the hilar lymph nodes is particularly important in Hodgkin's disease but may be useful with other tumors

Table 7-3
Recommended Imaging Strategies for Patients with Suspected Malignancies

I. *Central Nervous System*
  A. Intracranial Mass
    (1) MRI (if available) for both supratentorial and infratentorial lesions; obtain axial, coronal, and sagittal projections
    (2) Axial CT if MRI not available. Sagittal and/or coronal reconstructions useful, especially in region of sella
  B. Intraspinous Mass
    (1) MRI (if available) in axial and sagittal projections; coronal may be useful in selected circumstances
    (2) CT with intrathecal contrast material if MRI not available

II. *Thorax*
  A. Thoracic Cage
    (1) PA and lateral chest radiographs
    (2) CT of thorax
    (3) If mass is paraspinous, obtain spinal MRI or spinal CT with intrathecal contrast material to rule out intraspinous extension
  B. Intrathoracic Mass: PA and lateral chest radiographs
    (1) Anterior and/or middle mediastinum: chest CT with and without contrast enhancement
    (2) Posterior mediastinum
      (a) Chest CT with and without contrast enhancement
      (b) Spinal MRI or CT with intrathecal contrast to evaluate for intraspinous extension

III. *Abdominal Mass*
  A. Abdominal Plain Film
    (1) If gastrointestinal, obtain barium enema and/or upper-GI series
    (2) If not obviously gastrointestinal, obtain ultrasound
  B. Ultrasound
    (1) Retroperitoneal
      (a) Cystic renal: voiding cystourethrography, isotope renal scan, excretory urography, depending on ultrasound findings
      (b) Cystic suprarenal
        1. In infant, follow for resolution of adrenal hemorrhage
        2. In older child, CT to exclude cystic neuroblastoma
      (c) Solid renal: CT with and without contrast; value of MRI not yet documented
      (d) Solid suprarenal: CT with and without contrast; value of MRI not yet documented
      (e) Lymphadenopathy: LAG and CT if proven Hodgkin's disease; otherwise CT
    (2) Intraperitoneal
      (a) Intrahepatic solitary mass: radioisotope liver scan, CT with and without contrast; arteriography if surgery contemplated; MRI
      (b) Intrahepatic multiple lesions: Evaluate for primary tumor metastasizing to liver
      (c) Hepatobiliary cystic mass: Radioisotope scan of biliary tree
      (d) Splenomegaly: Evaluate for leukemia/lymphoma
      (e) Solid extrahepatic mass(es): CT with and without contrast; consider CT or ultrasound-guided percutaneous needle biopsy if surgical extirpation not required (*e.g.,* lymphoma)
      (f) Cystic extrahepatic mass: May or may not need CT, depending on surgeon's requirements

IV. *Skeletal Lesion: Plain Film*
  A. If obviously benign, no further studies usually needed
  B. If suspected malignancy: Radioisotope bone scan
    (1) If multiple lesions, evaluate for primary tumor metastasizing to bone
    (2) If solitary, obtain MRI (if available) or CT

also. CT evaluation of the hila has been a problem in the past, and several studies have suggested that MRI may be more sensitive.[45,46]

The anterior mediastinum is the compartment most frequently involved by malignant tumors, and these typically are leukemia or lymphoma. These diseases may cause anterior mediastinal lymphadenopathy or may produce infiltration of the thymus gland by malignant cells or a combination of the two. Plain film radiographic analysis of anterior mediastinal masses in children can be difficult because of the size of the normal thymus. Association with lymphadenopathy in other areas of the mediastinum, particularly the paratracheal, tracheobronchial, and hilar regions, may point toward tumor infiltration of the thymus. If only the thymus gland is involved, differentiation from normal thymus may be difficult in young children. On plain film, loss of the normal wavy contour of the

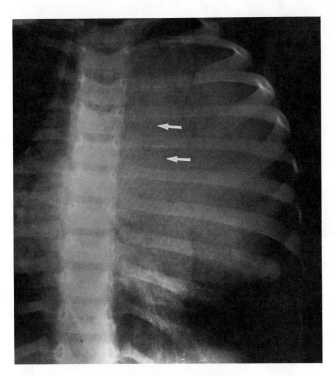

FIGURE 7-13. *Thoracic neuroblastoma.* Overpenetrated anteroposterior view of chest demonstrates large mediastinal mass with spreading of upper ribs, erosion of several posterior ribs, and speckled calcification (*arrows*).

thymus may suggest tumor infiltration. However, CT is more valuable than plain films in evaluating the thymus, although unfortunately, even CT may not provide this differentiation in all cases. The shape of the thymus gland on CT may be useful (Fig. 7-14). Contrast infusion is routinely used in mediastinal CT but has not been helpful in differentiating normal from abnormal thymus. Similarly, early experience with MRI has been disappointing, with the technique unable to date to differentiate normal and abnormal thymus.[47] A steroid challenge test is rarely useful since normal thymus, leukemia, and lymphomas all may respond.

Pleural involvement by malignant tumors is most typically from metastatic disease or lymphoma and is discussed below. Chest wall tumors may arise from the soft tissues, with the most common lesions being rhabdomyosarcoma and extraosseous Ewing's sarcoma. Although plain films may demonstrate the mass, CT is necessary to evaluate the extent of tumor, may be more sensitive for bony erosion, and may accurately determine the site of origin of tumors arising in unusual places such as the diaphragm (Fig. 7-15). Primary bone tumors, especially Ewing's sarcoma and a few osteogenic sarcomas, may arise from the ribs or thoracic vertebrae and present as chest masses. Again, CT evaluation may give specific diagnostic information as well as information concerning the extent of the tumor and possible pulmonary or mediastinal metastases.

Abdominal Masses

The plethora of diagnostic imaging examinations now available for the evaluation of abdominal masses in infants and children necessitates a logical and analytic approach to avoid

unnecessary expense, radiation, and morbidity. In the neonate, more than 85% of abdominal masses are nonmalignant.[48] A combination of plain films and abdominal ultrasound usually identifies the organ of origin and, if the mass is not solid, suggests its benign nature. Renal abnormalities account for more than half of palpable abdominal masses in the neonatal period, with hydonephrosis and cystic dysplastic kidney accounting for the majority of these (see Chap. 5). Ultrasound usually permits a specific diagnosis in these cases. The next most common cause of abdominal masses, pelvic masses in infant girls, is also readily amenable to ultrasound diagnosis. Ultrasound has been particularly useful in differentiating neonatal adrenal hemorrhage from adrenal neuroblastoma.[49] If a combination of plain film radiograph and ultrasound identifies a solid tumor arising from the retroperitoneum or liver, the probability of malignancy increases, and further evaluation is usually necessary (see below). The fact that a gastrointestinal lesion is accounting for the palpable mass is usually suggested by the plain film radiograph, which can then be followed by the appropriate gastrointestinal contrast examination.

In infants beyond the neonatal period and in children, the frequency of malignant abdominal tumors increases. Nevertheless, malignancy still accounts for less than half of palpable abdominal masses, and plain film radiography and ultrasound again should be the primary screening modalities. As in neonates, cystic or fluid-filled masses typically are benign, whereas solid masses must always be considered malignant until proved otherwise.

Several authors have approached the problem of the logical imaging evaluation of children with abdominal masses, and an algorithm has been developed that has proved useful.[48]

RETROPERITONEAL MASSES. The majority of ultrasonographically determined solid masses in infants and children arise from the kidney or adrenal gland. Mesoblastic nephroma accounts for the majority of renal masses in children under the age of 1 year but is indistinguishable from Wilms' tumor on imaging examinations (see Chap. 27). There is not yet sufficient information to know whether MRI has the ability to differentiate these two tumors. In children older than 1 year, nearly all solid tumors arising in the kidney will be Wilms' tumors. The combination of ultrasound and CT gives sufficient information about the size and location of the mass, vascular invasion or compromise, and lymph node and hepatic metastases for accurate presurgical evaluation.

Most nonrenal retroperitoneal solid tumors are neuroblastomas (see Chap. 28). As yet, no imaging modality can reliably distinguish neuroblastoma from ganglioneuroblastoma and from ganglioneuroma. Although some teratomas will be indistinguishable from neuroblastomas on imaging studies, most of them have sufficient evidence of multitissue origin on ultrasound and CT to suggest the correct diagnosis. Because many of these teratomas contain fat, MRI should be an excellent tool.

Both Wilms' tumors and neuroblastomas may be so large as to make accurate assessment of the organ of origin difficult by ultrasound, but CT with intravenous contrast enhancement is usually accurate for this purpose. Although the National Wilms' Tumor Study still calls for performance of excretory urograms, these examination really add little to the diagnosis and staging of patients with Wilms' tumors, neuroblastomas, or other suspected retroperitoneal tumors. However, if ultrasound suggests hydronephrosis or benign cystic lesions of the kidney, then excretory urography is a valuable adjunct.

Other retroperitoneal masses may be identified, but specific diagnoses may be difficult to make. Rhabdomyosarcoma, fibromatosis, fibrosarcoma, etc. do not have specific imaging characteristics, although precise evaluation of their location

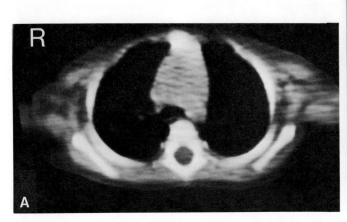

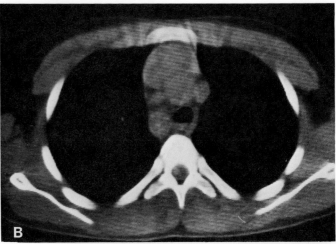

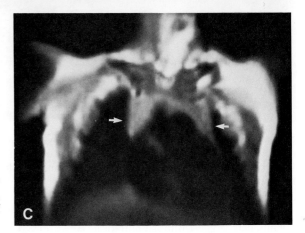

FIGURE 7-14. *Thymus gland.* **A.** CT through thymus shows normal triangular gland between heart and sternum. **B.** Rounded, tumor-infiltrated thymus is seen in 14-year-old girl with Hodgkin's disease. **C.** T1-weighted coronal scan of chest of 8-year-old boy demonstrates both lobes of thymus (*arrows*) to good advantage.

may suggest the correct diagnosis. Patients with lymphoreticular malignancies commonly have retroperitoneal lymphadenopathy, but other manifestations of the disease usually lead to the proper diagnosis.

INTRAPERITONEAL MASSES. Most intraperitoneal masses in infants and young children are related to the gastrointestinal tract, in which plain film and barium studies are usually diagnostic, or are cystic masses, in which ultrasound may suggest the organ of origin, the likelihood of malignancy, and, not infrequently, the specific diagnosis. Hepatic tumors and lymphoma account for most of the intraperitoneal abdominal masses identified as solid by ultrasound (Fig. 7-16). Occasionally, lymphomas appear relatively hypoechoic, mimicking fluid-filled masses, but careful ultrasound examination usually can determine correctly the solid nature of the mass and should be followed by abdominal CT scanning for staging purposes.

Solid hepatic masses identified on ultrasound should also be evaluated by contrast-enhanced CT scanning and a radionuclide scan. Whereas the combination of these two studies may suggest the proper diagnosis, hepatic angiography permits a definitive assessment of the hepatic vasculature and intrahepatic extension of tumor, critical pieces of information for the surgeon.[51] Recent reports of experience with MRI in hepatic tumors in children suggest that this procedure may be useful,[52] but careful evaluation is necessary before it can be considered a substitute for either CT or angiography.

PELVIC TUMORS. Rhabdomyosarcoma is the most common pelvic tumor in boys, whereas ovarian tumors and rhabdomyosarcomas must be considered primarily in girls (see Chaps. 30 and 35). Although cystography and excretory urography have been widely used in the past for evaluation of rhabdomyosarcomas arising in or near the urinary bladder, contrast-enhanced CT scanning allows evaluation of tumor masses in both intravesical and extravesical areas and usually supplies sufficient information about the primary tumor as well as about intra-abdominal metastases. Most ovarian tumors are cystic and benign and are identified as such by ultrasound. Teratomas may appear either echogenic or echolucent but frequently have mixed characteristics, which may suggest the correct diagnosis. Malignant ovarian tumors are uncommon in childhood. They are either solid on ultrasonographic examination or have mixed solid and cystic areas and should be more thoroughly evaluated by pelvic and abdominal CT.

MISCELLANEOUS ABDOMINAL MASSES. Malignant disease involving the spleen characteristically is infiltrative and causes splenomegaly rather than a discrete mass. This is especially true of leukemia. Lymphomatous involvement of the spleen can be infiltrative, discrete, or a combination of the two. Lymphoreticular malignancies confined to the spleen are extraordinary, and the diagnosis is usually apparent from other sources. Splenic cysts are typically hypoechoic, and careful ultrasonography usually obviates further studies.[17] Hepatic and splenic metastases from solid tumors and lymphomas can be

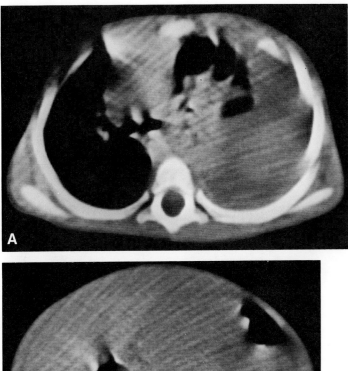

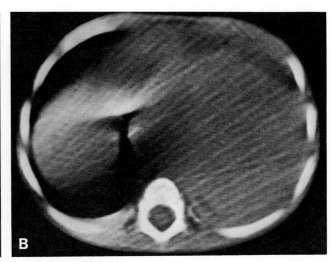

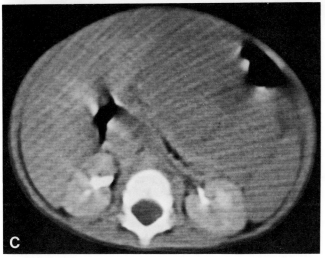

FIGURE 7-15. *Diaphragmatic rhabdomyosarcoma* in 3-year-old boy. Axial CT scans through lower part of chest (**A**), thoracoabdominal junction (**B**), and abdomen (**C**) demonstrate continuous mass extending from midchest to midabdomen. Diaphragm cannot be identified. These findings suggested the diagnosis, subsequently proved by biopsy.

identified by CT if they are at least 1 cm in size, although smaller masses frequently can be seen. Ultrasound and nuclear medicine can identify lesions 2 cm or larger, and ultrasound can often identify lesions of 1 cm. However, most patients with primary abdominal tumors will have a CT scan, and this examination is usually sufficient for evaluation of hepatosplenic metastases.

Although tumor-laden lymph nodes in the porta hepatis may cause biliary obstruction, most biliary masses in children are cystic and benign and are easily evaluated by ultrasound and nuclear medicine studies. Most pancreatic masses in children are cystic on ultrasound and require no further imaging studies. Rarely, solid masses in the pancreas can be found, from either metastatic disease, lymphoma, or rare endocrine tumors. Unless the patient already has a known primary, CT scanning should be used for better delineation of the mass.

Extremities

Osteogenic sarcoma and Ewing's sarcoma are the most common primary bone tumors of childhood, but the group of conditions known as the small round-cell tumors of childhood all must be considered in the differential diagnosis (see Chaps. 31 and 32). An algorithmic approach based on numerous criteria may narrow the differential diagnosis,[53] but an exact diagnosis is not always possible. Most osteogenic sarcomas make tumoral

bone and may be diagnosed on plain film radiography (see Fig. 7-4). Unfortunately, not all osteogenic sarcomas present with obvious malignant bone formation, and specific diagnosis is not always possible, especially in the earliest stages. Patients presenting with pain and unusual fractures should be evaluated for osteogenic sarcoma and other malignancies (Fig. 7-17). Small destructive lesions of bone associated with soft-tissue masses should also raise the possibility of early osteogenic sarcoma. The small round-cell tumors of childhood include metastases, especially from neuroblastoma, rhabdomyosarcoma and Wilms' tumor. Leukemia, lymphoma, histiocytosis X, and osteomyelitis should also be considered.

When a combination of clinical information and radiographic appearance make a primary tumor of bone likely, a CT or MRI scan should be obtained for further evaluation. CT has proved better for evaluation of the intramedullary extent of tumor and the extent of soft-tissue mass than is plain film radiography, conventional tomography, or radioisotope bone scan.[54] Early experience with MRI suggests that this technique may be even more sensitive than CT for intramedullary and soft-tissue extention[4] and has the added advantage of being able to demonstrate the lesion in sagittal and coronal as well as axial planes. Although more comparative studies need to be performed, at this early stage it seems that MRI of the extremity with the suspected primary bone tumor is the imaging modality of choice.

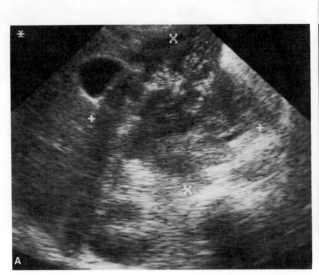 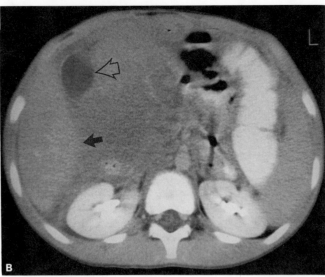

FIGURE 7-16. *Burkitt's lymphoma.* **A.** Transverse ultrasound examination of abdomen demonstrates large abdominal mass of mixed echogenicity (outlined by X and +). Mass is separate from liver (*straight arrow*) and normal gallbladder (*curved arrow*). **B.** Axial CT scan of abdomen at the same level demonstrates mass (*arrows*).

Staging

Imaging procedures are invaluable in the staging (see also Table 7-4) of most solid tumors and may come to play a role in the evaluation of acute leukemia. Although the staging procedures used depend on tumor type and location, the underlying principle is evaluation of the local and distant extent. Local extent is usually evaluated by the primary diagnostic modalities discussed above; this section will deal with the evaluation of common areas of metastatic disease.

Central Nervous System Metastases

Tumor metastatic to the brain, the spinal cord, and the meninges is usually evaluated by means of CT. However, as with primary brain tumors, MRI clearly is more accurate and offers better resolution than does CT. A significant advantage of MRI for metastatic lesions within the spinal canal is obviation of the intrathecal contrast material typically used in conjunction with CT scanning. Although there is fallout of signal from bone on MRI studies, metastatic involvement of adjacent vertebral structures usually can be identified by changes in marrow signal.

Pulmonary Metastases

Although metastases to the lung may be seen frequently on chest radiographs, CT is a far more valuable imaging modality for this purpose.[55] CT frequently identifies metastases 2 to 3 mm in diameter that may not be visible on plain chest films. In addition, CT can identify metastatic lesions at the periphery of the lungs, a problem area for plain films. Comparative studies have shown that CT is also more valuable than routine radiographic tomography and should be considered the modality of choice for evaluation of pulmonary metastases.[56] The principal disadvantage of CT has been its inability to differentiate metastases from benign lesions, especially granulomas, that may

Table 7-4
Recommended Imaging Evaluation for Metastatic Disease

CNS
  MRI if available; otherwise CT

Lungs and Mediastinum
  CT with and without contrast

Liver
  CT for primary evaluation; ultrasound for ease of follow-up

Retroperitoneal Lymph Nodes
  LAG for Hodgkin's disease or other tumor where focal therapy may be considered; otherwise CT

Skeletal
  Radioisotope bone scan
  Plain films of areas positive on bone scan
  Exceptions:
    Histiocytosis X: Radiographic bone survey
    Neuroblastoma: Radioisotope bone scan and radiographic bone survey

appear in the lungs.[57] However, children are far less likely to have granulomas than are adults, and nodular lesions in the lungs of children with known malignant solid tumors should be considered metastases until proved otherwise. As noted above, CT has been of arguable value in differentiating hilar masses from normal vascular structures, and MRI may play an important role in the detection of such masses.

Patients with pleural metastases frequently have large effusions that make evaluation of the underlying disease difficult by plain chest radiography. CT has the advantage of allowing imaging of underlying thoracic structures even in the presence

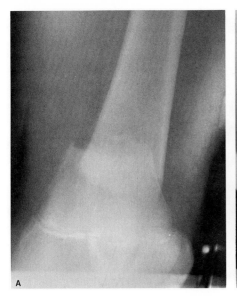
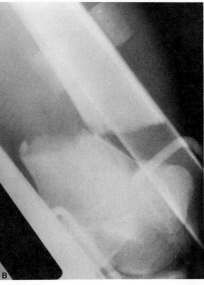
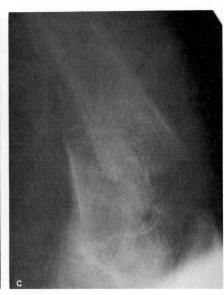

FIGURE 7-17. *Osteosarcoma* in 13-year-old boy. Anteroposterior (**A**) and lateral (**B**) views of distal femur show transverse fracture after trauma. Transverse fractures are unusual after infancy and are frequently secondary to an underlying pathologic process. Follow-up examination 3 weeks (**C**) later demonstrates irregular edges of fracture and tumoral new bone, suggesting malignant tumor.

of pleural effusion (Fig. 7-18). Because of this, CT-guided needle biopsy may obviate thoracotomy when tissue diagnosis is required. The imaging approach to mediastinal metastatic disease is the same as that for primary tumors.

Intra-abdominal Metastases

Metastases to the liver have traditionally been evaluated by scintigraphy. Using the newest equipment and techniques, radioisotope liver scans can certainly identify metastatic lesions greater than 2 cm in diameter and many lesions between 1 and 2 cm.[58] However, technical advances in both ultrasound and CT have made these imaging modalities more accurate as well. The sensitivity and resolution of ultrasound for liver metastases is comparable to, or slightly better than, that of isotope scans. CT appears able to identify 90% of lesions 1 cm or greater in size and many lesions that are even smaller.[59] Because hepatic metastases are most frequently found with primary intra-abdominal tumors, the liver can easily be evaluated during CT scans for evaluation of the primary tumor. The spleen, adrenal glands, and pancreas can similarly be evaluated at the time of initial CT. Although less sensitive than CT, ultrasound can be a valuable adjunct in the evaluation of the abdominal viscera and is particularly useful for short-interval follow-up studies where time, expense, and need for sedation or anesthesia may make CT less feasible.

The retroperitoneal lymph nodes (see Table 7-2) can be evaluated for metastases from nonlymphomatous tumors with 92% accuracy by lymphangiography and with 84% accuracy by CT.[60] As noted above, however, CT scanning is not able to differentiate lymph nodes enlarged because of benign processes from those enlarged because of tumor infiltration. CT also suffers from not being able to reveal when normal-size lymph nodes are infiltrated by tumor. Although reactive hyperplasia causes mild enlargement of lymph nodes, moderate to severe enlargement usually suggests infiltration by tumor. In such cases, CT may give sufficient diagnostic information. If more detailed information is required, lymphangiography

should be performed. Early studies of MRI suggest that this modality can identify the abnormally enlarged retroperitoneal lymph nodes. However, anatomic delineation is not improved over CT scanning.

Skeletal Metastases

Bony lesions can be found in patients with most types of solid tumors and may be seen in patients with lymphoreticular malignancies, including histiocytosis X. Radioisotope bone scans are more sensitive than plain film radiographs for the detection of metastatic disease.[61] Exceptions to this principle are found in histiocytosis X,[62] in which more than half the patients have false-negative bone scans, and in neuroblastoma,[63] in which both false-positive and false-negative bone scans have been reported (see Chaps. 23 and 28). Patients with histiocytosis X can be evaluated just with radiographs. However, patients with neuroblastoma should have both radioisotope bone scans and radiographs for adequate evaluation of the skeletal system. In general, CT scans offer little additional information when bony metastases are present but will better show the degree of bony involvement and associated soft-tissue masses if this information is needed.

Guide to Therapy

Accurate assessment of tumor volume and local extent is particularly important when surgery or radiation therapy is used. Generally, the imaging studies recommended for primary tumors described above and in the specific chapters will give adequate information for the surgeon or radiation therapist. In most instances, CT scanning of solid tumors will give adequate information, although, as noted, there are occasions when MRI may be more useful. Arteriography is rarely indicated other than in primary liver tumors, although it should be considered when questions of blood supply or preoperative vascular embolization are raised.

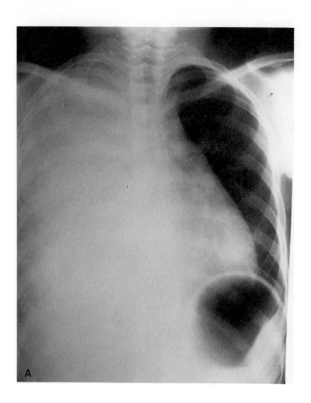

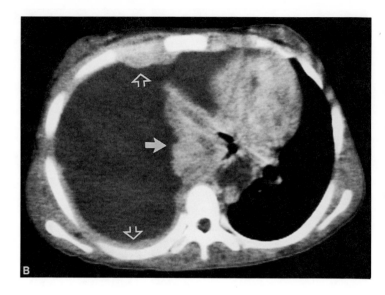

FIGURE 7-18. *Non-Hodgkin's lymphoma* in 13-year-old boy. Chest radiograph (**A**) shows large right pleural effusion of unknown etiology. CT scan (**B**) demonstrates collapsed lung (*closed arrow*) and pleural plaques of tumor (*open arrows*), one of which was biopsied for diagnosis.

Evaluation of Therapy

Typically, therapeutic response can be evaluated using the same imaging modalities used in evaluation of the primary tumor. In most instances, this will be CT. However, if ultrasound has been satisfactory in delineating the primary tumor, this method should be used for following response to therapy since it is cheaper and requires no sedation or anesthesia. Metastatic lesions are also best monitored using the same modality which demonstrated them at the time of presentation.

Detection of Recurrences

Recurrent disease can be defined as reappearance of tumor in its original location or as metastases in distant sites. The primary site is usually best followed with the imaging modality used for the initial tumor. Adequate evaluation for metastatic disease requires knowledge of the natural history of the tumor; chest films, head and chest CT, bone scans, and abdominal ultrasound and CT are all reasonably used, depending on the organ of origin of the original tumor.

The vexing problem that has yet to be resolved is how often follow-up studies should be obtained. A recently completed study of recurrent Hodgkin's disease in children showed that 56% of patients who relapsed did so within 2 years and 71% within 3 years of presentation (BR Parker, R Cohen, SS Donaldson et al: Unpublished data). However, an overall relapse rate of 48% in the years before 1970 has dropped to less than 10% since 1970, reflecting both inadequate staging in the early years and improved therapy and better staging in recent years. Thus, close-interval follow-up imaging procedures will detect recurrences, but the population at risk is small.

A recent study of the value of CT in the follow-up of abdominal neuroblastoma showed patients with stages III and IV disease to be at high risk for recurrence during the first 18 months after presentation.[64] The authors recommend close-interval follow-up with CT scans every 12 weeks during this high-risk period. Patients with stages I and II disease were at low risk of recurrence, and a single CT scan 12 weeks after surgery was recommended.

Statistical analyses of recurrent disease are complex, however.[65] Several studies using advanced statistical techniques have been published, with emphasis on bone tumors. These showed that patients with Ewing's sarcoma are at risk for bone metastases for 3 years with a truncal primary and for 4 years with an extremity primary.[66] However, therapeutic results have improved dramatically since this study was done, and the natural history of treated Ewing's tumor has certainly changed. A similar study of bone metastases in osteosarcoma demonstrated a linearly increasing risk for 5 to 29 months after diagnosis.[67]

Although these statistical analyses represent the best way to evaluate the appropriate frequency of follow-up studies, the changing natural history of most treated children's tumors makes accurate assessment of optimal timing difficult. Table 7-5 suggests a plan of follow-up that fits the present situation but is likely to change in the future.

Complications of Antitumor Therapy

All three primary modalities used in antitumor therapy—surgery, radiation, and chemotherapy—may lead to complications that can be defined and evaluated by imaging procedures. Most complications of surgery are not unique to cancer patients and will not be dealt with in this chapter.

Complications of radiation and chemotherapy can be described as direct effects, such as radio-osteonecrosis or cardiomyopathy, or as secondary, as in patients who develop infections or steroid-induced ulcers. From the point of view of the imaging specialist, most attention historically has been paid to the effects of radiation therapy.

Table 7-5
Recommended Follow-up Imaging Procedures

Leukemia
  A. Bone marrow MRI at completion of therapy, then every 3 months for 1 year, every 6 months during second year, then yearly for 3 years
  B. Gonadal ultrasound at completion of therapy

Hodgkin's Disease
  A. Chest radiographs monthly during therapy and for 18 months after therapy, then every other month for 1 year, every 6 months until 5 years after diagnosis, then yearly
  B. Chest and abdominal CT at completion of therapy and then semiannually until 3 years after diagnosis
  C. If LAG performed, monthly abdominal plain film until contrast material disappears

Non-Hodgkin's Lymphoma
  A. Imaging studies of affected areas monthly during therapy until resolution, then semiannually until 2 years after completion of therapy, then yearly

Wilms' Tumor
  A. Chest radiographs monthly until 1 year after completion of therapy, every other month for 1 year, semiannually for another year, then yearly
  B. Abdominal ultrasound every 3 months until 1 year after completion of therapy, then twice a year for 2 years, then yearly

Neuroblastoma
  A. Imaging study of primary area of involvement monthly until resolution, then every 3 months for 1 year, every 6 months for another year, then yearly
  B. Radioisotope bone scan at time of imaging studies of primary site

Bone Tumors
  A. Chest radiographs monthly until 2 years after completion of therapy, then every other month for 1 year, semiannually for another year, and yearly thereafter
  B. Chest CT at completion of therapy, every 3 months for 1 year, then semiannually until 5 years after diagnosis
  C. Radiographs of primary site monthly during therapy if not surgically removed
     Radiographs of residual bone every 2 months after surgery until 1 year after completion of chemotherapy, then semiannually for 1 year, then yearly until 5 years after diagnosis
  D. Radioisotope bone scan every third month until 1 year after completion of therapy, then semiannually for 1 year, then annually until 5 years after diagnosis

Radiation Complications

Children are more likely than adults to develop complications of radiation, since growing bone is more sensitive to irradiation than is the more stable adult bone (see Chaps. 11 and 50). Interference with normal bone growth may lead to shortening of an irradiated bone or to overall diminution in height from spinal irradiation.[68] In long bones, characteristic deformities similar to those seen in trauma and rickets have been described.[69] Loss of spinal height is best determined clinically, but radiographs typically show failure of maturation of the vertebral bodies in irradiated fields.[70] Spinal irradiation may also lead to scoliosis with secondary loss of height, but the average angle of radiation-induced scoliosis is less than 10°, infrequently leading to clinically apparent abnormalities. Other ways in which the impact of radiation on growth is seen frequently include hypoplasia of the clavicles and the iliac bones when they are included in treatment fields.

Depending on dose–time relations, the impact of radiation on mineralization ranges from mild osteoporosis to frank radio-osteonecrosis. Since profound bone necrosis has a radiographic pattern simulating small-cell infiltration, the differentiation between radiation effect and recurrent or metastatic disease can be difficult. However, radio-osteonecrosis does not cause rupture of the bony cortex and tends to be stable over successive examinations, whereas infiltrative bone disease usually breaks through the cortex into the subperiosteal region and shows progression over fairly short intervals of time. CT has the same problems as plain radiographs in this regard. There is as yet insufficient experience with MRI to determine if this modality will be better at differentiating necrosis from tumor. Nevertheless, the differentiation is usually made on plain films without great difficulty.

Radiation-induced tumors of bone are most commonly benign, with osteochondroma being the most frequent.[71] These osteochondromas typically arise from growth plates in non-weight-bearing bones (Fig. 7-19). However, they can arise in virtually any bone in which the growth plate is irradiated and have been described in patients receiving doses as small as 1200 cGy. Many of these lesions have been removed surgically and have been found to be benign. If not removed, they should be followed carefully with periodic examination, as any osteochondroma has the potential to undergo malignant degeneration.

Radiation-induced malignant tumors are a well-known phenomenon with osteosarcoma being the most common and chondrosarcomas and fibrosarcomas also being seen. The latent period for sarcoma development is 4.5 to 27 years, with a median of 11 years and a mean of 12 years.[72]

Radiation effects on nonosseous viscera are extensive and related to the particular organs involved. Irradiation of the brain, usually in combination with intrathecal chemotherapy, may lead to leukomalacia, which can be identified on CT scans[73] and MRI scans. Frank brain necrosis may occur with high doses. The thyroid gland is particularly susceptible to radiation damage, and thyroid cancers may be identified by nuclear medicine studies, by ultrasound, and by CT.

Acute radiation reaction in the lungs is well demonstrated on chest films, appearing as air space and interstitial infiltrates within a well-defined anatomic area corresponding to the radiation portals. Acute changes usually appear near the end of therapy or within a month of the completion of therapy and may last 2 to 9 months. If the dose is high enough, chronic interstitial fibrosis may develop, again well circumscribed within the radiation field. CT is more accurate than conventional chest radiographs in detecting the earliest changes of radiation fibrosis.[74]

The liver and kidneys are both susceptible to radiation damage. Radiation hepatitis has been well defined on radioisotope scans as areas of diminished activity corresponding to the radiation portals. Isotope liver scans may be abnormal in both acute and chronic phases. Since radiation hepatitis may mimic metastatic disease on scintigraphy, ultrasound or CT may be necessary to resolve a suspicious finding. The impact of radiation on the growing kidney is most likely to result in failure of normal growth.[75] Serial ultrasound examinations are excellent for determining and comparing renal size and in such cases will demonstrate a lack of growth over a period of several years.

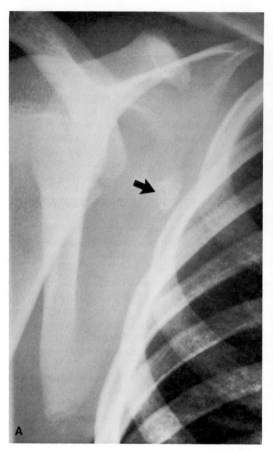
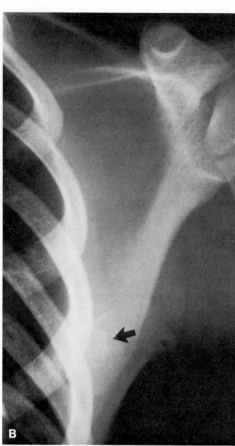

FIGURE 7-19. *Radiation-induced osteochondromas (arrows)* are seen in right (**A**) and left (**B**) scapulas in patient 13 years after treatment for metastatic Wilms' tumor. Both lungs received a radiation dose of 12 Gy; scapulas were included in the field.

The gastrointestinal mucosa is highly susceptible to radiation damage.[76] Barium studies are the best way to evaluate esophagitis and enterocolitis, as they show the mucosal changes and mesenteric thickening (see Fig. 7-3). CT and ultrasound can also show these changes, but the findings are not as specific.

Cartilage necrosis may occur when joints are included in the radiation field, and calcification of articular cartilage may then be identified on plain films. Similarly, ischemic necrosis of the humeral heads and femoral heads may be seen.[77] Muscle atrophy may be suggested on plain films but is easily evaluated on CT and, especially, MRI studies. MRI is particularly useful in identifying edema within fascial planes before the clinical effects are recognized.

Chemotherapy Complications

The direct adverse effects of chemotherapy can also be evaluated with imaging studies, depending on the organ involved (see Chaps. 9 and 50). Leukomalacia after intrathecal chemotherapy, usually in association with radiotherapy, has been defined on CT and MRI studies. Those drugs that have toxic effects on the lung lead to pulmonary fibrosis, which can be defined on plain films as volume loss and interstitial fibrosis.[78] However, these are late findings, and respiratory function studies are more sensitive than imaging studies in detecting early changes. Cardiomyopathy secondary to the anthracyclines causes cardiomegaly and pulmonary edema in later stages. However, early changes can be evaluated by calculating left ventricular ejection fractions on echocardiography or with radioisotopes.[79] MRI may identify the cardiac lesion very early, but appropriate studies have not yet been done.

Finally, the secondary effects of chemotherapy may be seen. The most common are infections secondary to immunosuppression (see Chap 39). The other common group of secondary effects is related to steroids and includes such radiographically demonstrable abnormalities as pseudotumor cerebri, retarded skeletal maturation, ischemic necrosis of the femoral heads, diffuse osteoporosis with compression fractures of vertebral bodies, abnormal fat deposition, and gastric and duodenal ulcers. The appropriate imaging study depends, of course, on the anatomic region involved.

FUTURE CONSIDERATIONS

A radiologist writing in 1958 would have known nothing of ultrasound, one in 1968 nothing of CT, and one in 1978 nothing of MRI. A radiologist in 1988, therefore, can only make predictions with a mixture of trepidation and bravado. Nonetheless, certain trends are already apparent, and exciting advances are clearly on the horizon.

Continuing technical advances are likely to make further improvements in the sensitivity and accuracy of the anatomic delineation of abnormalities by ultrasound, CT, and MRI. MRI, particularly, should undergo technologic advances in the 1990s similar to those made in CT in the 1970s and 1980s. MRI scans will continue to show improved resolution, will be done with greater rapidity, and should undergo a reduction in cost as patient throughput increases. Increased experience with smaller magnets may reduce the problems with examining patients on life-support apparatus and may reduce the capital cost of the equipment.

Increasing computer applications will improve the image quality of all the modalities. Digital radiography allows manipulation of plain film images as well as the more sophisticated modalities, so even this simplest of imaging procedures may become more accurate in the decade to come. The first of the computerized ultrasound units has already produced improved image resolution, and this will continue.

Resolution of CT images will also improve, and new software may make three-dimensional reconstruction useful for oncology patients, especially those undergoing radiation therapy. Scanning times may be reduced even further, making anesthesia and heavy sedation less necessary for children. The new nonionic contrast materials will further reduce the already small incidence of adverse contrast reactions.

The most exciting advances are likely to come as modalities now used primarily for anatomic information begin to produce physiological and even chemical information. PET scanning is already making available information about brain metabolism, and this may improve in the CNS as well as become available for other organ systems.

Much research activity is being done in the field of in vivo MR spectroscopy. Although early work has focused on phosphorous spectroscopy, technologic advances will permit identification and spectroscopic analysis of other atoms in their various biochemical states as well. Tissue characterization by such means is a likelihood, and the possibility of differentiating benign from malignant tissue by these methods may revolutionize oncologic diagnosis.

Tissue characterization by ultrasound has been an active field of research for some years. Although no clinically applicable results have yet been achieved, the potential still exists for a significant impact on oncologic problems, possibly at a substantially lower financial cost than with other modalities.

Finally, there is likely to be a change in the role of imaging specialists as they become a more integral part of the pediatric oncology team. The many imaging modalities now available for evaluation of children with malignancies require careful selection, performance, and interpretation to arrive at a correct diagnosis quickly and at least cost and patient discomfort. Not only should imaging specialists be involved in the evaluation of patients, but they should also play a role in the formulation of multi-institutional clinical research protocols. This ensures not only that the most advanced techniques are used properly, but that the relative efficacy of these procedures in diagnosis, staging, and follow-up is properly studied to enable the next generation of pediatric oncologic patients to obtain maximum benefit from the recent explosion in imaging technology.

REFERENCES

1. Sty JR, Wells RG, Starshak RJ, Schroeder BA: Imaging in acute renal infection in children. AJR 148:471–478, 1987
2. Majd M: Radionuclide imaging in pediatrics. Pediatr Clin North Am 32:1559–1579, 1985
3. Aisen AM, Martel W, Braunstein EM et al: MRI and CT evaluation of primary bone and soft tissue tumors. AJR 146:749–756, 1986
4. Boyko OB, Cory DA, Cohen MD et al: MR imaging of osteogenic and Ewing's sarcoma. AJR 148:317–322, 1987
5. Wells SK: The value of skull radiography in children with intracranial tumors. Clin Radiol 36:253–255, 1985
6. Osborn AG, Harnsberger HR, Smoker WRK: Base of the skull imaging. Semin Ultrasound CT MR 7:91–106, 1986
7. Norman D, Diamond C, Boyd D: Relative detectability of intracranial calcifications on computed tomography and skull radiography. J Comput Assist Tomogr 2:61–64, 1978
8. Han JS, Benson JE, Yoon YS: Magnetic resonance imaging in the spinal column and craniovertebral junction. Radiol Clin North Am 22:805–827, 1984
9. Siegel MJ, Jamroz GA, Glazer HS et al: MR imaging of intraspinal extension of neuroblastoma. J Comput Assist Tomogr 10:593–595, 1986
10. Reiman TAH, Siegel MJ, Shackelford GD: Wilms' tumor in children: Abdominal CT and US evaluation. Radiology 160:501–505, 1986
11. Miller JH, Greenspan BS: Integrated imaging of hepatic tumors in childhood. Radiology 154:83–90, 1985
12. Moss AA, Goldberg HI, Stark DD et al: Hepatic tumors: Magnetic resonance and CT appearance. Radiology 150:141–147, 1984
13. Marglin SI, Castellino RA: Selection of imaging studies for newly presenting patients with non-Hodgkin's lymphoma. Semin Ultrasound CT MR 7:2–8, 1986
14. Castellino RA, Musumeci R, Markovits P: Lymphography. In Parker BR, Castellino RA (eds): Pediatric Oncologic Radiology, pp 58–84. St Louis, CV Mosby, 1977
15. Dunnick NR, Parker BR, Castellino RA: Pediatric lymphography: Performance, interpretation, and accuracy in 193 consecutive children. Am J Roentgenol 129:639–646, 1977
16. Castellino RA, Hoppe RT, Blank N et al: Computed tomography, lymphography, and staging laparotomy: Correlations in initial staging of Hodgkin's disease. AJR 143:37–41, 1984
17. Bernardino ME, Thomas JL, Barnes PA et al: Diagnostic approaches to liver and spleen metastases. Radiol Clin North Am 20:469–485, 1982
18. Bekerman C, Port RB, Pang E et al: Scintigraphic evaluation of childhood malignancies by 67-Ga-citrate. Radiology 127:719–725, 1978
19. Gainey MA, McDougall IR: Diagnosis of acute inflammatory conditions in children and adolescents using 111-indium-oxine white blood cells. Clin Nucl Med 9:71–74, 1984
20. Haentjens M, Piepsza A, Schell-Frederick E et al: Limitations in the use of indium-111-oxine-labeled leucocytes for the diagnosis of occult infection in children. Pediatr Radiol 17:139–142, 1987
21. Munkner T: 131-I-meta-iodobenzyl-guanidine scintigraphy of neuroblastomas. Semin Nucl Med 15:154–160, 1985
22. Wieland DM, Brown LE, Tobes MC et al: Imaging the primate adrenal medullae with (I-123) and I-131) metaiodobenzylguanidine. J Nucl Med 22:358–364, 1981
23. Hattner RS, Huberty JP, Englestad BL et al: Localization of m-131-iodobenzylguanidine in neuroblastoma AJR 143:373–374, 1984
24. Dean JC, Carroll BA, Parker BR: Diagnostic ultrasound in pediatric oncology. Am J Pediat Hematol Oncol 7:270–282, 1985
25. Gooding CA, Berdon WE, Brodeur AE et al: Adverse reactions to intravenous pyelography in children. Am J Roentgenol 123:802–804, 1975
26. Bloch F: Nuclear induction. Physiol Rev 70:460–473, 1946
27. Purcell EM, Torrey HC, Pound RV: Resonance absorption by nuclear magnetic moments in a solid. Physiol Rev 69:127, 1946
28. Modic MT, Weinstein MA, Pavlicek W et al: Nuclear magnetic resonance imaging of the spine. Radiology 148:757–762, 1983
29. Weinstein MA: MRI of the spine and spinal cord. In Margulis AR, Gooding CA (eds): Diagnostic Radiology, pp 325–330. San Francisco, University of California–San Francisco, 1986
30. Gamsu G, Webb WR, Sheldon P et al: Nuclear magnetic resonance imaging of the thorax. Radiology 147:473–480, 1983
31. Siegel MJ, Nadel SN, Glazer HS et al: Mediastinal lesions in children: Comparison of CT and MR. Radiology 160:241–244, 1986
32. Fletcher BD, Kopiwoda SY, Strandjord SE et al: Abdominal neuroblastoma: Magnetic resonance imaging and tissue characterization. Radiology 155:699–704, 1985
33. Belt TG, Cohen MD, Smith JA et al: MRI of Wilms' tumor: Promise as the primary imaging method. AJR 146:955–961, 1986
34. Cohen MD, Klatte EC, Baehner R et al: Magnetic resonance imaging of bone marrow disease in children. Radiology 151:715–718, 1984
35. Olson DO, Shields AF, Scheurich CJ et al: Magnetic resonance imaging of the bone marrow in patients with leukemia, aplastic anemia, and lymphoma. Invest Radiol 21:540–546, 1986
36. Moore SG, Gooding CA, Brasch RC et al: Bone marrow in children with acute lymphocytic leukemia: MR relaxation times. Radiology 160:237–240, 1986
37. Kucharczyk W, Brant-Zawadzki M, Sobel D et al: Central nervous system tumors in children: Detection by magnetic resonance imaging. Radiology 155:131–136, 1985
38. Scott JA, Rosenthal DI, Brady TJ: The evaluation of musculoskeletal disease with magnetic resonance imaging. Radiol Clin North Am 22:917–924, 1984
39. Towbin RB, Strife JL: Percutaneous aspiration, drainage, and biopsies in children. Radiology 157:81–85, 1985

40. vanSonnenberg E, Wittich GR, Edwards DK et al: Percutaneous diagnostic and therapeutic interventional radiologic procedures in children: experience in 100 patients. Radiology 162:601–605, 1987

41. Norman D, Mills CM, Brant-Zawadzki M et al: Magnetic resonance imaging of the spinal cord and canal: Potentials and limitations. AJNR 5:9–14, 1984

42. Paushter DM, Modic MT, Masaryk TJ: Magnetic resonance imaging of the spine: Applications and limitations. Radiol Clin North Am 23:551–562, 1985

43. Bousvaros A, Kirks DR, Grossman H: Imaging of neuroblastoma: An overview. Pediatr Radiol 16:89–106, 1986

44. Siegel MJ, Nadel SN, Glazer HS et al: Mediastinal lesions in children: Comparison of CT and MR. Radiology 160:241–244, 1986

45. Cohen AM, Creviston S, LiPuma JP et al: NMR evaluation of hilar and mediastinal lymphadenopathy. Radiology 148:737–742, 1983

46. Levitt RG, Glazer HS, Roper CL et al: Magnetic resonance imaging of mediastinal and hilar masses: Comparison with CT. AJR 145:9–14, 1985

47. Cohen MD, Klatte EC, Smith JA et al: Magnetic resonance imaging of lymphomas in children. Pediatr Radiol 15:179–183, 1985

48. Kirks DR, Merten DF, Grossman H et al: Diagnostic imaging of pediatric abdominal masses: An overview. Radiol Clin North Am 19:527–545, 1981

49. Mettelstaedt CA, Volberg FM, Merten DF et al: The sonographic diagnosis of neonatal adrenal hemorrhage. Radiology 131:453–457, 1979

50. Miller JH, Greenspan BS: Integrated imaging of hepatic tumors in childhood I: Malignant lesions (primary and metastatic). Radiology 154:83–88, 1985

51. Wallace S: Primary liver tumors. In Parker BR, Castellino RA (eds): Pediatric Oncologic Radiology, pp 301–335. St Louis, CV Mosby, 1977

52. Moss AA, Goldberg HI, Stark DD et al: Hepatic tumors: Magnetic resonance and CT appearance. Radiology 150:141–147, 1984

53. Steinbach HL, Parker BR: Primary bone tumors. In Parker BR, Castellino RA (eds): Pediatric Oncologic Radiology, pp 378–406. St Louis, CV Mosby, 1977

54. Berger PE, Kuhn JP: Computed tomography of tumors of the musculoskeletal system in children: Clinical applications. Radiology 127:171–175, 1978

55. Muhm JR, Brown LR, Crowe JK et al: Use of computed tomography in the detection of pulmonary nodules. Mayo Clin Proc 52:345–348, 1977

56. Muhm JR, Brown LR, Crowe JK et al: Comparison of whole lung tomography and computed tomography for detecting pulmonary nodules. AJR 131:981–984, 1978

57. Schaner EG, Chang AE, Doppman JL et al: Comparison of computed and conventional whole lung tomography in detecting pulmonary nodules: A prospective radiologic–pathologic study. AJR 13:51–54, 1978

58. Chafetz N, Taylor A, Alazraki NP et al: The heterogeneous liver scan: Ultrasound correlation. Radiology 130:201–203, 1979

59. Snow JH, Goldstein HM, Wallace S: Comparison of scintigraphy, sonography, and computed tomography in the evaluation of hepatic neoplasms. AJR 132:915–918, 1979

60. Jing B, Wallace S, Zornoza J: Metastases to retroperitoneal and pelvic lymph nodes. Radiol Clin North Am 20:511–530, 1982

61. Gilday DL, Ash JM, Reilly BJ: Radionuclide skeletal survey for pediatric neoplasms. Radiology 123:399–406, 1977

62. Parker BR, Pinckney L, Etcubanas E: Relative efficacy of radiographic and isotopic bone surveys in the detection of the skeletal lesions of histiocytosis-X. Radiology 134:377–380, 1980

63. Kaufman RA, Thrall JH, Keyes JW Jr et al: False negative bone scans in neuroblastomas metastatic to the ends of long bones. AJR 130:131–135, 1978

64. Stark DD, Brasch RC, Moss AA et al: Recurrent neuroblastoma: The role of CT and alternative imaging tests. Radiology 148:107–112, 1983

65. Dwyer AJ, Doppman JL: Recurrent neuroblastoma: determining the frequency of follow-up examinations. Radiology 150:607, 1984

66. Dwyer AJ, Glaubiger DL, Ecker JG et al: Radiographic follow-up of patients with Ewing sarcoma: A demonstration of a general method. Radiology 145:327–331, 1982

67. McNeil BJ, Hanley J: Analysis of serial radionuclide bone images in osteosarcoma and breast carcinoma. Radiology 135:171–176, 1980

68. Probert JC, Parker BR: The effects of radiation therapy on bone growth. Radiology 114:155–162, 1975

69. DeSmet AA, Kuhns LR, Fayos JV et al: Effects of radiation therapy on growing long bones. Am J Roentgenol 127:935–939, 1976

70. Probert JC, Parker BR, Kaplan HS: Growth retardation in children after megavoltage irradiation of the spine. Cancer 32:634–639, 1973

71. Libshitz HI, Cohen MA: Radiation-induced osteochondromas. Radiology 142:643–647, 1982

72. Kim JH, Chu FC, Woodard HQ et al: Radiation-induced soft tissue and bone sarcoma. Radiology 129:501–508, 1978

73. Peylan Ramu N, Poplack DG, Pizzo PA et al: Abnormal CT scans of the brain in asymptomatic children with acute lymphocytic leukemia after prophylactic treatment of the central nervous system with radiation and intrathecal chemotherapy. N Engl J Med 298:815–818, 1978

74. Pagani JJ, Libshitz HI: CT manifestations of radiation-induced change in chest tissue. J Comput Assist Tomogr 6:243–248, 1982

75. Donaldson SS, Moskowitz PS, Canty EL et al: Radiation-induced inhibition of compensatory renal growth in the weanling mouse kidney. Radiology 128:491–495, 1978

76. Donaldson SS, Jundt S, Ricour C et al: Radiation enteritis in children: A retrospective review, clinicopathologic correlation and dietary management. Cancer 35:1167–1178, 1975

77. Libshitz HI, Edeiken BS: Radiotherapy changes of the pediatric hip. AJR 137:585–588, 1981

78. Alvarado CS, Boat TF, Newman AJ: Late onset pulmonary fibrosis and chest deformity in two children treated with Cytoxan. J Pediatr 92:443–446, 1978

79. Alexander J, Dainiak N, Berger HJ et al: Serial assessment of doxorubicin cardiotoxicity with quantitative radionuclide angiocardiography. N Engl J Med 300:278–283, 1979

eight

Biological Markers in Pediatric Cancer

Jorge A. Ortega and Stuart E. Siegel

The modern era of cancer markers began with the discovery of α-fetoprotein by G. I. Abelev in 1963.[1] Since then, there has been a growing interest in the production and release by cancer cells of cellular molecules that are more typical of embryonic or fetal cells than of differentiated cells. These biological markers are present in the cell or on the surface and are also secreted into body fluids, where they can be detected with sensitive assays. Determination of these biochemical markers has become increasingly important clinically, not only in diagnosis, but also in prognosis and treatment of different pediatric malignancies.

Biological markers have not as yet been identified for all pediatric malignancies, and although for some tumors they are extremely important in diagnosis and prognosis (neuroblastoma, germ cell tumors, hepatoblastoma), in others they are of questionable value or no use at all. The discovery of new markers suitable for clinical application and the elucidation of their pathophysiological behavior will enhance not only the follow-up of the pediatric cancer patient, but also the classification and diagnosis of childhood malignancies. Furthermore, as more specific markers become known, there will be new approaches for effective treatments. This chapter reviews the subject of markers in general and the known or possible markers for pediatric malignancies. Biological markers of lymphoproliferative disorders have been discussed in Chapter 4 and are excluded from this review.

CHARACTERISTICS OF BIOLOGICAL MARKERS IN PEDIATRIC MALIGNANCIES

The biochemical nature of the different biological markers of pediatric tumors so far identified varies markedly. Known markers include serum or tissue proteins (α-fetoprotein [AFP], ferritin), cell-surface antigens (carcinoembryonic antigen), hormones (human chorionic gonadotropin [hCG]), enzymes (alkaline phosphatase), oncogenes, and poietins. Table 8-1 summarizes the most widely recognized biological markers in pediatric malignancies along with their nature, normal values, and assay techniques. For the purpose of this review, biological markers have been grouped according to their biochemical nature.

Proteins

Several proteins have been identified as important markers for different types of pediatric malignancies and are widely used in pediatric oncology practice.

Alpha-Fetoprotein

AFP is a major serum protein synthesized by fetal liver cells, yolk sac, and, in trace amounts, by the fetal gastrointestinal tract.[2,3] It is similar in size, structure,

Table 8-1
Commonly Used Biological Tumor Markers

Marker	Nature	Specimen*	Normal Values	Technique†
AFP	Protein	S	<20 ng/ml	RIA
Alkaline phosphatase	Enzyme	S	38–125 U/liter	Spec
β-hCG	Hormone	S	5 mIu/ml	RIA
CEA	Antigen	S	2.5 ng/ml	RIA
Creatine kinase	Enzyme	S	M: 57–374 U/liter	Spec
			F: 35–230 U/liter	
Ferritin	Protein	S	7–150 µg/liter	EIA
HVA	Hormone	U	0–10 mg/24 h	HPLC
VMA	Hormone	U	2–10 mg/24 h	Spec
LDH	Enzyme	S	297–537 U/liter	Spec
NSE	Enzyme	S	15 ng/ml	RIA
Polyamines	Cationic molecules	CSF	58–278 pmol/nol	IEC
TAA	Antigen	S, U	Absent	CFT

* S = serum; U = urine; CSF = cerebrospinal fluid.

† RIA = radioimmunoassay; Spec = spectrophotometry; EIA = enzyme immunoassay; HPLC = high-pressure liquid chromatography; IEC = ion-exchange chromatography; CFT = complement-fixation test.

and amino acid sequence to serum albumin but is detectable in only minute amounts in the serum of normal adults.[4] The specific function of AFP during fetal development has not been clearly identified, but it appears to behave as a fetal albumin and possibly has the same osmotic and carrier functions in the fetus that albumin does in the adult.[5,6]

AFP is found in high concentration in fetal serum and the serum of children with hepatoblastoma, hepatocellular carcinoma, and teratocarcinomas (see Chaps. 26 and 33). The ability of a tumor to synthesize AFP usually reflects that of the fetal tissue from which its normal progenitor arises. Consequently, it is of no surprise to find extreme elevations of AFP, often exceeding 200,000 ng/ml, in children with hepatoblastoma, as the synthesis of AFP starts in the liver of the developing embryo as early as 6 weeks of gestation and stops at birth regardless of gestational age. The half-life of the protein in the circulation is between 4 and 9 days, and levels usually fall to the normal range within 4 to 6 weeks of complete resection of an AFP-producing tumor.

The amount of carbohydrate on AFP depends on the level of glycosylases in fetal and tumor tissue, and the activity of these enzymes differs in normal liver, yolk sac, and hepatocellular carcinomas. As a result, benign liver proliferation results in completely glycosylated AFP and hepatocellular carcinoma in less-glycosylated AFP.

Caution is required in interpreting AFP levels in infants, since slightly raised levels can be found in some children with disorders other than malignant hepatic and yolk sac tumors.[7] However, in practice, it is usually possible to exclude on clinical grounds the other conditions that might raise AFP (acute and chronic viral hepatitis and cirrhosis, inflammatory bowel diseases) when a hepatic or yolk sac tumor is suspected. Furthermore, these malignancies generally produce very high serum AFP levels, well beyond the physiologic range, thus permitting prediction of the histologic type of a tumor before surgery.

Ferritin

Ferritin is a soluble protein with a unique configuration: an outer shell and an inner core consisting of a variable amount of

iron deposited as a ferric hydroxyphosphate complex. This iron-storage compound is found mainly in the reticuloendothelial cells of the liver, spleen, and bone marrow, but it is also found in many parenchymal cells. For example, liver parenchymal cells contain variable amounts of ferritin. Organ-specific and species-specific isoferritins differing in electrophoretic mobility are now recognized.

Until recently, ferritin was considered an exclusively intracellular protein, but it is now known to occur in serum. With the development of sensitive techniques for serum ferritin assay, it has become apparent that small amounts circulate in normal subjects. Considerably higher concentrations may be found in many pathologic conditions, especially those in which there is necrosis or increased iron storage and in malignancies.[8,9] This finding stimulated many investigators to define the source of ferritin in serum of patients with different tumors. Ferritin is present in neuroblastoma tissue removed directly from patients[10] and is also produced by neuroblastoma cells *in vitro*.[11] Furthermore, human isoferritin has been identified in the serum of nude mice implanted with human neuroblastoma.[11] Increased ferritin levels have also been reported in patients with liver malignancies,[12] broadening the spectrum of this protein as a biological marker.

Hormones

Several hormones are being used as biological markers for specific tumors. Among them, the catecholamines and hCG have provided the most important tools in the identification and follow-up of different types of pediatric tumors.

Catecholamines

Tumor cells derived from the neural crest share similar biochemical properties; that is, the synthesis, uptake, and breakdown of catecholamines. Because neuroblastoma is a tumor of neural crest origin, it is not surprising that this tumor is frequently active in producing catecholamines and their metabolites. Under normal circumstances, the human adrenal gland contains less than 1 mg of catecholamines per gram of tissue, most of which is epinephrine. During emotional stress, pain, and hypoglycemia, the adrenal medulla discharges large quantities of epinephrine. The concentration of catecholamines in normal resting human blood plasma is extremely low and therefore difficult to determine. The catecholamines secreted into the blood are partly taken up and stored in granules in sympathetic nervous tissue and partly inactivated to the metanephrines. Figure 8-1 shows a schema of the catecholamine metabolism pathway.

Although the quantitation of urinary catecholamines and catabolites has been considered helpful by some investigators in the diagnosis of retinoblastoma and medulloblastoma, its efficiency has been questioned. In pheochromocytoma, the determination of urinary catecholamines and their metabolites, including normetanephrine and metanephrine, is essential, but pheochromocytoma is a rare tumor in the pediatric age group.

The most commonly assayed catabolites are vanillylmandelic acid (VMA) and homovanillic acid (HVA). Both catabolites have a short half-life (less than 8 hours). Many laboratories determine only VMA and use nonspecific colorimetric methods. However, this procedure is subject to interference by many exogenous and endogenous aromatic substances and requires the elimination of vanilla-rich foodstuffs from the diet for 3 days. VMA and HVA can be determined simultaneously by bidirectional paper chromatography,[13] a method that does not require dietary preparation of the patient. Moreover, rapid semiquantitative assessment of spots corresponding to several metabolites can be accomplished.[13] A significant difficulty still exists in comparing the normal values given by different authors, since results can be expressed either in terms of urine collection time or of the amount of urinary creatinine and must be normalized for age. To this problem has to be added the variable specificity of the multiple-assay methods used. Currently, the most accurate means of measuring urinary catecholamines is by high-pressure liquid chromatography (HPLC).

Human Chorionic Gonadotropin

Normally produced in the trophoblasts of the placenta, hCG is composed of two subunits of glycoprotein designated α and β. Whereas the former is similar to the α subunit of the pituitary hormones, the latter is uniquely different from the β subunit of the pituitary gonadotropins.[14] As a consequence of the development of the double-antibody radioimmunoassay, a sensitive measurement of the β subunit of hCG (β-hCG) is available.[15] The half-life of the hormone is 24 hours, and the normal serum level is less than 1 mg/ml.

Characteristically, tumors arising from trophoblastic elements are associated with elevated serum β-hCG. However, some nontrophoblastic pediatric tumors, such as embryonal carcinoma, commonly are associated with high concentrations of the hormone. In these patients, the production of hCG probably represents a primitive function of some neoplastic cells.[16]

Antigens

Antigenic phenotypes of different pediatric malignancies have been widely studied over the past 15 years, and significant evidence exists that antigenic changes are an essential feature of tumorigenesis (see Chap. 4). A critical issue in tumor immunology is that of tumor antigen specificity; that is, can tumors be recognized on the basis of the occurrence of specific antigen determinants? Tumor antigen identification is aimed not only at discerning differences between normal and malignant phenotypes in the specific host but also at defining antigen specificity according to distinct tumor tissue. It is clear that tumor-associated antigens (TAA) exist and that the malignant phenotype is as antigenically distinct from the original cellular phenotype as it is morphologically distinct. The main requirements for the use of TAA in diagnosis are reliability and ability to detect early-stage disease.

Carcinoembryonic Antigen

Carcinoembryonic antigen (CEA) is the most studied and the best known of the circulating TAA and can be measured by means of a radioimmunoassay. CEA is in fact a group of proteins detectable in patients with a variety of neoplasms, especially those of the gastrointestinal tract. This β-1 glycoprotein was first found as an apparently specific surface antigen associated with adenocarcinoma of the human colon. CEA has a molecular weight of approximately 180,000 daltons, and it is present in normal intestinal tissues; in various biological fluids such as urine, intestinal secretions, and pleural and peritoneal fluids; and in the cerebrospinal fluid.

Although about 70% of adult patients with gastrointestinal malignancies have raised CEA levels, CEA can also be high in patients with other cancers and in some nonmalignant conditions. Studies of serum CEA in children with different types of malignancies, mainly neuroblastoma, retinoblastoma, and germ cell tumors, suggest that CEA may act as a tumor marker in some cases.[17] However, it is not as specific as other biological markers and has a limited use in clinical pediatric oncology. Most investigators have concluded that CEA has its great-

FIGURE 8-1. Catecholamine metabolism pathway.

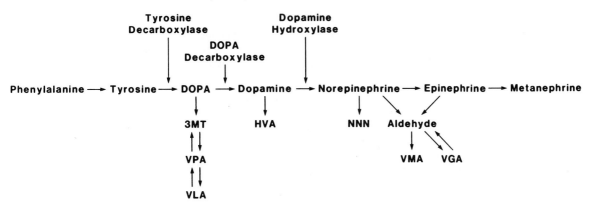

est usefulness in monitoring the response of malignant disease to therapy, that it should be used as an adjunctive diagnostic test, and that it has no place as a screening procedure.[18]

Tumor-Associated Antigens

The recent demonstration of TAA in a variety of human malignant neoplasms, including sarcomas of soft tissue or bone, has raised significant interest in them as potential biological markers. The introduction of a new method for preparing urine for testing by the complement-fixation technique[19] has further improved their measurement. The antigen detected in the complement-fixation assay has a high molecular weight (greater than 300,000 daltons). Normally, molecules of this size would be excluded from the urine by the glomerular basement membrane. However, the immune complexes probably damage the basement membrane of the glomerulus in such a way that high-molecular-weight antigens can pass through.[20] Even though there is limited experience with the determination of TAA in pediatric oncology patients, there is evidence of good correlation between the concentration in the urine and tumor activity, especially in bone and soft-tissue sarcomas.[19]

Utility of Monoclonal Antibodies

Major advances in human tumor immunology have come about as a result of the introduction of hybridoma technology and the development of highly specific monoclonal antibodies directed against tumor surfaces. Monoclonal antibodies have been made against a wide variety of tumor tissues using heterologous hosts (*e.g.,* mouse or rat). Although there are at present no antigens that define malignancy exclusively, there is a growing list of monoclonal antibodies against antigens that define malignant states when used appropriately. Panels of monoclonal antibodies are necessary to reach a definite diagnosis because of the heterogeneity in antigen expression among tumors of the same type.

An increasing number of monoclonal antibodies have been developed against tumor cell lines, including neural tumors, neuroepitheliomas, and rhabdomyosarcomas. The use of these panels of antibodies can help to distinguish different types of pediatric cancers accurately. However, the advantages of this technique are tempered by evidence that some antigens are denatured by fixation methods, whereas others are not detectable in fresh tissue. More detailed and extensive information on this subject can be found in Chapter 4.

Enzymes

Different enzymes have long been used as indicators of tumor activity; however, lack of specificity has hampered their use as biological markers. Nevertheless, continued efforts by different investigators have resulted in the identification of some specific human isoenzymes as tumor markers. It is well known that some tumor cells can release specific enzymes into the circulation, although the exact mechanism of release remains unclear.

Creatinine Kinase

Creatinine kinase is a widely distributed enzyme generally associated with the energy metabolism of contractile or transport systems. The enzyme is a dimer; the two subunits, designated M (muscle type) and B (brain type), form three different dimeric isoenzymes: MM, MB, and BB.

Skeletal muscle has the greatest concentration of creatinine kinase activity, almost exclusively the MM isoenzyme, followed by myocardial tissue. The concentrations of MM isoenzyme in other tissues are very low compared with those found in skeletal and cardiac cross-striated muscle. Creatinine kinase activity in the brain is attributable exclusively to the BB isoenzyme.

Immunohistochemical studies of small round-cell tumors in children have revealed both subunits in rhabdomyosarcomas and neuroblastomas, whereas Ewing's sarcomas contain only the B subunits.[21] Most recently, high plasma activity of the MB isoenzyme has been reported in association with rhabdomyosarcoma.[22] Although it is of limited use as a biological marker, creatinine kinase may prove to be of significant value in the differentiation of soft-tissue sarcomas of childhood (see Chaps. 30 and 31).

Alkaline Phosphatase

Following the initial reports by Kaplan[23] and Brozmanova and Skrovina[24] of increased serum levels of alkaline phosphatase in patients with osteogenic sarcoma, significant efforts have been made to determine the specific activity of this group of enzymes in primary tumor tissue and in pulmonary metastases (see Chap. 32). Several isoenzymes of alkaline phosphatase have been identified and named according to their tissue of origin as liver, bone, placenta, and gastrointestinal forms.[23] Different electrophoretic mobilities and in some cases antigenic differences allow isoenzyme identification and separation.[23]

Lactic Dehydrogenase (LDH)

An important enzyme, LDH reversibly catalyzes the oxidation of lactic to pyruvic acid. It is widely distributed in mammalian tissues, being abundant in myocardium, kidney, liver, muscle, and red cells. Because of this wide distribution, an elevated serum LDH concentration is of limited value in establishing the specific site of tissue damage. Such elevated concentrations have been found in patients with various pediatric malignancies such as leukemias, lymphomas, Ewing's sarcoma, rhabdomyosarcoma, and neuroblastoma. Changes in concentration are sometimes useful in monitoring response to therapy (see below).

Serum LDH is composed of at least five isoenzymes that can be separated by electrophoresis or other methods. The five isoenzymes have the same molecular weight, 135,000, but differ in the charge they carry. Each isoenzyme is a tetramer made up of subunits designated A and B. The isoenzymes consist of the five possible tetrameric combinations of monomers A and B.

Neuron-Specific Enolase (NSE)

A cytoplasmic marker was demonstrated recently in normal neural tissue. Marangos and Zomzely-Neurath have shown that this protein is an isoenzyme of the glycolytic enzyme enolase,[25] which is specifically localized to neurons and neuroendocrine cells.[26] There are three forms of enolase in the brain: neuron-specific enolase, non-neuronal enolase (NNE), and a hybrid form. These three forms are very different because their structural properties are unique, and antisera raised against one do not crossreact with the others.[27]

NSE is composed of two δ subunits, each of 39,000 daltons, whereas NNE is composed of two α subunits. Extensive immunochemical studies have provided evidence that the subunits are an excellent and specific marker for all neurons, and that the α subunit is present in all glial cells.[26] However, NNE is localized in glial cells within nervous tissue. Furthermore, the indicated cellular localizations of NSE and NNE are true only for fully differentiated tissue, since subunits appear only in differentiated cells.[27] Various endocrine tissues have been found to have significant levels of NSE; for example, the adrenal, pituitary, pineal, and thyroid glands. Therefore, NSE represents a marker for both neurons and neuroendocrine cells.

Sera from patients with tumors of neuroectodermal origin (medulloblastoma, primitive neuroectodermal tumor [PNET], retinoblastoma) may have increased NSE levels but usually less than 100 ng/ml. The ultimate value of NSE as a tumor marker requires further studies.

Poietins

Humoral regulators of human hematopoiesis have been found to be released into the circulation during the course of pediatric malignancies. Among these substances, erythropoietin and thrombopoietin have been reported to have value as biological markers. Even though neither of these regulators of human hematopoiesis has specificity for a given tumor, different lines of evidence indicate their release by tumor cells, suggesting utility in monitoring tumor burden.

Erythropoietin (EPO)

Erythropoietin is a glycoprotein with a molecular weight of about 34,000 daltons and a half-life of only a few hours. EPO is released by the kidneys and appears in very small amounts in human serum and urine. It plays a vital role in the regulation of erythropoiesis, acting as a true hormone. As one would expect, malignancies of the kidneys, especially Wilms' tumors, are the ones most likely to be associated with high serum and urine EPO. It is of interest that very few of the children with EPO-releasing malignancies have erythrocytosis. This finding suggests that in some patients, the tumor-derived EPO is biologically inactive or lacks specificity for the target early erythroid cell.

Different techniques have been used to measure EPO activity in different body fluids. The most commonly used are an *in vivo* assay using the exhypoxic polycythemic mouse, a hemagglutination technique, and a more recent radioimmunoassay. Each of these techniques has serious limitations, and the lack of an easy reproducible EPO assay hampers the use of the hormone as a potential clinical tumor marker.

Thrombopoietin

Thrombopoietin is a glycoprotein of about 35,000 to 37,000 daltons that has never been completely purified. The source(s) in humans has not been established. The hormone plays an important function in daily regulation of thrombopoiesis. A recent assay for thrombopoietin using platelet ^{35}S incorporation has made it feasible to measure its activity in serum; however, assay sensitivity and reproducibility have to be evaluated.

Marked thrombocytosis (platelet count greater than 1,000,000) has been reported in different pediatric malignancies, including neuroblastoma, lymphomas, sarcomas, and hepatoblastomas.[28] Hepatoblastoma is most commonly associated with thrombocytosis and consequently is the malignancy in which thrombopoietin is most likely to prove useful as a marker.

Cytogenetics and Oncogenes

The rapidly developing field of molecular tumor genetics has confirmed the prediction that genetic structures or rearrangements are associated at least with some pediatric malignancies (see Chaps. 2 and 3). Specific chromosomal deletions are associated with several pediatric tumors,[29] strongly suggesting that the genes located at the deleted region are involved in some aspect of tumorgenesis.

It is now thought that tumor formation is associated with activation of cellular genes called oncogenes. Activation can occur at the original chromosomal site or after translocation to other areas of the genome. Although cytogenetic abnormalities and expression of oncogenes have not been found uniformly in pediatric cancers, the increasing use of sophisticated techniques (cDNA probes for oncogenes, restriction endonuclease analysis) certainly has made oncogenes promising new biological markers. Two oncogenes have been associated with pediatric tumors, mainly neuroblastomas: N-*ras* and N-*myc*. In some adult tumors, oncogenes appear to provide prognostic information; this may eventually prove true in some pediatric malignancies also (see below).

Embryonic tumors have been the subject of many cytogenetic studies. Unlike the abnormalities observed in some carcinomas, the changes noted in these tumors represent constitutional changes; that is, the aberration generally exists in all somatic cells of the patient and is not confined to the tumor cells. This subject is covered more extensively in Chapter 3.

CLINICAL APPLICATIONS OF BIOLOGICAL MARKERS IN PEDIATRIC MALIGNANCIES

The development of sensitive assays for determination in the clinical laboratory of different tumor markers has become increasingly important for their application to diagnosis and staging, prognosis, evaluation of treatment response, development of investigational therapy, and, finally, understanding of the biology and etiology of pediatric malignancies. The availability of assays for these markers in clinical and research laboratories of pediatric cancer treatment centers has become increasingly necessary.

In this section, those pediatric tumor types for which biological markers have been established or reported and the clinical use and specificity of those markers will be discussed (see also Chap. 6).

Wilms' Tumor

The malignant neoplasm most common in children younger than 7 years is Wilms' tumor or nephroblastoma (see Chap. 27). It arises from embryonic nephrogenic tissue and often contains connective tissue elements. Wilms' tumor is usually diagnosed on the basis of a complex of clinical findings, including abdominal mass in association with an abnormal intravenous urogram, renal sonogram, or scan.

In 1967, Morse and Nussbaum isolated a mucopolysaccharide with the properties of hyaluronic acid from the sera of a patient with Wilms' tumor.[30] Subsequently, the presence of hyaluronic acid in the serum of patients with Wilms' tumor has been demonstrated by several other investigators (Table 8-2).[31-33] The presence of this mucopolysaccharide often causes serum hyperviscosity. The source has not been established in any of these patients; however, on the basis of histologic examinations and analysis of tumor extracts, it has been suggested that the tumor itself produces it.[23] The clinical course of the patients also suggests production of hyaluronic acid by the tumor, as its concentration decreases rapidly and dramatically upon initiation of specific therapy. Whether high concentrations of serum hyaluronic acid are a consistent finding in patients with Wilms' tumor requires further investigation. In addition, the development of a more sensitive technique to detect and measure the mucopolysaccharide is essential.

Elevated EPO levels have been described in the serum and urine of patients with Wilms' tumor. For example, Murphy and associates reported elevation of EPO in 37 patients with Wilms' tumors in various clinical stages without overt erythrocythemia.[34] Moreover, elevations of plasma and urine EPO persisted in patients with clinically manifest metastatic disease, whereas EPO levels abated within days following resection of the primary tumor in patients without metastatic disease. However, unexplained elevation of serum and urine EPO persisting after successful treatment of metastatic disease has cast some doubts on the specificity of the marker. As noted earlier, the lack of a sensitive and reproducible assay for EPO has further complicated its use as a tumor marker.

Raised CEA levels have been found by double-antibody techniques[7] in a few children with Wilms' tumor. However this finding has been neither expanded nor confirmed.

Cytogenetic studies of Wilms' tumor have often demonstrated a deletion of the short arm of chromosome 11.[35] The abnormality has been found primarily in patients with associated aniridia. It is expected that as the number of Wilms' tumor patients having cytogenetic studies increases, the frequency and significance of this karyotypic abnormality will become more recognizable.

Neuroblastoma

Neuroblastoma, one of the most common solid malignant tumors of childhood, has frequently been confused with other malignancies as well as with non-neoplastic diseases (see

Chap. 28). A significant number of biological markers have been identified for this malignancy, enhancing our knowledge of the disease (Table 8-3). The observation that neural crest tumors resulted in excretion of elevated quantities of catecholamines and their by-products led to development of biochemical tests aimed at detecting neuroblastoma. The tests are at present used for diagnostic purposes, as prognostic factors, and as parameters to evaluate disease response to therapy.

The initial reports of biochemical abnormalities in children with neuroblastoma referred to the excessive urinary excretion of epinephrine and norepinephrine.[36,37] Subsequently, it has been documented that, in fact, epinephrine and norepinephrine are normal or only minimally elevated in most patients with neuroblastoma. However, dopamine and its metabolites, mainly VMA, HVA, and 3-methoxy-4-hydroxyphenoglycol (MHPG), are often excreted in high amounts by neuroblastoma patients. There is an enormous variability in the quantitative excretion of these compounds, as well as a wide spectrum of the metabolites excreted. Furthermore, some neuroblastomas are cholinergic or inactive rather than adrenergic.

VMA and HVA are the most commonly assayed catabolites, and when both of them and MHPG are determined, positive findings are recorded in almost 100% of patients. Even though there is some discrepancy in the percentage of VMA excretors among reported series, ranging from 60%[38] to as high as 90%,[39] the differences most likely reflect variable specificity of the multiple-assay methods used rather than differences in the percentage of VMA excretors. Determination of HVA is the second most common catecholamine metabolite assay used for diagnostic purposes. However, HVA is less commonly elevated than is VMA in the urine of patients with neuroblastoma. Ninety-seven percent of neuroblastoma patients excrete MHPG in excess of three standard deviations above the mean.[39]

Catecholamine excretion has been correlated with histologic extent of tumor maturation, the patient's age at diagnosis, and the site of the primary tumor. Overall, it appears that as the tumor matures histologically, the amount of catecholamine excreted decreases. Thus, the less differentiated tumors are

---

Table 8-2
Biological Markers in Wilms' Tumor

Marker	Specimen	Specificity*	Use	Comments
Hyaluronic acid	Serum	Questionable	Follow-up	Advanced disease
EPO	Serum/urine	None	Diagnosis	Not a sensitive test
CEA	Serum	None	None	Not confirmed
Chromosome 11	Tumor cell	High	Diagnosis	Associated with aniridia

* See text for details.

Table 8-3
Biological Markers in Neuroblastoma

Marker	Specimen	Specificity	Use	Comments
Catecholamines	Serum/urine	High	Diagnosis, follow-up	HVA, VMA most commonly used
Cystathionine	Urine	None	Diagnosis	Questionable correlation to stage
Ferritin	Serum	None	Stage; prognosis	No correlation with serum iron
NSE	Serum	High	Prognosis	Stage III and IV
LDH	Serum	Low	Prognosis, follow-up	Easily available
N-*myc*	Tumor cells	High	Stage, prognosis	Amplification correlates with advanced disease
Monoclonal antibodies	Tumor cells	High	Diagnosis	Discriminates from other tumors

associated with the highest excretion.[40] The number of neurosecretory granules in the tumor appears to have a significant influence on the extent of catecholamine excretion; tumors with the greatest number of neurosecretory granules are usually associated with the highest concentration of VMA. Results have also suggested that the catecholamine excretion pattern correlates with age, with lower HVA and higher MHPG excretions in younger patients, especially those younger than 2 years of age. Normal catecholamine excretion has been found in primary neuroblastoma of the neck and throat. However, rather than the anatomic site of tumor origin, it appears that the major determinant is the involvement of the dorsal root ganglia, since these tumors rarely synthesize catecholamines.

Recent studies have suggested that the pattern of pretreatment urinary excretion of catecholamine metabolites may be of prognostic significance in patients with metastatic disease. Although Berontini-DeGutierrez-Moyano and associates[41] and Liebner and Rosenthal[42] found the prognosis to be unrelated to the initial urinary patterns of VMA, HVA, norepinephrine, and epinephrine, Labrosse and coworkers, in a larger study, found that high levels of HVA were associated with poor survival. These authors concluded that tumors favoring the production of norepinephrine–epinephrine catabolites had a better prognosis than did those producing primarily dopamine and its metabolites.[43] Gitlow and associates have also found that those patients who excrete large quantities of the dopamine catabolite HVA have a relatively poor prognosis compared to those who excrete lesser quantities.[44] Laug and Siegel reported that for patients with stage IV disease, the VMA/HVA ratio had statistically significant predictive values of disease outcome: the higher the value, the better the prognosis.[45] However, the VMA/HVA ratio does not consistently predict the outcome in other stages of the disease.

Although the prognostic value of initial catecholamine excretion still is questionable, it is evident that the return to normal of these biochemical markers following initial therapy correlates strikingly with disease response. Nevertheless, a return to a normal biochemical profile after therapy does not guarantee long-term survival.

Elevation of certain amino acids, mainly cystathionine and aminoisobutyric acid, has been reported in children with neuroblastoma. Cystathioninuria has been found in as many as 50% of children with neuroblastoma or ganglioneuroblastoma. However, its correlation with the stage of disease is controversial.[45,46] Furthermore, the urinary cystathionine assay, although sensitive, is not specific, as cystathionine can be elevated in many other conditions, including hepatic tumors. On the other hand, high urinary levels of aminoisobutyric acid are detected more uniformly in the urine of children with very malignant neuroblastomas.[45,47]

Ferritin is a useful marker for patients with neuroblastoma.[48] Neuroblastomas produce both basic and acidic ferritins and release them into the circulation, with the proportion of basic ferritin usually being higher.[49] Recent studies suggest that isoferritins from neuroblastomas have an adverse effect on a variety of host immune responses, including an inhibitory effect on rosette formation by T lymphocytes, a blocking effect on lymphocytes and lymphocyte response to mitogens, and depression of some granulocyte functions.[49] There is increasing evidence that serum ferritin levels at diagnosis are closely related to the patient's prognosis. Elevated levels are commonly seen in patients with active disease, with the exception of children with stage IVS, who have normal ferritin concentrations even when the tumor is growing. Ferritin levels can be used as a marker for disease burden following initiation of therapy, since levels return to normal with clinical remission. No correlation has been found between serum iron levels and serum ferritin concentrations at the time of diagnosis.

Neuron-specific enolase is a good marker for neuronal-cell derivation that is present in cell lines, tumor specimens, and histologic sections of neuroblastomas.[50,51] The sensitivity of the serum NSE assay appears to be high for stages III and IV tumor.[51] Recent data indicate that NSE is a prognostic marker for patients with stage IV disease identified before 1 year of age and for those with stage III disease diagnosed before age 2 years.[52] Patients with stage IVS disease seldom have NSE concentrations higher than 100 mg/ml, a significant difference from those with stage IV disease (Fig. 8-2). The reason for lower serum NSE in children with stage IVS is not known but does not appear to be related to tumor differentiation. It is of interest that normal ferritin levels are found in this patient population. Serum NSE levels correlate with response to therapy, but their sensitivity in predicting recurrence is questionable.

Lactic dehydrogenase is one of the most extensively studied enzymes released by necrotic and damaged tissue. Even though LDH lacks tumor specificity, it has been found useful as a marker in neuroblastoma patients for following disease activity.[53] Since serum LDH determination is easily available and inexpensive, it can be used for routine evaluations of therapy response. However, the lack of specificity limits considerably its values as a marker.

The observation that there are multiple copies of the N-*myc* oncogene (genomic amplification) in a large number of untreated primary neuroblastomas has attracted significant attention. The N-*myc* oncogene demonstrates partial homology with the well-known proto-oncogene c-*myc*. Amplification of the gene is found in more than 90% of cultured neuroblastoma

FIGURE 8-2. Serum neuron specific enolase activity in children with neuroblastoma according to stage. (Reproduced with permission from Zeltzer PM, Marangos PJ, Evans AE, Schneider SC: Serum neuron-specific enolase in children with neuroblastoma: Relationship to stage and disease course. Cancer 57:1230–1234, 1986)

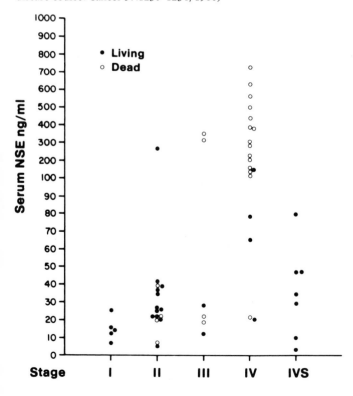

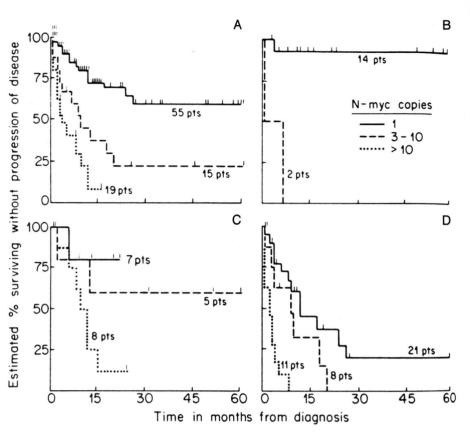

FIGURE 8-3. Relation between number of N-*myc* gene copies and progression-free survival in neuroblastoma. **A.** All patients (*p* = 0.0001). **B.** Patients with stage II tumors (*p* = 0.03; exact life-table test). **C.** Stage II tumors (*p* = 0.1). **D.** Stage IV tumors (*p* = 0.0002). In *D*, two patients with stage IV tumors and single copy of N-*myc* who have not suffered tumor progression after 27 and 62 months (*tick marks*) were found to have the disease before 1 year of age. (Reproduced with permission from Seeger RC et al: Association of multiple copies of the N-*myc* oncogene with the rapid progression of neuroblastoma. N Engl J Med 313:1114, 1985)

Table 8-4
Monoclonal Antibodies in Neuroblastoma and Cross-Reactivity with Other Common Pediatric Malignancies

	Cell Line			
Antibody	Neuroblastoma	Neuroepithelioma	Rhabdomyosarcoma	Ewing's Sarcoma
HSAN 1.2	++++	+	−	+
AB 459	++++	++	++	++
AB 390	++++	++	++++	+
P1 153/3	++++	++	−	++
A2 B5	+++	++	+	++
LEV 7	++++	+	−	+
BA 1	++++	+	−	−

cell lines but in only 38% of primary tumors.[54] Clinically, amplification is present only in tumors that already are widespread at diagnosis,[55] suggesting that amplification contributes to tumor progression. Amplification appears to be relatively specific for neuroblastomas, and the extent of the amplification seems to be bimodal: most patients have either a threefold to tenfold or a 100- to 300-fold amplification.[55] High-level amplification is more consistently observed in patients with advanced neuroblastoma. Furthermore, Seeger and associates have shown that the degree of amplification of N-*myc* may be associated with prognosis in patients with stage III or IV disease[55] (Fig. 8-3).

Other biological markers, mainly CEA and AFP, have been investigated in children with neuroblastomas. There are conflicting reports regarding CEA expression by neuroblastoma cells,[56,57] and, in general, CEA is considered of no value as a biological marker in this malignancy. Similarly, repeated studies have demonstrated that children with neuroblastoma do not have raised levels of AFP.[7]

The recent development of a panel of relatively specific monoclonal antibodies has made it possible to discriminate neuroblastoma from other childhood malignancies with which it can be confused.[58] Furthermore, such a panel may make it possible to differentiate neuroblastomas into groups of prognostic significance. Cell lines derived from typical neuroblastomas have shown a pattern of immunoreactivity with a panel of monoclonal antibodies raised against a variety of cell-membrane antigens that readily distinguishes them from other small round-cell neoplasias of childhood (Table 8-4). Among the antibodies, HSAN 1.2 appears to be the most specific neuroblastoma antibody of the panel[58] (see Chap. 6).

It has recently been suggested that quantitatively significant amounts of specific tumor-associated gangliosides are present in the circulation of patients with neuroblastoma.[59]

Subsequently, Schulz and associates have shown elevated levels of disialoganglioside (GD2) in sera of neuroblastoma patients compared to normal children and children with other tumors.[60] Further studies are required to define the potential diagnostic significance of the shedding of gangliosides by neuroblastoma cells.

Germ Cell Tumors

Germ cell tumors originate from the primordial germ cells and can be benign or malignant (see Chap. 33). The malignant tumors are divided into two major histologic subtypes: seminomas and nonseminomatous tumors. In children, the nonseminomatous group is the more frequent and is composed of embryonal carcinoma, endodermal sinus tumor (yolk sac tumor), teratocarcinoma, choriocarcinoma, and mixed tumors.

Biological markers have proved invaluable in identifying different types of germ cell tumors (Table 8-5). The demonstration of AFP synthesis by the human yolk sac and the establishment of an association between the presence of endodermal sinus tumor and AFP synthesis have established AFP as a useful tumor marker. AFP can be localized with immunoperoxidase staining to individual cells in such tumors. A positive immunoperoxidase stain for AFP in an endodermal sinus tumor (commonly called yolk sac carcinoma) is almost always associated with elevated serum levels of AFP. The normal serum level of AFP is below 20 ng/ml; however, in patients with yolk sac carcinoma levels may reach or exceed 100,000 ng/ml. Following surgical excision of a yolk sac tumor, there is a gradual decrease in serum AFP levels to normal values. Thus, persistence of elevated levels indicates residual primary tumor or metastasis, although, because of the long half-life of the protein (5 days), levels may remain elevated, but progressively decreasing, for several weeks after all tumor has been eradicated. The value of serum AFP in monitoring the results of therapy and assessing the presence of metastases and recurrence in patients with yolk sac tumors has been established.[61,62] The degree of elevation of serum AFP in different types of germ cell tumors depends on the extent of the endodermal sinus (yolk sac carcinoma) component. The significant value of AFP as a marker of germ cell tumors emphasizes the value of very sensitive methods for its determination in the diagnosis and follow-up of children with this tumor.

Human chorionic gonadotropin subunits are normally produced by the trophoblasts of the placenta. β-hCG may be elevated in patients with trophoblastic tumors, such as choriocarcinomas, or a variety of nontrophoblastic tumors, including embryonal carcinomas. β-hCG is detected in the serum of as many as 89% of patients with nonseminomatous germ cell

tumors[63] and indicates the presence of nongerminomatous cells such as yolk sac elements, embryonal carcinoma, or choriocarcinoma. Sustained or rising levels of hCG are almost always associated with persistent or recurrent tumors.

The relation between the histologic type of the tumor and the levels of hCG and AFP is well defined, and the determination of both markers can strongly suggest the type of malignancy. An elevated level of AFP is evidence of nonseminomatous cancer, whereas hCG may be elevated in patients with either nonseminomatous tumor or seminoma. Embryonal carcinoma, reflecting its potential for both somatic and placental differentiation, may produce either or both markers.

Several attempts have been made to determine the incidence of high CEA in children with germ cell tumors. However, CEA, which is usually found in the human embryo, has been found in only a few patients with teratocarcinoma, usually with an embryonal carcinoma component. In general, CEA has not been present in quantities readily analyzable and is detectable in fewer than 10% of these patients.[62]

Lactic dehydrogenase can be a useful marker for germ cell tumors, since about 10% of patients with metastatic tumors have elevated LDH as the only detectable evidence of active tumor with normal AFP and hCG.

Most recently, the use of monoclonal antibodies specific for neurofilament proteins, glial proteins, and myelin basic protein has allowed the identification of these neural antigens in human teratomas.[64] The presence of these antigens correlates with the presence of mature and immature elements and may have prognostic implications. Absence of all neural-specific antigens appears to be associated with malignant teratomas.

Hepatoblastoma–Hepatocellular Carcinoma

Normally, AFP is synthesized in the liver and yolk sac of the fetus. The synthesis of AFP stops at birth, and it disappears in the newborn with a half-life of 3 to 5 days. Elevated serum levels before 1 year of age can be associated with non-neoplastic liver disease, mainly hepatitis. However, an AFP concentration higher than 100 ng/ml usually indicates either a hepatoblastoma or a yolk sac tumor (Table 8-6) (see Chaps. 26 and 33).

Serum concentrations of AFP in adult patients with hepatocellular carcinoma have been extensively studied and reported elevated in 67% to 82% of patients.[65] Approximately one half of patients with this cancer can be identified by such elevation. Even though there is less information available on the AFP levels in hepatoblastoma, the most common hepatic malignancy in children, the data available strongly indicate an almost universal association between this malignancy and ele-

Table 8-5
Biological Serum Markers in Germ Cell Tumors

Marker	Specificity	Use	Comments
Seminoma			
hCG	High	Diagnosis, follow-up	Detectable in only 20% of patients
CEA	None	Limited value	Only occasionally elevated
Nonseminomatous tumors			
AFP	High	Diagnosis	Most commonly used
hCG	High	Diagnosis, follow-up	
CEA	None	Limited value	No correlation with disease activity
LDH	None	?	Indicates advanced disease

Table 8-6
Biological Markers in Liver Tumors

Marker	Specimen	Specificity	Use*	Comments
AFP	Serum	High	Diagnosis, follow-up	Excellent correlation with disease activity
Ferritin	Serum	None	?	Better use in hepatocellular cancer
Thrombopoietin	Serum/urine	None	?	No reliable assay available
EPO	Serum/urine	None	?	Not a sensitive test
hCG	Serum/urine	None	Diagnosis	Hepatoblastoma associated with precocious puberty

* See text for details.

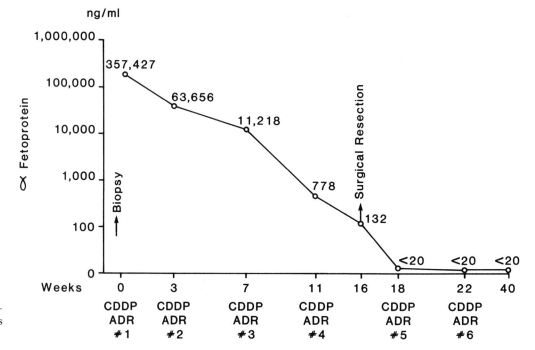

FIGURE 8-4. Decline and normalization of serum AFP levels after initiation of chemotherapy.

vated serum AFP.[7] Concentrations higher than 500,000 ng/ml are not unusual in children with hepatoblastoma. Failure of elevated serum AFP to return to normal after surgery is an indication either that the tumor was not completely resected or that there are metastases (Fig. 8-4). AFP content rises during the cell-regeneration phase after surgical resection of liver; however, this transient elevation is due to normal parenchymal regeneration and should not interfere with the expected decline of AFP following tumor resection.

Recently, it has been recognized that the amount of carbohydrate in AFP depends on the level of glycosylase in normal liver and tumor tissue. Benign liver proliferation results in completely glycosylated AFP, and new techniques may be able to capitalize on this difference to allow discrimination of benign from malignant liver disease.

At present, serial determinations of AFP constitute the most exact parameter to determine the effectiveness of therapy in children with hepatoblastoma.

The recent introduction of radioimmunodetection of tumors containing AFP with radiolabeled anti-AFP antibodies has broadened the scope of this biological marker for the detection and localization of liver and germ cell tumors.[66]

Serum ferritin has been found to be elevated in most patients with liver malignancies,[67] but its diagnostic role remains to be defined. However, serial estimation of serum ferritin may be valuable for monitoring the response to therapy, particularly in patients with hepatocellular carcinoma who have a normal AFP concentrations.

Thrombocytosis has long been recognized as a common finding in children with hepatoblastoma. Recently, two children with hepatoblastoma and thrombocytosis were documented to have elevated thrombopoietin levels in tumor extracts.[68] It is anticipated that the introduction of a sensitive and reproducible assay for thrombopoietin will enhance its role as a biological marker for hepatoblastoma. Increased EPO has also been reported in primary liver tumors.[69] However, it is not known how frequently this elevation occurs. Erythrocytosis is not a common finding in children with liver tumors.

The association of hepatoblastoma with precocious puberty is not uncommon. These patients have increased serum and urine chorionic gonadotropins simultaneously with increased AFP.[70] Most likely, virilizing hepatoblastomas secrete two different tumor markers, AFP and hCG, from different cells. It has been noticed that, unlike AFP levels, urine and serum hCG levels do not necessarily reflect the clinical course of the tumor.

Other biological markers, including increased transcobolamine I[71] and detection of des-r-carboxy (abnormal) prothrombin,[72] have recently been associated with hepatocellular carcinoma. Their clinical utility as markers is currently being evaluated.

Soft-Tissue Sarcomas

Skeletal muscle has the greatest concentration of creatinine kinase activity, almost exclusively the MM isoenzyme. Not surprising, creatinine kinase subunit M has proved useful for distinguishing poorly differentiated rhabdomyosarcomas from other types of small round-cell tumors in children[73] (Table 8-7) (see Chap. 30). Most recently, a patient with a rhabdomyosarcoma of the prostate has been reported to have a high plasma concentration of the creatinine kinase MB isoenzyme.[74] This preliminary experience will obviously encourage further studies of the value of creatinine kinase as a biological marker in rhabdomyosarcomas.

The detection of TAA in the urine of patients with various sarcomas has brought attention to these antigens, which probably are shed during the process of cell turnover. The results of Huth and associates indicate that postoperative measurement of TAA in sarcoma patients permits identification of those at high risk for recurrence.[75] Unfortunately, TAAs lack specificity, since they can be demonstrated in a variety of malignant neoplasms. Furthermore, the techniques for their detection are not widely available and require further standardization before TAA can become a useful tumor marker.

Although chromosome abnormalities, primarily aneuploidies, have been observed in rhabdomyosarcomas, a single, consistent abnormality associated with this tumor had not been found until preliminary studies revealed frequent alterations of chromosome 3 p14–21.[76] Rhabdomyosarcomas in children are divided into two major histologic subtypes, alveolar and embryonal, with the former being more resistant to therapy. The recent findings of a 2:13 translocation in an alveolar rhabdomyosarcoma may further facilitate the discrimination of the two subtypes.[77]

Recent work by Altmansberger and associates has demonstrated that desmin, an intermediate-filament protein, is a very useful marker for rhabdomyosarcoma.[78] This protein is readily characterized by an immunoperoxidase method that yields few, if any, false-positive or false-negative results in distinguishing rhabdomyosarcomas from other round-cell tumors of children.

Osteogenic Sarcoma

Serum levels of alkaline phosphatase are the only known biological marker for this bone malignancy (Table 8-8) (see Chap. 32). However, the enzyme concentration in the serum has not

---

Table 8-7
Biological Markers in Soft-Tissue Sarcomas

Marker	Specimen	Specificity	Use*	Comments
Creatinine	Serum	Low	Diagnosis	Scant information
TAA	Urine	None	?	Technique not widely available
Desmin	Tumor	High	Diagnosis	Different from other tumors
Chromosome 3	Tumor cells	?	Diagnosis	Embryonal rhabdomyosarcoma
Chromosome 2	Tumor cells t(2;13)	?	Diagnosis	Alveolar rhabdomyosarcoma

* See text for details.

Table 8-8
Biological Markers in Bone Tumors

Marker	Specimen	Specificity	Use*	Comments
Osteogenic sarcoma				
Alkaline phosphatase	Serum	Low	Prognosis, follow-up	Preoperative level might have prognostic value
Ewing's sarcoma				
LDH	Serum	Low	Prognosis	Questionable prognostic indicator
Chromosome 22 (structural changes)	Tumor cells	None	?	Has been found in other tumors

* See text for details.

been useful in most patients for determining tumor bulk or recurrence. Unfortunately, enzymatic changes occur mainly within tumor tissue and are expressed in the circulation only when the tumor is very large. The concentration of alkaline phosphatase in these tumors does not seem to bear any relation to the amount of calcification in the specimen, with heavily calcified lesions sometimes having lower specific activities than undifferentiated, uncalcified lesions.[79] To this day, the role of alkaline phosphatase in osteogenic sarcomas remains unclear. Interpretation of an elevated serum concentration can be complicated by the presence of other conditions such as liver disease, fracture, or even normal adolescent growth. However, the mean serum value in osteogenic sarcomas is far higher than that reported in other conditions. Furthermore, different studies seem to confirm the prognostic value of preoperative serum alkaline phosphatase determination[79-81] in that patients with tumors producing large amounts of alkaline phosphatase have a greater chance of recurrence than do those with lower values. In Levine and Rosenberg's study, patients whose tumor-tissue levels were higher than 0.6 mol/min per milligram had a high tumor recurrence rate.[79] Thus, determinations of alkaline phosphatase in patients with osteogenic sarcomas appear to have prognostic value.

Ewing's Sarcoma

A disease of young adolescents, Ewing's sarcoma occurs at a slightly earlier age than does osteogenic sarcoma (see Chap. 31). Unlike neuroblastoma, biological markers to date have not been specific for the diagnosis of Ewing's sarcoma (Table 8-8). Of all known tumor markers, only serum LDH has been of some value in the clinical management of patients. Pretreatment serum LDH levels were reported by Brereton and associates to have a significant relation to disease-free survival.[82] Subsequently, Glaubiger and coworkers found that normal serum LDH levels at presentation, distal site of primary disease, and absence of metastatic disease at diagnosis are the strongest indicators of a favorable prognosis.[83] Unfortunately, the influence of serum LDH levels in the analysis of end-results has not as yet been confirmed in large studies.

Recent cytogenetic studies performed on Ewing's sarcoma cells have shown frequent structural changes of chromosome 22.[84] Although an 11;22 translocation is the most frequent, autosome 22 also is involved in other translocations in this tumor.[85] The t(11;22) is not specific for Ewing's sarcoma since the same cytogenetic abnormality has been reported in neuroblastoma.

Tumors of the Central Nervous System

Biological markers in the blood and in cerebrospinal fluid (CSF) have a limited but growing role in the diagnosis of central nervous system (CNS) tumors (Table 8-9) (see Chap. 24). The polyamines are small molecules that are involved in nucleic acid metabolism and thus in cellular proliferation. Several lines of information suggest a relation between elevated polyamines in urine,[86] serum,[87] and CSF[88] and the presence of CNS tumors. Putrescine and spermine are the best known of the polyamines. These compounds are not tumor specific, and false-positive and false-negative results are extremely frequent. Nevertheless, the evaluation of putrescine and spermine as markers for CNS tumors, mainly medulloblastoma, has revealed that CSF polyamines in patients with medulloblastoma usually exceed the concentration in other CNS conditions.[89]

Elevation in the CSF of CEA in patients with leptomeningeal metastases from carcinomas has recently been reported.[90] However, the same study also demonstrated that CSF CEA was of no value as a marker of meningeal infiltration with lymphoma. In general, at present, the role of CSF CEA as a marker for both primary and metastatic CNS malignancies is at best questionable.

Most recently, NSE has received significant attention as a marker of neural crest tumors. Attention is being shifted to the use of this marker in primary brain tumors. Medulloblastomas, which are primitive neuroectodermal tumors, appear to have greater levels of NSE than do ependymomas, astrocytomas, and gliomas.[91]

Different human medulloblastoma cell lines have been used to raise monoclonal antibodies. However, most of them have shown variable reactivity, not only with medulloblastoma, but also with some other tumors.[92] At best, the use of monoclonal antibodies in the diagnosis of brain tumors is investigational.

Pituitary tumors, including adenomas and craniopharyngiomas, may cause elevation in serum prolactin through mechanical compression of the pituitary stalk (see Chap. 34). In addition, any other hormones that may be involved in the clinical syndrome should be measured (ACTH, growth hormone).

Table 8-9
Biological Markers in Brain Tumors

Marker	Specimen	Specificity	Use*	Comments
Medulloblastoma				
Polyamines	Serum/urine/ CSF	None	Detection of recurrence	Putrescine and spermine best known
NSE	Serum/CSF	High	Diagnosis	Requires further evaluation
Monoclonal antibodies	Tumor cells	?	?	?
Pituitary tumors				
Growth hormone	Serum	High	Diagnosis	Craniopharyngioma
ACTH	Serum	High	Diagnosis	Craniopharyngioma
hCG	Serum	High	Diagnosis	Carcinoma and dysgerminoma

* See text for details.

Pineal choriocarcinomas and dysgerminomas are usually associated with serum and CSF elevation of β-hCG and AFP, respectively. However, these markers have proved unreliable in defining disease activity or detecting recurrence.

CONCLUSION

The field of biological markers of cancer has been the focus of increasing interest for its applicability in diagnosis, prognosis, and therapy of pediatric malignancies. Although the clinical applications of some of the most-publicized markers have not fulfilled all the expectations, there is no doubt that biological markers have a definite role in pediatric oncology, and measurement of these markers by the clinical laboratory has become increasingly important in diagnosis and monitoring of childhood malignancies. An increasing number of markers associated with cancer are being identified, and, as new methods and techniques are developed, their clinical use is being defined. The introduction and increasing availability of new immunoassay and hybridoma technology obviously will enhance our ability to clarify the specificity of many of these markers.

Most recently, cytogenetic abnormalities and oncogenes have been added to the tumor cell-surface antigens, secreted proteins, hormones, enzymes, and isoenzymes previously recognized as markers. The observation of specific chromosomal abnormalities in specific pediatric malignancies not only constitutes a basic step in understanding the etiology of some tumors, but also permits a definite improvement in tumor-type identification. Furthermore, determinations *in utero* of some of these markers, mainly catecholamines and AFP, may prove useful for prenatal diagnosis. Discovery of the expression and amplification of oncogenes in some tumors constitutes one of the most promising recent advances in pediatric oncology for its application to tumor recognition and use as a marker. The increasing use of DNA probes for human oncogenes, and endonuclease analysis applied to DNA derived from pediatric tumors is rapidly becoming an important component of the diagnostic evaluation and "front-end" determination of prognosis. No doubt these exciting new developments in the field of biological markers will further stimulate the search for new markers and their application to modern clinical pediatric oncology.

REFERENCES

1. Abelev GI: α-Fetoprotein in oncogenesis and in association with malignant tumors. Adv Cancer Res 14:295–359, 1971
2. Gitlin D, Boesman M: Sites of serum α-fetoprotein synthesis in the human and in the rat. J Clin Invest 46:1010–1016, 1967
3. Ruoslahti E, Seppälä M: Alpha-fetoprotein in cancer and fetal development. Adv Cancer Res 29:275–346, 1979
4. Sell S, Becker FF: α-fetoprotein (guest editorial). J Natl Cancer Inst 60:19–24, 1978
5. Ruoslahti E, Pihko H, Seppälä M: α-fetoprotein: Immunochemical purification and chemical properties, expression in normal state and in malignant and non-malignant liver disease. Transplant Rev 20:39–60, 1974
6. Ruoslahti E, Terry WD: α-fetoprotein and serum albumin show sequence homology. Nature 260:804–807, 1976
7. Mann JR, Lakin GE, Leonard JC et al: Clinical applications of serum carcinoembryonic antigen and α-fetoprotein levels in children with solid tumors. Arch Dis Childh 53:366–374, 1978
8. Marcus DM, Zinberg N: Measurement of serum ferritin by radioimmunoassay: Results in normal individuals and patients with breast cancer. J Natl Cancer Inst 55:791–795, 1975
9. Jones PAE, Miller FM, Worwood M, Jacobs A: Ferritin-anaemia in leukaemia and Hodgkin's disease. Br J Cancer 27:212–217, 1973
10. Hann HL, Leitmeyer J, Evans AE, Hathaway A: Analysis of isoferritins from neuroblastoma tumors (abstr). Proc Am Assoc Cancer Res 22:188, 1981
11. Hann HL, Stahlhut NW, Millman I: Human ferritins in the sera of nude mice transplanted with human neuroblastoma or hepatocellular carcinoma. Cancer Res 44:3898–3901, 1984
12. Kew MC, Torrance JD, Derman D: Serum and tumour ferritins in primary liver cancer. Gut 19:294–299, 1978
13. Armstrong MD, McMillan A, Show K: 3-Methyoxy,4-hydroxy-D-mandelic acid, a urinary metabolite of nor-epinephrine. Biochim Biophys Acta 25:422–423, 1957
14. Vaitukitis JL: Human chorionic gonadotropin: Chemical and biological characterization. In Heberman RB, McIntire KR (eds): Immunodiagnosis of Cancer, pp 369–383. New York, Marcel Dekker, 1979
15. Vaitukaitis JL, Braunstein GD, Ross GT: A radioimmunoassay which specifically measures human chorionic gonadotropin in the presence of human luteinizing hormone. Am J Obstet Gynecol 113:751–758, 1972
16. Braunstein GD, Vaitukaitis JL, Carbone PP et al: Ectopic production of human chorionic gonadotropin by neoplasms. Ann Intern Med 78:39–45, 1973
17. Gold P, Freedman SO: Demonstration of tumour specific antigens in human colonic carcinomata by immunological tolerance and absorption techniques. J Exp Med 121:439–462, 1965
18. Hansen HJ, Synder JJ, Miller E et al: Carcinoembryonic antigen (CEA) assay. Hum Pathol 5:139–144, 1974
19. Rote NS, Gupta RK, Morton DL: Tumor associated antigens detected by autologous sera in urine of patients with solid neoplasms. J Surg Res 29:18–22, 1979
20. Huth JF, Gupta RK, Elber FR, Morton DL: A prospective postoperative evaluation of urinary tumor-associated antigens in sarcoma patients: Correlation with disease recurrence. Cancer 53:1306–1310, 1984
21. Wold LE, Li CY, Homburger HA: Localization of the B and M polypeptide subunits of creatinine kinase in normal and neoplastic tissues by an immunoperoxidase technic. Am J Clin Pathol 75:327–332, 1981
22. Hickman PE, Messina S, Trotter JM, Masarei JRL: High creatinine kinase MD isoenzyme activity associated with a rhabdomyosarcoma. Clin Chem 29:1549–1550, 1983
23. Kaplan M: Alkaline phosphatase. N Engl J Med 286:200–202, 1972
24. Brozmanova E, Skrovina B: Biochemical and haematological findings in malignant bone tumours. Neoplasma 21:75–82, 1974
25. Marangos PJ, Zomzely-Neurath C: Determination of characterization of neuron specific protein (NSP) associated with enolase activity. Biochem Biophys Res Commun 68:1309–1316, 1976
26. Schmechel DE, Marangos PJ, Brightman MW: Neuron specific enolase is a marker for peripheral and central neuroendocrine cells. Nature 76:834–837, 1979
27. Marangos PJ: Clinical studies with neuron specific enolase. Adv Neuroblastoma Res, pp 285–294. New York, Alan R. Liss, 1985
28. McDonald TP: A comparison of platelet size, platelet count and platelet 35S incorporation as assay for thrombopoietin. Br J Haematol 34:257–267, 1976
29. Yunis JJ: The chromosome basis of human neoplasia. Science 221:227–235, 1983
30. Morse BS, Nussbaum M: The detection of hyaluronic acid in the serum and urine of a patient with nephroblastoma. Am J Med 42:986–1002, 1967
31. Powers DR, Allerton SE, Boierle J, Buttler, BB: Wilms' tumor: Clinical correlation with circulating mucin in three cases. Cancer 29:1597–1605, 1972
32. Deutsch HF: Some properties of a human serum hyaluronic acid. J Biol Chem 224:767–774, 1972
33. Wu AHB, Parker OS, Ford L: Hyperviscosity caused by hyaluronic acid in serum in a case of Wilms' tumor. Clin Chem 30:914–916, 1984
34. Murphy GP, Allen JE, Staubitz WJ, Sinks LF, Mirand EA: Erythropoietin levels in patients with Wilms' tumor: Follow up evaluation. NY State J Med 72:487–489, 1972
35. Koufos A, Hansen MF, Lampkin BC et al: Loss of alleles at loci on human chromosomal 11 during genesis of Wilms' tumor. Nature 309:170–174, 1984
36. Mason GA, Hart-Mercer J, Millar EJ, Strang LB, Wynne NA: Adrenaline-secreting neuroblastoma in an infant. Lancet 2:322–325, 1957
37. Isaacs H, Medalic M, Politzer WM: Nor-adrenaline-secreting neuroblastomas. Br Med J 1:401–404, 1959
38. Voorhess ML, Gardner LI: Studies of catecholamine excretion by children with neural tumors. J Clin Endocrinol Metab 22:126, 1962
39. Gitlow SE, Bertani LM, Rausen A, Gribetz A, Dziedzic SW: Diagnosis of neuroblastoma by qualitative and quantitative determinations of catecholamine metabolites in urine. Cancer 25:1377–1383, 1980

40. Bore KE, McAdams AJ: Composite ganglioneuroblastoma: An assessment of the significance of histological maturation in neuroblastoma diagnosed beyond infancy. Arch Pathol Lab Med 105:325–330, 1978

41. Barontini-DeGutierrez-Moyano M, Bergada C, Becu L: Significance of catecholamine excretion in the follow up of sympathoblastomas. Cancer 27:228–232, 1971

42. Liebner EJ, Rosenthal EM: Serial catecholamines in the radiation management of children with neuroblastoma. Cancer 32:623–633, 1973

43. LaBrosse EH, Comoy E, Bohvon C: Catecholamine metabolism in neuroblastoma. J Natl Cancer Inst 57:633–638, 1976

44. Gitlow SE, Bertani L, Strauss L, Greenwood SM, Dziedzic SW: Biochemical and histological determinants in the prognosis of neuroblastoma. Cancer 32:898–905, 1973

45. Laug WE, Siegel SE, Shaw KNF, Landing B, Baptista J, Gutenstein M: Initial urinary catecholamine metabolite concentrations and prognosis in neuroblastoma. Pediatrics 62:77–83, 1978.

46. Geiser CF, Efron ML: Cystathioninuria in patients with neuroblastoma or ganglioneuroblastoma: Its correlation to vanillamandelic acid excretion and its value in diagnosis and therapy. Cancer 22:856, 1968

47. Gjessing LR: Cystathionuria and vanil-lactic-acid-uria In Bohuoun C (ed): Recent Results in Cancer Research: Neuroblastoma—Biochemical Studies. Vol 2, p 26. Berlin, Springer-Verlag, 1966

48. Hann HWL, Levy HM, Evans AE: Serum ferritin as a guide to therapy in neuroblastoma. Cancer Res 40:1411–1413, 1980

49. Hann HWL, Stahlhut BA, Evans AE: Serum ferritin as a prognostic indicator in neuroblastoma: Biological effects of isoferritins. Adv Neuroblastoma Res, pp 331–345. New York, Alan R. Liss, 1985

50. Ishiguro Y, Kato K, Ito T, Nagaya M, Yamada N, Sugito T: Neuron specific enolase in serum as a marker for neuroblastoma. Pediatrics 72:696–700, 1983

51. Zeltzer PM, Marangos PJ, Parma A: Raised neuron specific enolase in serum of children with metastatic neuroblastoma. Lancet 2:361–364, 1983

52. Zeltzer PM, Marangos PJ, Evans AE, Schneider SL: Serum neuron-specific enolase in children with neuroblastoma: Relationship to stage and disease course. Cancer 57:1230–1234, 1986

53. Quinn JJ, Altman AJ, Frantz CN: Serum lactic dehydrogenase: An indicator of tumor activity in neuroblastoma. J Pediatr 97:88–91, 1980

54. Schwab M, Varmus HE, Bishop JM et al: Chromosome localization in human normal cells and neuroblastomas of a gene related to c-myc. Nature 308:288–294, 1984

55. Seeger RC, Brodeur G, Sather H et al: Association of multiple copies of the n-myc oncogene with rapid progression of neuroblastoma. N Engl J Med 313:1111–1116, 1985

56. Frens DB, Bray PF, Wu JT, Lahey ME: The carcinoembryonic antigen assay: Prognostic value in neural crest tumors. J Pediatr 88:591–594, 1976

57. Ford CHJ, Gallant ME, Kaiser A: Immunocytochemical investigation of carcinoembryonic antigen expression in neuroblastomas with monoclonal and polyclonal antibodies. Pediatr Res 19:385–388, 1985

58. Donner L, Triche TJ, Israel MA, Seeger RC, Reynolds CP: A panel of monoclonal antibodies which discriminate neuroblastoma from Ewing's sarcoma, rhabdomyosarcoma, neuroepithelioma and hematopoietic malignancies. Progr Clin Biol Res 175:347–366, 1985

59. Ladisch S, Wu ZL: Circulating gangliosides as tumor markers. Progr Clin Biol Res 175:277–284, 1985

60. Schulz G, Cheresh DA, Varki NM et al: Detection of ganglioside G in tumor tissue and sera of neuroblastoma patients. Cancer Res 44:5914–5920, 1984

61. Talerman A, Haije WG: Alpha-fetoprotein and germ cell tumors: A possible role of yolk sac tumor in production of alpha-fetoprotein. Cancer 34:1722–1726, 1974

62. Bosl GL, Lange PH, Nochomovitz LE et al: Tumor markers in advanced nonseminomatous testicular cancer. Cancer 47:572–576, 1981

63. Perlin E, Engeler JE Jr, Edson M et al: The value of serial measurement of both human chorionic gonadotropin and alpha-fetoprotein for monitoring germ cell tumors. Cancer 37:215–219, 1976

64. Trojanowski JR, Hickey WF: Human teratomas express differentiated neural antigens: An immunohistochemical study with anti-neurofilament, anti-glial filament, and anti-myelin basic protein monoclonal antibodies. Am J Pathol 115:383–389, 1983

65. Bellet DH, Wands JK, Isselbacher KJ, Bohuon C: Serum α-fetoprotein levels in human disease: Perspective from a highly specific monoclonal radioimmunoassay. Proc Natl Acad Sci USA 81:3869–3873, 1984

66. Kim EE, Deland FH, Nelson MO et al: Radioimmunodetection of cancer with radiolabeled antibodies to α-fetoprotein. Cancer Res 40:3008–3012, 1980

67. Kew MC, Torrance JD, Derman D: Serum and tumour ferritins in primary liver cancer. Gut 19:294–299, 1978

68. Nickerson HJ, Silberman TL, McDonald TP: Hepatoblastoma, thrombocytosis, and increased thrombopoietin. Cancer 45:315–317, 1980

69. Mirand EA, Murphy GP: Erythropoietin alterations in human liver disease. NY State J Med 71:860–864, 1971

70. Nakagawara A, Keichi I, Isuneyoshi M, Daimuro Y, Enjoji M: Hepatoblastoma producing both alphafetoprotin and human chorionic gonadotropin: Clinical pathologic analysis of four cases and a review of the literature. Cancer 56:1636–1642, 1985

71. Wheeler K, Pritchard J, Luck W, Rosriter M: Transcobalamine 1 as a marker for fibrolamellar hepatoma. Med Pediatr Oncol 14:227–229, 1986

72. Liebman HA, Furie BC, Tang MH et al: Des-r-carboxy (abnormal) prothrombin as a serum marker of primary hepatocellular carcinoma. N Engl J Med 310:1427–1431, 1984

73. DeJong ASH, van Kessel M, Albus-Lutter CE, Voute PA: Creatinine kinase subunits M and B as markers in the diagnosis of poorly differentiated rhabdomyosarcomas in children. Hum Pathol 16:924–928, 1985

74. Hickman PE, Messina S, Trotter JM, Masarei JRL: High creatinine kinase MB isoenzyme activity associated with rhabdomyosarcoma. Clin Chem 29:1549–1550, 1983

75. Huth JF, Gupta RK, Eilber FR, Morton DL: A prospective postoperative evaluation of urinary tumor-associated antigens in sarcoma patients: Correlation with disease recurrence. Cancer 53:1306–1310, 1984

76. Trent J, Casper J, Meltzer P, Thompson F, Fogh J: Non-random chromosome alterations in rhabdomyosarcoma. Cancer Genet Cytogenet 16:189–197, 1985

77. Turc-Carel C, Lizard-Wacol S, Justrabo E et al: Consistent chromosomal translocation in alveolar rhabdomyosarcoma. Cancer Genet Cytogenet 19:361–362, 1986

78. Altmansberger M, Weber K, Droste R, Osborn M: Desmin is a specific marker for rhabdomyosarcomas of human and rat origin. Am J Pathol 118:85–95, 1985

79. Levine AM, Rosenberg SA: Alkaline phosphatase levels in osteosarcoma tissues are related to prognosis. Cancer 44:2291–2293, 1979

80. O'Hara J, Hutler R, Fotote F, Miller T, Woodard HQ: An analysis of thirty patients surviving longer than ten years after treatment for osteogenic sarcoma. J Bone Joint Surg 50A:335–354, 1968

81. Scranton P, DeCicco F, Totten R, Yunis E: Prognostic factors in osteosarcoma. Cancer 36:2170–2191, 1975

82. Brereton HD, Simon R, Pomeroy TC: Pretreatment serum lactate dehydrogenase predicting metastatic spread in Ewing's sarcoma. Ann Intern Med 83:352–354, 1975

83. Glaubiger DL, Makuch R, Schwarz J, Levine AS, Johnson RE: Determination of prognostic factors and their influence on therapeutic results in patients with Ewing's sarcoma. Cancer 45:2213–2219, 1980

84. Avrias A, Rimbaut C, Buffe D, Zucker JM, Masabraud A: Translocation involving chromosome 22 in Ewing's sarcoma: A cytogenetic study of four fresh tumors. Cancer Genet Cytogenet 12:21–25, 1984

85. Prieto F, Badia L, Montalar J, Massuti B: Translocation (11;22) in Ewing's sarcoma. Cancer Genet Cytogenet 17:87–89, 1985

86. Russell DH, Levy CC, Schimpf SC, Hawk IA: Urinary polyamines in cancer patients. Cancer Res 31:1555–1558, 1971

87. Nishioka K, Remsdahl MM: Elevation of putrescine and spermidine in sera of patients with solid tumors. Clin Chim Acta 57:155–161, 1974

88. Marton LJ, Hruby O, Levin VA et al: The relationship of polyamines in cerebrospinal fluid to the presence of central nervous system tumors. Cancer Res 36:973–977, 1976

89. Marton LJ, Edwards MS, Levin VA, Lubich WP, Wilson CB: Predictive values of cerebrospinal fluid polyamines in medulloblastomas. Cancer Res 39:993–997, 1979

90. Twijnstra A, Nooyen W, van Zanten AP, Hart AAM, Origerboer BW: Cerebrospinal fluid carcinoembryonic antigen in patients with metastatic and nonmetastatic neurological disease. Arch Neurol 43:269–272, 1986

91. Zeltzer PM, Schneider S, Marangos P, Zweig MH: Neuron specific enolase and creatinine kinase-BB are expressed by human brain tumors. J Neurol Oncol 2:264–267, 1984

92. Trojanowsk JQ, Lee VM-Y: Monoclonal and polyclonal antibodies against neural antigens: Diagnostic applications for studies of central and peripheral nervous system tumors. Hum Pathol 14:281–285, 1983

Principles
of Treatment

part

three

nine

General Principles of Chemotherapy

Frank M. Balis,
John S. Holcenberg, and
David G. Poplack

Oncologic chemotherapy has had its greatest impact in the treatment of childhood cancers. Since the introduction of drug therapy for childhood leukemia nearly four decades ago,[1] the overall prognosis of childhood cancer has improved dramatically. The 5-year survival rate for this group of diseases, once considered uniformly fatal in the predrug era, was 57% for all forms of cancer in children diagnosed between 1973 and 1981.[2] This striking increase in survival is directly related to the use of anticancer drugs along with surgery and radiotherapy as initial treatment.[3] In fact, many of the principles of the modern chemotherapy of cancer were derived in large part from empirical observations made in early clinical trials in children with drug-sensitive cancers such as acute lymphoblastic leukemia, Burkitt's lymphoma, and Wilms' tumor.[4]

The significantly higher response rates achieved by combining active agents into multidrug regimens were initially demonstrated in childhood acute lymphoblastic leukemia. Such *combination* chemotherapy improved both the remission rate and the duration of remission compared to single-agent therapy.[5] The treatment of Wilms' tumor serves as a model both for the use of a multidisciplinary or multimodal approach to the treatment of cancer and for the use of *adjuvant* chemotherapy in patients who are without clinical evidence of residual disease following local therapy with surgery or radiation but who are at high risk for recurrence. Most of the common pediatric solid tumors, such as rhabdomyosarcoma, lymphoma, Ewing's sarcoma, and osteosarcoma, are now managed using a multimodal approach combining surgery or radiotherapy for the primary tumor and early intensive adjuvant chemotherapy for control of micrometastases.[6] The recognition that lymphoblasts sequestered in a pharmacologic sanctuary such as the central nervous system were protected against the cytotoxic effects of systemically administered chemotherapy led to the development of *sanctuary* therapy, designed specifically to treat these cells with regional chemotherapy or local radiotherapy. Intrathecal chemotherapy was initially developed for the treatment of overt meningeal leukemia in children but is now an important component of central nervous system preventive therapy in childhood acute lymphoblastic leukemia.[7] Finally, the value of *neoadjuvant* (preoperative) chemotherapy has recently been demonstrated in the treatment of children with osteosarcoma (see Chap. 32).[8]

PROPERTIES OF ANTICANCER DRUGS

Pharmacodynamic and Pharmacokinetic Properties

Ideally, the quantitative aspects of both drug disposition (pharmacokinetics) and drug interaction at the target site (pharmacodynamics) are used to determine the optimal dose, schedule, and route of administration of a drug in order to achieve the maximum therapeutic benefit while minimizing toxicity. The sites of drug–

tumor cell interaction for the commonly used anticancer drugs are illustrated in Figure 9-1. Most of these agents are cytotoxins, and, in general, they produce their cytotoxic effects by interfering with the synthesis or function of DNA. In most instances, only actively proliferating cells are susceptible to the effects of these agents, and anticancer drugs are, therefore, most effective against tumors with a high growth fraction (a high percentage of actively proliferating cells). Because the growth fraction decreases as the size of a tumor increases, most anticancer drugs would be expected to be more effective against microscopic deposits of tumor cells than against bulk disease. Many of the cancers of the young have a rapid growth rate with a high growth fraction and early and extensive dissemination of micrometastases, which may explain, in part, why chemotherapy has had more of an impact in the treatment of childhood cancers than cancers of adults.

Despite the fact that these qualitative details of drug–tumor cell interactions have been defined for most anticancer drugs, the quantitative aspects of these interactions, such as the actual drug concentrations and exposure duration required to kill human tumor cells *in vivo,* have not been defined for most of these agents. These gaps in our knowledge of the quantitative aspects of anticancer drug pharmacodynamics have severely limited our ability to use these agents in a rational manner.[9] Without defined therapeutic and toxic drug concentrations, determination of drug dose and schedule has been relegated to empirical methods.

In contrast to the pharmacodynamics, the pharmacokinetic behavior of most of the commonly used agents has been studied, including quantitative aspects of drug absorption, distribution, biotransformation (metabolism), and excretion (see Table 9-1 for definition of pharmacokinetic terms). However, most of the studies have been performed in adults—the pharmacokinetics of many anticancer drugs have not been as extensively studied in children. Although these pharmacokinetic parameters are important for estimating the optimal dose, schedule, and route of administration, the discipline of pharmacokinetics has not played a significant role in the day-to-day management of the patient with cancer, despite the fact that anticancer drugs have pharmacologic characteristics, such as a low therapeutic index, severe toxicities, and wide interindividual variation in drug disposition, that could account for some of the variability observed in response and toxicity. Therapeutic drug monitoring, which has revolutionized drug therapy in other medical specialties, has been limited by the complexity of anticancer drug pharmacokinetics and the lack of well-defined therapeutic and toxic levels for most agents.[10] Instead, most anticancer drugs are administered in a standard starting

FIGURE 9-1. Schematic representation of site of action of commonly used anticancer drugs.

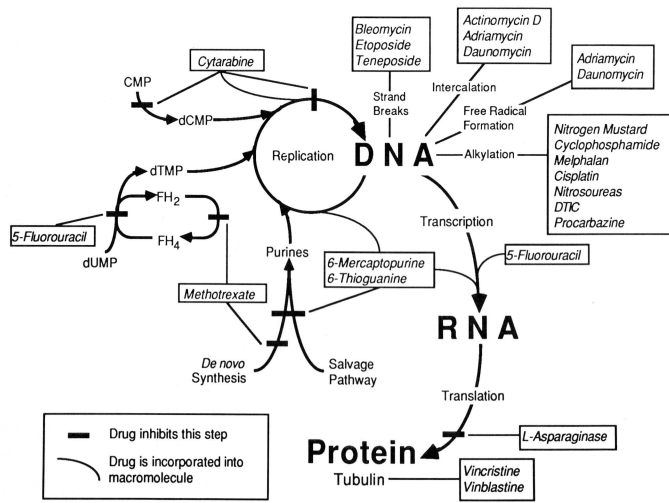

Table 9-1
Definition of Pharmacokinetic Terms Used in This Chapter

Term	Common Abbreviation	Units*	Definition
Clearance	Cl	Vol/time (ml/min)	Used to quantify the rate of drug elimination; expressed in terms of volume of plasma cleared of drug per unit of time. Total clearance is the sum of renal, metabolic, and biliary (fecal) elimination.
Half-life	t½	Time (h)	Time required to reduce the drug concentration by 50%. Plasma disappearance frequently has multiple phases with differing rates of disappearance (*e.g.,* rapid distribution phase, terminal or elimination phase). Half-lives listed for drugs in this chapter are the postdistributive (terminal, elimination) half-lives unless otherwise noted.
Area under the curve	AUC	Conc. × Time ($\mu M \cdot h$)	Quantitates total drug exposure; integral of drug conc. over time or the area under the plasma concentration–time curve. Used in calculation of clearance and bioavailability.
Volume of distribution	Vd; Vd_{ss}	Volume (liters)	Relates plasma conc. to total amount of drug in the body (volume required to dissolve the total amount of drug to give the final conc. found in plasma). A property of the drug rather than a real volume or physiologic compartment.
Bioavailability	F	Fraction (%)	Rate and extent of absorption of a drug. Frequently synonomous with the fraction of a dose absorbed when administered by some route other than intravenous.
Biotransformation	—	—	Enzymatic metabolism of a drug. May result in the activation of a prodrug, conversion to other biologically active intermediates, or inactivation of a drug.

* Conc. = concentration.

dose with subsequent dose modifications determined by the ensuing toxicities rather than by individualizing therapy on the basis of pharmacokinetic parameters.

Toxicities

Compared to other classes of drugs, the anticancer drugs are relatively nonselective. In therapeutic doses, actively dividing normal host tissues, such as bone marrow or mucosal epithelial cells, are sensitive to the cytotoxic effects of these agents. In fact, anticancer drugs have the lowest therapeutic index (ratio of toxic dose to therapeutic dose) of any class of drugs.[11] The acute toxicities of cancer chemotherapy are common and often predictable and frequently must be tolerated in order to administer effective doses of these agents. Acute toxicities common to many of the anticancer drugs include myelosuppression, nausea and vomiting, alopecia, mucositis, allergic or cutaneous reactions, and local ulceration from subcutaneous drug extravasation. Many drugs also have unique toxicities affecting various organs or tissues such as the cardiotoxicity associated with the anthracyclines. A considerable proportion of the oncologist's time is spent in providing supportive care for patients experiencing acute drug toxicities.[12]

The long-term side-effects of cancer chemotherapy are also of particular concern to the pediatric oncologist because of the high cure rates and the long life spans of successfully treated patients. The adverse effects of chemotherapy on growth, development, and reproductive function, as well as possible permanent cardiac, pulmonary, or renal damage and possible carcinogenic and teratogenic effects, are discussed in Chapter 50.

Drug Resistance

Whereas toxicities are usually predictable, the response of any given tumor to individual agents is not. Clinical resistance to anticancer drugs is the primary reason for treatment failure. It can be present at the outset of treatment or can develop under the selective pressure of drug exposure. The magnitude of the problem of drug resistance was appreciated early in cancer chemotherapy. When children with acute lymphoblastic leukemia were treated with single-agent therapy, at best only half achieved a remission, and nearly all of those who did respond eventually relapsed despite continuation of the drug that produced the remission.[4,13]

Recent evidence strongly suggests a genetic basis for the development of most forms of drug resistance.[14] The inherent genetic instability of tumor cells can effect the spontaneous generation of drug-resistant clones as a result of a mutation, deletion, gene amplification, translocation, or chromosomal rearrangement.[14] These genetic alterations are presumed to be random events, which may account, in part, for the variability in response observed in most clinical trials. Examples of biochemical mechanisms of resistance for the commonly used anticancer drugs are listed in Table 9-2. In many cases, these alterations in cellular metabolism can be related to an increase, a decrease, or an alteration in some gene product, such as the gene amplification identified in methotrexate-resistant cells

Table 9-2
Examples of Biochemical Mechanisms of Drug Resistance[15,29]

Mechanism	Drug
Impaired drug transport or uptake	Methotrexate, melphalan
Increased drug efflux from cell (decreased retention)	Anthracyclines, vinca alkaloids, dactinomycin
Impaired intracellular metabolic activation	6-Mercaptopurine, 5-fluorouracil
Increased intracellular metabolic inactivation	Cyclophosphamide, cytarabine
Detoxification by nonspecific pathways (glutathione)	Alkylating agents, anthracyclines
Increased levels of target enzymes	Methotrexate
Altered enzyme or target affinity for drug	Vincristine, methotrexate
Use of alternate metabolic pathways	6-Mercaptopurine
Repair of DNA damage	Alkylating agents

that results in overproduction of dihydrofolate reductase, the target enzyme of methotrexate.[16]

The phenomenon of multidrug (pleiotropic drug) resistance was recently described by Ling and colleagues.[17] Through a single mutation, tumor cells develop resistance to a variety of anticancer drugs primarily of natural origin such as the anthracyclines, dactinomycin, the vinca alkaloids, and the epipodophyllotoxins. The development of resistance to one of these agents following prolonged exposure of tumor cells *in vitro* is frequently associated with significant crossresistance to the other agents. Although several mechanisms for multidrug resistance may exist,[18-20] the multidrug-resistant phenotype has usually been associated with decreased intracellular drug accumulation and an increase in a plasma membrane glycoprotein (P-glycoprotein) that has the characteristics of an energy-dependent efflux pump protein.[19,20]

Gene amplification has been observed in cells expressing the multidrug-resistance phenotype. Elongated chromosomes with homogeneously staining regions, chromosomes with abnormally banding regions, or double-minute chromosomes have been identified in a high proportion of resistant tumor cell sublines *in vitro,* confirming the genetic origin of this form of resistance.[21] One amplified gene of interest, *mdr1,* has been identified *in vitro* in a multidrug-resistant human carcinoma cell line and subsequently cloned.[22] The gene product of *mdr1* appears to be the plasma membrane glycoprotein previously associated with multidrug resistance.[23] Expression of *mdr1* has been observed in human tumor specimens (Fig. 9-2) and in some normal human tissues from colon and kidney among others.[24] The degree of expression of *mdr1* is correlated with the level of resistance.[25]

Multidrug resistance can be partially reversed *in vitro* with calcium-channel blockers such as verapamil.[26,27] However, clinical trials with this approach have thus far failed to demonstrate any therapeutic advantage, because the cardiac toxicity of verapamil prevents the achievement of drug levels adequate to reverse Adriamycin resistance.[28]

PRINCIPLES OF CANCER CHEMOTHERAPY

Combination Chemotherapy

The selection of the drug(s) to be used in treating a child with cancer is made primarily on the basis of the histology of the tumor and the extent of the disease (the stage). The agents selected are those that have demonstrated activity against the

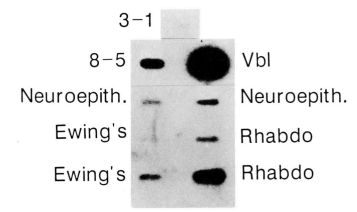

FIGURE 9-2. Expression of *mdr1* gene in selected pediatric tumors demonstated by slot blot analysis of RNA from six tumor specimens and three control cell lines. 3-1, negative control cell line; Vbl and 8-5, multidrug-resistant cell lines; Ewing, Ewing's sarcoma tumor specimens; Neuroepith, neuroepithelial tumor specimens; Rhabdo, rhabdomyosarcoma tumor specimen. Analysis shows variable expression of the *mdr1* gene in the tumor specimens. (Used with permission from Fojo AT et al: Expression of a multidrug resistance gene in human tumors and tissues. Proc Natl Acad Sci USA 84:265–269, 1987)

type of tumor being treated. However, even though a drug has been judged active in previous clinical trials, the incidence of natural (*de novo*) resistance to individual agents can be high, often exceeding 50%;[14,29] it is generally not possible to predict accurately whether a particular patient's tumor will respond to a given drug. To overcome this problem, active drugs are usually administered in combination to ensure a greater chance of achieving the maximum response. In addition to providing a broader range of coverage against naturally resistant cells, combination chemotherapy may also prevent or delay the development of acquired resistance in initially responsive tumors and results in additive or synergistic cytotoxic effects on tumor cells when agents with different mechanisms of action are used.

In the design of combination regimens, only drugs that have demonstrated single-agent activity against the type of tumor being treated should be incorporated. Recently, some drug combinations have also been designed to take advantage of interesting biochemical interactions between certain anticancer drugs, such as methotrexate and 5-fluorouracil or leucovorin and 5-fluorouracil. Obviously, the agents should not antagonize each other's antitumor effects as a result of pharmacokinetic or pharmacodynamic interactions. Each drug should be administered in its optimal dose with the shortest possible interval between courses of therapy. For this reason, it is desirable to select agents that do not have overlapping or additive toxicities.

Drug Dose and Schedule

The dose and schedule of drug administration are critical in achieving a maximum benefit from chemotherapy. Data from both experimental tumor models and clinical trials clearly demonstrate a steep dose–response curve in drug-sensitive tumors for the majority of anticancer drugs.[30] In vivo studies in rodent tumor systems, for example, have demonstrated a log-linear relation between drug dose and tumor-cell kill for some drugs, such as cyclophosphamide, in which a twofold increase in the dose resulted, in some tumors, in a tenfold increase in tumor-cell kill.[30] A similar dose–response relation has been noted in the clinic. In a randomized trial conducted in children with acute lymphoblastic leukemia, the influence of the dose of maintenance therapy on remission duration was evaluated. Patients who received full dosage had a median duration of hematologic remission that was significantly longer than that of the group randomized to half dosage (15 versus 6 months).[31] Similarly, in a retrospective analysis in patients with osteosarcoma treated with Adriamycin, those who received 75 mg/m² as prescribed by the treatment protocol had a relapse rate of 39% compared to 65% for those receiving less than 75% of the recommended dose.[32]

In designing and implementing treatment protocols, careful attention must be paid not only to administering drugs at the highest dose tolerated, but also to administering drug cycles at the shortest possible intervals, avoiding delays that could permit tumor regrowth.

Adjuvant Chemotherapy

In patients with no evidence of residual disease following local therapy with surgery or radiation, "prophylactic" or adjuvant chemotherapy is administered when the risk of recurrent disease at distant sites is high. The efficacy of adjuvant chemotherapy has been established for most of the common pediatric cancers, including Wilms' tumor, Ewing's sarcoma, lymphoma, rhabdomyosarcoma, astrocytoma, retinoblastoma, and osteosarcoma. The high risk of recurrence even after effective local therapy and the failure of chemotherapy to cure patients once the disease has recurred led to trials of adjuvant therapy. Theoretical and experimental evidence also support the use of adjuvant chemotherapy.[33] Microscopic foci of tumor should be more chemosensitive both on a cell-kinetic basis, because of a larger growth fraction, and because of the lower probability of natural resistance. The mathematical modeling experiments of Goldie and Coldman predict that the chance for cure is maximized if all available effective drugs are given simultaneously in the adjuvant setting, when there is minimal disease and the chances of drug resistance are lower.[14]

ROLE OF CLINICAL PHARMACOLOGY

The primary objective of the clinical pharmacologist is to increase the safety and efficacy of drug therapy by incorporating accumulated scientific knowledge about each drug and established pharmacologic principles into the design of treatment regimens. A wide range of factors must be considered. First, the mechanism of action of the drug may help predict which

(*Text continues on p. 172*)

Table 9-3
Some Physiologic Differences in Children (Compared to Adults) that May Influence Drug Disposition[34]

Organ or Compartment	Value at Birth*	Age Adult Values Are Reached†	Effect on Drug Disposition‡
Kidney			
Glomerular filtration	↓	1 yr	↓Renal excretion
Tubular function	↓	1 yr	↓Tubular secretion
Liver			
Oxidative metabolism	↓	6 mo	↓Metabolic clearance
Glucuronide conjugation	↓	2–3 yr	↓Metabolic clearance
Biliary excretion	↓	6 mo	↓Biliary excretion
Gastrointestinal			
Acid secretion	↓	2 yr	Altered drug absorption
Motility	↓	6 mo	Delayed absorption
Body composition			
Extracellular fluid	↑	6 mo	↑Distribution volume
Total body water	↑	6 mo	↑Distribution volume
Fat	↓	Adolescence	↓Distribution volume of lipophilic drugs
CSF volume	↑	3 yr	↑Distribution volume of intrathecal drugs

* ↓ = decreased; ↑ = increased.
† Compared to adult values and relative to body surface area.
‡ Refer to Table 9-4 to determine which drugs may be affected by alteration of renal, biliary, or metabolic function.

Table 9-4
Pharmacologic Properties of the Commonly Used Anticancer Drugs

Drug	Synonyms	Route*	Dose/m²	Schedule†	Mechanism of Action
Alkylating Agents					
Mechlorethamine	Mustargen, HN₂, nitrogen mustard	IV	6 mg	Weekly × 2, q 28 d	Alkylation; crosslinking
Cyclophosphamide	Cytoxan, CTX	IV PO	250–1800 mg 100–300 mg	Daily × 1–4 d, q 21–28 d Daily	(Prodrug) alkylation; crosslinking
Ifosfamide	IFOS	IV	1800 mg	Daily × 5, q 21–28 d	(Prodrug) alkylation; crosslinking
Melphalan	Alkeran, L-PAM	IV PO	10–35 mg 140–220 mg 4–20 mg	q 21–28 d Single dose (ABMT) Daily for 1–21 d	Alkylation; crosslinking
Lomustine	CeeNU, CCNU	PO	100–150 mg	Single dose, q 4–6 wk	Alkylation; crosslinking; carbamoylation
Carmustine	BiCNU, BCNU	IV	200–250 mg	Single dose, q 4–6 wk	Alkylation; crosslinking; carbamoylation
Cisplatin	Platinol, CDDP	IV	50–200 mg 20 mg	Over 4–6 h, q 21–28 d Daily × 5, q 21–28 d	Platination; crosslinking
Dacarbazine	DTIC	IV	250 mg	Daily × 5, q 21–28 d	(Prodrug) alkylation (monofunctional)
Procarbazine	Matulan, PCZ	PO	100 mg	Daily for 10–14 d	(Prodrug) alkylation; free-radical formation
Antimetabolites					
Methotrexate	MTX	PO, IM IV	7.5–30 mg 10–33,000 mg	Weekly or biweekly Bolus or CI (6–42 h)	Interferes with folate metabolism
6-Mercaptopurine	Purinethal, 6-MP	PO	75–100 mg	Daily	(Prodrug) incorporated into DNA and RNA; blocks purine synthesis, interconversion
6-Thioguanine	6-TG	PO	75–100 mg	Daily, 2 × day	(Prodrug) incorporated into DNA and RNA; blocks purine synthesis, interconversion
Cytarabine	Cytosine arabinoside	IV, SC	100–200 mg	q 12 h or CI for 5–7 d	(Prodrug) incorporated into DNA; inhibits DNA polymerase
	Cytosar, Ara-C	IV	3000 mg	q 12 h for 4 to 6 doses	
5-Fluorouracil	5-FU	IV	500 mg 800–1200 mg	Single or daily × 5 CI (24–120 h)	(Prodrug) inhibits thymidine synthesis; incorporated into RNA, DNA
Antibiotics					
Adriamycin	Doxorubicin, ADR	IV IV	75 mg 20 mg	Single, q 21 d Weekly	Intercalation; free-radical formation; membrane effects
Daunomycin	Daunorubicin, DNR	IV	30–45 mg	Daily × 3 or weekly	Intercalation; free-radical formation; membrane effects
Bleomycin	Blenoxane, BLEO	IV, IM, SC	10–20 units	Weekly	DNA strand breaks
Dactinomycin	Cosmegen, ACT-D, actinomycin D	IV	0.45 mg	Daily × 5, q 3–6 wk	Intercalation; DNA strand breaks
Plant Alkaloids					
Vincristine	Oncovin, VCR	IV	1.0–1.5 mg	Weekly × 3–6	Mitotic inhibitor; binds tubulin
Vinblastine	Velban, VLB	IV	3.5–6.0 mg	Weekly × 3–6	Mitotic inhibitor; binds tubulin
Etoposide	VePesid, VP-16, VP-16-213	IV	60–120 mg	Daily × 3–5, q 3–6 wk	DNA strand breaks
Teneposide	VM-26	IV	70–180 mg	Daily × 3	DNA strand breaks
Miscellaneous					
Prednisone	Deltasone, PRED	PO	40 mg	Daily	(Prodrug) receptor-mediated lympholysis
Prednisolone		PO, IV	40 mg	Daily	Receptor-mediated lympholysis
Dexamethasone	Decadron, DEX	PO, IV, IM	6 mg	Daily	Receptor-mediated lympholysis
L-Asparaginase	Elspar, L-ASP	IV, IM	6000 IU	3 times per wk	L-Asparagine depletion; ↓protein synthesis

* IV–intravenous; PO–oral; IM–intramuscular; SC–subcutaneous.
† d–day; wk–week; h–hour; CI–continuous infusion; ABMT–autologous bone-marrow transplant.
‡ M–myelosuppression; N & V–nausea and vomiting; A–alopecia; NT–neurotoxicity; GI–gastrointestinal toxicity; HD–high dose.
§ ↑–increased; ↓–decreased; GT–glutathione-S-transferase; IC–intracellular; dCTP–deoxycytidine triphosphate.

Toxicities‡	Antitumor Spectrum	Mechanisms of Resistance§
M, N & V, A, phlebitis, vesicant, mucositis; NT (HD)	Hodgkin's, brain tumors	↑GT, ↓Transport, ↑DNA repair
M, N & V, A, cystitis, water retention; cardiac (HD)	Lymphomas, leukemias, sarcomas, neuroblastoma	↑IC catabolism, ↑GT
M, N & V, A, cystitis, NT, renal	Sarcomas	
M, N & V; mucositis & diarrhea (HD)	Rhabdomyosarcoma; sarcomas, neuroblastoma and leukemias (HD)	↓Transport
M, N & V, renal & pulmonary toxicity	Brain tumors, lymphomas	↓Uptake, ↑IC catabolism, ↑DNA repair
M, N & V, renal & pulmonary toxicity	Brain tumors, lymphomas	↓Uptake, ↑IC catabolism, ↑DNA repair
M (mild), N & V, A, renal, NT	Testicular and other germ cell, osteosarcoma, brain tumors, neuroblastoma	↑DNA repair, ↑GT
M (mild), N & V, flu-like syndrome, hepatic	Neuroblastoma, sarcomas	
M, N & V, NT, rash, mucositis	Hodgkin's, brain tumors	
M (mild), mucositis, rash, hepatic; renal (HD), NT (HD)	Leukemia, lymphoma, osteosarcoma	↓Transport, ↑Target enzyme, ↓Polyglutamation
M, hepatic, mucositis	Leukemia (ALL, CML)	↓Activation, ↑IC degradation
M, N & V, mucositis, hepatic	Leukemia (ANL)	↓Activation, ↑IC degradation
M, N & V, mucositis, GI; NT, ocular, skin (HD)	Leukemia, lymphoma	↓Activation, ↓Transport, ↑dCTP, ↑IC degradation
M (bolus), mucositis, N & V, diarrhea	?	↓Activation, ↑target enzyme, altered target enzyme
M, mucositis, N & V, A, vesicant, cardiac (acute and chronic)	Leukemia (ALL, ANL), lymphoma, most solid tumors	Multidrug resistance
Same as Adriamycin	Leukemia (ALL, ANL)	Multidrug resistance
Lung, skin, hypersensitivity, Raynaud's	Lymphoma, testicular cancer	
M, N & V, mucositis, vesicant	Wilms', sarcomas	Multidrug resistance
NT, A, SIADH, hypotension, vesicant	Leukemia (ALL), lymphomas, most solid tumors	Multidrug resistance
M, A, mucositis, mild NT, vesicant	Histiocytosis, Hodgkin's, testicular	Mulidrug resistance
M, A, N & V, mucositis, mild NT, hypotension, allergic	Leukemias (ALL, ANL), lymphomas, neuroblastoma, sarcomas, brain tumors	Multidrug resistance
Same as etoposide	Same as etoposide	Multidrug resistance
Protean (see text)	Leukemia, lymphoma	Loss or defect in receptor
Protean (see text)	Leukemia, lymphoma	Loss or defect in receptor
Protean (see text)	Leukemia, lymphoma, brain tumors	Loss or defect in receptor
Allergic, coagulopathy, pancreatitis, hepatic, NT	Leukemia (ALL), lymphoma	↑IC asparagine synthase

* IV–intravenous; PO–oral; IM–intramuscular; SC–subcutaneous.
† d–day; wk–week; h–hour; CI–continuous infusion; ABMT–autologous bone-marrow transplant.
‡ M–myelosuppression; N & V–nausea and vomiting; A–alopecia; NT–neurotoxicity; GI–gastrointestinal toxicity; HD–high dose.
§ ↑–increased; ↓–decreased; GT–glutathione-S-transferase; IC–intracellular; dCTP–deoxycytidine triphosphate.

tumors will respond based on their biochemical and cytokinetic profiles. In addition, potential synergism or antagonism between drugs to be used in combination regimens may be predicted from the drugs' mechanisms of action. Second, the antitumor spectrum of various drugs delineated in single-agent studies in patients with recurrent disease determines which agents should be used. Drugs that can produce complete responses are obviously preferable to those that produce only partial responses.[29] Third, the optimal dosage range is defined in dose-finding studies as the highest dose that can be administered on a given schedule without unacceptable toxicity.

Fourth, special consideration for methods of calculating the dose must be made in children because of physiologic differences between children and adults (Table 9-3). A dose based only on weight or body surface area may not correlate with drug distribution or capacity for drug elimination. However, body surface area correlates better with cardiac output, renal and hepatic blood flow, and renal function than does body weight.[34] The degree of functional maturation of those organs primarily responsible for drug elimination (liver and kidney) should also be considered (see Chap. 12). Developmental differences may also exist in drug absorption, plasma protein or

Table 9-5
Pharmacokinetic Parameters of the Commonly Used Anticancer Drugs

Drug	Clearance (ml/min/m²)	Half-life*	Route of Elimination†	Volume of Distribution (liters/m²)‡	Protein Binding (%)	Bioavailability (% absorbed)	CSF:Plasma Ratio (%)§
Alkylating Agents							
Mechlorethamine		<1 min	D				
Cyclophosphamide							
Parent	45–95	2.5–6.5 h	M, r	13–22	20	90	50
Metabolites		4 h	M, R		50		10–20
Ifosfamide		4–7 h	M, R	30			30
Melphalan	200–300	1–2 h	D, r	20–30		32–100	10
CCNU	(Parent drug ND in plasma)		D, M		>90	50–>90	
BCNU	1500–2000	20–70 min	D, M	90	75		>90
Cisplatin							
Free drug	400–700	1.3 h	D, R			<10	
Total platinum		44 h	R		>95		<10
Dacarbazine	450	40 min	M, R	17	20	Variable	
Procarbazine		<10 min	M				
Antimetabolites							
Methotrexate	100	8–12 h	R, m	11	60	Variable	2–3
6-Mercaptopurine	800	<1 h	M	22	20	<20 (variable)	25
6-Thioguanine	2000	20 min	M			Variable	
Cytarabine	1000	2–3 h	M	30	10	<20	25
5-Fluorouracil							
Bolus dose	1200	12 min	M	13	<10	0–74 (variable)	48
Infusion	5000		M				10–20
Antibiotics							
Adriamycin	500–1200	30 h	B, M	750	75	Not absorbed	ND in CSF
Daunomycin	2000	14 h	B, M	1300		Not absorbed	ND in CSF
Bleomycin	40	3 h	R, m	10		Not absorbed	
Dactinomycin		36 h	R, B	Large			<10
Plant Alkaloids							
Vincristine	80	24 h	M, B	120	75	Poor	5
Vinblastine	400	24 h	M, B	800	75	Poor	
Etoposide	20–25	6–8 h	M, R	10	95	50 (variable)	<10
Teneposide	10–15	7–12 h	M, r	7–10	99		<5
Miscellaneous							
Prednisolone	250	2.5 h	M	50	70–>95	85	<10
Dexamethasone	200–250	4 h	M	50	70	85	15
L-Asparaginase	2¶	14–22 h	M	2.5¶		Not absorbed	ND in CSF**

* Postdistributive or terminal half-life; min–minutes; h–hours.
† D–spontaneous chemical decomposition; M–metabolism (biotransformation); R–renal excretion; B–biliary excretion; a lower case letter (d, m, r, b) indicates that this is a minor route for elimination of the drug.
‡ Volume listed is the steady-state volume of distribution.
§ ND–not detectable; CSF–cerebrospinal fluid.
¶ Calculated from a graph presented in Ref. 373.
** Although L-asparaginase is ND in CSF, CSF L-asparagine is depleted with systemic administration of L-asparaginase.

tissue binding, and distribution of drug in the various tissues of the body.[34] Fifth, the incidence and time course of toxicities are particularly important factors in designing optimal drug combinations or adjusting doses to avoid overlapping toxicities. Sixth, knowledge of the route of elimination is helpful in adjusting the dosage in patients with organ dysfunction.[35] Finally, clinicians must be aware of potential drug interactions on either a pharmacokinetic level[36] or a pharmacodynamic level to avoid unexpected or severe toxicities or antagonism that could diminish a drug's effectiveness. In other instances, these interactions can be used to increase the antitumor effects of the drugs being administered.

In practical terms, many of these factors are defined only many years after the drugs have entered clinical use, and the clinician must therefore rely on more empirical methods in designing treatment regimens. However, as the base of knowledge about a drug increases, it must be incorporated into treatment design so that the available drugs can be optimally used.

Because the primary role of the oncologist in the treatment of cancer is to plan and supervise the administration of anticancer drugs, an in-depth knowledge of the clinical pharmacology of this class of agents is essential. In the remainder of this chapter, the pharmacologic characteristics of the anticancer drugs currently in use to treat pediatric cancers are reviewed. Tables summarize the general pharmacologic properties (Table 9-4) and pharmacokinetic parameters (Table 9-5) of the commonly used anticancer drugs.

ALKYLATING AGENTS

The alkylating agents are an important group of anticancer drugs that have a broad range of clinical activity. In general, these drugs are chemically reactive compounds that exert their cytotoxic effect through the covalent bonding of an alkyl group to important cellular macromolecules (alkylation) (Fig. 9-3). Although a number of nucleophilic (electron-rich) molecules and their subunits are alkylated intracellularly, damage to the DNA template and inhibition of DNA synthesis appear to be the major determinants of cytotoxicity.[37] With the classical (bifunctional) alkylating agents that have two alkylating groups, this damage appears to result primarily from interstrand and intrastrand DNA–DNA and DNA–protein crosslinks.[38] However, the relative importance of these crosslinks and single alkylation reactions that can lead to DNA strand breaks has not been clearly established. Monofunctional agents such as procarbazine and dacarbazine have antitumor activity but do not produce DNA crosslinks.

The clinical pharmacology of the alkylating agents has been difficult to study, because the chemical reactivity and inherent instability of the active alkylating species make their measurement in biological fluids difficult. In most cases, spontaneous hydrolysis of alkylating agents or their active metabolites in solution is a major route of drug clearance. In addition, most alkylating agents undergo some degree of enzymatic metabolism, which can lead to both active and inactive metabo-

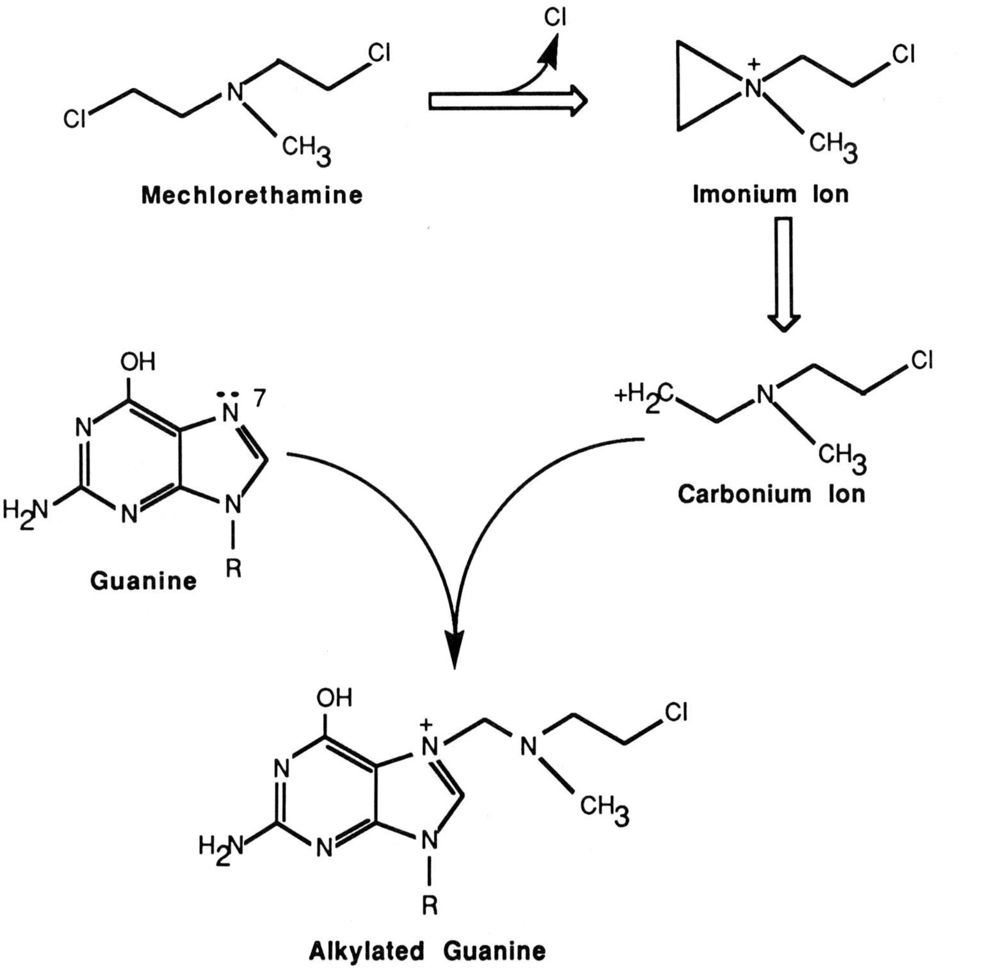

FIGURE 9-3. Alkylation of N-7 position of guanine by mechlorethamine, illustrating chemical reactions involved in the process of alkylation. The alkylating intermediates (imonium and carbonium ions) form spontaneously in solution. If the second chlorethyl group also reacts with another nucleotide base, a crosslink is formed.

lites. Some of the early pharmacologic studies performed by administering radiolabeled drugs to subjects produced misleading results because no attempt was made to separate the radioactivity present in plasma and other fluids into parent drug and metabolites.[39]

There are two general mechanisms of cellular uptake of the alkylating agents.[40] A carrier-dependent mechanism has been demonstrated for a group of water-soluble drugs such as mechlorethamine (choline carrier), melphalan (amino acid carriers), and cisplatin (amino acid carriers). Another group of lipid-soluble drugs, typified by the nitrosoureas and procarbazine, enters cells by passive diffusion and are carrier independent. These differences in cellular uptake have been related to differences in the cytotoxic properties of the drugs.[40] Drugs in the carrier-dependent group are more toxic to actively cycling cells, presumably as a result of enhanced transport at a time of active biosynthesis, whereas the carrier-independent agents are equally toxic to cycling and resting cells. Differences in cellular uptake may also explain the differences in hematologic toxicity. The carrier-independent agents are all associated with prolonged myelosuppression and cumulative, irreversible marrow damage.

Several mechanisms for the development of resistance to alkylating agents have been described, including a decrease in drug uptake or transport by the cell,[41,42] an increase in intracellular thiol compounds capable of detoxifying active alkylating species,[43,44] enhancement of intracellular enzymatic catabolism to inactive metabolites,[45] and an increase in the capability for repair of DNA damage produced by alkylation.[46] *In vitro* studies indicate that resistance to alkylating agents is difficult to induce despite protracted exposure of cells to the drugs, and that once resistance has been induced, it often is not stable in the absence of drug in the medium to create continuous selection pressure. In addition, crossresistance to these drugs is not frequent.[47–49] Certain combinations of alkylating agents (*e.g.,* thiotepa and cyclophosphamide) have actually been reported to be synergistic.[47]

Myelosuppression is the major dose-limiting toxicity for most of the commonly used alkylating agents. Since this toxicity can be overcome or reversed by bone-marrow transplantation, high doses of alkylating agents have been administered followed by an autologous or allogeneic bone-marrow transplant in order to take advantage of the steep dose–response curve characteristic of most alkylating agents.[50] Other common acute toxicities include nausea and vomiting, alopecia, allergic and cutaneous reactions, and gastrointestinal toxicity at high doses.

Of particular concern to the pediatric oncologist are the potential long-term effects of alkylator therapy. Alkylating agents can produce gonadal atrophy, permanently affecting reproductive function. The nitrogen mustards and the nitrosoureas have been linked to pulmonary fibrosis, and nephrotoxicity of the nitrosoureas can permanently impair renal function. These agents are also highly carcinogenic, mutagenic, and teratogenic.[51,52]

Of the various classes of alkylating agents, the nitrogen mustards and the nitrosoureas are most frequently used in the treatment of the childhood cancers. The chemical structures of these agents and several nonclassical alkylators are shown in Figure 9-4.

Nitrogen Mustards

The nitrogen mustards were the first type of alkylating agent used to treat cancer and remain the most widely used. Mechlorethamine (nitrogen mustard), introduced into clinical trials

in 1942, was the first drug demonstrated to be effective in the treatment of human cancers. A large number of synthetic analogues have since been screened for antitumor activity, and several with greater chemical stability and other pharmacologic advantages have largely supplanted mechlorethamine in clinical practice. Cyclophosphamide (and its isomer ifosfamide) and melphalan (phenylalanine mustard) are the most widely used in pediatric oncology.

Mechlorethamine

Although the role of mechlorethamine in the treatment of cancer has declined, it is still a model for the chemical reactions of bifunctional alkylators (Fig. 9-3). The spontaneously formed alkylating intermediates (imonium and carbonium ions) are highly reactive. They rapidly either undergo hydrolysis, leading to inactivation, or alkylate a wide variety of molecules with a propensity to react with the N-7 position on guanine. Because of this inherent instability even in aqueous solutions, mechlorethamine must be administered intravenously immediately after preparation to avoid significant loss of activity. In addition, precautions must be taken by those administering the drug, since direct contact with this reactive compound can be irritating to skin or mucous membranes.

Mechlorethamine is used primarily in combination with vincristine, prednisone, and procarbazine. This MOPP regimen remains frontline therapy for Hodgkin's disease[53] and has recently proved active in treating pediatric brain tumors (see Chaps. 21 and 24).[54,55] Topical mechlorethamine has been reported to be effective in treating the cutaneous lesions of histiocytosis.[56,57] The use of mechlorethamine as a sclerosing agent in the intracavitary therapy of pleural and pericardial effusions has declined with the advent of less-toxic agents such as tetracycline.

The pharmacokinetics of mechlorethamine in humans has not been well studied. In animals, the drug disappears from plasma in seconds.[58] In addition to its rapid spontaneous hydrolysis, mechlorethamine is rapidly metabolized (N-demethylated) in the liver.[58] As a result of this rapid degradation, renal excretion is not likely to play a role in drug clearance.

In addition to its major clinical toxicities—myelosuppression and nausea and vomiting—mechlorethamine has an anticholinergic effect, leading to diaphoresis, lacrimation, and diarrhea. It is a potent vesicant, producing a sclerosing thrombophlebitis above the site of administration and severe local tissue damage if it infiltrates. If mechlorethamine is extravasated, sodium thiosulfate should be injected into the area as rapidly as possible to neutralize the drug. Neurotoxicity in the form of an acute or delayed encephalopathy has been reported with the use of high doses of mechlorethamine.[59]

Oxazaphosphorines (Cyclophosphamide and Ifosfamide)

The oxazaphosphorines, cyclophosphamide and ifosfamide, are inactive prodrugs that require biotransformation by hepatic microsomal oxidative enzymes before expressing alkylating activity. Cyclophosphamide is one of the most widely used anticancer drugs, with a broad range of clinical activity that includes both the acute leukemias and a variety of solid tumors (Table 9-4). It is also used in preparative regimens prior to bone-marrow transplantation and as an immunosuppressant in non-neoplastic disorders. Ifosfamide remains an investigational agent in the United States, and its use in clinical practice is more limited. It has shown activity against the sarcomas.

BIOTRANSFORMATION. The chemical structures and metabolic pathways of cyclophosphamide and ifosfamide are shown in Figure 9-5. Cyclophosphamide is a true nitrogen mustard

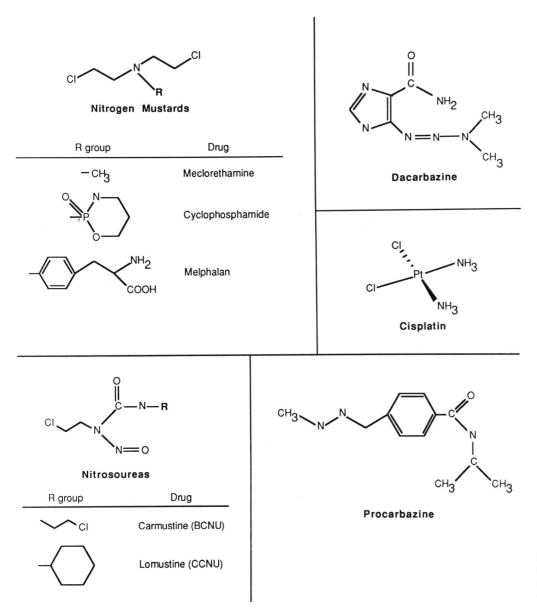

FIGURE 9-4. Chemical structures of alkylating agents commonly used to treat childhood cancers.

derivative with a bifunctional bischloroethylamine side chain. Ifosfamide is also bifunctional but has one chloroethyl group shifted to a ring nitrogen. The steps in the biotransformation of these two drugs are qualitatively identical. Hydroxylation of the 4-carbon position on the ring by hepatic microsomal mixed-function oxidases yields the primary 4-hydroxy metabolites, which are in spontaneous equilibrium with the open-ring aldehydes. Although not chemically reactive, these compounds are cytotoxic *in vitro* and are believed to be the transport forms of the active alkylating species, phosphoramide mustard and isofosfamide mustard, which are formed by spontaneous elimination of acrolein from the open-ring aldehydes. The biotransformation of these drugs leads to a variety of active chemicals that have significant biologic effects. Quantitatively, the rate of activation of cyclophosphamide is greater than that of ifosfamide, presumably due to the greater affinity of the activating enzymes for cyclophosphamide. This difference in the rate of activation accounts for the differences in clinical pharmacokinetics and maximally tolerated dose of the two isomers (see below).[60-63]

Further oxidation of the primary metabolites at the 4-carbon position by aldehyde dehydrogenase leads to inactivation. 4-Ketocyclophosphamide and carboxyphosphamide are the principal urinary metabolites of cyclophosphamide. The chloroethyl side chain can also be enzymatically cleaved (dechlorethylation). This pathway is more active with ifosfamide, leading to a greater rate of production of the potentially toxic product chloracetaldehyde.[62]

PHARMACOKINETICS. With the complexity of oxazaphosphorine metabolism and the number of active metabolites produced, the results of pharmacokinetic studies depend on which compounds are measured. Methods used to measure plasma drug concentrations have included measurement of total or fractionated radioactivity following administration of radiolabeled cyclophosphamide, total plasma alkylating activity following chemical derivatization, and inactive parent drug or specific metabolites following chromatographic separation. The first two assays are nonspecific, since the radioassay cannot distinguish between parent drug and active and inactive

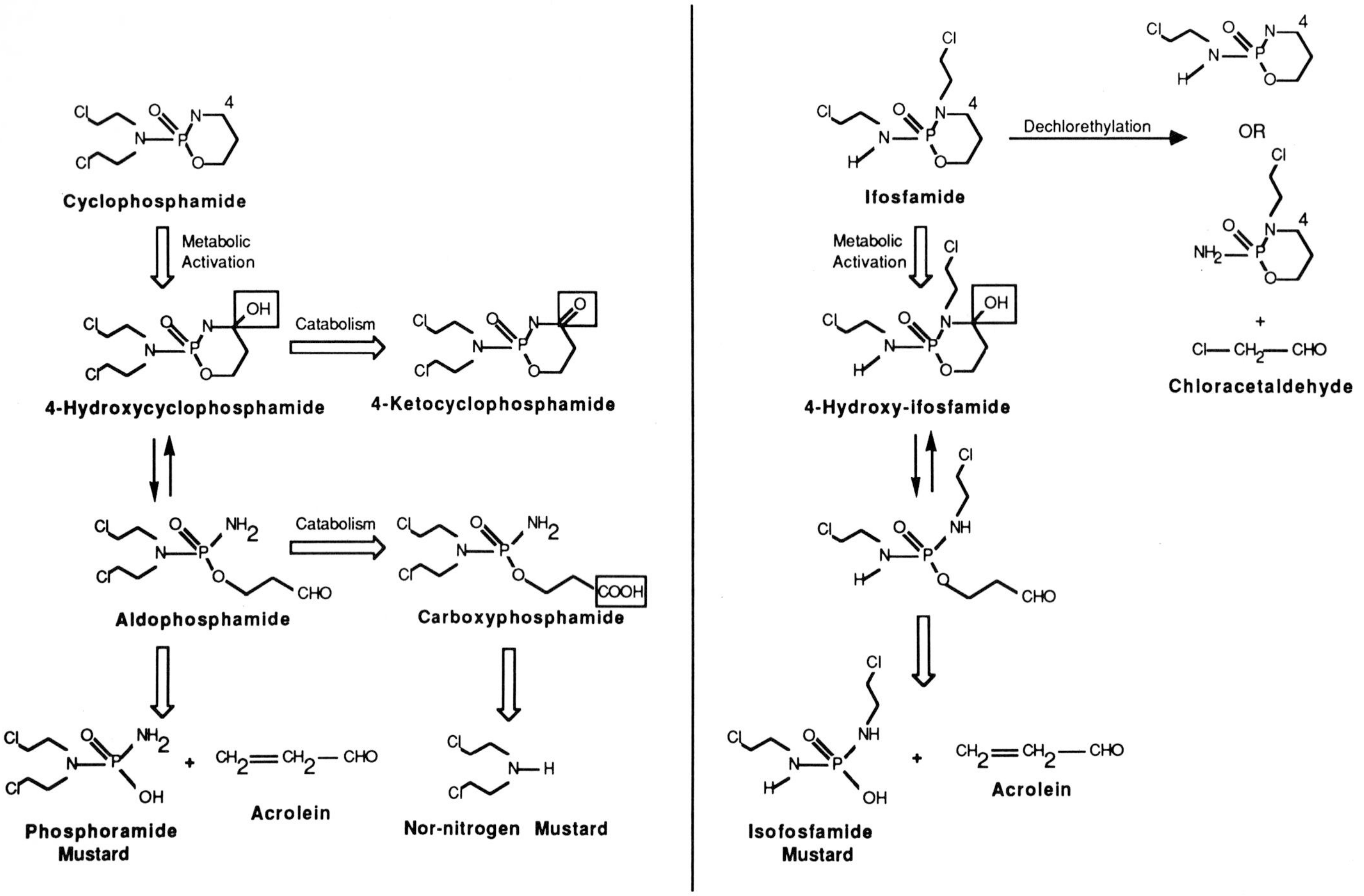

FIGURE 9-5. Metabolic pathways for the oxazaphosphorines, cyclophosphamide and ifosfamide. Both compounds must undergo hydroxylation at the 4 position before expressing cytotoxic activity; this reaction is catalyzed by hepatic microsomal enzymes. The 4-hydroxy metabolites are in spontaneous equilibrium with the open-ring aldehydes, which can in turn release acrolein and form the active alkylating mustards (phosphoramide mustard or isofosfamide mustard). Further oxidation at the 4 position of the primary metabolites (not shown for ifosfamide) leads to formation of inactive metabolites, which are excreted in the urine. Inactivation by dechlorethylation leads to formation of the potentially toxic by-product chloracetaldehyde. This is a minor pathway for cyclophosphamide but more active with ifosfamide.

metabolites and since chemical reactivity in the second assay may not correlate with cytotoxicity.[61] Although assays using gas chromatographic or high-pressure liquid chromatographic separation are more specific, it can be argued that describing the kinetic behavior of the inactive parent compound is not relevant to the drug's pharmacodynamics.

The pharmacokinetic behavior of unchanged cyclophosphamide has been well described; however, less is known about the disposition of the individual metabolites. When administered orally in low doses, cyclophosphamide is well absorbed (75%–95% of the dose absorbed).[64–66] The minimal first-pass metabolism following oral administration indicates that the hepatic extraction ratio for cyclophosphamide is low.

Cyclophosphamide and ifosfamide are eliminated primarily by hepatic biotransformation to both active and inactive metabolites, which are excreted mainly in the urine. Less than 20% of the dose is excreted unchanged in the urine,[65–70] and biliary excretion of unchanged drug is minimal.[67,71] The total body clearance in adults for the two drugs is 30 to 35 ml/min per square meter and 83 ml/min (approximately 55 ml/min per square meter) for cyclophosphamide[66,72] and ifosfamide,[62]

respectively. Renal clearance is low, accounting for less than 15% of total clearance[62,66] and indicating that there is substantial renal tubular reabsorption of cyclophosphamide. The parent drug can be efficiently extracted from plasma with hemodialysis.[73] Total clearance of cyclophosphamide in children (45 ml/min per square meter) appears to be higher than in adults.[74] The plasma half-life in children (4 hours)[74,75] is also reported to be shorter than that in adults (6–8 hours).[65–67,72] In two large studies, considerable interpatient variability was noted in the disposition of cyclophosphamide.[76,77]

The pharmacokinetics of cyclophosphamide are not dose dependent. Over a broad dosage range (100–3000 mg/m²), the proportion of drug converted to active metabolites appears to be constant, and there is no evidence of saturation of the activating enzymes.[67,77] However, with doses of ifosfamide greater than 2500 mg/m², the half-life is prolonged to 15 hours, and a much higher percentage of the drug is excreted in the urine unchanged, suggesting dose-dependent saturable metabolism of ifosfamide.[70]

The "activated" metabolites of cyclophosphamide and ifosfamide appear in plasma rapidly and have a half-life of approximately 4 hours. At equivalent doses, the plasma levels of alkylating metabolites of ifosfamide are approximately one third that generated from cyclophosphamide,[61-63] presumably due to a difference in the rate of enzymatic activation.

Patients with severe renal function impairment (creatinine clearance less than 20 ml/min) have been reported to have significantly higher plasma alkylating activity as measured by a nonspecific assay.[67,78] However, in a single anuric patient, Wagner and associates found no change in the disposition of cyclophosphamide and its activated metabolite.[79] In addition, the degree of hematotoxicity does not correlate with the severity of renal insufficiency.[61] There is no strong evidence to support dosage modifications in patients with renal dysfunction. Hepatic dysfunction may alter both the rate of drug activation and the rate of its elimination. With hepatic parenchymal damage, the half-life of cyclophosphamide is prolonged, and peak levels of "activated" cyclophosphamide are lower.[67]

TOXICITY.   Myelosuppression is the major dose-limiting toxicity of the oxazaphosphorines, but, unlike the lipid-soluble alkylating agents such as the nitrosoureas, they rarely cause cumulative marrow damage. Nausea, vomiting, and alopecia occur in most patients.

Hemorrhagic cystitis is a toxicity that appears to be unique to the oxazaphosphorines. It may range from mild dysuria and frequency to severe hemorrhage from severe bladder epithelial damage. The reported incidence of this complication ranges from 5% to 10% for cyclophosphamide and 20% to 40% for ifosfamide.[37,62] This toxicity is dose related and appears to be caused by the activated metabolites as well as by the biologically active by-products of breakdown such as acrolein (Fig. 9-5). The incidence and severity of this chemical cystitis can be lessened by aggressive hydration and frequent emptying of the bladder and by the concurrent administration of mesna (2-mercaptoethane sulfonate). Following administration, mesna is oxidized in plasma to a chemically stable and pharmacologically inert disulfide that is rapidly excreted by the kidneys and converted back to its reduced active form during tubular transport. It is therefore only active in urine and does not interfere with the antitumor effects of cyclophosphamide or ifosfamide.[80] Mesna also reduces the incidence of oxazaphosphorine-induced bladder cancers in rats,[62] a complication that also has been reported in humans.[81]

The oxazaphosphorines are nephrotoxic. Renal tubular damage has been reported with ifosfamide,[37] and cyclophosphamide can have a direct renal tubular effect that can result in water retention.[82] Other toxicities of ifosfamide include neurotoxicity characterized by somnolence, disorientation, and lethargy in about 20% of cases and, more rarely, coma and seizures.[83] The neurotoxicity is reversible. Transient hepatic dysfunction has also been reported with ifosfamide.[62] Cardiac toxicity has been observed in patients treated with high doses (more than 100–200 mg/kg) of cyclophosphamide, but there is no evidence of cumulative cardiotoxicity at standard doses.

RESISTANCE.   Mechanisms of resistance to cyclophosphamide involve intracellular inactivation of the activated metabolites. Elevated levels of glutathione, resulting from increased activity of the enzyme glutathione-S-transferase, can detoxify the biologically active metabolites of the drug.[84-86] Sensitivity to cyclophosphamide is also inversely correlated with intracellular levels of the enzyme aldehyde dehydrogenase, which oxidizes activated cyclophosphamide metabolites to inactive forms.[87] Intracellular levels of this enzyme can be estimated in tissue or tumor specimens by histochemical staining.

DRUG INTERACTIONS.   Compounds known to alter the activity of microsomal enzymes can affect the rate of activation and elimination of cyclophosphamide. Phenobarbital pretreatment enhances the rate of metabolism of cyclophosphamide and its activated metabolites in animals and in humans but does not affect the total quantity of alkylating metabolites formed in humans.[36] Cimetidine, which can interfere with the metabolic clearance of a number of compounds, increases concentrations of alkylating metabolites and prolongs the survival of tumor-bearing mice treated with cyclophosphamide.[88,89] This potential interaction has not been well studied in humans, but the authors suggest caution in combining these agents because of the possibility of exaggerated toxicities. Cyclophosphamide can also induce its own metabolism. With chronic dosing, there is a decrease in the plasma half-life.[65,75] Concurrent allopurinol appears to enhance the myelotoxicity of cyclophosphamide.[90] The mechanism of this interaction has not been elucidated.

Melphalan

Melphalan (L-phenylalanine mustard) is a rationally designed anticancer drug that has the bischloroethylamine moiety attached to the amino acid phenylalanine, with the intention that it would be taken up preferentially by melanin-producing cancers. This agent actually has a much broader range of clinical activity in adult cancers (multiple myeloma, melanoma, breast and ovarian cancers, and lymphoma), but, until recently, its use has been limited in the treatment of pediatric malignancies. The administration of bone-marrow ablative doses (180 mg/m^2) of melphalan followed by rescue with autologous bone-marrow transplant has resulted in high response rates in children with neuroblastoma (11 of 14 patients), Ewing's sarcoma (6 of 8 patients)[91,92] and acute leukemia (7 of 7 patients).[93] At more standard doses (35 mg/m^2), melphalan also appears to be active against rhabdomyosarcoma.[94]

Like other chemically reactive compounds, melphalan is rapidly cleared from the body. It is inactivated following spontaneous hydrolysis or alkylation reactions with plasma or tissue proteins. Melphalan does not appear to undergo any appreciable enzymatic degradation.[95] The absorption of melphalan following oral administration has been reported to be incomplete and highly variable;[95-98] the fraction of a dose absorbed usually ranges from 32% to 100%,[96,97] although patients with no detectable drug in plasma and urine following an oral dose have been reported.[98] In addition, the incidence of myelosuppression is lower with oral than with parenteral melphalan,[99] and poor therapeutic response may be attributable in part to poor absorption in individual patients.[98] The disposition following intravenous administration in children and adults is similar.[100] With standard parenteral doses, the terminal half-life ranges from 60 to 100 minutes,[96,97,101,102] with a total clearance of more than 200 ml/min per square meter.[96,101] Drug disposition in children is not dose dependent, since pharmacokinetic parameters in patients receiving high-dose therapy (up to 180 mg/m^2) are similar to those found at standard doses.[100,103-105] Renal excretion is a minor route of elimination, accounting for less than 20% of total drug clearance.[101] However, patients with renal dysfunction have a higher incidence of hematotoxicity,[106] and in nephrectomized animals the half-life of intravenous melphalan is prolonged and enhanced myelosuppression is observed.[107] Alberts and associates suggest a 50% dose reduction in patients with renal dysfunction based on these results.

At standard doses (5–35 mg/m^2), myelosuppression is the primary toxicity, and cumulative marrow damage has been observed with repeated doses.[37] At high doses with autologous bone-marrow reinfusion, gastrointestinal toxicity (mucositis, esophagitis, and diarrhea) becomes dose limiting.[91,92]

Nitrosoureas (Carmustine, Lomustine)

The nitrosoureas are a group of lipid-soluble alkylating agents (Fig. 9-4) that are highly active in experimental tumor models, including intracranially implanted tumors. Of the hundreds of nitrosourea compounds screened for antitumor activity, the most active agents are the series of 2-chloroethyl derivatives that includes carmustine (BCNU) and lomustine (CCNU), the nitrosoureas most widely used in pediatric oncology.[108,109] Rapid spontaneous chemical decomposition of these compounds in solution generates both an alkylating intermediate (chloroethyldiazohydroxide) and an isocyanate moiety that can carbamoylate amine groups on proteins. Alkylation, including crosslinking of DNA by both the monofunctional lomustine and the bifunctional carmustine,[46] is generally accepted as the primary mechanism of action of the nitrosoureas.[110,111] However, the isocyanates can inhibit DNA repair of alkylator damage and may contribute to both the antitumor activity and the toxicity of the nitrosoureas.[108,109]

The nitrosoureas have been used primarily to treat patients with brain tumors or lymphomas. However, the clinical utility of these agents in combination regimens is limited by delayed and cumulative myelosuppression and other serious long-term cumulative toxicities (*e.g.,* renal and pulmonary).

Biotransformation and Pharmacokinetics

In addition to their rapid spontaneous decomposition, nitrosoureas undergo significant hepatic metabolism.[112] The cyclohexyl ring of lomustine is hydroxylated to a number of isomeric derivatives that are more soluble and have greater alkylating activity than the parent drug.[108] Carmustine is inactivated by denitrosation through the action of microsomal enzymes. As a result of this rapid spontaneous and enzymatic degradation, the clearance of nitrosoureas from plasma is extremely fast. In early studies of carmustine[113] and lomustine,[114] parent drug could not be detected in plasma following intravenous or oral administration. With high-dose carmustine administered by intravenous infusion, the half-life was 22 minutes, with a clearance exceeding 2000 ml/min per square meter.[115] Similar results have been reported with more standard doses of the drug (half-life 70 minutes; clearance 1700 ml/min per square meter).[116] The nitrosoureas are well absorbed when administered orally. However, orally administered lomustine is nearly all converted to hydroxylated metabolites presystemically during its first pass through the liver.[117] These results confirm that the metabolites of lomustine are primarily responsible for the drug's antitumor activity. Although carmustine is also well absorbed, severe vomiting following oral administration frequently precludes adequate absorption.[118] The lipid-soluble nitrosoureas are widely distributed and readily penetrate into the central nervous system. Following equilibration, drug concentrations in the cerebrospinal fluid (CSF) approximate those in plasma,[114,119,120] which accounts for the activity of this group of drugs in treating brain tumors.

Toxicity

Gastrointestinal toxicity (nausea and vomiting) and cumulative delayed myelosuppression are the most consistent side-effects of the nitrosoureas. The nadir of blood counts occurs 4 to 5 weeks following administration, and the platelet count tends to be the most affected. With repeated dosing, chronic marrow hypoplasia develops.[108] With cumulative doses of more than 1500 mg/m^2, progressive renal atrophy has been reported.[121,122] Although in children this complication has been primarily associated with sesmustine (methylCCNU), it has also been reported following high cumulative doses of lomustine. Mitchell and Schein recommend that if nitrosourea therapy continues for more than 15 months or if cumulative doses of greater than 1000 mg/m^2 are reached, patients should be evaluated for nephrotoxicity and therapy discontinued if renal size or glomerular filtration rate is significantly decreased.[108] Similar cumulative doses (greater than 1500 mg/m^2) of carmustine are associated with progressive (and frequently fatal) pulmonary toxicity characterized by cough, dyspnea, tachypnea, and a restrictive-type ventilatory defect.[123,124] Central nervous system toxicity has been reported rarely.[108] High-dose carmustine (300–750 mg/m^2) can produce hypotension, tachycardia, flushing, and confusion.[116]

Drug Interactions

In an animal model, phenobarbital enhances the microsomal metabolism of the nitrosoureas and significantly reduces the antitumor activity of carmustine and, to a lesser extent, that of lomustine.[125] This potential interaction has not been well studied in humans.

Nonclassical Alkylating Agents

Cisplatin

Cisplatin (*cis*-diamminedichloroplatinum [II]) is a heavy-metal coordination complex (Fig. 9-4) that is not a true alkylating agent. However, it appears to exert its cytotoxic effects by platination, a mechanism analogous to alkylation. Through the formation of reactive (aquated) intermediates, cisplatin can directly and covalently bind to DNA, leading to the formation of intrastrand and interstrand DNA crosslinks.[126] Cisplatin is an effective agent for the treatment of testicular tumors[127] and has demonstrated activity against osteosarcoma, neuroblastoma, Wilms' tumor, germ cell tumors, and brain tumors.[128-130] The drug is administered intravenously on a variety of schedules including single dose (infused over an hour), divided dose (*e.g.,* daily for 5 days), and continuous (5-day) infusion. The divided dose and continuous-infusion schedules may lessen the gastrointestinal and renal toxicities.[127] Other strategies used to overcome the drug's dose-limiting nephrotoxicity include aggressive hydration and diuresis with mannitol,[131] the use of hypertonic sodium chloride solutions to promote chloruresis,[132] and the coadministration of sodium thiosulfate.[133]

PHARMACOKINETICS. The reactive intermediates of cisplatin are rapidly bound to protein and tissue and react with nucleophilic groups on protein to form covalent bonds.[134] Once protein bound, the aquated platinum intermediates are inactivated. Only the free (unbound) platinum species, which can be separated from the bound forms by ultrafiltration of plasma, are cytotoxic.[135,136] The interaction of platinum species with protein is a time-dependent reaction, and within 2 to 4 hours more than 90% of total platinum in plasma is protein bound.[137] This represents a major route of elimination of cytotoxic platinum intermediates.

The kinetic behaviors of bound and unbound (active) forms of cisplatin differ appreciably (Fig. 9-6). After an initial rapid decay, total platinum (more than 95% protein bound) persists in plasma and can be detected in urine for many days.

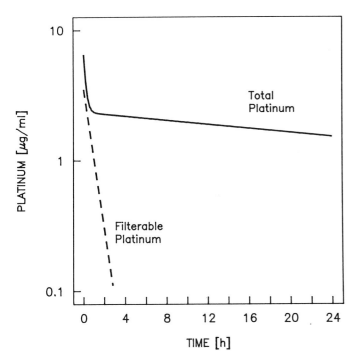

FIGURE 9-6. Plasma disappearance curves for different platinum species following a dose of cisplatin. Filterable, or unbound, platinum is believed to be the active form of the drug. Within 2 to 3 hours, most of the circulating total platinum is irreversibly protein bound and inactive.

The terminal half-life of total platinum ranges from 1 to 4 days.[135,137] In contrast, the unbound, active form has a much more rapid decline, with a terminal half-life of less than 1 hour.[135,138] In children, the half-lives of total and ultrafilterable (unbound) platinum are 44 hours and 1.3 hours, respectively.[129] Drug exposure (measured by the area under the plasma concentration–time curve) is not affected by the schedule of drug administration.[139,140]

Twenty-five percent to 75% of a dose of cisplatin is excreted in the urine as total platinum.[137,141] Initially, total platinum clearance equals or exceeds the creatinine clearance, but as protein binding proceeds, renal clearance of total platinum drops to only a small fraction of creatinine clearance.[135] The renal clearance of the non-protein-bound species of platinum is correlated with and actually exceeds creatinine clearance, suggesting tubular secretion.[139,142] Approximately 25% of unbound platinum species is excreted in the urine, and the degree of renal excretion is schedule dependent (greater with short infusions).[143] In a single patient with impaired renal function, the peak level of active, unbound platinum was elevated but the terminal half-life was not prolonged,[141] presumably due to the rapid reaction of these active species with plasma and tissue protein leading to inactivation. However, dosage reductions in patients with renal dysfunction are probably indicated, since the drug's nephrotoxic effects could further impair renal function.[35]

TOXICITY. Nephrotoxicity, manifested as azotemia and electrolyte disturbances (especially hypomagnesemia requiring supplementation), was the dose-limiting toxicity in the initial clinical trials with cisplatin. The exact mechanism of cisplatin nephrotoxicity is still not clear, but patients experience a reduction in renal blood flow and glomerular filtration rate as well as a loss of tubular function. Pathologic changes are noted primarily in the epithelium of the distal tubule and collecting ducts.[144] Although pretreatment hydration, diuresis, chloruresis, and less-toxic dose schedules have reduced the incidence and severity of this side-effect, moderate and permanent reductions in the glomerular filtration rate of patients receiving cisplatin have been documented.[145-147] As a result of its nephrotoxic effects, cisplatin can alter its own elimination rate as well as that of other drugs that rely on renal excretion, such as methotrexate.[148] In a recent series, the renal clearance of free platinum fell from nearly 500 ml/min with the first course to 150 ml/min by the fourth course in patients receiving repeated doses, probably as a result of decreased renal tubular secretion of the drug.[149] Higher renal cortical concentrations of platinum were found at autopsy in patients who had clinical renal toxicity than in patients without evidence of renal toxicity.[150]

As methods to prevent nephrotoxicity have allowed the administration of higher individual and cumulative doses of the drug, ototoxicity[151] and peripheral neuropathy[152] have become more prominent. The irreversible hearing loss is in the high-frequency range and appears to be related to a cumulative dose of cisplatin of greater than 400 mg/m^2.[151,153] Other toxicities include prominent nausea and vomiting, mild myelosuppression, Raynaud's phenomenon, and hypersensitivity reactions.[127]

DRUG INTERACTIONS. Giving cisplatin in combination with radiation and several other anticancer drugs, including cytarabine, 5-fluorouracil, and etoposide, results in synergistic cytotoxicity.[127] The plasma pharmacokinetics of cisplatin do not appear to be altered by agents used to reduce its nephrotoxicity (chloruresis,[154] sodium thiosulfate,[133] diuretics[141]).

Dacarbazine (DTIC)

Decarbazine is a triazene originally developed as an inhibitor of purine biosynthesis.[155] However, although its mechanism of action is not completely understood, it is clear that dacarbazine does not exert its antitumor effects as an antimetabolite. Instead, the compound appears to undergo microsomal metabolic activation (demethylation), presumably in the liver, to yield a reactive alkylating (methylating) species and the primary metabolite 5-aminoimidazole-4-carboxamide (AIC).[39] Dacarbazine is also light sensitive and undergoes photodecomposition to form cytotoxic derivatives, including the purine analogue azahypoxanthine.[39] Although this pathway may not be significant *in vivo,* commercial formulations can undergo decomposition if not protected from light,[156] and *in vitro* cytotoxicity of the drug can be enhanced by light exposure,[157] complicating interpretation of *in vitro* studies.

Dacarbazine is generally administered intravenously (150–250 mg/m^2) on a divided once-daily dosage schedule for 5 days. It is used primarily in the treatment of solid tumors (Table 9-4). Absorption following oral administration is slow, incomplete, and variable.[158] Following intravenous administration, the drug is rapidly cleared from the plasma, with a terminal half-life of 40 minutes and a total clearance of 450 ml/min per square meter. Half of the dose is excreted unchanged in the urine, and renal clearance exceeds the glomerular filtration rate, suggesting the drug is also eliminated by renal tubular secretion.[159] The remainder of the dose presumably undergoes biotransformation. The half-life and renal clearance of the metabolite AIC are similar to that of the parent drug.[159]

Gastrointestinal toxicity, consisting of moderate to severe nausea and vomiting, is the primary toxicity and is frequently dose limiting. Tolerance usually develops over the 5-day course of administration. At standard doses, myelosuppression is mild. Other side-effects include a flu-like syndrome with malaise, fever, and myalgias; mild hepatic dysfunction; and local pain at the site of intravenous injection. Rare cases of liver failure and death from veno-occlusive disease and hepatic vein thrombosis (Budd–Chiari syndrome) have been associated with the use of this drug.[160]

Procarbazine

Procarbazine is one of a group of methylhydrazine analogues that were originally synthesized as monoamine oxidase inhibitors but were discovered to have antitumor activity in animals. Procarbazine is currently used as part of the MOPP chemotherapy regimen for the treatment of Hodgkin's disease.[53] It is also active against brain tumors.[54,55,161] Like the other previously discussed alkylating agents, cyclophosphamide and dacarbazine, procarbazine appears to be a prodrug that requires metabolic activation *in vivo* to express its antitumor activity.[162] This activation yields both alkylating (methylating) and free-radical intermediates, which appear to produce the drug's antitumor effect.

The spontaneous chemical decomposition and biotransformation of procarbazine is complex and beyond the scope of this chapter. It has recently been reviewed.[162] Metabolic activation probably occurs in the liver and is catalyzed by the cytochrome P-450 enzyme complex.[163] In liver perfusion studies, procarbazine is extensively converted to its active azo metabolite.[164]

The disposition of procarbazine and its active intermediates has not been well characterized in humans. The drug is rapidly and completely absorbed from the gastrointestinal tract.[165] Along with the nearly complete first-pass conversion to cytotoxic metabolites, this probably accounts for the activity of the drug when administered orally. After intravenous administration, procarbazine is rapidly cleared from plasma via biotransformation, with a half-life of less than 10 minutes.[166] The metabolites of procarbazine are excreted primarily in the urine. Procarbazine or unidentified metabolites enter the CSF readily.[166] Drugs such as phenobarbital and phenytoin that are capable of inducing hepatic microsomal enzymes can increase the rate of procarbazine activation.[162] On the other hand, procarbazine can inhibit the biotransformation of the barbiturates, phenothiazines, and other sedatives, resulting in potentiation of their sedative effects. The inhibition of monoamine oxidase by procarbazine can put patients at risk for hypertensive reactions from foods high in tyramine (*e.g.,* bananas, wine, cheese).

The primary toxicities of procarbazine include nausea and vomiting and myelosuppression. Some patients develop evidence of neurotoxicity consisting of paresthesias, somnolence, depression, or agitation. Neurotoxicity is prominent with high-dose intravenous administration.[167] Patients are also at risk for the long-term toxicities (including carcinogenesis) discussed in the introductory remarks.

ANTIMETABOLITES

The antimetabolites are close structural analogues of vital intermediates in the biosynthetic pathways of nucleic acids and proteins. By acting as fraudulent substrates for the enzymes in these various pathways, antimetabolites either inhibit synthesis of cellular macromolecules and their building blocks or are incorporated into the macromolecules, resulting in a defective product. Antimetabolites important in the treatment of pediatric cancers include the folate analogue methotrexate, the purine analogues 6-mercaptopurine and 6-thioguanine, and the

pyrimidine analogues cytarabine and 5-fluorouracil. The structures of these antimetabolites and their naturally occurring counterparts are shown in Figure 9-7.

In general, the clinical pharmacology of these agents is similar to that of the endogenous compounds they structurally resemble. The absorptive, metabolic, and excretory pathways are frequently shared by both the normal metabolite and the antimetabolite, and the rate of elimination is very rapid for most of the antimetabolites. Most of the antimetabolites are prodrugs that require metabolic activation to express their cytotoxic effects. The purine and pyrimidine analogues, for example, usually require intracellular conversion to nucleotides, which are the active forms of these drugs. Since most antimetabolites interfere directly with DNA synthesis, they are cell-cycle and S-phase specific; that is, the maximal cytotoxic effect occurs in cells that are synthesizing DNA. This, in part, explains the highly schedule-dependent nature of this class of anticancer drugs, since more prolonged drug exposure increases the chance of exposing a higher proportion of the cell population to the drugs during active DNA replication.

Methotrexate

Methotrexate is the most widely used antimetabolite in pediatric oncology. It is effective in the treatment of acute lymphoblastic leukemia, non-Hodgkin's lymphoma, the histiocytoses, and osteosarcoma. Methotrexate is administered on an intermittent schedule by a variety of routes, including orally, intramuscularly, subcutaneously, intrathecally, and intravenously. With intravenous therapy, an extraordinarily wide range of doses has been employed, ranging from a 10-mg bolus to 33,000 mg/m² as a 24-hour infusion. Doses above 100 to 300 mg/m², which are usually administered by continuous infusion, must be followed by a course of the rescue agent leucovorin (5-formyl-tetrahydrofolate) to prevent the development of severe toxicities. The loading and infusion doses required to achieve a desired steady-state plasma concentration ($[MTX]_{plasma}$) can be estimated from the following formulas:[168]

$$\text{Loading dose (mg/m}^2) = (1.5 \times 10^7) \cdot ([MTX]_{plasma})$$

$$\text{Infusion dose (mg/m}^2/\text{hr}) = (3 \times 10^6) \cdot ([MTX]_{plasma})$$

To achieve a steady state plasma level of 10 μM (1×10^{-5} M), the loading dose would be 150 mg/m² followed by an infusion of 30 mg/m² per hour. The clinical pharmacology of methotrexate has been extensively studied, and it is probably the best understood anticancer drug.[169]

Mechanism of Action

Methotrexate is a structural analogue of folic acid, a required cofactor for the synthesis of both purines and the pyrimidine, thymidine. As a result of the substitution of an amino group for the hydroxyl group at the 4 position on the pteridine ring of folic acid (Fig. 9-7), methotrexate is a tight-binding inhibitor of dihydrofolate reductase, the enzyme responsible for converting folates to their active chemically reduced (tetrahydrofolate) form.[170] In the presence of an excess of methotrexate, intracellular tetrahydrofolate pools become depleted, leading to depletion of DNA precursors and inhibition of DNA synthesis. In addition, the accumulation of partially oxidized dihydrofolic acid, resulting from the inhibition of dihydrofolate reductase, appears to contribute to the inhibition of *de novo* purine synthesis.[171,172] Critical determinants of methotrexate cytotoxicity include (1) the rate of thymidylate synthesis, since

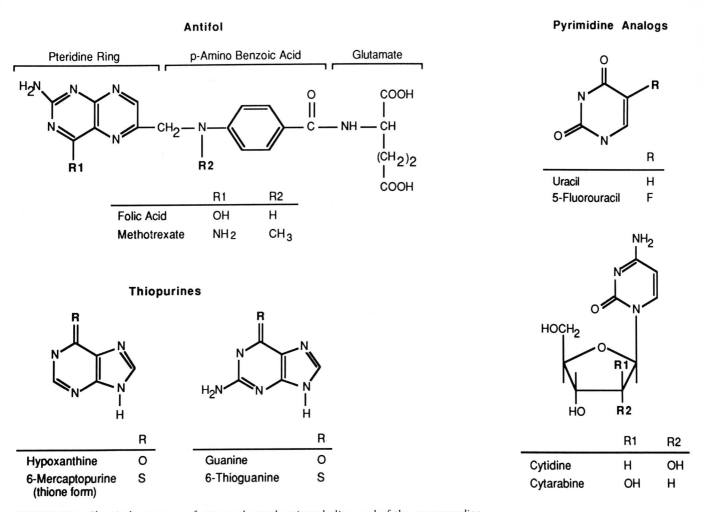

FIGURE 9-7. Chemical structures of commonly used antimetabolites and of the corresponding endogenous compounds of which they are analogues.

the synthesis of thymidylate from uridylate is the only reaction that oxidizes the folate cofactor to the inactive dihydrofolate form[173]; and (2) the presence of intracellular methotrexate concentrations in excess of dihydrofolate reductase binding sites, since intracellular levels of this target enzyme are 20- to 30-fold higher than required to maintain tetrahydrofolate pools.[170,174]

Methotrexate shares membrane-transport processes and intracellular metabolic pathways with the naturally occurring folates. It competes with the tetrahydrofolates for an energy-dependent transport system for cell entry. Upon entry, methotrexate is rapidly and tightly bound to the target enzyme, and uptake is unidirectional until the enzyme binding sites are saturated, allowing for even greater intracellular accumulation of drug.[170] With the accumulation of free intracellular drug in excess of enzyme binding sites, methotrexate, like the naturally occurring folates, is metabolized to polyglutamate derivatives, which cannot efflux from the cell. Methotrexate polyglutamate formation enhances the cytotoxicity of the drug by allowing even greater accumulation of free intracellular drug and retention of the drug within the cell even after extracellular drug disappears. Methotrexate polyglutamates are also more potent inhibitors of dihydrofolate reductase and are capable of directly inhibiting other enzymes in the synthetic pathways for thymidine (thymidylate synthase) and purines.[173,175,176] Methotrexate polyglutamate formation is optimal

in vitro when cells are exposed to high concentrations for long periods.

Pharmacokinetics

At standard oral doses of 7.5 to 20 mg/m², the rate and extent of absorption of methotrexate is highly variable.[177-180] Peak levels can occur from 0.5 to 5 hours after administration. The portion of the dose that is absorbed ranges from 5% to 97%. Absorption is also saturable so that as the dose is increased, the fraction absorbed declines.[181-183] Therefore, simply increasing the dose in patients who have low plasma levels following standard oral doses, may not overcome poor bioavailability. Several studies have suggested that the poor and variable absorption of methotrexate in some patients might influence the outcome of therapy in acute lymphoblastic leukemia.[184,185] The bioavailability of oral methotrexate can also be significantly reduced when administered with food.[186] When administered intramuscularly or subcutaneously, methotrexate is completely absorbed.[182,187,188]

The disposition of methotrexate in children differs from that in adults.[189,190] In one study, children had lower plasma concentrations of methotrexate and excreted the drug in the urine more rapidly following a 6-hour infusion than did adults.[191] The volume of distribution was also greater in children. The plasma disappearance of methotrexate is multiphasic, with a terminal half-life of 8 to 12 hours.[190] Retention of the drug in large extravascular fluid collections such as ascites or pleural fluid is associated with prolongation of the half-life as a result of slow release of retained drug into the circulation.[169] This prolonged exposure to the drug can result in more severe toxicity.

Methotrexate is eliminated primarily by renal excretion, undergoing glomerular filtration and both renal tubular reabsorption and secretion.[192,193] Approximately 70% to 90% of a dose is excreted unchanged in the urine, most within the first 6 hours. The renal clearance of methotrexate can exceed the rate of creatinine clearance. In patients with significant renal dysfunction, methotrexate clearance is delayed, resulting in prolonged exposure and severe toxicities. High-dose methotrexate thus should not be given to patients with a creatinine clearance of less than 50% to 75% of normal. Low-dose therapy should be withheld in patients with a serum creatinine level greater than 2 mg/dl. Any patient suspected of having renal dysfunction who receives methotrexate should have the plasma levels closely monitored and receive leucovorin if drug clearance is delayed.[10]

Methotrexate is also metabolized in the liver to 7-hydroxy-methotrexate.[194] Although this is a minor route of elimination, plasma concentrations of 7-hydroxy-methotrexate are frequently equivalent to or exceed those of methotrexate following high-dose infusions,[195,196] presumably due to the slower clearance of the metabolite. 7-Hydroxy-methotrexate may compromise the cytotoxicity of methotrexate by competing with it for cell transport and polyglutamation. However, once polyglutamated, 7-hydroxy-methotrexate appears to be able to bind to and inhibit dihydrofolate reductase.[170] Methotrexate clearance is not significantly altered with hepatic dysfunction. However, modification of the methotrexate dose in patients with abnormal liver function tests may be indicated to avoid further hepatic damage.

Total methotrexate clearance (renal + metabolic) is approximately 100 ml/min per square meter, but may differ widely among patients.[169,197] In patients with normal creatinine clearance, there is not a good correlation between methotrexate clearance and creatinine clearance.[198] Renal tubular dysfunction, not measured by creatinine clearance, may account for this disparity. A small test dose of methotrexate can more accurately predict the kinetics and steady-state level of a high-dose infusion.[198] Optimal management dictates that each course of high-dose methotrexate be closely monitored by following renal function and plasma methotrexate concentration to determine the dose and duration of leucovorin rescue.

Toxicity

The primary toxicities of methotrexate are myelosuppression and orointestinal mucositis, which occur 5 to 14 days after the dose. The development of toxic reactions is related to both the concentration of drug and the duration of exposure.[168] In patients receiving a 6-hour infusion of methotrexate, a 48-hour methotrexate concentration above 1 μM was associated with the development of significant toxicity. These toxicities can be prevented by the timely administration of the tetrahydrofolate leucovorin. With the use of careful therapeutic drug monitoring and continuation of leucovorin rescue until plasma methotrexate concentration has fallen below 0.1 μM, the toxicity of high-dose methotrexate can be avoided in most patients.[168,169]

Nephrotoxicity observed with high-dose methotrexate can delay methotrexate clearance and markedly enhance the drug's other toxicities.[199] The renal damage may be related to precipitation of methotrexate or 7-hydroxy-methotrexate in acidic urine or to direct toxic effects on the renal tubule.[169]

Drug precipitation can be prevented by vigorous intravenous hydration and alkalinization of the urine. The development of renal dysfunction during high-dose methotrexate is a medical emergency. Patients must be closely monitored and the leucovorin dose increased in proportion to the plasma methotrexate concentration (see recommendations by Bleyer[200]). Hemodialysis and hemoperfusion have not been useful for drug removal in patients with renal dysfunction.[201–203]

Hepatic toxicity consisting of transient transaminasemia and, less commonly, hyperbilirubinemia has been associated with both standard and high doses of methotrexate but is more common and more severe with higher doses. Hepatic fibrosis has been observed primarily in patients receiving chronic low-dose methotrexate.[190] Other side-effects include a dermatitis characterized by erythema and desquamation,[204] allergic reactions, and acute pneumonitis.[205] High-dose methotrexate can also produce acute, subacute, and chronic neurotoxicity, particularly in association with cranial irradiation.[206,207]

Resistance

Mechanisms of resistance to methotrexate identified experimentally include decreased membrane transport, increased levels of the target enzyme dihydrofolate reductase, altered affinity of dihydrofolate reductase for methotrexate, decreased polyglutamation of methotrexate, and decreased thymidylate synthase activity.[173] Increases in target enzyme levels have been associated with gene amplification of the sequence encoding for the enzyme,[19,208] a phenomenon that has also been documented in lymphoblasts from a patient whose tumor was clinically resistant to methotrexate.[209]

Drug Interactions

A number of drugs have been associated with an increase in toxicity when coadministered with methotrexate.[36] The most significant interactions involve agents that interfere with methotrexate excretion, primarily by competing for renal tubular secretion. The list of such drugs includes probenecid, salicylates, sulfisoxazole, penicillins, and the nonsteroidal anti-inflammatories indomethacin and ketoprofen. Nephrotoxic drugs such as the aminoglycosides and cisplatin may also alter the clearance of methotrexate.[36] Pharmacodynamic interactions resulting in synergistic cytotoxic effects have been reported with methotrexate and 5-fluorouracil, methotrexate and cytarabine, and methotrexate and L-asparaginase.[210]

Purine Analogues

The two purine antimetabolites used in the treatment of pediatric cancers, 6-mercaptopurine and 6-thioguanine, are thiol-substituted derivatives of the naturally occurring purine bases hypoxanthine and guanine (Fig. 9-7). Both agents are prodrugs and must be converted intracellularly to ribonucleotides before expressing antitumor activity.

6-Mercaptopurine

6-mercaptopurine has been used in the treatment of acute lymphoblastic leukemia for more than three decades, initially as an induction agent but now primarily for the maintenance of remission. It is also used in the treatment of chronic myelogenous leukemia and histiocytosis. In standard maintenance regimens, 6-mercaptopurine is administered orally at a dose of 75 to 100 mg/m² per day. Recently, high-dose (50 mg/m² per hour for 48 hours) continuous-infusion therapy was evaluated in an attempt to circumvent the limited bioavailability and the low and variable plasma levels observed with oral dosing.[211] The common toxicities of 6-mercaptopurine include myelosuppression, hepatic dysfunction (elevated transaminases and cholestatic jaundice), and mucositis. The exact mechanism of action of 6-mercaptopurine is still unclear, but following intracellular activation it interferes with *de novo* purine synthesis and purine ribonucleotide interconversion. In the form of 6-thioguanylate, 6-mercaptopurine is also incorporated into DNA and RNA.[212,213]

BIOTRANSFORMATION. 6-Mercaptopurine is extensively metabolized *in vivo* (Fig. 9-8). The primary degradative pathway is conversion to the inactive metabolite 6-thiouric acid by the enzyme xanthine oxidase. In addition, 6-mercaptopurine can be methylated on the thiol group and then undergo oxidation leading either to 6-methylthiouric acid or to the hydroxylated derivative, which is then conjugated with glucuronide prior to excretion.[212] Intracellular activation involves conversion to the ribonucleotide derivative by the enzyme hypoxanthine:guanine phosphoribosyltransferase. The active intracellular metabolites are thought to be 6-thioinosine, 6-methylthioinosine, 6-thioxanthosine, and 6-thioguanosine.[212]

PHARMACOKINETICS. Specific methods have recently been developed that can quantitate 6-mercaptopurine and distinguish it from its major metabolites. Using these methods, Zimm and coworkers found that, in contrast to earlier reports, a standard oral dose of 6-mercaptopurine is poorly (less than 20%) absorbed and that the resulting plasma drug levels are also highly variable.[214] Moreover, in that study, only one third of these patients achieved plasma concentrations of the drug above the minimal *in vitro* cytotoxic concentration of 1 μM.[215] Significant interpatient variability following oral dosing has been confirmed by other investigators.[216,217] Significant intraindividual variability has also been noted in patients monitored following multiple doses over the course of maintenance therapy (Balis FM: Unpublished data). The bioavailability of 6-mercaptopurine is apparently limited by the extensive first-pass metabolism of the drug by xanthine oxidase in the liver and intestinal mucosa. When 6-mercaptopurine is coadministered with the xanthine oxidase inhibitor allopurinol, the fraction of the dose absorbed increases fivefold.[218]

6-Mercaptopurine is eliminated primarily by biotransformation. However, renal excretion of unchanged drug does become quantitatively significant (20%–40%) with high intravenous doses.[211,219] Elimination is rapid, with a total clearance rate of 800 ml/min per square meter and a half-life of less than 1 hour.[214,218] The intravenous infusion of 50 mg/m² per hour achieves steady-state plasma drug concentrations in excess of 5 μM and CSF concentrations greater than 1 μM, well above concentrations of the drug known to be cytotoxic *in vitro*.

DRUG INTERACTIONS. The classic example of a drug interaction in cancer chemotherapy is the effect of allopurinol on the catabolism of 6-mercaptopurine to thiouric acid. When these two agents are administered concurrently, the hemato-

FIGURE 9-8. Metabolic pathways for 6-mercaptopurine, including intracellular activation to ribonucleotides (active intracelluar metabolites are 6-thioinosine, 6-metylthioinosine, 6-thioxanthosine, and 6-thioguanosine) and degradation, primarily to thiouric acid. Enzymes catalyzing reactions are shown in *italics*. 6-MP, 6-mercaptopurine; 6-methylMP, 6-methylmercaptopurine; PRPP, phosphoribosylpyrophosphate.

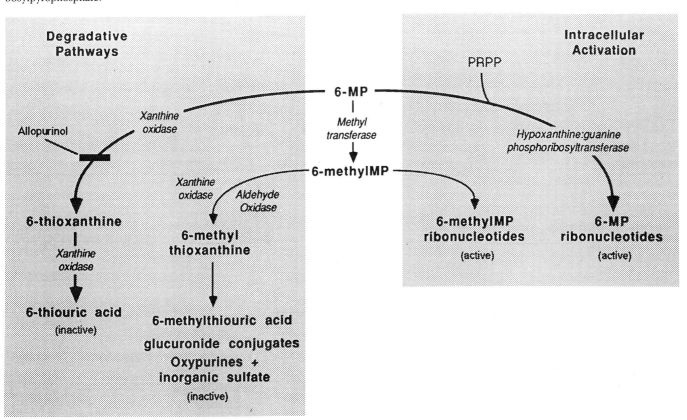

logic toxicity of 6-mercaptopurine is significantly enhanced.[220] As mentioned earlier, allopurinol pretreatment results in a fivefold increase in the fraction of the dose of 6-mercaptopurine that passes into the systemic circulation following oral administration.[218] However, the disposition of intravenously administered 6-mercaptopurine is not affected by the coadministration of allopurinol (Fig. 9-9).[211,218,219] This differential effect is due to the inhibition of first-pass metabolism of 6-mercaptopurine by allopurinol.[218] The dose of oral 6-mercaptopurine should be reduced by 75% when administered to patients receiving allopurinol, but intravenous 6-mercaptopurine doses need not be modified unless the patient has renal dysfunction. (The renal excretion of unchanged 6-mercaptopurine increases from 20% to more than 40% of the dose in patients receiving the drug by intravenous infusion and also receiving allopurinol.[211]) Although allopurinol enhances the bioavailability of 6-mercaptopurine, it has not been shown to augment the antileukemic effect of the drug[36] and may actually antagonize the antitumor effects on a pharmacodynamic level.[218] Methotrexate and folates also inhibit xanthine oxidase, and methotrexate can minimally enhance 6-mercaptopurine bioavailability.[220]

6-Thioguanine

The use of 6-thioguanine in pediatric oncology has been limited to the therapy of the nonlymphocytic leukemias. The drug is administered orally in doses of 75 to 100 mg/m² daily or twice daily. Myelosuppression is the primary toxicity. Mucositis and hepatotoxicity are less common than with 6-mercaptopurine. The pathways for intracellular activation are similar to those for 6-mercaptopurine, and, once converted to a ribonucleotide, 6-thioguanine also inhibits purine biosynthesis and interconversion and is incorporated into both DNA and RNA. The catabolism of 6-thioguanine, however, differs from that of 6-mercaptopurine.[213] The primary pathway is methylation of the thiol group followed by oxidation and elimination of inorganic sulfate. 6-Thioguanine is also deaminated to the inactive metabolite 6-thioxanthine, which is then oxidized by xanthine oxidase to 6-thiouric acid.[213] Although allopurinol interferes with this last step, this is a minor pathway, and the substrate that accumulates (6-thioxanthine) is inactive. Thus the coadministration of allopurinol and 6-thioguanine does not require a dose modification.

The bioavailability of oral 6-thioguanine is poor, and plasma levels are variable, with a 30-fold range in peak plasma concentration after a 100-mg/m² dose.[222,223] In most patients studied, plasma concentrations were below that required *in vitro* to produce maximal cytotoxicity.[223] The bioavailability was diminished further in nonfasting patients and patients experiencing nausea and vomiting. Intravenous administration has been evaluated on a single-dose[224] and a daily-for-5-days schedule.[225] With standard doses (less than 100 mg/m²), the drug is cleared rapidly. Total clearance is greater than 2000 ml/min per square meter, and the terminal half-life is 20 minutes.[224] However, a reduced clearance rate (320 ml/min per

FIGURE 9-9. Effect of allopurinol on plasma levels of 6-mercaptopurine (75 mg/m²) after intravenous (**A**) and oral (**B**) administration. Points represent the mean and standard error of five patients studied both with and without allopurinol pretreatment. (Used with permission from Zimm S et al: Inhibition of first-pass metabolism in cancer chemotherapy: Interaction of 6-mercaptopurine and allopurinol. Clin Pharmacol Ther 34:810–817, 1983)

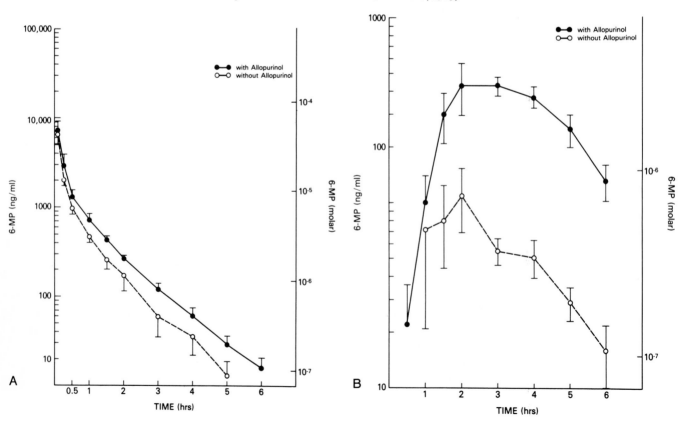

square meter) and a longer terminal half-life (2–6 hours) at doses exceeding 700 mg/m^2 indicate that the pharmacokinetics of this drug are dose dependent.[224,225] 6-Thioguanine is cleared primarily by biotransformation, with only small amounts of the drug excreted unchanged in the urine.[226] Saturation of the degradative enzymes at high doses probably accounts for the dose-dependent kinetics.

Pyrimidine Analogues

Cytarabine (Cytosine arabinoside; Ara-C)

Cytarabine is an arabinose nucleoside analogue of deoxycytidine (Fig. 9-7) that is highly active in the treatment of the acute leukemias and lymphoma. Once activated intracellularly, cytarabine interferes with DNA replication and repair through inhibition of DNA polymerase and, more importantly, through incorporation into DNA.[227,228] Depending on the dose and schedule of cytarabine used, incorporation into DNA is thought to inhibit chain elongation, result in chain termination or reinitiation at sites of previously replicated segments, or cause DNA strand breaks.[227] A wide range of doses and schedules of cytarabine have been employed. The standard dose is 100 to 200 mg/m^2 either as a bolus injection every 12 hours or by continuous infusion, and it is usually administered daily for 5 to 7 days. High-dose regimens (3–9 g/m^2 either every 12 hours for 4 to 12 doses or as a continuous infusion) have also been implemented with the intention of overcoming resistance mechanisms.[229,230] Low-dose cytarabine regimens (5–20 mg/m^2 per day over several weeks) are purported to induce differentiation of leukemic cells.[231]

BIOTRANSFORMATION. After entering cells via the carrier-mediated nucleoside-transport system, cytarabine is converted to the active nucleotide cytosine arabinoside triphosphate (ara-CTP) by three sequential phosphorylations catalyzed by intracellular kinases (Fig. 9-10). Ara-CTP then competes with the natural substrate deoxycytidine triphosphate (dCTP) for DNA replicative and repair enzymes. Alternatively, inactivating

enzymes (deaminases) found in high concentrations within the cell can catabolize cytarabine and ara-CMP to the inactive by-products uridine arabinoside (ara-U) and ara-UMP.[232] Cytidine deaminase is a ubiquitous enzyme, and the catabolism of cytarabine to ara-U is the primary route of elimination for the drug. Alterations in these various steps can result in drug resistance, including a decrease in membrane transport, a decrease in activation by deoxycytidine kinase, an increase in degradation by cytidine deaminase, and an increase in the competing natural substrate, dCTP.[229]

PHARMACOKINETICS. The pharmacokinetic characteristics of cytarabine are directly related to the activity of the major degradative enzyme, cytidine deaminase. Less than 20% of an oral dose of cytarabine reaches the systemic circulation because of the high levels of this enzyme in gastrointestinal epithelium and liver, which catabolize the drug presystemically.[233] The hepatic extraction ratio is estimated to be as high as 80%.[234] Cytarabine is completely absorbed when administered subcutaneously.[235]

Drug elimination is rapid with intravenous dosing. Total clearance is generally reported to be 1000 ml/min per square meter or greater, and the postdistributive half-life is 2 to 3 hours.[230,233,235–237] Metabolism to ara-U accounts for 80% to 90% of total cytarabine clearance, whereas renal clearance accounts for less than 10% of total clearance. The ara-U formed is excreted in the urine. Because of the ubiquity of cytidine deaminase (liver, gastrointestinal tract, plasma, leukocytes, and other tissues), hepatic dysfunction will not significantly alter the rate of elimination of cytarabine. With high-dose prolonged intravenous infusions, steady-state plasma concentration of cytarabine was 5 μM at a dose of 2 g/m^2 per day, and the steady-state concentration of ara-U was tenfold higher (60 μM).[230] In these patients, plasma clearance appeared to decrease with increasing dose, suggesting saturation of deaminases at the higher dose levels.[230,238] In children receiving an infusion of 5 g/m^2 daily, total clearance was 555 ml/min per square meter.[238]

The cellular pharmacokinetics of ara-CTP, the active intracellular metabolite of cytarabine, have been characterized in the leukemic blasts of patients receiving high-dose cytarabine.

FIGURE 9-10. Metabolic pathways for cytarabine (Ara-C), including intracellular activation to the deoxyribonucleotide triphosphate Ara-CTP by cellular kinases and degradation by deaminases to the inactive metabolites Ara-U and Ara-UMP. Enzymes catalyzing reactions are shown in *italics*.

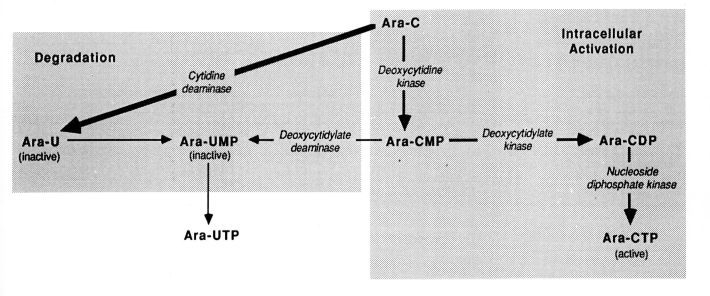

Following a 3-g/m² dose administered as a short infusion, there was considerable interpatient variability in the degree of accumulation of ara-CTP in these cells. In addition, there was no correlation between the pharmacokinetic parameters of cytarabine and the cellular concentrations of ara-CTP.[239,240] Patients responding to the drug had a significantly slower rate of elimination of ara-CTP ($t\frac{1}{2}$ of 5.6 hours in responding patients and 3.2 hours in resistant patients) and significantly higher trough levels (196 μM versus 23 μM).[239] This is consistent with earlier studies demonstrating greater ara-CTP formation *in vitro* in the leukemic cells of patients achieving a complete remission on cytarabine therapy compared to nonresponders.[241] In a current trial, the dose of cytarabine is based on the accumulation of ara-CTP in the patient's leukemic cells following a test dose of cytarabine. The pharmacokinetic parameters of the active intracellular metabolite appear to be of more predictive value than plasma levels of the parent drug.

TOXICITY. The primary toxicities of cytarabine are myelosuppression, nausea and vomiting, and gastrointestinal mucosal damage, including life-threatening bowel necrosis.[242,243] A syndrome of high fever, malaise, myalgias, joint or bone pain, and, less frequently, rash, conjunctivitis, and chest pain has also been reported in children receiving cytarabine in standard doses.[244] Coadministration of corticosteroids appears to relieve these symptoms. With high-dose regimens, neurotoxicity, primarily in the form of cerebellar dysfunction, becomes prominent.[245,246] Symptoms include ataxia, dysarthria, nystagmus, and somnolence. Pathologically, the patients experience a loss of Purkinje cells and gliosis in the cerebellum, as well as nerve cell loss in the dentate nucleus. In many instances, this toxicity has been irreversible. It appears to be dose related. The risk increases in patients receiving total doses exceeding 24 g/m².[247] The drug should be immediately withdrawn if there is nystagmus or ataxia. Skin and ocular toxicity have also been observed on high-dose regimens.

5-Fluorouracil

The fluorinated pyrimidine 5-fluorouracil (Fig. 9-7) is one of the few rationally designed anticancer drugs. It has been widely used in the treatment of carcinomas of the gastrointestinal tract, breast, ovary, and head and neck but to date has only limited application in the treatment of pediatric cancers. The cellular pharmacology of 5-fluorouracil has been extensively studied. This compound is a prodrug and must be converted intracellularly to nucleotides before expressing cytotoxicity.[248,249] There are several possible pathways for the anabolism of 5-fluorouracil to active forms, and the activity of each pathway may differ in different tissues and tumors.[250] The deoxyribonucleotide 5-FdUMP is a potent inhibitor of thymidylate synthase (leading to depletion of the DNA precursor thymidine), and the ribonucleotide 5-FUTP is incorporated into RNA. 5-FdUTP is also apparently incorporated into DNA in low levels, but mechanisms in the mammalian cell designed to block the incorporation of uridine into DNA also limit the incorporation of fluoropyrimidines. Mechanisms of resistance to 5-fluorouracil include a decrease in the activity of activating enzymes and an increase in levels of the target enzyme thymidylate synthase.[251] A mutant thymidylate synthase with decreased affinity for 5-FdUMP has also been described.[252]

PHARMACOKINETICS. 5-Fluorouracil is administered intravenously as a bolus injection (500 mg/m²) or a long-term infusion (800–1200 mg/m² over 24 hours). Bioavailability following oral administration is highly variable, in part due to a saturable first-pass elimination process.[253,254] In one study of 13 patients, 2 had undetectable plasma drug levels following an oral dose of 750 mg, and the fraction of the dose absorbed ranged from 0 to 74%.[254] Because of this variability and the unpredictability of absorption, 5-fluorouracil should not be administered by the oral route.

5-Fluorouracil is eliminated primarily by biotransformation. The degradative pathway is the same as that for the naturally occurring pyrimidines uracil and thymine.[248] Less than 10% of the drug is excreted unchanged in the urine. With standard bolus dosing, the elimination of 5-fluorouracil is rapid. The half-life is 12 minutes, and total clearance is greater than 1000 ml/min.[255] With a continuous infusion schedule, the pharmacokinetics differ significantly, with clearance values as high as 5000 ml/min. This is consistent with a dose-dependent or saturable clearance process.[255-257] Although the liver is generally said to be the principal site of drug catabolism, these clearance values with infusions markedly exceed the rate of hepatic blood flow, indicating that biotransformation must also be taking place in other organs.[255]

TOXICITY. The incidence and severity of clinical toxicities of 5-fluorouracil are, in part, dependent on the dosing schedule. With intravenous bolus dosing, myelosuppression is the primary toxicity, but when the drug is given as a continuous infusion (doses up 14,000 mg over 24 hours), myelosuppression is minimal to mild and gastrointestinal toxicity becomes dose limiting. This difference appears to be directly related to a difference in the concentration of 5-fluorouracil achieved in the bone marrow, which is equivalent to the plasma concentration following an intravenous bolus but only 0.1% to 2% of the plasma concentration with slow infusion.[253] Neurologic symptoms (somnolence, cerebellar ataxia, headache), ocular toxicity (conjunctivitis, ectropion), and dermatitis are also reported.

DRUG INTERACTIONS. A number of compounds alter both the pharmacokinetics and the pharmacodynamics of 5-fluorouracil. The combinations of methotrexate followed by 5-fluorouracil (pretreatment with methotrexate enhances the intracellular activation of 5-fluorouracil) and 5-fluorouracil and leucovorin (folates are required for the stable binding of 5-FdUMP to thymidylate synthase) are synergistic in experimental systems, and these combinations are currently being tested in clinical trials.[258,259] Thymidine delays the clearance and enhances the toxicity of 5-fluorouracil by competing for the enzyme that catabolizes the drug.[260]

ANTITUMOR ANTIBIOTICS

Most of the antitumor antibiotics in current use are naturally occurring substances that were originally isolated from the microbial broth of a variety of species of the group of soil-inhabiting microorganisms known as *Streptomyces*. The agents from this class of anticancer drugs that are used in the treatment of pediatric cancers include the anthracyclines, dactinomycin, and bleomycin.

Anthracyclines (Doxorubicin, Daunomycin)

The anthracyclines, Adriamycin (doxorubicin) and daunomycin (daunorubicin), are the most widely used antitumor antibiotics. Structurally, these highly pigmented compounds are composed of a planar tetracyclic anthraquinone nucleus linked

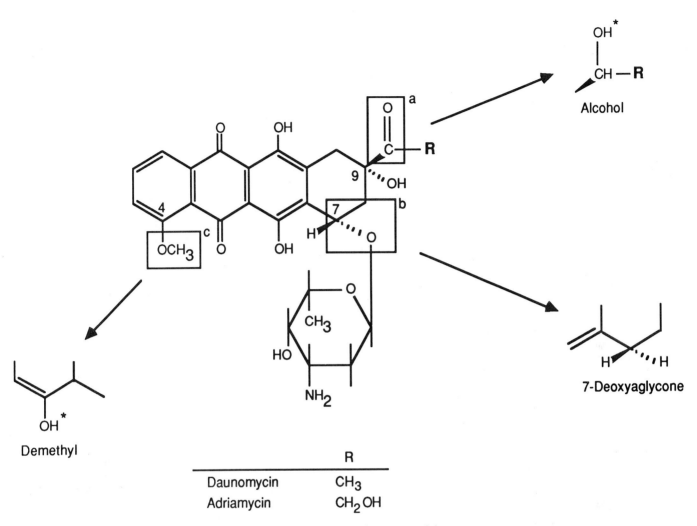

FIGURE 9-11. Chemical structure of anthracycline antitumor antibiotics Adriamycin and daunomycin (daunorubicin). The two drugs differ only in the presence or absence of a hydroxyl group on the carbonyl side chain at ring position 9. Sites on the molecule that are subject to biotransformation are enclosed in boxes. Reduction of the carbonyl group at the 9 position (*a*) leads to formation of the alcohols adriamycinol and daunomycinol, which retain cytotoxic activity. Methoxy group at the 4 position can also be demethylated (*b*). Resultant hydroxyl groups (denoted by an *) may then be conjugated with glucuronide or sulfate, which detoxifies the drugs. Free-radical formation yields the inactive deoxyglycone metabolite (*c*) following rearrangement and transfer of electrons.

to the amino sugar daunosamine (Fig. 9-11). Adriamycin has a wide range of clinical activity against pediatric cancers, including the acute leukemias, lymphomas, sarcomas of soft tissue and bone, Wilms' tumor, neuroblastoma, and hepatoblastoma. The use of daunomycin is currently limited to the acute leukemias. Traditionally, the anthracyclines have been classified as intercalating agents, which insert into and bind to the DNA double helix, interfering with DNA replication, transcription, and repair.[261] However, these drugs can also undergo chemical reduction by a wide range of intracellular flavin-dependent enzyme systems yielding highly reactive free radicals.[262,263] Transfer of an electron from these unstable radicals to molecular oxygen yields superoxide radicals that can cause oxidative damage to cellular macromolecules. These reactive intermediates can also covalently bind (alkylate) DNA.[264] Anthracyclines also appear to exert a cytotoxic effect by reacting directly with the cell membrane.[265] The anthracyclines are subject to multidrug resistance, which is discussed in the introduction to this chapter.

Biotransformation

The anthracyclines are extensively metabolized to both active and inactive metabolites (Fig. 9-11). The principal active metabolites are the corresponding alcohols, adriamycinol and daunomycinol, which are the result of the chemical reduction of the carbonyl side chain by aldoketoreductase.[266,267] The free radicals of anthracyclines are formed by one- or two-electron reduction catalyzed by microsomal or other enzymes systems. These unstable intermediates undergo rearrangements followed by cleavage of the sugar moiety.[263] After the rapid transfer of electrons to molecular oxygen, the remaining byproducts are the deoxyaglycones. Although these compounds are of no biological significance, their presence indicates that the anthracyclines existed *in vivo* in the free-radical state. The final step in anthracycline catabolism is their conjugation with a sulfate or glucuronide group, either at the reduced carbonyl (alcohol) or following demethylation of the methoxy group at the 4 position on the ring (Fig. 9-11).

Pharmacokinetics

Because of the complexity of anthracycline metabolism, the study of drug disposition *in vivo* has been technically difficult. However, the recent development of high-pressure liquid chromatographic techniques has allowed the separation and quantitation of both parent drug and active metabolites.[268,269] Currently, this is the only valid methodology for studying these agents.

The anthracyclines are administered intravenously, either as a bolus injection or by infusion. The instability of these compounds in an acid environment prevents their oral administration, and their severe vesicant properties prohibit intramuscular or subcutaneous administration. Following an intravenous injection, there is an initial rapid decline in plasma concentration,[269–271] which is generally attributed to the rapid and avid binding of these drugs by tissues (initial half-life is 10 minutes). This extensive binding also accounts for the very large volumes of distribution (greater than 500 liters/m^2) reported for these agents (Table 9-5). The initial distributive phase is followed by a long terminal phase, with half-lives greater than 24 hours for both daunomycin and Adriamycin.[267,269,271] Despite the fact that drug concentrations at the start of the terminal phase are $\frac{1}{50}$ the peak concentrations, 75% of the total drug exposure occurs during this terminal phase.[271]

The anthracyclines are eliminated by biotransformation (primarily in the liver) and biliary excretion. Renal excretion accounts for only 10% of total drug clearance.[267,270] The total plasma clearance generally exceeds 1000 ml/min per square meter, and, in children, when clearance is corrected for body surface area, it is independent of the age of the child.[270] In addition, the pharmacokinetics of Adriamycin are linear over a wide range of dosage schedules (3-minute bolus injection to 16-hour infusion).[272]

Dosage modifications are not required in patients with renal dysfunction, even in patients with severe insufficiency or those on hemodialysis.[273] However, delayed clearance of Adriamycin associated with an increase in toxicity has been reported in both adult and pediatric patients with hepatic dysfunction.[270,274] Unfortunately, there are no good correlations between abnormal liver function tests and impaired Adriamycin clearance.[275,276] The best current recommendation is that dose reduction be reserved for patients with multiple liver-function test abnormalities or direct bilirubin elevations greater than 2.0 mg/dl,[276,277] although this guideline may significantly underdose some patients.[278]

The primary anthracycline metabolites, adriamycinol and daunomycinol, are cytotoxic but less active than their respective parent drugs.[279] Exposure to adriamycinol as measured by the area under the plasma concentration–time curve is approximately half that of Adriamycin on both the bolus and infusion schedules.[271,280] In contrast, daunomycinol exposure appears to be threefold to fourfold higher than daunomycin, and the metabolite has a longer terminal half-life (23 to 40 hours).[267,269] However, measurement of these compounds is complicated by the fact that daunomycin is metabolized to daunomycinol *in vitro* in whole blood incubated at 37°C.[269]

Toxicity

The acute toxicities of the anthracyclines include myelosuppression, mucositis (less with daunomycin[281]), nausea and vomiting, and alopecia.[282] Extravasation of these agents leads to severe local tissue damage and deep ulcerations, which heal very slowly and are difficult to skin graft. Extravasation is usually managed with ice packs and local injection of cortico-steroids and sodium bicarbonate. At best, these measures will only ameliorate, not prevent, the reaction; in animal models, only marginal benefit can be demonstrated with these methods. In severe cases, early surgical excision of affected tissue followed by full-thickness skin graft or skin flap coverage should be considered.[283] Dimethyl sulfoxide (DMSO) and a combination of α-tocopherol (10%) in DMSO effectively reduces the skin necrosis in rats.[284] The anthracyclines can also potentiate radiation reactions in many tissues, including, skin, liver, esophagus, lungs, and heart; thus concurrent use of these two modalities should be avoided. A radiation recall phenomenon can also be observed when these drugs are administered in the postirradiation period.[282]

Both acute and chronic cumulative cardiac toxicity are associated with the use of anthracyclines. The acute form is characterized most frequently by arrhythmias and conduction abnormalities, but there is also an acute drop in left ventricular function, reaching a nadir at 24 hours followed by variable recovery.[285] Rarely, this may be clinically manifest as the myocarditis–pericarditis syndrome, which, in its severest form, is characterized by the rapid onset of congestive failure associated with pericarditis.[286] In general, the acute asymptomatic cardiac changes are transient and do not prevent the further use of anthracyclines.

The chronic late cardiomyopathy is related to the cumulative dose of anthracyclines. The incidence of clinically apparent cardiac toxicity starts increasing significantly after cumulative doses exceed 550 mg/m^2 for Adriamycin or 600 mg/m^2 for daunomycin.[282] However, more sensitive cardiac indices suggest that the myocardial damage accumulates steadily with the dose.[286] The primary pathologic change in the myocardium as a result of drug-induced cardiomyopathy is the destruction and loss of myofibrils.[287] The mechanism of myocardial damage may be either a direct effect on the myocardial cell membrane or drug-induced free-radical formation within the cell.[286] Neither hypothesis can completely explain the pathophysiology of anthracycline cardiac toxicity.

Patients with overt cardiac toxicity usually present within a few months of their last dose with the typical features of congestive heart failure. Although some patients with this complication can be managed medically, the mortality rate is 50%.[286] Factors reported to increase the risk for the development of a cardiomyopathy include prior or concurrent mediastinal irradiation and the concurrent administration of cyclophosphamide or mitomycin C.[286] Children appear to be at higher risk for cardiac toxicity,[282] and patients younger than 5 years are at higher risk than older ones.[288] Dose rate is also an important factor in all age groups, with cardiac toxicity observed more commonly in patients receiving individual doses of 50 mg/m^2 or greater.[286,288]

Several approaches have been used to assess the degree of anthracycline-induced cardiomyopathy. The most sensitive and direct method is the evaluation of pathologic changes in the myocardium by endomyocardial biopsy.[287] The results correlate well with cardiac function measured at cardiac catheterization, but the technique has the disadvantage of being an invasive, technically demanding procedure. Unfortunately, noninvasive functional studies, such as the ECG, echocardiogram, and radionuclide cineangiography, may not demonstrate abnormalities until a critical degree of myocardial injury has occurred. However, serial measurement of cardiac function is of some value in monitoring patients on anthracycline therapy.[282] Radionuclide cineangiography appears to be the most sensitive and accurate technique.[289] A new device capable of instantaneously measuring respiratory sinus arrhythmia has recently been applied to monitoring anthracycline cardiac toxicity with promising results.[290]

Current approaches to the prevention of anthracycline cardiac toxicity include altering the schedule of drug administration, coadministration of agents that protect the myocardium from the toxic effects of anthracyclines, and the development of less cardiotoxic anthracycline analogues such as idarubicin. Lowering peak concentrations of anthracycline by administering the drugs on a lower-dose weekly schedule or by continuous infusion appears to reduce the cardiotoxic effects without compromising the antitumor effect.[291,292] Several cardioprotective agents have been evaluated in preclinical studies. The most promising, ICRF-187, is a chelating agent currently in clinical trials.[263] Free-radical scavengers such as α-tocopherol have also been protective in animal models.[286]

Bleomycin

Bleomycin is a structurally and pharmacodynamically unique antibiotic that is actually a mixture of low-molecular-weight (1500 daltons) glycopeptides. The major species, bleomycin A2, which accounts for 70% of the commercial preparation, consists of an S-peptide that binds to DNA and a nitrogen-rich segment at the opposite end of the molecule that chelates heavy metals such as iron and copper.[293,294] After binding to DNA, bleomycin produces single- and double-strand breaks by a metal ion (Fe^{2+}, Cu^{2+})-catalyzed free-radical reaction.[295] The exact mechanisms of resistance to bleomycin have not been elucidated, but the primary determinants of bleomycin cytotoxicity are cellular uptake, DNA repair activity, and level of activity of bleomycin hydrolase, the major intracellular catabolic enzyme.[296]

Dosage and Toxicity

Bleomycin can be administered intravenously by bolus or infusion, intramuscularly, or subcutaneously at doses of 10 to 20 units/m². (A unit is a measure of the drug's antimicrobial activity and is equivalent to about 1.5 mg of peptide.) The drug is active against Hodgkin's disease, the lymphomas, and testicular cancer and other germ cell tumors.

Unlike most other anticancer drugs, bleomycin is not myelosuppressive. The dose-limiting toxicity is an interstitial pneumonitis that can lead to pulmonary fibrosis. Patients with this toxicity present with cough and dyspnea that can progress to hypoxia and death.[294] Below a total cumulative dose of 450 units, sporadic cases of pulmonary toxicity are reported, with an incidence of 3% to 5%. At doses above 450 units, the incidence increases with the dose.[297] However, subclinical changes in pulmonary function can be detected at lower doses in many patients.[298] Both pulmonary radiation and use of supplemental oxygen enhance the chances for the development of pulmonary toxicity in patients previously treated with bleomycin.[299] In one report, all five patients previously treated with bleomycin who were exposed to oxygen concentrations greater than 40% during anesthesia developed fulminant respiratory distress and died.[300] The pathologic changes in the lung include edema and cellular infiltration in the perivascular interstitial space followed by damage to alveolar lining cells and formation of hyaline membranes and fibrosis. These changes may worsen even after withdrawal of the drug. At the first sign of lung damage, bleomycin therapy should be discontinued. High-dose corticosteroids may be of value in decreasing fibroblast activity, although this recommendation is based only on anecdotal experience.[299] If patients require anesthesia, oxygen concentration should be kept below 25% when possible. Pulmonary function should be closely monitored in patients receiving this agent.

Cutaneous reactions to bleomycin are also common. Hyperpigmentation and areas of eythema, induration, and desquamation are most commonly seen. Other side-effects include fever, hypersensitivity reactions, and Raynaud's phenomenon.

Pharmacokinetics

Bleomycin is not administered orally and would most likely be digested by intestinal peptidases. Absorption following intramuscular and subcutaneous injection is nearly complete,[301,302] and plasma concentrations with a continuous subcutaneous infusion closely simulate those after an intravenous infusion.[302] With intravenous bolus dosing in children, the drug has a biphasic plasma disappearance curve with a terminal half-life of 3 hours. Total clearance was 41 ml/min per square meter, and renal clearance accounted for 65% of total drug clearance.[303] Patients with renal failure have prolonged terminal drug half-lives and higher steady-state plasma concentrations when the drug is administered by continuous infusion.[304,305] A 75% dosage reduction has been recommended for patients with a creatinine clearance of less than 25 ml/min.[306] In patients undergoing hemodialysis, bleomycin was not detected in the dialysate.

Dactinomycin (Actinomycin D)

Dactinomycin was one of the first drugs demonstrated to have significant antitumor effect in humans, and it has been in clinical use for more than 30 years. It continues to have a role in the treatment of Wilms' tumor, Ewing's sarcoma, rhabdomyosarcoma, and other soft-tissue sarcomas, even though it has been supplanted by the anthracyclines in some recent protocols. Structurally, dactinomycin is composed of a planar tricyclic ring chromophore (phenoxazone) to which two identical cyclic polypeptides are attached.[307] The drug binds to DNA by intercalation and blocks the replication and transcription of the DNA template.[307] Dactinomycin can also cause single-strand breaks in DNA.

Despite three decades of clinical use, there is limited information on the clinical pharmacology of dactinomycin. The drug is administered intravenously, traditionally on a daily-for-5-days schedule (0.45 mg/m² per day). However, a single bolus dose of 1.5 to 2 mg/m² appears to be as effective.[308,309] After an intravenous bolus injection, dactinomycin has an initial rapid disappearance as a result of its rapid and avid tissue binding.[310,311] This is followed by a long elimination phase with a half-life of 36 hours.[310] The drug is eliminated by both renal and biliary excretion, although only 30% of the dose is recovered in the urine and stool over the week following the dose. Only a small fraction of the dose appears to be metabolized.[310] Dactinomycin is concentrated in nucleated cells in blood and bone marrow.

The primary toxicities of dactinomycin are myelosuppression, orointestinal mucositis, and severe nausea and vomiting. Extravasation of this drug can result in severe local tissue damage and ulceration. Dactinomycin is a radiation sensitizer, and it can enhance the local toxicity of radiation therapy when administered concurrently. It can also cause a radiation recall effect when administered up to 2 years after irradiation.[312]

PLANT ALKALOIDS

Plant products have been used in the treatment of a variety of diseases for hundreds of years and are still an important source of both medically useful and illicit drugs. It has been estimated that in recorded history more than 3000 species of plants have been used as some form of cancer treatment. However, despite extensive screening in the modern era of cancer treatment, only a few clinically active anticancer drugs have been derived from the higher plants.[313,314] The only agents with applications in the treatment of childhood cancers are the vinca alkaloids, derived from leaf extracts of the periwinkle plant, and the epipodophyllotoxins, semisynthetic derivatives of podophyllotoxin, which was extracted from the roots and rhizomes of the mandrake. As with other "natural" drugs, these compounds have novel and complex chemical structures (Fig. 9-12) and potent biological properties.[314] The biotransformation of these drugs is also complex; and the metabolic pathways have only been partially defined.

Vinca Alkaloids (Vincristine, Vinblastine)

The vinca alkaloids, vincristine and vinblastine, are structurally similar alkaloids composed of two multiring subunits, vindoline and catharanthine (Fig. 9-12). Despite their structural similarity, vincristine and vinblastine have very distinct clinical and toxiciologic properties. These drugs are members of the class of drugs that act as mitotic inhibitors (spindle poisons). They exert their effect by binding to tubulin, a dimeric protein that polymerizes to form microtubules.[315] The resulting disruption of the intracellular microtubular system interferes with a number of vital cell functions, including mitosis, maintenance of the cytostructure, and movement and transport of solutes such as neurotransmitters (in neuronal axons) and hormones and proteins (in secretory cells).[316] The cytotoxic effect of these agents is primarily related to their ability to inhibit mitotic spindle formation, causing metaphase arrest during mitosis. However, cells in culture are killed by these compounds during all of the phases of the cell cycle, an observation that is not completely compatible with the tubulin-binding effects of these drugs. The vinca alkaloids are subject to multidrug resistance, as discussed earlier.

Vincristine has a very wide spectrum of clinical activity and is currently used in the treatment of acute lymphoblastic leukemia, Hodgkin's and non-Hodgkin's lymphomas, rhabdomyosarcoma and other soft-tissue sarcomas, osteosarcoma, Ewing's sarcoma, Wilms' tumor, brain tumors, and neuroblastoma. Vinblastine has been used in the treatment of histiocytosis, testicular cancer, and Hodgkin's disease.

FIGURE 9-12. Chemical structures of the plant alkaloids commonly used in treatment of childhood cancers, including the vinca alkaloids and the semisynthetic podophyllotoxin derivatives.

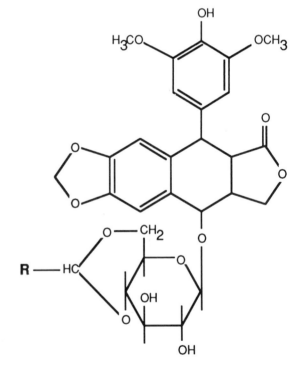

Vinca Alkaloids	R
Vincristine	CHO
Vinblastine	CH$_3$

Epipodophyllotoxins	R
Etoposide (VP-16)	CH$_3$
Teniposide (VM-26)	(thiophene)

Pharmacokinetics

Definitive pharmacokinetic study of the vinca alkaloids has been difficult because of a lack of sensitive and specific drug assays. Much of the available pharmacokinetic information comes from studies using radiolabeled drug, although recently more specific chromatographic techniques, a radioimmunoassay, and an enzyme-linked immunoabsorbent assay have been developed.[317-319] The vinca alkaloids are poorly absorbed when administered orally and for this reason are administered intravenously as a bolus injection. Slow infusions have also been investigated.[320,321] After bolus administration, the vinca alkaloids manifest a triphasic disappearance pattern in plasma. After a rapid initial decline (initial half-life is less than 5 minutes), these agents have a long terminal half-life of approximately 24 hours.[322-325] The long terminal half-life and the large steady-state volume of distribution (Table 9-5) are consistent with avid and extensive tissue binding characteristic of these drugs. Nelson and associates reported a marked difference in the clearance rate and volume of distribution of vincristine and vinblastine, with vinblastine being cleared at a sevenfold greater rate and having a threefold larger volume of distribution.[325] For vincristine, there are no significant differences in the disposition of the drug according to age, with clearance values of 84 ml/min per square meter and 82 ml/min per square meter reported for children and adults, respectively.[322,323] Studies in both nonhuman primates and man have demonstrated that vincristine enters the CSF following intravenous administration, although the levels are only 3% to 5% of the corresponding plasma levels.[326,327]

Hepatic metabolism and biliary excretion are the principal routes for elimination of vincristine. From 70% to 75% of the radioactivity from a radiolabeled dose of vincristine appears in the feces by 72 hours, whereas slightly more than 10% of the radioactivity is excreted in the urine.[324,328,329] There is some evidence that glucuronide conjugation plays an important role in the hepatic metabolism of vincristine. However, the structures of the various vincristine and vinblastine metabolites remain to be identified.

Dosage modifications of the vinca alkaloids are generally recommended in infants and in patients with delayed biliary excretion as evidenced by an elevated direct bilirubin. However, because definitive pharmacokinetic data are lacking, these guidelines are empirically derived. Infants do appear to manifest increased toxicity with standard doses of vincristine based on body surface area. Infants and younger children have a relatively larger ratio of body surface area to weight. Therefore, many pediatric protocols determine vincristine dosage in infants and younger children on the basis of weight (0.03–0.05 mg/kg) rather than body surface area.

The standard dose for vincristine is 1.0 to 1.5 mg/m^2 administered every 1 to 3 weeks. Because early studies suggested that total doses greater than 2 mg led to increased toxicity (primarily neurotoxicity), especially when administered on a weekly basis, many protocols have limited the total single dose to 2 mg. Recently, this practice has been questioned on the basis that neurotoxicity correlates with the area under the plasma concentration–time curve and that substantial interindividual variation occurs in the plasma pharmacokinetics of vincristine, with a greater than tenfold variation in the area under the curve.[330,331] Escalation of the dose beyond the 2 mg maximum may therefore be well tolerated in some patients. Vinblastine doses range from 3.5 to 6.0 mg/m^2, administered in 1- to 3-week cycles.

The administration of the vinca alkaloids by continuous infusion has theoretical advantages in that this approach takes advantage of the dependence of cell kill on duration of drug exposure.[320,321,332] However, this schedule appears to be more toxic, and the overall clinical utility of this strategy, which has not been studied in children, remains to be demonstrated.

Toxicity

Neurotoxicity is the dose-limiting toxicity for vincristine. It is related to the cumulative dose and is more common on a weekly schedule. Manifestations of the peripheral sensory and motor neuropathy include loss of deep tendon reflexes, neuritic pain (such as muscular cramping and jaw pain), paresthesias, and wrist and foot "drop." Occasionally, cranial motor nerves may be affected, and autonomic nerve involvement may be responsible for paralytic ileus or urinary retention. In most cases, these symptoms are reversible upon withdrawal of the drug. Accidental intrathecal administration of vincristine has been reported and is usually fatal. Other toxicities associated with vincristine include alopecia, inappropriate antidiuretic hormone syndrome, seizures, and orthostatic hypotension. Nausea and vomiting and myelosuppression are encountered relatively rarely.

In contrast, myelosuppression is the dose-limiting toxicity for vinblastine, which also frequently causes mucositis. Neurotoxicity with vinblastine therapy is minimal. Both vincristine and vinblastine are vesicants; extreme care must be taken to avoid extravasation during their administration.

Epipodophyllotoxins (Etoposide, Teniposide)

Etoposide (VP16) and the investigational agent teniposide (VM26) are active analogues with a unique mechanism of action that is different from the parent drug podophyllotoxin, which is a tubulin binder. Neither etoposide nor teniposide binds to tubulin.[333] Instead, both of these structurally similar compounds (Fig. 9-12) exert their principal antitumor effect through an interaction with DNA that leads to an inhibition of DNA synthesis. These compounds appear to induce single- and double-strand DNA breaks in intact cells only, a process that is mediated through type II topoisomerase, an enzyme that reversibly cleaves DNA.[334-336] The epipodophyllotoxins can also be metabolized to reactive phenoxy radical intermediates that could play a role in the mechanism of action of these drugs.[337,338]

The clinical activity of the epipodophyllotoxins against childhood cancers is still being defined. To date, teniposide has been used more frequently in pediatrics, whereas etoposide has been tested primarily in adults. Thus far, there are no major differences in the antitumor spectra of these drugs. Activity has been observed against the acute leukemias, Hodgkin's and non-Hodgkin's lymphomas, neuroblastoma, rhabdomyosarcoma and other soft-tissue sarcomas, Ewing's sarcoma, germ cell (including testicular) cancer, and brain tumors.[339-342] The pharmacology of these agents has recently been reviewed in detail.[338]

Dosage and Toxicity

The solubility of the epipodophyllotoxins in water is poor, so both are supplied in nonaqueous formulations. Prior to intravenous administration, these agents are diluted in 5% dextrose in water or 0.9% saline and infused over 30 to 60 minutes to avoid the hypotension noted with rapid injections. Etoposide is usually administered on a daily schedule for 3 to 5 days at a dose of 60 to 120 mg/m^2 per day, although there is no convincing evidence of schedule dependence of this drug. Teniposide is administered at a dose of 70 to 180 mg/m^2. Both agents have also been administered on a single high-dose schedule (up to 800 mg/m² of etoposide and up to 1000 mg/m² of teniposide).

The major dose-limiting toxicity of both drugs is myelosuppression. Other toxicities include alopecia, nausea and vomiting, phlebitis, mild peripheral neuropathy, hepatocellular enzyme elevations, and mucositis. Arrhythmias are relatively rare. Hypersensitivity reactions, ranging from bronchospasm to anaphylaxis, occur less frequently with etoposide than with teniposide (less than 1% versus up to 10% of cases).[343,344] A severe skin rash has also been reported with high-dose teniposide.[345]

Pharmacokinetics

The disposition of the epipodophyllotoxins is characterized by a significant degree of intrapatient and interpatient variability. The bioavailability of oral etoposide is approximately 50% but ranges from 10% to 80%.[346,347] There is also considerable dose-to-dose variation within a patient.[348,349] Bioavailability is also nonlinear—with increasing dose, the fraction absorbed decreases.[350] Because oral absorption is erratic and this route of administration has been associated with increased toxicity, its clinical usefulness is limited.[342,351]

The epipodophyllotoxins are extensively metabolized, although specific details of the metabolic pathways have yet to be elucidated. Some of these metabolites retain cytotoxic activity.[352] The major metabolites identified in urine are the hydroxy acid derivatives.[353] Glucuronide and sulfate conjugates have also been detected.[338] Renal clearance accounts for 30% to 40% of the total systemic clearance of etoposide[348,354,355] but only 10% of teniposide clearance.[356,357] This difference probably reflects the difference in the degree of protein binding of the two drugs (Table 9-5). Biliary excretion is not a major route of elimination for etoposide (accounting for less than 10% of total elimination in most studies).[338] Initial studies in adults showed that teniposide had a slower rate of clearance and a longer terminal half-life than etoposide; however, studies in children have demonstrated that the disposition of these drugs is more similar than previously thought.[339] The pharmacokinetic parameters are independent of the dose in doses up to 1,000 mg/m².[355,356] Penetration of the epipodophyllotoxins into the CSF is poor.

The pharmacokinetics of etoposide have been evaluated in patients with hepatic and renal dysfunction.[358,359] Etoposide clearance was significantly lowered and the terminal half-life prolonged in patients with renal insufficiency, putting them at higher risk for toxicity. Overall, a good correlation was found between creatinine clearance and etoposide clearance in both studies, suggesting that etoposide dose modifications should be based on the creatinine clearance. Etoposide clearance was not delayed in patients with abnormal hepatic function, indicating that dose adjustments are not necessary in these patients.

MISCELLANEOUS AGENTS

Corticosteroids (Prednisone, Prednisolone, Dexamethasone)

Although they are not generally thought of as anticancer drugs because of the diversity of their other clinical uses, the corticosteroids play a significant role in the treatment of acute lymphoblastic leukemia, lymphoma, and Hodgkin's disease and have been incorporated into treatment regimens for histiocytosis and brain tumors. In addition, they are useful in managing some of the complications of cancer, including hypercalcemia, increased intracranial pressure, anorexia, and chemotherapy-induced nausea and vomiting. The mechanism of the lympholytic effect of corticosteroids is not clearly defined, but it appears to be mediated through glucocorticoid receptors. Glucocorticoid receptor content in leukemic blasts correlates with the response to corticosteroid therapy both *in vitro* and *in vivo*,[360] and a loss of or defect in the glucocorticoid receptor can lead to drug resistance *in vitro*.[361]

The chemical structures of the most commonly used synthetic analogue of cortisol, prednisone, prednisolone, and dexamethasone are shown in Figure 9-13. The addition of the 1,2 double bond in prednisolone and dexamethasone increases the glucocorticoid and anti-inflammatory potency fourfold while decreasing mineralocorticoid activity. Further addition of the fluorine at position 9 in dexamethasone enhances the activity another fivefold. Prednisone is an inactive prodrug analogous to cortisone and requires chemical reduction of the ketone group at position 11 to a hydroxyl group, yielding prednisolone. This activation occurs in the liver.[362] Both prednisolone and dexamethasone are eliminated by the catabolic enzymes that inactivate cortisol either by reduction of the 4,5 double bond (hepatic and extrahepatic) or reduction of the 3-ketone to a hydroxyl group followed by conjugation with a sulfate or glucuronide (hepatic).

Pharmacokinetics

The absorption of orally administered prednisone, prednisolone, and dexamethasone is nearly complete (greater than 80%).[362,363] Prednisone is rapidly converted to prednisolone, which is the predominant form (fourfold to tenfold higher) in plasma after an oral dose of prednisone.[362] In children, variability in the absorption of prednisone has been reported.[364] The elimination half-lives are 2.5 hours for prednisolone[364,365] and 4 hours for dexamethasone,[366] reflecting differences in the rate of catabolism resulting from the different modifications to cortisol. Hepatic metabolism is the primary route of elimination; renal clearance accounts for 10% or less of total clearance.[367,368] The clearance of prednisolone is dose dependent and increases with increasing dose. This appears to be related in part to concentration-dependent binding of prednisolone to plasma proteins.[368] At low concentrations, prednisolone, like cortisol, is highly (more than 95%) bound to transcortin, but with increasing concentration this specific carrier protein is saturated, and the relative amount of free drug available for metabolic degradation increases. Dexamethasone is not bound to transcortin, and the degree of protein binding is concentration independent.[369]

Toxicity

The corticosteroids have some effect on almost every organ and tissue in the body; thus the side-effects of these agents are protean. Significant common toxicities include increased appetite, centripedal obesity, immunosuppression, myopathy, osteoporosis, aseptic necrosis, peptic ulceration, pancreatitis, psychiatric disorders, cataracts, hypertension, precipitation of diabetes, growth failure, amenorrhea, impaired wound healing, and atrophy of subcutaneous tissue.[370]

L-Asparaginase

L-Asparaginase is an enzyme that provides selective nutritional therapy for a limited range of pediatric cancers, specifically acute lymphoblastic leukemia and lymphomas. This enzyme

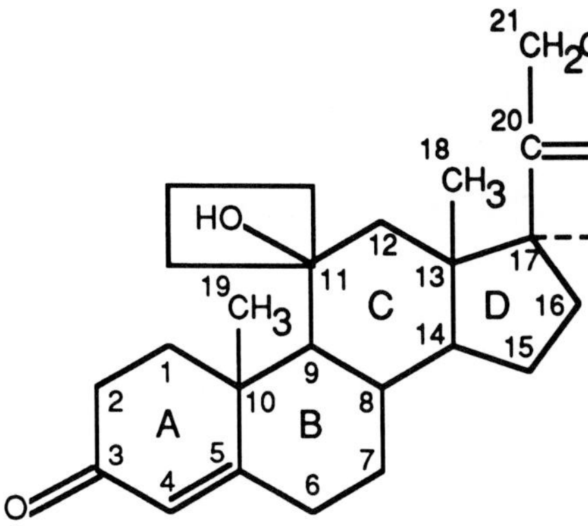

Cortisol
(Hydrocortisone)

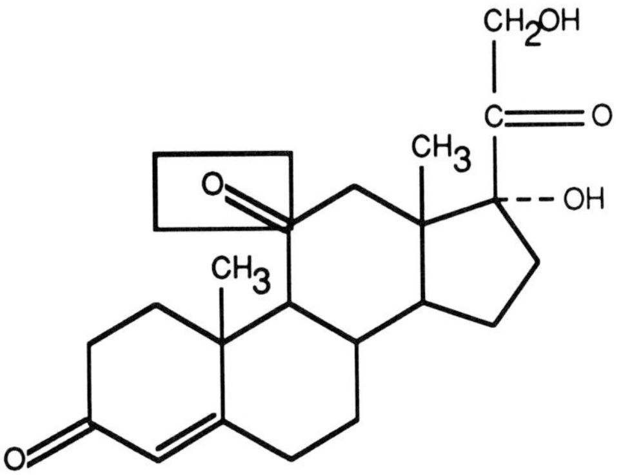

Cortisone
(Inactive)

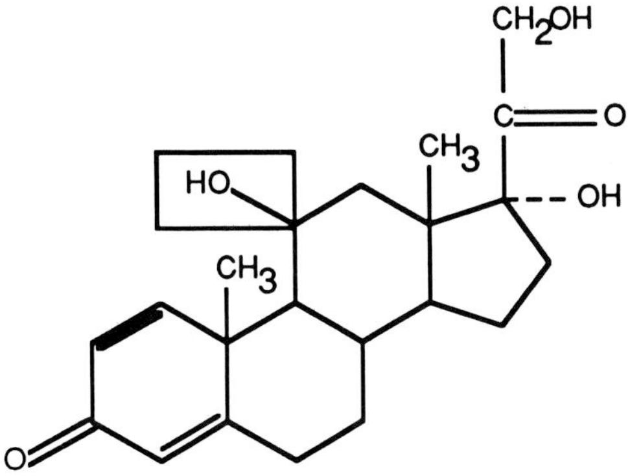

Prednisolone

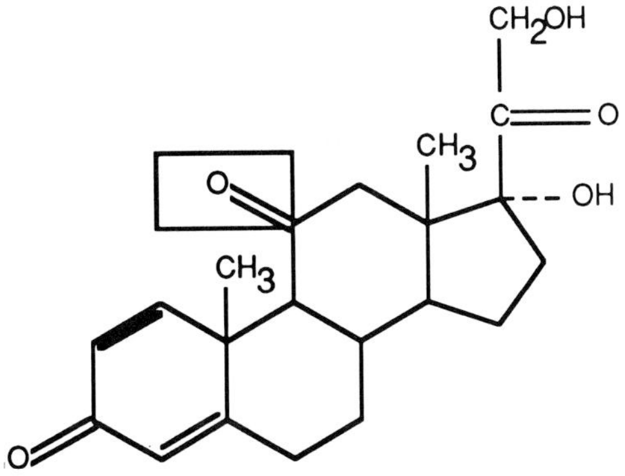

Prednisone
(Inactive)

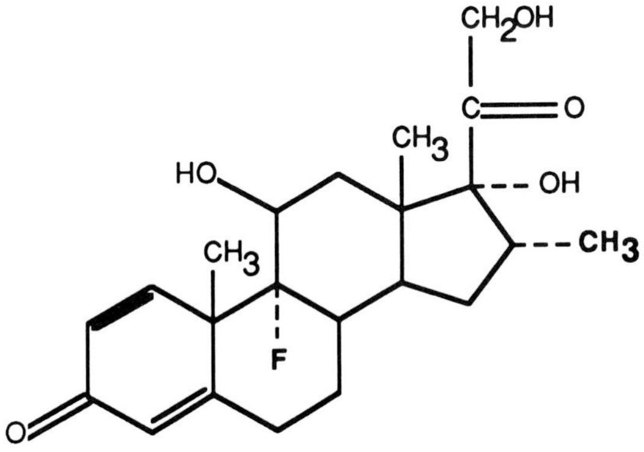

Dexamethasone

FIGURE 9-13. Chemical structures of the naturally occurring and synthetic corticosteroids commonly used in treatment of childhood cancers. Reduction of the keto group (cortisone, prednisone) to a hydroxyl group (cortisol, prednisolone) at the 11 position is necessary for activity. Addition of the 1,2 double bond (prednisolone, dexamethasone) and the fluorine group at the 9 position (dexamethasone) increases glucocorticoid activity. Changes in synthetic compounds are shown in **boldface.**

catalyzes the conversion of the amino acid L-asparagine to aspartic acid and rapidly depletes the circulating pool of L-asparagine. In most tissues, this nonessential amino acid can be synthesized from aspartic acid and glutamine by the enzyme asparagine synthase. However, levels of this synthetic enzyme are low in the sensitive lymphoid malignancies, which thus are dependent on the circulating pool of L-asparagine that is depleted by L-asparaginase, accounting for the selective antileukemic effect of this drug.[370,371] Depletion of L-asparagine within leukemic cells results in inhibition of protein synthesis, which accounts for the cytotoxicity of this agent. Resistant cells have high inducible levels of asparagine synthase.

The affinity constant of L-asparaginase for L-asparagine is approximately tenfold higher than the minimal concentration of the amino acid required *in vitro* to support cell growth. Because of this and the continual production and release of L-asparagine by normal tissues, an excess of the enzyme is necessary to lower the concentration of L-asparagine to critical levels.[370,372] L-Asparaginase is currently derived from bacterial sources (*E. coli, Erwinia carotovora*) and is administered intravenously or intramuscularly at a dose of 6000 international units (IU)/m² on an intermittent schedule (usually three times a week).

Pharmacokinetics

Oral administration of this drug is impractical due to denaturation and peptidase digestion within the intestinal tract. With intravenous administration, peak levels of the enzyme are dose related, and the plasma half-life is 14 to 22 hours. Daily administration results in significant accumulation of L-asparaginase.[373] Peak levels with intramuscular injection are approximately half those measured after intravenous dosing. Patients who develop antibody to L-asparaginase have a rapid fall in the plasma levels of the enzyme,[374] indicating that the antibody can interfere with the therapeutic effects of L-asparaginase. Plasma levels of the target amino acid, L-asparagine, fall rapidly and remain low for up to 10 days after the enzyme is no longer detectable. The enzyme distributes primarily within the intravascular space, but its effects are more wide reaching. For example, even though L-asparaginase cannot be detected in the CSF after systemic administration, CSF levels of L-asparagine are depleted for long periods.[375]

Toxicity

The principal side-effects of L-asparaginase are related to either immunologic sensitization to a bacterial protein or decreased protein synthesis.[370] Hypersensitivity reactions range from urticaria to laryngeal edema, bronchospasm, and anaphylaxis. Diphenhydramine, epinephrine, and other resuscitative measures must be available when administering this agent, even with the initial dose. Skin testing is frequently performed to identify patients who may be allergic to the drug but is not completely reliable. Detection of a specific IgG4 antibody in plasma may also be predictive of allergic reactions.[376] The incidence of hypersensitivity reactions is lower (10%) in patients receiving combination chemotherapy than in those receiving it as a single agent (40%), presumably as a result of the immunosuppressive effects of the other drugs in the regimen.[376,377] Since the two available preparations of L-asparaginase (*E. coli* and *Erwinia*) are not crossreactive, patients experiencing hypersensitivity reactions to one should be switched to the other.

Coagulopathies resulting from deficiencies or, more importantly, from imbalances in coagulation factors (fibrinogen, II, V, VII, VIII-X, antithrombin II, and protein C) can lead to both clotting and hemorrhagic complications, including stroke. Decreased serum albumin, insulin, and lipoproteins are frequently observed. Other toxicities include an encephalopathy characterized by somnolence, disorientation, seizures, and coma, which has been related to hyperammonemia in some patients;[378] acute pancreatitis, which can progress to hemorrhagic pancreatitis; and hepatotoxicity. Myelosuppression and gastrointestinal toxicity (with the exception of nausea and vomiting) are generally not observed.

Drug Interactions

When administered after large doses of methotrexate or cytarabine, L-asparaginase can rescue patients from the toxic effects of these agents. The sequential combinations of methotrexate–L-asparaginase and cytarabine–L-asparaginase have proved effective in the treatment of children with relapsed leukemia.[379,380] The rescue effect is usually attributed to a decrease

in protein synthesis in normal tissue. Antagonism has been observed when the drugs are given in the opposite sequence (L-asparaginase followed by methotrexate).[381]

CENTRAL NERVOUS SYSTEM PHARMACOLOGY OF ANTICANCER DRUGS

The distribution or penetration of the various anticancer drugs into the central nervous system (CNS) is of particular concern to the pediatric oncologist both because primary and metastatic tumors of the brain or meninges are common in children and because current treatment regimens are associated with acute and chronic neurotoxicity. With the exception of the nitrosoureas and some of the antimetabolites, penetration of the anticancer drugs across the blood–brain barrier is limited (Table 9-5). The degree of penetration is determined by several factors, including (1) the physicochemical properties of the drug (lipophilicity, molecular size, and degree of ionization); (2) protein and tissue binding, which determine free drug concentration; and (3) affinity of the drug for carriers that facilitate the transport of endogenous compounds into the CNS. Recently, an effort has been made to design small, lipophilic drugs, such as diaziquone (AZQ), that are specifically targeted for the treatment of CNS tumors.

The influence of protein and tissue binding can be seen in the poor access of extensively bound drugs such as the vinca alkaloids and anthracyclines to the CNS. A difference in the effectiveness of the synthetic corticosteroids in preventing the development of meningeal leukemia may also be due to differences in protein binding.[382] The concentration of prednisolone and dexamethasone in the CSF is approximately equivalent to the free drug concentration in plasma. However, because prednisolone, unlike dexamethasone, is tightly and extensively bound to transcortin at low concentrations, its free plasma and CSF levels are lower at equipotent doses.[382]

Intrathecal Chemotherapy

One approach taken to circumvent the limited access of drugs into the CNS is direct injection into the CSF. Intrathecally injected chemotherapy (methotrexate, cytarabine) is highly efficacious both as primary and as preventive therapy for meningeal leukemia and lymphoma. As a form of regional chemotherapy, intrathecal administration has the advantage of delivering very high drug concentrations to the CSF and meninges with low doses and therefore minimal systemic toxicity.[383] However, there are several disadvantages to intralumbar injections. Repeated lumbar punctures are painful and inconvenient. In 10% of intralumbar injections, the drug is not delivered into the subarachnoid space but is instead injected or leaks into the subdural or epidural space.[384] Because of the slow unidirectional flow of the CSF, distribution of drugs within it, specifically to the ventricles, is poor. Ventricular methotrexate levels are highly variable and less than 10% of simultaneous lumbar levels with an intralumbar dose.[385] In addition, the depth of penetration of effective levels into the parenchyma is limited to only a few millimeters for the commonly used agents.[386] Finally, intrathecal therapy is associated with unique toxicities, such as chemical arachnoiditis.

The distribution of drug to the ventricles can be significantly improved by positioning the patient prone or supine for at least 30 minutes after intralumbar injection. In an animal model, ventricular levels of methotrexate were as much as 1000-fold higher in animals placed in the supine or Trendelenburg position after drug administration than in those kept upright.[387] Most of the problems associated with intralumbar injection can also be overcome with direct intraventricular administration. This approach entails the surgical placement of a catheter into the lateral ventricle which is then attached to a subcutaneously implanted reservoir for access.[388] Administration of drugs directly into the ventricle via this reservoir is more convenient and less painful and is amenable to more frequent injections. Intraventricular therapy ensures that the drug is actually delivered to the subarachnoid space and results in much better drug distribution throughout the CSF.[385] The improved drug distribution may be the reason for the improved therapeutic results noted with intraventricular therapy over intralumbar dosing in the treatment of overt meningeal leukemia.[389]

Currently, there are only a few agents that are routinely administered intrathecally. The most commonly used agents are the antimetabolites methotrexate and cytarabine and the alkylator thiotepa. Recently, promising results have also been reported with intrathecal diaziquone.[390]

Methotrexate

Intrathecal methotrexate has been in clinical use for nearly three decades, primarily for the treatment of the meningeal spread of cancer, especially leukemia and lymphoma. It is also administered prophylactically to patients with newly diagnosed leukemia. Acute and delayed neurotoxic reactions to intrathecal methotrexate have been reported. An acute chemical arachnoiditis characterized by headache, nuchal rigidity, vomiting, fever, and a CSF pleocytosis can present several hours to days after a dose. A subacute encephalopathy, which may be irreversible in some patients, presents with extremity paresis and cranial-nerve palsies, ataxia, visual impairment, seizures, and coma. This syndrome is associated with elevated CSF drug levels.[391] A chronic, progressive demyelinating encephalopathy that appears months to years after intrathecal methotrexate consists of dementia, spastic paralysis, seizures, and coma in more advanced cases. Severe, often fatal reactions can result from the inadvertent administration of excessive doses of methotrexate or the administration of the wrong agent (*e.g.,* vincristine) intrathecally. Great care must be taken by clinicians administering drugs by this route.[392]

Methotrexate clearance from the CSF after intrathecal injection is biphasic, with a terminal half-life of 14 hours.[385] Methotrexate is eliminated by bulk resorption of CSF and a nonspecific active transport system in the choroid plexus. Conditions associated with delayed clearance of methotrexate from the CSF include the presence of meningeal leukemia, communicating hydrocephalus, or the lumbar puncture syndrome.[385] The systemic exposure to an intrathecal dose of methotrexate is longer than from the equivalent dose administered intravenously. Plasma levels of methotrexate remain above 0.01 μM twofold longer with the intrathecal dose.[393]

When methotrexate is administered intrathecally, the volume of the CSF becomes the primary initial volume in which the drug is distributed. The initial concentration of drug is determined by this volume. In young children, CSF volume increases much more rapidly than the body surface area, reaching the adult volume by the age of 3 years.[394] Therefore, an intrathecal dose based on body surface area would be expected to underdose young children and overdose adolescents. Bleyer and colleagues have recommended an intrathecal dosage schedule for methotrexate based on age instead of body surface area (Table 9-6).[394] This regimen has been less neurotoxic, and, since this dosing scheme was incorporated

Table 9-6
Pharmacokinetically Derived Dosing Schedule for Intrathecal Methotrexate[394]

Age (yr)	Dose (mg)
<1	6
1	8
2	10
≥3	12

into frontline leukemia protocols, the CNS relapse rate has declined significantly, from 12% to 7%.[395] The greatest decline was observed in the youngest patients, the group in whom the intrathecal methotrexate dosage was increased with the new regimen.

Cytarabine

Intrathecally administered cytarabine is also of value in the treatment and prevention of meningeal leukemia. The clinical pharmacology of intrathecal cytarabine is quite different from that seen with systemic administration. With an intraventricular dose of 30 mg, peak levels exceed 2 mM and remain above 1 μM (the minimal cytotoxic concentration *in vitro*) for 24 hours.[396,397] Levels of cytidine deaminase, the enzyme that metabolizes cytarabine to ara-U, are very low in brain and CSF,[398] and metabolism to ara-U is therefore only a minor pathway of elimination. The ratio of ara-U to cytarabine in the CSF is only 0.08. The terminal half-life of cytarabine is 3.5 hours, and the clearance is 0.42 ml/min, similar to the CSF bulk flow rate.[396] Plasma levels following an intrathecal 30 mg dose are less than 1 μM.

High-Dose Systemic Therapy for Meningeal and CNS Tumors

Limited CNS penetration of some anticancer agents can be overcome by administering high doses of the drugs systemically. This approach has been successful with methotrexate and cytarabine. The advantages of the systemic approach over intrathecal therapy include (1) more uniform distribution of drug throughout the neuraxis, independent of the rate or direction of CSF flow; (2) CSF levels that can be sustained longer with prolonged intravenous infusions; and (3) better drug penetration into the deep perivascular spaces and brain parenchyma. The obvious disadvantage is the potential for severe systemic toxicity.

After an intravenous dose, the ratio of methotrexate concentration in CSF to plasma is low (0.03). However, with the use of leucovorin rescue, very high systemic methotrexate levels can be achieved safely, and therapeutic levels of methotrexate can be attained in the CSF. A regimen consisting of a 33,600 mg/m^2 dose administered over 24 hours as a loading dose (6000 mg/m^2) followed by a continuous infusion (1200 mg/m^2 per hour for 23 hours) results in CSF methotrexate concentrations of 30 to 40 μM.[399] With this regimen, the remission induction rate in patients with overt meningeal leukemia is 80%. This regimen has also been successful as preventive therapy for meningeal leukemia in patients with acute lymphoblastic leukemia (see Chap. 16).[400]

The CSF-to-plasma ratio of cytarabine is more favorable but is dose dependent. The ratio in one study decreased from 0.33 to 0.18 with an increase in the dose from 4000 to 18,000 mg/m^2 administered as a 72-hour infusion.[401] However, the standard 3000 mg/m^2 dose given every 12 hours results in persistent cytotoxic concentrations of cytarabine in the CSF, in part because the elimination half-life of cytarabine in CSF is eightfold longer than in plasma due to the low levels of cytidine deaminase in brain and CSF.[402] High-dose intravenous cytarabine appears to be efficacious for the treatment of CNS leukemia and lymphoma[403,404] but is associated with significant systemic toxicity.

Other agents in which the systemic approach may be applicable include 6-mercaptopurine, cyclophosphamide, and thiotepa. When administered as a high-dose infusion (50 mg/m^2 per hour over 48 hours), cytotoxic levels of 6-mercaptopurine can be achieved and maintained in the CSF.[211] The activity of high-dose 6-mercaptopurine is currently being tested in pediatric brain tumors. Cyclophosphamide in high doses (80 mg/m^2 per day for 2 days) appears to be active against brain tumors.[405] The CSF and CNS kinetics of the active metabolites of cyclophosphamide have not been well characterized to correlate with this clinical activity. Finally, a recent study indicates that the systemic approach may also be more appropriate for thiotepa,[406] a drug that has been administered intrathecally for menigeal cancer. Intrathecally administered thiotepa is rapidly cleared from the CSF at a rate tenfold higher than CSF bulk flow. As a result, with an intraventricular dose, drug exposure in the lumbar region is only 5% of that in the ventricles. After intravenous administration, plasma and CSF drug levels are equivalent, and significant levels of the active metabolite, tepa, are also seen in CSF. The clearance of tepa is much slower, resulting in a greater exposure to alkylators in the CSF. Tepa is not formed in measurable concentrations with an intrathecal dose. The authors concluded that there was no relative advantage to the intrathecal administration of thiotepa.[406]

DRUG DEVELOPMENT

A national effort to develop new, effective, and less toxic anticancer drugs was undertaken in 1955 under the auspices of the National Cancer Institute (NCI). At its peak in the early 1970s, up to 40,000 compounds a year were screened for antitumor activity.[29] The process of developing a new drug, which may take from 10 to 12 years, starts with the acquisition of prospective agents from a variety of sources, ranging from the NCI intramural program and other research institutes to the pharmaceutical industry. These compounds may be chemically synthesized (including analogues of known active agents) or natural products usually derived from microorganisms or higher plants.[407] The potential drugs are then screened for antitumor activity in model tumor systems. Initial screening is performed in a transplantable murine leukemia model, and active agents are then tested *in vivo* against a panel of murine tumors (both leukemia and solid tumors) and against human tumor xenografts that are transplanted into immunodeficient nude mice.[29,407,408] Compounds that are active in other systems can bypass the initial screen and proceed directly to the tumor panel. A new screening procedure, which is based on *in vitro* activity against cell lines derived from human solid tumors is also currently being tested by the NCI.[409]

A compound judged to be active in the tumor panel is then tested to determine whether an adequate formulation for human use can be produced in large scale. Formulation and production are especially a problem with highly unstable or hydrophobic compounds and complex products extracted from natural sources.[29] Before testing in humans, toxicology studies are performed in several animal species to define qualitatively the drug's toxic effects and help determine a safe starting dose for the human studies.[410]

The initial stage of human testing (Phase I trial) is designed [1] to determine the maximally tolerated dose (MTD) of the new drug in humans using several schedules; [2] to define qualitatively the types of toxicities that may occur; and [3] to study the clinical pharmacology of the agent. This first phase of testing is done in a small group (15–30) of patients with refractory cancer and is not intended to determine the drug's therapeutic effect. Separate Phase I trials are usually conducted in children because children with solid tumors tend to have a greater dose tolerance than adults for most previusly tested agents.[411] Because of this, the NCI recommends that the starting dose in pediatric Phase I trials by 80% of the adult MTD and that the dose be escalated in subsequent patients by a fixed 20% increment.[411]

Once the optimal dose and schedule for the new drug have been defined, the second stage of testing (Phase II trial) defines the spectrum of activity and response rate in various human cancers. These disease-specific single agent studies are conducted on groups of 35 to 50 patients with early termination of the trial if the first 14 patients have no response.[412] Responses are usually defined as a greater than 50% reduction in the volume of all measurable sites of tumor. Although patients entered on these trials are also refractory to conventional therapy, heavily pretreated patients should not be entered because they are more likely to have highly resistant (multidrug-resistant) tumors. Half of the evaluable drugs tested in Phase II setting since 1970 have been deemed active in at least one form of cancer.[413] However, most responses have occurred in patients with lymphoma or leukemia, and the response rates for the more refractory solid tumors are low. This may reflect either the greater responsiveness of the hematologic malignancies to chemotherapy or the failure of current screening procedures to detect drugs that are potentially effective for the solid tumors. New screening procedures using human solid tumor cell lines may remedy this trend.

If efficacy is demonstrated in Phase II studies, the drug is then moved into the frontline treatment of newly diagnosed patients and compared to standard therapy, usually in large randomized clinical trials. Only one or two agents out of the initial 15,000 screened per year make it through the entire drug testing procedure and are released for use in humans.

There has been an emphasis in recent years on the development of biologic response modifiers. These agents produce their antitumor effect by modulating the host's response to the tumor or by causing differentiation in the tumor. The optimal design of preclinical screening studies and clinical trials has yet to be established, but these agents do not fit the mold of the classic anticancer drugs.[414]

The ethical issues involved in conducting these investigational studies are particularly complex in children and have received public attention.[407] In offering new agent studies, especially Phase I trials, to these terminally ill patients, the physician must consider the emotional and psychosocial status of the patient and family. In addition, the realistic expectations for therapeutic benefit and lack of curative potential should be presented before entering a child on one of these studies.

Because of the known biologic differences between adult and pediatric malignancies and the physiologic differences affecting drug distribution and elimination, it is important to define separately the optimal dose and schedule and the spectrum of activity of new agents in children with cancer. Future progress in the treatment of pediatric cancer will in large part be dependent on the identification of new active agents. For this reason, clinicians should consider enrolling patients with refractory disease on Phase I and Phase II new agent studies when clinically and ethically indicated.

FUTURE PERSPECTIVES

Despite the great strides made in the chemotherapy of childhood cancer over the past three decades, many challenges lie ahead. Although a high proportion of children with certain types of cancer are being cured, there are still too many who either fail to respond or relapse after a good initial response. These treatment failures may be due to *de novo* or acquired resistance to the drugs being used or to inadequate therapy as a result of improper dosage modifications, interindividual differences in drug disposition with poor absorption or more rapid drug clearance in a subgroup of patients, or dose limitations necessitated by acute and chronic toxicities that limit the dosage and frequency that drugs can be administered. Each of these issues poses a challenge to the pediatric oncologist.

The incidence of *de novo* resistance of newly diagnosed tumors to "active" drugs may be as high as 50%. Thus, many patients receive drugs in standard combination regimens that are ineffective against their tumor and produce undesirable side-effects. Human-tumor clonogenic or colony-forming assays have been extensively studied as a means of defining a drug sensitivity profile for individual tumors, similar to the sensitivity testing routinely performed with bacterial isolates.[415,416] This approach is appealing since it might allow individualized treatment planning that would include only truly active drugs. However, serious drawbacks limit the practical value of this technique. First, in many patients, sufficient tumor specimens are not readily accessible, and, when they are available, adequate *in vitro* growth is achieved in only a small proportion of specimens (28% of a series of pediatric tumors[416]). Second, to date, there are no rigorous prospective correlations using these assays to compare *in vitro* responses of tested tumors to single agents or combination regimens with the clinical response in the patient to the same agents.[415,416] Measurement of biochemical (*e.g.,* increased target enzyme or altered transport capacity) or genetic (*e.g., mdr1* gene) markers of drug resistance in tumor specimens is a promising potential means of quantitating drug sensitivity[415]; however, the clinical applicability and usefulness of this approach have yet to be demonstrated. Overcoming drug resistance, particularly in multidrug-resistant tumors, is perhaps the greatest challenge. Once the exact mechanism of resistance is defined, methods of reversing these cellular changes can be sought, such as the use of calcium-channel blockers to reverse the decreased cellular uptake of drugs in multidrug resistance.[26] Biochemical alterations that result in resistance to one agent may also make these resistant cells more sensitive to the effects of a second drug. An example of this phenomenon, termed *collateral sensitivity,* is the increased sensitivity of 6-mercaptopurine-resistant murine leukemia lines to methotrexate.[417] When such a situation exists, it provides the clinician with a potential opportunity to exploit selectively the alterations in these resistant cells.

Current dosing modifications used in most treatment regimens are empirical. For example, the practice of defining a standard starting dose that is modified on the basis of ensuing toxicities does not take into account possible individual variability in drug disposition that could result in serious underdosing or overdosing of some patients. A more rational approach, basing drug dose and schedule on plasma drug concentration (*therapeutic drug monitoring*), has already been adopted in most other medical specialties. This strategy has also been successful in conjunction with high-dose methotrexate therapy.[418] Although therapeutic and toxic drug concentrations are not known for most anticancer drugs, simply defining the average plasma concentration after a standard drug dose might help to identify outliers and result in more rational dose modifications in patients with organ dysfunction. Knowledge of the pharmacokinetics of a drug is also useful in determining the most appropriate schedule of drug administration. Continuous-infusion schedules of cytarabine, based in part on the drug's rapid clearance and short half-life, are known to be the most efficacious schedule of administration for conventional doses of the drug.

Finally, the search for new, more selective, and less toxic agents and for more effective drug combinations must continue. As our knowledge about the molecular aspect of malignant transformation and tumor progression grows, agents specifically designed to interfere with the critical steps in these processes can be developed. In addition, the use of *biochemical modulation* (the administration of a drug as a modulating agent to alter the pharmacokinetics or pharmacodynamics of another cytotoxic agent and enhance its cytotoxic effect; *e.g.,* sequential methotrexate/5-fluorouracil) has shown promise in experimental systems.

To overcome these challenges, a greater effort must be made to incorporate the advances made in the basic science of cancer and pharmacology into the design and use of chemotherapeutic treatment modalities.

REFERENCES

1. Farber S, Diamond LK, Mercer RD et al: Temporary remissions in acute leukemia in children produced by folic acid antagonist 4-amethopteroylglutamic acid (aminopterin). N Engl J Med 238:787–793, 1948
2. Young JL, Ries LG, Silverberg E et al: Cancer Incidence, survival, and mortality for children younger than age 15 years. Cancer 58(Suppl):598–602, 1986
3. Hammond GD: Keynote address: The cure of childhood cancers. Cancer 58(Suppl):407–413, 1986
4. Bleyer WA: Antineoplastic agents. In Yaffe SJ (ed): Pediatric Pharmacology: Therapeutic Principles in Practice, pp 349–377. New York, Grune & Stratton, 1980
5. Henderson EH, Samaha RJ: Evidence that drugs in multiple combinations have materially advanced the treatment of human malignancies. Cancer Res 29:2272–2280, 1969
6. Hammond GD, Bleyer WA, Hartmann JR et al: The team approach to the management of pediatric cancer. Cancer 41:29–35, 1978
7. Pochedly C: Prophylactic CNS therapy in childhood acute leukemia. Am J Pediatr Hematol Oncol 1:119–126, 1979
8. Rosen G, Caparros B, Huvos AG et al: Neoadjuvant chemotherapy for osteogenic sarcoma: A model for the treatment of other highly malignant neoplasms. Recent Results Cancer Res 103:148–157, 1986
9. Collins JM, Dedrick RL: Pharmacokinetics of anticancer drugs. In Chabner B (ed): Pharmacologic Principles of Cancer Treatment, pp 77–99. Philadelphia, WB Saunders, 1982
10. Balis FM, Holcenberg JS, Bleyer WA: Clinical pharmacokinetics of commonly used anticancer drugs. Clin Pharmacokinet 8:202–232, 1983
11. Spiegel RJ: The acute toxicities of chemotherapy. Cancer Treat Rev 8:197–207, 1981
12. Perry MC, Yarbro JW (eds): Toxicity of Chemotherapy. Orlando, Grune & Stratton, 1984
13. Frei E, Freireich EJ, Gehan E et al: Studies of sequential and combination antimetabolite therapy in acute leukemia—6-mercaptopurine and methotrexate. Blood 18:431–454, 1961
14. Goldie JH, Coldman AJ: The genetic origin of drug resistance in neoplasms: Implications for systemic therapy. Cancer Res 44:3643–3653, 1984
15. Seeber S: Cellular mechanisms of anticancer drug resistance. J Cancer Res Clin Oncol 103(Suppl):A51, 1982
16. Biedler JL, Spengler BA: Metaphase chromosome anomaly: Association

with drug resistance and cell-specific products. Science 191:185–187, 1976

17. Ling V, Kartner N, Sudo T et al: Multidrug resistant phenotype in Chinese hamster ovary cells. Cancer Treat Rep 67:869–874, 1983

18. Batist G, Tulpule A, Sinha BK et al: Overexpression of a novel anionic glutathione transferase in multidrug-resistant human breast cancer cells. J Biol Chem 261:15544–15549, 1986

19. Gerlach J, Kartner N, Bell D, Ling V: Multidrug resistance. Cancer Surv 5:89–94, 1986

20. Biedler JL, Patterson RHF: Altered plasma membrane glycoconjugates of Chinese hamster cells with acquired resistance to actinomycin D, daunorubicin and vincristine. In Sartorelli AC, Lazlo JS, Bertino JR (eds): Molecular Actions and Targets for Cancer Chemotherapeutic Agents, pp 453–482. New York, Academic Press, 1981

21. Scotto KW, Biedler JL, Melera PW: Amplification and expression of genes associated with multidrug resistence in mammalian cells. Science 232:751–755, 1986

22. Roninson IB, Chin JE, Choi K: Isolation of human *mdr* DNA sequences amplified in multidrug-resistant KB carcinoma cells. Proc Natl Acad Sci USA 83:4538–4542, 1986

23. Ueda K, Cornwell MM, Gottesman MM et al: The *mdr* 1 gene, responsible for multidrug-resistance, codes for P-glycoprotein. Biochem Biophys Res Comm 141:956–962, 1986

24. Fojo AT, Ueda K, Slamon DJ et al: Expression of a multidrug resistance gene in human tumors and tissues. Proc Natl Acad Sci USA 84:265–269, 1987

25. Shen D-W, Fojo A, Chin JE: Human multidrug-resistant cell lines: increased *mdr* 1 expression can precede gene amplification. Science 232:643–645, 1986

26. Beck WT: Cellular pharmacology of multiple drug resistance and its circumvention. Adv Enzyme Reg 22:207–227, 1984

27. Willingham MC, Cornwell MM, Cardarelli CO et al: Single cell analysis of daunomycin uptake and efflux in multidrug-resistant and -sensitive KB cells: Effects of verapamil and other drugs. Cancer Res 46:5941–5946, 1986

28. Ozols RF, Cunnion RE, Klecker RW et al: Verapamil and Adriamycin in the treatment of drug-resistant ovarian cancer patients. J Clin Oncol 5:641–647, 1987

29. DeVita VT: Principles of chemotherapy. In DeVita VT, Hellman S, Rosenberg SA (eds): Cancer Principles and Practice of Oncology, pp 257–285. Philadelphia, JB Lippincott, 1985

30. Frei E, Canellos GP: Dose: A critical factor in cancer chemotherapy. Am J Med 69:585–594, 1980

31. Pinkel D, Hernandez K, Borella L et al: Drug dosage and remission duration in childhood lymphocytic leukemia. Cancer 27:247–256, 1971

32. Cortes EP, Holland JF, Glidewell O: Adjuvant treatment of primary osteosarcoma: Cancer and Leukemia Group B experience. Recent Results Cancer Res 68:16–24, 1979

33. Martin DS: The scientific basis for adjuvant chemotherapy. Cancer Treat Rev 8:169–189, 1981

34. Ames MM: Pharmacokinetics of antitumor agents in children. In Ames MM, Powis G, Kovach JS (eds): Pharmacokinetics of Anticancer Agents in Humans, pp 400–431. Amsterdam, Elsevier, 1983

35. Powis G: Effects of disease states on pharmacokinetics of anticancer drugs. In Ames MM, Powis G, Kovach JS (eds): Pharmacokinetics of Anticancer Agents in Humans, pp 365–397. Amsterdam, Elsevier, 1983

36. Balis FM: Pharmacokinetic drug interactions of commonly used anticancer drugs. Clin Pharmacokinet 11:223–235, 1986

37. Colvin M: The alkylating agents. In Chabner B (ed): Pharmacologic Principles of Cancer Treatment, pp 276–308. Philadelphia, WB Saunders, 1982

38. Kohn KW: Molecular mechanisms of crosslinking by alkylating agents and platinum complexes. In Sartorelli AC, Lazlo JS, Bertino JR (eds): Molecular Actions and Targets for Cancer Chemotherapeutic Agents, pp 3–16. New York, Academic Press, 1981

39. Farmer PB, Newell DR: Alkylating agents. In Ames MM, Powis G, Kovach JS (eds): Pharamcokinetics of Anticancer Agents in Humans, pp 77–111. Amsterdam, Elsevier, 1983

40. Byfield JE, Calabro-Jones PM: Carrier-dependent and carrier-independent transport of anti-cancer alkylating agents. Nature 294:281–283, 1981

41. Wolpert MK, Ruddon RW: A study on the mechanisms of resistance to nitrogen mustard in Ehrlich ascites tumor cells: Comparison of uptake of HN_2-^{14}C into sensitive and resistant cells. Cancer Res 29:873–879, 1969

42. Redwood WR, Colvin M: Transport of melphalan by sensitive and resistant L1210 cells. Cancer Res 40:1144–1149, 1980

43. Calcutt G, Connors TA: Tumour sulphhydryl levels and sensitivity to the nitrogen mustard Merophan. Biochem Pharmacol 12:839–845, 1963

44. Arrick BA, Nathan CF: Glutathione metabolism as determinant of therapeutic efficacy: A review. Cancer Res 44:4224–4232, 1984

45. Sladek NE: Bioassay and relative cytoxic potency of cyclophosphamide metabolites generated *in vitro* and *in vivo*. Cancer Res 33:1150–1158, 1973

46. Ewig RAG, Kohn KW: DNA damage and repair in mouse leukemia L1210 cells treated with nitrogen mustard, 1,3-bis(2-chloroethyl)-1-nitrosourea, and other nitrosoureas. Cancer Res 37:2114–2122, 1977

47. Schabel FM, Trader MW, Laster WR et al: Patterns of resistance and therapeutic synergism among alkylating agents. Antibiot Chemother 23:200–215, 1978

48. Teicher BA, Cucchi CA, Lee JB et al: Alkylating agents: *In vitro* studies of cross-resistance patterns in human cell lines. Cancer Res 46:4379–4383, 1986

49. Frei E, Cucchi CA, Rosowsky A et al: Alkylating agent resistence: *In vitro* studies with human cell lines. Proc Natl Acad Sci USA 82:2158–2162, 1985

50. Postmus PE, de Vries EGE: Intensive chemotherapy and autologous bone marrow transplantation for solid tumors. Monogr Ser Eur Organ Res Treat Cancer 14:77–96, 1984

51. Connors TA: Alkylating drugs, nitrosoureas and dimethyltriazenes. In Pinedo HM (ed): Cancer Chemotherapy (Annual 3), pp 32–74. New York, Elsevier, 1981

52. Mirkes PE: Cyclophosphamide teratogenesis: A review. Teratogen Carcinogen Mutagen 5:75–88, 1985

53. Cramer P, Andrieu JM: Hodgkin's disease in childhood and adolescence: Results of chemotherapy–radiotherapy in clinical stages IA–IIB. J Clin Oncol 3:1495–1502, 1985

54. van Eys J, Cangir A, Coody D, Smith B: MOPP regimen as primary chemotherapy for brain tumors in infants. J Neurooncol 3:237–243, 1985

55. Cangir A, Ragab AH, Steuber P et al: Combination chemotherapy with vincristine (NSC-67574), procarbazine (NSC-77213), prednisone (NSC-10023) with or without nitrogen mustard (NSC-762) (MOPP vs OPP) in children with recurrent brain tumors. Med Pediatr Oncol 12:1–3, 1984

56. Monk BE, McKee PH, du Vivier A: Histiocytosis X of the scalp and face responding to topical nitrogen mustard. J R Soc Med 78(Suppl 11):6–7, 1985

57. Wong E, Holden CA, Broadbent V, Atherton DJ: Histiocytosis X presenting as intertrigo and responding to topical nitrogen mustard. Clin Exp Dermatol 11:183–187, 1986

58. Nadkarni MV, Trams EG, Smith PK: Observations on the rapid disappearance of radioactivity from blood after intravenous triethylenemelamine–C^{14}. Proc Am Assoc Cancer Res 2:136, 1956

59. Shapiro WR, Young DF: Neurological complications of antineoplastic therapy. Acta Neurol Scand 100(Suppl):125–132, 1984

60. Grochow LB, Colvin M: Clinical pharmacokinetics of cyclophosphamide. Clin Pharmacokinet 4:380–394, 1979

61. Grochow LB, Colvin M: Clinical pharmacokinetics of cyclophosphamide. In Ames MM, Powis G, Kovach JS (eds): Pharmacokinetics of Anticancer Agents in Humans, pp 135–154. Amsterdam, Elsevier, 1983

62. Brade WP, Herdrich K, Varini M: Ifosfamide—pharmacology, safety and therapeutic potential. Cancer Treat Rev 12:1–47, 1985

63. Colvin M: The comparative pharmacology of cyclophosphamide and ifosfamide. Semin Oncol 9(Suppl):2–7, 1982

64. Wagner T, Fenneberg K: Pharmacokinetics and bioavailability of cyclophosphamide from oral formulations. Arzneimittelforschung 34:313–316, 1984

65. D'Incalci M, Bolis G, Facchinetti T et al: Decreased half life of cyclophosphamide in patients under continual treatment. Eur J Cancer 15:7–10, 1979

66. Juma FD, Rogers HJ, Trounce JR: Pharmacokinetics of cyclophosphamide and alkylating activity in man after intravenous and oral administration. Br J Clin Pharmacol 8:209–217, 1979

67. Bagley CM, Bostick FW, DeVita VT: Clinical pharmacology of cyclophosphamide. Cancer Res 33:226–233, 1973

68. Jardine I, Fenselau C, Appler M et al: Quantitation by gas chromatography–chemical ionization mass spectrometry of cyclophosphamide, phosphoramide mustard, and nornitrogen mustard in the plasma and urine of patients receiving cyclophosphamide therapy. Cancer Res 38:408–415, 1978

69. Wagner T, Heydrich D, Jork T et al: Comparative study on human pharmacokinetics of activated ifosfamide and cyclophosphamide by a modified fluorometric test. J Cancer Res Clin Oncol 100:95–104, 1981

70. Allen LM, Creaven PJ, Nelson RL: Studies on the human pharmacokinetics of ifosfamide (NSC-109724). Cancer Treat Rep 60:451–458, 1976

71. Dooley JS, James CA, Rogers HJ, Stuart-Harris R: Biliary elimination of cyclophosphamide in man. Cancer Chemother Pharmacol 9:26–29, 1982

72. Juma FD, Rogers HJ, Trounce JR: Effect of renal insufficiency on the pharmacokinetics of cyclophosphamide and some of its metabolites. Eur J Clin Pharmacol 19:443–445, 1981

73. Wang LH, Lee CS, Majeske BL et al: Clearance and recovery calculations in hemodialysis: Application to plasma, red blood cell and dialysate measurements for cyclophosphamide. Clin Pharmacol Ther 29:365–372, 1981

74. Juma FD, Koech DK, Kasili EG et al: Pharmacokinetics of cyclophosphamide in Kenyan African children with lymphoma. Br J Clin Pharmacol 18:106–107, 1984

75. Sladek NE, Priest J, Doeden D et al: Plasma half-life and urinary excretion of cyclophosphamide in children. Cancer Treat Rep 64:1061–1066, 1980

76. Slee PH, de Bruijin EA, Driessen OM et al: Pharmacokinetics of the cytostatic drugs used in the CMF-regimen. Anticancer Res 3:269–271, 1983

77. Wilkinson PM, O'Neill PA, Thatcher N: Pharmacokinetics of high-dose cyclophosphamide in patients with metastatic bronchogenic carcinoma. Cancer Chemother Pharmacol 11:196–199, 1983

78. Bramwell V, Calvert RT, Edwards G et al: The disposition of cyclophosphamide in a group of myeloma patients. Cancer Chemother Pharmacol 3:253–259, 1979

79. Wagner T, Heydrich D, Bartels H et al: The influence of damaged liver parenchyma, renal insufficiency and hemodialysis on the pharmacokinetics of cyclophosphamide and its activated metabolites. Arzneimittelforschung 30:1588–1592, 1980

80. Burkert H: Clinical overview of mesna. Cancer Treat Rev 10(Suppl):175–181, 1983

81. Samra Y, Hertz M, Lindner A: Urinary bladder tumors following cyclophosphamide therapy. A report of two cases with a review of the literature. Med Pediatr Oncol 13:86–91, 1985

82. Bode U, Seif SM, Levine AS: Studies on the antidiuretic effect of cyclophosphamide: Vasopressin release and sodium excretion. Med Pediatr Oncol 8:295–303, 1980

83. Pratt CB, Green AA, Horowitz ME et al: Central nervous system toxicity following the treatment of pediatric patients with ifosfamide/mesna. J Clin Oncol 4:1253–1261, 1986

84. Gurtoo HL, Hipkens JH, Sharma SD: Role of glutathione in the metabolism-dependent toxicity and chemotherapy of cyclophosphamide. Cancer Res 41:3584–3591, 1981

85. McGown AT, Fox BW: A proposed mechanism of resistance to cyclophosphamide and phosphoramide mustard in a Yoshida cell line in vitro. Cancer Chemother Pharmacol 17:223–226, 1986

86. Crook TR, Souhami RL, Whyman GD et al: Glutathione depletion as a determinant of sensitivity of human leukemia cells to cyclophosphamide. Cancer Res 46:5035–5038, 1986

87. Hilton J, Colvin M: The role of aldehyde dehydrogenase activity in cyclophosphamide sensitivity of hematopoietic and leukemic cell populations (abstr). Proc Am Assoc Cancer Res 25:339, 1984

88. Dorr RT, Alberts DS: Cimetidine enhancement of cyclophosphamide antitumor activity. Br J Cancer 45:35–43, 1982

89. Dorr RT, Soble MJ, Alberts DS: Interaction of cimetidine but not ranitidine with cyclophosphamide in mice. Cancer Res 46:1795–1799, 1986

90. Boston Collaborative Drug Surveillance Program: Allopurinol and cytotoxic drugs. JAMA 227:1036–1040, 1974

91. Graham-Pole J, Lazarus HM, Herzig RH et al: High-dose melphalan for the treatment of children with refractory neuroblastoma and Ewing's sarcoma. Am J Pediatr Hematol Oncol 6:17–26, 1984

92. Lazarus HM, Herzig RH, Graham-Pole J et al: Intensive melphalan chemotherapy and cryopreserved autologous bone marrow transplantation for the treatment of refractory cancer. J Clin Oncol 1:359–367, 1983

93. Maraninchi D, Abecasis M, Gastaut JA et al: High-dose melphalan and autologous bone marrow transplantation for relapsed leukaemia. Cancer Chemother Pharmacol 10:109–111, 1983

94. Horowitz M, Etcubanas E, Christensen M et al: Melphalan: A clinically effective agent for rhabdomyosarcoma as predicted by the xenograft model (abstract). Proc Am Soc Clin Oncol 5:205, 1986

95. Alberts DS, Chang SV, Chen HS et al: Comparative pharmacokinetics of chlorambucil and melphalan in man. Recent Results Cancer Res 74:124–131, 1980

96. Woodhouse KW, Hamilton P, Lennard A et al: The pharmacokinetics of melphalan in patients with multiple myeloma: An intravenous/oral study using a conventional dose regimen. Eur J Clin Pharmacol 24:283–285, 1983

97. Bosanquet AG, Gilby ED: Pharmacokinetics of oral and intravenous melphalan during routine treatment of multiple myeloma. Eur J Cancer Clin Oncol 18:355–362, 1982

98. Alberts DS, Chang SY, Chen HS et al: Oral melphalan kinetics. Clin Pharmacol Ther 26:737–745, 1979

99. Brox L, Birkett L, Belch A: Pharmacology of intravenous melphalan in patients with multiple myeloma. Cancer Treat Rev 6(Suppl):27–32, 1979

100. Ardiet C, Tranchand B, Biron P et al: Pharmacokinetics of high dose intravenous melphalan in children and adults with forced diuresis: Report in 26 cases. Cancer Chemother Pharmacol 16:300–305, 1986

101. Christensen ML, Sinkule JA, Horowitz M et al: Clinical pharmacokinetics of melphalan, L-phenylalanine mustard (PAM), in patients with refractory solid tumors (abstr). Proc Am Assoc Cancer Res 25:366, 1984

102. Alberts DS, Chang SY, Chen H-SG et al: Kinetics of intravenous melphalan. Clin Pharmacol Ther 26:73–80, 1979

103. Hersh MR, Ludden TM, Kuhn JG et al: Pharmacokinetics of high dose melphalan. Invest New Drugs 1:331–334, 1983

104. Tahal A, Ahmad RA, Rogers DW et al: Pharmacokinetics of melphalan in children following high-dose intravenous injection. Cancer Chemother Pharmacol 10:212–216, 1983

105. Gouyette A, Hartmann O, Pico JL: Pharmacokinetics of high-dose melphalan in children and adults. Cancer Chemother Pharmacol 16:184–189, 1986

106. Cornwell GG, Pajak TF, McIntyre OR et al: Influence of renal failure of myelosuppressive effects of melphalan: Cancer and Leukemia Group B experience. Cancer Treat Rep 66:475–481, 1982

107. Alberts DS, Chen HS, Benz D et al: Effect of renal dysfunction in dogs on the disposition and marrow toxicity of melphalan. Br J Cancer 43:330–334, 1981

108. Mitchell EP, Schein PS: Contributions of nitrosoureas to cancer treatment. Cancer Treat Rep 70:31–41, 1986

109. Ames MM, Powis G: Pharmacokinetics of nitrosoureas. In Ames MM, Powis G, Kovach JS (eds): Pharmacokinetics of Anticancer Agents in Humans, pp 113–134. Amsterdam, Elsevier, 1983

110. Kann HE: Comparison of biochemical and biological effects of four nitrosoureas with differing carbamoylating activities. Cancer Res 38:2363–2366, 1978

111. Tew KD, Sudhakar S, Schein PS, Smulson ME: Binding of chlorozotocin and 1-(2-chloroethyl)-3-cyclohexyl-1-nitrosourea to chromatin and nucleosomal fractions of HeLa cells. Cancer Res 38:3371–3378, 1978

112. Schein PS, Heal J, Green D, Wooley PV: Pharmacology of nitrosourea antitumor agents. Antibiot Chemother 23:64–75, 1978

113. DeVita VT, Denham C, Davidson JD, Oliverio VT: The physiological disposition of the carcinostatic 1,3-bis(2-chloroethyl)-1-nitrosourea (BCNU) in man and animals. Clin Pharmacol Ther 8:566–577, 1967

114. Sponzo RW, DeVita VT, Oliverio VT: Physiologic disposition of 1-(2-chloroethyl)-3-cyclohexyl-1-nitrosourea (CCNU) and 1-(2-chloroethyl)-3-(4-methyl cyclohexyl)-1-nitrosourea (MeCCNU) in man. Cancer 31:1154–1159, 1973

115. Levin VA, Hoffman W, Weinkam RJ: Pharmacokinetics of BCNU in man: A preliminary study of 20 patients. Cancer Treat Rep 62:1305–1312, 1978

116. Henner WD, Peters WP, Eder JP et al: Pharmacokinetics and immediate effects of high-dose carmustine in man. Cancer Treat Rep 70:877–880, 1986

117. Lee FY, Workman P, Roberts JT, Bleehen NM: Clinical pharmacokinetics of oral CCNU (lomustine). Cancer Chemother Pharmacol 14:125–131, 1985

118. Weiss RB, Issell BF: The nitrosoureas: Carmustine (BCNU) and lomustine (CCNU). Cancer Treat Rev 9:313–330, 1982

119. Walker MD, Hilton J: Nitrosourea pharmacodynamics in relation to the central nervous system. Cancer Treat Rep 60:725–728, 1976

120. Levin VA, Weinkam RJ, Hoffman W, Wilson CB: Pharmacokinetics of BCNU in humans (abstr). Proc Am Assoc Cancer Res 18:76, 1977

121. Harmon WE, Cohen HJ, Schneeburger EE: Chronic renal failure in children treated with methyl CCNU. N Engl J Med 300:1200–1203, 1979

122. Ellis ME, Weiss RB, Kuperminc M: Nephrotoxicity of lomustine: A case report and literature review. Cancer Chemother Pharmacol 15:174–175, 1985

123. Aronin PA, Mahaley MS, Rudnick SA et al: Prediction of BCNU pulmonary toxicity in patients with malignant gliomas: An assessment of risk factors. N Engl J Med 303:183–191, 1980

124. Weinstein AS, Diener-West M, Nelson DF, Pakuris E: Pulmonary toxicity of carmustine in patients treated for malignant glioma. Cancer Treat Rep 70:943–946, 1986

125. Levin VA, Sterns J, Byrd A et al: The effect of phenobarbital pretreatment on the antitumor activity of 1,3-bis(2-chloroethyl)-1-nitrosourea (BCNU), 1-(2-

chloroethyl)-3-cyclohexyl-1-nitrosourea (CCNU) and 1-(2-chloroethyl)-3-(2,6-dioxo-3-piperidyl)-1-nitrosourea (PCNU), and on the plasma pharmacokinetics and biotransformation of BCNU. J Pharmacol Exp Ther 208:1–6, 1979

126. Zwelling LA: Cisplatin and new platinum analogs. In Pinedo HM, Chabner BA (eds): Cancer Chemotherapy (Annual 8), pp 97–116. New York, Elsevier, 1986

127. Loehrer PJ, Einhorn LH: Cisplatin. Ann Intern Med 100:704–713, 1984

128. Jaffe N, Knopp J, Chuang VP et al: Osteosarcoma: Intra-arterial treatment in the primary tumor with cis-diamminedichloroplatinum (II) (CDP): Angiographic, pathologic, and pharmacologic studies. Cancer 51:402–407, 1983

129. Pratt CB, Hayes A, Green AA et al: Pharmacokinetic evaluation of cisplatin in children with malignant solid tumors: A phase II study. Cancer Treat Rep 65:1021–1026, 1981

130. Kahn AB, D'Souza B, Wharam M et al: Cisplatin therapy in recurrent brain tumors. Cancer Treat Rep 66:2013–2020, 1982

131. Chary KK, Higby DJ, Henderson ES, Swinerton KD: Phase I study of high-dose cis-dichlorodiammineplatinum (II) with forced diuresis. Cancer Treat Rep 61:367–370, 1977

132. Corden BJ, Fine RL, Ozols RF, Collins JM: Clinical pharmacology of high-dose cisplatin. Cancer Chemother Pharmacol 14:38–41, 1985

133. Pfeifle CE, Howell SB, Felthouse RD et al: High-dose cisplatin with sodium thiosulfate protection. J Clin Oncol 3:237–244, 1985

134. LeRoy AF, Lutz RJ, Dedrick RL et al: Pharmacokinetic study of cis-diamminedichloroplatinum (II) (DDP) in the beagle dog: Thermodynamic and kinetic behavior of DDP in a biologic milieu. Cancer Treat Rep 63:59–71, 1979

135. Gormley PE, Bull JM, LeRoy AF, Cysyk R: Kinetics of cis-dichlorodiammineplatinum. Clin Pharmacol Ther 25:351–357, 1979

136. Patton TF, Himmelstein KJ, Belt R et al: Plasma levels and urinary excretion of filterable platinum species following bolus injection and IV infusion of cis-dichlorodiammineplatinum (II) in man. Cancer Treat Rep 62:1359–1362, 1978

137. DeConti RC, Toftness BR, Lange RC, Creasy WA: Clinical and pharmacologic studies with cis-diamminedichloroplatinum (II). Cancer Res 33:1310–1315, 1973

138. Himmelstein KJ, Patton TF, Belt RJ et al: Clinical kinetics of intact cisplatin and some related species. Clin Pharmacol Ther 29:658–664, 1981

139. Vermorken JB, van der Vijgh WJ, Klein I et al: Pharmacokinetics of free and total platinum species after rapid and prolonged infusions of cisplatin. Clin Pharmacol Ther 39:136–144, 1986

140. Patton TF, Repta AJ, Sternson LA, Belt RJ: Pharmacokinetics of intact cisplatin in plasma: Infusion versus bolus dosing. Int J Pharm 10:77–85, 1982

141. Belt RJ, Himmelstein KJ, Patton TF et al: Pharmacokinetics of non-protein-bound platinum species following administration of cis-dichlorodiammineplatinum (II). Cancer Treat Rep 63:1515–1521, 1979

142. Jacobs C, Kalman SM, Tretton M, Weiner MW: Renal handling of cis-diamminedichloroplatinum (II). Cancer Treat Rep 64:1223–1226, 1980

143. Reece PA, Stafford I, Davy M, Freeman S: Disposition of unchanged cisplatin in patients with ovarian cancer (abstr). Proc Am Assoc Cancer Res 28:193, 1987

144. Gonzalez-Vitale JC, Hayes DM, Cvitkovic E, Sternberg SS: The renal pathology in clinical trials of cis-platinum (II) diamminedichloride. Cancer 39:1362–1371, 1977

145. Meijer S, Sleijfer DT, Mulder NH et al: Some effects of combination chemotherapy with cisplatinum on renal function in patients with nonseminomatous testicular carcinoma. Cancer 51:2035–2040, 1983

146. Womer RB, Pritchard J, Barratt TM: Renal toxicity of cisplatin in children. J Pediatr 106:659–663, 1985

147. Fjeldborg P, Srensen J, Helkjaer PE: The long-term effect of cisplatin on renal function. Cancer 58:2214–2217, 1986

148. Crom WR, Pratt CB, Green AA et al: The effect of prior cisplatin therapy on the pharmacokinetics of high-dose methotrexate. J Clin Oncol 2:655–666, 1984

149. Reece PA, Stafford I, Russell J, Gill PG: Reduced ability to clear ultrafilterable platinum with repeated courses of cisplatin. J Clin Oncol 4:1392–1398, 1986

150. Stewart DJ, Mikhael N, Nanji A et al: Human tissue cisplatin pharmacology: Clinical implications (abstract). Proc Annu Meet Am Assoc Cancer Res 26:154, 1985

151. McHaney VA, Thibadoux MA, Hayes FA et al: Hearing loss in children receiving cisplatin chemotherapy. J Pediatr 102:314–317, 1983

152. Legha SS, Dimery IW: High-dose cisplatin administration without hypertonic saline: Observation of disabling neurotoxicity. J Clin Oncol 3:1373–1378, 1985

153. Schaefer SD, Post JD, Close LG, Wright CG: Ototoxicity of low and moderate-dose cisplatin. Cancer 56:1934–1939, 1985

154. Bajorin DF, Bosl GJ, Alcock NW et al: Pharmacokinetics of cis-diamminedichloroplatinum (II) after administration in hypertonic saline. Cancer Res 46:5969–5972, 1986

155. Chabner BA: DTIC (dacarbazine). In Chabner B (ed): Pharmacologic Principles of Cancer Treatment, pp 350–354. Philadelphia, WB Saunders, 1982

156. Stevens MF, Peatey L: Photodegradation of solutions of the antitumor drug DTIC (proceedings). J Pharm Pharmacol 30:47P, 1978

157. Gerulath AH, Loo TL: Mechanism of action of 5-(3,3-dimethyl-1-triazeno)imidazole-4-carboxamide (NSC-45388) in mammalian cells in culture. Biochem Pharmacol 21:2335–2343, 1972

158. Loo TL, Luce JK, Jardine JH, Frei E III: Pharmacologic studies of the antitumor agent 5-(dimethyltriazeno)imidazole-4-carboxamide. Cancer Res 28:2448–2453, 1968

159. Breithaupt H, Dammann A, Aigner K: Pharmacokinetics of dacarbazine (DTIC) and its metabolite 5-aminoimidazole-4-carboxamide (AIC) following different dose schedules. Cancer Chemother Pharmacol 9:103–109, 1982

160. Paschke R, Heine M: Pathophysiological aspects of dacarbazine-induced human liver damage. Hepatogastroenterology 32:273–275, 1985

161. Kumar AR, Renaudin J, Wilson CB et al: Procarbazine hydrochloride in the treatment of brain tumors. J Neurosurg 40:365–371, 1974

162. Weinkam RJ, Shiba DA: Procarbazine. In Chabner B (ed): Pharmacologic Principles of Cancer Treatment, pp 340–349. Philadelphia, WB Saunders, 1982

163. Dunn DL, Lubet RA, Prough RA: Oxidative metabolism of N-isopropyl-α-(2-methylhydrazino)-p-toluamide hydrochloride (procarbazine) by rat liver microsomes. Cancer Res 39:4555–4563, 1979

164. Baggiolini M, Dewald B, Aebi H: Oxidation of p-(N¹-methylhydrazinomethyl)-N-isopropylbenzamide to the methylazo derivative and oxidative cleavage of the N²–C bond in the isolated perfused rat liver. Biochem Pharmacol 18:2187–2196, 1969

165. Oliverio VT, Denham C, DeVita VT, Kelley MG: Some pharmacologic properties of a new antitumor agent, N-isopropyl-α-(2-methylhydrazino)-p-toluamide hydrochloride (NSC-77213). Cancer Chemother Rep 42:1–7, 1964

166. Raaflaub J, Schwartz DE: Über den metabolismus einer cytostatisch wirksamen Methylhydrazin-derivates (Natulan). Experientia 21:44–45, 1965

167. Chabner BA, Sponzo R, Hubbard S et al: High-dose intermittent intravenous infusion of procarbazine. Cancer Chemother Rep 57:361–363, 1973

168. Bleyer WA: The clinical pharmacology of methotrexate. Cancer 41:36–51, 1978

169. Chabner BA: Methotrexate. In Chabner B (ed): Pharmacologic Principles of Cancer Treatment, pp 229–255. Philadelphia, WB Saunders, 1982

170. Goldman ID, Matherly LH: The cellular pharmacology of methotrexate. Pharmacol Ther 28:77–102, 1985

171. Allegra CJ, Fine RL, Drake JC, Chabner BA: Effect of methotrexate on intracellular folate pools in human MCF breast cancer cells. J Biol Chem 261:6478–6485, 1986

172. Baram J, Allegra CJ, Fine RL et al: Effect of methotrexate on intracellular folate pools in purified myeloid precursor cells from normal human bone marrow. J Clin Invest 79:692–697, 1987

173. Jolivet J, Cowan KH, Curt GA et al: The pharmacology and clinical use of methotrexate. N Engl J Med 309:1094–1104, 1983

174. White JC: Reversal of methotrexate binding to dihydrofolate reductase by dihydrofolate: Studies with purified enzyme and computer modelling using network thermodynamics. J Biol Chem 254:10889–10895, 1979

175. Allegra CJ, Chabner BA, Drake JC et al: Enhanced inhibition of thymidylate synthetase by methotrexate polyglutamates. J Biol Chem 260:9720–9726, 1985

176. Chabner BA, Allegra CJ, Curt GA et al: Polyglutamation of methotrexate. J Clin Invest 76:907–912, 1985

177. Kearney PJ, Light PA, Preece A, Mott MG: Unpredictable serum levels after oral methotrexate in children with acute lymphoblastic leukaemia. Cancer Chemother Pharmacol 3:117–120, 1979

178. Balis FM, Savitch JL, Bleyer WA: Pharmacokinetics of oral methotrexate in children. Cancer Res 43:2342–2345, 1983

179. Pinkerton CR, Welshman SG, Kelly JG et al: Pharmacokinetics of low-dose methotrexate in children receiving maintenance therapy for acute lymphoblastic leukaemia. Cancer Chemother Pharmacol 10:36–39, 1982

180. Pinkerton CR, Welshman SG, Bridges JM: Serum profiles of methotrexate after its administration in children with acute lymphoblastic leukaemia. Br J Cancer 45:300–303, 1982

181. Henderson ES, Adamson RH, Oliverio VT: The metabolic fate of tritiated methotrexate II: Absorption and excretion in man. Cancer Res 25:1018–1024, 1965

182. Campbell MA, Perrier DG, Dorr RT et al: Methotrexate: Bioavailability and pharmacokinetics. Cancer Treat Rep 69:833–838, 1985

183. Smith DK, Omura GA, Ostroy F: Clinical pharmacology of intermediate-dose oral methotrexate. Cancer Chemother Pharmacol 4:117–120, 1980

184. Craft AW, Rankin A, Aherne W: Methotrexate absorption in children with acute lymphoblastic leukemia. Cancer Treat Rep 65(Suppl 1):77–81, 1981

185. The Medical Research Council's Working Party on Leukaemia in Childhood: Medical Research Council leukaemia trial, UKALL VII. Arch Dis Childh 60:1050–1054, 1985

186. Pinkerton CR, Glasgow JFT, Welshman SG, Bridges JM: Can food influence the absorption of methotrexate in children with acute lymphoblastic leukaemia? Lancet 2:944–946, 1980

187. Edelman J, Biggs DF, Jamali F, Russell AS: Low-dose methotrexate kinetics in arthritis. Clin Pharmacol Ther 35:382–386, 1984

188. Balis FM, Lester C, Murphy R et al: Pharmacokinetics of subcutaneous methotrexate (abstr). Proc Am Assoc Cancer Res 27:169, 1986

189. Wang YM, Fujimoto T: Clinical pharmacokinetics of methotrexate in children. Clin Pharmacokinet 9:335–348, 1984

190. Bleyer WA: Cancer chemotherapy in infants and children. Pediatr Clin North Am 32:557–574, 1985

191. Wang YM, Kim PY, Latin E et al: Degradation and clearance of methotrexate in children with osteosarcoma receiving high-dose infusion. Med Pediatr Oncol 4:221–229, 1978

192. Huffman DH, Wan SH, Azarnoff DL, Hoogstraten B: Pharmacokinetics of methotrexate. Clin Pharmacol Ther 14:572–579, 1973

193. Liegler DG, Henderson ES, Hahn MA, Oliverio VT: The effect of organic acids on renal clearance of methotrexate in man. Clin Pharmacol Ther 10:849–857, 1969

194. Jacobs SA, Stoller RG, Chabner BA et al: 7-Hydroxy methotrexate as a urinary metabolite in human subjects and Rhesus monkeys receiving high-dose methotrexate. J Clin Invest 57:534–538, 1976

195. Lankelma J, van der Klein E: The role of 7-hydroxy methotrexate during methotrexate anticancer chemotherapy. Cancer Lett 9:133–142, 1980

196. Erttmann R, Bielack S, Landbeck G: Kinetics of 7-hydroxy-methotrexate after high-dose methotrexate therapy. Cancer Chemother Pharmacol 15:101–104, 1985

197. Evans WE, Crom WR, Stewart CF et al: Methotrexate systemic clearance influences probability of relapse in children with standard-risk acute lymphoblastic leukemia. Lancet 1:359–362, 1984

198. Stoller RG, Hande KR, Jacobs SA et al: Use of plasma pharmacokinetics to predict and prevent methotrexate toxicity. N Engl J Med 297:630–634, 1977

199. Abelson HT, Fasburg MT, Beardsley GP et al: Methotrexate-induced renal impairment: Clinical studies and rescue from systemic toxicity with high-dose leucovorin and thymidine. J Clin Oncol 1:208–216, 1983

200. Bleyer WA: Therapeutic drug monitoring of methotrexate and other antineoplastic drugs. In Baer DM, Dita WR (eds): Interpretations in Therapeutic Drug Monitoring, pp 169–181. Chicago, American Society of Clinical Pathology, 1981

201. Langleben A, Hollomby D, Hand R: Case report: Management of methotrexate toxicity in an anephric patient. Clin Invest Med 5:129–132, 1982

202. Gibson TP, Reich SD, Krumlovsky FA et al: Hemoperfusion for methotrexate removal. Clin Pharmacol Ther 23:351–355, 1978

203. Winchester JF, Rahman A, Tilstone WJ et al: Will hemoperfusion be useful for cancer chemotherapeutic drug removal? Clin Toxicol 17:557–569, 1980

204. Doyle LA, Berg C, Bottino G, Chabner BA: Erythema and desquamation after high-dose methotrexate. Ann Intern Med 98:611–612, 1983

205. Sostman HD, Matthay RA, Putman C, Smith GJW: Methotrexate-induced pneumonitis. Medicine 55:371–388, 1976

206. Bleyer WA: Neurologic sequelae of methotrexate and ionizing radiation: A new classification. Cancer Treat Rep 65(Suppl 1):89–98, 1981

207. Packer RJ, Grossman RI, Belasco JB: High dose methotrexate-associated acute neurologic dysfunction. Med Pediatr Oncol 11:159–161, 1983

208. Curt GA, Carney DN, Cowan KH et al: Unstable methotrexate resistance in human small-cell carcinoma associated with double minute chromosomes. N Engl J Med 308:199–202, 1983

209. Horns RC, Dower WJ, Schimke RT: Gene amplification in a leukemic patient treated with methotrexate. J Clin Oncol 2:2–7, 1984

210. Schornagel JH, McVie JG: The clinical pharmacology of methotrexate. Cancer Treat Rev 10:53–75, 1983

211. Zimm S, Ettinger LJ, Holcenberg JS et al: Phase I and clinical pharmacologic study of mercaptopurine administered as a prolonged intravenous infusion. Cancer Res 45:1869–1873, 1985

212. Van Scoik KG, Johnson CA, Porter WR: The pharmacology and metabolism of the thiopurine drugs 6-mercaptopurine and azathioprine. Drug Metab Rev 16:157–174, 1985

213. McCormack JJ, Johns DG: Purine antimetabolites. In Chabner B (ed): Pharmacologic Principles of Cancer Treatment, pp 213–228. Philadelphia, WB Saunders, 1982

214. Zimm S, Collins JM, Riccardi R et al: Variable bioavailability of oral mercaptopurine. N Engl J Med 308:1005–1009, 1983

215. Poplack DG, Balis FM, Zimm S: The pharmacology of orally administered chemotherapy. Cancer 58(Suppl):473–480, 1986

216. Lennard L, Keen D, Lilleyman JS: Oral 6-mercaptopurine in childhood leukemia: Parent drug pharmacokinetics and active metabolite concentrations. Clin Pharmacol Ther 40:287–292, 1986

217. Sulh H, Koren G, Whalen C et al: Pharmacokinetic determinants of 6-mercaptopurine myelotoxicity and therapeutic failure in children with acute lymphoblastic leukemia. Clin Pharmacol Ther 40:604–609, 1986

218. Zimm S, Collins JM, O'Neill D et al: Inhibition of first-pass metabolism in cancer chemotherapy: Interaction of 6-mercaptopurine and allopurinol. Clin Pharmacol Ther 34:810–817, 1983

219. Coffey JJ, White CA, Lesk AB et al: Effect of allopurinol on the pharmacokinetics of 6-mercaptopurine (NSC 755) in cancer patients. Cancer Res 32:1283–1289, 1972

220. Brooks RJ, Dorr RT, Durie BGM: Interaction of allopurinol with 6-mercaptopurine and allopurinol. Biomedicine 36:217–222, 1982

221. Balis FM, Holcenberg JS, Zimm S et al: The effect of methotrexate on the bioavailability of oral 6-mercaptopurine. Clin Pharmacol Ther 41:384–387, 1987

222. LePage GA, Whitecar JP: Pharmacology of 6-thioguanine in man. Cancer Res 31:1627–1631, 1971

223. Brox LW, Birkett L, Belch A: Clinical pharmacology of oral thioguanine in acute myelogenous leukemia. Cancer Chemother Pharmacol 6:35–38, 1981

224. Konits PH, Egorin MJ, Van Echo DA et al: Phase II evaluation and plasma pharmacokinetics of high-dose intravenous 6-thioguanine in patients with colorectal carcinoma. Cancer Chemother Pharmacol 8:199–203, 1982

225. Kovach JS, Rubin J, Creagan ET et al: Phase I trial of parenteral 6-thioguanine given on 5 consecutive days. Cancer Res 46:5959–5962, 1986

226. Lu K, Benvenuto JA, Bodey GP et al: Pharmacokinetics and metabolism of β-2'-deoxythioguanosine and 6-thioguanine in man. Cancer Chemother Pharmacol 8:119–123, 1982

227. Kufe DW, Spriggs DR: Biochemical and cellular pharmacology of cytosine arabinoside. Semin Oncol 12(Suppl 3):34–48, 1985

228. Kufe D, Spriggs D, Egan EM, Munroe D: Relationship among ara-C pools, formation of (ara-C)DNA, and cytotoxicity of human leukemic cells. Blood 64:54–58, 1984

229. Capizzi RL, Yang J, Rathmell JP et al: Dose-related pharmacologic effects of high-dose Ara-C and its self-potentiation. Semin Oncol 12(Suppl 3):65–75, 1985

230. Donehower RC, Karp JE, Burke PJ: Pharmacology and toxicity of high-dose cytarabine by 72-hour continuous infusion. Cancer Treat Rep 70:1059–1065, 1986

231. Cheson BD, Jasperse DM, Simon R, Friedman MA: A critical appraisal of low-dose cytosine arabinoside in patients with acute non-lymphocytic leukemia and myelodysplastic syndromes. J Clin Oncol 4:1857–1864, 1986

232. Chabner BA, Hande KR, Drake JC: Ara-C metabolism: Implications for drug resistance and drug interactions. Bull Cancer 66:89–92, 1979

233. Ho DHW, Frei E: Clinical pharmacology of 1-β-arabinofuranosyl cytosine. Clin Pharmacol Ther 12:944–954, 1971

234. Weiss G, Phillips J, Von Hoff D: A clinical–pharmacological comparison of hepatic arterial and peripheral vein infusion of cytarabine for liver cancer (abstr). Proc Am Soc Clin Oncol 5:34, 1986

235. Slevin ML, Piall EM, Aherne GW et al: The pharmacokinetics of cytosine arabinoside in the plasma and cerebrospinal fluid during conventional and high-dose therapy. Med Pediatr Oncol 1(Suppl):157–168, 1982

236. Wan SH, Huffman DH, Azarnoff DL et al: Pharmacokinetics of 1-β-arabinofuranosylcytosine in humans. Cancer Res 34:392–397, 1974

237. Capizzi RL, Yang J-L, Cheng E et al: Alterations of the pharmacokinetics of

high-dose ara-C by its metabolite, high ara-U in patients with acute leukemia. J Clin Oncol 1:763–771, 1983

238. Ochs J, Sinkule JA, Danks MK et al: Continuous infusion high-dose cytosine arabinoside in refractory childhood leukemia. J Clin Oncol 2:1092–1097, 1984

239. Plunkett W, Iacoboni S, Estey E et al: Pharmacologically directed ara-C therapy for refractory leukemia. Semin Oncol 12(Suppl 3):20–30, 1985

240. Liliemark JO, Plunkett W, Dixon DO: Relationship of 1-β-D-arabinofuranosyl-cytosine in plasma to 1-β-D-arabinofuranosylcytosine 5′-triphosphate levels in leukemic cells during treatment with high-dose 1-β-D-arabinofuranosylcytosine. Cancer Res 45:5952–5957, 1985

241. Chou T-C, Arlin Z, Clarkson BD et al: Metabolism of 1-β-D-arabinofuranosylcytosine in human leukemic cells. Cancer Res 37:3561–3570, 1977

242. Jones GT, Abramson N: Gastrointestinal necrosis in acute leukemia: A complication of induction therapy. Cancer Invest 1:315–320, 1983

243. Johnson H, Smith TJ, Desforges J: Cytosine arabinoside-induced colitis and peritonitis: Nonoperative management. J Clin Oncol 3:607–612, 1985

244. Castleberry RP, Crist WM, Holbrook T et al: The cytosine arabinoside (ara-C) syndrome. Med Pediatr Oncol 9:257–264, 1981

245. Herzig RH, Lazarus HM, Herzig GP et al: Central nervous system toxicity with high-dose cytosine arabinoside. Semin Oncol 12(Suppl 3):233–236, 1985

246. Barnett MJ, Richards MA, Ganesan TS et al: Central nervous system toxicity of high-dose cytosine arabinoside. Semin Oncol 12(Suppl 3):227–232, 1985

247. Herzig RH, Wolff SN, Lazarus HM et al: High-dose cytosine arabinoside therapy for refractory leukemia. Blood 62:361–369, 1983

248. Myers CE: The pharmacology of the fluoropyrimidines. Pharmacol Rev 33:1–15, 1981

249. Chabner BA: Pyrimidine antagonists. In Chabner B (ed): Pharmacologic Principles of Cancer Treatment, pp 183–200. Philadelphia, WB Saunders, 1982

250. Heidelberger C, Danenberg PV, Moran RG: Fluorinated pyrimidines and their nucleosides. Adv Enzymol 54:58–119, 1983

251. Jolivet J, Curt GA, Clendeninn NJ et al: Antimetabolites. In Pinedo HM, Chabner BA (eds): Cancer Chemotherapy (Annual 5), pp 1–29. New York, Elsevier Science, 1983

252. Jastreboff MM, Kedzierska B, Rode W: Altered thymidylate synthetase in 5-fluorodeoxyuridine-resistant Ehrlich ascites carcinoma cells. Biochem Pharmacol 32:2259–2267, 1983

253. Fraile RJ, Baker LH, Buroker TR et al: Pharmacokinetics of 5-fluorouracil administered orally, by rapid intravenous and by slow infusion. Cancer Res 40:2223–2228, 1980

254. Christophidis N, Vajda FJE, Lucas I et al: Fluorouracil therapy in patients with carcinoma of the large bowel: A pharmacokinetic comparison of various rates and routes of administration. Clin Pharmacokinet 3:330–336, 1978

255. Collins JM, Dedrick RL, King FG et al: Nonlinear pharmacokinetic models for 5-fluorouracil in man: Intravenous and intraperitoneal routes. Clin Pharmacol Ther 28:235–246, 1980

256. Wagner JG, Gyves JW, Stetson PL et al: Steady-state nonlinear pharmacokinetics of 5-fluorouracil during hepatic arterial and intravenous infusions in cancer patients. Cancer Res 46:1499–1506, 1986

257. McDermott BJ, van den Berg HW, Murphy RF: Nonlinear pharmacokinetics for the elimination of 5-fluorouracil after intravenous administration in cancer patients. Cancer Chemother Pharmacol 9:173–178, 1982

258. Sequential methotrexate and 5-FU in the management of neoplastic disease (symposium proceedings). Semin Oncol 10(Suppl 2):1–39, 1983

259. The current status of 5-fluorouracil–leucovorin calcium combination (symposium proceedings). In Bruckner HW, Rustum YM (eds): Advances in Cancer Chemotherapy, pp 1–88. New York, John Wiley & Sons, 1984

260. Au JL-S, Rustum YM, Ledesma EJ et al: Clinical pharmacological studies of concurrent infusion of 5-fluorouracil and thymidine in treatment of colorectal carcinomas. Cancer Res 42:2930–2937, 1982

261. Pigram WJ, Fuller W, Amilton LDH: Stereochemistry of intercalation: Interaction of daunomycin with DNA. Nature 235:17–19, 1972

262. Handa K, Sato S: Generation of free radicals of quinone group containing anticancer chemicals in NADPH–microsome system as evidenced by initiation of sulfite oxidation. Gann 66:43–47, 1975

263. Myers C: Anthracyclines. In Pinedo HM, Chabner BA (eds): Cancer Chemotherapy (Annual 8), pp 52–64. New York, Elsevier Science, 1986

264. Bachur NR, Gee MV, Friedman RD: Nuclear catalyzed antibiotic free radical formation. Cancer Res 42:1078–1081, 1982

265. Goormaghtigh E, Ruysschaert JM: Anthracycline glycoside–membrane interactions. Biochim Biophys Acta 779:271–288, 1984

266. Takahashi S, Bachur NR: Adriamycin metabolism in man: Evidence from urinary metabolites. Drug Metab Dispos 4:79–87, 1976

267. Riggs CE: Clinical pharmacology of daunomycin in patients with acute leukemia. Semin Oncol 11(Suppl 3):2–11, 1984

268. Israel M, Pegg WJ, Wilkerson PJ, Garnick MB: Liquid chromatographic analysis of Adriamycin and metabolites in biological fluids. J Liq Chromatogr 1:795–809, 1978

269. Rahman A, Goodman A, Foo W et al: Clinical pharmacology of daunorubicin in phase I patients with solid tumors: Development of an analytical methodology for daunorubicin and its metabolites. Semin Oncol 11(Suppl 3):36–44, 1984

270. Evans WE, Crom WR, Sinkule JA et al: Pharmacokinetics of anticancer drugs in children. Drug Metab Rev 14:847–886, 1983

271. Greene RF, Collins JM, Jenkins JF et al: Plasma pharmacokinetics of Adriamycin and adriamycinol: Implications for the design of in vitro experiments and treatment protocols. Cancer Res 43:3417–3421, 1983

272. Eksborg S, Strandler HYS, Edsmyr F et al: Pharmacokinetic study of I.V. infusions of Adriamycin. Eur J Clin Pharmacol 28:205–212, 1985

273. Speth PA, Linssen PC, Haanen C: Adriamycin chemotherapy in patients with severe renal insufficiency and during hemodialysis. Third European Conference on Clinical Oncology and Cancer Nursing June 16–20, 1985, Stockhom, Sweden, p 77, 1985

274. Benjamin RS, Wiernik PH, Bachur NR: Adriamycin chemotherapy: Efficacy, safety and pharmacologic basis of an intermittent single high-dosage schedule. Cancer 35:19–27, 1974

275. Brenner DE, Wiernik PH, Wesley M, Bachur NR: Acute doxorubicin toxicity: Relationship to pretreatment liver function, response and pharmacokinetics in patients with acute non-lymphocytic leukemia. Cancer 53:1042–1048, 1984

276. Kaye SB, Cummings J, Kerr DJ: How much does liver disease affect the pharmacokinetics of Adriamycin? Eur J Cancer Clin Oncol 21:893–895, 1985

277. Chang PC, Brenner DE, Riggs CE et al: Adriamycin toxicity: Preliminary guidelines for dosage reduction (abstr). Clin Res 27:382A, 1979

278. Sulkes A, Collins JM: Reappraisal of some dosage adjustment guidelines. Cancer Treat Rep 71:229–233, 1987

279. Ozols RF, Willson JKV, Weltz MD et al: Inhibition of human ovarian cancer colony formation by Adriamycin and its major metabolites. Cancer Res 40:4109–4112, 1980

280. Riggs CE, Tipping SJ, Angelou JE et al: Human pharmacokinetics of continuous infusion Adriamycin (abstr). Proc Am Soc Clin Oncol 2:32, 1983

281. Yates JW, Glidwell O, Wiernik P, Holland JF: A study of Daunomycin versus Adriamycin induction, and monthly versus bimonthly maintenance in acute myelocytic leukemia, from CALGB (abstr). Proc Am Assoc Cancer Res 22:487, 1981

282. Wong KY, Lampkin BC: Anthracycline toxicity. Am J Pediatr Hematol Oncol 5:93–97, 1983

283. Bowers DG, Lynch JB: Adriamycin extravasation. Plast Reconstr Surg 61:86–92, 1978

284. Svingen BA, Powis G, Appel PL, Scott M: Protection against Adriamycin induced skin necrosis in the rat by dimethyl sulfoxide and α-tocopherol. Cancer Res 41:3395–3399, 1981

285. Singer JW, Narahara KA, Ritchie JL et al: Time- and dose-dependent changes in ejection fraction determined by radionuclide angiography after anthracycline therapy. Cancer Treat Rep 62:945–948, 1978

286. Myers CE, Kinsella TJ: Cardiac and pulmonary toxicity. In DeVita VT, Hellman S, Rosenberg SA (eds): Cancer Principles and Practice of Oncology, pp 2022–2032. Philadelphia, JB Lippincott, 1985

287. Mason JW, Bristow MR, Billingham ME et al: Invasive and noninvasive methods of assessing Adriamycin cardiotoxic effects in man: Superiority of histopathologic assessment using endomyocardial biopsy. Cancer Treat Rep 62:857–864, 1978

288. Sallan SE, Clavell LA: Cardiac effects of anthracyclines used in the treatment of childhood acute lymphoblastic leukemia: A 10-year experience. Semin Oncol 11(Suppl 3):19–21, 1984

289. Alexander J, Dainiak N, Berger HJ et al: Serial assessment of doxorubicin cardiotoxicity with quantitative radionuclide angiocardiography. N Engl J Med 300:278–283, 1979

290. Hrushesky WJM, Fader D: Non-invasive, instantaneous quantification of doxorubicin-induced heart damage (abstr). Proc Am Soc Clin Oncol 4:41, 1985

291. Chlebowski RT, Parloy WS, Pugh RT et al: Adriamycin given as a weekly schedule without a loading course—clinically effective with reduced incidence of cardiotoxicity. Cancer Treat Rep 64:47–51, 1980

292. Legha SS, Benjamin RS, Mackay B et al: Reduction of doxorubicin cardiotoxicity by prolonged continuous intravenous infusion. Ann Intern Med 96:133–139, 1982

293. Sikic BI: Clinical pharmacology of bleomycin. In Sikic BI, Rozencweig M, Carter SK (eds): Bleomycin Chemotherapy, pp 37–43. New York, Academic Press, 1985

294. Chabner BA: Bleomycin. In Chabner B (ed): Pharmacologic Principles of Cancer Treatment, pp 377–386. Philadelphia, WB Saunders, 1982

295. Hecht SM: DNA strand scission by activated bleomycin group antibiotics. Fed Proc 45:2784–2791, 1986

296. Ozawa S, Tamura A, Suzuki H et al: Mechanisms affecting peplomycin sensitivity of Chinese hamster cell lines. J Antibiot (Tokyo) 38:1257–1265, 1985

297. Blum RH, Carter SK, Agre K: A clinical review of bleomycin—a new antineoplastic agent. Cancer 31:903–914, 1973

298. Comis RL, Kuppinger MS, Ginsberg SJ et al: Role of single-breath carbon monoxide-diffusing capacity in monitoring the pulmonary effects of bleomycin in germ cell tumor patients. Cancer Res 39:5076–5080, 1979

299. Eigen H, Wyszomierski D: Bleomycin lung injury in children. Am J Pediatr Hematol Oncol 7:71–78, 1985

300. Goldiner PL, Schweizer O: The hazards of anesthesia and surgery in bleomycin-treated patients. Semin Oncol 6:121–124, 1979

301. Oken MM, Crooke ST, Elson MK et al: Pharmacokinetics of bleomycin after IM administration in man. Cancer Treat Rep 65:485–489, 1981

302. Harvey VJ, Slevin ML, Aherne GW et al: Subcutaneous infusions of bleomycin: A practical alternative to intravenous infusion. J Clin Oncol 5:648–650, 1987

303. Yee GC, Crom WR, Lee FH et al: Bleomycin disposition in children with cancer. Clin Pharmacol Ther 33:668–673, 1983

304. Crooke ST, Comis RL, Einhorn LH et al: Effects of variation in renal function on the clinical pharmacology of bleomycin administered as an IV bolus. Cancer Treat Rep 61:1631–1636, 1977

305. Holoye PY, Broughton A, Strong JE, Bedrossian CW: Bleomycin pharmacokinetics of continuous intravenous infusion (abstr). Proc Am Assoc Cancer Res 18:70, 1977

306. Petrilli ES, Castaldo TW, Matutat RJ et al: Bleomycin pharmacology in relation to adverse effects and renal function in cervical cancer patients. Gynecol Oncol 14:350–354, 1982

307. Selman A Waksman Conference on Actinomycins: Their Potential for Cancer Chemotherapy. Cancer Chemother Rep 58:1–123, 1974

308. Blatt J, Trigg ME, Pizzo PA, Glaubiger D: Tolerance to single-dose dactinomycin in combination chemotherapy for solid tumors. Cancer Treat Rep 65:145–147, 1981

309. Carli M, Pastore G, Paolucci G et al: High single doses versus 5 day divided doses of dactinomycin in childhood rhabdomyosarcoma: Preliminary results (abstr). Proc Am Soc Clin Oncol 2:76, 1983

310. Tattersall MHN, Sodergren JE, Sengupta SK et al: Pharmacokinetics of actinomycin D in patients with malignant melanoma. Clin Pharmacol Ther 17:701–708, 1975

311. Brothman AR, Davis TP, Duffy JJ, Lindell TJ: Development of an antibody to actinomycin D and its application for the detection of serum levels by radioimmunoassay. Cancer Res 42:1184–1187, 1982

312. Glaubiger D, Ramu A: Antitumor antibiotics. In Chabner B (ed): Pharmacologic Principles of Cancer Treatment, pp 402–407. Philadelphia, WB Saunders, 1982

313. Creasy WA: Plant alkaloids. In Becker FA (ed): Cancer: A Comprehensive Treatise, vol 5, pp 379–425. New York, Plenum Press, 1977

314. Cassady JM, Douros JD (eds): Anticancer Agents Based on Natural Product Models. New York, Academic Press, 1980

315. Owellen RJ, Hartke CA, Dickerson RM, Hains FO: Inhibition of tubulin-microtubule polymerization by drugs of the vinca alkaloid class. Cancer Res 36:1499–1502, 1976

316. Bender RA, Chabner BA: Tubulin binding agents. In Chabner B (ed): Pharmacologic Principles of Cancer Treatment, pp 256–268. Philadelphia, WB Saunders, 1982

317. Hacker MP, Dank JR, Ershler WB: Vinblastine pharmacokinetics measured by a sensitive enzyme-linked immunosorbent assay. Cancer Res 44:478–481, 1984

318. Sethi VS, Burton SS, Jackson DV: A sensitive radioimmunoassay for vincristine and vinblastine. Cancer Chemother Pharmacol 4:183–187, 1980

319. Castle MC, Mead JAR: Investigation of the metabolic fate of tritiated vincristine in the rat by high-pressure liquid chromatography. Biochem Pharmacol 27:37–44, 1978

320. Jackson DV, Sethi VS, Spurr CL et al: Pharmacokinetics of vincristine infusion. Cancer Treat Rep 65:1043–1048, 1981

321. Zeffren J, Yagod A, Kelson D, Winn R: Phase I trial of a 5-day infusion of vinblastine (abstr). Proc Am Assoc Cancer Res 21:178, 1980

322. Sethi VS, Kimball JC: Pharmacokinetics of vincristine sulfate in children. Cancer Chemother Pharmacol 6:111–115, 1981

323. Sethi VS, Jackson DV, White DR et al: Pharmacokinetics of vincristine sulfate in adult cancer patients. Cancer Res 41:3551–3555, 1981

324. Owellen RJ, Root MA, Hains FO: Pharmacokinetics of vindesine and vincristine in humans. Cancer Res 37:2603–2607, 1977

325. Nelson RL, Dyke RW, Root MA: Comparative pharmacokinetics of vindesine, vincristine, and vinblastine in patients with cancer. Cancer Treat Rev 7(Suppl):59–63, 1980

326. Jackson DV, Castle MC, Poplack DG et al: Pharmacokinetics of vincristine in the cerebrospinal fluid of sub-human primates. Cancer Res 40:722–724, 1980

327. Jackson DV, Sethi VS, Spurr CL et al: Pharmacokinetics of vincristine in the cerebrospinal fluid of humans. Cancer Res 41:1466–1468, 1981

328. Bender RA, Castle MC, Margileth DA, Oliverio VT: The pharmacokinetics of [3H]-vincristine in man. Clin Pharmacol Ther 22:430–435, 1977

329. Jackson DV, Castle MC, Bender RA: Biliary excretion of vincristine. Clin Pharmacol Ther 24:101–107, 1978

330. Van den Berg HW, Desai, ZR, Wilson R et al: The pharmacokinetics of vincristine in man: Reduced drug clearance associated with raised serum alkaline phosphatase and dose-limited elimination. Cancer Chemother Pharmacol 8:215–219, 1982

331. Desai ZR, Van den Berg HW, Bridges JM et al: Can severe vincristine neurotoxicity be prevented? Cancer Chemother Pharmacol 8:211–214, 1982

332. Yap H-Y, Blumenschein GR, Hortobagyi GN et al: Continuous 5-day infusion vinblastine in the treatment of refractory advanced breast cancer (abstr). Proc Am Assoc Cancer Res 20:334, 1979

333. Brewer CF, Loike JD, Howritz SB et al: Conformational analysis of podophyllotoxin and its congeners: Structure–activity relationship in microtubule assembly. J Med Chem 22:215–221, 1979

334. Yalowich JC, Goldman ID: Analysis of the inhibitory effects of VP-16-213 (etoposide) and podophyllotoxin on thymidine transport and metabolism in Ehrlich ascites tumor cells in vitro. Cancer Res 44:984–989, 1984

335. Ross W, Rowe T, Glisson B et al: Role of topoisomerase II in mediating epipodophyllotoxin-induced DNA cleavage. Cancer Res 44:5857–5860, 1984

336. Gellert M: DNA topoisomerases. Annu Rev Biochem 50:879–910, 1981

337. Haim N, Roman J, Nemec J, Sinha BK: Peroxidative free radical formation and O-demethylation of etoposide (VP-16) and teniposide (VM-26). Biochem Biophys Res Commun 135:215–220, 1986

338. Clark PI, Slevin ML: The clinical pharmacology of etoposide and teniposide. Clin Pharmacokinet 12:223–252, 1987

339. Evans WE, Stewart CF, Christensen ML, Crom WR: Clinical pharmacology of anticancer drugs in children: Differences and similarities between children and adults. In Poplack DG, Massimo L, Cornaglia-Ferraris P (eds): The Role of Pharmacology in Pediatric Oncology, pp 29–71. Boston, Martinus Nijhoff, 1987

340. O'Dwyer PJ, Leyland-Jones B et al: Etoposide (VP16-213): Current status of an active anticancer drug. N Engl J Med 312:692–700, 1985

341. O'Dwyer PJ, Alonso MT, Leyland-Jones B, Marsoni S: Teniposide: A review of 12 years of experience. Cancer Treat Rep 68:1455–1466, 1984

342. Schmoll H: Review of etoposide single-agent activity. Cancer Treat Rev 9(Suppl):21–30, 1982

343. Weiss RB, Bruno S: Hypersensitivity reactions to cancer chemotherapeutic agents. Ann Intern Med 94:66–72, 1981

344. Johnson DH, Greco FA, Wolff SN: Etoposide-induced hepatic injury: A potential complication of high-dose therapy. Cancer Treat Rep 67:1023–1024, 1983

345. de Vries EG, Mulder NH, Postmus PE et al: High–dose teniposide for refractory malignancies: A phase I study. Cancer Treat Rep 70:595–598, 1986

346. Cunningham D, McTaggart L, Soupkop M et al: Etoposide: A pharmacokinetic profile including an assessment of bioavailability. Med Oncol Tumor Pharmacother 3:95–99, 1986

347. Stewart DJ, Nundy D, Maroun JA et al: Bioavailability, pharmacokinetics,

and clinical effects of an oral preparation of etoposide. Cancer Treat Rep 69:269–273, 1985

348. Harvey VJ, Slevin ML, Joel SP et al: Variable bioavailability following repeated oral doses of etoposide. Eur J Cancer Clin Oncol 21:1315–1319, 1985

349. Smythe RD, Pfeffer M, Scalzo A, Comis RL: Bioavailability and pharmacokinetics of etoposide (VP-16). Semin Oncol 12(Suppl 1):48–51, 1985

350. Harvey VJ, Slevin ML, Joel SP et al: The effect of dose on the bioavailability of oral etoposide. Cancer Chemother Pharmacol 16:178–181, 1986

351. Brunner KW, Sonntag RW, Ryssel HJ, Cavalli F: Comparison of the biologic activity of VP-16-213 given IV and orally in capsules or drink ampules. Cancer Treat Rep 60:1377–1379, 1976

352. Evans WE, Sinkule JA, Crom WR et al: Pharmacokinetics of VM26 and VP16 in children with cancer. First International Symposium on the Podophyllotoxins in Cancer Therapy, July 8–9, 1981, Southhampton, England, Mead Johnson, p 51, 1981

353. Strife RJ, Jarrdine I, Colvin M: Analysis of the anticancer drugs VP16-213 and VM-26 and their metabolites by high-performance liquid chromatography. J Chromatogr 182:211–220, 1980

354. Allen LM, Creaven PJ: Comparison of the human pharmacokinetics of VM-26 and VP-16, two antineoplastic epipodophyllotoxin glucopyranoside derivatives. Eur J Cancer 11:697–707, 1975

355. Hande KR, Wedlund PJ, Noone RM et al: Pharmacokinetics of high-dose etoposide (VP-16-213) administered to cancer patients. Cancer Res 44:379–382, 1984

356. Holthuis J, de Vries E, Postmus P et al: Pharmacokinetics of high dose teniposide (VM 26) (abstr). Proc Am Assoc Cancer Res 27:177, 1986

357. D'Incalci M, Rossi C, Sessa C et al: Pharmacokinetics of teniposide in patients with ovarian cancer. Cancer Treat Rep 69:73–77, 1985

358. Arbuck SG, Douglass HO, Crom WR et al: Etoposide pharmacokinetics in patients with normal and abnormal organ function. J Clin Oncol 4:1690–1695, 1986

359. D'Incalci M, Rossi C, Zucchetti M et al: Pharmacokinetics of etoposide in patients with abnormal renal and hepatic function. Cancer Res 46:2566–2571, 1986

360. Lippman ME, Konior GS, Leventhal BG: Clinical implications of glucocorticoid receptors in human leukemia. Cancer Res 38:4251–4256, 1978

361. Thompson EB, Harmon JM, Zawydiwski R: Corticosteroid effects on an acute lymphoblastic leukemic cell line: A model for understanding steroid therapy. In Murphy SB, Gilbert JR (eds): Leukemia Research: Advances in Cell Biology and Treatment, pp 157–169. New York, Elsevier Science, 1983

362. Pickup ME: Clinical pharmacokinetics of prednisone and prednisolone. Clin Pharmacokinet 4:111–128, 1979

363. Duggan DE, Yeh KC, Matalia N et al: Bioavailability of oral dexamethasone. Clin Pharmacol Ther 18:205–209, 1975

364. Green OC, Winter RJ, Kawahara FS et al: Pharmacokinetic studies of prednisolone in children. J Pediatr 93:299–303, 1978

365. Rose JQ, Nickelsen JA, Ellis EF et al: Prednisolone disposition in steroid-dependent asthmatic children. J Allergy Immunol 67:188–193, 1981

366. Richter O, Ern B, Reinhardt D, Becker B: Pharmacokinetics of dexamethasone in children. Pediatr Pharmacol 3:329–337, 1983

367. Tsuei SE, Moore RG, Ashley JJ, McBride WG: Disposition of synthetic glucocorticoids I: Pharmacokinetics of dexamethasone in healthy adults. J Pharmacokinet Biopharm 7:249–264, 1979

368. Rose JQ, Yurchak AM, Jusko WJ: Dose dependent pharmacokinetics of prednisone and prednisolone in man. J Pharmacokinet Biopharm 9:389–405, 1981

369. Melby JC: Clinical pharmacology of systemic corticosteroids. Annu Rev Pharmacol Toxicol 17:511–527, 1977

370. Liu Y-P, Chabner BA: Enzyme therapy: L-Asparaginase. In Chabner B (ed): Pharmacologic Principles of Cancer Treatment, pp 435–443. Philadelphia, WB Saunders, 1982

371. Capizzi RL, Cheng YC: Therapy of neoplasms with asparaginase. In Holcenberg J, Roberts J (eds): Enzymes as Drugs, pp 1–24. New York, Wiley-Interscience, 1981

372. Haley EE, Fischer GA, Welch AD: The requirement for L-asparagine of mouse leukemia cells L5178Y in culture. Cancer Res 21:532–536, 1961

373. Ohnuma T, Holland JF, Freeman A, Sinks LF: Biochemical and pharmacological studies with asparaginase in man. Cancer Res 30:2297–2305, 1970

374. Peterson RG, Handschumacher RE, Mitchell MS: Immunological responses to L-asparaginase. J Clin Invest 50:1080–1089, 1971

375. Riccardi R, Holcenberg JS, Glaubiger DL et al: L-Asparaginase pharmacokinetics and asparagine levels in cerebrospinal fluid of Rhesus monkeys and humans. Cancer Res 41:4554–4558, 1981

376. Cheung NK, Chau IY, Coccia PF: Antibody response to Escherichia coli L-asparaginase: Prognostic significance and clinical utility of antibody measurement. Am J Pediatr Hematol Oncol 8:99–104, 1986

377. Oettgen HF, Stephenson PA, Schwartz MK et al: Toxicity of E. coli L-asparaginase in man. Cancer 25:253–278, 1970

378. Leonard JV, Kay JDS: Acute encephalopathy and hyperammonaemia complicating treatment of acute lymphoblastic leukaemia with asparaginase. Lancet 1:162–163, 1986

379. Wells RJ, Feusner J, Devney R et al: Sequential high-dose cytosine arabinoside–asparaginase treatment in advanced childhood leukemia. J Clin Oncol 3:998–1004, 1985

380. Baum E, Nachman J, Ramsey N et al: Prolonged second remissions in childhood acute lymphocytic leukemia: A report from the Children's Cancer Study Group. Med Pediatr Oncol 11:1–7, 1983

381. Capizzi RL: Schedule-dependent synergism and antagonism between methotrexate and L-asparaginase. Biochem Pharmacol 23:151–161, 1974

382. Balis FM, Lester CM, Chrousos GP et al: Differences in cerebrospinal fluid penetration of corticosteroids: Possible relationship to the prevention of meningeal leukemia. J Clin Oncol 5:202–207, 1987

383. Collins JM: Regional therapy: An overview. In Poplack DG, Massimo L, Cornaglia-Ferraris P (eds): The Role of Pharmacology in Pediatric Oncology, pp 125–135. Boston, Martinus Nijhoff, 1987

384. Larson SM, Schall GL, DiChiro G: The influence of previous lumbar puncture and pneumoencephalography on the incidence of unsuccessful radioisotope cisternography. J Nucl Med 12:555–557, 1971

385. Bleyer WA, Poplack DG: Clinical studies on the central-nervous-system pharmacology of methotrexate. In Pinedo HM (ed): Clinical Pharmacology of Anti-Neoplastic Drugs, pp 115–131. Amsterdam, Elsevier/North-Holland Biomedical, 1978

386. Blasberg RG, Patlak C, Fenstermacher JD: Intrathecal chemotherapy: Brain tissue profiles after ventriculo-cisternal perfusion. J Pharmacol Exp Ther 195:73–83, 1975

387. Echelberger CK, Riccardi R, Bleyer A et al: Influence of body position on ventricular cerebrospinal fluid methotrexate concentration following intralumbar administration (abstr). Proc Am Soc Clin Oncol 22:365, 1981

388. Ommaya AK: Implantable devices for chronic access and drug delivery to the central nervous system. Cancer Drug Deliv 1:169–179, 1984

389. Bleyer WA, Poplack DG: Intraventricular versus intralumbar methotrexate for central-nervous-system leukemia: Prolonged remission with the Ommaya reservoir. Med Pediatr Oncol 6:207–213, 1979

390. Zimm S, Holcenberg J, Balis F et al: Intrathecal diaziquone: A new, clinically useful agent for the treatment of meningeal neoplasia (abstr). Proc Am Assoc Cancer Res 28:190, 1987

391. Bleyer WA, Drake JC, Chabner BA: Neurotoxicity and elevated cerebrospinal-fluid methotrexate concentration in meningeal leukemia. N Engl J Med 289:770–773, 1973

392. Poplack DG: Massive intrathecal overdose: "check the label twice!" N Engl J Med 311:400–402, 1984

393. Bleyer WA: Intrathecal methotrexate versus central nervous system leukemia. Cancer Drug Deliv 1:157–167, 1984

394. Bleyer WA: Clinical pharmacology of intrathecal methotrexate II: An improved dosage regimen derived from age-related pharmacokinetics. Cancer Treat Rep 61:1419–1425, 1977

395. Bleyer WA, Coccia PF, Sather HN et al: Reduction in central nervous system leukemia with a pharmacokinetically derived intrathecal methotrexate dosage regimen. J Clin Oncol 1:317–325, 1983

396. Zimm S, Collins JM, Miser J et al: Cytosine arabinoside cerebrospinal fluid kinetics. Clin Pharmacol Ther 35:826–830, 1984

397. Ho DHW, Frei E: Clinical pharmacology of 1-β-D-arabinofuranosylcytosine. Clin Pharmacol Ther 12:944–954, 1971

398. Ho DHW: Distribution of kinase and deaminase of 1-β-D-arabinofuranosylcytosine in tissues of man and mouse. Cancer Res 33:2816–2820, 1973

399. Balis FM, Savitch JL, Bleyer WA et al: Remission induction of meningeal leukemia with high-dose intravenous methotrexate. J Clin Oncol 3:485–489, 1985

400. Poplack DG, Reaman GH, Bleyer WA et al: Central nervous system preventive therapy with high dose methotrexate in acute lymphoblastic leukemia: A preliminary report (abstr). Proc Am Soc Clin Oncol 3:204, 1984

401. Donehower RC, Karp JE, Burke PJ: Pharmacology and toxicity of high-dose cytarabine by 72-hour continuous infusion. Cancer Treat Rep 70:1059–1065, 1986

402. Lopez JA, Nassif E, Vannicola P et al: Central nervous system pharmacokinetics of high-dose cytosine arabinoside. J Neurooncol 3:119–124, 1985

403. Frick J, Ritch PS, Hansen RM, Anderson T: Successful treatment of meningeal leukemia using systemic high-dose cytosine arabinoside. J Clin Oncol 2:365–368, 1984

404. Frick JC, Hansen RM, Anderson T, Ritch PS: Successful high-dose intravenous cytarabine treatment of parenchymal brain involvement from malignant lymphoma. Arch Intern Med 146:791–792, 1986

405. Allen JC, Helson L: High-dose cyclophosphamide chemotherapy for recurrent CNS tumors in children. J Neurosurg 55:749–756, 1981

406. Strong JM, Collins JM, Lester C, Poplack DG: Pharmacokinetics of intraventricular and intravenous N,N′,N″-triethylenethiophosphoramide (thiotepa) in Rhesus monkeys and humans. Cancer Res 46:6101–6104, 1986

407. Frei E: The National Cancer Chemotherapy Program. Science 217:600–606, 1982

408. Venditti JM: Preclinical drug development: Rationale and methods. Semin Oncol 8:349–361, 1981

409. Shoemaker RH: New approaches to antitumor drug screening: The human tumor colony-forming assay. Cancer Treat Rep 70:9–12, 1986

410. Grieshaber CK, Marsoni S: Relation of preclinical toxicology to findings in early clinical trials. Cancer Treat Rep 70:65–72, 1986

411. Marsoni S, Ungerleider RS, Hurson SB, et al: Tolerance to antineoplastic agents in children and adults. Cancer Treat Rep 69:1263–1269, 1985

412. Simon R: How large should a phase II trial of a new drug be? Cancer Treat Rep 71:1079–1085, 1987

413. Marsoni S, Hoth D, Simon R, et al: Cliinical drug development: An analysis of phase II trials, 1970–1985 Cancer Treat Rep 71:71–80, 1987

414. Talmadge JE, Herberman RB: The preclinical screening laboratory: Evaluation of immunomodulatory and therapeutic properties of biologic response modifiers. Cancer Treat Rep 70:171–182, 1986

415. Sikic BI: Anti-cancer drug sensitivity testing: Current role and future prospects. In Kimura K, Yamada K, Krakoff IH, Carter SK (eds): Cancer Chemotherapy: Challenges for the Future, pp 48–57. Tokyo, Excerpta Medica, 1986

416. Morris GL, Zeltzer PM, Schneider SL, Von Hoff DD: Cloning of pediatric malignancies for drug sensitivity testing in the human tumor cloning assay. Am J Pediatr Hematol Oncol 8:52–57, 1986

417. Strobel-Stevens JD, El Dareer SM, Trader MW, Hill DL: Some biochemical characteristics of L1210 cell lines resistant to 6-mercaptopurine and 6-thioguanine and with increased sensitivity to methotrexate. Biochem Pharmacol 31:3133–3137, 1982

418. Erlichman C, Donehower RC, Chabner BA: The practical benefits of pharmacokinetics in the use of antineoplastic agents. Cancer Chemother Pharmacol 4:139–145, 1980

ten

General Principles of Surgery

Daniel M. Hays

During the past decade, improvements in survival in one pediatric tumor system or another could be expected annually. These changes required surgeons constantly to reevaluate the procedures performed in conjunction with advances in chemotherapeutic management or radiotherapy techniques. It is an oversimplification to state that surgeons are moving in the direction of more radical or more conservative surgery. Operative procedures such as limb salvage with vascular grafts or hepatic trisegmentectomy are either radical or conservative depending on your point of view, but they are more extensive procedures than have been carried out previously. Less-extensive surgery is now performed for a number of tumors in which chemotherapy/radiotherapy responsiveness has been established and in which the procedures formerly used routinely, such as pelvic exenteration or hemipelvectomy, appear to make a significant change in the patient's ability to appreciate life fully.[1,2] Unfortunately, complete surgical excision is still associated with the highest survival rates in these situations.[3,4]

There continue to be pediatric tumors in which the traditional surgical approaches are the most important factors influencing survival, such as hepatomas, fibrosarcomas, stages I and II neuroblastomas, synovial sarcomas, and some rarer tumors. However, these now represent a minority of the pathologic tumor types seen by surgeons concerned with pediatric oncology. In the larger group of children, surgery is now an integral part of combined programs of surgery, chemotherapy, and radiotherapy, each modality playing a role at a specific point, the timing of which is highly dependent on the effects of the other(s). Far from eliminating surgery in the management of children with solid tumors, this approach has actually increased the volume of surgery carried out in almost all centers where pediatric tumors are treated. Categories of patients formerly never seriously considered for extirpative or even exploratory surgery are now subjected to such procedures routinely, when control of dissemination or significant reductions in tumor volume are achieved.

Procedures for "palliation" represent a sizable portion of the operations performed in adult oncology, but the word seems largely absent from the pediatric vocabulary. Huge extremity tumors with ulceration and possibly fractures are amputated and bypass procedures carried out for disseminated abdominal disease in pediatric patients with known distant metastases. Even in these instances, hope of permanent chemotherapy effect is harbored.

RESPONSE OF THE PEDIATRIC PATIENT TO SURGICAL PROCEDURES

Metabolic Alterations Resulting from Surgery

Major surgery, like any equivalent trauma, produces a homeostatic response that, within certain limits, is predictable. This process is usually described as consisting of four phases. The first of these may involve an initial epinephrine response with vascular and splenic contraction. This is rapidly supplemented by a complex adrenal response that includes the release of aldosterone, catecholamines, antidiuretic hormone, and other mineralocorticoids and glucocorticoids. This output results in protein breakdown, water and sodium retention, potassium loss, and many other secondary and less significant changes. Its duration is directly related to the degree of trauma but is ordinarily 2 to 4 days. The second phase is a withdrawal of the intensive adrenal-mediated corticosteroid stimulus and a reversal of the secondary derangements it has produced, with water and sodium excretion a prominent feature. This also is usually several days in length. The third phase is a spontaneous anabolic reaction with the formation of new proteins, assuming appropriate calories, protein, and vitamins are provided. The fourth phase, which may require months, is a restoration of depleted fat stores.

All humans, including the infant and child, follow a response pattern similar to that seen in the adult.[5,6] The entire process, including its recovery phase, may be accelerated in younger patients. In the infant, this process is complicated by negative phosphorus balance produced by growing bone (also see Chap. 12). To achieve a positive nitrogen balance (phase three), the infant requires a higher ratio of calories to nitrogen intake: 230 kCal/g N versus adult levels of less than 150 kCal/g N (see Chap. 40).[7]

This section describes the several unique characteristics of the pediatric patient's response to surgery. There are many exceptions, including (1) categories of neonatal patients with different gestational ages and birthweights; (2) infants with anomalies or nutritional and hemolytic diseases; and (3) children with diabetes, cystic fibrosis, and the like—all in addition to a neoplastic process. These factors may make them *not* conform to the patterns described.

The Neonatal Patient

The current frequent use of ultrasonography during pregnancy has resulted in the discovery of fetal tumors.[8,9] These have been primarily sacrococcygeal teratomas without apparent malignant elements, but malignant neoplasms have also been identified (see Chap. 33). Tumor rupture, as well as increased risk of dissemination, would seem probable during a prolonged or difficult vaginal delivery. Therefore, when any type of large solid tumor is identified antenatally, cesarean-section delivery is usually indicated. In the neonatal period, patients require major surgery for sacrococcygeal and other teratomas; neck and mediastinal tumors of any type that obstruct the major bronchi or trachea; and, occasionally, hepatoblastomas, nephroblastomas, or neuroblastomas.[10–13] Previously unrecognized large abdominal or cervical and, particularly, tumors attached to the cranium may produce dystocia and may be ruptured during vaginal delivery, leading to massive hemorrhage.[14]

The characteristics of the neonatal infant as a candidate for surgery include unique features (see Chap. 12). Red blood cell volume is at its lifetime peak, particularly if placental blood has been infused. The pulmonary arterioles are unusually muscular and reactive, with vasoconstriction the common reaction to hypoxia or acidosis.[15,16] This may result in a return to a partial fetal circulation, with opening of the foramen ovale and ductus arteriosis; that is, the lungs may be bypassed. Renal glomerular filtration and tubular function are both significantly below childhood (or adult) levels, with decreased concentrating ability and reduced reserve in the excretion of hydrogen ions and sodium.

The energy expenditure of the neonate by weight is also at its lifetime height, with 38 to 42 kCal/kg required for maintenance and an approximately equal amount needed to sustain growth. Despite this need, the glycogen reserves of the infant are rapidly depleted and must be constantly renewed; otherwise, hypoglycemia develops. Four to six hours without replacement of energy sources may result in protein and fat catabolism and acidosis. Shivering is not possible in the neonate, and during the entire first month the infant makes little effort to restore a falling temperature in response to a cold environment. Brown fat is utilized for energy, increasing oxygen requirements.

Relative to resistance to infection, the skin and mucous membranes of some neonates (particularly preterm infants) appear to provide a deficient barrier to the entry of bacteria. Smaller infants also have a decreased production of surfactant and relatively immature alveoli. Overall complement activity appears to be reduced by approximately 50% in the neonate. Immunoglobin M is absent and granulocyte function impaired.[17] Although neonates have immunologically competent plasma cells, they have received little antigenic challenge and appear in some instances to have a delayed response to bacterial invaders.

With respect to selection of the form of therapy for cancer (if one has a choice), the late effects of irradiation on the neonate are devastating, and chemotherapy may be difficult to control in this age group,[18] leaving surgery as the preferred modality when it can be applied effectively.[13]

The Infant and Child

The basic responses of the older infant, child, and adult to major surgery are similar. Several features are peculiar to infants, including a lower percentage of body fat for insulation, so that heat loss can be rapid and large amounts of energy can be expended simply in maintaining body temperature. The insensible water loss through skin and mucous membrane surfaces is greater in infants than in older children. Some of the factors relative to possible susceptibility to infection in the neonate persist into the postneonatal period.[19]

The wound-healing potential of infants and children is similar, and possibly more rapid, than that seen in young adults and clearly faster than the same process in older adults. During the initial 6 to 8 weeks of life, both hepatic and renal function are immature, and intensive chemotherapy provokes a more unpredictable response and is more difficult to monitor. This has resulted in a high therapy-related mortality rate during this period.[20] Thereafter, the tolerance of older infants and children to the adverse effects of chemotherapy may be superior to that of adults if drugs are used that have myelosuppression as the major element in toxicity.[21] Children usually tolerate other forms of toxicity as well as adults. Their regenerative response following extensive hepatic resection is more rapid than that following the same degree of stimulus (resection) in adults. The relative immaturity of kidney, liver, and lung that persists into later infancy is rarely a factor in clinical cancer management. The child's overall cardiac status is superior to that of most adults with cancer, and their dependent venous tributaries rarely thrombose or produce venous emboli. Thus, in most respects, the child is an ideal subject for the major surgery that may be required to manage some pediatric solid tumors.

PRINCIPLES OF MANAGEMENT

Evaluation of Pediatric Patients in Preparation for Surgery

General Problems in Evaluation

Evaluation of the pediatric patient prior to major surgery for cancer is dissimilar to the same type of evaluation in adults.

The parents' contribution is a major one with respect to possible familial or congenital problems and medications being taken (see also Chap. 46). At a minimum, the surgeon and anesthesiologist must approach the following areas before any major surgical procedure for cancer: (1) elicit any family history of inheritable disease (particularly dystrophies, myotonia, or hemolytic diseases); (2) consider the possibility of unrecognized congenital anomalies (particularly cardiac or pulmonary); (3) investigate anemias and determine the presence or absence of coagulation defects; (4) screen the patient for incipient acute infections of the upper or lower respiratory tract and for exposures (or early signs) of contagious disease; (5) determine the status of the upper airway (particularly in infants) with respect to malformations of the tongue or larynx that would interfere with adequate ventilation; (6) survey renal and hepatic function; and (7) have a general concept and record of the attainment of the major developmental milestones in younger children.

In patients who have previously been treated for a neoplasm, the effects of irradiation and specific chemotherapeutic agents on the cardiopulmonary system require detailed evaluation before administration of a general anesthetic. The status of all pediatric patients is classified by physical state according to criteria of the American Society of Anesthesiologists prior to surgery (Table 10-1).

Nutritional Status at Diagnosis

The incidence of apparent nutritional depletion at diagnosis as a result of chronic caloric or protein deficiencies is less common in children than in adults with cancer, in whom neoplasms frequently directly affect gastrointestinal function. Children with relatively large tumors such as nephroblastomas, which may comprise as much as 15% of total body weight, may have well-preserved general nutrition by standard measurements. However, more refined techniques usually reveal deficiencies.[22]

When malnutrition *is* apparent at the onset of therapy, it is unquestionably beneficial to restore the patient to a reasonable nutritional status before carrying out major surgery, and the most expeditious means by which this can be accomplished should be used (see section on Techniques of Nutritional Support as well as Chap. 40). If major surgery is to be the initial event in a patient's course, the nutritional repletion should be carried out in a relatively emergency program of enteral and parenteral realimentation.

Table 10-1
Physical Status Classification Used in Pediatric Anesthesia

Class 1: No organic, physiologic, biochemical, or psychiatric disturbance
Class 2: Mild to moderate systemic abnormalities, caused either by the disease to be treated surgically or by another pathophysiologic process
Class 3: Severe systemic abnormality from any cause
Class 4: Immediately life-threatening, severe systemic disorder
Class 5: Moribund patient who is submitted to operation in desperation
E: Any patient in one of the classes above who is operated on in an emergency receives the letter ''E'' beside the numerical classification; *e.g.,* 2E.

(American Society of Anesthesiologists, Sakad M: Grading Patients for surgical procedures. Anesthesiology 2:281–284, 1941)

EFFECT OF NUTRITIONAL SUPPORT ON OUTCOME IN CANCER PATIENTS. Among patients who have a relatively normal nutritional profile at diagnosis, it has been difficult to demonstrate that the addition of abundant protein, calories, and vitamins—"hyperalimentation"—during therapy has made a significant difference in the outcome.[23,24] Several authors have shown that the amount of chemotherapy tolerated by the patient can be increased if his or her status can be raised from one of malnutrition to adequate nutrition.[25,26] It has not been shown, however, that marrow recovery from the effects of myelosuppressive agents is more rapid in a state of total parenteral nutrition-induced repletion.

When an intensive chemotherapy regimen is in progress, the surgeon's concern is that the patient may require a secondary surgical procedure at any time, either by plan (second-look procedure) or in connection with an emergency resulting from therapy. It is advantageous to have such patients as close to a normal nutritional status as possible during the entire period of intensive therapy from the point of view of this potential or planned surgery. This ordinarily involves continuous, well-monitored total parenteral nutrition but may be accomplished enterally under favorable circumstances.

RATIONALE AND INDICATIONS FOR INTENSIVE NUTRITIONAL SUPPORT. The nutritional well-being of the child with cancer is threatened equally by the effects of the neoplasm and by the effects of therapy. The incidence of malnutrition among children on cancer therapy regimens is high. Fortunately, the most advanced forms and techniques of nutritional support can be safely provided for the pediatric patient with cancer.[27] The aim of all of the procedures described subsequently is to provide a reliable route for the introduction of nutrients into the gastrointestinal tract or the systemic venous system without undue risk. If at the time of operation or during the course of cancer therapy, routine oral nutrition must be interrupted for any reason that is not readily remediable or will lead to the use of intravenous fluids for nutrition for more than 1 week, it is preferable to initiate a nutritional support system at once, without waiting for the development of indications of malnutrition. Some intensive therapy regimens require nutritional support routinely, and this can be anticipated.

Anesthesia for Pediatric Cancer Surgery

Characteristics of Pediatric Anesthesia

Pediatric anesthesiology, in general, has distinct characteristics, including (1) relatively infrequent use of local and regional anesthetics; (2) employment of a wide range of sizes of all types of equipment to administer anesthesia, including tubes, rebreathing chambers with dead-space limits, ventilators, and fluid pumps; (3) accommodation to the unique difficulties in arterial and venous access and of temperature maintenance in younger patients; and (4) recognition of the special respiratory and metabolic problems of the neonate and infant. Anesthesiologists recognize the peculiar susceptibility to apnea in premature and low-birth-weight infants and those with a history of respiratory distress syndrome, which may continue for years. The proportion of patients in which an endotracheal tube is used to administer an inhalation anesthetic or to assist breathing is much greater than in adult anesthesiology, exceeding 80% in some pediatric institutions. The use of inflammable gases has largely been replaced, permitting the extensive use of cautery and electrical devices. All pediatric patients received a Physical Status Classification (Table 10-1) before surgery.

Two problems have been of particular significance in pediatric anesthesiology. First, malignant hyperthermia, a condition of unknown etiology, is more prevalent in childhood and includes the sudden development of tachycardia followed by extreme hyperthermia in an otherwise stable anesthetized patient.[28] This condition is so menacing that ordinarily the operative procedure is terminated, if possible, and all measures directed toward resuscitation and termination of the hyperthermia. The second problem concerns the administration of succinylcholine to patients with unrecognized congenital pseudocholinesterase deficiency, which may produce muscular paralysis for many hours or even days.[29,30] This can be avoided by the use of other muscle-relaxing agents.

The psychological aspects of the administration of a general anesthetic to the child are complex and unique and have received widespread attention. In many institutions, the child now visits the hospital prior to elective surgery, and members of the anesthesiology staff demonstrate the use of the masks and machines that will be used and attempt to establish a trustful relationship with the child to be anesthetized (see Chap. 46). Anesthesiologists visit the child and family before operation to further discuss the procedure and attempt to allay anxiety.

Anesthesia for Cancer Surgery

The special problems in maintenance of anesthesia presented by pediatric patients with solid tumors may be grouped as (1) tumor effects on respiratory mechanics; (2) massive blood and fluid losses; and (3) effects of specific endocrine products released by tumors (Table 10-2).

The tracheobronchial airway may be distorted or partially occluded by cervical and mediastinal tumor masses. Children with mediastinal tumors may develop patterns of voluntary elevation of the thorax or head movements that result in reasonably satisfactory respiratory efforts when they are conscious but which may leave the unconscious patient with obstruction of the airway (see Chap. 37). Large subdiaphragmatic tumors elevate and reduce the mobility of the diaphragm and compress the intrathoracic contents. In such patients, it is important that an adequate airway be ensured before and after the administration of muscle relaxants. For this reason, the patient is ordinarily induced and carried down to a relatively deep plane with an inhalation anesthetic. Once this is achieved, breathing can be controlled and relaxants administered. Achieving rapid and complete control of the respiratory effort is essential in these patients.

Blood loss during surgery is particularly apparent in removing hepatic tumors but may be seen in the mobilization and excision of any of the large solid tumors of the thorax, abdomen, or pelvis. Hypoxia secondary to acute anemia can rapidly produce a state of decompensation in multiple organs.

The single endocrinologically active tumor seen in childhood that produces major problems in anesthesia is pheochromocytoma (see Chap. 35). These tumors are rarely malignant.[31] In childhood, in contrast to adults, pheochromocytomas are frequently familial,[32] occur predominantly in females, and produce hypertension that is usually sustained rather than episodic.[33-35] The mean patient age is approximately 9 years. The basic practical problems in anesthesia for removal of these tumors are controlling the hypertension before tumor removal and controlling hypotension after its removal. In the past, the period immediately following devascularization of this tumor was frequently one of fatal and near-fatal episodes. Although there is no long-range medical treatment for pheochromocytoma, a period of preparation for surgery of several weeks is desirable, during which the blood pressure is reduced. In most centers, this effect is produced by using alpha-blocking agents, which obstruct the receptors for epinephrine or norepinephrine, from the time of diagnosis. Immediately before surgery, these may be supplemented with beta-adrenergic blockers. The latter are also used intraoperatively to control tachycardia and prevent arrhythmias, which may result from the effects of the alpha-adrenergic blockade. The long-range effects of the pheochromocytoma produce a hypovolemic state with plasma volume reduced by about 15%. This is ordinarily partially replaced in the 12 hours prior to surgery. Careful monitoring preoperatively and postoperatively is necessary to allow the uneventful expansion of the vascular system following tumor removal. Hypotension that follows a division of the blood supply from the tumor may require additional transfusion and the use of norepinephrine or angiotensin.

Neuroblastoma and nephroblastoma are both, at times, associated with mild hypertension, but the condition is not ordinarily labile and has not resulted in problems in the administration of anesthesia. The other tumors in the APUD system occur infrequently in childhood, and their endocrine function is not ordinarily a significant factor in the administration of anesthesia.

Hemodilution, Induced Hypotension, and Hypothermia During Anesthesia

Three special techniques are used to reduce blood loss or minimize the effects of a decrease in circulating red blood cell volume: (1) acute normovolemic hemodilution; (2) deliberate hypotension; and (3) hypothermia.

Table 10-2
Pediatric Solid Tumors That Present Special Problems in Anesthetic Management

Tumor	Problems
Cervical and mediastinal tumors adjacent to trachea and major bronchi	Asphyxia, arrest, aspiration, pneumothorax. Induction problems associated with paralytic agents. Postexcision problems include the above plus tracheobronchial malasia
Hepatic tumors; large upper-abdominal tumors (neuroblastoma, nephroblastoma); phrenic nerve involvement	Elevation and immobilization of the diaphragm; blood loss with hypovolemia, acidosis, shock, asphyxia
Neuroblastoma	Hypertension (unusual); large-vessel occlusion/injury
Pheochromocytoma	Hypertension (usual)
Sacrococcygeal teratomas	Blood loss with secondary effects (see above); prolonged immobilization in the prone position required for excision may compromise respiratory efforts in the neonate

Acute normovolemic hemodilution has been used more extensively in pediatric solid-tumor surgery than have the other techniques. Although originally developed to facilitate cardiac surgical procedures, and then operations on patients with Jehovah's Witnesses' religious beliefs, it has more recently been employed in many types of patients in which significant blood loss can be anticipated. Normovolemic hemodilution utilizes the technique of autologous blood transfusion, although donor blood may be used in the final replacement. In summary, the patient's blood is withdrawn at room temperature to reduce the patient's hematocrit to approximately 20%, with simultaneous replacement of the blood with a larger volume of an electrolyte solution or colloid. Originally, a colloid, dextran, was used, but, more recently, solutions of lactated Ringer's solution containing magnesium have been preferred. Mean arterial pressure is maintained at approximately 40 to 50 mm Hg. In the system used by Schaller for the resection of pediatric hepatic tumors, the temperature is allowed to fall to 32°C during the procedure.[36] Blood lost during the hepatic resection contains relatively few red cells. After the dissection is complete, the patient's blood is reinfused and a diuretic administered to assist in eliminating the excess fluid from the extravascular compartment. Most patients in whom this general type of procedure has been used require no bank blood for a standard hepatic lobectomy.

The second technical device is the deliberate induction of a hypotensive state.[37,38] This reduces myocardial work and clearly decreases blood loss. When systolic and diastolic pressures are reduced by less than 40% of normal range for age, no ill effects are apparent relative to coronary perfusion or cerebral blood flow under most circumstances. Many different agents have been used to reduce pressure, including nitroprusside and related drugs, usually combined with propranolol to prevent reflex tachycardia and to decrease the amount of drug required to maintain moderate hypotension. An adverse effect of hypotension produced by sodium nitroprusside is increased intracranial pressure.

The third technique used to reduce blood loss or minimize the effects of organ ischemia is hypothermia.[39] This is frequently graded from "mild" to "severe" and produced by many different techniques. The significant advantage of hypothermia is the drastic decrease in organ oxygen consumption and requirement; this decrease is at a rate of approximately 5% to 7% per each fall of 1°C. In the ideal function of a hypothermia system, the oxygen demands never exceed the oxygen supply as temperature drops. Less anesthetic agent is required for patients on hypothermia regimens. When temperatures fall below 31° to 32°C, the patient may require active rewarming to prevent further drift. A complication of this technique is the development of ventricular fibrillation, which usually is readily reversible by appropriate drugs or electrical DC countershock. Forms of moderate and deep hypothermia require the provision for cardiopulmonary bypass and are not ordinarily employed in the resection of tumors except those involving the heart, such as the extensions of nephroblastoma into the left atrium with attachment.

Additional methods of reducing operative blood loss include tumor embolization, which is also used as a therapeutic technique. Its use during the immediate preoperative period to reduce tumor volume and hemorrhage is controversial.[40,41] Techniques to prevent sequestration in the distal venous systems, to shunt caval and portal blood around the liver, and to minimize blood loss during hepatic lobectomy are described in Chapter 26.

Monitoring Standards

Minimal monitoring equipment for a patient during any procedure under anesthesia includes (1) a precordial or esophageal stethoscope; (2) a blood pressure cuff; (3) a continuous electrocardiogram; and (4) a temperature monitor (usually rectal). In more extensive procedures, additions to this core of monitoring aids include the arterial catheter (blood gases), central venous pressure recording, pulmonary wedge pressure, urine output, blood loss measures, and others. At present, tissue and organ probes of various types are being developed that will measure oxygen use and availability in many sites.

STAGING OF PEDIATRIC SOLID TUMORS

Development of Staging Systems

The original concept of "stage" in solid tumors was a system designed to describe only the extent of disease at one point in the course, usually at diagnosis. A shorthand form was used, condensing the multiple types of possible extension of the disease into four or five categories, exemplified by the TNM (T = tumor; N = nodes; M = metastases) system first employed in 1944. In the prechemotherapy era, staging systems were useful in determining at what "stage" detection occurred and which forms of cancer advanced most rapidly. They indicated which patients went to surgery or received irradiation and what type or dose. Surgeons, radiotherapists, and pathologists frequently modified (for different tumor types) the TNM staging system, and these modifications received the endorsement of national (American Joint Committee on Cancer) and international (UICC) organizations. In some tumor systems, the TNM classification was divided into a clinical stage (before surgery) and pathologic stage (after surgery and histologic examination), and this continues to be employed in many adult tumors.

In the era of effective chemotherapy, the staging of solid tumors is an absolute necessity for comparing multi-institutional therapy trials. There are at least three features that make the TNM system less useful to pediatric, as opposed to adult, oncologists. First, it is based on the premise that tumors originate from a single localized focus, a concept not always obvious in pediatric tumors. Second, there is a concentration of interest on the extent of lymph node disease, which again is not as prominent a feature in most pediatric tumors except lymphomas, which have unique staging systems. Third, it cannot readily be applied to the variants of neuroblastoma or of highly chemotherapy-sensitive tumors.

Staging in Pediatric Intergroup Studies

The initial two staging systems developed by the pediatric cancer cooperative groups clearly reflected different approaches. The system developed for the study of Wilms' tumor, which was initially sponsored by the American Academy of Pediatrics and evolved into the National Wilms' Tumor Study (NWTS), was based (with the exception of stage IV) on what the surgeon could or did accomplish at the initial operation (see Chap. 27).[42] Whether the tumor was "completely resected" or not was a determinate of stages I, II, and III. In contrast, the staging system developed for neuroblastoma by Evans and associates and used by Children's Cancer Study Group (CCSG) defines stage only in terms of the extent of disease.[43] Although it is hard to conceive of a stage I neuroblastoma that would not be excised, it was quite possible for a stage III neuroblastoma to be either completely excised, incompletely excised, or simply biopsied. Staging systems for neuroblastoma that stress node involvement and histologic factors are being evaluated (see Chap. 28).

The Intergroup Rhabdomyosarcoma Study (IRS) Staging System was modeled, to a degree, after the NWTS system, depending clearly on the extent of initial surgery (see Chap. 30).[44] The prognostic significance of the distinction between Clinical Groups I–II, III, and IV has been clearly demonstrated, but the distinctions relative to outcome between Clinical Groups I and II are, in some sites, not clear. This seems to reflect both the fact that in some sites, clinical lymph node involvement *per se* is not a major factor in survival and that "microscopic residual disease" is an ill-defined concept.

The concept of "microscopic residual disease" has several applications in pediatric solid-tumor staging and management. When introduced into the IRS in 1972 this concept was simply stated: "The surgeon believes that the tumor has been totally excised but the pathologist finds tumor present microscopically in the margin of the specimen."[45] Thus, by this definition, if the surgeon believed that there was microscopic residual there was *gross* residual, not microscopic residual. The concept of microscopic residual may represent an area of misunderstanding between the pathologist and the clinician and probably has less significance in soft-tissue sarcomas than it may have in cutaneous and other adult carcinomas. When the line of resection is positive, residual tumor exists. No other inferences are well established.

Histologic Differentiation and Staging

The question of whether the degree of histologic differentiation of the malignant cells should be an integral part of staging is a major concern in several pediatric tumor systems. In adult cancers, the TNM system is supplemented by "G" ("grade") of histologic differentiation in several classifications, notably for soft-tissue sarcomas. Histologic distinctions, which might be summarized by the letter "G" in a "TNMG" system, would reflect differences in outcome in several pediatric tumors such as neuroblastoma, some categories of rhabdomyosarcoma, and perhaps malignant germ cell tumors.

The NWTS committee has approached this problem by defining and separating a group of distinctly unfavorable tumor types within the original study group and excluding one form (rhabdoid) completely (see Chaps. 6 and 27). Thus, in the NWTS, grade is separate from stage, age, or other clinical features. A contrasting approach is that of Shimada, whose classification of neuroblastoma includes histologic features along with clinical variables to develop a stage that reflects overall prognosis from both points of view (see Chap. 28).[46,47]

For rhabdomyosarcomas, pathologists differ on the weight that should be given to a number of histologic features. Palmer's system of classification had powerful predictability but excluded from consideration a sizable group of tumors that were believed to be rhabdomyosarcomas by most pathologists (see Chaps. 6 and 30).[48]

Tsokos and associates have found that there is a spectrum of alveolar rhabdomyosarcomas, with those that have the most strikingly alveolar features having the most favorable prognosis; that is, the "solid" alveolar rhabdomyosarcoma is associated with the least favorable outlook.[49] In the IRS, the basic distinction–alveolar versus nonalveolar histology—is a significant predictor of outcome in patients in clinical group I with extremity lesions. In patients in clinical group II, it is of marginal significance, and in patients in clinical groups III and IV it appears to have no influence on outcome. An international panel of pathologists is currently (1988) evaluating the classification systems for rhabdomyosarcoma.

Prospective studies to validate the predictive value of staging systems of the NWTS and IRS have been made repeatedly and, in general, have been confirmatory. Low tumor inci-

dence has not made this possible for malignant germ cell or hepatic tumors.

Pretherapy Staging Systems

The concept that a strictly pretherapy staging system would be desirable for rhabdomyosarcoma,[50] neuroblastoma,[51] and possibly other pediatric tumors is now prevalent among pediatric oncologists, surgeons, and pathologists. Specific areas in the IRS may illustrate this need. It would appear, from careful review of study records, that patients with rhabdomyosarcomas with precisely the same site, size, and degree of extension (as closely as one can determine) will be placed in clinical group I, II, or III by the surgeon and consultants depending on the procedure elected and performed. Recognition of this fact has made many believe that there should be a system of staging carried out at that time when all noninvasive studies have been performed, including biopsy in some instances, but prior to any therapy. At present, in the IRS, such a system is being evaluated, although strictly as a study; that is, it is not used to direct therapy. This again raises the complex question of whether grade should be a part of the pretherapy, as well as the postsurgical, staging system. It *is* ordinarily known prior to any therapy.

Staging in Other Pediatric Tumors

With respect to the malignant germ cell tumors of childhood, the system of staging has in general followed the pattern of adult oncology groups (see Chap. 33). In regard to nongonadal malignant germ cell tumors, it is not known how well this system reflects prognosis. In the last CCSG study, inclusion of patients was determined by histology and site (all of the poorest prognostic groups were included), and stage did not determine therapy.

Surgical oncologists who treat sizable groups of malignant hepatic tumors in adults do not ordinarily use complicated staging systems, instead referring to these tumors as either localized (to the liver) or disseminated and, within the liver, as confined to specific lobes or segments. The staging system employed by CCSG and the Pediatric Oncology Group (POG) was developed on an empirical basis, and except for the distinction between resected and nonresected tumors or the presence of distant spread, it has yet to be demonstrated to be an indicator of outcome. Recent studies suggest that histologic features are of major prognostic significance in hepatoblastoma (see Chap. 26).

With the exception of rhabdomyosarcoma, the soft-tissue sarcomas of childhood have, in general, been placed in stage by adult criteria and often included in the same series. The division of extremity sarcomas into disseminated, intracompartmental, and extracompartmental groups is used in some centers, largely by orthopedic surgeons. Its validity as a predictor of outcome is probable.

Although there may be many controversial issues involving staging, there is universal agreement that the comparison of therapeutic results would be tremendously facilitated by a single widely recognized staging system for each specific tumor type. Such a system might be modified as therapeutic needs develop and its strength in prediction repeatedly verified. Because of its early origin, use of the NWTS classification of Wilms' tumor has become almost worldwide. The IRS staging system is also widely used for rhabdomyosarcomas and for other soft-tissue sarcomas not included in the original studies. There is no suggestion, however, of a universal staging system for neuroblastoma, with at least four classifications systems currently in widespread use.

Laparotomy For Staging

Hodgkin's Disease

Traditional laparotomies for the staging of Hodgkin's disease continue to be used in some pediatric institutions and not in others. Its use in patients in clinical stages I and II (A or B) continues to be controversial (see Chap. 21). In the minds of some investigators, accurate staging by laparotomy is of more significance in children than it is in adults because the adverse effects of unnecessary radiotherapy or intensive chemotherapy are more significant. Laparotomy should not be used unless it will influence therapeutic decisions, and in institutions in which almost all patients are treated by regimens of intensive chemotherapy, its usefulness might be limited to the identification of stage IV disease in the liver, which can frequently be accomplished by simpler procedures. The probability of change in clinical stage by a standard laparotomy procedure continues to be approximately 30%, and there is little indication at present that this can be greatly reduced by the extensive use of lymphangiography, computed tomography (CT), or other imaging studies. Removal of the extensively involved spleen, which eliminates the need for irradiation of right-upper-quadrant structures (kidney and right lower lobe) and the ability to transpose or reposition the ovaries in girls are obvious secondary benefits of laparotomy in some patients (see Chap. 11). The susceptibility of the splenectomized child to lethal hyperacute infections secondary to encapsulated organisms appears to have been remarkably reduced by the current use of pneumococcal vaccine, prophylactic antibiotics, and early recognition and energetic therapy when such episodes occur (also see Chap. 39).[52] The adequacy of a partial splenectomy in staging Hodgkin's disease is controversial.[53,54]

With respect to node biopsies, the laparotomy for the staging of Hodgkin's disease, no matter how apparently limited or localized it appears to be to the surgeon, should be complete,[55] or the results will be more confusing than helpful. When the number of node biopsies obtained during the laparotomy is limited, that is, an incomplete laparotomy, the procedure will fail to identify patients who should be placed in stage III and result in inadequate therapy and increased rates of relapse.[56] A complete laparotomy is also of particular significance in the staging of advanced disease. Current treatment protocols may require substages of IIIA to be established (IIIA$_1$, IIIA$_2$, IIIA$_3$), and this clearly requires a sampling of all designated node groups (see Chap. 21). Laparotomy is also used in patients with advanced disease to establish hepatic involvement and to identify the presence of recurrent abdominal disease after therapy.[57]

Non-Hodgkin's Lymphoma (NHL)

There are large series of staging laparotomies carried out in adult patients with non-Hodgkin's lymphoma,[58,59] but few elective staging laparotomies have been performed in children. These procedures in adults have demonstrated that extensive involvement of the retroperitoneal space and intestinal mesentery is common in NHL, in contrast to Hodgkin's disease. In childhood NHL, ordinarily it is possible to demonstrate the presence of widespread disease without a laparotomy. The occasional patient with isolated cervical disease might make consideration of staging laparotomy reasonable, but, since most therapy regimens for pediatric NHL would be minimally influenced by the findings of such a procedure, it is rarely carried out.

On the other hand, when a patient is explored for an acute abdominal condition or for an unidentified abdominal mass and NHL is diagnosed (or presumed) for the first time at laparotomy, in addition to an attempt to excise the mass, a thorough examination of the abdominal contents with hepatic and lymph node biopsies is helpful in predicting outcome and may influence the stage and management decisions.

Laparoscopy (Peritoneoscopy)

Laparoscopy is occasionally useful in clearly identifying metastatic abdominal (peritoneal) implants or metastases on the liver surface (Fig. 10-1).[60] If a general anesthetic is to be employed, more information can frequently be obtained with a minilaparotomy in the area of interest. Laparoscopy is used in children with demonstrated stage III Hodgkin's disease to obtain percutaneous liver biopsies,[61] and in this context it is regarded as a substitute for staging laparotomy. Laparoscopy is carried out in some adult clinics under local anesthesia, but, in pediatric patients this approach usually would not permit adequate inspection of the surfaces of the liver.

Many types of endoscope have been employed for this procedure, including the new flexible fiberoptic instruments. The procedure begins with the introduction of pneumoperitoneum with either carbon dioxide or nitrous oxide. The peritoneal cavity is opened through a single subumbilical incision with an optional second incision in the supraumbilical area to

FIGURE 10-1. Laparoscopy: tumor visible on liver surface. Protrusion of a hepatoblastoma to the surface of the left hepatic lobe as seen with a laparoscope in a 2-year-old boy. All other hepatic surfaces were normal in appearance, suggesting that the tumor was resectable, which proved to be the case at laparotomy. The bright object to the left (running vertically) is a metal cannula passed through the abdominal wall to perform a biopsy of the lesion. (Courtesy of Dr. Stephen Gans)

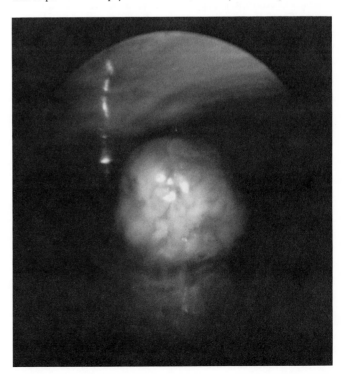

improve the exposure of the diaphragmatic surface of the liver. The inferior surface of the liver can best be observed through the subumbilical opening and the superior surface of the liver through the upper opening. Biopsy of abnormal areas on the hepatic surface is usually carried out with a needle passed percutaneously under direct vision from the endoscope. In the absence of any abnormality of the hepatic surfaces, two deep needle biopsies are obtained from each lobe.

A contraindication to laparoscopy is any form of intestinal obstruction that makes the intestinal tract susceptible to perforation. Patients who are excessively obese present mechanical problems and are undesirable candidates.

A negative laparoscopy for hepatic involvement must be qualified, because, in rare instances, positive biopsies have been obtained at laparotomy following a negative laparoscopy. Techniques of laparoscopy are usually standardized in institutions in which the procedure is carried out frequently.[60]

BIOPSIES AND PRIMARY SURGICAL PROCEDURES

Intraoperative Consultations and Biopsies

Traditionally, this type of consultation almost always involved the pathologist and usually the performance of a rapid-section histologic study, that is, the "frozen section." Currently, it may involve almost any member of the multidisciplinary group concerned with the patient's care.

Rapid-section techniques for histologic diagnosis and for the identification of tumor margins play a less important part in pediatric solid-tumor management than in the surgery of the carcinomas of adults. In the rapid diagnosis of adult tumors, a pathologist may achieve an error rate (the correlation of the rapid-section and the permanent-section diagnoses) of 1% to 2%, including both positive and negative errors, but in pediatric tumors this rate would undoubtedly be considerably higher. In respect to sarcomas, few pathologists are willing to make a more specific diagnosis than "malignant tumor," and even fewer will attempt a diagnosis of a specific lymphoma on the basis of rapid-section techniques. Familiarity with and confidence in rapid-section techniques is extremely variable among institutions, however; in some, the statements above would not apply. The special techniques that are essential for the precise identification of the solid tumors of childhood usually must be preceded by routine stains and require special techniques that are not available in the operating room situation (see Chap. 6). Thus, in pediatric oncology it is relatively rare for a precise diagnosis to be made on the basis of a rapid-section examination in the operating room. In general, intraoperative decisions must be made on the basis of an established diagnosis of malignancy and a presumed diagnosis of some specific entity.

In adult oncology, the pathologist may be called to the operating room to determine whether the specimen margins are "clear." This is uncommon in pediatric oncology, as it is recognized that most of the sarcomas of childhood have microscopic extensions that would make such an impression on the basis a few rapid sections inaccurate.

The concept that the pathologist comes to the operating room simply to perform rapid sections and give "yes" or "no" answers is archaic. The presence in the operating room of a pathologist familiar with pediatric solid tumors is an indispensable aid to the surgeon in making intraoperative decisions. These may involve whether a specific lesion is benign or malignant. For example, if an inflammatory mass is found involving the distal ilium, is this Crohn's disease or a lymphoma? Is an intrahepatic lesion neoplastic or granulomatous? Does a small renal tumor represent a synchronous bilateral nephroblastoma or a renal anomaly?

A different approach to rapid histologic diagnosis involves the use of fine-needle aspiration, either in the operating room or on the ward. In some institutions, this technique has completely changed the practice of histopathology as it relates to oncology. Although this technique has been used for a half a century, the development of improved techniques in Europe during the past decade has reestablished its common use on a worldwide basis. Success with this technique depends on a cooperative and enthusiastic pathologic specialist, namely, a cytologist. Its use in pediatric neoplasms is less developed than in the identification of adult tumors.[62] In most childhood tumors, a diagnosis of "malignancy" is the most ambitious goal to which one can aspire. Its use in establishing the presence of tumor recurrence is more straightforward.[63] When performed with modern fine-needle techniques, directed, when deep tumors are concerned, by CT and ultrasonography, the complication rate following such procedures is minimal (see Chaps. 6 and 7).[63] The accuracy of identifying malignant versus nonmalignant tissue should be greater than 90% in clearly solid tumors but not in lymph nodes. The aspiration procedure itself, in different institutions, may be performed by surgeons, pathologists, or others on the wards, but it also is frequently a part usually the initial step of a more involved surgical procedure.

The appearance of the radiation oncologist in the operating theater may be of great aid in planning subsequent therapy. This may be superior to, and surely would supplement, the use of metallic marking devices to indicate tumor margins or sites of involvement. The radiation therapist is an essential part of the operating team in the placement of tubes for brachytherapy, and it is vital that he or she be present at the placement of any devices (*e.g.,* tubes and molds) used in local radiotherapy techniques of any type.

The presence of the pediatric oncologist in the operating room is a more recent development but may also be essential in arriving at correct decisions for overall therapy. This member of the team has the clearest perception of what chemotherapy can be expected to accomplish in a given tumor type, and this expectation may indicate whether the procedure in progress should be an attempt to excise totally or a simple biopsy with reoperation in prospect after an anticipated response.

The team approach to pediatric tumor management clearly extends into the operating room!

Biopsy Techniques

Solid-Tumor Biopsies

These procedures are traditionally divided into excisional biopsies, in which the entire tumor, at least that apparent at operation, is included in the specimen, and incisional biopsies, which include only a portion of the tumor.

Nephroblastomas have traditionally been excised without biopsy, as it was believed that any breach of the tumor capsule would promote intraperitoneal spread (see Chap. 27). The effectiveness of chemotherapy has probably made this rationale moot, but the policy continues, since the risk of performing an unnecessary nephrectomy under these circumstances is practically nil. All of the neoplastic and infectious processes that might simulate a nephroblastoma ordinarily require nephrectomy.

The diagnosis of neuroblastoma is frequently made by other studies before exposure of the primary tumor (see Chap.

28). However, some neuroblastomas are not disseminated and markers are not definite, so that a distinction between neuroblastoma and other tumors in the abdomen or mediastinum is needed. Recognition that the lesion is a lymphoma may be of importance in limiting the extent of surgery. If the diagnosis lies between neuroblastoma, nephroblastoma, or hepatoblastoma, the extent of the excision may not be greatly influenced by a precise diagnosis, although hepatic lobectomies rarely need to be performed for locally invasive neuroblastoma but are routinely carried out for hepatoblastoma (see Chap. 26).

The diagnosis of rhabdomyosarcoma is usually made by a direct open biopsy, since there are no helpful markers or specific identifying imaging studies (see Chap. 30). Among rhabdomyosarcomas, the pathologist is expected to identify the histologic subgroups to allow adequate staging and direct therapy (see Chap. 6). For this purpose, several grams of tissue for study are desirable at a minimum. Genitourinary rhabdomyosarcomas are frequently biopsied through an endoscope. Although these are predominantly embryonal in subtype, here, also, larger biopsies are helpful to the pathologist. The needle biopsies performed to establish the diagnosis of prostatic rhabdomyosarcoma are difficult to interpret and must include several cores. Trunk and extremity rhabdomyosarcomas should be approached by either excisional or incisional biopsy techniques, with the incision placed so that it will not interfere with the incision required for a subsequent wide local excision. This almost always means a vertical incision in extremities.

Ovarian solid tumors, in which the diagnosis is frequently suspected or indicated by markers, may be biopsied or an oophorectomy performed for biopsy purposes if the tumor involves a major part of an ovary (see Chap. 35). If a malignant or teratoid tumor is identified by this procedure, the other ovary is inspected and biopsied or incised longitudinally for inspection of its interior, with biopsy of apparently abnormal areas. Potential tumor implants or omental nodules should be biopsied in this as in all abdominal procedures for neoplasia. When a solid testicular tumor is identified by biopsy, the cord vessels, which have been previously occluded, are divided and the testicle and cord structures up to the internal inguinal ring removed for examination.

Teratomas and other germ cell tumors, either gonadal or extragonadal, represent major risks in sampling error relative to the identification of malignant elements. Therefore, when feasible, excisional biopsies are recommended to allow the pathologist to examine multiple sites within the tumor (see Chap. 33).

Isolated deep intrahepatic masses present special problems in biopsy. Although needle biopsy cores may not provide a precise diagnosis, if they clearly indicate the presence of a malignant neoplasm confined to a resectable portion of the liver, formal lobectomy is ordinarily performed at the same procedure. In some institutions, if it is thought that the tumor is a hepatoblastoma whose resectability may be increased by initial chemotherapy, attempt at resection is delayed.

Soft-tissue sarcomas of the trunk and extremities are best managed by excisional biopsy when this is feasible. A precise diagnosis, including histologic grade, is of importance in directing management. In most instances, wide local excision will follow the excisional biopsy of all except grade I tumors. Tumors of low-grade malignancy, such as well-differentiated fibrosarcomas, fibromatoses (desmoids), and ganglioneuromas, are managed by an initial excisional biopsy except when large (see Chap. 33). Histologic distinctions here are extremely difficult, and relatively extensive surgery may or may not be indicated. Except in the most experienced hands, rapid histologic diagnosis is hazardous. The malignant bone tumors of childhood are ordinarily diagnosed by direct open biopsy for similar reasons.

The many studies that may be carried out on solid-tumor specimens, such as electron microscopy, histochemistry, and chromosomal analysis, make it important to preserve portions of the specimen in different ways, including freezing.

Lymph Node and Marrow Biopsies

Peripheral lymph-node biopsies are standard procedures for patients with potential lymphomas, neuroblastomas, and extremity (and usually trunk) rhabdomyosarcomas, fibrosarcomas, and other soft-tissue sarcomas.

In Hodgkin's disease, it is important to excise the largest of any group of apparently involved peripheral lymph nodes, since this is the most likely to be unequivocally positive. Adjacent smaller nodes, although simpler to excise, may be negative or reveal only confusing secondary features. In the biopsy of lymphomas, it is important when possible to excise an entire node, which allows examination of the capsule and its infiltration by the tumor. The processing of lymph nodes for identification of different pediatric neoplasms is not uniform, and the presence of a knowledgeable pathologist in the operating room during the procedure is essential. In these tumor systems, "touch" preparations and needle biopsies are frequently used and may augment the pathologist's ability to identify the tumor, although they rarely can be relied on for definitive diagnosis.

The use of trephine and aspiration marrow biopsies has largely eliminated the need for formal surgical biopsy. Occasionally, in patients with little marrow or in which the neoplastic pattern is of particular significance, cubes of marrow are removed from the iliac crest or sternum.

Primary Excisions

The traditional concept that cure for the patient with cancer was largely dependent on the surgeon's ability to excise the primary lesion completely, preferably with a margin of normal tissue surrounding it, must be modified when applied to several pediatric solid tumors. In other pediatric tumors, however, this basically remains the situation today. Included in this group would be most soft-tissue sarcomas, including rhabdomyosarcomas arising in the trunk and extremities; some osteosarcomas; malignant teratoid tumors; and, to some extent, hepatoblastomas and hepatocellular carcinomas. The group of tumors that are on the border between benign and malignant neoplasms, such as ganglioneuromas, fibromatoses, and low-grade fibrosarcomas, must also be listed among those in which surgical resection is the most important factor in therapy.

In other pediatric solid tumors, the concept of primary excision requires modification (Table 10-3). The extent of the desirable envelope of normal tissue surrounding the tumor is often hard to determine in pediatric sarcomas. "Pseudoencapsulation" simply means that projections of tumor tissue extend beyond what appears grossly to be the maximum extent of the tumor. Thus, survival following many excisions that are believed to be complete is actually dependent on the effects of ancillary chemotherapy or irradiation on microresidual tumor. These deposits may be local, regional, or systemic, and their presence can be illustrated in many tumor systems. One example is the striking increase in survival among patients with "completely excised" hepatoblastomas when they began receiving chemotherapy after surgery. Similarly, in many sites of rhabdomyosarcoma, a striking improvement in survival was noted in patients in clinical group I (completely resected

Table 10-3
Initial Versus Delayed Excision of the Primary in Pediatric Solid Tumor Management

Nephroblastoma

Unilateral	In the US, almost all nephroblastomas are excised without biopsy prior to institution of chemotherapy regimens even in the presence of dissemination; patients with encasement of midline vessels are the only sizable group in whom this is not recommended. In Europe, use of presurgery chemotherapy without tissue diagnosis is common, with delayed nephrectomy at 6–10 weeks or time of maximum response.
Bilateral	Traditional approach has been initial nephrectomy on the side with the larger tumor and heminephrectomy (or extent of resection required) on the side with the smaller tumor. This might still be recommended if one tumor was quite small and peripheral. Otherwise, the current approach would be initial bilateral biopsy, chemotherapy, and delayed attempt at tumor resection bilaterally (see Chap. 27).

Neuroblastoma

Stages I, II, and resectable III	Initial resection is routine.
Stage III (Evans)	Total excision is possible in a *minority* of patients and has been carried out either during initial exploratory laparotomy or thoracotomy or at a second-look procedure after intensive chemotherapy. There is a demonstrated increase in survival when excision can be accomplished. Chemotherapy results in a resectable state in some tumors.
Stage IV	Initial excision of the primary does not increase survival duration. When clinical complete response has been achieved by chemotherapy, delayed excision of the primary is performed when feasible.
Stage IV$_s$	Excision of primary, either initial or delayed, cannot be demonstrated to affect survival. When tumor mass remains after metastatic foci have been eliminated (unusual), excision of the primary is usually carried out.

Rhabdomyosarcoma

Paratesticular, extremity, trunk, and superficial head and neck sites	Primary excision of resectable tumors is standard.
Bladder–prostate, vaginal sites	Primary chemotherapy ± radiotherapy is ordinarily employed, with delayed resection usually required.
Orbital, parameningeal	Primary excision is not ordinarily attempted (paraminengeal) or required to achieve high rates of survival (orbital).

Malignant Hepatic Tumors

Hepatoblastoma or hepatocellular carcinoma	Primary excision by lobectomy of resectable tumors is standard. Tumors deemed unresectable in some series have been reduced by chemotherapy and subsequently resected with survival.

Malignant Germ-Cell Tumors

Resectable ovarian, testicular, or extragonadal sites	Primary excision is standard.
Huge pelvic tumors with unlikely resectability	Biopsy, intensive chemotherapy, and delayed attempt at excision or debulking is standard.

tumors) with the use of chemotherapeutic agents following surgery. Thus, there is an increasing group of tumors in which it appears that gross resection of the tumor, always combined with intensive chemotherapy or chemotherapy/radiotherapy regimens, is the most effective form of management. In these situations, the role of surgery is no more essential than that of other modalities, all being required in most cases for successful treatment. This includes almost all patients with neuroblastoma and ganglioneuroblastoma[51] except those in stages I and II; rhabdomyosarcomas of many sites, including bladder, prostate, vagina, paratesticular tissues, or retroperitoneum; most malignant germ cell tumors; and nephroblastoma (unfavorable and possibly even with favorable histology).

It is for this group that the concept of initial chemotherapy courses followed by a delayed attempt at surgical excision is prevalent. In rhabdomyosarcoma, malignant germ cell tumors, neuroblastoma, osteosarcoma, and hepatic tumors, such an approach is based on an initial tissue diagnoses (or at least marrow diagnoses, in neuroblastoma). In the current management of nephroblastoma in most European clinics, the diagnosis is based only on clinical studies.

A final group of patients are those in whom excision of the primary tumor is of little significance or is less important than other modalities. This includes patients with stage IVS neuroblastoma, usually Ewing's sarcoma, localized lymphomas, and possibly forms of nephroblastoma with favorable histology, as illustrated by the results of treatment of bilateral disease by chemotherapy in patients in whom the tumor is never completely resected.

Debulking of Pediatric Solid Tumors

The rationale for debulking, or cytoreductive surgery, is logical, but the conversion of this concept into an increase in patient survival or duration of survival has been uncertain. Among adult patients with carcinoma, there has been relatively little beneficial effect of such procedures except in ovarian tumors and NHL.[64]

Debulking for neuroblastoma has a long history, with Koop at The Children's Hospital of Philadelphia being an early advocate (Table 10-4).[65] There has never been a randomized

Table 10-4
Indications for Cytoreductive Surgery (Debulking Procedures) in Pediatric Patients with Solid Tumors

Tumor Type	Criterion and Procedures
Malignant germ-cell tumors	In patients with extensive and apparently unresectable pelvic or pelvic–lower abdominal tumors, subtotal and partial excisions are employed, including omentectomy and excision of large discrete peritoneal implants. Following demonstration of responsiveness of these tumors to multiagent chemotherapy regimens, such procedure are now frequently delayed except when total or near-total excision appears feasible at the time of the initial approach.
Non-Hodgkin's lymphoma	Cytoreductive procedures have been used in some institutions in patients with massive, relatively localized abdominal disease to permit reduction in radiation dosage, sparing the vertebral marrow from intensive exposure.
Neuroblastoma	These procedures are used in patients with Stage III, apparently unresectable abdominal disease before or, more frequently, after chemotherapy–radiotherapy regimens. In patients with stage IV disease who have localized massive abdominal involvement, debulking may be employed as a part of the BMT regimen, permitting reduction in the volume and dosage of local irradiation or possibly eliminating the need for local irradiation. Otherwise, debulking in stage IV disease does not extend survival.
Rhabdomyosarcoma	Not ordinarily performed as an elective procedure. May be carried in course of BMT regimens, as noted under neuroblastoma.
Nephroblastoma	Not ordinarily performed.*
Hepatoblastoma, hepatocellular carcinoma	Not ordinarily performed.*
Hodgkin's disease	Not ordinarily employed.

* Many resections for nephroblastoma and malignant hepatic and other tumors become, in effect, cytoreductive surgery because of incomplete tumor excision, but this is due to circumstances encountered at surgery and was not the preoperative intent.

trial evaluating this type of procedure, and there is such variation in technique associated with its use for neuroblastoma that it is doubtful whether it is possible to evaluate this question in an inter-institutional group (see Chap. 28). All large pediatric tumor services include a number of patients in whom extensive debulking procedures for neuroblastoma have resulted in long-range survival even when it is obvious that the tumor was not completely resected. These cases are not confined to the very young, and in these cases it is difficult to ascribe the results to other factors.

At present, debulking procedures are being performed in patients with widespread abdominal neuroblastoma and rhabdomyosarcoma during preparation for total body irradiation (TBI) or high-dose chemotherapy to be followed by bone-marrow transplantation. These operations are performed after induction and before the tumor-cell (and marrow) "wipe-out" procedure.

If debulking includes patients in whom the tumor is reduced to microscopic residual, this approach has had at least limited success in patients with rhabdomyosarcoma (stages IIA and IIC) in the IRS (see Chap. 30). As noted previously, a sizable number of these patients actually have gross residual tumor, and their survival rates must be attributed partially to the subtotal tumor excision. The relapse rates in these patients are lower than those in roughly comparable patients in clinical group III with unresected (biopsy only) or gross residual disease despite the less intensive chemotherapy they receive.[66]

Another form of debulking is the removal of extensive intra-abdominal disease in children with NHL (see Chap. 20). At the Memorial Hospital for Cancer and Allied Diseases, this procedure was performed routinely (1978–1984) following the initial courses of chemotherapy; that is, at approximately 8 weeks.[67] The purpose was either to eliminate the necessity for irradiation or to reduce the necessary dosage to nodal areas over the vertebral column and thus spare the spinal marrow, permitting more intensive chemotherapy.[68]

With respect to hepatoblastoma, a number of patients have survived after excision of the primary tumor with the exception of a small margin of obvious residual neoplasm (subtotal excisions) (see Chap. 26). These patients have been treated with chemotherapy and well-localized radiotherapy to the site of remnant tumor. However, most of the patients in this category of incompletely resected hepatic tumors ultimately have lethal local recurrence or dissemination.

Prophylactic Lymph-Node Dissections

Defined as dissections carried out in patients without clinical evidence of node involvement, prophylactic lymph-node dissections are widely practiced in adult oncologic surgery. In adults with carcinoma, these procedures are regarded as being of major therapeutic and prognostic significance, and their value justifies the occasional upper-extremity edema and the more frequent healing problems, including occasional skin-flap necrosis, associated with groin dissections.

In pediatric oncology, the use of these procedures is much more limited (Table 10-5). Retroperitoneal lymph-node dissections are performed routinely in most, but not all,[69] institutions for paratesticular rhabdomyosarcoma and for some testicular tumors (see Chap. 30). These dissections are either confined to the side of the primary tumor or cross the midline only above the origin of the inferior mesenteric artery. The same procedure carried out in a large series of adults has not resulted in impotence, although retrograde ejaculation into the bladder has been reported. Attempts to replace retroperitoneal node dissection with noninvasive procedures such as pedal lymphagiogram, CT, and ultrasound have not been strenuously pursued, but there have been a sizable group of errors noted in the limited series reported in which these studies were followed by a confirmatory dissection (see Chap. 7). Most investigators believe that if the retroperitoneal node dissection re-

Table 10-5
Prophylactic (No Clinically Apparent Disease) Lymph-Node Dissections* in Management of Pediatric Tumors

Tumor Type	Criterion and Procedures
Paratesticular rhabdomyosarcoma	Unilateral or high-crossover retroperitoneal node dissection is recommended. If negative, abdominal irradiation is unnecessary. Operation has been eliminated in some European series in patients with negative lymphangiograms and negative scanning studies of retroperitoneal tissues.
Testicular tumors	Similar node dissections are used for malignant testicular tumors, including embryonal carcinoma, teratocarcinoma, choriocarcinomia, and, in some clinics, endodermal sinus tumors. The procedure is not usually carried out in infants and, in some clinics, not in younger children or in children with pure endodermal sinus tumor histology. In the latter group, node dissection is delayed pending the failure of α-fetoprotein to return to normal levels in some clinics.
Extremity and trunk rhabdomyosarcoma; soft-tissue sarcomas	Axillary and inguinofemoral node dissection is recommended for staging purposes. If the node dissection is positive, retroperitoneal dissection is performed. These procedures should precede any major amputation that would rarely be carried out if they are positive.
Head and neck rhabdomyosarcoma	Radical neck dissections as performed in adults are rarely indicated. Obviously involved nodes may be removed.

* The en bloc node dissection with wide skin flap elevation, performed in the groin and (at times) axilla of adults, is not commonly used in children. Gross removal of all visible nodal tissue is the usual aim of the procedure in pediatric tumor management.

veals no tumor, abdominal irradiation can be omitted. The incidence of recurrence in the retroperitoneal space in patients with paratesticular rhabdomyosarcoma is extremely small in the IRS, either with or without node dissection,[70] although in other series it is larger.[69]

The iliofemoral node dissections carried out in pediatric patients are usually regarded as extensive sampling procedures, with no attempt to remove all tissues within the boundaries of the femoral triangle, as is the aim in the adult iliofemoral node (groin) dissection. Skin flaps are not extensively dissected, and problems of necrosis are rare. The axillary dissections that are carried out for rhabdomyosarcoma or other soft-tissue sarcomas of the upper extremity include removal of all apparent nodes, usually by en bloc dissection but without myectomies. In children, this has not resulted in a significant incidence of arm edema.

Retroperitoneal node inspection and sampling, if not dissection, are indicated in patients with lower-extremity sarcomas in which the iliofemoral nodes are positive. This will lead to determination of a correct stage and direct radiotherapy. Extensive pelvic retroperitoneal lymph-node dissections are carried out in association with pelvic exenteration procedures and in the management of the more malignant pelvic germ cell tumors.

Radical cervical lymph-node dissection, one of the frequent procedures in adult surgery, is rarely indicated in children. Most rhabdomyosarcomas of the head and neck have a low incidence of clinical node metastases, and the incidence of microscopically positive lymph nodes in early series that were biopsied was low. If chemotherapy is able to produce a significant response in the primary tumor (which is rarely resected in these sites), it is apparently also able to eliminate microscopic metastatic disease in the regional nodes.

Pelvic Exenterations and Urinary and Intestinal Diversions

Pelvic Exenteration and Urinary Diversion

These procedures are performed primarily in patients with rhabdomyosarcoma of the distal genitourinary tract although

occasionally for other solid tumors that involve and obstruct the ureters or bladder outlet.

Relatively acute obstructions of the ureters are frequently seen in patients with rhabdomyosarcoma of the prostate or bladder, usually secondary to displacement of structures by the tumor rather than direct invasion. Relief of obstruction may be required on one or both sides and is achieved by the introduction of fine catheters into the renal pelvis through the ureter or flank, by more permanent tube nephrostomies, or occasionally by ureterocutaneous stomas. Bladder outlet obstruction may be relieved by cystostomy. These procedures may provide an interval during which tumor size can be reduced by chemotherapy, if necessary supplemented by irradiation.

Patients with vaginal primary tumors are now successfully treated without anterior pelvic exenteration.[71] Similar success with primary chemotherapy or chemotherapy/radiotherapy has not been achieved in most patients with bladder/prostate rhabdomyosarcoma,[72] and at least 40% of these will ultimately require exenteration if they are to survive. As a salvage procedure following failure of chemotherapy/radiotherapy, anterior pelvic exenteration is effective, with a 75% long-range rate of survival.[73] Total pelvic exenteration is rarely required for rhabdomyosarcoma in any site. In the female patient, anterior exenteration includes removal of the uterus and upper vagina, although it is sometimes possible to remove the bladder without including the uterus. The ovaries are almost always retained.

Reestablishment of a functional urinary tract after cystectomy was originally dependent on uretero-intestinal anastomosis, ordinarily to the distal sigmoid colon. This operation was supplanted by one in which isolated ileal segments connected the ureters to the skin of the abdominal wall; that is, the ileal loop. Subsequently, a segment of colon has been used, making it possible to create antireflux "valves" in the conduit wall. During the past 5 years, many of the surviving patients with ileal and colon loops have been converted by Kock pouch procedures to drainage not requiring a permanent bag. However, the Kock procedure is not usually done during the initial operation to remove a neoplasm.

Because the average adult undergoing a urinary diversion procedure for cancer is of a relatively advanced age, the insidious recurrent pyelonephritis associated with ureterointestinal transplants and other diversions is usually not a significant consideration. In contrast, in the child with cancer renal decompensation frequently develops sometime between the 10th and 20th year of urinary diversion. After diversion into the colon, few patients have lived beyond their 40th year. Ileal loop diversion would appear to have a better record, although more secondary surgery of various types is required; in general, these patients require some type of operation at approximately 5-year intervals, usually because of stomal stenosis, prolapse or development of redundancy in the loop. It is not possible to create an effective antireflux "valve" in the wall of the ileum. The colon loop provides the latter feature, but the colonic mucosa, constantly exposed to urine (or urine and feces), appears to have an increased incidence of secondary carcinoma. The long-range effects of the Kock pouch diversion are unknown.

Intestinal Diversion

Permanent colostomies are rarely performed for childhood tumors, although they have occasionally been required in the management of huge tumors of the pelvis, primarily rhabdomyosarcomas and teratomas. Temporary colostomies have been used more frequently, usually to relieve obstruction of the distal colon or rectum secondary to the same tumors or to alleviate irradiation colitis.

Carcinoma of the colon or rectum secondary to either familial polyposis or chronic ulcerative colitis of long duration requires total colectomy and frequently permanent ileostomy. The procedure for ulcerative colitis is done primarily to prevent carcinoma (Table 10-6). At times, a small segment of rectum has been retained in patients with either disease and intestinal continuity restored by an ileorectal pull-through or similar procedure.[74] In such cases, the small distal rectal segment must be monitored frequently; the development of subsequent polyposis or ulcerative colitis makes its resection mandatory.[75]

REPETITIVE SURGERY

Surgery necessitated by the appearance of specific postoperative complications is frequently carried out during the initial 48 hours following major surgical procedures for solid tumors (see section on complications). This section will discuss only repetitive surgery directly associated with the management of the neoplasm, whether planned or elective (Table 10-7).

Early Secondary Surgery

Procedures to Remove Known or Presumed Residual Tumor at the Primary Site

The decision to perform this type of surgery is common in the management of soft-tissue sarcomas of the trunk or extremities and is usually associated with one of several clinical situations: (1) the initial clinical impression has been that the tumor was benign and it was excised without the margins that would have been taken for a malignant tumor; (2) appraisal of the margins of the tumor specimen by a pathologist reveals microscopic tumor; or (3) reappraisal of the situation following the establishment of a precise histologic diagnosis suggests the desirability of more extensive surgery. In the most common situation, the original surgeon has designed the operation to remove a benign tumor such as lipoma or fibroma that is subsequently found to be malignant. When this occurs, if there is a possibility of completely or even grossly excising the tumor with wider margins, this approach is standard. When a patient is transferred from one hospital to another (possibly one country to another) after the initial procedure and there is uncertainty about precisely what was done at the initial operation, although a diagnosis of sarcoma was established and histologic slides are available, reexcision of the entire area, when feasible, is the accepted procedure.

Determination of the completeness of surgical excision by microscopic study of the margins of a large sarcoma is associated with a tremendous sampling error. Negative margins are only suggestive in dealing with the sarcomas of childhood. In many institutions, it is assumed that if a wider excision is feasible without undue loss of function, it should be carried out. When the patient is received in transfer by a secondary–tertiary care center, recognizable sarcoma is found in the second specimen in a relatively high percentage of cases in which early secondary surgery is performed. Even in cases in which it is not detected, it is a reasonable assumption that it exists.[76]

If there is demonstrated residual tumor, as indicated by examinations of the margins of the specimen, the decision whether to perform early secondary surgery rests entirely on its feasibility and on the type and extent of tumor involved. The decision to withhold secondary surgery in such cases might be

---

Table 10-6
Surgical Procedures or Related Conditions in Children Associated with Increased Cancer Incidence in Adulthood

Predisposing Conditions in Infancy or Childhood	Neoplasms Seen in Late Childhood or Adults	Interval to Neoplasia (yr)	Means of Prevention of Neoplasms
Chronic ulcerative colitis for >10 yr	Adenocarcinoma of colon	10–20	Total colectomy for ulcerative colitis
Familial polyposis coli, Gardner's syndrome	Adenocarcinoma of colon	10–30	Total colectomy for both conditions
Urinary diversion to colon (ureterointestinal transplants)	Adenocarcinoma of colon	25–50	Cutaneous or ileal loop urinary diversions; Kock pouch procedure
Unresected idiopathic choledochal dilatation ("choledochal cyst")	Adenocarcinoma, choledochus	20–40	Excision rather than drainage of idiopathic dilatations of the choledochus
Biliary atresia and other forms of infantile cholestasis; glycogen storage disease; childhood cirrhosis of uncertain etiology	Hepatocellular carcinoma	5–20	Early surgery for biliary atresia, available therapy for other conditions when possible

Table 10-7
Indications for Delayed or Elective Secondary Surgical Procedures in Patients with Pediatric Solid Tumors

Type of Surgical Procedure	Nephroblastoma	Neuroblastoma	Rhabdomyosarcoma (RMS) and Soft-Tissue Sarcomas (STS)	Malignant Germ-Cell Tumors*	Malignant Hepatic Tumors
Delayed definitive surgery following biopsy and intensive chemotherapy and possibly irradiation	Occasionally used in large tumors or those with involvement of midline vessels. Common practice (without biopsy) in Europe	Extensively used in patients with stage III–IV disease after chemotherapy response. Not in patients with stage I–II tumors	Standard for bladder, prostate, and vaginal sites in RMS and for initially unresectable (stage III) RMS and STS. Use in potentially resectable RMS in other sites is controversial	Frequently after biopsy only; initial excision is preferred when tumor is resectable	Possibly. Used in several series in both unresectable and probably also resectable tumors. Initial excision of resectable tumors by lobectomy is standard procedure
Second-look procedures after initial excisions of localized disease to evaluate chemotherapy response and possibly excise residual or recurrent tumor	Not usually done. Patients followed by noninvasive studies	Yes in stage III with complete response to chemotherapy	Yes in RMS and STS if initial excision was incomplete and clinical complete or partial response achieved or retained on chemotherapy–radiotherapy regimens	Yes; may be indicated by elevation in markers (AFP, hCG)	Yes except in stage I; *i.e.,* completely resected tumors. May be dictated by marker (AFP) response
Second-look procedures in patients with stage IV (disseminated) disease following complete or partial response to chemotherapy or irradiation	Rarely. Patients followed by non-invasive studies	Yes	Yes	Yes but not usually applicable	Yes, but response rarely achieved in stage IV disease
Regional lymph-node dissections or sampling (at sites of no clinical involvement)	Not as separate procedure. (Hilar and para-aortic node sampling at initial surgery)	Not as separate procedure. (Regional nodes excised with specimen at initial procedure)	Yes when not performed as part of initial surgery. Axillary and ileofemoral procedures for trunk and extremity RMS and STS. Rarely cervical node sampling	Not as separate procedure. (Pelvic and periaortic node dissection usual during excision of primary tumor)	Not as separate procedure. (Local porta hepatis sampling at initial surgery)
Early secondary surgery (with no interval chemotherapy or irradiation) in cases of demonstrated (microscopic residual) or assumed incomplete initial excision	No	No	Frequently for trunk–extremity sites of both RMS and STS. Procedure may be associated with regional node dissection	No	Rarely feasible

* Excluding testicular (see Table 10-5).

based on the undesirability of removing or of injuring adjacent normal structures or on the tumor histology. The latter situation particularly involves patients with nephroblastomas (favorable histology), in which the responsiveness of the tumor to chemotherapy may make the presence of microscopic residual tumor relatively unimportant, or to neuroblastoma, in which, because of proximity to the aorta and other structures, complete excision may be an unrealistic goal. It rarely applies to apparently localized soft-tissue sarcomas.

The standard procedure for removing microscopic residual tumor is a wide local excision, removing an envelope of apparently normal tissue around the tumor in all directions, not simply the area where the "residual" was presumed to be. This is because localization of microscopic residual tumor is imprecise.

Node Dissections

Early secondary surgery also includes the lymph node dissections performed after a diagnosis has been established by excision of the primary tumor (Table 10-6). The most common procedure in this category is the retroperitoneal node dissection performed in boys with paratesticular rhabdomyosarcoma (see prior section) and some types of primary testicular tumors. This dissection may be performed at the time of the orchidectomy but usually is not because of uncertainty regarding the precise diagnosis. The utility of this procedure in paratesticular rhabdomyosarcoma is questioned at present,[69] but it is employed as an indicator of the need or absence of need for abdominal irradiation.

In boys older than 2 years with the more malignant forms of testicular germ-cell tumors—that is, embryonal carcinoma and choriocarcinoma—retroperitoneal node dissections are commonly performed. In others (yolk sac tumors), if the serum α-fetoprotein concentration is elevated before excision of the tumor and rapidly falls to normal levels after surgery, node dissection may be deferred and the marker levels closely monitored for evidence of relapse (see Chaps. 8 and 33).[77] In boys less than 2 years of age, relapse is uncommon.

In patients with rhabdomyosarcomas or other soft-tissue sarcomas of the trunk and extremities, axillary dissections or iliofemoral node sampling is standard as a secondary procedure if it was not performed at the time of the primary excision. When an excisional biopsy of such tumors has been the first procedure, usually performed without a histologic diagnosis, once the diagnosis is established, a secondary wide local excision and an associated regional node evaluation (iliofemoral) or complete dissection (axillary) are routine.

Types of Second-Look Procedures

The first second-look operations were recommended in 1964 by Gilbertson and Wangenstein,[78] who performed a secondary exploratory procedure at a predetermined interval following curative resections for ovarian or gastrointestinal cancer. This concept was refined by the use of carcinoembryonic antigen (CEA) as an indicator of the probability of recurrence in patients with colon cancer. The principle behind this approach was the belief that if recurrent cancer could be detected when it was relatively localized, survival would be increased. In most areas of adult oncology, the use of second-look operations has remained controversial (ovarian cancer excepted), but in pediatric oncology variations of this concept have been widely adopted in different tumor systems. In children, it has rarely been performed after apparent total tumor excision, and the purposes of the procedure are usually broader.

There has been extensive experience with second-look procedures in children with neuroblastoma in CCSG, POG,

and cancer centers[79] as well as in those with malignant germ-cell tumors[80] and rhabdomyosarcoma (Table 10-6) (see Chaps. 28, 30, and 33). In 1978, CCSG began protocols that included a procedure of this type in patients with stage IV and unresectable stage III neuroblastoma who achieved a chemotherapy response. The same studies included a large group of patients who had delayed primary laparotomies; that is, those in whom the diagnosis was made and therapy begun without biopsy of the primary tumor. Patients in whom second-look surgery was performed had received a chemotherapy regimen for 18 to 20 weeks, achieving a complete or partial response. Compliance with this directive was far from complete, but more than 60 patients had such procedures performed. The survival rate in this group was lower than that in patients in the same series in which initial biopsy and delayed primary excision, also after 18 to 20 weeks of chemotherapy, were the sequence.

In the case of rhabdomyosarcoma, during IRS-II, approximately 60 patients from selected institutions were subjected to a second-look procedure between 1982 and 1984.[81] These were patients in clinical group III (localized, unresected tumor) or IV (disseminated, with pulmonary and/or bone marrow metastases only) with a complete or partial response to intensive chemotherapy. The purpose of this procedure was to observe the effects of chemotherapy and the resection of residual tumor to the extent possible. A tertiary surgical procedure, described in a subsequent protocol, was designed to observe the effects of subsequent irradiation and alternate forms of chemotherapy in patients achieving a partial response as observed at the initial second-look. An additional aim was to resect residual tumor when this was feasible. The results of this project are under study, but the observations at the second-look procedures are diverse and the specimens obtained of interest. In some patients, no identifiable tumor was found in either the primary or metastatic sites, whereas in others the tumor is more widespread than at the first procedure. In still others, tumor cells that could be identified had undergone significant histologic changes, presenting an appearance suggestive of immature muscle cells.

Approximately 100 second-look procedures have been performed during the trial of a six-drug regimen for malignant germ cell tumors, gonadal (ovarian only) and extragonadal, by CCSG. An initial survey suggests that these operations have not been therapeutically helpful in patients with ovarian tumors, but in the children with germ cell tumors in nongonadal sites, reexcision may be complete at the time of secondary surgery, and this may influence survival.

The current recommendations of the NWTS for the management of most synchronous bilateral nephroblastomas constitute a series of second-look procedures. This regimen begins with a biopsy of both tumors. After several courses of chemotherapy, if response is apparent, a second laparotomy with an attempt to perform bilateral "tumorectomies" is done. If this cannot be accomplished at the second procedure, additional chemotherapy, possibly plus irradiation, is instituted. This is followed by a third laparotomy, again with an attempt to preserve some renal tissue bilaterally.

The overall results of the second-look procedures are difficult to evaluate statistically, but it appears that the operation may be useful in neuroblastoma, rhabdomyosarcoma,[82] some germ cell tumors, and bilateral and some other forms of nephroblastoma.[83]

Surgery for Local or Regional Relapse

It is probable that during the course of many solid tumors, local relapse precedes distant relapse but is unrecognized. Autopsy studies from the IRS suggest that local relapse is usually present in association with distant relapse, although in this case whether it preceded the distant relapse is uncertain.[84] However, when local relapse is identified without evidence of distant relapse, an energetic therapeutic approach using all modalities is indicated.[85] This is also true in some instances when localized regional relapse is apparent, particularly in patients who have been untreated for an extended interval. Isolated local relapse in most tumor systems is treated in the same fashion as an untreated localized primary tumor, but surgery is more extensive (when it is possible), chemotherapy more intensive, and irradiation administered to more extended fields, when this is feasible. Commonly, the initial procedure for local relapse is to confirm its presence, although this may have been done by prior incisional or aspiration biopsy.

In NWTS-2, 3.8% of 259 patients in clinical groups II and III (irradiated patients) had an initial clinical recurrence at the operative site or elsewhere in the abdomen excluding the liver and opposite kidney.[86] Unfavorable histology, the use of contracted irradiation fields, and delay in irradiation (more than 10 days postoperatively) increased this local relapse rate. In the International Society of Pediatric Oncology (SIOP) trials (1042 patients), the abdominal relapse rate was 8% (see Chap. 27).[87]

Recurrent nephroblastoma in the renal fossa is managed by as wide a local excision as is feasible, conserving vital structures.[85] If the local recurrence is at a site in which resection is difficult, intensive chemotherapy is frequently used, followed by a second attempt at excision weeks or months later. Carefully directed radiation therapy may be used if irradiation has been included in the original therapy and more extensive irradiation if it has not. Local recurrence of stage I or II neuroblastoma is managed similarly, ordinarily omitting irradiation.

Isolated localized recurrence of most soft-tissue sarcomas of the extremities (including rhabdomyosarcoma) when initial therapy has been adequate suggests that amputation will be required for survival. Recurrent rhabdomyosarcomas of the trunk, retroperitoneal space, and pelvic viscera are treated by wider local excisions followed by irradiation (when possible) and chemotherapy.

In patients on a primary chemotherapy or primary chemotherapy/radiotherapy regimen, local recurrence is defined as progressive increase in tumor size after an initial response. In rhabdomyosarcomas of the bladder and prostate, this is ordinarily treated by total cystectomy or anterior pelvic exenteration. Recurrent vaginal rhabdomyosarcomas have frequently been successfully managed by hysterectomy/vaginectomy or vaginectomy (in distal lesions), with retention of the bladder and rectum.[71] These patients have already received intensive chemotherapy as well as irradiation, and the management of local relapse with experimental chemotherapy regimens ordinarily leads to dissemination and fatality. Anterior pelvic exenteration as a salvage procedure following local relapse in patients with bladder, prostate, or vaginal rhabdomyosarcomas is associated with an approximately 75% survival rate when carried out before dissemination has occurred (also see Chap. 30).[73]

Local recurrence of hepatoblastoma is rarely observed and suggests a tumor that is not prone to metastasize. Laparotomy and a second local excision should be attempted if this is technically feasible. Isolated local recurrence of osteosarcoma suggests a need for extremity amputation or excision of the involved bone in trunk sites.

In general, patients with local or local/regional recurrence who have received minimal chemotherapy and no local irradiation have the highest survival rates.[88] Local relapse occurring months or even years after the end of a nonintensive chemotherapy regimen has a similarly favorable outlook. Certain tumor varieties and sites are associated with relatively frequent salvage after local relapse, including vaginal or paratesticular rhabdomyosarcoma, favorable-histology nephroblastoma, neuroblastoma in younger patients with recurrence in soft-tissue sites, and some teratomas.[89] In contrast, patients who suffer local relapse early in the course of an intensive chemotherapy regimen have little chance of survival. Relapse that appears to be localized to an area of "geographic miss"—that is, at the margin of an irradiation field—may be treated successfully by wide local excision, selective irradiation, and intensive chemotherapy. Isolated local relapse in tumors that usually are widely disseminated suggests a unique biological behavior of this specific tumor and supports an approach of energetic local therapy in addition to systemic chemotherapy.

SURGERY OF METASTATIC DISEASE

Metastatic Disease Present at Diagnosis

The presence of pulmonary metastases in patients with nephroblastoma is frequently ignored initially. The primary is excised, and the metastases and the tumor bed are treated with systemic chemotherapy postoperatively. Only massive pulmonary involvement would reverse this sequence in North American clinics. In the NWTS, a standard nephrectomy has been followed by a two- or three-drug chemotherapy regimen for 15 months in almost all patients with pulmonary metastases at diagnosis, and the survival rate is 66% (74% with favorable histology) among the 236 patients treated from 1969 to 1983 (see Chap. 27).[90] In rare instances, in children with nephroblastoma or hepatoblastoma, it has been possible to excise metastatic lesions at the time of resection of the primary. These have been situations in which an abdominothoracic incision is used to remove the primary tumor, and metastatic lesions are readily removed through the same incision.

In other tumors, when metastatic disease is present at diagnosis, the initial surgical procedure is ordinarily reduced in scope to biopsy of the primary tumor or of a metastasis. Opportunities for secondary (delayed) resection of the primary tumor and of the metastases, with long-range survival, have been seen in children with neuroblastoma, rhabdomyosarcoma, hepatoblastoma, osteogenic sarcoma, and other tumors (Table 10-8). The surgical techniques are reviewed in the following section.

Surgery of Distant Relapse

Pulmonary Metastasis

The extreme chemotherapy sensitivity of nephroblastoma makes it unique among solid tumors. Most long-range reports on the management of metastatic pulmonary nephroblastoma include patients who have been treated successfully by surgery alone, radiotherapy alone, or combinations of both modalities, with and without adjunctive chemotherapy. At present, in most patients with this form of dissemination, the pulmonary lesions will be completely cleared solely by chemotherapy. Areas of persistent disease following a series of courses of chemotherapy are treated with surgical excision or radiotherapy. Prophylactic irradiation of the entire lung fields may be performed after the excision or localized treatment of individual metastatic nodules. Except when required by the presence of metastases among the hilar structures, excisions for metastatic pulmonary nephroblastoma are not lobectomies but segmental

Table 10-8
Surgical Resection of Metastatic Disease in the Management of Pediatric Solid Tumors

	Pulmonary Metastasis	Hepatic Metastasis	Other Metastases
Nephroblastoma	Excision is usually preceded by chemotherapy ± irradiation. May be regarded as a substitute for radio-therapy or to remove irradiation-resistant lesions. Pulmonary tissue is conserved. In relapse, may be necessary to establish lesions as neoplastic	Used when control of all extrahepatic lesions has been achieved and localized hepatic foci are apparent by US, CT, *etc.* Only for a small number of hepatic lesions, permitting removal by lobectomy or tumorectomy	
Neuroblastoma	Rarely used, since response to chemotherapy when it occurs is usually complete. Feasible if all extrapulmonary disease is controlled with persistent pulmonary lesions	Not in patients with disseminated foci or stage IVS disease. In older patients with a late solitary hepatic recurrence persistent after intensive chemotherapy	
Rhabdomyosarcoma	Indicated in patients in whom control of primary and all disseminated disease by chemotherapy ± radiotherapy has been achieved, but with persistence of pulmonary lesions that can be resected without major compromise in pulmonary function. May be necessary for diagnosis.	As in nephroblastoma	Solitary CNS metastasis in frontal and parietal lobes have been excised with extended survival
Hepatoblastoma	Resection of isolated metastasis has been accomplished with long-range survival after resection of primary and chemotherapy ± radiotherapy	May be part of initial procedure. Solitary recurrent nodules in remnant lobe(s) after initial resection	
Osteosarcoma	Resection of pulmonary metastatic lesions is standard except in cases with lack of local tumor control, extrapulmonary metastasis, or rapid appearance of multiple lesions. Pulmonary tissue conserved	Not ordinarily site of metastasis	
Soft-tissue sarcomas	As in rhabdomyosarcoma, has been particularly successful in chondrosarcomas and fibrosarcomas	As in rhabdomyosarcoma	CNS lesions may be resected, as in rhabdomyosarcoma

resections or simple tumor enucleations. This type of procedure may be repeated if metastases recur.

Currently, the most widely used major excisional procedures for pulmonary metastases are carried out for osteosarcoma.[91] The technical procedures performed for this condition are relatively unique, although they have been used for other metastatic sarcomas in some centers (see Chap. 32). The preservation of the maximum amount of lung tissue is a major aim. Neither lobectomies nor segmental resections are ordinarily included in the procedure; instead, the individual metastatic nodules are enucleated or excised with a minimal margin of surrounding lung tissue. Emphasis is on locating all of the lesions in both lungs and removing them, leaving a relatively intact volume of pulmonary tissue. The response to this type of procedure in series of selected cases has been favorable, and in some the operation has been repeated as many as three or four times on each side. The indications for this approach among patients with osteosarcoma have been expanded. At present,

the contraindications are usually (1) failure of local control of the primary; (2) extrapulmonary dissemination; or (3) metastatic lesions so numerous and appearing so rapidly that complete excision of visible metastases would appear to be impossible.

Pulmonary metastatic lesions associated with hepatoblastoma have at times receded and been eliminated by chemotherapy in cases in which the primary tumor was also responsive and was resected. In such cases, long-range survival is possible.

Hepatic Metastasis

Isolated metastases of nephroblastoma in the liver have frequently been resected, with subsequent survival. Currently, these lesions would be treated with intensive chemotherapy before and following excision (see Chap. 27). At times, multiple hepatic lesions have also been approached in this way. The most favorable situation for such a procedure is when hepatic relapse occurs late in the course in a patient who has not previously received intensive therapy and is currently off all chemotherapy. The presence of one or two relatively large hepatic metastases with no other suspicious areas at this stage suggests that tumor dissemination may not be a continuing process.

The hepatic involvement of stage IVS neuroblastoma ordinarily consists of relatively diffuse nodules throughout both lobes, and surgical excision is not required or helpful (see Chap. 28). Involvement of the liver in older patients with neuroblastoma, particularly in late recurrence, may be discrete and amenable to resection when control of the generalized disease is possible. Such lesions may be reduced in size with chemotherapy before surgery. A similar approach has been used in patients with isolated hepatic metastases from rhabdomyosarcoma and other soft-tissue sarcomas.

Other Metastatic Sites

Isolated residual metastatic lesions in bone secondary to Ewing's sarcoma, neuroblastoma, and other sarcomas have occasionally been excised, but this has usually been carried out with the aim of confirming the histology of the tumor. The sites are then irradiated, and chemotherapy is usually reinstituted.

The usual operative procedures for metastatic intracerebral neoplasms are decompressions. However, isolated metastatic lesions in the frontal and parietal lobes in children with rhabdomyosarcoma have been excised, with long-term survival. Again, the most favorable situation for success is the isolated lesion occurring a significant interval after the end of a chemotherapy regimen.

Distant (as opposed to regional) metastatic neuroblastoma in lymph nodes or other soft tissues is frequently excised for histologic examination, and there are numerous long-range survivors, particularly among younger patients. The general dictum that metastasis of neuroblastoma to soft tissue, as opposed to bone, presents a more favorable situation for intensive multidisciplinary therapy appears to be borne out by the experience of most institutions.[92] Distant metastatic disease in lymph nodes and other soft tissues (usually breast) in rhabdomyosarcoma and other soft-tissue sarcomas is rarely treated successfully, and surgery is used largely for identification of sites of relapse.

SPECIALIZED TECHNIQUES REQUIRING SURGERY

Regional Chemotherapy: Perfusion and Infusion Techniques

Perfusions are procedures in which a body segment is isolated, with both the arterial and venous connections controlled, and blood or other fluids containing the antitumor drug are circulated through the segment with an external pump. Infusion implies delivery of high concentrations of the therapeutic agent into the arterial supply of the organ or area to be treated or, occasionally, into the portal venous system in hepatic tumors. The use of perfusion and infusion techniques in various body sites, primarily in adult patients, was reported during the 1960s and 1970s. Since that time, interest has concentrated on infusion techniques for primary or metastatic liver tumors and less frequently on infusion therapy for extremity sarcomas (see Chaps. 26 and 32).

Perhaps the largest group of adult patients receiving infusion therapy at present have mestastatic colon carcinoma. This form of therapy was initiated by ligation of the hepatic artery.

When it was established that this could be accomplished safely, although with questionable therapeutic results, small catheters were introduced at surgery through branches of the hepatic artery to deliver agents to one or both hepatic lobes. These catheters were then connected with chambers that could be carried by an ambulatory patient during a continuous infusion. Ultimately, chambers were implanted subcutaneously for continuous outpatient therapy. Agents that have been infused include vincristine, cyclophosphamide, and 5-fluorouracil. Some surgeons believe that the therapeutic results can be duplicated simply by excising metastatic hepatic lesions when they are few, and other investigators find it difficult to demonstrate that this technique using 5-fluorouracil is more efficacious than systemic intravenous therapy.[93]

In pediatric patients, isolation perfusion systems were used in the 1960s and subsequently have been replaced almost entirely by infusion systems. The use of the hepatic arterial system for infusion has been reported periodically,[94] and the infusion of trunk and extremity lesions even less frequently, during the past decade. There are a number of reasons for this. First, the hepatic arterial system is small in patients the age of those with hepatoblastoma and may readily thrombose, ending therapy. Also, in the case of large hepatic tumors, the arteries required for infusion may be completely buried beneath a mass of tumor extending inferiorly over the porta hepatis, so that a relatively large tumor resection is required before the catheter can be placed in the optimum site.

In respect to extremity lesions, regional perfusion and infusion techniques have been employed in children since 1950. A more recent innovation has been the tourniquet infusion technique, in which the arterial inflow and venous outflow are temporarily occluded following injection of the chemotherapeutic agent. This provides a relatively static circulation in the isolated area temporarily. Perfusion systems have been employed occasionally in treating extremity sarcomas and may have been useful in converting unresectable to resectable lesions.

Organ Transplantation

The initial results of renal transplantation when used for unresectable bilateral nephroblastoma were disappointing because most of these patients suffered tumor relapse soon after beginning immunosuppressive regimens. Survival is now more common following renal transplantation, apparently as a result of revised policies in overall management, including (1) longer intervals on dialysis between the nephrectomies and transplantation, with an increased exposure to cancer chemotherapeutic agents, as oncologists have become more conversant with the problems of administering agents to the anephric patient; (2) earlier nephrectomies, before wide extension of the tumor in the retroperitoneal areas has occurred; and (3) more effective local irradiation.[95]

Similarly, most early liver transplantation procedures for neoplasms failed because of tumor recurrence, and this problem continues to the extent that some large transplant services rarely accept a patient with cancer of any type. The exception may be the patient with a small, well-defined tumor surrounding the porta hepatis without evidence of nodal or distant dissemination. Patients with the fibrolamellar variant of hepatocellular carcinoma may also be a relatively favorable group for transplantation, with a 50% survival rate reported.[96] The advent of cyclosporin therapy has greatly increased the rate and duration of survival among liver transplant patients generally, but this has not yet been apparent in the few patients in whom transplantation has been performed for neoplasia.

Intraoperative Radiotherapy

The use of intraoperative radiotherapy (IOR) is under consideration for pediatric patients with abdominal neuroblastoma and possibly other tumors. Operating room facilities to make this feasible are available in a few institutions, where it is apparent that pediatric patients will be included in the use of this form of therapy.

IOR was reintroduced into modern medicine in 1971.[97] The aim of the current procedure is to deliver a single high-dose exposure to an unresected segment of a tumor or total tumor identified under direct vision. Thus, the margins of the tumor and hence the radiation portals can be determined with precision. The technique of maintaining anesthesia and physiologic support with both the operating and the anesthesia teams momentarily out of the operating room presents problems. The surgical techniques are standard (Fig. 10-2). The intraoperative treatment cones are introduced as sterile instruments directly into the surgical field. Scatter from such therapy can be strictly limited. Current experience involves adults with pancreatic, bladder, or widespread colorectal cancer.[98]

Animal studies suggest that irradiation doses must be limited to 1500 to 2000 rad if intestine is in the field, but, if the intestine can be excluded, large vessel walls will tolerate single doses exceeding 3000 rad. Both supervoltage and orthovoltage techniques have been used.

TECHNIQUES TO PROVIDE NUTRITIONAL SUPPORT

Short-Term Central Venous Catheterization

The original central catheters, made of polyvinylchloride or Silastic, were introduced by pericutaneous needles or though small incisions into the subclavian or jugular veins or, at times, the saphenofemoral system. These small-bore catheters were employed in all sizes of patients, including neonates, and ordinarily provided solely for the introduction of solutions for total parenteral nutrition.[99] Blood drawing was rarely possible, and the system was opened as infrequently as possible. This technique did not meet the multiple needs of children with cancer on intensive therapy regimens and is rarely used in such patients today.

Indwelling Silastic Catheters for Long-Term Parenteral Nutrition

These techniques use large-bore catheters designed for multipurpose function (see also Chap. 40). They are made for long-term use with cuffs to prevent dislodgment and of a size permitting blood withdrawal as well as continuous or intermittent infusion of nutrients, antineoplastic agents, antibiotics, anticoagulants, and other solutions. These catheters are placed by direct exposure in the cephalic, external or internal jugular, or saphenous systems or they have been placed pericutaneously via the subclavian vein (Fig. 10-3). The Hickman catheter was a modified version of the original Broviac[100] made of barium-impregnated silicone rubber and providing a larger diameter and a cuff designed to incite fibrosis in the surrounding subcutaneous tissues.

Currently, there are many different types of catheters, including single, double, and triple lumens for use in larger patients. The smallest single-lumen catheter is 4F, and the smallest double-lumen catheter is 7F. These are placed in the appropriate vein under direct vision and advanced into the right atrium. The catheter is then "tunneled" subcutaneously to its exit, ordinarily on the lower anterior chest wall. This site is distant from oral–nasal secretions, free from the influence of neck motion, and readily available to those caring for the patient without unnecessary body movement. The catheter tip is placed in the right atrium under fluoroscopic control, or its position is ascertained by roentgenograms in the operating room. Right-sided insertion is preferable because access to the atrium is more reliable from this side. Catheter patency is maintained by daily flushes of heparin or by continuous administration of heparin as a component of other solutions. Success in the placement of these catheters is dependent on aseptic technique, rigorously controlled catheter care, and careful preparation and technique in the delivery of all infused elements.

FIGURE 10-2. Intraoperative radiotherapy (IOR): surgical aspects. **A.** Sterile applicator is inserted through an abdominal incision to the site of the tumor. **B.** Applicator has been surrounded by sterile drapes and "docked" to a linear accelerator for therapy. Surgical equipment such as metal retractors is standard. (Courtesy of Dr. Stephen M. Stowe)

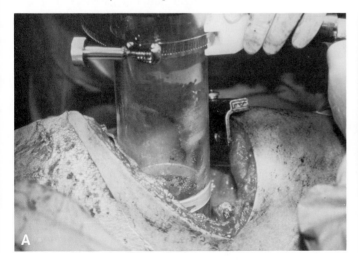

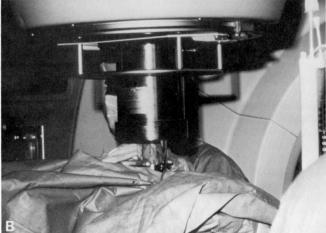

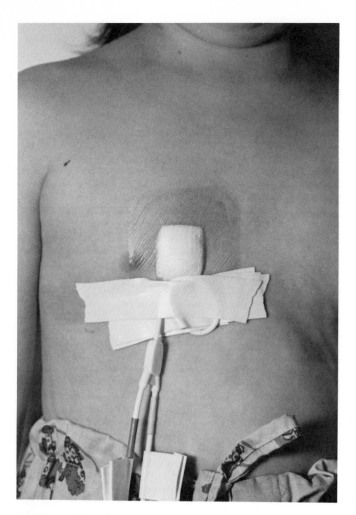

FIGURE 10-3. Long-range infusion therapy. Double-lumen Hickman catheter is in place. It had been inserted through a neck-line incision, which is healed. The larger lumen is usually used for blood removal and the smaller lumen for all types of infusion or medication. (Courtesy of Dr. James B. Atkinson)

Totally Implanted Silastic Catheters

Totally implanted catheters are a modification of the Broviac/Hickman technique in which peripheral access to the intravenous system is via a chamber that is completely skin covered.[101,102] The access to the central venous system is similar to that provided by the catheters described previously, but because the chamber is not exposed, no dressings are required. Needles are passed through the skin and a Silastic septum into this chamber. A special needle is provided (Huber point); with this needle, it is asserted that the septum can be punctured as many as 2000 times without malfunction. The size of the equipment makes this system more appropriate for children weighing 8 kg or more.

Enteral Nutritional Support

Although enteral support is the oldest way of providing nutritional supplements for the patient with cancer, the concepts and techniques for effecting it have been completely altered during the past decade. The traditional large tubes passed through the mouth or nose, which were used to transmit kitchen-blended formulas to the stomach, have been replaced with fine-bore catheters that are well tolerated by most patients and by curd-free nutritional solutions that will readily pass through them (see Chap. 40).[103] Current feeding tubes are not only small (5F to 8F) but radiopaque and end-weighted. After being guided through the pharynx with a trocar, whether they are placed in the stomach or intestine depends on the state of the patient and of gastrointestinal function. Gastric feedings have the advantage of using the physiologic mixing reservoir with adjustments of tonicity before the feedings pass, in increments, into the duodenum. This advantage may be offset by an increased risk of regurgitation or vomiting and aspiration. When the feedings are introduced distally, the tonicity of the solution must be more finely adjusted and the volume and caloric content of feedings advanced more slowly. This position of the tube has the advantage of permitting simultaneous gastric suction if this is desirable.

Modern enteral feeding formulas are prepared to specification and represent optimum nutritional support. However, they still must be increased in increments and the patient monitored for distention or problems associated with intestinal overload. Even in the event of vomiting or anorexia secondary to cancer chemotherapeutic agents or radiation therapy, the jejunum may accept low-calorie isotonic solutions with effective absorption of the nutrients.

Modern catheters are manufactured from soft silicone rubber or polyurethane, making ulceration of the nasal passages uncommon, although continual observation is still mandatory. The position of the end of the catheter should be determined roentgenographically before feedings are begun.

Invasive Approaches for Enteral Nutrition

Gastrostomies carried out for the feeding of pediatric patients with cancer are rarely of the permanent type with a complete mucosal-lined passageway. They are ordinarily of the vertically constructed (Stamm) variety or a horizontal tube with a tunnel created in the gastric wall (Witzel). These gastrostomy openings will close spontaneously on removal of the tube.

Gastrostomy feedings have all of the advantages and disadvantages described for inlying gastric tubes. Inability to tolerate a nasal tube would appear to be the principal indication for their use. However, in the patient in whom it is important to have both gastric suction and a jejunal feeding tube, this is most effectively carried out through a gastrostomy.

Several techniques of introducing gastrostomy tubes through the abdominal wall without a laparotomy have been described.[104,105] These are carried out under gastroscopic control with the stomach inflated and a guide suture passed through the abdominal and stomach walls into the inflated stomach pouch. This is followed by dilation and catheter insertion.

Small-tube feeding jejunostomies may readily be created at the time of laparotomy. These are usually situated immediately distal to the ligament of Treitz with the jejunum firmly anchored to the abdominal wall and the feeding tube brought into it through a tunnel. This results in spontaneous closure without fistula when the tube is no longer required. In contrast to the early large jejunostomy tubes previously placed in position at laparotomy, this small catheter will not produce intestinal obstruction, and complications associated with dislodgment or peritonitis are rare. Some authors will not use this technique in patients who have received abdominal irradiation for fear of creating an enterocutaneous fistula.[106] Immunosuppressed patients are at increased risk of abdominal wall infections, and the exit and entry sites of the catheter must be closely observed. The greatest benefit to be derived from the use of an inserted small-catheter jejunal feeding tube is elimination of the need for intravenous total parenteral nutrition. Special tubes have been devised to provide better fixation within the abdominal wall.

In summary, major recent advances have been made with regard to both parenteral and enteral nutritional support.[106] Enteral support is associated with fewer complex problems relative to the solutions, is not difficult to monitor, and is more economical. Parenteral nutrition can provide more complex variations in nutritional support and, ordinarily, more calories and protein. It also provides access to the central venous system for withdrawal of blood and the introduction of other therapeutic solutions and agents.

COMPLICATIONS AND SEQUELAE REQUIRING SURGERY

Early Acute Complications

Secondary hemorrhage; wound infection; pelvic, abdominal, and subdiaphragmatic abscess; evisceration; and the effects of inadvertent injury to major vessels[107] are common to patients in all age groups following major tumor surgery. Several complications, however, are more common in the pediatric age group.

Intestinal Obstruction and Intussusception

Once the initial paralytic ileus associated with laparotomy has subsided, development of intestinal obstruction early in the postoperative course presents a differential diagnosis almost confined to intussusception, volvulus with ischemia, or the release of a localized collection of septic fluid into the general peritoneal cavity. Volvulus is rarely found as early in the postoperative course as is intussusception, and intra-abdominal collections are usually associated with fever, rarely seen in the patient with intussusception.

Intussusception is seen with unusual frequency following abdominal surgical procedures of all types in childhood and even after some operative procedures adjacent to the peritoneal cavity (see Chap. 37).[108] Children with resected abdominal tumors were included in all of the early series of patients with postoperative intussusception, and subsequent reports were confined to children with abdominal tumors.[109] It was thought by some oncologists that the effect of cancer chemotherapeutic agents, particularly vincristine, was a predisposing factor in postoperative intussusception.

These intussusceptions are not confined to infants and are primarily of an intestinal segment rarely involved in conventional forms of intussusception; that is, they are ileoileal rather than ileocolic. Signs and symptoms are also dissimilar to those found in idiopathic infantile intussusceptions and are basically those of any distal small-intestinal obstruction. Occasionally, these intussusceptions progress into the colon and produce more classic signs. The clinical appearance of these patients is relatively uniform. After surgery, there is an obvious return of active intestinal function, followed by the sudden onset of a second period of ileus, usually within 5 to 14 days after the procedure. The diagnosis usually can be made only by colon contrast studies if a major effort is made to fill the ileum.

Once the diagnosis of intussusception is probable, a laparotomy should be carried out because the results of hydrostatic reduction of intussusceptions confined to the small intestine are unpredictable. At surgery, manual reduction is usually possible, but resections may be required. The etiology of these

episodes is unknown, but it can be demonstrated that the small intestine undergoes a phase of disorganized peristalsis, with antiperistalsis common, after laparotomy.

Additional oncology-related intussusceptions are the result of tumor masses in the intestinal wall, primarily lymphomas (see Chap. 20).[110]

Localized Intestinal Necrosis

Localized intestinal necrosis is usually associated with the response to chemotherapy seen in the childhood forms of non-Hodgkin's lymphoma.[111] The destruction of tumor nodules in the intestinal wall in such cases is so rapid that the formation of scar tissue or even the walling off of the necrotic tissue by surrounding intestinal loops or the omentum does not occur. Free perforation into the peritoneal cavity is a common sequela. In other situations, a vessel may be eroded, resulting in a hemorrhage into either the peritoneal cavity or the intestinal tract. Perforation in this instance is a clear indication for laparotomy and intestinal resection; if perforation occurs in the distal intestinal tract, exteriorization may be used.

Acute Abdominal Conditions in Immunosuppressed or Neutropenic Patients

In addition to the specific conditions described in other sections, patients who are on immunosuppressive therapy or severely neutropenic frequently show the signs and symptoms of either actual or simulated conditions that might require abdominal surgery (Table 10-9). The most frequent underlying disease is acute leukemia, in which more than 5% of the patients develop an acute abdominal condition at some time during their course. Among 286 pediatric patients with acute leukemia reported from Memorial–Sloan Kettering Cancer Institute, 6 developed typhlitis, 6 appendicitis, and 1 each intussusception, intestinal obstruction, pancreatitis, and liver abscess (see also Chaps. 37 and 39).[112] Seven patients were treated without surgery, and all died. Five of nine patients treated surgically survived, but these appear to have been patients who were beginning to achieve remission at the time of the surgical procedure. In a more recent report, five leukemic children with appendicitis all survived appendectomy. Typhlitis is seen most frequently in children with acute leukemia

---

Table 10-9
Conditions Producing Acute Abdominal Signs and Symptoms in Immunosuppressed or Neutropenic Children on Antineoplastic Therapy

- Small-intestinal intussusception, primarily ileoileal, usually without intramural intestinal tumor involvement but may be led by tumor nodule
- Intestinal-wall tumor lysis with necrosis, perforation, or hemorrhage (common in NHL)
- Typhlitis, enterocolitis (nonspecific), leukemic cecal infiltration
- Aspergillosis or mucormycosis infections
- Lower-lobe pneumonia
- Hepatic or splenic abscesses; subdiaphragmatic, subhepatic, or pelvic septic collections; portal vein thrombosis
- Splenic infarcts
- Hemoperitoneum or retroperitoneal hematoma secondary to coagulation defects or tumor rupture
- Primary peritonitis
- Diseases common to children without neoplasms; *i.e.,* acute appendicitis, abdominal manifestations of viremias, *etc.*

and consists of inflammation of the bowel wall, usually with well-demarcated ulcers, which are filled with organisms but a relative lack of inflammatory cells. More than 70% of such patients have septicemia, 35% involving multiple organisms. The most common of these are forms of *Klebsiella* and *Pseudomonas,* with *Candida* and *Clostridium* also seen.

The differential diagnosis of abdominal disease in patients in this category is uniquely difficult. There may be an astonishing lack of a inflammatory response, and peritonitis may exist without significant muscular guarding or rebound tenderness. Abdominal pain and diminished or absent peristaltic sounds are usual features. If the patient is receiving steroid therapy, fever associated with infection may be absent. Roentgenograms may reveal evidence of paralytic ileus and, if typhlitis is present, a lack of gas in the right lower quadrant and minimal distention of the terminal ileum. Thickening of the bowel wall may be recognized, and contrast studies of the colon may reveal mucosal irregularities, rigidity, and a loss of haustral markings in the region of the cecum.

The initial therapy of a patient with the differential diagnostic problem outlined above consists of nasogastric suction, analgesics, intravenous fluids, and parenteral broad-spectrum antibiotics. Generalizations are difficult, but it would appear that a carefully selected group of these patients will benefit from surgical intervention to determine the source of the abdominal symptoms.

In addition to appendicitis, typhlitis, and intussusception, a number of conditions may be recognized first in the setting of the apparent acute abdomen. Abscesses of the liver and spleen can ordinarily be recognized by CT or ultrasound and are primarily sites of *Candida* infection. These collections are ordinarily treated conservatively, although antibiotics may be introduced into the cavities.

Hemoperitoneum occurs in patients with serious coagulation defects, most frequently in patients with severe thrombocytopenia. It may originate in tears of the spleen or rupture of necrotic masses in the intestinal wall. Nonsurgical causes of a simulated acute abdominal condition include lower-lobe pneumonias irritating the diaphragmatic surfaces and the effects of the vinca alkaloids on intestinal function.

Central Nervous System Complications

Perforation of a tumor into the epidural space or through the dura is an additional indication for emergency surgery. In most pediatric patients, however, this occurs in sites such as the base of the skull in rhabdomyosarcoma that make urgent removal of the tumor almost impossible. Spinal cord compression producing paraplegia or paraparesis is an indication for emergency surgery under most circumstances, in patients of any age (see also Chap. 37).[113] Viability of the distal cord cells may still be dependent on relief of pressure within hours once a level of transsection has developed.

Infection

The major role infection plays as the cause of death in patients with leukemia is described in other chapters. Among children with solid tumors, it is also the principal cause of death. The several reasons for the increased susceptibility of the cancer patient to infection and the prophylactic measures designed to decrease the impact of these factors are discussed in Chapter 39. Surgical aspects of this problem include both infections following operative procedures or following complications associated with surgery and surgical procedures indicated in the management of infections.

Wound Infection

In operative procedures for cancer, the use of prophylactic antibiotic regimens is standard for all procedures that involve opening the obstructed intestinal or urinary tract and is frequent in other situations in which wide areas of tissue are exposed for long periods. Wound infections are more prevalent in patients with oncologic diseases than in those undergoing surgery for other conditions;[114] this is attributable to the extent of the dissection; the duration of exposure of dissected areas, which is frequently longer in cancer-related procedures; contamination by infected fluids; and the reduction of the patient's defense mechanisms against infection. However, procedures on patients with relatively intact mechanisms to combat infection and which are not associated with contamination, such as the staging laparotomies for clinical stages I and II Hodgkin's disease, carry extremely low rates of wound infection. Prophylactic antibiotics in such patients are not required for the procedure and may be detrimental in assessing developments in the postoperative course. Heavily contaminated wounds in patients with cancer are only partially closed at the skin level or left completely open to the depth of the fasciae.

Other Local Infections

Of particular concern among local infections are those of the perianal region, which are found in more than 10% of patients with leukemia at autopsy. These infections produce intense local pain and are accompanied by induration and mucosal ulceration. When they occur in severely neutropenic patients, they do not produce the well-localized abscesses adjacent to the rectum seen in patients with normal tissue reactions. Thus, perianal drainage of abscesses is relatively uncommon but may have to be done as recovery from neutropenia is established. The most frequent organism is *Pseudomonas aeruginosa,* and bacteremias are common (see Chaps. 37 and 39). Most of these patients are best managed without surgery, although extensive bleeding and a slough of the perirectal tissues may dictate a temporary colostomy, particularly if the patient is recovering homeostatic mechanisms and remission is anticipated.

Subdiaphragmatic, subhepatic, and pelvic abscesses can frequently be controlled by antibiotics so that their drainage, when required, ordinarily can be performed on a semielective basis. Needle draining with the introduction of antibiotics may be an alternative, or may precede open drainage.

Unique surgical problems are encountered with certain types of fungal infections, particularly aspergillosis, in patients who have received steroid therapy and long-term broad-spectrum antibacterial antibiotics.[115] These secondary infections frequently occur at the sites of prior bacterial infection and are characterized by thrombosis, infarction, and necrosis of tissue, particularly in the lung. They are treated primarily with amphotericin B and similar agents. Superficial infections may require debridement. If the patient's general condition permits, the resection of residual cavities in the lung, which cannot be effectively treated with antifungal agents, may be done.

Open Lung Biopsy

Persistent interstitial pneumonitis in an immunocompromised patient is one of the untoward developments associated with successful chemotherapy for neoplasms. The most common organism is *Pneumocystis carinii*.[116,117] Such patients have, in general, been treated with intensive broad-spectrum antibacterial antibiotics without resolution of the pneumonitis. This type of therapy may be continued or a specific diagnosis attempted. A continued symptomatic state or progression of the lesions mandates the latter approach. Bronchoscopic techniques are used in an attempt to obtain material for cultures, particularly in older patients. Techniques of needle aspiration or the use of cutting-needle biopsies have been widely used. Needle aspiration at times produces pneumothorax, but the general complication rate is low, as is the rate of identifying the specific organism: less than 30% in most series. The use of larger-bore cutting needles to obtain biopsy material has a significantly higher complication rate, including both pneumothorax and interstitial hemorrhage, and the diagnostic yield is usually no greater than 35%.

Open lung biopsy, in contrast, provides a specific diagnosis in more than 90% of patients in whom it is employed.[116,117] Actual changes in treatment, however, are confined to less than half of these patients, and a significant influence on outcome in probably obtained in less than 25%. These disappointing results have led some to question the utility of open lung biopsy in these patients, particularly as the use of prophylactic trimethoprim–sulfamethoxazole has altered the relative composition of this group of patients (see Chap. 39).[118]

Open lung biopsy is performed through a small right or left anterolateral thoracotomy, with removal of a wedge of lung tissue several centimeters in diameter that should include an area of maximum involvement. A small chest catheter is left in the thorax for several days, but complications such as pneumothorax or hemorrhage are uncommon.

COMPLICATIONS OF CHEMOTHERAPY AND IRRADIATION REQUIRING SURGERY

Chemotherapy Effects

When peripheral veins are used to administer cancer chemotherapeutic agents, infiltration may result in inflammation and necrosis of skin and subcutaneous tissue. The immediate measures to be taken in this situation are discussed in Chapters 37 and 46. When necrosis results, it is frequently in sites overlying tendons, where prolonged infection is most undesirable. If the patient's condition permits, early repeated debridement, followed if necessary by early skin grafting, is indicated. When the patient is on intensive chemotherapy regimens, however, early removal of necrotic tissue by a combination of mechanical and enzymatic debridement is standard management, with grafting deferred.

Ischemia of the cecum or the ascending colon, which may progress to infarction and perforation and is probably the end-stage of typhlitis, constitutes a unique complication of intensive chemotherapy for neoplasms or polycythemia (see Chap. 39). It is usually associated with neutropenia. This phenomenon has been linked with specific agents, notably methotrexate. Its localization to this segment of the colon is unexplained. Emergency resection of the cecum or right colectomy is the ideal management, but because of the precarious status of many of these patients, simple drainage or diversion may be the compromise procedure selected.

Hemorrhagic cystitis may be a chronic or acute problem after chemotherapy (particularly with cyclophosphamide), occurring with increased frequency if the bladder has been irradiated (see Chaps. 9 and 11). Prophylaxis is discussed in Chapter 37. When prolonged and severe, this form of cystitis may require urinary diversion. Sclerotics have been introduced into the bladder, which makes the probability of retaining a normally functional bladder at the conclusion of therapy unlikely. Cystectomy has been performed in some cases, either early in the course for acute bleeding, or later for malfunction

of the bladder resulting from inflammatory changes and scarring of the bladder wall.

Acute or chronic pancreatitis is associated with therapy that includes the enzyme L-asparaginase (see Chap. 9). The initial management of this condition is similar to that used in idiopathic or obstructive pancreatitis, with an attempt to minimize the stimulatory effect of gastrointestinal function and content with gastrointestinal suction and appropriate medications. Chronic forms of this disease occur, including the development of pancreatic pseudocysts, which may ultimately require surgical excision or drainage.

Pericarditis has been associated with the administration of Adriamycin, dactinomycin, and other agents, frequently combined with irradiation of the pericardium. The irradiation effect is dose related. Ultimately, pericardectomy has been required in a few patients.

Complications of Irradiation

The most common of these conditions seen in pediatric patients is irradiation enteritis; less frequent is colitis.[119] Irradiation enteritis is frequently observed when a segment of intestine in the irradiated field is fixed by adhesions, the result of prior surgery. As abdominal irradiation frequently follows a major surgical procedure, this combination of an intestinal (usually small bowel) loop attached in the area of prior surgery is common. In an abdomen without adhesions, the general mobility of the intestine appears to protect individual segments from extensive damage. Irradiation enteritis has an acute phase associated with abdominal pain and transient ileus. It is more commonly recognized as a form of chronic low-grade intestinal obstruction or malabsorption developing months after the end of irradiation.[120] Although there may be initial changes in the mucosa, the residual disease is largely intramural, consisting of extensive fibrosis and obstruction of lymphatics. The gross appearance of such intestinal segments is strikingly similar to that seen in Crohn's disease. Irradiation colitis is much more common in adults, particularly those with gynecological tumors, than in children.

A similar histologic picture is seen in the distal esophagus, usually in patients treated with both intensive chemotherapy and irradiation. Here, a superimposed acute or subacute infection, which is commonly fungal, may exacerbate the inflammatory process in the esophageal wall, ultimately resulting in obstruction.

The operative correction of these irradiation-induced conditions is usually conservative in scope until a remission is well established and the patient's homeostatic status is relatively normal. When this stage is reached, if the intestinal segment involved is limited and obstruction per se is a problem, intestinal resection is useful. To avoid the development of intestinal fistulas, the surgical dictum requires that the anastomosis associated with such resections for irradiation effects be between two "normal" segments of intestine, at times an unattainable goal.[121] Bypass procedures are also employed. If the involved segments are longer and the obstruction is tolerable, resection may simply increase the malabsorptive aspects of the course. Severe strictures of the distal esophagus in their acute or subacute phases are treated by gastrostomy or forms of nutritional support with gastric suction. After an established remission and return to a relatively normal hematologic and nutritional status, resection or bypass of the stenotic esophageal segments can be considered. This can be accomplished with an isolated segment of intestine or by upward mobilization of a gastric "tube." Acute perforations of the esophagus are ordinarily managed by nonoperative techniques in this situation, but if the patient's general condition permits, temporary cervical esophagostomy or early replacement of the esophagus may be considered.

MULTI-INSTITUTIONAL TRIALS AND THE SURGEON

The incidence of many childhood solid tumors is so low that institutional studies evaluating treatment programs, including surgery, are impossible. Because of their striking response to therapy, however, studies of some of these tumors that are of particular interest to surgeons indicate new channels of clinical research activity and are of far greater significance than their numbers suggest. In the analysis of regimens designed for these relatively uncommon solid tumors, cooperative group studies always have the inherent advantage of numbers.

Several of the more common solid tumors (nephroblastoma, neuroblastoma stage I–II), when locally resected and treated by relatively simple chemotherapy regimens, have very low relapse rates. In studies of these tumors, large groups of patients are required to demonstrate any significant differences in outcome. This would also be true in the case of comparative trials of almost all of the new modalities of therapy such as temperature alterations with surgery and laser surgery. Thus, here also, multi-institutional trials are essential.

Some solid tumors of childhood are almost routinely disseminated at the time of diagnosis but are responsive to multimodality regimens, including chemotherapy for the control of disseminated disease followed by radiotherapy and surgery for the evaluation of therapy and the elimination of residual tumor. These tumors may be sensitive to alterations in chemotherapy regimens, and frequent evaluation of the effects of therapy is a significant factor in management. The successful use of a protocols of this type requires cooperation and compliance by institutional surgeons. Evaluation of these studies and the associated surgical procedures would be impossible without the numbers of patients available in cooperative groups.

A significant aspect of cooperative trials is the review by a central pathology committee or an individual pathologist of all of the tissue sections obtained. This may include all of the surgical and autopsy specimens among the rarer solid tumors of childhood and has provided a concentration of pathologic material on these tumors that has not been available previously. In contrast to the excellent prior collections of material on unusual tumors, such as those of the Armed Forces Institute of Pathology, these studies include the tumor specimens from a group of patients treated currently and usually by the same regimens. The impact of these pathology reviews on surgical practice in pediatric oncology has been immense.

REFERENCES

1. Voute PA, Vos A, de Kraker J: Chemotherapy as initial treatment in rhabdomyosarcoma (abstr). Proc Am Soc Clin Oncol 3:87, 1984
2. Flamant F, Rodary C, Voute PA et al: Primary chemotherapy in the treatment of rhabdomyosarcoma in children: Trial of the International Society of Pediatric Oncology (SIOP) preliminary results. Radiother Oncol 3:227–236, 1985
3. Fleming ID, Etcubanas E, Patterson R et al: The role of surgical resection when combined with chemotherapy and radiation in the management of pelvic rhabdomyosarcoma. Ann Surg 199:509–514, 1984
4. Ghavimi F, Herr H, Jereb B et al: Treatment of genitourinary rhabdomyosarcoma in children. J Urol 132:313–319, 1984
5. Knutrud O: The water and electrolyte metabolism of the newborn child after major surgery. Oslo, Norwegian Monographs on Medical Science, 1965
6. Rickham PR: The Metabolic Response to Neonatal Surgery. Cambridge, MA, Harvard University Press, 1957
7. Benner JW, Coran AG, Weintraub WH et al: The importance of different calorie sources in the intravenous nutrition of infants and children. Surgery 86:429–433, 1979
8. Holzgreve W, Mahony BS, Glick PL et al: Sonographic demonstration of fetal sacrococcygeal teratoma. Prenatal Diagn 5:245–57, 1985
9. Flake AW, Harrison M, Adzick NS et al: Fetal sacrococcygeal teratoma. J Pediatr Surg 21:563–566, 1986
10. Hrabovsky EE, Otherson BH, deLorimier A Jr et al: Wilms' tumor in the neonate: A report from the National Wilms' Tumor Study. J Pediatr Surg 21:385–387, 1986
11. Fraumeni F Jr, Miller RW: Cancer deaths in the newborn. Am J Dis Child 117:186–189, 1969
12. Bader JL, Miller RW: US cancer incidence and mortality in the first year of life. Am J Dis Child 133:157–159, 1979
13. Gale GB, D'Angio GJ, Uri A et al: Cancer in neonates: The experience at the Children's Hospital of Philadelphia. Pediatrics 70:409–413, 1982
14. Hays DM, Mirabal VQ, Karlan MS et al: Fibrosarcomas in infants and children. J Pediatr Surg 5:176–183, 1970
15. Scopes JE, Ahmed I: Minimal rates of oxygen consumption in sick and premature newborn infants. Arch Dis Childh 41:407, 1966
16. Peckham GJ, Fox WW: Physiologic factors affecting pulmonary artery pressure in infants with persistent pulmonary hypertension. J Pediatr 93:1005, 1978
17. Shieoka AO, Santos JI, Hill HR: Functional analysis of neutrophil granulocytes from healthy, infected and stressed neonates. J Pediatr 95:454, 1979
18. Siegel SE, Moran RG: Problems in the chemotherapy of cancer in the neonate. Am J Pediatr Hematol Oncol 3:287–296, 1981
19. Mollith DL: Age dependent variation in lymphocyte function in the post-operative child. J Pediatr Surg 21:633–635, 1986
20. Stephenson SR, Cook BA, Mease AD et al: The prognostic significance of age and pattern of metastases in stage IV-S neuroblastoma. Cancer 58:372–375, 1986
21. Glaubiger DL, Von Huff DD, Holcenberg JS et al: The relative tolerance of children and adults to anti-cancer drugs. Front Radiat Ther Oncol 16:42–49, 1982
22. Donaldson SS, Wesley MN, DeWys WD et al: A study of the nutritional status of pediatric cancer patients. Am J Dis Child 135:1107–1112, 1981
23. Ghavini F, Shils ME, Scott RN et al: Comparison of morbidity in children requiring abdominal radiation and chemotherapy with and without total parenteral nutrition. J Pediatr 101:530–537, 1982
24. Van Eys J: Nutrition and cancer: Physiological interrelationships. Annu Rev Nutr 5:435–461, 1985
25. Ramirez I, Van Eys J, Carr D et al: Malnutrition in children with malignancies (abstract). Proc Am Assoc Cancer Res 21:378, 1980
26. Rickard KA, Loghmani ES, Grosfeld JL et al: Short- and long-term effectiveness of enteral and parenteral nutrition in reversing or preventing protein–energy malnutrition in advanced neuroblastoma: A prospective randomized study. Cancer 56:2881–2897, 1985
27. Rickard KA, Detamore CM, Coates TD et al: Effect of nutrition staging on treatment delays and outcome in stage IV neuroblastoma. Cancer 52:587–598, 1983
28. Britt BA: Etiology and pathophysiology of malignant hyperthermia. Fed Proc 38:44, 1979
29. Kalow W, Benst K: A method for the detection of atypical forms of human serum cholinesterase. Can J Biochem Phys 35:339, 1957
30. Cook DR, Fisher BH: Neuromuscular blocking effects of succinylcholine in infants and children. Anesthesiology 42:662, 1975
31. Quissel B, Mohammad A, Bauer JH et al: Malignant pheochromocytoma in childhood: Report of a case with familial neurofibromatosis. Med Pediatr Oncol 7:327–333, 1979
32. Marshall DG: Two boys with four pheochromocytomas each. J Pediatr Surg 21:815–817, 1986
33. Bloom DA, Fonkalsrud EW: Surgical management of pheochromocytoma in children. J Pediatr Surg 9:179–184, 1974
34. Scott HW Jr, Dean RH, Oates JA et al: Surgical management of pheochromocytoma. Am Surgeon 47:8–13, 1981
35. Heikkinen ES, Akerblom HK: Diagnostic and operative problems in multiple pheochromocytomas. J Pediatr Surg 12:157–163, 1977
36. Schaller RT Jr, Schaller J, Furman EB: The advantages of hemodilution anesthesia for major liver resection in children. J Pediatr Surg 19:705–710, 1984
37. Thompson GF, Miller RD, Stevens WC et al: Hypotensive anesthesia for total hip arthroplasty: A study of blood loss and organ function (brain, heart, liver and kidney). Anesthesiology 48:91, 1978
38. Lindop MJ: Complications and morbidity of controlled hypotension. Br J Anaesth 47:799, 1975
39. Mitchenfelder JD, Uihlein A, Daw EF: Moderate hypothermia in man, haemodynamic and metabolic effects. Br J Anaesth 37:738, 1965

40. Gauthier F, Valayer J, Thai BL et al: Hepatoblastoma and hepatocarcinoma in children: Analysis of a series of 29 cases. J Pediatr Surg 21:424–429, 1986

41. Horton JA, Hrabovsky E, Klingberg WG et al: Therapeutic embolization of a hyperfunctioning pheochromocytoma. AJR 140:987–988, 1983

42. Beckwith JB, Palmer NF: Histopathology and prognosis of Wilms' tumor: Results of the first National Wilms' Tumor Study. Cancer 41:1937–1948, 1978

43. Evans AE, D'Angio GJ, Randolph JG: A proposed staging for children with neuroblastoma. Cancer 27:374, 1971

44. Maurer HM (For the IRS Committee): The Intergroup Rhabdomyosarcoma Study (NIH): Objectives and clinical staging classification. J Pediatr Surg 10:977–978, 1975

45. Protocol of the Intergroup Rhabdomyosarcoma Study, 1972

46. Shimada H, Chatten J, Newton WA Jr: Histopathologic prognostic factors in neuroblastic tumors: Defintion of subtypes of ganglioneuroblastoma and an age-linked classification of neuroblastoma. JNCI 73:405–416, 1984

47. Shimada H, Aoyama C, Chiba T: Prognostic subgroups for undifferentiated neuroblastoma. Hum Pathol 16:471–476, 1985

48. Palmer N, Sachs N, Foulkes M: Histopathology and prognosis in rhabdomyosarcoma (IRS-1) (abstr). Proc Am Soc Clin Oncol 1:170, 1982

49. Tsokos M, Miser A, Wesley R et al: Solid variant alveolar rhabdomyosarcoma: A primitive rhabdomyosarcoma with poor prognosis and distinct histology. SIOP Abstracts, pp 71–74, 1985

50. Donaldson S, Belli JA: A rational clinical staging system for childhood rhabdomyosarcoma. Clin Oncol 2:135–139, 1984

51. LeTourneau JN, Bernard JL, Hendren WH et al: Evaluation of the role of surgery in 130 patients with neuroblastoma. J Pediatr Surg 20:244–249, 1985

52. Hays DM, Ternberg JL, Chen TT: Postsplenectomy sepsis and other complications following staging laparotomy for Hodgkin's disease in childhood. J Pediatr Surg 21:628–632, 1986

53. Boles ET Jr, Hasse GM, Hamoudi AB: Partial splenectomy in staging laparotomy for Hodgkin's disease. J Pediatr Surg 13:581–585, 1978

54. Dresser RK, Golomb HM, Ultman JE et al: Prognostic classification of Hodgkin's disease: Risk of false negative results. N Engl J Med 299:345–346, 1978

55. Hays DM: Operative staging of Hodgkin's disease and non-Hodgkin's lymphoma. In Rob C. Smith R (eds): Operative Surgery, pp 220–224 London, Butterworths, 1978

56. Sullivan MP, Fuller LM, Chen T et al: Intergroup Hodgkin's disease in children, study of stages I and II: A preliminary report. Cancer Treat Rep 66:937–947, 1982

57. Coker DD, Morris DM, Coleman JJ et al: Restaging laparotomy for Hodgkin's disease. Am Surgeon 197:79–83, 1983

58. Chabner BA, Johnson RE, Young RC et al: Sequential nonsurgical and surgical staging of non-Hodgkin's lymphoma. Ann Intern Med 85:149–154, 1976

59. Goffinet DR, Warnke R, Dunnick NR et al: Clinical and surgical (laparotomy) evaluation of patients with non-Hodgkin's lymphomas. Cancer Treat Rep 61:981–991, 1977

60. Coupland GAE, Townend MB, Martin CJ: Peritoneoscopy: Use in assessment of intra-abdominal malignancy. Surgery 89:645–649, 1981

61. DeVita VT, Bagley CM, Goodell B et al: Peritoneoscopy in the staging of Hodgkin's disease. Cancer Res 31:1746–1750, 1971

62. Taylor SR, Nunez C: Fine-needle aspiration biopsy in a pediatric population: Report of 64 consecutive cases. Cancer 54:1449–1453, 1984

63. Schaller RT Jr, Schaller JF, Buschmann C et al: The usefulness of percutaneous fine-needle aspiration biopsy in infants and children. J Pediatr Surg 18:398–405, 1983

64. Silberman AW: Surgical debulking of tumors. Surg Gynecol Obstet 155:577–585, 1982

65. Koop CE, Johnson DG: Neuroblastoma: Assessment of therapy in reference to staging. J Pediatr Surg 6:595, 1971

66. Maurer HM, Donaldson M, Gehen EA et al (For the IRS Committee): The Intergroup Rhabdomyosarcoma Study: Update November 1978. Natl Cancer Inst Monogr 56:61–68, 1981

67. Exelby P: Malignant lymphomas in children. World J Surg 4:49–62, 1980

68. Wollner N, Wachtel AE, Exelby PR et al: Improved prognosis in children with intraabdominal non-Hodgkin's lymphoma following LSA₂-L₂ protocol chemotherapy. Cancer 45:3034–3039, 1980

69. Olive D, Flamant F, Zucker JM: Paraaortic lymphadenectomy is not necessary in the treatment of localized paratesticular rhabdomyosarcoma. Cancer 54:1283–1287, 1984

70. Raney RB, Hays DM, Lawrence W et al: Paratesticular rhabdomyosarcoma in childhood. Cancer 42:729–736, 1978

71. Hays DM, Crist W, Shimada H et al: Sarcomas of the vagina and uterus: The Intergroup Rhabdomyosarcoma Study (IRS). J Pediatr Surg 20:718–724, 1985

72. Raney B, Hays D, Maurer H et al: Primary chemotherapy ± radiation therapy (RT) and/or surgery for children with localized sarcoma of the prostate, bladder, or vagina: Preliminary results of the Intergroup Rhabdomyosarcoma Study (IRS-II) (abstr). International Soc Pediatr Oncol, p 93, 1985

73. Hays DM, Raney RB Jr, Lawrence W et al: Bladder and prostatic tumors in the Intergroup Rhabdomyosarcoma Study (IRS I): Results of therapy. Cancer 50:1472–1482, 1982

74. Sarre RG, Jangelman DG, McGannon E et al: Colectomy with iliorectal anastomosis for familial adenomatous polyps: The risk of rectal cancer. Surgery 101:21–26, 1987

75. Stryker SJ, Telander RL, Perrault J: Anorectal evaluation after colectomy and endorectal ileoanal anastomosis in children and young adults. J Pediatr Surg 20:656–660, 1985

76. Giuliano AE, Eilber FR: The rationale for planned reoperation after unplanned total excision of soft-tissue sarcomas. J Clin Oncol 3:1344–1348, 1985

77. Flamont F, Nihoul-Fekete C, Patte C et al: Optimal treatment of stage I yolk sac tumor of the testes in children. J Pediatr Surg 21:108–111, 1986

78. Gilbertson VA, Wangensteen OH: A summary of thirteen years with the second look program. Surg Gynecol Obstet 114:438, 1964

79. Rosen EM, Cassady JR, Frantz CN et al: Improved survival in neuroblastoma using multimodality therapy. Radiother Oncol 2:189–200, 1984

80. Billmire DF, Grosfeld JL: Teratomas in childhood: Analysis of 142 cases. J Pediatr Surg 21:548–551, 1986

81. Crist W, Raney B, Ragab A et al (for the IRS Committee): Intensive chemotherapy including cis-platin with or without etoposide for children with soft tissue sarcomas. Med Pediatr Oncol 15:51–57, 1987

82. Etcubanas E, Kun L, Pratt C et al: Patterns of failure in the treatment of childhood rhabdomyosarcoma: A review of prospective studies at St. Jude Hospital. SIOP Abstracts, pp 95–97, 1985

83. Tucker OP, McGill CW, Pokorny WJ et al: Bilateral Wilms' tumor. J Pediatr Surg 21:1110–1113, 1986

84. Gaiger AM, Soule EH, Newton WA Jr (for the IRS Committee): Pathology of rhabdomyosarcoma: Experience of the Intergroup Rhabdomyosarcoma Study, 1972–1978. Natl Cancer Inst Monogr 56:19–27, 1981

85. Grosfeld JL, West KW, Weber TR: Second look laparotomy for Wilms' tumor: Indications and results in 19 patients. J Pediatr Surg 20:145–149, 1985

86. Patrick RM, Thomas MT, Farewell VT et al: Abdominal relapses in irradiated second National Wilms' Tumor Study patients. J Clin Oncol 2:1098–1101, 1984

87. Burgers JMV, Tournade MF, Bey P et al: Abdominal recurrences in Wilms' tumours: A report from the SIOP Wilms' tumour trials and studies. Radiother Oncol 5:175–182, 1986

88. Raney RB, Crist WM, Maurer HM et al (for the IRS Committee): Prognosis of children with soft tissue sarcoma who relapse after achieving a complete response: A report from the Intergroup Rhabdomyosarcoma Study. Cancer 52:44–50, 1983

89. Lack EE, Travis WD, Welch KJ: Retroperitoneal germ cell tumors in childhood. Cancer 56:602–608, 1985

90. Breslow NE, Churchill G, Nesmith B et al: Clinicopathologic features and prognosis for Wilms' tumor patients with metastases at diagnosis. Cancer 58:2501–2511, 1986

91. Telander RL, Pairolero PC, Pritchard DJ et al: Resection of pulmonary metastatic osteogenic sarcoma in children. Surgery 84:335–341, 1978

92. Rosen EM, Cassady JR, Frantz CN et al: Stage IV-N: A favorable subset of children with metastatic neuroblastoma. Med Pediatr Oncol 13:194–198, 1985

93. Vaughn CB, Chapman J, Zaks J et al: Hepatic arterial and systemic chemotherapy for the treatment of primary and secondary malignancies of the liver. Cancer Drug Deliv 2:119–125, 1985

94. Golladay ES, Mollitt DL, Osteen PK et al: Conversion to resectability by intraarterial infusion chemotherapy after failure of systemic chemotherapy. J Pediatr Surg 20:715–717, 1985

95. Sheldon CA, Elick B, Najarian JS et al: Improving survival in the very young renal transplant recipient. J Pediatr Surg 20:622–626, 1985

96. Starzl TE, Iwatsuki S, Shaw BW Jr et al: Treatment of fibrolamellar hepatoma with partial or total hepatectomy and transplantation of the liver. Surg Gynecol Obstet 162:145–148, 1978

97. Abe M, Fukada M, Yamono K: Intraoperative irradiation in abdominal and cerebral tumors. Acta Radiol 10:408–416, 1971

98. Gunderson L, Tepper J, Biggs P et al: Intraoperative plus or minus external beam irradiation. Curr Probl Cancer Treat 7:1–69, 1983

99. Newman BM, Jewett TC, Karp MP et al: Percutaneous central venous catheterization in children: First line choice for venous access. J Pediatr Surg 21:685–688, 1986

100. Weber TR, West KW, Grosfeld JL: Broviac central venous catheterization in infants and children. Am J Surg 145:202–204, 1983

101. McGovern B, Solenberger R, Reed K et al: A totally implantable venous access system for long-term chemotherapy in children. J Pediatr Surg 20:725–727, 1985

102. Golladay ES, Mollitt DL: Percutaneous placement of a venous access port in a pediatric patient population. J Pediatr Surg 21:683–684, 1986

103. Andrassy RJ, Page CP, Feldtman RW et al: Continual catheter administration of an elemental diet in infants and children. Surgery 82:205–210, 1977

104. Gauderer MWL, Ponsky LJ, Izant RJ: Gastrostomy without laparotomy: A percutaneous endoscopic technique. J Pediatr Surg 15:872–875, 1980

105. Strodel WE, Lemmer JL, Eckhauser F et al: Early experience with endoscopic percutaneous gastrostomy. Arch Surg 118:449–453, 1983

106. Andrassy RJ: Surgical techniques for nutritional support of the pediatric oncology patient. In Hays DM (ed): Pediatric Surgical Oncology, pp 269–286. Orlando, Grune & Stratton, 1986

107. Azizkhan RG, Shaw A, Chandler JG: Surgical complications of neuroblastoma resection. Surgery 97:514–517, 1985

108. Hays, DM: Intussusception as a postoperative complication in pediatric surgery. Surg Gynecol Obstet 112:583–589, 1961

109. Dudgeon DL, Hays DM: Intussusception complicating the treatment of malignancy in childhood. Arch Surg 105:52–56, 1972

110. Ein SH, Stephens CA, Shandling B et al: Intussusception due to lymphoma. J Pediatr Surg 21:786–788, 1986

111. Meyers PA, Potter VP, Wollner N et al: Bowel perforation during initial treatment for childhood non-Hodgkin's lymphoma. Cancer 56:259–261, 1985

112. Exelby PR, Ghandchi A, Lansigan N et al: Mangement of the acute abdomen in children with leukemia. Cancer 35:826–829, 1975

113. Massad M, Haddad F, Slim M et al: Spinal cord compression in neuroblastoma. Surg Neurol 23:657–572, 1985

114. Sharma LK, Sharma PK: Postoperative wound infection in a pediatric surgical service. J Pediatr Surg 21:889–891, 1986

115. Shamberger RC, Weinstein HJ, Grier HE et al: The surgical management of fungal pulmonary infections in children with acute myelogenous leukemia. J Pediatr Surg 20:840–844, 1985

116. Hiatt JR, Gong H, Mulder DG et al: The value of open lung biopsy in the immunosuppressed patient. Surgery 92:285–291, 1982

117. Imoke E, Dudgeon DL, Colombani P et al: Open lung biopsy in the immunocompromised pediatric patient. J Pediatr Surg 18:816–821, 1983

118. Doolin EJ, Luck SR, Sherman JO et al: Emergency lung biopsy: Friend or foe of the immunosuppressed child? J Pediatr Surg 21:485–487, 1986

119. Donaldson SS, Jundt S, Ricour C et al: Radiation enteritis in children. Cancer 35:1167–1178, 1985

120. Beer WH, Fan A, Halsted CH: Clinical and nutritional implications of radiation enteritis. Am J Clin Nutr 41:85–91, 1985

121. Marks G, Mohiudden M: The surgical management of the radiation-injured intestine. Surg Clin North Am 63:81–96, 1983

eleven

General Principles of Radiation Therapy

Laurence E. Kun and John E. Moulder

The use of radiation to treat cancer was first reported within a year of Röntgen's discovery of x-rays in 1895. Initial "caustic" applications of this new physical modality evolved over two to three decades to fractionated, protracted courses of irradiation capable of achieving a differential effect on tumor cells biologically while relatively sparing adjacent normal structures.[1,2] Improvements in available sources of radiations together with knowledge of the interactions of radiations and matter provided a physical basis for concentrating the radiation dose in the identified target volume, again limiting the effects in the intervening tissues. Current investigations of the time–dose relationship, radiation sensitizers and protectors, and interactions with tumor immunology and basic cellular biology reflect the increasing application of laboratory radiation biology to understanding of the potential applications of radiation therapy.

Radiation therapy in pediatric malignant diseases requires detailed attention to physical and biological principles to maximize efficacy in a setting of heightened concern regarding potential late toxicities. The central role of this modality in the curative management of most types of childhood cancer demands an understanding of its language, scientific basis, and clinical practice in the context of multidisciplinary pediatric oncology.

THE BIOLOGICAL BASIS OF RADIOTHERAPY

The goal of therapeutic irradiation is to achieve a favorable *therapeutic ratio* by causing the death of all tumor cells that are capable of indefinite division without producing unacceptable damage to adjacent normal tissues. This favorable therapeutic ratio is not based on an inherent difference between the radiosensitivity of tumor cells and normal cells; rather, it is based on differences between the tissue kinetics of tumors and normal tissues.

Interaction of Radiation with Biological Material

The cell killing effects of radiation (as well as the mutagenic and carcinogenic effects of radiation) are a result of DNA damage. DNA may be affected directly, but more frequently the DNA damage is an indirect effect mediated through free radicals produced by radiation ionization of water. Because radiation damage is an indirect chemical event, the chemical state of the cell at the time of irradiation is an important determinant of how much DNA damage is produced. The presence of compounds that increase the reactivity or lifespan of free radicals (*e.g.,* molecular oxygen and certain nitroimidazoles) sensitizes cells to radiation, whereas the presence of compounds that scavenge free radicals (*e.g.,* sulfhydryls) protects cells from radiation damage.[3]

Radiosensitivity of Mammalian Cells

Radiation-induced cell death rarely occurs immediately (Fig. 11-1). Cell death results from the inability of the damaged cells to reproduce indefinitely; cell death becomes apparent only after subsequent cellular division(s).[4,5] This reproductive death of cells has important consequences for radiotherapy. First, it means that cells that divide regularly (*e.g.,* bone-marrow stem cells, intestinal crypt cells, basal cells of the epidermis) are very radiosensitive; that is, they show a rapid decrease in numbers following irradiation. In contrast, cells that do not divide (*e.g.,* mature muscle and nerve cells) are radioresistant, showing little or no decrease in numbers following irradiation. Second, it means that slowly dividing cells (*e.g.,* endothelial cells) will be slow to show radiation effects. These two facts explain why the radiation tolerance of certain tissues is relatively low (*e.g.,* bone marrow, growing bone, gastrointestinal tract) whereas the tolerance of other tissues is relatively high (*e.g.,* mature bone, brain) and why rapidly proliferating tissues (bone marrow, oral mucosa, skin) respond to irradiation within days or weeks whereas tissues with slow cell turnover (*e.g.,* kidney, spinal cord, lung) show responses months to years after irradiation.

After irradiation of a population of mammalian cells, there is a decrease in the proportion of cells capable of continued replication (Fig. 11-2). The cell survival (S) is generally represented by either a linear quadratic equation of the form

$$S = e^{-(\alpha D + \beta D^2)}$$

FIGURE 11-1. Pedigree of a mouse L cell after irradiation with 2.16 Gy of x-rays. Pyknotic (degenerating) cells (X) are common 40 to 150 hours after irradiation, and some nondividing cells (■) are produced; an abnormal multi-polar division is seen at 45 hours. Nevertheless, 190 hours after irradiation, three daughter cells remain that appear to be clonogenic (□). (Adapted from Thompson LH, Suit HD: Int J Radiat Biol 15:347–362, 1969)

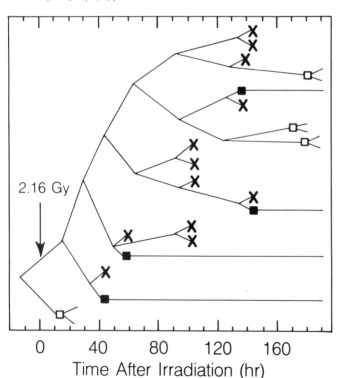

where D is the dose and α and β are fitting parameters, or by the target theory formula

$$S = 1 - (1 - e^{-D/D_0})^n$$

where n is the number of targets and D_0 is the mean dose required to inactivate a target. The two formulas are difficult to distinguish in practice (Fig. 11-2). They differ theoretically in that the target theory equation presumes a model for cell inactivation whereas the linear quadratic does not.

Typically, the dose–response curve for radiation cell killing has a shoulder region that reflects the ability of irradiated cells to accumulate and repair sublethal damage after small doses of irradiation (Fig. 11-2). Increasing doses beyond the shoulder region result in exponential cell death. The rate of exponential cell destruction is a measure of the true radiosensitivity of the irradiated cell population and varies relatively little for most cell lines. Somewhat greater fluctuations have been noted in the shoulder region (either n or α, depending on the model used), suggesting that some of the variability in response to irradiation may depend on factors that affect this portion of the survival curve.[6,7]

Sublethal radiation damage is repaired with a half-life of 1 to 2 hours, so that radiation doses separated by even a few hours have less effect than a large dose given all at once. In addition, because repair of radiation damage can occur even during irradiation, low-dose-rate irradiation (where a dose is spread over hours or days, as in brachytherapy) is less effective at killing cells than is high-dose-rate irradiation. Despite the lower cell killing efficacy of low-dose rate irradiation, there is evidence of a differential response of tumors and normal tissues to low-dose-rate irradiation, such that lowering the dose rate appears to enhance the therapeutic ratio.[8]

Radiosensitivity and the Cell Cycle

Cellular radiation sensitivity differs with the position in the cell cycle.[9] The variation is relatively independent of cell line, with the sensitivity greatest for cells in mitosis (M) and early in the DNA synthesis (S) phase and least for cells late in S phase and early in the gap between DNA synthesis and mitosis (G_2). Normally proliferating cells are randomly distributed in the cell cycle (also see Chap. 3). Irradiation will preferentially kill the cells in the sensitive phases of the cycle, so that the surviving cells will be concentrated in the less-sensitive phases of the cycle, resulting in partial replicative synchronization. This synchronization would affect the response of the cell population to subsequent treatments with radiation or cell-cycle-specific drugs if the surviving cells progress in unison through subsequent sensitive and resistant phases of the cell cycle. Attempts to utilize synchrony to increase differentially the proportion of tumor cells in sensitive phases of the cycle have not proved useful clinically, in part because cells do not remain synchronized for very long *in vivo* and in part because we lack sufficient knowledge of human tumor and normal tissue kinetics.[10]

Oxygen and Radiosensitivity

One of the major factors influencing the shape of the survival curve after irradiation is the oxygen concentration. With photon irradiation (x-rays or gamma rays), the reduction of oxygen tensions below those normally present in tissue leads to a substantial reduction in cell kill both *in vivo* and *in vitro* (Fig. 11-3). The *oxygen enhancement ratio* (OER) is the radiation dose necessary to produce a given surviving fraction in the

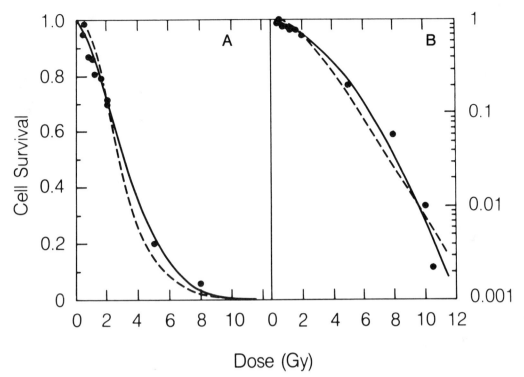

FIGURE 11-2. Radiation survival curves for Chinese hamster ovary (CHO) cells irradiated *in vitro* under fully oxygenated conditions. Data are plotted on both a linear (**A**) and a semilog (**B**) scale and are fitted with both a linear-quadratic survival curve (*solid line*), with $\alpha = 0.095$ Gy^{-1} and $\beta = 0.04$ Gy^{-2}, and with a multi-target single-hit survival curve (*dashed line*), with $n = 3.5$ and $D_0 = 1.63$ Gy. (Adapted from Palcic and Skarsgard: Radiat Res 100:328–339, 1984)

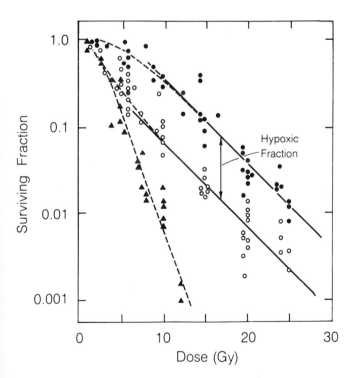

FIGURE 11-3. Radiation survival curves for EMT6 tumor cells irradiated *in vitro* under fully oxygenated (▲) and fully hypoxic conditions (●), and for cells irradiated *in vivo* in unanesthetized air-breathing mice (○). (Adapted from Moulder JE, Rockwell S: Cancer Metastasis Rev 5:313–341, 1987)

reduced oxygen (hypoxic) population divided by that required to produce the same effect in the normally oxygenated environment. The OER for most mammalian cell lines is 2.5 to 3;

that is, hypoxic tissue requires about three times the radiation dose to achieve the same degree of cell kill seen in normally oxygenated tissues.

There are numerous lines of evidence that tumors contain zones of cells that are hypoxic enough to be radioresistant but which remain viable.[11] These hypoxic areas are caused both by transient deficiencies in tumor blood flow and by chronic vascular insufficiency. When animal tumors are irradiated, the cell survival curve generally reveals a radiation-resistant subpopulation with a radiosensitivity similar to that of hypoxic cells (Fig. 11-3). In addition, the histologic pattern seen in many human tumors suggests that tumor growth is limited by oxygen diffusion, and measured tumor oxygen tensions are generally lower than those found in normal tissue.[11] The relative radioresistance and subsequent proliferation of the surviving hypoxic cells are believed to be a significant mechanism for tumor radioresistance.

Relative Biological Effectiveness

The cell killing effectiveness of radiation depends in part on the type (quality) of radiation.[12] The quality of radiation is determined by the density of ionizations along the path of the radiation photon; this density of ionization is measured by the *linear energy transfer* (LET). Radiations with high LET (*e.g.,* neutrons, pions, heavy charged particles) produce more cell killing per unit of absorbed dose than do low-LET radiations (x-rays, gamma rays, electrons) (Fig. 11-4).

The difference in the measured biological effect of different types of radiation is characterized by the parameter known as the *relative biological effectiveness* (RBE). RBE is experimentally determined as the ratio of the dose of a standard type of radiation (usually 250 kVp x-rays) to the dose of a test radiation that produces the same biological effect. RBEs range from slightly less than one (*e.g.,* 0.9 for ^{60}Co) to considerably greater than one (*e.g.,* 1.2–2.5 for neutrons). High-LET radiations produce cell survival curves with smaller shoulder regions (Fig.

11-4); as a result, the RBE depends on the radiation dose, becoming larger at small doses.

Interest in radiotherapy with high-LET radiation[13,14] is based in part on the decreased OER observed for high-LET radiations (Fig. 11-4). Radiation cell killing is less oxygen-dependent for neutron (OER of 1.5–2.5) and heavy charged particles (OER of 1.0–2.0) irradiation than for photon irradiation. To date, clinical trials with neutron therapy have not demonstrated a quantitative improvement in the response of most forms of cancer.[15]

Radiosensitization and Radioprotection

An attractive approach to improving the therapeutic ratio is to use chemicals to radiosensitize the tumor or to radioprotect the critical normal tissues.[3] Recent efforts to radiosensitize tumors have been based, for the most part, on electron-affinic drugs (*e.g.,* misonidazole and metronidazole), which preferentially radiosensitize hypoxic cells.[16,17] Clinical use of the nitroimidazole radiosensitizers has been limited by their cumulative neurotoxicity. At the doses that can be tolerated by humans, misonidazole can sensitize hypoxic cells *in vitro* by a factor of 1.2 to 1.6 and can sensitize tumors *in vivo* to single doses of radiation by a factor of 1.1 to 1.4 (Fig. 11-5). However, when misonidazole is used in fractionated radiotherapy of rodent tumors at drug doses that would be tolerated in humans, enhancement factors do not exceed 1.15 (Figs. 11-5 and 11-6). Despite the limitation on the dose of misonidazole, several trials have shown significant benefits with its use.[17] Clinical trials with more effective and less toxic agents are in progress.[3,17]

Numerous other strategies also have been employed in attempts to minimize the effects of tumor hypoxia, including transfusion of anemic patients, modifications of standard radia-

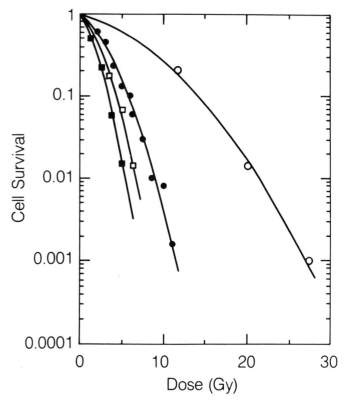

FIGURE 11-4. Radiation survival curves for R-1 rhabdomyosarcoma cells irradiated *in vitro* with 300 kV x-rays (●,○) and 15 MeV neutrons (■,□) under oxic (■,●) and hypoxic (○,□) conditions. The neutron cell survival curves show more killing per rad, smaller shoulders, and a lower OER. (Adapted from Barendsen GW, Broerse JJ: Eur J Cancer 5:373–391, 1969)

FIGURE 11-5. Misonidazole radiosensitization projected for clinical trials on the basis of *in vitro* radiosensitization of hypoxic cells (▲); *in vivo* sensitization of rodent tumors with single-dose irradiation (□); and *in vivo* sensitization of rodent tumors with fractionated irradiation (●). Misonidazole doses are in mg/ml for the *in vitro* data and in mg/g tumor concentration for the *in vivo* data. Tumor concentrations achieved in the clinical trials are shown at the top.

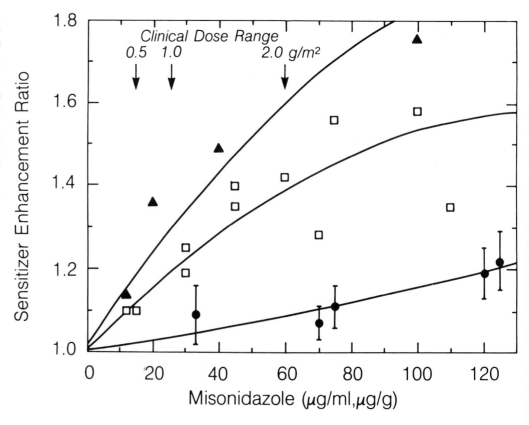

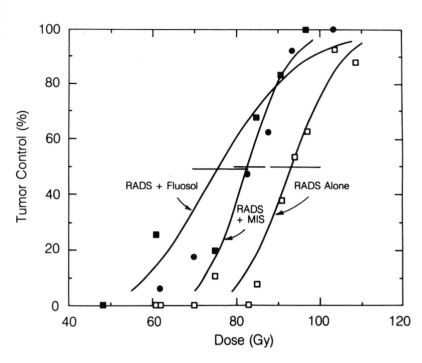

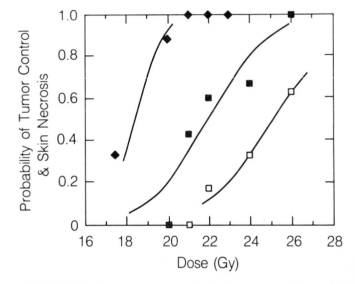

FIGURE 11-6. Tumor control dose-response curves for rat sarcomas treated with fractionated irradiation, showing the effects of treatment with misonidazole or with a perfluorochemical emulsion plus carbogen (95% O_2 plus 5% CO_2) breathing. BA1112 rhabdomyosarcomas were irradiated three times per week (Mon-Wed-Fri) for 4 to 5 weeks. Tumors were treated with radiation only (□), with 15 mg/kg Fluosol-DA 20% (IV) plus carbogen 30 minutes before and during the Monday irradiations (■), or with 400 mg/kg misonidazole 30 minutes before the Monday irradiations (●).

tion schedules, radiotherapy with hyperbaric oxygen, and irradiation with particles (neutrons, pions, heavy charged particles) that have lower OERs.[11] Several of these approaches have shown marginal clinical efficacy in large trials. A new approach to solving the problem of hypoxic cells is the use of perfluorochemical emulsions plus oxygen breathing to increase the oxygen-carrying capacity of the blood (Fig. 11-6).[18]

Efforts to protect normal tissues have been based on sulfhydryl compounds such as the cysteamine analogue WR-2721.[3] These compounds can radioprotect cells *in vitro* and a variety of tissues and tumors *in vivo*. Attempts to improve the therapeutic ratio (*i.e.,* to protect normal tissues specifically) with these agents are based on both decreased drug uptake by tumors and on decreased radioprotection under hypoxic conditions. Clinical trials of WR-2721 are in progress.[3]

Tumor Dose–Response Relationships

The dose of radiation administered to the tumor correlates with the probability of achieving local control.[19] The dose–control relationship is a sigmoid curve (Figs. 11-6 and 11-7), demonstrating significant improvement in local tumor control with small increments of dose in the midportion of the dose–response curve. The total dose required to achieve tumor control depends on the type and size of the tumor (Figs. 11-7 and 11-8) and on the fractionation schedule (Figs. 11-8 and 11-9).

Radiation Fractionation

The most important variables influencing the therapeutic ratio in clinical radiation oncology are the total dose, the number of radiation fractions (and hence the dose per fraction), and the interval between radiation fractions (and hence the overall treatment time).[20–24] The application of radiation therapy evolved rapidly to *fractionated, protracted treatment* based on early radiobiological experiments and clinical observations.[20,25] Fractionated treatment using small daily doses of radiation (1.8–2.2 Gy per day) over 5 to 7 weeks to total doses of

FIGURE 11-7. Dose-response curve for local tumor control after single dose radiotherapy of skin cancers 0.5 to 1 cm in diameter (♦) or 3 to 4 cm in diameter (■), and for skin necrosis (□). (Adapted from Trott KR et al: Radiother Oncol 2:123–129, 1984)

50 to 70 Gy produced local control of many epithelial carcinomas in adults with relative sparing of normal tissues.

The relation between the radiation fractionation schedule and the tumor control dose has been established clinically in certain neoplasms in which tumor control doses have been measured for different fractionation schedules.[19,26] Figure 11-8 illustrates the typical positive slope in the relation of the tumor control dose to overall treatment time for control of epithelial carcinomas. In contrast, the relation for some radiosensitive tumors (*e.g.,* Hodgkin's disease, lymphoma, seminoma) is relatively independent of the fractionation schedule (Fig. 11-8).

Multiple small radiation fractions separated by at least 4 hours (typically 24 hours) permit the repair of sublethal dam-

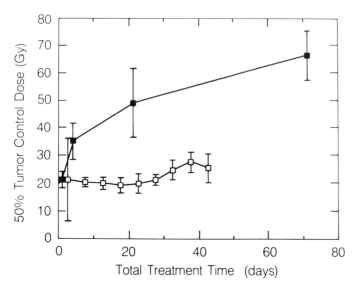

FIGURE 11-8. Relation of the 50% tumor control dose to the length of the fractionation schedule for conventional fractionated irradiation of 3- to 4-cm diameter skin tumors (■) and for Hodgkin's disease (□). Skin tumor data are adapted from Trott and associates[19]; Hodgkin's data are adapted from Fischer and Fischer.[26] All data shown with 95% confidence intervals.

age. Because each radiation fraction provides another opportunity for sublethal damage to be repaired, both tumors and tissues become more resistant to irradiation as the number of radiation fractions increases (Fig. 11-9). It has been argued that tumors might repair damage less well than normal tissues because the hypoxic cells in tumors are repair deficient, but there is little direct evidence to support this hypothesis. There is evidence that late-responding normal tissues accumulate and repair more sublethal damage than do tumors or rapidly responding normal tissues; this finding is the basis of trials with larger-than-conventional numbers of smaller-than-usual radiation fractions (*hyperfractionation*).[22]

Prolonging the overall treatment time may allow a portion of the hypoxic tumor cells to reoxygenate and become more radiosensitive. Reoxygenation of hypoxic (radiation-resistant) tumor cells appears to occur rapidly after the start of a course of radiation.[27] Although neither the kinetics nor the mechanisms underlying reoxygenation are clearly known, it appears that this phenomenon is an important reason for the increased efficacy of fractionated radiation therapy.

Protraction of irradiation will also allow the more rapidly proliferating normal tissues and tumors to *repopulate*. Repopulation during the course of fractionated radiotherapy is a significant cause of the apparent radioresistance of rapidly proliferating tissues such as skin (Fig. 11-9), gut, and oral mucosa. Rapid repopulation is not a factor for tissues such as lung, spinal cord, or kidney (Fig. 11-9). Repopulation can also increase the radioresistance of tumors if the growth rate is sufficiently high and the radiation schedule is sufficiently prolonged.[21] For example, it has been postulated that the apparent radioresistance of Burkitt's malignant lymphoma is due to the rapid proliferation of the tumor (doubling time of less than 24 hours) between radiation fractions (see Chap. 20).

During protracted irradiation, cells may *redistribute* through the cell cycle as populations become partially synchronized by radiation. In addition, cells that were nonproliferating (quiescent) may be *recruited* into proliferation. Redistribution and recruitment of cells occur in both tumors and normal tissues and may be a factor in fractionated radiotherapy. However, we currently lack the detailed knowledge of cell kinetics required to exploit redistribution and recruitment.[10]

Unconventional Radiation Fractionation

In practice, most radiation therapy is delivered once a day, 5 days per week, with daily doses of 1.8 to 2.2 Gy; such a course is now termed *standard* or *conventional* fractionation (Table 11-1). A number of other schedules have been tried. Clinical trials over the past few decades have generally shown that *hypofractionation* (fewer, larger radiation fractions) and *split-course* radiotherapy (where a break of 1–4 weeks is planned near the middle of an otherwise conventional schedule) produce poor clinical results.[23,24]

Some clinical and laboratory data support the concept of dividing the daily dose into two or three smaller treatments, the hyperfractionated schedule (Table 11-1).[22] Laboratory studies suggest that late-responding normal tissues are spared more by fractionation than either tumors or acutely responding tissues.[28] Hyperfractionation allows larger numbers of fractions to be given without the problems associated with prolonging treatment. These hyperfractionated treatments must be separated by at least 3 hours to ensure repair of sublethal damage in normal tissues between fractions. Clinical trials indicate that daily doses of 2 Gy can be replaced with twice-daily doses of 1.2 to 1.3 Gy (to total doses 20%–30% higher than those used in conventional fractionation), without exceeding late normal tissue tolerance, although these schedules often produce increased acute normal tissue reactions. It is not yet clear whether the hyperfractionated schedules are enhancing tumor response.

Because of the variation in daily doses and radiation schedules encountered in clinical practice, attempts have been

FIGURE 11-9. Effect of fractionation on the radiation response of tumors and normal tissues in the rat. Isoeffect curves are shown for tumor control dose for BA1112 rat rhabdomyosarcomas treated in conventional (■) and hypofractionated (▲) schedules; for skin tolerance in conventional (□) and hypofractionated (△) schedules; and for renal tolerance in conventional (○) schedules. All data shown with 95% confidence intervals. (Adapted from Rockwell S, Moulder JE: Biological factors of importance in split-course radiotherapy. In Paliwal BR et al [eds]: Optimization of Cancer Radiotherapy, pp 171–182. New York, American Institute of Physics, 1985)

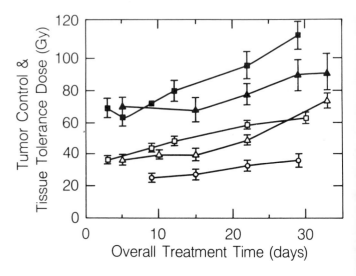

Table 11-1
Patterns of Radiation Fractionation*

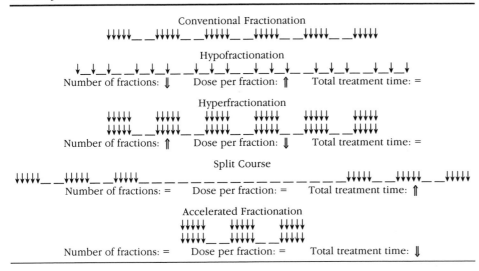

* Days with radiation treatments are shown by arrows. The size of the arrow is proportional to the daily dose; two arrows indicate multiple treatments per day.

made to develop models or formulas for equating different schedules. The best known of these models are the nominal standard dose (NSD or ret) model proposed by Ellis[29] and the more recent α/β model.[28,30] Despite widespread interest in this approach, neither NSD, α/β, nor any of the alternative models is accurate enough, or sufficiently general in scope, to be used to calculate tolerance doses or tumor control doses in nonstandard schedules.

PHYSICAL BASIS OF RADIATION THERAPY

Ionizing Radiations

Biologically effective radiations produce energetic charged particles in tissue. This property of ionizing radiations results in direct and indirect ionization of intracellular molecules and attendant biological effects. Ionizing radiations include x-rays and gamma rays, electromagnetic waves with sufficient energy to eject orbital electrons within the absorbing medium. X-rays and gamma rays are identified both as wave forms and as discrete packets of energy called photons. Ionizing particulate radiations include neutrons, electrons, charged pi-mesons, and heavy particles (*e.g.,* protons, alpha particles, or stripped nuclei). Particulate radiations ionize directly by electron ejection or indirectly by interacting with atomic nuclei, the resultant emissions of nuclear particles ultimately ejecting orbital electrons (Table 11-2).

X-rays (or roentgen rays) and gamma rays are considered together as photons, with identical physical and biological properties. X-rays are produced when electrically accelerated electrons are stopped rapidly, converting electrical energy into a beam of x-rays. Gamma rays are spontaneously and continuously emitted by the nuclei of radioactive elements during the process of nuclear decay.

Photons interact with matter by three major processes (Fig. 11-10). In *photoelectric absorption,* the incident photon ejects an inner orbital electron; the photon "disappears" as it loses all of its energy to the ejected photoelectron. Photoelec-

tric absorption predominates in the low-energy range of 10 to 50 keV (keV = 1000 electron volts). The photoelectric effect is uniquely dependent on the atomic number of the absorbing material to the third power (Z^3), explaining the increased absorption in bone relative to soft tissue for low- or intermediate-energy x-rays up to 60 to 90 keV.[31]

In *Compton absorption,* the incident photon loses only part of its energy in ejecting an outer orbital electron. The remainder proceeds as a scattered photon of lower energy along a path at an angle to the incident beam. The scattered photon is capable of further interactions. Compton scatter predominates in the energy range commonly used for radiation therapy: between 100 keV and 10 MeV (MeV = million electron volts). Compton interaction is virtually independent of Z, with essentially identical absorption tissues of different densities.[31]

The third type of photon absorption is *pair production.* In response to strong nuclear forces, an incident photon of greater than 1.02 MeV is converted into a positive and a negative electron pair. The positive electron (or positron) is subsequently anihilated by combining with a free electron, resulting in two photons (energy = 0.51 MeV each) traveling in opposite directions. Pair production accounts for 30% to 50% of absorption in the high therapeutic energy range of 10 to 20 MeV. Pair production is dependent on Z to the first power, resulting in a minor increase in energy deposition in bone.[31]

Electrons interact by direct collision with outer orbital electrons. Serial interactions cause the electron to slow down and change directions, ultimately losing energy over a finite range in tissue.

For heavy charged particles, the density of interactions is directly proportional to the charge and inversely proportional to the velocity of the particle. Protons, alpha particles (stripped helium atoms), and stripped nuclei of helium and carbon interact directly with the orbital electrons, producing a large number of ionizations along a given length of the incident beam. This physical property has been defined as high LET.[31]

The initial event in neutron absorption is nuclear capture of the incident particle. Nuclear stability is regained by ejec-

(*Text continues on p. 242*)

Table 11-2
Characteristics of Medically Useful Radiations

Type	Source	Physical Properties	Depth-Dose Curve	Biological Characteristics	Use
Photons Gamma rays X-rays	Cobalt-60 teletherapy Linear accelerator (4–48 MeV)	Skin-sparing; slow fall-off in dose with depth; absorption independent of tissue density; linear accelerator offers superior beam definition*	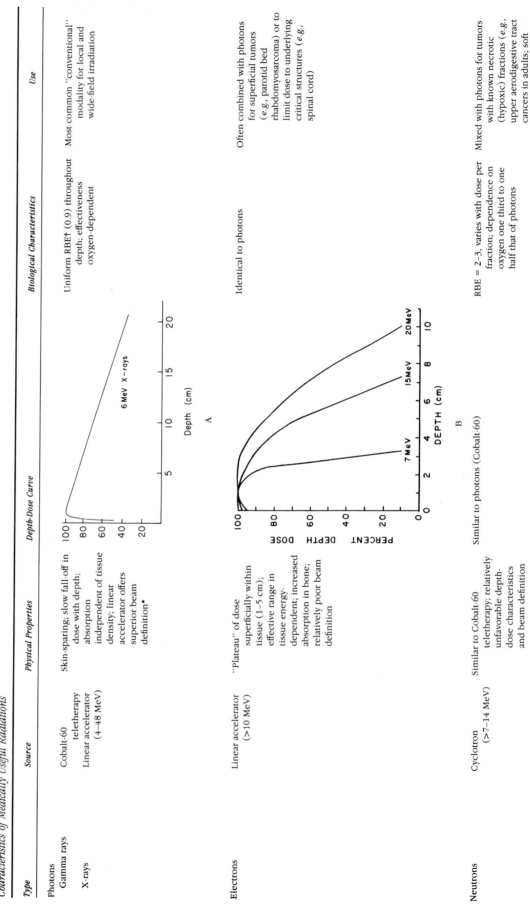	Uniform RBE† (0.9) throughout depth; effectiveness oxygen-dependent	Most common "conventional" modality for local and wide-field irradiation
Electrons	Linear accelerator (>10 MeV)	"Plateau" of dose superficially within tissue (1–5 cm); effective range in tissue energy-dependent; increased absorption in bone; relatively poor beam definition		Identical to photons	Often combined with photons for superficial tumors (*e.g.*, parotid bed rhabdomyosarcoma) or to limit dose to underlying critical structures (*e.g.*, spinal cord)
Neutrons	Cyclotron (>7–14 MeV)	Similar to Cobalt-60 teletherapy; relatively unfavorable depth-dose characteristics and beam definition	Similar to photons (Cobalt-60)	RBE = 2–3, varies with dose per fraction; dependence on oxygen one third to one half that of photons	Mixed with photons for tumors with known necrotic (hypoxic) fractions (*e.g.*, upper aerodigestive tract cancers in adults; soft tissue sarcoma)

| Protons | High-energy cyclotron (>160–250 MeV) | Plateau dose distribution with physical (Bragg) peak; depth of peak and range in tissue distinct and energy-dependent; absorption independent of tissue density; excellent beam definition | RBE = 1.1; relative oxygen-independence similar to neutrons | Focal concentration of high physical dose limits use to small volumes (*e.g.,* pituitary adenoma, basisphenoid chordoma, ocular melanoma) |
| Heavy charged particles ("stripped nuclei" of carbon, neon, argon) | High-energy cyclotron-synchrotron (>5000 MeV) | Similar to protons | RBE 1.5–3; Bragg peak RBE for hypoxic cells 2.5–5; oxygen independence similar to neutrons | Focal tumors (*e.g.,* ocular lesions); deep-seated tumors with potential hypoxic foci and/or potential dosimetric gain re photon therapy (*e.g.,* cancers of the pancreas, colon, prostate, thyroid) |

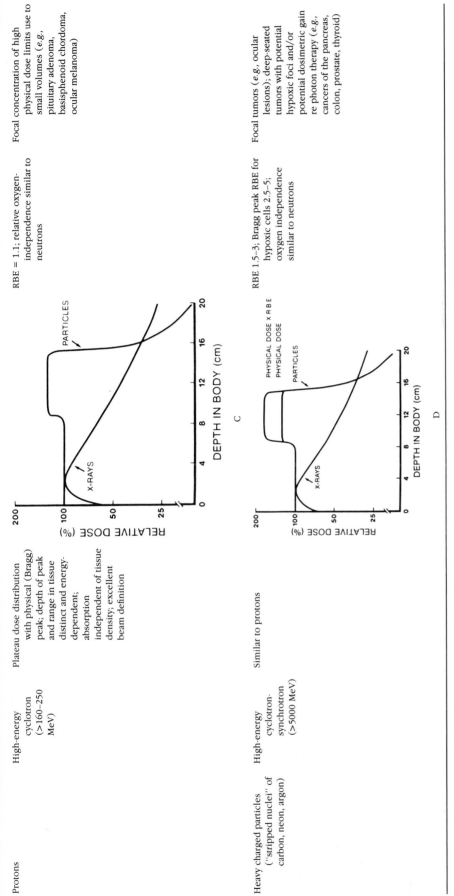

(Figure *A* is used with permission from Hendee WR: Medical Radiation Physics. Chicago, Year Book Medical Publishers, 1970. Figures *B, C,* and *D* are used with permission of The Committee for Radiation Oncology Studies [CROS]. Cancer Clin Trials 1:153–208, 1978)

* Beam definition refers to the sharpness of field margins in tissue.

† RBE = relative biological effectiveness (RBE = 1 for 250 kV orthovoltage X-rays).

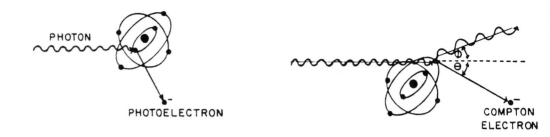

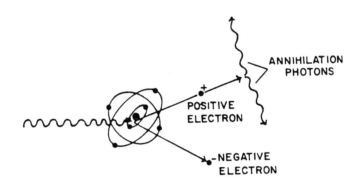

FIGURE 11-10. Interactions of photons (x-rays or γ-rays) with matter. Photoelectric effect (**top left**) predominates below 100 keV; Compton (**top right**), from 100 keV to 10 MeV; pair production (**bottom**), above 10 to 20 MeV (see text). (Johns HE, Cunningham JR [eds]: The Physics of Radiology, pp 133–166. Springfield, IL, Charles C Thomas, 1983)

tion of a proton, alpha particle, or gamma ray. Neutron capture may result in fission of the nucleus. The resultant heavy charged particles interact secondarily in the same way as the other high-LET particles described above.

Units of Measurement

The *absorbed dose* is the amount of energy imparted per unit mass. The International System of Units (SI units) identifies the *gray* (Gy) as the unit of measurement, equivalent to one joule (energy)/kg (mass). The Gy has both theoretical and practical advantages over the rad; one Gy is equivalent to 100 rad.[32] The standard definition of the rad (100 ergs/g tissue) approximated the energy absorbed in tissue from 1 roentgen air exposure (see below). The term centigray (cGy) is commonly used, equivalent to 1/100 Gy (or 1 rad).

The *roentgen* (R) is a unit of exposure, or ionization produced in air. For x-ray and gamma-ray exposures in the therapeutic range, one R is roughly equivalent to 0.95 cGy (or rad) in soft tissue. The SI unit for exposure is coulomb (charge)/kg (mass of air).

The *activity* of radioactive elements is most simply expressed as the number of disintegrations per second. The standard unit of radioactivity for decades was the *curie* (Ci), equivalent to 3.7×10^{10} disintegrations per second (the decay of 1 g of radium). The SI unit replacing the Ci is the *becquerel* (Bq), defined as $\sec^{-1}$. One Ci equals 3.7×10^{10} Bq.

A unit of radiation protection recognizes the physical absorbed dose (Gy) and a qualifying factor (Q), defined by the LET (for protection) or the radiobiologic effectiveness (RBE). The rem (rad × Q) has been superseded by the SI unit, the *sievert* (Sv); 1 Sv is equivalent to 100 rem.[33]

External-Beam Irradiation

Radiation therapy is broadly divided into *external-beam irradiation* and *brachytherapy*. In external-beam therapy, a well-defined x-ray or gamma-ray beam is directed to a specified anatomic volume. In brachytherapy, radioactive sources are applied directly within or around a given tumor site as discussed below. In pediatric oncology, virtually all radiation therapy is administered as external-beam irradiation.

Photon-Beam Therapy

Photon beams have been used in radiation therapy since Röntgen's discovery of x-rays produced from a cathode ray tube. The maximal energy of the beam defines the quality of irradiation: *orthovoltage* (100–400 keV) or *supervoltage* (greater than 1 MeV; synonymous with megavoltage). *Cobalt teletherapy* units direct emitted gamma rays from the continuous decay of a radioactive ^{60}Co source. The energy level is 1.2 MeV. *Linear accelerators* use high-energy electrons, accelerated along a waveguide to 4 to 48 MeV, to produce x-rays with rather precise beam definition.

The dose distribution of photon irradiation in tissue is dependent on the energy of the beam. Figure 11-11 compares the relative depth dose in tissue or water for several different beam energies. Orthovoltage beams deliver 100% of the energy on the surface, losing energy quickly below the superficial tissues; by 3 to 4 cm depth, the dose is 50% of the maximal dose. With ^{60}Co or 4 MeV x-rays, there is a *skin-sparing effect*: less than 60% of the maximal dose is deposited at the surface, the superficial dose building to the 100% dose level at a depth of 0.5 to 1.0 cm (Fig. 11-11B). The dose in tissue diminishes less rapidly with ^{60}Co or 4 MeV photons than with orthovoltage: 50% of the maximal dosage is reached 12 to 14 cm below the surface. With higher-energy photons, one sees an increase in the depth of maximal dosage and more effective penetration: 20 MeV linear-accelerator x-rays, for example, achieve a maximal dose level at 4.5 cm; the surface dose is less than 20%, and the dose is diminished to 50% of maximal at 23 to 24 cm depth.

The dose distribution in tissue is displayed as a depth dose curve or isodose plot. A single beam delivers a diminishing dose at depths beyond maximal build-up (Fig. 11-12). Modern techniques identify an isocenter (fixed for a specific treatment

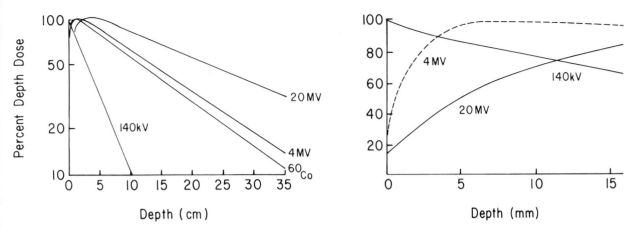

FIGURE 11-11. Dose distribution of photons in tissue. **Left.** Comparison of orthovoltage x-rays (140 keV) with ^{60}Co teletherapy, low-energy (4 MeV), and high-energy (20 MeV) linear accelerators (see text). **Right.** Graph magnifies the dose build-up and absorption in the entry region, indicating the "skin-sparing effect" of supervoltage beams. (Johns HE, Cunningham JR [eds]: The Physics of Radiology, pp 133–166. Springfield, IL, Charles C Thomas, 1983)

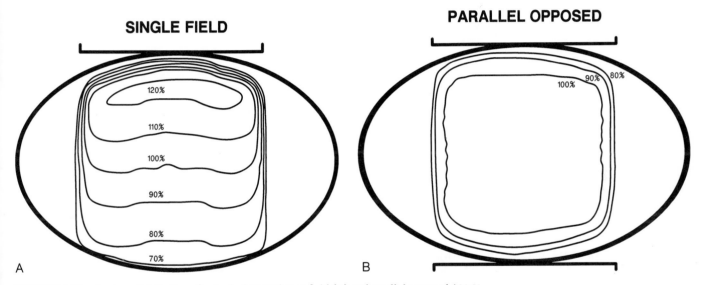

FIGURE 11-12. Isodose distribution of a single 4 MeV photon field (**A**) and parallel opposed 4 MeV fields (**B**). The distribution is normalized to the geometric center of the treated volume, with 100% encompassing this point. The uniform distribution with parallel opposed fields contrasts with the single beam.

unit) at which two or more fields may focus, entering from different directions (Fig. 11-12). *Parallel opposed* fields enter from 180° opposing angles, most often anterior and posterior or right and left lateral in position. The dose distribution in parallel opposed arrangements is relatively uniform throughout the irradiated volume.

Electron-Beam Therapy

Electron-beam irradiation provides relatively uniform doses within 1 to 5 cm of the surface, the depth of penetration varying directly with the energy of the electron beam (Table 11-2). The unique depth dose characteristic of electrons is a relatively flat region of nearly uniform dosage (80%–100%) with rapid fall-off beyond the 80% depth. With 18 MeV electrons, for example, the dose between entry and 5 cm is uniformly between

80% and 100% of maximum; at 8 cm depth, the dose is less than 10%.[34] There is little skin sparing with electron irradiation. The LET of electrons is equivalent to that of photons. Caution is necessary in areas of tissue inhomogeneity; bones absorb electrons preferentially (with increased dose within bone and decreased dose deep to bone), whereas air cavities (*e.g.,* sinuses) transmit electrons, resulting in deeper penetration of the incident beam. Electron beams are available from intermediate- or high-energy (10 MeV or greater) linear accelerators.

Neutron Irradiation

Neutrons are most commonly produced by cyclotrons, with depth dose characteristics for 7 to 14 MeV neutrons being similar to those of ^{60}Co.[35] Neutrons are high-LET radiations and are of interest because of the relative lack of oxygen dependence

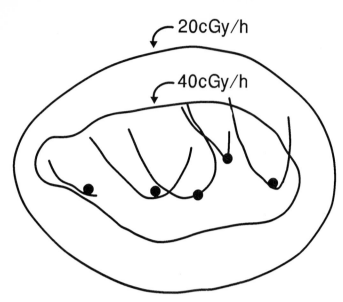

FIGURE 11-13. Brachytherapy dose distribution, representing an implant of 5 cm transverse diameter. The high-dose level (40 cGy/h) adjacent to the sources is diminished by 50% (20 cGy/h) within 1 to 2 cm. This distribution is from the implant pictured in Figure 11-14, the dots representing the center of the linear sources visualized from a transverse section through the implanted volume.

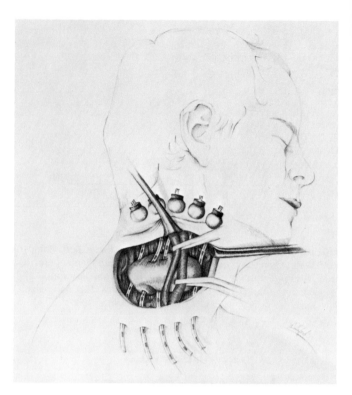

FIGURE 11-14. Interstitial brachytherapy application showing Silastic tubes inserted along a residual desmoid tumor in the neck. Afterloading ^{192}Ir wires are illustrated within the tubes.

as summarized above. Initial neutron trials resulted in disastrous late effects owing to a lack of data regarding the differences in RBE with small fraction sizes.[36,37] In recent studies using appropriately adjusted RBE values, there has been evidence of various degrees of effectiveness for specific tumor sites (*e.g.,* soft-tissue sarcomas, advanced squamous cell carcinomas of the upper aerodigestive tract).[35] In childhood cancer, the potential use of neutrons is limited due to concerns about added late toxicities, both somatic and carcinogenic.[38]

Heavy-Particle Irradiation

High-energy cyclotrons produce energetic charged particles of potential value in radiation therapy. Protons, for example, yield a discrete volume of increased dose at a depth that varies with the energy of the incident proton beam (Table 11-2). The dose distribution is characterized by a *Bragg peak* resulting from relatively dense nuclear reactions as the particle loses velocity. Therapeutically useful proton energies (*e.g.,* 160 MeV) have an RBE only slightly higher than that of photons.[39] Other particles (*e.g.,* high-energy carbon, neon, or argon ions) have a similar dose distribution. In addition, the LET of the latter particles is increased in the region of peak physical dosage, resulting in an even greater biological dose differential at the depth of the Bragg peak (Table 11-2).[39] Protons have produced intriguing results in focal intraocular tumors such as choroidal melanoma and in pituitary adenomas.[40]

Brachytherapy

Direct application of radioactive materials to localized accessible tumor sites is termed brachytherapy. The principal types of brachytherapy include *intracavitary* applications (within body cavities such as the vagina or nasopharynx), *interstitial* implants (directly into tissue), and mold applications (adjacent to tumor sites such as skin or eye). Brachytherapy has been used

in adults for decades, most often for cancers of the female genital tract, upper aerodigestive tract, breast, and soft tissues.[41] Pediatric applications have been described more recently, primarily for retinoblastoma and soft-tissue tumors (see Chap. 25).[42,43,44]

The primary advantage of brachytherapy is the ability to achieve a concentrated high dose volume with relative sparing of adjacent normal tissues. The dose distribution in brachytherapy is governed largely by the inverse square law. Figure 11-13 shows a typical dose distribution of interstitial therapy with high dose levels near the sources and rapid fall-off. By geometric planning, one can achieve a dose distribution encompassing the desired target volume with far less irradiation of surrounding normal tissues than can be achieved with external-beam irradiation. To assure relative dose homogeneity within the target volume, brachytherapy applications are used primarily for tumors less than 5 cm in greatest diameter.

Initial experience with brachytherapy used ^{226}Ra or ^{222}Rn sources. Rigid needles or tubes limited attainable geometry, while handling the radioactive sources for direct implantation created radiation safety problems for personnel. Current practice most commonly uses ^{129}Ir, an artificially produced radionuclide imbedded in wire or seeds that can be *afterloaded* into hollow Silastic tubes (Fig. 11-14). Interstitial placement of the tubes is performed by direct positioning or by stereotactic localization using computed tomographic (CT) guidance. The geometry of the implant can be planned before insertion, confirmed by radiographs during the procedure, and altered if necessary; when it is satisfactory, the tubes are loaded with the radioactive sources. This sequence allows greater accuracy while limiting exposure of medical personnel. The implant remains in place for a calculated period of time, typically 2 to 5 days, and is subsequently removed with little difficulty. Problems of radiation safety are magnified in children, but procedures to assure personnel and parental exposures within established limits can be achieved even in young children.

Iodine-125 sources have the advantage of emitting lower-energy photons, simplifying radiation safety procedures. Iodine-125 has been used predominantly in permanent low-activity implants in adults, small seeds remaining in place with gradual decay over several months. The lack of data regarding potential somatic and carcinogenic effects of long-term exposure to low-dose irradiation in children limits consideration of permanent implants for pediatric cancer. High-activity ^{125}I has recently been introduced for use in removable implants with potential advantages in pediatrics due to the limited penetration of the lower-energy photons beyond the immediate implant volume.[45]

Brachytherapy also has potential radiobiological advantages compared with external-beam irradiation. Dose rates in brachytherapy are generally 30 to 100 cGy/hour in comparison to 100 to 300 cGy/minute with external therapy. Low dose rates appear to achieve reduction in tumor cell proliferation while permitting repair of sublethal damage in normal tissues.[46,47] In addition, low-dose-rate irradiation has a much lower OER compared with acute exposures during external-beam therapy.

Pediatric brachytherapy experience has been well documented in retinoblastoma, with use of both ^{137}Cs and ^{192}Ir plaques applied directly to focal areas of retinal involvement (see Chap. 25).[42,48] Recent series document successful applications of both intracavitary and interstitial brachytherapy in soft-tissue sarcomas (see Chap. 31).[44] The technique may be most applicable in vaginal rhabdomyosarcoma. Brachytherapy for primary central nervous system tumors has proved quite effective in the more typical adult malignant gliomas; applications in both low-grade and malignant tumors in children are now being studied.[49]

TECHNIQUES OF RADIATION THERAPY

Basic Procedures

Treatment Planning

The initial process in planning radiation therapy is to identify the *target volume*. For curative irradiation, the target volume usually includes the primary tumor site and immediately adjacent area(s) of potential microscopic extension. Inclusion of adjacent or regional lymph nodes is dependent on tumor type and extent. Data from clinical examination, radiographic studies, and operative assessment may be used to define the target volume. Knowledge of the natural history of specific tumor presentations is critical in determining the appropriate irradiation volume.

Once the target volume has been determined, an interactive process of patient simulation and dosimetry defines the treatment plan. Simulation permits accurate localization of the target volume from one or several directions; the simulator is a diagnostic-quality x-ray unit structured to mimic the treatment machine geometrically. The position and divergence of the photon beam are identical to those of the linear accelerator, allowing the radiation oncologist to plan accurately treatment strategies that have been identified by and may be later confirmed by computerized dosimetry. Planning seeks to maximize dose homogeneity within the target volume and permit appropriate dose limitation for critical normal structures.

Dosimetry provides a detailed analysis of the dose distribution within a given plane. CT-based treatment planning ac-

curately displays the dose relation based on the planned field configuration. The simplest technique to provide homogeneous dosage is a parallel opposed pair of treatment fields. Such uniformity is ideal when treating the cranium (to encompass the subarachnoid space), the abdomen (especially when treating the entire peritoneal cavity), or more localized central anatomic areas (such as the nasopharynx or mediastinum). The energy of the photon beam determines the depth of maximal dosage and the distribution, specific indications often requiring low-energy (*e.g.,* treatment of the subarachnoid space) or high-energy (*e.g.,* para-aortic) megavoltage beams.[51]

More complex field arrangements are often desirable, concentrating the high-dose volume or limiting doses to specific structures (Fig. 11-15). In addition, blocks are customarily used to define the treatment volume. Customized blocks are fabricated from a lead alloy that provides precise beam definition to limit the irradiation volume to the desired anatomic region (Fig. 11-16).

With treatment volumes extending beyond one body cavity, one must use adjoining-field configurations such as mantle and para-aortic fields in Hodgkin's disease (Fig. 11-17). Field junctions require exquisite attention to avoid areas of overdosage and underdosage, which may be associated with local recurrence or unnecessary toxicity.

Immobilization

Immobilization is critical for proper simulation and daily treatment. Infants and children younger than 2 or 3 years old may require sedation. Most older children can be reassured with appropriate explanations, gaining sufficient confidence to maintain the necessary position unattended for the 30- to 90-second period of each treatment field. For anatomic sites other than the torso, specific devices are often used to achieve stabilization and reproducibility, including headholders (chin sup-

FIGURE 11-15. Complex isodose distribution illustrating doses within an axial section of the central abdomen from a combination of opposed anterior–posterior and right–left lateral fields. Blocks (*b*) have been inserted in each field at predetermined times to limit the dose to the kidneys and to achieve a high dose localized to the left midabdomen while delivering tolerated doses to the remainder of the treated volume. The case depicted achieved 47 Gy to the target volume in a child treated postoperatively for a large retroperitoneal soft tissue sarcoma.

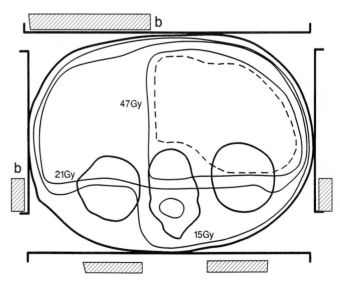

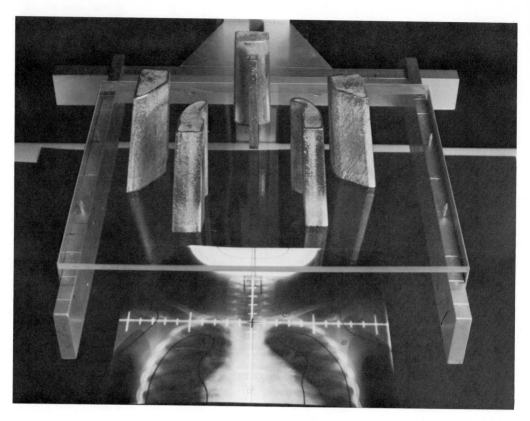

FIGURE 11-16. Individually fabricated treatment blocks are composed of Cerrubend, a lead alloy with a relatively low melting point. Blocks are constructed to precisely preclude normal structures as outlined by the radiation oncologist on the simulation film. The blocks are mounted on a Lucite tray as shown.

ports, fixed mesh casts) and removable casts to assure consistent positioning of an extremity.

For neuraxis therapy, a cast or mold is necessary to support the patient in a reproducible prone position. Plaster or self-setting acrylics may be used (Fig. 11-18).

Sedation

Infants can usually be treated while napping or swaddled; when treatment involves the head and neck region, sedation may be necessary. Children between 9 to 12 months and 2½ to 3 years often require sedation.

The safest means to achieve daily sedation is chloral hydrate. Oral doses of 50 to 65 mg/kg are effective in at least 75% of children, producing adequate levels of sedation after 20 to 25 minutes; children usually awaken rather promptly after treatment. When chloral hydrate is ineffective, the most prudent course is daily use of ketamine, a parenteral general anesthetic administered by an anesthesiologist.

Less predictable sedation may be achieved with Nembutal (5 mg/kg given intramuscularly or intravenously over several minutes) or a combination of meperidine (Demerol) (1.7 mg/kg), promethazine (0.5–1 mg/kg), and chlorpromazine (0.3–0.5 mg/kg) given together by the intramuscular or intravenous route.

Specific Techniques

Cranial Irradiation

The goal of cranial irradiation for acute lymphoblastic leukemia is to deliver tumoricidal doses to the entire intracranial subarachnoid space (see Chap. 16). The target volume includes the extension of the subarachnoid space around the

optic nerve, in practice incorporating the orbital apex and the posteriormost aspect of the retina.

Particular attention is necessary to include the subfrontal region down to the cribriform plate and the temporal fossa (Fig. 11-19A). Inclusion of the cribriform plate demands precision field alignment to allow appropriate blocking of the anterior eye and lens. To correct for divergence in the opposed lateral field configuration, it is necessary to angle the entrance beams posteriorly to achieve parallel rays at the level of the orbital rims (Figs. 11-19B and C).[51]

The lower margin has been arbitrarily established at the second cervical vertebra to assure coverage of the base of the skull. It is important to extend the field just beyond the skull to achieve dose homogeneity in the peripherally located subarachnoid space.[50] Ideal dosimetry is obtained with low-energy linear accelerators (4–6 MeV).[50]

Craniospinal Irradiation

Craniospinal irradiation is one of the most technically demanding techniques in radiotherapy. The goal is homogeneous irradiation of the subarachnoid space, including the brain and the spinal canal. The target volume for the cranium is identical to that discussed above for acute lymphoblastic leukemia; inclusion of the posterior orbit for primary central nervous system tumors appears to be necessary only to the degree that it ensures adequate margins around the cribriform plate. Failure at the latter site has been documented all too commonly in medulloblastoma, highlighting the need to address this region (see Chap. 24).[52]

The most consistently accurate technique for craniospinal irradiation utilizes a prone position with an immobilizing cast (Fig. 11-20). Lateral craniocervical fields encompass the brain, including the intracranial and upper cervical subarachnoid spaces. Minimizing inhomogeneity at the junction with an ad-

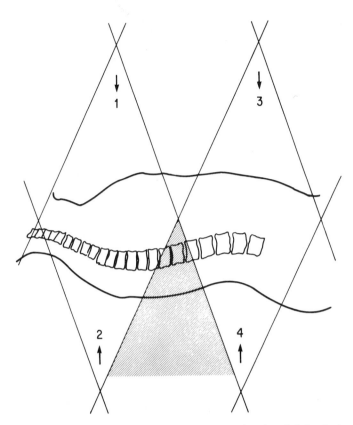

FIGURE 11-17. Adjoining supradiaphragmatic (*1, 2*) and abdominal (*3, 4*) fields illustrating the junction of divergent photon beams. A "gap" on the surface allows the anterior fields (*1, 3*) to join at the midfrontal plane. Opposed posterior fields (*2, 4*) achieve a mirror image configuration, a "cold" area (*shaded*) posterior to the midplane from fields 2 and 4 compensating for the overlap in this region as fields 1 and 3 exit.

joining posterior spinal field requires correction for the divergence in three planes. A detailed plan of calculated field angles and gaps at this junction follows carefully outlined guidelines (Fig. 11-20).[53] To compensate for potential inhomogeneity, the spinal level of the craniocervical–spinal junction is changed every five to seven fractions, distributing any potential overdosage or underdosage in space.

An alternative technique utilizes a prone position with the head rotated to the side.[54] The use of a single blocked field that includes the cranium and spine avoids the problem of a field junction but invites problems because of a lack of precise parallelism of the skull. Coverage of the cribriform plate and exclusion of the contralateral orbit are more difficult with this technique.

Photon irradiation is conventionally employed for the spinal field because of the accuracy of the field junction and the certainty of dose distribution in the spine. Electron-beam irradiation has been advocated by several centers, the limited penetration of 15- to 20-MeV electrons potentially resulting in less hematosuppression and diminishing the exit dose (especially to the thyroid, heart, and gastrointestinal tract). One would expect relatively little advantage in limiting spinal growth disturbances. Potential concerns about the junction with craniocervical photon fields and shadowing the spinal canal due to greater absorption in the overlying posterior spinal processes are currently being investigated.[55]

Abdominal Irradiation

For presentations requiring whole-abdominal irradiation, such as Wilms' tumor, malignant lymphoma, and ovarian neoplasms, it is important to include the entire peritoneal cavity (see Chaps. 20, 27, 35). The treatment volume extends from above the diaphragm superiorly to the midobturator foramen inferiorly. Customized blocks permit shielding toward the cardiac apex in addition to the acetabulum and femoral head regions. In reality, whole-abdominal irradiation is limited by

FIGURE 11-18. An immobilizing cast used for craniospinal irradiation. The entrance of the lateral craniocervical fields is outlined.

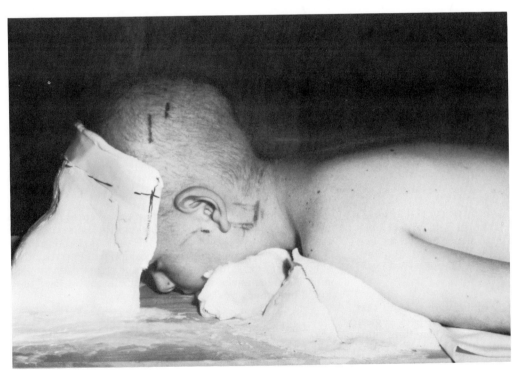

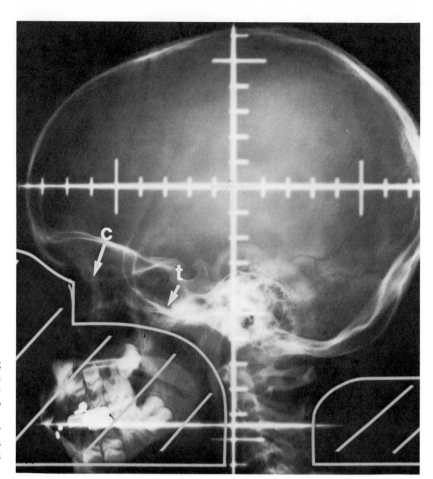

FIGURE 11-19. Cranial irradiation for ALL, picturing the treatment field (**A**), which encompasses the region of the cribriform plate (*c*) and inferior margin of the temporal fossa (*t*). The use of posterior beam angles to correct for divergence is illustrated (**B, C**). Directly opposed fields (**B**) result in divergence of the anterior margins (*a.m.*) into the contralateral eye. Angled fields (**C**) achieve virtually parallel anterior beam margins (*a.m.*) with nonparallel central rays (*c.r.*).

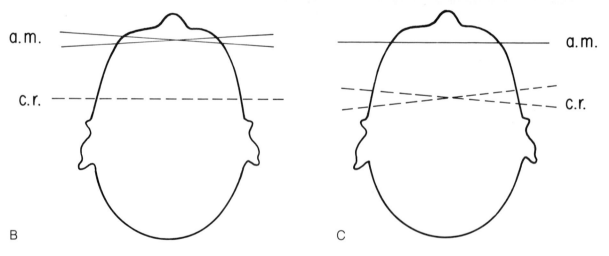

the need to block the kidneys at 14 to 18 Gy and at least a portion of liver at 18 to 24 Gy. Complex field arrangements allow higher doses to specific target volumes beyond the general tolerance of the entire abdomen (see Fig. 11-15).

Extremity Irradiation

Irradiation of extremity lesions is often more difficult than complex field arrangements for the head and neck region. Treatment fields must encompass the tumor region, often along with a considerable length of the extremity. It is critical to exclude a strip of tissue at least 1 to 2 cm wide along the entire length of the irradiated extremity, as dermal lymphatics may be obliterated following irradiation if the entire circumference of the extremity is subtended. Fastidious attention to immobilization and daily treatment positioning often requires a special cast or customized device. Accuracy in treatment planning and techniques improves the likelihood of later functional integrity.[56]

Lung Irradiation

The important factors in whole-lung irradiation include volume definitions and prior abdominal irradiation. The treat-

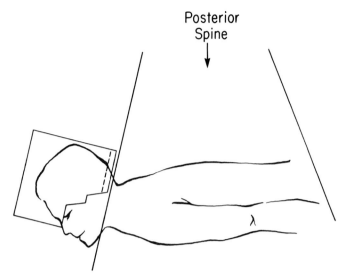

Posterior
Spine

FIGURE 11-20. Field alignment for craniospinal irradiation. Lateral craniocervical fields adjoin a posterior spinal field. The junction is moved at regular intervals, the dotted line representing the new lower border of the lateral fields to which the posterior spinal field will be matched.

ment fields should extend to cover the lung bases inferiorly, usually to the level of the 11th or 12th thoracic vertebra. Caution must be exercised in children previously treated to the abdomen, noting the limits of liver and kidney tolerance depending on the previous irradiation volume, the presence of one or both kidneys, and time interval since previous therapy.

Head and Neck Irradiation

Radiation therapy for tumors of the head and neck region differs with the tumor site and histology. Careful definition of treatment volume usually requires detailed CT imaging. For most pediatric applications (*e.g.,* rhabdomyosarcoma, other soft-tissue sarcomas, nasopharyngeal lymphoepithelioma), tumoricidal doses to the tumor volume exceed the normal tolerance of the spinal cord. The target volume often includes tissues adjacent to the orbit(s) or base of skull. Multiple treatment fields and coordinated use of photons and electrons are necessary to achieve necessary doses within the target volume while observing normal tissue tolerance. Prospective dosimetry including CT-based plans is essential to successful irradiation in these instances (Fig. 11-21).

COMBINATIONS OF SURGERY AND IRRADIATION

The combined use of surgery and radiation therapy has been a basic principle of cancer management since the early 1900s.[57] The rationale for preoperative or postoperative irradiation has been based on the failure patterns of the two modalities. Recurrence after local or radical surgical excision implies residual microscopic disease at the operative margins; recurrence after radiation therapy in general relates to large tumor volume, with an excess of clonogenic tumor cells beyond the number that can be destroyed by locally tolerated doses of radiation.[58] The presence of hypoxic foci increases with tumor size; even a small proportion of hypoxic cells substantially affects the dose necessary to eradicate the clonogenic population.[59]

With combined therapy, the goal of surgery is to remove all macroscopic disease, reducing the proportion of clonogenic cells (by approximately three logarithms) and eliminating the hypoxic cell fraction. Radiation therapy seeks to eradicate peripheral extensions of disease beyond the operative margins, destroying the normally oxygenated microscopic foci. Planned surgery and postoperative irradiation must include a reasonable likelihood of complete surgical resection of macroscopic disease; little is gained by debulking if surgery removes only a portion of the identifiable tumor, thereby reducing the clonogenic cells by less than one or two logarithms, introducing tumor cells into a broader area by contaminating the entire operative bed, and altering vascularity of the residual tumor, thus potentially increasing the number of hypoxic cells.[52,60] A laboratory model of rhabdomyosarcoma has confirmed the clinical observation that surgery contributes to local control only if complete resection of macroscopic disease is achieved (Fig. 11-22).[61]

Preoperative irradiation is often preferable to postoperative therapy. Irradiation is more effective with intact vascularity; in practice, preoperative doses are generally 75% to 80% of postoperative doses. In addition, preoperative treatment reduces the likelihood of surgical implantation or dissemination.[62] In Wilms' tumor, for example, preoperative irradiation diminishes the frequency of intraoperative tumor rupture, decreasing both abdominal recurrence and disease-related mortality (see Chap. 27).[63] In some tumor systems, preoperative irradiation may reduce the volume of normal tissue necessarily resected to assure adequate tumor removal. Suit and associates have shown excellent local tumor control with preoperative

FIGURE 11-21. Multiple fields are used for tumors in the head and neck region. For nasopharyngeal rhabdomyosarcoma, for example, opposed lateral fields incorporate wedges (*hatched*) to balance the dose from the anterior field. The hatched rectangles depicted at the posterior aspect of the fields (lateral to the wedges) indicate spinal cord blocks to limit dose levels to the sensitive cervical cord.

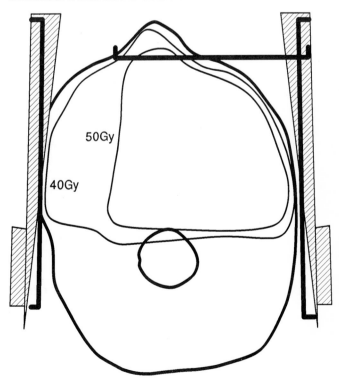

50Gy

40Gy

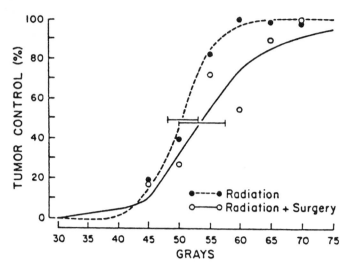

FIGURE 11-22. Effect of surgery on local tumor control with radiation therapy. The rat rhabdomyosarcoma model clearly shows no benefit with partial (50%) tumor resection. The laboratory model actually suggests a paradoxical effect requiring a higher radiation dose to obtain equivalent control rates ≥50% to 70%. (Fischer JJ et al: The effect of subtotal resection on the dose of radiation required to cure the rat rhabdomyosarcoma BA1112. Surg Gynecol Obstet 156:189–192, 1983)

irradiation and wide local resection of extremity soft-tissue sarcomas using irradiation doses below those indicated for postoperative management and avoiding amputation.[64]

Combined surgery and radiation therapy may be utilized solely to address regional lymph-node metastases. In several tumor systems, such as ovarian dysgerminoma, testicular seminoma, or, potentially, paratesticular rhabdomyosarcoma, surgery is used for the primary tumor with radiation therapy employed to eradicate microscopic foci in regional nodes.[60]

Intraoperative irradiation has recently engendered considerable interest (also see Chap. 10).[65] Direct irradiation of the tumor bed during the operative procedure offers theoretical advantages in localization and immediate treatment of residual microscopic deposits. In practice, large electron fields are used to deliver 15 to 20 Gy in one fraction to the operative bed, most often for intra-abdominal cancers in adults (*e.g.*, those of the pancreas, stomach, rectum, and retroperitoneum).[66] Problems include the technical availability of irradiation in the operative amphitheater and assurance of appropriate field alignment with limited visual exposure. In addition, radiobiological data indicate that single large radiation fractions are limited in achieving tumor sterilization by the presence of hypoxic cell fractions.[67] Late effects on hollow viscera (biliary tract, bowel, ureter) and peripheral nerves appear to be the dose-limiting phenomena in regard to normal tissue tolerance.[68] Potential applications in childhood cancer are large retroperitoneal sarcomas or locally resected malignant lesions of long bones. Concerns about late soft-tissue changes mandate caution in the pediatric age group.

COMBINATIONS OF CHEMOTHERAPY AND IRRADIATION

The coordinated use of irradiation and chemotherapy is fundamental to modern cancer management, especially in children. The interactions between radiation therapy and cytotoxic chemotherapy are complex. Improvement in the therapeutic ratio results from combined effects categorized by Steel, as shown in Table 11-3.[69,70] Diminution in the therapeutic ratio can occur with combined therapy, defined by Fu either as *inhibition* (combined effect less than that of the more-active modality alone) or *antagonism* (combined effect less than that achieved by the less-active agent alone).[71]

It is difficult to prove true radiosensitization when combining cytotoxic drugs with irradiation; increased radiation cell kill per dose level is more easily identified as an effect of chemical agents that cannot destroy tumor cells themselves (*e.g.*, hypoxic-cell sensitizers).[71,72]

Spatial cooperation is readily apparent in pediatric oncology, best typified by irradiation of sanctuaries in acute lymphoblastic leukemia and by combined-modality therapy for apparently localized or metastatic presentations, including Wilms' tumor, Ewing's sarcoma, and rhabdomyosarcoma. Additive effects are also apparent in the latter group of solid tumors, both radiation therapy and chemotherapy reducing the local clonogenic tumor-cell population. There is a variable degree of chemotherapy-induced enhancement of radiation damage to normal tissues. Improvement of the therapeutic ratio by additive local interactions may be limited by overlapping toxicities, necessitating dose reductions or interruption depending on the target tissues, the agent(s) used, and the time between chemotherapy and irradiation.[70,73]

Several mechanisms explain the potential enhancing interactions of chemotherapy combined with irradiation. *Increased slope of the radiation dose–response curve* (the classic definition of "radiosensitization") has been noted with DNA intercalating agents such as dactinomycin and cisplatin.[71,73] Dactinomycin also typically *inhibits repair of sublethal damage,* enhancing tumor and normal tissue effects equally during fractionated irradiation.[71,74] Adriamycin has similar clinical interactions; in the laboratory, it seems to affect predominantly the accumulation of sublethal damage rather than its repair.[73]

Chemotherapy-induced *alterations in cell kinetics* may produce synchronization toward the more radiation-sensitive phases of the cell cycle; hydroxyurea has most often been used in this manner, although a differential effect between tumor and normal tissue has not been confirmed.[75] *Preirradiation tumor reduction* has potential effects beyond additive clono-

---

Table 11-3

*Interactions of Chemotherapy and Radiation Therapy
That Potentially Improve the Therapeutic Ratio*

1. Spatial cooperation—independent actions of local irradiation and systemic chemotherapy, the latter addressing occult or overt disease beyond the irradiated volume; no true "interaction" is apparent in this mechanism, typifying the term "adjuvant chemotherapy."
2. Additive antitumor effects—independent tumor cell kill in excess of that achieved by either modality alone, different mechanisms affecting the same tissue; toxicities of the two modalities must not overlap to a degree requiring significant dose reduction in either radiation therapy or chemotherapy.
3. Enhancement of tumor response—"true interaction," resulting in a combined antitumor effect greater than would be achieved by simple addition of the tumor cell kill of each modality if used separately.
4. Protection of normal tissues—use of drugs to protect against irradiation effects on normal tissues with little or no similar protection against tumor cell kill. (Modified from Steel[73], Fu[72])

genic cell kill, decreasing the hypoxic cell fraction and recruiting intermitotic cells into the more sensitive proliferative phase along with the reduction in tumor volume.[59,71]

Protection of normal tissue has been described following time-dependent preirradiation administration of cytarabine, cyclophosphamide, or methotrexate.[70,76,77] Laboratory evidence of bone-marrow sparing in this setting has been difficult to confirm in the clinic.[70]

To enhance the therapeutic ratio, combinations of radiation therapy and chemotherapy must potentiate antitumor effects selectively with quantitatively less increase in normal tissue effects. It has been difficult, for example, to show an improved therapeutic ratio with dactinomycin or Adriamycin, the noted sensitization being shared equally by normal tissues and tumors.[71,73,78] Increased normal tissue reactions have been quantified in the laboratory, Phillips and Fu defining the dose–effect factor (DEF) as the radiation dose divided by the radiation dose in the presence of drug to produce the same biological effect.[78] Normal tissue interactions may be site specific (*e.g.,* increased bladder toxicity with cyclophosphamide and irradiation, methotrexate–irradiation interactions in the central nervous system). Additive normal-tissue effects may be secondary to similar effects on the target tissue (*e.g.,* bleomycin and irradiation effects on lung) or different tissue changes affecting the same organ (*e.g.,* cardiac effects of Adriamycin on the myocyte and indirect effects of irradiation on cardiac function secondary to vascular changes).[78]

NORMAL-TISSUE EFFECTS

The effects of radiation therapy on normal tissues have been variously described as "radiophysiology" or "radiation pathology," best reflecting the *anticipated acute effects* and *potential late effects,* respectively.[1,79] Temporally, one may describe normal-tissue reactions as acute (occurring during the course of fractionated irradiation), subacute (occurring within the first 3–6 months after treatment), and late (onset later than 6 months after irradiation).

Radiation effects depend both on inherent cellular radiosensitivity and on tissue kinetics. With notable exceptions, such as small lymphocytes, cellular radiosensitivity varies little within human cell lines. It is the rapidly proliferating tissues that express acute radiation injury, differences in tissue effects largely reflecting the kinetics of the target tissue.[80–82] Acutely responding tissues include the skin, mucous membranes, spermatogonia, and hematopoietic cells. Acute changes follow depletion of the actively proliferating stem cells and depend on the size of the stem-cell compartment and the response of the cell renewal system to injury. The latter responses include recruitment of noncycling uncommitted or committed stem cells into the proliferating pool and reduction in the mean cell cycle time. The difference in tissue effects is typified by the laboratory observations of jejunal and testicular changes following a single fraction of 10 Gy: despite identical dose–survival curves for jejunal crypt cells and spermatogonia, the jejunum is histologically normal within 10 to 14 days of irradiation, whereas the testis continues to show progressive hypoplasia, the sperm count remaining low for months if not permanently.[82]

Acute radiation reactions depend to some degree on the fraction size, dose rate, and interval between fractions. Total dose is not relevant beyond recognized thresholds of clinically apparent changes. Subacute and late reactions are dependent on both time–dose factors and the total cumulative dose.[80,82] Slowly proliferating tissues evidence subacute radiation changes, typified by the vascular connective tissues such as

pericardium and small blood vessels of the kidney and liver.[81] Late responding tissues are frequently nonproliferative; radiation effects have been attributed to parenchymal depletion secondary to endothelial changes in small blood vessels or, alternatively, to direct depletion of parenchymal or stromal cells as an effect of radiation exposure.[79,81–83] The dose–survival relation for late effects differs from that of acute responses: injury to slowly responding tissues is more dependent on fraction size (Fig. 11-23).[28] The relation is most easily summarized by the divergence in acute and late effects of the same tissue (*e.g.,* small bowel, skin, or mucous membranes) with increasing dose per fraction. For example, skin and small bowel show nearly equivalent acute reactions with fractions of 150 to 350 cGy but far more serious late changes as the fraction size increases within that range.[28,84]

Acute effects of irradiation are expected reactions, differing to some degree according to individual susceptibility. Combinations of irradiation and prior or concurrent chemotherapy may enhance acute reactions; for instance, epithelial reactions are heightened with concurrent dactinomycin or, less predictably, prior cisplatin. It is important to recognize the *lack* of correlation between acute reactions and late visceral effects of irradiation.[81] Acute changes require supportive management and should not affect planned therapy unless they are so severe as to force undesirable interruptions in treatment.

Late irradiation effects are the dose-limiting factors in curative irradiation. Interactions with other modalities often define or limit the dose of irradiation from otherwise curative levels. Prior or subsequent surgery increases the risks of adhesions, stricture, fistulas, and tissue necrosis. Chemotherapy during, before, or after irradiation may reduce the tolerance of

FIGURE 11-23. Isoeffect curves for acute (*dotted lines*) and late (*solid lines*) effects of irradiation. Note the relatively steep slope of the late effects, indicating a quantitatively greater increase in late effects with larger doses per fraction. The acute effects show relatively less incremental change with increase in dose per fraction. (Thames HD et al: Changes in early and late radiation responses with altered dose fractionation: Implications for dose–survival relationships. Int J Radiat Oncol Biol Phys 8:219–226, 1982)

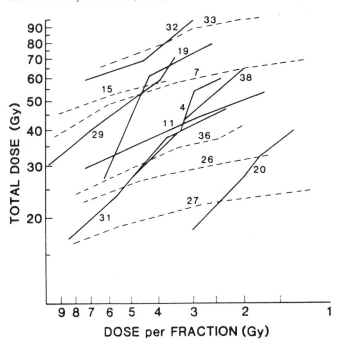

the brain, liver, heart, lungs, or kidneys to irradiation.[81,85] Attention to late visceral effects defines tolerance doses for anatomic regions, challenging both the physical (dosimetric) and biological (fractionation) principles of therapeutic irradiation.

Acute Reactions

Immediate radiation reactions include transient cutaneous erythema (a little-noticed, mild erythema lasting several hours after the initial fraction), sialadenitis (often occurring within several hours of the first two or three fractions and resolving spontaneously thereafter), and xerostomia (symptomatically noted within several days of irradiation encompassing the salivary glands). Fatigue accompanies wide-field irradiation. Appetite suppression, nausea, and vomiting occur unpredictably, related both to objective factors (best expressed as the *integral dose,* defined as the dose/fraction multiplied by the volume subtended) and emotional reactions (most evident in adolescents).

Progressive erythema or hyperpigmentation begins during the second or third week of fractionated irradiation. With supervoltage irradiation, reactions are generally limited to dry radioepidermitis, with transient flaking and hyperpigmentation resolving over several weeks. Tangentially irradiated surfaces show more intense reactions, the build-up effect of supervoltage occurring within the epidermis due to beam entry essentially perpendicular to the curved surface. Similarly, cutaneous folds such as the intergluteal fold or groins show greater reactions as the epidermis is "buried" beneath the lower-dose entry volume. Moist radioepidermitis may occur in such areas at doses above 30 to 40 Gy and is marked by incomplete or total denudation of the dermis. The lack of skin-sparing with electrons results in similar moist reactions with doses above 30 to 40 Gy. In moist reactions, repopulation occurs from the periphery as well as from central foci of apparently radioresistant epidermal cells, covering the ulcerated areas with pale, thin epidermis even during therapy. Moist radioepidermitis heals with permanently hypopigmented atrophic skin and telangiectasis. To promote healing, dry radioepidermitis is best managed by lanolin-based lubricants; symptomatic areas of locally intense reactions respond to rinsing with dilute hydrogen peroxide and regular applications of moisturing ointments.

Radioepithelitis of the mucous membranes occurs slightly earlier than cutaneous changes. A tumor false membrane of superficial mucosal ulceration and fibrinous exudate may appear over or within primary tumors of the upper aerodigestive tract during the first week of treatment. The normal mucosa shows diffuse enanthema by the 15th to 21st day, which progresses to focal or confluent superficial ulceration with or without an overlying pseudomembrane of fibrinous debris. Frequent rinsing with dilute hydrogen peroxide will clear much of the thick mucus and superficial debris. Symptomatic treatment with analgesics, liquid antacids, and local anesthetics must be initiated early to encourage adequate oral nutrition. The addition of anticandidal agents may be needed; close observation is required to identify candidal superinfection (see Chap. 39). With treatment fields including much of the upper alimentary tract, a nasogastric feeding tube (if tolerated) or intravenous hyperalimentation may be necessary.

Hair loss is noted during the third week of therapy. Return begins 3 to 4 months after irradiation; with supervoltage, hair regrowth occurs almost uniformly below doses of 45 to 50 Gy. Tangentially irradiated regions (*e.g.,* the occipital region with posterior fossa irradiation) may show less or no regrowth at such doses.

Hematologic Effects of Irradiation

The acute effects of irradiation on the bone marrow often limit the continuity of wide-field irradiation or intensive combined chemotherapy–radiation therapy. Abdominal or thoracic irradiation includes at least 15% to 25% of the active bone marrow in children. More than 25% to 30% of the proliferating marrow in children younger than 5 years is in the extremities; by adolescence, the active marrow concentrates in the pelvis, vertebrae, ribs, and sternum. The calvarium accounts for approximately 10% by age 20 years.[86,87]

Radiation therapy produces rapid pronounced lymphopenia (Fig. 11-24). Described even with limited-volume treatment, the effects on lymphocytes have been most extensively studied during wide-field conventionally fractionated irradiation (*e.g.,* craniospinal and total nodal irradiation). Measurable lymphopenia occurs within 1 to 3 days of starting therapy; by day 5 or 6, the total lymphocyte count is one fourth of the initial value.[87] The rapid fall in lymphocytes is the result of unique intermitotic cell death in addition to delayed lethality with cellular division.[88] Both B cells and T cells fall rapidly with irradiation; the proportional reduction in B lymphocytes is greater. The small, resting lymphocytes are more sensitive to irradiation than the large, transformed cells.[88] Among the T-cell population, the inducer T cells are most affected; T-cell lymphopenia relatively spares the suppressor T-cell population.[89] Postirradiation recovery is noted within 1 to 3 months for B cells; reduction in T-cell numbers and function persists for more than 1 to 5 years after extended-field irradiation.[90,91]

Neutrophils decline after the first week of irradiation, reaching a nadir 2 to 3 weeks into therapy. Absolute neutrophil counts will frequently plateau at 35% to 40% of initial levels; prior chemotherapy or irradiation results in a more pronounced fall.[79,87] Recovery of peripheral neutrophil counts is noted 1 to 2 months postirradiation.

A quantitatively variable reduction in platelet counts generally parallels that of neutrophils; previously untreated patients often show little thrombocytopenia even with extensive irradiation.[79,87] With sequential supradiaphragmatic and infradiaphragmatic irradiation in Hodgkin's disease, platelets usually fall to one third of initial levels only during the latter treatment.[87,92]

Monocytes decrease acutely, evidencing rapid recovery during a course of radiation therapy.[87] Occasional instances of absolute eosinophilia have been documented.

The effect of irradiation is largely on the uncommitted stem cells (CFU$_s$).[93] The committed unipotential stem cells (CFU$_c$) tend to be less radiosensitive.[94] With wide-volume irradiation, stem cell activity increases in the unirradiated hematopoietic marrow.[86] Repopulation occurs from migration of stimulated stem cells into the irradiated volume.[95,96] The extent of recovery depends on dose and volume: the degree of regeneration is inversely related to the volume of marrow irradiated. With limited fields (*e.g.,* local mediastinal irradiation), it is unusual to see repopulation after doses above 35 to 40 Gy.[97,98] Local regeneration is more common after wide-field irradiation; recovery beyond 1 year is noted in 50% of patients receiving 40 Gy in 4 weeks to supradiaphragmatic and infradiaphragmatic fields for Hodgkin's disease.[99,100] Further regeneration and expansion of the active marrow into sites such as the proximal humerus or femur occur as long as 3 years after such therapy.[99,100]

The degree of bone-marrow regeneration is greater in young children. Sacks and colleagues, using radionuclide marrow imaging to quantify hematopoietic function, ascertained that relative activity at or beyond 1 year following 30 to 40 Gy to wide marrow fields is 1.5-fold greater in children than it is in

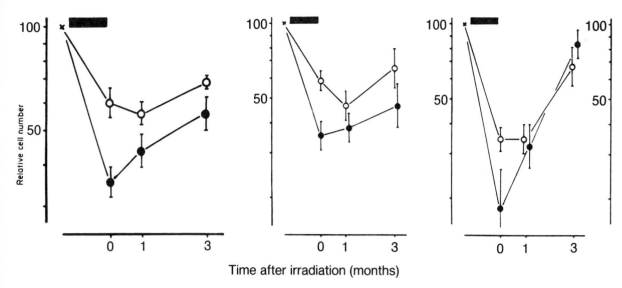

FIGURE 11-24. Changes in circulating lymphocytes after regional radiation therapy. Relative decrease in total lymphocyte (**left**), T-cell (**middle**), and B-cell (**right**) populations are shown following "local" (*open circles*) and "extended" (*closed circles*) irradiation for breast cancer. T-cell reduction is quantitatively less, but recovery is prolonged beyond 3 to 24 months. B-cell reduction is more rapid and pronounced, but complete recovery is usually evident within 3 months after therapy. (Idestrom K et al: Changes of the peripheral lymphocyte population following radiation therapy to extended and limited fields. Int J Radiat Oncol Biol Phys 5:1761–1766, 1979)

20- to 40-year-old adults and two times greater in adults older than 40 years.[100] With doses above 40 Gy, the differential recovery is twofold and threefold for the respective age groups.[100]

Bone-marrow failure is the cause of death after acute total-body irradiation exposures between 5 Gy and 10 Gy. Following total-body exposure to 5 Gy, 50% of people die within 30 days from the secondary effects of neutropenia or thrombocytopenia. At 10 Gy, 100% of individuals die from secondary consequences of bone-marrow failure within 30 days.

Visceral Effects

Postirradiation pneumonitis is a subacute reaction occurring 1 to 3 months after treatment (Table 11-4). Radiographic findings (early alveolar or subacute interstitial densities confined to the irradiated volume) are often the only sign (Fig. 11-25); less than 5% to 10% of patients present with cough, dyspnea, and low-grade fever. Postirradiation pneumonitis is usually self-limited. Corticosteroids are effective only in ameliorating symptoms; cautious use of these drugs is indicated in cases with progressive symptoms.

With irradiation to more than 20% to 30% of the lung volume, subacute pneumonitis occurs with increasing frequency following doses in excess of 25 to 30 Gy. In conjunction with chemotherapy (especially dactinomycin or bleomycin), there is an estimated 5% likelihood of pneumonitis at 20 Gy and 50% at 24 Gy using 150- to 200-cGy fractions.[101] Tolerance for whole-lung irradiation is estimated at 18 to 20 Gy in 10 to 12 fractions.[81] In children also receiving chemotherapy, whole-lung irradiation is usually limited to 15 to 18 Gy in 100 to 150-cGy fractions. Following single-fraction whole-lung irradiation, such as with total-body irradiation, there is a threshold of recognizable pulmonary effects at 7.0 Gy, with a rapid increase in the frequency of clinically significant pneumonitis to 100% fatality above 11 to 12 Gy.[102] The pathophysiology of pneumonitis is immediate injury to alveolar type II cells.[103] In animal models, capillary endothelial changes are identifiable ultrastructurally within 5 days, preceding by several weeks the histologic changes that correlate with the clinical syndrome.[104]

Late pulmonary changes are most apparent as decreased lung compliance secondary to interstitial fibrosis (also see Chap. 50). Changes are most marked following significant subacute pneumonitis, resolving with "fibrosis of substitution."[1] Decreases in total lung capacity, vital capacity, and diffusion have been described beyond 6 to 12 months after doses in excess of 30 to 35 Gy.[105–107] In children treated for pulmonary metastases, a 25% to 30% reduction in total lung capacity and compliance has been described.[108,109] Significant chronic effects in general are limited to changes in residual lung volume and a decrease in diffusion capacity, dependent both on the volume of lung irradiation and on the combined use of chemotherapy.[110]

Postirradiation pericarditis has been documented in 3% to 7% of patients after mediastinal irradiation.[111,112] Pericardial effusion is apparent on imaging studies; 50% to 80% of patients experience symptoms of pain, fever, or dyspnea.[112,113] Onset has been documented between 2 months and 2.5 years postirradiation; the median time of onset has ranged from 6 to 18 months. The disease is usually self-limited; corticosteroids are indicated to relieve progressive symptoms or for objective signs of constrictive pericarditis, which infrequently progresses to cardiac tamponade. A small proportion of cases evolve to late chronic pericarditis.[114] The incidence of postirradiation pericarditis in patients receiving treatment to more than 50% of the cardiac volume increases with dose and fraction size.[111] Above 50 Gy, there is an estimated 20% frequency of documented pericarditis.[111] Previous radiotherapy techniques for Hodgkin's disease delivered excessive anterior mediastinal doses (greater than 50–55 Gy); follow-up studies have shown a 25% to 28% incidence of pericarditis in this population.[112,113]

Late cardiac effects include diffuse myocardial fibrosis and potential coronary artery thrombosis. Rabbit models of cardiac

Table 11-4
Radiation Dose Toxicity Levels for Subacute and Late Visceral Effects

Organ	Toxicity	Whole Organ Irradiation			Partial Organ Irradiation				Chemotherapy Effect
		5–10% Incidence	Dose*	>25–50% Incidence	Volume	<5–10% Incidence	Dose*	>25–50% Incidence	
Lung	Subacute pneumonitis or late fibrosis	18–20 Gy 15–18	(CTx−)† (CTx+)‡	24–25 Gy 21–24	<30% of one lung	25–30 Gy <20	(CTx−)† (CTx+)‡	45–50 Gy >35	++
Heart	Subacute pericarditis	35–40		>50	<50%	40–50		60–70	+/−
	Late cardiomyopathy	45–50 30–40	(CTx−) (CTx+)	>60 >50	<25%	<40 30–40	(CTx−) (CTx+)	>70 >50	+++
Liver	Subacute hepatopathy	25–30 20–25	(CTx−) (CTx+)	>40 >35	<60%	NA§		NA	+
Kidney	Subacute or late nephropathy	18–20 16–18	(CTx−) (CTx+)	24–28 22–26	>50%	20–24		>30	+
	Late hypertension	Similar to subacute levels			>50%	20–25		>35	+/−
Small bowel	Subacute enteropathy	15–25		>40	<50%	20–25		>60	+
Brain	Late necrosis	54–60		>65	<50%	Equal to whole brain			+
Spinal cord	Subacute-late myelopathy	40–45		>50	<15	45–50		>55	−

* Dose assumes conventional fractionation (150–200 cGy one daily, 5 days per week).
† (CTx−) implies without prior, concurrent, or subsequent chemotherapy.
‡ (CTx+) implies interaction with one or more chemotherapeutic agent(s) in any sequence.
§ NA = not applicable.

injury show a primary radiation effect on capillary endothelial cells, with subsequent ischemia due to altered microvascularity resulting in late myocardial fibrosis.[83,115] Pericardial thickening, morphologic changes of the aortic and mitral valves, and ventricular dysfunction have been described in as many as 10% of patients studied more than 5 years after cardiac irradiation to doses exceeding 40 Gy.[116] Only in series using outdated anterior mediastinal techniques or repeat courses of irradiation for Hodgkin's disease has the incidence of major functional abnormalities been significant, approaching 50% in two such series.[116,117] Despite altered capacities on functional studies, to date only 10% of patients in the latter series have had symptoms or signs of cardiac disease.[118] Coronary artery disease has been attributed to radiation therapy.[119] Although it is difficult to differentiate this event from naturally occurring arterial disease, the few cases of young Hodgkin's-disease survivors developing myocardial infarction indicate a possible connection between irradiation and coronary artery occlusions.[119,120]

Postirradiation hepatopathy is a subacute syndrome more often manifest by morphologic and biochemical changes than in clinical signs of hepatic dysfunction. Abnormal radionuclide or CT imaging reflects relative changes in liver function limited to the irradiated volume (Fig. 11-26). Transient elevation of alkaline phosphatase is often the only biochemical reflection of asymptomatic postirradiation changes.[121,122] Clinical hepatopathy occurs within 1 to 3 months, usually following doses to the entire liver exceeding 30 to 35 Gy. Hepatomegaly, jaundice, and ascites accompany pronounced biochemical findings, thrombocytopenia, and diffuse alterations in liver morphology on radionuclide study.[123] The incidence of clinical postirradiation hepatopathy in routine pediatric radiotherapy is relatively low: liver dysfunction was noted in 9% of children following hepatic irradiation in the second National Wilms' Tumor Study (NWTS-2).[124] Clinical and chemical signs are usually self-limited, resolving over several months with supportive medical management.[121] Ensuing chronic hepatic dysfunction has been rare.[123,125] Fatal hepatic failure occurs

rarely; three cases were reported in NWTS-2, representing less than 1% of all children with abdominal irradiation and 2% of those with whole-liver irradiation.[124] Life-threatening hepatopathy has usually followed irradiation with prior or concurrent liver damage (*e.g.,* malnutrition, parenchymal liver metastases), concurrent multiagent chemotherapy, or partial hepatectomy.[121,126] It has been suggested that children tolerate liver irradiation with less likelihood of overt injury than adults, although the use of combined chemotherapy–irradiation requires appropriate caution during treatment to the entire liver volume.

Treatment-related hepatopathy is a veno-occlusive phenomenon. Clinical and laboratory studies show a primary endothelial reaction in the central veins followed by a pattern of centrilobular congestion, secondary sinusoidal congestion, and hepatocyte atrophy.[81,125,127] Chronic changes are marked by various degrees of fibrosis involving the central veins and hepatic portal regions.[125]

Postirradiation nephropathy presents as a subacute or late renal reaction. "Acute radiation nephritis" is a subacute syndrome appearing 6 to 12 months after treatment exceeding 24 to 28 Gy in 3 to 5 weeks to more than 50% of the functioning renal volume. Clinically, signs mimic the nephrotic syndrome, with hypertension, edema, proteinurea, and azotemia. With medical management, there is resolution to a chronic phase of various degrees of renal dysfunction and hypertension.[128,130,131]

Chronic postirradiation nephropathy represents either the late effects of the acute syndrome or, more commonly, *de novo* mild-to-moderate hypertension, proteinuria, and azotemia occurring 2 to 3 years after treatment. Late effects may be limited to hypertension, the more common "benign" hypertension noted 3 to 7 years postirradiation. More significant "malignant" hypertension occurs less often, usually with onset 18 to 24 months after therapy.

The pathophysiology of radiation-induced nephropathy has classically been related to a primary arteriolonephrosclerosis.[79] Obliterative endothelial changes in the glomerular arte-

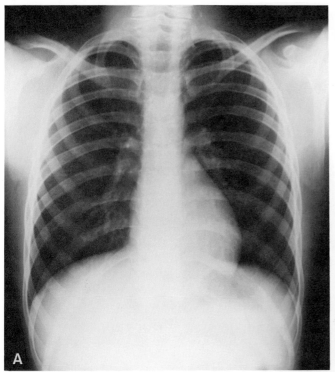

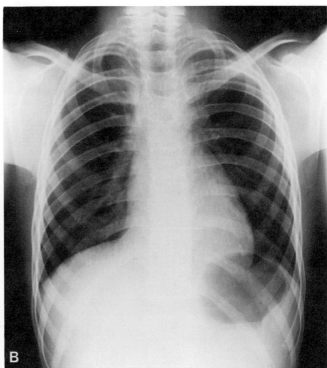

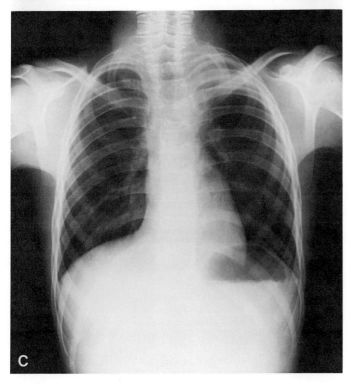

FIGURE 11-25. Serial radiographic changes follow mantle field irradiation for Hodgkin's disease. Note negative mediastinum preirradiation (**A**), with appearance of interstitial infiltrates in the superior mediastinum 3 months after irradiation (**B**) associated with minor respiratory symptoms. Late fibrosis (**C**) is seen in a distribution limited to the region of the subacute resection.

rioles have been noted in animal models, preceding a secondary decrease in renal tubular epithelium. A second hypothesis of primary vascular damage implicates direct effects on the capillaries, with subsequent glomerular sclerosis and delayed tubular disruption.[132] Conflicting recent reports suggest a primary effect on the regenerating tubular epithelium rather than the renal vessels; it may not be feasible to identify the initiating event in humans, as the late effects of secondary hypertension with consequent arteriolar changes obscure the inciting tissue

change.[133] Combinations of chemotherapy and irradiation further limit the tolerance levels in children (Table 11-4).[134] With dactinomycin or Adriamycin, renal tolerance is estimated at 16 to 18 Gy to the entire renal volume. Unilateral renal irradiation to levels of 22 Gy in 5 to 6 weeks has been associated with a 50% likelihood of decreased glomerular filtration rate, progressive atrophy, and late benign hypertension; functional changes are usually transitory and self-limited.[135] The kidney is more sensitive to irradiation during the compensatory hyper-

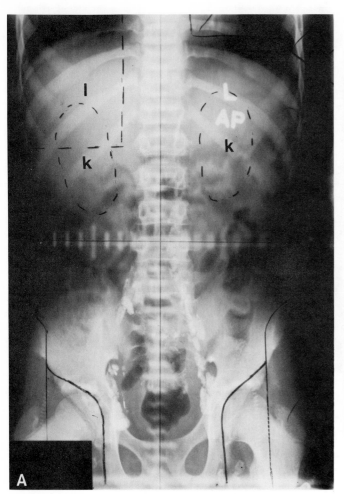

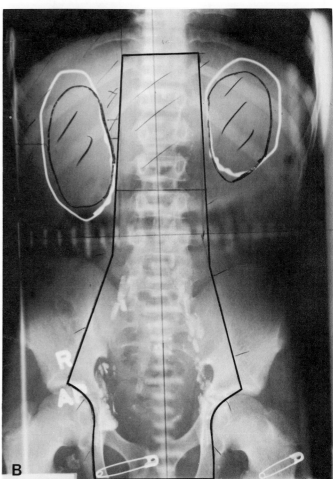

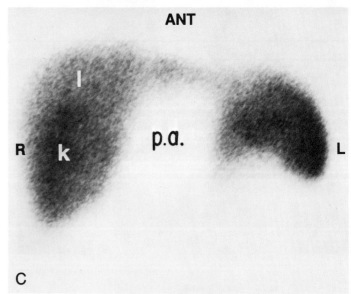

FIGURE 11-26. Irradiation-induced changes in radionuclide liver scan. Whole abdominal irradiation (**A**) incorporated kidney blocks (*k*, at 16 Gy) and a block to the right lobe of the liver (*l*, at 21 Gy). Following 30 Gy to the wide abdominal fields, reduced fields to the para-aortic and pelvic regions (**B**) received a total of 45 Gy. Liver scan 2 months after irradiation (**C**) shows graded reduction in uptake corresponding to individual dose levels under the kidney (*k*) and liver (*L*) blocks; little activity is apparent within the geometric region corresponding to the high-dose para-aortic fields (*p.a.*).

trophy phase following contralateral nephrectomy; doses to the remaining kidney are limited to 14 to 15 Gy in this setting.[136,137]

Subacute or late enteropathy occurs in as many as one fourth to one third of children following abdominal surgery, irradiation, and chemotherapy.[138] Doses as low as 15 Gy have

been associated with focal small-bowel obstruction, often requiring simple lysis of adhesions to relieve edematous obstruction at the level of prior surgical resection.[138]

Postirradiation changes in endocrine function are largely delayed effects, noted months to years after treatment to fields that include the hypothalamic–pituitary region or the thyroid gland. Following cranial irradiation at 24 Gy in 12 to 16 fractions for acute lymphoblastic leukemia, there is a measurable reduction in stimulated growth hormone levels.[139] Linear growth remains relatively unaffected at this dose.[140] A more significant long-term reduction in growth-hormone secretion occurs in children after 45 to 55 Gy, associated with a significant fall-off in linear growth.[141–143] Although they are more apparent in children, reduced growth-hormone levels are also apparent in adults after more than 50 Gy.[144] Thyroid-stimulating hormone (TSH) levels measured after stimulation with releasing hormones are subnormal after pituitary–hypothalamic irradiation in children.[145] Hyposecretion of other hypothalamic–pituitary hormones has been noted less often; reduced adrenocorticotropic hormone (ACTH) response, follicle-stimulating hormone (FSH), and luteinizing hormone have been reported in addition to hypersecretion of prolactin.[144,146]

Direct effects on the thyroid gland result in a dose-related incidence of chemical hypothyroidism, most frequently described in children treated for Hodgkin's disease. With doses below 25 to 26 Gy, isolated elevation of TSH has been reported in approximately 20% of children.[147] At doses of 25 to 40 Gy, more than 75% of children have elevated TSH levels at a median of 18 to 30 months; one fourth of those with high TSH values have subnormal levels of T_4. Recovery of thyroid function beyond 3 to 5 years has been documented in a few cases.[147]

Although relatively resistant to irradiation in adults, Leydig cells in boys appear to be fairly sensitive to irradiation. Decreased testosterone and elevated FSH levels occur after testicular doses of approximately 24 Gy; the degree of later recovery is uncertain.[148,149] Alterations in ovarian endocrine dysfunction are apparent in more than 50% of adolescents and young women after doses as low as 250 to 400 cGy. Temporary amenorrhea or irregular menses are noted within 1 to 4 months after treatment.[150] Recovery is age related, permanent amenorrhea and infertility occurring in approximately 30% of younger women after 400 cGy compared to 100% of women older than 40 years.[151]

Central Nervous System Effects

Acute effects on the central nervous system are uncommon. With conventional fractionation, one occasionally sees exaggeration of existent neurologic signs in the presence of a space-occupying intracranial lesion. Following single fractions of 750 to 1000 cGy, acute neurologic deterioration occurs in as many as 50% of patients with known intracerebral pathology.[152] Early death following radiation exposure of 10,000 cGy or more (*e.g.*, nuclear accident) is due to immediate central nervous system reactions.

Subacute reactions are relatively mild, transient effects on the brain and spinal cord. A postirradiation syndrome has been documented in 30% to 50% of patients treated for acute lymphoblastic leukemia; it presents as somnolence, anorexia, nausea, and sometimes fever 4 to 8 weeks after irradiation (see Chap. 16).[153] With primary intracranial neoplasms, it is common to see transient exacerbation of local neurologic signs in addition to the malaise and appetite suppression that mark the subacute period.[154] A similar phenomenon following spinal cord irradiation presents as Lhermitte's syndrome with shock-like paresthesias of the extremities during neck flexion. Subacute reactions are generally self-limited, only occasionally requiring treatment (corticosteroids for pronounced symptoms). The pathophysiology is believed to be related to a transient demyelination.[155,156] Perhaps the most important factor in clinical management is the recognition of subacute postirradiation

phenomena and the knowledge that such changes do not correlate either with progression of the primary disease or with later development of cerebral necrosis or myelopathy.[156,157]

Late effects on the central nervous system often limit both the volume and the intensity of treatment. The most pronounced cerebral effect is postirradiation necrosis, a well-defined entity occurring 6 months to many years after treatment, most often between 6 months and 2 years.[157] Symptoms and signs of focal neurologic dysfunction accompany CT or magnetic resonance imaging (MRI) changes confirming injury to the white matter.[158,159] The diagnosis is easily rendered after incidental cerebral irradiation for extraneural malignancies, whereas the condition is often difficult to differentiate from recurrent or progressive tumor following treatment of primary intracranial neoplasms.[158,160] Management of clinically significant cerebral necrosis may be conservative (with corticosteroids) or interventive (with surgery to establish the diagnosis and, potentially, resect the necrotic focus when location and extent permit).[161] In most reported instances, this complication has ultimately proved fatal. The pathophysiology appears to relate primarily to reparative changes in the endothelium of small vessels, with scattered focal or confluent areas of ischemic, coagulative brain necrosis.[81,162] Direct effects on glial tissue are believed to contribute to late cerebral changes.[157,162] With conventional fractionation (*i.e.*, daily doses of 150–220 cGy), postirradiation cerebral necrosis has rarely been documented below cumulative doses of 60 to 70 Gy.[157] A threshold

FIGURE 11-27. Subacute and late leukoencephalopathy following postirradiation systemic methotrexate. Paraventricular areas of decreased white-matter attenuation (*a*) are typical of leukoencephalopathy superimposed upon late post-treatment calcifications (*b*) in the region of the gray–white matter junction.

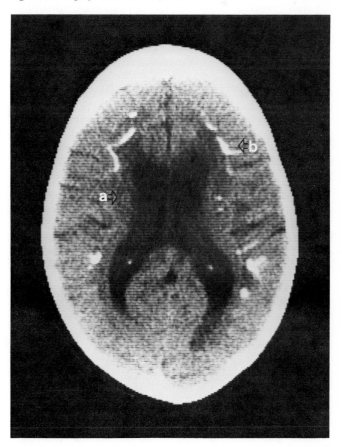

level of 54 Gy has been reported.[163] The most critical determinant is dose per fraction; virtually all cases reported after total doses of less than 60 Gy followed treatment with more than 250 to 300 cGy per fraction.[157,164] An incidence of 0.04% to 0.4% has been estimated following 50 to 54 Gy at 180 to 200 cGy per fraction.[157] Postirradiation myelopathy is similarly related to fraction size and the length of the spinal cord subtended.[165] Clinically presenting most often as a Brown–Sequard syndrome, myelopathy occurs with rapidly increasing incidence at doses above 45 to 50 Gy using conventional fractionation.

An interaction of chemotherapy and irradiation in central nervous system effects has been difficult to define except with methotrexate (see Chaps. 9 and 16). Necrotizing leukoencephalopathy is a subacute syndrome of lethargy, seizures, perceptual changes, and cerebellar dysfunction with characteristic white-matter changes on CT and MRI (Fig. 11-27).[166] It has been noted almost exclusively in the setting of high-dose intravenous methotrexate following otherwise-tolerated doses of irradiation (*i.e.*, 24 Gy/12 to 16 fractions).[166,167] Cerebral atrophy and calcifications related histologically to mineralizing microangiopathy appear to follow low-dose cranial irradiation in conjunction with intrathecal or systemic methotrexate.[168–170]

An age relationship has been suggested both for mineralizing microangiopathy and postirradiation cerebral necrosis.[162,168] The age effect has been documented only in primate studies to date, with increased focal necrosis and significant neurologic signs in prepubertal monkeys.[162] The most important age-related clinical correlation has been with neuropsychologic effects. Deficits in intellectual function have been noted both in survivors of acute lymphoblastic leukemia and in brain tumor populations.[142,171–175] Alterations in IQ scores and memory appear to be most pronounced in children younger than 4 to 6 years at the time of irradiation.[171,172,175,176] Although the incidence and degree of neuropsychologic dysfunction are as yet poorly documented, the occurrence of identifiable learning difficulties beyond 1 to 3 years after treatment appears to relate to supratentorial irradiation.[175,177,178]

Reproductive Effects

Azoospermia is apparent within 6 to 8 weeks following fractionated doses as low as 200 cGy.[179] Recovery is dose related, with gradually improving oligospermia documented 3 to 5 years after doses of 200 to 500 cGy.[179] The dose scattered to the testes during full dose (35–40 Gy) "inverted-Y" irradiation for Hodgkin's disease results in 200 to 400 cGy cumulatively; as many as 25% of men show residual oligospermia 5 years after treatment.[180,181] The radiation effect is directly on the mitotically active spermatogonia. Irradiation effects appear to be less pronounced in prepubertal testes.[182]

Infertility in females is believed to be secondary to direct effects on the ovarian follicles rather than on the postmitotic oocytes. A clear dose–response relation for permanent amenorrhea and infertility has not been established; in adolescents and young women, successful pregnancy has occurred in nearly 60% after doses of 250 to 650 cGy to the ovaries.[150] Despite morphologic changes (severe follicular depletion) and elevated FSH after irradiation for Wilms' tumor with estimated doses exceeding 1000 to 3000 cGy, subsequent fertility has been noted in a proportion of prepubertal girls.[183–185]

Somatic Effects

Changes in bone growth and soft-tissue development are the most readily identifiable consequences of irradiation in young children. Alterations in bone growth are dependent on age,

dose, and type of radiations. Qualitative changes in vertebral development are noted almost uniformly following irradiation in children younger than 13 to 15 years of age. Classic effects include horizontal growth-arrest lines, irregular vertebral flattening, and distorted contour.[186] Scoliosis has been most apparent in young children treated with orthovoltage irradiation to fields extending to the midline, resulting in asymmetric irradiation of the two vertebral growth centers. Scoliosis often is noted only after the adolescent growth spurt.[187] The degree of scoliosis in the orthovoltage experience was dose dependent: mild radiographic angulation (0–25°) noted after approximately 25 to 32 Gy and significant scoliosis (greater than 25°) after doses exceeding 32 to 36 Gy.[187] Vertebral abnormalities are less pronounced with supervoltage. With supervoltage fields intentionally encompassing the full vertebral width, it is uncommon to note significant scoliosis below 35 Gy.[188,189] Significant reduction in vertebral height has been seen primarily in children treated before age 6 years or during the pubertal growth spurt (Fig. 11-28).[189]

Irradiation of the epiphyseal growth centers of long bones results in age-dependent reduction in linear growth. With doses of only 6 to 10 Gy, measurable changes approximating 2 cm have been noted in infants.[190] At more than 40 Gy, discrepancies in bone growth may exceed 2 to 12 cm, proportional to the amount of residual growth normally expected in the affected bone.[190] Similar dose levels produce delay or arrest of tooth development following mandibular exposure.[191]

Effects on muscle and soft-tissue development with supervoltage often exceed those on growing bone. Hypoplastic muscle development is commonly apparent after treatment of preadolescent children.[192]

FIGURE 11-28.   Changes in vertebral bodies 6 years after abdominal irradiation (24 Gy) for Wilms' tumor was done in a patient at age 4 years. Note decreased height at the vertebrae below T10, scalloped contour, and irregular decrease in bone density.

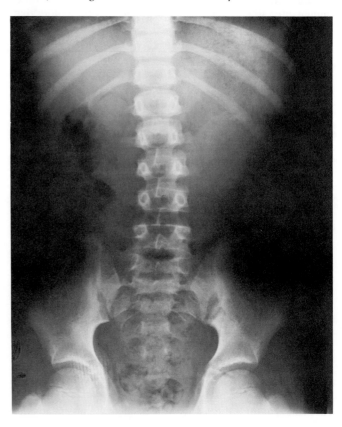

Carcinogenesis

Radiation carcinogenesis has been well documented in population studies.[193] The frequency of secondary cancer is one of the most important determinants of the risk:benefit ratio of radiation in children. Following orthovoltage irradiation, the actuarial incidence of treatment-related tumors was 14% in long-term survivors in a large pediatric series.[194] Although correlated to both radiation therapy and alkylating agents, 90% of the tumors occurred within the irradiated volume, with a median time to onset of 9 years.[194] The occurrence following supervoltage exposure has not been well quantified. In a single-institution series of 330 cases followed 5 to 30 years (median = 14 years), the incidence of secondary malignant tumors was 1% within the treated volume and 0.7% "out of field."[195] A similar frequency (4 of 426) of irradiation-related malignant tumors has been reported from the Intergroup Rhabdomyosarcoma Study in longer-than-5-year survivors.[196] Secondary benign tumors (e.g., osteochondroma, meningioma) occur with twice the frequency of malignant tumors.[195,197]

The risk of radiation-related neoplasms is higher in children with genetically determined disorders (e.g., neurofibromatosis, xeroderma pigmentosum).[198] Specific childhood cancers such as genetic forms of retinoblastoma and nevoid basal-cell carcinoma are associated with a marked incidence of secondary tumors, exceeding 15% to 20% after supervoltage irradiation for retinoblastoma.[199,200] A single report estimating a 90% risk of secondary tumors following irradiation for retinoblastoma has not been confirmed in other series.[201] In a major multi-institutional survey of carcinogenic effects in children, fully one third of cases occurred in the survivors of the relatively uncommon genetically related cancers.[198]

REFERENCES

1. del Regato JA, Spjut HJ, Cox JD: Cancer: Diagnosis, Treatment, and Prognosis, pp 59–92. St Louis, CV Mosby, 1985
2. Coutard H: Principles of X-ray therapy of malignant disorders. Lancet 2:1–12, 1934
3. Brown JM: Sensitizers and protectors in radiotherapy. Cancer 55:2222–2228, 1985
4. Thompson LH, Suit HD: Proliferation kinetics of X-irradiated mouse L cells studied with time-lapse photography II. Int J Radiat Biol 15:347–362, 1969
5. Hopwood LE, Tolmach LJ: Manifestations of damage from ionizing radiation in mammalian cells in the postirradiation generations. Adv Radiat Biol 8:317–362, 1979
6. Malaise EP, Fertil B, Chavaudra N, Guichard M: Distribution of radiation sensitivities for human tumor cells of specific histologic types: Comparison of in vitro to in vivo data. Int J Radiat Oncol Biol Phys 12:617–624, 1986
7. Weichselbaum RR, Little JB: X-ray sensitivity and repair in human tumour cells. In Steel GG, Adams GE, Peckham MJ (eds): The Biological Basis of Radiotherapy, pp 113–121. Amsterdam, Elsevier, 1983
8. Hall EJ: Radiation dose-rate: A factor of importance in radiobiology and radiotherapy. Br J Radiol 43:81–97, 1972
9. Sinclair WK: Cell cycle dependence of the lethal radiation response in mammalian cells. Curr Topics Radiat Res 7:264–285, 1972
10. Steel GG: Growth Kinetics of Tumours. Oxford, Clarenden Press, 1977
11. Moulder JE, Rockwell S: Tumor hypoxia: Its impact on cancer therapy. Cancer Metastasis Rev (in press)
12. Barendsen GW, Broerse JJ: Experimental radiotherapy of a rat rhabdomyosarcoma with 15 MeV neutrons and 300 kV X-rays. Eur J Cancer 5:373–391, 1969
13. Withers HR: Biologic basis for high-LET radiotherapy. Radiology 108:131–137, 1973
14. Tobias CA: The future of heavy-ion science in biology and medicine. Radiat Res 103:1–33, 1985
15. Broerse JJ, Batterman JJ: Fast neutron radiotherapy: For equal or for better. Med Phys 8:751–760, 1981
16. Brown JM: Clinical trials of radiosensitizers: What should we expect? Int J Radiat Oncol Biol Phys 10:425–429, 1984
17. Dische S: Chemical sensitizers for hypoxic cells: A decade of experience in clinical radiotherapy. Radiother Oncol 3:97–115, 1985
18. Rose C, Lustig R, McIntosh N, Teicher B: A clinical trial of Fluosol DA 20% in advanced squamous cell carcinoma of the head and neck. Int J Radiat Oncol Biol Phys 12:1315–1318, 1986
19. Trott KR, Maciejewski B, Preuss-Bayer G, Skolyszewski J: Dose–response curve and split-dose recovery in human skin cancer. Radiother Oncol 2:123–129, 1984
20. Trott KR: Experimental results and clinical implications of the four R's in fractionated radiotherapy. Radiat Environ Biophys 20:159–170, 1982
21. Fowler JF: Potential for increasing the differential response between tumors and normal tissues: Can proliferation rate be used? Int J Radiat Oncol Biol Phys 12:641–645, 1986
22. Withers HR: Biologic basis for altered fractionation schemes. Cancer 55:2086–2095, 1985
23. Rockwell S, Moulder JE: Biological factors of importance in split-course radiotherapy. In Paliwal BR, Herbert DE, Orton CG (eds): Optimization of Cancer Radiotherapy, pp 171–182. New York, American Institute of Physics, 1985
24. Cox JD: Large-dose fractionation: Hypofractionation. Cancer 55:2105–2111, 1985
25. Fletcher GH: Key note address: The scientific basis of the present and future practice of clinical radiotherapy. Int J Radiat Oncol Biol Phys 9:1073–1082, 1983
26. Fischer JJ, Fischer DB: The determination of time–dose relationships from clinical data. Br J Radiol 44:785–792, 1971
27. Kallman RF: The phenomena of reoxygenation and its implications for fractionated radiotherapy. Radiology 105:135–142, 1972
28. Thames HD, Withers HR, Peters LJ, Fletcher GH: Changes in early and late radiation responses with altered dose fractionation: Implications for dose–survival relationships. Int J Radiat Oncol Biol Phys 8:219–226, 1982
29. Ellis F: Dose, time and fractionation: A clinical hypothesis. Clin Radiol 20:1–7, 1969
30. Moulder JE, Dutreix J, Rockwell S, Siemann DW: Applicability of animal tumor data to cancer therapy in humans. Int J Radiat Oncol Biol Phys (submitted)
31. Johns HE, Cunningham JR (eds): The Physics of Radiology, pp 133–166. Springfield, IL, Charles C Thomas, 1983
32. Bjarngard BE: Radiation therapy and SI units. Int J Radiat Oncol Biol Phys 7:283–285, 1981
33. Johns HE, Cunningham JR (eds): The Physics of Radiology, pp 532–534. Springfield, IL, Charles C Thomas, 1983
34. Tapley NV: Electron beam. In Fletcher GH (ed): Textbook of Radiotherapy, pp 40–60. Philadelphia, Lea & Febiger, 1980
35. Catterall M: The assessment of the results of neutron therapy. Int J Radiat Oncol Biol Phys 8:1573–1580, 1982
36. Stone RS, Larkin JC: The treatment of cancer with fast neutrons. Radiology 39:608–614, 1942
37. Duncan W: Current thoughts on fast neutron therapy. Br J Radiol 51:943–952, 1978
38. Mole RH: Late effects of radiation: Carcinogenesis. Br Med Bull 29:78–83, 1973
39. Hall EJ: The particles compared. Int J Radiat Oncol Biol 8:2137–2140, 1982
40. Munzenrider JE, Shipley WU, Verhey LJ: Future prospects of radiation therapy with protons. Semin Oncol 8:110–114, 1981
41. Pierquin BL: Past, present and future of interstitial radiation therapy. Int J Radiat Oncol Biol Phys 9:1237–1242, 1983
42. Stallard HB: Eye and orbit. In Fletcher GH (ed): Textbook of Radiotherapy, pp 419–425. Philadelphia, Lea & Febiger, 1973
43. Gerbaulet A, Panis X, Flamant F, Chassagne D: Iridium afterloading curietherapy in the treatment of pediatric malignancies. Cancer 56:1274–1279, 1985
44. Goffinet DR, Martinez A, Pooler D, Palos B, Donaldson SS: Pediatric brachytherapy. In George FW III (ed): Modern Interstitial and Intracavitary Radiation Management, pp 57–70. New York, Masson Publishing, 1983
45. Goffinet DR, Cox R, Clarke DH, Fu KK, Hilaris B, Ling C: Brachytherapy. Am J Clin Oncol (in press)
46. Hall EJ: The biological basis of endocurietherapy: The Henschke Memorial Lecture, 1984. Endocurie Hyper Oncol 1:141–152, 1985
47. Pierquin B, Chassagne D, Baillet F, Paine CH: Clinical observations on the time factor in interstitial radiotherapy using iridium 192. Clin Radiol 24:506–510, 1973
48. Bedford MA, Bedotto C, MacFaul PA: Retinoblastoma: A study of 139 cases. Br J Ophthalmol 55:17–27, 1971

49. Gutin PH, Edwards MSB, Wara WM et al: Preliminary experience with ^{125}I-brachytherapy of pediatric brain tumors. Concepts Pediatr Neurosurg 5:187–206, 1985

50. Gillin MT, Kline RW, Kun LE: Cranial dose distribution. Int J Radiat Oncol Biol Phys 5:1903–1906, 1979

51. Kline RW, Gillin MT, Kun LE: Cranial irradiation in acute leukemia: Dose estimate in the lens. Int J Radiat Oncol Biol Phys 5:117–121, 1979

52. Jereb B, Reid A, Ahuja RK: Patterns of failure in patients with medulloblastoma. Cancer 50:2941–2947, 1982

53. Kun LE, Camitta BM, Mulhern RK et al: Treatment of meningeal relapse in childhood acute lymphoblastic leukemia: I. Results of craniospinal irradiation. J Clin Oncol 2:359–364, 1984

54. Glasgow GP, Marks JE: The dosimetry of a single "hockey stick" portal for treatment of tumors of the cranio-spinal axis. Med Phys 10:672–675, 1983

55. Muller-Runkel R, Vijayakumar S: Spinal axis irradiation with electrons: Measurements of attenuation by the spinal processes. Med Phys 13:539–544, 1986

56. Jentzsch K, Binder H, Cramer H et al: Leg function after radiotherapy for Ewing's sarcoma. Cancer 47:1267–1278, 1981

57. Moss WT: The integration of irradiation and surgery as the treatment for selected cancers. Int J Radiat Oncol Biol Phys 8:1373–1378, 1982

58. Fletcher GH: Combination of irradiation and surgery. Int Adv Surg Oncol 2:55–98, 1979

59. Stanley JA, Shipley WU, Steel GG: Influence of tumor size on hypoxic fraction and therapeutic sensitivity of Lewis lung tumor. Br J Cancer 36:105–113, 1977

60. Fletcher GH: Basic principles of the combination of irradiation and surgery. Int J Radiat Oncol Biol Phys 5:2091–2096, 1979

61. Fischer JJ, Martin DF, Cardinale F, Fischer DB, Neaderland M: The effect of subtotal resection on the dose of radiation required to cure the rat rhabdomyosarcoma BA1112. Surg Gynecol Obstet 156:189–192, 1983

62. Powers WE, Palmer LA: Biologic basis of preoperative radiation treatment. Am J Roentgenol Radiat Ther Nucl Med 102:176–192, 1968

63. Lemerle PA, Voute PA, Tournade MF et al: Effectiveness of preoperative chemotherapy in Wilms' tumor: Results of an International Society of Paediatric Oncology (SIOP) clinical trial. J Clin Oncol 1:604–609, 1983

64. Suit HD, Proppe KH, Mankin HJ, Woods WC: Preoperative radiation therapy for sarcoma of soft tissue. Cancer 47:2269–2274, 1981

65. Tepper J, Sindelar W: Summary of the Workshop on Intraoperative Radiation Therapy. Cancer Treat Rep 65:911–918, 1981

66. Abe M, Takahashi M: Intraoperative radiotherapy: The Japanese experience. Int J Radiat Oncol Biol Phys 7:863–868, 1981

67. Sindelar WF, Tepper JE, Travis EL, Terrill R: Tolerance of retroperitoneal structures to intra-operative radiation. Ann Surg 196:601–608, 1982

68. Kinsella TJ, Sindelar WF, DeLuca AM et al: Tolerance of peripheral nerve to intraoperative radiotherapy (IORT): Clinical and experimental studies. Int J Radiat Oncol Biol Phys 11:1579–1585, 1985

69. Steel GG, Peckham MJ: Exploitable mechanisms in combined radiotherapy–chemotherapy: The concept of additivity. Int J Radiat Oncol Biol Phys 5:85–91, 1979

70. Steel GG: The combination of radiotherapy and chemotherapy. In Steel GG, Adams GE, Peckham MJ (eds): The Biological Basis of Radiotherapy, pp 239–248. Amsterdam, Elsevier, 1983

71. Fu KK: Biological basis for the interaction of chemotherapeutic agents and radiation therapy. Cancer 55:2123–2130, 1985

72. Steel GG: Terminology in the description of drug–radiation interactions. Int J Radiat Oncol Biol Phys 5:1145–1150, 1979

73. Trott KR: Radiation–chemotherapy interactions. Int J Radiat Oncol Biol Phys 12:1409–1413, 1986

74. D'Angio GJ, Farber S, Maddock DL: Potentiation of X-ray effects by actinomycin-D. Radiology 73:175–177, 1959

75. Elkind MM: Keynote address: Modifiers of radiation response in tumor therapy: Strategies and expectations. Int J Radiat Oncol Biol Phys 8:89–100, 1982

76. Millar JL, Hudspith BN: Sparing effect of cyclophosphamide (NSC-26271) pretreatment on animals lethally treated with γ-radiation. Cancer Treat Rep 60:409–414, 1976

77. Millar JL, Blackett NM, Hudspith BN: Enhanced post-irradiation recovery of the haemopoietic system in animals pretreated with a variety of cytotoxic agents. Cell Tissue Kinet 11:543–553, 1978

78. Phillips TL, Fu KK: The interaction of drug and radiation effects on normal tissues. Int J Radiat Oncol Biol Phys 4:59–64, 1978

79. Rubin P, Casarett GW: Clinical Radiation Pathology, pp 1–61. Philadelphia, WB Saunders, 1968

80. Bloomer WD, Hellman S: Normal tissue responses to radiation therapy. New Engl J Med 293:80–83, 1975

81. Rubin P: The Franz Buschke Lecture: Late effects of chemotherapy and radiation therapy: A new hypothesis. Int J Radiat Oncol Biol Phys 10:5–34, 1984

82. Withers HR, Thames HD, Peters LJ, Fletcher GH: Keynote Address: Normal tissue radioresistance in clinical radiotherapy. In Fletcher GH, Nervi C, Withers HR (eds): Biological Bases and Clinical Implications of Tumor Radioresistance, pp 139–152. Chicago, Year Book Medical Publishers, 1983

83. Trott KR: Chronic damage after radiation therapy: Challenge to radiation biology. Int J Radiat Oncol Biol Phys 10:907–913, 1984

84. Withers HR, Peters LJ, Thames HD, Fletcher GH: Hyperfractionation. Int J Radiat Oncol Biol Phys 8:1807–1809, 1982

85. Withers HR: Predicting late normal tissue responses. Int J Radiat Oncol Biol Phys 12:693–698, 1986

86. Rubin P, Scarantino CW: The bone marrow organ: The critical structure in radiation–drug interaction. Int J Radiat Oncol Biol Phys 4:3–23, 1978

87. Plowman PN: The effects of conventionally fractionated, extended portal radiotherapy on the human perpheral blood count. Int J Radiat Oncol Biol Phys 9:829–839, 1983

88. Anderson RE, Warren NL: Ionizing radiation and the immune response. Adv Immunol 24:215–235, 1976

89. Posner MR, Reinherz E, Lane H, Mauch P, Hellman S, Schlossman SF: Circulating lymphocyte populations in Hodgkin's disease after mantle and paraaortic irradiation. Blood 61:705–708, 1983

90. Idestrom K, Petrini B, Blomgren H, Wasserman J, Wallgren A, Baral E: Changes of the peripheral lymphocyte population following radiation therapy to extended and limited fields. Int J Radiat Oncol Biol Phys 5:1761–1766, 1979

91. Fuks Z, Strober S, Bobrove AM, Sasazuki T, McMichael A, Kaplan HS: Long term effects of radiation on T and B lymphocytes in peripheral blood of patients with Hodgkin's disease. J Clin Invest 58:803–814, 1976

92. Johnson RE, Kun LE, Belladonna JA, Johnson SK, Brereton HD, Cohen GA: Hematologic recovery and deterioration after "successful" radiotherapy for Hodgkin's disease. Ann Intern Med 80:213–216, 1974

93. Till JE, McCulloch EA: A direct measurement of the radiation sensitivity of normal mouse bone marrow cells. Radiat Res 14:213–222, 1961

94. Senn JS, McCulloch EA: Radiation sensitivity of human bone marrow cells measured by a cell culture method. Blood 35:56–60, 1970

95. Maloney MA, Patt HM: Migration of cells from shielded to irradiated marrow. Blood 39:804–808, 1972

96. Tubiana M, Frindel E, Croizat H, Parmentier C: Effects of radiations on bone marrow. Pathol Biol 27:326–334, 1979

97. Sykes MP, Chu FCH, Savel H, Bonadonna G, Mathis H: The effects of varying dosages of irradiation upon sternal-marrow regeneration. Radiology 83:1084–1088, 1964

98. Hill DR, Benak SB, Phillips TL, Price DC: Bone marrow regeneration following fractionated radiation therapy. Int J Radiat Oncol Biol Phys 6:1149–1155, 1980

99. Rubin P, Landman S, Mayer E, Keller B, Ciccio S: Bone marrow regeneration and extension after extended field irradiation in Hodgkin's disease. Cancer 32:699–711, 1973

100. Sacks EL, Goris ML, Glatstein E, Gilbert E, Kaplan HS: Bone marrow regeneration following large field radiation: Influence of volume, age, dose, and time. Cancer 42:1057–1065, 1978

101. Phillips TL, Margolis L: Radiation pathology and the clinical response of lung and esophagus. In Vaeth JM (ed): Frontiers of Radiation Therapy and Oncology, pp 254–273. Baltimore, University Park Press, 1972

102. Keane TJ, VanDyk J, Rider WD: Idiopathic interstitial pneumonia following bone marrow transplantation: The relationship with total body irradiation. Int J Radiat Oncol Biol Phys 7:1365–1370, 1981

103. Rubin P, Shapiro DL, Finkelstein JN, Penney DP: The early release of surfactant following lung irradiation of alveolar type II cells. Int J Radiat Oncol Biol Phys 6:75–77, 1980

104. Phillips TL: An ultrastructural study of the development of radiation injury in the lung. Radiology 87:49–54, 1966

105. Host H, Yale JR: Lung function after mantle field irradiation for Hodgkin's disease. Cancer 32:328–332, 1973

106. Lokich JJ, Bass H, Eberly FE, Rosenthal DS, Moloney WC: The pulmonary effect of mantle irradiation in patients with Hodgkin's disease. Radiology 108:397–402, 1973

107. doPico GA, Wiley AL, Dickie HA: Pulmonary reaction to upper mantle radiation therapy for Hodgkin's disease. Chest 75:688–692, 1979

108. Littman P, Meadows AT, Polgar G, Borns PF, Rubin E: Pulmonary function in survivors of Wilms' tumor: Patterns of impairment. Cancer 37:2773–2776, 1976

109. Wohl MEB, Griscom NT, Traggis DG, Jaffe N: Effects of therapeutic irradiation delivered in early childhood upon subsequent lung function. Pediatrics 55:507–516, 1975

110. Watchie J, Coleman CN, Raffin TA et al: Minimal long-term cardiopulmonary dysfunction following treatment for Hodgkin's disease. Int J Radiat Oncol Biol Phys 13:517–524, 1987

111. Stewart JR, Fajardo LF: Dose response in human and experimental radiation-induced heart disease. Radiology 99:403–408, 1971

112. Mill WB, Baglan RJ, Kurichety P, Prasad S, Lee JY, Moller R: Symptomatic radiation-induced pericarditis in Hodgkin's disease. Int J Radiat Oncol Biol Phys 10:2061–2065, 1984

113. Byhardt R, Brace K, Ruckdeschel J, Chang P, Martin R, Wiernik P: Dose and treatment factors in radiation-related pericardial effusion associated with the mantle technique for Hodgkin's disease. Cancer 35:795–802, 1975

114. Applefeld MM, Cole JF, Pollock SH et al: The late appearance of chronic pericardial disease in patients treated by radiotherapy for Hodgkin's disease. Ann Intern Med 94:338–341, 1981

115. Fajardo LF, Stewart R: Pathogenesis of radiation-induced myocardial fibrosis. Lab Invest 29:244–257, 1973

116. Perrault DJ, Levy M, Herman JD et al: Echocardiographic abnormalities following cardiac radiation. J Clin Oncol 3:546–551, 1985

117. Gottdiener JS, Katin MJ, Borer JS, Bacharach SL, Green MV: Late cardiac effects of therapeutic mediastinal irradiation. N Engl J Med 308:569–572, 1983

118. Hancock EW: Heart disease after radiation. N Engl J Med 308:588, 1983

119. Kopelson G, Herwig KJ: The etiologies of coronary artery disease in cancer patients. Int J Radiat Oncol Biol Phys 4:895–906, 1978

120. Stewart JR: Cancer and coronary artery disease. Int J Radiat Oncol Biol Phys 4:915–916, 1978

121. Tefft M, Mitus A, Das L, Vawter GF, Filler RM: Irradiation of the liver in children: Review of experience in the acute and chronic phases, and in the intact normal and partially resected. Am J Roentgenol Radiat Ther Nucl Med 108:365–385, 1970

122. Poussin-Rosillo H, Nisce LZ, D'Angio GJ: Hepatic radiation tolerance in Hodgkin's disease patients. Radiology 121:461–464, 1976

123. Ingold JA, Reed GB, Kaplan HS, Bagshaw MA: Radiation hepatitis. Am J Roentgenol Radiat Ther Nuc Med 93:200–208, 1965

124. Thomas PRM, Tefft M, D'Angio GJ, Morgan ED, Baum E, Breslow NE, Takashima J for the National Wilms' Tumor Study Committee: Radiation associated toxicities in the Second National Wilms' Tumor Study (NWTS-2) (abstr). Int J Radiat Oncol Biol Phys 10:88, 1984

125. Lewin K, Millis RR: Human radiation hepatitis: A morphologic study with emphasis on the late changes. Arch Pathol 96:21–26, 1973

126. Kun LE, Camitta BM: Hepatopathy following irradiation and Adriamycin. Cancer 42:81–84, 1978

127. Farjardo LF, Colby TV: Pathogenesis of veno-occlusive liver disease after radiation. Arch Pathol Lab Med 104:584–588, 1980

128. Luxton RW: Radiation nephritis. Q J Med 22:215–242, 1953

129. Luxton RW: Radiation nephritis: A long-term study of 5 patients. Lancet 2:1221–1224, 1961

130. Luxton RW, Kunkler PB: Radiation nephritis. Acta Radiol 2:169–178, 1964

131. Mair JG: Effects of radiations on kidney, bladder, and prostate. Front Radiat Ther Oncol 6:196–227, 1972

132. Glatstein E, Fajardo LF, Brown JM: Radiation injury in the mouse kidney: I. Sequential light microscopic study. Int J Radiat Oncol Biol Phys 2:933–943, 1977

133. Withers HR, Mason KA, Thames HD: Late radiation response of kidney assayed by tubule-cell survival. Br J Radiol 59:587–595, 1986

134. Moskowitz PS, Donaldson SS, Canty EI: Chemotherapy-induced inhibition of compensatory renal growth in the immature mouse. AJR 134:491–496, 1980

135. Kim TH, Somerville PJ, Freeman CR: Unilateral radiation nephropathy: The long-term significance. Int J Radiat Oncol Biol Phys 10:2053–2059, 1984

136. Donaldson SS, Moskowitz PS, Canty EL, Efron B: Radiation-induced inhibition of compensatory renal growth in the weanling mouse kidney. Radiology 128:491–495, 1978

137. Jongejan HTM, van der Kogel AJ, Provoost AP, Molenaar JC: Radiation nephropathy in young and adult rats. Int J Radiat Oncol Biol Phys 13:225–232, 1987

138. Donaldson SS, Jundt S, Ricour C, Sarrazin D, Lemerle J, Schweisguth O: Radiation enteritis in children: A retrospective review, clinicopathologic correlation, and dietary management. Cancer 35:1167–1178, 1975

139. Shalet SM, Beardwell CG, Morris-Jones PH, Pearson D: Pituitary function after treatment of intracranial tumours in children. Lancet 2:104–107, 1975

140. Swift PGF, Kearney PJ, Dalton RG, Bullimore JA, Mott MG, Savage DCL: Growth and hormonal status of children treated for acute lymphoblastic leukaemia. Arch Dis Childh 53:890–894, 1978

141. Shalet SM, Beardwell CG, Aarons BM, Pearson D, Morris-Jones PH: Growth impairment in children treated for brain tumours. Arch Dis Childh 53:491–494, 1978

142. Danoff BF, Cowchock FS, Marquette C, Mulgrew L, Kramer S: Assessment of the long-term effects of primary radiation therapy for brain tumors in children. Cancer 49:1580–1586, 1982

143. Duffner PK, Cohen ME, Anderson SW et al: Long-term effects of treatment on endocrine function in children with brain tumors. Ann Neurol 14:528–532, 1983

144. Samaan NA, Vieto R, Schultz PN et al: Hypothalamic, pituitary and thyroid dysfunction after radiotherapy to the head and neck. Int J Radiat Oncol Biol Phys 8:1857–1867, 1982

145. Oberfield SE, Allen JC, Pollack J, New MI, Levine LS: Long-term endocrine sequelae after treatment of medulloblastoma: Prospective study of growth and thyroid function. J Pediatr 108:219–223, 1986

146. Mechanick JI, Hochberg FH, LaRocque A: Hypothalamic dysfunction following whole-brain irradiation. J Neurosurg 65:490–494, 1986

147. Constine LS, Donaldson SS, McDougall R, Cox RS, Link MP, Kaplan HS: Thyroid dysfunction after radiotherapy in children with Hodgkin's disease. Cancer 53:878–883, 1984

148. Delic JI, Hendry JH, Morris ID, Shalet SM: Leydig cell function in the pubertal rat following local testicular irradiation. Radiother Oncol 5:29–37, 1986

149. Brauner F, Czernichow P, Cramer P, Schaison G, Rappaport R: Leydig-cell function in children after direct testicular irradiation for acute lymphoblastic leukemia. N Engl J Med 309:25–28, 1983

150. Horning SJ, Hoppe RT, Kaplan HS, Rosenberg SA: Female reproductive potential after treatment for Hodgkin's disease. N Engl J Med 304:1377–1382, 1981

151. Ash P: The influence of radiation on fertility in man. Br J Radiol 53:271–278, 1980

152. Young DF, Posner JB, Chu F, Nisce L: Rapid-course radiation therapy of cerebral metastases: Results and complications. Cancer 34:1069–1076, 1974

153. Freeman JE, Johnston PGB, Voke JM: Somnolence after prophylactic cranial irradiation in children with acute lymphoblastic leukaemia. Br Med J 4:523–525, 1973

154. Boldrey E, Sheline G: Delayed transitory clinical manifestations after radiation treatment of intracranial tumors. Acta Radiol Ther 5:5–10, 1966

155. Jones A: Transient radiation myelopathy (with reference to Lhermitte's sign of electrical paresthesia). Br J Radiol 37:727–744, 1964

156. Hoffman WF, Levin VA, Wilson CB: Evaluation of malignant glioma patients during the postirradiation period. J Neurosurg 50:624–628, 1979

157. Sheline GE, Wara WM, Smith V: Therapeutic irradiation and brain injury. Int J Radiat Oncol Biol Phys 6:1215–1228, 1980

158. Mikhael MA: Dosimetric considerations in the diagnosis of radiation necrosis of the brain. In Gilbert HA, Kagen AR (eds): Radiation Damage to the Nervous System, pp 59–91. New York, Raven Press, 1980

159. Packer RJ, Zimmerman RA, Bilaniuk LT: Magnetic resonance imaging in the evaluation of treatment-related central nervous system damage. Cancer 58:635–640, 1986

160. Burger PC, Dubois PJ, Schold SC et al: Computerized tomographic and pathologic studies of the untreated, quiescent, and recurrent glioblastoma multiforme. J Neurosurg 58:159–169, 1983

161. Edwards M, Wilson C: Treatment of radiation necrosis. In Gilbert HA, Kagen AR (eds): Radiation Damage to the Nervous System, pp 129–143. New York, Raven Press, 1980

162. Caveness WF: Experimental observations: Delayed necrosis in normal monkey brain. In Gilbert HA, Kagen AR (eds): Radiation Damage to the Nervous System, pp 1–38. New York, Raven Press, 1980

163. Marks JE, Baglan RJ, Prassad SC, Blank WF: Cerebral radionecrosis: Incidence and risk in relation to dose, time, fractionation and volume. Int J Radiat Oncol Biol Phys 7:243–252, 1981

164. Kramer S, Southard ME, Mansfield CM: Radiation effect and tolerance of the central nervous system. Front Radiat Ther Oncol 6:332–345, 1972

165. Abbatucci JS, Delozier T, Quint R, Roussel A, Brune D: Radiation myelopathy

of the cervical spinal cord: Time, dose and volume factors. Int J Radiat Oncol Biol Phys 4:239–248, 1978

166. Price RA, Jamieson PA: The central nervous system in childhood leukemia II: Subacute leukoencephalopathy. Cancer 35:306–318, 1975

167. Bleyer WA: Neurologic sequelae of methotrexate and ionizing radiation: A new classification. Cancer Treat Rep 65:89–98, 1981

168. Price RA, Birdwell DA: The central nervous system in childhood leukemia: III. Mineralizing microangiopathy and dystrophic calcification. Cancer 42:717–728, 1978

169. Peylan-Ramu N, Poplack DG, Pizzo PA, Adornato BT, Di Chiro G: Abnormal CT scans of the brain in asymptomatic children with acute lymphocytic leukemia after prophylactic treatment of the central nervous system with radiation and intrathecal chemotherapy. N Engl J Med 298:815–818, 1978

170. Ochs JJ, Parvey LS, Whitaker JN et al: Serial cranial computed-tomography scans in children with leukemia given two different forms of central nervous system therapy. J Clin Oncol 1:793–798, 1983

171. Eiser C: Intellectual abilities among survivors of childhood leukaemia as a function of CNS irradiation. Arch Dis Childh 53:391–395, 1978

172. Meadows AT, Massari DJ, Fergusson J, Gordon J, Littman P, Moss K: Declines in IQ scores and cognitive dysfunctions in children with acute lymphocytic leukaemia treated with cranial irradiation. Lancet 2:1015–1018, 1981

173. Rowland JH, Glidewell OJ, Sibley RF, Holland JC, Tull R, Berman A, Brecher ML, Harris M, Glicksman AS, Forman E, Jones B, Cohen ME, Duffner PK, Freeman AI for the Cancer and Leukemia Group B: Effects of different forms of central nervous system prophylaxis on neuropsychologic function in childhood leukemia. J Clin Oncol 2:1327–1335, 1984

174. Kun LE, Mulhern RK, Crisco JJ: Quality of life in children treated for brain tumors. J Neurosurg 58:1–6, 1983

175. Mulhern RK, Crisco JJ, Kun LE: Neuropsychological sequelae of childhood brain tumors: A review. J Clin Child Psychol 12:66–73, 1983

176. Jannoun L: Are cognitive and educational development affected by age at which prophylactic therapy is given in acute lymphoblastic leukaemia? Arch Dis Childh 58:953–958, 1983

177. Williams JM, Davis KS: Central nervous system prophylactic treatment for childhood leukemia: Neuropsychological outcome studies. Cancer Treat Rev 13:113–127, 1986

178. Li FP, Winston KR, Gimbrere BA: Follow-up of children with brain tumors. Cancer 54:135–138, 1984

179. Rowley MJ, Leach DR, Warner GA, Heller CG: Effect of graded doses of ionizing radiation on the human testis. Radiat Res 59:665–678, 1974

180. Pedrick TJ, Hoppe RT: Recovery of spermatogenesis following pelvic irradiation for Hodgkin's disease. Int J Radiat Oncol Biol Phys 12:117–121, 1986

181. Thachil JV, Jewett MAS, Rider WD: The effects of cancer and cancer therapy on male fertility. J Urol 126:141–145, 1981

182. Delic JI, Hendry JH, Morris ID, Shalet SM: Seminiferous epithelial function in the pubertal rat following local testicular irradiation. Radiother Oncol 5:39–45, 1986

183. Himelstein-Braw R, Peters H, Faber M: Influence of irradiation and chemotherapy on the ovaries of children with abdominal tumours. Br J Cancer 36:269–275, 1977

184. Shalet SM, Beardwell CG et al: Ovarian failure following abdominal irradiation in childhood. Br J Cancer 33:655–658, 1976

185. Li FP, Gimbrere K, Gelber RD et al: Adverse pregnancy outcome after radiotherapy for childhood Wilms' tumor (abstr). Proc Am Soc Clin Oncol 5:202, 1986

186. Neuhauser EBD, Wittenborg MH, Berman CZ, Cohen J: Irradiation effects of roentgen therapy on the growing spine. Radiology 59:637–650, 1952

187. Riseborough EJ, Grabias SL, Burton RI, Jaffe N: Skeletal alterations following irradiation for Wilms' tumor, with particular reference to scoliosis and kyphosis. J Bone Joint Surg [Am] 58:526–536, 1976

188. Thomas PRM, Griffith KD, Fineberg BB, Perez CA, Land VJ: Late effects of treatment for Wilms' tumor. Int J Radiat Oncol Biol Phys 9:651–657, 1983

189. Probert JC, Parker BR: The effects of radiation therapy on bone growth. Radiology 114:155–162, 1975

190. Gonzalez DG, Breur K: Clinical data from irradiated growing long bones in children. Int J Radiat Oncol Biol Phys 9:841–846, 1983

191. Jaffe N, Toth BB, Hoar RE, Ried HL, Sullivan MP, McNeese MD: Dental and maxillofacial abnormalities in long-term survivors of childhood cancer: Effects of treatment with chemotherapy and radiation to the head and neck. Pediatrics 73:816–823, 1984

192. Oliver JH, Gluck G, Gledhill RB, Chevalier L: Musculoskeletal deformities following treatment of Wilms' tumour. Can Med Assoc J 119:459–464, 1978

193. Mettler FA, Moseley RD: Medical Effects of Ionizing Radiation. Orlando, Grune & Stratton, 1985

194. Li FP, Cassady JR, Jaffe N: Risk of second tumors in survivors of childhood cancer. Cancer 35:1230–1235, 1975

195. Potish RA, Dehner LP, Haselow RE, Kim TH, Levitt SH, Nesbit M: The incidence of second neoplasms following megavoltage radiation for pediatric tumors. Cancer 56:1534–1537, 1985

196. Heyn R, Newton WA, Ragab A, Tefft M, Mauer HM, Beltangady M: Second malignant neoplasms in patients treated on the Intergroup Rhabdomyosarcoma Study I–II (IRS I–II) (abstr). Proc Am Soc Clin Oncol 5:215, 1986

197. Jaffe J, Ried HL, Cohen M, McNeese MD, Sullivan MP: Radiation induced osteochondroma in long-term survivors of childhood cancer. Int J Radiat Oncol Biol Phys 9:665–670, 1983

198. Meadows AT, Baum E, Fossati-Bellani F et al: Second malignant neoplasms in children: An update from the Late Effects Study Group. J Clin Oncol 3:532–538, 1985

199. Rubin CM, Robison LL, Cameron JD et al: Intraocular Retinoblastoma Group V: An analysis of prognostic factors. J Clin Oncol 3:680–685, 1985

200. Lueder GT, Judisch F, O'Gorman TW: Second nonocular tumors in survivors of heritable retinoblastoma. Arch Ophthalmol 104:372–373, 1986

201. Abramson DH, Ellsworth RM, Kitchin FD, Tung G: Second nonocular tumors in retinoblastoma survivors: Are they radiation-induced? Ophthalmology 91:1351–1355, 1984

twelve

Special Considerations for the Infant with Cancer

Gregory H. Reaman

The diagnosis and management of cancer in children pose many difficult challenges to the multidisciplinary care team. Particularly in infants, the potential long-term sequelae of multimodality therapy are of major concern. The unique problems associated with the delivery of aggressive and potentially toxic treatment are further magnified in the management of newborns with cancer.

Cancer in the first year of life, and particularly during the first 4 weeks, is relatively rare.[1] However, the distribution frequencies of malignant tumors observed in infancy differ considerably from those in older children.[2] Identifiable differences in clinical features at presentation and in response to therapy also have been reported in infants compared to older children with the same disease. These findings may provide significant biological insights into the distinctly different outcomes observed for various malignancies in infants.

The effect of very young age at diagnosis on prognosis varies greatly depending on the specific diagnosis. The prognosis for acute lymphoblastic leukemia (ALL) is decidedly worse in infants than in older children.[3-5] On the other hand, infants with neuroblastoma, even those with distant dissemination, or with Wilms' tumor have improved long-term survival compared to older children with these tumors.[6-8] The diagnosis of cancer in the newborn and young infant provides important insights into early human developmental oncobiology and suggests an intimate relationship between oncogenesis and teratogenesis.[9] The fact that many fetal and neonatal malignant tumors that are clinically manifested in the first few months of life tend to spontaneously regress or cytodifferentiate has led to speculations about the expression of oncogenes by embryonal cells and their modulation in the intrauterine milieu.[10]

This chapter reviews differences in the incidence of tumor types in newborns and infants and provides some background and guidelines for professionals faced with the challenge of treating these patients. Also reviewed herein are some of the biological differences that may have prognostic and therapeutic implications for infants with the types of cancer most frequently observed in this age group.

EPIDEMIOLOGY

The first population-based measure of cancer incidence by tumor type in newborns (<30 days) and infants (<1 year) in the United States[2] has extended to a full decade the neonatal cancer mortality data that had been recorded previously for shorter intervals.[11,12] Data from the Third National Cancer Survey[13] indicate that the incidence of malignant neoplasms is 183.4 per million live births per year in infants and 36.5 per million live births per year in neonates.[2] Unlike the overall experience in childhood, there are no significant differences in incidence between male and female neonates. Death certificates for all children younger

Table 12-1

Incidence and Mortality Rates of Malignant Tumors in Newborns and Infants in the United States*

Tumor Type	Incidence		Mortality	
	Newborns	*Infants*	*Newborns*	*Infants*
Leukemia	4.7	31.8	2.6	20.8
Neuroblastoma	19.7	62.7	1.8	7.8
CNS	0.9	14.0	0.3	6.6
Kidney	4.7	19.7	0.5	3.6
Reticuloendotheliosis	0	2.8	0.2	3.4
Sarcoma	3.7	17.8	0.7	3.3
Liver	0	7.5	0.4	2.6
Lymphoma	0.9	1.9	<0.1	1.5
Teratoma	0	2.8	0.3	0.7
Carcinoma	0.9	5.6	0.2	0.5
Germ cell, excluding teratoma	0	0	0	0.2
Retinoblastoma	0	15.9	<0.1	0.1
Other	0.9	0.9	0.5	1.6
Total	36.5	183.4	7.6	52.7

(Adapted from Bader JL, Miller RW: U.S. cancer incidence and mortality in the first year of life. Am J Dis Child 133:157–159, 1979)

* Incidence determined from Third National Cancer Survey (10% sample of U.S. population), 1969–1971; mortality determined from U.S. death certificates, 1960–1969. Rates are per million live births per year.

than 1 year who died of cancer in the United States from 1960 to 1969 were analyzed to compare the incidence of tumor types using mortality as an indicator of frequency and, more importantly, to construct incidence:mortality ratios.

As shown in Table 12-1, the frequency rankings of tumor types in both newborns and infants differ substantially when assessed by incidence rather than mortality (see Chap. 1). Neuroblastoma ranks first in incidence, followed by leukemia, kidney tumors (Wilms' tumor or its infantile congeners),[14] sarcomas (rhabdomyosarcoma, malignant mesenchymoma, fibrosarcoma, synovial sarcoma, liposarcoma, hemangiosarcoma, osteosarcoma, and undifferentiated), retinoblastoma, central nervous system (CNS) tumors (80% glial in origin), and liver tumors (67% hepatoblastoma).

As shown in Table 12-2, there is a distinct difference in the rank order of distribution frequencies of tumor types in infants compared to all children younger than 15 years.[15] Neuroblastoma accounts for more than 50% of cancers in the newborn; acute leukemia, Wilms' tumor, and sarcomas each account for another 12%.

Each year, approximately 653 malignancies are diagnosed in infants in the United States; 130 of these are observed in the neonatal period, and 65 are apparent on the first day of life.

DIAGNOSIS

Symptoms and Signs

Recognizing symptoms without having the benefit of subjective patient complaints in this particular age group presents a challenge. In young infants, particularly in newborns, the nonspecific findings of lethargy, somnolence, irritability, feeding difficulties, vomiting, fever or hypothermia, and failure to thrive require a high index of suspicion of significant pathology. Although these signs or symptoms are rarely accounted for by the diagnosis of a malignancy, they may be associated with cancer in the infant (see Chap. 5).

More often, because of the distribution of tumor types

Table 12-2

Differences in Distribution Frequencies of the Major Forms of Cancer in Newborns, Infants, and Children

Tumor Type	Newborns	Infants	Children <15 Years
Leukemia	13	18	31
ALL		8	20.4
Other		10	10.5
CNS	3	8	18
Neuroblastoma	54	35	8
Lymphoma	0.3	1	14
Wilms' tumor	13	11	6
Sarcoma (soft tissue and bone)	11	10	11
Liver		4	1.3
Teratoma		2	0.4
Retinoblastoma		9	4
Other	5.7	2	6.3

observed in infants, there are obvious abnormalities on physical examination that assist in formulating a differential diagnosis which may include a malignancy. Here again, however, the relative infrequency of cancer and the more common occurrence of developmental anomalies or nonmalignant conditions result in difficulties in distinguishing benign from possibly malignant lesions. Table 12-3 summarizes some clinical and laboratory abnormalities commonly associated with cancer or with the more frequent nonmalignant conditions observed in neonates and infants.

Laboratory and Diagnostic Studies

Laboratory techniques that require the minimum amount of whole blood, serum, and plasma have reduced the difficulties associated with removing relatively large volumes of blood to

Table 12-3
Differential Diagnosis of Malignant and Nonmalignant Conditions in Infancy

Feature	Malignancy	Nonmalignant Condition
Skin nodules	Neuroblastoma Acute leukemia Reticuloendothelioses	Congenital viral infections Vasculitis Fibromatosis Neurofibromatosis Xanthoma

Head and neck masses	Rhabdomyosarcoma
	  Orbital
	  Cervical
	Nasopharyngeal
	Neuroblastoma
	Lymphoma
		Brachial cleft cyst
		Thyoglossal duct cyst
		Cystic hygroma
		Fibromatosis
		Hemangioma
		Abscess
		Cellulitis
		Reactive hyperplasia of cervical nodes
		Granulomatous lesions (*e.g.,* atypical
		    tuberculosis)

Abdominal or pelvic masses	Neuroblastoma Wilms' tumor Sarcomas Malignant teratomas Lymphoma Germ cell	Polycystic kidneys Hydronephrosis Benign teratoma Urinary retention Gastrointestinal duplication Intussusception Chordoma Meningomyelocele Horseshoe kidney Splenomegaly Hepatomegaly
Hepatomegaly	Neuroblastoma Acute leukemia Hepatoblastoma	Congenital viral infections Storage diseases Cavernous hemangioma Hemangioendothelioma

Signs/symptoms of
  increased inracranial
  pressure
	Brain tumors
	Acute leukemia
	Retinoblastoma
		Intracranial hemorrhage
		Communicating hydrocephalus
		Dandy–Walker malformation
		Vascular malformations

Anemia	Acute leukemia
	Neuroblastoma
	  (disseminated)
		Acute/chronic blood loss
		Hypoproliferative anemia (nutritional,
		    congenital)
		Dyserythropoietic anemias
		Transient erythroblastopenia

Pancytopenia	Acute leukemia
	Neuroblastoma
	  (disseminated)
	Retinoblastoma
	  (disseminated)
		Congenital viral infections
		Immune-mediated neutropenia and
		    thrombocytopenia
		Congenital and acquired aplastic anemias

perform such diagnostic examinations as complete blood counts and chemistries to assess specific organ dysfunction and the existence of specific tumor markers. Radiographic investigations, including ultrasonography, computed tomography, magnetic resonance imaging, and radionuclide scans, are best performed in specialized pediatric centers (see Chap. 7). Such centers provide technical and interpretive expertise in the diagnosis and management of infants and newborns. These radiographic studies can guide the pediatric surgeon in determining the nature and extent of the operative procedure (biopsy or resection) required to establish a definitive diagnosis.

Pathologic Considerations

The ultimate histopathologic diagnosis of cancer in infants requires the expertise of the pediatric pathologist. Specialized cytochemical, ultrastructural, and immunocytochemical techniques required to establish accurate diagnoses are discussed in Chapter 6. Although the pathologic findings of certain tumor types are not unique to this age group, one potential pitfall in the pathologic diagnosis of soft tissue malignancies warrants brief mention here.

Fibrous proliferations in childhood and particularly in infancy are often difficult to evaluate because their histologic features do not always correlate well with clinical behavior. In such lesions, increased cellularity, high mitotic index, infiltrative growth pattern, and poor differentiation do not always indicate aggressive clinical behavior.[16–18] Although fibromatosis appears to lend itself more to description than to definition,[19] it has been defined as a group of nonmetastasizing fibrous tumors that tend to invade locally and to recur following surgical excision.[20,21] Such lesions, which may result in confusion in distinguishing benign from malignant soft tissue tumors in infancy, include fibrous hamartoma of infancy,[22] infantile myofibromatosis,[23] fibromatosis colli,[24] infantile digital fibromatosis,[25] giant cell fibroblastoma,[26] cranial fasciitis,[27,28] lipoblastoma,[29] fetal rhabdomyoma,[30] and infantile hemangiopericytoma.[31,32]

MANAGEMENT

Surgery

The surgical management of the infant with cancer encompasses two major facets of care: fastidious attention to metabolic and physiological details, and adaptation of the extent of the surgical procedure to the unique biological behavior of the specific tumor in this age group. Surgical care during the preoperative, operative, and postoperative period must focus on such physiological considerations as temperature regulation, blood volume, fluid and electrolyte control (including calcium and phosphate), gestational development in the case of newborns, and the integrity of cardiac, pulmonary, and renal function.[33] Surgical care must be integrated into the overall treatment plan with regard to preoperative and postoperative chemotherapy and radiation therapy, which can alter nutritional status, wound healing, and immune function (also see Chap. 10).

Maintenance of fluid and caloric intake is imperative. Feeding should be sustained as long as possible without interruption. If the infant is to be kept *non per os,* an intravenous glucose solution with maintenance sodium and potassium should be supplied. The rate of infusion should provide somewhat higher than maintenance fluid requirements to ensure good renal function, particularly when hyperosmolar contrast materials have been used for radiographic studies.

Strict attention to the integrity of the coagulation system is also required in the young infant. Although vitamin K is routinely given at birth, additional doses may be needed to establish normal levels of vitamin K-dependent clotting factors (see Chap. 38).

In newborns, particularly those who are premature or small for gestational age, hypoglycemia, hypocalcemia, and environmental temperature must be observed and regulated. The infant's relatively thin skin, with a diminished layer of insulating subcutaneous fat, and the proportionately large surface-area-to-weight ratio create a pronounced vulnerability to large heat losses.[34] Metabolic acidosis, vasoconstriction, and depleted plasma volume can result from increased metabolic rate induced by hypothermic stress. Temperature regulation requires avoidance of heat loss and may necessitate transporting infants on beds with overhead servo-controlled heating units.

In the operating room, the infant should be placed on a heated mattress or heating lights should be used, and those skin areas that can be covered should be wrapped. Another potential source of heat loss is the evaporated water from the respiratory tract. Effective temperature exchange from endotracheal ventilation during anesthesia (required for most major operative procedures in infants) can be used to control evaporative water and heat loss. A heated nebulizer should be used to saturate the ventilated gases with water vapor and to maintain the temperature of the inhaled gases. This also avoids dehydration of airway secretions and injury to the respiratory epithelium. Intravenous fluids and transfused blood should also be warmed.

Adequate venous access must be ensured. If significant pulmonary compromise or metabolic acidosis is apparent or anticipated or if significant blood loss is likely, an indwelling temporal, radial, or tibial artery cannula should be placed to monitor arterial blood gases and possible hypotension.

During the course of surgery, blood loss must be monitored closely. Sponges should not be wetted so that they can be weighed to estimate their blood content. The volume of blood loss from suction should be collected in a reservoir, which should be placed close to the operating table in ready view of the anesthesiologist. The volume of "dead space" in the suction tubing between the patient and the calibrated measuring container should be minimized to provide greater accuracy of the blood loss estimate.[33] Hypocalcemia can occur as a result of the citrate in transfused blood, and effective levels of ionized calcium can also be lowered during administration of sodium bicarbonate to correct metabolic acidosis.[33] Prolonged operative procedures require an indwelling urinary catheter to monitor more closely urinary output and to avoid overdistention of the bladder.

When large serosal surfaces, such as the thorax or abdomen, are exposed during the operation, a significant volume of serous fluid is sequestered into the "third space." Replacement with 5% dextrose and Ringer's lactate approximates the composition of serum lost into the wound. The rate of infusion ranges from 5 to 15 ml/kg/hour, depending on the magnitude of loss. Rates 150% to 200% of those used for maintenance fluids may be required.[33] The appropriate use of colloid solutions may also be required.

The status of volume replacement postoperatively should be determined by assessing tissue perfusion. If there is concern, monitoring of central venous pressure should be done as well. After major abdominal, thoracic, and neurosurgical procedures, most infants recover to their preoperative status by the fifth postoperative day, with the resolution of ileus following abdominal surgery, return to oral feedings, and the beginning of wound healing.[33]

Radiation Therapy

Radiation therapy plays a major role in the management of most pediatric cancers. Because of the potential for acute and chronic side-effects, radiation must be used cautiously in young infants. The severity of the side-effects is generally assumed to be inversely related to the age of the child and directly related to dose.[35] Acute morbidity, such as gastrointestinal dysfunction, bone marrow suppression, and skin reactions, is seldom a limiting factor when radiation therapy is used alone, and the changes produced are generally reversible. However, pronounced late effects are not readily reversible. Very little published data exist on side-effects unique to infants and newborns. Estimates of potential damaging effects, generated from established specific tissue dose tolerances (see Chaps. 11 and 50), and guidelines formulated to avoid these effects are based on evidence derived from animal studies and experience with older children.

A major late effect of radiation is growth disturbance. Numerous investigators have shown in animal models that growing bone is very sensitive to ionizing radiation.[36] The possibility of bone and soft tissue deformity in children secondary to radiation therapy is well recognized, but the normal growth pattern of any organ or structure in the young child can be severely disrupted by therapeutic doses of radiation. Specific examples include mental retardation, aortic arch dysgenesis, and agenesis of the female breasts following radiation of relevant structures.[37] The oncogenetic effect of therapeutic radiation has recently emerged as a major problem.[38] At this point, there are no data to suggest that infants are particularly vulnerable to this effect.

It is generally believed that because of ongoing development, radiation sensitivity of certain structures and organs in infants is increased. One such organ is the brain. By the end of the first year of life, 90% of adult brain weight has been reached, but the brain of the young infant is still immature. There is a very high mitotic activity of spongioblasts, and many of the major nerve tracts have not been myelinated, particularly in the frontal lobes.[39] It has been reported that patients treated at a young age with radiation for brain tumors have a very high incidence of mental retardation.[40] Other major organ systems may also be particularly vulnerable to damage, including the skeleton, kidney, liver, and lung. Skeletal growth has been shown to be more severely affected, dose for dose, with younger age.[41,42] By extrapolation, it could be assumed that the young infant would be most affected. Acute and chronic nephropathy can be caused by relatively low-dose radiation therapy given at any age.[43] The kidney of the newborn may be even more sensitive to irradiation because of its immaturity, as demonstrated by low glomerular filtration rates during the first 6 months of life. In addition, the cortex-to-medullary-volume ratio of the kidney remains low during the first several months of life, not reaching the 3:1 ratio of the adult until 6 months of age.[44] Radiation damage to the liver can result in acute and chronic changes that may prove lethal. The liver's limited ability to conjugate bilirubin during the first week of life demonstrates immaturity, which suggests an increased radiation sensitivity.[45,46] Radiation therapy would also be expected to reduce the potential for normal development of the lung of the young infant and newborn. It can again be assumed that susceptibility to chronic pulmonary insufficiency increases with decreasing age at treatment.[47]

Pediatric tumors are generally quite radiosensitive; thus, relatively low total doses may be utilized. Protraction of therapy, using low-dose fractions and split-course techniques, coupled with alternating or simultaneous courses of chemotherapy, may be useful in preventing some of the late effects.[35] The total dose, daily dose, and duration of treatment given to infants and newborns must be based on the natural history of the specific disease process. Chemotherapy given for systemic benefit will probably provide an element of local tumor control as well, which may permit a significant reduction in total dose of radiotherapy required.[35]

Obvious technical difficulties exist in ensuring immobility during treatment planning and delivery. Physical restraints, sedation, and even short-term general anesthesia may be required.

The volume irradiated should be kept as small as possible, and beam-shaping blocks, electron therapy, and other technical maneuvers should be used to avoid irradiating especially sensitive structures and to decrease the risk of long-term sequelae. In tumors that tend to regress spontaneously, such as Stage IV-S neuroblastoma, it may not always be necessary to include the entire implicated volume to achieve the desired therapeutic results. "Shrinking fields" are also advantageous in other clinical situations. This method minimizes the volume that receives the highest dose and thus can avoid the delivery of damaging doses of radiation to vulnerable structures. Surgical procedures can be performed after preliminary courses of chemotherapy or after administration of part of the total planned radiation dose. This provides time during which relatively normal growth and development can occur. Reexploration permits accurate localization of the tumor volume that must be irradiated. In some situations, a second-look operation may allow direct implantation of radioactive materials into residual tumor, thus further minimizing the volume treated (see Chap. 10).[35]

Chemotherapy

The rationale for the use of cancer chemotherapeutic agents in the newborn and infant is no different than that for older children with disseminated solid tumors and acute leukemia (see Chap. 9).[48] However, because of the difficulties associated with surgery and radiotherapy in infants, chemotherapy plays an important role in reducing the size of massive tumors that clinically appear local. Such chemotherapeutic "debulking" may make these tumors more amenable to surgical or radiotherapeutic ablation, as well as preventing systemic spread or suppressing the growth of occult micrometastatic disease present at diagnosis.[49-51]

This is not to suggest that chemotherapy is without its own unique challenges in infants with cancer. Reports in the literature of specific toxicities in infants are very sparse. Several reports have demonstrated that infants experience excessive vincristine-related neurotoxicity, manifested in extreme cases by hypotonia, poor cry, inability to feed, and fatal flaccid paralysis.[3,52,53] Increased myelosuppression resulting in excessive toxicity in infants with Wilms' tumor given regimens containing vincristine, dactinomycin, and Adriamycin was seen in the Second National Wilms' Tumor Study, which resulted in the recommendation that dosages of all drugs be reduced by 50% in infants younger than 1 year (see Chap. 27).[54,55] This dosage reduction has not resulted in an increased rate of recurrence or metastasis.[56] These guidelines, which have been also adopted by the Intergroup Rhabdomyosarcoma Study Committee, appear to be rational recommendations for the management of solid tumors in an adjuvant setting where life-threatening toxicity due to myelosuppression must be considered (see Chap. 30). The same principles have also been used with intensive myeloablative regimens for the treatment of acute nonlymphoblastic leukemia (ANLL).[57] However, in a large series of infants with ALL, excessive chemotherapy-related toxicity, other than vincristine neurotoxicity, was not observed, and reduction of induction dosages for anticipated toxicity had an unfavorable impact on rates of remission induction and on remission duration (see Chap. 16).[3]

Reduction of initial dosages in an attempt to prevent toxicity does not lessen the need for continued vigilance in monitoring possible toxicity. To maximize therapeutic efficacy, judicious incremental increases of subsequent doses should be considered if toxicity has not developed. Chemotherapy-induced toxicity to specific organ systems (liver, lung, heart, kidney, CNS) has rarely been reported in infants. In the few cases of hepatotoxicity, the use of multiple chemotherapeutic agents or of simultaneous radiation therapy to the target organ makes it difficult to implicate specific drugs.[53,54,56]

Data are lacking on the clinical pharmacology of chemotherapeutic agents in newborns and infants (see Chap. 9). The optimal use of chemotherapy in this age group might best be accomplished with pharmacokinetic monitoring. However, there are distinct technical difficulties in monitoring small infants, and the rapid changes in physiological parameters that affect pharmacokinetics, particularly in the newborn, make such investigations difficult. Virtually every aspect of the distribution, excretion, and metabolism of anticancer drugs might be expected to be quantitatively and qualitatively altered in the newborn and young infant. Aspects unique to the pharmacology of the neonate include the rapid change in relative volume of fluid compartments that occurs after birth; different rates of hepatic metabolism; decreased efficiency of renal excretion; decreased protein-binding capacity; increased volume of cerebrospinal fluid, brain, and spinal cord relative to body surface area; increased permeability of blood–brain barrier; and erratic gastrointestinal absorption.[58]

Rapid changes in the volumes of body water compartments occur during the first 9 months of life. In newborns, total body water constitutes almost 80% of body weight, whereas values similar to those in adults (50%–55%) are seen in the older child.[59] Extracellular water volume is approximately 45% of body weight at birth but decreases to 20% in older children. However, the volumes of total body water and extracellular water are virtually constant when calculations are based on surface area. Most of the drugs used in cancer chemotherapy are distributed either in total body water or extracellular water. The convention of using body surface area in determining drug dosage results in a standardization of the concentration of chemotherapeutic agent originally in the drug's volume of distribution.[60] However, this method may not be appropriate for the very small infant (less than 6.0 kg), in whom calculations of dosage based on body weight may be more physiologic.[61]

The renal function of very young infants is less than would be predicted on the basis of body weight or surface area. Renal blood flow is lower in newborns, and the ability of the renal tubules to concentrate or acidify the urine is restricted.[62] The glomerular filtration rate is low at birth and changes rapidly during early development.[62-64] Even more significant for neonatal pharmacology is the underdevelopment of the organic ion transport system for active tubular secretion. The lower urinary pH of the newborn may result in an increased reabsorption rate of weakly acidic drugs. The maturation of various renal functions proceeds at different rates. Glomerular filtration attains the value seen in childhood (per unit of surface area) at 10 to 30 weeks of age.[64] In contrast, renal tubular secretion is not fully developed until about 7 months.[64,65] Chemotherapeutic agents that are not extensively metabolized and depend on renal excretion for elimination will be cleared slowly in the newborn and very young infant. This may result in prolonged plasma half-lives, with an increased risk of toxicity.

It has been demonstrated that at birth infants can metabolize a number of drugs and that the ability of hepatic tissue to metabolize different drugs matures at different rates.[66,67] The cytocrome P-450-dependent mixed-function oxidase system appears to develop early in infancy, as demonstrated by the fact that the clearance of phenobarbital changes from twice the adult level during the first 5 days of life to about half of that level at 1 month.[67] The rate of activation of cyclophosphamide would be expected to change in proportion to the activity of the hepatic mixed-function oxidase system.[68] There are wide interindividual variations in plasma clearance of specific drugs during the first few days of life. Thus, knowledge of the statistical mean rate of metabolism might be of little value to the clinician in choosing a drug dosage and regimen for a given infant.[58]

Because of the lower concentration of plasma proteins, the presence of a qualitatively different (fetal) albumin, high serum concentrations of competing substances such as bilirubin and free fatty acids, and lower blood pH,[63,69] the binding of drugs by plasma proteins is lower in the neonate, resulting in a higher volume of distribution.

Intrathecally administered methotrexate and cytarabine (ara-C) are widely used for the treatment or prevention of meningeal leukemia. It has been demonstrated that age-related pharmacokinetic differences exist and that body surface area does not accurately reflect the volume of the CNS.[70] An improved regimen for intrathecal methotrexate therapy has been proposed in which dosage is calculated according to the volume of the CNS, resulting in uniform cerebrospinal fluid (CSF) concentrations of drug. The substantially greater ability of drugs to enter the CNS of the newborn compared to the adult has been thought to reflect incomplete myelination. Increased CSF levels of methotrexate, despite normal renal clearance, have been demonstrated in infants receiving very high-dose systemic infusions of methotrexate when compared with older children.[71]

The absorption of drugs from the gastrointestinal tract is largely dependent on pH-related diffusion and gastric emptying time. Low gastric pH and prolonged gastric emptying time in infants[72] may result in relative inefficiency of orally administered chemotherapeutic agents. Diminished bile acid metabolism due to hepatic immaturity[73] may also result in prolonged clearance of those chemotherapeutic agents normally excreted in bile and thus in unanticipated toxicity.

Recommendations for dosage modifications in situations in which excessive myelosuppression should be avoided in newborns and young infants are provided in Table 12-4. These guidelines are based on the limited data available, and must be applied within the context of the specific cancer being treated and the individual clinical situation. Unless otherwise stated, "decreased dose" implies a 50% reduction of the reference dose for older children when calculated on the basis of body surface area. For infants weighing less than 6.0 kg, doses calculated on a mg/kg basis, using reference doses in milligrams derived for a 1 m^2 individual divided by 30 (assuming that a 1 m^2 individual weighs 30 kg), result in approximately the same 50% reduction.

Supportive Care

For the reasons already cited, management of the infant with cancer is best accomplished in a specialized pediatric tertiary care setting, wherein the unique medical, surgical, anesthesia, blood-banking, and nutritional requirements of seriously ill newborns and infants can be met readily.

Because venous access often becomes a problem very early in the management of infants, the elective placement of a tunneled indwelling right atrial (Hickman or Broviac) catheter[74,75] should be considered to facilitate the administration of parenteral alimentation, blood products, and chemotherapy. Cannulation of the external jugular vein rather than the usual cephalic vein is generally recommended for infants.[74] The use of other subcutaneous implantable devices for intravenous infusion is being evaluated in infants. Specific guidelines to prevent and treat the infectious and thrombotic occlusive complications of these indwelling catheters are presented elsewhere (see Chaps. 10 and 46).

Early empiric institution of nutritional support by nasogastric/jejunal feeding should be considered before the initiation of intensive therapies (see Chap. 48). Because there is growing suspicion that a malnourished state impairs host ability to tolerate anticancer therapy, possibly decreasing response to treatment,[76-78] the early use of parenteral alimentation is warranted when less invasive approaches are precluded by gastrointestinal dysfunction. This is necessary to prevent added morbidity of multimodality therapy until it is safely established that normal weight gain and growth can be accomplished without such supplementation.

Table 12-4
*Dosage Modifications of Chemotherapeutic Agents in Infants and Newborns**

Drug	Reason for Modification	Dose Modification
Vincristine	Decreased biliary excretion	Decrease by 50%; further decrease necessary in presence of jaundice
Actinomycin D	Decreased biliary excretion	
Adriamycin/Daunomycin	Decreased biliary excretion	Consider full dose of daunomycin after 3–6 mo of age in ALL
Cyclophosphamide	Hepatic activation decreased at birth	Decrease by 50% until >1–2 mo
Prednisone	Protein binding decreased in newborn	Decrease until 1 mo, particularly in presence of hyperbilirubinemia
Methotrexate (IV or PO)	Renal excretion and renal tubular secretion decreased until 6–8 mo	Decrease proportionately to decrease in GFR (assuming normal of 75–100 ml/min); monitor plasma clearance closely for high-dose regimens
Methotrexate (IT)	Relative difference in CSF volume	<3 mo, 3 mg; 4–11 mo, 6 mg; 12–23 mo, 8 mg
Ara-C	Clearance dependent on levels of cytidine deaminases; possible increased CSF levels with high-dose regimens	Decrease by 50%, particularly in high-dose regimens
Ara-C (IT)	Relative difference in CSF volume	<3 mo, 7.5 mg; 4–11 mo, 15 mg; 12–23 mo, 30 mg
DTIC	Decreased renal excretion	Decrease proportionately to decrease in GFR
Cisplatin	Decreased renal excretion and renal tubular secretion (until 6 mo)	Decrease proportionately to decrease in GFR
VP-16/VM-26	Decreased biliary excretion in neonatal period	Decrease by 50%; decrease further if jaundice is present
6-Mercaptopurine	Clearance dependent on levels of hepatic enzymes; decreased until 3 mo	Decrease by 50% until >3 mo

* Many of these modifications have been derived empirically and are not based on detailed pharmacokinetic studies.

Table 12-5
Neuroblastoma: Age-Related Differences in Disease Stage at Diagnosis

Evans Stage	Infants (%)	Children >12 Months of Age (%)
I	20	15
II	20	12.5
III	5	12.5
IV	25	55
IV-S	30	5

Of great importance is the immediate availability of blood products with the lowest possible shelf-life and of methodologies to provide maximal transfusion support without risk of excessive volume overload and unnecessarily increased donor exposures (*e.g.,* infant quadpacks and quintpacks, quadruple or quintuple blood collection systems, centrifugation of platelet-rich plasma, plateletpheresis, and directed donor programs) (see Chap. 38).[79] All blood products administered to infants receiving intensive chemotherapy should be irradiated (at least 1500 cGy) to prevent graft-versus-host disease.[80]

Potential long-term, organ-specific, treatment-related toxicities, anticipated to occur with increased frequency in infants with cancer, warrant the early institution of a coordinated, longitudinal evaluation of growth and specific organ (lung, skeletal, liver, kidney) function to identify subclinical problems that may respond to early therapeutic intervention (see Chap. 50). Most importantly, longitudinal assessment of neuropsychological development in infants at risk for neurotoxic sequelae might delineate early signs predictive of learning disabilities that could benefit from early remedial intervention.

SPECIFIC NEOPLASMS IN INFANCY

Neuroblastoma

Neuroblastoma accounts for more than one third of the malignancies observed in the first year of life and more than half of those in the neonatal period.[2] It is estimated that 21% to 35% of all neuroblastomas occur in infants younger than 1 year of age.[7,81] A provocative finding is that small neuroblastomas are found incidentally during routine necropsies of young infants dying of other causes with a frequency 40 times greater than expected for clinically overt neuroblastoma.[82] Recently, preterm birth has been found to be associated with a relatively lower risk for neuroblastoma, whereas low birth weight in term infants is associated with increased risk. These findings suggest a critical role for timing of exposure during gestation and the consequent relationship between teratogenesis and carcinogenesis.[83,84]

The primary site of neuroblastoma in infants is not different from that observed for older children: more than half of neuroblastomas in infants present in the abdomen, presumably originating in the adrenal (see Chap. 28).

Differences in extent of disease at diagnosis, demonstrated by the most widely used staging system, exist when data on infants are compared to those for older children,[6,85,86] as shown on Table 12-5. Only 25% of infants present with widespread metastases at diagnosis (Stage IV) and 30% of infants have Stage IV-S disease, known to be associated with a very favorable prognosis.[85,87–90] Stage IV-S patients are a unique group of infants who have seemingly localized primary tumors that do not cross the midline but also have evidence of distant spread to liver, skin, bone marrow, or combinations of these sites, without radiographic evidence of bone metastases.

The independent variables of age and stage have a dramatic impact on outcome in neuroblastoma. The overall disease-free survival for all infants with neuroblastoma approximates 75%, and survival rates ranging from 40% to 90% for infants with Stage IV disease have been reported.[88-91]

Although age and stage have important prognostic implications, these two variables alone cannot predict outcome. Other important prognostic variables in infants include serum levels of neuron-specific enolase (NSE),[92,93] serum ferritin,[94] cellular DNA content,[95] histopathology,[96] and amplification of the N-*myc* oncogene.[97,98] Infants with Stage III disease and favorable histopathology, less than ten copies of N-*myc,* and normal ferritin have a 3-year progression-free survival in excess of 70%, compared to less than 30% for infants with unfavorable histopathology, increased ferritin, and more than ten copies of N-*myc.*[98] Similarly, infants with Stage IV disease and NSE less than 100 ng/ml have a 70% progression-free survival rate compared to 30% for those with Stage IV disease and higher levels.[92] Such determinations should be considered in formulating treatment plans for infants with advanced-stage neuroblastoma.

The management of infants with Stage I or Stage II neuroblastoma consists of surgery alone if there is no residual tumor. Infants with Stage II neuroblastoma are likely to have posterior mediastinal primaries, and radiation therapy in doses of 900 to 1800 cGy has been used to treat intraspinal disease, with minimal toxicity,[99,100] if there is a risk of prohibitive morbidity with surgical excision.

Few other clinical situations in pediatric oncology are as controversial as the management of infants with Stage IV-S neuroblastoma. The finding of hyperdyploid cells by flow microfluorometric DNA analysis[95] provides convincing evidence that this is a malignant lesion rather than a hyperplastic proliferation resulting from a one-mutation (one hit) event in germinal cells, as previously proposed.[101]

Among 165 Stage IV-S patients for whom adequate follow-up data are available in the recent literature, the survival rate is 77%.[88-90] Only 24% of the deaths in this group resulted from progression of disease to Stage IV. The remainder were due to respiratory compromise secondary to massive hepatomegaly, coagulopathy, or therapy-related complications. More than 50% of these patients received some form of chemotherapy and some received radiotherapy. Of those who received no chemotherapy, 80% exhibited spontaneous regression of tumor. In the recently published 7-year Children's Cancer Study Group (CCSG) experience with 44 infants with Stage IV-S neuroblastoma,[90] the only deaths occurred in 3 patients younger than 2 months old at diagnosis, and the 2-year disease-free survival for infants aged 3 to 12 months was 97%. No significant influence of therapy (chemotherapy or radiotherapy) on ultimate survival could be demonstrated. A recent report of a nonrandomized study by the Pediatric Oncology Group demonstrated that chemotherapy consisting of cyclophosphamide and Adriamycin accelerated tumor regression but had no impact on overall survival.[102] The rate of spontaneous regression (30%) was decidedly lower in this series than in previous reports.[90,103]

Resolution of the controversy requires reexploration of the definition of Stage IV-S neuroblastoma.[104] Most importantly, the recently reported biological variables that have demonstrated prognostic significance in neuroblastoma (NSE, ferritin, N-*myc* amplification, and histopathology) must be evaluated in this group of patients. At present, because chemotherapy does accelerate tumor regression, treatment with cyclophosphamide 5 mg/kg/day for 5 days[107] or the sequentially scheduled regimen of cyclophosphamide 150 mg/m² for 7 days and Adriamycin 35 mg/m² on day 8[106] would seem warranted to initiate regression and certainly to prevent life-threatening complications related to mass disease. Radiotherapy in doses of 450 cGy (150 cGy daily fractions using lateral opposing fields) has also been effective.[35,103] Research is needed to identify those infants who may require more intensive therapy.

Wilms' Tumor

Kidney tumors account for 11% of cancers in infants. Although Wilms' tumor occurs in infants—16% of patients entered on the Second National Wilms' Tumor Study (NWTS-II) were younger than 12 months at diagnosis—the more frequent renal neoplasms in newborns and infants are infantile congeners of Wilms' tumor,[10] listed in Table 12-6. The most common is the congenital mesoblastic nephroma, delineated by Bolande and colleagues as a distinct entity.[12] In the past, this growth was confused with Wilms' tumor, which may account, in part, for the more favorable reported prognosis of Wilms' tumor in infants. Mesoblastic nephroma (also known as mesenchymal hamartoma of the kidney) is not encapsulated and infiltrates into normal renal parenchyma. Complete surgical excision, with meticulous nephrectomy, is required. Local recurrence

Table 12-6
Infantile Congeners of Wilms' Tumor

Renal Neoplasm	*Histologic and Clinical Characteristics*
Congenital mesoblastic nephroma	Fibromyomatoid tumor; usually benign; often congenital; most common in infants < 6 mo
Well-differentiated epithelial nephroblastoma	Closely packed, well-differentiated tubules; usually benign
Polycystic nephroblastoma or multiocular cystic nephroma	Macrocysts lined by flattened epithelium and fibrous septae; usually benign
Fetal rhabdomyomatous nephroblastoma	Predominantly in skeletal muscle; one third bilateral; usually benign
Nodular and blastema—nephroblastomatosis complex	Nodular or confluent subcortical masses of hamaratoid, hyperplastic epithelium; precursor of Wilms' tumor, particularly bilateral, hereditary type

occurs following inadequate resection, and close follow-up is recommended. Only sparse reports of metastatic spread exist.[106] Recently, a potentially aggressive variant has been described that is identified by foci of hemorrhage and necrosis, involvement of adjacent structures, and high cellularity and mitotic index and is associated with invasion of adjacent structures or organs, multiple recurrences, and metastases.[107] It is speculated that this lesion represents an intermediate between congenital mesoblastic nephroma and clear cell sarcoma of the kidney in the spectrum of infantile renal mesenchymal tumors originating from the premetanephric stromagenic stage of renal blastema.[108,109]

The clinical presentation and management of infants with Wilms' tumor are no different than in the older child (see Chap. 27). However, toxic deaths were reported in 6% of infants with group I or II disease in NWTS-II, presumably related to excessive hematologic toxicity.[55] Modifications in therapy for infants, consisting of a 50% reduction in the dosage of all chemotherapeutic agents were subsequently implemented and resulted in significant reduction in the severity and frequency of toxicity, with no deaths. Reduction in dosage did not jeopardize therapeutic efficacy of adjuvant therapy. There was no significant difference in relapse rates between infants treated with full doses of vincristine and actinomycin (with or without Adriamycin) and those treated with 50% lower doses.[57] Similar management has produced no excess toxicity or relapse in NWTS-III.

Acute Lymphoblastic Leukemia

Infants account for approximately 3% of all children with ALL and experience the worst prognosis of any group of children with this disease (Fig. 12-1).[3,4] In recent clinical trials of the CCSG, fewer than 25% of patients survived without relapse at 3 years from diagnosis. Infants present with a constellation of clinical features associated with a poor prognosis (Table 12-7). In addition, the blasts of infants with ALL more frequently have a common ALL antigen (CALLA)-negative phenotype which

also has important prognostic implications (see Chap. 16).[4] More recently, increased frequencies have been reported for cytogenetic abnormalities: pseudodiploidy and hypodiploidy, and translocations involving a break at the 11q23 region, the site of the c-*ets* 1 oncogene.[110] The relationship between cytogenetic abnormalities and outcome in this group is being investigated.

The poor outcome of infants with ALL and the high frequency of the CALLA-negative phenotype have raised questions as to whether this disease is truly of lymphoid origin. Phenotypic analysis of blast cells using monoclonal antibodies against lymphoid, myeloid, stem cell, and megakaryocytic determinants suggests that this disease originates from lymphoid cells at the earliest stages of B-cell commitment.[111] In addition, distinct differences in the ordered, hierarchical association of phenotype and genomic rearrangements have been observed in infants when compared to older children.[112] These unique biological differences may partially explain the poor outcome of ALL in infants.

Early treatment failure, characterized by systemic as well as extramedullary relapse, rather than excessive therapy-related toxicity with conventional treatments, explains the poor outcome of infants with ALL. Improved disease-free survival without excessive toxicity can be achieved in infants by using intensive therapy regimens that have proved successful for other ALL patients at high risk for early treatment failure.[113] A CNS relapse rate in excess of 20% despite CNS preventive therapy with whole brain irradiation and intrathecal methotrexate has been observed in infants.[3] Debilitating neuropsychological sequelae, presumably related to CNS irradiation, have been observed in 50% of the small number of long-term survivors.

The need for therapeutic strategies specifically designed for infants is obvious. Attempts to mitigate the disastrous neuropsychological sequelae associated with cranial irradiation by using very high-dose systemic methotrexate infusions[114] with intensive intrathecal chemotherapy are being explored in a CCSG study of ALL in infants. Further intensification of chemotherapy regimens and the use of alternative modalities, including transplantation, require investigation.

Acute Nonlymphocytic Leukemia

In contrast to ALL, the outcome for infants with ANLL is not significantly different than that for older children (see Chap. 17).[57] An excess of the French–American–British classification

FIGURE 12-1. Childhood ALL: survival from start of therapy, by age at diagnosis. (Reaman G, Zeltzer P, Bleyer WA et al: Acute lymphoblastic leukemia in infants less than one year of age: A cumulative experience of the Children's Cancer Study Group. J Clin Oncol 3:1513–1521, 1985. Copyright © 1985 Grune & Stratton)

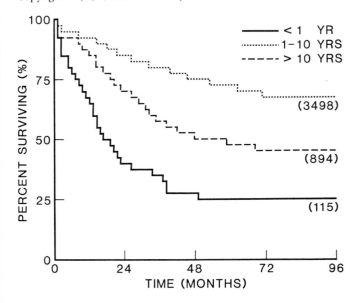

Table 12-7
Biological Characteristics That Are More Frequent in Infants Than in Older Children With ALL*

Characteristic	p Value
Elevated leukocyte count	<0.0001
Hepatomegaly	<0.0001
Splenomegaly	<0.0001
CNS leukemia at diagnosis	<0.0001
Hypogammaglobulinemia	<0.0001
Day 14 bone marrow M3 or M4	<0.0001
Thrombocytopenia	<0.05

(Reaman G, Zeltzer P, Bleyer WA et al: Acute lymphoblastic leukemia in infants less than one year of age: A cumulative experience of the Children's Cancer Study Group. J Clin Oncol 3:1513–1521, 1985. Copyright © 1985 Grune & Stratton)
* Based on analysis of 115 infants and 4392 children (>1 year) with ALL.

M4 and M5 (myelomonocytic and monoblastic) subtypes, which are associated with a less favorable prognosis,[115] has been observed in infants with ANLL. Among infants with ANLL entered on a recent CCSG study, hyperleukocytosis, CNS leukemia at diagnosis, and skin infiltration were found to occur significantly more often than among older children with this disease.[57] CNS leukemia at diagnosis was observed in 25.7% of infants compared to 5.3% of older children. Skin infiltration was observed in one third of infants younger than 3 months. Despite the marked differences in these clinical and laboratory features, no differences in either complete remission rate or survival at 3 years have been observed between infants younger than 1 year and children older than 2 years.

Rhabdomyosarcoma

Soft tissue sarcomas are relatively rare in infants, and this age group account for only 5% of patients in the Intergroup Rhabdomyosarcoma studies (see Chap. 30).[116] No differences in sex ratio or clinical groupings (stage) were observed. The significant differences in clinical presentation and response are shown in Table 12-8. Unlike neuroblastoma and Wilms' tumor, rhabdomyosarcoma occurring before 1 year of age is not associated with a more favorable outcome. Infants were noted to receive less chemotherapy and radiotherapy. Review of the radiotherapy data for infants with embryonal rhabdomyosarcoma demonstrated an increased risk of local recurrence in those given total doses below 4000 cGy in an attempt to reduce morbidity. In orbital rhabdomyosarcoma, effective local control was achieved with doses between 3000 and 4000 cGy; reduction of radiation doses to less than 3000 cGy to minimize acute and long-term side-effects in infants with soft tissue sarcomas may jeopardize local tumor control.[117]

Brain Tumors

Primary tumors of the CNS account for approximately 8% of cancer in infants and 3% of malignant tumors observed in newborns (see Chap. 24). The most common presenting feature is rapidly expanding head size and bulging fontanelle. Because of the expandability of the cranial vault, symptoms referrable to increased intracranial pressure, other than vomiting, are rare in infants. Papilledema is rarely observed. Other clinical signs observed with greater frequency include paresis, seizures, cranial nerve palsies, lethargy, and nuchal rigidity.[40] In contrast to the experience in older children, an increased

frequency of supratentorial, rather than infratentorial tumors, has been observed in infants,[40,118] in part because of an increased relative frequency of cerebral hemispheric tumors. Medulloblastoma and ependymal tumors account for approximately 50% of the histologic subtypes. Also, infants, unlike older children, show nearly equal sex distributions in the occurrence of brain tumors (see Chap. 24).

The primary treatment for brain tumors in children is radiation therapy. Because of the doses employed, serious sequelae are almost a certainty in infants with these tumors. Chemotherapy using vincristine and cisplatin, vincristine, nitrogen mustard, and procarbazine,[119] or cisplatin and VP-16,[120] with radiotherapy delayed until patients are 18 to 36 months old, has demonstrated efficacy without excessive toxicity in early follow-up. Further investigations of these and other preradiotherapy chemotherapy regimens, including the 8-in-1 regimen,[121] hopefully will provide a reasonable approach to the management of infants with brain tumors.

CONCLUSION

Improved survival can be achieved with intensive therapy, and the awareness of treatment-related toxicity in this patient population has significantly increased. The most important challenges that remain include continued investigation of the biological differences of certain tumor types in infants, the unique pharmacology of chemotherapeutic agents in the infant population, particularly in newborns, and the design of specific therapeutic strategies that provide adequate or increased disease control while lessening potential acute and long-term toxicities of therapy. It is expected that meeting these challenges will result in further improvements in the treatment of cancer in infants.

Table 12-8
Intergroup Rhabdomyosarcoma Studies I and II: Clinical Features and Outcome of Infants and Older Children

	Infants (n = 78)	Children >1 Year of Age (n = 1,561)
Tumor Type		
Undifferentiated sarcoma	26%	7%
Botryoid pathology	10%	4/%
Pelvic (bladder, prostate, vagina) primary	24%	10%
Clinical Group III Patients		
Mortality	54%	40%
Local recurrences	48%	16%

REFERENCES

1. Young JL, Miller RW: Incidence of malignant tumors in U.S. children. J Pediatr 86:254–258, 1975
2. Bader JL, Miller RW: U.S. cancer incidence and mortality in the first year of life. Am J Dis Child 133:157–159, 1979
3. Reaman G, Zeltzer P, Bleyer WA et al: Acute lymphoblastic leukemia in infants less than one year of age: A cumulative experience of the Children's Cancer Study Group. J Clin Oncol 3:1513–1521, 1985
4. Crist W, Pullen J, Boyett J et al: Clinical and biologic features predict a poor prognosis in acute lymphoid leukemias in infants: Pediatric Oncology Group Study. Blood 67:135–140, 1986
5. Finklestein JZ, Higgins GR, Rissman E et al: Acute leukemia during the first year of life. Presentation, chemotherapy and clinical course. Clin Pediatr 11:236–240, 1972
6. Evans AE, D'Angio GJ, Randolph J: A proposed staging for children with neuroblastoma. Cancer 27:374–378, 1971
7. Breslow NE, McCann B: Statistical estimation of prognosis for children with neuroblastoma. Cancer Res 31:2098–2103, 1971
8. Breslow NE, Palmer MF, Hill LR et al: Wilms' tumor: prognostic factors for patients without metastases at diagnosis. Cancer 41:1577–1589, 1978
9. Bolande RP: Neoplasia of early life and its relationship to teratogenesis. Perspect Pediatr Pathol 3:145–151, 1976
10. Bolande RP: Models and concepts derived from human teratogenesis and oncogenesis in early life. J Histochem Cytochem 32:878–884, 1984
11. Miller RW: Prenatal origins of cancer in man: epidemiologic evidence. In Tomatis L, Mohr U, Davis W (eds): Transplacental Carcinogenesis, pp 175–180. Lyon, France, International Agency for Research on Cancer, Scientific publication no. 4, 1973
12. Fraumeni JF Jr, Miller RW: Cancer deaths in the newborn. Am J Dis Child 117:186–189, 1969
13. Cutler SJ, Young JL Jr: Third National Cancer Survey: Incidence Data. Natl Cancer Inst Monogr 41:75–787, 1975
14. Bolande RP: Congenital mesoblastic nephroma of infancy. In Rosenberg HS, Bolande RP (eds): Perspectives in Pediatric Pathology, vol 1, pp 227–242. Chicago, Year Book Medical Publishers, 1973

15. Hanson MR, Mulvihill JH: Epidemiology of cancer in the young. In Levine AS (ed): Cancer in the Young, pp 3–11. New York, Masson Publishing, 1982

16. Chung EB: Pitfalls in diagnosing benign soft tissue tumors in infancy and childhood. Pathol Annu 20:323–386, 1985

17. Enzinger FM, Weiss SW: Fibrous proliferations of infancy and childhood. In Enzinger FM, Weiss SW (eds): Soft Tissue Tumors, pp 77–101. St Louis, CV Mosby, 1983

18. Soule EH, Mahour GH, Mills SD et al: Soft tissue sarcomas of infants and children: A clinical pathologic study of 135 cases. Mayo Clin Proc 43:313–316, 1968

19. Rosenberg, HS, Steenbeck WA, Spjut HJ: The fibromatoses of infancy and childhood. Perspect Pediatr Pathol 4:269–348, 1978

20. Allen PW: The fibromatoses. The clinical pathologic classification based on 140 cases: I. Am J Surg Pathol 1:255–268, 1977

21. Allen PW: The fibromatoses. The clinical pathologic classification based on 140 cases: II. Am J Surg Pathol 1:305–311, 1977

22. Mitchell ML, DiSant'Aagnese PA, Gerber JE: Fibrous hamartoma of infancy. Hum Pathol 13:586–588, 1982

23. Chung EB, Enzinger FM: Congenital fibromatosis (abstr). Lab Invest 40:246, 1979

24. Beatty EC Jr: Congenital generalized fibromatosis in infancy. Am J Dis Child 103:128–132, 1962

25. Iwasaki H, Kikuchi M, Ohtuski I et al: Infantile digital fibromatosis. Identification of actin filaments in cytoplasmic inclusions by heavy meromyosin binding. Cancer 52:1653–1657, 1983

26. Shmookler BM, Enzinger FM: Giant cell fibroblastoma: A peculiar childhood tumor (abstr). Lab Invest 46:76A, 1982

27. Allen PW: Recurring digital fibrous tumors of childhood. Pathology 4:215–217, 1972

28. Lauer DH, Enzinger FM: Craniofasciitis of childhood. Cancer 45:401–409, 1980

29. Shmookler BM, Enzinger FM: Giant cell liposarcoma occurring in children. An analysis of 17 cases and review of the literature. Cancer 52:567–572, 1983

30. Gardner DG, Corio RL: Fetal rhabdomyoma of the tongue with discussion of the two histologic variants of this tumor. Oral Surg 56:293–296, 1983

31. Campbell JS: Congenital capillary hemangiomas of the parotid gland. A lesion characteristic of infancy. N Engl J Med 254:56–61, 1956

32. Eimoto T: Ultrastructure of an infantile hemangiopericytoma. Cancer 40:2161–2163, 1977

33. de Lorimier AA, Harrison, MR: Surgical treatment of tumors in the newborn. Am J Pediatr Hematol Oncol 3:271–277, 1981

34. Sinclair JC: Thermal control of premature infants. Annu Rev Med 23:129–133, 1972

35. Littman P, D'Angio GJ: Radiation therapy in the neonate. Am J Pediatr Hematol Oncol 3:279–285, 1981

36. Engel D: Experiments in the production of spinal deformities by radium. Am J Roentgenol 42:217–224, 1939

37. Littman P, D'Angio GJ: Growth considerations in the radiation therapy of children with cancer. Annu Rev Med 30:405–415, 1979

38. Meadows AT, D'Angio GJ, Evans AE, et al: Spontaneous and treatment-related second malignant neoplasms in children. In Severi L (ed): Perugia Quadrennial International Conference on Cancer, pp 45–49. Monteluce, Italy, 1978

39. Yakovlev PI, Lecours AR: The myelogenetic cycles of regional maturation of the brain. In Minkowsky A (ed): Regional Development of the Brain in Early Life, pp 3–71. Oxford, Blackwell, 1967

40. Farwell J, Dohrmann GJ, Flannery JT: Intracranial neoplasms in infants. Arch Neurol 35:533–557, 1978

41. Neuhauser EBD, Wittenborg M, Berman L et al: Irradiation effects of roentgen therapy on the growing spine. Radiology 59:637–650, 1952

42. Probert JC, Parker BR: The effects of radiation therapy on bone growth. Radiology 114:155–162, 1975

43. Maier JG: Effects of radiation on kidney, bladder and prostate. In Vaeth JM (ed): Frontiers of Radiation Therapy and Oncology, vol 6, pp 196–207. Basel, Karger, 1972

44. Tina LU, Papadopoulon ZL, Jose P, Calcagno PL: Renal diseases. In Avery GB (ed): Neonatology. Pathophysiology and Management of the Newborn, pp 661–700. Philadelphia, JB Lippincott, 1981

45. Kraut JW, Bagshaw MA, Glatstein E: Hepatic effects of irradiation. In Vaeth JM (ed): Frontiers of Radiation Therapy and Oncology, vol 6, pp 182–195. Basel, Karger, 1972

46. Maisels MJ: Neonatal jaundice. In Avery GB (ed): Neonatology. Pathophysiology and Management of the Newborn, pp 473–544. Philadelphia, JB Lippincott, 1981

47. Rubin P, Van Houtte P, Constine L: Radiation sensitivity and organ tolerances in pediatric oncology: A new hypothesis. In Vaeth JM (ed): Frontiers of Radiation Therapy, vol 16, pp 62–82. Basel, Karger, 1982

48. Bleyer WA: Cancer chemotherapy in infancy and children. Pediatr Clin North Am 32:557–574, 1985

49. Siegel SE, D'Angio DJ, Evans AE, Breslow N et al: The treatment of Wilms' tumor: Results of the National Wilms' Tumor Study. Cancer 38:633–647, 1976

50. Ortega JA, Rivard GE, Isaacs H et al: Influence of chemotherapy on the diagnosis of rhabdomyosarcoma. Med Pediatr Oncol 1:227–234, 1975

51. Siegel MM, Siegel SE, Isaacs H et al: Primary chemotherapeutic management of unresectable and metastatic hepatoblastoma in children. Med Pediatr Oncol 4:294–304, 1978

52. Allen JC: The effects of cancer therapy on the nervous system. J Pediatr 93:903–909, 1978

53. Wood WG, O'Leary M, Nesbit ME: Life-threatening neuropathy and hepatotoxicity in infants during induction therapy for acute lymphoblastic leukemia. J Pediatr 98:642–645, 1981

54. Jones B, Breslow N, Takashima J: Toxic deaths in the Second National Wilms' Tumor Study. J Clin Oncol 2:1028–1033, 1984

55. Informational Bulletin, National Wilms' Tumor Study II, February 16, 1977

56. Morgan E, Baum E, Breslow N et al: Chemotherapy-related toxicity in infants treated according to the Second National Wilms' Tumor Study. J Clin Oncol (in press)

57. Lampkin B, Buckley J, Nesbit N et al: Clinical and laboratory findings and response to therapy in infants less than one year of age with acute non-lymphocytic leukemia (ANLL) (abstr). Proc Am Soc Clin Oncol 785, 1984

58. Siegel SE, Moran RG: Problems in the chemotherapy of cancer in the neonate. Am J Pediatr Hematol Oncol 3:287–295, 1981

59. Friis-Hansen B: Body water compartments in children: Changes during growth and related changes in body composition. Pediatrics 28:169–181, 1961

60. Pinkel D: The use of body surface area as a criterion of drug dosage in cancer chemotherapy. Cancer Res 18:853–856, 1958

61. Shirkey HC: Pediatric clinical pharmacology and therapeutics. In Avery GS (ed): Drug Treatment: Principles and Practice of Clinical Pharmacology and Therapeutics, pp 97–157. Sydney, Adis Press, 1980

62. Hook JB, Bailie MD: Perinatal renal pharmacology. Annu Rev Pharmacol Toxicol 19:491–509, 1979

63. Morselli PI: Clinical pharmacokinetics in neonates. Clin Pharmacol 1:81–86, 1976

64. West JR, Smith HW, Chasis H: Glomerular filtration rate, effective renal blood flow and maximal tubular excretory capacity in infancy. J Pediatr 32:10–18, 1948

65. Gladtke E, Heimann G: The rate of development of elimination functions in kidney and liver of young infants. In Morselli, A Garattine B, Sereni C (eds): Basic and Therapeutic Aspects of Perinatal Pharmacology, pp 393–402. New York, Raven Press, 1976

66. Neims AH, Warner M, Loughman PM et al: Developmental aspects of the hepatic cytochrome P-450 monooxygenase system. Rev Pharmacol Toxicol 16:427–445, 1976

67. Done AK, Cohen SN, Strebel L: Pediatric clinical pharmacology and the "therapeutic orphan." Rev Pharmacol Toxicol 17:561–573, 1977

68. Grochow LB, Colvin M: Clinical pharmacokinetics of cyclophosphamide. Clin Pharmacokinet 4:380–394, 1979

69. Ehrenbo M, Agurell S, Jalling B et al: Age difference in drug binding by plasma proteins; studies on human fetuses, neonates and adults. Eur J Clin Pharmacol 3:189–193, 1971

70. Bleyer WA: Clinical pharmacology of intrathecal methotrexate: II. An improved dosage regimen derived from age related pharmacokinetics. Cancer Treat Rep 61:1419–1425, 1977

71. Bleyer A, Reaman G, Poplack D et al: Central nervous system (CNS) pharmacology of high dose methotrexate (HDMTX) in infants with acute lymphoblastic leukemia (ALL) (abstr). Proc Am Soc Clin Oncol 3:199, 1984

72. Yaffes SJ, Juchau MR: Perinatal pharmacology. Rev Pharmacol Toxicol 14:219–238, 1974

73. Murphy GM, Singer E: Bile acid metabolism in infants and children. Gut 15:151–162, 1974

74. Heimback DM, Ivey TD: Techniques for placement of a permanent home hyperalimentation catheter. Surg Gynecol Obstet 143:635–636, 1976

75. Hickman, RO, Buckner CD, Clift RA et al: A modified right atrial catheter for access to the venous system in marrow transplant recipients. Surg Gynecol Obstet 148:871–875, 1979

76. Donaldson SS, Wesley MN, Ghavimi F et al: A prospective randomized

clinical trial of total parenteral nutrition in children with cancer. Med Pediatr Oncol 10:129–139, 1982

77. Van Eys J, Wesley MM, Cangir A et al: The safety of intravenous hyperalimentation in children with malignancies. J Parenter Enter Nutr 6:291–294, 1982
78. Brennan MF: Total parenteral nutrition in the cancer patient. N Engl J Med 305:375–382, 1981
79. Luban NLC: Blood groups and blood component transfusion in Miller DR, Baehner RL, McMillan CW (eds): Blood Diseases of Infancy in Childhood, pp 46–93. St Louis, CV Mosby, 1984
80. Woods WG, Lubin BH: Fatal graft versus host disease following a blood transfusion in a child with neuroblastoma. J Pediatr 67:217–221, 1981
81. Voute PA: Neuroblastoma. In Sutow WW, Fernbach DJ, Vietti TJ (eds): Clinical Pediatric Oncology, pp 559–587. St Louis, CV Mosby, 1984
82. Beckwith JB, Perrin EV: In situ neuroblastoma; a contribution to the natural history of neural crest tumors. Am J Pathol 43:1089–1104, 1963
83. Johnson CC, Spitz MR: Neuroblastoma: Case control analysis of birth characteristics. JNCI 74:789–792, 1985
84. Johnson CC, Spitz MR: Prematurity and risk of childhood cancer (letter). JNCI 76:2, 1986
85. Evans AE, Chatten J, D'Angio GJ et al: Review of 17 IV-S neuroblastoma patients at the Children's Hospital of Philadelphia. Cancer 45:833–839, 1980
86. Evans AE: Staging and treatment of neuroblastoma. Cancer 45:1799–1802, 1980
87. D'Angio GJ, Evans AE, Koop CE: Special pattern of widespread neuroblastoma with a favorable prognosis. Lancet 1:1046–1049, 1971
88. Rosen EM, Cassidy JR, Frantz CN et al: Neuroblastoma: The Joint Center for Radiation Therapy/Dana-Farber Cancer Institute/Children's Hospital experience. J Clin Oncol 2:719–732, 1984
89. Nitschke R, Humphrey GB, Sexauer CL et al: Neuroblastoma: Therapy for infants with good prognosis. Med Pediatr Oncol 11:154–158, 1983
90. Nickerson HJ, Nesbit ME, Grosfeld JL et al: Comparison of stage IV and IV-S neuroblastoma in the first year of life. Med Pediatr Oncol 13:261–268, 1985
91. Kretschmer CS, Frantz CN, Rosen EM et al: Improved prognosis for infants with stage IV neuroblastoma. J Clin Oncol 2:799–803, 1984
92. Zeltzer PM, Parma AM, Dalton A et al: Raised neuron-specific enolase in serum of children with metastatic neuroblastoma. Lancet 2:361–363, 1983
93. Zeltzer PM, Marangos PS, Sather H et al: Prognostic importance of serum neuron-specific enolase in local and widespread neuroblastoma. In Evans AE, D'Angio GJ, Seeger RC (eds): Advances in Neuroblastoma Research, pp 319–329. New York, Allen R Liss, 1985
94. Hann HWL, Evans AE, Siegel SE et al: Prognostic importance of serum ferritin in patients with stage III and IV neuroblastoma: The Children's Cancer Study Group experience. Cancer Res 45:2843–2847, 1985
95. Look AT, Hayes FA, Nitschke R et al: Cellular DNA content as a predictor of response to chemotherapy in infants with unresectable neuroblastoma. N Engl J Med 311:231–235, 1984
96. Shimada H, Chatten J, Newton WA et al: Histopathologic prognostic factors in neuroblastic tumors: definition of subtypes of ganglioneuroblastoma and an age-linked classification of neuroblastomas. JNCI 73:405–416, 1984
97. Brodeur GM, Seeger RC, Schwab M et al: Amplification of N-myc in untreated human neuroblastoma correlates with advanced disease stage. Science 224:1121–1124, 1984
98. Seeger R, Brodeur HG, Sather H et al: Multiple copies of the N-myc oncogene in neuroblastomas are associated with rapid tumor progression. N Engl J Med 313:1111–1116, 1985
99. Jacobson HM, Marcus RB, Thor TL et al: Pediatric neuroblastoma: Postoperative radiation therapy using less than 2,000 rad. Int J Radiat Oncol Biol Phys 9:501–505, 1983
100. McGuire WA, Simons DL, Grosfeld JL et al: Should stage II neuroblastoma receive irradiation? Proc Am Soc Clin Oncol 3:80, 1984
101. Knudson AG, Meadows AT: Regression of neuroblastoma IV-S: A genetic hypothesis. N Engl J Med 302:1254–1256, 1980
102. McWilliams NB, Hayes FA, Smith IE et al: IV-S neuroblastoma (NBL): chemotherapy (CT) vs observation (O). Proc Am Soc Clin Oncol 5:830, 1986
103. Evans AE, Baum E, Chard R: Do infants with stage IV-S neuroblastoma need therapy? Arch Dis Child 56:271–274, 1981
104. McWilliams NB: IV-S neuroblastoma: treatment controversy revisited. Med Pediatr Oncol 14:41–44, 1986
105. Green AA, Hayes FA, Hustu HO: Sequential cyclophosphamide and doxorubicin for induction of complete remission in children with disseminated neuroblastoma. Cancer 48:2310–2317, 1981
106. Snyder HM, Lack EE, Chetty-Baktavizian A et al: Congenital mesoblastic nephroma: Relationship to other renal tumors of infancy. J Urol 126:513–516, 1981
107. Beckwith JB, Weeks DA: Congenital mesoblastic nephroma. When should we worry? Arch Pathol Lab Med 110:98–99, 1986
108. Joshi VV, Kasznica J, Walters TR: Atypical mesoblastic nephroma. Pathological characteristics of a potentially aggressive variant of conventional congenital mesoblastic nephroma. Arch Pathol Lab Med 110:100–106, 1986
109. Haas JE, Bonadio JF, Beckwith JB: Clear cell sarcoma of the kidney with emphasis on ultrastructural studies. Cancer 54:2978–2987, 1984
110. Carroll AJ, Frankel LS, Pullen DJ, Crist WM: Acquired cytogenetic abnormalities in blast cells of infants with acute lymphoblastic leukemia (abstr). Blood 69(Suppl):252A, 1986
111. Dinndorf PA, Reaman GH: Acute lymphocytic leukemia in infants: evidence for B cell origin of disease by use of monoclonal antibody phenotyping. Blood 68:975–978, 1986
112. Felix C, Reaman GH, Korsmeyer SJ, et al: Immunoglobulin and T cell receptor gene configuration in acute lymphoblastic leukemia of infancy. Blood 70:536–544, 1987
113. Reaman G, Steinherz P, Gaynon P et al: Improved survival of infants less than one year of age with acute lymphoblastic leukemia treated with intensive multiagent chemotherapy Cancer Treat Rep 71:1033–1039, 1987
114. Poplack D, Reaman G, Bleyer W et al: Central nervous system (CNS) preventive therapy with high dose methotrexate (HDMTX) in acute lymphoblastic leukemia (ALL): A preliminary report. Proc Am Soc Clin Oncol 3:204, 1984
115. Weinstein HJ, Mayer RJ, Rosenthal DS et al: Chemotherapy for acute myelogenous leukemia in children and adults. VAPA update. Blood 62:315–319, 1983
116. Ragab A, Heyn R, Tefft M et al: Infants under one year of age with soft tissue sarcomas: a report from the Intergroup Rhabdomyosarcoma Study (IRS) Committee (abstr). Proc Am Soc Clin Oncol 5:807, 1986
117. Tefft M, Wharam M, Gehan E: Radiation therapy and embryonal rhabdomyosarcoma: local control in children less than one year of age and in children with tumors of the orbit. A report from the Intergroup Rhabdomyosarcoma Study (IRS). Proc Am Soc Clin Oncol 5:803, 1986
118. Cangir A, Shallenberger RG, Chorossy M: Malignant neoplasms in neonatal period (abstr). Proc Am Soc Clin Oncol 6:215, 1987
119. Kretschmer C, Flummerfelt-Rappaport P, Tarbell N et al: Preradiation chemotherapy for infants and children with malignant tumors of the CNS. Proc Am Soc Clin Oncol 5:813, 1986
120. Strauss LC, Killmond T, Maria BL et al: Primary chemotherapy with cisplatin and VP16 in children under 36 months old with brain tumors. Proc Am Soc Clin Oncol 5:832, 1986
121. Zeltzer P, Odom L, Priest J: Pilot study of pre- and post-radiation therapy (XRT) chemotherapy using eight drugs in one day (8 in 1) for high risk medulloblastoma: Effect on XRT delivery and toxicity (abstr). Proc Am Soc Clin Oncol 5:829, 1986

thirteen

Cancer Clinical Trials: Design, Conduct, Analysis, and Reporting

Richard S. Ungerleider and
Susan S. Ellenberg

The major concern of pediatric oncologists is the cure of children with malignancy. The past three decades have witnessed a remarkable improvement in the life expectancy of children diagnosed with cancer, which has occurred as the cumulative result of many typically modest advances. Demonstration of the benefit of these advances largely relies on the systematic use of therapeutic clinical trials. A clinical trial is an experiment that attempts to answer a medical question, most often regarding the effect of a therapeutic intervention on the outcome of a disease. As an experiment, it is carried out under conditions determined in advance by the investigator, who uses a specified methodology to test the hypothesis of interest. A valuable experiment is one that addresses a nontrivial question in such a way as to provide results that are unambiguous, reliable, and easily interpretable. This chapter discusses the requirements of a valuable clinical trial in terms of design, analysis, and subsequent reporting, with attention to the particular problems in applying clinical trials methodology to the study of cancer in children. Our intention is to provide information of use both in mounting clinical trials and in reviewing the published efforts of others.

The rationale for conducting clinical trials in pediatric oncology goes beyond the demonstrated utility of the approach to date. It is more importantly based on the need to reach accurate conclusions regarding the benefit of toxic and expensive therapies. Nonexperimental research, in which reasoning rather than observation is used to reach conclusions, or flawed experimental research, in which the therapeutic intervention is inconsistent or uncontrolled, can severely restrict progress toward the cure of childhood cancer by erroneously supporting the value of what is actually a useless or harmful treatment.

Cancer clinical trials are conventionally categorized into three types,[1] derived from usage adopted by the National Cancer Institute (NCI) drug development program. A Phase I trial investigates the toxicities associated with a particular agent and determines the maximum tolerated dose (MTD) for a given schedule and route of administration.[2] A Phase II trial estimates the activity of the agent against individual tumor types.[3] A Phase III trial assesses the activity of the agent in a comparative fashion, with reference to either the natural history of the disease or standard therapy.[4] The application of these concepts now extends beyond new drug development to include the evaluation of any new therapeutic approach, but the progression (from assessment of toxicity through estimation of efficacy and finally to establishment of superiority, equivalence, or inferiority through direct comparison) remains constant. When clinical trials are used to evaluate a treatment regimen rather than an individual agent, Phases I and II are sometimes combined and referred to as a pilot study.[5]

PLANNING THE CLINICAL TRIAL

The process of planning a clinical trial culminates in the generation of a protocol, or written guide to the experiment to be conducted. The impact of the protocol on the conduct of the clinical trial is obvious: as a procedural guide, it helps ensure that the investigation is carried out uniformly. An equally vital role is to ensure that the investigators develop a precise, well-justified, and practical approach to the study. Adherence to the organizational requirements of a well-constructed protocol should guide the investigator through the planning process so that the resultant clinical trial is significant, feasible, and has a high likelihood of providing a definitive answer to an important question.

The components of a typical protocol are listed in Table 13-1. The eventual success of any clinical trial depends heavily on the care and skill devoted to the consideration of each of these items. Given the substantial investment in time, effort, and expense required from participants (collaborators *and* patients) during the trial and the potential damage associated with an incorrect result, the responsibility of critical protocol development cannot be overemphasized. Proper attention to these requirements helps to maximize the value of the experiment and its probability of impact on the medical community.

Objectives

The first protocol requirement is a statement of objectives. This should be limited to the actual research question, such as, "in Stage I Wilms' tumor, to determine whether 6 months of postoperative treatment with vincristine and actinomycin D (dactinomycin) results in disease-free survival equivalent to that observed with 15 months of vincristine and actinomycin D." Less exact versions, such as, "to reduce the vicissitudes of treatment of Wilms' tumor," should be rejected. The inability to set down a sharply defined objective is indicative of a poorly developed research plan, as is commonly seen when a patient-management guide masquerades as a clinical trials protocol. A precise statement of the objective focuses the investigator on the conditions required to conduct the chosen experiment and allows him or her to assess the feasibility of the trial in terms of the available resources.

It is particularly important in pediatric clinical trials to limit the number of study objectives because the available patient population is not sufficiently large to provide answers to numerous experimental questions. Ideally, the objectives should reflect the most important hypotheses that require evaluation, although this is not always possible. The restrictions imposed by limited patient numbers generally necessitate multi-institutional collaborations. Although such arrangements do increase patient availability, they often cause difficulty in arriving at a common research plan because of the multiplicity of opinions involved.

It is advisable to select objectives that will provide useful information regardless of whether the study results are positive

Table 13-1
Typical Protocol Headings

1. Objectives
2. Background
3. Patient Eligibility Criteria
4. Design
5. Treatment Plan
6. Drug Information
7. Criteria for Evaluating Treatment Effect
8. Clinical and Laboratory Data to be Accessioned
9. Statistical Considerations
10. Informed Consent
11. References
12. Appendices

or negative. This is possible when a biological hypothesis is tested in a carefully controlled manner.[6]

Background

The Background section provides the underpinnings for the entire protocol by presenting the arguments for conducting the clinical trial and for selecting the specific experimental conditions enumerated in subsequent sections. As a crystallization of the thoughts that led to the proposal's existence, it should provide adequate justification for mounting what will be a difficult, time-consuming, and costly exercise. This section is generally a review of the pertinent medical literature, presented in such a way as to convince the reader that the question is compelling, has not previously been answered, and can feasibly be addressed with existing resources. The plausibility of the hypothesis must be supported through documentation of its biological or experiential basis. Information on prognostic factors pertinent to patient selection should be reviewed and material relevant to design considerations included. Discussion of the significance of the proposed trial should be within the perspective provided by previous clinical trials. Background information for Phase I protocols should include preclinical (*in vitro* and animal) data, as well as results of human trials with the experimental agent. The rationale for using the agent in children should be presented, along with justifications for the chosen schedule and starting dose. Phase II protocols should additionally include a summary of available toxicity data in adults and children and a justification of the choice of malignancies against which the agent will be assessed. Phase III protocols require extensive Background sections that establish the basis and significance of the protocol within the framework of previously ascertained results.

Patient Eligibility Criteria

The protocol should clearly define the characteristics of the patient population to be studied, including such factors as diagnosis, extent of disease (stage), age restrictions, allowable prior therapy, physiological and performance status, and any other conditions the investigator wishes to specify, such as the expression of particular immunologic markers by malignant cells. In the United States, informed consent must be obtained from patients or parents (depending on patient age) to establish eligibility (see Chaps. 15 and 46). The population defined by these criteria will be the one to which the study results clearly apply; thus, the criteria must be carefully chosen and precisely defined.

Although it may be desirable to restrict study entry to a homogeneous patient population, the realities of biological variability preclude this; until all factors affecting prognosis are elucidated, study populations will consist of mixtures of patient groups, each of which may behave differently under the conditions of the experiment. The relatively small number of pediatric patients available to enter clinical trials presents further problems, in that overly restrictive criteria can result in insufficient entries to answer the study question. It is often difficult, and sometimes impossible, to reach the proper balance. It should be realized that some studies simply are not feasible. Diluting the study population is not a solution, and the investigator should resist the temptation to widen eligibility merely to satisfy accrual requirements. One should attempt to exclude groups of patients who *a priori* may not be comparable with the others in terms of potential benefit from therapy, as their inclusion will diminish the sensitivity of the study.

Although this may lead to results that are valid for only a small percentage of the patient population, the gain in interpretability offsets the cost of limited applicability.

Phase I protocols generally specify patients who have failed conventional therapy yet have sufficiently intact organ function for accurate assessment of toxicity. At least 1 month should have elapsed since the most recent antitumor therapy to ensure that acute effects of that treatment have subsided. Patients with solid tumors should not have bone marrow dysfunction, so that toxic effects on normally functioning marrow can be assessed. This criterion does not apply to patients with leukemia. Patients with any histologic type of cancer are usually eligible for Phase I studies, although solid tumor and leukemia patients must be evaluated separately to determine the maximum tolerated dose.[2] Patients with leukemia commonly tolerate higher doses of myelosuppressive agents; moreover, marrow suppression is sought in leukemia patients[7,8] but avoided in solid tumor patients. Regardless of tumor type, life expectancy sufficient to permit assessment of drug-related effects should be specified.

Phase II studies are ideally conducted with previously untreated patients to avoid the problems of acquired drug resistance and diminished tolerance associated with prior treatment. However, because most childhood cancers are potentially curable at diagnosis with conventional therapies, Phase II studies in children generally specify that patients must have failed standard therapy and often a retrieval therapy as well. There has been increasing use of Phase II evaluation prior to definitive therapy ("experimental window") in certain clinical situations, such as Stage III or Stage IV neuroblastoma in children older than 1 year, where the outcome of conventional therapy is dismal and a delay in such therapy to evaluate new agents is not deemed unethical. The value of this approach has not yet been determined, but the response rates in previously untreated patients are expected to be more reliable than those in patients who have undergone multiple pretreatments.

Phase II protocols additionally specify histologic diagnoses acceptable for entry because the endpoint, tumor shrinkage, is often dependent on tumor type. Patients are also generally required to have measurable disease so that antitumor response can be reliably assessed.

Design

The Design section of the protocol provides a brief overview of the study's structure, describing the methods by which the objectives are to be met. The minimum requirements for this section include the plans for patient allocation and the criteria by which the experimental effect is to be evaluated (*i.e.,* study endpoints). In our previous example of a Phase III clinical trial in Stage I Wilms' tumor, where the endpoint of interest is relapse, the design would specify that after surgical removal of the tumor and 6 months of adjuvant chemotherapy with vincristine and actinomycin D, patients are to be randomly allocated to no further therapy versus an additional 9 months of chemotherapy, with subsequent tabulation of relapses on both regimens.

Phase I studies in children typically employ a standardized design in which cohorts of three patients with solid tumor and three with leukemia are treated with identical dosages of the experimental agent and then observed for acute toxicity. In the absence of dose-limiting toxicity (DLT), an additional cohort is treated with an increased dosage level and observed. This procedure continues until DLT occurs in one or more patients. If the DLT is nonhematologic, an additional three patients are treated at the preceding dosage level to verify that it is a safe starting dosage for Phase II trials; the trial then ceases. If the DLT is hematologic, the trial is closed only for solid tumor patients; cohorts of leukemia patients continue to receive escalated dosages until nonhematologic DLT occurs and the preceding level is verified as safe. Although patients treated at low dosages may be subsequently retreated at a higher level, the analysis to determine a safe dosage should be based on cohorts that have not previously been treated with the study drug to avoid mistaking cumulative toxicity for acute effects.

The starting dosage, in the absence of data derived from adult Phase I trials, is based on animal toxicology studies and generally is one tenth of the dosage lethal to 10% of a cohort of mice, expressed in mg/m^2 ($\frac{1}{10}$ $MELD_{10}$).[9] If data from Phase I trials in adults are available, it is more efficient to start children's trials at 75% to 80% of the adult Phase II dosage, bypassing levels that are presumably safe in children but are unlikely to be of benefit. Escalation should continue, in the absence of DLT, beyond the Phase II dosage established for adults, because children often display greater tolerance to chemotherapy,[8] and one generally wants to deliver the highest safe dosage of a new agent in efficacy trials.

In Phase I trials, the stepwise dosage increases are prespecified in the protocol. When the starting dosage is based on animal data, a modified Fibonacci scheme[10] is often used to determine the escalations for successive cohorts: the starting dosage is increased by 100% in the first escalation, and subsequent dosages are increased by adding 67%, 50%, 40%, and finally 33% of the dosage established by the preceding cohort. The diminution of the escalations reflects increasing caution as one gets farther from the starting dosage. Starting dosages derived from the adult MTD are presumably close to the childhood MTD, and escalation should proceed cautiously, using 20% increases over the preceding dosage level.[8]

The conventional objective of Phase II trials is to determine whether a new agent, or any new treatment strategy, appears sufficiently active to warrant further study. "Activity" is usually defined by objective tumor responses, although laboratory endpoints such as immune parameters and cytogenetic normalization are of increasing interest because of the advances in understanding of the malignant process. It is generally desirable to limit Phase II studies to small numbers of patients to permit testing of the maximum number of agents or programs that require evaluation. Sample sizes for Phase II studies have traditionally been set at 25 to 40 patients. Such patient numbers, however, do not permit accurate estimation of tumor response rate. For example, if 5 responses are observed in 25 patients, the 90% confidence interval around the observed rate of 20% is [10%, 36%]. With 40 patients and 8 responses, the 90% confidence interval around the same observed rate of 20% is [11%, 31%]—narrower, but still too wide to permit reliable distinction between uninteresting and moderate levels of activity. Thus, typical designs have been geared toward identifying regimens whose response rates appear consistent with interesting levels of activity, rather than obtaining accurate estimates of response rates.

Phase II Trials: Specific Designs

The simplest and perhaps most widely used Phase II design was suggested by Gehan[11] in 1961. Gehan proposed a two-stage design, with the sample size in the first stage dependent on the minimum response rate of interest and the total sample size dependent on the expected variability of the estimate of the response rate (standard error). A sample size of 25 patients will produce an estimate of response rate with a standard error no greater than ten percentage points. The purpose of the two-stage design is to permit early termination when the activity level observed is clearly inconsistent with the minimum level of interest ($p < 0.05$). For example, in a disease for which many agents are reasonably active, a new agent might be of interest only if it were associated with a true response rate of 25% or more. If this agent were given to 11 consecutive patients without a response, one would probably want to discontinue its use because a drug with a "true" 25% response rate would show such a negative result less than 5% of the time. In a disease for which few active agents have been identified, the threshold response rate of interest may be as low as 15%, or even 10%. Table 13-2 shows the required first-stage sample size for different response rates of interest. The total sample size should generally be at least 25, and larger samples are needed when small response rates are of interest.

A related design was proposed by Fleming[12] in 1982. This design uses two or more stages and allows for early termination when one can be fairly certain that the activity level is either too low or adequately high. To implement a Fleming design, one first selects the upper limit of the "definitely uninteresting" range of response rates and the lower limit of the "definitely interesting" range. (The midpoint between the two limits would be considered the "indifference point".) One can then select a sample size to minimize the probability of "accepting" a truly uninteresting drug while also minimizing the probability of "rejecting" a truly interesting drug. For example, consider a situation in which one would not be interested in a new drug with a response rate of 10% or less but would be very interested in one with a response rate of 30% or more. A typical two-stage Fleming design in this case would be as follows:

Stage 1: Enter 20 patients. If 2 or fewer responses are observed, stop and conclude that the response rate is unlikely to be as great as 30%. If 6 or more responses are observed, stop and conclude that the response rate is unlikely to be as low as 10%. If 3, 4, or 5 responses are observed, proceed to the second stage.

Stage 2: Enter an additional 15 patients. If the total number of responses in all 35 patients is 6 or less, conclude that the activity level is uninteresting. If 7 or more responses are observed, the drug warrants further investigation.

With this design, one has a 5% chance of incorrectly rejecting a true 30% drug and an 8% chance of incorrectly accepting a true 10% drug. (A drug with a true response rate of 20% has an approximately equal chance of being accepted or rejected.) In addition, when the true rate is as low as 10% or as high as 30%, the probability of early termination is about one third. The calculations required to construct Fleming designs are complex; sample two-stage designs for some situations of interest are shown in Table 13-3. (The example discussed above is summarized in the fifth line of this table.) Additional designs, including three-stage designs, may be found in Fleming's article.[12]

Other designs for Phase II trials have been proposed. Herson's design[13] incorporates prior information about therapeutic efficacy into the decision rules. Sylvester and Staquet[14] have developed designs based on decision-theoretical concepts. Their approach is to quantify the ethical "cost" of treating patients with inferior therapy and then to select a sample size that minimizes this cost over the current as well as the future patient population. Lee and coworkers[15] have proposed a design that allows for an inconclusive result as well as "positive" and "negative" outcomes.

When patient accrual is expected to be relatively rapid and multiple new agents are available for study, a randomized Phase II design, as discussed by Simon and associates,[16] has some advantages over the sequential study of one treatment arm at a time. A randomized Phase II study is simply the simultaneous implementation of two or more Phase II studies. It does not permit formal statistical comparisons between the arms because sample sizes are too small for such comparisons to be done reliably. However, the randomization does ensure that no systematic bias is operating in the selection of study patients to receive each treatment. Thus, results from a randomized Phase II study can be more reliably ordered in setting priorities for future studies than results from sequentially conducted studies, in which patient selection patterns may have differed.

Phase III Trials: Eligibility and Choice of Controls

Phase III trials compare the efficacy of an experimental therapy with that of a standard or control therapy. Because these trials are intended to determine definitively whether a new therapeutic strategy should be adopted, the results must be sufficiently precise so that both false-positive and false-negative results are unlikely. In the study of pediatric cancer, Phase III trials are usually feasible only in the cooperative group or multicenter settings because of the relative scarcity of patients.

There has been much debate in the past concerning acceptable control groups for Phase III studies. One approach is a two-arm study, in which one group of patients receives the control therapy and the other receives the experimental therapy; alternatively, all patients can be treated with the experimental therapy, with results eventually compared to those achieved with a previous group of patients given what is currently considered the control therapy. This use of "historical controls" appeals to many physicians because it sharply reduces the number of patients required for study, and because a nonrandomized study in which all patients receive the same therapy is obviously easier to explain to potential subjects. However, these studies are inherently unreliable because there is no protection against the possibility that different types of patients were treated with the two therapies.

As an example, suppose standard therapy for a particular category of patients is purely palliative, and a new, potentially curative therapy is being tried for these patients. The investigators elect to treat a series of patients with the new therapy, and then compare the survival in these patients with that of a historical series treated with the palliative therapy. There are several clear sources of potential bias in this situation. First,

Table 13-2
First-Stage Sample Sizes for Gehan Phase II Trial Design

Minimal Response Rate of Interest (%)	First-Stage Sample Size*
5	59
10	29
15	19
20	14
25	11
30	9
40	6
50	5

* If no responses are observed in these patients, the trial may be terminated with the conclusion that the true response rate is unlikely to be at or above the specified minimal level. If any responses are observed, additional patients are accrued.

Table 13-3
Two-Stage Fleming Designs for Phase II Trials

Preselected Response Ranges* and Total (n)	Stage 1 (n)	Stage 2 (n)	Early Stopping Points†		Final Decision Point‡	α§	β‖	Probability of Early Stop#	
			S_{low}	S_{high}				Lower RR	Higher RR
5% Versus 20%									
20	10	10	0	3	3	0.02	0.40	0.74	0.61
30	15	15	0	4	3	0.06	0.13	0.47	0.39
40	20	20	0	4	4	0.05	0.08	0.38	0.60
10% Versus 30%									
25	15	10	1	5	5	0.04	0.19	0.56	0.52
35	20	15	2	6	6	0.05	0.08	0.69	0.62
20% Versus 40%									
25	15	10	3	7	8	0.05	0.28	0.67	0.48
35	20	15	4	9	11	0.04	0.20	0.64	0.45
50	25	25	4	11	15	0.03	0.10	0.43	0.42

* The first percentage is the upper limit of the "definitely uninteresting" range and the second is the lower limit of the "definitely interesting" range. See text for details.
† If number of responses at first stage is no greater than S_{low}, stop and conclude activity level is uninteresting. If number of responses is at least as great as S_{high}, stop and conclude activity level is interesting.
‡ If total responses are equal to or greater than this, conclude activity level is interesting.
§ Probability of incorrectly accepting a low-activity drug.
‖ Probability of incorrectly rejecting a high-activity drug.
RR = response rate.

certain eligibility criteria will be established for patients receiving the new therapy. Thus, patients who appear close to death, show evidence of organ dysfunction, have received intensive prior therapy, or refuse consent may not be treated with the new therapy. The historical series may not have been constructed with these, or any, eligibility criteria, and thus may include some extremely poor prognosis patients who are not comparable to any patients treated with the new therapy. (Even if the same eligibility criteria were applied, changes in diagnostic techniques might affect patient selection.) Second, there will be patients considered for the new therapy who meet all the eligibility criteria but who, for one reason or another, are not entered on the study. Several such circumstances can be envisioned: perhaps the patient appears to be in worse condition than the required tests indicate; perhaps there is a reluctance to enter infants even though they are technically eligible; perhaps the parents' English is poor, or they appear intellectually ill-equipped to understand the concept of a clinical study and thus cannot provide truly "informed" consent; perhaps the new therapy is expensive (*e.g.*, bone marrow transplant), and only relatively affluent patients are ultimately entered. Certain types of patients may then appear in different proportions in the historical and the experimental series. The comparison of survival or other outcome between these two series of patients is likely to be heavily biased if such patient characteristics are correlated with prognosis. Finally, changes in supportive care procedures may improve survival apart from any fundamental population differences. There is no way to adjust for this type of effect.

Thus, if differences in outcome are found—for example, if the average survival on the experimental therapy is substantially longer than on the palliative (historical control) therapy —it will be difficult to know how much of the difference to attribute to the new treatment, and how much to fundamental differences in the patient populations or to changes in suppor-

tive care. Although statistical methods to "adjust" comparisons for such differences have been developed and are quite useful in many situations (see Analysis section), one cannot measure and record all patient characteristics that affect prognosis. Many such characteristics undoubtedly remain to be identified. Thus, observed differences in outcome in historically controlled studies are always potentially attributable, in part or in total, to non-treatment-related causes, and hence will always be suspect.

The most reliable way to generate unbiased comparisons between treatments is to allocate patients to treatment by randomization. A randomized trial is unquestionably the procedure of choice for the definitive evaluation of an experimental therapy. Large randomized studies do not always seem feasible, but they can sometimes be *made* feasible when investigators pool their efforts and develop a cooperative trial. Occasionally, however, even the multicenter approach is insufficient. For example, there are very few cases of acute monocytic leukemia diagnosed in infants each year, and a randomized trial in this patient population would probably be unrealistic. In such cases, a carefully done historically controlled trial, however imperfect, may be the only way to evaluate a new therapy.

Phase III Trials: Sample Size

The required sample size for a randomized Phase III study depends on [1] the minimum difference in outcome considered important to detect, [2] the levels of Type I and Type II error considered acceptable, and [3] the expected outcome with standard therapy. Type I (alpha) error is the conclusion that the new treatment is better than the standard when in fact it is not. The probability of a Type I error is the *significance level* of the experiment and is denoted by α. Type II (beta) error is the failure to conclude that the new treatment is superior to the standard when it actually is. The probability of a Type II error is denoted by β; its complement $(1 - \beta)$ is called the *power* of the experiment.

The specifics of the sample size calculation also depend on the type of endpoint of primary interest. A complete discussion of sample size determination for binary endpoints ("yes/no" variables such as response), along with extensive tabulations of sample size requirements according to the above parameters, has been published by Fleiss.[17] Sample size considerations for time variables (survival time, remission duration) are well discussed by George and Desu[18] and by Rubinstein and colleagues.[19] Both of these papers deal with the problem of "censored data"—survival times for patients who remain alive at the time of study reporting. However, these methods assume that the risk of an adverse event such as death or relapse is constant over time for any given patient. In many instances, particularly with pediatric tumors, a substantial cure rate can be anticipated, so that the risk of an adverse event should essentially disappear once a patient has been event-free for a certain period of time. Sposto and Sather[20] have developed methods for determining sample sizes in this situation. Finally, for those cases in which the use of historical controls may be unavoidable, sample size considerations are addressed by Makuch and Simon.[21]

Conventionally, the Type I error for testing results from Phase III studies is set at 5% and the Type II error is set between 10% and 20%. This is done because it is generally considered a more serious error to incorrectly abandon a standard treatment, with which there may be extensive experience, than to fail to identify an experimental treatment that affords a moderate advantage. In general, the relative seriousness of the two types of error will depend in part on characteristics of the treatments other than efficacy. A small α relative to β is very appropriate when the experimental therapy is highly toxic, logistically difficult (*e.g.,* requiring extensive hospitalization or multiple clinic visits), or very costly, whereas the standard therapy is relatively benign, simple, and inexpensive. In some circumstances, however, it may be more appropriate to set α and β more nearly equal. For example, when the new therapy is less intensive than the standard, one would want to adopt the new therapy only if it did not lead to a worse outcome on average. In this case, one would worry as much if not more about failing to detect reduced efficacy than falsely concluding that the standard, more intensive therapy was superior.

The size of the difference one is interested in detecting must be carefully considered, since the required sample size is extremely sensitive to this difference. For example, if one wanted to be 80% certain of observing a statistically significant ($p < 0.05$) difference in event rates associated with two thera-

pies when the true event rates were 20% and 40%, 91 patients per arm would be required. However, for event rates of 20% and 30%, the required sample size would be 313 per arm, and for rates of 20% and 25%, 1134 per arm. Thus, detection of very small differences, while possibly desirable, will not be an achievable goal for most pediatric studies. On the other hand, one must make sure that the specified difference is small enough so that a study resulting in "no statistically significant difference" will be convincingly negative. If a study enters only enough patients to reliably detect very large differences, smaller differences that may be clinically meaningful will be unlikely to produce statistically significant results. As an example, consider the following hypothetical data:

Complete Response	Treatment	
	Drug A	Drug B
Yes	15 (50%)	9 (30%)
No	15	21
Total Patients	30	30

The difference in complete response (CR) rates appears impressive: 50% versus 30%. However, the p value for this difference is 0.147—suggestive, but far from conventional significance. Such data would have to be considered inconclusive. The observed difference is too large to conclude comfortably that the two drugs are equivalent, but the numbers are too small to exclude chance as the basis for the difference.

Specialized Designs for Randomized Clinical Trials

SEQUENTIAL DESIGNS. A sequential design is one in which the total sample size is not fixed at the beginning but depends instead on the data accumulated as the trial progresses. Historically, the motivation for the use of sequential designs was the desire for efficiency, achieved by terminating an experiment as soon as the answer is "known." In the context of clinical trials, the motivation also relates to ethical considerations. When early results indicate that one treatment is producing substantially improved outcomes, it becomes difficult to justify the continued randomization of patients to the study. However, the application of simple monitoring plans, such as stopping the study as soon as the p value reaches 0.05, has been shown to lead to a far greater frequency of Type I errors (false positives) than the nominal 0.05 level would indicate. For example, McPherson[22] points out that if the data

Table 13-4

Group Sequential Designs for Phase III Trials with Five Analyses: Nominal p *Value Required to Declare Significance at Overall* p $= 0.05$*

Design	Analysis				
	1	2	3	4	5
Pocock	0.0158	0.0158	0.0158	0.0158	0.0158
O'Brien/Fleming	0.5×10^{-6}	0.0013	0.0005	0.0228	0.0417
Fleming/Harrington/O'Brien					
(1)	0.0024	0.0030	0.0035	0.0043	0.0458
(2)	0.0051	0.0061	0.0073	0.0089	0.0402

* Four interim analyses and one final analysis (see text for details).

are reviewed 10 times during the course of a study in which the true efficacies of the treatments are identical, the probability of observing a p value of 0.05 or less at least once is about 20%. Thus, the true Type I error in this context is actually 0.20, not 0.05. The Type I error will increase with more frequent interim monitoring.

To deal with the problem of inflating Type I error by frequent evaluation of study results, several different approaches have been developed. All of them, of course, require the use of more stringent significance criteria than the usual 0.05 level. The most practical of these are called "group sequential designs" because they are based on analysis of data at regular intervals, often semiannually, as "groups" of data are accumulated. Three such designs are presented in Table 13-4. The basis for these designs is that one must compensate for the extra opportunities to declare significance (and possibly make a Type I error in so doing) by reducing the significance level of each test so that, over the entire course of the trial, the probability of Type I error remains at 5%. The first design, proposed by Pocock[23,24] is the simplest. It uses the same significance level at each test, with the particular level calculated as a function of the number of interim tests as well as the desired overall significance level and power. O'Brien and Fleming[25] proposed an alternative approach (O–F design). They suggested that the final test should be done at a level close to the usual 0.05, and that the earlier tests therefore be done at much more extreme levels. Their design uses a sequence of p values: the first is exceptionally small, with the remainder gradually increasing so that the final p value is close to the conventional level. A variation of this design was later published by Fleming, Harrington, and O'Brien (F–H–O design).[26] This design is intermediate between the first two in that the final test is done at a significance level close to 0.05, but the p values for the four interim tests increase much more gradually; there is a much larger gap between the p values used for test 4 and test 5 than in the original O–F design. One selects a particular F–H–O design by specifying the proportion (R) of the desired overall α to be used as the significance level of the final test. The first F–H–O design in Table 13-4 represents an R of 0.92; that is, the final α is 0.0458, approximately equal to 0.92×0.05. The second F–H–O design uses an R of 0.80, resulting in an α of 0.0402.

Clearly, since the Pocock design uses higher p values for the early tests, it would permit more trials to be stopped early. This efficiency is offset to a degree by the requirement of somewhat larger maximum sample sizes (should early termination not occur) to achieve power equivalent to the other designs. The major disadvantage of the Pocock design is that results that may look impressive at the end of a trial, with a nominal p value of 0.02 or 0.03, will not be considered significant at the 0.05 level. Although there is a valid probabilistic basis for this, many researchers would not find it appealing to have their conclusion at the final test depend so heavily on the number of times the data were tested. The O–F and F–H–O designs are also dependent on the frequency of testing, but the p values used for the final test remain close to the conventional 0.05 level. Thus, with these procedures, the overall Type I error is kept stable by reducing the probability of early termination still further.

The above designs allow for the possibility of early termination only in the case where one treatment appears markedly superior to the other. However, it is frequently the case in randomized clinical trials that, as the data accumulate, the two treatments appear similar or the experimental treatment appears worse than the standard. Just as an intuitive but nonrigorous approach to early termination in the face of large differences inflates the Type I error, such an approach in the face of small or no differences can inflate the Type II error. However, designs are available that allow for early termination of apparently negative trials while maintaining high power to detect reasonable differences if they do exist. DeMets and Ware[27] have proposed an asymmetric design that allows early trial termination not only when there are large advantages to the experimental therapy, in the manner of O'Brien and Fleming, but also when the new therapy appears equivalent to or worse than the standard. As with the other designs, the number of planned analyses must be specified in advance, and the termination criteria for each analysis can then be determined. Whitehead and Stratton[28] have developed a design based on similar considerations. A somewhat simpler design, developed by Ellenberg and Eisenberger,[29] addresses only the issue of early termination when the results are negative. This is not a group sequential design, but a two-stage design in which the study is terminated with a negative conclusion if, at the end of the first stage, the experimental therapy is producing outcomes equivalent to or worse than the standard therapy. The sample size for the trial, should it not be terminated early, is determined in the standard way for fixed sample size Phase III trials; the sample size for the first stage is calculated to ensure that a result of equivalence or inferiority of the experimental treatment at that stage would be very unlikely if the experimental therapy truly afforded a substantial improvement over the standard. The loss of power incurred by allowing for the possibility of early termination is negligible.

Sequential designs are desirable because they permit valid analyses of significance levels even though a trial does not complete its full accrual. However, they are not readily applicable to all clinical trial situations. When observation of the endpoint may be substantially delayed—for example, when survival time is the endpoint and average survival time is a year or more from study entry—it may not be practical to implement a sequential design because patient accrual may be almost complete by the time sufficient events have been observed to justify even an early interim analysis. However, when response is the primary endpoint, or when survival is the endpoint in the context of a rapidly fatal disease, sequential designs may be considered.

FACTORIAL DESIGNS. In a factorial design, two or more questions are addressed in the same cohort of patients by multiple randomization. For example, if both a surgical question and an adjuvant chemotherapy question are of interest in a given population, a double randomization would allocate the patients to treatment as shown below.

	Surgical Technique A	Surgical Technique B	
Adjuvant Therapy A	$n/4$	$n/4$	$n/2$
Adjuvant Therapy B	$n/4$	$n/4$	$n/2$
Total	$n/2$	$n/2$	n

In this illustration, n is the total number of patients to be studied. If the effect of each factor can be considered to operate independently of the other (*i.e.,* the difference in efficacy of the adjuvant therapy regimens does not depend on which surgical technique was used, and *vice versa*), then each question can be evaluated by collapsing over the categories of the other question. Thus, the n patients accrued may be used to evaluate two maneuvers rather than one. Factorial designs can clearly improve the efficiency of clinical trials in situations where the assumption of independent effects is reasonable. This assumption must be carefully considered; if the data cast doubt on its validity, categories would not be collapsible, and the power of the study to detect differences would be drastically reduced. If one of the maneuvers to be tested affects the administration of the other (*e.g.,* if both questions involve cytotoxic drugs, and the dosages may vary among the four possible combinations), the assumption of independence is clearly violated and a factorial design would not be appropriate. Examples of studies with factorial designs are the National Wilms' Tumor Study-III, in which early-stage patients were randomized between postoperative radiotherapy and no postoperative radiotherapy and also between two different chemotherapy regimens;[30] and a study of adjuvant therapy for colon cancer, in which patients were randomized to receive or not receive chemotherapy and to receive or not receive immunotherapy.[31] Various aspects of factorial designs are discussed by Byar and Piantadosi.[32]

RANDOMIZED CONSENT DESIGN. In the late 1970s, Zelen[33] proposed a new type of design in which randomization would occur prior to informed consent. Patients would be assessed for eligibility, and those who appeared eligible would then be randomized. As initially proposed, patients randomized to "standard therapy" would not be subject to the informed consent procedure because they would be receiving the best available treatment. Only those randomized to receive the experimental treatment would be given the formal opportunity to consent or refuse their allocated treatment. A modified version of this design in which all patients would undergo an informed consent procedure was later proposed.[34]

The primary motivation for this design was to help overcome the discomfort many physicians feel about asking patients to participate in a study wherein their treatment will be decided not by the physician but by some random mechanism. It was speculated that there would be much less resistance to the informed consent process if physicians could tell the patients their assigned treatment at the time they described the study and offered participation. This in turn would lead to a greater willingness on the part of physicians to enter patients on randomized studies.

The randomized consent design, often referred to as "prerandomization," has a great deal of intuitive appeal. Many physicians do have problems with the process of obtaining informed consent and may refrain from participating in clinical trials because of these problems.[35] However, the randomized consent design introduces new difficulties (discussed in detail by Ellenberg[36]). These include analysis of those patients who refuse their allocated treatment; the surprisingly larger sample sizes required to compensate for these refusals; and the loss of assurance that the patient will be fully informed about the study and all treatment alternatives. The limited experience with the randomized consent design has not demonstrated any major effect on patient accrual patterns.

Treatment Plan

The treatments to be delivered on protocol should be precisely and thoroughly defined to ensure uniformity of conditions throughout the experiment. Variations in therapeutic intervention can reduce or destroy the interpretability of the results. All aspects of therapy should be set forth, including surgical procedures to be employed and supportive care guidelines. Provisions for treatment modifications in the event of toxicity should be specified. It is particularly useful in complex protocols to include a schema that shows the temporal relationships of chemotherapy and other treatment modalities from study entry, through various treatment phases (induction, consolidation, maintenance), to discontinuation of therapy. Schematics quickly convey information to medical personnel not directly involved in the development of the protocol.

Drug Information

This section serves as a reference for participants by supplying specifics regarding mechanism of action, animal and human toxicology data, and pharmaceutical information for each of the drugs used in the clinical trial.

Criteria for Evaluating Treatment Effect

The parameters for assessing the effects of treatment on individual patients are generally referred to as endpoints. An endpoint is a medical event that may represent benefit (complete remission) or harm (relapse, death). The results of the clinical trial will be based on analyses of the accumulation of endpoint assessments, the criteria for which were predetermined by the investigator. A well-constructed protocol incorporates endpoints that are objective, practical, and relevant to the clinical situation being studied. By defining endpoints, the researcher indicates precisely which measures of treatment outcome will reliably meet the objectives of the protocol. These will, in turn, assist in clarifying what clinical and laboratory data need to be obtained during the trial and will provide the basis for statistical analysis.

The endpoints of Phase I and Phase II trials have become fairly standardized. In Phase I trials, the endpoints are the degree and duration of changes in organ function following exposure to the experimental agent. It is useful to include in this section of the protocol a table that defines increasing degrees of toxicity for various organ systems and indicates the level of toxicity that is deemed unacceptable. Phase II endpoints, and subsidiary Phase I endpoints, are concerned with the evidence for, and duration of, response to the investigational agent. (These endpoints are considered subsidiary in Phase I trials because the agent will be administered to the majority of patients at suboptimal dosages.) Complete response is widely defined as the total disappearance of all clinically detectable malignant disease for at least 4 weeks, and partial response as a 50% or greater decrease in the sum of the products of the longest perpendicular diameters of all measurable lesions, with no increase in size of any lesions and no appearance of new lesions. Progressive disease denotes appearance of new lesions or enlargement of existing ones.[37]

When an untoward event (death, progression, relapse) is the endpoint of interest, it is generally useful not only to tabulate how many patients experienced that event but to measure the time elapsed from entry to endpoint. This provides a more sensitive basis for comparison of the therapies because additional information is incorporated into the analysis.[38]

As untreated malignancies are almost always fatal, the ultimate merit of a therapy resides in its ability to prevent the patient's death. Thus, an endpoint of unarguable interest is survival time. This is often an impractical choice, however, as death from disease may be considerably removed from onset of therapy, and results of the trial correspondingly delayed or confused by intervening events. Alternative endpoints are often chosen that are presumed to be early signals of long-term survival, such as the disappearance of detectable tumor or the absence of metastases at 3 years. Alternative endpoints may not always reflect survival, however, as in situations where salvage therapies are effective irrespective of prior treatment failure; the influence of an adverse event during the first treatment will be abrogated by the successful second treatment. Demonstration of patient benefit in terms of survival is hampered not only by the logistics of follow-up but by problems in analysis introduced when subsequent therapies are nonuniform.

An alternative endpoint that has been advocated for use as a standard endpoint in trials of childhood ALL is "event-free survival." This is defined by Mastrangelo and associates[39] as "the first occurrence of the major events that represent initial treatment failure: failure to achieve remission (*i.e.,* death in the induction period or nonresponse), relapse at any site following successful remission achievement, and death in remission without preceding relapse." This endpoint, also termed "failure-free survival" or "time to first event," would be meaningful for studies in any disease population but is especially appropriate for trials in which most patients achieve remission and many achieve long-term survival. Mastrangelo and co-workers have urged that event-free survival always be evaluated in studies of pediatric ALL (along with any other endpoints believed to be of interest), with the purpose of enhancing the comparability of study results in this population.

Ancillary endpoints may pertain to quality of life; these are frequently highly subjective and not easily quantified. However, increasingly valuable in studies of children are endpoints regarding adverse effects of treatment, such as the occurrence of second malignancies, growth disturbances, or neuropsychological impairment attributed to therapy.

Clinical and Laboratory Data to Be Accessioned

The data set required for determination of eligibility and evaluation of treatment effect must be presented. This set includes pretreatment, on-treatment, and posttreatment evaluations, indicating specific clinical and laboratory assessments and their timing. These schedules are often presented in tabular form. In comparative trials, it is essential that the frequency and nature of these assessments be identical for the regimens being compared to avoid an unbalanced increase in the likelihood of detecting real or chance differences due to differences in medical surveillance.

Clinical trials are also used to provide systematic information regarding the natural history of the disease independent of therapeutic intervention, as when patient characteristics are recorded at presentation and subsequently correlated with outcome.[38] The details of acquiring such data should be included in this section.

Statistical Considerations

Statistical considerations for each objective of the study are included in this section of the protocol. The estimated number of patients required, the anticipated rate of patient accrual, and the expected duration of the trial (including follow-up) are given along with the description of the proposed analysis of outcome data. In planning the study, the availability of patients should be documented, whenever possible, to determine whether the study objectives are realistic. Such documentation might be based on accruals to previous protocols for a similar patient population, or on data from surveys of collaborating institutions that establish the frequency of the required patient characteristics. Conducting a study that accrues too few patients and thereby provides uninterpretable results is a major

waste of resources, as is accruing more patients than necessary to provide accurate results.

Informed Consent

All research projects that involve human subjects and are conducted or supported in part or entirely by the U.S. Department of Health and Human Services (DHHS) are subject to regulations regarding the protection of those subjects (see Chaps. 15 and 53).[40] Documentation that research subjects have given prior informed consent to participate is an absolute requirement of cancer clinical trials supported by DHHS research funds administered through NCI. A study-specific sample of the informed consent document should be included in all clinical trials protocols for use by investigators and for purposes of review by local Institutional Review Boards (IRBs) and by NCI. Local versions of multiclinic protocols must contain all federally required elements. The federally required elements of informed consent are presented in Table 13-5 in the checklist format used by NCI staff to evaluate such documents.

The DHHS has prescribed additional protections specifically for children who are subjects of clinical research.[41] Children are defined as persons who have not reached the legal age for consent to treatments or procedures involved in the research; legal age is determined by the applicable law of the jurisdiction in which the research will be conducted. DHHS regulations require IRB assurances that adequate provisions are made for obtaining the assent (affirmative agreement) of children capable of providing assent; failure to object is not construed as assent. The IRB may, however, waive the requirement for assent under certain circumstances. When the IRB determines that assent is required, it also determines whether and how assent must be documented. In addition, the IRB must ensure that adequate provisions are made for obtaining permission from both parents or guardians unless one parent is deceased, unknown, incompetent, or not reasonably available, or when only one parent has legal custody of the child.[41] The provisions concerning informed consent apply to the process of obtaining permission from parents.

MANAGING THE CLINICAL TRIAL

Registration

Every study patient should be formally registered as a study participant before receiving any protocol-directed intervention. Registration for a nonrandomized study simply refers to the entry of a patient's name or hospital number into a paper or computer log. Pretreatment registration ensures that all patients who begin treatment can be identified for reporting purposes at the end of the study. In addition, the process of registration can be used to verify that the patient meets the eligibility criteria. Registration is important, even in studies conducted within a single institution, as a quality control measure to prevent the inadvertent loss of "problem patients"— early deaths and progressions, or refusals of further treatment after minimal therapy—from the reporting process. In randomized studies, the process of randomization usually ensures the recording of all patients entering the study. Studies in which randomization follows an interval during which all patients are treated uniformly (*e.g.,* a study of maintenance therapy in which all patients receive the same induction therapy) should require registration before the initial treatment interval to

Table 13-5
Informed Consent Checklist—Required Elements

1. Clearly state that the study involves research.
    State which drugs, treatments, or delivery techniques are experimental.
    Clarify the study purpose(s) in layman's terms.
    State the patient's expected duration of participation in study (*e.g.,* "the patient will be treated until there is evidence that therapy is no longer effective").
    Describe briefly the procedures to be performed to monitor the patient during study (*e.g.,* radiographs, laboratory evaluation). An exhaustive list is not necessary.
    Describe briefly the experimental aspects or new delivery techniques of the study.
    State in specific terms the route of administration of each drug (*e.g.,* intravenous, oral, continuous infusion).
    State estimated time required for the delivery of each drug or time of procedure.

2. State the risks that are attributed to specific drugs or procedures.

3. Clarify and describe expected benefits to be derived from participation in this study (*e.g.,* tumor shrinkage, improved quality of life).

4. Discuss, in general terms, alternative treatments to participation in this study (*e.g.,* conventional chemotherapy, irradiation, hormonal therapy).

5. State the extent to which confidentiality of records will be maintained. State that a qualified representative of the FDA and/or NCI may inspect patient/study records.

6. State whether compensation for study-related injury will be provided by the institution or other insurer.
    State whether emergency treatment of injury will be provided by the institution.

7. List the names and phone numbers of contact persons for research-related questions.
    List names and phone numbers of contact persons (not involved in the research) for questions of patient rights.

8. Clearly state that participation is voluntary. State that refusal to participate will involve no loss of benefits or penalize the patient's care. State that discontinuation of participation in the study will involve no loss of benefits to which the patient is entitled.

---

identify any selection patterns that might affect the generalizability of trial results.

Randomization

The purpose of randomization is to avoid systematic bias in the allocation of patients to treatment. Bias will almost surely be present if an investigator knows the next treatment assignment before he or she decides whether to offer participation in the study to the next available patient. It is important, then, to select a method of randomization that will not permit prediction of treatment assignments. *Ad hoc* methods, such as assigning alternate patients to each of two treatment groups or assigning patients on the basis of birthdate (*e.g.,* odd numbers assigned to one group, even numbers to the other) do not provide adequate protection against predictability and should be avoided.[42]

Perhaps the most widely used mechanism is the random number table, either in published form or as generated by a computer program. In using a published table, one begins at some "randomly chosen" entry in the table and uses the sequence of numbers beginning with that entry to determine successive treatment assignments. For example, in the case of two treatment groups, the parity of the number (odd or even) could determine the associated treatment assignments. Alternatively, computer programs that generate series of random numbers may be used to generate treatment assignment lists.* Such lists clearly must not be accessible to physicians participating in the trial.

When subgroups of patients with identifiably different prognoses are studied in the same trial, a stratified randomization plan may be considered. The purpose of stratification is to ensure that patients with a better or worse prognosis will not be overrepresented in a particular treatment group. The simplest way to stratify at randomization is to generate a separate allocation list for each subgroup. Thus, if three factors, each with two possible levels, were to be used for stratification, one would need eight separate lists, one for each possible combination of factor levels. An alternative method involves determining, for each new patient, the treatment allocation that would result in the best "balance" overall with regard to the factors of interest. Patients are then either directly assigned to that treatment (deterministic method) or are assigned to treatment by a random mechanism that yields a high probability (but not 100%) that they will be allocated to the treatment resulting in best balance (random method). Detailed calculations are required to determine the balance for each possible

---

* Computer-generated random numbers cannot be said to be truly random, since they will repeat eventually. However, the number of patients on any given trial is very small relative to the cycle of repetition, so that computer-generated lists should be acceptably random for practical purposes.

allocation; a computer program is the only practical method when more than two or three stratification factors are used. This method of treatment assignment, usually referred to as "adaptive allocation," has become fairly popular in multicenter trial settings despite its complexity. Adaptive allocation methods have been described by several authors.[43–45] Deterministic adaptive allocation is not actually a form of randomization, because the allocation is determined by the distribution of prognostic factors both for the new patient and for the series of patients already entered. Nevertheless, the allocation is for all practical purposes not predictable because of the complexity of the required calculations. Hence, it may be considered an unbiased allocation, even though it is not strictly random.

To protect the validity of randomization, it is essential to establish procedures that are not susceptible to "tampering." Envelope randomization is less desirable than telephone randomization because envelopes can be opened and resealed, and the decision to randomize or not to randomize a patient may depend on the contents of the envelope. A randomization list, monitored by a central data manager or randomization clerk and accessible only in response to a request to randomize a specifically named patient, provides greater security.

The timing of randomization is important. Patients should generally be randomized as close in time as possible to the point at which the treatment programs begin to differ. It is unwise to randomize patients several weeks or even several days before beginning therapy. When patients change their minds and withdraw from the study before receiving treatment, or undergo changes in their condition such that it would no longer be appropriate for them to receive their allocated therapy, serious problems arise in analyzing the results. Similarly, if all patients are treated uniformly for a certain period of time and treatments diverge only after this initial period, randomization should be delayed until it is time to begin the second treatment interval. For example, a study question may relate to maintenance therapy, with all patients scheduled to receive the same induction therapy. Randomization should then be done at the end of induction, just before maintenance therapy begins. If randomization were done before induction, a subset of patients would be randomized who would never receive the allocated maintenance therapy. Some would die or progress during the induction interval, and others would refuse further therapy in general or the regimen assigned at the end of the induction period. If these patients were included in the analysis, the comparison would be diluted because some patients would not have received the assigned treatment. However, their exclusion could introduce bias if the nondelivery of treatment were related to the particular treatment assigned—for instance, if patients with good prognosis tended to refuse the more intensive treatment and those with poor prognosis tended to refuse the less intensive treatment. To avoid these problems, one should register all patients before induction therapy, explaining the future randomization at that time. The randomization itself would be carried out only after the successful completion of induction, and informed consent would be obtained at that time. Some patients may refuse randomization at this time, but the comparison based on all who do agree to randomization will be unbiased and undiluted.

Data Collection

The design of data forms is not a trivial task, and requires the input of clinician, statistician, data manager, and computer programmer. One must ensure that all data items necessary to meet the objectives of the protocol are included, that items

unlikely to be of interest are eliminated, that the items are unambiguously presented, that coding procedures are consistent and straightforward, that the form is structured for maximum efficiency in entering and then keying the data, and that the format of the data will allow for efficient analysis.

Determining the required data items is not always as simple as it might seem. One must go through the protocol step by step and carefully consider what information must be collected to answer the questions addressed. It is important to be selective. The collection and computer entry of excessive, nonessential data will waste valuable hours of the data manager's time.

It is almost impossible to compose a perfect data form on the first attempt. Ideally, the forms should be "piloted," perhaps on nonstudy patients, before they are used to collect study data. Only by actually using the forms can errors and ambiguities be discovered. Instructions should be contained within the form to the extent possible. For very complicated forms, a special coding manual may be required. Often, institutions or cooperative groups develop general instructional manuals for completing data forms, which are used in a variety of studies. The advantage of shortening the form by removing instructional material must be balanced against the advantage of having the instructions immediately available.

Forms should be designed with ease of completion as a primary consideration. Errors are more likely to be made when the form is filled out than at any other point in the data management process. Ease of data entry is also very important, and experienced data managers and data entry personnel should be consulted when new forms are being designed. The efficiency of forms with regard to computer programming and data analysis is also important but is secondary to the previous considerations.

A schedule for collection of data forms should be established, publicized to the investigators, and enforced by the data management offices. When completion of data forms is delayed, the potential increases for errors and for missing data that may become unretrievable. Because data managers are often nurses with clinical as well as administrative responsibilities, sufficient time must be allotted for them to complete and submit forms on the required schedule. Proper monitoring of a study cannot be reliably accomplished without a continually current data base.

The explosion of microcomputer technology has led to experimentation with direct data entry onto computer files, potentially eliminating the need for paper forms. This procedure may already be common for studies within a single institution, where the same person manages both the collection and computer entry of the data, but it is not yet widely used in multicenter trials. The technology does exist to support such "distributed data entry" systems. Data can be keyed onto floppy diskettes at each institution and then mailed to the central data center; even more efficient is electronic transmission of data over phone lines. Completed data forms would then be printed out after the data were entered for purposes of internal editing and medical review. It seems inevitable that such systems will increase in popularity as clinical and data management staff become as familiar and comfortable with the computer as they are with pencil and paper.

Quality Control

"Quality control" refers to all the checks and reviews of data over the course of the study that are designed to make sure the protocol is being appropriately followed and the data being submitted are accurate. Quality control considerations should affect every step of the protocol, from patient entry through final follow-up. Much of the responsibility for quality control during the course of the study will fall to the central data management personnel.

Checklists should be used at the time of patient registration or randomization to ensure that the patient really is eligible and willing to participate before he or she is formally entered on the study. Data entry procedures should be developed to minimize errors in transposing data from the form to the computer file. Many data centers require two independent keyings of every form, with software designed to catch discrepancies and thus identify keypunch errors. Many centers have also developed software to simulate the data form on the computer screen, with the cursor moving automatically from one field to the next. Such capabilities should increase the efficiency of entry and control the error rate. Computer programs must be written (and thoroughly pretested) to detect errors and missing information in the data that are entered. A system must be devised to notify physicians or data managers about errors, to request corrected or updated information, and to flag cases for which errors remain. For multicenter studies, or even single-institution studies with multiple participants, it is often worthwhile to conduct training sessions for staff who will be responsible for completing data forms and submitting them to a central office. Of course, the value of training sessions is not confined to data managers. Complex protocols often require initial training sessions for surgeons, radiotherapists, pathologists, and others who may need more instruction in the experimental procedures than can be reliably transmitted in the written protocol.

Many aspects of the protocol must be subject to medical review. For example, when radiotherapy is an important part of an experimental treatment program, centralized quality assurance review of the port films is mandatory to ensure that the treatments are being administered according to the protocol. Such review must be prompt, especially at the beginning of a study, so that problems can be corrected before they affect a large proportion of the study population. Pathology and surgical reports must be reviewed for final determination of patient eligibility. Again, such reviews must be performed promptly because a high ineligibility rate signals the need for some modification of the patient entry procedures. Reports of responses, relapses, or other events of interest may also require review. The responsibility for these data reviews is generally shared among the study chairperson, data management staff, and treatment specialists.

Follow-up

Ideally, all patients enrolled in clinical trials of cancer treatment should receive regular follow-up throughout the remainder of their lives. There are two major purposes of extended follow-up. The first is to maintain a check on the treatment comparisons by detecting any late crossing of survival curves and obtaining better estimates of possible cure rates. The second is to detect any late adverse effects of the treatment that may not be evident at the time the trial results are initially reported. In pediatric trials, such known adverse affects include second malignancies, sterility, and cognitive dysfunction. Although data are not often available to demonstrate clearly that such effects are sequelae of radiotherapy or chemotherapy rather than the disease process itself, there is often a strong biological basis for assuming that these effects are primarily the result of cytotoxic therapy. Follow-up forms should specifically request information concerning known or

suspected adverse effects of the therapies used and the disease studied, and should also solicit information on any other adverse effects noted, regardless of whether an association between the effect and prior treatment appears plausible.

The desirable frequency of follow-up reporting varies with the time since study entry. Patients should be reported on frequently, preferably three or four times a year, as long as the study is in an active stage (*i.e.,* before reporting of results). Without frequent follow-up, it is impossible to monitor the study results reliably. Extreme differences observed relatively early in a study may lead to consideration of early termination, but without current follow-up on all patients one would not know to what extent the observed difference might be an artifact of delayed reporting.

After study results have been reported, a large proportion of surviving patients may be expected to be long-term survivors. It may then be reasonable to request follow-up reporting only on a semi-annual or yearly basis, with the understanding that any deaths, relapses, or adverse effects should be reported as soon as they are observed.

Interim Analysis

The data from clinical trials must be monitored on a regular basis to check for problems in implementing study procedures, unexpectedly severe toxicity, or early evidence related to treatment effects that might require early termination of the study. As discussed previously, it is preferable that the design of the study account for the possibility of early termination due to strong early results. However, a procedure has been developed that permits early termination on a valid statistical basis even when a sequential design was not used initially. The procedure, "stochastically curtailed testing,"[47–49] essentially permits termination when it can be shown that the probability of reversing the currently observed result is very small. Stochastically curtailed testing will not allow termination at early stages in the study, since the possibility of reversal when most of the patients remain to be entered or observed can never be discounted. (An exception is when accrual is much slower than anticipated; stochastically curtailed testing may then be used to calculate the achievable power based on continued accrual at the observed rate for a fixed interval.) However, it may permit some reduction in the accrual requirement toward the end of the trial, and may also allow acceleration of data reporting. As with the analysis of sequentially designed trials, stochastically curtailed testing is most appropriate when the endpoint is observed relatively soon following study entry, since the possibility of reversal depends on the number of observed events rather than the number of patients entered. Because this procedure has only recently been presented in the statistical literature, it is not yet in widespread use in clinical trials. However, the technique has been used in at least one major clinical trial, in which it contributed to the decision to terminate early.[50] General issues regarding study monitoring and interim analysis are discussed by Green and colleagues[51] and by Geller and Pocock.[52]

ANALYSIS

The most efficient, most sophisticated statistical analysis cannot compensate for major errors in the design or conduct of a clinical trial. This does not in any way diminish the importance of proper selection and use of analytic procedures. Before discussing specific procedures that are useful in cancer clinical trials, it may be worthwhile to consider some general issues that are relevant to the analysis of clinical trials data.

Avoidance of Bias

A "bias" is the effect on a study result of some systematic aspect of study design, data collection, or analysis that is unrelated to the actual effect of the treatment under study. For example, a comparison of a medical treatment with a surgical procedure in which treatment assignment depended on a patient's health status (*e.g.,* the patients who receive medical treatment are those whose poor condition precludes their undergoing the surgical procedure) would clearly be biased. The surgically treated patients would be in better shape from the beginning; if their outcome were better on average, there would be no way to know how much, if any, of this superiority was attributable to treatment. This may seem an extreme and obvious example of bias that could have been avoided by randomizing patients to treatment. However, bias can find its way into even the most meticulously randomized trial. The most common cause of bias at the analysis stage of clinical trials is the improper exclusion of patients from analysis. This can affect not only comparisons between treatments but estimates of the effect of a single regimen. A good rule of thumb is that patients who meet the eligibility criteria, are entered on the study, and begin treatment should be included in the analysis of study data. An unbiased estimate of the probability of response to a treatment regimen in a given patient population requires the inclusion of all patients in that population who were treated with the regimen. "Problem patients," such as those who die or refuse further therapy after only one or two doses of drug, are representative of some fraction of the overall population who might be eligible for this regimen but who would not benefit from it because their disease was too advanced or because they found the treatment intolerable. Such patients are frequently classified as "inevaluable" and are excluded from study analysis. However, a response rate has a clear meaning only when the numerator is the number of patients who respond, and the denominator is the total number treated. The proportion of responders among patients who receive "adequate" treatment (as defined by each investigator) may have some secondary interest but is not readily interpretable by the medical community at large. A response rate based on a denominator reduced by exclusion of "inevaluable" patients is a biased estimate of the proportion of the patient population that would be expected to experience tumor regression if this regimen were administered to the entire population.

In a randomized study, improper exclusions can clearly bias the treatment comparison. Consider a population of children who have achieved complete response to induction therapy and are then randomized to receive either maintenance therapy or no further treatment. The protocol requires that maintenance therapy begin within 14 days of completion of induction therapy. For some patients, initiation of maintenance therapy is delayed; several other patients progress or die in this interval; and a few patients refuse maintenance therapy despite their prior agreement. Some investigators would exclude such patients from the analysis on the basis that the maintenance therapy may be ineffective if delayed too long (and certainly cannot be effective if not given). However, it may also be true that patients with poorer prognoses are more likely to present these kinds of problems. Also, patients randomized to "no further therapy" obviously will not be excluded on the basis of treatment delay or inadequate courses of therapy. Thus, the exclusions may bias the comparison in favor of the mainte-

nance treatment. (Additional discussion of this topic is provided by Gail.[53])

Multiple Comparisons and Subsets

If a box contains 19 black balls and 1 red ball, the probability of selecting the red ball on any one draw is $\frac{1}{20}$ or 0.05. However, the probability of selecting the red ball *at least once* is 0.23 if one draws five times and 0.40 if one draws 10 times. In a clinical trial, if one subjects the data to multiple tests of hypothesis, the probability of at least one spuriously positive result increases rapidly beyond the nominal 0.05 level of each individual significance test. There is no totally satisfactory way around this dilemma. It does not seem realistic to limit the exploration of data that were obtained at great expense of time and money; nor does it seem reasonable to require that all tests be done at very strict significance levels to ensure that the overall significance level be protected, at the cost of severely reducing the power to detect important effects. An intermediate approach might be to consider all questions other than the primary focus of the trial as exploratory questions. Tests could be done at the usual 0.05 or 0.01 level, but a "significant" result would be interpreted as a suggestive observation requiring confirmation rather than a definitive result. This general approach has been suggested by several authors.[54-56]

An important example of the multiple-comparisons problem in clinical trials is the analysis of data within patient subsets. It is not unreasonable to speculate that treatment effects may be limited to, or more pronounced in, some subgroups of patients, but confirming such speculation is difficult without extraordinarily large sample sizes. When multiple subsets are considered, the chances are considerably increased that either a uniformly ineffective therapy will appear effective in one or more subsets or a uniformly effective therapy will appear ineffective in one or more subsets. In randomized studies, one can test for the significance of interactions between treatment and covariates; that is, differential effects in subsets beyond what might be expected by chance. However, the power for detecting interactions in a clinical trial of moderate size is low. "Qualitative interactions" (beneficial effect in one subset, harmful effect in the other) are of special concern,[57] but are no less difficult to detect reliably. Thus, when apparent differences in subset-specific treatment effects are observed in a clinical trial, it is impossible (except when the differences are extreme) to determine with confidence whether they are real or spurious. The most sensible approach seems to be to base conclusions on the overall result. The overall result is the most stable, and the study population presumably was defined on the basis of an expected homogeneity of treatment effect. Differences in subset-specific treatment effects, if suggestively large, should be independently confirmed before they are accepted.

Analysis of Phase II Studies

Phase II studies are generally concerned with response rates. Thus, the observed response rate (number of responders/number of patients treated) is usually the statistic of primary interest. Although this is our best estimate of the *true* response rate—the proportion of patients who would demonstrate response in an infinite patient population—one cannot assume on the basis of findings in 30 to 40 patients that the estimate is precise. To evaluate how close the estimate is likely to be to the true response rate, a *confidence interval* is constructed around the estimate. A confidence interval can be defined as that set of possible rates that includes, with specified probability, the true response rate.

The most widely used method to calculate a confidence interval for a proportion p observed in a sample of size *n* is based on the normal approximation to the binomial distribution. The formula for calculating the upper and lower limit of the confidence interval for p is given in Table 13-6A. The point on the tail of the standard normal curve (centered at 0, standard deviation of 1) beyond which only a (specified) small portion of the distribution lies is *z*. A few commonly used *z* values are given in Table 13-6B, and an example of the actual calculation of confidence limits is given in part C.

Although this is a simple method, it is based on an approximation that is reasonably accurate only when p is in the middle range ($0.3 < p < 0.7$) *and* when *n* is about 30 or more. For smaller sample sizes, or when proportions closer to 0 or 1 are being estimated, there is a better approximation that is only slightly more complicated to calculate (see 13-6D).[58]

The estimation of survival time parameters is somewhat more complicated. If all patients have died, so that all survival times are known exactly, one can directly calculate the median survival and the proportion surviving at various time points. The median of the observed survival times is the halfway point in an ordered listing of all survival times. It is preferable to the mean as a central measure for this type of data because the mean can be drawn away from the center of the distribution by one or two very large observations, as can be seen in the example in Table 13-7. This example also demonstrates that the central measure, whether median or mean, is often insufficient to adequately summarize the data. For the data used in the table, the range of values would be essential to a useful summary description.

When data are censored—that is, some patients are still alive, so that their survival times are known only to be longer than the current follow-up time—estimation of survival parameters is more difficult. Some parameters can still be measured directly; for example, if more than 1 year has elapsed since patient entry was terminated, and if follow-up is current on all patients, the proportion of patients surviving 1 year can be directly estimated by dividing the number who survived at least 1 year by the total number of patients who entered the study. If the censored survival times are all in the upper half of the distribution when the times are ordered, the median will still be the central observation. However, when some data are censored at relatively early points, we can no longer estimate the median or the year-by-year survival rates by ordering the observations and counting. In these situations, life table methods are required to provide valid and maximally informative estimates. The Kaplan–Meier procedure,[59] which provides probabilities of survival at each point in time at which a death occurred, is probably the most commonly used in cancer studies, and should always be used when the number of deaths is relatively small. The other type of procedure, often referred to as the actuarial method,[60] calculates probabilities at fixed points in time (*e.g.,* 6-month intervals). With this procedure, there is some loss of information, since the ordering of deaths within any given interval is ignored. However, if the number of deaths is large, and the size of the interval is chosen sensibly, the loss of information should not be too serious. The latter procedure requires less computation; however, with the availability of computer programs to perform these procedures, this has become less of an issue.

Life table survival probabilities are frequently presented graphically as survival curves. Figure 13-1 shows the Kaplan–Meier plot of survival probabilities for the data set shown in Table 13-8. These hypothetical data represent a clinical situation in which 30 patients were entered on a study over a period of

Table 13-6
Calculating Confidence Limits for Proportions

(A) Approximation to upper and lower confidence limits

$$p \pm z\sqrt{p(1-p)/n}$$

(B) Commonly used *z* values

Confidence Interval	*z*
99%	2.58
95%	19.6
90%	1.645

(C) Example of calculating confidence interval

Number of patients (n) = 30
Observed responses = 9
Observed response rate (p) = 9/30 = 30%

For a 90% confidence interval, $z = 1.645$.
Confidence limits are calculated as follows:

$$0.30 \pm 1.645\sqrt{(0.30 \times 0.70)/30}$$
$$= 0.30 \pm 0.14$$
$$= (0.16, 0.44)$$

(D) Better approximation to confidence limits

$$[p + A/2 \pm z\sqrt{p(1-p)/n + A/4n}]/(1+A),$$

where $A = z^2/n$.

Table 13-7
Centrality Estimates for Survival Times*

Observed survival times (months)	1, 1, 1, 1, 2, 2, 2, 2, 3, 3, 4, 5, 5, 20, 30
Mean survival time	5.5
Median survival time	2

* See text for details.

FIGURE 13-1. Plot of life-table probabilities. Tick marks indicate censored observations.

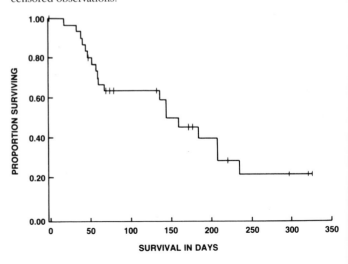

Table 13-8
Patient Entry and Survival Times

Patient	Day of Entry	Status at Day 365	Survival Time*
1	11	Dead	53
2	23	Dead	41
3	36	Dead	208
4	37	Dead	208
5	39	Alive	326+
6	44	Alive	321+
7	56	Dead	60
8	68	Alive	297+
9	79	Dead	137
10	85	Dead	184
11	88	Dead	160
12	91	Dead	235
13	94	Dead	48
14	124	Dead	145
15	139	Dead	145
16	144	Alive	221+
17	188	Alive	181+
18	191	Dead	58
19	193	Alive	172+
20	205	Dead	61
21	208	Dead	68
22	217	Dead	34
23	232	Alive	133+
24	248	Dead	45
25	261	Dead	18
26	282	Dead	39
27	285	Alive	80+
28	290	Alive	75+
29	295	Alive	70+
30	297	Alive	68+

* A "+" indicates a censored survival time (see text for details).

Table 13-9
*Kaplan–Meier Life Table Probabilities**

Days from Study Entry	Proportion Surviving
18	0.967
34	0.933
39	0.900
41	0.867
45	0.833
48	0.800
53	0.767
58	0.733
60	0.700
61	0.667
68	0.633
137	0.588
145	0.543
145	0.498
160	0.452
184	0.396
208	0.339
208	0.283
235	0.212

* See text for details.

300 days, with follow-up continuing until day 365. The plot "steps down" at each point in time at which a death was observed. The tick marks on the plot correspond to the survival times with a "+" in Table 13-8, indicating data censoring at those points. For example, the survival time for patient 5 in Table 13-8 is given as 326+ days. The experience of this patient is represented by the rightmost tick mark on the survival plot. The estimated median survival, as well as probabilities of survival at particular points, may be approximated from the plot or, more easily, from the table that produced the plot (Table 13-9). In this case, the median survival is 145 days; the probabilities of 3-, 6-, and 9-month survival are 63%, 45%, and 21%, respectively. The actual calculation of Kaplan–Meier life table probabilities is well described by Peto and colleagues[61]; both procedures are described by Lee.[62] Methods for calculating confidence intervals for survival parameters are discussed by Simon.[58]

Evaluating the effect of therapy on patient survival is difficult in the context of a Phase II study. Objective tumor shrinkage is generally accepted as being attributable to the treatment administered because the frequency of spontaneous tumor regression in untreated patients is thought to be very low. However, without a control group, it is impossible, except in very dramatic circumstances, to demonstrate that survival benefit is attributable to a particular treatment. Although it can reasonably be assumed that a tumor response would not have oc-

curred had the patient not been treated, it cannot so readily be assumed that a patient who survives for a given number of months following treatment would have survived for a shorter period without treatment. (The exception would be the "dramatic circumstance" of a substantial proportion of patients achieving long-term survival in a disease that previously was uniformly fatal within a short interval.) It has been a common practice among investigators reporting results of Phase II studies to compare the survival experience of responders with that of nonresponders and to view a prolonged survival of the responders as evidence of survival benefit attributable to the treatment. The fallacious reasoning behind this type of analysis has been widely discussed.[63-65] The fundamental problem is that an association between response and survival cannot be assumed to be a causal association. Patients will show variable survival times whether they are treated or not; those patients who are destined to survive longer because of more favorable baseline characteristics may be the ones who exhibit tumor shrinkage when treated with anticancer therapies. Thus, effects of treatment on survival may be reliably demonstrated only with the use of appropriate control groups.

Analysis of Phase III Studies

Most of the methods discussed in this section are directed at the comparison of treatment effects, which is the major objective of Phase III trials. However, we also consider other analyses, such as the identification of prognostic factors. Estimates of survival and response parameters are obtained using the methodology described in the previous section. The larger sample sizes available in Phase III trials permit more reliable estimates of these parameters.

The general approach in statistical testing is to consider a null hypothesis (no difference in treatment effect) against an alternative hypothesis (unequal effects). When the data demonstrate a sufficiently large difference in patient outcome, the null hypothesis may be rejected. The p value associated with the statistical test of the null hypothesis can be interpreted as follows: if the null hypothesis were true—that is, if there were truly no difference in treatment effect—the probability of an *observed* difference as large or larger than this one is equal to p. Thus, if p is small, the observed data may be considered sufficiently inconsistent with the null hypothesis to warrant its rejection. It should be noted that failure to reject the null hypothesis does not in any way demonstrate that the null hypothesis is true. If the sample sizes are large enough, however, failure to reject may indicate inconsistency with a true treatment difference that is of clinical importance.

Comparison of Proportions

When the endpoint is binomial—that is, there are only two outcome possibilities—the data can be represented in a 2×2 table, as depicted in Table 13-10A. Unless an unbalanced randomization scheme is used, $a + b$ and $c + d$ will each be approximately equal to $n/2$. If there is no association between treatment group and the likelihood of a success, then $a/a + b$ and $c/c + d$ should be approximately equal. The most commonly used test of the null hypothesis of no association is the chi-square test. This test is based on approximating the distribution of the binomial outcome variable with a normal distribution (bell-shaped curve), and therefore should be used only when the sample size is relatively large and the proportions of successes are neither extremely low nor extremely high. A good rule of thumb in the case of equal numbers in the two treatment groups is that the chi-square test is appropriate when the total number of successes $(a + c)$ is no less than 10 and no more than $n - 10$. The formula for the chi-square statistic is given in Table 13-10B. The value $n/2$, subtracted inside the squared term in the numerator, provides an adjustment, or "correction," to account for the application of normal distribution theory to binomial data. When the value of chi-square is

large, the null hypothesis may be rejected at a significance level that depends on the magnitude of the statistic. Some commonly used values are given in Table 13-10C; more extensive tables can be found in many standard textbooks.[66,67]

When the data are such that the chi-square test may not be appropriate, the Fisher–Irwin test (or Fisher's exact test) may be performed. This test requires more extensive computation, but is available in many statistical software packages. Alternatively, extensive tables for use with this test have been published.[68] The calculations required to perform the Fisher–Irwin test are described by Fleiss.[17]

Comparison of Survival Times

In many, if not most, Phase III trials in cancer, the primary endpoint is survival. In comparing survival (or similar endpoints, such as event-free survival), the use of proportions is not entirely satisfactory. The construction of a table as described in the previous section, using "alive/dead" as the outcome variable, could be misleading if the follow-up reporting tended to be more delayed on one treatment arm than on the other (as may occur when one treatment requires more frequent contact with the clinic). If we standardize follow-up by modifying the outcome variable to "alive/dead at 3 years following study entry," we lose information on patients who entered the study fewer than 3 years before the analysis, and we gain no information from deaths after the 3-year point. To improve the efficiency of survival comparisons, methods have been developed that use all of the information available for every patient and allow comparison of the overall distributions of survival time rather than focusing on a particular point in time. These methods also accommodate censored data. Two methods that can be recommended in most situations are the log rank test and the test based on the Cox proportional hazards model. Instruction in the use of these procedures is beyond the scope of this chapter; in any case, they are most safely implemented with a well-validated computer program. (Programs for these procedures are available in most large statistical software packages for mainframe computers, and in many packages for microcomputers.) An excellent discussion of the actual mechanics of the log rank test is given by Peto and colleagues[61]; Lee[62] discusses these and other methods for survival analysis in relatively nontechnical terms, and provides many excellent examples to illustrate the calculations.

A word about "proportional hazards." This often-used term means that the relative superiority (with respect to prolonging survival) of one treatment over another remains constant over time. The assumption of proportional hazards is the basis of the Cox procedure, and while it is not formally required by the log rank test, a marked nonproportionality of hazards would severely limit the interpretability of test results. There are many circumstances in which hazards would not necessarily be expected to be proportional. One example is the comparison of a highly toxic regimen versus one that is less toxic. The more toxic regimen may result in more treatment-related deaths early on, but may provide a better chance for long-term survival, even with the excess of early deaths taken into account. In these circumstances, an overall test of survival may obscure the appropriate interpretation of the data. In many instances, particularly with pediatric patients, treatment to improve the chance of long-term survival may be the appropriate strategy, even though the risk of early death due to acute toxicity may be greater. However, the additional early deaths may prevent the more toxic regimen from demonstrating a statistically superior survival advantage overall. An excellent discussion of this problem and suggested analyses to demonstrate the

Table 13-10
Chi-square Test for Comparison of Proportions

(A) Representation of data

Outcome	Treatment A	Treatment B	Total
Success	a	c	a + c
Failure	b	d	b + d
Total	a + b	c + d	a+b + c+d = (n)

(B) Chi-square statistic with correction for continuity

$$\chi^2 = \frac{n(|ad - bc| - n/2)^2}{(a + b)(c + d)(a + c)(b + d)}$$

(C) Significance levels for the chi-square statistic

p Value	χ^2
0.10	2.71
0.05	3.84
0.025	5.02
0.01	6.63
0.005	7.88
0.001	10.83

nonproportionality of hazards is provided by Stablein and co-workers.[67]

Identification of Prognostic Factors

There is an extensive statistical literature concerning the identification of baseline factors that are associated with the eventual patient outcome. The methodology most suited to determining which of a set of factors are important in predicting outcome is the regression model. Such models are used to develop prediction equations for outcome, based on the values of the known factors. Because the outcome of interest in cancer studies is usually binary (e.g., response/nonresponse) or a time variable that may be censored, specialized models must be chosen that accommodate such outcomes. With a binary outcome, one is essentially trying to calculate the probability of the outcome of interest; with a time-interval outcome, one is trying to predict the length of survival or event-free survival. For binary outcomes, the procedure of logistic regression is probably the most appropriate technique for evaluating the relative importance of baseline factors; the Cox regression model is widely used for outcomes such as survival time, where some of the data may be censored. In building either type of model, parameters reflecting the contribution of each factor to the accurate prediction of the outcome are estimated. When these parameters differ significantly from zero, one can infer that the factors have some prognostic value. Of course, when many factors are evaluated, the probability that at least one will differ significantly from zero, even if none has any effect on outcome (the multiple-comparisons problem), is not negligible. Thus, the results of such analyses must be interpreted cautiously. It is also important to realize that the significance levels resulting from these analyses are very much dependent on the sample size. Weak associations may attain significance when large data sets are analyzed; conversely, strong associations may not be demonstrated at conventional levels of significance in small samples. The identification of several "significant" prognostic factors is therefore no guarantee of a highly predictive model. For detailed discussions of the use of regression models to identify prognostic factors in cancer studies, the reader is referred to recent articles by Harrell and colleagues,[70] Simon,[71] and Sather.[72]

Adjustment for Covariates

Randomization ensures that no systematic bias will affect the treatment comparison, but it cannot ensure that the two treatment groups will be identical with regard to prognosis. It may happen by chance that more of the poor-prognosis patients are assigned to one of the treatments. To prevent this type of imbalance from influencing the treatment comparison, one can perform an analysis that accounts for the effects of important prognostic factors, or covariates. The most common method of adjustment is to perform a separate analysis for each level of the covariate (or for each possible combination of levels, when multiple covariates are considered simultaneously) and then statistically aggregate the results. For example, in a clinical trial of childhood ALL, one might want to adjust for age by considering outcomes separately for infants (<1 year), children ages 1 to 10 years, and those over 10—groups that have been shown to have differing prognoses. Even if there are no imbalances, it has been shown that this type of adjusted, or stratified, analysis is somewhat more efficient than an unadjusted analysis; by comparing outcomes within homogeneous subgroups, the variability of the overall result is slightly reduced.[73] Both adjusted and unadjusted analyses should generally be performed

and reported whenever important prognostic factors have been identified for the patient population under study. A more complete discussion of the rationale and methodology for adjustment of comparative analyses can be found in the text by Friedman and colleagues[74] and in articles by Simon.[71,75]

Meta-Analysis

Meta-analysis is generally defined as a quantitative summary of research in a particular area. What differentiates a meta-analysis from the more familiar review of the literature is the construction of an overall summary result that is obtained by statistically aggregating the results of the reviewed studies. Formal meta-analysis, also referred to as an "overview," is relatively new to oncologic research, although this technique is becoming more common in other medical research areas and has been widely used in the social sciences for many years. Many scientists believe that meta-analysis is proving to be a useful, perhaps even essential, tool in reaching reliable conclusions from the mixed assortment of studies that may have addressed the same research question. Others have expressed concerns about the validity of combining data from separate investigations, and about whether the questions that can be properly addressed by these methods are of sufficient interest to warrant the effort they entail.[76] Much of the controversy centers around the issue of "combinability" of studies. The question of which studies are sufficiently similar—with regard to treatment, patient population, and methods of determining endpoints—must be dealt with in planning any meta-analysis. If one considers only randomized clinical trials, it seems unlikely that meta-analysis will come to play a major role in pediatric cancer research, because there are rarely multiple studies comparing similar regimens in the same disease population. The aggregation of nonrandomized studies may be more feasible in terms of patient numbers, but this approach is even more problematic because the selection biases that inevitably arise in uncontrolled studies may be multiplied if the results of such studies are formally combined.

REPORTING RESULTS OF CLINICAL TRIALS

Ineffective reporting seriously compromises the value of well-conceived and expertly conducted clinical trials. These complex, time-consuming, and expensive investigations are conducted to increase the therapeutic information available to a medical community that is heavily reliant on the medical literature. Meaningful communication is therefore a critical component of the clinical trials process; without it, much, if not all, of the value of the investment in clinical trials is lost. Indeed, the publication of ambiguous or misleading results can be medically harmful and scientifically counterproductive.

The need for systematic investigation to identify advances in cancer treatment is widely accepted, and sophistication regarding issues of design and analysis in clinical trials has increased—yet the methodology of reporting these trials has not received the attention it merits. With the recognition that reliable comparisons among results of clinical trials can be made only in the presence of standardized reporting procedures, the World Health Organization in 1979 published recommendations for uniform approaches to assessment and reporting. These recommendations were developed and endorsed by an international assemblage of representatives of cancer clinical trials organizations.[37,77] Although they provide a useful starting point, these recommendations proved ineffective in circumventing the methodologic deficiencies increasingly noted in the clinical trials literature.[63,78–81] Various suggestions have been directed toward medical journal contributors and editors[82–86] in an effort to enhance the utility of reported results. A recent useful development is the adoption by the editorial board of *Cancer Treatment Reports* of a set of methodologic guidelines for clinical trials reporting[87]; these guidelines have been endorsed by editors of the *Journal of Clinical Oncology*[88] and *Cancer*[89] and are under consideration by other journals as well.[90] Attention to such principles will help ensure the quality of future clinical trials publications, and undoubtedly will have an important influence on the planning process that precedes the actual clinical investigation.

The value of any clinical trials publication is obviously related to the value of the experiment it reports. A useful publication is accurate, medically informative, and convincing to the reader. Accuracy is largely predetermined by the validity of the experimental design, the quality of its execution, and the legitimacy of the statistical analysis. The degree to which a paper is medically informative is dependent on the importance of the study question and the appropriateness of the experimental conditions. The ability to persuade the reader, however, relates largely to the information the author chooses to communicate. Although the general structure of research papers (background, methods, results, conclusions) is widely known, the detail presented is often insufficient to persuade a critical readership of the validity or applicability of the conclusions. Even when the design and conduct of the study and the analysis of results are impeccable, an inadequate description of these features prevents meaningful interpretation by the experienced audience for whom it is intended. This may delay the acceptance of an important advance or, more commonly, as in small studies with limited power, may suggest the acceptance or rejection of a concept based on what in reality is an equivocal result that requires further investigation.[78,90]

To be maximally effective, then, the author of a clinical trials report should write from the perspective of a critical reader. In evaluating the manuscript, a reader will initially want to know the scientific motivation for the study, particularly the specific hypothesis being addressed and the reasons for its plausibility and pertinence. A detailed methods section permits an assessment of the strengths of the design and provides an opportunity to replicate the effort, if warranted. This section should clearly describe the experimental conditions, including the specifics of patient registration procedures, inclusion and exclusion criteria, description of the target patient population, the details of the treatment regimen(s) and any modifications thereof, the schedule of follow-up evaluations, the procedures used to assess major endpoints (including whether the person making the endpoint evaluation was "blinded" to the treatment assignment), and, in comparative trials, the nature of the control group and the specific methods used for treatment assignment. It should be noted whether the treatment allocation was by randomization. A description of the specific methods used to guarantee random treatment assignment and their timing relative to patient entry on study should be provided.[91] A brief description of quality control procedures will assure the reader that the information reported is complete and accurate. Finally, some discussion of the statistical procedures used to analyze the data will be useful to the reader in assessing the reliability of the reported results. This description includes identification of analytic procedures used, along with explanatory material for techniques likely to be unfamiliar to the journal readership. References to articles or books describing all but the simplest and most standard techniques should be provided.

The results section presents the outcome of the experi-

ment; clear and detailed exposition is crucial. A complete description of the patients entered on study, including age, disease characteristics, nature and amount of prior therapy, and other items considered important in determining eligibility or establishing prognosis should be included. Toxicity and compliance information should be included, and outcomes for all patients entered should be reported. Confining information to patients deemed evaluable prevents accurate comparisons across studies whose policies regarding evaluability may differ.[85,87] When feasible, as with small studies, lists of individual endpoint determinations are of interest.

It is important to define endpoints carefully in reports of clinical trials. Commonly used phrases such as "disease-free survival" are not necessarily defined in the same way by all investigators. The adoption of standard definitions and analyses, as proposed by Mastrangelo and associates[39] for pediatric leukemia studies, would facilitate the interpretation of study results and the comparison of results across studies.

Clinical trials reports usually conclude with the author's interpretations of the study results. If the data have been analyzed appropriately, the conclusions are generally self-evident. Potential sources of bias, the need for independent confirmation, and any other caveats should be included in the discussion. Claims of patient benefit should be circumspect and based on the demonstrated difference in outcome between the experimental and control groups, whose characteristics have been well-described. Claims of nonbenefit should be accompanied by either a confidence interval around the observed difference, or a calculated probability (power) that a clinically important difference would have been detected with the sample size at hand.[92] Further generalizations to a wider population should be made cautiously.

The authors thank Ms. Anna Pannell for her able assistance in the preparation of this manuscript.

REFERENCES

1. Muggia FM, Carter SK, MacDonald JS: The Cancer Therapy Evaluation Program of the National Cancer Institute. Semin Oncol 8:394–402, 1981
2. Von Hoff DD, Kuhn J, Clark GM: Design and conduct of phase I trials. In Buyse M, Staquet M, Sylvester R (eds): Cancer Clinical Trials: Methods and Practice, pp 210–220. London, Oxford University Press, 1983
3. Carter SK: Clinical aspects in the design and conduct of phase II trials. In Buyse M, Staquet M, Sylvester R (eds): Cancer Clinical Trials: Methods and Practice, pp 223–238. London, Oxford University Press, 1983
4. Marsoni S, Wittes R: Clinical development of anticancer agents—A National Cancer Institute perspective. Cancer Treat Rep 68:77–85, 1984
5. Livingstone RB, Carter SK: Experimental design and clinical trials: Clinical perspectives. In Carter S, Glatstein E, Livingstone RB (eds): Principles of Cancer Treatment. New York, McGraw-Hill, 1982
6. Simon R: The design and analysis of clinical trials. In Levine A (ed): Cancer in the Young, pp 391–402. New York, Masson Publishing, 1982
7. Karon M, Sieger L, Leimbrock S, Finkelstein J, Nesbit MF, Swaney JJ: Azacytidine: A new active agent for the treatment of acute leukemia. Blood 42:359–365, 1973
8. Marsoni S, Ungerleider RS, Hurson SB, Simon RM, Hammershaimb LD: Tolerance to antineoplastic agents in children and adults. Cancer Treat Rep 69:1263–1269, 1985
9. Grieshaber CK, Marsoni S: Relation of preclinical toxicology to findings in early clinical trials. Cancer Treat Rep 70:65–72, 1986
10. Collins JM, Zaharko DS, Redrick RL, Chabner BA. Potential roles for preclinical pharmacology in phase I clinical trials. Cancer Treat Rep 70:73–80, 1986
11. Gehan EA: The determination of the number of patients required in a preliminary and follow-up trial of a new chemotherapeutic agent. J Chron Dis 13:346–353, 1961
12. Fleming TR: One-sample multiple testing procedure for phase II clinical trials. Biometrics 38:143–151, 1982

13. Herson J: Predictive probability early termination plans for phase II clinical trials. Biometrics 35:775–783, 1979
14. Sylvester RJ, Staquet MJ: An application of decision theory to phase II clinical trials in cancer. In Tagnon HJ, Staquet MJ (eds): Recent Advances in Cancer Treatment, pp 1–11. New York, Raven Press, 1977
15. Lee YJ, Staquet MJ, Simon R, Catane R, Muggia F: Two stage plans for patient accrual in phase II cancer clinical trials. Cancer Treat Rep 63:1721–1726, 1979
16. Simon R, Wittes RE, Ellenberg SS: Randomized phase II clinical trials. Cancer Treat Rep 69:1375–1381, 1985
17. Fleiss JL: Statistical Methods for Rates and Proportions, 2nd ed. New York, John Wiley & Sons, 1981
18. George SL, Desu MM: Planning the size and duration of a clinical trial studying the time to some critical event. J Chron Dis 27:15–24, 1974
19. Rubinstein LV, Gail MH, Santner TJ: Planning the duration of a comparative clinical trial with loss to follow-up and a period of continued observation. J Chron Dis 34:469–479, 1981
20. Sposto R, Sather HN: Determining the duration of comparative clinical trials while allowing for cure. J Chron Dis 38:683–690, 1985
21. Makuch RW, Simon R: Sample size requirements for non-randomized comparative studies. J Chron Dis 33:175–181, 1980
22. McPherson K: Statistics: The problem of examining accumulating data more than once. N Engl J Med 290:501–502, 1974
23. Pocock SJ: Group sequential methods in the design and analysis of clinical trials. Biometrika 64:191–199, 1977
24. Pocock SJ: Interim analyses for randomized clinical trials; the group sequential approach. Biometrics 38:153–162, 1982
25. O'Brien PC, Fleming TR: A multiple testing procedure for clinical trials. Biometrics 35:549–556, 1979
26. Fleming TR, Harrington DP, O'Brien PC: Designs for group sequential tests. Controlled Clin Trials 5:348–361, 1984
27. DeMets DL, Ware JH: Asymmetric group sequential boundaries for monitoring clinical trials. Biometrika 69:661–663, 1982
28. Whitehead J, Stratton I: Group sequential clinical trials with triangular continuation regions. Biometrics: 39:227–236, 1983
29. Ellenberg SS, Eisenberger MA: An efficient design for phase III studies of combination chemotherapies. Cancer Treat Rep 69:1147–1154, 1985
30. D'Angio GJ, Evans AE, Breslow N et al: Results of the third National Wilms' Tumor Study. Proc Am Assoc Cancer Res 25:183, 1984
31. Gastrointestinal Tumor Study Group: Adjuvant therapy of colon cancer—Results of a prospectively randomized trial. N Engl J Med 310:737–743, 1984
32. Byar DP, Piantadosi S: Factorial designs for randomized clinical trials. Cancer Treat Rep 69:1055–1062, 1985
33. Zelen M: A new design for randomized trials. N Engl J Med 300:1242–1245, 1979
34. Zelen M: Alternatives to classic randomized trials. Surg Clin North Am 61:1425–1432, 1981
35. Taylor KM, Margolese RG, Soskolne C: Physicians' reasons for not entering eligible patients in a randomized clinical trial of surgery for breast cancer. N Engl J Med 310:1363–1367, 1984
36. Ellenberg SS: Randomization designs in comparative clinical trials. N Engl J Med 310:1404–1408, 1984
37. Miller AB, Hoogstraten B, Staquet M, Winkler A: Reporting results of cancer treatment. Cancer 47:207–214, 1981
38. Peto R, Pike MC, Armitage P, Breslow NE, Cox DR, Howard SV, Mantel N, McPherson K, Peto J, Smith PG: Design and analysis of randomized clinical trials requiring prolonged observation of each patient: I. Introduction and design. Br J Cancer 34:585–612, 1976
39. Mastrangelo R, Poplack D, Bleyer A, Riccardi R, Sather H, D'Angio G: Report and recommendations of the Rome Workshop Concerning Poor-Prognosis Acute Lymphoblastic Leukemia in Children: Biologic bases for staging, stratification and treatment. Med Pediatr Oncol 14:191–194, 1986
40. US Department of Health and Human Services, Public Health Service, National Institutes of Health, Office for Protection from Research Risks: National of Human Subjects, Title 45, Code of Federal Regulations, Part 46, revised as of March 8, 1983. OPRR Reports, Washington, DC, US Government Printing Office
41. 45 CFR Part 46. Additional protections for children involved as subjects in research. Federal Register 48:9814–9820, March 8, 1983
42. Chalmers TC, Celano P, Sacks HS, Smith H Jr: Bias in treatment treatment assignment in controlled clinical trials. N Engl J Med 309:1358–1361, 1983
43. Simon R, Pocock SJ: Sequential treatment assignment with balancing for prognostic factors in the controlled clinical trial. Biometrics 31:103–115, 1975
44. Simon R: Adaptive treatment assignment methods and clinical trials. Biometrics 33:743–749, 1977
45. Taves DR: Minimization: A new method of assigning patients to treatment and control groups. Clin Pharmacol Ther 15:443–453, 1974
46. Begg CD, Iglewicz B: A treatment allocation procedure for sequential clinical trials. Biometrics 36:81–90, 1980
47. Halperin M, Lan KKG, Ware JH, Johnson NJ, DeMets DL: An aid to data monitoring in long-term clinical trials. Controlled Clin Trials 3:311–323, 1982
48. Lan KKG, Simon R, Halperin M: Stochastically curtailed testing in long-term clinical trials. Communications in Statistics 1:207–219, 1982
49. Anderson PK: Conditional power calculations as an aid in the decision whether to continue a clinical trial. Controlled Clin Trials 8:67–74, 1987
50. DeMets DL, Hardy R, Friedman LM, Lan KKG: Statistical aspects of early termination in the beta blocker heart attack trial. Controlled Clin Trials 5:362–372, 1984
51. Green SJ, Fleming TR, O'Fallon JR: Policies for study monitoring and interim reporting of results. J Clin Oncol 5:1477–1484, 1987
52. Geller NL, Pocock SJ: Interim analysis in randomized clinical trials: Ramifications and guidelines for practitioners. Biometrics 43:213–223, 1987
53. Gail MH: Eligibility exclusions, losses to follow-up, removal of randomized patients and uncounted events in cancer clinical trials. Cancer Treatment Rep 69:1107–1112, 1985
54. Simon R: Patient subsets and variation in therapeutic efficacy. Br J Clin Pharmacol 14:473–482, 1982
55. Sather HN: Statistical evaluation of prognostic factors in ALL and treatment results. Med Pediatr Oncol 14:158–165, 1986
56. Armitage P: Importance of prognostic factors in the analysis of data from clinical trials. Controlled Clin Trials 1:347–353, 1981
57. Gail MH, Simon R: Testing for qualitative interactions between treatment effects and patient subsets. Biometrics 41:361–372, 1985
58. Simon R: Confidence intervals for reporting results of clinical trials. Ann Intern Med 105:429–435, 1986
59. Kaplan E, Meier P: Nonparametric estimation from incomplete observations. J Am Stat Assoc 53:457–481, 1958
60. Cutler SJ, Ederer F: Maximum utilization of the life table method in analyzing survival. J Chron Dis 8:699–712, 1958
61. Peto R, Pike M, Armitage P, et al: Design and analysis of randomized clinical trials requiring prolonged observation of each patient: II. Analysis and examples. Br J Cancer 35:1–39, 1977
62. Lee ET: Statistical Methods for Survival Data Analysis. Belmont, CA, Wadsworth, 1980
63. Anderson JR, Cain KC, Gelber RD: Analysis of survival by tumor response. J Clin Oncol 1:710–719, 1983
64. Weiss GB, Bunce H III, Hokanson JA: Comparing survival of responders and nonresponders after treatment: A potential source of confusion in interpreting cancer clinical trials. Controlled Clin Trials 4:43–52, 1983
65. Mantel N: Responder versus nonresponder comparisons: Daunorubicin plus prednisone in treatment of acute nonlymphocytic leukemia. Cancer Treat Rep 67:315–316, 1983
66. Snedecor GW, Cochran WG: Statistical Methods, 7th ed. Ames, Iowa State University Press, 1980
67. Armitage P: Statistical Methods in Medical Research. London, Blackwell Scientific Publications, 1971
68. Pearson ES, Hartley HO (eds): Biometrika Tables for Statisticians, vol 1, 3rd ed. Cambridge, England, Cambridge University Press, 1970
69. Stablein DM, Carter WH, Novak JW: Analysis of survival data with nonproportional hazard functions. Controlled Clin Trials 2:149–159, 1981
70. Harrell FE, Jr, Lee KL, Matchar DB, Reichert TA: Regression models for prognostic prediction: Advantages, problems, and suggested solutions. Cancer Treat Rep 69:1071–1078, 1985
71. Simon R: Use of statistical regression models. In Buyse ME, Sylvester RJ, Staquet MJ (eds): Cancer Clinical Trials: Design, Practice, and Analysis. London, Oxford University Press, 1984
72. Sather HN: The use of prognostic factors in clinical trials. Cancer 58:461–467, 1986
73. Green SB, Byar DP. The effect of stratified randomization on size and power of statistical tests in clinical trials. J Chron Dis 31:445–54, 1978
74. Friedman LM, Furberg CD, DeMets DL: Fundamentals of Clinical Trials. Littleton, MA, John Wright & Sons, 1983
75. Simon R. Heterogeneity and standardization in clinical trials. In Tagnon HJ,

Staquet MJ (eds): Controversies in Cancer, pp 37–49. New York, Masson Publishing 1979

76. Yusuf S, Simon R, Ellenberg SS (eds): Proceedings of a workshop on overviews of randomized clinical trials. Statistics in Medicine 6:217–409, 1987

77. WHO Handbook for Reporting Results of Cancer Treatment. WHO Offset Publication No. 48. Geneva, World Health Organization, 1979

78. DerSimonian R, Charette LJ, McPeek B, Mosteller F: Reporting on methods in clinical trials. N Engl J Med 306:1332–1337, 1982

79. Tonkin K, Tritchler D, Tannock I: Criteria of tumor response used in clinical trials of chemotherapy. J Clin Oncol 3:870–875, 1985

80. Liberati A, Himel HN, Chalmers TC. A quality assessment of randomized controlled trials of primary treatment of breast cancer. J Clin Oncol 4:942–951, 1986

81. Anderson JR, Davis RB: Letter. J Clin Oncol 4:115–117, 1986

82. Makuch RW: Statistical guidelines for medical research reports. Cancer Treat Rep 66:217–219, 1982

83. O'Fallon JR, Dubey SD, Salsburg DS, Edmonson JH, Soffer A, Colton T: Should there be statistical guidelines for medical research papers? Biometrics 34:687–695, 1978

84. Altman DG, Gore SM, Gardner MJ, Pocock SJ. Statistical guidelines for contributors to medical journals. Br Med J 286:1489–1493, 1983

85. Zelen M: Guidelines for publishing papers on cancer clinical trials; responsibilities of editors and authors. J Clin Oncol 12:164–169, 1983

86. George SL: Statistics in medical journals: A survey of current policies and proposals for editors. Med Pediatr Oncol 13:109–112, 1985

87. Simon R, Wittes RE: Methodologic guidelines for reports of clinical trials. Cancer Treat Rep 69:1–3, 1985

88. Bertino JR: Guidelines for reporting clinical trials. J Clin Oncol 4:1, 1986

89. Simon R, Wittes RE: Methodologic guidelines for reports of clinical trials. Cancer 58:212–214, 1986

90. Wittes RE: How we know what we (think we) know. J Clin Oncol 4:827–829, 1986

91. Byar DP, Simon RS, Friedewald WT, Schlesselman JJ, DeMets DL, Ellenberg JH, Gail MH, Ware JH: Randomized clinical trials. Perspective on some recent ideas. N Engl J Med 295:74–80, 1976

92. Freiman JA, Chalmers TC, Smith H Jr, Kuebler RR: The importance of beta, the type II error and sample size in the design and interpretation of the randomized control trial: survey of 71 "negative" trials. N Engl J Med 299:690–694, 1978

fourteen

Biologics and Biological Response Modifiers

Maryann Roper

Biologics are substances of natural, often human, origin. Biological response modifiers (BRMs) are those agents or methods that can modify a biological or immune response in the host toward a therapeutic advantage against the host's tumor. Not all biologics are BRMs, and not all BRMs are biologics. Ideally, BRMs act on the host's own immune response or on the cancer cell, either to stimulate the body's immune system to kill the tumor or to modify the cancer cell in such a way as to make it more susceptible to destruction. A BRM might selectively reconstitute an element of the immune system, hyperinduce an otherwise normal activity, or selectively eliminate or suppress a specific type of cell. In any case, the antitumor effect will be maximal when the mechanism of action is optimal. Ideally, a biological approach to cancer treatment would have minimal toxicity to the patient and maximal toxicity to the tumor. It should not be surprising, however, that when biological agents are used as cytotoxics in large doses, appreciable side-effects can occur.

Although the idea of using the body's own immune system as a treatment for cancer dates back to the turn of the century,[1-3] only recently have large-scale clinical trials of biologics been undertaken. As the understanding of the immune system has increased, so have attempts to manipulate it in the effort to eliminate cancer cells (see Chap. 4). In 1979, the National Cancer Institute (NCI) established the Biological Response Modifiers Program to address the challenge of using biological agents in cancer therapy.[4] Many agents identified as being of interest in the planning stages of that program are still with us, in varying stages of clinical development and usefulness for cancer treatment.

In the last decade, therapy with biologics and BRMs has taken a giant leap forward, mainly because of recombinant DNA[5] and monoclonal antibody (MoAb)[6] technologies (see Chaps. 3 and 4). The ability to "mass produce" large quantities of highly purified proteins has taken treatment with biological agents out of the realm of one-time laboratory experiments and into the clinical arena. With the availability of adequate quantities of biological agents, carefully controlled clinical studies using large numbers of patients can now be performed, permitting valid conclusions concerning the toxicities and antitumor activities of these agents.

Despite the growing body of literature on biologics and BRMs in adult cancers, the use of these agents in pediatric oncology patients has been limited.

OVERVIEW OF RELEVANT BIOLOGICS

Biologics and BRMs encompass a wide range of types of agents and putative mechanisms of action (Table 14-1). Biologics can be classified according to their cellular origin or their function. A common denominator is thought in most cases to be the presence of a specific receptor on the surface of the cell directly affected by the agent. This appears to be the case for cytokines, antibodies and

Table 14-1
Categories of Biologics and Biological Response Modifiers

Immunomodulating Agents
   Microorganisms or microbial/fungal products
      BCG, *Corynebacterium parvum,* Lentinan, Glucan
   Synthetic compounds
      Levamisole, poly ICLC, isoprinosine, bestatin, prostaglandin E
         inhibitors, tuftsin
   Anticancer Drugs
      Cyclophosphamide, Adriamycin, vincristine, vinblastine,
         6-mercaptopurine
Cytokines
   Interferons (alpha, beta, gamma)
   Lymphokines
      Interleukin-2, macrophage activation factor
   Toxins (produced by either lymphocytes or macrophages)
      Lymphotoxin, tumor necrosis factor
   Growth and differentiation factors
      Colony-stimulating factors, transforming growth factor (TGF),
         bombesin, epidermal growth factor (EGF), tumor
         angiogenesis factor
Monoclonal Antibodies
Adoptive Transfer of Cells
   Lymphocyte-activated killer cells (LAK), tumor infiltrating
      lymphocytes (TIL)

complement, and growth and differentiation factors. It may not be the case for immunomodulatory agents, which may directly affect intracellular mechanisms rather than working through a surface receptor.[7]

BRMs frequently act by influencing the activity of cells. In contrast, cytotoxic agents generally affect the synthesis or function of DNA. Biologics (except differentiation factors) cause cytotoxicity either by direct killing of tumor cells or by setting into action a chain of cellular events that results in tumor cell death.

Cytokines and Lymphokines

Interferons

Originally described as antiviral agents, interferons are glycoproteins produced by cells in response to stimulation by a variety of mitogens or antigens. Interferon-alpha is induced from leukocytes and lymphoblastoid cell lines; interferon-beta is induced from foreskin fibroblasts; and interferon-gamma is produced exclusively by T-lymphocytes.[8] Interferons are 140 to 165 amino acids in length, with molecular weights of 17 to 25 kD. Interferon-alpha and interferon-beta share approximately 30% sequence homology, whereas the amino acid sequence of interferon-gamma is significantly different from these varieties. Interferons have been shown to mediate a wide spectrum of effects *in vivo* and *in vitro,* including induction of many substances (proteins, enzymes, prostaglandins, histoincompatibility antigens) that may in turn mediate interferon's activity; antiviral activity; and immunomodulatory effects.[8] The mechanism of interferon's antitumor activity has not been clearly defined. Dose–response information suggests that higher doses result in increased responses, leading to the conclusion that the mechanism of action is a direct cytostatic antitumor effect rather than an immunomodulatory one.[9] Since 1981, recombinant forms of all types of interferons have been produced and are being used in clinical trials.[10,11]

Constitutional symptoms—fever, chills, myalgias, arthralgias, headaches, and fatigue—are the most frequent therapy-limiting toxicities of interferon.[12,13] Additional toxicities are listed in Table 14-2. Minor variations in toxicities occur according to the type of interferon used and the dose, route, and schedule of administration.

Interferon-alpha (IFN-α) has shown activity in patients with hairy cell leukemia, non-Hodgkin's lymphoma (NHL), myeloma, chronic myelogenous leukemia (CML), melanoma, renal cell carcinoma, Kaposi's sarcoma, and CNS tumors (Table 14-3).[14–22] Interferon-gamma (IFN-γ) is active in chronic myelogenous leukemia.[23] An interesting recent laboratory observation of IFN-γ activity in a mouse tumor system may suggest a reason for the generally poor antitumor activity seen with IFN-γ in clinical studies to date. Talmadge and associates reported that the maximum tolerated dose of IFN-γ in tumor-

Table 14-2
Interferon Toxicities

Constitutional:	Fever*, chills*, myalgias*, arthralgias, anorexia*, fatigue†, weakness†, weight loss*
Cardiovascular:	Hypertension, hypotension, arrhythmias (atrial and ventricular), myocardial infarction
Gastrointestinal:	Nausea, vomiting, diarrhea
Renal/Metabolic:	Hypocalcemia, hyperkalemia, azotemia, proteinuria, interstitial nephritis
Hematologic:	Neutropenia†, thrombocytopenia*, anemia, coagulation abnormalities
Hepatic:	Elevated transaminases†
CNS:	Headache, lethargy*, confusion, decreased concentration*, mood alterations, EEG abnormalities, seizures, peripheral neuropathy
Other:	Hair loss, antibodies to IFN, oral herpes simplex

(Krown SE: Interferons and interferon inducers in cancer treatment. Semin Oncol 13:207–217, 1986)
* Common side-effects.
† Dose-limiting toxicities.

Table 14-3
Interferon-Alpha Antitumor Activity in Adult Malignancies*

Response Rates

>30%	10%–30%	<10%
Hairy cell leukemia	Multiple myeloma	Breast cancer
CML	CLL	Colon cancer
NHL (low grade)	Melanoma	Lung cancer
CTCL	Renal cell carcinoma	Brain tumors
Kaposi's sarcoma (AIDS-related)	Ovarian carcinoma	
Carcinoid		
Bladder tumors (local therapy for superficial tumors)		

(Adapted from Reference 22)
* CML = chronic myelogenous leukemia; NHL = non-Hodgkin's lymphoma; CTCL = cutaneous T-cell lymphoma; CLL = chronic lymphocytic leukemia.

bearing mice was not the most effective dose in killing tumors,[24] suggesting a bell-shaped rather than a linear dose–response curve. A clinical trial to test this observation is being planned. Studies with interferon-beta (IFN-β) are in progress, but it is too early to assess the spectrum of antitumor activity. The interferons generally have not been effective in the treatment of solid tumors.[10]

The experience with interferon in children has not been as extensive as that in adults (Table 14-4). In the 1970s, the Cantell interferon,[25] a naturally extracted product, was used in clinical trials in patients with osteogenic sarcoma.[26] Initially, the patients treated with interferon were said to show improvement, as compared to historical controls. The study was then expanded to a three-arm trial comparing interferon versus chemotherapy (including doxorubicin and methotrexate) versus an untreated control group. All three arms showed improved survival when compared to historical controls. There were no significant differences in outcome between the treated patients (interferon or chemotherapy) and the untreated control group. In a subsequent study, no responses were seen in 11 patients with metastatic osteogenic sarcoma who received up to 10×10^6 units/day for a minimum of 30 days.[27]

A limited number of interferon studies have been conducted in children with hematologic malignancies. Although one patient with T-cell acute lymphoblastic leukemia (ALL) experienced a complete remission that lasted approximately 1 year,[28] most patients showed only transient responses or no effect.[26–30]

Because of its activity in melanoma and NHL, clinical trials combining IFN-α with agents known to be active in those dis-eases have been designed to determine the contribution of IFN to existing therapies. In the trials in progress,[31–33] the IFN-α dose used in each combination was the highest dose that could be given without compromising the administration of known effective doses of cytotoxic agents. The outcome of these studies is pending. Studies of IFN-α are also planned for children with chronic myelogenous leukemia (CML) because this agent has shown activity in adults with CML.

Interleukin-2

Initially described as a T-cell growth factor, interleukin-2 (IL-2) is a 15 kD glycoprotein produced by T-helper lympho-cytes (OKT4+, LEU3+, or CD4+ in humans).[34] IL-2 can maintain the long-term growth of T-lymphocytes in culture and can mediate a wide range of *in vitro* and *in vivo* immunologic effects, including induction of cytotoxic T-cells, induction of T-helper cells, enhancement of natural killer (NK) cell activity, and restoration of allograft responsiveness.[35]

For purposes of anticancer therapy, the most notable effect of IL-2 is its ability to generate immune lymphoid cells that can lyse fresh, noncultured, NK cell-resistant primary and metastatic tumor cells, but cannot lyse normal cells. Removed from the host, incubated *ex vivo* with IL-2, and retransfused into the host, lymphokine-activated killer (LAK) cells can produce antitumor effects alone or in combination with additional doses of IL-2, both in animals and in humans.[35] Early experiments with LAK cells and IL-2 were conducted in animal models of lung metastases. When tumors were well established, the animals were treated with LAK cells and concomitant IL-2. In a characteristic experiment (Table 14-5), the maximal antitumor

Table 14-4
Interferon: Pediatric Clinical Trials

Reference	Dose and Schedule*	Toxicities	Responses†
26	3×10^6	Fever, chills, lethargy, malaise, weight loss	PR in osteogenic sarcoma
27	10×10^6 Daily $\times$ 30 IM	Fever, chills, lethargy, leukopenia, thrombocytopenia	No responses seen (11 osteosarcoma; 1 chondrosarcoma)
28	50×10^6 Daily $\times$ 14; SC $\times$ 3 mo	Fever, chills, malaise, anorexia, seizure, elevated transaminases, thrombocytopenia, coagulation abnormalities	CR in T-cell ALL OR in NHL
29	30×10^6 Daily IV	Fever, chills, malaise	Transient decrease in circulating blasts in 5/5 ALL, 2/3 AML
30	30×10^6 Daily $\times$ 10 d CI	Malaise, hepatotoxicity, coagulation abnormalities, fever, fatigue, lethargy, nausea, chills, headache, hypotension, seizures	Transient decrease in circulating blasts in 5/12 ANLL patients

* Dose is expressed in U/m². The dose listed is the maximum dose utilized in the trial.
† CR = complete response; PR = partial response; OR = objective response.

effect was noted when animals received both IL-2 and LAK cells.[36] Additional biological features of LAK cells are summarized in Table 14-6.[35]

The use of a cytokine (IL-2) to generate an effector cell (LAK cell), and the activity of that cell in producing clinical antitumor responses, represents a major step forward in the cellular therapy of cancer. The first clinical trial using this approach was reported by Rosenberg and associates at NCI in 1985.[37] In that study, 25 patients with advanced cancer who had failed standard therapy were treated with IL-2 (100,000 U/kg every 8 hours on days 1–5 and 12–16) and infusions of autologous LAK cells (on days 12, 13, and 15) obtained from five daily leukaphereses (on days 8–12) (Table 14-7). Objective tumor regression was noted in 11 of the 25 patients. One melanoma patient experienced a complete response; partial responses were seen in 10 other patients (3 patients with melanoma, 3 with colorectal cancer, 3 with renal cell cancer, and 1 with lung adenocarcinoma).

Based on these promising observations, additional Phase II studies using high doses of IL-2 in combination with LAK cells were initiated in melanoma, renal cell cancer, and colorectal cancer patients. Preliminary results show response rates of interest in patients with melanoma and renal cell cancer (Table 14-8).[38,39] Further studies by Rosenberg and colleagues support the initial observations of activity in these tumor types.[40] Antitumor activity using this regimen has also been observed in two patients with NHL.[40] Because of the recent nature of the studies, the duration of responses is short. Even so, several responses of greater than 6 months' duration have been seen. One melanoma patient has maintained a complete response for over 22 months.

In addition to the clinical responses seen with IL-2 plus LAK cells, both complete (renal cell) and partial (melanoma) responses have been reported following therapy with IL-2 alone.[40] These observations have led to the design of clinical trials in which patients are randomized to receive either IL-2 alone or IL-2 with LAK cells to determine the contribution of LAK cells to the treatment outcome.

In clinical trials using high doses of IL-2 (100,000 U/kg thrice daily, or a total dose of approximately 12 million U/m^2/day), considerable toxicity has been noted (Table 14-9), with many patients requiring intensive care unit (ICU) support.[40,41] In most cases, the toxicities were readily reversible. There have, however, been four therapy-related deaths among the 180 courses of treatment delivered. The dramatic toxicities observed with this therapy have led some investigators to sug-

Table 14-5

Immunotherapeutic Effect of LAK Cells and rIL-2 on Established Pulmonary Sarcoma Metastases

	Mean Number of Metastases at Day 13	
Cells*	HBSS	rIL-2
None	228	152
Cultured splenocytes	183	156
Fresh splenocytes	214	191
LAK cells	200	20†

(Mule JJ et al: The antitumor efficacy of lymphokine activated killer cells and recombinant interleukin-2 in vivo. J Immunol 135:646–652, 1985)

* 1 × 10^8 splenocytes cultured for 3 days without IL-2; fresh splenocytes or LAK cells were injected intravenously on days 3 and 6 after tumor injection (3 × 10^5 MCA sarcoma cells). Each group consisted of 6 mice. rIL-2 (15,000 U/dose) or Hank's balanced salt solution (HBSS) was injected intraperitoneally every 8 hours on days 3 through 8 after tumor injection.[28]

† LAK cells + rIL-2 versus rIL-2 alone, $p < 0.01$.

Table 14-6

Interleukin-2 and LAK Cells: Characteristics of Therapy in Murine Lung and Liver Metastases

Established metastases can be inhibited by treatment with IL-2 and LAK cells. Both LAK cells and IL-2 are required for optimal activity; either alone is less effective.

A dose–response relationship exists between the number of LAK cells administered and the therapeutic effect observed.

A dose–response exists between the amount of IL-2 administered and the therapeutic effect observed.

Incubation of splenocytes for 3 days in culture appears optimal for the generation of LAK cells with maximal activity after reinfusion *in vivo*.

IL-2/LAK cell immunotherapy is effective in hosts suppressed by total body irradiation or cyclophosphamide treatment.

Allogeneic LAK cells are effective in conjunction with IL-2.

Irradiated LAK cells (3000 cGy) are less effective than nonirradiated cells.

LAK cells can be generated from the splenocytes of tumor-bearing mice.

The precursor of LAK cells that is effective *in vivo* is a non-T-cell (Thy-1−).

Metastases that persist after IL-2/LAK cell therapy remain sensitive to LAK cell lysis both *in vitro* and in subsequent *in vivo* experiments.

Administration of IL-2 leads to *in vivo* proliferation of transferred LAK cells.

(Rosenberg SA. Adoptive immunotherapy of cancer using lymphokine activated killer cells and recombinant interleukin-2. In DeVita VT Jr, Hellman S, Rosenberg SA [eds]: Important Advances in Oncology 1986, pp 55–91. Philadelphia, JB Lippincott, 1986)

Table 14-7
*Interleukin-2 and LAK Cells: Clinical Protocol**

Procedure	Day															
	1	2	3	4	5	6	7	8	9	10	11	12	13	14	15	16
IL-2	I	I	I	I	I							I	I	I	I	I
Pheresis								Ph	Ph	Ph	Ph	Ph				
LAK Cells												L	L		L	

* Interleukin-2 is administered at 100,000 U/kg as a 20–30 minute infusion thrice daily. Patients are leukapheresed on days 8 through 12. Pheresed cells from days 8 and 9 are combined and reinfused, after culture, on day 12; cells from day 10 are infused on day 13, and cells from days 11 and 12 are reinfused on day 15.

Table 14-8
Interleukin-2 plus LAK Cells: Results of Clinical Trials

Reference	Diagnosis	Evaluable Patients	CR	PR	CR + PR	Duration CR (mo)
37	Renal cell	32	2	3	5 (16%)	7+, 4+
38	Melanoma	32	1	5	6 (19%)	7+
39	Renal cell	36	5	8	12 (34%)	6, 8+, 5+, 4+, 3+
39	Melanoma	26	2	4	6 (23%)	22+, 2+
39	Colorectal	26	1	2	3 (12%)	8+
39	NHL	2	1	1	2 (100%)	10

Table 14-9
*Toxicities Reported with High-Dose IL-2**

Toxicity	Frequency (%)
Nausea and vomiting	85
Diarrhea	85
Anemia	83
Elevated creatinine	81
Hyperbilirubinemia	79
Hypotension (requiring pressors)	68
Chills	67
Weight gain (≥10% body weight)	61
Thrombocytopenia (≤60,000/mm³)	46
Disorientation	36
Oliguria	35
Somnolence	14
Arrhythmias	13
Central line sepsis	13
Respiratory distress (requiring intubation)	9
Coma	5
Mucositis	4
Pleural effusion	3
Hepatitis A	3
Myocardial infarction	2
Death	2

* 100,000 U/kg thrice daily on days 1–5 and 12–16.

gest that its risks may outweigh its benefits.[42] An analogy might be drawn with the early days of bone marrow transplantation (BMT): both approaches can cause death (with perhaps a greater risk for the early BMT) and both demonstrate high-grade toxicities (the majority of which are reversible), for which many patients require ICU treatment. But in both cases, the intensity of the approach may be necessary in order to achieve complete responses.[43]

Other clinical trials, using lower doses of IL-2 administered on different schedules with or without LAK cells, are in progress (Table 14-10).[40,44-50] The toxicities in these studies vary. Rosenberg and colleagues treated 38 patients with lower doses of IL-2 (10,000 U/kg or 30,000 U/kg thrice daily) but continued to administer IL-2 until toxicity precluded further treatment. In regimens using 100,000 U/kg of IL-2, a median of 20 doses could be delivered; for regimens of 30,000 U/kg or 10,000 U/kg, medians were 27 and 68 doses, respectively.[40] West and coworkers treated 48 patients with an intravenous continuous infusion (CI) of IL-2 in doses up to 5 million U/m²/day, in combination with LAK cells, in 5-day cycles.[44] In the 40 patients who could be evaluated, 13 partial responses were observed. Toxicities were similar to those seen in the high-dose studies, but ICU support was required for only 6 of the 40 evaluable patients. Sarwal and associates described a regimen in which IL-2 was administered 3 times a week as a 5-minute intravenous bolus.[45] At doses up to 8 million U/m²/day, side-effects included intolerable chills and fever, malaise, and hypotension, but the majority of patients could be treated in an outpatient setting. Several partial responses were noted, particularly in patients with melanoma.

In the studies reported to date, only one patient younger than 20 years has been treated with IL-2.[40] Several Phase I trials are planned or in progress in pediatric patients, but results are not yet reportable. Because of the activity of both IL-2 alone and IL-2 with LAK cells in patients with melanoma and because neuroblastoma has reported antigenic similarities to melanoma, neuroblastoma may be an excellent target for IL-2 and LAK cell therapy. With several responses having been seen in NHL, clinical trials in hematologic malignancies are also of interest.

Table 14-10
*Summary of IL-2 Clinical Trials**

Reference*	Dose and Schedule†	Toxicities	Responses
44	5×10^6 IV Daily × 5 (+LAK cells)	Fever, fatigue, anemia, hypoalbuminemia, rash, eosinophilia, nausea and vomiting, diarrhea, stomatitis, elevated creatinine, hypotension, dyspnea, weight gain, hyperbilirubinemia	CR—none PR—renal, lung, melanoma, parotid, Hodgkin's disease, NHL
45	14×10^6 IV M,W,F × 4 wk	Rigors, fever, malaise, hypotension, lymphocytosis, eosinophilia	CR—none PR—melanoma
46	10^7 IV bolus/CI Daily × 7	Hypotension, fever, nausea, diarrhea, rash, fatigue, weight gain, arrhythmia, confusion, anemia	None
47	5×10^7 IP M,W,F	Fever, diarrhea	Too early (Ovarian)
48	$>1 \times 10^6$ SC Daily × 5	Fatigue, fever, nausea, elevated creatinine, eosinophilia, thrombocytopenia	Too early (Renal cell)
49	3×10^6 IV and SC Daily × 5 (+CYT)	Fatigue, malaise, nausea, lymphocytosis, eosinophilia, elevated creatinine	MR—renal
50	5×10^6 SC M, W, F (+IFN-β)	Fatigue, fever, malaise	OR—melanoma, carcinoid

* Most trials are Phase I; two are Phase I–II (Refs. 44 and 48).
† Dose is expressed in units/m². The dose listed is the maximum dose delivered in each study.
MR = mixed response; CYT = cyclophosphamide.

Laboratory experiments are exploring the possibility of improving the efficacy of IL-2 while decreasing its toxicity. To test the effects of these agents on IL-2-induced toxicity, cyclophosphamide, doxorubicin, and BCNU were given to non-tumor-bearing mice receiving IL-2. Doxorubicin and BCNU had no impact on the survival of IL-2-treated normal animals, but cyclophosphamide significantly prolonged their survival time.[51] In mice with pulmonary metastases from the MCA-105 sarcoma, the addition of a single dose of cyclophosphamide to the treatment regimen significantly increased survival time as compared to those treated only with IL-2. Another line of investigation uses IL-2 to generate a new class of lytic cells from lymphocytes infiltrating tumor specimens. These tumor infiltrating lymphocytes (TIL) are 50 to 100 times more effective in their ability to kill tumors in mice than are LAK cells.[52] Clinical trials to explore the potential of these laboratory observations are in progress.

Tumor Necrosis Factor

The concept of treating cancer patients with endotoxin, of which tumor necrosis factor (TNF) is a component, dates back to the turn of the century, when Dr. William Coley observed that a sarcoma patient underwent a spontaneous regression of his tumor following a life-threatening episode of erysipelas.[2] This observation prompted Coley to intentionally infect other cancer patients to determine whether serious infection would

have the same effect on their tumors. Responses were seen,[2,3] leading Coley to conclude that this approach had a role in cancer therapy.

Little else was done with endotoxin therapy until the 1970s, when a clinical trial using a crude preparation made according to Coley's specifications was attempted in NHL patients.[53] All patients initially received the same chemotherapy and were subsequently randomized to receive either no further treatment or a vaccine mixture of heat-killed *Streptococcus pyogenes* and *Serratia marcescens*. After the first 5 years of follow-up, all 22 patients in the vaccine group were alive, whereas 7 of the 25 patients in the other group had died. Both the complete remission rate and the durations of remissions were longer in the vaccinated patients. With additional follow-up, however, differences between the two groups disappeared. This study has not been repeated.

In 1976, Carswell and colleagues induced a serum factor in mice that could cause hemorrhagic necrosis and regression of mouse tumors.[54] Tumor necrosis factor (TNF) is a 17 kD glycoprotein produced by macrophages conditioned by *bacillus Calmette-Guerrin* (BCG) or other stimulating agents and triggered by endotoxin, and more recently produced by recombinant DNA techniques.[55–57] TNF has been isolated from the serum of laboratory animals and, in minute quantities, from humans.[58,59] In several series of laboratory experiments, TNF caused a dose-dependent hemorrhagic necrosis of established tumors in mice (primarily sarcomas and leukemias) with no toxic effects on the animals,[54] leading to the hope of a tumor-specific cytotoxic agent. *In vitro,* TNF exhibits both cytotoxic and cytostatic effects on tumor cells.[60] Its mechanism of action is not conclusively defined; observations regarding possible contributions to the antitumor activity of TNF are summarized in Table 14-11.[61–67] TNF also has a wide range of immunologic effects (Table 14-12).[68–70] Also of interest is the observation that the amino acid sequence of TNF is virtually identical to that of cachectin,[71] a protein hormone that causes aberrations in lipoprotein metabolism, possibly resulting in the wasting syndrome frequently observed in cancer patients.

In combination with IFN-γ, TNF shows marked synergistic antitumor activity *in vitro.*[72] In assays of 22 fresh tumor samples, the addition of small amounts of IFN-γ, which by itself was inactive, caused significant decreases in the amounts of TNF required for cytotoxicity. The median TNF dose required to reduce colony formation to 50% of the control was 2200 units in the absence of IFN-γ, but only 163 units after IFN-γ was added. TNF also shows increased activity *in vitro* when used in combination with cytotoxic drugs, such as actinomycin D[60] and adriamycin.[73]

Recombinant TNF is currently in Phase I clinical testing at several centers (Table 14-13).[74–78] Although plans for pediatric trials are underway, TNF studies to date have focused on adult cancer patients. In these initial studies, TNF has been administered subcutaneously, intramuscularly, or intravenously on twice-weekly or alternate-day schedules. Whereas no toxicity had been seen in the early studies in mice, clinical side-effects in Phase I trials include fever, headache, severe rigors, hypotension, fatigue, and anorexia. Laboratory studies show transient neutropenias (occurring and resolving within 3 hours after treatment) and sporadic elevations in hepatic enzyme analyses.[76] Although there is a report of a partial response in a colon cancer patient,[77] the spectrum of tumor types sensitive to TNF has not yet been defined in an appropriately designed series of Phase II clinical trials.

Growth Factors

Colony-Stimulating Factors

Hematopoietic precursor cells cannot survive or proliferate in a culture system unless specifically stimulated by a group of regulatory glycoproteins, called colony-stimulating factors (CSFs) because they stimulate precursor cells to form colonies of progeny cells.[79] The most thoroughly characterized CSFs are those controlling granulocyte (G) and macrophage (M) populations (G-CSF and GM-CSF). These substances have clinical relevance to the treatment of cancer patients in that they might [1] protect the bone marrow from the potentially lethal effects of chemotherapy or radiation, allowing higher doses of effec-

Table 14-11
Possible Mechanisms of TNF Antitumor Activity

Effects cell-cycle specific events[61]
Does not require cell division for cytotoxicity[62]
Requires internalization for maximal activity[63]
Results in extensive vascular changes[64]
Kills tumors in macrophage-depleted animals[65]
May require host T-cells for cytotoxicity[66]
Reduces c-*myc* expression[67]

Table 14-12
Immunologic Effects of TNF

Substitutes for T-helper cells[68]
Inhibits T-cell or B-cell response to mitogens[69]
Induces B-cell maturation[69,70]
Inhibits Concanavalin A-induced suppression[69]
Supports antibody production by mouse spleen cell cultures[69]

Table 14-13
Early Clinical Trials of TNF

Reference	Dose and Schedule*	Toxicities	Responses†
74	200 µg/m² Alt. SC/IV Twice weekly × 4 wk	Severe rigors, hypertension, fatigue, tenderness at injection site, hypercoagulability	TE
75	125 µg/m² Alt. IM/IV Twice weekly × 4 wk	Severe chills, fever	TE
76	250,000 U/kg IV Alternate days	Fever, nausea/vomiting, headache, malaise, fatigue, elevated liver transaminases, neutropenia, joint pain	AGL
77	125 µg/m² IV Thrice weekly	Severe rigors, chills, fatigue, nausea/vomiting, headache, hypotension, dyspnea	Colon (PR)
78	125 µg/m² IV Daily × 5, every 21 days	Severe chills, fever, fatigue, headache, nausea/vomiting, thrombocytopenia	TE

* The dose listed is the maximum dose administered on the study. "Alt." indicates alternating routes of administration.
† TE = too early; AGL = acute granulocytic leukemia.

Table 14-14
Human Colony-Stimulating Factors

Reference	Name	Molecular Weight	Activity
80, 81	GM-CSF (CSF-α)	22,000	Stimulates granulocyte or macrophage colony formation (peak at 14 days)
			Stimulates eosinophil colony formation
			Potentiates erythroid and multipotential (GEMM) colony formation, in combination with erythropoietin
82	G-CSF (CSF-β)	$\approx$30,000	Preferentially stimulates mature granulocyte precursors
			Induces differentiation of murine WEHI-3B leukemia cells
83, 84	Urine CSF	45,000	Indirectly stimulates GM colony formation by stimulating adherent accessory cells to produce CSFs
85	Pluripoietin	18,000	Combines the activities of CSF-α and CSF-β

tive agents to be delivered, [2] cause terminal differentiation of cancer cells, and [3] stimulate the functional activity of preexisting cells, which would be particularly valuable in instances of life-threatening sepsis and neutropenia.

Four human CSFs have been identified: GM-CSF,[80,81] G-CSF,[82] human urine CSF,[83,84] and pluripoietin[85] (Table 14-14). In addition to colony-stimulating activities, the CSFs can stimulate several functions of mature granulocytes, eosinophils, and macrophages, including survival, phagocytic activity, antibody-dependent cytotoxicity, and the expression of various membrane markers.[79] Human myeloid leukemia cells express receptors for G-CSF,[86] suggesting the possibility that G-CSF could induce terminal differentiation in myeloid leukemias and therefore prove valuable in suppressing this malignancy. With the development of recombinant CSFs and the availability of larger amounts of these agents, clinical trials are underway.

Tumor Growth Factors

The growth and differentiation of normal and malignant tissue appear to be at least partially controlled by a series of peptide growth factors. Several such factors have been described and their activity characterized.[87] For purposes of cancer therapy, it is possible that agonists to cancer cell growth factors, or to their cellular receptors, could block the self-stimulating effects of these molecules on tumor growth. For example, bombesin, an autocrine growth factor for small cell lung cancers, is also a mitogen for these tumor cells.[88] MoAbs have been raised against bombesin that can inhibit the growth of lung cancer cells *in vitro.* Clinical trials using this approach are in progress.

Angiogenesis Factor

Laboratory experiments have demonstrated that increasing angiogenic activity is acquired in normal cells as they progress to a preneoplastic state. Angiogenic peptides are present in many normal tissues and in tumors undergoing neovascularization.[89] Solid tumors are angiogenesis-dependent. To exploit this feature of tumors, a new class of angiostatic steroids that inhibit angiogenesis and tumor growth when administered with heparin, has been discovered which specifically induce dissolution of the basement membranes of growing capillaries. This loss of basement membranes results in endothelial cell rounding, cell death, and subsequent capillary involution. Such pharmaco-

Table 14-15
Estimated Rates of MoAb Toxicity in a Series of Clinical Trials

Toxicity	Estimated Frequency (%)
Fever	15
Diaphoresis	16
Rigors/chills	14
Pruritis	12
Urticaria	8
Dyspnea	7
Nausea	4
Vomiting	3
Diarrhea	2
Bronchospasm	2
Hypotension	1
Anaphylaxis	0.5

(Dillman RO et al: Toxicities and side effects of murine monoclonal antibodies. J Biol Response Mod 5:73–84, 1986)

logic manipulation could kill tumor cells not by direct cytotoxicity, but by shutting down their blood supply. Efforts are under way to produce adequate quantities of the specific steroid and heparin fractions for use in clinical trials.

Monoclonal Antibodies

As recombinant DNA technology has revolutionized the use of cytokines in cancer therapy, so has the work of Kohler and Milstein, who described a technique for producing MoAbs, revolutionized serotherapy.[6] Yet, despite this advance, MoAbs have not proven to be the "magic bullets" of cancer treatment. The potential benefit of MoAb treatment is tumor-specific cell killing with minimal host toxicity. Although most clinical trials of MoAbs have resulted in minimal toxicity (Table 14-15),[90] antitumor responses have been few and transient (Table 14-16).[91–104]

Early attempts at monoclonal antibody therapy in children used the J5 antibody (detecting the CALLA antigen) to treat leukemia patients[93] or to treat their harvested bone marrows prior to autologous transplant.[94] Four children with ALL received multiple infusions of varying doses of J5. All patients had transient decreases and then rebound of their peripheral blast counts. Patients whose marrows were purged with the J5 antibody had a better outcome, and 12 of 33 achieved complete remissions (median duration = 22 months).

More recently, tumor responses to monoclonal antibodies have been seen in patients with melanoma and neuroblastoma.[95,104] Complete and partial responses were reported in pediatric neuroblastoma patients receiving 3F8, an antibody directed against the ganglioside antigen GD2.[95] Complete and partial responses have also been seen in adult melanoma patients treated with R24, an antibody that detects the GD3 ganglioside antigen.[104] Both GD2 and GD3 are present on neuro-blastoma cells, so a therapeutic trial combining these two active antibodies could be considered.

Because of the complex immunologic problems involved in MoAb therapy, this field has yet to reach its full potential (Table 14-17). Technology that permits more ready production of human monoclonals may avoid the problems related to administering relatively large amounts of mouse protein to human patients. At this time, however, the human nonsecretor cell lines used as fusion partners to make human–human hybridomas do not fuse as readily as do mouse nonsecretor lines. In addition, most human secretor cells produce IgM antibodies, which are generally of low titer and weak affinity.[22] The technology to make human IgG antibodies is not yet routinely available.

Table 14-16
Antitumor Responses to MoAbs Seen in Patients with Hematologic Malignancies or Melanoma

Reference	Tumor Type	Antibody/Antigen	Human Antimouse Ig+	Tumor Regression
Pediatric Trials				
93	ALL	J5/CALLA	NR*	0/4
95	Neuroblastoma	3F8/GD2	(Most)	3/8
Adult Trials				
96	T-cell ALL	Leu-1/T65, and others	1/3	1/6
97	CLL	T101/T65	0/6	2/6
98	CLL	T101/T65	0/4	0/4
99	CLL	T101/T65	0/13	0/13
96	CTCL	Leu-1/T65	4/8	6/7
98	CTCL	T101/T65	2/4	0/4
100	CTCL	T101/T65	4/4	4/7
101	B-cell lymphoma	Anti-idiotype	5/10	6/10
102	Melanoma	96.5/p97 48.7/gp240	4/5	0/5
103	Melanoma	9.2.27/gp240	3/8	0/8
104	Melanoma	R24/GD3	12/12	5/12
95	Melanoma	3F8/GD2	(Most)	4/9

* Not reported.

Table 14-17
Monoclonal Antibodies: Problems with Therapy

Problem	Possible Solutions
Antigenic modulation	Not all antibodies cause modulation Use "cocktails" containing several antibodies recognizing the same antigen (different epitopes) or different antigens Choose a different antigen to target for subsequent therapy
Circulating free antigen	Plasmapheresis
Antimouse Ig+/anaphylaxis	Human monoclonal antibodies Drug-induced immunosuppression Plasmapheresis with immunospecific absorption Alteration in antibody dose and schedule Induction of tolerance
Transient nature of tumor responses	Repeated intermittent MoAb conjugated to drugs, toxins, or isotopes Infuse MoAbs attached to cells

DEVELOPMENT, APPLICATION, AND EVALUATION OF CLINICAL TRIALS

Clinical trials with biologics can be designed to study the agent either as a direct mediator of cell death (a cytotoxic) or as a modulator of a selected immunologic effect (a biological response modifier) (Table 14-18).[11] In the first case, in which biologics are intended to directly kill tumor cells, the approach to clinical studies is similar to that used for classic chemotherapeutic agents. Most cytotoxics are tested to define their maximum tolerated dose (MTD), the highest dose that can be administered to human patients with tolerable side effects. The MTD is also the dose that generally produces the most tumor kill.

In a clinical study of a BRM, the trial is directed at determining a dose and schedule that will optimize the desired biological effect. BRMs do not have to be administered at the MTD; they need only be given at doses capable of producing the intended immunomodulatory response. This dose could be lower than the MTD and thus might result in fewer or milder side-effects. To date, most biologics that have shown clinical antitumor effects have been administered at or near the MTD.

Preclinical Screening

Preclinical screening of biologics is more complex than the screening of classic cytotoxic agents.[105,106] The NCI's chemotherapy screening program has been organized to evaluate large numbers of agents (approximately 10,000 annually). In contrast to this extensive but necessarily superficial approach, the BRM screening program develops an in-depth evaluation of only a few agents (10–20) each year. The goals of the preclinical screening process are [1] to verify the BRM or antitumor effects of an agent that may have been previously described, [2] to determine the predictive value of the screen's immunomodulation assays for the ability to monitor cancer patients by using the same assays, [3] to determine the predictive value of the screen for an agent's antitumor activity, and [4] to attempt to determine the best dose and schedule for the administration of a biologic or BRM so as to provide some guidance for the design of clinical trials.

Because of the diversity of biologics and BRMs, no single screening approach can be planned. For agents that act on cells of the rodent immune system, a "common-track" set of assays has been developed (Table 14-19).[106] The endpoint by which BRM activity is assessed is the effect on an intermediary cell that, in turn, kills the tumor cell. Because more than one class of effector cells can kill tumor cells, a wide range of cellular assays must be performed (B-cell, T-cell, NK cells, macrophages) to completely assess the activity of each BRM. But for agents that are species-specific, such as certain human cytokines, MoAbs, and differentiation factors, "special-track" screens are being developed to include the use of human tumor xenografts in nude mice and in vitro evaluations of normal and malignant human cells. Additional studies useful in the screening of BRMs are listed in Table 14-20. As with cytotoxic agents, biologics and BRMs must also be tested for antitumor activity in classic in vitro and animal tumor systems.

Clinical Trials

Phase I clinical studies are intended to define the toxicities of a new agent, to determine its pharmacokinetics, and to find a dose and schedule of administration that can safely be admin-

---

Table 14-18
Objectives of Clinical Trials with Biologics

Used as a Cytotoxic	Used as a Biological Response Modifier
General Objective of Clinical Trials	
To achieve tumor cytotoxicity	To achieve tumor killing by modification of a specific biological response
Preclinical Screening	
To assess cytotoxicity in cell cultures and in animal models	To assess alterations in biological responses either *in vitro* or in animal models
	To assess cytotoxicity in cell cultures and in animal models
To determine the dose and schedule that will result in maximum tumor killing	To determine the dose and schedule that will optimize the desired biological response in animal models
Phase I Clinical Trials	
To determine toxicity	To determine toxicity
To determine pharmacokinetics	To determine pharmacokinetics
To define the MTD	To define the dose and schedule that will optimize the desired biological effect
Phase II Clinical Trials	
To identify tumors sensitive to the MTD	To identify tumors sensitive to the optimal biological dose
Phase III Clinical Trials	
To determine the role of the agent in the overall approach to therapy of the malignancy	

(Adapted from Reference 11)

Table 14-19
*BRMs: "Common Track" Preclinical Screening**

| Macrophages | Cellular Targets of Testing | | | |
	NK Cells	T Cells	B Cells
Culture with BRM for 24 h; 72 h cytotoxicity assay of ^{125}IUdR-labeled tumor cells and/or 18 h ^{111}In-labeled tumor cells	Culture with BRM for 24 h; 4 h cytotoxicity assay against ^{51}Cr-labeled YAC tumor target cells	Test for allogeneic MLR blastogenesis; MLTR-CMC allogeneic and/or syngeneic	
Inject BRM IV, harvest alveolar macrophages, and test for tumoricidal activity	Inject BRM IV; measure NK activity as above; IFN stimulation	Immunize against TSTA, CTL	Test for stimulation of specific antibody production
	Test for prevention of metastases in 3-week-old mice (fibrosarcoma)	Immunize against TSTA, SC challenge for alteration of tumor growth in UV-irradiated mice after immunization	
Study kinetics of activation	Study kinetics of activation; induction of hyporesponsiveness		Assay duration of response

(Talmadge JE, Herberman RB: The preclinical screening laboratory: Evaluation of immunomodulatory and therapeutic properties of biological response modifiers. Cancer Treat Rep 70:171–182, 1985)
* IUdR = iododeoxyuridine; MLR = mixed lymphocyte response; MLTR-CMC = mixed lymphocyte tumor response followed by cell-mediated cytotoxicity; TSTA = tumor-specific transplantation antigen; CTL = cytotoxic T-cells.

Table 14-20
Biological Response Modifiers: Nonroutine Analyses Useful in Preclinical Screening

Characterization of *in vitro* effector cell populations by:
  Depletion
  Antiserum sensitivity
  Purification of effector cells
Examination of synergistic actions of BRMs
  Combination chemoimmunotherapy
  Combination of BRMs
Direct cytotoxic activity
Stimulation of cytokine production
Immunomodulation in tumor-bearing animals
Induction of helper or suppressor cells
Compartmentalization, cell number, and differential of induced effector cells
Therapy parameters: dose, route, schedule, duration
Pharmacokinetics and biodistribution
Toxicity

(Talmadge JE, Herberman RB: The preclinical screening laboratory: Evaluation of immunomodulatory and therapeutic properties of biological response modifiers. Cancer Treat Rep 70:171–182, 1985)

istered to patients in subsequent clinical trials. For trials of BRMs, appropriate immunologic monitoring is incorporated into the study to determine whether, at a dose that can be administered safely, the desired biological effect will be achieved. Following the determination of the best dose and schedule of administration for a biological agent, Phase II clinical trials are initiated to determine the efficacy of that agent in a wide range of tumor types. Phase III studies are

undertaken to determine the significance of this agent in the overall therapy of tumors shown responsive in Phase II (see Table 14-18).

Limitations to this approach can be seen in a review of the clinical development of IFN-α.[10] Because an optimal immunomodulatory dose could not be defined in preclinical and Phase I studies, a number of different doses and schedules were taken into Phase II testing. Sensitive malignancies, such as hairy cell leukemia, respond to low doses of interferon (2–4 million U/m² daily or thrice weekly). Higher doses, up to 20 million U/m², were necessary to achieve tumor responses in renal cell carcinoma and melanoma. These results could reflect differing sensitivities of tumors to the antiproliferative effects of interferon. Alternatively, different tumors may be killed by different types of effector cells, which in turn require varying doses of interferon for *in vivo* activation.

Immunologic Monitoring in Clinical Trials

The problem of immunologic monitoring in clinical trials of BRMs deserves mention.[105,106] First, it is generally not practical to repeat the wide variety of immunologic studies that are done *in vitro* as part of the preclinical screen on each patient in a clinical trial. The major limiting factors to this approach are patient safety and cost. It is therefore necessary to select carefully the appropriate immunologic parameters to be assessed. Assuming that an agent is brought to clinical trial only after an extensive series of preclinical studies, this choice is aided by examining the existing laboratory data. It is yet another step in the hypothesis to assume that the immune parameter selected for study is critical to the process of tumor cytotoxicity.

Other variables to be considered in the choice of immunologic monitoring include patient-to-patient variation, day-to-day variability within individual patients, the time of sampling relative to the administration of the agent, the possibility of other medications altering the immunologic function under observation, the effect of the patient's underlying malignancy, and correct selection of the source of the sample (*i.e.*, marrow, blood, or lymph node). When a "negative" result is obtained in a clinical trial designed to modify a biological response, particularly if that clinical trial is based on positive preclinical results, a possible explanation could be inadequate attention to these variables.

DEVELOPING COMBINATION THERAPY

As additional biologics and BRMs are found to be active *in vitro* and in animal tumor models, the next challenge will be to design effective combinations of biologics or combinations of biologics with chemotherapeutic agents.[107] Knowledge of the pharmacokinetics, mechanism of action, and toxicities of an agent can be used to design combinations for testing *in vitro* and in animal models. With an infinite number of possible combinations of agents, dose, and schedule, a good "litmus test" for any combination is its activity in the preclinical setting. Combination therapy can be designed to increase the antitumor activity of an agent (additive or synergistic) or to decrease clinical toxicity without reducing potency.

APPROACH TO PEDIATRIC CLINICAL TRIALS

Traditionally, clinical testing of a new agent in children has followed the successful use of that agent in adults. This is because of the relatively smaller numbers of pediatric cancer patients, the effectiveness of traditional chemotherapy in the more common pediatric tumors, and the smaller numbers of patients who might be eligible and available for Phase I clinical trials.

Phase I pediatric studies of a new agent frequently begin at 75% of the adult MTD. With agents known to be highly toxic in adults, the starting dose can be lowered to ensure patient safety. In most cases, an agent's MTD for children is not significantly different from the adult dose.

FUTURE CONSIDERATIONS

Biological approaches to cancer therapy are rapidly becoming the hope of the future for cancer treatment. With the availability of mass production techniques, promising new agents can be brought to clinical trials much more rapidly than in the past, permitting clinical testing of large numbers of agents for a wide variety of indications. As more positive results are obtained in trials using biologics or BRMs in adult cancer patients, the challenge for pediatric oncologists will lie in recognizing potentially effective agents and acting to bring those agents into the clinic quickly and safely.

REFERENCES

1. Ehrlich P: On immunity with special reference to cell life. Proc R Soc Lond 66:424–448, 1900
2. Coley WB: The treatment of malignant tumors by repeated inoculations of erysipelas: With a report of ten original cases. Am J Med Sci 105:487–511, 1893
3. Coley WB: Contributions to the knowledge of sarcoma. Ann Surg 14:199–220, 1891
4. Biologic Response Modifiers: Subcommittee Report. Natl Cancer Inst Monogr 63: 1983
5. Emery AEH: Recombinant DNA technology. Lancet 2:1406–1409, 1981
6. Kohler G, Milstein C: Continuous culture of fused cells secreting antibody of predefined specificity. Nature 256:495–496, 1975
7. Mihich E: Future perspectives for biological response modifiers: A viewpoint. Semin Oncol 13:234–254, 1986
8. Borden EC, Ball LA: Interferon: Biochemical, cell growth inhibitory, and immunologic effects. In Brown ER (ed): Progress in Hematology, pp 299–399. New York, Grune & Stratton, 1981
9. Golomb HM: Interferons: Present and future use in cancer therapy. J Clin Oncol 4:123–125, 1986
10. Kirkwood JM, Ernstoff MS: Interferons in the treatment of cancer. J Clin Oncol 2:336–352, 1984
11. Hawkins MJ, Hoth DF, Wittes RE: Clinical development of biological response modifiers: Comparison with cytotoxic drugs. Semin Oncol 13:132–140, 1986
12. Krown SE: Interferons and interferon inducers in cancer treatment. Semin Oncol 13:207–217, 1986
13. Quesada JR, Talpaz M, Rios A et al: Clinical toxicity of interferons in cancer patients. A review. J Clin Oncol 4:234–243, 1986
14. Quesada JR, Reuben JR, Manning JT et al: Alpha interferon for induction of remission in hairy cell leukemia. N Engl J Med 310:15–18, 1984
15. O'Connell MJ, Colgan JP, Oken MM et al: Clinical trial of recombinant leukocyte interferon A as initial therapy of favorable histology non-Hodgkin's lymphomas and chronic lymphocytic leukemia. J Clin Oncol 4:128–136, 1985
16. Quesada JR, Alexanian R, Hawkins M et al: Treatment of multiple myeloma with recombinant alpha-interferon. Blood 67:275–278, 1986
17. Talpaz M, McCredie KB, Mavligit GM et al: Leukocyte-interferon induced cytoreduction in chronic myelogenous leukemia. Blood 62:689–692, 1983
18. Kirkwood JM, Ernstoff MS, Davis CA: Comparison of intramuscular and intravenous recombinant alpha-2-interferon in melanoma and other cancers. Ann Intern Med 103:32–36, 1985
19. Quesada JR, Rios A, Swanson D et al: Antitumor activity of recombinant derived interferon alpha in metastatic renal cell carcinoma. J Clin Oncol 3:1522–1528, 1985
20. Krown SE, Real FX, Cunningham-Rundles S et al: Preliminary observations on the effect of leukocyte A interferon in homosexual men with Kaposi's sarcoma. N Engl J Med 308:1071–1076, 1983
21. Mahaley M, Urso M, Whaley R et al: Immunology of primary intracranial tumors: IV. Phase I study of human lymphoblastoid interferon. J Biol Response Mod 3:19–25, 1984
22. Fauci AF, Rosenberg SA, Sherwin SA et al: Immunomodulators in clinical medicine. Ann Intern Med 106:421–433, 1987
23. Kurzrock R, Talpaz M, Kantarjian H et al: Phase II study of recombinant interferon gamma in chronic myelogenous leukemia. Blood 68(Suppl 1):225a, 1986
24. Talmadge JE, Tribble HR, Pennington RW, et al: Immunomodulatory and immunotherapeutic properties of recombinant gamma interferon and recombinant tumor necrosis factor in mice. Cancer Res 47:2563–2570, 1987
25. Cantell K, Hirvonen S: Preparation of human leukocyte interferon for clinical use. Tex Rep Biol Med 35:138–144, 1977
26. Strander H, Aparisi T, Brostrom L et al: Adjuvant treatment of osteosarcoma with human interferon-alpha. In Zoon KC, Noguchi PO, Liu T-Y (eds): Interferon: Research, Clinical Application and Regulatory Considerations, pp 247–254. New York, Elsevier, 1984
27. Caparros B, Rosen G, Cunningham-Rundles S: Phase II trial of interferon (IFN) in metastatic osteogenic sarcoma. Proc Am Assoc Cancer Res 23:121, 1982
28. Ochs J, Abromowitch M, Rudnick S et al: Phase I-II study of recombinant alpha-2 interferon against advanced leukemia and lymphoma in children. J Clin Oncol 4:883–887, 1986
29. Hill NO, Pardue A, Kahn A et al: High-dose human leukocyte interferon trials in leukemia and cancer. Med Pediatr Oncol 9:132–149, 1981
30. Mirro J, Dow L, Kalwinsky D et al: A phase I-II study of continuous infusion high-dose human lymphoblastoid interferon for nonlymphocytic leukemia. Cancer Treat Rep 70:363–376, 1986
31. Cooper MR, Fefer A, Thompson J et al: Alpha-2 interferon, melphalan, and prednisone in the treatment of newly diagnosed multiple myeloma. Proc Am Soc Clin Oncol 4:216, 1985
32. Hawkins MJ, O'Connell MJ, Schiller JH et al: Phase I evaluation of recombinant A interferon alpha in combination with COPA chemotherapy. Proc Am Soc Clin Oncol 4:229, 1985
33. Hawkins MJ: Evaluation of recombinant alpha interferons in Phase III cooperative group trials. Interferon Letter 2:3, 1985

34. Morgan DA, Ruscetti FW, Gallo R: Selective *in vitro* growth of lymphocytes from normal human bone marrows. Science 193:1007, 1976

35. Rosenberg SA: Adoptive immunotherapy of cancer using lymphokine activated killer cells and recombinant interleukin-2. In DeVita VT Jr, Hellman S, Rosenberg SA (eds): Important Advances in Oncology 1986, pp 55–91. Philadelphia, JB Lippincott, 1986

36. Mule JJ, Shu S, Rosenberg SA: The anti-tumor efficacy of lymphokine activated killer cells and recombinant interleukin-2 in vivo. J Immunol 135:646–652, 1985

37. Rosenberg SA, Lotze MT, Muul LM et al: Observations on the systemic administration of autologous lymphokine-activated killer cells and recombinant interleukin-2 to patients with metastatic cancer. N Engl J Med 313:1485–1492, 1985

38. Fisher RI, Coltman CA, Doroshow JH et al: Phase II clinical trial of Interleukin-2 plus lymphokine activated killer cells in metastatic renal cancer. Proc Am Soc Clin Oncol 6:244, 1987

39. Dutcher J, Creekmore R, Weiss G et al: Phase II study of high dose interleukin-2 and lymphokine activated killer cells in patients with melanoma. Proc Am Soc Clin Oncol 6:246, 1987

40. Rosenberg SA, Lotze MT, Muul LM et al: A progress report on the treatment of 157 patients with advanced cancer using lymphokine-activated killer cells and interleukin-2 or high dose interleukin-2 alone. N Engl J Med 316:889–897, 1987

41. Margolin K, Rayner A, Hawkins M et al: Toxicity of interleukin-2 and lymphokine-activated killer cell therapy. Proc Am Soc Clin Oncol 6:251, 1987

42. Moertel CG: On lymphokines, cytokines and breakthroughs. JAMA 256:3141–3142, 1986

43. DeVita VT, Roper M: The emergence of biologicals as cancer treatment: The good news and the bad. Hosp Pract 22:15–21, 1987

44. West WH, Taver KW, Yannelli JR et al: Constant-infusion recombinant interleukin-2 in adoptive immunotherapy of advanced cancer. N Engl J Med 316:898–905, 1987

45. Sarwal AN, Hersh EM, Murray JL et al: Phase I study of therapy with recombinant DNA produced IL-2 (rIL-2) in cancer patients. Proc Am Assoc Cancer Res 27:321, 1986

46. Kohler PC, Hank J, Hong D et al: Phase I trial of recombinant interleukin-2. Proc Am Soc Clin Oncol 5:221, 1986

47. Chapman PB, Hakes T, Gabrilove JL et al: A phase I pilot study of intraperitoneal rIL-2 in ovarian cancer. Proc Am Soc Clin Oncol 5:231, 1986

48. Whitehead RP, Hemstreet GP, Bradley EC: Phase I-II trial of subcutaneous recombinant human interleukin-2 in disseminated renal cell carcinoma. Proc Am Soc Clin Oncol 5:234, 1986

49. Kolitz JE, Merluzzi VJ, Welte K et al: A Phase I trial of recombinant interleukin-2 and cyclophosphamide in advanced malignancy. Proc Am Soc Clin Oncol 5:235, 1986

50. Krigel R, Poiesz B, Comis R et al: A Phase I study of recombinant interleukin-2 plus recombinant beta-ser-17 interferon. Proc Am Soc Clin Oncol 5:225, 1986

51. Papa M, Vetto J, Shiloni E et al: Synergistic effects of chemotherapy and interleukin-2 in the therapy of mice with advanced pulmonary tumors. J Immunol (in press)

52. Rosenberg SA, Speiss P, Lafreniere R: A new approach to the adoptive immunotherapy of cancer using tumor infiltrating lymphocytes. Science 223:1318–1321, 1986

53. Kempin S, Cirrincione C, Myers J et al: Combined modality therapy of advanced nodular lymphomas: The role of non-specific immunotherapy (MBV) as an important determinant of response and survival. Proc Am Soc Clin Oncol 22:514, 1981

54. Carswell EA, Old LJ, Kassel RL et al: An endotoxin-induced serum factor that causes necrosis of tumors. Proc Natl Acad Sci USA 72:3666–3670, 1975

55. Pennica D, Nedwin GE, Hayflick JS et al: Human tumor necrosis factor: precursor structure, expression and homology to lymphotoxin. Nature 312:724–729, 1984

56. Shirai T, Yamaguchi H, Ito H et al: Cloning and expression of the gene for human tumor necrosis factor. Nature 313:803–806, 1985

57. Wang AM, Creasey AA, Ladner MB et al: Molecular cloning of the complementary DNA for human tumor necrosis factor. Science 228:149–154, 1985

58. Matthews N: Tumor necrosis factor from the rabbit. II. Production by monocytes. Br J Cancer 44:418–424, 1981

59. Matthews N: Production of anti-tumor cytotoxin by human monocytes. Immunology 44:135–142, 1981

60. Oettgen HF, Old LJ: Tumor necrosis factor. In DeVita VT Jr, Hellman S, Rosenberg SA (eds): Important Advances in Oncology 1987, pp 105–130. Philadelphia, JB Lippincott, 1987

61. Darzynkiewicz Z, Williamson B, Carswell EA, Old LJ: Cell-cycle specific effects of tumor necrosis factor. Cancer Res 44:83–90, 1984

62. Suyama K, Goldstein J, Green S: Effects of murine tumor necrosis factor on Friend erythroleukemia cells. Exp Cell Biol 53:85–92, 1985

63. Kull FC, Cuatrecasas P: Possible requirement of internalization in the mechanism of in vitro cytotoxicity in tumor necrosis serum. Cancer Res 41:4885–4890, 1981

64. Bloksma N, Hofhuis FM, Willers JM: Role of mononuclear phagocyte function in endotoxin-induced tumor necrosis. Eur J Cancer Clin Oncol 20:397–403, 1984

65. Green S, Dobrjanski A, Chiasson MA: Action of tumor necrosis factor on mouse myelomonocytic leukemia (WEHI/3) in vitro and in vivo. Proc Am Assoc Cancer Res 22:284, 1981

66. Haranaka K, Satomi N, Sakuri A: Antitumor activity of murine tumor necrosis factor against transplanted murine and heterotransplanted human tumors in nude mice. Int J Cancer 34:263–267, 1984

67. Yarden A, Kimshi A: Tumor necrosis factor reduces c-myc expression and cooperates with interferon-gamma in HeLa cells. Science 234:1419–1423, 1986

68. Hoffman MK, Green S, Old LJ et al: Serum containing endotoxin-induced tumour necrosis factor substitutes for helper T cells. Nature 263:416–417, 1976

69. Hoffman MK, Oettgen HF, Old LJ et al: Induction and immunological properties of tumor necrosis factor. J Reticuloendothel Soc 23:307–319, 1978

70. Hoffman MK, Oettgen HF, Old LJ et al: Endotoxin-induced serum factor controlling differentiation of bone marrow-derived lymphocytes. Proc Natl Acad Sci USA 74:1200–1203, 1977

71. Beutler B, Cerami A: Cachectin: More than a tumor necrosis factor. N Engl J Med 316:379–385, 1987

72. Salmon SE, Young L: Antitumor effect of tumor necrosis factor is markedly enhanced by gamma interferon. Proc Am Soc Clin Oncol 5:222, 1986

73. Regenass U, Muller M, Curschellas E, Matter A: Anti-tumor effects of tumor necrosis factor in combination with chemotherapeutic agents. Int J Cancer 39:266–273, 1987

74. Chapman PB, Lester TJ, Caspar ES et al: Phase I study of recombinant tumor necrosis factor. Proc Am Soc Clin Oncol 5:231, 1986

75. Blick MB, Sherwin SA, Rosenblum MG et al: A phase I trial of recombinant tumor necrosis factor in cancer patients. Proc Am Soc Clin Oncol 5:14, 1986

76. Khan A, Pardue A, Aleman C et al: Phase I clinical trial with recombinant tumor necrosis factor (TNF). Proc Am Soc Clin Oncol: 5:226, 1986

77. Trump DL, Grem JL, Bertie D et al: A clinical trial of recombinant tumor necrosis factor administered three times weekly. Proc Am Assoc Cancer Res (in press)

78. Creagan E, Kovach J, Moertel L et al: A Phase I clinical trial of human recombinant tumor necrosis factor. Proc Am Soc Clin Oncol (in press)

79. Metcalf D: The molecular biology and functions of the granulocyte-macrophage colony stimulating factors. Blood 67:257–267, 1986

80. Gasson JC, Weisbart RH, Kaufman SE et al: Purified human granulocyte-macrophage colony stimulating factor: Direct action on neutrophils. Science 226:1339–1342, 1984

81. Wong GG, Witek J, Temple PA et al: Human GM-CSF: Molecular cloning of the complementary DNA and purification of the natural and recombinant proteins. Science 228:810–815, 1985

82. Begley CG, Metcalf D, Lopez AF, Nicola NA: Fractionated populations of normal human narrow cells respond to both human colony-stimulating factors with granulocyte-macrophage activity. Exp Hematology 13:956–962, 1985

83. Kawasaki ES, Ladner MB, Wang AM: Molecular cloning of a complimentary DNA encoding human macrophage-specific colony stimulating factor (CSF-1). Science 230:291–296, 1985

84. Motoyoshi K, Takaku F, Mizoguchi H et al: Purification and some properties of colony stimulating factor from normal human urine. Blood 52:1012–1016, 1978

85. Welte K, Platzer E, Lu L et al: Purification and biochemical characterization of human pluripotent hematopoietic colony-stimulating factor. Proc Natl Acad Sci USA 82:1526–1530, 1985

86. Nicola NA, Begley CG, Metcalf D: Identification of the human analogue of a regulator that induces differentiation in murine leukemia cells. Nature 314:625–628, 1985

87. Sporn MB, Roberts AB, Wakefield LM et al: Transforming growth factor-beta: Biological function and chemical structure. Science 233:532–534, 1986

88. Cuttitta F, Carney DN, Mulshine J et al: Autocrine growth factors in human small cell lung cancer. Cancer Surveys 4:707–727, 1985

89. Folkman J: Angiogenesis and its inhibitors. In DeVita VT Jr, Hellman S, Rosenberg SA (eds): Important Advances in Oncology 1985, pp 42–62. Philadelphia, JB Lippincott, 1985

90. Dillman RO, Beauregard JC, Halpern SE, Clutter M: Toxicities and side effects of murine monoclonal antibodies. J Biol Response Mod 5:73–84, 1986

91. Oldham RK: Monoclonal antibodies in cancer therapy. J Clin Oncol 1:582–590, 1983

92. Houghton AN, Scheinberg DA: Monoclonal antibodies: Potential applications to the treatment of cancer. Semin Oncol 13:165–179, 1986

93. Ritz J, Schlossman SF: Utilization of monoclonal antibodies in treatment of leukemia and lymphoma. Blood 59:1–11, 1982

94. Ritz J, Sallan SE, Bast RC et al: Autologous bone marrow transplantation in CALLA-positive acute lymphoblastic leukemia after in vitro treatment with J-5 monoclonal antibody and complement. Lancet 2:60–63, 1982

95. Cheung N-K, Berger N, Coccia P et al: Murine monoclonal antibody specific for GD2 ganglioside: A phase I trial in patients with neuroblastoma, melanoma and osteogenic sarcoma. Proc Am Assoc Cancer Res 27:318, 1986

96. Levy R, Miller RA, Stratte PT et al: Therapeutic trials of monoclonal antibody in leukemia and lymphoma: Biologic considerations. In Boss BD, Langman R, Trowbridge I et al (eds): Monoclonal Antibodies and Cancer, pp 5–16. Orlando, FL, Academic Press, 1983

97. Dillman RO, Shawler DL, Dillman JB et al: Therapy of chronic lymphocytic leukemia and cutaneous T-cell lymphoma. J Cell Biochem 9A:108, 1985

98. Dillman RO, Shawler DL, Dillman JB et al: Therapy of chronic lymphocytic leukemia and cutaneous T cell lymphoma with T101 monoclonal antibody. J Clin Oncol 2:881–891, 1984

99. Foon KA, Schroff RW, Bunn PA et al: Effects of monoclonal antibody therapy in patients with chronic lymphocytic leukemia. Blood 64:1085–1093, 1984

100. Foon KA, Schroff RW, Mayer D et al: Monoclonal antibody therapy of chronic lymphocytic leukemia and cutaneous T-cell lymphoma: Preliminary observations. In Boss BD, Langman R, Trowbridge I (eds): Monoclonal Antibodies and Cancer, pp 39–52. Orlando, FL, Academic Press, 1983

101. Meeker TC, Lowder J, Maloney DG et al: A clinical trial of anti-idiotype therapy for B cell malignancy. Blood 65:1349–1363, 1985

102. Goodman GE, Beaumier P, Hellstrom I et al: Pilot trial of murine monoclonal antibodies in patients with advanced melanoma. J Clin Oncol 3:340–352, 1985

103. Oldham RK, Foon KA, Morgan C et al: Monoclonal antibody therapy of malignant melanoma: In vivo localization in cutaneous metastases after intravenous administration. J Clin Oncol 2:1235–1244, 1984

104. Houghton AN, Mintzer D, Cordon-Cardo C et al: Mouse monoclonal antibody detecting GD3 ganglioside: A phase I trial in patients with malignant melanoma. Proc Natl Acad Sci USA 82:1242–1246, 1985

105. Fidler IJ, Berendt M, Oldman RK: Rationale for and design of a screening procedure for the assessment of biological response modifiers for cancer treatment. J Biol Response Mod 1:15–26, 1982

106. Talmadge JE, Herberman RB: The preclinical screening laboratory: Evaluation of immunomodulatory and therapeutic properties of biological response modifiers. Cancer Treat Rep 70:171–182, 1985

107. Borden EC, Hawkins MJ: Biologic response modifiers as adjuncts to other therapeutic modalities. Semin Oncol 13:144–152, 1986

fifteen

Ethical Considerations in Pediatric Oncology

John C. Fletcher,
Jan van Eys, and
Lorah D. Dorn

Ethics involves the study and recommendation of bodies of guidance—rules, norms, and principles—that help to resolve difficult problems of moral choice.

At a basic level, an ethical problem involves a conflict of widely accepted moral duties or obligations. What are the basic criteria of ethical reasoning? We must first assume that decision makers have available the best of medical and social facts and have identified the ethical problems in a given case. They must then make choices about the best approach to the problem. The facts are not the source of ethics. Human beings choose among various forms of practical guidance to resolve ethical problems. Many physicians claim to approach ethics on a case-by-case basis, as if ethical guidance had to be created anew for each problem. This claim likely rests on unexamined ideas; systematic studies of what physicians actually do when faced with ethical problems of clinical research[1] and surgery[2] indicate that they rely on complex sets of ethical beliefs and practices.

In our view, the selection of ethical guidance involves two interdependent claims. First, ethical guidance should be judged by the consequences of following it. Second, the consequences should be examined in terms of ethical principles widely accepted across cultural, philosophical, and religious lines. People who differ in their moral beliefs can still cooperate to resolve ethical problems. Cooperation requires choices about which principles are crucial, what weight should be assigned to those principles, and how they should be applied to the problem at hand. Also, coercion must be avoided in practical ethics.[3] Otherwise, ethical differences too easily degenerate into power struggles or cynicism.

Wherever possible, selection of ethical guidance should be supported by well-documented studies of the benefits or detriments of following such guidance. Some approaches to ethical problems in pediatric oncology have been well studied (*e.g.*, the consequences of disclosing the diagnosis of cancer to children). Others, such as the degree of understanding of children and their parents regarding participation in Phase I/II trials, have been neglected.

Against this brief background about our approach to ethics we note three special concerns. First, pediatric oncologists treat both children and adolescents. Age-related differences can pose problems related to the dependence of young children on adults as contrasted with the adolescent's struggle for independence. The greater maturity and different needs of adolescents with cancer have increasingly led oncologists to differentiate their care from that of young children.[4,5]

Second, every member of the care team has an *obligation* to raise ethical questions. In a pediatric oncology unit, ethics is everyone's business. Cooperation and open communication are vital to resolving an ethical problem before it becomes detrimental to the care of the child and to the parents. Third, hospitals should provide specialized consultation for health professionals and families who face complex ethical problems. Many hospitals in the United States and Canada now make available consultation provided by an identified ethics consultant, a team, or by a hospital ethics committee.[6]

SPECIFIC AREAS OF ETHICAL PROBLEMS

Ethical problems arise in several phases and aspects of care of children and adolescents with cancer, including [1] the initial meeting with patient and family, [2] parental permission and children's assent for treatment, [3] confidentiality, [4] refusal of therapy, [5] participation in Phase I/II trials, and [6] terminal care. Each of these potential problem areas is discussed and an approach understood to be "dominant" (*i.e.*, generally accepted by practitioners in pediatric oncology) is recommended. Ethical objections, if any, to the preferred approach are delineated and discussed.

The primary source of ethical guidance for the practice of pediatric oncology is a set of five ethical principles, discussed at length elsewhere[7,8] and listed in Table 15-1. These principles provide general criteria to guide the decision making of all involved in the struggle against childhood cancer. Below, we describe the dominant approach to six ethical problem areas in pediatric oncology. The practical guidance embodied in an "approach" is a bridge between general ethical principles and particular judgments. An approach contains various rules and norms that, when followed, have proven beneficial. Dominant approaches must be critically examined in the light of ethical principles and reformulated when they are no longer beneficial. Different societies will rank the ethical principles differently in such evaluations because of the influence of socioeconomic realities and cultural traditions.

INITIAL DISCUSSION WITH PATIENT AND FAMILY

What are the ethical issues surrounding the oncologist's initial discussion with the patient and family? When parents are informed that their child has cancer, many preconceptions and fears are aroused. The initial dialogue is often one of the most crucial points in the overall treatment course. The perceptions that parents and patient retain from that first encounter will determine many of the subsequent choices they make.

Ethical issues arise in choices about who should be present, what should be communicated, and what should be done about the information presented. The degree of trust and cooperation among the care team is also ethically relevant. Studies show that attention to the emotional needs of the care team strengthens them to respond more appropriately to the anxiety in families and patients.[9,10] Although the question

needs study, attention to emotional needs probably encourages the raising of ethical questions and increases cooperation in resolving ethical problems.

Before effective therapies were developed for many types of cancer, disclosure of a cancer diagnosis to patients, especially to children, was seen as harmful by most physicians.[11] Therapeutic advances and cultural change favoring less paternalism among health care professionals have led to a virtual reversal in favor of full disclosure.[12] In a study of 116 long-term survivors of childhood cancer and their parents that spanned these two periods, Slavins and others examined the mental health consequences of nondisclosure and early disclosure of the diagnosis of cancer to children.[13] The patients' age at diagnosis ranged from birth to 18 years (mean = 5.7 years) and age at follow-up evaluation ranged from 5.8 to 36 years (mean = 18.04 years). Would survivors who learned of their diagnosis early on be "better adjusted" than those who had not been told, or had learned about their cancer long after diagnosis? A psychiatrist and psychologist independently interviewed the survivors and gave several standardized tests. The incidence of symptoms of emotional problems was significantly higher in those who were informed late or were self-informed, compared with those whose parents risked being open with them despite the physician's advice not to disclose.

Inclusion of the Child: The Dominant Approach

Gradually, the goal in most centers became inclusion of the child at the major decision points in the treatment process, beginning with the initial meeting.[14-16] The pace of this inclusion will be affected by [1] the developmental stage of the child, [2] the oncologist and care team, and [3] the parents and their capacity to manage the forces working upon them.[17] The benefits of initial honesty between physicians, parents, and children have been documented in several personal interview and questionnaire studies since 1965.[18-20] Adolescent patients may already know their diagnosis before the initial meeting. In 1984, Pfefferbaum and others found that 39% of 63 adolescent cancer patients had been told their diagnosis by their hometown physician and that 33% of them suspected the diagnosis before it was given.[21] Thus, it is important for physicians to clarify in the initial meeting what the adolescent patient already knows or suspects.

Table 15-1
Ethical Principles for the Practice of Pediatric Oncology

Respect for persons: the duty to respect the self-determination and choices of autonomous persons, as well as to protect persons with diminished autonomy (*e.g.*, young children, mentally retarded persons, and those with other mental impairments).

Beneficence: the obligation to secure the well-being of persons by acting positively on their behalf and, moreover, to maximize the benefits that can be attained.

Nonmaleficence: the obligation to minimize harm to persons and, wherever possible, to remove the causes of harm altogether.

Proportionality: the duty, when taking actions involving risks of harm, to so balance risks and benefits that actions have the greatest chance to result in the least harm and the most benefit to persons directly involved.

Justice: the obligation to distribute benefits and burdens fairly, to treat equals equally, and to give reasons for differential treatment based on widely accepted criteria for just ways to distribute benefits and burdens.

(Material adapted from the National Commission for the Protection of Human Subjects of Biomedical and Behavioral Research: The Belmont Report,[7] and Beauchamp TL, Childress JF: Principles of Biomedical Ethics, 3rd ed[8])

Ethical Objections

The contemporary literature in pediatric oncology and biomedical ethics has no defenses of nondisclosure. O'Connor[22] and Kearney[23] warn against "blunt honesty," and Kearney recommends an indirect, gradual approach in which "the pace of revelation can be determined by the patient." O'Connor suggests that the discussion of leukemia begin "about anemia, low platelets, abnormal cells. The child or . . . adult will usually let the physician . . . know how much more they want to hear by how much they probe. If they continue to probe, gradually more explicit answers can be given. If the direct question is asked, 'Do I have leukemia?,' the answer can be, 'Yes, you do have leukemia.' " Kearney warns that an overly direct approach can "profoundly and irreversibly upset young adolescents if the challenge to their equilibrium is beyond their limited emotional reserves." Neither author cites studies or clinical examples to support these warnings. Both favor looking for "cues" from patients, presumably to avoid the possible harms of forcing painful information on those who do not want to know it. This objection can be grounded in the principle of nonmaleficence, which is the source of the physician's duty to prevent or take every precaution to minimize harm.

Response to Objections

Ethical arguments against nondisclosure or partial disclosure are based in beneficence, respect for persons, and justice. First, the well-being and security of the child is served by a disclosure of cancer from caring and supportive parents and physicians working together. This approach avoids the likelihood (more common in a previous era) that a child will be told of the diagnosis by someone other than his or her parents and physicians. Avoiding the isolation, confusion, fear, and stigmatization that can be caused by such experiences is a strong reason to include children in disclosure. Second, although young children and early adolescents are not autonomous, they benefit from respect for their capacity to express their desires, for their feelings, and for their potential for self-determination. Third, optimal disclosure of the diagnosis requires

---

Table 15-2
Additional Ethical Considerations in the Initial Meeting

1. Physician must be knowledgeable.
   a. Accurate information should proceed from what is known to what is unknown.
   b. Misinformation should be corrected without judgments of other physicians.
2. The following information is to be communicated.
   a. Provide diagnosis.
   b. Explain disease.
   c. Discuss prognosis.
   d. Outline additional tests.
   e. Explain immediate therapeutic plans.
   f. Discuss availability of physician day and night.
3. Binding decisions must not be exacted precipitously.
4. Ample opportunity to consider choices and ask questions must be given.
5. The patient's and family's native language must be used.
   a. If the physician is not fluent, an interpreter should be present for accurate and exact statements.
6. Refusal of therapy should be dealt with as discussed in text.

(Material drawn from van Eys[28,32] and Greenberg and associates.[24])

---

scientific and medical expertise, and exclusion of the child from this benefit is unfair.

The O'Connor–Kearney position appears to be directed against a rigid policy of full disclosure of the diagnosis in every situation, rather than against disclosure itself. We know of no study addressing the question of whether children are harmed by disclosure of a cancer diagnosis in the context of family and care team support. In studies cited above,[18-20] parents and children expressed relief to researchers that they knew what the problem was and what to expect. However, these studies were not primarily searching for harmful effects of disclosure.

The physician's responsibility to explain the diagnosis to parents and child, if the child can understand it, is nontransferable. Concerns about the "fragility" of a patient (*e.g.,* depression or suicidality) should be assessed professionally before disclosure of the diagnosis, so that agreement can be reached about the potential for harm. In the absence of psychiatric contraindications to full disclosure, the moral danger of the O'Connor–Kearney approach is unjustified paternalism. Protection of the vulnerable patient is justified when a clear danger of harm creates an exception to the duty of disclosure until the problem of harm can be addressed. With this exception, a clear, timely statement of the diagnosis of cancer is owed to the patient.

Response to Parental Refusal

A diagnosis of cancer is painful to anticipate, especially for parents. What is the physician's responsibility if parents do not want the child or adolescent to know the diagnosis? If a child's developmental stage permits inclusion, the physician can arrange a preliminary meeting to help the parents deal with their objections and fears about including the child. If needed, a mental health professional can also be present. A preliminary meeting preserves the goal of inclusion and respects the parents' need to guard against anxiety. Disagreements about the rules of communication, in which the parents insist on shielding the child from knowledge, should be worked out without the child's presence. Such disagreements can usually be resolved by the physician's willingness to tell the child about a cancer diagnosis. Family members with a key role in child's care should be invited to the meetings, including siblings who are old enough to help.

The overriding responsibility of the pediatric oncologist is to the patient. The child's well-being can be increased with treatment and care, and the child must not be shielded from knowledge of the difficulties and side-effects of treatment. The goal of the initial meeting should be to convey to the child, with kindness and support, what is known and unknown about the diagnosis and treatment. Table 15-2 summarizes additional considerations for the initial meeting. As many meetings as needed to attain these goals should be held.

PARENTAL PERMISSION AND CHILDREN'S ASSENT

The major ethical issues of informed consent with adult subjects capable of choice are information, comprehension, and voluntariness.[7,8] The immaturity of children and the role of permission by parental proxies call for a reversed order of these issues:

1. How "voluntary" should choices about research participation for children be? Should children be given the right to veto research? How can coercion and undue pressure on children and their parents be avoided?

2. Can children with cancer participate in an assent process and understand information about research? If not, an objection to assent can be made on empiric grounds.
3. In choices about what information to give to children, which "elements of assent" should have ethical priority?

Voluntariness in Assent and Parental Permission

Physicians may not ethically or legally treat children without the permission of parents, except in emergencies. The term "permission" distinguishes between what a person may do autonomously (consent) and what one may do for another (give permission). Use of the term "assent" was suggested in the mid-1970s by a national commission to distinguish a child's agreement to treatment from a legally valid consent.[25] The commission recommended that assent to research be required when children are 7 years of age or older and that "a child's objection to participation in research should be binding unless the intervention holds out a prospect of direct benefit that is important to the health or well-being of the child and is available only in the context of the research." This position was modified in federal regulations issued in 1983 to protect children in research (see also Chap. 53).[26] The regulations require that an Institutional Review Board (IRB) "determine that adequate provisions are made for soliciting the assent of the children, when in the judgment of the IRB the children are capable of providing assent" (45 CFR 46. 408). The regulations also authorize IRBs to waive assent for the reason of direct benefit, defined by the commission, and for incapacity due to age, immaturity, or psychological state. Assent is defined as a "child's affirmative agreement to participate in research; mere failure to object should not, absent affirmative agreement, be construed as assent" (45 CFR 46. 402[b]). Although the regulations give IRBs functional authority over the practice of assent, they presume that, with some exceptions, a child should be given the voluntary choice to assent or object to research participation.

No study has been done since the federal regulations appeared of how completely pediatric oncologists agree with the premise of voluntary choice. In 1982, before the regulations were issued, Kapp surveyed IRB chairmen in 70 children's hospitals and 123 medical schools about assent practices.[27] Usable responses were obtained from 70 institutions (34%). The study found that 41 of the IRBs (59%) approached each study on an *ad hoc* basis, deferring to the judgment of the investigator about whether assent should be sought. Of the 29 institutions (41%) that had written specific guidelines about age and assent, 11 (16%) agreed with the commission's recommendation that assent should be required from children aged 7 or older; ages of assent ranged from 2 to 16 years in the other 18 institutions. Kapp concluded that the study showed "a strong bias toward expecting the investigator to obtain the child's assent when deemed feasible." The patterns and frequency of IRB waiver of assent since 1983 have not been studied.

A new study needs to be done of oncologists' practices in seeking assent from children aged 4 to 18 to participate in research. The question to be investigated would be whether the dominant approach among oncologists and care teams is that assent must always be obtained from children.[28] This approach is based on respect for persons and justice. If children's feelings are similar to those of adults, they should be treated in similar ways to adults being asked to consent to research. It follows that researchers should not do invasive and often painful procedures for the benefit of others as well as the child without seeking the child's prior assent.

Ethical Objections to Voluntarism

Not all pediatric oncologists agree that the voluntaristic principle is beneficial in assent to research. The IRB of the National Cancer Institute waives the assent requirement on each pediatric cancer project with therapeutic intent. All therapies in the Clinical Center of the National Institutes of Health are available only in the context of research. A strenuous effort is made to inform parents and children about the nature of each project. Children under 14 are not routinely asked to assent to therapeutic cancer research but are thoroughly informed along with their parents. A position of "inform but no assent" is drawn from principles of beneficence, nonmaleficence, and truthfulness. The position makes two claims. First, the child's and parents' well-being is served and harm to the child prevented by avoiding the risk that a child's refusal to participate in therapeutic research will be painfully overridden by parents and physicians. Second, it is untruthful and inauthentic to invite a child make a voluntary choice if one does not intend to respect a refusal.

Response to Objections

This position is vulnerable to criticism based on the principle of respect for persons, which encourages respect for the feelings and potential for self-determination of children. Also, objection can be made that refusal of research is not identical with refusal of an established therapy for cancer that is available elsewhere, if such exists.

A further objection to the voluntaristic premise in the context of nontherapeutic research was made by Ackerman.[29] He argued that a strict interpretation of voluntarism was an evasion of adults' duty to guide children to make the best choice. This may be an especially important consideration when the child is ill and preoccupied with many physical and emotional problems. Ackerman stressed a duty to enhance the personal development of a child, based in the beneficence principle. Adults, in his view, are required to guide children who object to research participation in a manner that is consistent with the goal of a child's becoming the "right kind of person" as an adult. However, Ackerman makes an exception for an "intractable" objection based on anxiety or fear that cannot be allayed.

Avoiding Coercion in Assent and Permission

Ackerman's arguments could be misused to influence unduly or coerce a child capable of assent to submit to nontherapeutic research. Federal guidelines do not permit waiver of assent for nontherapeutic research, except for reasons of age, immaturity, or psychological condition. In addition to inappropriate parental pressure, two other sources of coerciveness need to be noted.

First, researchers exert undue influence if they present research to parents and children with the assumption that experimental therapy is the best therapy. This position is not true *a priori*. Research addresses cancer as a problem. The outcomes of therapies are judged statistically, and the individual patient is seen as a case with the appropriate eligibility criteria. In contrast, therapy addresses a unique patient with a disease and individualizes management for that patient. That there is a common ground does not change the fundamental premise. The research aspect of the proffered intervention must not be downplayed by emphasizing the therapeutic benefits that are foreseen.

Second, coerciveness can be implied when permission and assent are requested too soon after disclosure of diagnosis. It is advised that, when possible, time to recover from the emotional shock of hearing a cancer diagnosis should precede such a request.[30,31] In the psychic shock that follows the diagnosis, "the problem may be seen as only a choice between refusal and consent, rather than between consent and some possible alternative." (ref. 30, p. 424).

In addition to emotional incapacity to give permission voluntarily, one or both may also be impaired by mental retardation, illness, or other handicaps. Assessment of a parent's capacity to give permission involves the same procedures used to determine the capacity of the adult patient who is impaired. Physicians are well-advised to seek psychiatric consultation when in doubt about parenteral capacity, especially when only one parent is available or is the single, legally authorized decision-maker but is impaired.

Capacity to Assent and Parents' Comprehension of Research

Success in the treatment of some childhood cancers has been gained through systematic investigation of empirically derived strategies. Such treatment strategies are complex. Because a referral to a pediatric cancer center is also a referral to participation in research, the consent process is ethically more complex than for conventional therapies.[32]

Do children have a capacity for assent to such complex choices? What is known about the process of parental permission for pediatric research?

Need for Empiric Studies

Although the dominant approach is to seek assent, there have been few empiric studies of children's capacity to assent to clinical research or whether assent benefits them in any way. No research other than a study in progress has examined pediatric cancer patients' understanding of participation, once they have assented.[33] In contrast, much understanding has been gained by studies, reviewed by Meisel and Roth,[34] of problems in adult consent. Such studies are relevant to issues of parental permission for research.

Many studies found adults, including cancer patients, to be ill-informed about research participation.[35–39] However, other studies showed that the consent process was improved in terms of the subject's recall and other outcome measures when brief, simply worded consent documents were used,[40] when the consent document was sent to the home before the procedure,[41] and when a family member was involved with the patient in the consent process.[42] These studies also support the concept that consent or permission is an ongoing process rather than a single event.

Four exploratory studies have described children's or parents' comprehension of research. McCollum and Schwartz[43] interviewed parents (140 mothers, 33 fathers) of 140 children admitted to a pediatric research center for a variety of disorders, including childhood cancers. Parents were asked what they understood as the purpose of admission: 61 parents said that admission was for diagnosis and therapy, 60 added "research" to these two purposes, 9 said that research was primary, 6 cited "pure" research, and 4 responses were unclassified. The investigators did not explain why 44% of parents did not refer at all to "research." One answer could be that physicians had not explained the difference between therapeutic research and proven therapy. Alternately, the explanations may have been too complex, or the parents' concern and worry about their child's illness may have interfered with their comprehension.

Schwartz[44] studied 50 hospitalizations of 36 children (ages 2–18 years) in a pediatric research center to learn whether children understood the research purpose of their admission. Of the 36 children, 26 were admitted for studies of short stature. None of the 17 children younger than 11 years of age knew about research, and only 6 of the 19 children older than 11 displayed such knowledge. Of these 6, 5 showed symptoms of "overwhelming anxiety." Four of the 6 saw the hospital as combining research and therapy. The 2 subjects who viewed their hospitalization as involving "pure research" signed out of the hospital and refused to continue. The study does not say what the subjects were told about research, if anything. The main contribution of this study, like that of McCollum and Schwartz, is to describe the state of understanding of the young research subject and parents in the 1960s and early 1970s.

A third study[45] reported on a series of classroom consent discussions with a total of 213 school children (ages 6–9) invited to participate in an experimental trial of swine influenza vaccine. The children's questions, scientists' answers, and subsequent discussion were taped. The study concluded that young children can be meaningfully involved in the consent process but did not explore what the children who eventually participated actually knew about the risks and benefits of the trial.

Weithorn and Campbell[46] used hypothetic situations to compare capacity to consent in 96 healthy, normal volunteers, divided evenly among four age groups of 24 subjects each (9-, 14-, 18-, and 21-year-olds). Capacity to consent was assessed in terms of four recognized legal standards: evidence of choice, ability to make a "reasonable" choice that envisions outcomes, ability to use "rational" reasons, ability to understand risks and benefits of alternatives. Four scenarios were put to these subjects. Two concerned medical problems (diabetes and epilepsy); and two psychiatric problems (depression and enuresis). The 14-year-olds did not differ significantly from 21-year olds in capacity. The 9-year-olds were less capable than 18- and 21-year olds of understanding information but equally capable of expressing reasonable treatment preferences. These conclusions cannot be generalized to cancer patients. However, IRBs and oncologists might use Weithorn's methodology to assess the capacity of children with cancer to assent to research.[47]

Results of a study of 20 pediatric cancer patients (ages 7–20) have been analyzed to examine relations of stages of cognitive development, control over illness, and anxiety upon reasoning about illness, when compared with 24 patients treated for obesity (ages 7–17.3 years) and 23 healthy children and adolescents (ages 7–19).[48] No statistically significant differences in any of these factors was found between these groups. This finding supports researchers who assume that children and adolescents with cancer have the capacity to assent. It is noteworthy that the mean level of anxiety was not high in any of these groups, nor was anxiety directly related to an understanding of illness. Thus, the capacity to understand appears not to be impaired by anxiety.

Developmental issues are clearly central to the assent process.[49] Young children lack abstract reasoning, which is necessary to comprehend some aspects of research participation. However, children can clearly participate in the assent process. The *way* they are informed should be different from the way adults are informed.

Elements of Assent and Consent

Physician investigators are responsible for the informed consent process in pediatric oncology. In choices about which information to emphasize and how much information to give, what elements should receive ethical priority? How much information is adequate from an ethical standpoint?

Federal regulations codify information to be given to prospective research subjects. Mandated are eight "elements of informed consent," subdivided into 19 separate items, plus six additional elements to be given "when appropriate" (45 CFR 46.16). Table 15-3 shows the required elements of informed consent and suggested elements of assent.

The dominant approach to giving information to parents is essentially the same as that for adult research subjects: [1] to prepare a written document that adequately covers the required elements of consent, which is evaluated for its ease of comprehension by an IRB, [2] to give an oral explanation of the most important elements, with ample opportunity for ques-

---

Table 15-3
Elements of Informed Consent and Assent

Elements of Informed Consent
1. State and describe
   a. Research of nature of study
   b. Purpose of study
   c. Duration of participation
   d. Procedures to be followed
   e. Which procedures are experimental
2. Describe
   f. Reasonably foreseeable risks
   g. Discomforts
3. Describe
   h. Benefits to the subject
   i. Benefits to others
4. Disclose
   j. Alternative procedures or treatments
5. Describe
   k. Confidentiality of records identifying the subject
6. Explain if the project involves more than minimal risk
   l. Policy on compensation for injuries due to research
   m. Availability of medical treatment for such injuries
   n. Source of further information
7. Explain
   o. Whom to contact for questions about the research, or
   p. In event of research injury
8. State
   q. Participation is voluntary
   r. No loss of benefits on withdrawal
   s. May withdraw at any time

Elements of Assent
1. Purpose of study
2. Duration
3. Procedures
4. Role of child
5. Knowledge of research participation
6. Risks/side-effects
7. Benefits to self
8. Benefits to others
9. Alternative treatments
10. Confidentiality
11. Freedom to ask questions
12. Voluntary participation
13. Freedom to withdraw

(Material drawn from 45 Code of Federal Regulations 46. 116; Susman and colleagues.[33])

---

tions, and [3] to evaluate the parents' comprehension of information. Some centers use "assent forms" to explain research to children and ask for assent. Presumably, the steps in giving information to children are similar to those taken with adults, although practices regarding assent forms probably vary widely.

Ethical Objections to Informed Consent and Assent

Ingelfinger objected to rising legal and federal pressures for informed consent and assent to research with adults and children,[50] citing a trend toward trivialization of the consent process. Specifically, he objected to the excessive amounts of information to be conveyed, which obscured the most ethically relevant aspects of informed consent. Also, he doubted that most patients were able to comprehend the information, and suggested that this created a climate of unreality and legalism around consent.

Although Ingelfinger did not base his objections on the ethical principle of proportionality, he could easily have done so. If the time and effort of preparing consent documents and conducting the consent process is wasted, the research enterprise is harmed. If patients are given consent documents without help in evaluating the elements that are most and least important in terms of ethical priorities, they lose significant benefits. Planning for the consent process requires that actions be taken to achieve the greatest benefits of understanding with the least amount of harm (*e.g.,* wasted effort, misunderstandings, and focusing on the least important matters).

Ingelfinger did not object to the duty to inform but to the imposition of a disproportionate amount of information on that duty. No fundamental objections to the obligation to inform prospective research subjects, whether adults or children, appear in the medical ethics literature. The major issue is how best to select and give information.

Response to Objections

Careful study would probably show Ingelfinger's critique to be valid. The dominant approach to informed consent may be counterproductive because of excessive technical detail given in a vacuum of ethical priorities about how the subject, whether adult or child, should weigh choices about participation. More research is needed to understand the dominant approach to information giving and to determine whether it requires reform. Levine[51] extensively reviews the contemporary approach to consent in research and describes some studies of the comprehensibility of consent documents.

Today, investigators are free to decide what information is given to the child and how it is given. Moral choice is involved in selecting and emphasizing information. At a minimum, care teams should examine the suggested elements of assent in Table 15-3, rank them in terms of ethical importance, and adjust their information giving accordingly. It is likely that most care teams would assign the highest ranks to the elements of benefit and risk. Federal regulations should eventually be improved by adding "basic elements of assent" to guide researchers who have this responsibility.

CONFIDENTIALITY

The issues of confidentiality in pediatric cancer care are no different ethically from those of any other medical encounter, despite the difficulties involved.[52] The child's status as a minor or developmentally immature person is not an ethically acceptable reason to disregard the duty of confidentiality owed to any patient. Two issues arise frequently: [1] protection of sensitive information volunteered by patients during routine history taking so that it does not become available to third parties with no medically justified reason to know; and [2] conflicts between patient, family, and social interests that raise the question of whether confidentiality can be breached to benefit or protect others.

Protection of Privacy: The Dominant Approach

Protection of the patient's privacy and of sensitive information is more difficult in large teaching hospitals, where cancer protocols are subject to oversight by many people. Information about the child's and parents' social and sexual history, child abuse, and drug and alcohol abuse emerges in interviews with child and family. How can a distinction be made and preserved between information necessary for proper care and treatment and information that is private and confidential? No studies comparing approaches to improve confidentiality have been published in pediatric oncology. The literature on medical confidentiality is general, abounds with problems, and lacks practical, well-studied recommendations.

Despite many difficulties, the dominant approach is to place the responsibility with the primary attending physician. This responsibility begins with the patient's chart.

The chart is the mode of communication among the members of the care team. Teams are very large, and the concept of team-wide confidentiality is untenable. Even an occasional lapse by each member of the team threatens a total breakdown in confidentiality. The number of persons who might read a given chart in a tertiary teaching center can exceed 100.[53] In addition, the chart is seen by third-party payers, utilization review agencies, research oversight teams, and quality assurance teams. The greatest source of protection, therefore, is the physician's limitation of information in the chart to that necessary for proper care and communication among professionals.

In a tertiary treatment center, teaching activities can also threaten confidentiality, because much privileged information is often conveyed. Every professional and paraprofessional group has trainees who are assigned to patients. Maintaining patient anonymity in such conditions is impossible. Rigorous attention to confidentiality and correction of errors is required.

Research records can also represent uncontrolled documentation of sensitive information on patients. The records may be reviewed, discussed, filed, and disseminated widely. Patients' names are usually withheld, but current quality assurance review by teams from government and cooperative groups insists on matching chart and flowsheet to assess accuracy and veracity. The total amount of information so disseminated is enormous. If the physician exercises no restraint on the information included, confidentiality can break down completely.

Issues with the Adolescent

Troubling conflicts arise between the responsibility to adolescent patient confidentiality, parental interests, and protection of the welfare of others. Information given by adolescents to physicians about sexual relationships, abortions, or drug use may be unknown to parents. The potential clash between knowledge about the sexual relationships of unemancipated minors and the interests of parents can constitute serious problems.

A hypothetic example of such a conflict would be an adolescent cancer patient who lives at home and tests positive for human immunodeficiency virus (HIV) antibody. The patient reveals to physicians the identity of his sexual partner. The patient's parents are unaware of the sexual relationship, and the patient refuses to inform the sexual partner or parents of the test results. Should physicians breach confidentiality to protect the welfare of the possibly infected lover? Must the parents also be informed?

In similar cases,[54] disclosure to the sexual partner has been recommended, over the patient's objections if necessary. This is assumed to be the dominant and ethically desirable practice, although it is probably not being followed in many centers. There are three ethical reasons to support disclosure over the objections of the adolescent: a duty to warn potential victims of a serious risk to them, based on the principle of nonmaleficence; benefits to the third party from knowledge and care by physicians, grounded in beneficence; and protection of the public health, a duty that combines features from both principles. A California court that weighed the duty to warn third parties against the duty of confidentiality held that once the therapist determines that a patient poses a serious danger to others, he bears a duty to exercise reasonable care to protect the foreseeable victim of that danger."[55,56]

Does the physician have a duty to inform the parents of HIV infection if the patient refuses? In the hypothetic case, the patient resides with parents. This creates a higher legal duty to inform parents. Ethically, the desirable approach, especially if the physician practiced full disclosure of diagnosis and clinical information, is to inform them and to help the family and patient deal with this additional burden.

Physicians can avoid some confidentiality dilemmas with adolescents (and other patients) by not making an absolute commitment from the outset. When a patient asks, "Can you keep a secret?" the answer is "It depends on the circumstances; physicians cannot make absolute promises to keep every secret, but we do everything possible to protect your welfare." Once the physician learns the facts, the answer must be honest—"yes" if secrecy is ethically justifiable and "no" if it is objectionable under the circumstances. If information must be conveyed to the parents, the physician should tell the adolescent *before* that disclosure.

REFUSAL OF TREATMENT

The recommended approach to parental refusal of proven therapy is less ethically complex than refusals of or withdrawal from treatment by adolescents. As discussed by Macklin, the *prima facie* right of parents to decide for their minor children can be taken away in some circumstances, especially if exercise of that right will result in harm or death to the child.[57] The ethical and legal grounds for overriding parents' preferences have been well developed by authoritative national ethics commissions,[58] in the medical ethics literature,[59–61] and in legal commentary[62,63] and court cases, especially two decisions in the Chad Green case (see also Chap. 53).[64–66]

Parental Refusal of Treatment for a Child

The main ethical issue in parental refusal of therapy is depriving the child of life-sustaining benefits. Thus, the success rate of the refused therapy becomes crucial. If physicians can offer a reasonable case for treatment, the claims for parental autonomy must not override the duties created by beneficence and nonmaleficence to protect the best interests of the child. If the therapy has little hope of even palliation, refusal would generally be considered appropriate. However, if the proffered therapy can promise almost certain cure (*e.g.,* in Stage I Wilms' tumor), outside arbitration should be sought, whether from an ethics committee, the local child-protective agency, or a court of law. In our view, only the refusal of an accepted cancer therapy demands further review. Parental or patient refusal of participation in research should be respected, and the issue should be changed quickly to offering an accepted therapy, if one is available. Parents inclined to refuse treatment are generally unlikely to give permission for research.

Refusal of Treatment by Adolescents

Refusal of cancer therapy by adolescents is a more complex ethical problem, especially when parents disagree with the refusal. The closer the patient is to adulthood, the greater should be the respect shown for personhood and autonomous choice. Legal definitions of an emancipated minor reflect this principle and generate rules to define independent decision making as a legal right. The legal markers of emancipation are [1] separate residence from parents, with or without their consent; [2] economic self-support, without regard to source of income; and [3] self-management of financial affairs.[67] Adolescents with cancer rarely fall in this category. More pertinent is whether they are "mature minors," a category that bases their authority to consent or refuse in developmental maturity and knowledge. Psychological and cognitive capacity to dissent from treatment was examined by Leiken,[68] who recommended the following approach: if the adolescent has a sound knowledge of the disease, refusal of treatment should be taken very seriously and attempts made to reconcile disagreements between parents and patient. If such attempts fail, resort to external help and arbitration is required to protect all concerned.

RESEARCH ETHICS IN CHILDHOOD CANCER

The major ethical issues in Phase I/II trials involve questions about [1] the basis of the trial (*i.e.,* whether it ought to be done), [2] the adequacy of children's and parents' understanding of the trial, and [3] the vulnerability of patients at the threshold of deciding about participation.

Phase I Trials

Pure Phase I trials (*i.e.,* a child is the first human to receive a drug) do not occur in pediatric oncology (see also Chap. 13). The introduction of a new agent in children is dependent on satisfactory experience with that agent in adults. Children are generally as tolerant or more tolerant of new drugs than are adults. However, Phase I trials need to be done in children for the same reasons they are warranted in adults. Many Phase I research risks have been avoided in pediatric oncology because of the higher risks accepted by adult cancer patients.

When should a new cancer drug or other approach to therapy be studied in children for the first time? The urgency and scientific merit of the research question should be the determining factors. However, selection of patients is an ethical factor equal to scientific merit. No protection for the patient and researcher exceeds the scientific and ethical review provided by an effective IRB. The work of the IRB involves applying all five ethical principles to the proposed research (see Table 15-1), but the proportionality principle may be the most central in answering the question, "Should this study be done?" Assessment of the risks and benefits of the trial and ensuring the protection of the welfare and rights of the subjects are the key tasks of the IRB.

The primacy of therapeutic intent in relation to Phase I trials is a matter of controversy. Lipsett[69] argued that "therapeutic intent" must *always* be the primary justification of the trial. This aim is based on beneficence. The second purpose of a Phase I trial, according to his view, is the understanding of drug dynamics, metabolism, toxicity, and maximum tolerated dose. Selection of subjects is also a crucial ethical consideration in Phase I trials. Patients should have extensive metastatic disease but have a reasonable life expectancy, lest there be "no therapeutic potential and no opportunity to establish maximum tolerated dose and toxic effects" (ref. 69, p. 941). Lipsett acknowledged the vulnerability of patients with advanced cancer to pressure to participate in Phase I trials, but argued that safeguards of "family or friends . . . peer judgment inherent in the academic clinical research setting, and the judgments of the IRBs" were generally sufficient.

This view of a Phase I study has two dangers: falsely raising hopes about therapy,[70] and a too-easy conscience about the protection given to vulnerable Phase I subjects in the absence of data on what children or adults understand about their participation in Phase I studies.[71]

Substantive ethical objections to Phase I trials do not appear in the literature. Objections usually point to potentially exploitative and harmful misuses of research because of the vulnerability of children.[72,73]

Phase II Cancer Studies: A New Approach

When children with cancer do not respond to standard therapy, they become candidates for Phase II trials of new anticancer agents. The prospect for therapeutic intent is greater than in Phase I trials. An objection to Phase II trials is overusing them to manage patients in end-stage cancer and presenting a trial as if there were no choice but to participate.[74]

Nitschke and others[75] reported an innovative but controversial practice aimed to safeguard voluntariness and increase knowledge about Phase II trials—a "final-stage" conference in which patients older than 5 participated and chose either research participation or supportive care. Of 44 families asked to participate, only one refused. Of the remaining 43 families, the parents were offered the choice of having the physician explain the difference between Phase II drugs and supportive care to the child in their presence, or explaining this privately to the child after their discussion with the physician. The group conference was chosen by 36 parents and privacy by 7. The authors reported that "the majority of children made the decision"; 14 chose Phase II trials and 28 supportive care. One adolescent did not make a choice and was lost to follow-up. Of the 18 patients who chose supportive care and stayed at home, only 2 showed severe depression and behavioral problems. The authors comment that a gradual decrease in the number of patients choosing research as the study progressed was unexplainable. However, they stopped mentioning benefits to medicine and future patients because one noncompliant patient finally stated that he wanted to refuse therapy but did not do so to please his physicians, who needed more information about the drug. There could well be a cause and effect relationship between this change and the drop-off in patients who chose research drugs.

Some practitioners object to allowing young children to make decisions about therapy, because they think that children younger than 11 do not have an adequate understanding of disease and illness. Another objection, based on what may be the dominant view (although the practice may be changing), states that it is the physician's responsibility to make a recommendation about terminal care, "considering the potential value of the drug to this patient and to future patients, the dangers and discomfort inherent in its use, and most important, the feelings and attitudes of this particular child and his or her family."[76,77] In short, the physician bears most of the responsibility for the final decision. It is assumed that this approach reduces abnormal grief and the anguish of doubt and regret about possibly having made the wrong choice. Nitschke replied to these objections by noting that a follow-up showed that no parents had expressed guilt or regret about permitting their child to participate in the choice.[78] He defended the approach of including the child by using the norms of informed consent. These conflicts between alternate practices involve tensions between the principle of respect for persons and duties created by nonmaleficence.

TERMINAL CARE

Three ethical questions arise most frequently in terminal care of children with cancer:

1. Should physicians acquiesce to the patient's or family's desire for no further treatment, or for more treatment when the best medical view is that treatment should be tempered or withheld?
2. Should physicians recommend forgoing life-sustaining treatment, either by withholding or withdrawing it?
3. Is euthanasia justifiable under any circumstances?

A report of the President's Commission for the Study of Ethical Problems in Medicine and Biomedical and Behavioral Research[79] has addressed these issues and will be followed closely in this discussion. The commission's recommendations may well embody the dominant approaches to these problems in adults and infants. However, very little is actually known about the benefits or detriments of following such guidance, especially in pediatrics. Very few empiric studies have been done of the decision-making process in end-stage pediatric cancer. There has been no study of the consequences of following the recommendations of the President's commission as applied to decisions to forgo the treatment of children with cancer. In contrast to information gained from empiric studies of end-of-life issues in adults and newborns, including costs of the last year of life in large populations,[80,81] a significant gap exists in knowledge about such questions involving children. An exception is a study that compared outcomes and costs of children with cancer dying at home or in the hospital, described below.

Conflicts with Patient's and Family's Desires

Physicians may ethically and legally refuse to acquiesce to the patient's or family's stated or written desires for nontreatment when predictable harm might result for the patient (see also Chap. 49). The physician's refusal to comply must be balanced by the duty not to abandon the patient who consistently refuses life-sustaining treatment while arrangements are being made to refer or transfer the patient to another setting.[82]

If patient or family desire more medical treatment when the physician's judgment is that treatment should be tempered or withheld, the physician should take the following steps: [1] give a clear recommendation about the lack of benefit of the desired treatment, [2] assure all concerned that the patient will receive all other supportive care, and [3] request consultation from a bioethicist or ethics committee. If the patient or family then persist, the physician can withdraw from the case and refer care to another physician. This latter step is especially indicated if the desired treatment is expensive or burdensome.

The physician's duty not to acquiesce completely to patient's or family's desires in either situation is grounded in the principle of nonmaleficence, because acting on these desires would lead to harm. The principle of respect for the autonomous choices of persons is an ethical cornerstone of the practice of medicine as applied to consent and refusal of treatment, but it can clearly be limited by the stronger moral claims to prevent harm, even when further treatment is strongly desired by patient and family. Such ethical conflicts between the physician and the patient and family are opportunities to request consultation.

Forgoing Life-Sustaining Treatment

Life-sustaining treatments encompass all means to increase the life span of critically ill children. These include cardiopulmonary resuscitation (CPR), antibiotics, and special means of feeding and hydration. Should physicians, although committed to sustaining life, ever recommend that such treatments be withheld or withdrawn?

The crucial distinction to use in these cases, as recommended by the President's commission, is the degree to which the patient will benefit from or be burdened by a proposed treatment. This criterion ought to apply whether the choice is not to start treatment or to withdraw it.[83] The older distinction between "ordinary and extraordinary" care to differentiate the obligatory and the optional has been irreparably blurred. There is little difference, in practice, between the ethical significance of "ordinary" treatments, such as parenteral nutrition and hydration, and "extraordinary" interventions, such as CPR and hemodialysis. If physicians have sound reasons to predict that a possibly life-sustaining treatment will not benefit the patient and is likely to add burden and increase suffering, they have a duty to make their assessment known to the patient and family. The duty arises from the principles of beneficence and nonmaleficence, as well as the practice of full disclosure to patients and families.

Do not resuscitate (DNR) orders provide a clear example. The DNR order means that in the event of an acute cardiac or respiratory arrest, CPR will not be initiated. The commission recommended that hospitals have explicit policies and procedures for DNR decisions to protect the interests of patients and families. The guidelines shown in Table 15-4, compatible with the recommendations of the President's commission, are used by some hospitals and state medical societies and have been adapted to pediatric oncology. These guidelines can serve as a model for recommending that any life-sustaining treatment is optional when its burdens outweigh its benefits.

The reasons for including the capable child in decision making at the end of life are consistent with those that support inclusion in disclosure of diagnosis, assent to treatment, and other turning points of therapy. Respect for the child's feelings and desires, especially if the practice has been inclusionary, creates a strong reason to be open with the child about DNR recommendations or decisions to forgo other life-sustaining treatments.

Many physicians and nurses believe that deciding to withdraw a life-sustaining treatment once it has begun is ethically more difficult than deciding not to begin such treatment at all. This reasoning is usually fallacious. Greater justification

Table 15-4
Guidelines for Writing DNR Orders

1. A significant evaluation of the patient's medical condition is required before consideration of DNR orders.
2. The attending physician, in consultation with the care team, should determine the appropriateness of DNR orders.
3. When the patient is capable of participation, the DNR order should be written only after the physician sees the child with parents and they agree. If the child lacks capacity to participate, the parents should be consulted. If disagreement by child or parents exists, a DNR order must not be implemented; the progress notes should document the facts of the interaction, stating that CPR should only be tried until a review can occur.
4. The DNR order shall be written by the attending physician, who has the responsibility to ensure that it is discussed with the care team.
5. DNR orders compatible with maximal therapeutic care.
6. The attending physician shall record the facts and reasons for the DNR order in the progress notes.
7. The order should be reviewed regularly and may be rescinded at any time.

(Material drawn from the President's Commission for the Study of Ethical Problems in Medicine and Biomedical and Behavioral Research,[79] the Minnesota Medical Society,[82] and Fletcher[83])

should be required for not beginning a treatment than for discontinuing it. Until a therapy is actually tried, its benefits and burdens are more difficult to know with certainty. After a limited trial, physicians have more data. If the results are negative, no ethical reason can be posed against discontinuation.

Strong ethical objections to discontinuing the feeding and hydration of terminally ill patients have been made to protect the principle of sanctity of life. Also, fears are expressed that stopping feeding and hydration erodes bonds of elemental kindness between humans and creates precedents for euthanasia.[84,85] However, a clear direction in law and ethics is emerging that treats such technology on the same basis as any other life-sustaining treatment.[86]

Questions at the end of life for children are more poignant than for adults, and ethical analysis is harder to separate from emotion (see Chap. 49). Neither children nor their parents can give advance directives for terminal care in a "living will." The dominant ethos of pediatric oncology favors an assumption to sustain life, unless no rational grounds exist for giving cancer therapy. Thus, the dominant approach to decisions about life-sustaining treatment is medical in nature, tempered by concern for the quality of life of the patient. When no curative therapy is available and the patient is terminally ill, the best alternative may be pediatric hospice care.[87] Hospice care can be given either on an inpatient basis or at home, and is designed to optimize quality of life when curative measures are exhausted.

Martinson and others[88] studied the benefits and detriments of a program of nurse-directed home care for 64 children dying of cancer who were referred by physicians to the program. Children were required to be younger than 17 years and to have no hospitalization planned at the time of referral. With physician consultation, each family chose the degree of intensity of supportive measures to be given at home. Of the 58 children who had died at time of publication, 46 died at home; 11 died in the hospital and 1 died en route to the hospital by ambulance. One month after death, parents of the 46 children who died at home were asked if they would choose home care if they had to choose again. Only 2 (2.7%) of 73 parents were uncertain about choosing home care again. Twelve months later, 56 of the 58 parents said they would choose home care again. Moldow and others[89] compared the costs of home care of the 46 children who died at home with costs for a sample of 12 children eligible for home care who died in the hospital

with only comfort care at the end of life. Costs of hospital care were found to be 22% to 207% higher.

Euthanasia

Euthanasia involves acting directly (*e.g.,* by an injection of air or strychnine), to cause the death of a terminally ill patient with the intent of relieving suffering.[90] The dominant approach is to cast moral blame on such actions, especially with voiceless and dying children. Reasons to support this position, including laws that punish euthanasia, include preserving trust in the physician–patient relationship that physicians will not harm; preventing possible abuse, even in an ideal system of requested beneficent euthanasia; and preventing the desensitization to killing that would occur in those who carried out euthanasia. However, medical treatment of severe pain with drugs at a dosage known to hasten death is permitted if relief of pain cannot be attained by other measures.

Society permits a moral line to be drawn between giving morphine, which relieves pain, and giving agents like strychnine, which can only cause death (ref. 79, pp 80–81). The rule that physicians should follow is to give drugs for pain in terminal illness with due care and judgment.

William H. Boley, a student in the doctoral program in Religious Studies, University of Virginia, participated in planning and research for this chapter and made valuable comments on early drafts. Contributions by the third author were made, in part, through support from the Department of Health and Human Services, National Research Service Award #1-F31-NR05965-01 from the National Center for Nursing Research.

REFERENCES

1. Fox RC: Experiment Perilous. Glencoe, IL, Free Press, 1959
2. Bosk C: Forgive and Remember: Managing Medical Failure. Chicago, University of Chicago Press, 1979
3. Englehardt HT: Foundations of Bioethics, pp 49–56. New York, Oxford University Press, 1986
4. Tebbi CK: Care for adolescent oncology patients. In Highby DJ (ed): Supportive Care in Cancer Therapy, pp 281–303. Boston, Martinus Nijhoff, 1983
5. Tebbi CK, Stern M: Burgeoning speciality of pediatric oncology. Cancer

Bulletin of the University of Texas M.D. Anderson Hospital and Tumor Institute at Houston 36:265–272, 1984

6. Fletcher JC: Goals and process of ethics consultation in health care. BioLaw 2:37–47, 1986
7. National Commission for the Protection of Human Subjects of Biomedical and Behavioral Research: The Belmont Report. Washington, DC, US Government Printing Office, GPO 887-809, 1983
8. Beauchamp TL, Childress JF: Principles of Biomedical Ethics, 3rd ed. New York, Oxford University Press (in press)
9. Gibbons MB, Boren H: Stress reduction. Nurs Clin North Am 20:98, 1985
10. Mount BM: Dealing with our losses. J Clin Oncol 4:1133, 1986
11. Oken D: What to tell cancer patients: A study of medical attitudes. JAMA 175:1120–1128, 1961
12. Novack DH, Plumer R, Smith RL et al: Changes in physicians' attitudes toward telling the cancer patient. JAMA 241:897–900, 1979
13. Slavins LA, O'Malley JE, Koocher GP, Foster DJ: Communication of the cancer diagnosis to pediatric patients: Impact on long-term adjustment. Am J Psychiatry 139:179–183, 1982
14. Donaldson MH: The multidisciplinary approach to the care of children with cancer. In Donaldson MH, Seydel HG (eds): Trends in Childhood Cancer, pp 9–10. New York, John Wiley & Sons, 1976
15. Taylor G: Helping families cope when a child has cancer. Medical Times 109:24S, 1981
16. Moore IM, Kramer RF, Perin G: Care of the family with a child with cancer: Diagnosis and early stages of treatment. Cancer Nurs Perspect 13:64, 1986
17. Boverman H, Bivalic L: Personal communication, December 30, 1986
18. Vernick J, Karon M: Who's afraid of death on a leukemia ward? Am J Dis Child 109:393, 1965
19. Spinetta JJ: Adjustment and adaptation in children with cancer. In Spinetta JJ, Deasy-Spinetta P (eds): Living with Childhood Cancer, pp 5–17. St Louis, CV Mosby, 1981
20. Koocher GP: Psychosocial issues during the acute treatment of pediatric cancer. Cancer 58:468–472, 1986
21. Pfefferbaum B, Levenson PM, van Eys J: Comparison of physician and patient perceptions of communication issues. South Med J 75:1080–1083, 1982
22. O'Connor PA: Truth telling in pediatrics—by degrees. Prog Clin Biol Res 139:189–194, 1983
23. Kearney PJ: Ethics, cancer and children. Med Hypotheses 3:174–179, 1977
24. Greenberg LW, Jewett LS, Luck RS et al: Giving information for a life-threatening diagnosis. Am J Dis Child 138:649–653, 1984
25. National Commission for the Protection of Human Subjects of Biomedical and Behavioral Research: Report and Recommendations. Research Involving Children, vol 1, pp 12–13. DHEW Publ. No. OS 77-0004, Washington, DC, US Government Printing Office, 1977
26. 45 Code of Federal Regulations 46. Subpart D—Additional protections for children involved as subjects in research. Federal Register 48:9818, March 8, 1983
27. Kapp M: Children's assent for participation in pediatric research protocols. Clin Pediatr 22:275–278, 1983
28. van Eys J: Children as decision makers. J Assoc Pediatr Oncol Nurses 3:18–30, 1986
29. Ackerman TF: Fooling ourselves with child autonomy and assent in non-therapeutic clinical research. Clin Res 27:345–348, 1979
30. Leiken SL: Beyond proforma consent for childhood cancer research. J Clin Oncol 3:420–428, 1985
31. Koocher GP, O'Malley JE: The Damocles Syndrome, p 14. New York, McGraw-Hill, 1981
32. van Eys J: Clinical research and clinical care: Ethical problems in the "war on cancer." Am J Pediatr Hematol Oncol 4:419–423, 1982
33. Susman EJ, Dorn LD, Fletcher JC: Informed assent in children's participation in biomedical research (unpublished manuscript)
34. Meisel A, Roth LH: What we do and do not know about informed consent. JAMA 246:2473–2477, 1981
35. Schultz AL, Pardee GP, Ensinck JW: Are research subjects really informed? West J Med 123:76–80, 1975
36. Kennedy BJ, Lillehaugen T: Patient recall of informed consent. Med Pediatr Oncol 7:173–178, 1979
37. Muss HB, White DR, Michielutte R et al: Written informed consent in patients with breast cancer. Cancer 43:7549–7556, 1979
38. Cassileth BR, Zupkis RV, Sutton-Smith K et al: Informed consent: Why are its goals imperfectly realized? N Engl J Med 302:896–700, 1980
39. Rimer BK, Jones WL, Keintz MK et al: Cancer patients' recall of important information. Prog Clin Biol Res 156:153–159, 1984
40. Epstein LC, Lasagna L: Obtaining informed consent. Arch Intern Med 123:682–688, 1969
41. Morrow G, Gootnick J, Schmale A: A simple technique for increasing cancer patients' knowledge of informed consent to treatment. Cancer 42:793–799, 1978
42. Fletcher JC, Boverman M: Involving a family member in the informed consent process. Paper presented to the American Psychological Association, Toronto, 1980
43. McCollum AT, Schwartz AH: Pediatric research hospitalization: Its meaning to parents. Pediatr Res 3:199–204, 1969
44. Schwartz AH: Children's concepts of research hospitalization. N Engl J Med 287:589–592, 1972
45. Lewis CE, Lewis MA, Ifekwunique M: Informed consent by children and participation in an influenza vaccine trial. Am J Publ Health 68:1079–1082, 1978
46. Weithorn LA, Campbell SB: The competency of children and adolescents to make informed treatment decisions. Child Dev 53:1589–1598, 1982
47. Weithorn LW: Children's capacities to decide about participation in research. IRB; Rev Human Subjects Res 5:1–5, March–April, 1983
48. Susman EJ, Dorn LD, Fletcher JC: Reasoning about illness in ill and healthy children and adolescents: Cognitive and emotional development aspects. J Devel Behav Pediatr 8:266–273, 1987
49. Grisso T, Vierling L: Minors' consent to treatment: A developmental perspective. Prof Psychol 9:413–427, 1978
50. Ingelfinger FJ: The unethical in medical ethics. Ann Intern Med 83:264–269, 1975
51. Levine RJ: Ethics and Regulation of Clinical Research, 2nd ed, pp 95–153. Baltimore, Urban & Schwarzenberg, 1986
52. van Eys J: Confidentiality of medical records in pediatric cancer care is a myth. In Truman JT, van Eys J, Pochedly C (eds): Human Values in Pediatric Hematology/Oncology, pp 67–81. New York, Praeger, 1986
53. Siegler M: Confidentiality in medicine, a decrepit concept. N Engl J Med 307:1518–1521, 1982
54. Smith PS, Goldman DS: Care of the young hemophiliac: New socioeconomic demands and the changing physician-patient relationship. In Truman JT, van Eys J, Pochedly C (eds): Human Values in Pediatric Hematology/Oncology, pp 145–142. New York, Praeger, 1986
55. Tarasoff v. Regents of the University of California, 551 p. 2nd 334 (Cal Sup Ct 1976)
56. Beauchamp TL, Childress JF: Principles of Biomedical Ethics. 2nd ed, pp 281–284. New York, Oxford University Press, 1984
57. Macklin R: Consent, coercion, and conflict of rights. Perspect Biol Med 20:365, 1977
58. President's Commission for the Study of Ethical Problems in Medicine and Biomedical and Behavioral Research: Making Health Care Decisions, vol 1, p 183. Washington DC, US Government Printing Office, 1982.
59. Ackerman TF: The limits of beneficence: Jehovah's Witnesses and childhood cancer. Hastings Center Rep 10:13–14, August 1980
60. Relman AS: Treating children without parental consent. Prog Clin Biol Res 76:109–114, 1981
61. Truman JT, Brant J: Ethical and legal issues in the treatment of children with cancer. Am J Pediatr Hematol/Oncol 6:313–317, 1984
62. Holder AR: Legal Issues in Pediatrics and Adolescent Medicine, 2nd ed. New Haven, Yale University Press, 1985
63. Morrisey JM, Hofmann AD, Thrope JC: Consent and Confidentiality in the Health Care of Children and Adolescents, pp 97–101. New York, Free Press, 1986
64. Custody of a Minor (Chad Green I), 375 Mass 733, 379 NE 2nd 1053 (1978)
65. Custody of a Minor (Chad Green II), 378 Mass 732, 393 NE 2nd 836 (1979)
66. Truman JT: Custody of a minor: the Chad Green case in historical perspective. In Truman JT, van Eys J, Pochedly C (eds): Human Values in Pediatric Hematology/Oncology, pp 83–89. New York, Praeger, 1980
67. Morrisey JM, Hofmann AD, Thrope JC: Consent and Confidentiality in the Health Care of Children and Adolescents, p 34. New York, Free Press, 1986
68. Leiken SL: Minors' assent or dissent to medical treatment. In President's Commission for the Study of Ethical Problems in Medicine and Biomedical and Behavioral Research: Making Health Care Decisions, vol 3. Appendices. Studies on the Foundations of Informed Consent, pp 185–186. Washington DC, US Government Printing Office, 1982
69. Lipsett MB: On the nature and ethics of phase I trials. JAMA 248:941–942, 1982

70. Capron AM: Ethics of phase I trials (letter). JAMA 249:882–883, 1983

71. Ackerman TF, Strong CM: Ethics of phase I trials (letter). JAMA 249:883, 1983

72. Krant MJ, Cohen-JL, Rosenbaum C: Moral dilemmas in clinical cancer experimentation. Med Pediatr Oncol 3:141–147, 1977

73. Cogliano-Shutta NA: Pediatric phase I clinical trials: Ethical issues and nursing considerations. Oncol Nurs Forum 13:29–32, 1986

74. van Eys J: Randomized clinical trials in pediatric oncology (letter). N Engl J Med 300:1115, 1979

75. Nitschke MD, Humphrey GB, Sexauer CL et al: Therapeutic choices made by patients with end-stage cancer. J Pediatr 101:471–476, 1982

76. Leiken SL, Connell K: Therapeutic choices by children with cancer (letter). J Pediatr 103:167, 1983

77. Shumway: Therapeutic choices by children with cancer (letter). J Pediatr 103:168, 1983

78. Nitschke MD: Letter. J Pediatr 103:169, 1983

79. President's Commission for the Study of Ethical Problems in Medicine and Biomedical and Behavioral Research. Deciding to Forego Life-Sustaining Treatment, pp 43–90. Washington, DC, US Government Printing Office, 1983

80. Lubitz J, Prihoda R: The use and costs of Medicare services in the last 2 years of life. Health Care Finance Rev 5:117–131, 1984

81. US Congress, Office of Technology Assessment: Case Study #10: The costs and effectiveness of neonatal intensive care (341-844/1016). Washington, DC, US Government Printing Office, 1981

82. Minnesota Medical Association: Do not resuscitate (DNR) guidelines. MMA Board of Trustees, Health Association Center, Suite 400, 2221 University Ave, SE, Minneapolis, MN 55414

83. Fletcher JC: Ethical issues. In Parrillo JE (ed): Current Therapy in Critical Care, pp 341–344. Philadelphia, BD Decker, 1987

84. Callahan D: On feeding the dying. Hastings Center Rep 13:22, 1983

85. Meilaender G: On removing food and water: Against the stream. Hastings Center Rep 14:11–13, December 1984

86. Lynn J (ed): By No Extraordinary Means: The Choice to Forego Life-Sustaining Food and Water. Bloomington, IN, Indiana University, 1986

87. Corr CA, Corr DM: Pediatric hospice care. Pediatrics 76:774–780, 1985

88. Martinson IM, Moldow DG, Armstrong GD et al: Home care for children dying of cancer. Res Nurs Health 9:11–16, 1986

89. Moldow DG, Armstrong GD, Henry SF, Martinson IM: The cost of home care for dying children. Med Care 20:1154–1160, 1982

90. Fletcher JC: Is euthanasia ever justifiable? In Wiernik PH (ed): Controversies in Oncology, pp 297–321. New York, John Wiley & Sons, 1982

Management of Common Cancers of Childhood

part

four

sixteen

Acute Lymphoblastic Leukemia

David G. Poplack

The therapeutic experience of acute lymphoblastic leukemia (ALL) is one of the true success stories of modern clinical oncology. Over the past 40 years, the prognosis has dramatically improved for children with this disease. Before effective antileukemic therapy, ALL was uniformly fatal, with most children surviving only 2 to 3 months from diagnosis. Currently, however, about 60% of children with this disease achieve prolonged disease-free survival (>5 years from diagnosis), and most of these patients are considered to be cured. This extraordinary treatment success results from a series of treatment advances that began with the identification of effective single-agent chemotherapy in the late 1940s, followed by the development of combination chemotherapy and subsequently maintenance chemotherapy, in the 1950s and early 1960s. In addition, the introduction of central nervous system preventive therapy in the late 1960s and, most recently, the strategies of tailoring therapy according to "risk" factors and intensifying therapy, particularly for "poor risk" patients, have also contributed to treatment success. Other therapeutic innovations, such as allogeneic bone marrow transplantation, have evolved within the setting of childhood ALL treatment, emphasizing that this disease has served as a paradigm for the development of treatment strategies for other malignancies, both pediatric and adult. This chapter reviews the pathophysiology and biology of ALL, discusses current therapeutic approaches, and highlights those unresolved treatment issues that pose a major challenge for the future.

EPIDEMIOLOGY

Acute leukemia is the most common malignancy in children. Each year about 2000 cases are diagnosed in the United States, accounting for almost one-third of the cases of childhood cancer (see Chap. 1). The incidence of childhood ALL in the United States is approximately 4 per 100,000 children younger than 15 years. ALL accounts for approximately three-fourths of all cases of childhood leukemia.[1-3]

The peak incidence of ALL occurs at approximately 4 years of age (Fig. 16-1).[4,5] This young age peak historically has appeared at different times in different countries. It initially occurred in Great Britain in the 1920s, in the United States in the 1940s, and in Japan in the 1960s.[6,7] The times of appearance of these peaks correspond to major periods of industrialization in these countries, suggesting that they reflect different periods of exposure to new environmental leukemogens.[4]

Among children in the United States, ALL is more common in whites than in blacks. This may be owing to the fact that the increased early peak incidence of ALL, noted above, occurs in whites but has not been observed in blacks.[8] It has been hypothesized that this phenomenon reflects either a difference in susceptibility or in exposure to whatever environmental influences might be responsible for the early age peak in whites.[9,10]

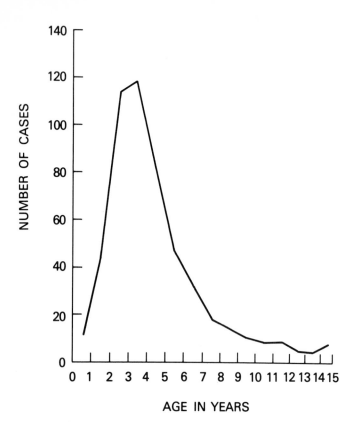

FIGURE 16-1.   Age distribution of 527 children with acute lympho-blastic leukemia. (Fraumeni JF Jr, Manning MD, Mitus WJ: Acute childhood leukemia: Epidemiological study by cell type of 1263 cases at the Children's Cancer Research Foundation in Boston, 1947–1965. J Natl Cancer Inst 46:461–470, 1971)

Males have a higher incidence of ALL than females; the difference is greatest among pubertal children.[9,11,12] Despite speculation regarding a possible role for sex hormones in leukemogenesis, no link has been definitively established.[9]

There appear to be geographic differences in the frequency and age distribution of ALL (see also Chap. 54). For example, in North Africa and the Middle East, ALL is relatively rare; non-Hodgkin's lymphoma is the most common childhood malignancy. Although in India and China ALL is somewhat more common, its incidence is also considerably less than in the industrialized West.[13] This geographic variation may, in part, reflect differences in the incidence of the various immunologic subtypes of ALL.[14] For example, there appears to be a lower incidence of common ALL in developing countries and a higher incidence of T-cell ALL than in more industrialized countries. The reason for this is unclear. Although it has been hypothesized that this results from underdiagnosis of common ALL in developing countries, it also has been suggested that children in industrialized countries are exposed to the leukemogens that specifically cause common ALL.[14–16] Therefore, the pronounced young age peak in ALL observed in developed countries can be largely explained on the basis of a higher incidence of common ALL.

Over the years, there has been considerable interest in the reported occurrence of so-called leukemic clusters, the observation of a greater than expected number of leukemia cases within a given geographic area or time period.[17–23] The documentation of *bona fide* leukemic clusters would have profound epidemiologic implications, potentially permitting identification of common infectious or environmental exposures. Under careful scrutiny, however, most purported clusters have not been substantiated, in part because of difficulties in defining the population at risk.[9,13,24,25]

GENETICS

Genetic factors are presumed to play a significant role in the etiology of acute leukemia, including ALL (see also Chaps. 2 and 3). Evidence for this relationship is based on several observations, including the association between various constitutional chromosomal abnormalities and childhood ALL, the occurrence of familial leukemia, the high incidence of leukemia in identical twins, and the demonstration of karyotypic abnormalities in leukemic cells of children with this disease.

The association between constitutional chromosomal abnormalities and childhood leukemia is well known. Children with trisomy 21 (Down's syndrome) have up to 15 times the risk of developing leukemia compared with normal children.[26] Although both ALL and acute nonlymphocytic leukemia (ANLL) are observed, ALL predominates in all but the neonatal age group.[27] Fibroblasts from patients with Down's syndrome are more readily transformable *in vitro* by oncogenic SV-40 virus than are fibroblasts of normal individuals.[28,29] This suggests that the increased risk of leukemia in children with Down's syndrome reflects the presence of an inherently unstable genome susceptible to the effects of extrinsic leukemogenic agents such as viruses.[9]

The incidence of acute leukemia in Bloom's syndrome and Fanconi's anemia is well documented.[30–32] These rare, recessively transmitted disorders are characterized by increased chromosomal fragility. Although ANLL is most common in Bloom's syndrome, ALL also occurs.[30,33] Patients with Bloom's syndrome manifest short stature and photosensitive telangiectatic erythema.[34] There is some evidence that the development of leukemia in these patients is a consequence of genetic recombination which occurs in somatic cell chromosomes.[33] Fanconi's constitutional aplastic anemia is characterized by short stature and various congenital abnormalities, including skeletal and renal anomalies, hyperpigmentation, deafness, mental retardation, and microcephaly.[35] As in Down's syndrome, the fibroblasts of patients with this disorder manifest increased *in vitro* susceptibility to SV-40 viral transformation.[36,37] Fanconi's anemia is most frequently associated with the development of acute myelomonocytic leukemia (AMML), rather than with ALL.[4,37]

Lymphoid malignancies, including ALL, have been reported in patients with ataxia telangiectasia, an autosomal recessive disorder also characterized by increased chromosomal fragility (see also Chap. 4).[38,39] Abnormalities of the group D chromosomes, particularly translocation or inversion of chromosome 14, and chromosome 7 have been observed. It is of interest that the loci of the three rearranging T-cell receptor genes—gamma, beta (chromosome 7), and alpha (chromosome 14)—are located at chromosomal positions susceptible to breakage and rearrangement in ataxia telangiectasia.[16] The extent to which the associated immunodeficiency present in ataxia telangiectasia is involved in the development of malignancy in these apparently genetically predisposed individuals is unknown.

A variety of other less common preexisting chromosomal abnormalities have been linked to isolated reports of leukemia.[5,40,41] Included among these are children with Kleinfelter's syndrome and trisomy G syndrome.[42] An increased risk of childhood leukemia has been reported in association with increasing maternal age, presumably reflecting the increased incidence of subtle karyotypic abnormalities in older mothers.[9,43,44] Several studies have suggested a link between maternal reproductive history and the risk of ALL.[45-47] A higher risk has been associated with a history of fetal loss. It is unclear whether this reflects genetic predisposition, an abnormal intrauterine environment, or a common environmental exposure. Higher birth weights also appear to be associated with a greater risk of ALL, but the biologic basis for this observation is unknown.[48,49]

Multiple cases of leukemia within families have been reported, including aggregates among siblings, others in the same generation, or multiple individuals in several generations.[50-53] The frequency of leukemia is higher than expected in families of patients with leukemia[54,55]: siblings of children with leukemia, including ALL, have approximately a twofold to fourfold greater risk of developing the disease than do unrelated children in the general population.[40,56] Although these observations appear to imply an inherent genetic risk, it is also possible that the occurrence of multiple cases of leukemia within a family indicates a common exposure to unknown environmental leukemogens. The possibility that familial cases might indicate the presence of an underlying inherited immunodeficiency disorder has also been suggested.[20,57]

The occurrence of leukemia in identical twins has been used to support the role of genetic factors in the etiology of acute leukemia.[40] The concordance of acute leukemia in monozygotic twins is estimated to be as high as 25%.[58] This risk, highest in infancy, diminishes with age such that after 7 years of age, the risk to the unaffected twin is similar to that for individuals within the general population.[40,53] Although the high concordance rate among younger twins suggests a genetic predisposition,[9] it may also be the result of simultaneous exposure to a common prenatal or postnatal leukemogenic event.[59] Another possibility is that a leukemogenic event occurs *in utero* in one twin and the malignant cells migrate to the second through shared placental circulation.[60-62] Thus, the extent to which the occurrence of leukemia in identical twins implicates a genetic susceptibility is not clear.

The presence of karyotypic abnormalities in the leukemic cells of patients with this disease also suggests genetic factors in childhood ALL. These chromosomal abnormalities are detailed in the cytogenetics section (see below).

PATHOGENESIS

In addition to genetic factors, several other possible predisposing factors have been examined, including environmental factors, viral infection, and immunodeficiency and leukemia.

Environmental Factors

Ionizing radiation and certain toxic chemicals may predispose one to acute leukemia (see also Chaps. 2 and 3). The high incidence of leukemia among survivors of the atomic bomb explosions in Japan during World War II is well documented.[63-65] The risk of leukemia was greatest for individuals closest to the explosion.[66,67] In individuals who received exposure doses greater than 100 R, the dose–response relationship for the production of leukemia was linear.[68] The type of leukemia observed was related to the age at exposure: ALL was seen more frequently in children, and ANLL was more common in adults. Among survivors of the atomic bomb, there was no increase in the incidence of leukemia in children exposed to radiation *in utero*. This experience contrasts with other studies, which indicate that there is an increased risk of leukemia in children exposed to diagnostic radiation *in utero*, particularly during the first trimester.[69,70] In a study by the National Academy of Sciences, a fivefold increased risk of all childhood cancers was found in children exposed to radiation during the first trimester; when exposure occurred during the second and third trimester, the risk was 1.5 times normal. Leukemias made up approximately one-half of the cancers noted in that study; the increased risk for leukemia extends through 12 years of age.[71] A significant leukemogenic effect has been reported in children exposed *in utero* to doses of 0.3 to 0.8 cGy.[72] The risk of developing leukemia from *ex utero* diagnostic radiation has been difficult to determine. A recent study suggested that about 1% of all cases of adult leukemia can be assumed to be a result of exposure to diagnostic radiography.[73] No such data are available on the development of leukemia during childhood.

Therapeutic radiation has been associated with a higher risk of acute leukemia in some individuals, including patients with ankylosing spondylitis treated with relatively high dose radiation and neonates administered thymic radiation (once used to treat enlargement of the thymus).[74,75] An increased leukemic mortality was also observed in one study in which children received scalp irradiation for treatment of tinea capitis.[76] The development of nonlymphoid leukemias in adults has been linked to the use of certain radionuclides such as ^{32}P treatment for polycythemia vera.[77]

Although the potential of ionizing radiation to cause leukemia is well appreciated, the actual percentage of leukemia cases directly attributable to radiation is presumed to be small. Controversy persists regarding the risks from exposure to ionizing radiation from routine emissions from nuclear power plants or as a result of fallout from atmospheric nuclear testing.[73,78,79]

Chronic chemical exposure (*e.g.,* benzene) has been associated with the development of ANLL in adults.[80,81] Direct evidence linking such exposure to the development of childhood ALL, however, does not exist. There is substantial evidence that chemotherapy, particularly with alkylating agents, has leukemogenic potential. In a recent study of more than 9000 2-year survivors of childhood cancer, a 14-fold excess of leukemia was observed, primarily attributable to therapy with alkylating agents.[82] Most of these cases, however, were ANLL.

Other factors studied for possible association with ALL include exposure to electromagnetic fields, herbicides, and pesticides and maternal use of alcohol, contraceptives, diethylstilbestrol, or cigarettes.[47,83-86] Definitive links between these factors and the risk of childhood ALL have not been confirmed.

Viral Infection

There is intense interest in the possible role played by viral infection in the etiology of human leukemia. Certain RNA viruses are known to cause leukemia in murine, avian, bovine, feline, and nonhuman primate species.[87] Study of these vertically transmitted viruses in the murine system have demonstrated that the development of leukemia in that species could be influenced by a number of factors, including the amount of virus, the environment, and the genetic background, hormonal status, age, and immunologic status of the host.

Study of the murine model led to the "viral–oncogene hypothesis," which has been proposed as a model for the viral etiology of human leukemia.[88] According to this hypothesis, the viral DNA of RNA tumor viruses is incorporated into the genomes of vertebrate cells. These "virogenes" are then vertically transmitted. Although their normal expression is presumably repressed, it is theorized that derepression by a variety of endogenous or exogenous factors (*e.g.,* chemical carcinogens, ionizing radiation) occurs, leading to the development of leukemia.

Although this hypothesis is attractive, until recently evidence directly linking viruses to the development of human acute leukemia primarily has been circumstantial and has included the rare finding of "virus-like" particles in human leukemic cells and in the bone marrow, plasma, and urine of patients with leukemia, and the demonstration of reverse transcriptase and 70S high molecular weight RNA in human leukemia cells.[89–93] Recently, however, the human T-cell leukemia-lymphoma virus (HTLV-I) has been definitively linked to the development of adult T-cell leukemia-lymphoma, a disorder prevalent in several specific geographic regions, including the Caribbean basin, southeastern United States, and parts of Japan.[94,95] Attempts to identify evidence of HTLV-I infection in children with ALL, however, have been unsuccessful.[96] Nevertheless, the role apparently played by HTLV-I in the production of adult T-cell lymphoma-leukemia confirmed, for the first time, the role of retroviruses in human leukemogenesis.

The Epstein–Barr virus (EBV), a DNA virus widespread in humans, is associated with Burkitt's lymphoma and thus presumably with the L3 subtype of ALL (see Immunology section). EBV infection and its relationship to c-*myc* proto-oncogene expression and to the t8;14 translocation is discussed in detail in Chapter 21.

At one time a possible relationship between feline leukemia virus (FeLV) and human acute leukemia was proposed.[97] Although this virus can propagate within human cells *in vitro* and other feline tumor viruses can produce tumors in subhuman primates, epidemiologic studies have failed to link exposure to cats with the development of leukemia in humans.[5,98–101]

Immunodeficiency and Leukemia

Children with various congenital immunodeficiency diseases, including Wiscott–Aldrich syndrome, congenital hypogammaglobulinemia, and ataxia telangectasia, have an increased risk of developing lymphoid malignancy (see also Chap. 4).[32] Although ALL may occur in patients with these disorders, it is not common. It has been hypothesized that impairment of immune surveillance is responsible for the eventual development of malignancy in these conditions. As noted previously, however, patients with ataxia-telangiectasia have increased chromosomal fragility and frequent abnormalities of chromosomes 14 and 7, suggesting that in this disorder, genetic mechanisms are important.

The chronic use of immunosuppressive drugs is also associated with an increased risk of lymphoid malignancy (see Chap. 22); however, ALL is not common.[102]

Abnormalities of the immune system are occasionally observed in newly diagnosed patients with ALL.[103,104] Abnormally low serum immunoglobulin levels have been noted in up to 30% of newly diagnosed patients. Whether such abnormalities precede the development of leukemia or are a consequence of the disease is not clear. T-cell leukemic lymphoblasts with a suppressor cell immunophenotype, which suppress immunoglobulin biosynthesis *in vitro,* have been described.[105] However, this phenotype occurs infrequently and is unlikely to account for the observed incidence of low serum immunoglobulin levels in newly diagnosed patients.

ALL as a Clonal Disease

ALL, like other lymphoid malignancies, is believed to develop as a consequence of malignant transformation of a single abnormal progenitor cell, which has the capability to expand by indefinite self-renewal. Evidence for the clonal origin of ALL derives from studies of glucose-6-phosphate-dehydrogenate (G-6PD) types and from chromosomal molecular biologic analysis of leukemic lymphoblasts. Studies of girls, heterozygous for the X-chromosome linked G-6PD enzyme, have demonstrated that at diagnosis, leukemic lymphoblasts manifest a single G-6PD type, indicating the presence of clonal disease. The same G-6PD type is also found in leukemic cells obtained at relapse or from extramedullary sites.[106] In contrast, both enzyme types are found in morphologically normal blood cells and in other normal tissue obtained from these patients. This indicates that ALL is a clonally derived disease in which expression of differentiation by the progenitor cell is limited to the lymphoid pathway. Additional support for the "clonal expansion" theory comes from cytogenetic studies, which have documented the same karyotype present in leukemic cells at diagnosis and at relapse.[107–109]

Rearrangement of immunoglobulin and T-cell receptor genes also have been studied as a marker of clonality in ALL of pre-B-cell lineage.[110] These studies have confirmed that, in most cases, identical patterns of immunoglobulin and T-cell receptor gene rearrangement are observed in leukemic cells obtained at diagnosis and upon relapse. Infrequently, clonal variations in such serial samples have suggested the presence of biclonal disease. In these cases, however, the observation that these cells share at least one identical immunoglobulin gene rearrangement implies that the cells had a common clonal origin and were not truly biclonal.[110] The fact that immunoglobulin and T-cell receptor gene markers are involved in the process of cell differentiation and are sequentially expressed during lymphoid differentiation suggests that the evolution of subclones within a malignant cell population is not surprising.

BIOLOGY/PATHOLOGY

Childhood ALL—A Heterogeneous Disorder

In recent years morphologic, immunologic, cytogenetic, and biochemical characterization of leukemic lymphoblasts have confirmed that ALL is a biologically heterogeneous disorder. This heterogeneity, detailed below, reflects the fact that the leukemia may develop at any point during the multiple stages of normal lymphoid differentiation.

Morphologic Classification

There have been a number of attempts to subclassify ALL cells morphologically using criteria such as cell size, nuclear: cytoplasmic ratio, nuclear shape, number and prominence of nucleoli, character and intensity of cytoplasmic staining, presence of cytoplasmic granules, and inclusions and character of nuclear chromatin.[111–116] Most of these efforts have been unsuccessful, either because they were technically difficult to reproduce or lacked meaningful clinical correlation.[117–124] One system, however, proposed by the French–American–British (FAB) Cooperative Working Group has now become universally accepted (Table 16-1).[125,126] The FAB system (Table 16-1 and Fig. 16-2) divides lymphoblasts into three categories. L1 lymphoblasts are usually smaller and have scanty cytoplasm and inconspicuous nucleoli. Cells of the L2 variety are larger, demonstrate considerable heterogeneity in size, and have prominent nucleoli and more abundant cytoplasm. Lymphoblasts of the L3 type, notable for their deep cytoplasmic basophilia, are large, frequently display prominent cytoplasmic vacuolation, and are identical cytomorphologically to Burkitt's lymphoma cells. Approximately 85% of children with ALL have

Table 16-1
FAB Classification of Lymphoblastic Leukemia[126]

Cytologic Features	L1	L2	L3
Cell size	Small cells predominate	Large, heterogeneous in size Variable, heterogeneous in any one case	Large and homogeneous
Nuclear chromatin	Homogeneous in any one case		Finely stippled and homogeneous
Nuclear shape	Regular, occasional clefting or indentation	Irregular, clefting and indentation common	Regular—oval to round
Nucleoli	Not visible or small and inconspicuous, more vesicular	One or more present, often large	Prominent, one or more
Amount of cytoplasm	Scanty	Variable, often moderately abundant	Moderately abundant
Basophilia of cytoplasm	Slight or moderate, rarely intense	Variable, deep in some	Very deep
Cytoplasmic vacuolation	Variable	Variable	Often prominent

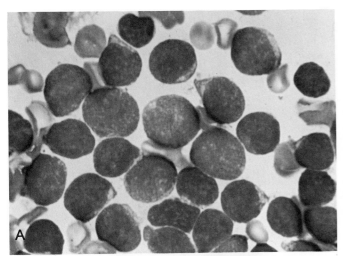

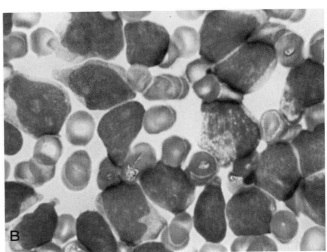

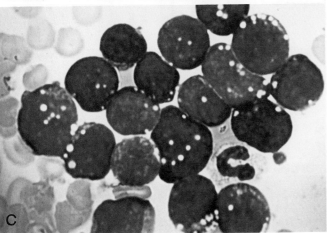

FIGURE 16-2. Morphologic appearance of ALL cells classified according to the FAB system. **A.** L1 morphology. **B.** L2 morphology. **C.** L3 morphology.

predominant L1 morphology, 14% have L2, and 1% have L3.[127,128] The L2 subtype is more common in adults.[129] Lymphoblasts of the L3 type possess cell surface immunoglobulin and other characteristic B-cell markers. There is, however, no apparent correlation between the FAB L1 and L2 morphologic types and immunologic cell surface markers.[127,130,131] Concor-

dance among investigators using the FAB system is relatively high.[128,132,133] Since its original description, refinements to the system have been proposed.[127,133]

Various studies have demonstrated that the FAB classification has prognostic value.[127,128,132–135] L1 morphology is associated with a higher remission induction rate and a better

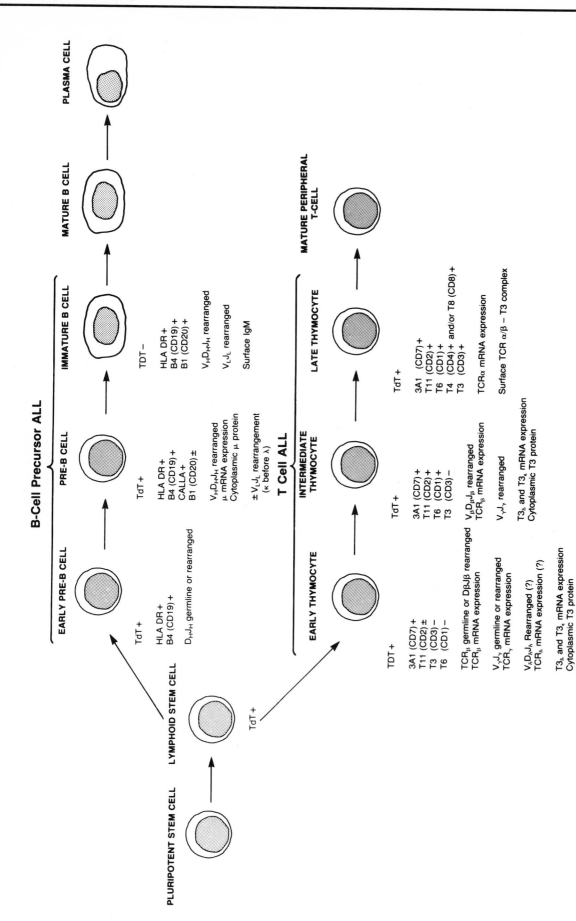

FIGURE 16-3. Schematic representation of stages of lymphoid differentiation found in acute lymphoblastic leukemia of infancy and childhood. Schematic shows stages delineated on the basis of terminal deoxynucleotidyl transferase activity, reactivity with commonly used monoclonal antibodies, and immunoglobulin and T-cell receptor gene rearrangement and their protein products (see text and Refs. 16, 150, 151, 155, 161, 170, 172, and 173 for details).

event-free survival than the L2 morphology. L2 morphology has been found by some investigators to convey a poor prognosis, independent of other prognostic variables such as initial leukocyte count and age at diagnosis. Patients with the L3 morphology have the worst overall prognosis.[136,137] Although the FAB classification system appears to have value as a prognostic indicator (see prognostic factors), no biologic basis for the morphologic differences delineated by this system has been identified.

Immunology/Molecular Biology

Studies of the immunobiology of ALL have confirmed that leukemic transformation and clonal expansion can occur at different stages of maturation in the process of lymphoid differentiation (Fig. 16-3). In the early 1970s when the first surface markers were used to characterize ALL in terms of its cell of origin and stage of differentiation, three immunologic subsets of ALL were delineated. Using receptors for sheep erythrocytes, approximately 20% of patients were found to have T lymphoblasts.[138–141] Cell surface immunoglobulin and complement receptors identified ALL of B-cell origin in 1% to 2% of patients, whereas, using these older immunologic methods of characterization, the majority of patients had no detectable cell surface markers and were considered to have non-T, non-B cell leukemia.[139,142] The development of heterologous antisera, and subsequently monoclonal antibodies, directed against a human leukemia associated antigen indicated that approximately 80% of patients formerly presumed to have had non-T, non-B cell ALL had a common ALL antigen (CALLA) on their cell surface.[143–146] This subset was referred to as "common" ALL to differentiate it from the CALLA negative, non-T and non-B cell group with null cell ALL.

Subsequently, using more sophisticated immunologic techniques, it has been shown that the overwhelming majority of leukemias previously determined to be of the non-T, non-B cell type are actually of B-cell lineage. The demonstration of intracytoplasmic immunoglobulin in some of these cells, their reactivity with monoclonal antibodies specific for B-cell associated antigens, and their ability to differentiate *in vitro* into cells with mature B-cell markers has confirmed that approximately 80% to 85% of childhood ALL cases develop as a result of the monoclonal proliferation of B-cell precursors.[147–152] The presence of cytoplasmic immunoglobulin (C_{Ig}) has been a useful marker to determine the level of differentiation of leukemic cells of B-cell lineage. Cells that possess C_{Ig}, so called pre-B cells, represent an intermediate cell in the process of B-cell differentiation. They are more mature than cells that do not synthesize C_{Ig}, called early pre-B cells, but not as mature as those demonstrating surface immunoglobulin.[151,153,154] C_{Ig} is present in approximately 20% to 30% of cases of B-cell precursor ALL.

Using a panel of monoclonal antibodies specific for various stages of B-cell differentiation, along with information on the presence or absence both of cytoplasmic and surface immunoglobulin, investigators have classified B-lineage ALL into discrete stages according to the degree of differentiation/maturation (Fig. 16-3).[155,156] Although such classification schemes run the risk of oversimplification, each of the stages of differentiation outlined in Figure 16-3 has been observed in normal adult and fetal bone marrow. There are prognostic differences between the various precursor B ALL subgroups. As noted previously, mature B-cell ALL has an extremely poor prognosis; patients with pre-B cell ($C_{Ig}+$) ALL reportedly do worse than those with early pre-B ALL ($C_{Ig}-$) (Fig. 16-4).[151,157] Patients with B-cell precursor ALL whose lymphoblasts manifest the CALLA antigen have a more favorable prognosis.[151,157,158]

The application of recombinant DNA technology has added further to the understanding of ALL (Figs. 16-3, 16-5, 16-6). Normal B-cell precursors are believed to proceed through a hierarchical process of immunoglobulin gene rearrangement as they evolve into antibody producing cells. Identification of immunoglobulin gene rearrangement has been helpful in confirming the B-cell precursor lineage of ALL cells otherwise devoid of other B or pre-B-cell markers.[151,158,159] Investigators have also proposed the existence of a hierarchy of immunoglobulin gene rearrangements in B-cell precursor ALL that mirrors different stages of normal B-cell differentiation (Fig. 16-3).[151,152] In this proposed hierarchy, heavy chain rearrangement precedes κ light chain rearrangement, which in turn precedes λ light chain rearrangement.[152,156,159,160] As shown in Figure 16-3, it is possible to relate the pattern of immunoglobulin gene rearrangement to the discrete stages of differentiation identified among B-cell precursor ALL using monoclonal

FIGURE 16-4. Duration of complete remission for patients with "early pre-B," T, pre-B, and B-cell acute lymphoblastic leukemia (see text for details).[151]

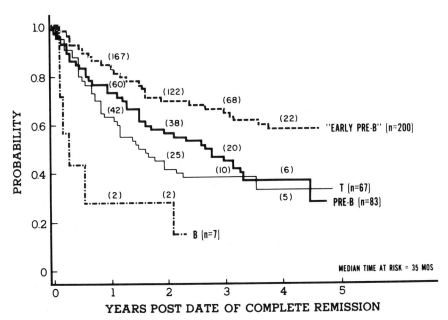

YEARS POST DATE OF COMPLETE REMISSION

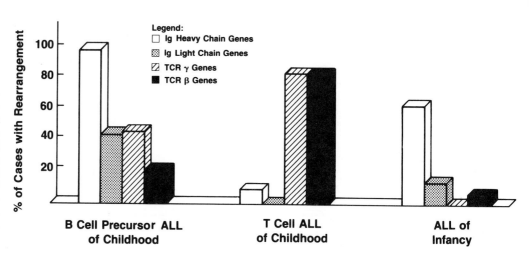

FIGURE 16-5. Relative incidence of immunoglobulin and T-cell receptor gene rearrangement and expression in acute lymphoblastic leukemia of childhood and infancy. Summary of data on more than 60 children analyzed by Southern blot analysis.[150,161,163] (Adapted from Kirsch IR: Molecular biology of the leukemias. Pediatr Clin North Am 35:693–722, 1988)

antibodies to the different B-cell differentiation antigens.[156,160] Notably, however, heavy chain gene rearrangement has also been observed in approximately 10% of T-cell ALL cases (Fig. 16-5).[161] The latter observation indicates that the presence of heavy chain rearrangement alone is not a sufficient basis for assigning B-cell lineage.[159,161,162] This phenomenon of "lineage spillover" also has been observed in T-cell ALL (see below) (Fig. 16-5). B-cell precursor ALL devoid of immunoglobulin (or T-cell receptor) rearrangement has been described. This "germ-line" configuration appears to be a characteristic of some cases of B-cell precursor ALL of infancy (Fig. 16-6).[163]

T-cell ALL is noted for its distinctive clinical features. It frequently occurs in older males who present with high initial leukocyte counts and often have a mediastinal mass. Approximately one-half of children with T-cell ALL have mediastinal masses, and from one-third to one-half have initial leukocyte counts greater than 100,000/mm³.[2,164] Patients with T-cell leukemia reportedly have a higher incidence of CNS leukemia.[165] T-cell ALL historically has been characterized by significantly shorter remission durations and overall survival, although there is evidence that the outcome for such patients on more recent intensive chemotherapy regimens is improved.[166,167] Because of the frequent occurrence of T-cell disease in older patients with high initial leukocyte counts, the degree to which T-cell ALL is a significant independent prognostic variable is unclear (see prognostic factors).[158,167,168] T-cell ALL has been further subclassified using monoclonal antibodies, which detect surface antigens present from discrete stages in the process of normal T-cell differentiation/maturation.[155,170–172] Three stages of normal intrathymic differentiation have been proposed: early (Stage I), intermediate (Stage II), and late (Stage III) (Fig. 16-3). Although T-cell maturation involves a continuum of phenotypic changes, T cells can be identified that are presumably derived from each of these different stages of differentiation.[171–173] Most studies have indicated that the majority of T-cell ALL cases are derived from the early thymocytic stage. In contrast, malignant cells from patients with T-cell lymphoma generally manifest an intermediate or mature phenotype.[151,171,172] Subclassification of T-cell ALL into stages of differentiation has furthered our biologic understanding of T-cell disease. Its clinical relevance, however, remains unclear, and meaningful clinical correlations among these three subgroups of T-cell ALL remain to be identified.

Recombinant DNA techniques also have been used to explore the biology of T-cell ALL (see Chap. 3). Molecular genetic analysis of the genes encoding the T-cell receptor provides a useful molecular marker of T-cell lineage commitment and the stage of T-cell differentiation. Study of the antigen specific α, β, and γ T-cell receptor genes in T-cell ALL reveals a rough hierarchy of T-cell receptor activation events that can be correlated, to some extent, with T-cell surface antigen expression in a fashion analogous to the hierarchy of immunoglobulin gene rearrangement found in B-cell precursor ALL (Fig. 16-3).[156,159,161,174] In this sequence, rearrangement of the γ and β T-cell receptor loci is an early developmental event in T-cell ALL ontogeny, followed by the later step of αmRNA expression (Fig. 16-3). Other events, such as rearrangement of the Δ chain of the T-cell receptor, also occur early in normal T-cell ontogeny.[175] Studies of the time of appearance and the incidence of Δ chain activation in ALL are underway. Although these markers can provide insight into the developmental state of T-cell ALL, use of molecular markers alone to designate T-cell lineage is not appropriate. Gamma and β T-cell receptor rearrangements are known to occur in B-cell precursor ALL even more frequently than the occurrence of immunoglobulin gene rearrangement in T-cell ALL (Fig. 16-5).[161] Such "lineage spillover" may represent leukemias derived from cells at an early stage of lymphoid development when both T-cell receptor and immunoglobulin genes are accessible to a common recombinase enzyme.[16,161,176] Cases of T-cell ALL, putatively derived from the earliest stages of differentiation, have been observed in which neither immunoglobulin nor T-cell receptor rearrangements can be identified.

Although lymphoid leukemia cells generally adhere to lineage "fidelity," there are now numerous reports of situations in which typing with a panel of monoclonal antibodies has demonstrated reactivity with antibodies specific for different lineages.[177–180] Lineage infidelity, or biphenotypy, usually refers to cases in which leukemia cells manifest markers of more than one cell type on the same cell. Many such cases reflect the use of monoclonal antibodies that lack specificity. There are, however, examples that suggest that in some cases the leukemia develops from precursor cells that normally manifest dual markers at some time during their development. Simultaneous expression of lymphoid and myeloid markers appears to occur more commonly than previously believed. The incidence of this phenomenon was reported to be 13% in one study of childhood ALL; in adults with ALL the incidence may be even higher.[178,179] The clinical importance of this observation in childhood ALL is not clear, however, the presence of myeloid antigen expression in adult ALL is associated with a lower remission induction rate and, in those cases expressing B-cell lineage antigens, a shorter overall survival.[179] More information on the biological basis and clinical significance of lineage infidelity in childhood ALL is needed. The occurrence of lineage spillover in molecular markers (discussed above)

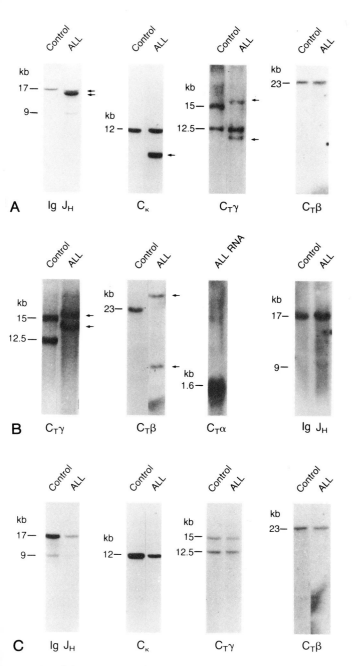

FIGURE 16-6. Examples of various patterns of immunoglobulin and T-cell receptor gene rearrangement in acute lymphoblastic leukemia of childhood shown by Southern and Northern analysis. (Reproduced with permission from Carolyn Felix, M.D.) **A.** B-cell precursor ALL. This case demonstrates rearrangement of both alleles of the immunoglobulin heavy chain gene, one allele of the κ light chain gene, and both alleles of the T-cell receptor gamma gene. The T-cell receptor beta gene remains in germ-line configuration. **B.** T-cell ALL. This case illustrates rearrangement of both alleles of the T-cell receptor γ and β chain genes and T-cell receptor α-messenger RNA expression. Germ-line configuration of the immunoglobulin heavy chain gene is shown. **C.** ALL of infancy (B-cell precursor). This case demonstrates the germ-line configuration both of immunoglobulin heavy and light chain genes and of the γ and β T-cell receptor genes. Rearrangements are indicated by arrows and germ-line bands by dash marks.

and co-expression of presumed lineage specific-cell surface antigens suggests, however, that some features of the traditional methods of lineage classification may be too restrictive.

Changes in blast cell immunophenotype have been noted at relapse; however, most patients retain their original immunophenotype.[181,182] The presence of a different cell lineage at the time of relapse, so-called lineage switch (*e.g.,* lymphoid to myeloid), is a rare event. The explanation for this phenomenon is not clear, but several theories have been suggested, including chemotherapeutic eradication of one clone and subsequent expansion of a second clone of an originally biclonal leukemia, chemotherapy-induced modulation of the original leukemic clone (or its associated cell surface antigens), the occurrence of a second leukemogenic event, and the occurrence of a leukemogenic event affecting more than one precursor cell. As discussed below, certain chromosomal abnormalities occur more frequently in association with specific immunophenotypes.

Cytogenetics

With the advent of improved chromosomal banding techniques and advances in cell culture methodology, cytogenetic analysis has increasingly contributed to the understanding of the biology and treatment of ALL (see Chaps. 2, 3, and 17). Using newer methods of chromosomal analysis, abnormalities can be recognized in the leukemia cells of more than 90% of cases of ALL.[183,184] Abnormalities exist in both chromosomal number (ploidy) and structure. Many of the observed abnormalities appear to have prognostic import.[185-191]

Ploidy can be determined either directly by the classic method of counting the modal number of chromosomes in a metaphase karyotype preparation or by an alternative indirect method that measures DNA content by flow cytometry.[186,189] In contrast to ANLL, in which hypodiploidy is most common, most cases of ALL exhibit diploidy or hyperdiploidy. The ploidy of ALL karyotypes has been shown to be a prognostic determinant.[186,189,192,193] Children with higher ploidy (>50 chromosomes), who account for approximately 30% of children with ALL, have the best prognosis, in contrast to those in the pseudodiploid category who have a relatively poor prognosis. Patients in the hyperdiploid group generally share a number of the more important good prognostic features (see prognostic factors), including a favorable age, low initial leukocyte count and a B-cell precursor phenotype often displaying the CALLA antigen.[186,189] The worst prognosis occurs in the rare group of patients with near-haploid ALL.[189,194]

When structural chromosomal abnormalities occur in ALL, they are limited to the leukemic cells, a finding consistent with the presumed clonal nature of the disease.[195-197] Of the structural abnormalities encountered, translocations are the most common, occurring in about 40% of cases. They are most frequent in the pseudodiploid group, occurring with approximately equal frequency in the other abnormal ploidy groups. Translocations convey a poor prognosis and have been associated with a high rate of both induction failure and relapse.[185,187,192] The high incidence of translocations in the pseudodiploid group appears to explain their poor prognosis.[184] The most common translocations seen in childhood ALL are noted in Table 16-2. Of these, the t(8;14), t(9;22), t(4;11), and t(1;19) are associated with a high rate of early treatment failure.

There appears to be an association between certain translocations and immunophenotype. The t(8;14) (q24;q32) seems to be specific and can be identified in virtually every case of B-cell ALL.[192,198] The molecular mechanism associated with this translocation in B-cell ALL, involving rearrangement and abnormal expression of the *myc* oncogene and the immu-

Table 16-2
Distribution of Chromosomal Translocations in Childhood ALL

Chromosomal Translocation	Immunophenotype	Number of Patients	Percentage
t(8;14) (q24;q23)	B	10	2.4
t(9;22) (q23;q11)*	Variable	18	4.4
t(1;19) (q23;p13.3)	Pre-B	21	5.1
t(11;14) (p13;q13)	T	5	1.2
t(4;11) (q21;q23)	Early pre-B	6	1.5
t(12;v) (p;v)	Early pre-B and pre-B	26	6.3
Random	Variable	90	22.0
None	Variable	234	57.0
Total		410	100.0

Data on 410 patients treated at the St. Jude Children's Cancer Research Hospital. (Reproduced with permission of Thomas A. Look, MD.)
* One patient with the t(9;22) also had the t(1;19).

noglobulin heavy chain gene, is similar to that observed in Burkitt's lymphoma and is consistent with the hypothesis that B-cell ALL represents a disseminated form of that disease (see Chap. 20).[189] B-cell ALL responds extremely poorly to conventional ALL treatment but fares somewhat better on therapy similar to that used for Burkitt's lymphoma.

The t(1;19) (q23;p13.3) has been found in approximately one-third of cases of pre-B-cell ALL (C$_{Ig}$+).[199,200] It is not yet clear whether those pre-B-cell cases that possess this translocation have a different prognosis than other cases of pre-B-cell ALL.

The t(4;11) (q21;q23) is observed in patients with early pre-B-cell ALL (C$_{Ig}$-). Although morphologically consistent with ALL, these cells may manifest some cytochemical and ultrastructural features of monocytes and thus may have biphenotypic characteristics.[192,201] The t(4;11) occurs with a disproportionate frequency in infants with ALL.[191,202]

The t(11;14) (p13;q13) is observed in ALL with a T-cell phenotype of the intermediate stage. These translocations have been demonstrated to bisect the gene encoding the alpha chain of the T-cell receptor on chromosome 14.[200,203]

As noted in Table 16-2, translocations involving the short arm of chromosome 12 are also observed. Most of these cases are of B-cell precursor phenotype.

The finding of Ph^1 positive ALL has stimulated considerable controversy. This abnormality is more frequent in adult ALL but occurs in about 5% of children with this disease.[204] The typical translocation, t(9;22) (q34;q11), is similar to that observed in chronic myelogenous leukemia (CML). In the past, it had been suggested that Ph^1 positive ALL actually represented CML that lacked a chronic phase and presented in blast crisis. It is now evident, however, that both cytogenetic and molecular differences can distinguish Ph^1 positive ALL from CML. In Ph^1 positive ALL, unlike in CML, the translocation cannot be detected in multiple cell lineages. The Ph^1 chromosome is not detectable during remission in successfully treated Ph^1 positive ALL patients, whereas it is present in the remission or chronic phase of CML.[191] At a molecular level, in CML the c-*abl* gene on chromosome 9 is translocated to a 5.8 kilobase span of chromosome 22 known as the "break-point cluster region" (*bcr*).[205] In Ph^1 positive ALL, however, the pattern may be different, the break points on chromosome 22 occurring outside the *bcr*.[189,206] There also appears to be a difference in the *abl* gene products expressed in the two diseases. In Ph^1 positive ALL, a unique p180 protein with tyrosine kinase activity has

been observed that is distinct from the typical p210 protein encoded by the chimeric *bcr-abl* message in CML (see Chap. 18).[207] The Philadelphia chromosome has been observed in both B-cell precursor ALL and in T-cell ALL. Clinically, patients with Ph^1 positive ALL respond poorly to therapy, having a distinctly lower remission induction rate, a higher frequency of CNS leukemia, and early recurrence of their disease.[204] It has been suggested that this group of patients requires alternative therapy to conventional ALL treatment, possibly bone marrow transplantation.[204]

Another translocation that occurs in ALL involves chromosome 12. This t(12;v) (p;v) abnormality commonly occurs in patients with CALLA-positive B-cell precursor disease.[200]

In addition to the consistently observed translocations noted above, unique translocations observed in single cases make up approximately one-half of the chromosomal translocations in this disease.[189] Whether all translocations are intimately involved in the leukemogenic process is unknown. It does appear possible, however, that at a molecular level, at least some translocations, through induction of altered gene expression, confer a growth advantage on cells of a particular phenotype.

Chromosomal studies of bone marrow obtained during remission in ALL are karyotypically normal. The presence of aneuploidy during remission reportedly heralds relapse.[197,198]

At relapse, in most patients, the leukemic clone is karyotypically identical to that observed at diagnosis. As noted previously, this information is consistent with the suggestion that relapse in ALL signifies the recurrence of original leukemia rather than the development of a new leukemic clone.[197]

Biochemical Characterization

Various biochemical markers have been studied in ALL. Some have been found to be useful in the diagnosis and classification of the disease; others have been evaluated as potential avenues for selective therapy. Terminal deoxynucleotidyl transferase (TdT) is an unusual DNA polymerizing enzyme that catalyzes the polymerization of deoxynucleoside monophosphates into a single-strand DNA "primer" without the need for template instruction.[208,209] TdT is found in the nucleus and is believed to play a role in immunoglobulin and T-cell antigen receptor rearrangement, thus influencing the generation of immunologic diversity.[210] TdT activity can be demonstrated by use of a quantitative enzyme assay, by an indirect immunofluorescent technique, or by radioimmunoassay. The first two methods are usually preferred because they permit identification of activity within individual cells. Significant TdT activity is not present in normal lymphocytes but is detectable in normal cortical thymocytes and in leukemic lymphoblasts of both T-cell and B-cell precursor lineage. In true B-cell ALL, TdT activity is usually not present.[211] Determination of TdT activity may be helpful in the diagnosis of ALL and in differentiating ALL from AML, in which TdT activity is rarely present.[212,208] In cases in which the Ph^1 chromosome is identified, the presence of TdT activity helps confirm the lymphoid nature of the process. Detection of TdT activity may help identify sanctuary relapses (*e.g.,* testes), particularly in cases in which routine pathology yields equivocal results. Because TdT positive cells may be present in increased numbers in patients recovering from chemotherapy or bone marrow transplantation, it cannot be used as a sole indicator of bone marrow relapse.[213] Serial measurement of TdT activity in peripheral blood lymphocytes obtained during remission does not permit the earlier detection of bone marrow relapse.[214]

Purine pathway enzymes are known to play an important role in normal lymphocyte function. This pathway has been extensively studied in ALL.[215] A unique pattern of three enzymes (adenosine deaminase, 5′-nucleotidase, and purine nucleoside phosphorylase) has been observed in ALL.[209,216-218] Abnormal lymphocyte function and either absence or reduction of the activity of each of these enzymes is a characteristic of certain immunodeficiency disorders. Among the acute leukemias, the activity of adenosine deaminase, which catalyzes the conversion of adenosine to inosine, is highest in ALL. The highest levels are found in T-cell ALL, which is also characterized by decreased 5′-nucleotidase and purine nucleoside phosphorylase activity, when compared with non-T-cell ALL.[209,216-219] Investigators have attempted to take advantage of the unique biochemical enzyme profile of T-cell ALL. 2′-Deoxycoformycin, a potent inhibitor of ADA, has demonstrated activity against ALL in clinical trials. This agent has also been evaluated as an *in vitro* bone marrow purging agent.[220,221]

The activity of another purine pathway enzyme, inosine monophosphate dehydrogenase, may be elevated in ALL and in AML when compared with normal bone marrow, although the significance of this finding is not clear.[209] Tyrosine protein kinase activity is reportedly low in both ALL and AML.[222] Whether this enzyme activity plays a role in the leukemic process is not clear; however, both the relationship of tyrosine kinase activity to several retroviral oncogenes and its increased activity in Ph[1] positive leukemias associated with c-*abl* translocation are intriguing.

Abnormalities in various lysozomal enzymes also have been observed in ALL. Isoenzyme I, one of three isoenzymes of the acid hydrolase hexosaminidase, is elevated in common and pre-B-cell ALL.[223] The ratio of isoenzyme I to isoenzyme A has been used as an adjunctive diagnostic tool by some investigators.[224] Abnormalities in other lysozomal hydrolases also occur.[209,225] Elevated serum lactate dehydrogenase (LDH) has been observed in ALL at diagnosis.[226,227] LDH levels reportedly normalize during remission and increase again at relapse. The degree of LDH elevation at diagnosis appears to correlate with prognosis (longer remission durations occurring in patients with lower initial serum LDH activity).[227]

Glucocorticoid receptors have been identified on leukemic lymphoblasts, and the distribution of glucocorticoid receptor number appears to differ significantly among each of the major immunologic subtypes of ALL. The greatest number of receptor sites per cell is seen in early pre-B-cell ALL, followed by pre-B-cell ALL. T-cell ALL has significantly lower receptor numbers, and B-cell ALL has the fewest.[228-231] Glucocorticoid receptor content correlates with sensitivity to steroid treatment *in vitro,* and there have been attempts to correlate receptor number with response to therapy *in vivo.* Lower receptor number has been associated with poorer responses to induction therapy and shorter remission durations.[130,231-234] It is not clear, however, whether glucocorticoid receptor number is an independent prognostic variable that provides more information than the technically less complex, more conventional prognostic factors (see Prognostic Factors).

Cytokinetics

H3-thymidine labeling indices and flow cytometry have been used to evaluate cell kinetics in newly diagnosed patients with ALL.[235-239] There appears to be a correlation between lymphoblast proliferative capacity and prognosis. Several investigators have shown a relationship between high proliferative activity and shorter remission duration, suggesting that the kinetic characteristics of leukemic blasts underlies the clinical responsiveness of children with ALL. It has even been suggested that both the H3-labeling index and the percentage of cells in S-phase are independent prognostic variables.[236-238] This has not

been a consistent finding, however, and awaits further confirmation. Lymphoblast proliferative activity has been demonstrated to vary with immunophenotype; higher H3-thymidine labeling indices and a higher percentage of cells in the S phase of the cell cycle have been observed in both T-cell ALL and B-cell ALL.[237,238]

Cytochemistry

Cytochemical stains have also been studied with respect to their ability to differentiate between various clinical and immunologic subsets of ALL. The PAS, acid phosphatase, beta glucuronidase, and acid alpha naphthyl acetate esterate reactions have all been evaluated in this regard.[240-248] Although some correlations appear strong (strong focal paranuclear acid phosphatase activity appears to be more common in T-cell disease), the practical use of this type of information is limited and has been supplanted by more sophisticated immunophenotyping techniques such as fluorescence activated cell sorting.

Clinical Presentation and Differential Diagnosis

ALL is a disorder characterized by the uncontrolled growth and proliferation of immature lymphoid cells. As such, the signs and symptoms of the child presenting with ALL reflect the degree of bone marrow infiltration with leukemic cells as well as the extent of extramedullary disease spread. The most common symptoms and clinical findings (Table 16-3) are usually manifestations of the underlying anemia, thrombocytopenia, and neutropenia, which reflect the failure of normal hematopoiesis. Pallor, fatigue, petechiae, purpura, bleeding, and fever are often present (see also Chap. 5). Lymphadenopathy, hepa-

Table 16-3
Clinical and Laboratory Features at Diagnosis in Children with ALL[168]

Clinical and/or Laboratory Feature	Percentage of Patients
Symptoms and Physical Findings	
Fever	61
Bleeding (*e.g.,* petechiae or purpura)	48
Bone pain	23
Lymphadenopathy	50
Splenomegaly	63
Hepatosplenomegaly	68
Laboratory Features	
Leukocyte count (mm³)	
<10,000	53
10,000–49,000	30
>50,000	17
Hemoglobin (g/dL)	
<7.0	43
7.0 to 11.0	45
>11.0	12
Platelet count (mm³)	
<20,000	28
20,000–99,000	47
>100,000	25
Lymphoblast morphology	
L1	84
L2	15
L3	1

tomegaly, and splenomegaly are manifestations of extramedullary leukemic spread. Hepatosplenomegaly occurs in approximately two-thirds of the patients and is usually asymptomatic. Lymphadenopathy, usually painless, may be localized or generalized. The duration of symptoms in children presenting with ALL may vary from days to weeks, or in some cases, even months. Anorexia is common; significant weight loss is infrequent. Bone pain, particularly affecting the long bones, is common and reflects leukemic involvement of the periosteum and bone. Not infrequently, young children in particular present with a limp or refusal to walk. These symptoms and the presence of arthralgias, which may result from leukemic infiltration of a joint, may make the delineation between ALL and nonmalignant disorders such as juvenile rheumatoid arthritis and osteomyelitis difficult. Bone tenderness is frequently observed.

Signs or symptoms of central nervous system involvement rarely are present at the time of initial diagnosis.

A number of presenting clinical features and laboratory findings have prognostic importance. These are discussed more fully in the sections on Prognostic Factors and Treatment.

Because the child with ALL typically presents with various nonspecific symptoms, ALL may mimic a variety of nonmalignant conditions from which it must be differentiated (Table 16-4). These include infectious mononucleosis, idiopathic thrombocytopenic purpura, acute infectious lymphocytosis, pertussis and parapertussis, and certain viral illnesses (such as those resulting from cytomegalovirus and EBV), all of which may have similar features to their clinical presentation. ALL must also be differentiated from aplastic anemia, which usually presents with pancytopenia. Rarely, ALL itself may initially present with an aplastic picture.[249] Definitive diagnosis of ALL requires a bone marrow aspirate (see below).

Clinicians must also consider ALL among the differential diagnoses of patients presenting with hypereosinophilia. A number of cases have been reported of ALL occurring in association with symptomatic hypereosinophilia, and, in rare instances, eosinophilia has preceded the diagnosis of ALL by many months.[250] In symptomatic patients with eosinophilia, the classic findings of the hypereosinophilic syndrome (Loeffler's syndrome—hypereosinophilia, pulmonary infiltrates, cardiomegaly, and congestive failure) have been observed. The pathogenesis of ALL occurring with hypereosinophilia is not clear. A recent report indicates that some patients with this syndrome have a characteristic translocation t(5;14) (see Cytogenetics section).[251] ALL presenting with hypereo-

sinophilia must be differentiated from eosinophilic leukemia and ANLL presenting with hypereosinophilia. The latter also has a characteristic chromosomal abnormality (structural rearrangements of chromosome 16).[252]

Childhood ALL also must be distinguished from other pediatric malignancies that may present with bone marrow involvement, including neuroblastoma, rhabdomyosarcoma, retinoblastoma, and non-Hodgkin's lymphoma (see Chaps. 20, 25, 28, and 30). Neuroblastoma, in particular, may be difficult to distinguish morphologically, under light microscopy, from ALL, especially if typical neuroblastoma pseudorosettes are not present. Additional laboratory and clinical evaluation should permit differentiation of these two disorders (see Chap. 28).

Leukemia or Lymphoma?

Acute lymphoblastic leukemia and childhood non-Hodgkin's lymphoma are closely related disorders; distinguishing between the two is difficult (see also Chap. 20). Many patients who present with features "characteristic" of a lymphoma, such as an anterior mediastinal mass or massive lymphadenopathy, or both, have bone marrow involvement. Cytomorphologically, the malignant T cells of lymphoblastic lymphoma are indistinguishable from those of T-cell ALL, and those of Burkitt's lymphoma are similar to those from children with B-cell ALL. As noted previously (see Immunology/Molecular Biology section) B-cell ALL shares immunologic and molecular features of Burkitt's lymphoma and is considered to be a disseminated form of that disease. Most institutions treat patients with these B-cell disorders with similar chemotherapy regimens. The distinction between T-cell ALL and T-cell lymphoblastic lymphoma is also ill defined. There is some evidence that these disorders arise from different stages of T-cell differentiation and thus have immunophenotypes reflecting different stages of T-cell maturation (see Immunology/Molecular Biology section). Because this distinction does not apply in every case, however, it does not provide a reliable basis for delineating between the two diseases. Whether molecular phenotyping will eventually distinguish more definitively between these entities is not clear.

In the absence of more refined biologic criteria, the percentage of blasts in the bone marrow has been used to distinguish between T-cell ALL and T-cell non-Hodgkin's lymphoma. This arbitrary method is confounded by the fact that different criteria are used by different institutions and study groups. For some, greater than 25% blast cells in bone marrow signifies leukemia; for others, any evidence of abnormal bone marrow infiltration, regardless of percentage, is used to define leukemia. Because of these differences, meaningful comparison of treatment results obtained by different groups is often difficult.

Laboratory Findings

An elevated leukocyte count (>10,000/mm^3) occurs in approximately one-half of patients with ALL; in approximately one-fifth of patients, the initial leukocyte count is greater than 50,000/mm^3 (Table 16-3). An increased leukocyte count at diagnosis is the single most important predictor of prognosis in ALL (see Prognostic Factors). Neutropenia (<500 granulocytes/mm^3) is a frequent phenomenon and is associated with an increased risk of serious infection.[253] Anemia (hemoglobin <10 g/dL) is present in approximately 80% of patients at diagnosis. Even when the anemia is severe, the reticulocyte count is usually low and the erythrocytes usually manifest a normo-

---

Table 16-4
Differential Diagnosis of Childhood ALL

Nonmalignant conditions
  Juvenile rheumatoid arthritis
  Infectious mononucleosis
  Idiopathic thrombocytopenic purpura
  Pertussis; parapertussis
  Aplastic anemia
  Acute infectious lymphocytosis
Malignancies
  Neuroblastoma
  Lymphoma
  Retinoblastoma
  Rhabdomyosarcoma
Unusual Presentations
  Hypereosinophilic syndrome

cytic, normochromic pattern. Thrombocytopenia occurs in the majority of patients. Approximately three-fourths have fewer than 100,000 platelets/mm³. The severity and the degree of bleeding correlate with the degree of thrombocytopenia.²⁵⁴ Severe hemorrhage is rare with platelet counts less than 20,000/mm³, unless fever and infection (both of which can affect platelet survival) are present (see Chap. 38).²⁵⁴

To establish definitively the diagnosis of leukemia, a bone marrow aspirate is necessary. Although leukemia cells may be present in the peripheral blood at diagnosis, attempts to establish the diagnosis on the basis of morphologic assessment of these cells alone may be misleading. Under most circumstances, a bone marrow aspirate provides sufficient material to establish the diagnosis. Occasionally bone marrow biopsy may be required. Although the presence of greater than 5% lymphoblasts in the bone marrow indicates leukemia, most centers require a minimum of 25% blast cells before the diagnosis is confirmed. Usually most cells in the marrow aspirate are leukemic lymphoblasts. In some cases, for example to differentiate an aplastic presentation of ALL from aplastic anemia, multiple aspirates and biopsy specimens may be required. Definitive diagnosis of the specific leukemic cell type requires morphologic assessment of bone marrow aspirate slides stained with Romanofsky dye as well as the use of several special histochemical stains, including myeloperoxidase or Sudan black, periodic acid-Schiff (PAS), and nonspecific esterase stains using the naphthol-ASD chloroacetate substrates.²⁵⁵ Use of these special stains usually will permit differentiation of ALL from ANLL and establish a definitive diagnosis. (Table 16-5). In addition, most centers routinely perform TdT analysis and immunophenotyping using a panel of monoclonal antibodies. Cytogenetic analysis may reveal evidence of chromosomal translocations typical for certain subtypes of ALL (e.g., t(8;14) in B-cell ALL) and provide important prognostic information (see Cytogenetics and Prognostic Factors). Despite the use of these various techniques, rare cases may defy classification and may require a more extensive work-up (e.g., ultrastructural cytochemistry, molecular phenotyping).

Other Laboratory Studies and Findings

In addition to the hematologic abnormalities discussed above, other abnormal laboratory studies frequently are observed in the newly diagnosed patient with ALL. Many of these findings

Table 16-5
Morphologic and Cytochemical Characteristics of ALL and ANLL*

	ALL	ANLL
Nuclear: cytoplasmic ratio	High	Low
Nuclear chromatin	Clumped	Spongy
Nucleoli	0–2	2–5
Granules	Absent	Present
Auer rods	Absent	May be present
Cytoplasm	Blue	Blue-gray
Cytochemical reaction		
Peroxidase	−	+
Sudan black B	−	+
Periodic-acid-schiff	+	−
Naphthol ASD chloroacetate esterase	−	+
α-Naphthyl acetate esterase	−	+

* General characteristics that help differentiate ALL from ANLL are summarized. Wide morphologic variation exists in both groups, and more refined criteria to define subgroups (e.g., FAB classification) exist.

and their degree of abnormality reflect the leukemic cell burden, the extent of extramedullary spread, or the excessive proliferation and destruction of the leukemic cells.

Increased serum uric acid levels, most common in patients with a large leukemic cell burden, reflect increased anabolism and catabolism of purines. A major complication of hyperuricemia is uric acid nephropathy and subsequent renal failure. The risk of this complication is greatest immediately after the start of treatment, when leukemic cell lysis releases large quantities of uric acid. Adequate hydration and alkalinization, together with the use of the xanthine oxidase inhibitor allopurinol, are required to prevent this potentially serious complication (see Supportive Care section and Chap. 37).

The kidneys may be infiltrated with leukemic cells and are often enlarged at diagnosis.²⁵²,²⁵⁶,²⁵⁷ Various metabolic abnormalities may be encountered, including elevated serum levels of calcium, potassium, and phosphorus. These abnormalities are more frequent in patients with extensive lymphadenopathy and hepatosplenomegaly and high initial leukocyte counts.²⁵⁸ Hypercalcemia may be due to leukemic infiltration of bone, although release of a parathormone-like substance from lymphoblasts has been reported.²⁵⁷ Elevated serum phosphorous levels can occur as a result of leukemic cell lysis and may induce hypocalcemia.²⁶⁰

Liver function abnormalities, presumably the result of leukemic spread, may be present but usually are mild. Leukemic cell lysis may also be associated with elevation of serum LDH, which is reported to correlate with prognosis, as noted previously. Chest radiographs will reveal an anterior mediastinal mass in approximately 5% to 10% of newly diagnosed patients (Table 16-3). A variety of other radiologic changes may be demonstrated. Bony changes, particularly in the long bones, are most frequent and include transverse radiolucent metaphyseal bands, periosteal elevation with reactive subperiosteal cortical thickening, osteolytic lesions, diffuse osteoporosis, and transverse metaphyseal "growth arrest" lines.²⁶¹⁻²⁶⁴ Radiologically documented bone changes may be seen in patients who are asymptomatic. When bone pain is present, it usually rapidly disappears following initiation of antileukemic therapy. Rarely ALL may masquerade as osteomyelitis.²⁶⁵

Serum immunoglobulin levels are low in approximately 30% of children with ALL at diagnosis, as noted earlier.²⁶⁶⁻²⁶⁸ In some studies, decreased immunoglobulin levels have been linked to a poor prognosis (see Prognostic Factors).²⁶⁶,²⁶⁸ The presence of low serum immunoglobulins at diagnosis in most cases probably reflects relative depletion of normal mature B cells or mature T helper cells, or both, in the circulation.²⁶⁹,²⁷⁰ Impairment of terminal differentiation of normal peripheral B cells into immunoglobulin secreting cells or suppression of immunoglobulin biosynthesis by suppressor T lymphoblasts are other possible explanations.²⁶⁹

Clotting abnormalities may be observed in some patients with ALL. In general, however, coagulation abnormalities are not a feature of the disease, and at presentation disseminated intravascular coagulation is encountered infrequently (see Chap. 38). A more frequently recognized complication of treatment is a coagulopathy primarily associated with L-asparaginase therapy that may produce thromboses or hemorrhagic infarction, or both.²⁷¹

Patterns of Spread

Extramedullary spread is a common feature in ALL. Extramedullary involvement may be readily detectable clinically or demonstrable solely by invasive diagnostic procedures. Extramedullary disease is significant both because it may cause morbidity at a localized site and because extramedullary relapse frequently heralds a subsequent bone marrow relapse, presumably the result of "seeding" from the involved extramedullary site to the bone marrow. Most patients have some evidence of extramedullary involvement at diagnosis (Table 16-3); however, the incidence of occult extramedullary spread in patients assumed clinically to be in complete remission is difficult to determine. Estimates vary from approximately one-third to one-half of these patients.[272–275] The most common sites of extramedullary spread are the CNS, testes, liver, kidneys, and spleen. From a clinical point of view, the two most important sites of extramedullary relapse are the CNS and the testes.

CNS Leukemia

The potential clinical impact of central nervous system leukemia did not become fully apparent until the late 1950s and early 1960s when, with improved systemic therapy and longer survival, the CNS became the most frequent site of initial relapse.[276] By the late 1960s and early 1970s, the incidence of CNS leukemia in some studies ranged as high as 80% to 85%.[276,277] The significance of this increasing rate of CNS relapse was twofold. First, CNS leukemia was difficult to eradicate. CNS remissions of short duration could be obtained in most patients; however, CNS recurrence was frequent.[278] Second, and perhaps more important, in most cases CNS relapse was followed by the rapid development of bone marrow disease.[279] Thus, most patients who experienced a CNS relapse during this pre-CNS preventive therapy era died as a consequence of marrow relapse rather than from the morbidity of CNS disease. The recognition of this phenomenon led to the development of effective CNS preventive therapy (see CNS preventive therapy section), a strategy in part responsible for the improved prognosis of children with this disease (see treatment section).

CNS leukemia is believed to develop as a result of leukemic metastases. Cytogenetic studies have documented karyotypic similarity between leukemic cells in the cerebrospinal fluid (CSF) and those in the bone marrow.[280] CNS leukemia may result from hematogenous spread of circulating lymph leukemia cells or by direct extension from involved cranial bone marrow.[281–283] Hematogenous spread may occur by means of migration of circulating leukemia cells through venous endothelium or as a consequence of petechial hemorrhages in cases of severe thrombocytopenia.[285] The choroid plexus, with its abundant capillaries, is often a frequent site of leukemic infiltration.[286] Direct extension of leukemia cells may occur from involved cranial bone marrow through bridging veins to the superficial arachnoid. Eventually infiltration of the deep arachnoid, the pia-glial membrane, and the brain parenchyma itself may occur. Direct spread from involved cranial bone marrow may also occur along the perineurium.

The signs and symptoms of clinically overt central nervous system leukemia are shown in Table 16-6. Headache, nausea and vomiting, lethargy, irritability, nuchal rigidity, papilledema, and other manifestations of increased intracranial pressure are most commonly seen. Cranial nerve involvement, most frequently of the seventh, third, fourth, and sixth cranial nerves, may be present either together with other symptoms or as an isolated event. Facial nerve and ocular motor palsies, infiltration of the optic nerve, and eighth cranial nerve involvement, manifested by hyperacusis, tinnitus, vertigo, and even deafness, may occur. More unusual manifestations of CNS leukemia include the hypothalamic-obesity syndrome in which destruction of the ventromedial nucleus of the hypothalamus, the "satiety center," results in hyperphagia, pathologic weight gain, and diabetes insipidus. Both leukemic subdural involvement and spinal epidural leukemia occurring with spinal cord compression have been observed. Intracranial leukemic cell masses occur relatively rarely. The numerous neurologic manifestations of overt CNS leukemia make it obligatory for clinicians to investigate exhaustively any neurologic signs or symptoms in the child with ALL to exclude the possibility of CNS leukemia.

CNS leukemia at diagnosis occurs in less than 5% of children with ALL.[287] With the institution of central nervous system preventive therapy, surveillance lumbar punctures have become an integral part of most ALL treatment protocols (see CNS preventive therapy section). As a consequence, symptomatic CNS disease is observed less frequently and the diagnosis is most often made in the asymptomatic patient. Diagnosis of CNS leukemia requires cytologic confirmation of the presence of leukemic cells in cerebrospinal fluid (CSF). CSF obtained by lumbar puncture must be examined after cytocentrifugation of the CSF specimen, a procedure that concentrates the leukemic cells and increases diagnostic sensitivity.[288–290] In symptomatic patients, CSF pressure is usually increased; elevated CSF protein and hypoglycorrhachia are frequent. With CNS leukemia now more frequently diagnosed in the asymptomatic patient, CSF pressure may be normal, CSF leukemic cell counts relatively low, and abnormalities in CSF chemistry determinations absent. In situations in which a significant pleocytosis is

Table 16-6
Signs and Symptoms in CNS Leukemia[287,288]

Description	Percentage	Symptoms and Signs
Increased intracranial pressure	95	Vomiting, headache, papilledema, lethargy, irritability, seizures, coma
Visual disturbances	30	Diplopia, blurred vision, blindness, photophobia
Myelopathy	23	Nuchal rigidity, hemiparesis, paraplegia
Cranial nerve palsy	20	Seventh and sixth nerve palsies
Hypothalamic syndrome	10	Hyperphagia, sleep–wake disturbances, pathologic weight gain
Vertigo	10	
Auditory disturbances	9	
Cerebellar dysfunction	6	
Hallucinations	5	
Hyperpnea	5	
Proptosis	5	

absent, the diagnosis of meningeal leukemia is more problematic.[291] In suspicious but equivocal cases, TdT determination has been advocated as a means of aiding confirmation of the diagnosis. The use of monoclonal antibodies to identify lymphoblasts in CSF may also have some value.[292,293] The role of other techniques, such as determination of CSF beta-2-microglobulin, is more controversial and requires further evaluation.[294–296] Other studies such as cranial computed tomography, electroencephalography, plain skull radiographs, and nuclear magnetic resonance imaging may occasionally be abnormal with CNS leukemia but usually are not. None of these methods have sufficient diagnostic sensitivity to be indicated for routine use. Analysis of initial clinical features in children who have developed CNS leukemia has identified certain factors that correlate with an increased risk for the development of this complication (see CNS preventive therapy section).

Testicular Leukemia

The incidence of testicular leukemia paradoxically has increased with the improved survival of children with ALL; clinically evident testicular relapse was extremely rare before the development of effective chemotherapy.[297] More recently, in males receiving chemotherapy, the incidence of overt testicular relapse has been reported to be as high as 16%, although in most studies the actual figure is probably less than 10%.[298–305] In boys who have successfully completed a full course of chemotherapy for their disease, testicular recurrence is a principal cause of late relapse. The reported incidence in this setting varies but has been as high as 40%.[306]

Clinically overt testicular involvement usually appears as painless testicular enlargement, most often unilateral. The diagnosis must be established by testicular biopsy. Bilateral biopsies are indicated because disease is frequently present in the contralateral testis.[303] Wedge biopsies are the preferred diagnostic technique because this procedure may be less likely to result in sampling error. Histologic interpretation, however, is frequently difficult. The incidence of false-negative results from testicular biopsies obtained during maintenance therapy or before stopping all treatment approaches 10%.[307–309] Although it has been suggested that TdT determination may help discriminate between leukemic lymphoblasts and reactive lymphocytes in equivocal biopsy specimens, a recent study suggests that TdT determination is not helpful.[310] When testicular relapse occurs, disease is usually located within the interstitial spaces; in advanced cases, leukemic infiltration of the tubules may occur.[299] A number of factors are associated with an increased likelihood of developing testicular relapse, including a high initial leukocyte count (>20,000/mm^3), T-cell disease, prominent lymphadenopathy and splenomegaly, and significant thrombocytopenia (<30,000/mm^3).[270,311–315] The time to development of overt testicular relapse ranges from 2 months to several years.[301,316,317]

Clinically demonstrable testicular disease is rarely present at initial diagnosis; however, occult testicular disease has been diagnosed in one-fourth of newly diagnosed boys.[318] Occult testicular involvement also occurs in up to 15% of asymptomatic boys undergoing biopsies after completion of an apparently successful course of chemotherapy.[297,298,301,312] This phenomenon is consistent with the relatively high incidence of late overt testicular relapses. The possibility of occult testicular disease, together with the fact that testicular recurrence is frequently followed by systemic relapse, had prompted a number of centers to advocate routine bilateral testicular biopsy either at some time during maintenance chemotherapy or immediately before its cessation. This practice recently has been

questioned because of studies indicating that testicular biopsies at diagnosis, after induction, during maintenance, or before cessation of chemotherapy are associated with a significant false-negative rate and do not accurately predict eventual testicular relapse.[302,307,308,319] Noninvasive screening for occult testicular disease using transscrotal ultrasound and magnetic resonance imaging has been evaluated; neither technique is sufficiently sensitive.[320]

The occurrence of isolated testicular relapse has led many to consider the testes, like the CNS, a "sanctuary site" of extramedullary disease. It has been suggested that leukemic testes are protected from therapeutic concentrations of systemically administered chemotherapy by the "blood–testes" barrier.[321] Animal studies, however, have questioned the role of the blood–testes barrier in the development of testicular leukemia.[322] The demonstration of leukemia in the liver, spleen, and abdominal lymph nodes in patients studied by exploratory laparotomy at the time of a presumed isolated testicular relapse raises the possibility that "isolated" testicular relapse may be a misnomer, an artifact related to the relative ease with which overt disease is clinically detected at this anatomic site.[323] Some evidence indicates that the incidence of testicular relapse may be somewhat lower on treatment regimens using more aggressive therapy, although this contention has been questioned recently.[302,323–325]

Although some investigators have advocated the use of prophylactic testicular radiation to prevent testicular disease, this approach has not gained wide acceptance.[326,327] The treatment of overt testicular leukemia is discussed later (see Treatment of Relapse section).

Other Extramedullary Sites

The CNS and testes are the most common sites of clinically overt extramedullary disease; however, leukemic infiltration of other anatomic sites does occur. Involvement of the liver, spleen, and lymph nodes is common at initial presentation; their size is an indirect measure of the degree of leukemic cell burden. Studies have documented a clear-cut relationship between the extent of disease in these sites and either remission duration or survival; massive enlargement is associated with a poor prognosis. Mediastinal involvement at diagnosis is frequent in patients with T-cell ALL. Although some studies have suggested that the presence of a mediastinal mass has significant prognostic import, it does not appear to be an independent prognostic variable. The prognostic impact of extramedullary involvement is discussed more fully in the section on prognostic factors.

The clinical incidence of kidney involvement is difficult to assess. It is usually manifest by kidney enlargement rather than by renal dysfunction. Kidney enlargement may be noted at initial clinical presentation or during the course of the disease. Intravenous pyelography typically reveals enlargement with cortical thickening; caliceal changes may also be present. Renal involvement requiring therapeutic intervention is rare. When treatment is required, radiotherapy is used.

Leukemic infiltrates can occur throughout the gastrointestinal tract; large bowel involvement is most frequent. In some patients, a necrotizing enteropathy may develop in which necrosis and hemorrhage of the bowel wall result in perforation. This complication, which commonly involves the cecum, is known as "typhlitis" (see Chap. 37).

Isolated pulmonary relapse has been reported.[328] Leukemic pulmonary infiltrates may be present as an interstitial pneumonia, difficult to distinguish from other interstitial pneumonias that occur in children with ALL (*e.g., Pneumo-*

cystis carinii, cytomegalovirus). The infiltrates may be diffuse or nodular and can produce alveolocapillary block.[329] Lung biopsy is required to make a definitive diagnosis.

The ovary is an infrequent site of localized relapse; when it occurs other pelvic tissues, including the uterus and vagina, may be involved.[330,331] Localized relapse in the eye may involve the iris, hypopyon, or the anterior chamber.[332,333]

Prognostic Factors

Certain clinical and laboratory features exhibited at diagnosis by patients with ALL have prognostic value, providing a potential means of delineating patients into subgroups, which predictably will have relatively favorable or unfavorable prognoses. The identification of prognostic factors has become an essential element in the design and analysis of current therapeutic trials. It is now common practice for treatment centers to assign patients on the basis of prognostic factors into different risk groups and to "tailor" specific treatment accordingly. A variety of characteristics have been proposed as having prognostic import, including the initial leukocyte count, age at diagnosis, sex, race, cytogenetics, degree of organomegaly and lymphadenopathy, presence of a mediastinal mass, initial hemoglobin level, initial platelet count, FAB morphologic classification, immunophenotype, serum immunoglobulin levels, the presence or absence of CNS disease at diagnosis, the length of time to attainment of remission status (*e.g.,* the response to initial treatment), glucocorticoid receptor levels, and HLA type.[127,133,167,169,334–348]

The initial leukocyte count is perhaps the most significant prognostic factor identified, in most cases retaining its importance after adjustment for other criteria. There is a linear relationship between the initial leukocyte count and outcome in children with ALL: children with the highest leukocyte counts tend to have a poor prognosis (Fig. 16-7).[167,169,334,341,346–352] Although there is no sharp dividing line, patients with an initial leukocyte count more than 50,000 cells/mm³ (approximately 20% of children with ALL) are universally recognized as having

a particularly poor prognosis. The biological basis for higher initial leukocyte counts is unclear, although there are definite associations between certain biological features and this pattern of presentation. Patients with T-cell ALL often have a high initial leukocyte count and, as noted previously, increased lymphoblast proliferative activity (see Cytokinetics Section).

There is also a clear relationship between age at diagnosis and outcome.[339,340,346,349] Patients who are young when diagnosed (<2 years of age) and older patients (>10 years of age) have a relatively poor prognosis in contrast to children in the intermediate age group (Fig. 16-8). The worst prognosis is for infants younger than 1 year of age at diagnosis.[353] This group of patients are the most resistant to current treatment, and their disease appears to be biologically unique (see below).

Because they are readily available and relatively independent predictors of prognosis, the parameters of initial leukocyte count and age at diagnosis are commonly used and appear to provide a reliable basis for patient stratification.

As noted in Table 16-7, a number of other features have been associated with prognosis. Their relative value as prognostic indicators varies. When subjected to appropriate multivariate statistical analysis, many of these features function as dependent rather than independent prognostic determinants. A recent review of the relative order of significance and interrelationship of prognostic factors for event-free survival in a group of 1419 patients treated between 1978 and 1983 by the Childrens Cancer Study Group revealed that the factors of greatest multivariate prognostic importance were the initial leukocyte count, sex (girls have a more favorable prognosis), presence of a mediastinal mass, day 14 marrow response, age, platelet count, hepatomegaly, and FAB morphologic subtype (Table 16-8).[169,354] The prognostic importance of many of these variables was associated with the initial leukocyte count.[169]

The predictive value of the various prognostic factors may differ among different studies; not all studies confirm the same factors as having prognostic significance. In addition to initial leukocyte count and age, a number of other features have prognostic import in most studies. Cytogenetic abnormalities, both in chromosomal number and structure, appear to have

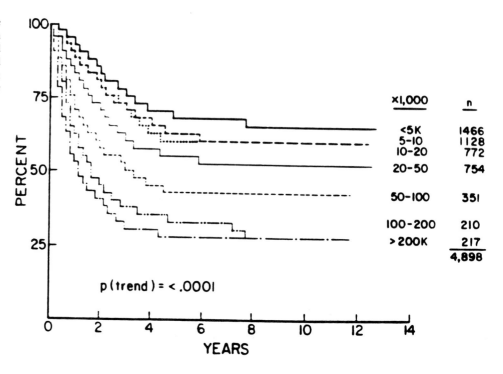

FIGURE 16-7. Continuous complete remission duration of children with acute lymphoblastic leukemia, stratified according to their initial white blood cell count. Data from 4898 children treated by the Childrens Cancer Study Group.[340]

×1,000	n
<5K	1466
5-10	1128
10-20	772
20-50	754
50-100	351
100-200	210
>200K	217
	4,898

p(trend) = <.0001

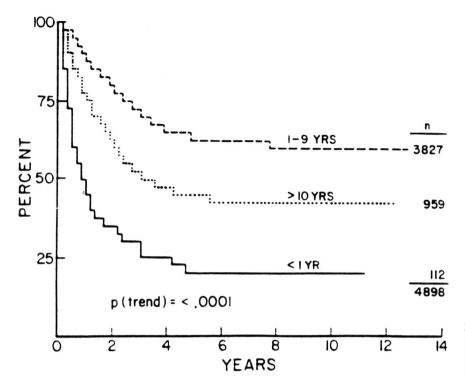

FIGURE 16-8. Continuous, complete remission duration of children with acute lymphoblastic leukemia stratified into three age groups. Data from Childrens Cancer Study Group.[340]

Table 16-7
Factors That Have Been Associated with Prognosis in ALL

Initial WBC
Age at diagnosis
Sex
Cytogenetics/ploidy
Immunologic subtype
FAB morphology
Mediastinal mass
Organomegaly and lymphadenopathy
Hemoglobin level
Race
Platelet count
Serum immunoglobulins
Rapidity of leukemic cytoreduction

prognostic significance. As noted previously, patients with hyperdiploidy tend to have a relatively favorable prognosis; hypodiploidy or pseudodiploidy are associated with a poor outcome, and individuals with near-haploid ALL have the worst prognosis. Certain chromosomal translocations are also associated with a high rate of induction failure and early relapse. These include the t(8;14), t(9;22), t(4;11), and t(1;19) abnormalities (see Cytogenetics Section).

The prognostic importance of sex has been well documented.[339,340,349,354-356] In most studies, girls have a better prognosis than boys. This appears to be due both to the development of testicular relapse and to the higher incidence of T-cell disease, which tends to occur in older males who often present with a high initial leukocyte count, significant organomegaly, lymphadenopathy, and mediastinal masses.

Immunophenotype also correlates with prognosis (see Immunology/Molecular Biology section). Patiénts with B-cell ALL have the worst prognosis. T-cell ALL has been associated with a poor prognosis in many studies, although after adjustment for its association with the initial leukocyte count, which has greater prognostic influence, T-cell phenotype does not appear to be a strong independent predictor of treatment outcome. Several studies have demonstrated that with more intensive treatment protocols, the prognostic influence of T-cell phenotype is lost.[166,167,169,342,357]

Among the patients with B-cell precursor ALL, those with the early pre-B-cell phenotype have a more favorable prognosis compared with patients with the pre-B-cell phenotype (Fig. 16-4), who fare relatively poorly. Among the total group of B-cell-precursor ALL patients, those whose blast cells are CALLA positive have a more favorable outcome. CALLA negativity occurs in approximately 10% of patients with pre-B-cell or early pre-B-cell ALL.[358] Among patients with early pre-B-cell ALL, those who are CALLA negative have a higher induction failure rate; CALLA negativity is not, however, an adverse prognostic factor in early pre-B-cell ALL once complete remission has been obtained.[358] A relatively small subset of patients with T-cell ALL have leukemia cells that express the CALLA antigen.[344] Preliminary data suggest that patients with CALLA negative T-cell ALL are less likely to achieve a complete remission and tend to have a decreased duration of event-free survival when compared with CALLA positive T-cell ALL patients.[344]

Low serum levels of IgG have been shown to be a strong predictor of induction failure. Low levels of all three of the major immunoglobulin subclasses (IgG, IgM, and IgA) are associated with a poor event-free survival; the association with low IgM levels appears to be most significant (see Clinical Presentation/Differential Diagnosis section).[266-268] A relationship between certain human leukocyte antigen (HLA) types and prognosis has been suggested but has not been demonstrated in most major studies.[266,343,350,359]

The association of FAB morphologic classification with prognosis was addressed earlier. The association of the L3 subtype with B-cell ALL, a diagnosis that carries an exceptionally poor prognosis, is well accepted. The relative value of distinguishing between the L1 and L2 subtypes as an indicator of prognosis is somewhat controversial.

Table 16-8
Relative Importance of Factors Predicting Event-Free Survival
(As Determined by Multivariate Analysis* with All Variables Considered Simultaneously)

Order of Importance	Standardized χ^2 Value	p Value
1 WBC	39.3	<0.0001
2 Sex	37.4	<0.0001
3 Mediastinal mass	21.6	<0.0001
4 Day 14 bone marrow	18.3	<0.0001
5 Age	14.2	<0.0001
6 Platelet count	13.1	0.0003
4 Liver size	11.7	0.0006
8 FAB blast morphology	7.8	0.0004
9 Serum IgM level	2.8	0.09
10 Spleen size	1.7	0.19
11 Serum IgA level	1.0	0.31
12 Race	0.9	0.34
13 Serum IgG level	0.4	0.42
14 T-Cell leukemia	0.3	0.53
15 Hemoglobin level	0.3	0.58
16 Node enlargement	0.3	0.59
17 CNS leukemia at diagnosis	0.1	0.72

* Analysis of 1490 patients on Childrens Cancer Study Group studies between 1978 and 1983.[169] Chromosomal studies were not performed. As noted in the text, chromosomal status has been shown by others to be an important indicator of prognosis.

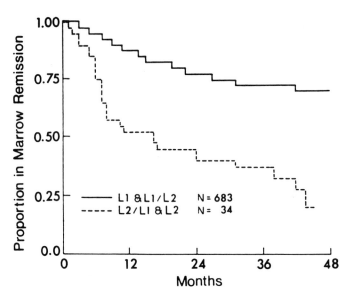

FIGURE 16-9. FAB morphologic classification and hematologic remission duration ($p = 0.001$). L1 = 90% to 100% L1 lymphoblasts; L1/L2 = 75% to 89% L1 lymphoblasts; L2/L1 = 50% to 74% L1 lymphoblasts; L2 = >50% L2 lymphoblasts.[127]

Numerous investigators have demonstrated an association between the L2 morphologic subtype and a poor prognosis (Fig. 16-9).[127–129,132–135,169,344,356] The Childrens Cancer Study Group analyzed the classification of 3500 ALL patients according to FAB morphologic criteria and found that patients with 10% or more L2 lymphoblasts had less favorable outcomes than did those with predominantly L1 blast morphology.[133,169] The effect of L2 morphology was found to be continuous in that patient outcome was worse as the percentage of L2 lymphoblasts increased over 10%. In that study, blast cell morphology was found to be an independent variable not linked to the initial leukocyte count. Similar findings have recently been reported by other investigators.[344,356] In contrast, other studies, while confirming the association between L2 morphology and an increased likelihood of induction failure, have determined that the impact of L2 morphology on duration of complete remission is either greatly reduced or not significant after adjusting for other independent risk factors.[167,345] In one study, L2 morphology failed to add prognostic information after leukocyte count, age, race, and leukemic cell ploidy were considered.[167] Some of the differences noted among various studies may be related to differences in the methods of FAB classification.

An unusual morphologic variant of ALL is the so-called hand-mirror cell variant in which leukemic cells are characterized by a hand-mirror shape caused by the presence of a handle-shaped uropod.[360,361] The characteristic amoeboid configuration of these lymphoblasts is believed to reflect their dynamic state of cell motility. Earlier, small studies suggested that hand-mirror cells either had no prognostic import or were associated with a favorable outcome.[361,362] A more recent, larger study indicates that this morphologic variant, which occurs in up to 5% of childhood ALL cases, is an independent, unfavorable prognostic factor associated with a significantly

worse disease-free survival rate.[363] The suggestion that the hand-mirror cell variant is associated with the development of CNS disease has not been confirmed.[364,365]

Race is also a prognostic factor. Black children reportedly have a significantly lower remission induction rate and higher rate of marrow recurrence.[366–368] The difference in prognosis for blacks does not appear to be related to differences in medical care.[368] It appears that blacks with ALL present with a different constitution of clinical and biologic features, including a higher frequency of elevated initial leukocyte counts, mediastinal masses, and L2 morphology. The "common ALL" phenotype and hyperdiploidy appear to be less frequent in black ALL patients.[366] Some studies indicate that the predictive value of race becomes insignificant when adjustment is made for the initial leukocyte count; others, however, demonstrate that the predictive value of race cannot be totally accounted for by initial leukocyte count, FAB morphologic characteristics, or leukemic cell ploidy.[167,354,366] The hypothesis that differences in drug absorption or metabolism may contribute to the poor outcome of black children with ALL has not been substantiated.[366]

In addition to the initial leukocyte count, leukemic cell burden can be assessed indirectly by evaluation of the extent of extramedullary disease. In particular, the degree of hepatosplenomegaly and lymphadenopathy have each emerged in most univariate analyses as important prognostic variables.[169] Although multivariate analyses reveal that some of these features, like a mediastinal mass, may tend to be dependent variables in some studies, others retain significance even after adjustment for other independent features such as the initial leukocyte count.[169] The German Berlin–Frankfurt–Münster (BFM) study group uses a measurement of hepatosplenomegaly along with the initial leukocyte count to compute a "risk factor index," which forms a basis for treatment stratification according to prognosis.[369]

The predictive value of most prognostic factors is lost with progressively increasing periods of complete remission. Patients in complete remission for 18 to 24 months after diagnosis have an equal probability of subsequent relapse regardless of their sex, age at presentation, or initial leukocyte count. With the exception of the male sex, and possibly older age (>10 years), other recognized adverse prognostic factors lose their significance by 2 years from diagnosis and no longer influence the chance for long-term survival.[356,370]

Although not a true "front-end" factor, response to treatment has emerged as an important indicator of prognosis. Patients who do not achieve remission status within the usual 4- to 6-week induction period have a high rate of relapse and shortened survival.[350] In one study, patients who eventually achieved a complete remission but had less than 50% cytoreduction 5 days after the administration of induction therapy had a significantly reduced remission duration and survival rate (Fig. 16-10). Recent studies indicate that the presence of residual leukemia on the day 14 bone marrow is an important predictor of event-free survival (see Induction Therapy section).[169,350,366]

Infants

Infants (younger than 12 months of age) with ALL have an extremely poor prognosis, worse than virtually any other patient group (see Chap. 12).[353,372–376] Although their complete remission rate appears to be no different from that of older children, the event-free survival and disease-free survival for patients in this age group are extremely poor, the consequence of a high incidence of early bone marrow and extramedullary relapse (Fig. 16-8). The CNS relapse rate in infants is also inordinately high. Infants with ALL have an increased incidence of poor prognostic features, including high initial leukocyte count, massive organomegaly, thrombocytopenia, CNS leukemia at diagnosis, hypogammaglobulinemia, and failure to achieve complete remission status by day 14 of induction therapy.[353] ALL of infancy also appears to be biologically unique. Leukemic cells from these children generally arise from a very early stage of commitment to B-cell differentiation. They usually express the HLA-DR antigen, are CALLA negative, and do not express mature B-cell antigens.[377] Studies of immunoglobulin and T-cell receptor gene configuration in these patients confirm that ALL in infancy represents an earlier stage of B-cell development than that found in the B-cell precursor ALL of older children. Infants with ALL also have an increased incidence of chromosomal abnormalities that are associated with a poor prognosis; structural abnormalities of chromosome 11—for example, t(4;11) and t(q32)—are frequently observed.[353,372] Because of their exceedingly poor prognosis, infants are often stratified separately for treatment purposes.

As the above discussion illustrates, certain prognostic factors (*e.g.,* age at diagnosis, initial leukocyte count) are universally accepted as having prognostic import, but there are conflicting data regarding the value of many of the other variables studied (*e.g.,* FAB morphologic classification, immunophenotype). Differences in the predictive ability of these prognostic factors, which themselves have been retrospectively derived from different studies, may be due to a number of factors, including variation in the representativeness and size of the patient population in a study and differences in the treatment received. Ultimately, the type of treatment received is the most important prognostic factor. Several recent studies have demonstrated that the impact of a number of prognostic features (*e.g.,* immunophenotype) can be overridden by the use of intensive therapeutic strategies.[166,167,169,342,357] In analyzing the predictive value of any prognostic factor, it is important to perform a multifactorial analysis to determine the relative degree to which it functions as an independent variable.

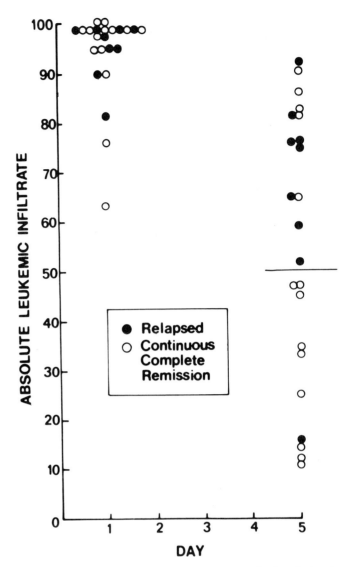

FIGURE 16-10. Effect of induction treatment on absolute leukemic infiltrate of bone marrow, measured before induction therapy and on Day 5 of therapy. All patients eventually achieved complete remission, however, continuous remission status correlated with the extent of initial cytoreduction. Relapse occurred in only 10% of patients who had greater than 50% cytoreduction at 5 days. Median follow-up in this study was 42 months.[371]

As noted above, most current treatment protocols assign patients into different risk groups on the basis of prognostic factors, treating each group according to the relative risk of failure. Patients with poor risk features are generally treated with more aggressive, intensive therapy. Patients in more favorable risk categories, with a higher likelihood of cure, are treated with therapy designed to be equally effective but less intensive, in the hope of avoiding potentially deleterious treatment-associated sequelae. No single method of stratifying patients according to prognostic variables is universally accepted. The initial leukocyte count and age at diagnosis form the basis for most current methods of prognostic stratification. In recent years, efforts to refine the criteria upon which risk group assignment is made, and thus the homogeneity of patient subgroups defined, have led to the development of more sophisticated systems of "staging" children with ALL. The Childrens Cancer Study Group, for example, uses an algorithm based on initial leukocyte count, age at diagnosis, FAB classification, extent of bulk disease, E-rosette positivity, sex, and platelet count to assign patients to one of five currently recognized risk groups (Fig. 16-11).[169,347] In addition to defining three risk categories (good, average, and poor), primarily on the basis of initial leukocyte count, age at diagnosis, and FAB morphology, this system identifies two additional risk group categories—one for infants, the other for patients with lymphomatous features at presentation.[347,378]

Patients whose clinical and laboratory features identify them as having this lymphomatous presentation (leukemia/lymphoma syndrome), while not a homogeneous population, have a relatively poor event-free survival and a high risk for extramedullary relapse, particularly CNS recurrence.[378,379] As noted above, the West German BFM study group has used a risk factor index based on initial leukocyte count and degree of organomegaly to stratify patients into four different treatment groups. In current BFM studies, lack of responsiveness to initial corticosteroid therapy is used to define a population thought to be at a particularly high risk for early treatment failure.[380]

Although stratification of ALL patients into different prognostic subgroups is a mechanism for optimizing treatment for patients with relatively homogeneous prognostic features, this strategy has confounded comparative analysis of treatment results. Many therapeutic trials use different eligibility criteria, making comparison of end results difficult. A recent international workshop has suggested the use of common criteria both for defining the population of ALL patients included in a particular clinical trial and for reporting treatment results.[348]

TREATMENT

The recognition that ALL is a heterogeneous disease and that children can be stratified into various risk groups has had a profound impact on therapy. In general, treatment has become more sophisticated. Although combination chemotherapy remains the primary therapy, it is no longer appropriate, in the context of current biological knowledge, for all patients with ALL to be treated on a uniform or "standard" treatment regimen. The initial evaluation of the patient with ALL requires sophisticated laboratory techniques to derive appropriate cytogenetic, immunologic, or biochemical information. Paradoxically, as understanding of the disease has improved, the approach to its treatment has become more complex. This circumstance, coupled with the increased intensity of many current treatment regimens, emphasizes the need for children with ALL to be treated in established pediatric cancer centers where state-of-the-art treatment protocols are available. Although the specific approaches to patients in various risk groups may be somewhat different, all modern ALL treatment regimens divide therapy into four main treatment elements: remission induction, CNS preventive therapy, consolidation, treatment, and maintenance therapy.

Induction Therapy

The initial aim of ALL treatment is induction of remission. By definition, individuals in remission have no evidence of leukemia when evaluated both by physical examination and by hematologic assessment of bone marrow and peripheral blood. Peripheral blood values must be within the defined range of normality and the bone marrow must be of normal cellularity with less than 5% lymphoblasts.[381,382] Complete remission status also assumes the absence of detectable CNS or extramedullary disease.[383] Achievement of complete remission is a basic premise of antileukemic treatment and a known prerequisite for prolonged survival.[384] In clinically overt ALL, the leukemic cell burden is estimated to be approximately 10^{12} leukemic cells (Fig. 16-12).[385,386] To induce a complete remission, chemotherapy must reduce the total number of leukemic cells by 99% (10^{-2}) such that fewer than 10^{10} blasts are present.[387]

FIGURE 16-11. Outcome of 2600 children with acute lymphoblastic leukemia stratified according to prognostic groups and treated by the Childrens Cancer Study Group. (Reproduced with permission of WA Bleyer, MD, and H Sather, PhD.)

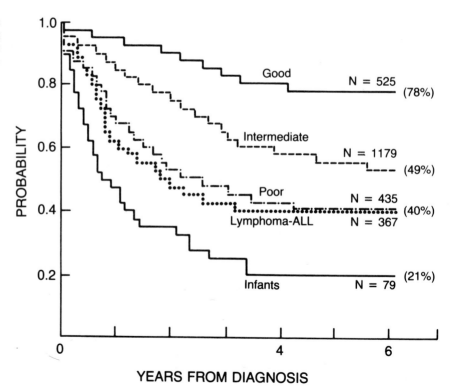

In the 1950s and 1960s, a number of single agents were identified that could induce complete remissions in patients with ALL. However, because of relatively low remission induction rates and the likelihood of early relapse, the concept was conceived of using combination chemotherapy, multiple agents with different modes of action, to produce an additive antileukemic effect. Although the basic two-drug combination of vincristine and prednisone induces remissions in approximately 85% of children with ALL, the addition of L-asparaginase or an anthracycline, or both, improve the remission induction rate to approximately 95%.[324,350,388–393] The addition of a third agent to vincristine and prednisone also significantly prolongs remission duration.[371,394–395] Whether the added leukemic cell kill theoretically achieved by including a fourth induction agent leads to improvement in remission duration is controversial. The results of one randomized study indicated that adding daunomycin to the three-drug combination of vincristine, prednisone, and L-asparaginase did not improve remission duration.[396] More recent protocols, however, using this four-drug induction combination, together with intensive consolidation and maintenance therapy, uniformly demonstrate improved overall remission duration, even in high risk patients.[166,335,369,397,398]

Because the use of a fourth drug or additional drugs may increase the incidence of toxicity during induction therapy, most centers reserve the use of drug combinations employing four or more agents for patients in the higher risk groups.

As noted earlier (see Prognostic Factors section), the rapidity of leukemic cytoreduction during induction has prognostic significance. Patients in whom less than 50% cytoreduction has occurred by day 5 or who have more than 25% lymphoblasts in their day 14 bone marrow, have a significantly reduced remission duration and survival rate. (Fig. 16-10). Patients not in complete remission at the end of the usual induction period have a shortened survival and, if a remission is eventually achieved, a higher rate of relapse.[350]

In addition to high initial leukocyte count and unfavorable age at diagnosis, a number of other features have been associated with a lower remission induction rate, including L3 morphology, CNS disease at diagnosis, chromosomal translocations, low serum IgG, and an M3 bone marrow on day 14.[185,187,192,350] Although one study reported a lower remission

induction rate in infants, this has not been a uniform finding.[346,372,375,376] Failure of induction therapy is a relatively rare event, occurring in less than 5% of children with ALL treated on most current regimens. Improved supportive care has decreased mortality during induction therapy to approximately 3% or less.[270]

Central Nervous System Preventive Therapy

The recognition that CNS recurrence constituted a major obstacle to overall treatment success (see CNS leukemia section) stimulated efforts to prevent CNS disease. The concept of CNS preventive therapy is based on the premise that the central nervous system acts as a "sanctuary site" where leukemic cells, undetected at diagnosis, reside protected by the blood–brain barrier from therapeutic concentrations of systemically administered antileukemic therapy. According to this view, the prevention of CNS relapse is more appropriately termed "presymptomatic CNS therapy" rather than "CNS prophylaxis," a term widely used.

One of the earliest attempts at CNS preventive therapy involved the administration of intrathecal aminopterin or methotrexate immediately following the attainment of complete remission and monthly thereafter. Although this approach significantly lowered the rate of CNS relapse compared with an untreated control group, the overall remission durations in this group of patients were too brief to allow definitive conclusions regarding the benefits of CNS preventive therapy.[384] Another early study demonstrated that administration of a single intrathecal methotrexate dose delayed the onset of CNS leukemia but ultimately did not decrease its frequency.[399]

The use of CNS irradiation as CNS preventive therapy was based on murine studies that demonstrated cures of L1210 leukemia when cranial radiation was added to systemic treatment with cyclophosphamide.[400] The first documentation of the value of CNS preventive therapy in patients evolved from a series of studies performed at the St. Jude Children's Research Hospital (Table 16-9). Although relatively low doses of craniospinal radiation (500 or 1200 cGy) demonstrated no preventive effect (studies I–III), the administration of either 2400 cGy cranial radiation plus five concurrent doses of intrathecal

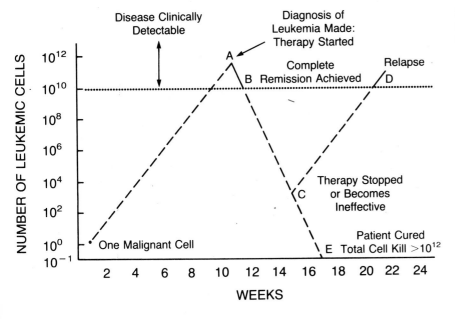

FIGURE 16-12. Schematic representation of the results of therapy in a patient with leukemia. (Adapted from Reference 597)

methotrexate or 2400 cGy of craniospinal radiation alone (studies V–VII) reduced the incidence of CNS relapse to approximately 10%.[401,402] Because craniospinal radiation is associated with excessive myelosuppression and retards spinal growth, cranial radiation (2400 cGy) plus intrathecal methotrexate became the standard form of CNS preventive therapy. Although this approach was universally adopted in the 1970s, concerns subsequently developed regarding the apparent adverse effects of this form of CNS preventive therapy. The identification of CT brain scan abnormalities, altered intellectual and psychomotor function, and neuroendocrine dysfunction in patients treated with 2400 cGy cranial radiation and intrathecal chemotherapy prompted a reappraisal of CNS preventive therapy strategies and stimulated the search for alternative methods of CNS preventive therapy that are equally effective but less toxic (see Late Effects section).[403–422] The use of a lower dose of cranial radiation (1800 cGy) with intrathecal methotrexate appears to be as effective as 2400 cGy and is currently used in most CNS preventive therapy regimens that continue to administer cranial radiation.[288,357,423] It is not yet clear, however, whether the use of 1800 cGy plus intrathecal methotrexate will result in a lower incidence of adverse CNS sequelae.[421,423] In addition to using lower doses of radiation, other approaches are being evaluated in the search for alternative methods of CNS preventive therapy. These include the use of triple intrathecal chemotherapy (methotrexate, cytarabine, and hydrocortisone) alone; intermediate dose methotrexate, either alone or with concomitant intrathecal methotrexate; intrathecal methotrexate alone; or high dose systemic methotrexate.[423–432]

A variety of patient characteristics are associated with an increased risk of CNS leukemia, including a high initial leukocyte count, T-cell disease, very young age, thrombocytopenia, lymphadenopathy, hepatomegaly or splenomegaly, and black race.[288] The highest rates of CNS relapse occur in infants and patients with extremely high leukocyte counts or lymphomatous presentations.[288,353,379] Although no single factor or group of factors can predict with absolute certainty whether an individual patient is not at risk for CNS relapse, the recognition that patients differ in their risk for developing CNS leukemia has permitted investigators to successfully modify CNS preventive therapy accordingly. It is now clear that cranial radiation is not necessary for patients with a good prognosis; intrathecal methotrexate alone, given periodically throughout maintenance chemotherapy, provides adequate CNS preventive therapy for these patients.[288] Maintenance intrathecal triple chemotherapy, the combination of intrathecal and moderate dose intravenous methotrexate, and high dose intravenous methotrexate alone all appear to provide equivalent protection to that offered by cranial radiation and intrathecal methotrexate for patients at an intermediate risk of CNS relapse.[424,426–428] For example, the Pediatric Oncology Group has used triple intrathecal chemotherapy (methotrexate, cytarabine, and hydrocortisone) during induction, consolidation, and in maintenance to prevent meningeal relapse. This approach appears to be as effective as 2400 cGy of cranial radiation plus intrathecal methotrexate in children with ALL without lymphomatous presentations or T-cell disease.[426] Whether intrathecal methotrexate alone, administered from the start of treatment throughout maintenance therapy, is equivalent to the use of 1800 cGy of cranial radiation plus intrathecal methotrexate is a question currently being studied in average risk patients by the Childrens Cancer Study Group.

The desirability of avoiding cranial radiation in CNS preventive therapy regimens derives from concerns that radiotherapy is in large part responsible for many of the long-term adverse CNS sequelae observed in patients treated with cranial radiation and IT chemotherapy (see Late Effects section). Currently, however, patients at low and intermediate risks of CNS relapse may receive equally effective therapy with the alternatives to radiation noted above, but most centers continue to administer cranial radiation plus intrathecal methotrexate to patients at high risk for CNS relapse. Preliminary results of a recent randomized study comparing intravenous high dose methotrexate infusions alone to cranial radiation plus intrathecal methotrexate demonstrated equivalent CNS protection in both average and high risk patients, suggesting that the use of cranial radiation for high risk patients may eventually be replaced by aggressive chemotherapeutic approaches.[424] In that study, a progressive decline in verbal IQ and significantly impaired academic achievement were observed in patients treated with cranial radiation (2400 cGy) plus intrathecal

Table 16-9
Prevention of CNS Leukemia—Early Studies of St. Jude Children's Research Hospital

Study and Year	Preventive CNS Therapy	Number of Patients	Initial CNS Relapse (%)	Time at Risk*
I–III (1962–65)	500–1200 rad craniospinal	37	40	19 months
IV (1965–67)	None	42	60	19 months
V (1967–68)	2400 rad cranial + intrathecal methotrexate	31	10	10 years
VI (1968–70)	2400 rad craniospinal or None	45	4	8 years
		49	67	4 years
VII (1970–71)	2400 rad cranial + intrathecal methotrexate or 2400 rad craniospinal	45	7	
		49	6	

(Adapted and modified from References 598, 599, and 600)

* Efficacy of preventive therapy also depends on time at risk for this complication. This figure indicates median duration of initial hematologic remission for each group.

methotrexate.[433,434] In view of the various therapeutic strategies currently in use, additional clinical trials evaluating both efficacy and relative toxicity are needed before the optimal mode of CNS preventive therapy for each of the various patient prognostic subgroups can be identified.

In addition to delayed forms of neurotoxicity (discussed in the section on Late Effects of Antileukemic Therapy), CNS preventive therapy may be associated with acute or subacute neurotoxic sequelae. Both intrathecal methotrexate and cranial radiation alone can produce a wide spectrum of neurotoxicities.[435] Intrathecal methotrexate may be associated with an acute arachnoiditis that occurs 12 to 24 hours after intrathecal injection and is characterized by headaches, nausea and vomiting, meningismus, and other signs of increased intracranial pressure.[436,437] These reactions are usually not severe, are self-limited, and have been reduced in frequency by the use of an intrathecal methotrexate dosing schedule based on the relationship of age to CNS volume (see Chap. 9).[432] A subacute form of methotrexate neurotoxicity characterized by encephalopathy and myelopathy has been observed more rarely.[438,439] In addition, from 5 to 7 weeks after cranial radiation some patients develop a subacute neurotoxic reaction characterized by somnolence, lethargy, anorexia, fever, and irritability. This "somnolence syndrome," which may be accompanied by EEG abnormalities and CSF pleocytosis, usually reverses within 1 to 3 weeks.[440,441] It is unclear whether the somnolence syndrome correlates with the development of other late sequelae seen with CNS preventive therapy employing cranial radiation. Secondary CNS tumors have been reported in some children with ALL following CNS preventive therapy with cranial radiation and intrathecal therapy (see Late Effects Section).

Consolidation and Maintenance Therapy

Once complete remission has been achieved, additional maintenance or continuation therapy is required. Early clinical studies demonstrated that without additional therapy, most patients will relapse within a median of 1 to 2 months, the actual time of unmaintained remission varying with the intensity and duration of induction therapy.[442,443] As shown in Figure 16-12, patients in complete remission theoretically have a leukemic cell burden in the range of 10^{10}. Thus, although successful induction may have produced a 99% (two log) or greater reduction in the number of leukemia cells, a significant amount of additional therapy is necessary before the leukemia will be totally eradicated. The presence of occult leukemic disease during apparent remission has been documented by biopsy (see Patterns of Spread section). In addition, at relapse, lymphoblasts often demonstrate chromosomal and immunoglobulin gene rearrangement patterns identical to those obtained at the time of original diagnosis.[110,444–446] Several mechanisms have been proposed to explain this persistence of leukemic cells during remission: the development of biochemical drug resistance, the residence of leukemic cells in physiologic or pharmacologic "sanctuary" sites (e.g., CNS and testes), and maintenance of a population of leukemia cells in a kinetic state (G0) in which they are less vulnerable to chemotherapy.

To be effective in preventing relapse, maintenance therapy must not only suppress leukemic growth, but also provide continuing leukemic cytoreduction without permitting the emergence of a drug-resistant clone.

In early clinical studies, a variety of single agents were evaluated as maintenance agents.[384,447–450] Drugs particularly effective during induction were found not to be optimal for maintenance therapy. For example, continued treatment with vincristine and prednisone did not prolong remission duration. In contrast, maintenance treatment with methotrexate and 6-mercaptopurine substantially prolonged remission length.[393,449,451–453] The combination of methotrexate and 6-mercaptopurine, administered continuously, has been used most widely and constitutes the principal element in most maintenance therapy regimens. The optimal schedule of administration of these two drugs is different. Methotrexate is more effective administered intermittently, whereas daily 6-mercaptopurine appears optimal. In recent years, various combinations have been studied in which other agents are added to the standard 6-mercaptopurine and methotrexate regimen. Addition of intermittent pulses of vincristine and prednisone to 6-mercaptopurine and methotrexate maintenance chemotherapy appears to have prolonged remission duration for some patients, although the value of this approach after intensive induction therapy is unclear.[454–459] Other approaches studied include repeated pulses of multidrug combinations and sequential, intensive multiagent therapy.[166,357,391,397,460,461] A recent study has suggested that weekly administration of L-asparaginase adds to the effectiveness of maintenance therapy.[461]

The choice of appropriate maintenance chemotherapy appears to differ according to risk group. Whereas 6-mercaptopurine and methotrexate may provide adequate maintenance therapy for certain low-risk patients, more intensive maintenance therapy appears to be more effective for high-risk patients.

Consolidation therapy, a period of intensified treatment administered immediately after remission induction, is now a common component of many therapy protocols, particularly those treating high-risk patients.[166,357,397,427,430,459,461–467] A number of these regimens use agents and schedules designed to minimize the development of drug cross-resistance. The evidence that intensification of this type has improved treatment success, even in patients with a poor prognosis, is substantial.[166,357,397,398,463,468–470] The West German BFM study group, using both intensive induction and consolidation and "reinduction" and "reconsolidation" phases of therapy early in maintenance, reports prolonged event-free survival in approximately 65% to 70% of patients, including those with high-risk features.[357,398,471] Similar results have been obtained in high-risk patients using a Childrens Cancer Study Group protocol that incorporates many of the features of the LSA-2 lymphoma regimen and uses alternating non-cross-resistant combination chemotherapy.[166] A regimen using periodic pulses of "reinduction-type" chemotherapy also has produced close to a 70% event-free survival in higher risk patients.[424]

Although the recent use of more intensive treatment regimens has been associated with a modest increase in therapy-associated toxicity, the advantages of such treatment, particularly for patients in the higher risk groups, are clear.

Drug dosage is an important factor in maintenance chemotherapy. The existence of a definite relationship between chemotherapy dose and therapeutic response in leukemia was originally documented in animal studies.[473] Its influence during maintenance was demonstrated in an early randomized study in which patients receiving chemotherapy with 6-mercaptopurine, methotrexate, and cyclophosphamide at full dose had significantly longer remission durations then did patients receiving therapy at one-half the dose.[474] Subsequent clinical studies have confirmed this finding.[472,473,475] The frequency of drug administration also appears to influence the length of remission.[472,476] Patients who receive maintenance therapy on a more continual rather than an interrupted schedule have longer remission durations.[472,475,476]

Recent studies of the clinical pharmacology of orally administered 6-mercaptopurine and methotrexate have documented that their bioavailability following oral administration may be limited and is highly variable, suggesting a possible explanation for treatment failures that occur during oral maintenance therapy with these agents (see Chap. 9).[477-479] Compliance problems also may adversely impact on the efficacy of maintenance therapy.[480] The possible problems associated with oral administration of 6-MP and methotrexate theoretically could be circumvented by parenteral administration. However, data regarding the relative effectiveness of parenteral versus oral maintenance therapy are conflicting. Results of a recent Medical Research Council leukemia trial (UKALL VII) indicated a significantly longer actuarial relapse-free survival for patients who received methotrexate intramuscularly compared with those given the drug orally.[481] In another study, which randomized children with non-T-cell ALL to receive methotrexate during maintenance either as a single oral dose or as an intramuscular injection, the route of administration appeared to have no real influence on the relapse rate.[482]

Duration of Treatment

The optimal length of maintenance chemotherapy has not been clearly defined. Most centers treat patients for a total of approximately 2.5 to 3 years. Data from several studies support this approach.[481,483-486] An early study by the Southwestern Oncology Group found no difference in the outcome of patients treated for 3 versus 6 years.[483] Two more recent randomized Childrens Cancer Study group studies also indicate no advantage for 5 years of maintenance over 3 years.[484,485] A study by the British Medical Research Council also examined the effect of variation in length of treatment on duration of remission and demonstrated that 19 months of therapy was less effective in preventing relapse than was 3 years of treatment.[486] The optimal duration of treatment for girls may be different than that for boys. A more recent MRC study demonstrated that 1.5 years of therapy was sufficient for girls but inadequate for boys.[487] The tendency for a greater percentage of males to relapse following cessation of chemotherapy was observed in a long-term follow-up study of patients treated on the Childrens Cancer Study Group 141 protocol. In that study, patients in complete continuous remission for 3 years were randomized to discontinue therapy, to receive a 4-week course of reinduction chemotherapy and then discontinue therapy, or to continue therapy for a total of 5 years. No significant difference was noted in disease-free survival between the different treatment regimens. However, a higher incidence of late relapse occurred among males, even after excluding patients with occult testicular disease.[485] This is consistent with other studies which, as noted previously, have demonstrated that sex is a significant predictor of late relapse, even when isolated testicular relapse is excluded.[304,313,488]

Investigators at the St. Jude Children's Research Hospital have demonstrated that after successful completion of 2.5 years of therapy, approximately 80% of patients will remain disease-free.[489] Most of the 20% of patients who eventually relapsed did so in the first year off therapy. In the second through the fourth year after cessation of chemotherapy, the risk of relapse was only about 2% to 3% per year. Recurrence after 4 years from the cessation of therapy was not encountered.[489] Similar results were observed in a recent study from Great Britain that concluded that patients alive 6 years from diagnosis without relapse have a high likelihood of prolonged survival and cure.[482]

It is likely that the intensity of therapy has a bearing on the optimal duration of therapy. The current practice of treating patients for 2.5 to 3 years of maintenance chemotherapy is derived from studies in which patients were treated with a variety of chemotherapeutic regimens, many of which incorporated fewer agents and were less intensive than those currently in use. For this reason, conclusions about the duration of maintenance based on those studies may not be directly applicable to current treatment programs. Whether patients receiving more intensive therapy earlier in their course of treatment ultimately will require a shorter overall duration of therapy is an important question for future study. In this regard, the experience of the West German BFM study group, which has used a maintenance regimen of 2 years' duration with excellent results, is of interest.

TREATMENT OF RELAPSE

Bone Marrow Relapse

Bone marrow relapse is the principal form of treatment failure in patients with ALL. Depending on the type of chemotherapy used, complete remissions can be induced in most patients who experience an initial marrow relapse. The combination of vincristine, prednisone, and L-asparaginase produces complete remissions in approximately 70% to 75% of patients treated for an initial bone marrow relapse; the addition of daunorubicin increases the reinduction rate to from 80% to 90%.[490-498] Administration of an intensive course of cytarabine and VM-26 reportedly induces complete remissions in approximately one-third of patients not achieving complete responses with the highly effective four-drug reinduction regimen of L-asparaginase, vincristine, daunorubicin, and prednisone.[498,499]

A number of factors influence the ability to achieve a second remission. Patients who relapse at some point after having successfully completed a previous chemotherapy regimen are more likely to achieve a second complete remission if the relapse occurs while they are receiving maintenance chemotherapy.[500-503] For patients who relapse on therapy, the prognosis for remission induction is less favorable and is influenced by the length of their first remission; longer initial remissions are associated with a greater likelihood of successful remission induction.[497,503-505] Other factors purported to predict for less successful second remission induction, such as a high initial leukocyte count or unfavorable age at time of original diagnosis, appear to be less important and have not been reported consistently to have predictive value.[497,503,506] The nature and intensity of previous therapy appears to be important; patients previously treated with suboptimal primary induction and maintenance therapy have a higher reinduction rate.[507-510] In patients experiencing multiple relapses, the reinduction rate with most regimens declines with each successive relapse, presumably a result of the development of drug resistance.[490,493,511]

The eventual outcome of children who achieve a second remission is influenced by a variety of factors. Patients relapsing after completion of a previous chemotherapy regimen have a better chance both of achieving and maintaining a prolonged second remission than do those relapsing while receiving chemotherapy.[500-502,512] The overall survival of patients who relapse off therapy is better than that for patients who relapse on therapy (Fig. 16-13). In addition, the prognosis of patients who relapse off treatment is inversely proportional to the interval from the time of discontinuation of therapy to relapse. Children whose first relapse occurs later than 6 months after cessation of therapy have significantly longer second remis-

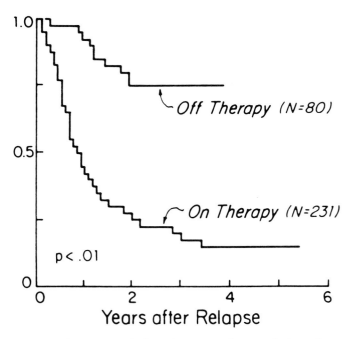

FIGURE 16-13. Survival after relapse according to whether relapse occurred during therapy or after its discontinuation. Initial treatment was the same for all patients.[512]

sions.[500-502] A recent analysis of 165 patients who suffered an initial marrow relapse off treatment indicated that, with respect to survival, the primary dividing point was 3 months after discontinuation of therapy.[512] In that study, patients who relapsed between 3 and 6 months after cessation of treatment had a relatively good prognosis, similar to those who relapsed between 6 and 12 months after therapy. The best overall survival was observed in patients who had relapsed more than 12 months after discontinuation of therapy (Fig. 16-13).

The length of previous remission duration also appears to be a factor with predictive value for remission duration.[497,513-515] Children whose initial bone marrow remission was greater than 18 months have a significantly better prognosis than do those with shorter first remission durations. A recent review of 600 children in second remission treated with chemotherapy documented prolonged second remissions in less than 5% of children who relapsed within 18 months of achieving first remission. In contrast, sustained second remissions were observed in approximately 25% of children whose relapse occurred after 18 months.[513] In addition to duration of first remission, other features have been found in some studies to be associated with the likelihood of achieving a prolonged second remission, including a low leukocyte count (<20,000/mm³) at initial diagnosis and relapse and unfavorable age (<2 years or >10 years) at initial diagnosis.[497,503]

A bone marrow relapse portends a poor prognosis for most patients. With aggressive treatment, however, long-term second remissions are being achieved in an increasing number of relapsed patients.[497,502,516-519] A small percentage will successfully complete a second course of chemotherapy and continue in prolonged, disease-free remission. As noted above, more favorable outcomes are likely to be observed in patients who have relapsed at some point after completion of their initial chemotherapy. The results of recent studies suggest that prolonged second remissions (>2 years) can be obtained with aggressive chemotherapy in approximately 10% to 25% of pa-

tients who relapse on therapy and in up to one-third of patients who relapse after elective cessation of therapy.[497,502,513,516,517,519]

The chemotherapeutic approach to the relapsed patient should include aggressive multiple drug reinduction therapy followed by intensive systemic consolidation and maintenance chemotherapy. The need for a second course of CNS preventive therapy for patients in second remission is well established; without it nearly 50% will suffer a CNS relapse.[507] In patients who received cranial radiation as part of their initial CNS prophylaxis, intrathecal chemotherapy is usually employed as the second form of CNS preventive therapy (see CNS Relapse section).[497,502]

Bone Marrow Transplantation

The use of bone marrow transplantation as a therapeutic approach for ALL patients who have suffered a bone marrow relapse has increased in recent years. This approach, discussed in detail in Chapter 48, involves the administration of intensive cytoreductive therapy, usually employing total body irradiation and high-dose chemotherapy in doses lethal to normal bone marrow, and subsequent hematopoietic "rescue" with intravenously infused bone marrow obtained from an appropriately compatible donor. The initial interest in bone marrow transplantation was generated to some degree by the generally unfavorable treatment results obtained in relapsed patients treated with conventional chemotherapy. The earliest experiences with bone marrow transplantation involved multiply relapsed patients, refractory to conventional chemotherapy, who were usually transplanted in relapse. Results in this group of patients generally were disappointing; approximately 10% of those receiving marrow from an HLA-matched sibling achieved a prolonged disease-free survival.[520,521] Significantly better results are obtained in patients transplanted during remission than in those transplanted either in relapse or in partial remission. In an earlier study, the Seattle transplant group demonstrated that 27% of patients transplanted in second or subsequent remission and 15% of patients transplanted in relapse were alive and disease-free, with a minimum follow-up of more than 5 years.[522] A more recent analysis, from the same institution, of children in second remission who received a marrow transplant from an HLA-identical sibling demonstrated that with a median follow-up of more than 4 years, the probability of disease-free survival was 40%, with a plateau extending from 2.5 to 10.4 years.[523] Similar results, from studies with shorter follow-up, have been reported by other centers.[524-527] Recently the Memorial Sloan–Kettering Cancer Center reported an estimated disease-free survival at 5 years of 64% in a group of children in second remission, transplanted from HLA-identical sibling donors using preparative therapy with hyperfractionated total-body irradiation followed by cyclophosphamide (Fig. 16-14).

In most studies patients transplanted in earlier remissions fare significantly better than patients transplanted after multiple relapses.[513,528] The length of first remission and the presence of high risk features at diagnosis also have been reported to be predictive factors.[513] Patients with shorter initial remissions and those with high-risk features at diagnosis fare poorer when transplanted in second remission. Nevertheless, for patients in second bone-marrow remission who relapsed initially while undergoing chemotherapy (or within 3 months of its completion) and who have a histocompatible sibling, bone marrow transplantation is considered the treatment of choice.[512,513,528]

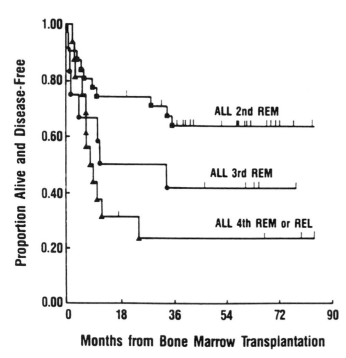

FIGURE 16-14. Disease-free survival of children receiving transplants for ALL. Patients were stratified according to their disease status at the time of transplantation. REM = remission; REL = relapse. (Brochstein JA, Kernan NA, Groshen S et al: Allogeneic bone marrow transplantation after hyperfractionated total body irradiation and cyclophosphamide in children with acute leukemia. N Engl J Med 317:1618–1624, 1987)

At present, however, routine allogeneic bone-marrow transplantation is limited to the approximately one-third of relapsed patients who have an HLA-identical sibling. In an effort to circumvent this problem, a number of alternative approaches are being studied, including transplantation from partially matched, related donors or from unrelated donors matched with the help of comprehensive tissue typing banks. Techniques such as T-cell depletion of donor marrow (to decrease the incidence and severity of graft-versus-host disease) and the development of improved cytoreductive regimens may make transplantation from histoincompatible donors more feasible in the future.

Studies of autologous transplantation are currently in progress. In this approach, pretransplant "preparative" therapy is followed by infusion of remission marrow treated with either drugs or leukemia-specific monoclonal antibodies to remove potentially "contaminating" leukemic cells. A recent study from the University of Minnesota, with a relatively short follow-up period, indicated that relapse-free survival can be achieved in approximately 20% of relapsed patients using this strategy.[529]

Extramedullary Relapse

CNS Relapse

Despite the success of CNS preventive therapy in dramatically reducing the incidence of CNS recurrence, CNS relapse remains a significant cause of treatment failure in ALL. CNS relapse may occur either as an isolated event or together with a bone marrow relapse or recurrence at another extramedullary

site, such as the testes. Currently CNS recurrence is observed in less than 10% of patients. The outcome for patients after CNS relapse is generally poor. Although CNS remissions can be induced in greater than 90% of patients, the median duration of remissions is usually relatively short, ranging from 1 to 2 years. The majority of patients eventually encounter either a subsequent CNS relapse or a recurrence at other sites such as the bone marrow or testes, or both.[288,530,531] The most successful treatment regimens have used intrathecal chemotherapy for CNS remission induction followed by consolidation therapy with either craniospinal radiation or maintenance chemotherapy.[532–537] Intrathecal methotrexate alone induces CNS remissions in more than 90% of patients; however, unless followed by maintenance intrathecal therapy or craniospinal irradiation, relapse occurs in 3 to 4 months.[278,539,540] Cranial radiation alone has little value in the treatment of overt CNS disease because it does not adequately treat sites of disease along the spinal axis. Further, when cranial radiation is combined with intrathecal methotrexate, it appears to increase toxicity and does not appear to prolong remission duration.[279,540,541] Craniospinal radiation alone, administered in adequate doses (2400 cGy), can induce complete remissions and prolong disease-free survival. Most centers, however, do not use craniospinal radiation alone because the higher spinal radiation dose required to achieve equivalent disease control, when intrathecal therapy is omitted, is associated with prolonged bone-marrow suppression. As discussed below, craniospinal radiation, at doses of 2400 to 3000 cGy to the cranial vault and 1200 to 1800 cGy to the spinal axis, is usually administered after successful induction of CSF remission.[288,532–536,542] Other therapeutic approaches studied include intrathecal chemotherapy with maintenance intrathecal therapy, intraventricular chemotherapy, and intraventricular chemotherapy with low-dose craniospinal irradiation.[288,533,535,543,545,546] A summary of the major randomized trials in overt CNS leukemia is shown in Table 16-10.

To some extent, the choice of therapy for the patient with overt CNS leukemia is guided by the type of CNS preventive therapy received previously. For example, approximately one-third of patients whose initial CNS preventive therapy did not include cranial radiation will achieve prolonged disease-free survival when craniospinal irradiation is administered following reinduction of CSF remission at the time of an initial CNS relapse.[530,534] In contrast, the role of craniospinal radiation to treat CNS recurrence in a patient who originally received cranial radiation as part of CNS preventive therapy is less clear. Results from the British Medical Research Council Concord and UKALL I trials demonstrated a continuous complete remission rate of less than 10% in such patients.[534] More recently, other investigators have demonstrated substantially better results with this approach.[535] However, craniospinal radiation administered in this setting is known to pose a significantly greater risk for delayed neurotoxicity.[535,547]

A number of attempts have been made to improve on the use of intrathecal methotrexate. "Triple therapy" consisting of simultaneously administered intrathecal cytarabine, hydrocortisone, and methotrexate has been advocated but, on careful review, has been shown to produce remission durations similar to those achieved with methotrexate alone.[288] The use of intraventricular chemotherapy, administered by means of an intraventricular subcutaneous reservoir, has been evaluated. This approach more completely distributes drug within the CNS, minimizes patient discomfort, and avoids the problems of inadequate delivery of drug into the CSF which may occur with unsuccessful lumbar punctures. Studies comparing this approach have demonstrated longer remission durations and fewer CNS relapses with intraventricular than with intralumbar therapy.[547,548]

Table 16-10
Randomized Trials in Overt CNS Leukemia[287,288]

Trial	Year	Reference	Number of Patients	Randomization*	Median Remission Duration (months)	p Value
1	1971	278	47	IT M → Maintenance IT M / Maintenance IV BCNU / No maintenance	16 / 3 / 4	<0.01
2	1973	540	31	IT M + maintenance IT M → Cr 24 Gy / 0 Gy	4 / >8	<0.05
3	1975	601	66	Craniospinal 20–25 Gy / IT M × 8 / IT M + maintenance IT M	7 / 4 / 8	0.041 / 0.001
4	1976	534	17	IT M → Cr 25 Gy + spinal 10 Gy / Cr 25 Gy	>24 / 4	<0.01
5	1975	602	32	IT M/DXM → Maintenance IT M/DXM / Maintenance radiocolloid	18 / 12	NS
6	1977	533	65	IT + maintenance IT → M/HC/A / M/HC	16 / 12	NS
7	1977	603	68	IT M/A/HC / IT A/HC IT M/HC → Maintenance + IT TT	15 / 13	NS
8	1978	547	18	Induction + maintenance intraventricular M → Single dose / C × T	11 / 12	NS
9	1985	536	49	IT M/A/HC → Cr 24 Gy / Cr 24 Gy + spinal 14 Gy	12–24 / 24–36	<0.02

* M, methotrexate; A, ara-C; DXM, dexamethasone; HC, hydrocortisone; IT TT, "triple therapy" with M + A + HC; NS, not significant; C × T, concentration × time; CR, cranial radiation.

Several other treatment approaches have been advocated to control meningeal leukemia. High-dose systemic methotrexate infusions will induce CSF remissions in the majority of patients.[549] The feasibility or effectiveness of this approach in maintaining CNS remissions is not known and its applicability may be limited, particularly in patients receiving CNS irradiation, because of concerns about delayed neurotoxicity.[288,546] Systemic high-dose cytarabine also has been demonstrated to produce remissions in patients with overt CNS leukemia.[550,551] Its use, however, may be limited by its attendant myelosuppression and neurotoxic potential. New intrathecal agents are also being developed. Preliminary results of an ongoing phase I–II study of intrathecal diaziquone (AZQ) indicate that this agent can produce complete CSF remissions in patients with refractory CNS leukemia.[552]

A number of factors, in addition to therapy, influence the outcome after a CNS recurrence. Patients with a low initial leukocyte count (<20,000/mm^3) who received CNS preventive therapy that did not include cranial radiation or who developed their CNS relapse a relatively long period after their original diagnosis have a better prognosis following CNS recurrence.[512,553,554] Children whose initial relapse was a CNS relapse that occurred after all chemotherapy had been completed have the best overall prognosis. In those who have isolated CNS relapses on therapy, survival is inversely proportional to the interval from discontinuation of therapy to relapse.[288,512]

As noted previously, an isolated CNS relapse frequently precedes a bone marrow recurrence. It has been hypothesized that this phenomenon results from "re-seeding" of the bone marrow by leukemic cells from the CNS. Alternatively it has been suggested that CNS relapse is merely an early harbinger of more widespread disease, indicating an increased likelihood of relapsing in other sites, such as the bone marrow.[542,554] In any case, because CNS relapse often precedes marrow relapse, administration of additional systemic "reinforcement" chemotherapy at the time of an isolated CNS relapse is advocated. Many centers administer reinduction chemotherapy similar to that given for a systemic recurrence.[542]

Testicular Relapse

Optimal therapy for testicular relapse includes both the administration of local radiotherapy and the use of systemic chemotherapy. Radiation dose appears to be a crucial factor in local control. Doses less than 1200 cGy are generally suboptimal; doses of 2400 cGy to both testes have been considered adequate.[298,555] Reports of local recurrence in patients treated with 2400 cGy, however, suggest that higher doses may be more optimal.[556] Bilateral testicular radiotherapy is indicated for all patients; unilateral treatment may be followed by relapse in the contralateral testis.[301,321] Radiation therapy adversely affects normal testicular function. Sterility is an expected consequence at the radiation doses used.[298,557,558] Recent studies also indicate that testicular endocrine function may be impaired at doses of 2400 cGy. Elevated follicle stimulating hormone (FSH) and luteinizing hormone (LH) levels, decreased testosterone levels, and delayed sexual maturation have all been observed following gonadal radiation. For this reason, such patients must be carefully followed up for signs of delayed sexual maturation and may require androgen and replacement therapy.[559-561]

The impact of a testicular relapse on prognosis depends on whether it was overt (clinically detectable) or occult (detected on routine testicular biopsy) and whether the recurrence was an isolated event or accompanied by a simultaneous hematologic relapse.[301,512] The prognosis is better when the relapse is occult or occurs as an isolated event.[301] Isolated testicular relapse is observed more frequently than with a concurrent bone marrow relapse, although, as noted previously (see Patterns of Spread section), many patients who present with isolated testicular relapses probably have occult intraabdominal disease. Isolated testicular relapse frequently heralds a systemic relapse.[298,299,301,316] Consequently, when an isolated testicular relapse is diagnosed, treatment must include intensification of systemic therapy in addition to bilateral testicular radiation. Most centers "reinduce" patients who suffer an overt testicular relapse with intensive systemic chemotherapy. This strategy has dramatically improved the prognosis for patients with testicular relapse.[303,562-565]

Other Sites of Relapse

Recurrence of leukemia may occasionally occur at other sites (*e.g.,* ovary, eye). If feasible, the appropriate treatment should include local measures for disease control (*e.g.,* radiation therapy) and intensification of systemic chemotherapy.

LATE EFFECTS OF ALL TREATMENT

The improved survival of children with ALL has focused attention on the late effects of antileukemic therapy. A number of adverse sequelae have been identified (see also Chap. 50).

Those affecting the central nervous system have been of greatest concern. Despite early reports suggesting that CNS preventive therapy with cranial radiation and intrathecal chemotherapy was devoid of significant long-term side effects, as noted earlier a large body of evidence has accumulated that indicates that this treatment may produce abnormal CT brain scans, impaired intellectual and psychomotor function, and neuroendocrine abnormalities.[421,546,566-577]

Four neuropathologically distinct forms of delayed CNS toxicity have been identified in patients with ALL: subacute leukoencephalopathy, mineralizing microangiopathy, subacute necrotizing leukomyelopathy, and cortical atrophy.[546]

Necrotizing leukoencephalopathy, a particularly severe form of delayed neurotoxicity, is relatively uncommon. It occurs most frequently in patients who have received large cumulative doses of cranial radiation and intrathecal and systemic methotrexate (*e.g.,* for treatment of recurrent meningeal leukemia).[578,579] Its development after CNS preventive therapy regimens that use conventional cranial radiation (2400 or 1800 cGy) and intrathecal methotrexate is relatively unusual. Leukoencephalopathy is characterized pathologically by multifocal demyelination. Patients with this syndrome may present with a variety of clinical findings that range from poor school performance and mild confusion to lethargy, dysarthria, dysphasia, ataxia, spasticity, and progressive dementia.[580-582]

Mineralizing microangiopathy, a degenerative mineralizing disorder of small vessels, is accompanied by dystrophic calcification of brain tissue, primarily gray matter.[572] It also occurs more frequently in patients who have received greater cumulative doses of cranial radiation and intravenous methotrexate, particularly in younger children (less than 6 years of age). The intracerebral calcifications of mineralizing microangiopathy can be demonstrated on CT scan.

Acute necrotizing myelopathy, characterized by necrotizing lesions of the spinal cord, is a pathologic finding first detected on routine autopsy examination of a group of children who died with ALL.[546,572] Its clinical significance and true incidence are unclear.

The most common histopathologic manifestation of CNS treatment, cortical atrophy, is a well-recognized delayed toxic-

FIGURE 16-15. Late development of intracerebral calcifications following CNS-preventive therapy with cranial radiation and intrathecal chemotherapy. **A.** Normal CT brain scan obtained 3 years after initiation of CNS treatment. **B.** Abnormal scan from the same patient obtained 7 years after the start of CNS preventive therapy demonstrating presence of intracerebral calcification.[418]

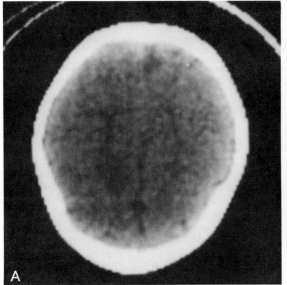
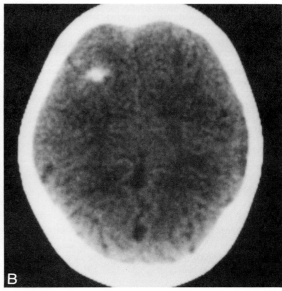

ity of whole brain radiation. Radiation produces multiple microscopic areas of focal necrosis that eventually cause the loss of cortical tissue and generalized cortical atrophy.[416,573]

A number of studies have demonstrated abnormal CT brain scans in asymptomatic ALL patients who have received CNS preventive therapy, particularly with cranial radiation and intrathecal chemotherapy. Abnormal CT scan findings include ventricular dilatation and widening of the subarachnoid spaces (cerebral cortical atrophy), decreased attenuation coefficient (hypodensity of white matter indicating localized edema or demyelination, or both), and intracerebral calcifications (representing mineralizing microangiography).[416] The incidence of these abnormalities appears to be related to the intensity of CNS preventive therapy. For example, the highest incidence of CT scan abnormalities occurred in patients who received 2400 cGy of cranial radiation plus maintenance intrathecal chemotherapy.[546] Although the eventual clinical significance of the CT brain scan changes observed in asymptomatic ALL patients who have received CNS preventive therapy is unknown, recent studies have documented a significant association between these abnormalities and neuropsychological dysfunction.[405,406,546] The observation that CT scan lesions may first appear as late as 7 years after initiation of CNS preventive therapy is of concern and emphasizes the importance of long-term CT scan follow-up examination (Fig. 16-15).[418]

Initial studies failed to reveal evidence of lasting behavioral or intellectual impairment in survivors of childhood ALL. Recent studies, however, using more sophisticated techniques have demonstrated significant functional deficits in both intellectual and perceptual motor function in some patients. In addition to significantly impaired academic achievement, decreased IQ scores, increased distractability, and abnormalities in memory and frontal lobe functions have been documented.[405,406,408-410,412,413,415,421,433,434,444,546] The confirmation of functional impairment of the CNS has been the major impetus behind the search for alternative approaches to CNS preventive therapy (see below and CNS Preventive Therapy section).

Neuroendocrine abnormalities, primarily involving the hypothalamic pituitary axis, also have been documented in children who have received cranial radiotherapy with CNS preventive therapy. The principal finding is decreased growth hormone output measured either by response to provocative stimuli or by analysis of basal pulsatile growth hormone secretion.[403,414,420] The incidence of impaired growth hormone responses to provocative stimuli may be as high as 50%, or even greater.[414,420] Blunted spontaneous basal pulsatile secretion of growth hormone is also a consistent finding in children with ALL who have received 2400 cGy of cranial radiation and intrathecal methotrexate (Fig. 16-16).[403]

Short stature occurs in some children with ALL, although there is disagreement as to its frequency.[420,546,574] In most children "catch-up growth" occurs after discontinuation of therapy; others have persistent short stature. Although abnormal growth hormone output resulting from cranial radiation may explain the short stature in some children, others have normal hypothalamic–pituitary function, suggesting that growth delay in children with ALL may be multifactorial.[403,420,546] Nevertheless, the development of short stature following cranial radiation requires comprehensive endocrine evaluation. If its deficiency is documented, growth hormone replacement may be warranted.

There appears to be a prevalence of obesity in children who have successfully completed therapy for ALL.[575] Although it has been suggested that cranial radiation is associated with this phenomenon, the validity of this relationship requires additional confirmation. The possible mechanism for this phenomenon is unclear.

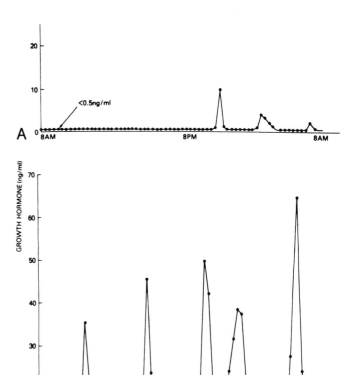

FIGURE 16-16. Spontaneous pulsatile growth hormone secretion in (**A**) a patient with acute lymphoblastic leukemia who had received CNS-preventive therapy with 2400 cGy cranial radiation and intrathecal methotrexate and (**B**) a representative normal child.[403]

There is considerable information indicating that the incidence of the CNS sequelae, documented above, is a function of the intensity of CNS treatment.[546] Most of these abnormalities were observed in patients who received 2400 cGy of cranial radiation and concomitant intrathecal chemotherapy, the standard form of CNS preventive therapy administered to patients in the 1970s. In an attempt to avoid these sequelae, a major thrust of ALL treatment has been the development of alternative methods of CNS preventive therapy that are equally effective but less toxic (see CNS preventive therapy section). Although there is some preliminary evidence suggesting that less intensive CNS preventive therapy may avoid some of these adverse effects, there is little information in the literature to date on the incidence of these abnormalities with the various alternative methods of CNS preventive therapy currently being evaluated. In one nonrandomized study, the psychometric test results of patients who received either 2400 cGy or 1800 cGy of cranial radiation plus intrathecal methotrexate were compared with those of a group of patients who received intrathecal methotrexate alone. Significantly lower scores were found in both groups of radiated patients compared with those who received only intrathecal therapy.[421] These results must be considered only suggestive; more detailed information regarding patients receiving lower doses of cranial radiation is needed. As noted earlier, in one of the few prospective randomized studies assessing intellectual function longitudinally, patients treated with 2400 cGy of cranial radiation plus intrathecal methotrexate showed a progressive decline in verbal IQ and significantly impaired academic achievement, findings not observed in patients randomly allocated to receive the alternative mode of CNS preventive therapy studied, high-dose protracted systemic methotrexate infusions.[433,434]

Although new approaches may offer the possibility of reducing and even preventing adverse CNS sequelae, currently a large number of patients being followed by pediatric oncologists are at risk of developing late CNS toxicity. Such children should be closely monitored. Periodic CT brain scans (every 2–3 years) are recommended for patients who have received cranial radiation and, in particular, for those very young (<8 years of age) at the time of diagnosis.[546] Periodic follow-up with comprehensive neuropsychometric testing, performed at the same intervals, may permit early identification of developing deficits and possibly allow therapeutic intervention. Comprehensive neuroendocrine assessment is appropriate for individuals who demonstrate abnormally decreasing linear growth.

In addition to adverse sequelae affecting the CNS, other late effects of antileukemic treatment may occur. Chemotherapy may produce long-term side-effects in some children. Patients receiving maintenance treatment frequently have elevated liver function test findings, primarily a reflection of methotrexate hepatotoxicity. When chemotherapy stops, however, in most patients liver function returns to normal; persistent liver function abnormalities are rare. Many current protocols, particularly intensive regimens used to treat patients with high-risk features, use anthracyclines. Treatment with these agents carries the potential risk of cardiomyopathy, however, because the total cumulative doses of these agents in most protocols is considerably lower than 550 mg/m^2, clinically significant cardiomyopathy in this population of patients is a relatively rare occurrence. A number of other toxicities associated with the variety of antileukemic agents currently used may occur. Entities such as hemorrhagic cystitis and bladder fibrosis with cyclophosphamide treatment, avascular necrosis secondary to steroid treatment, and significant sequelae of L-asparaginase-induced thrombosis and hemorrhagic infarction are encountered relatively infrequently in patients with ALL. These and other drug-related toxicities are discussed in more detail in Chapters 9 and 50.

The reproductive capacity of patients with ALL treated with prolonged chemotherapy has been studied. Although cyclophosphamide therapy is known to impair reproductive function, little detailed information exists on the reproductive status of patients treated with other commonly used chemotherapies. There is some evidence that in the majority of cases, girls with leukemia retain intact reproductive function. However, the timing of chemotherapy in relationship to puberty may be important.[575,576] A study of boys who received chemotherapy for ALL, not including cyclophosphamide, also revealed no evidence of significant gonadal dysfunction.[577] Although this preliminary evidence is encouraging, additional information on a larger number of patients treated in the periods before, during, and after puberty is required before definitive conclusions regarding the reproductive capacity of these patients can be drawn. More information is also needed on the outcome of pregnancy following treatment for leukemia. While our knowledge of the teratogenicity and mutagenicity of antileukemic therapy is incomplete, some data indicate that normal births occur in the majority of cases in which women receive chemotherapy before gestation or after the first trimester.[578] Likewise, available information suggests that chemotherapy administered to males at or before the time of insemination does not appear to result in fetal damage. Although available information appears to be reason for cautious

optimism, additional long-term follow-up of offspring of survivors of childhood leukemia is needed.

The risk of second malignancy in children with ALL appears to be very low. Slightly more than 100 second malignancies occurring in ALL patients have been reported in the literature.[579-586] Most have involved the hematopoietic system, although solid tumors have been reported. Recently there have been an increasing number of secondary brain tumors reported, most of which have been observed in children who have received cranial radiation as part of CNS preventive therapy.[580,581,583,584] Most of these brain tumors have been gliomas. Although a causal relationship between the development of secondary brain tumors and cranial radiation is suggested, CNS tumors have also been reported in a small number of patients who have not received cranial radiation.

The psychosocial status of long-term survivors of ALL has appropriately become an area of concern. It has been reported that, when compared with matched groups of controls or with siblings, survivors of ALL are likely to have more behavioral problems, lower levels of life satisfaction, impaired attainment of social skills, and poorer school performance.[587,588] To what extent some of these problems are preventable in the future through modification of treatment (e.g., alternative methods of CNS preventive therapy) is not clear. Despite the fact that many children with ALL have tolerated their treatment well and may not experience significant late sequelae, the medical community must be aware of the special problems and needs that children with ALL may incur as they are reincorporated into the mainstream of society. In addition to being sensitive to the possibility of late effect of treatment, care givers must also be cognizant of the special problems that these patients may encounter as they grow up in a society in which misapprehension and fears regarding cancer in general and leukemia in particular are still widespread, and where acceptance of patients into normal community activities is not always enthusiastic.

Supportive Care

Optimal management of the child with ALL requires appropriate attention to several areas of supportive care, including the rationale use of blood component therapy, an aggressive approach to detection and treatment of infectious complications, careful attention to the metabolic and nutritional needs of the patient, and comprehensive, continuous psychosocial support for both patient and family. Detailed discussions of these topics are presented in Chapters 37 to 47 and will be discussed only briefly in this section.

The problems and complications encountered by children undergoing ALL treatment are unique and frequently complex. For this reason, experienced personnel and specialized resources are required to provide optimal supportive care. Patients treated outside a children's cancer center and not according to an organized treatment protocol reportedly have a poorer overall prognosis.[589] This may reflect in part the difficulty in providing the specialized supportive care needs required by children with ALL in a setting other than that of a specialized children's cancer center.

The importance of adequate hematologic supportive care cannot be overemphasized. Before the systematic use of platelet transfusions, hemorrhage was the leading cause of death in patients with this disease. The use of prophylactic platelet transfusions and aggressive platelet transfusion support has markedly reduced the incidence of significant bleeding. Erythrocyte transfusions are frequently required to treat anemia and, as with all blood products, must be appropriately screened to exclude the possibility of contamination with hepatitis B or HIV infection. The use of granulocyte transfusions in the febrile, neutropenic patient has been controversial (see Chap. 38). The granulocytopenia that occurs as a consequence of therapy-induced marrow hypoplasia or with disease progression places patients at risk for serious, potentially life-threatening infection.

An aggressive approach to diagnosis and rapid empiric therapeutic intervention are important principles for the successful management of the severely neutropenic (<500 granulocytes/mm^3) patient. The empiric use of broad spectrum antibiotics in such individuals has dramatically reduced overall mortality. (see Chap. 39). Granulocytopenia, chemotherapy induced immunosuppression, disruption of normal anatomic barriers by invasive procedures, or therapy-induced complications (*e.g.*, mucositis) all increase susceptibility to bacterial, fungal, viral, and parasitic infections. Although the risk of bacterial and secondary fungal infections may be greater in patients undergoing intensive induction or reinduction therapy, the child with leukemia is susceptible to various forms of infections while undergoing maintenance chemotherapy. *Pneumocystis carinii* pneumonia is a serious, potentially life-threatening complication that commonly affects children undergoing maintenance chemotherapy. The prophylactic use of trimethoprim-sulfamethoxasole dramatically reduces the incidence of this type of infection and is used routinely in many centers.[590] The leukemic child undergoing treatment is also at risk for disseminated varicella if exposure to an infected individual occurs. Immediate administration of zoster immune globulin to such patients (within 72–96 hours) appears to have a protective effect.[591] Other viral infections also place the leukemic child at risk. Measles tends to run a more complicated, atypical course in a leukemic host.[592] Nonimmunized children exposed to the measles virus should be treated with gamma globulin. Because of the risk of dissemination, immunization against measles or the use of any vaccines containing a live virus is contraindicated in patients receiving chemotherapy.

A variety of metabolic abnormalities may be observed in children with ALL, usually occurring either during induction or in the presence of progressive disease (see Clinical Presentation and Treatment sections). Hyperuricemia, which frequently accompanies hyperleukocytosis in newly diagnosed patients, requires immediate and vigorous hydration and the administration of allopurinol to minimize uric acid deposition in the kidneys and to prevent renal failure (see Chap. 37).

Adequate nutrition also becomes a concern for the patient with leukemia. When normal parenteral alimentation is prevented by an unforeseen therapeutic complication, intravenous hyperalimentation may be indicated (see Chap. 40). Children in remission also require an adequate diet. Some patients undergoing chemotherapy undergo a decrease in body growth.[593,594] Whereas this may, in part, be the consequence of chemotherapy or CNS radiation, nutritional factors may play a role. This area is deserving of further study.

Psychosocial support for both patient and family is needed on an ongoing basis. The diagnosis of leukemia places profound stress on both patient and family. The maintenance of strong psychosocial support is a crucial element in the treatment process (see Chaps. 41 and 42). Depending on their age and level of understanding, children need reassurance in dealing with the diagnosis and with the changes in life-style that are likely to accompany treatment. Fears and concerns regarding the possibility of death, anxieties relating to changes in body habitus, and general disquiet over prospects for the future are concerns common to many patients. Parents need assistance in dealing both with their own fears and with the impact of the diagnosis on their child, siblings, and other family members. Interpersonal and marital relationships and even familial economic stability may be threatened. Concerns may differ according to different stages of the illness. Optimal support of both patient and family requires a coordinated effort involving physicians, nurses, social workers, clergy, and other skilled health care personnel on a continuing basis.

FUTURE CHALLENGES

Despite the dramatic treatment advances achieved over the past four decades, approximately 40% of children with ALL will eventually die of their disease. The challenge that ALL presents to the pediatric oncologist remains formidable, and significant obstacles remain before a cure will become a reality for all children with this disease. Future clinical trials and laboratory studies must focus on a number of unresolved, critical treatment issues.

The major challenge is to improve therapy significantly for those children at high risk of relapse. Although in recent years intensification of treatment has increased the event-free survival of this group of patients, further progress is needed. Because many current protocols treating high-risk patients are accompanied by significant myelosuppression, further intensification of treatment under present conditions may not be feasible. Recently molecularly cloned hematopoietic growth factors, such as GM-CSF and G-CSF, have been developed that are able to shorten the duration and severity of chemotherapy induced myelosuppression.[595] The use of these agents may provide a potential means for intensifying treatment in the future.

Greater biological understanding of the disease that affects patients at high risk of relapse is required. Current evidence suggests that there is significant biological heterogeneity among these patients, with substantial differences in clinical presentation and in the immunologic, cytogenetic, and molecular features of their disease. The recent application of molecular genetic techniques to the study of lymphoid leukemia has improved our understanding of the process of lymphoid differentiation and maturation. Whether these methods can be used to uncover biological differences that can be exploited therapeutically remains to be seen. The study of the molecular biology of drug resistance is an example of one area that may ultimately provide valuable information on the mechanisms underlying treatment failure (Fig. 16-17).

Future clinical studies also must focus on the causes of treatment failure. For example, the majority of patients failing current therapy do so during maintenance therapy. Recent studies suggesting that variation and limitation in drug bioavailability may be a mechanism of treatment failure in some patients require confirmation.[479]

Further refinement in the criteria upon which risk groups are delineated is needed. A substantial percentage of patients with so-called good risk features fail current therapy. Enhancement in the ability to identify such patients at diagnosis would permit their stratification into more intensive treatment regimens. In addition, more accurate methods for determining patients at high risk for extramedullary relapse (*e.g.,* CNS recurrence) should help to design more selective therapy. Patients with an exceedingly low risk of CNS relapse, for example, would receive less intensive, and presumably less neurotoxic, therapy, whereas individuals at high risk for CNS recurrence would be treated on regimens more aggressively focusing on the prevention of CNS disease.

More sensitive methods for detecting residual disease are needed. Molecular biological techniques, such as assessment of immunoglobulin and T-cell receptor gene rearrangement, may provide better methods of identifying residual leukemia in otherwise morphologically normal marrows. Although this approach has been demonstrated to be feasible with current methodology, further technical refinements, perhaps incorpo-

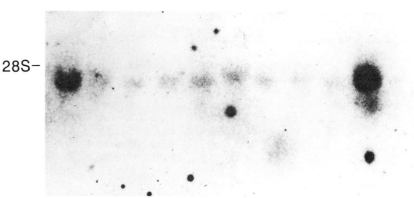

FIGURE 16-17. Multidrug-resistance gene (mdr1) expression in peripheral blood lymphoblasts from ten patients with acute lymphoblastic leukemia. Samples were obtained from patients at the time of initial presentation (I) or at the time of relapse (R) after treatment with regimens that included vincristine and daunomycin. Lane at the left contains RNA from a multidrug-resistant KB cell line as a positive control. The strong signal seen in the relapsed sample (second from the right) indicates a high level of expression of the multidrug-resistance gene. (Courtesy of Dr. A. Fojo)

rating techniques such as *in situ* hybridization, may be required.[110]

Attention must also focus on developing more effective therapy for relapsed patients. New antileukemic agents, effective by both systemic and intra-CSF routes of administration, are needed. With improvements in the techniques of bone marrow transplantation, the applicability of this approach is likely to increase. Recent successes in the use of partially mismatched donors have made the possibility of totally crossing the "HLA barrier" more realistic. In addition, recent promising results using autologous bone marrow transplantation suggest that the role of this approach may expand as newer methods of *in vitro* purging (*e.g.*, radiolabeled monoclonal antibodies, biologicals) become available. In addition to being applied in the setting of relapse, this approach conceivably could be used to treat high risk patients during their initial remission.

The observation that some forms of adult leukemia respond to certain types of interferons has stimulated the investigation of the role of biologicals as a possible means of treating lymphoid leukemia. Clinical studies of interferon in childhood ALL are ongoing. Recent studies with interleukin-2 have demonstrated maturation and cytotoxicity of leukemic lymphoblasts cultured *in vivo* with this agent.[596] *In vivo* studies of this approach are underway. Because their mechanisms of action are different from standard antineoplastic chemotherapy, the therapeutic potential of biologicals such as interferon and interleukin is appealing. Further investigation of the potential of these and other biological response modifiers such as antileukemic agents is likely to continue.

Finally, as cure becomes a reality for greater numbers of patients, concerns over the late effects of ALL treatment have increased. Future clinical trials must focus on minimizing adverse sequelae without compromising therapeutic efficacy.

Ultimately, the effectiveness in addressing the major unsolved treatment issues in ALL will depend on the ability both to design innovative clinical trials and to aggressively pursue basic research focused on increasing the understanding of this biologically complex disease.

REFERENCES

1. Pierce MI, Borges WH, Heyn R, Wolff JA, Gilbert ES: Epidemiological factors and survival experience in 1770 children with acute leukemia treated by members of Children's Study Group A between 1957 and 1964. Cancer 23:1296–1304, 1969
2. Committee on Leukemia and Working Party on Leukemia in Childhood: Duration of survival of children with acute leukaemia. Br Med J 4:7–9, 1971
3. Tivey H: The natural history of untreated acute leukemia. Ann NY Acad Sci 60:322–358, 1954
4. Miller RW: Epidemiology of leukemia. In Neth R, Gallo RC, Hufschneider PH, Mannweiler K (eds): Modern Trends in Human Leukemia. New York, Springer-Verlag, 1979
5. Fraumeni JF Jr, Miller RW: Epidemiology of human leukemia: Recent observations. J Natl Cancer Inst 38:593–605, 1967
6. Miller RW: Ethnic differences in cancer occurrence: Genetic and environmental influences with particular reference to neuroblastoma. In Mulvihill JJ, Miller RW, Fraumeni JF Jr (eds): Genetics of Human Cancer. New York, Raven Press, 1977
7. Miller RW: Cancer epidemics in the People's Republic of China. J Natl Cancer Inst 60:1195–1203, 1978
8. Court Brown WM, Doll R: Leukemia in childhood and young adult life. Trends in mortality in relation to aetiology. Br Med J 1:981–988, 1961
9. Gunz F, Baikie AG: Leukemia, 3rd ed. New York, Grune & Stratton, 1974
10. Hanson MR, Mulvihill JJ: Epidemiology of childhood cancer. In Levine AS (ed): Cancer in the Young, pp 3–12. New York, Masson, 1980
11. Fraumeni JF Jr, Wagoner JK: Changing sex differentials in leukemia. Public Health Rep 79:1093–1100, 1974
12. Cook JV: Incidence of acute leukemia in children. JAMA 119:547–550, 1942
13. Pendergrass TW: Epidemiology of acute lymphoblastic leukemia. Semin Oncol 12(2):80–91, 1985
14. Greaves MF, Pegram SM, Chan LC: Collaborative group study of the epidemiology of acute lymphoblastic leukaemia subtypes: Background and first report. Leuk Res 9:715–733, 1985
15. Magrath I: Appendix: Selected epidemiological data pertinent to topics discussed in this volume. In Magrath IT, O'Conor GT, Ramot B (eds): Pathogenesis of leukemias and lymphomas: Environmental Influences, pp 379–386. New York, Raven Press, 1984
16. Greaves MF: Differentiation-linked leukemogenesis in lymphocytes. Science 234:697–704, 1986
17. Heath CW, Hasterlik RJ: Leukemia among children in a suburban community. Am J Med 34:796–812, 1963
18. Gunz FW, Spears GFS: Distribution of acute leukaemia in time and space. Studies in New Zealand. Br Med J 4:604–608, 1968
19. Evatt BL, Chase GA, Heath CW: Time-space clustering among cases of acute leukemia in two Georgia counties. Blood 41:265–272, 1973
20. Till MM, Jones JH, Pentycross CR, Hardisty RM, Lawler SD, Harvey BAM, Soothill JF: Leukaemia in children and their grandparents: Studies of immune function in six families. Br J Haematol 29:575–586, 1975
21. Schwartz SO, Greenspan I, Brown ER: Leukemia clusters in Niles, Ill. Immunologic data on families of leukemia patients and others. JAMA 186:106–108, 1963
22. Dowsett EGH: Leukemia in Kingston, Surrey, 1958–64: An epidemiologic study. Br J Cancer 20:16–31
23. Heath CW Jr, Mannery MD, Zelkowitz L: Case clusters in the occurrence of leukaemia and congenital malformations. Lancet 2:136–137, 1964
24. Caldwell GG, Heath CW Jr: Case clustering in cancer. South Med J 69:1598–1602, 1976
25. Morgan KZ: Radiation-induced health effects. Science 195:344–348, 1977

26. Miller RW: Neoplasia and Down's syndrome. Ann NY Acad Sci 171:637–644, 1970

27. Rosner F, Lee SL: Down's syndrome and acute leukemia: Myeloblastic or lymphoblastic? Am J Med 53:203–218, 1972

28. Miller RW, Todaro GJ: Viral transformation of cells from persons at high risks of cancer. Lancet 1:81–82, 1969

29. Todaro GJ, Martin GM: Increased susceptibility of Down's syndrome fibroblasts to transformation by SV40. Proc Soc Exp Biol Med 124:1232–1236, 1967

30. Sawitsky A, Bloom D, German J: Chromosomal breakage and acute leukemia in congenital telangiectatic erythema and stunted growth. Ann Intern Med 65:487–495, 1966

31. Sasaki MS, Tonomura A: A high susceptibility of Fanconi's anemia to chromosome breakage by DNA cross-linking-agents. Cancer Res 33:1829–1836, 1973

32. Miller RW: Relation between cancer and congenital defects: An epidemiologic evaluation. J Natl Cancer Inst 40:1079–1085, 1968

33. Festa RS, Meadows AT, Boshes RA: Leukemia in a black child with Bloom's syndrome: Somatic recombination as a possible mechanism for neoplasia. Cancer 44:1507–1510, 1978

34. Bloom D: The syndrome of congenital telangietatic erythema and stunted growth. J Pediatr 68:103–113, 1966

35. Fanconi G: Familial constitutional panmyelocytopathy, Fanconi's anemia. Semin Hematol 4:233–240, 1967

36. Dosik H, Hsu LY, Todaro GJ, Lee SL, Hirschhorn K, Selirio E, Atter AA: Leukemia in Fanconi's anemia: Cytogenetic tumor virus susceptibility studies. Blood 36:341–352, 1970

37. Garriga S, Crosby WH: The incidence of leukemia in families of patients with hypoplasia of the marrow. Blood 14:1008–1014, 1959

38. Gotoff SO, Amirmokri E, Liebner EJ: Ataxia-telangiectasia: Neoplasia, untoward response to x-irradiation, and tuberous sclerosis. Am J Dis Child 11:617–625, 1967

39. Hecht F, Koler RD, Rigas DA, Dahnke GS, Case MP, Tisdal V: Leukaemia and lymphocytes in ataxia-telangiectasia. Lancet 2:1193, 1966

40. Miller RW: Persons with exceptionally high risk of leukemia. Cancer Res 27:2420–2423, 1967

41. Zuelzer WW, Mastrangelo R: Evidence for a genetic factor related to leukemogenesis and congenital abnormalities: Chromosomal observations in pedigree of an infant with partial D trisomy and leukemia. J Pediatr 72:367–376, 1968

42. Muts–Homshma SJM, Muller HP, Geracost JPM: Klinefelter's syndrome and acute non-lymphocytic leukemia. Blut 44:15–20, 1981

43. Stark CR, Mantel N: Maternal-age and birth order effects in childhood leukemia: Age of child and type of leukemia. J Natl Cancer Inst 42:857–866, 1969

44. Stark CR, Mantel N: Effects of maternal age and birth order on the risk of mongolism and leukemia. J Natl Cancer Inst 37:687–698, 1966

45. Gibson RW, Broiss IDJ, Graham S et al: Leukemia in children exposed to multiple risk factors. N Engl J Med 279:906–909, 1968

46. Robison LL, Buckley J, Daigle A et al: Childhood acute nonlymphocytic leukemia (ANLL): Association with in vitro marijuana exposure. Proc Am Soc Clin Oncol 6:231, 1987

47. Van Steensel–Moll HA, Valkenburg HA, Vandenbroucke JP et al: Are maternal fertility problems related to childhood leukemia? Int J Epidemiol 14:555–559, 1985

48. Daling JR, Starzyk P, Olshan AF et al: Birth weight and the incidence of childhood cancer. J Natl Cancer Inst 72:1039–1041, 1984

49. Robison LL, Codd M, Gunderson P et al: Birth weight as a risk factor for childhood acute lymphoblastic leukemia. Pediatr Hematol Oncol 4:63–72, 1987

50. Videback A: Familial leukemia. Acta Pathol Microbiol Scand 44:372–376, 1958

51. Gunz FW, Gunz JP, Veale AMO, Chapman CJ, Hoosto IB: Leukemia: A study of 909 families. Scand J Haematol 15:117–131, 1975

52. Heath CW Jr, Molone WC: Familial leukemia. Five cases of acute leukemia in three generations. N Engl J Med 272:882–887, 1965

53. Zuelzer WW, Cox DE: Genetic aspects of leukemia. Semin Hematol 6:228–249, 1969

54. Gunz FW, Veale AMO: Leukemia in close relatives—accident or predisposition? J Natl Cancer Inst 42:517–524, 1969

55. Miller RW: Deaths from childhood leukemia and solid tumors among twins and other sibs in the United States 1960–1962. J Natl Cancer Inst 46:203–209, 1971

56. Draper GJ, Heaf MM, Kennier–Wilson LM: Occurrence of childhood

cancers among sibs and estimation of familial risks. J Med Genet 14:81–90, 1977

57. Till M, Rapson N, Smith PG: Family studies in acute leukemia in childhood: A possible association with autoimmune disease. Br J Cancer 49:62–71, 1979

58. MacMahon B, Levy MA: Prenatal origin of childhood leukemia: Evidence from twins. N Engl J Med 270:1082–1085, 1964

59. Keith L, Brown E: Epidemiologic study of leukemia in twins (1928–1969). Acta Genet Med Geneol (Rome) 20:9–22, 1971

60. Clarkson BD, Boyse EA: Possible explanation of the high concordance for acute leukemia in monozygous twins. Lancet 1:699–701, 1971

61. Chaganti RS, Miller DR, Meyers PA, German J: Cytogenetic evidence of the intrauterine origin of acute leukemia in monozygotic twins. N Engl J Med 300:1032–1034, 1979

62. Hartley SE, Sainsbury C: Acute leukemia and the same chromosome abnormality in monozygotic twins. Hum Genet 58:408–410, 1981

63. Bizzozzero OJ Jr, Johnson KG, Ciocco A: Radiation-related leukemia in Hiroshima and Nagasaki, 1946–64: I. Distribution, incidence and appearance in time. N Engl J Med 274:1095–1101, 1966

64. Folley JH, Borges W, Yamawaki T: Incidence of leukemia in survivors of the atomic bomb in Hiroshima and Nagasaki, Japan. Am J Med 13:311–321, 1952

65. Moloney WC: Leukemia in survivors of atomic bombing. N Engl J Med 253:88–90, 1955

66. Tomonaga M: Statistical investigation of leukemia in Japan. NZ Med J 65:863–869, 1966

67. Wald N: Leukemia in Hiroshima City atomic bomb survivors. Science 127:699–700, 1958

68. Brill AB, Tomonaga M, Heyssel RM: Leukemia in man following exposure to ionizing radiation. Ann Intern Med 56:590–609, 1962

69. Jablon S, Kato H: Childhood cancer in relation to prenatal exposure to atomic bomb radiation. Lancet 2:100–103, 1970

70. Smith PG: Current assessment of "case clustering" of lymphomas and leukemias. Cancer 42:1026–1034, 1978

71. National Academy of Sciences: Biological Effects of Atomic Radiation. Washington DC, National Research Council, 1980

72. Morgan KZ: Radiation-induced health effects. Science 195:344–348, 1977

73. Evans JS, Wennberg JE, McNeil BJ: The influence of diagnostic radiography on the incidence of breast cancer and leukemia. NEJM 315:810–815, 1986

74. Court Brown WM, Doll R: Mortality from cancer and other causes after radiotherapy for ankylosing spondylitis. Br Med J 5474:1327–1332, 1965

75. Murray R, Heckel P, Hempelmann LH: Leukemia in children exposed to ionizing radiation. N Engl J Med 261:585–589, 1959

76. Davies AM, Modan B, Djaldetti M, DeVries A: Epidemiological observations on leukemia in Israel. Arch Intern Med 108:86–90, 1961

77. Modan B, Litienfield A: Polycythemia vera and leukemia. The role of radiation therapy. Medicine (Baltimore) 44:305–344, 1965

78. Miller RW, Boice JD Jr: Radiogenic cancer after prenatal or childhood exposure. In Upton AC, Albert RT, Burns FJ, Shore RE (eds): Radiation Carcinogenesis, pp 379–438. New York, Elsevier, 1986

79. Black D: New evidence on childhood leukaemia and nuclear establishments. Br Med J 294:591–592, 1987

80. Vigliani EC, Sarta G: Benzene and leukemia. N Engl J Med 271:872–876, 1964

81. Aksoy M, Erdem S, Dincol G: Types of leukemia in chronic benzene poisoning. A study of thirty-four patients. Acta Haematol 55:65–72, 1976

82. Tucker MA, Meadows AT, Boice JD Jr, Stovall M, Oberlin O, Stone BJ, Birch J, Voute PA, Hoover RN, Fraumeni JF Jr: Leukemia after therapy with alkylating agents for childhood cancer. JNCI 78:459–464, 1987

83. Stjernfeldt M, Ludvigsson J, Berglund K et al: Maternal smoking during pregnancy and risk of childhood cancer. Lancet 1:1350–1532, 1986

84. McKinney PA, Stiller CA: Response to "Maternal smoking during pregnancy and the risk of childhood cancer (Stjernfeldt, 1986). Lancet 2:519, 1986

85. Zeltzer PM: Acute lymphoblastic leukemia in the offspring of a mother exposed to diethylstilbestrol in utero. Am J Pediatr Hematol Oncol 5:315–316, 1983

86. Greenberg RS, Shuster JL: Epidemiology of cancer in children. Epidemiol Rev 7:22–48, 1985

87. Gallo C, Wong–Staal F: Retroviruses as etiologic agents of some animal and human leukemias and lymphomas and as tools for elucidating the molecular mechanism of leukemogenesis. Blood 60:545–557, 1982

88. Todaro GJ, Huebner RJ: The viral oncogene hypothesis: New evidence. Proc Natl Acad Sci USA 69:1009–1015, 1972

89. Gallo RC, Saxinger RC, Gallagher RE et al: Some ideas on the origins of leukemia in man and recent evidence for the presence of type C viral-related information. In Watson JD, Winsten JA (eds): Origins of Human Cancer, Cold Spring Harbor Conference, vol 4, pp 1253–1286. Cold Spring Harbor, New York, Cold Spring Harbor Laboratory, 1977

90. Cawley TC, Karpas A: The ultrastructural demonstration of virus-like particles in human leukemia cells. Eur J Cancer 10:559–562, 1974

91. Gallo RC, Yang SS, Ting RC: RNA dependent DNA polymerase of human acute leukemia cells. Nature 228:927–929, 1970

92. Baxt WG, Hehlmann R, Speigelman S: Human leukaemic cells contain reverse transcriptase associated with a higher molecular weight virus-related RNA. Nature 240:72–75, 1972

93. Inoue M, Yano S, Tanaka H et al: Cytoplasmic inclusions in virus like particles and blast cells in acute lymphoblastic leukemia, Acta Pathol Jpn 36:1231–1239, 1986

94. Poiesz BJ, Ruscetti FW, Gasdar AF et al: Detection and isolation of type C retrovirus particles from fresh and cultured lymphocytes of a patient with cutaneous T-cell lymphoma. Proc Natl Acad Sci USA 77:7415–7419, 1980

95. Bunn PA, Schechter GP, Jaffee ES et al: Clinical course of retrovirus-associated adult T-cell lymphoma in the United States. N Engl J Med 309:257–264, 1983

96. Williams DL, Ragab AH, McDougal JS: HTLV-1 antibodies in childhood leukemia. JAMA 253:2496, 1985

97. Levy SB: Cat leukemia: A threat to man? N Engl J Med 290:513–514, 1974

98. Deinhardt F, Wolfe LG, Theilen GH, Snyder SP: ST-feline fibrosarcoma virus: Induction of tumors in Marmoset monkeys. Science 167:881, 1970

99. Schneider R, Dorn CR, Klauber MR: Cancer in households: A human cancer retrospective study. J Natl Cancer Inst 41:1285–1292, 1968

100. Hanes B, Gardner MB, Loosli CG, Heidbreder G, Kogan B, Marylander H, Huebner RJ: Pet association with selected human cancers: A household questionnaire survey. J Natl Cancer Inst 45:1155–1162, 1970

101. Gardner MB: Current information on feline and canine cancers and relationship or lack of relationship to human cancer. J Natl Cancer Inst 46:281–289, 1971

102. Penn I: Second malignant neoplasms associated with immunosuppression medications. Cancer 37:1024–1032, 1976

103. Konior GS, Leventhal BG: Immunocompetence and prognosis in acute leukemia. Semin Oncol 3:283–288, 1976

104. Hersh EM, Whitecar JP, McCredie KB, Bodey GP, Freireich EJ: Chemotherapy, immunocompetence, immunosuppression and prognosis in acute leukemia. N Engl J Med 285:1211–1216, 1971

105. Broder S, Poplack DG, Whang-Peng J, Durm M, Goldman C, Muul L, Waldmann TA: Characterization of a suppressor-cell leukemia: Evidence for the requirement of a two T cell interaction in the development of human suppressor effector cells. N Engl J Med 298:66–72, 1978

106. Dow LW, Martin P, Moohr J, Greenberg M, Macdougall LG, Najfeld V, Fialkow PJ: Evidence for clonal development of childhood acute lymphoblastic leukemia. Blood 66:902–907, 1985

107. Zuelzer WW, Inoue S, Thompson RI, Ottenbreit MJ: Long-term cytogenetic studies in acute leukemia of children: The nature of relapse. Am J Hematol 1:143–190, 1976

108. Whang-Peng J, Knutsen T, Ziegler J, Leventhal B: Cytogenetic studies in acute lymphocytic leukemia: Special emphasis on long-term survival. Med Pediatr Oncol 2:333–351, 1976

109. Williams DL, Raimondi SC, Rivera G: Most cases of acute lymphoblastic leukemia (ALL) undergo marked karyotypic shift from diagnosis to relapse. Blood 62(suppl 1):741a, 1984

110. Wright JJ, Poplack DG, Bakhski A, Reaman G, Cole D, Jensen JP, Korsmeyer SJ: Gene rearrangements as markers of clonal variation and minimal residual disease in acute lymphoblastic leukemia. J Clin Oncol 5:735–741, 1987

111. Mathe G, Pouillart P, Sterescu M, Amiel JL, Schwarzenberg L, Schneider M, Hayat M, Hayat M, DeVassal F, Jasmin C, Lafleur M: Subdivision of classical varieties of acute leukemia: Correlation with prognosis and cure expectancy. Eur J Clin Biol Res 16:554–560, 1971

112. Mathe G, Belpomme D, Dantchev D, Pouillart P, Navares L, Hauss G, Schlumberger JR, Lafleur M: Search for correlation between cytological types and therapeutic sensitivity of acute leukemias. Blood Cells 1:37–52, 1975

113. Jacquillat C, Weil M, Auclerc G, Gemon MF: Cytologie et prognostic des leucemies aigues lymphoblastiques. Actual Hematol 7:42–50, 1973

114. Bennett JM, Klemperer MR, Segal GB: Survival prediction based on morphology of lymphoblasts. Recent Results Cancer Res 43:23–27, 1973

115. Flandrin G, Daniel MT, Couderc O: Classification cytologique des leucemies aigues lymphoblatiques: Incidences cliniques et prognostiques. Actual Hematol 7:25–32, 1973

116. Pantazopoulos N, Sinks LF: Morphological criteria for prognostication of acute lymphoblastic leukemia. Br J Haematol 31:95–102, 1975

117. Oster MW, Margileth DA, Simon R, Leventhal BG: Lack of prognostic value of lymphoblast size in acute lymphoblastic leukemia. Br J Haematol 33:131–135, 1976

118. Murphy S, Borella L, Sen L, Mauer A: Lack of correlation of lymphoblast cell size with presence of T-cell markers or with outcome in childhood acute lymphoblastic leukemia. Br J Haematol 31:95–101, 1975

119. Shaw MT, Humphrey GB, Lawrence R, Fischer DB: Lack of prognostic value of the periodic-acid-Schiff reaction and blast cell size in childhood acute lymphocytic leukemia. Am J Hematol 2:237–243, 1977

120. Janka GE, Teige-Singer S, Haas RJ, Lau BM: Lymphoblast cell size and prognosis in acute lymphoblastic leukemia in childhood. Blut 37:89–94, 1978

121. Scheer U, Shellong G: The prognostic value of measuring cell size in acute lymphoblastic leukemia in childhood. Klin Paediatr 191:127–132, 1979

122. Wagner VM, Baehner RL: Lack of correlation between blast cell size and length of first remission in acute lymphocytic leukemia in childhood. Med Pediatr Oncol 3:373–377, 1977

123. Lee SL, Kopel SS, Glidewell O: Cytomorphological determinants of prognosis in acute lymphblastic leukemia of children. Semin Oncol 3:209–217, 1976

124. Flandrin G, Bernard J: Cytological classification of acute leukemias. A survey of 1400 cases. Blood Cells 1:7–15, 1975

125. Bennett JM, Catovsky D, Daniel MT et al: French-American-British (FAB) Cooperative Group proposals for the classification of acute leukemias. Br J Haematol 33:451–458, 1976

126. Bennett JM, Catovsky D, Daniel MT et al: French-American British (FAB) Cooperative Group: The morphological classification of acute leukemias—concordance among observers and clinical correlation. Br J Haematol 47:553–561, 1981

127. Miller DR, Leikin S, Albo V et al: Prognostic importance of morphology (FAB classification) in childhood acute lymphoblastic leukemia. Br J Haematol 48:199–206, 1981

128. Lilleyman JS, Hamm IM, Stevens RF, Eden OB, Richards SM: French American British (FAB) morphological classification of childhood lymphoblastic leukaemia and its clinical importance. J Clin Pathol 39:998–1002, 1986

129. Brearly RL, Johnson SAN, Lister TA: Acute lymphoblastic leukemia in adults: Clinicopathological correlations with the French-American-British (FAB) Cooperative Group classification. Eur J Cancer 15:909–914, 1979

130. Morphologic, Immunologic, and Cytogenetic (MIC) working classification of acute lymphoblastic leukemias. Report of the Workshop held in Leuven, Belgium, April 22–23, 1985. First MIC Cooperative Study Group. Cancer Genet Cytogenet 23(3):189–197, 1986

131. Palmer MK, Hann IM, Jones PM, Evans DIK: A score at diagnosis for predicting length of remission in childhood acute lymphoblastic leukaemia. Br J Cancer 42:841–849, 1980

132. Viana MB, Maurer HS, Ferenc C: Sub-classification of acute lymphoblastic leukemia in children: Analysis of the reproducibility of morphologic criteria and prognostic implications. Br J Haematol 44:383–388, 1980

133. Miller DR, Krailo M, Bleyer WA, Lukens JN, Siegel SE, Coccia PR, Weiner J, Hammond D: Prognostic implications of blast cell morphology in childhood acute lymphoblastic leukemia: A report from the Childrens Cancer Study Group. Cancer Treat Rep 69:1211–1221, 1985

134. Keleti J, Revesz T, Schuler D: Morphologic diagnosis in childhood leukemia. Br J Haematol 40:501–502, 1978

135. Wagner VM, Baehner RL: Correlation of the FAB morphologic criteria and prognosis in acute lymphocytic leukemia of childhood. Am J Pediatr Hematol Oncol 1:103–106, 1979

136. Wolff LJ, Richardson ST, Neiburger JB, Neiburger RG, Irwin DS, Baehner RL: Poor prognosis of children with acute lymphocytic leukemia and increased B cell markers. J Pediatr 89:956–958, 1976

137. Magrath IT, Ziegler JL: Bone marrow involvement in Burkitt's lymphoma and its relationship to acute B cell markers. Leuk Res 4:33–59, 1979

138. Gupta S, Good RA: Markers of human lymphocyte subpopulations in primary immunodeficiency and lymphoproliferative disorders. Semin Hematol 17:1–29, 1980

139. Brouet JC, Preud'homme JL, Seligmann M: The use of B and T membrane markers in the classification of human leukemias, with special reference to acute lymphoblastic leukemia. Blood Cells 1:81–90, 1975

140. Kersey J, Nesbit M, Hallgren H, Sabad A, Yunis E, Gajl–Peczalska K: Evidence for origin of certain childhood acute lymphoblastic leukemias and lymphomas in thymus-derived lymphocytes. Cancer 36:1348–1352, 1975

141. Sen L, Borella L: Clinical importance of lymphoblasts with T markers in childhood acute leukemias. N Engl J Med 292:828–832, 1975

142. Brouet JC, Seligmann M: The immunological classification of acute lymphoblastic leukemias. Cancer 42:817–827, 1978

143. Chessells JM, Hardisty RM, Rapson NT, Greaves MF: Acute lymphoblastic leukemia in children: Classification and prognosis. Lancet 2:1307–1309, 1977

144. Billing R, Clark B, Guidera K, Minowada J: Heteroantisera against acute lymphocytic leukemia raised to the lymphoblastoid cell line NALM-1. Int J Cancer 22:694–699, 1978

145. Pesando JM, Ritz J, Lazarus H, Costello SB, Sallan S, Schlossman SF: Leukemia-associated antigens in ALL. Blood 54:1240–1248, 1979

146. Ritz J, Pesando JM, Notis–McConarty J, Lazarus H, Schlossman, SF: A monoclonal antibody to human acute lymphoblastic leukemia antigen. Nature 283:583–585, 1980

147. Vogler LB, Crist WM, Bockman DC et al: Pre-B-cell leukemia; A new phenotype of childhood lymphoblastic leukemia. N Engl J Med 298:872–878, 1978

148. Cossman J, Neckers LM, Arnold A: Induction of differentiation in the primitive B-cells of common, acute lymphoblastic leukemia. N Engl J Med 307:1251–1254, 1982

149. Nadler LM, Ritz J, Bates MP et al: Induction of human B-cell antigens in non-T-cell acute lymphoblastic leukemia. J Clin Invest 70:433–442, 1982

150. Vogler LB, Crist WM, Sarrif AM et al: An analysis of clinical and laboratory features of acute lymphocytic leukemia with emphasis on 35 children with pre-B-leukemia. Blood 58:135–140, 1981

151. Crist WM, Grosse CE, Pullen J, Cooper MD: Immunologic markers in childhood acute lymphocytic leukemia. Sem Oncol 12:105–121, 1985

152. Korsmeyer SJ, Hieter PA, Ravetch JV et al: A hierarchy of immunoglobulin gene rearrangements in human leukemic pre-B cells. Proc Natl Acad Sci USA 78:2096–7100, 1981

153. Pullen DJ, Falletta MJ, Crist WM et al: Southwest Oncology Group experience with immunological phenotyping in acute lymphocytic leukemia of childhood. Cancer Res 41:4802–4809, 1981

154. Brouet JC, Preud'homme JL, Penit C, Valensi F, Rouget P, Seligmann M: Acute lymphoblastic leukemia with pre-B-cell characteristics. Blood 54:269–273, 1979

155. Foon KA, Todd RF III: Immunologic classification of leukemia and lymphoma. Blood 68:1–31, 1986

156. Nadler LM, Korsmeyer SJ, Anderson KC, Boyd AW, Slaughenhoupt B, Park E, Jensen J, Coral F, Mayer RJ, Sallan SE, Ritz J, Schlossmann SF: B cell origin of non-T cell acute lymphoblastic leukemia. A model for discrete stages of neoplastic and normal pre-B cell differentiation. J Clin Invest 74:332–340, 1984

157. Crist WM, Boyett J, Roper M et al: Pre B-cell leukemia responds poorly to treatment: A Pediatric Oncology Group Study. Blood 63:407–414, 1984

158. Greaves MF, Janossy G, Peto J et al: Immunologically defined subclasses of acute lymphoblastic leukemia in children: Their relationship to presentation features and prognosis. Br J Haematol 48:179–197, 1981

159. Korsmeyer SJ, Arnold A, Bakshi A et al: Immunoglobulin gene rearrangement and cell surface antigen expression in acute lymphocytic leukemias of T cell and B-cell precursor origins. J Clin Invest 71:301–313, 1983

160. Waldmann TA, Korsmeyer SJ, Bakshi A et al: Molecular genetic analysis of Human Lymphoid Neoplasms. Immunoglobulin genes and the c-myc oncogene. Ann Intern Med 102:497–510, 1985

161. Felix CA, Wright JJ, Poplack DG, Reaman GH, Cole D, Goldman P, Korsmeyer SJ: T cell receptor α-, β-, and γ-genes in T cell and pre-B cell acute lymphoblastic leukemia. J Clin Invest 80:545–556, 1987

162. Tawa A, Hozumi N, Minden M, Mak TW, Gelfand EW: Rearrangement of the T-cell receptor B-chain gene in non-T-cell, non-B-cell acute lymphoblastic leukemia of childhood. N Engl J Med 313:1033–1037, 1985

163. Felix CA, Reaman GH, Korsmeyer SJ, Hollis GF, Dinndorf PA, Wright JJ, Kirsch IR: Immunoglobulin and T cell receptor gene configuration in acute lymphoblastic leukemia of infancy. Blood 70:536–541, 1987

164. Bowman WP, Melvin S, Mauer AM: Cell markers in lymphomas and leukemias. In Stollerman GH (ed): Advances in Internal Medicine, vol 25, pp 391–425. Chicago, Year Book Medical Publishers, 1980

165. Sallan SE, Ritz J, Pesando J, Gelber R, O'Brien C, Hitchcock S, Coral F, Schlossman SK: Cell surface antigens: Prognostic implications in childhood acute lymphoblastic leukemia. Blood 55:395–402, 1980

166. Steinherz PG, Gaynon P, Miller DR, Reaman G, Bleyer A, Finkelstein J, Evans RG, Meyers P, Steinherz LJ, Sather H, Hammond D: Improved disease-free survival of children with acute lymphoblastic leukemia at high risk for early relapse with the New York regimen—a new intensive therapy protocol: A report from the Childrens Cancer Study Group. J Clin Oncol 4:744–752, 1986

167. Kalwinsky DK, Roberson P, Dahl G, Harber J, Rivera G, Bowman WP, Pui C-H, Ochs J, Abromowitch M, Costlow ME, Melvin SL, Stass S, Williams DL, Murphy SB: Clinical relevance of lymphoblast biological features in children with acute lymphoblastic leukemia. J Clin Oncol 3:477–484, 1985

168. Miller DR: Acute lymphoblastic leukemia. Pediatr Clin North Am 27:269–291, 1980

169. Hammond GD, Sather H, Bleyer WA, Coccia P: Stratification by prognostic factors in the design and analysis of clinical trials for acute lymphoblastic leukaemia. Haematology and blood transfusion. In Buchner T, Schellong G, Hiddemann W, Urbanitz D, Ritter J (eds): Acute Leukemias, pp 161–166. Berlin, Springer-Verlag, 1987

170. Reinherz EL, Kung PC, Goldstein G, Levey RH, Schlossman SF: Discrete stages of human intrathymic differentiation: Analysis of normal thymocytes and leukemic lymphoblasts of T-cell lineage. Proc Natl Acad Sci USA 77:1588–1592, 1980

171. Weiss LM, Bindl JM, Picozzi VJ, Link MP, Warnke RA: Lymphoblastic lymphoma: An immunophenotype study of 26 cases with comparison to T cell acute lymphoblastic leukemia. Blood 67:474–478, 1986

172. Roper M, Crist WM, Metzgar R et al: Monoclonal antibody characterization of surface antigens in childhood T-cell lymphoid malignancies. Blood 61:830–837, 1983

173. Reinherz EL, Schlossman SF: Derivation of human T-cell leukemias. Cancer Res 41:4767–4770, 1981

174. Mirro J Jr, Kitchingman G, Behm FG, Murphy SB, Goorha RM: T cell differentiation states identified by molecular and immunologic analysis of the T cell receptor complex in childhood lymphoblastic leukemia. Blood 69:908–912, 1987

175. Chien Y-Y, Iwashima M, Wettstein DA et al: T cell receptor Delta gene rearrangements in early thymocytes. Nature 330:722–727, 1987

176. Kitchingman GR, Rovigatti U, Mauer AM, Melvin S, Murphy SB, Stass S: Rearrangement of immunoglobulin heavy chain genes in T cell acute lymphoblastic leukemia. Blood 65:725–729, 1985

177. Dinndorf PA, Andrews RG, Benjamin D, Ridgway D, Wolff L, Bernstein ID: Expression of normal myeloid-associated antigens by acute leukemia cells. Blood 67:1048–1053, 1986

178. Mirro J, Zipf TF, Pui C, Kitchingman G, Williams D, Melvin S, Murphy SB, Stass S: Acute mixed lineage leukemia: Clinicopathologic correlations and prognostic significance. Blood 65:1115–1123, 1985

179. Sobol RE, Mick R, Royston I, Davey FR, Ellison RR, Newman R, Cuttner J, Griffin JD, Collins H, Nelson D, Bloomfield CD: Clinical importance of myeloid antigen expression in adult acute lymphoblastic leukemia. N Engl J Med 316:1111–1117, 1987

180. Stass S, Mirro J: Lineage heterogeneity in acute leukemia: Acute mixed-lineage leukemia and lineage switch. Clin Haematol 15:811–827, 1986

181. Greaves M, Paxton A, Janosay G, Pain C, Johnson S, Lister TA: Acute lymphoblastic leukemia associated antigen III. Alterations in expression during treatment and in relapse. Leuk Res 4:1–14, 1980

182. Borella L, Casper JT, Lauer SK: Shifts in expression of cell membrane phenotypes in childhood lymphoid malignancies at relapse. Blood 54:64–71, 1979

183. Yunis JJ, Brunning RD: Prognostic significance of chromosomal abnormalities in acute leukaemias and myelodysplastic syndromes. Clin Haematol 15:597–620, 1986

184. Williams DL, Raimondi S, Rivera G et al: Presence of clonal chromosome abnormalities in virtually all cases of acute lymphoblastic leukemia. N Engl J Med 310:640–641, 1985

185. Bloomfield CD, Goldman AE, Alimena G, Berger R, Borgstrom GH et al: Chromosomal abnormalities identify high-risk and low-risk patients with acute lymphoblastic leukemia. Blood 67:415–420, 1986

186. Look AT, Roberson PK, Williams DL, Rivera G, Bowman WP et al: Prognostic importance of blast cell DNA content in childhood acute lymphoblastic leukemia. Blood 65:1079–1086, 1985

187. Williams DL, Harber J, Murphy SB, Look AT, Kalwinski DK et al: Chromosomal translocations play a unique role in influencing prognosis in childhood acute lymphoblastic leukemia. Blood 68:205–212, 1986

188. LeBeau MM, Rowley JD: Chromosomal abnormalities in leukemia and lymphoma: Clinical and biological significance. Adv Human Genet 15:1–54, 1986

189. Look AT: The emerging genetics of acute lymphoblastic leukemia: Clinical and biologic implications. Semin Oncol 12:92–104, 1985

190. Hossfeld DK: Chromosomes in acute lymphocytic leukemia. Cancer Genet Cytogenet 26:59–64, 1987

191. Sandberg AA: The chromosomes in human leukemia. Semin Hematol 23:201–217, 1986

192. Third International Workshop on Chromosomes in Leukemia: Chromosomal abnormalities and their clinical significance in acute lymphoblastic leukemia. Cancer Res 43:868–873, 1983

193. Secker–Walker LM, Lowler SD, Hardisty RM: Prognostic implications of chromosomal findings in acute lymphoblastic leukaemia at diagnosis. Br Med J 2:1529–1530, 1978

194. Brodeur GM, Williams DL, Look AT et al: Near-haploid acute lymphoblastic leukemia: A unique subgroup with a poor prognosis? Blood 58:14–19, 1981

195. Rowley JD: The cytogenetics of acute leukaemia. Clin Haematol 7:385–406, 1978

196. Reisman LE, Mitani M, and Zuelzer WW: Chromosome studies in leukemia: I. Evidence for the origin of leukemic stem lines from aneuploid mutants. N Engl J Med 270:591–597, 1974

197. Look AT: The cytogenetics of childhood leukemia: Clinical and biologic implications. Pediatr Clin North Am 35:723–742, 1988

198. Berger R, Bernheim A, Brouet JC, Daniel MT, Flandrin G: t(8:14) translocation in a Burkitt's type of lymphoblastic leukaemia (L3). Br J Haematol 43:87–90, 1979

199. Carroll AJ, Crist WM, Parmley RT et al: Pre-B cell leukemia associated with chromosome translocation 1;19. Blood 63:721–724, 1984

200. Williams DL, Look AT, Melvin SL, Roberson PK, Dhal G, Flake T, Stass S: New chromosomal translocations correlate with specific immunophenotypes of childhood acute lymphoblastic leukemia. Cell 36:101–109, 1984

201. Parkin JL, Arthur DC, Abramson CS et al: Acute leukemia associated with the t(4;11) chromosome rearrangement: Ultrastructural and immunologic characteristics. Blood 60:1321–1331, 1982

202. Kocova M, Kowalczyk JR, Sandberg AA: Translocation 4;11 acute leukemia: Three case reports and review of the literature. Cancer Genet Cytogenet 16:21–32, 1985

203. Erikson J, Williams DL, Finan J, Nowell PC, Croce CM: Locus of the α-chain of the T-cell receptor is split by chromosome translocation in T-cell leukemias. Science 229:784–786, 1985

204. Ribeiro RC, Abromowitch M, Raimondi SC, Murphy SB, Behm F, Williams DL: Clinical and biologic hallmarks of the Philadelphia chromosome in childhood acute lymphoblastic leukemia. Blood 70:948–953, 1987

205. Groffen J, Stephenson JR, Heisterkamp N, deKlein A, Bartram CR, Grosveld G: Philadelphia chromosomal breakpoints are clustered within a limited region, bcr, on chromosome 22. Cell 36:93, 1984

206. Cannizzaro LA, Nowell PC, Belasco JB, Croce CM, Emanuel BS: The breakpoint in 22q11 in a case of Ph-positive acute lymphocytic leukemia interrupts the immunoglobulin light chain gene cluster. Cancer Genet Cytogenet 18:173, 1985

207. Clark SS, McLaughlin J, Crist WM, Champlin R, Witte ON: Unique forms of the abl tyrosine kinase distinguish Ph¹-positive CML from Ph¹-positive ALL. Science 235:85–88, 1987

208. McCaffrey R, Smoler DF, Baltimore D: Terminal deoxynucleotidyl transferase in a case of childhood acute lymphoblastic leukemia. Proc Natl Acad Sci USA 70:521–525, 1973

209. Hoffbrand AF, Drexler HG, Ganeshaguru K, Piga A, Wickremasinghe RG: Biochemical aspects of acute leukaemia. Clin Haematol 15:669–694, 1986

210. Desiderio SV, Yancopoulos DG, Paskind M et al: Insertion of N regions into heavy chain genes is correlated with expression of terminal deoxynuclotidyl transferase in B cells. Nature 311:752–755, 1984

211. Drexler HG, Messmore HL, Menom M, Monowada J: Incidence of TdT-positivity in cases of leukemia and lymphoma. Acta Haematol 75:12–17, 1986

212. Hutton JJ, Coleman MS, Moffett S et al: Prognostic significance of terminal transferase activity in childhood acute lymphoblastic leukemia: A prospective analysis of 164 patients. Blood 60:1267–1276, 1982

213. Janossy G, Bollum FJ, Bradstock KF et al: Terminal transferase positive human bone marrow cells exhibit the antigenic phenotype of common acute lymphoblastic leukemia. J Immunol 123:1525–1529, 1979

214. Barr RD, Koekebakiker M, Sarin PS: Early relapse of acute lymphoblastic leukemia is not predictable by serial biochemical assays of terminal transferase activity in cells from peripheral blood. Leuk Res 8:351–354, 1984

215. Poplack DG, Blatt J, Reaman G: Purine pathway enzyme abnormalities in acute lymphoblastic leukemia. Cancer Res 41:4821–4823, 1981

216. Smyth JF, Poplack DG, Holiman BJ, Leventhal BG, Yarbro G: Correlation of adenosine deaminase activity with cell surface markers in acute lymphoblastic leukemia J Clin Invest 62:710–712, 1978

217. Reaman GH, Levin N, Muchmore A, Holiman BJ, Poplack DG: Diminished lymphoblast 5'-nucleotidase activity in acute lymphoblastic leukemia with T-cell characteristics. N Engl J Med 300:1374–1377, 1979

218. Blatt J, Reaman G, Levin N, Poplack DG: Purine neucleoside phosphorylase activity in acute lymphoblastic leukemia. Blood 56:380–382, 1980

219. Smyth JF, Harrap KR: Adenosine deaminase activity in leukaemia. Br J Cancer 31:544–549, 1975

220. Poplack DG, Sallan SE, Rivera G: Phase I study 2'-deoxycoformycin in acute lymphoblastic leukemia. Cancer Res 41:3343–3346, 1981

221. Russell NH, Hoffbrand AV, Bellingham AJ: Potential use of purine nucleosides and enzyme inhibitors for selective depletion of Thy-lymphoblasts from human bone marrow. Leuk Res 10:325–329, 1986

222. Wickremasinghe RG, Piga A, Mire AR et al: Tyrosine protein kinases and their substrates in human leukaemia cells. Leuk Res 9:1443–1450, 1985

223. Ellis RB, Rapson NT, Patrick AD, Greaves MF: Expressions of hexosaminidase isoenzymes in childhood leukemia. N Engl J Med 298:476–480, 1978

224. Greaves MJ: Analysis of the clinical and biological significance of lymphoid phenotypes in acute leukemia. Cancer Res 41:4752–4766, 1981

225. Besley GTN, Broadhead DM, Bain AD, Dewar AE, Eden OB: Enzyme markers in acute lymphoblastic leukaemia. Lancet 2:1311, 1978

226. Kornberg A, Polliack A: Serum lactic dehydrogenase (LDH) levels in acute leukemia: Marked elevations in lymphoblastic leukemia. Blood 56:351–355, 1980

227. Pui HJ, Parwaresch MR, Kulenkampff C, Staudinger M, Stein H: Lysosomal acid esterase: Activity and isoenzymes in separated normal human blood cells. Blood 55:891–897, 1985

228. Quddus FF, Leventhal BG, Boyett JM, Pullin DJ, Crist WM, Borowitz MJ: Glucocorticoid receptors in immunological subtypes of childhood acute lymphocytic leukemia cells: A Pediatric Oncology Group study. Canc Res 45:6482–6486, 1985

229. Lippman ME, Barr R: Glucocorticoid receptors in purified subpopulations of human peripheral blood lymphocytes. J Immunol 118:1977–1981, 1977

230. Konior GS, Lippman ME, Johnson GE, Leventhal BG: Glucocorticoid receptors in subpopulations of childhood acute lymphocytic leukemia. Cancer Res 37:2688–2695, 1977

231. Lippman ME, Konior GS, Leventhal BG: Clinical implications of glucocorticoid receptors in human leukemia. Cancer Res 38:4251–4256, 1976

232. Mastrangelo R, Malandrino R, Riccardi R, Longo P, Ranelletti FO, Iacobelli S: Clinical implications of glucocorticoid receptors studied in childhood acute lymphoblastic leukemia. Blood 56:1036–1040, 1980

233. Iacobelli S, Marchetti P, DeRosi G, Mandelli F: Glucocorticoid receptors and steroid sensitivity of human acute lymphoblastic leukemia. In Hormones and Cancer, pp 235–246. New York, Alan R Liss, 1984

234. Pui C-H, Ochs J, Kalwinsky DK, Costlow ME: Impact of treatment efficacy on the prognostic value of glucocorticoid receptor levels in childhood acute lymphoblastic leukemia. Leuk Res 8:345–350, 1984

235. Murphy SB, Aur RBJ, Simone JV, George S, Mauer AM: Pretreatment cytokinetic studies in 94 children with acute leukemia. Relationship to other variables at diagnosis and outcome of standard treatment. Blood 49:683–691, 1977

236. Scarffe JH, Hann IM, Evans DI, Morris Jones P, Palmer MK, Lilleyman SJ, Crowther D: Relationship between the pretreatment proliferative activity of marrow blast cells and prognosis of acute lymphoblastic leukaemia of childhood. Br J Cancer 41:764–771, 1980

237. Look AT, Melvin SL, Williams DL, Brodeur GM, Dahl GV, Kalwinsky DK, Murphy SB, Mauer AM: Aneuploidy and percentage of S-phase cells determined by flow cytometry correlate with cell phenotype in childhood acute leukemia. Blood 60:959–967, 1982

238. Dow LW, Change LJA, Tsiatis AA, Melvin SL, Bowman WP: Relationship of pretreatment lymphoblast proliferative activity and prognosis in 97 children with acute lymphoblastic leukemia. Blood 59:1197–1202, 1982

239. Gavosto F, Masera P: Different cell proliferation models in myeloblastic and lymphoblastic leukemia. Contribution of cell kinetics to the classification of acute leukaemias. Blood Cells 1:217, 1975

240. McKenna RW, Byrnes RK, Nesbit ME, Bloomfield CD, Kersey JH, Spangers

E, Brunning RD: Cytochemical profiles in acute lymphoblastic leukemia. Am J Pediatr Hematol Oncol 1:263–274, 1979

241. Catovsky D, Galetto J, Okos A, Miliani E, Galton DAG: Cytochemical profile of B and T leukemic lymphocytes with special reference to acute lymphoblastic leukemia. J Clin Pathol 27:767–771, 1979

242. Fledges AJ, Aur RJA, Verzosa MS, Daniels S: Periodic acid-Schiff reaction, a useful index of duration of complete remission in acute childhood lymphocytic leukaemia. Acta Haematol 52:8–13, 1974

243. Ascari E, Marini G, Invernizzi R, Ippolita G, Casirotia G, Fontana G, Rizzo SC: On the usefulness of PAS reaction for the prognosis of acute lymphoblastic leukemia. Haematologica 60:300–307, 1975

244. Lilleyman JS, Mills V, Sugden PJ, Britton JA: Periodic acid-Schiff reaction and prognosis in lymphoblastic leukemia. J Clin Pathol 32:158–161, 1979

245. Humphrey GB, Nesbit ME, Brunning RD: Prognostic value of the periodic acid-Schiff (PAS) reaction in acute lymphoblastic leukemia. Am J Clin Pathol 61:393–397, 1974

246. Ritter J, Gaedicke G, Winkler K, Landbeck G: Immunological Oberflachenmarker von Lymphoblastin bei der saure Phosphatase-positiven akuten Leukamie. Z Kinderbeilk 120:211–215, 1975

247. Huhn D, Rodt H, Thiel E: Acid phosphatase in acute lymphoblastic leukemia (ALL). In Thierfelder S, Rodt H, Thiel E (eds): Immunological Diagnosis of Leukemias and Lymphomas, pp 169–170. Berlin, Springer-Verlag, 1977

248. Knowles DM, Halper JP, Machin GA, Sherman W: Acid a-naphthyl acetate esterase activity in human neoplastic lymphoid cells. Am J Pathol 96:257–277, 1979

249. Melhorn DK, Gross S, Newman AJ: Acute childhood leukemia presenting as aplastic anemia. The response to corticosteroids. J Pediatr 77:647–652, 1970

250. Nelken RP, Stockman JA: The hypereosinophilic syndrome in association with acute lymphoblastic leukemia. J Pediatr 89:771–773, 1976

251. Hogan TF, Koss W, Murgo AJ, Amato RS, VanScoy FL: Acute lymphoblastic leukemia with chromosomal 5;14 translocation and hypereosinophilia: Case report and literature review. J Clin Oncol 5:382–390, 1987

252. Testa JR, Hogge DE, Misawa S et al: Chromosome 16 rearrangements in acute myelomonocytic leukemia with abnormal eosinophils. N Engl J Med 310:468–469, 1984

253. Bodey GP, Buckley M, Sathe US: Quantitative relationships between circulating leukocytes and infections in patients with acute leukemia. Ann Intern Med 64:328–340, 1966

254. Gaydos LA, Freireich EJ, Mantel N: The quantitative relation between platelet count and hemorrhage in patients with acute leukemia. N Engl J Med 266:905–909, 1962

255. Gralnick HR, Galton DAG, Catovsky D, Sultan C, Bennett JM: Classification of acute leukemia. Ann Intern Med 87:740–753, 1977

256. Kushner DC, Weinstein HJ, Kirkpatrick JA: The radiological diagnosis of leukemia and lymphoma in children. Semin Roentgenol 115:316–334, 1980

257. Hann IM, Lees PD, Palmer MK et al: Renal size as a prognostic factor in childhood acute lymphoblastic leukemia. Cancer 48:207–209, 1981

258. Bunin NJ, Pui Ch: Differing complications of hyperleukocytosis in children with acute lymphoblastic or acute nonlymphoblastic leukemia. J Clin Oncol 3:1590–1595, 1985

259. Ramsey NKC, Brown DM, Nesbit ME, Cercia PF, Krivit W, Krutzik S: Autonomous production of parathyroid hormone by lymphoblastic leukemia cells in culture. J Pediatr 94:623–625, 1979

260. Zasman J, Brown DM, Nesbit ME: Hyperphosphatemia, hyperphosphaturia and hypocalcemia in acute leukemia. N Engl J Med 289:1335–1340, 1973

261. Wilson JKU: The bone lesions of childhood leukemia: A survey of 140 cases. Radiology 72:672–681, 1959

262. Aur RJA, Westbrook W, Riggs W Jr: Childhood acute leukemia: Initial radiological bone involvement and prognosis. Am J Dis Child 124:653–654, 1972

263. Masera G, Carnelli U, Ferraci M, Recchia M, Bellini F: Prognostic significance of radiological bone involvement in childhood acute lymphoblastic leukemia. Arch Dis Child 52:530–533, 1977

264. Thomas LB, Forkner CE, Frei E, Besse BE, Stabenan JR: The skeletal lesions of acute leukemia. Cancer 14:608–621, 1961

265. Sitarz AL, Berdon WE, Wolff JA, Baker DH: Acute lymphocytic leukemia masquerading as acute osteomyelitis. Pediatr Radiol 9:33–35, 1980

266. Leiken S, Miller DR, Sather H et al: Immunologic evaluation in the prognosis of acute lymphoblastic leukemia. A report from Childrens Cancer Study Group. Blood 58:5601, 1981

267. Khalifa AS, Take H, Cejka J, Zuelzer WW: Immunoglobulins in acute leukemia in children. J Pediatr 85:788, 1974

268. Hann IM, Morris-Jones PH, Evans DIK et al: Low IgG or IgA: A further indicator of poor prognosis in childhood acute lymphoblastic leukaemia. Br J Cancer 41:317, 1980

269. Banker D, Pahwa R, Miller DR et al: Immunoregulatory properties of childhood leukemias. J Clin Immunol 2:230, 1982

270. Miller LP, Miller DR: Acute lymphoblastic leukemia in children: Current status, controversies, and future perspective. Crit Rev Oncol Hematol 1:129–197, 1986

271. Priest JR, Ramsay NKC, Steinherz PG, Tubergen DG, Cairo MS, Sitarz AL, Bishop AJ, White L, Trigg ME, Levitt CJ, Cich JA, Coccia PF: A syndrome of thrombosis and hemorrhage complicating L-asparaginase therapy for childhood acute lymphoblastic leukemia. J Pediatr 100:984–989, 1982

272. Mathe G, Schwarzenberg L, Mery AM, Cattan A, Schneider M, Amiel JL, Schlumberger JR, Poisson J, Wajener G: Extensive histological and cytological survey of patients with acute leukaemia in "complete remission." Br Med J 1:640–642, 1966

273. Nies BA, Bodey GP, Thomas LB, Brecher G, Freireich EJ: The persistence of extramedullary leukemic infiltrates during bone marrow remission of acute leukemia. Blood 26:133–141, 1965

274. Simone JV, Holland E, Johnson W: Fatalities during remission of childhood leukemia. Blood 39:759–770, 1972

275. Sharp HL, Nesbit MF, D'Angio GJ, Krivit W: Addition of local radiation after bone marrow remission in acute leukemia in children. Cancer 20:1403–1404, 1967

276. Evans AW, Gilbert ES, Zandstra R: The increasing incidence of central nervous system leukemia in children. Cancer 26:404–409, 1970

277. Hardisty RM, Norman PM: Meningeal leukemia. Arch Dis Child 42:441–447, 1967

278. Sullivan MP, Vietti TJ, Haggard ME, Donaldson MA, Krall JM, Gehan EA: Remission maintenance therapy for meningeal leukemia: Intrathecal methotrexate versus intravenous bis-nitrosourea. Blood 38:680–688, 1971

279. Gribbon MA, Hardisty RM, Chessells JM: Long-term control of central nervous system leukemia. Arch Dis Child 52:673–678, 1977

280. Mastrangelo R, Zuelzer WW, Ecklund PS, Thompson RI: Chromosomes in the spinal fluid. Evidence for metastatic origin of meningeal leukemia. Blood 35:227–235, 1970

281. Thomas LB: Pathology of leukemia in the brain and meninges: Postmortem studies of patients with acute leukemia and of mice given inoculations of L1210 leukemia. Cancer Res 25:1555–1571, 1965

282. Thomas LB, Chirigos MA, Humphreys SR, Golden A: Pathology of the spread of L1210 leukemia in the central nervous system of mice and effect of treatment with cytoxan. J Natl Cancer Inst 28:1355–1389, 1962

283. Price RA, Johnson WW: The central nervous system and childhood leukemia: I. The arachnoid. Cancer 31:530–533, 1973

284. Azzarelli B, Roesmann U: Pathogenesis of central nervous system infiltration in acute leukemia. Arch Pathol Lab Med 101:203–205, 1977

285. West RJ, Grayham-Pole J, Hardisty RM, Pike MC: Factors in pathogenesis of central nervous system leukaemia. Br Med J 3:311–314, 1972

286. de Quirroz A, Ribeiro DA: Alteracoaes encephalicas nos leucemias. Aspectos histopatologicos do envolvimento dos plexos coroides. Arq Neuro Psiquiatr 36:332–339, 1978

287. Bleyer WA: Central nervous system leukemia. Pediatr Clin North Am 35:789–814, 1988

288. Bleyer WA, Poplack DG: Prophylaxis and treatment of leukemia in the central nervous system and other sanctuaries. Semin Oncol 12(2):131–1148, 1985

289. Bleyer WA: Central nervous system leukemia. In Gunz FW, Henderson ES (eds): Leukemia, 4th ed, pp 865–911, New York, Grune & Stratton, 1983

290. Davey DD, Foucar K, Giller R: Milipore filter versus cytocentrifuge for detection of childhood central nervous system leukemia. Arch Pathol Lab Med 110:705–708, 1986

291. McIntosh, Ritchey AK: Diagnostic problems in cerebrospinal fluid of children with lymphoid malignancies. Am J Pediatr Hematol Oncol 8:28–31, 1986

292. Veerman AJ, Huismans LD, van Zantwijk IC: Diagnosis of meningeal leukemia using immunoperoxidase methods to demonstrate common acute lymphoblastic leukemia cells in cerebrospinal fluid. Leuk Res 9:1195–200, 1985

293. van Leeuwen EF, Pinkster T, Behrendt H, Tetteroo PAT, Kinderziekenhuis E: A micro-assay for early detection of central nervous system (CNS) leukemia. Fourth International Symposium on Therapy of Acute Leukemias, Rome, p 283, 1987

294. Nagelkerke AF, vanKamp GJ, Veerman AJ, deWaal FC: Unreliability of beta-2-microglobulin in early detection of central nervous system relapse in

acute lymphoblastic leukemia. Eur J Cancer Clin Oncol 21:659–663, 1985

295. Marra R, Pagano L, Storid S, Sica S, Leone IG, Bizzi B: Beta 2 microglobulin in cerebrospinal fluid of patients affected by acute leukemia. Fourth International Symposium on Therapy of Acute Leukemias, Rome, p 351, 1987

296. Seidenfeld J, Martin LJ: Biochemical markers of central nervous system tumors measured in cerebrospinal fluid and their potential use in diagnosis and patient management: A review. JNCI 63:919–931, 1979

297. Watson EM, Sauer HR, Sadugor MG: Manifestations of the lymphoblastomas in the genito-urinary tract. J Urol 61:626–642, 1949

298. Stoffel TJ, Nesbit ME, Livitt SH: Extramedullary involvement of the testes in childhood. Cancer 35:1203–1211, 1975

299. Kuo TT, Tschang TP, Chu JY: Testicular relapse in childhood acute lymphocytic leukemia during bone marrow remission. Cancer 38:2604–2612, 1976

300. Fengler R, Henze G, Langermann H-J et al: Haufigkeit und Behandlungseigebnisse testikularer Rezidive bie der akuten lymphoblastischen Leukamie in Kindesalter. Klin Padiatr 194:204–208, 1982

301. Hustu HO, Aur RJA: Extramedullary leukaemia. Clin Haematol 7:313–337, 1978

302. Russo A, Schiliro G: The Enigma of testicular leukemia: A critical review. Med Pediatr Oncol 14:300–306, 1986

303. Bowman WP, Aur RJA, Hustu HO, Rivera G: Isolated testicular relapse in acute lymphocytic leukemia of childhood: Categories and influence on survival. J Clin Oncol 2:924–929, 1984

304. Sather H, Miller D, Nesbit M, Heyn R, Hammond D: Differences in prognosis for boys and girls with acute lymphoblastic leukaemia. Lancet 1:739–743, 1981

305. Eden OB, Rankin A, Kay HEM: Isolated testicular relapse in acute lymphoblastic leukemia of childhood. Arch Dis Child 58:128–132, 1983

306. Baum ES, Land VJ, Joo P, Starling K, Leiken S, Miale T, Krivit, W, Miller D, Chard R, Nesbit M, Sather H, Hammond D: Cessation of chemotherapy during complete remission of childhood acute lymphoblastic leukemia. Proc Am Soc Clin Oncol 18:290, 1977

307. Hudson MM, Frankel LS, Mullins J, Swanson DA: Diagnostic value of surgical testicular biopsy after therapy for acute lymphocytic leukemia. J Pediatr 107:50–53, 1985

308. Pui C-H, Dahl GB, Bowman WP, Rao BN, Abromowitch M, Ochs J, Rivera G: Elective testicular biopsy during chemotherapy for childhood leukaemia is of no clinical value. Lancet 2:410–412, 1985

309. Chessells JM: Diagnostic value of testicular biopsy in acute lymphoblastic leukemia. J Pediatr 108:331–332, 1986

310. Chessells JM, Pincott J, Janossy G: TdT+ cells in routine testicular biopsy; significance and relation to histology and clinical outcome. Br J Haematol 58:184–185, 1984

311. Eden OB, Hardisty RM, Innes EM et al: Testicular disease in acute lymphoblastic leukaemia in childhood. Br Med J 1:334–338, 1978

312. Wong KY, Ballard ET, Strayer FH et al: Clinical and occult testicular leukemia in long-term survivors of acute lymphoblastic leukemia. J Pediatr 96:569–574, 1980

313. Baum E, Sather H, Nachman J et al: Relapse rate following cessation of chemotherapy during complete remission of acute lymphocytic leukemia. Med Pediatr Oncol 7:25–34, 1979

314. Nesbit ME, Robison L, Ortega JA et al: Testicular relapse in childhood acute lymphoblastic leukemia: Association with pretreatment patient characteristics and treatment. A report for Children's Cancer Study Group. Cancer 45:2009–2016, 1980

315. Kay HEM: Testicular infiltration in acute lymphoblastic leukaemia. Br J Haematol 53:537–542, 1983

316. Givler RL: Testicular involvement in leukemia and lymphoma. Cancer 23:1290–1295, 1969

317. Sarontz HI, Gilchrist GS, Smithsen WA, Burgent EO, Cupps RF: Testicular relapse in childhood leukemia. Mayo Clin Proc 53:212–216, 1978

318. Kim TH, Hargreaves HK, Byrnes RK et al: Pretreatment testicular biopsy in childhood acute lymphocytic leukemia. Lancet 2:652–658, 1981

319. Kim TH, Hargreaves HK, Chan WC, Brynes RK, Alvarado C, Woodard J, Ragab A: Sequential testicular biopsies in childhood acute lymphocytic leukemia. Cancer 57:1038–1041, 1986

320. Klein EA, Kay R, Norris DG, George CR, Richmond B: Noninvasive testicular screening in childhood leukemia. J Urol 136:864–866, 1986

321. Finklestein JZ, Dyment PG, Hammond D: Leukemic infiltration of the testes during bone marrow remission. Pediatrics 43:1042–1045, 1969

322. Riccardi R, Vigersky R, Barnes S et al: Methotrexate levels in the interstitial space and seminiferous tubule of rat testis. Cancer Res 42:1617–1619, 1982

323. Baum E, Heyn R, Nesbit M, Tilford D, Hachman J: Occult abdominal involvement with apparently isolated testicular relapse in children with acute lymphocytic leukemia. Am J Pediatr Hematol Oncol 6:343–346, 1984

324. Haghbin M: Chemotherapy of acute lymphoblastic leukemia in children. Am J Hematol 1:201–209, 1976

325. Brecher ML, Weinberg V, Boyett JM, Sinks LLF, Jones B, Glicksman A, Holland JF, Freeman AI: Intermediate dose methotrexate in childhood acute lymphoblastic leukemia resulting in decreased incidence of testicular relapse. Cancer 58:1024–1028, 1986

326. Kay H, Rankin A: Testicular irradiation in leukaemia. Lancet 2:1115, 1981

327. Nesbit ME, Sather H, Robinson LL, Donaldson M, Littman P, Ortega JA, Hammond GD: Sanctuary therapy: A randomized trial of 724 children with previously untreated acute lymphoblastic leukemia. Cancer Res 42:674–680, 1982

328. Georgitis J, Eiger H, Provisor D, Baehner RL: Isolated pulmonary leukemic relapse following successful bone marrow transplant in a child with acute lymphoblastic leukemia. Pediatrics 64:913–917, 1979

329. Ross JS, Ellman L: Leukemia infiltration of the lungs in the chemotherapy era. Am J Clin Pathol 61:325, 1974

330. Eden OB: Extramedullary leukaemia. In Willoughby M, Siegel SE (eds): Hematology and Oncology, p 47. London, Butterworths, 1982

331. Bunin NJ, Pui C-H, Hustu O, Rivera GK: Unusual extramedullary relapses in children with acute lymphoblastic leukaemia. J Pediatr 109:665–668, 1986

332. Ninane J: The eye as a sanctuary in acute lymphoblastic leukaemia. Lancet 1:452, 1980

333. Jankovic M, Masera G, Uderzo C, Cattorelli G, Conter V, Ceppellini C, Miglior M, Lasagni F, Lambertenghi E, Parravicini C et al: Recurrences of isolated leukemic hypopyon in a child with acute lymphoblastic leukemia. Cancer 57:380–384, 1986

334. Simone JV, Verzosa MS, Rudy JA: Initial features and prognosis in 363 children with acute lymphocytic leukemia. Cancer 36:2099–2108, 1975

335. Pendergrass TW, Hoover R, Godwin JD: Prognosis of black children with acute lymphoblastic leukemia. Med Pediatr Oncol 1:143–148, 1975

336. Miller DR, Leikin S, Albo V et al: The use of prognostic factors in improving the design and efficiency of clinical trials in childhood leukemia. Cancer Chemother Rep 64:381–392, 1980

337. Rogentine C, Rapani R, Yankee R et al: HLA antigens in acute leukemia. Tissue Antigens 3:470–476, 1973

338. Kersey J, Coccia P, Bloomfield C: Surface markers define human lymphoid malignancies with differing prognoses. Hematol Blood Transfus 20:17–24, 1977

339. Sather HN: Age at diagnosis of childhood acute lymphoblastic leukemia. Med Pediatr Oncol 14:166–172, 1986

340. Hammond D, Sather H, Nesbit M, Miller D, Coccia P, Bleyer A, Lukens J, Siegel S: Analysis of prognostic factors in acute lymphoblastic leukemia. Med Pediatr Oncol 14:124–134, 1986

341. Sather HN: Statistical evaluation of prognostic factors in ALL and treatment results. Med Pediatr Oncol 14:158–165, 1986

342. Henze G, Langermann HG, Kaurmann U et al: Thymic involvement and initial white blood count in childhood acute lymphoblastic leukemia. Am J Pediatr Hematol Oncol 3:369, 1981

343. Revesz T, Banczur M, Gyodi E et al: The association of HLA-DR5 antigen with longer survival in childhood leukaemia. Br J Hematol 48:508, 1981

344. Lilleyman JS, Hann IM, Stevens RF: The clinical significance of blast cell morphology in childhood lymphblastic leukemia. Med Pediatr Oncol 14:144–147, 1986

345. van Eyes J, Pullen J, Head D, Boyett J, Crist W, Falletta J, Humphrey GB, Jacoson J, Riccardi V, Brock B: The French-American-British (FAB) classification of leukemia. The Pediatric Oncology Group experience with lymphocytic leukemia. Cancer 57:1046–1051, 1986

346. Zuelzer WW, Flatz G: Acute childhood leukemia: A ten-year study. Am J Dis Child 100:886–907, 1960

347. Bleyer WA, Sather H, Coccia P, Lukens J, Siegel S, Hammond GD: The staging of childhood acute lymphoblastic leukemia: Strategies of the Childrens Cancer Study Group and a three-dimensional technique of multivariate analysis. Med Pediatr Oncol 14:271–280, 1986

348. Mastrangelo R, Poplack D, Bleyer WA, Riccardi R, Sather H, D'Angio G: Report and recommendations of the Rome Workshop concerning poor-prognosis acute lymphoblastic leukemia in children: Biologic bases for staging, stratification, and treatment. Med Pediatr Oncol 14:191–194, 1986

349. Robison L, Sather H, Coccia P et al: Assessment of the interrelationship of

prognostic factors in childhood acute lymphoblastic leukemia. Am J Pediatr Hematol Oncol 2:3–5, 1980

350. Miller DR: Prognostic factors in childhood acute lymphoblastic leukemia. J Pediatr 87:672–676, 1974

351. George S, Fernbach D, Vietti I, Sullivan MP, Lane DM, Haggard ME, Berry DH, Lonsdale D, Komp D: Factors influencing survival in pediatric acute leukemia. Cancer 32:1542–1553, 1973

352. Hardisty R, Till M: Acute leukemia 1959–64: Factors affecting prognosis. Arch Dis Child 43:107–115, 1968

353. Reaman G, Zeltzer P, Bleyer WA, Amendola B, Level C, Sather H, Hammond D: Acute lymphoblastic leukemia in infants less than one year of age: A cumulative experience of the Childrens Cancer Study Group. J Clin Oncol 3:1513–1521, 1985

354. Harousseau JL, Tobelem G, Schaison G et al: High risk acute lymphocytic leukemia: A study of 141 cases with initial white blood counts over 100,000/cu. mm. Cancer 46:1996–2003, 1980

355. Baumer JH, Mott MG: Sex and prognosis in childhood acute lymphoblastic leukaemia. Lancet 2:128–129, 1978

356. Chessells JM, Hardisty RM, Richards S: Long survival in childhood lymphoblastic leukaemia. Br J Cancer 55:315–319, 1987

357. Riehm H, Gadner H, Henze G, Kornhuber B, Niethammer D, Schellong G: The five therapy trials ALL-BFM 1970–1986: A synopsis of results (abstract). Am Soc Clin Oncol, 1987

358. Pullen J, Boyett J, Borowitz M, Dowell B, Falletta J, Krejmas N, Sexauer C, Crist W: How important is common acute lympyocytic leukemia antigen (CALLA) negativity as a prognostic factor in children excluding infants with B-precursor acute lymphocytic leukemia (ALL): A Pediatric Oncology Group (POG) study. Proc Am Soc Clin Oncol 6:151, 1987

359. Davey FR, Lachant NA, Dock NL et al: HLA antigens and childhood acute lymphocytic leukaemia. Br J Haematol 47:211, 1981

360. Sjogren U: Amoeboid movement configuration and mitotic indices of lymphoid cells from children with acute lymphoblastic leukemia. Lymphology 9:69–71, 1976

361. Schumacher HR, Chambion JE, Thomas WJ, Pitts LL, Stass SA: Acute lymphoblastic leukemia-hand mirror variant. An analysis of a large group of patients. Am J Hematol 7:11–17, 1979

362. Sjogren U, Garwicz S: Prognostic significance of amoeboid movement configuration in lymphoid cells from children with acute lymphoblastic leukaemia. Scand J Haematol 24:335–339, 1980

363. Miller DR, Steinherz PG, Fuer D, Sather H, Hammond D: Unfavorable prognostic significance of hand mirror cells in childhood lymphocytic leukemia. Am J Dis Child 137:346–350, 1983

364. Glassy EF, Sun NCJ, Okun DB: Hand-mirror cell leukemia: Report of nine cases and a review of the literature. Am J Clin Pathol 74:651–656, 1980

365. Hogeman PHG, Veerman AJP, Huismans DR, Van Zantwijk C, Bezemer PD, Stamtwis IH, DeWaal FC: Handmirror cells and central nervous system relapse in childhood acute lymphoblastic leukaemia. Acta Haematol 72:181–189, 1984

366. Kalwinsky DK, Rivera G, Dahl GV, Roberson P, George S, Murphy SB, Simone JV: Variation by race in presenting clinical and biologic features of childhood acute lymphoblastic leukaemia: Implications for treatment outcome. Leuk Res 9:817–823, 1985

367. Sklo M, Gordis L, Tonascia J, Kaplan E: The changing survivorship of white and black children with leukemia. Cancer 42:59–66, 1978

368. Walters TR, Bushmore M, Simone J: Poor prognosis in Negro children with acute lymphoblastic leukemia. Cancer 29:210–214, 1972

369. Riehm H, Gadner H, Henze G et al: The Berlin childhood acute lymphoblastic leukemia therapy study, 1970–1976. Am J Pediatr Hematol Oncol 2:299–306, 1980

370. Sather H, Coccia P, Nesbit M et al: Disappearance of the predictive value of prognostic variables in childhood acute lymphocytic leukemia. Cancer 48:370–376, 1981

371. Frei E III, Sallan SE: Acute lymphoblastic leukemia: Treatment. Cancer 42:828–838, 1978

372. Frankel LS, Ochs J, Shuster J, Duboyw R, Bowman P, Hockenberry M, Leventhal B, Carroll AJ, Pullen J: Pilot protocol improves remissions for infant leukemia and provides detailed laboratory characterization. Proc Am Soc Clin Oncol 6:161, 1987

373. Leiper AD, Chessells J: Acute lymphoblastic leukaemia under 2 years. Arch Dis Child 61:1007–1012, 1986

374. Pui C-H, Raimondi SC, Murphy SB, Ribeiro RC, Kalwinski DK, Dahl GV, Crist WM, Williams DL: An analysis of leukemic cell chromosomal features in infants. Blood 69:1289–1293, 1987

375. Leverger G, Bancillon A, Schaison G, Alby N, Boiron M: Acute lymphoblastic leukemia in very young children. Am J Pediatr Hematol Oncol 8:213–219, 1986

376. Crist W, Pullin J, Boyett J, Falletta J, van Eyes J, Borowitz M, Jackson J, Dowell B, Frankel L, Quddus F et al: Clinical and biologic features predict a poor prognosis in acute lymphoid leukemias in infants: A Pediatric Oncology Group Study. Blood 67:135–140, 1986

377. Dinndorf PA, Reaman GH: Acute lymphoblastic leukemia in infants: Evidence for B cell origin of disease by use of monoclonal antibody phenotyping. Blood 68:975–978, 1986

378. Steinherz P, Siegel S, Bleyer A, Coccia P, Leikin S, Lukens J, Miller D, Nesbit M, Reaman G, Sather H, Hammond D: Lymphomatous presentation of acute lymphoblastic leukemia (abstract #599). Proc Am Soc Clin Oncol 5:153, 1986

379. Reaman GH, Poplack DG, Wesley R, Bleyer WA, Miser J, Feusner J, Hammond D: Prognostic factors for central nervous system (CNS) relapse in acute lymphoblastic leukemia (ALL) of childhood (abstract #C-787). Proc Am Soc Clin Oncol 3:202, 1984

380. Schrappe M, Henze G, Ludwig R, Reiter A, Ritter J, Wehinger H, Riehm H: The in vivo corticosteroid response and its prediction for early therapy failure in childhood ALL: A report from the BFM Study Group (abstract #62). Proceedings of the 4th International Symposium on Therapy of Acute Leukemia. Rome, February 1982

381. Bisel HF: Criteria for the evaluation of response to treatment in acute leukemia. Blood 11:676–677, 1956

382. Hewlett JS, Battle JD, Bishop RC, Fowler WM, Schwartz SO, Hagen PS, Louis J: Phase II study of A-8104 (NSC-25154) in acute leukemia in adults. Cancer Chemother Rep 42:25–28, 1964

383. Pinkel D: Five-year follow-up of "total therapy" of childhood lymphocytic leukemia. JAMA 216:648–652, 1971

384. Frei E, Karon M, Levin RH, Freireich EJ, Taylor RS, Hananian J, Selawry O, Holland JF, Hoogstraten B, Wolman IJ, Abin E, Sawitsky A, Lee S, Mills SD, Burgert EO, Spurr CL, Patterson RB, Ebaugh FG, James GW, Moon JH: The effectiveness of combinations of antileukemia agents in inducing and maintaining remission in children with acute leukemia. Blood 26:642–656, 1965

385. Frei E III, Freireich EJ: Progress and perspectives in the chemotherapy of acute leukemia. Adv Chemother 2:269–298, 1965

386. Skipper HE, Perry SE: Kinetics of normal and leukemic leukocyte populations—relevance to chemotherapy. Cancer Res 30:1883–1897, 1970

387. Hart JS, Shirkawa S, Trujillo J, Frei E III: The mechanism of induction of complete remission in acute myeloblastic leukemia in man. Cancer Res 29:2300–2307, 1969

388. Ortega JA, Nesbit ME, Donaldson MH, Hittle RE, Weiner J, Karon M, Hammond D: L-Asparaginase, vincristine, prednisone and Daunomycin in acute lymphocytic leukemia. Cancer Res 37:535–540, 1977

389. Vietti TJ, Starling K, Wilbur K, Lonsdale D, Lane DM: Vincristine, prednisone and Daunomycin in acute leukemia of childhood. Cancer 27:602–607, 1971

390. Mathe G, Hayat M, Schwarzenberg L, Amiel JL, Schneider M, Cattan A, Schlumberger JR, Jasmin C: Acute lymphoblastic leukemia treated with combination of prednisone, vincristine and rubidomycin: Value of pathogen-free rooms. Lancet 2:380–382, 1967

391. Sallan S, Camitta BM, Cassady JR, Nathan DG, Frei E III: Intermittent combination chemotherapy with Adriamycin for childhood acute lymphoblastic leukemia: Clinical results. Blood 51:425–433, 1978

392. Henderson ES: Combination chemotherapy of acute lymphocytic leukemia of childhood. Cancer Res 27:2570–2572, 1967

393. Aur RJA, Simone JV, Verzosa M, Hustu HO, Barker LF, Pinkel DP, Rivera G, Dahl GV, Wood A, Stagner S, Mason C: Childhood acute lymphocytic leukemia: Study VIII. Cancer 42:2123–2134, 1978

394. Mauer AM: Treatment of acute leukemia in children. Clin Haematol 7:245–258, 1978

395. Pinkel D: Treatment of acute leukemia. Pediatr Clin North Am 23:117–130, 1976

396. Aur R, Simone J, Hustu O, Rivera G, Dahl G, Bowman P, George S: Multiple combination therapy for childhood acute lymphocytic leukemia (ALL) (abstract). Blood 52:238, 1978

397. Henze G, Langermann JH, Bramswig J et al: Ergebnisse der Studie BFM 76/79 zur Behandlung der akuten lymphoblastichen Leukämie bei Kindern und Jugendichen. Klin Padiatr 193:145–154, 1981

398. Henze G, Langermann HJ, Fengler R et al: Therapiestudie BFM 79/81 zur Behandlung der akuten lymphoblastichen Leukämie bei Kindern und Jugendi-

chen: Intensivierte Reinduktionstherapie für Patientengruppen mit unterschied-lichem Rezidvrisiko. Klin Padiatr 194:195–203, 1982

399. Melhorn DK, Gross S, Fisher EJ, Newman AJ: Studies on the use of prophylactic, intrathecal amethopterin in childhood leukemia. Blood 36:55–60, 1970

400. Johnson RE: An experimental therapeutic approach to L1210 leukemia in mice: Combined chemotherapy and central nervous system irradiation. J Natl Cancer Inst 32:1333–1340, 1964

401. Aur RJA, Simone JV, Husto HO, Verzosa MS: A comparative study of central nervous system irradiation and intensive chemotherapy early in remission of childhood acute lymphocytic leukemia. Cancer 29:381–391, 1972

402. Aur RJA, Simone JV, Husto HO, Walters T, Borella L, Pratt C, Pinkel D: Central nervous system therapy and combination chemotherapy of childhood lymphocytic leukemia. Blood 37:272–281, 1971

403. Blatt J, Bercu BB, Gillin JC, Mendelson WB, Poplack DG: Reduced pulsatile growth hormone secretion in children after therapy for acute lymphoblastic leukemia. J Pediatr 104:182–196, 1984

404. Bode U, Oliff A, Bercu BB et al: Absence of CT brain scan and endocrine abnormalities with less intensive CNS prophylaxis. Am J Pediatr Hematol Oncol 2:21–24, 1985

405. Brouwers P, Riccardi R, Poplack D, Fedio P: Attentional deficits in long-term survivors of childhood acute lymphoblastic leukemia. J Clin Neuropsychol 6:325–336, 1984

406. Brouwers P, Riccardi R, Fedio P, Poplack DG: Long-term neuropsychological sequelae of childhood leukemia: correlation with CT brain scan abnormalities. J Pediatr 106:723–730, 1985

407. Carli M, Perilongo G, Lavarda AM et al: Risk factors for cerebral calcifications in patients treated with conventional CNS prophylaxis. Paper presented at Third International Symposium on Therapy of Acute Leukemias Rome, December 1982

408. Eiser C: Effects of chronic illness on intellectual development: A comparison of normal children with those treated for childhood leukemia and solid tumors. Arch Dis Child 55:766–770, 1980

409. Eiser C, Lansdown R: Retrospective study of intellectual development in children treated for acute lymphoblastic leukemia. Arch Dis Child 52:525–529, 1977

410. Goff J, Anderson H, Cooper P: Distractability and memory deficits in long-term survivors of acute lymphoblastic leukemia. Dev Behav Pediatr 1:158–163, 1980

411. Habermalz E, Habermalz HJ, Stephani U et al: Cranial computed tomography of 64 children in continuous complete remission of leukemia: I. relations to therapy modalities. Neuropediatrics 14:144–148, 1983

412. Meadows A, Massari D, Fergusson J et al: Declines in IQ scores and cognitive dysfunction in children with acute lymphocytic leukemia treated with cranial irradiation. Lancet 1:1015–1018, 1981

413. Moss H, Nannis E, Poplack DG: The effect of prophylactic treatment of the central nervous system on the intellectual functioning of children with acute lymphoblastic leukemia. Am J Med 71:47–52, 1981

414. Oliff A, Bode U, Bercu BB et al: Hypothalamic-pituitary dysfunction following CNS prophylaxis in acute lymphocytic leukemia: Correlation with CT scan abnormalities. Med Pediatr Oncol 7:141–151, 1979

415. Pavlovsky S, Fisman N, Arizaga R et al: Neuropsychological study in patients with ALL. Am J Pediatr Hematol Oncol 5:79–86, 1983

416. Peylan–Ramu N, Poplack DG, Pizzo PA, Adornato BT, Di Chiro G: Abnormal CT scans of the brain in asymptomatic children with acute lymphocytic leukemia after prophylactic treatment of the central nervous system with radiation and intrathecal chemotherapy. N Engl J Med 298:815–819, 1978

417. Ochs J, Mulhern RK: Late effects of antileukemic treatment. Pediatr Clin North Am 35:815–834, 1988

418. Riccardi R, Brouwers P, Di Chiro G, Poplack DG: Abnormal computed tomography brain scans in children with acute lymphoblastic leukemia: Serial long-term follow-up. J Clin Oncol 3:12–19, 1985

419. Scotti G, Bracchi M, Masera G et al: Prophylactic treatment of the central nervous system in acute lymphoblastic leukemia. CT findings in 45 children off therapy. Ital J Neurol Sci 2:361–365, 1981

420. Shalet SM, Price DA, Beardwell CG, Twomey JA, Morris–Jones PH, Pearson D: Normal growth despite abnormalities of growth hormone secretion in children treated for acute leukemia. J Pediatr 94:719–722, 1979

421. Tamaroff M, Salwen R, Miller DR, Murphy ML, Nir Y: Neuropsychological sequelae in irradiated (1800 RADS(r) and 2400(r) and non-irradiated children with acute lymphoblastic leukemia (ALL). Proc Am Soc Clin Oncol 4:165, 1985

422. Ochs J, Mulhern RK: Late effects of antileukemic treatment. Pediatr Clin North Am 35:815–834, 1987

423. Nesbit ME Jr, Sather HN, Robison LL et al: Presymptomatic central nervous system therapy in previously untreated childhood acute lymphoblastic leukaemia: Comparison of 1800 rad and 2400 rad. A report for Children's Cancer Study Group. Lancet 1:461–466, 1981

424. Poplack DG, Reaman GH, Bleyer WA et al: Central nervous system preventive therapy with high-dose methotrexate in acute lymphoblastic leukemia: A preliminary report (abstract). Proc Am Soc Clin Oncol 3:204, 1984

425. Haghbin M, Tan CT, Clarkson BK et al: Treatment of acute lymphoblastic leukemia in children with "prophylactic" intrathecal methotrexate and intensive systemic therapy. Cancer Res 35:807–811, 1975

426. Sullivan MP, Chen T, Dyment PG et al: Equivalence of intrathecal chemotherapy and radiotherapy as central nervous system prophylaxis in children with acute lymphatic leukemia: A Pediatric Oncology Group Study. Blood 60:948–958, 1982

427. Freeman AI, Weinberg V, Brecher ML et al: Comparison of intermediate-dose methotrexate with cranial irradiation for postinduction treatment of acute lymphocytic leukemia in children. N Engl J Med 308:477–484, 1983

428. Murphy SB, Dahl GV, Look AT, Ochs J, Abromowitch M, Pui C–H, Bowman WP, Simone JV, Kalwinski DK, Evans WE, George S, Mirro J, William D, Dow L, Rivera G: Recent results from total therapy study X for standard and high risk acute lymphoblastic leukemia in children: Recognition of new clinical and biologic risk features. In Neth, Gallo, Greaves, Janka (eds): Modern Trends in Human Leukemia: VI. Haematology and Blood Transfusion, vol 29, pp 787–781. Berlin, Springer-Verlag, 1985

429. Komp DM, Fernandez C, Falletta JM et al: CNS prophylaxis in acute lymphoblastic leukemia. Cancer 50:1031–1036, 1982

430. Moe PJ, Wesenberg F, Kolmannskog S: Methotrexate infusions in poor prognosis acute lymphoblastic leukemia: II. High-dose methotrexate (HDM) in acute lymphoblastic leukemia in childhood: A pilot study from April 1981. Med Pediatr Oncol 14:189–190, 1986

431. Schrappe M, Beck J, Brandeis WE et al: Treatment of acute lymphoblastic leukemia in childhood and adolescence: Results of the multicenter therapy study ALL-BFM81. Klin Padiatr 199(3):151–160, 1987

432. Abramowitch M, Ochs J, Pui CH et al: Efficacy of high-dose methotrexate in childhood acute lymphocytic leukemia: Analysis by contemporary risk classifications. Blood 71:866–869, 1988

433. Brouwers P, Moss H, Reaman G, McGuire T, Trupin E, Libow J, Tarnowski K, Bleyer W, Feusner J, Ruymann F, Miser J, Hammond D, Poplack D: Central nervous system preventive therapy with systemic high dose methotrexate versus cranial radiation and intrathecal methotrexate: Longitudinal comparison of effects of treatment on intellectual function of children with acute lymphoblastic leukemia. Proc Am Soc Clin Oncol 6:C-622, 1987

434. Brouwers P, Moss H, Reaman G, McGuire T, Trupin E, Libow J, Tarnowski K, Bleyer W, Feusner J, Ruymann F, Miser J, Hammond D, Poplack D: Central nervous system preventive therapy with systemic high dose methotrexate versus cranial radiation and intrathecal methotrexate: Longitudinal comparison of effects of treatment on academic achievement of children with acute lymphoblastic leukemia. Proc Am Soc Clin Oncol 6:176, 1988

435. Pizzo P, Poplack DG, Bleyer WA: Neurotoxicities of current leukemia therapy. Am J Pediatr Hematol Oncol 1:127–138, 1979

436. Geiser CF, Bishop Y, Jaffe N, Furman L, Traggis D, Frei E III: Adverse effects of intrathecal methotrexate in children with acute leukemia in remission. Blood 45:189–195, 1975

437. Mott MG, Stevenson P, Wood CB: Methotrexate meningitis (letter). Lancet 2:6565, 1972

438. Saiki JG, Thompson S, Smither F, Atkinson R: Paraplegia following intrathecal chemotherapy. Cancer 29:370–374, 1972

439. Gagliano R, Costani J: Paraplegia following intrathecal methotrexate; report of a case and review of the literature. Cancer 37:1663–1668, 1976

440. Freeman JE, Johnston PGB, Boke JM: Somnolence after prophylactic cranial irradiation in children with acute leukemia. Br Med J 4:523–525, 1973

441. Aronson S, Elmquist D: Somnolence in children with acute leukemia. Br Med J 3:344, 1974

442. Frei E III: Progress in treatment for the leukemias and lymphomas. Cancer 18:1580–1584, 1965

443. Lonsdale D, Gehan EEA, Fernbach DJ, Sullivan MP, Lane D, Ragab AH: Interrupted vs continued maintenance therapy in childhood leukemia. Cancer 336:342–352, 1975

444. Whang-Peng J, Knutsen T: Lymphocytic leukaemias, acute and chronic. Clin Haematol 9:87–127, 1980

445. Whang–Peng J, Freireich EJ, Oppenheim JJ, Frei E III, Tijo JH: Cytogenetic studies in 45 patients with acute lymphocytic leukemia. J Natl Cancer Inst 42:881–897, 1969

446. Secker-Walker LM, Swansbury GJ, Lawler SD, Hardisty RM: Bone marrow chromosomes in acute lymphoblastic leukemia: A long-term study. Med Pediatr Oncol 7:371–385, 1979

447. Karon M, Freireich ER, Frei E III, Wolman IJ, Djerassi I, Stanley LL, Sawitsky A, Hananian J, Selawry O, James D Jr, George P, Patterson RB, Burgert O Jr, Haunrani FI, Oberfield RA, Macy CT, Hoogstraten B, Bloom J: The role of vincristine in the treatment of childhood acute leukemia. Clin Pharmacol Ther 7:332–339, 1966

448. Howard JP, Albo V, Newton WA Jr: Cytosine arabinoside: Results of a cooperative study in acute childhood leukemia. Cancer 21:341–345, 1968

449. Freireich EJ, Gehan E, Frei E III, Schroeder LR, Wolman IJ, Anbari R, Burget EO, Mills SE, Pinkel D, Selawry OS, Moon JH, Gendel BR, Spurr CL, Storis R, Haurani F, Hoogstraten B, Lee W: The effect of 6-mercaptopurine on the duration of steroid induced remission in acute leukemia: A model for evaluation of other potentially useful therapy. Blood 21:699–716, 1963

450. Hyman CB, Borda E, Brubaker C, Hammond D, Sturgeon P: Prednisone in childhood leukemia. Comparison of interrupted and continuous therapy. Pediatrics 24:1005–1008, 1959

451. Mauer AM, Simone JV: The current status of the treatment of childhood acute lymphoblastic leukemia. Cancer Treat Rev 3:17–41, 1976

452. Holland JV, Glidewell OA: Chemotherapy of acute lymphocytic leukemia of childhood. Cancer 30:1480–1487, 1972

453. Frei E III: Acute leukemia in children. Model for the development of scientific methodology for clinical therapeutic research in cancer. Cancer 53:2013–2025, 1984

454. Simone JV: Factors that influence haematological remission duration in acute lymphocytic leukemia. Br J Haematol 32:465–472, 1976

455. Leikin S, Albo V, Lee S et al: Reinduction and pulse therapy in acute lymphocytic leukemia. Proc Am Soc Clin Oncol 1:486, 1981

456. Selawry OS: New treatment schedule with improved survival in childhood leukemia: Intermittent parenteral vs daily oral administration of methotrexate for maintenance of induced remission JAMA 194:75–81, 1965

457. Niemeyer CM, Hitchcock–Bryan S, Sallan SE: Comparative analysis of treatment programs for childhood acute lymphoblastic leukemia. Semin Oncol 12:122–130, 1985

458. Chessells JM: Acute leukemia in children. Clin Hematol 15:727–753, 1986

459. Rivera GK, Mauer AM: Controversies in the management of childhood acute lymphoblastic leukemia: Treatment intensification, CNS leukemia, and prognostic factors. Semin Hematol 24:12–26, 1987

460. Haghbin M, Tan CC, Clarkson BD, Mike V, Burchenal JH, Murphy ML: Intensive chemotherapy in children with acute lymphoblastic leukemia. (L-2) protocol. Cancer 33:1491–1498, 1974

461. Clavell LA, Gelber RD, Cohen HJ, Hitchcock–Bryan S, Cassady R, Tarbell NJ, Blattner SR, Tantravahi R, Leavitt P, Sallan SE: Four-agent induction and intensive asparaginase therapy for treatment of childhood acute lymphoblastic leukemia. N Engl J Med 315:657–663, 1986

462. Gaynon P, Steinherz P, Bleyer WA, Ablin A, Albo V, Finklestein J, Grossman N, Littman P, Novak L, Pyesmany A, Reaman G, Sather H, Hammond GD: Superiority of intensive therapy for children with previously untreated acute lymphoblastic leukemia (ALL) and unfavorable prognostic features (UPF). Proc of Am Soc Clin Oncol 5:162, 1986

463. Moe PJ, Seip M, Finne PH et al: Intermediate dose methotrexate in childhood acute lymphocytic leukemia. Eur Paediatr Haematol Oncol 1:113–118, 1984

464. Rivera GK, George SL, Williams DL et al: Early results of intensified remission induction chemotherapy for childhood acute lymphocytic leukemia. Med Pediatr Oncol 14:177–181, 1986

465. Camitta B, Lauer S, Casper J: Early intensive rotating therapy for higher risk childhood acute lymphocytic leukemia (CALL). Fourth International Symposium on Therapy of Leukemia, Rome, p 187, 1987

466. Fujimoto T, Mimay J, Utumi J, Sasaki K: Early consolidation therapy for children with high risk (HR) acute lymphoblastic leukemia (ALL). Am Soc Clin Oncol 3:#C-751, p 193, 1984

467. Pinkerton CR, Bowman A, Holtzel H, Chessells JM: Intensive consolidation chemotherapy for acute lymphoblastic leukemia (UKALL X pilot study). Arch Dis Child 62:12–18, 1987

468. Haghbin M, Murphy ML, Tan CC et al: A long-term clinical follow-up of children with acute lymphoblastic leukemia treated with intensive chemotherapy regimens. Cancer 46:241–252, 1980

469. Rivera G, Dahl GU, Murphy SB et al: The epipodophyllotoxin VM 26 in treatment of high-risk acute lymphoblastic leukemia: Rationale and early results. In Murphy SB, Gilbert JR (eds): Leukemia Research: Advances in Cell Biology and Treatment, pp 213–220. New York, Elsevier Biomedical, 1983

470. Pullen DJ, Sullivan MP, Falletta JM et al: Modified LSA2-L2 treatment in 53 children with E-rosette-positive T-cell leukemia: Results and prognostic factors (a Pediatric Oncology Group study). Blood 60:1159–1167, 1982

471. Riehm H, Gadner H, Henze G et al: Acute lymphoblastic leukemia: Treatment results in three BFM studies (1970–1981) In Murphy SB, Gilbert JR (eds): Leukemia Research: Advances in Cell Biology and Treatment, pp 251–263. New York, Elsevier Biomedical, 1983

472. Gaynon P, Bleyer WA, Steinherz P, Finklestein J, Miller D, Reaman G, Sather H, Hammond GD: Impact of treatment dose and delay on the disease free survival (DFS) of children with acute lymphoblastic leukemia (ALL) and unfavorable prognostic features (UPF) (abstract). Proc Am Soc Clin Oncol 6:156, 1987

473. Skipper HE, Schabel FM, Wilcox WS: Experimental evaluation of potential anticancer agents: XIII. On the criteria and kinetics associated with "curability" of experimental leukemia. Cancer Chemother Rep 35:1–111, 1964

474. Pinkel D, Hernandez K, Borella L, Holton C, Aur R, Samoy G, Pratt C: Drug dosage and remission duration in childhood lymphocytic leukemia. Cancer 27:247–256, 1971

475. Improvement in treatment for children with acute lymphoblastic leukaemia. The Medical Research Council UKALL Trials, 1972–84. Report to the Council by the Working Party on Leukaemia in Childhood. Lancet 1:408–411, 1986

476. Medical Research Council Leukaemia Trial: UKALL V: An attempt to reduce the immunosuppressive effects of therapy in childhood acute lymphoblastic leukaemia. Report to the Council by the Working Party on Leukaemia in Childhood. J Clin Oncol 4:1758–1764, 1986

477. Zimm S, Collins JM, Riccardi R et al: Variable bioavailability of oral mercaptopurine: Is maintenance chemotherapy in acute lymphoblastic leukemia being optimally delivered? N Engl J Med 308:1005–1009, 1983

478. Balis FM, Savitch JL, Bleyer WA: Pharmacokinetics of oral methotrexate in children. Cancer Res 43:2342–2345, 1983

479. Poplack DG, Balis FM, Zimm S: The pharmacology of orally administered chemotherapy. A reappraisal. Cancer 58:473–480, 1986

480. Kamen BA, Holcenberg JS, Turo K, Whitehead VM: Methotrexate and folate content of erythrocytes in patients receiving oral vs intramuscular therapy with methotrexate. J Pediatr 104:131–133, 1984

481. Medical Research Council Leukaemia Trial: UKALL VII: A Report to the Council by the Working Party on Leukaemia in Childhood. Arch Dis Child 60:1050–1054, 1985

482. Chessells JM, Leiper AD, Tiedemann K et al: Oral methotrexate is as effective as intramuscular in maintenance therapy of acute lymphoblastic leukemia. Arch Dis Child 62:172–176, 1987

483. Land VJ, Berry DH, Herson J et al: Long term survival in childhood acute leukemia: "Late" relapses. Med Pediatr Oncol 7:19–24, 1979

484. Nesbit ME, Sather HN, Robinson LL et al: Randomized study of 3-years versus 5-years of chemotherapy in childhood acute lymphoblastic leukemia. J Clin Oncol 1:308–316, 1983

485. Miller D, Leiken S, Albo V, Sather H, Hammond D: Duration of therapy (DT) in childhood acute lymphoblastic leukemia (ALL) (abstract). Am Soc Clin Oncol 5:#609, p 156, 1986

486. Working Party on Leukaemia in Childhood: Treatment of acute lymphoblastic leukaemia: Effect of variation in length of treatment on duration of remission. Br Med J 2:495–497, 1977

487. Medical Research Council Working Party on Leukaemia in Childhood: Duration of chemotherapy in childhood acute lymphoblastic leukaemia. Med Pediatr Oncol 10:511–520, 1982

488. Evan's DI, Jones P, Hann IM, Palmer MK: Sex and prognosis in childhood acute lymphoblastic leukaemia. Lancet 2:522–523, 1978

489. George SL, Aur SRJA, Mauer AM, Simone JV: A reappraisal of the results of stopping therapy in childhood leukemia. N Engl J Med 300:269–273, 1979

490. Lane DM, Haggarad ME, Lonsdale D, Starling K, Sullivan MP: Remission induction in childhood leukemia with second course vincristine (NSC-67574) and prednisone (NSC-10023) therapy. Cancer Chemother Rep 54s:113–118, 1970

491. Howard JP: Response of acute leukemia in children to repeated courses of vincristine (NSC 67574). Cancer Chemother Rep 51:465–469, 1967

492. Sutow WW, Vietti TJ, Fernbach DJ, Lane DM, Donaldson MH, Berry DH:

Combination of vincristine and prednisone in therapy of acute leukemias in children. J Pediatr 73:426–430, 1968

493. Sutow WW, Garcia F, Starling SK, Williams TE, Lane DM, Geham EA: L-asparaginase therapy in children with advanced leukemia. Cancer 28:819–824, 1971

494. Kung FH, Nyhan WL, Cuttner J, Falkson G, Lanzkowsky P, De Ouka V, Nawabi IV, Koch K, Pluess H, Freeman A, Burgert EO, Leone LA, Ruymann F, Patterson RB, Degnan T, Hakami N, Pajak TF, Holland J: Vincristine, prednisone and L-asparaginase in the induction of remission in children with acute lymphoblastic leukemia following relapse. Cancer 41:428–434, 1978

495. Chessells JM, Cornbleet M: Combination chemotherapy for bone marrow relapse in childhood lymphoblastic leukemia. Med Pediatr Oncol 6:359–365, 1979

496. Reaman GH, Ladisch S, Echelberger C, Poplack DG: Improved treatment results in the management of single and multiple relapses of acute lymphoblastic leukemia. Cancer 45:3090–3094, 1980

497. Rivera GK, Buchanan G, Boyett JM et al: Intensive retreatment of childhood acute lymphoblastic leukemia in first bone marrow relapse. N Engl J Med 325:273–278, 1986

498. Buchanan GR, Boyer JM, Rivera GK: Reinduction therapy in 173 children with acute lymphoblastic leukemia (ALL) in first bone marrow (BM) relapse: A pediatric Oncology Group Study (abstract). Proc Am Soc Clin Oncol 6:146, #574, 1987

499. Rivera G, Aur RJ, Dahl GV et al: Combined VM-26 and cytosine arabinoside in treatment of refractory childhood lymphocytic leukemia. Cancer 45:1284–1288, 1980

500. Rivera G, Aur RJA, Dahl GV et al: Second cessation of therapy in childhood lymphocytic leukemia. Blood 53:1114–1120, 1979

501. Chessells JM, Breatnach F: Late marrow recurrences in childhood acute lymphoblastic leukaemia. Br Med J 283:749–757, 1981

502. Rivera G, George SL, Bowman WP: Second central nervous system prophylaxis in children with acute lymphoblastic leukemia who relapse after elective cessation of therapy. J Clin Oncol 1:471–476, 1983

503. Nachman J, Baum E, Ramsay N, Weetman R, Neerhout R, Sather H, Hammond D: Prognostic factors for reinduction and duration of second remission in children with acute lymphocytic leukemia. Proc Am Soc Clin Oncol 5:200, 1986

504. Pinkel D: Patterns of failure in acute lymphocytic leukemia. Cancer Treat Symp 2:259–266, 1983

505. Henze G, Buchmann S, Fengler R, Hartmann R: The BFM relapse studies in childhood ALL: Concepts of two multicenter trials and results after 2½ years. In Buchner T, Schellong G, Hiddemann W, Urbanitz D, Ritter J (eds): Acute Leukemias: Prognostic Factors and Treatment Strategies. Haematol Blood Transfusion 30:147–155, 1987

506. Herson J, Starling KA, Dyment PG, Humphrey GB, Pullen J, Vats T: Vincristine and prednisone vs vincristine, L-asparaginase and prednisone for second remission induction of acute lymphocytic leukemia in children. Med Pediatr Oncol 6:323–327, 1979

507. Rivera G, Pratt CB, Aur RJA, Verzosa M, Husto HO: Recurrent childhood lymphocytic leukemia following cessation of therapy. Treatment and response. Cancer 37:1679–1686, 1976

508. Jacquillat CL, Weil M, Gemon MJ, Israel V, Schaison G, Auclerc G, Ablin AR, Flandrin G, Tanzer J, Bussel A, Weisgerber C, Dresch C, Najean Y, Goudemand M, Seligmann M, Bernard B, Bernard J: Evaluation of 216 four year survivors of acute leukemia. Cancer 32:286–293, 1973

509. Leventhal BG, Levine AS, Graw RG, Simone R, Freireich EJ, Henderson ES: Long-term second remissions in acute lymphocytic leukemia. Cancer 35:1136–1140, 1975

510. Cornbleet MA, Chessels JM: Bone marrow relapse in acute lymphoblastic leukemia in childhood. Br Med J 2:104–106, 1978

511. Starling K, Lane DM, Sutow WW, Mento RW, Thurman WG: Third and fourth remission with prednisone (NSC-67564) and vincristine (NSC-67574) in children with acute leukemia. Cancer Chemother Rep 54:293–294, 1970

512. Bleyer WA, Sather H, Hammond GD: Prognosis and treatment after relapse of acute lymphoblastic leukemia and non-Hodgkin's lymphoma: 1985. Cancer 58:590–594, 1986

513. Butturine A, Rivera GK, Bortin MM, Gale RP: Which treatment for childhood acute lymphoblastic leukaemia in second remission? Lancet 1:429–432, 1987

514. Rossi MR, Amadori S, Bagnulo S et al: Randomized multicenter Italian study on two treatment regimens for marrow relapse in childhood acute lymphoblastic leukemia. Pediatr Hematol Oncol 3:101–120, 1986

515. Sallan SE, Hitchcock–Bryan S: Relapse in childhood acute lymphoblastic leukemia after elective cessation of initial treatment: Failure of subsequent treatment with cyclophosphamide, cytosine arabinoside, vincristine and prednisone (COAP). Med Pediatr Oncol 9:455–462, 1981

516. Poplack DG, Reaman GH, Wesley R: Treatment of acute lymphoblastic leukemia in relapse: Efficacy of a four-drug reinduction regimen. Cancer Treat Rep 54(4):93–96, 1981

517. Baum E, Nachman J, Ramsay N et al: Prolonged second remissions in childhood acute lymphocytic leukemia: A report from the Children's Cancer Study Group. Med Pediatr Oncol 11:1–7, 1983

518. Fengler R, Hartmann R, Buchmann S, Bender–Gotze C, Bode U, Dopfer R, Gerein V, Graf N, Jurgens H, Mertens R, Rath B, Verheyer G, Wustemann M, Zerfab B, Henze G: Induction therapy for early bone marrow relapse of childhood acute lymphoblastic leukemia—results of 2 multicentric trials. Proceedings of the Fourth International Conference on Treatment of Acute Leukemia, p 403. Rome, February 1987

519. Creutzig U, Schellong G: Treatment of relapse in acute lymphoblastic leukemia of childhood [in German]. Dtsch Med Wochenschr 105:1109–1112, 1980

520. Thomas ED, Buckner CD, Banaji M, Clift RA, Fefer A, Flournoy M, Goodell BW, Hickman RO, Lerner KG, Neiman PE, Sale GE, Sanders JE, Singer J, Stevens M, Storb R, Weiden PL: One hundred patients with acute leukemia treated by chemotherapy, total body irradiation, and allogeneic marrow transplantation. Blood 49:511–522, 1977

521. Blume KG, Beutler E, Bross KJ, Chiller RK, Ellington OB, Fahey JL, Farbstein MJ, Forman SJ, Schmidt GM, Scott EP, Spruce WE, Turner MA, Wolf JL: Bone marrow ablation and allogeneic marrow transplantation in acute leukemia. N Engl J Med 302:1041–1046, 1980

522. Thomas ED, Sanders JE, Flowinoy N et al: Marrow transplantation for patients with acute lymphoblastic leukemia: A long-term follow-up. Blood 62:1139–1141, 1983

523. Sanders JE, Thomas ED, Buckner CD, Doney K: Marrow transplantation for children with acute lymphoblastic leukemia in second remission. Blood 70:324–326, 1987

524. O'Reilly RJ: Allogeneic bone marrow transplantation: Current status and future directions. Blood 67:941–964, 1983

525. Johnson FL, Thomas ED, Clark BS et al: A comparison of bone marrow transplantation to chemotherapy for children with acute lymphoblastic leukemia in second and subsequent remission. N Engl J Med 305:846–851, 1981

526. Dinsmore R, Kirkpatrick D, Flomenberg N et al: Allogeneic bone marrow transplantation for patients with acute lymphoblastic leukemia. Blood 62:381–388, 1983

527. Woods WG, Nesbit ME, Ramsay NK et al: Intensive therapy followed by bone marrow transplantation for patients with acute lymphocytic leukemia in second or subsequent remission: Determination of prognostic factors (a report from the University of Minnesota Bone Marrow Transplantation Team). Blood 61:1182–1189, 1983

528. Bleyer WA, Coccia PF, Sather HN, Level C, Lukens J, Niebrugge DJ, Siegel S, Littman PS, Leikin SL, Miller DR, Chard RL Jr, Hammond GD: Reduction in central nervous system leukemia with a pharmacokinetically derived intrathecal methotrexate dosage regimen. J Clin Oncol 1:317–325, 1983

529. Kersey JH, Weisdorf D, Nesbit ME, LeBien TW, Woods WG, McGlave PB, Kim T, Vallera DA, Goldman AI, Bostrom B, Hurd D, Ramsay NK: Comparison of autologous and allogeneic bone marrow transplantation for treatment of high-risk refractory acute lymphoblastic leukemia. N Engl J Med 317:461–467, 1987

530. Bast RC Jr, Sallan SE, Reynolds C, Lipton J, Ritz J: Autologous bone marrow transplantation for CALLA-positive acute lymphoblastic leukemia: An update. In Dicke KA, Spitzer G, Zander AR (eds) Autologous Bone Marrow Transplantation, pp 3–6. Houston, The University of Texas—M.D. Anderson Hospital and Tumor Institute, 1985

531. George SL, Ochs JJ, Mauer AA et al: The importance of an isolated central nervous system relapse in children with acute lymphoblastic leukemia. J Clin Oncol 3:776–781, 1985

532. Willoughby MLN: Treatment of overt meningeal leukaemia in children: Results of second MRC Meningeal Leukaemia Trial. Br Med J 1:864–867, 1976

533. Sullivan MP, Moon TE, Trueworthy R et al: Combination intrathecal therapy for meningeal leukemia: Two versus three drugs. Blood 50:471–479, 1977

534. Willoughby MLN: Treatment of overt CNS leukemia. In Mastrangelo R, Poplack DG, Riccardi R (eds): Central Nervous System Leukemia: Prevention and Treatment, pp 113–122. Boston, Martinus-Nijhoff, 1983

535. Kun LE, Camitta BM, Mulhern RK, Lauer SJ, Kline RW, Casper JT, Kamen BA,

Kaplan BM, Barber SW: Treatment of meningeal relapse in childhood acute lymphoblastic leukemia: I. Results of craniospinal irradiation. J Clin Oncol 2:359–364, 1984

536. Land VJ, Thomas PRM, Boyett JM, Glicksman AS, Culbert S, Castleberry RP, Berry DH, Vats T, Humphrey GB: Comparison of maintenance treatment regimens for first central nervous system relapse in children with acute lymphocytic leukemia. A Pediatric Oncology Group study. Cancer 56:81–87, 1985

537. Steinherz P, Jereb B, Galicich J: Therapy of CNS leukemia with intraventricular chemotherapy and low-dose neuraxis radiotherapy. J Clin Oncol 3:1217–1226, 1985

538. Sullivan MP, Humphrey GB, Vietti TJ, Haggard ME, Lee E: Superiority of conventional intrathecal methotrexate therapy with maintenance over intensive intrathecal methotrexate therapy, unmaintained, or radiotherapy (2000–2500 rads tumor dose) in treatment for meningeal leukemia. Cancer 35:1066–1073, 1975

539. Sullivan MP, Vietti TJ, Fernbach DJ, Griffith KM, Haddy TB, Watkins WL: Clinical investigations in the treatment of meningeal leukemia: Radiation therapy regimens vs conventional intrathecal methotrexate. Blood 34:301–319, 1969

540. Duttera MJ, Bleyer WA, Pomeroy TC, Leventhal CM, Leventhal BG: Irradiation, methotrexate toxicity, and the treatment of meningeal leukaemia. Lancet 2:703–707, 1973

541. Moe PJ, Finne PN: Central-nervous-system leukemia in children. Tidsskr Nor Laegeforen 95:874–876, 1975

542. Nesbit M, Sather H, Ortega J et al: Effect of isolated central nervous system leukaemia on bone marrow remission and survival in childhood acute lymphoblastic leukaemia. Lancet 1:1386–1389, 1981

543. Bleyer WA, Poplack DG, Simon RM: "Concentration × time" methotrexate via a subcutaneous reservoir: A less toxic regimen for intraventricular chemotherapy of central nervous system neoplasms. Blood 51:835–842, 1978

544. Green DM, West Cr, Brecher ML et al: The use of subcutaneous cerebrospinal fluid reservoirs for the prevention and treatment of meningeal relapse of acute lymphoblastic leukemia. Am J Pediatr Hematol Oncol 4:147–154, 1982

545. Haghbin M, Galicich JH: Therapy of CNS leukemia, continued use of the Ommaya reservoir in the prevention and treatment of CNS leukemia. Am J Pediatr Hematol Oncology 1:111–119, 1979

546. Poplack DG, Brouwers P: Adverse sequelae of central nervous system therapy. Clin Oncol 4:263–285, 1985

547. Bleyer WA, Poplack DG: Intraventricular versus intralumbar methotrexate for central-nervous-system leukemia. Med Pediatr Oncol 6:207–213, 1979

548. Shapiro WR, Posner JB, Ushio Y, Chernik NL, Young DF: Treatment of meningeal neoplasms. Cancer Treat Rep 61:733–743, 1977

549. Balis F, Savitch J, Bleyer WA et al: Remission induction of meningeal leukemia with high-dose intravenous methotrexate (abstract). Proc Am Soc Clin Oncol 3:202, 1984

550. Amadori S, Papa G, Avvisati G, Petti MC, Motta M, Salvagnini M, Meloni G, Martelli M, Monarca B, Mandelli F: Sequential combination of systemic high-dose Ara-C and asparaginase for the treatment of central nervous system leukemia and lymphoma. J Clin Oncol 2:98–101, 1984

551. Frick J, Ritch PS, Hansen RM et al: Successful treatment of meningeal leukemia using systemic high-dose cytosine arabinoside. J Clin Oncol 1:365–368, 1984

552. Zimm S, Holcenberg J, Balis F, Doherty K, Poplack DG: Intrathecal (IT) diaziquone (AZQ): A new, clinically useful agent for the treatment of meningeal neoplasia. Proc Am Assoc Cancer Res 28:190, #755, 1987

553. Hutchinson R, Heyn R, Waskerwitz M: Long-term remission of central nervous system leukemia. Proc Am Soc Clin Oncol 21:388, 1980

554. Bleyer WA: Intrathecal methotrexate versus central nervous system leukemia. Cancer Drug Delivery 1:157–167, 1984

555. Steinfeld AD: Radiation therapy in the treatment of leukemic infiltrates of the testes. Radiology 120:681–682, 1976

556. Mirro J, Wharam MD, Karzer H et al: Testicular leukemic relapse: Rate of regression and persistent disease after radiation therapy. J Pediatr 99:439–440, 1981

557. Land VJ, Askin FB, Ragab AH, Starling KM, Vats T, Wondmiller J: "Late" overt or occult testicular leukemia—incidence and prognosis. Proc Am Soc Clin Oncol 20:378, 1979

558. Speider B, Rubin P, Casarret G: Aspermia following lower truncal irradiation in Hodgkins' disease. Cancer 32:692–698, 1973

559. Blatt J, Sherins RJ, Niebrugge D, Bleyer WA, Poplack DG: Leydig cell function in boys following treatment for testicular relapse of acute lymphoblastic leukemia. J Clin Oncol 3:1227–1231, 1985

560. Shalet SM, Hoerner A, Ahmed SR, Morris–Jones PH: Leydig cell damage after testicular irradiation for lymphoblastic leukemia. Med Pediatr Oncol 13:65–68, 1985

561. Brauner R, Czernichow P, Cramer P et al: Leydig-cell function in children after direct testicular irradiation for acute lymphoblastic leukemia. N Engl J Med 309:25–28, 1983

562. Culbert S, Doering E, Jeleden G et al: Testicular leukemic relapse: A treatable entity (abstract). Proc Am Soc Clin Oncol 2:79, 1983

563. Fengler R, Henze G, Langermann HJ et al: Favourable treatment results after testicular relapse of childhood acute lymphoblastic leukemia: A report of the BFM Study Group (abstract). In Mandelli F (ed): Abstracts from Third International Symposium on Therapy of Acute Leukemias, p 156, Rome, 1983

564. Frankel LS, Provisor A, Kletzel M et al: Successful therapy for overt testicular relapse in childhood acute lymphocytic leukemia (abstract). Proc Am Soc Clin Oncol 3:192, 1984

565. Tiedemann K, Chessells JM, Sandlund RM: Isolated testicular relapse in boys with acute lymphoblastic leukemia treatment and outcome. Br Med J 285:1614–1616, 1982

566. Poplack DG: Evaluation of adverse sequelae of central nervous system prophylaxis in acute lymphoblastic leukemia. In Mastrangelo R, Riccardi R, Poplack DG (eds): Central Nervous System Leukemia Prevention and Treatment. Boston, Martinus-Nijhoff, 1983

567. Bleyer WA: Current state of intrathecal chemotherapy for meningeal neoplasms. Natl Cancer Inst Monogr 46:171–178, 1977

568. Bleyer A, Griffin T: White matter necrosis, mineralizing microangiopathy, and intellectual abilities in survivors of childhood leukemia: Associations with central nervous system irradiation and methotrexate therapy. In Gilbert A, Kagan AR (eds): Radiation Damage to the Nervous System, pp 155–174, New York, Raven Press, 1980

569. Kay HEM, Knapton PJ, O'Sullivan JP, Wells DG, Harris RF, Innes EM, Stuart J, Schwartz CM, Thompson EN: Encephalopathy in acute leukemia associated with methotrexate therapy. Arch Dis Child 47:344–354, 1972

570. Price RA, Jamieson PA: The central nervous system in childhood leukemia: II. Subacute leukoencephalopathy. Cancer 35:306–318, 1975

571. Rubinstein LJ, Heran MM, Long JF, Wilber JR: Disseminated necrotizing leukoencephalopathy; a complication of treated central nervous system leukemia and lymphoma. Cancer 35:291–305, 1975

572. Price RA: Therapy related central nervous system diseases in children with acute lymphocytic leukemia. In Mastrangelo R, Poplack DG, Riccardi R (eds): Central Nervous System Leukemia: Prevention and Treatment. Boston, Martinus-Nijhoff, 1983

573. Caveness WF: Experimental observations: Delayed necrosis in normal monkey brain. In Gilbert HA, Kagan AR (eds): Radiation Damage to the Nervous System, pp 1–28. New York, Raven Press, 1980

574. Fisher JN, Aur RJA: Endocrine assessment in childhood acute lymphocytic leukemia. Cancer 49:145–151, 1982

575. Siris ES, Leventhal BG, Vaitukaitis JL: Effects of childhood leukemia and chemotherapy on puberty and reproduction function in girls. N Engl J Med 294:1143–1146, 1976

576. Pasqualini T, Escobar ME, Domene H, Muriel FS, Pavlovski S, Rivarola MA: Evaluation of gonadal function following long-term treatment for acute lymphoblastic leukemia in girls. Am J Pediatr Hematol Oncol 9:15–22, 1987

577. Blatt J, Poplack DG, Sherins RJ: Testicular function in boys following chemotherapy for acute lymphoblastic leukemia. N Engl J Med 304:1121–1124, 1981

578. Blatt J, Mulvihill JJ, Ziegler JL et al: Pregnancy outcome following cancer chemotherapy. Am J Med 69:828–832, 1980

579. Zarrabi MH, Rosner F, Grunwald HW: Second neoplasms in acute lymphoblastic leukemia. Cancer 52:1712–1719, 1983

580. Malone M, Lumley H, Erdohazi M: Astrocytoma as a second malignancy in patients with acute lymphoblastic leukemia. Cancer 57:1979–1985, 1986

581. Albo V, Muller P, Leiken S et al: Nine brain tumors as a late effect in children "cured" of acute lymphoblastic leukemia from a single protocol (abstract). Proc Am Soc Clin Oncol 4:172, 1985

582. Anderson JR, Treip CS: Radiation-induced intracranial neoplasms. A report of three possible cases. Cancer 53:426–429, 1984

583. Chung CK, Stryker JA, Cruse R et al: Glioblastoma multiforme following prophylactic cranial irradiation and intrathecal methotrexate in a child with acute lymphoblastic leukemia. Cancer 47:2563–2565, 1981

584. McWhirter WR: Cerebral astrocytoma as a complication of acute lymphoblastic leukemia. Med J Aust 145(2):96–97, 1986

585. Meadows AT, Baum E, Fossati–Bellani et al: Second malignant neoplasms in

children: An update from the Late Effects Study Group. J Clin Oncol 3:532–538, 1985

586. Meadows AT, D'Angio GJ, Mike V et al: Patterns of second malignant neoplasms in children. Cancer 40(suppl):1903–1911, 1977

587. Koocher GP, O'Malley J: The Damocles Syndrome: Psychosocial Consequences of Surviving Childhood Cancer. New York, McGraw-Hill, 1981

588. Sawyer M, Crettenden A, Toogood I: Psychological adjustment of families of children and adolescents treated for leukemia. Am J Pediatr Hematol Oncol 8:200–207, 1986

589. Meadows AT, Kramer S, Hopson R et al: Survival in childhood acute lymphocytic leukemia (ALL): The influence of protocol and place of treatment. Cancer Invest 1:49–55, 1983

590. Hughes WT: Pneumocystis carinii pneumonia. N Engl J Med 297:1381–1383, 1977

591. Ellis R: Zoster immune globulin—an assessment. Morbib Mortal Weekly Rep 26:59, 1977

592. Murphy JV, Yunis EJ: Encephalopathy following measles infection in children with chronic illness. J Pediatr 88:937–942, 1976

593. Verzosa MS, Aur RJA, Simone JV, Husta HO, Pinkel DP: Five years after central nervous system irradiation of children with leukemia. Int J Radiat Oncol Biol Phys 1:209–215, 1976

594. Griffin NK, Wadsworth J: Effect of treatment of malignant disease on growth in children. Arch Dis Child 55:600–603, 1980

595. Metcalf D: The molecular biology and functions of the granulocyte-macrophage colony-stimulating factors. Blood 67:257–267, 1986

596. Colamonici OR, Cole D, Trepel JB, Poplack DG, Neckers LH: Induction of functional and prototypic differentiation in immature T cell leukemias by treatment with Il-2. Fourth International Symposium on Therapy of Acute Leukemias, p 332, Rome, 1987

597. Valeriote F, Vietti TJ: Cellular kinetics and conceptual basis of chemotherapy. In Sutow WW, Vietti TJ, Fernbach DJ (eds): Clinical Pediatric Oncology, pp 1182–1196. St. Louis, CV Mosby, 1977

598. Poplack DG: Acute lymphoblastic leukemia and less frequently occurring leukemias in the young. In Levine AS (ed): Cancer in the Young, pp 405–460. New York, Masson, 1982

599. Husto HO, Aur RJA, Verzosa MS, Simone JV, Pinkel D: Prevention of central nervous system leukemia by irradiation. Cancer 32:585–597, 1973

600. Simone JV: Childhood leukemia as a model for cancer research. Cancer Res 39:4301–4307, 1979

601. Frankel LS et al: The curative potential of CNS relapse in childhood acute lymphocytic leukemia. Proc Am Soc Clin Oncol 1:124, 1982

602. Muriel FS, Schere D, Barengals A et al: Remission maintenance therapy for meningeal leukemia: Intrathecal methotrexate and dexamethasone versus intrathecal craniospinal irradiation with radiocolloid. Br J Haematol 34:119–127, 1976

603. Humphrey GB, Krons HF, Filler J et al: Treatment of overt CNS leukemia. Am J Pediatr Hematol Oncol 1:37–47, 1972

seventeen

Acute Nonlymphocytic Leukemia

Holcombe E. Grier and Howard J. Weinstein

Acute nonlymphocytic leukemia (ANLL) represents approximately 15% to 20% of all leukemia seen in childhood. During the last decade, technologic advances in *in vitro* bone marrow culture and cytogenetics and the development of monoclonal antibodies have greatly increased our understanding of the biology of ANLL. There has also been progress in therapy. Modern intensive chemotherapy, bone marrow transplantation for those patients with histocompatible donors, and advances in supportive care have contributed to the improved outlook for children with ANLL. Nevertheless, further gains are necessary because, despite these achievements, only 30% to 40% of newly diagnosed children with ANLL can be expected to remain in long-term remission and hopefully be cured of their disease.

EPIDEMIOLOGY

There are approximately 2500 newly diagnosed cases of childhood leukemia in the United States each year.[1] The ratio of ANLL to acute lymphoblastic leukemia (ALL) throughout childhood is approximately 1:4, with the exception of congenital leukemia (leukemia in the first 4 weeks of life), which is most often ANLL.[2] There is no evidence that the incidence of ANLL has changed over time. The incidence of ANLL remains stable from birth through age 10; the peak occurrence of childhood leukemia at age 4 is entirely due to patients with ALL. The incidence then increases slightly during the teenage years and remains stable until a progressive increase is noted beginning at approximately 55 years of age. Unlike ALL, ANLL is equally distributed among racial groups. There is no sex-related difference in incidence.

GENETICS

There is no obvious familial predisposition to ANLL. The strongest evidence for a genetic predisposition to acute leukemia is the occurrence of this disease in identical twins.[3,4] If one identical twin develops leukemia before 6 years of age, the risk of disease in the other twin is 20%. The concordance is highest in the first year of life. Certain inherited disorders and congenital conditions associated with chromosome instability predispose patients to develop ANLL (Table 17-1). Primary among the inherited disorders is trisomy 21, or Down's syndrome (see Chap. 2). Children with Down's syndrome are 20 times more likely to develop acute leukemia. The cell types of leukemia in these children follow the usual distribution for this age group, but the age peak is nearly 3 years earlier than expected.[5]

   Neonates with trisomy 21 may show a transient uncontrolled proliferation of blasts (usually myeloblasts). This transient myeloproliferative syndrome is clinically and hematologically indistinguishable from congenital leukemia.[2] Affected

Table 17-1
Predisposing Factors Associated with ANLL

Trisomy 21 (Down's syndrome)
Fanconi's anemia
Bloom's syndrome
Kostmann's syndrome
Diamond–Blackfan anemia
Certain drugs (benzene, alkylating agents, nitrosoureas)
Ionizing radiation
Myelodysplastic syndromes (monosomy 7)

Table 17-2
Correlates of Consistent Chromosome Abnormalities in ANLL

Chromosome Change	Morphology or Clinical Characteristics
t(8;21)	M2 (AML with differentiation)
t(15;17)	M3 (promyelocytic leukemia)
inv(16) or 16q	M4 with dysplastic eosinophils
t(1;11), t(9;11)	M4 or M5 (monocytic or myelomonocytic leukemia)
−7 or 7q−	Therapy-related ANLL, myelodysplastic syndrome
trisomy 8	M2, M4, M5
inv(3) or t(3;3)	M1, M2 with abnormal thrombopoeisis

neonates may have a markedly increased leukocyte count, signs and symptoms of bone marrow failure, and, occasionally, leukemia cutis (multiple skin nodules formed by myeloblastic infiltration). Neonates with trisomy 21 mosaicism who lack the typical stigmata of Down's syndrome are also susceptible to this condition.[6-9] Interestingly, in these infants the blast cells have the trisomy 21 karyotype.

In contrast to congenital leukemia, this myeloproliferative syndrome spontaneously regresses within weeks to months, and *in vitro* growth of bone marrow at diagnosis is normal. These findings argue against this syndrome being a "true" leukemia. However, clonal cytogenetic abnormalities like those seen in leukemia (see below) have been noted in the bone marrow cells of children with constitutional trisomy 21 who had myeloproliferative syndromes that spontaneously remitted.[10,11] Further, at least one patient with trisomy 21 has been reported who developed ANLL 19 months after the spontaneous resolution of a transient myeloproliferative syndrome.[12] Newborns who have Down's syndrome and an increase in blasts should probably be observed over at least several weeks for signs of spontaneous remission before any specific antileukemic therapy is instituted.

Two other congenital disorders that predispose patients to ANLL are Fanconi's anemia and Bloom's syndrome (see Chap. 2).[1] These disorders are characterized by an abnormality in DNA repair. The exact link between the molecular defects in these diseases and the increased risk of leukemia is unknown. Rarely, patients with congenital disorders of myelopoiesis such as Kostmann's syndrome and Diamond–Blackfan anemia may develop ANLL.

Cytogenetics

Studies using newer techniques of short-term culture, cell synchronization, and quinacrine or Giemsa banding identify clonal cytogenetic abnormalities in more than 80% of patients

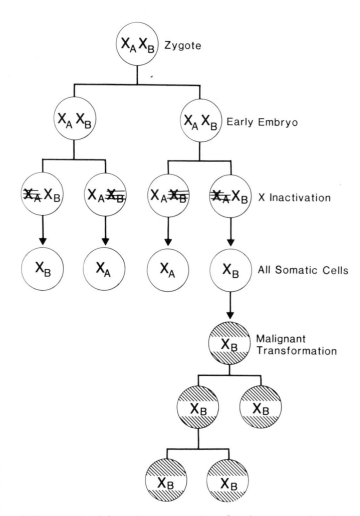

FIGURE 17-1. Schematic representation of X chromosome inactivation (Lyon hypothesis). Inactivation occurs randomly in each cell during early embryogenesis. The malignant cells all derive from one transformed cell (clonal) and hence all have the same active X chromosome.

with ANLL.[13-15] These chromosome changes are acquired and therefore are present only in the malignant cells. The bone marrow karyotype returns to normal during hematologic remissions, and the same clone usually reappears at relapse.

Moreover, specific chromosome abnormalities correlate with particular French–American–British (FAB) subtypes of ANLL (Table 17-2).[16-23] The percentage of patients with an abnormal karyotype also correlates with morphologic subtype, and the chromosome pattern shows a relationship with age.[24,25] In 1979, the Children's Cancer Study Group (CCSG) began an extensive study of the chromosomal abnormalities in a group of uniformly treated children with ANLL. The most frequent abnormalities observed were trisomy 8, t(8;21), t(15;17), and the loss of a sex chromosome.[26] There are many reports correlating chromosome abnormalities and remission rate, remission duration, or survival (see Prognostic Factors).

BIOLOGY

The molecular basis of the malignant change in ANLL is unknown. It is thought that in most cases of ANLL a single progenitor capable of indefinite self-renewal undergoes malignant transformation, giving rise to poorly differentiated precursors (blasts). These blasts have a decreased capacity to differentiate in response to normal physiological stimuli and gradually become the predominant cell in the bone marrow. Studies over the last decade have supported the clonal origin of the acute and chronic leukemias. Investigations of cell surface antigens, biochemical markers, *in vitro* bone marrow culture patterns, chromosomes, and oncogenes have also provided a better understanding of the biology of ANLL. The molecular events associated with normal myeloid maturation and malignant transformation are beginning to be examined (see Chap. 19).

Clonal Origin

Abundant evidence exists that most, if not all, cases of ANLL are clonal (derived from one cell). The evidence is based on cytogenetic analyses of bone marrow blast cells, as previously discussed, and the study of female patients with ANLL who are heterozygous for two electrophoretically distinct forms of the X-linked enzyme glucose-6-phosphate dehydrogenase (G6PD). According to the Lyon hypothesis, early in embryogenesis one of the X chromosomes becomes inactive (Fig. 17-1). Inactivation is random, and the same X chromosome remains inactive through all subsequent divisions. Blasts from patients with ANLL who are heterozygous for G6PD contain only a single isoenzyme type, whereas normal cells express both types.[27,28] A similar analysis can be made using molecular biologic techniques that examine X chromosome-linked DNA polymorphisms sensitive to the DNA methylation that occurs with X inactivation.[29] The leukemic blasts in all cases of ANLL

that have been studied with these techniques have been clonal.[27-30]

Cellular Level of Origin

The transforming event in ANLL could theoretically occur in any cell along the pathway from a pluripotent stem cell to committed precursors cells such as the myeloblast (Fig. 17-2). G6PD and cytogenetic analyses show that the cellular level of origin of ANLL is heterogeneous. In some patients, the clonal marker is noted in committed erythroid and myeloid precursors and their progeny, implying involvement of a multipotent progenitor. In other patients, the leukemia is expressed in cells restricted to granulocytic and macrophage lineage, suggesting involvement of a more committed granulocyte-macrophage progenitor (see Fig. 17-2).[27,28,30-32] Involvement of B-lymphocytes in a patient with ANLL has been suggested by a disproportionate representation of a single G6PD isoenzyme in Epstein–Barr virus (EBV)-transformed B-cell clones.[33]

Most patients in remission have mature granulocytes, erythrocytes, and platelets of both G6PD isoenzyme types (nonclonal cells). Recent studies of peripheral blood cells have shown that some patients with ANLL in apparent remission continue to have clonal hematopoiesis.[29,34] The bone marrow in these patients is morphologically and cytogenetically in remission. These data indicate a possible multistep process of leukemogenesis in which the two central features are [1] the emergence of a clone of hematopoietic preleukemic precursors capable of normal differentiation, and [2] clonal evolution as defined by the development of a cytogenetic ab-

ACUTE MYELOGENOUS LEUKEMIA—MULTIPOTENT MYELOID OR GRANULOCYTE—MACROPHAGE INVOLVEMENT

FIGURE 17-2. Stem cell diagram showing sites of malignant transformation in ANLL (*shaded*) and CML (*stippled*). Colony-forming unit (*CFU*) represents single cells that can form colonies when bone marrow is grown *in vitro*.

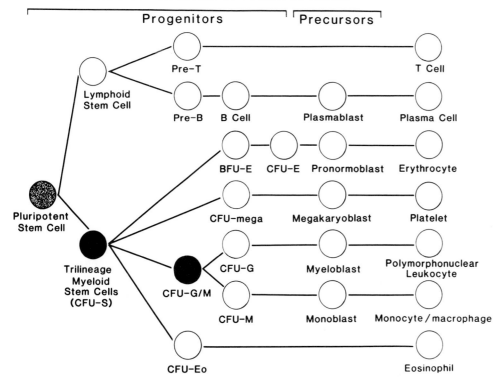

THE PROGENITOR BASIS OF HEMATOPOIESIS

normality, leading to overt blast disease. These exciting findings also question the definition of complete remission as conventionally used. One can no longer assume that the return of normal peripheral counts concomitant with <5% blasts in the bone marrow is reflective of polyclonal hematopoiesis.

Although the clonal expansion hypothesis is well established, there are rare but important cases in which acute leukemia arises in the donor cells after a bone marrow transplant from a histocompatible sibling, suggesting that extracellular leukemic factors may play an important role in certain patients.[35]

Bone Marrow Growth *in Vitro*

In vitro culture of bone marrow from patients with ANLL provides a method to study the proliferative capacity and differentiation potential of blast cell precursors. Normal marrow contains progenitors for all the hematopoietic lineages. These progenitors are difficult to identify morphologically, but give rise to characteristic colonies if plated on semisolid media in the presence of exogenously provided growth factors (colony-stimulating factors, or CSF). These normal colonies are rarely seen in bone marrow specimens from patients with leukemia. Instead, one observes small clusters of cells with blast-like morphology without maturation to granulocytes (reviewed in ref. 36). The suppression of normal hematopoiesis may be due to either physical displacement of stem cells by leukemic cells or production of inhibitory humoral factors, such as acid isoferritins.[37] With the alteration of culture conditions, large numbers of CFU-L (colonies that contain leukemic blasts and are generally smaller than the typical CFU-GM colony) can be grown from the bone marrow of patients with ANLL.[35] The cell surface phenotypes of the clonogenic cells that give rise to CFU-L often differ from the phenotypes of bone marrow leukemic blasts.[38,39] It is not known if the CFU-L actually function as the "stem cell" for the leukemia.

Previous data suggested that leukemic blasts and CFU-L were relatively unresponsive to the various CSFs produced by lymphocytes and other accessory cells. Recently, however, it has been shown that the blasts from some patients with ANLL are susceptible to the influence of some CSFs.[40] In addition, leukemic blasts from a subset of patients with ANLL produce biologically active GM-CSF (also termed CSF-1). These data may implicate, at least in some cases, an autocrine basis for the uncontrolled growth of leukemic blasts. Several investigators have attempted to correlate the patterns of *in vitro* colony growth at diagnosis with prognosis in ANLL.[41–43] The colony pattern, unlike colony number, reverts to normal following successful remission induction.[44]

Oncogenes

Many proto-oncogenes or cellular oncogenes have been implicated in different types of tumorigenesis (see Chap. 3). No specific oncogene has been implicated in the genesis of ANLL. Proto-oncogenes are expressed in normal cells and tissues and may help to control the growth and development of cells and organisms. One class of oncogenes codes for growth factor-like molecules, another class codes for protein kinases, and a third class may be linked with cell-cycle regulation and DNA replication. Proto-oncogenes are thought to confer malignant potential by one of several mechanisms: increased expression secondary to amplification of genomic material, increased transcription of a single gene, or expression of an abnormal product.[45] Chromosomal translocations may move a proto-on-

cogene from one chromosome to another and thus alter the expression of the oncogene. Examples of this include Burkitt's lymphoma and chronic myelogenous leukemia. In the t(8;14) translocation of Burkitt's lymphoma, the translocated c-*myc* is transcriptionally activated by enhancer elements associated with immunoglobulin loci (see Chap. 20).[46] In the t(9;22) or Philadelphia chromosome in CML, c-*abl* translocates to a restricted region, (the breakpoint cluster region, or bcr), on chromosome 22, and an aberrant c-*abl* protein is found because of the fusion of the bcr and *abl* genes (see Chap. 18).[47]

Mutated *ras* oncogenes, predominantly the N-*ras* gene, have been observed in several cases of ANLL.[48] The *ras* family of cellular oncogenes are the most frequently identified transformation-inducing genes in solid tumors.[49,50] Activation of cellular *ras* (c-*ras*) genes is caused by single base mutations, resulting in a single base substitution that yeilds a p21 species with increased transforming ability.[51–53] The role of mutated *ras* p21 in malignant myelopoiesis is unknown.

PATHOGENESIS AND NATURAL HISTORY

The etiology of ANLL in humans is unknown, but certain predisposing factors are well established (see Table 17-1). People who were exposed to radiation during the nuclear bombings of Hiroshima and Nagasaki have an increased incidence of leukemia. Those who were exposed in childhood had a higher incidence of leukemia, with a shorter latency period. The mix of ANLL and CML was similar across all age groups; ALL was not seen.[54]

Certain drugs and chemicals have been associated with leukemia. Exposure to benzene increases the risk of ANLL.[55] The most frequent cause of secondary ANLL in childhood is prior exposure to cytotoxic drugs, particularly the alkylating agents used to treat cancer. Patients treated with alkylating agents for Hodgkin's disease, Langerhans' cell histiocytosis, and other solid tumors have an increased incidence of ANLL.[56–58] These patients may manifest a myelodysplastic syndrome before developing leukemia, and abnormalities of chromosome 7 are common (see Chap. 19).[58–60] Secondary leukemia is particularly refractory to chemotherapy agents (see below).[61,62] The incidence of secondary leukemia peaks at approximately 6 years and appears to be time-limited, with no occurrences after 11 years in one study of adults treated with alkylating agents for Hodgkin's disease.[57] The vast majority of children with ANLL have no obvious predisposing factors.

CLASSIFICATION

Morphology

In 1976, the French–American–British (FAB) committee divided the acute nonlymphocytic leukemias into six subtypes.[63] An updated proposal was offered in 1982 to further define the FAB subtypes of the myelodysplastic syndromes (formerly called preleukemia) and to clarify the differences between the myelodysplastic disorders and ANLL, particularly the M6 subtype.[64] In 1987, the group added the M7 (megakaryocytic leukemia) subtype and made some refinements in the overall classification system.[65,66] The FAB system is widely accepted and has been extremely useful for reporting and standardizing data.[67] The classification identifies sub-groups of patients based on morphologic considerations and histochemical staining and has been shown in several studies to be of prognostic importance.

Table 17-3

French–American–British Classification of ANLL and Frequency in Childhood

FAB Class	Common Name	Histochemistry*	Age <2	Age ≥2
M1	Acute myeloblastic leukemia without differentiation	MP+	4 (17%)	32 (25%)
M2	Acute myeloblastic leukemia with differentiation	MP+	—	34 (27%)
M3	Acute promyelocytic leukemia	MP+	—	6 (5%)
M4	Acute myelomonocytic leukemia	MP+ NSE+	7 (30%)	33 (26%)
M5	Acute monocytic leukemia	NSE+	12 (52%)	20 (16%)
M6	Erythroleukemia (D:G)	MP+ (myeloblasts) PAS+ (erythroid precursors)	—	3 (2%)
M7	Acute megakaryoblastic leukemia	PPO+	—	—

* MP = myeloperoxidase; NSE = nonspecific esterase; PAS = periodic acid-Schiff; PPO = platelet peroxidase (by electron microscopy).

† M7 not included in FAB at time of study. Data for FAB age distribution are from Creutzig U, Schaaff A, Ritter J, et al: Acute myelogenous leukemia in children under 2 years of age: Studies and treatment results in 23 children in the AML therapy study BFM-78. Klin Padiatr 196(3):130–134, 1984.

Table 17-4

ANLL Surface Antigen Expression

Surface Antigen	Least Mature Normal Precursor Expressing Antigen*	Antigen Expression by FAB Type†
Ia (HLA-DR)	CFU-GEMM	M1, M2, M4, M5
MY9 (CD16)	CFU-GEMM	M1–M6
PM-81	CFU-GM (day 14)	M1–M6
AML-2-23	CFU-GM (day 7)	M1, M2, M4–M6
MY7 (CD13)	CFU-GM (day 7)	M1–M4, M6
MY8	Myeloblast	M4, M5
Mo1 (CD11)	Myeloblast	M4, M5
MY4 (CDw14)	Promonocyte, monocyte	M4, M5

* CFU-GEMM = mixed lineage progenitor cell; CFU-GM = day 7 and day 14 granulocyte/monocyte colony forming cells.

† Antigen considered associated with FAB type if >50% of ANLL samples tested were positive.

A minimum of 30% blasts is required for the diagnosis of ANLL.[65] Table 17-3 presents the FAB classification of ANLL along with the frequency of the subtypes in childhood. Monocytic leukemia (M5) is particularly common in children younger than 2 years. Acute megakaryocytic leukemia (M7) is strongly associated with myelofibrosis or increased bone marrow reticulin. The blast morphology and histochemical stains may not distinguish M7 from ALL (especially L2) or the M5 subtype of ANLL. Consequently, unlike other FAB subtypes, the diagnosis of M7 leukemia requires confirmation by electron microscopy (presence of platelet peroxidase) or the presence of platelet-specific cell surface markers (platelet glycoproteins Ib, IIb/IIIa, or factor VIII-related antigen).[65] The M7 subtype was associated with abnormalities of chromosome 21 in five pediatric cases reviewed by Sariban and associates.[68]

Cell Surface Markers

The heterogeneity of ALL has been demonstrated by studies of cell surface phenotype and gene rearrangements.[69–71] These evaluations confirm the lineage fidelity of most acute leukemias and are of prognostic and therapeutic significance. The immunoglobulin and T-cell receptor gene rearrangements and cell surface antigens that define immunologic subtypes of ALL are not limited to lymphoid cells. For example, the sheep red blood cell (SRBC) receptor (T11 or CD2) has been identified on a small percentage of malignant myeloblasts.[72] In addition, at least partial rearrangements or transcription of immunoglobulin heavy chain genes (or both) can occur in some myeloid cells.[73] However, the blasts from most patients with ANLL do not have T-lymphocyte surface antigens or early B-cell surface antigens, including CALLA (the common acute lymphoblastic leukemia antigen). Specifically they do not react with B1 (CD20), B4 (CD19), J5 (CALLA or CD10), T11 (SRBC receptor or CD2), and T101 (CD5).

A series of monoclonal antibodies have been developed that recognize determinants expressed on normal and leukemic myeloid cells.[74] These antibodies recognize myeloid surface antigens during normal marrow myelopoiesis (Table 17-4) and can be helpful in classifying the unusual case of acute undifferentiated leukemia.[75]

Significant differences in antigen expression have been observed among FAB groups.[74,76–78] Expression of Ia is uncommon in M3. Expression of several antigens was correlated with M4 and M5 (Ia, MY4, MY8, Mo1, Mo2, PM-81, and AML-2-23). In general, the M1 and M2 cases tend to express early antigens, whereas expression of later antigens such as MY8 and Mo1 is more common in M2, M4, and M5. These immunologically determined subgroups of ANLL are also of potential clinical significance (see Prognostic Factors).

Biochemical Markers

Muramidase, or lysozyme, is a hydrolytic enzyme that is present in the primary granules of primitive granulocytes and monocytes. Elevated serum and urine levels of this enzyme are present in ANLL, and levels are especially high in the monocytic and myelomonocytic subtypes (M5 and M4).[79] Increased blood and urine lysozyme levels have been associated with renal tubular dysfunction and subsequent hypokalemia in some patients.

Terminal deoxynucleotidyl transferase (TdT) is a unique enzyme (DNA polymerase) that may have a role in the generation of immunologic diversity. In normal tissue, TdT is restricted to cortical thymocytes and a small percentage of bone marrow lymphoid cells. Approximately 95% of cases of ALL are TdT positive, whereas fewer than 10% of cases of ANLL are positive.[80] One third of patients patients with chronic myelogenous leukemia (CML) in blast crisis have TdT-positive cells.[81]

Acute Mixed Lineage Leukemia

With the use of multiple techniques for analyzing the phenotypic and genotypic lineage-associated characteristics of leukemic blasts, cases of acute leukemia are being reported as biclonal or of mixed lineage. Mixed lineage leukemia can take one of three forms: [1] the blast cells can each express surface antigens of different lineages, [2] two disparate populations of blasts with distinct morphology or surface antigens can coexist, or [3] an apparent conversion of the leukemia from lymphoid to myeloid (or the reverse) can occur.[82] Mirro and colleagues estimate that approximately 25% of cases diagnosed as ANLL will possess lymphoid-associated surface antigens, and 13% of those that appear to be typical ALL will have surface markers common to the myeloid lineage.[83] This phenomenon may reflect the lack of lineage specificity of the markers used, aberrant gene expression resulting from the leukemogenic event, or a leukemia arising from a pluripotent progenitor.[84,85] Coexpression of lymphoid and myeloid markers by the same cell and the lack of chromosomally documented independent clones favor the latter two possibilities.

The clinical significance of acute mixed lineage leukemia is still unclear. Preliminary data from St. Jude Children's Research Hospital, however, indicate that children with ANLL whose blasts express the E-rosette antigen have a poor response to daunorubicin and cytosine arabinoside (ara-C).[72] Lineage conversion may occur in upwards of 5% of children with acute leukemia within 1 to 4 years from diagnosis.[86] In some cases, the original blast cell karyotype is replaced by an entirely different karyotype. It is not clear whether some of these cases represent second malignancies or chemotherapy-induced clonal selection.

CLINICAL AND LABORATORY FEATURES

The child with ANLL may present with very few symptoms; alternatively, the first signs of leukemia may be life-threatening sepsis or hemorrhage. It is estimated that there are an average of 10^{12} leukemic cells present at diagnosis. The presenting signs and symptoms generally reflect diminished production of erythrocytes, granulocytes, and platelets, leading to anemia, infection, and hemorrhage (Table 17-5). Extramedullary infiltration of the skin (leukemia cutis) is often the first sign of leukemia in the neonate.

Fatigue, pallor, headache, tinnitus, dyspnea, and congestive heart failure can all indicate anemia. The initial hemoglobin ranged from 2.7 to 14.3 g/dl (median = 7 g/dl) in one large series of children with ANLL.[87] The anemia is usually normocytic and normochromic. The peripheral blood smear frequently contains teardrop forms and nucleated erythrocytes.

Thrombocytopenia is the usual cause of hemorrhage in patients with ANLL. Petechiae, bruising, epistaxis, and gingival bleeding are the most common symptoms. Approximately 50% of newly diagnosed children with ANLL have platelet counts below 50,000/mm[3].[87] Disseminated intravascular coagulation (DIC) may occur in any FAB subtype but is extremely common in M3 leukemia because of thromboplastin activity contained in the promyelocytic granules.[88] The DIC frequently accelerates when cells lyse with the initiation of therapy, and many investigators advocate the use of prophylactic low-dose heparin during induction therapy for any patient with acute promyelocytic leukemia.[89,90]

The absolute neutrophil count (ANC: a sum of the polymorphonuclear and band forms) of patients with ANLL is frequently depressed (<1000/mm[3]), and lingering bacterial infections of the lung, sinuses, gingiva, teeth, perirectal area, and

Table 17-5
Signs and Symptoms at Presentation in ANLL

Sign or Symptom	Percentage of Patients
Fever	34
Pallor	25
Anorexia, weight loss	22
Weakness, fatigue	19
Sore throat	18
Other respiratory symptoms	23
Bleeding	
Cutaneous	18
Mucosal	10
Menorrhagia*	5
Bone or joint pain	18
Lymphadenopathy	14
Gastrointestinal symptoms	13
Neurologic signs or symptoms	10
Swollen gingiva	8
Chest pain	5
Recurrent infection	3

(Data from Choi SI, Simone JV: Med Pediatr Oncol 2:119, 1976)
* Thirty percent of postmenopausal females had menorrhagia.

skin may be the first sign of leukemia. Fever or infection is common when the ANC is less than 200/mm[3]. After appropriate culturing, empiric antibiotics are indicated for the patient with fever and an ANC <500/mm[3] (see Chap. 39). Infections are even more common when the bone marrow reveals monosomy 7, because the granulocytes of some of these patients have defects in chemotaxis.[91] This defect may only occur in cases where the malignant cells are able to differentiate to neutrophils, as defined by the presence of only one chromosome 7 in the mature cell.[92,93]

The leukocyte count at presentation in childhood ANLL can be quite variable. On occasion, the peripheral blood may contain few or no blasts, despite a bone marrow that is hypercellular, with 80% to 90% blasts. Approximately one fourth of children with ANLL will have a leukocyte count >100,000/mm[3].[94]

Hepatomegaly or splenomegaly occurs in over half of children with ANLL.[87] Massive enlargement of lymph nodes is present at diagnosis in fewer than 25% of patients and is most commonly seen in leukemias with a monocytic component (M4 or M5). Chloromas or myeloblastomas are localized tumors seen in patients with ANLL that may appear green on the cut surface because of the enzyme myeloperoxidase. Myeloblastomas are rare. They may arise in bones or soft tissues and are frequently seen in the epidural area and around the orbits.[95] These tumors are more common in infants with M4 and M5 subtypes, and are also associated with the 8;21 translocation. Chloromas may appear before an increase in blasts is detectable in the bone marrow or they may herald relapse.[95] The lesions of leukemia cutis appear colorless or slightly purple ("blueberry muffin") and are most commonly observed in neonates with acute monocytic leukemia. The testicles are a relatively uncommon site of extramedullary ANLL.

Central nervous system (CNS) involvement in ANLL can manifest either as the rare CNS (parenchymal) chloroma or typical meningeal infiltration. At presentation, cytocentrifuged specimens of cerebrospinal fluid (CSF) are positive for blasts in 5% to 15% of ANLL patients, a higher percentage than in ALL.[94,96–98] Only approximately 2% of patients present with symptoms referable to the CNS, such as headaches, nausea, vomiting, photophobia, papilledema, and cranial nerve palsies.[96] Seizures are very uncommon. A review of two consecutive protocols at St. Jude Children's Research Hospital found that the presence of CNS disease at diagnosis correlated with a high initial leukocyte count and with age less than 2 years.[96] Other investigators have noted that children with monoblastic[94] or myelomonoblastic[94,98] leukemia are more likely to have CSF leukemic blasts at diagnosis.

METHODS OF DIAGNOSIS

The definitive diagnosis of leukemia is made by examination of the bone marrow aspirate. Wright–Giemsa and special histochemical stains of the aspirate provide a clear diagnosis in the majority of patients. In most cases, the marrow is hypercellular, with 50% to 100% blasts. According to the new recommendations of the FAB group, acute leukemia can be diagnosed when the marrow has >30% blasts.[65] A British study reported that morphology and histochemistry failed to identify the type of acute leukemia in one of every five patients.[75] In these instances, bone marrow cytogenetics and cell surface markers may help to differentiate between lymphoid and nonlymphoid leukemia. Severe infections, hemolysis, and other marrow infiltrations may lead to a leukoerythroblastic peripheral blood picture that can mimic leukemia (especially CML). The bone marrow aspirate should differentiate between these processes. If questions remain, treating the underlying problem and repeating the bone marrow in 7 to 10 days should clarify the situation.

PROGNOSTIC FACTORS

Consensus exists regarding important clinical and laboratory prognostic variables in childhood ALL.[99] In ANLL, however, similar analyses of many pediatric and adult studies have failed to identify consistent prognostic factors.[100] Some factors are reported to influence remission rate, and others appear to influence remission duration. In addition, the influence of these prognostic factors may vary according to the type and effectiveness of the therapy administered. The major elements of several pediatric ANLL studies are listed in Table 17-6.

The prognostic significance of several pretreatment factors has been evaluated in children and adults with ANLL (Table 17-7). These data are quite controversial.[100] A high leukocyte count and liver enlargement were predictive of a decreased remission induction rate for patients treated on the BFM study (Table 17-6).[98] A retrospective review of VAPA (vincristine, Adriamycin, prednisone, and ara-C) and 80-035 (Table 17-6) failed to identify clinical or laboratory variables that influenced the rate of complete remission. However, monocytic or myelomonocytic leukemia, leukocyte count >100,000/mm³, and age less than 2 years at diagnosis all predicted an increased risk of relapse and decreased overall survival in a univariate analysis.[94] FAB subtype and high leukocyte count continued to predict an increased risk of relapse in multivariate analyses; only the M5 subtype independently predicted poor overall survival. High leukocyte counts and younger age have also been predictive of short remissions in other studies of childhood ANLL.[100,101] Other investigators have not uniformly confirmed the negative prognostic influence of the M4 and M5 subtypes.[98,101,102]

A study from St. Jude Children's Research Hospital noted that a decreased platelet count, a higher labeling index (>10% at diagnosis), and a spleen size greater than 5 cm below the right costal margin were all related to a poor outcome (Table 17-6).[102] A high S-phase index of bone marrow is reported to be favorable in some but not all studies. There have also been attempts to correlate clinical response to the *in vitro* sensitivity of clonogenic leukemia cells to chemotherapy. A recently reported study did find a significant correlation between *in vitro* sensitivity to daunorubicin and ara-C (cytarabine) and successful remission induction.[103]

Data from a CCSG protocol indicated that a more rapid induction of remission correlated with a better chance for long-term continuous remission.[104] In some adult ANLL studies, patients who develop hepatitis (a defined by elevated hepatic transaminases) after remission induction are reported to have longer remissions or survival than those who do not develop hepatitis.[105,106]

Several studies of ANLL in adults have reported a correlation between initial karyotype and remission rate, remission duration, or survival. Data from the Fourth International Workshop on Chromosomes in Leukemia showed that the highest complete remission rate was in patients with t(8;21) and the lowest in those with hyperdiploidy or abnormalities of chromosome 7. The chromosome pattern at presentation (all normal chromosomes, a mixture of normal and abnormal, or all abnormal) did not predict complete remission. However, patients with all abnormal metaphases, abnormalities of chromosome 5, or a translocation involving band 11q23 all had significantly shorter remissions.[107] Structural abnormalities of chromosome 16 (pericentric inversion or partial deletion of the long arm) have been consistently identified in children and adults with acute myelomonocytic leukemia and abnormal eosinophils.[19–21] Adult patients in this specific subgroup have a favorable prognosis despite a tendency to develop CNS leukemia.[108,109] These findings have not been corroborated in children with ANLL.

The largest study correlating cytogenetic findings and prognosis in children with ANLL was reported by the CCSG.[26] Patients with normal karyotypes did not have a higher remission rate than patients with clonal chromosomal abnormalities. Specific cytogenetic changes, however, were prognostically important. Trisomy 8 and t(8;21) were associated with a high complete remission (CR) rate (>90%), whereas abnormalities of chromosome 7 were associated with a low CR rate (28%). In addition, t(15;17) was associated with excessive induction toxicity.[26]

Patients with therapy-linked leukemia or occupational exposure to potentially leukemogenic agents and those with myelodysplastic syndromes have an increased frequency of abnormalities involving chromosomes 5, 7, or both, and a relatively poor response to chemotherapy.[61,62,110,111] The use of surface marker analysis to predict outcome of ANLL has not been extensively investigated. In a recent study of adult ANLL patients, two myeloid antigens (MY4 and MY7) predicted a low rate of CR, and HLA-DR, MY8, and Mo1 were associated with a decreased remission duration.[78]

TREATMENT

The goal of therapy in ANLL is to achieve a long-term remission and hopefully a cure. The initial step is induction of a complete remission, defined as the reduction of leukemia cells to undetectable levels (<5% myeloblasts in bone marrow), return of both normal marrow function and peripheral blood counts,

Table 17-6
*Major Elements of Several Pediatric ANLL Regimens**

Phase/Feature	Study Designations				
	VAPA	*AML-76*	*AML BFM-78*	*80-035*	*CCSG-241 A*
Remission induction	VCR 1.5 mg d 1, 5 Dox 30 mg d 1, 2, 3 Pred 40 mg d 1–5 Ara-C 100 mg d 1–7	VCR 1.5 mg d 1 DNR 25 mg d 1 Ara-C 150 mg d 4–7 6-AZ 15 g d 5–7	VCR 1.5 mg/wk × 4 Dox 25 mg/wk × 4 Pred 60 mg × 28 d Ara-C 75 mg × 16 d 6-TG 60 mg × 28 d	DNR 45 mg d 1–3 Ara-C 200 mg d 1–7	DNR 30 mg × 3 d 5-aza 100 mg × 4 d Ara-C 75 mg × 4 d Pred 40 mg × 4 d VCR 1.5 mg × 1 d
	Second induction— repeat course for shorter period	Repeated weekly until hypoplasia occurs	Phase II Dox 25 mg wk 2, 4 Ara-C 75 mg × 16 d CTX 500 mg wk 1, 3, 5	Second induction with decreased duration	Repeated every 2 wk for minimum of 4 and maximum of 7 courses
Remission rate	74%	72%	79%	70%	63% (73% if include marrows with <15% blasts)
Intensification	Sequential administration: Courses 1–4 Dox 45 mg d 1 Ara-C 200 mg d 1–5 Courses 5–8 Dox 30 mg d 1 5-aza 150 mg d 1–5 Courses 9–12 VCR 1.5 mg d 1 Pred 800 mg d 1–5 6-MP 500 mg d 1–5 MTX 7.5 mg d 1–5 Courses 13–16 Ara-C 200 mg d 1–5	None	None	Sequential administration: Courses 1–4 DNR 45 mg d 1 Ara-C 200 mg d 1–5 6-TG 200 mg d 1–5 Courses 5–7 DNR 30 mg d 1 5-aza 150 mg d 1–5 Courses 8–11 Ara-C 200 mg d 1–5 6-TG 200 mg d 1–5	None
Maintenance	None	VCR 1.5 mg wk 1 CTX 200 mg wk 1 Dox 20 mg wk 1 6-MP 50 mg/d wk 2–4 Ara-C 150 mg wk, 2, 3, 4	Dox 25 mg every 8 wk × 1 yr Ara-C 40 mg × 4 d every mo 6-TG 40 mg daily	None	6-TG 75 mg × 28 d 5-aza 100 mg × 4 d Ara-C 75 mg × 4 d CTX 75 mg × 4 d VCR 1.5 mg × 1 d
(Duration)		(Monthly for 30 mo)	(2 years)		(Monthly × ≥2 years)
Late intensification	None	Two courses Pred 100 mg × 5 d VCR 2 mg d 1 MTX 7.5 mg × 5 d 6-MP 500 mg × 5 d	None	None	None
CNS prophylaxis	None	IT MTX monthly × 6 mo then every 3 mo	CNS irradiation with concurrent IT MTX	Intermittent IT ara-C	IT MTX monthly × 6 mo
3-year CCR	50%	29%	50%	50%	33% (at 30 mo)

* All doses are per square meter (m²). VCR = vincristine; Pred = prednisone or methylprednisolone; Ara-C = cytosine arabinoside; Dox = doxorubicin; 6-MP = 6-mercaptopurine; MTX = methotrexate; DNR = daunorubicin; 6AZ = 6-azouridine; 6TG = 6-thioguanine; CTX = cyclophosphamide; 5-AZA = 5-azacytidine; IT = intrathecal; CCR, continuous complete remission. References for studies: VAPA, Ref. 122; AML-76, Ref. 102; 80-035, Ref. 43; CCSG-241a, Ref. 134.

resolution of hepatosplenomegaly and lymphadenopathy, and return to a normal performance status. Once remission is achieved, the objective is to prevent recurrence of leukemia. This is most often attempted by continued administration of chemotherapy, but bone marrow transplantation is being used increasingly for children with histocompatible donors.

Immediate Therapy at Diagnosis

The initial hours of therapy should be directed toward recognition and prevention or treatment of life-threatening complications. Bleeding, infection, the tumor lysis syndrome, and leukostasis are all potentially fatal complications.

Table 17-7
*Prognostic Factors in Pediatric ANLL**

Variable	Influence on:		Reference
	Remission Rate	Remission Duration	
Presenting features			
Age <2 years	None	Negative	94
FAB M4, M5	None	Negative	94
CNS leukemia at diagnosis	None	None	94, 98
High initial leukocyte count	Negative/none	None/negative	98/94
Platelet count >100,000/mm³	Positive/none	None	102
Splenomegaly >5 cm	None	Negative	102
Hepatomegaly ≥5 cm	Negative	None	98
High labeling index	None	Negative	98
Cytogenetics			
Monosomy 7, 7q−	Negative	None	26, 107
Abnormalities of			
chromosome 11*	None	Negative	107
All abnormal metaphases*	None	Negative	107
inv 16*	None	Positive	108, 109
Surface antigens			
MY4, MY7*	Negative	None	78
HLA-DR, MY8, Mo1*	None	Negative	78

* Not yet confirmed in pediatric studies.

Bleeding

Bleeding in ANLL is usually secondary to thrombocytopenia. Spontaneous bleeding in a normal host rarely occurs until the platelet count is below 20,000/mm³. However, concomitant conditions such as infection may predispose to hemorrhage at higher platelet counts. We recommend prophylactic platelet transfusions to maintain platelet counts above 20,000/mm³ in all patients. A higher target platelet count should be used for patients with bleeding or infection. If there is laboratory evidence of DIC, aggressive replacement of clotting factors with fresh frozen plasma is recommended in addition to platelet transfusions (see Chap. 38). The M3 and M5 subtypes of ANLL are particularly associated with DIC, and the coagulopathy usually worsens with cytotoxic therapy. As noted earlier, many investigators recommend the prophylactic use of low-dose heparin (50 U/kg every 6 hours) for patients with promyelocytic leukemia.[89,90] This approach remains controversial, and some investigators suggest that remission induction can be accomplished without heparin.[112]

Fever and Infection

Fever is seen at diagnosis in 30% to 40% of patients with ANLL. Although infection is usually suspected, it is documented in only 50% of cases. Nevertheless, febrile, neutropenic patients should receive empiric antibiotics after appropriate cultures have been obtained.[113] A semisynthetic penicillin and an aminoglycoside are generally recommended. Enteric gram-negative bacilli and gram-positive bacteria (*e.g., Staphylococcus epidermidis*) are responsible for the majority of infections (see Chap. 39).

Tumor Lysis Syndrome

The tumor lysis syndrome encompasses the metabolic consequences of the release of the cellular content of dying leukemia cells—hyperuricemia with subsequent renal failure; hyperkalemia and hyperphosphatemia from the release of intracellular potassium and phosphorus, respectively, and secondary hypocalcemia. Renal failure is preventable in the majority of cases. Careful hydration, alkalinization of the urine with intravenous bicarbonate, and administration of allopurinol should be promptly instituted in all children (see Chap. 37). Close monitoring of serum electrolytes (especially potassium, calcium, and phosphate), urine output, and serum creatinine is imperative.[114,115]

Leukostasis

Leukostasis is the term used to describe intravascular clumping of blasts, with subsequent hypoxia, hemorrhage, and infarction of the affected tissue. Leukostasis rarely occurs in ANLL unless the leukocyte count is greater than 200,000/mm³. The brain and lungs are the most commonly symptomatic organs. Lung involvement is heralded by tachypnea and falling partial pressure of arterial oxygen. CNS symptoms may include somnolence, stroke, and coma.[116–118] As soon as metabolic parameters are stabilized, prompt initiation of therapy is imperative for any patient with a high leukocyte count (>200,000/mm³) and ANLL. Extreme caution should be taken with these patients. Oral doses of hydroxyurea are safe and effective in this situation.[119] Leukophoresis or exchange transfusion lowers the leukocyte count rapidly but only transiently and should be used for symptomatic patients (*i.e.,* those with tachypnea or CNS signs) until the cytotoxic therapy begins to lyse leukemia cells.[120] No firm data support CNS irradiation for leukostasis, although some investigators suggest its use. In any case, preventive measures are the best therapy: once leukostasis begins, tissue damage is inevitable.

In the BFM study, children with M5 leukemia, leukocyte counts > 100,000/mm³, and specific organ involvement with leukemia had a particularly high incidence of fatal hemorrhage.[98]

Remission Induction

Once the patient has been stabilized, remission induction should begin without delay. Clinical trials in ANLL have consistently demonstrated two important principles of induction therapy: combinations of two agents are more effective than single agents, and drug dosages must be high enough to achieve bone marrow aplasia for best results. The most effective drugs for remission induction are the anthracyclines (daunorubicin or doxorubicin) and ara-C.[100] Most remission induction regimens consist of a 7-day course (continuous infusion or twice daily injections) of ara-C plus 3 days of an anthracycline, with or without the addition of 6-thioguanine. A review of the adult ANLL remission induction literature does not show a higher remission rate when 6-thioguanine is added to anthracycline and ara-C.[121] With these regimens, 70% to 85% of children with ANLL will achieve a remission (see Table 17-6).[94,98,102,122]

The drug dosages necessary to kill leukemic blasts come dangerously close to destroying normal marrow cells and cause prolonged bone marrow hypoplasia. With the exception of some patients with promyelocytic (M3) leukemia, all ANLL patients must go through a period of severe bone marrow hypoplasia to achieve remission.[123] Most protocols call for a bone marrow aspirate and biopsy 14 days after the initiation of therapy. Persistence of blasts usually implies resistant leukemia rather than early recovery of normal cells and indicates a second course of induction therapy. A hypoplastic marrow with fewer than 5% blasts often heralds a remission. The severe pancytopenia during induction persists for an average of 21 to 30 days from the start of therapy, with longer durations in patients requiring a second remission induction cycle.

Gastrointestinal toxicity, manifested as diarrhea and oral mucositis, is common during remission induction. Ara-C causes a predictable mucosal change in the intestine.[124] Diarrhea, sometimes massive, is quite common. A particularly severe manifestation of this toxicity has been referred to as ileocecitis or "typhlitis."[125,126] Heralded by right lower quadrant pain, typhlitis may proceed to abdominal distention, vomiting, lower GI bleeding, fever, and even septic shock. Management is primarily medical and includes bowel rest, intravenous fluids, and broad-spectrum antibiotics. Surgery is reserved for intestinal perforation, abdominal wall fasciitis, massive bleeding, or uncontrollable septic shock.[127] Typhlitis may be more common in children; its incidence is reduced in regimens using daunorubicin rather than doxorubicin (see Chaps. 37 and 39).[128,129]

Remission induction fails in 20% to 30% of children with ANLL. Approximately half of these patients have drug-resistant leukemia cells; the others die of hemorrhage, infection, or leukostasis. Patients with resistant leukemia may be treated with any of several active combinations of drugs (see Treatment of Relapsed Patients). The choice of regimen will depend on the drugs used for remission induction. Attaining higher initial remission induction rates will depend on the development of new or more effective chemotherapeutic agents with an improved therapeutic index.

Continuation Therapy

Successful remission induction results in an approximately 2 to 3 log leukemia cell kill (from 10^{12} to 10^{9}). However, as in ALL, significant numbers of leukemic blasts remain in remission marrows at a level below the detectability of current histologic, biochemical, cytogenetic, and immunologic methods. Without further treatment after standard induction therapy, more than 90% of patients will relapse by 1 year. A study from Johns Hopkins Hospital used an intensive 10-day kinetically based induction without continuation therapy. The median remission duration was 31 weeks, and 12% of patients remained in remission at 5 years.[130] In a subsequent cohort of 25 adults given a second course of intensive induction, the median duration of remission was extended from 9 to 30 months, with 58% in remission at 2 years.[131]

Therapy beyond remission is beneficial, but the intensity and duration of continuation therapy remain controversial, as does the appropriate selection of patients for bone marrow transplantation in first remission. Several therapeutic strategies have been used during the postremission period: [1] "maintenance" therapy, which can be defined as postremission treatment that is less myelosuppressive than induction therapy, [2] "consolidation," used to describe regimens that are essentially the same as those used for induction, both in terms of drugs and doses used, and [3] "intensification," defined as therapy with the same drugs used in induction but at higher doses or with myelosuppressive doses of "non-cross-resistant" active agents not administered in induction.

Long-term follow-up (>5 years) of clinical studies using maintenance therapy for childhood ANLL show leukemia-free survival plateaus of 20%. These were outpatient trials and therefore were intended not to induce severe myelosuppression (nadirs with neutrophils >500/mm^3 and platelets >100,000/mm^3).[102,104] The merit of early intensification or consolidation therapy in ANLL is under investigation. Results from one study (VAPA) have suggested a high proportion of long-term survivors following intensive postremission chemotherapy (see Table 17-6).[122,132] In this study, patients received 14 months of intensive sequential combination chemotherapy after the remission induction period. The intensification was based on the steep dose–response curve observed for some of the chemotherapeutic agents in experimental animal leukemia models. In addition, combinations of drugs believed to be non-cross-resistant were used sequentially to circumvent the problem of drug resistance. In this study, 74% of children achieved a complete remission, and 45% of these remain in continuous remission at 5 years. The successor study to VAPA also used a similar approach and achieved comparable results (Fig. 17-3).[94] The value of intensification therapy requires confirmation in larger prospective controlled clinical trials.

The BFM cooperative study used a different approach in treating childhood ANLL (see Table 17-6).[98] The initial therapy consisted of an intensive induction and consolidation regimen, given over 8 weeks, using seven different drugs and cranial irradiation. This was followed by maintenance therapy for 2 years. Complete remission was achieved in 79% of patients, and 52% of that group remain in continuous remission at 5 years.

Other studies have evaluated immunotherapy or splenectomy during the maintenance phase of ANLL. The CCSG found no advantage for immunotherapy (bacillus Calmette-Guerin, BCG) and allogeneic acute myelomonocytic leukemic cells and chemotherapy compared to chemotherapy alone in maintaining remission.[133] A successor protocol with intensified maintenance therapy but without immunotherapy showed an improved continuous complete remission rate (see Table 17-6).[134] The addition of splenectomy to chemotherapy did not prolong the duration of remission of children with ANLL in a St. Jude Children's Research Hospital study.[102]

The value of maintenance therapy has been questioned in many adult ANLL studies. Several adult studies have produced conflicting results regarding the benefit of maintenance

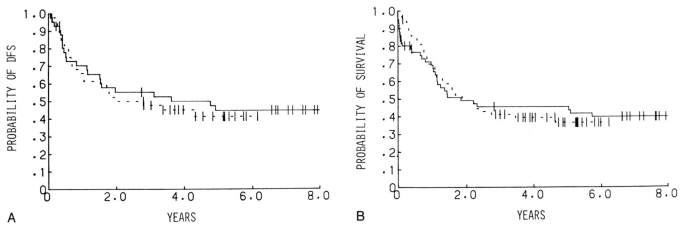

FIGURE 17-3. Kaplan–Meier estimates for probability of disease-free survival (*DFS*) (**A**) for patients entering remission and for survival (**B**) for all patients treated on VAPA (*solid line*) or 80-035 (*dashed line*).

chemotherapy after either intensification or consolidation therapy.[121] A CCSG controlled trial that is in progress hopefully will answer this question for children with ANLL.

Etoposide (VP-16) and tenoposide (VM-26) are active in ANLL. Odom and Gordon noted a remarkable response to the epipodophyllotoxins VM-26 and VP-16 in infants with monocytic leukemia.[135] One infant had leukemia cutis only, but four others had widespread disease at the start of therapy. Four of the five infants were off therapy at times ranging from 11 months to 6 years. These results are extremely interesting, but verification in a larger group of infants is necessary.

Bone Marrow Transplantation

Bone marrow transplantation (BMT) is being used increasingly to treat children with ANLL in first remission. However, estimates based on family size in the United States indicate that fewer than 40% of potential candidates for BMT will have an HLA-compatible donor. (The principles of BMT are reviewed in Chap. 48.)

Marrow grafting for children with ANLL is usually performed within several months after a complete remission is achieved. Most studies have used cyclophosphamide (120 mg/kg) plus total body irradiation (750–1400 cGy) to prepare patients for transplantation. Published data from single-center and cooperative group trials indicate 5-year leukemia relapse rates of approximately 20% and actuarial leukemia-free survival ranging from 55% to 70%.[136–140] Graft-versus-host disease (GVHD) and interstitial pneumonitis account for most of the deaths after transplant. This is in contrast to marrow grafting for ALL in second or third remission, in which relapse accounts for a large fraction of the failures.

Although these results are encouraging, controversy continues over the relative efficacy of chemotherapy versus marrow transplantation in first remission. It is difficult to compare uncontrolled trials of BMT and chemotherapy because of the selection criteria for transplantation and the possibility of relapse before a patient arrives at a transplant center. The CCSG has reported the only prospective controlled study of transplantation versus chemotherapy for pediatric patients with ANLL in first remission. This was a biologically assigned trial (treatment was based on the availability of a histocompatible sibling donor). Patients undergoing BMT were prepared by administration of cyclophosphamide (60 mg/kg on 2 days) followed by total body irradiation (750–1320 cGy). Patients

without HLA-compatible donors were randomized to one of two chemotherapy regimens. At 3 years from initial remission, BMT is associated with a significantly better disease-free survival rate than chemotherapy (49% versus 36%, *p* = 0.03). The VAPA and BFM studies, however, have achieved results with chemotherapy that are comparable to the CCSG transplant data.[94,98]

Conflicting results have been reported in adult ANLL studies comparing BMT and chemotherapy in first remission.[142–144] There is a trend toward a leukemia-free survival advantage for the transplanted patients, but this difference was not statistically significant in two of the three studies. Because most failures after BMT are secondary to toxicity, salvage is unlikely. For patients relapsing after continuation chemotherapy, subsequent transplantation remains a possibility. Transplantation in second remission or early relapse yields long-term survivals of 20% to 45%.[139,145] As with transplantation in first remission, the majority of deaths are due to GVHD or interstitial pneumonitis.

Because of the controversial data on marrow transplantation in ANLL in first remission, reserving BMT for patients who relapse is a reasonable alternative strategy. In this situation, it is not clear whether one should first attempt to induce a second remission or proceed directly to BMT. There are few reports that address this issue. Retrospective analysis of data from the Seattle transplant experience indicate similar outcomes for patients transplanted in second remission or early relapse.[146] The poorest outcome was observed in patients who failed to enter a second remission after induction chemotherapy and then underwent BMT.

Are there factors predictive of relapse after chemotherapy that might be used to select children for BMT? As previously discussed, consistent prognostic factors are difficult to identify, but may include the M4 and M5 subtypes of ANLL.[94,101] Unfortunately, several transplant studies have also reported that M4 and M5 ANLL have an adverse influence on transplant outcome.[139,140]

There is less controversy about the merits of BMT for patients with myelodysplastic syndromes and therapy-linked ANLL. If such children have histocompatible siblings, we currently recommend transplantation as primary therapy (without attempts to induce a remission with chemotherapy). The Fred Hutchinson Transplant Center has obtained excellent results using this approach in young adults and children with myelodysplastic syndromes.[147]

Several groups have explored autologous marrow transplantation in patients with ANLL.[148] *Ex vivo* drug or antibody

Table 17-8
Central Nervous System Prophylaxis

Study	CNS Leukemia at Diagnosis	CNS Prophylaxis	CNS Relapses/ Total Relapses	Actuarial 3-Year CCR	Reference
St. Jude AML-76	14/81 (17%)	IT MTX	3/50	0.29	102
AML-BFM-78	14/151 (9%)	Cranial RT; IT MTX	1/47	0.50	98
VAPA	No initial LP performed	None	8/22	0.50	94
80-035	11/64 (17%)	IT ara-C	3/20	0.50	94

treatment of autologous marrow assumes a differential toxicity of the leukemic stem cells and normal pluripotent stem cell; transplantation of untreated marrow presupposes a differential effect of freezing, a minimal dose of leukemic cells below which relapse will not occur, an autologous graft-versus-leukemia effect, or a combination of the three. In contrast to auto-transplantation for ALL, immunologic approaches for purging marrow have been limited by cross-reactivity of most anti-ANLL monoclonal antibodies with normal hematopoietic progenitors and precursors.[74] However, several ANLL autotransplant protocols using anti-ANLL monoclonals and complement are currently under way. As an alternative approach, pharmacologic purging of leukemic cells from remission marrow has been attempted. Preliminary data from an autotransplant study using 4-hydroperoxycylophosphamide (4-HC) to treat marrow harvested from children and adults with ANLL in second or third remission have been encouraging.[149] The actuarial relapse rate was 46% and actuarial survival at 2 years was 43%. As in autologous BMT for ALL, it is not possible to measure the efficacy of *ex vivo* purging in this setting.

Other centers have recently been evaluating purged or nonpurged autologous BMT for patients with ANLL in first remission.[148] Marrow is harvested and cryopreserved in early first remission, usually after several months of consolidation chemotherapy. The patient then receives supralethal preparatory therapy and reinfusion of autologous marrow. This procedure may be viewed as another course of intensive consolidation therapy. Results are too preliminary for a fair evaluation of this treatment method.

Central Nervous System Prophylaxis

CNS prophylaxis became an intregal part of ALL therapy when it became clear that treatment of this sanctuary site prolonged overall disease-free survival.[150] Without specific CNS therapy, isolated CNS relapse occurs in up to 20% of children with ANLL.[97,132] The majority of patients with CNS relapse will develop a subsequent bone marrow relapse.

As in ALL, it appears that CNS prophylaxis for children with ANLL is effective in decreasing subsequent isolated CNS relapse (Table 17-8). Intrathecal methotrexate or cranial irradiation combined with intrathecal methotrexate was effective CNS prophylaxis in the BFM and St. Jude Children's Research Hospital studies, respectively.[98,102] However, it has not been demonstrated by clinical trial technique that effective CNS prophylaxis contributes to better disease-free survival. The successor to the VAPA protocol, 80-035, incorporated intrathecal ara-C for CNS prophylaxis. Although there were fewer CNS relapses, this did not lend to an improvement in the overall disease-free survival.[94] The value of CNS prophylaxis may not become apparent until durations of bone marrow remission

Table 17-9
Useful Regimens in Resistant ANLL

Drugs/Schedule*	CR/Patients Treated	Reference
VP-16 200 mg d 1–3 5-aza 300 mg d 4, 5 Regimen repeated after 1–2 days until marrow hypoplasia or progressive leukemia develops	10/22 (45%)	152
Ara-C 3 g h 0, 12, 24, 36 Asparaginase 6,000 u h 42 Regimen repeated d 8	8/19 (42%)	155
Methotrexate 100 mg d 1 Asparaginase 500 u/kg d 2 (max. = 20,000 u) (24 h after MTX) Regimen repeated weekly × 2–3	2/6 (33%)	157
Ara-C 3 g every 12 h × 12 doses†	12/24 (50%)†	158
VM-26 200 mg d 1–3 AMSA 100 mg d 1–3 Repeat on d 7 if residual leukemia	5/7 (71%)	159

* All doses per square meter (m²) except as noted. AMSA = amsacrine; other abbreviations as in Table 17-6.
† Study of adult patients.

become significantly longer. CNS relapse occurs much less often in adults than in children with ANLL; other factors predicting an increased incidence of CNS relapse include monocytic and myelomonocytic leukemia (M4 and M5) and, in one study, age less than 2 years or a leukocyte count > 25,000/mm³ at diagnosis.[96,132,151]

Treatment of Relapsed Patients

Success is limited in treating children who relapse or who fail initial induction attempts. However, outcome is somewhat dependent on the initial therapy and the timing of relapse. In the VAPA experience, 25% of children who relapsed while receiving intensive sequential chemotherapy achieved a subsequent remission, whereas those who relapsed after elective cessation of therapy had a greater than 50% likelihood of entering a second remission (Weinstein, personal communication). Several active relapse regimens exist for children with ANLL (Table 17-9).[152–159] High-dose ara-C, with or without L-asparaginase, produces remissions in a substantial proportion of patients who have failed conventional doses of ara-C.[155,158] Many of these active agents are currently included in trials of initial continuation therapy for children with ANLL.

Second remissions maintained with chemotherapy are invariably shorter than the initial remission and, with very rare exceptions, are of relatively brief duration. Autologous or allogeneic BMT in second remission does offer the potential for long-term survival (see above).

FUTURE CONSIDERATIONS

Despite the advances outlined above, the range of overall survival of children with ANLL does not yet approach that seen in ALL. Complete remission is now achieved in 75% to 85% of children with ANLL; 30% to 60% of these children remain free of disease following marrow grafting or further chemotherapy. It is clear that some form of postremission treatment is necessary, but whether this should include maintenance or intensification (consolidation) chemotherapy or autologous or allogeneic BMT remains open to investigation.

The low relapse rate after BMT makes this approach particularly attractive. Removal of T-lymphocytes or other mediators of graft versus host disease may decrease toxicity for those patients with a histocompatible sibling and extend the procedure to patients without a complete match.[160-163] However, there is some evidence that the graft versus leukemia phenomenon contributes to the cure rate in BMT; theoretically, abrogation of GVHD with T-cell depletion could actually decrease overall disease-free survival for patients with ANLL.[164,165] Autologous transplant techniques have produced impressive results in relapsed patients with ANLL.[148,149,166] Studies are already under way to evaluate the efficacy of autotransplants in first remission.

Several other approaches are possible. Imaginative use of old drugs (*e.g.*, high-dose ara-C) coupled with newer agents may improve survival for patients with ANLL. Recent studies have demonstrated the ability of various agents (*e.g.*, retinoic acid, phorbol esters, low doses of ara-C) to induce differentiation of ANLL blasts *in vitro*.[167,168] There have been several clinical studies using these drugs in patients with preleukemia, smoldering leukemia, and *de novo* ANLL. Preliminary clinical results have been variable, and there has been little or no documentation of *in vivo* differentiation of leukemic blasts. Understanding the growth factor requirements for clonogenic leukemic cells will provide further information about their potential to differentiate normally.

REFERENCES

1. Li FP, Bader JL: Epidemiology of cancer in childhood. In Nathan DG, Oski FA (eds): Hematology of Infancy and Childhood, vol 2, p 918. Philadelphia, WB Saunders, 1987
2. Weinstein HJ: Congenital leukemia and the neonatal myeloproliferative disorders associated with Down's syndrome. Clin Hematol 7:147, 1978
3. Miller RW: Persons with exceptionally high risk of leukemia. Cancer Res 27:2420, 1967
4. Zuelzer WW, Cox DE: Genetic aspects of leukemia. Semin Hematol 6:228, 1969
5. Rosner F, Lee SL: Down's syndrome and acute leukemia: Myeloblastic or lymphoblastic? Am J Med 53:203, 1972
6. Brodeur GM, Dahl GV, Williams DL et al: Transient leukemoid reaction and trisomy 21 mosaicism in a phenotypically normal infant. Blood 55:691, 1980
7. Heaton DC, Fitzgerald PH, Fraser CJ et al: Transient leukemoid proliferation of the cytogenetically unbalanced +21 cell line of a constitutional mosaic boy. Blood 57:883, 1981
8. Weinberg AG, Schiller G, Windmiller J: Neonatal leukemoid reaction—An isolated manifestation of mosaic trisomy 21. Am J Dis Child 136:310, 1982
9. Seibel NL, Sommer A, Miser J: Transient neonatal leukemoid reactions in mosaic trisomy 21. J Pediatr 104:251, 1984
10. Lazarus KH, Heerema NA, Palmer CG et al: The myeloproliferative reaction in a child with Down syndrome: Cytological and chromosomal evidence for a transient leukemia. Am J Hematol 11:417, 1981
11. Lai JL, Zandecki M, Weill J et al: Leucoblastose et dysmegacaryocytopoiese transitoires avec clone 46,XX+21, t(5;7), chez un nouveau-ne trisomique 21. Nouv Rev Fr Hematol 25:363, 1983
12. Morgan R, Hecht F, Cleary ML et al: Leukemia with Down's syndrome: Translocation between chromosomes 1 and 19 in acute myelomonocytic leukemia following transient congenital myeloproliferative syndrome. Blood 66:1466, 1985
13. Yunis JJ, Bloomfield CD, Ensrud K: All patients with acute nonlymphocytic leukemia may have a chromosomal defect. N Engl J Med 305:135, 1981
14. Kaneko Y, Rowley JD, Maurer HS et al: Chromosome pattern in childhood acute nonlymphocytic leukemia. Blood 60:389, 1982
15. Bernstein R, Macdougall LG, Pinto MR: Chromosome patterns in 26 South African children with acute nonlymphocytic leukemia. Cancer Genet Cytogenet 11:199, 1984
16. Second International Workshop on Chromosomes in Leukemia: Cytogenetic, morphologic, and clinical correlations in acute nonlymphocytic leukemia with t(8q−;21q+). Cancer Genet Cytogenet 2:99, 1980
17. Larson RA, Kondo K, Vardiman JW et al: Evidence for a 15;17 translocation in every patient with acute promyelocytic leukemia. Am J Med 76:827, 1984
18. Berger R, Bernheim A, Weh H-J et al: Cytogenetic studies on acute monocytic leukemia. Leuk Res 4:119, 1980
19. Arthur DC, Bloomfield CD: Partial deletion of the long arm of chromosome 16 and bone marrow eosinophilia in acute nonlymphocytic leukemia: A new association. Blood 61:994, 1983
20. Le Beau MM, Larsen RA, Bitter MA et al: Association of inv(16) (p13q22) with abnormal marrow eosinophils in acute myelomonocytic leukemia: A unique cytogenetic-clinicopathologic association. N Engl J Med 309:630, 1983
21. Tantravahi M, Schwenn M, Hankle C et al: A pericentric inversion of chromosome 16 is associated with dysplastic marrow eosinophils in acute myelomonocytic leukemia. Blood 63:800, 1984
22. Sweet DL, Golomb HW, Rowley JD et al: Acute myelogenous leukemia and thrombocythemia associated with an abnormality of chromosome no. 3. Cancer Genet Cytogenet 1:33, 1979
23. Bernstein R, Pinto MR, Behr A et al: Chromosome 3 abnormalities in acute nonlymphocytic leukemia (ANLL) with abnormal thrombopoiesis: Report of three patients with a "new" inversion anomaly and a further case of homologous translocation. Blood 3:613, 1982
24. Rowley JD, Alimena G, Garson OM et al: A collaborative study of the relationship of the morphological type of acute nonlymphocytic leukemia with patient age and karyotype. Blood 59:1013, 1982
25. Brodeur GM, Williams DL, Kalwinsky DK et al: Cytogenetic features of acute nonlymphoblastic leukemia in 73 children and adolescents. Cancer Genet Cytogenet 8:93, 1983
26. Woods WG, Nesbit ME, Buckley J et al: Correlation of chromosome abnormalities with patient characteristics, histologic subtype, and induction success in children with acute nonlymphocytic leukemia. J Clin Oncol 3:3, 1985
27. Fialkow PJ, Singer JW, Adamson JW et al: Acute nonlymphocytic leukemia: Expression is restricted to granulocytic and monocytic differentiation. N Engl J Med 301:1, 1979
28. Fialkow PJ, Singer JW, Adamson JW et al: Acute nonlymphocytic leukemia: Heterogeneity of stem cell origin. Blood 57:1068, 1981
29. Fearon ER, Burke PJ, Schiffer CA et al: Differentiation of leukemia cells to polymorphonuclear leukocytes in patients with acute nonlymphocytic leukemia. N Engl J Med 315:15, 1986
30. Ferraris AM, Canepall L, Mareni C et al: Reexpression of normal stem cells in erythroleukemia during remission. Blood 62:177, 1983
31. Reid MM, Tantravahi R, Grier HE et al: Detection of leukemia-related karyotypes in granulocyte/macrophage colonies from a patient with acute myelomonocytic leukemia. N Engl J Med 308:1324, 1983
32. Grier HE, Weinstein HJ, Revesz T et al: Cytogenetic evidence for involvement of erythroid progenitors in a child with therapy linked myelodysplasia. Br J Haematol 64:513, 1986
33. Ferraris AM, Raskind WH, Bjornson BH et al: Heterogeneity of B cell involvement in acute nonlymphocytic leukemia. Blood 66:342, 1985

34. Jacobson RJ, Temple MJ, Singer JW et al: A clonal complete remission in a patient with acute nonlymphocytic leukemia originating in a multipotent stem cell. N Engl J Med 310:1513, 1984

35. Elfenbein GJ, Brogaonkar DS, Bias WB et al: Cytogenetic evidence for recurrence of acute myelogenous leukemia after allogeneic bone marrow transplantation in donor hematopoietic cells. Blood 52:627, 1978

36. Griffin JD, Lowenberg B: Clonogenic cells in acute myeloblastic leukemia. Blood 68:1185, 1986

37. Broxmeyer HE, Bognacki J, Dorner MH et al: The identification of leukemia-associated inhibiting activity (LIA) as acidic isoferritins: A regulatory role for acidic isoferritins in the production of granulocytes and macrophages. J Exp Med 153:1426, 1981

38. Lange B, Ferrero D, Pessano S et al: Surface phenotype of clonogenic cells in acute myeloid leukemia defined by monoclonal antibodies. Blood 64:693, 1984

39. Sabbath KD, Ball ED, Larcom P et al: Heterogeneity of clonogenic cells in acute myeloblastic leukemia. J Clin Invest 75:746, 1985

40. Young DC, Wagner K, Griffin JD: Constitutive expression of the granulocyte-macrophage colony-stimulating factor gene in acute myeloblastic leukemia. J Clin Invest 79:100, 1987

41. Moore MAS, Spitzer G, Williams N et al: Agar culture studies in 127 cases of untreated acute leukemia: The prognostic value of reclassification of leukemia according to in vitro growth characteristics. Blood 44:1, 1974

42. Spitzer G, Dicke KA, Gehan EA et al: A simplified in vitro classification for prognosis in adult leukemia: The application of in vitro results in remission-predictive models. Blood 48:795, 1976

43. Browman G, Goldberg J, Gottlieb AJ et al: The clonogenic assay as a reproducible in vitro system to study predictive parameters of treatment outcome in acute nonlymphoblastic leukemia. Am J Hematol 15:227, 1983

44. Moore MAS, Williams N, Metcalf D: In vitro colony formation by normal and leukemic human hematopoietic cells: Characterization of the colony-forming cells. J Natl Cancer Inst 50:603, 1973

45. Bishop JM: The molecular genetics of cancer. Science 235:305, 1987

46. Croce CM, Nowell PC: Molecular basis of human B cell neoplasis. Blood 65:1, 1985

47. Stam K, Heisterkamp N, Grosveld G et al: Evidence of a new chimeric bcr/c-abl mRNA in patients with chronic myelocytic leukemia and the Philadelphia chromosome. N Engl J Med 313:1429, 1985

48. Bos JL, Verlaan-de Vries M, van der Eb AJ et al: Mutations in N-ras predominate in acute myeloid leukemia. Blood 69:1237, 1987

49. Bishop JM: Cellular oncogenes and retroviruses. Annu Rev Biochem 52:301, 1983

50. Land H, Parada LF, Weinberg RA: Cellular oncogenes and multistep carcinogenesis. Science 222:771, 1983

51. Reddy EP, Reynolds RK, Santos E et al: A point mutation is responsible for the acquisition of the transforming properties by T24 human bladder carcinoma oncogene. Nature 300:149, 1982

52. Taparowsky E, Suard Y, Fasano O et al: Activation of the T24 Bladder carcinoma transforming gene is linked to a single amino acid change. Nature 300:762, 1982

53. Tabin CJ, Bradley SM, Bargmann CI et al: Mechanism of actination of a human oncogene. Nature 300:143, 1982

54. Kamada N, Kimio T: Cytogenetic studies of hematological disorders in atomic bomb survivors. In Ishihara T, Sasaki MS (eds): Radiation-induced Chromosome Damage in Man. New York, Alan R Liss, 1983

55. Rinsky RA, Smith AB, Hornung R et al: Benzene and leukemia: An epidemiologic risk assessment. N Engl J Med 316:1044, 1987

56. Tucker MA, Meadows AT, Boice JD et al: Secondary leukemia after alkylating agents for childhood cancer (abstr). Proc Am Soc Clin Oncol 3:85, 1984

57. Blayney DW, Longo DL, Young RC et al: Decreasing risk of leukemia with prolonged follow-up after chemotherapy and radiotherapy for Hodgkin's disease. N Engl J Med 316:710, 1987

58. Pedersen-Bjergaard J, Philip P, Mortensen BT et al: Acute nonlymphocytic leukemia, preleukemia, and acute myeloproliferative syndrome secondary to treatment of other malignant diseases. Clinical and cytogenetic characteristics and results of in vitro culture of bone marrow and HLA typing. Blood 57:712, 1981

59. Rowley JD, Golomb HM, Vardiman JW: Nonrandom chromosome abnormalities in acute leukemia and dysmyelopoietic syndromes in patients with previously treated malignant disease. Blood 58:759, 1981

60. Nowell R, Wilmoth D, Lange B: Cytogenetics of childhood preleukemia. Cancer Genet Cytogenet 10:261, 1983

61. Preisler HD, Lyman GH: Acute myelogenous leukemia subsequent to therapy for a different neoplasm: Clinical features and response to therapy. Am J Hematol 3:209, 1977

62. Cadman EC, Capizza RL, Bertino JR: Acute nonlymphocytic leukemia: A delayed complication of Hodgkin's disease therapy: Analysis of 109 cases. Cancer 40:1280, 1977

63. Bennett JM, Catovsky D, Daniel MT et al: Proposals for the classification of the acute leukemias. Br J Haematol 33:451, 1976

64. Bennett JM, Catovsky D, Daniel MT et al: Proposals for the classification of the myelodysplastic syndromes. Br J Haematol 51:189, 1982

65. Bennett JM, Catovsky D, Daniel MT et al: Proposed revised criteria for the classification of acute myeloid leukemia. Ann Intern Med 103:626, 1985

66. Bennett JM, Catovsky D, Daniel M-T et al: Criteria for the diagnosis of acute leukemia of megakaryocyte lineage (M7). A report of the French–American–British cooperative group. Ann Intern Med 103:460, 1985

67. Bloomfield CD, Brunning RD: The revised French–American–British classification of acute myeloid leukemia: Is new better? Ann Intern Med 103:614, 1985

68. Sariban E, Oliver C, Corash L et al: Acute megakaryoblastic leukemia in childhood. Cancer 54:1423, 1984

69. Nadler LM, Ritz J, Griffin JD et al: Diagnosis and treatment of human leukemias and lymphomas utilizing monoclonal antibodies. In Brown EB (ed): Progress in Hematology, vol 12, p 187. New York, Grune & Stratton, 1981

70. Korsmeyer SJ, Arnold A, Bakhshi A et al: Immunoglobulin-gene rearrangement and cell surface antigen expression in acute lymphocytic leukemias of T cell and B cell precursor origins. J Clin Invest 71:301, 1983

71. Minden M, Toyonaga B, Ha K et al: Somatic rearrangement of the T-cell antigen receptor gene in human T-cell malignancies. Proc Natl Acad Sci USA 81:1224, 1985

72. Mirro F, Antoun GR, Zipf TF et al: The E-rosette-associated antigen of T-cells can be identified on blasts from patients with acute myeloblastic leukemia. Blood 65:363, 1985

73. Rovigatti U, Mirro J, Kitchingman G et al: Heavy chain immunoglobulin gene rearrangement in acute nonlymphocytic leukemia. Blood 63:1023, 1984

74. Griffin JD, Ritz J, Nadler LM et al: Expression of myeloid differentiation antigens on normal and malignant myeloid cells. J Clin Invest 68:932, 1981

75. Chan LC, Pegram SM, Greaves MF: Contribution of immunophenotype to the classification and differential diagnosis of acute leukaemia. Lancet 1:475, 1985

76. Ball ED, Fanger MW: The expression of myeloid-specific antigens on myeloid leukemia cells: Correlations with leukemia subclasses and implications for normal myeloid differentiation. Blood 61:456, 1983

77. van der Reijden HJ, van Rhenen DJ, Lansdorp PM et al: A comparison of surface marker analysis and FAB classification in acute myeloid leukemia. Blood 61:443, 1983

78. Griffin JD, Davis R, Nelson DA et al: Use of surface marker analysis to predict outcome of adult acute myeloblastic leukemia. Blood 68:1232, 1986

79. Wiernik PH, Serpick AA: Clinical significance of serum and urinary muramidase activity in leukemia and other hematologic malignancies. Am J Med 46:330, 1969

80. Kung PC, Long JC, McCaffrey RP et al: Terminal deoxynucleotidyl transferase in the diagnosis of leukemia and malignant lymphomas. Am J Med 64:788, 1978

81. Marks SM, McCaffrey R, Rosenthal DS et al: Blastic transformation in chronic myelogenous leukemia: Experience with 50 patients. Med Pediatr Oncol 4:159, 1978

82. Miller KB, Harris NL: Case records of the Massachussetts General Hospital: Case 13-1987. N Engl J Med 316:767, 1987

83. Mirro J, Zipf TF, Pui CH et al: Acute mixed lineage leukemia: Clinicopathologic correlations and prognostic significance. Blood 66:1115, 1985

84. McCulloch EA: Stem cells in normal and leukemic hemopoiesis (Henry Stratton Lecture, 1982). Blood 62:1, 1983

85. Smith LJ, Curtis JE, Messner HA et al: Lineage infidelity in acute leukemia. Blood 61:1138, 1983

86. Stass S, Mirro J, Melvin S et al: Lineage switch in acute leukemia. Blood 64:701, 1984

87. Choi S-I, Simone JV: Acute nonlymphocytic leukemia in 171 children. Med Pediatr Oncol 2:119, 1976

88. Groopman J, Ellman L: Acute promyelocytic leukemia. Am J Hematol 7:395, 1979

89. Gralnick HR, Bagley J, Abrell E: Heparin treatment for the hemorrhagic diathesis of acute promyelocytic leukemia. Am J Med 52:167, 1972

90. Drapkin RL, Gee TS, Dowlings MD et al: Prophylactic heparin therapy in acute promyelocytic leukemia. Cancer 41:2484, 1978

91. Borgstrom GH, Teerenhovi L, Vuopio P et al: Clinical implications of monosomy 7 in acute nonlymphocytic leukemia. Cancer Genet Cytogenet 2:115, 1980

92. Pedersen-Bjergaard J, Vindelov L, Philip P et al: Varying involvement of peripheral granulocytes in the clonal abnormality −7 in bone marrow cells in preleukemia secondary to treatment of other malignant tumors: Cytogenetic results compared with results of flow cytometric DNA analysis and neutrophil chemotaxis. Blood 60:172, 1982

93. Kere J, Ruutu T, de la Chapelle A: Monosomy 7 in granulocytes and monocytes in myelodysplastic syndrome. N Engl J Med 316:499, 1987

94. Grier HE, Gelber RD, Camitta BM et al: Prognostic factors in childhood acute myelogenous leukemia. J Clin Oncol 5:1026–1032, 1987

95. Wiernik P, Serpick AA: Granulocytic sarcoma (chloroma). Blood 35:361, 1970

96. Pui C-H, Dahl GV, Kalwinsky DK et al: Central nervous system leukemia in children with acute nonlymphoblastic leukemia. Blood 66:1062, 1985

97. Dahl GV, Simone JV, Hustu HO et al: Preventive central nervous system irradiation in children with acute nonlymphocytic leukemia. Cancer 42:2187, 1978

98. Creutzig U, Ritter J, Riehm H et al: Improved results in childhood acute myelogenous leukemia: A report of the German cooperative study AML BFM 78. Blood 65:298, 1985

99. Niemeyer CM, Hitchcock-Bryan S, Sallan SE: Comparative analysis of treatment programs for childhood acute lymphoblastic leukemia. Semin Oncol 12:122, 1985

100. Lampkin BC, Woods W, Strauss R et al: Current status of the biology and treatment of acute non-lymphocytic leukemia in children (Report from the ANLL Strategy Group of the Children's Cancer Study Group). Blood 61:215, 1983

101. Chessels JM, Callaghan UO, Hardisty RM: Acute myeloid leukaemia in childhood: clinical features and prognosis. Br J Haematol 63:555, 1986

102. Dahl GV, Kalwinsky DK, Murphy S et al: Cytokinetically based induction chemotherapy and splenectomy for childhood acute nonlymphocytic leukemia. Blood 60:856, 1982

103. Dow LW, Dahl GV, Kalwinsky DK et al: Correlation of drug sensitivity in vitro with clinical responses in childhood acute myeloid leukemia. Blood 68:400, 1986

104. Baehner RL, Kennedy A, Sather H et al: Characteristics of children with acute non-lymphocytic leukemia in long-term continuous remission: A report for Children's Cancer Study Group. Med Pediatr Oncol 9:393, 1981

105. Barton JC, Conrad ME: Beneficial effects of hepatitis in patients with acute myelogenous leukemia. Ann Intern Med 90:188, 1979

106. Foon KA, Yale C, Clodfelter K et al: Posttransfusion hepatitis in acute myelogenous leukemia. JAMA 244:1806, 1980

107. Fourth International Workshop on Chromosomes in Leukemia 1982 (1984): Clinical significance of chromosomal abnormalities in acute nonlymphoblastic leukemia. Cancer Genet Cytogenet 11:332, 1984

108. Holmes R, Keating MJ, Cork A et al: A unique pattern of central nervous system leukemia in acute myelomonocytic leukemia associated with inv(16)(p13q22). Blood 65:1071, 1985

109. Larson RA, Williams SF, Le Beau MM et al: Acute myelomonocytic leukemia with abnormal eosinophils and inv(16) or t(16;16) has a favorable prognosis. Blood 68:1986

110. Koeffler HP: Myelodysplastic syndromes (preleukemia) Semin Hematol 23:284, 1986

111. Keating MJ, Smith TL, Gehan EA et al: A prognostic factor analysis for use in development of predictive models for response in adult acute leukemia. Cancer 50:457, 1982

112. Goldberg MA, Ginsburg D, Mayer RJ et al: Is heparin administration necessary during induction chemotherapy for patients with acute promyelocytic leukemia? Blood 69:187, 1987

113. Pizzo PA: Infectious complications in the child with cancer: I. Pathophysiology, II. Management, III. Prevention. Pediatrics 98:341, 513, 534, 1981

114. O'Regan, Carson S, Chesney RW et al: Electrolyte and acid-base disturbances in the management of leukemia. Blood 49:345, 1977

115. Cohen LF, Balow JE, Magrath IT et al: Acute tumor lysis syndrome: A review of 37 patients with Burkitt's lymphoma. Am J Med 68:486, 1980

116. Dearth JC, Fountain KS, Smithson WA et al: Extreme leukemic leukocytosis (blast crisis) in childhood. Mayo Clin Proc 53:207, 1978

117. Lichtman MA, Rowe JM: Hyperleukocytic leukemias: Rheological, clinical and therapeutic considerations. Blood 60:279, 1982

118. Bunin NJ, Pui C-H: Differing complications of hyperleukocytosis in children with acute lymphoblastic or acute nonlymphoblastic leukemia. J Clin Oncol 3:1590, 1985

119. Grund FM, Armitage JO, Burns CP: Hydroxyurea in the prevention of the effects of leukostasis in acute leukemia. Arch Intern Med 37:1246, 1977

120. Cuttner J, Holland JF, Norton L et al: Therapeutic leukapheresis for hyperleukocytosis in acute myelocytic leukemia. Med Pediatr Oncol 11:76, 1983

121. Mayer RJ: Current chemotherapeutic treatment approaches to the management of previously untreated adults with de novo acute myelogenous leukemia. Semin Oncol (in press)

122. Weinstein HJ, Mayer RJ, Rosenthal DS et al: Treatment of acute myelogenous leukemia in children and adults. N Engl J Med 303:473, 1980

123. Stone RM, Maguire ME, Goldberg MA et al: Acute promyelocytic leukemia (APL): Complete remission (CR) can occur without bone marrow aplasia (abstr 720). Blood 66:209a, 1985

124. Slavin RE, Dias MA, Saral R: Cytosine arabinoside induced gastrointestinal toxic alterations in sequential chemotherapeutic protocols: A clinical-pathologic study of 33 patients. Cancer 42:1747, 1978

125. Lea JW, Masys DR, Shackford SR: Typhilitis: A treatable complication of acute leukemia therapy. Cancer Clin Trials 3:355, 1980

126. Abramson SJ, Berdon WE, Baker DH: Childhood typhlitis: Its increasing association with acute myelogenous leukemia. Radiology 146:61, 1983

127. Shamberger RC, Weinstein HJ, Delorey MJ et al: The medical and surgical management of typhlitis in children with acute myelogenous leukemia. Cancer 57:603, 1986

128. Yates J, Glidewell O, Wiernik P et al: Cytosine arabinoside with daunorubicin or adriamycin for therapy of acute myelocytic leukemia: A CALGB Study. Blood 60:454, 1982

129. Delorey M, Pearl B, Grier H et al: Typhlitis during induction chemotherapy for childhood acute myelogenous leukemia (AML) (abstr). Proc Am Soc Clin Oncol 4:269, 1985

130. Vaughan WP, Karp JE, Burke PJ: Long chemotherapy-free remissions after single cycle timed-sequential chemotherapy for acute myelocytic leukemia. Cancer 45:859, 1980

131. Vaughan WP, Karp JE, Burke PJ: Two-cycle timed-sequential chemotherapy for adult acute nonlymphocytic leukemia. Blood 64:975, 1984

132. Weinstein HJ, Mayer RJ, Rosenthal DS et al: Chemotherapy for acute myelogenous leukemia in children and adults: VAPA update. Blood 62:315, 1983

133. Baehner RL, Bernstein ID, Sather H et al: Improved remission induction rate with D-ZAPO but unimproved remission duration with addition of immunotherapy to chemotherapy in previously untreated children with ANLL. Med Pediatr Oncol 7:127, 1979

134. Baehner RL, Bernstein ID, Sather H et al: Contrasting benefits of two maintenance programs following identical induction in children with acute nonlymphocytic leukemia: A report from the Children's Cancer Study Group. Cancer Treat Rep 68:1269, 1984

135. Odom LF, Gordon EM: Acute monoblastic leukemia in infancy and early childhood: Successful treatment with an epipodophyllotoxin. Blood 64:875, 1984

136. Santos GW, Tutschka PJ, Brookmeyer R et al: Marrow transplantation for acute nonlymphocytic leukemia after treatment with Busulfan and cyclophosphamide. N Engl J Med 309:1347, 1983

137. Brochstein JA, Kernan N, Emanuel D et al: Marrow transplantation for acute leukemia after hyperfractionated total body irradiation (HFTBI) and cyclophosphamide (CTX) (abstr). Blood 68(Suppl 1):271a, 1986

138. Sanders JE, Thomas ED, Buckner CD et al: Marrow transplantation for children in first remission of acute nonlymphocytic leukemia. An update. Blood 66:460, 1985

139. Zwaan FE, Hermans J, Barrett AJ et al: Bone marrow transplantation for acute nonlymphoblastic leukemia: A survey of the European Group for bone marrow transplantation (E.G.B.M.T.). Br J Haematol 56:645, 1984

140. Bostrom B, Brunning RD, McGlave P et al: Bone marrow transplantation for acute nonlymphocytic leukemia in first remission. Analysis of prognostic factors. Blood 65:1191, 1985

141. Nesbit M, Buckley J, Lampkin B et al: Comparison of allogeneic bone marrow transplantation (BMT) with maintenance chemotherapy in previously untreated childhood acute nonlymphocytic leukemia (ANLL) (abstr). Proc Am Soc Clin Oncol 6:163, 1987

142. Powles RL, Morgenstern G, Clink HM et al: The place of bone marrow transplantation in acute myelogenous leukaemia. Lancet 1:1047, 1980

143. Appelbaum FR, Dahlberg S, Thomas ED et al: Bone marrow transplantation vs. chemotherapy maintenance for acute myelogenous leukemia: A prospective study. Ann Intern Med 101:581, 1984

144. Champlin RE, Ho WG, Gale RP et al: Treatment of acute myelogenous

leukemia. A prospective controlled trial of bone marrow transplantation vs. consolidation chemotherapy. Ann Intern Med 102:28, 1985

145. Thomas ED: Marrow transplantation for malignant disease (Karnofsky Memorial Lecture). J Clin Oncol 1:517, 1983

146. Applebaum FR, Clift RA, Badner CD et al: Allogeneic marrow transplantation for acute non-lymphoblastic leukemia after first relapse. Blood 61:949, 1983

147. Applebaum FR, Storb R, Ramberg RE et al: Treatment of preleukemic syndromes with marrow transplantation. Blood 69:92, 1987

148. Linch DC, Burnett AK: Clonal studies of ABMT in acute myeloid leukemia. Clin Haematol 15:167, 1986

149. Yeager AM, Kaiser H, Santos G et al: Autologous bone marrow transplantation in patients with acute nonlymphocytic leukemia, using ex vivo marrow treated with 4-hydroperoxycyclophosphamide. N Engl J Med 315:141, 1986

150. Mauer AM: Therapy of acute lymphoblastic leukemia in childhood. Blood 56:1, 1980

151. Mayer RJ, Weinstein HJ, Coral FS et al: The role of intensive postinduction chemotherapy in the management of patients with acute myelogenous leukemia. Cancer Treat Rep 66:1455, 1982

152. Look AT, Dahl GV, Kalwinsky D et al: Effective remission induction of refractory childhood acute nonlymphocytic leukemia by VP-16-213 plus azacitidine. Cancer Treat Rep 65:995, 1981

153. Ochs J, Sinkule A, Danks MK et al: Continuous infusion high-dose cytosine arabinoside in refractory childhood leukemia. J Clin Oncol 2:1092, 1984

154. Krischer J, Land VJ, Civin CI et al: Evaluation of AMSA in children with acute leukemia. Cancer 54:207, 1984

155. Wells RJ, Feusner J, Devney R et al: Sequential high-dose cytosine arabinoside-asparaginase treatment in advanced childhood leukemia. J Clin Oncol 3:998, 1985

156. Kalwinsky DK, Dahl GV, Mirro J et al: Cyclophosphamide/Etoposide: Effective reinduction therapy for children with acute nonlymphocytic leukemia in relapse. Cancer Treat Rep 69:887, 1985

157. Harris RE, McCallister JA, Provisor DS et al: Methotrexate/L-asparaginase combination chemotherapy for patients with acute leukmia in relapse: A study of 36 children. Cancer 46:2004, 1980

158. Herzig RH, Wolff SN, Lazarus HM et al: High-dose cytosine arabinoside therapy for refractory leukemia. Blood 62:361, 1983

159. Mirro J, Dahl GV, Kalwinsky D et al: A phase II study of simultaneous continuous infusions of teniposide (VM-26) and m-AMSA in relapsed acute leukemia (abstr). Proc Am Soc Clin Oncol 5:154, 1986

160. Kersey JH, Le Bien T, Vallera D et al: Allogeneic and autologous marrow transplantation: Ex vivo purging with monoclonal antibody or immunotoxins to remove leukemic cells or to prevent graft versus host disease. In Hagenbeek A, Lowenberg B (eds): Minimal Residual Disease in Acute Leukemia. pp 275–281. Boston, Martinus Nijhoff Publishers, 1986

161. O'Reilly RJ, Keinan N, Collins N et al: Abrogation of both acute and chronic GVHD following transplant of lectin-agglutinated, E-rosette depleted (SBA-E-) marrow for leukemia (abstr). Blood 68(Suppl 1):291a, 1986

162. Smith BR, Burakoff SJ, Weinstein H et al: Differential outcome of histocompatible versus histoincompatible Leu-1 depleted bone marrow transplants (abstr). Blood 68(Suppl 1):292a, 1986

163. Prentice HG, Blacklock HA, Janossy G et al: Depletion of T lymphocytes in donor marrow prevents significant graft versus host disease in matched allogeneic leukemic marrow transplant recipients. Lancet 1:474, 1984

164. Apperley JS, Jones L, Arthur C et al: Incidence of relapse after T-cell depleted marrow transplant for chronic granulocytic leukemia (CGL) in 1st chronic phase (CP) (abstr). Blood 68(Suppl 1):270a, 1986

165. Gale RP, Champlin R: How does bone marrow transplantation cure leukemia? Lancet 1:2, 1984

166. O'Reilly RJ: New promise for autologous marrow transplants in leukemia. N Engl J Med 315:186, 1986

167. Desforges JE: Cytarabine: Low-dose, high-dose, no dose? N Engl J Med 309:1637, 1983

168. Koeffler HP: Induction of differentiation of human acute myelogenous leukemia cells: Therapeutic implications. Blood 62:709, 1983

eighteen

Chronic Leukemias of Childhood

Arnold J. Altman

Chronic leukemias are myeloproliferative disorders characterized by a predominance of relatively mature cells. In contrast to the acute leukemias, they are relatively indolent, with a natural history usually spanning several years. Some subtypes, however, may have a rapidly progressive clinical course.

Chronic leukemias are rare in childhood. The most common type, chronic myelocytic leukemia, accounts for less than 5% of all childhood leukemias. Other chronic leukemias discussed in this chapter include juvenile chronic myelocytic leukemia, familial chronic myelocytic leukemia, chronic myelomonocytic leukemia, and chronic lymphocytic leukemia.

CHRONIC MYELOCYTIC LEUKEMIA

Chronic myelocytic leukemia (CML) is a clonal panmyelopathy involving all of the hemic lineages and at least some of the lymphoid lines. It is characterized by myeloid hyperplasia of the bone marrow, extramedullary hematopoiesis, expansion of the total body granulocyte pool, elevation of the leukocyte count, with appearance of the complete range of granulocyte precursor cells in the peripheral blood, and a specific cytogenetic marker, the Philadelphia (Ph[1]) chromosome.

Historical Background

CML was the first form of leukemia to be recognized as a distinct clinical entity. Donné[1] described the characteristic hematologic changes in 1844; in 1845, Bennett,[2] Craigie,[3] and Virchow[4] independently described the clinical features and autopsy findings. These early observers were impressed by the marked splenic enlargement and peculiar changes in the color and consistency of the blood. On microscopic examination, the blood was found to contain a predominance of colorless corpuscles similar to those found in small numbers in normal blood and in large numbers in pus. Although he could find no focus of inflammation, Bennett attributed the hematologic findings to "the presence of purulent matter." Virchow used the descriptive term "white blood," which, translated into Greek, became "leukemia." Virchow subsequently subdivided leukemia into two categories: splenic and lymphatic.

In 1870, Neumann[5] suggested that the marrow, rather than the spleen, was the source of the excess colorless corpuscles in splenic leukemia; subsequent authors referred to splenic leukemia as myeloid leukemia. In 1889, Ebstein[6] recognized the clinical distinction between acute and chronic leukemias, and 1 year later Ehrlich[7] introduced techniques for staining blood cells that permitted the morphologic distinction between myeloid and lymphoid leukemias.

The earliest form of therapy for CML was the use of potassium arsenate (Fowler's solution) by Lissauer in 1865;[8] this produced limited and temporary improvement. Radiotherapy, introduced by Pusey in 1902,[9] produced better and more predictable effects with much less toxicity and became the standard therapy until the introduction of busulfan in 1953.

The cytogenetic hallmark of CML, the Ph[1] chromosome, was described by Nowell and Hungerford in 1960.[10] This was also the first specific chromosomal abnormality associated with a human malignancy, and its discovery inaugurated the era of cancer cytogenetics.

Epidemiology

CML is primarily a disease of middle age; the peak incidence is seen in the fourth and fifth decades. Although it has been diagnosed in infants as young as 3 months,[11] more than 80% of pediatric CML cases are diagnosed after age 4 years and 60% after age 6.[12,13] There is no significant racial or sexual predilection and no demonstrable hereditary component.

The only environmental factor implicated in the etiology of CML is radiation. An increased incidence of CML has been reported in radiologists, survivors of atomic bomb explosions, and individuals exposed to therapeutic radiation for treatment of ankylosing spondylitis and other disorders. However, only 5% to 7% of all CML cases have a documented exposure to excessive radiation, and radiation is rarely implicated in pediatric CML. No infectious agent has been related to the pathogenesis of CML.

Genetics

The Ph[1] chromosome is a chromosome 22 that has lost most of its long arm. Careful cytogenetic analysis[14] has shown that the "missing" portion is actually translocated to the distal long arm of chromosome 9 as part of the reciprocal translocation t(9;22) (q34;q11) (Fig. 18-1). The position of the breakpoint on chromosome 9 is variable from patient to patient, but breaks on chromosome 22 are restricted to a specific 5.8 kilobase (kb)

sequence termed the breakpoint cluster region (bcr).[15] As a consequence of the t(9;22), two proto-oncogenes, c-*abl* and c-*sis*, exchange chromosomes.[16-18]

C-*abl*, the human homologue of the Abelson B-cell murine leukemia virus oncogene (v-*abl*), is transposed from chromosome 9 to the bcr of chromosome 22. This results in a profound alteration in both structure and expression of this gene. The normal c-*abl* gene is universally active in hematopoietic cells at all stages of differentiation and encodes messenger RNA (mRNA) species of 6 and 7 kb whose translation product is a 145 kilodalton (kD) protein of unknown function. The t(9;22) creates a fusion gene whose 5' end is derived from bcr sequences and whose 3' end represents c-*abl* sequences. This *bcr*/c-*abl* gene encodes a novel mRNA of 8 kb whose translation product is a 210 kD protein (p210) with tyrosine kinase activity.[19,20] p210 is not found in normal cells, but is similar in its structure and function to the transforming protein encoded by v-*abl*. This tyrosine kinase protein is involved in the v-*abl*-induced malignant transformation of a variety of murine lymphohematopoietic cell lineages, possibly through interaction with growth factors.[21] The precise role of p210 in the pathogenesis of human CML remains to be defined.

C-*sis*, the human homologue of the Simian sarcoma virus oncogene (v-*sis*), is transposed from chromosome 22 to chromosome 9. Normally, it encodes sequences of the β chain of platelet-derived growth factor (PDGF).[22] Although neither the structure nor the expression of c-*sis* is demonstrably altered by the translocation event, it is possible that a subtle transformation of this fibroblast-stimulating gene may be responsible for the myelofibrosis seen in some CML patients.

Variant Translocations

Although the classic t(9;22) is found in approximately 90% of CML cases, in some instances other types of translocations may be found.[23-25] Approximately 3% of CML patients have translocations of 22q11 to regions other than 9q34. Another 3% have

FIGURE 18-1. Anatomy of the (9;22) (q34;q11) translocation with formation of the Ph[1] chromosome (22q−) and the hybrid *bcr*/c-*abl* gene (see text for further explanation).

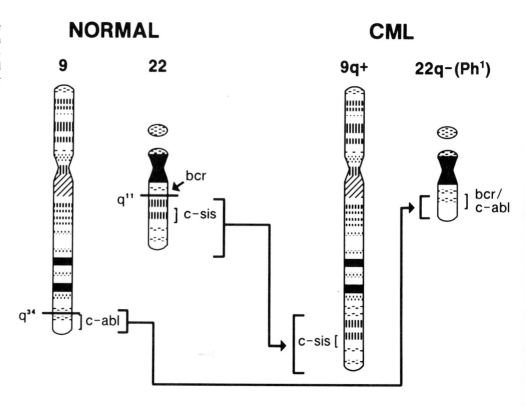

complex translocations involving three or more chromosomes; such translocations virtually always involve band 9q34. Other patients may have an undetected or "masked" Ph[1] chromosome (see Ph[1]-negative CML). A small percentage will have, in addition to the Ph[1] chromosome, other visible karyotypic abnormalities such as a second Ph[1] chromosome, isochromosome 17, or an extra chromosome 8 or 18—secondary changes that appear to represent a mechanism of tumor progression and are found with increased frequency as the disease evolves to a more aggressive phase.

Ph[1]-Negative CML

Approximately 5% to 10% of patients with otherwise typical CML do not manifest the Ph[1] chromosome. In some of these cases, the Ph[1] chromosome may be masked by translocation of additional genetic material to the 22q11 region.[25] In other cases, there may be rearrangements or breaks in the 9q34 region without the reciprocal break at 22q11.[26,27] In general, Ph[1]− cases have a poorer prognosis than do Ph[1]+ cases.

Ph[1]-Positive Acute Leukemia

Although characteristic of CML, the Ph[1] chromosome is not exclusive to it, being found in approximately 3% to 10% of childhood acute leukemias, 2% to 3% of adult acute myeloid leukemias, and 25% to 33% of adult acute lymphoid leukemias.[28-30] These Ph[1]+ acute leukemias have no antecedent CML features and are clinically and hematologically indistinguishable from other acute leukemias except for a relatively poorer prognosis.

Some Ph[1]+ acute leukemias may represent blastic presentations of CML, whereas others are apparently true *de novo* acute leukemias. There are few clinical or hematologic features that distinguish between these two entities, although cases associated with basophilia or marked splenomegaly are more likely to be associated with CML. To confuse the issue further, classic chronic phase CML has developed after a period of hematologic and cytogenetic remission in a patient who initially presented with apparent *de novo* Ph[1]+ acute leukemia.[31]

Differences between blastic phase CML and *de novo* Ph[1]+ acute leukemia are more apparent at the cytogenetic and molecular levels. Ph[1]+ acute leukemias usually do not manifest the specific nonrandom chromosomal aberrations (discussed above) that are characteristic of CML as it evolves into blastic phase. Further, the marrow karyotype of the *de novo* acute Ph[1]+ leukemia case usually reverts to normal after therapy, whereas the Ph[1] chromosome persists in the marrow of the CML patient. The bcr rearrangement with production of p210 characteristic of CML is found inconsistently in acute Ph[1]+ leukemias. Instead, approximately half of these cases show rearrangements outside the bcr region and formation of a novel 190 kD protein (p190) with tyrosine kinase activity similar to that of p210.[30]

Biology

Clonal Nature of CML

Independent lines of evidence derived from cytogenetic and isoenzyme studies indicate that CML is an acquired disorder of unicellular origin and that the target of neoplastic transformation is a multilineage stem cell with the potential for generating all of the hemic cells (erythrocytes, neutrophils, basophils, eosinophils, monocytes, megakaryocytes) and at least some of the lymphoid lineages. This multilineage potential helps to explain the cytologic heterogeneity of the blastic phase of CML (discussed in the Natural History section).

CYTOGENETIC EVIDENCE. The Ph[1] chromosome has proved useful in defining the malignant population in CML. It is an acquired abnormality that is demonstrable in virtually all proliferating erythroid, granulocytic, monocytic, and megakaryocytic precursor cells but not in fibroblasts or other somatic cells.[32,33] A similar pattern of clonal restriction can be demonstrated for other karyotypic markers, for example, in CML patients with coincident sexual mosaicism or Down's syndrome.[34-36] Routine karyotypic studies do not indicate the presence of the Ph[1] chromosome in the lymphocytes of CML patients. However, the phenomenon of lymphoblastic transformation in some CML patients suggests that at least some lymphoid lineages are involved in the malignant process. This is supported by demonstration of the Ph[1] chromosome in a small proportion of B-lymphocytes and T-lymphocytes when CML blood is cultured *in vitro*[37]; other studies have documented the presence of Ph[1]+ B- and T-lymphocytes in multilineage colonies derived from CML precursor cells.[38] In comparison with hemic cells, lymphoid cells are relatively long-lived, and therefore most of those present at diagnosis of CML probably antedate the neoplastic transformation event; this may explain the relatively small fraction involved in the malignant clone.

C-band polymorphism analysis exploits the staining characteristics of the highly repetitive DNA found in constitutive heterochromatin. These so-called C-band areas are present at all centromeres and are particularly prominent near the centromeres of chromosomes 1, 9, and 16. Since chromosome 9 is involved in the t(9;21), analysis of C-band polymorphism can be used to document clonality of the hematopoietic population in CML.[39,40]

ISOENZYME EVIDENCE. In accordance with the Lyon hypothesis, random inactivation of one X-chromosome occurs in each cell during early embryogenesis; the progeny of each of these cells will subsequently manifest the same pattern of X-chromosome inactivation in a clonal fashion. Because approximately half of the cells will express one X-chromosome and half the other X-chromosome, females who are heterozygous for an X-linked enzyme should have roughly equal proportions of the two isoenzymes in each tissue. On the other hand, a neoplastic clone arising from a single cell should manifest only a single isoenzyme pattern. Studies of females with CML who are heterozygous for the X-linked enzyme glucose-6-phosphate dehydrogenase (G6PD) have demonstrated that the normal somatic tissues show the expected double isoenzyme distribution, whereas the Ph[1]+ hemic lineages contain a single (clonal) isoenzyme phenotype.[41,42] The demonstration that Ph[1]+ B-lymphocytes also manifest a clonal pattern of G6PD distribution provides confirmatory evidence that this lineage is also derived from the CML stem cell[43,44]; this has important implications with regard to the initial transformation event in CML (discussed below).

The Initial Transformation Event

Although clearly germane to the pathogenesis of CML, the formation of the Ph[1] chromosome may not be the primary event in the neoplastic sequence. There are documented cases in which the typical clinical and hematologic abnormalities of CML antedated the appearance of the Ph[1] chromosome[45,46]; in other cases, the Ph[1] chromosome disappeared during therapy while the clinical and hematologic features of CML persisted.[47] Isoenzyme studies that indicate clonality of some Ph-lymphoid populations also imply a transformation event preceding the 9;22 translocation.[40,44] It has been suggested that a rearrangement or break in the 9q34 band (the locus of c-*abl*) may be the critical initiating step in the evolution from benign to malignant hematopoiesis.[27]

The expansion of the CML clone from a single transformed cell to predominance in marrow and blood is dramatic evidence of its ability to overgrow the normal hemic elements. The mechanisms by which it achieves preeminence have been of great interest to students of the disease. Some clues have been provided by analysis of proliferative kinetics and *in vitro* colony production; these studies suggest *an expansion of the pool of committed granulocyte/monocyte stem cells (CFU-GM), a relative insensitivity to regulatory molecules,* and *the production of molecules that are inhibitory to normal hematopoietic stem cells.*

Growth Advantage of the CML Clone

A topic of major importance for understanding the pathogenesis of CML is the means by which the neoplastic clone overgrows the normal hemic population. This question has been studied by using cell kinetic techniques and *in vitro* growth assays. The definitive answer remains elusive, but there is now evidence to suggest several mechanisms, including expansion of the pool of committed granulocyte/monocyte stem cells (CFU-GM), a relative insensitivity to regulatory molecules, and the production of molecules that are inhibitory to normal hematopoietic stem cells.

CELL KINETICS. In chronic phase CML, there is a threefold to 30-fold increase in peripheral blood band and segmented neutrophils and a tenfold to 100-fold increase in the total blood granulocyte pool (TBGP).[48-53] These leukocytes freely exchange between the peripheral blood, bone marrow, and spleen. The average half-life (T½) of granulocytes in the blood is five to ten times longer in CML patients than in normal persons; this is partially a reflection of the large number of immature forms, but even the relatively mature granulocytes of CML have a peripheral blood T½ that is twofold to fourfold longer than normal.[53] This increased blood transit time contributes to the expansion of the TBGP. Of greater significance, however, is the markedly increased granulocyte production rate.

The hyperproduction of myeloid cells in CML is not attributable to a relatively rapid rate of cell division; indeed, measurements of mitotic activity, DNA synthesis, and generation time indicate that CML cells may actually divide more slowly than normal hemic precursor cells.[48-53] That there is, however, an overproduction of committed myeloid precursor cells can be demonstrated by assays of the granulocyte/monocyte colony forming unit (CFU-GM).[54-59] CFU-GM are quantitated by counting the number of GM colonies produced when a blood or marrow sample is suspended in a semisolid medium (*e.g.,* agar) containing appropriate stimulatory factors. Bone marrow suspensions from chronic phase CML patients generate 10 to 20 times the number of GM colonies produced by normal marrow. The disparity is even more striking when peripheral blood is studied. Whereas normal blood contains relatively few CFU-GM, blood from CML patients may have an even greater proportion of these precursor cells than does marrow. The majority of these circulating CFU-GM may be generated in the spleen.[60] Nonetheless, colony production is qualitatively normal (in chronic phase); mature GM forms are produced and the process is dependent on the same colony-stimulating fac-

tors (CSF) that are obligatory for *in vitro* colony formation by normal CFU-GM.

Following chemotherapy or splenic irradiation, the TBGP and the T½ return to normal values coincident with reduction in marrow cellularity, decreased marrow and peripheral blood CFU-GM, and disappearance of immature cells from the peripheral blood. This suggests that most of the kinetic abnormalities found in chronic phase CML do not reflect an intrinsic maturational defect of the neoplastic cells, but are a consequence of the premature release of immature cells from the marrow due to the mechanical pressure of an increased granulocytic cell mass. The primary abnormality appears to be an overproduction of CFU-GM.

As the disease progresses to blast phase, defects in maturation become more conspicuous. Myeloblasts become abundant in the marrow and peripheral blood, while the relative and absolute number of polymorphs declines. There is an inverse correlation between the percentage of myeloblasts in the marrow and the fraction of these cells in DNA synthesis.[61] This decline in proliferative and maturational potential is reflected in absent or reduced GM colony production *in vitro.*

ABNORMALITIES IN FEEDBACK REGULATION. Under normal circumstances, myelopoiesis is regulated by at least three negative feedback molecular species: lactoferrin (LF), prostaglandin E (PGE), and acidic isoferritins (AIF) (Fig. 18-2). LF, the product of mature polymorphonuclear leukocytes (PMN), down-regulates granulocytopoiesis by reducing monocyte/macrophage production of CSF.[62,63] PGE and AIF, which are derived from subpopulations of monocytes and macrophages, inhibit proliferation of normal granulocyte/monocyte precursor cells;[63-65] their inhibitory actions appear to be restricted to those cells that express HLA-DR (Ia) antigens.[66-68]

CML cells appear to be relatively insensitive to feedback inhibition for a variety of reasons, including deficient LF production by the PMN, decreased responsiveness of the monocyte/macrophage to regulation by LF,[69-72] and decreased sensitivity of progenitor cells to PGE and AIF. The PGE and AIF resistance may reflect deficient HLA-DR antigen expression by CML cells[68,69] or a decreased proportion of sensitive target cells.[68] CML cells may augment their proliferative advantage by releasing humoral factors to which they are resistant, but which suppress normal hemopoietic precursor cells.[70,73]

Multistep Pathogenesis

The evolution of CML may be visualized as a multistep process that can be summarized as follows:

1. An initial transformation event (possibly rearrangement of c-*abl*) occurs in a multipotent progenitor cell. This results in production of a clone of "premalignant" hemic (and possibly lymphoid) cells.
2. At some point in the evolution of the disease, a recognizable cytogenetic alteration (the Ph[1] chromosome) appears in the transformed clone. The translocation of c-*abl* to chromosome 22 and its fusion with the bcr unmasks or deregulates tyrosine kinase activity. The Ph[1]+ clone acquires a growth advantage over normal hemic stem cells, and there is initially an overproduction of relatively mature cells, particularly those of the granulocytic series.
3. As the disease progresses, there is sequential evolution of progressively more abnormal stem cell clones from the original Ph[1]+ clone; new cytogenetic alterations appear, and there is an increasing dissociation between proliferation and differentiation. The newly evolved

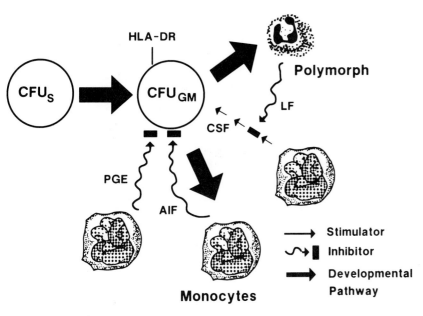

FIGURE 18-2. Positive and negative feedback loops regulating myelopoiesis. In this postulated schema, progeny of the pluripotent stem cells (*CFU-S*) become committed granulocyte/monocyte precursor cells (*CFU-GM*). CFU-GM are induced to proliferate and produce polymorphs and monocytes by colony-stimulating factors (*CSF*). CFU-GM are inhibited from proliferating by lactoferrin (*LF*) (which inhibits generation of CSF) and by acidic isoferritins (*AIF*) and prostaglandin E (*PGE*) (which act directly on CFU-GM bearing HLA-DR antigens). In CML, the neoplastic clone may derive its growth advantage by modifications of these regulatory pathways.

clones suppress the proliferation of normal stem cells as well as the cells of the preceding leukemic clone. Eventually, immature (blast) cells predominate and the process terminates in an acute leukemia.

Natural History

The natural history of CML is divided into the chronic, accelerated, and blast phases. These phases represent the progressive shift in the nature of the disorder from one of hyperproliferation, with production of mainly mature hemic elements, to one characterized by a differentiation arrest, with production of predominantly immature (blast) cells.

Chronic Phase

The chronic phase is characterized by marked expansion of the hematopoietic pools; morphologically mature blood cells are produced that show only subtle functional abnormalities. Generally, the neoplastic cells are restricted to the bone marrow, liver, spleen, and peripheral blood. Therefore, symptomatology is related to organ infiltration, hyperviscosity, and the metabolic consequences of hyperproliferation, all of which are relatively easy to control. On the average, the chronic phase lasts about 3 years.

SYMPTOMS. Patients usually present with relatively nonspecific complaints, such as fever, night sweats, weakness, left upper quadrant pain or fullness, or bone pain. Neurologic dysfunction, respiratory distress, visual difficulties, or priapism may complicate cases in which there is marked hyperleukocytosis.

PHYSICAL FINDINGS. The usual physical findings in this phase of CML are pallor, low-grade fever, ecchymoses, hepatosplenomegaly, and sternal tenderness. Signs relating to leukostasis (neurologic abnormalities, papilledema, retinal hemorrhages, and tachypnea) are seen in patients with hyperleukocytosis.

LABORATORY FINDINGS. A mild normochromic, normocytic anemia, marked leukocytosis with "shift to the left," and thrombocytosis are common laboratory findings. The mean hematocrit at presentation in children (25 ml/dl) is significantly less than that seen in adults.[13,74] The leukocyte count at diagnosis ranges from approximately 8000 to 800,000/mm^3; the median count in children (approximately 250,000/mm^3) is higher than that seen in adults.[10,11,66] Extreme hyperleukocytosis (>500,00/mm^3) is also more common in children. The peripheral smear shows myeloid cells at all stages of differentiation; myeloblasts and promyelocytes generally comprise less than 15% of the differential count, and there is no hiatus leukemicus in maturation (Fig. 18-3). There is also an absolute increase in the numbers of basophils and eosinophils. The mean platelet count in children is approximately 500,000/mm^3, which is not significantly higher than that in adults.[74]

The bone marrow is hypercellular, mainly reflecting granulocytic (and often megakaryocytic) hyperplasia; there is orderly granulocyte maturation, eosinophilia, and basophilia. Myelofibrosis, which occurs in 30% to 40% of patients during the course of the disease, is relatively uncommon in the chronic phase.[75,76] The bone marrow and spleen occasionally contain lipid-laden histiocytes that resemble Gaucher cells or sea-blue histiocytes.

Characteristic serologic findings include elevation of uric acid, lactic dehydrogenase (LDH), vitamin B$_{12}$, and vitamin B$_{12}$ binding protein (transcobalamin 1).

The most significant abnormality of the granulocyte population is a reduction in leukocyte alkaline phosphatase (LAP) activity, a diagnostically useful cytochemical finding that does not appear to adversely affect PMN function. Recent evidence suggests that the low LAP activity is not an intrinsic defect of the PMN but results from the relatively decreased monocyte mass (monocytes normally secrete a factor that induces LAP activity).[77] LAP activity increases with infection, reduction of the granulocyte count following chemotherapy, or progression to a more acute phase of the disease. Subtle functional abnormalities of PMN adherence, chemotaxis, and bactericidal activity can be demonstrated in chronic phase CML; however, the PMNs are sufficiently effective to prevent infectious complications.[78–80] PMN function deteriorates progressively with evolution of the disease.

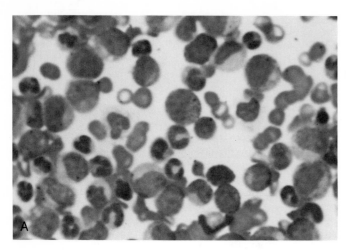
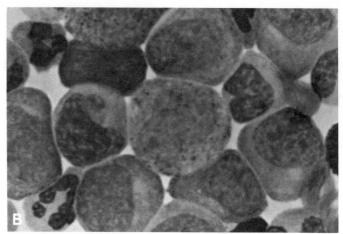

FIGURE 18-3. Peripheral blood smear of chronic phase CML. **A.** Low-power magnification showing marked leukocytosis. **B.** High-power magnification showing the entire range of myeloid cells from myeloblast to mature PMN.

DIFFERENTIAL DIAGNOSIS. The differential diagnosis of chronic phase CML includes leukemoid reaction, juvenile CML, and other myeloproliferative disorders. The combination of low LAP score and presence of the Ph[1] chromosome usually distinguishes CML from these disorders.

In leukemoid reactions, splenomegaly is usually not marked, the LAP score is high, the Ph[1] chromosome is absent, and there is often a demonstrable inflammatory focus. In juvenile CML, the LAP may be low, but the Ph[1] chromosome is absent; leukocytosis and splenomegaly are less marked than in CML and there is a greater involvement of skin, lymphoid tissue, and the monocytic lineage. CML can be distinguished from other myeloproliferative disorders by the disproportionate involvement of the granulocyte series and the presence of the Ph[1] chromosome.

Metamorphosis

After an average of about 3 years, the chronic phase of CML undergoes a metamorphosis into a more aggressive phase; this may occur gradually or abruptly. In about 5% of cases, the evolution is explosive, with a rapidly increasing blast cell population in the peripheral blood and concurrent neutropenia and thrombocytopenia ("blast crisis"). About 50% of patients develop a progressive maturation defect resulting in a hematologic picture similar to *de novo* acute leukemia; the remaining 45% have the gradual evolution of a myeloproliferative syndrome.

The onset of metamorphosis is characterized by progressive systemic symptoms (fever, night sweats, weight loss), increasing leukocyte counts with a high proportion of immature cells, basophilia, and increasing resistance to chemotherapy. Along with these features the cytogenetic picture undergoes karyotypic evolution, with development of new abnormalities—most commonly, duplication of the Ph[1] chromosome, isochromosome 17, or trisomy 8. Occasionally, the first manifestation of metamorphosis is extramedullary (*i.e.,* meningeal leukemia or a chloroma arising in soft tissue or bone); such findings usually herald the imminent blast transformation of the marrow.

Blast Phase

The blast phase is characterized by loss of the leukemic clone's capacity to differentiate. As a consequence, the clinical picture resembles that of an acute leukemia, with anemia, thrombocytopenia, and increased numbers of blast cells in both the peripheral blood and bone marrow. A marrow blast percentage of 30% or more is diagnostic of blast phase. The signs and symptoms are those of a *de novo* acute leukemia; if basophilia is extreme, there may also be hyperhistaminemic symptoms (pruritis, cold urticaria, gastric ulceration). When the absolute blast count exceeds $100,000/mm^3$, the patient is at risk for hyperleukocytosis syndrome with leukostasis.

CYTOLOGIC HETEROGENEITY. As a reflection of the pluripotent nature of the leukemic stem cells in CML, blast transformation may involve any of the lymphohematopoietic lineages. In approximately 60% to 70% of cases, the blast cell morphology is myeloblastic; however, the blast cells are usually peroxidase-negative and rarely have Auer rods. Careful analysis using lineage-specific markers such as glycophorin-A, platelet peroxidase, and monoclonal antibodies will identify some of these blast transformations as erythroid, monocytic, or megakaryocytic.[81,82] Approximately one third of cases have blast cells with lymphoid morphology. These cells generally express a phenotype corresponding to an early B-cell; in rare cases, blast cells may express T-lineage markers.[81–83] In some patients, the blast cells manifest features of more than one myeloid line or have mixed myeloid-lymphoid features.

The cytologic nature of blast transformation may be related to secondary cytogenetic changes occurring in conjunction with karyotypic evolution. For example, rearrangements involving chromosome 7 (the site of the T-cell receptor β-chain gene) have been associated with T-lymphoblastic conversion, whereas involvement of region q21 of chromosome 3 (the putative locus of a gene regulating thrombopoiesis) has been seen in patients with megakaryoblastic conversion.[83a,83b]

DIFFERENTIAL DIAGNOSIS. Since most instances of blast phase CML occur following a well-documented chronic phase, the diagnosis is usually clear-cut. However, the rare patient who presents in blast phase without a recognized preceding chronic phase may pose diagnostic difficulty. The combination of marked splenomegaly, basophilia, and the Ph[1] chromosome distinguishes blast phase CML from most types of *de novo* acute leukemia; the distinction between blast phase CML and *de novo* Ph[1]+ acute leukemia was discussed earlier.

Prognostic Considerations

The median survival in CML is 3 to 4 years from diagnosis; fewer than 30% of patients survive 5 years. Since patients generally die within months of transformation to accelerated or blast phase, the major determinant of survival is the duration of the chronic phase, which can be highly variable. For adults, factors at diagnosis that are predictive of early transformation include splenomegaly (>15 cm below costal margin), hepatomegaly (>6 cm below costal margin), thrombocytopenia (<150,000/mm^3), thrombocytosis (>500,000/mm^3), marked leukocytosis (>100,000/mm^3), or high proportions of blast cells or immature granulocytes (>1% or >20%, respectively). These prognostic factors can be used to divide adult CML patients into groups with a poor, average, or good prognosis (median survivals = 3, 4, or 5 years, respectively).[84,85] The role of these factors in the prognosis of pediatric CML patients is less clear; in one study, only peripheral blood and marrow blast counts at presentation were of prognostic significance.[12]

Once patients have entered the blast phase, the only parameters that correlate with survival are blast cell phenotype and cytogenetic findings. In general, lymphoblastic phenotype and minimal karyotypic evolution augur a more favorable response to therapy.[86]

Therapy

Achievement of true remission in CML would require destroying all Ph^1+ cells and replacing them with cytogenetically normal precursors. This is rarely accomplished with conventional therapeutic approaches, but bone marrow transplantation has achieved apparent cure for a significant minority of patients. In general, the goal of treatment for patients in chronic phase has been to provide symptomatic relief by ameliorating leukocytosis and organomegaly. For patients in accelerated or blast phase, the goal is reversion to chronic phase. Before initiating any specific antileukemic therapy, consideration must be given to metabolic, leukostatic, and meningeal complications that pose management problems.

Special Management Problems

METABOLIC. Metabolic consequences of rapid cytolysis (*e.g.,* hyperuricemia, hyperkalemia, hyperphosphatemia) should be anticipated and treated appropriately with hydration, alkalinization, and allopurinol.[87] A detailed discussion of metabolic management is found in Chapter 37.

HYPERLEUKOCYTOSIS. The extremely high leukocyte count associated with some cases of CML can cause leukostatic complications in several organs, especially the brain, lung, retina, and penis.[74,88,89] Since leukocytes are less deformable than erythrocytes, the viscosity of the blood increases dramatically as the fractional volume of leukocytes (leukocrit) increases. Myeloblasts, which are larger and more rigid than other leukocytes, contribute disproportionately to viscosity; thus, the patient with myeloblastic transformation is at particularly high risk. If hyperleukocytosis is symptomatic or extreme (leukocytes > 200,000/mm^3 or blast count >50,000/mm^3), it should be treated with the simultaneous use of cytotoxic drugs (*e.g.,* hydroxyurea 50–75 mg/kg/day by IV infusion) and leukapheresis (or exchange transfusion)[90]; erythrocyte transfusions (which increase blood viscosity) should be avoided if possible.

PRIAPISM. Persistent painful penile erection may result from sludging and mechanical obstruction by leukemic cells, coagulation within the corpora cavernosa secondary to thrombocytosis, or impingement by the spleen on abdominal veins and nerves. Treatment includes analgesia, hydration, application of warm compresses, radiotherapy (to penis or spleen), and initiation of high-dose chemotherapy (*e.g.,* hydroxyurea 50–75 mg/kg/day IV).[89,90]

MENINGEAL LEUKEMIA. Meningeal leukemia is almost unknown in the chronic phase of CML and is rare in blast phase. The incidence may increase with improved survival of patients with blast transformation. The usual neurologic signs are cranial nerve palsies and papilledema; the diagnosis is confirmed by demonstrating pleocytosis, with blast cells in the spinal fluid. Intrathecal methotrexate is effective therapy,[91] but most patients eventually succumb to the hematologic consequences of the blast transformation. The role of prophylactic CNS therapy is undefined as yet.[92]

Cytoreduction in Chronic Phase

SINGLE-AGENT CHEMOTHERAPY. Single-agent chemotherapy (busulfan[93] or hydroxyurea[94]) is the standard approach to chronic phase CML. The goal is to achieve symptomatic relief by lowering the white blood cell count and reducing liver and spleen size. However, it is rare for a true remission to be achieved; in most cases, the bone marrow continues to manifest granulocyte hyperplasia and Ph^1+ metaphases even after the blood count has normalized and organomegaly has resolved. Therefore, even though symptomatic relief is achieved, there is no delay of blast crisis or prolongation of survival.

Busulfan. Busulfan an alkylating agent, is cell-cycle phase nonspecific; it is characterized by delayed onset and prolonged duration of effect. The usual dosage is 0.06 to 0.1 mg/kg/day PO (adult dose, 4 mg/day). Once treatment is initiated, there is a lag of 10 to 14 days before the leukocyte count falls significantly and the differential count begins to normalize. Splenic regression lags behind the peripheral blood response, and it may be 3 months before the spleen is no longer palpable. The dosage should be reduced by 50% when the leukocyte count reaches 30,000 to 40,000/mm^3 and the drug discontinued when counts fall to 20,000/mm^3 or less. The leukocyte count will continue to fall for another 2 to 3 weeks after the last dose. Failure to stop therapy *before* the count normalizes may result in severe (and possibly irreversible) marrow aplasia. The average patient requires 4 to 6 weeks of busulfan therapy to attain clinical remission; once the leukocyte count has leveled off, the patient may be given continuous maintenance therapy with low-dose busulfan, or intermittent couses when the leukocyte count exceeds 30,000/mm^3.[95] In addition to its myelosuppressive effects, busulfan may produce pulmonary fibrosis or an Addisonian-like syndrome characterized by hyperpigmentation, wasting, and hypotension.

Hydroxyurea. Hydroxyurea inhibits ribonucleoside diphosphate reductase, an enzyme essential for DNA synthesis, and is therefore specific for cells in S-phase of the cell cycle. Unlike busulfan, it is relatively short-acting; however, its control of the leukocyte count is less reliable and it must be used daily for prolonged periods. The recommended beginning dose is 10 to 20 mg/kg/day,[90] and dosages must be adjusted according to the hematologic response. Hydroxyurea appears to be as effective as busulfan in controlling chronic phase CML,[96,97] while providing a greater margin of hematologic safety and less systemic toxicity.

MULTIAGENT CHEMOTHERAPY. In rare cases, busulfan-induced marrow hypoplasia has produced reversion to Ph[1]− status or to stable Ph[1]+/Ph[1]− mosaicism followed by prolonged remission.[98–101] Following up on this observation, several groups have employed aggressive multiagent chemotherapy regimens (sometimes in conjunction with splenctomy) in an effort to ablate the Ph[1]+ clone.[102–104] In approximately half of patients so treated, cytogenetic conversion of the marrow is achieved. However, the effect is usually of short duration and does not exert a significant impact on duration of chronic phase or survival.

SPLENIC IRRADIATION. Irradiation of the spleen in patients with chronic phase CML reduces splenomegaly, lowers the peripheral leukocyte count, and also reduces the number of immature cells and the mitotic index at sites distant from the spleen (e.g., bone marrow). This distant (abscopal) effect has been postulated to result from the release of an inhibitor into the plasma[105] or an interruption of the flow of CFU-GM from the splenic parenchyma into the circulation.[60] Before the introduction of busulfan, splenic irradiation was the main treatment for chronic phase CML. Although symptomatic relief was achieved, disease control was generally short-lived (4–6 months), and there was little impact on survival. Splenic irradiation was replaced by chemotherapy as the first-line treatment when a prospective controlled clinical trial showed that intermittent splenic irradiation was inferior to busulfan in achieving consistent control of the leukocyte count and in prolonging survival.[106] Splenic irradiation may be considered for transient palliation of the symptoms produced by massive splenomegaly in patients refractory to systemic chemotherapy, but this is generally ineffective and may result in profound myelosuppression.

SPLENECTOMY. The enlarged spleen of the patient with CML contains a substantial burden of leukemic cells, and, in some cases, blast transformation may originate in the spleen.[107] It has been proposed that removal of this pool of cells might delay metamorphosis. However, several large controlled trials have failed to demonstrate any benefit from splenectomy in prolonging chronic phase or survival.[108,109] Splenectomy may be of benefit in selected patients with hypersplenism or painful splenomegaly; it may also be useful in reducing the leukemic burden in patients about to undergo ablative therapy prior to bone marrow transplant. However, these potential benefits must be weighed against the risk of overwhelming postsplenectomy sepsis syndrome and extreme thrombocytosis.

Management of Blast Phase

Chemotherapy using regimens developed for the treatment of acute myelogenous leukemia (AML) has proved disappointing in blast phase CML, even when very aggressive combination chemotherapy regimens were used (Table 18-1).[110–122] Patients with myeloblastic morphology have a median survival of 3 months after blast transformation. The subset of patients with lymphoblastic transformation is more sensitive to chemotherapy; approximately two thirds of such patients will revert to chronic phase following treatment with vincristine/prednisone regimens.[81] Unfortunately, the response is of short duration (median < 6 months) and fewer than 20% of patients survive 1 year. The use of more intensive ALL regimens, such as the Memorial Hospital L10 or L10M protocols, may extend the median survival to 15 months.[116]

A promising new approach using alternate-day plicamycin (mithramycin) and daily hydroxyurea has shown efficacy in converting myeloid blast phase back to chronic phase.[122] The fact that treatment is not associated with an initial period of aplasia suggests the intriguing possibility that the plicamycin/hydroxyurea combination exerts its effects by inducing differention of the blast population rather than by cytotoxicity; this

Table 18-1
Results of Treatment of Blast Phase CML

Regimen*	Number of Patients	Complete Responses (%)†	Partial Responses (%)‡	Reference
VCR/pred	10 (myeloid)	0	NR	81
	11 (lymphoid)	67	NR	
TRAMPCOL	19	42	9	112
HD ara-C	21	24	13	113
HU/6-MP/pred				
± VCR/DNR	202	12	22	114
HU/6-MP/VP-16	5	20	NR	115
L-10/L-10M	15 (lymphoid)	67	NR	116
5-aza/VP-16	27	4	56	117
Mitoxantrone	13 (myeloid)	0	31	118–120
DATA	30	0	13	121
Plica/HU	6 (myeloid)	100	NR	122
	3 (lymphoid)	33	NR	

* VCR = vincristine, pred = prednisone, 6-TG = 6-thioguanine, HD ara-C = high-dose cytosine arabinoside, MTX = methotrexate, CTX = cyclophosphamide, L-asp = L-asparaginase, 5-aza = 5-azacytidine, HU = hydroxyurea, 6-MP = 6-mercaptopurine, plica = plicamycin, DNR = daunorubicin, DXR = doxorubicin. Regimens: TRAMPCOL = 6-TG/DNR/ara-C/MTX/pred/CTX/VCR/L-asp; L-10/L-10M = VCR/pred/DXR/CTX/MTX/ara-C/L-asp/TG; DATA = DNR/5-aza/6-TG/ara-C.
† Reversion to chronic phase.
‡ Decline in blast count; NR = not reported.

hypothesis is supported by *in vitro* studies documenting the ability of these agents to induce morphologic differentiation and to alter expression of oncogenes in CML blast cells.[123]

New Approaches

BONE MARROW TRANSPLANTATION. The theoretical and technical aspects of bone marrow transplantation (BMT) are discussed in Chapter 48. Three sources of hematopoietic stem cells have been used for transplantation in CML patients: autologous peripheral blood or bone marrow cells, syngeneic bone marrow from an identical twin, or allogeneic bone marrow, usually from an HLA-identical sibling.

Autologous Transplantation. In this approach, large quantities of circulating or marrow stem cells are collected from the patient during chronic phase and stored until metamorphosis begins. At that point, the patient receives myeloablative chemotherapy or radiotherapy, followed by infusion of the chronic phase cells. The objective is to restore a second chronic phase. This is, at best, a temporizing approach because the marrow is reconstituted with cells of the Ph[1]+ clone. Usually, the blast phase cells are resistant to even the most intensive regimens and the second chronic phase is brief (median duration = 4 months); fewer than 30% of patients treated in this fashion survive for 1 year.[124,125]

A promising new approach to autologous transplantation may derive from the observation that certain long-term culture techniques deplete the marrow of Ph[1]+ progenitor cells while augmenting the Ph[1]– population.[126,127] Theoretically, these Ph[1]– progenitor cells could be used to reconstitute the patient's marrow following myeloablative chemotherapy or radiotherapy. The curative potential of such an approach would require that the Ph[1]– cells represent normal hematopoietic stem cells rather than an early stage in the evolution of the CML clone.

Syngeneic or Allogeneic Transplantation. Unlike autologous transplantation, these approaches do offer the possibility of cure. Disease status at the time of transplant is the most powerful predictor of survival. The best results have been obtained in patients transplanted in first chronic phase (49%–70% long-term survival); the chances for long-term survival become progressively worse when transplants are done in second chronic phase (30%–58%), accelerated phase (15%–35%), or blast phase (10%–20%).[128,129]

About one third of patients die of transplantation-related complications soon after BMT; these deaths are mainly due to acute graft-versus-host disease (GVHD) and interstitial pneumonitis.[130] About one fourth of long-term survivors have the stigmata of chronic GVHD.[131] Despite these risks, most authorities recommend performing the procedure soon after the diagnosis for CML patients who have HLA-matched siblings. This approach seeks to avoid the risk of transformation into accelerated or blast phase; further, chronic phase patients who undergo BMT within 1 year of diagnosis may have better results than those who have the procedure after a longer interval.[128]

BIOLOGICAL RESPONSE MODIFIERS. Interferon (IFN). IFN preparations have significant antiproliferative activity against both normal and CML myeloid progenitor cells; they may also modify expression of HLA-DR antigens and of *c-abl* in CML cells.[132–134] Clinical trials have indicated that both alpha and gamma IFN can induce hematologic remission in chronic phase CML; in some cases, there has even been partial or complete suppression of the Ph[1]+ clone.[132,135,136] Further studies are needed to define the role of IFN in the management of CML (see also Chap. 14).

Inducers of Differentiation. Certain molecules known to induce differentiation of leukemic cells *in vitro* are being used in clinical trials to determine whether they can prevent or delay the development of blast crisis. Among these are retinoic acid and low-dose cytosine arabinoside (ara-C).[137]

JUVENILE CHRONIC MYELOCYTIC LEUKEMIA

Juvenile chronic myelocytic leukemia (JCML), like classic adult CML, is a clonal panmyelopathy associated with elevated leukocyte count, splenomegaly, and decreased LAP.[138–141] Among the features that distinguish JCML from the adult form are onset in infancy or early childhood, cutaneous manifestations, lymphadenopathy, thrombocytopenia with hemorrhagic diathesis, elevated fetal hemoglobin level, immunologic deficiency, prominent involvement of the monocytic series, a relatively rapid course, and absence of the Ph[1] chromosome (Table 18-2).

Pathogenesis

There are two intriguing clues to the pathogenesis of JCML. One of these is an association with neurofibromatosis[141–143] and the other is an association with persistent Epstein–Barr virus (EBV) infection.[143,144]

Biology

Hematologic and limited cytogenetic evidence suggests that there is clonal involvement of the erythroid, myeloid, monocytic, and megakaryocytic lineages in JCML.[140,145] However, the predominant cell in the bone marrow and blood appears to be a primitive monocytic precursor.[140,145–147]

Clinical Features

Most patients with JCML are diagnosed before the age of 2 years. Presenting physical findings include cutaneous lesions (eczema, xanthomata, and café-au-lait spots), lymphadenopathy, hepatosplenomegaly, and hemorrhagic manifestations. Respiratory symptoms (chronic tachypnea, cough, expiratory wheezing) may be prominent.

Laboratory Features

The peripheral blood picture is characterized by anemia, leukocytosis, and thrombocytopenia. The leukocytosis is generally not as pronounced as it is in adult CML and is associated with a relatively high proportion of blasts (including normoblasts), lymphocytes, and monocytes. The bone marrow shows both erythroid and myeloid hyperplasia; immature cells of the monocytic series are prominent and megakaryocytes are infrequent.

The erythrocytes show many features characteristic of fetal-type erythropoiesis, including high hemoglobin (Hgb) F level, fetal glycine/alanine ratio in the gamma chain of Hgb F,

Table 18-2
Differences Between Adult and Juvenile Forms of CML

Finding	Adult Form	Juvenile Form
Chromosome studies	Ph^1-positive	Ph^1-negative
Age at onset	Usually >2 years old	Usually <2 years old
Physical findings		
Facial rash	Absent	Present
Lymphadenopathy	Occasional	Frequent, with tendency to suppuration
Splenomegaly	Marked	Variable
Hemorrhagic manifestations	Absent	Frequent
Hematologic findings		
Leukocyte count at onset	Usually >100,000	Usually <100,000
Monocytosis of peripheral blood and bone marrow	Absent	Usually present
Thrombocytopenia	Uncommon at onset	Frequent at onset
Erythrocyte abnormalities		
Ineffective erythropoiesis	Absent	Present
I antigen on erythrocyte	Normal	Reduced
Fetal hemoglobin levels	Normal	15%–50%
Normoblasts in peripheral blood	Unusual	Frequent
Other laboratory findings		
Urinary and serum muramidase	Slightly elevated	Markedly elevated
Immunologic abnormalities	None	Strikingly high immunoglobulin levels, high incidence of antinuclear antibodies (52%) and anti-IgG antibodies (43%)
Nature of colonies produced *in vitro* from peripheral blood	Predominantly granulocytic	Almost exclusively monocytic
Response to busulfan	Uniformly good	Poor
Median survival	2½–3 years	<9 months

(Altman AJ, Baehner RL: In vitro colony forming characteristics of chronic granulocytic leukemia in childhood. J Pediatr 86:221, 1975)

fetal-type glycolytic enzyme pattern, and low I antigen expression.[148,149] The LAP score is low. Immunologic abnormalities include stikingly high immunoglobulin levels, high incidence of antibodies to nuclear antigen and IgG,[150] and possible inability to control EBV infection.[144]

Cytogenetic Features

The cytogenetic pattern of JCML is heterogeneous, the only consistent feature being absence of the Ph^1 chromosome. The majority of patients have a normal karyotype. Abnormalities, when found, most commonly involve chromosomes 7 and 8.[140,143,151]

Natural History

Median survival time for patients with JCML is less then 9 months. Most patients succumb to infection and do not manifest a terminal blast phase. Occasionally, JCML terminates in a erythroleukemia-like phase, characterized by anemia, erythroblastosis, and megaloblastic erythroid hyperplasia of the bone marrow.[152]

Therapy

Generally chemotherapy has been of limited value in JCML. Oral 6-mercaptopurine, either alone or in combination with subcutaneous ara-C, has produced symptomatic relief in some

patients,[138,153] but supportive care was as effective as vigorous chemotherapy in most cases. In some cases, intensive multiagent chemotherapy (as used for treatment of acute nonlymphoid leukemias) has produced clinical remissions lasting as long as 27+ months.[154] However, to date, bone marrow transplantation has been curative.[155]

FAMILIAL CHRONIC MYELOCYTIC LEUKEMIA

A familial form of CML has been reported in at least three pairs of infant siblings.[156,157] This disorder is indistinguishable from JCML by standard clinical and laboratory criteria; however, its evolution is less predictable. In each of the families studied, one sibling died of progressive leukemia and the other had long-term asymptomatic survival.

CHRONIC MYELOMONOCYTIC LEUKEMIA

Chronic myelomonocytic leukemia (CMML) is a rare disorder of childhood characterized by recurrent upper respiratory and pulmonary infections, anemia, unexplained monocytosis, neutropenia, thrombocytopenia, and progressive splenomegaly.[158-160] Atypical monocytoid cells with unipolar hairy projections are seen in the peripheral smear, and the bone marrow is hypercellular with a high proportion of young myeloid and monocytoid forms. In some cases the course may be relatively indolent, and aggressive chemotherapy may actually shorten survival by producing severe pancytopenia. Low-dose ara-C has achieved complete remissions in some adults with CMML.[161]

CHRONIC MONOCYTIC LEUKEMIA

Chronic monocytic leukemia (CMoL) is characterized by anemia, neutropenia, and thrombocytopenia in association with an increased number of mature monocytic elements in the blood and bone marrow. There may also be involvement of extramedullary tissues, such as skin, gums, and viscera. Only a few cases of childhood CMoL have been reported, and some of these may actually represent cases of acute monocytic leukemia, histiocytosis, or JCML.[162,163]

CHRONIC LYMPHOCYTIC LEUKEMIA

Chronic lymphocytic leukemia (CLL) is a monoclonal neoplasm of relatively mature lymphocytes. In the vast majority of cases, the B-cell lineage is affected. CLL is a disease primarily of elderly adults; only rare cases have been reported in children.[164-168]

Clinical and Laboratory Features

Presenting features include pallor, hepatosplenomegaly, and generalized lymphadenopathy. Hematologic findings include anemia, lymphocytosis, and infiltration of the bone marrow with small mature lymphoid cells. Lymph node architecture is obliterated by a diffuse population of small lymphocytes.

Functional immunologic defects of both the B- and T-cell populations are demonstrable. These include hypogammaglobulinemia, inadequate antibody response to antigenic stimuli, and decreased responsiveness to mitogens.

Monoclonality of the lymphoid population is demonstrable by analysis of membrane immunoglobulins and of immunoglobulin gene rearrangement. However, these techniques have been applied to only a handful of pediatric cases.[164-166]

Cytogenetics

Common nonrandom cytogenetic abnormalities in adult CLL include trisomy 12, 14q+ translocations, trisomy 3, and abnormalities of chromosome 6.[171,172] In one pediatric case, t(2;14)(p13;q32) with breakpoints at or near the kappa light-chain and heavy-chain loci was reported.[164]

Therapy

Adult CLL cases are usually treated with chlorambucil and sometimes steroids. Only two reported pediatric cases[164,167] have been treated in this fashion, and both patients responded well. At least two others[165,169] have had stable courses without any chemotherapy.

REFERENCES

1. Donné A: Cours de Microscopie Complementaire des Études Medicales. Paris. Balliere, 1844
2. Bennett JH: Two cases of disease and enlargement of the spleen in which death took place from the presence of purulent matter in the blood. Edinburgh Med Surg J 64:413–423, 1845
3. Craigie D: Case of disease of the spleen in which death took place in consequence of the presence of purulent matter in the blood. Edinburgh Med Surg J 64:400–412, 1845
4. Virchow R: Weisses blut. Frorlep's Notizen 36:151–156, 1845
5. Neumann E: Ein fall von leukamie mit erkrankung des knochenmarkes. Arch Heilk 11:1–14, 1870
6. Ebstein W: Ueber die acute leukamie und pseudoleukamie. Dtsch Arch Klin Med 44:343–396, 1888–1889
7. Ehrlich P: Farbenanalytisch Untersuchungen zur Histologie une Klinik des Blutes. Berlin, Hirschwald, 1891
8. Lissauer: Zwei falle von leucaemie. Berl Klin Wschr 2:403, 1865
9. Pusey WA: Report of cases treated with roentgen rays. JAMA 38:911, 1902
10. Nowell PC, Hungerford DA: A minute chromosome in human chronic granulocytic leukemia. Science 132:1497–1498, 1960
11. Altman AJ: Unpublished data
12. Castro-Malespina H, Schaison G, Briere J et al: Philadelphia chromosome-positive chronic myelocytic leukemia in children. Survival and prognostic features. Cancer 52:721–727, 1983
13. Homans AC, Young PC, Dickerman JD, Land ML: Adult-type CML in childhood: Case report and review. Am J Pediatr Hematol Oncol 6:220–224, 1984
14. Rowley JD: A new consistent chromosomal abnormality in chronic myelogenous leukemia identified by quinacrine fluorescence and giemsa staining. Nature 243:290–303, 1973
15. Heisterkamp N: Structural organization of the bcr gene and its role in the Ph[1] translocation. Nature 315:758–61, 1985
16. Heisterkamp N, Stephenson JR, Groffen et al: Localization of c-abl oncogene adjacent to a translocation breakpoint in chronic myelogenous leukaemia. Nature 306:239–242, 1983
17. Groffen J, Heisterkamp N, Stephenson JR et al: C-sis is translocated from chromosome 22 to chromosome 9 in chronic myelocytic leukemia. J Exp Med 158:9–15, 1983
18. Bartram CR, de Klein A, Hagemeijer A et al: Localization of the human c-sis oncogene in Ph[1]-positive and Ph[1]-negative chronic myelocytic leukemia by in situ hybridization. Blood 63:223–225, 1984
19. Konopka JB, Watanabe SM, Singer J et al: Cell lines and clinical isolates derived from Ph[1]-positive chronic myelogenous leukemia patients express c-abl proteins with a common structural alteration. Proc Natl Acad Sci USA 82:1810–1814, 1985
20. Konopka JB, Watanabe SM, Witte ON: An alteration of the human c-abl oncogene in K562 leukemia cells unmasks associated tyrosine kinase activity. Cell 37:1035–1042, 1984
21. Witte ON: Functions of the abl oncogene. Cancer Surveys 5:183–197, 1986
22. Doolittle RF, Humkapiller MW, Hood LE et al: Simian sarcoma virus gene, v-sis, is derived from the gene (or genes) encoding a platelet derived growth factor. Science 221:275–277, 1983
23. Rowley JD: Identification of the constant chromosome regions involved in human hematologic malignant disease. Science 216:749–751, 1982
24. Sandberg AA: Chromosomes and causation of human cancer and leukemia: XI. The Ph[1] and other translocations in CML. Cancer 46:2221–2226, 1986
25. Lessard M, Duval S, Fritz A: Unusual translocation and chronic myelocytic leukemia: "Masked" Philadelphia chromosome (Ph[1]). Cancer Genet Cytogenet 4:237–244, 1981
26. Lewis JP, Jenke H, Lazerson J: Philadelphia chromosome-negative chronic myelogenous leukemia in a child with t(8;9) (p11 or 12;q34). Am J Pediatr Hematol Oncol 5:265–269, 1983
27. Lewis JP: Evidence that 9pter → q34::q34 → qter is the initial DNA lesion converting benign to malignant hematopoiesis in chronic myelogenous leukemia (CML). Clin Res 31:88A, 1983
28. Priest JR, Robison LL, McKenna RW et al: Philadelphia chromosome positive childhood acute lymphoblastic leukemia. Blood 56:15–22, 1980
29. Bloomfield CD, Lindquist LL, Brunning RE et al: The Philadelphia chromosome in acute leukemia. Virchow's Arch 29:81–91, 1978
30. Kurzrock R, Shtalrid M, Kloetzer WS, Gutterman JU: Expression of c-abl in Philadelphia-positive acute myelogenous leukemia. Blood 70:1584–1588, 1987
31. Beard MEJ, Durrant J, Catovsky D et al: Blast crisis of chronic myeloid leukemia (CML). I. Presentation simulating acute lymphoid leukaemia (ALL). Br J Haematol 34:167–178, 1976
32. Clein GP, Flemens RJ: Involvement of the erythroid series in blastic crisis of chronic myeloid leukemia. Further evidence for the presence of Philadelphia chromosome in erythroblasts. Br J Haematol 12:754–758, 1966
33. Golde DW, Burgaleta C, Sparkes RS et al: The Philadelphia chromosome in human macrophages. Blood 49:367–370, 1977
34. Tough IM, Court Brown WM, Baikie AG et al: Cytogenetic studies in chronic myeloid leukaemia and acute leukaemia associated with mongolism. Lancet 1:411–417, 1961

35. Fitzgerald PH, Pickering AF, Elby JR: Clonal origin of the Philadelphia chromosome and chronic myeloid leukaemia: Evidence from a sex chromosome mosaic. Br J Haematol 21:473–480, 1971

36. Fialkow PJ, Gartler SM, Yoshida A: Clonal origin of chronic myelocytic leukemia in man. Proc Natl Acad Sci USA 58:1468–1471, 1967

37. Bernheim A, Berger R, Preud'homme JL et al: Philadelphia chromosome positive blood B lymphocytes in chronic myelocytic leukemia. Leukemia Res 5:331–339, 1981

38. Fauser AA, Kanz L, Bross KJ, Lohr GW: T cells and probably B cells arise from the malignant clone in chronic myelogenous leukemia. J Clin Invest 75:1080–1082, 1985

39. Rajasekariah P, Garson OM: C-banding studies in patients with Ph^1+ chronic granulocytic leukaemia. Pathology 13:197–203, 1981

40. Sadamori N, Sandberg AA: The clinical and cytogenetic significance of c-banding on chromosome #9 in patients with Ph^1-positive chronic myeloid leukemia. Cancer Genet Cytogenet 8:235–241, 1983

41. Fialkow PJ, Jacobson RJ, Papayannopoulou T: Chronic myelocytic leukemia: clonal origin in a stem cell common to the granulocyte, erythrocyte, platelet, and monocyte/macrophage. Am J Med 63:125–130, 1977

42. Barr RD, Fialkow PJ: Clonal origin of chronic myelocytic leukemia. N Engl J Med 289:308–308, 1973

43. Fialkow PJ, Denman AM, Jacobson RA et al: Chronic myelocytic leukemia. Origin of some lymphocytes from leukemic stem cells. J Clin Invest 62:815–823, 1978

44. Fialkow PJ, Martin PJ, Najfeld V et al: Evidence for a multistep pathogenesis of chronic myelogenous leukemia. Blood 58:158–163, 1981

45. Lisker R, Casas L, Mutchinick O et al: Late appearing Philadelphia chromosome in two patients with chronic myelogenous leukemia. Blood 56:812–814, 1980

46. Goldman J, Lu D-P: New approaches in chronic granulocytic leukemia. Origin, prognosis and treatment. Semin Hematol 19:241–256, 1982

47. Hagemeijer A, Smit E, Lowenberg B, Abels J: Chronic myeloid leukemia with permanent disappearance of the Ph^1 chromosome and development of new clonal subpopulation. Blood 53:1–14, 1979

48. Ogawa M, Fried J, Sakai Y et al: Studies of cellular proliferation in human leukemia. The proliferative activity, generation time, and emergence time of neutrophilic granulocytes in chronic granulocytic leukemia. Cancer 25:1031–1049, 1970

49. Chervenick PA, Boggs DR: Granulocyte kinetics in chronic myelocytic leukaemia. Ser Haematol 1:24–37, 1968

50. Stryckmans P, Debusscher L, Peltzer T, Socquet M: Variations of the proliferative activity of leukemic myeloblasts related to the stage of the disease. In Bessis M, Brecher G (eds): Unclassifiable Leukemias, pp 239–248. New York, Springer Verlag, 1975

51. Cronkite EP, Vincent PC: Granulocytopoiesis. In Stohlman F Jr (ed): Hemopoietic Cellular Proliferation, pp 211–222. New York, Grune & Stratton, 1970

52. Galbraith PR, Abu-Zahra HT: Granulopoiesis in chronic granulocytic leukaemia. Br J Haematol 22:135–143, 1972

53. Athens JW, Raab SO, Haab OP et al: Leukokinetic studies. X. Blood granulocyte kinetics in chronic myelocytic leukemia. J Clin Invest 44:765–777, 1965

54. Goldman JM, Th'ng KH, Lowenthal RM: In vitro colony forming cells and colony stimulating factor in chronic granulocytic leukaemia. Br J Cancer 30:1–12, 1974

55. Moberg C, Olofsson T, Olsson I: Granulopoiesis in chronic myeloid leukaemia. I. In vitro cloning of blood and bone marrow cells in agar culture. Scand J Haematol 12:381–390, 1974

56. Altman AJ, Baehner RL: In vitro colony forming characteristics of chronic granulocytic leukemia in childhood. J Pediatr 86:221–224, 1975

57. Moore MAS: In vitro culture studies in chronic granulocytic leukemia. Clin Hematol 6:97–112, 1977

58. Moore MAS: Agar culture studies in CML and blastic transformation. Ser Haematol 8:11–27, 1977

59. Moore MAS, Mertelsmann R, Pelus LM: Phenotypic evaluation of chronic myeloid leukemia. Blood Cells 7:217–236, 1981

60. Morris TCM, Vincent PC, Gunz FW et al: Evidence following splenic radiotherapy for a highly dynamic traffic of CFU-GM between the spleen and other organs in chronic granulocytic leukaemia. Leukemia Res 11:109–117, 1987

61. Gavosto F: Granulopoiesis and cell kinetics in chronic myeloid leukaemia. Cell Tissue Kinet 7:151–163, 1974

62. Broxmeyer HE, Smithyman A, Eger RR et al: Identification of lactoferrin as the granulocyte-derived inhibitor of colony-stimulating activity production. J Exp Med 148:1052–1067, 1978

63. Pelus LM, Broxmeyer HE, Kurland JI, Moore MAS: Regulation of macrophage and granulocyte proliferation: specificities of prostaglandin E and lactoferrin. J Exp Med 150:277–292, 1979

64. Broxmeyer HE, Gentile P, Cooper S et al: Functional activities of acidic isoferritins and lactoferrin in vitro and in vivo. Blood Cells 10:397–426, 1984

65. Kurland JI, Broxmeyer HE, Pelus LM et al: Role for monocyte-macrophage-derived colony-stimulating factor and prostaglandin E in the positive and negative feedback control of myeloid stem cell proliferation. Blood 52:388–407, 1978

66. Broxmeyer HE: Relationship of cell cycle expression of Ia-like antigenic determinants on normal and leukemia human granulocyte-macrophage progenitor cells to regulation in vitro by acidic isoferritins. J Clin Invest 69:631–642, 1982

67. Pelus LM, Saletan S, Silver R, Moore MA: Expression of Ia antigens on normal and chronic myeloid leukemic human granulocyte-macrophage colony forming cells is associated with the regulation of cell proliferation by prostaglandin E. Blood 59:284–292, 1982

68. Cannistra SA, Hermann F, Davis R et al: Relationship between HLA-Dr expression by normal myeloid progenitor cells and inhibition of colony growth by prostaglandin E. Implication for prostaglandin E resistance in chronic myeloid leukemia. J Clin Invest 77:13–20, 1986

69. Pelus LM, Broxmeyer HE, Clarkson BD, Moore MAS: Abnormal responsiveness of granulocyte-macrophage committed colony-forming cells from patients with chronic myeloid leukemia to inhibition by prostaglandin E. Cancer Res 40:2512–2515, 1980

70. Broxmeyer HE, Mendelsohn N, Moore MAS: Abnormal granulocyte feedback regulation of colony forming and colony stimulating activity-producing cells from patients with chronic myelogenous leukemia. Leukemia Res 1:3–12, 1977

71. Aglietta M, Piacibello W, Gavosto F: Insensitivity of chronic myeloid leukemia cells to inhibition of growth by prostaglandin E. Cancer Res 40:2507–2511, 1980

72. Broxmeyer HE, Frossbard E, Jacobsen N, Moore MAS: Evidence for a proliferative advantage of human leukemia colony-forming cells in vitro. J Natl Cancer Inst 60:513–521, 1978

73. Oloffson T, Olsson I: Suppression of normal granulopoiesis in vitro by a leukemia-associated inhibitor (LAI) of acute and chronic leukemia. Blood 55:975–982, 1980

74. Rowe JM, Lichtman MA: Hyperleukocytosis and leukostasis: Common features of childhood chronic myelogenous leukemia. Blood 63:1230–1234, 1984

75. Gralnick HR, Harbor J, Vogel C: Myelofibrosis in chronic granulocytic leukemia. Blood 37:152–162, 1971

76. Clough V, Geary CG, Hashmi K et al: Myelofibrosis in chronic granulocytic leukaemia. Br J Haematol 42:515–526, 1979

77. Matsuo T: In vitro modulation of alkaline phosphatase activity in neutrophils from patients with chronic myelogenous leukemia by monocyte-derived activity. Blood 6:492–497, 1986

78. Cramer E, Auclair C, Hakim J et al: Metabolic activity of phagocytizing granulocytes in chronic granulocytic leukemia. Arch Int Med 50:93–106, 1977

79. Anklesaria PN, Advani SH, Bhisey AN: Defective chemotaxis and adherence in granulocytes from chronic myeloid leukemia (CML) patients. Leukemia Res 9:641–648, 1985

80. Baker MA, Taub RN, Whelton CH, Hindenburg A: Aberrant sialylation of granulocyte membranes in chronic myelogenous leukemia. Blood 63:1194–1197, 1984

81. Griffin JD, Todd RF III, Ritz J et al: Differentiation patterns in the blastic phase of chronic myeloid leukemia. Blood 61:85–91, 1983

82. Griffin JD, Tantravahi R, Canelos GP: T-cell surface antigens in a patient with blast crisis of chronic myeloid leukemia. Blood 61:640–644, 1983

83. Bakhshi A, Minowada J, Arnold A et al: Lymphoid blast crises of chronic myelogenous leukemia represent stages in the development of B-cell precursors. N Engl J Med 309:826–831, 1983

83a. Yasukawa M, Iwasama K, Kawamura S, et al: Phenotypic and genotypic analysis of chronic myelogenous leukemia with T-lymphoblastic and megakaryoblastic mixed crisis. Br J Haematol 66:331–336, 1987

83b. Bernstein R, Bagy A, Pinto M, et al: Chromosome 3q21 abnormalities associated with hyperactive thrombopoiesis in acute transformation of chronic myeloid leukemia. Blood 68:652–657, 1986

84. Tura S, Boccarani M, Corbelli G et al: Staging of chronic myeloid leukemia. Br J Haematol 47:105–119, 1981

85. Sokal JE, Cox EB, Baccarani M: Prognostic discrimination in "good-risk" chronic granulocytic leukemia. Blood 63:789–799, 1984

86. Sadamori N, Gomez SA, Sandberg AA: Therapeutic and prognostic value of initial chromosomal findings at the blastic phase of Ph^1-positive chronic myeloid leukemia. Blood 61:935–939, 1983

87. Allegretta GJ, Welsman SJ, Altman AJ: Oncologic emergencies I: Metabolic and space-occupying consequences of cancer and cancer treatment. Pediatr Clin North Am 32:601–612, 1985

88. Lichtman MA, Rowe JM: Hyperleukocytic leukemias: Rheological, clinical, and therapeutic considerations. Blood 60:279–283, 1982

89. Graw RG Jr, Skeel RT, Carbone PP: Priapism in a child with chronic granulocytic leukemia. J Pediatr 74:788–790, 1969

90. Schwartz JH, Canellos GP: Hydroxyurea in the management of the hematologic complications of chronic granulocytic leukemia. Blood 46:11–16, 1975

91. Schwartz JH, Canellos GP, Young RC, DeVita VT: Meningeal leukemia in the blastic phase of chronic granulocytic leukemia. Am J Med 59:819–828, 1975

92. Smith AG, Prentice AG, Lucie NP, Dagg JH: Meningeal relapse in Ph^1-positive acute lymphoblastic and lymphoid blast crisis of chronic granulocytic leukemia. Is CNS prophylaxis indicated? Cancer 51:2031–2034, 1983

93. Haut A, Abbott WS, Wintrobe MM, Cartwright GE: Busulfan in the treatment of chronic myelocytic leukemia. Blood 17:1–19, 1961

94. Kennedy BJ: Hydroxyurea therapy in chronic myelogenous leukemia. Cancer 29:1052–1056, 1972

95. Galton DAG: Chemotherapy of chronic myelocytic leukemia. Semin Hematol 6:323–343, 1969

96. Rushing D, Goldman A, Gibbs G et al: Hydroxyurea versus busulfan in the treatment of chronic myelogenous leukemia. Am J Clin Oncol 5:307–313, 1982

97. Bolin RW, Robinson WA, Sutherland J et al: Busulfan versus hydroxyurea in the long term therapy of chronic myelogenous leukemia. Cancer 50:1683–1686, 1982

98. Finney R, McDonald GA, Baikie AG et al: Chronic granulocytic leukaemia with Ph^1-negative cells in bone marrow and a ten year remission after busulphan hypoplasia. Br J Haematol 23:283–288, 1972

99. Speed SE, Lawler SD: Chronic granulocytic leukaemia. The chromosomes and the disease. Lancet 1:403–407, 1964

100. Brandt L, Mitelman F, Panani A et al: Extremely long duration of chronic myeloid leukaemia with Ph^1-negative and Ph^1-positive bone marrow cells. Scand J Haematol 16:321–325, 1976

101. Golde DW, Bersch NL, Sparkes RS: Chromosomal mosaicism associated with prolonged remission in chronic myelogenous leukemia. Cancer 37:1849–1852, 1976

102. Cunningham I, Gee T, Dowling M et al: Results of treatment of Ph^1 chronic myelogenous leukemia with an intensive treatment regimen (L-5 protocol). Blood 53:375–379, 1979

103. Kantarjian HM, Vellekoop L, McCredie KB et al: Intensive combination chemotherapy (ROAP 10) and splenectomy in the management of chronic myelogenous leukemia. J Clin Oncol 3:192–200, 1985

104. Sokal JE, Gomez GA: The Philadelphia chromosome and Philadelphia chromosome mosaicism in chronic myelogenous leukemia. J Clin Oncol 4:104–111, 1986

105. Li JG: The leukocytopenic effect of focal splenic X-irradiation in leukaemic patients. Radiology 80:471–476, 1963

106. Medical Research Council's Working Party for Therapeutic Trials in Leukaemia: Chronic granulocytic leukaemia: Comparison of radiotherapy and busulfan therapy. Br Med J i:201–208, 1968

107. Neiman F, Brandt L, Nilsson PG: Cytogenetic evidence for splenic origin of blastic transformation in chronic myelogenous leukaemia. Scand J Haematol 13:87–92, 1973

108. Italian Cooperative Group on Chronic Myeloid Leukemia: Results of a prospective study of early splenectomy in chronic myeloid leukemia. Cancer 54:333–338, 1984

109. Medical Research Council's Working Party for Therapeutic Trials in Leukaemia: Randomized trial of splenectomy in Ph^1-positive chronic granulocytic leukaemia, including an analysis of prognostic factors. Br J Haematol 54:415–530, 1983

110. Koeffler HP, Golde DW: Chronic myelogenous leukemia-new concepts. N Engl J Med 304:1201–1209, 1269–1274, 1981

111. Hayes D, Ellison R, Glidewell O et al: Chemotherapy for the terminal phase of chronic myelocytic leukemia. Cancer Chemother Rep 58:233–247, 1974

112. Spiers ASD, Goldman JM, Catovsky D et al: Multiple-drug chemotherapy for acute leukemia: the TRAMPCOL regimen: Results in 86 patients. Cancer 40:20–29, 1977

113. Iacoboni SJ, Plunkett W, Kantarjian HM et al: High-dose cytosine arabinoside: treatment and cellular pharmacology of chronic myelogenous leukemia blast crisis. J Clin Oncol 4:1079–1088, 1986

114. Coleman M, Silver RT, Pajek TF et al: Combination chemotherapy for terminal-phase chronic granulocytic leukemia: Cancer and Leukemia Group B studies. Blood 55:29–36, 1980

115. Donadio D, Marty M, Navarro M et al: Hydroxyurea, 6MP and VP-16 in the accelerated phase or in blastic transformation of CML. Proceedings of the 3rd International Symposium on Therapy for Acute Leukemia, p 333, 1982

116. Jain K, Arlin A, Mertelsmann R et al: Philadelphia chromosome and terminal transferase positive acute leukemia. Similarity of terminal phase of chronic myelogenous leukemia and de novo acute leukemia. J Clin Oncol 1:669–676, 1983

117. Schiffer CA, deBellis R, Kasdorf H, Wiernik PH: Treatment of blast crisis of chronic myelogenous leukemia with 5-azacytidine and VP16-213. Cancer Treat Rep 66:267–271, 1982

118. Schulman P, van Echo D, Budman D et al: Phase II trial of mitoxantrone (DHAD NSC 301739) in blastic phase in chronic myelogenous leukemia (B-CML) (abstr). Blood 60 (Suppl 1): 558, 1982

119. Hulhoven R, Prentice G, Michaux JL et al: A phase I/II study of mitoxantrone in acute myelogenous leukemia. Proceedings of the 3rd International Symposium for Therapy of Acute Leukemia, p 383, 1982

120. Paciucci P, Ohnuma T, Cuttner J et al: Phase I-II evaluation of mitoxantrone in patients with refractory leukemia. Proceedings of the 3rd International Symposium for Therapy of Acute Leukemia, p 382, 1982

121. Winton EF, Miller D, Vogler WR: Intensive chemotherapy with daunorubicin, 5-azacytidine, 6-thioguanine, and cytarabine (DATA) for the blastic transformation of chronic granulocytic leukemia. Cancer Treat Rep 65:389–392, 1981

122. Koller CA, Miller DM: Preliminary observations on the therapy of the myeloid blast phase of chronic granulocytic leukemia with plicamycin and hydroxyurea. N Engl J Med 315:1433–1438, 1986

123. Koller CA, Campbell VW, Polansky DA et al: In vivo differentiation of blast-phase chronic granulocytic leukemia: Expression of c-myc and c-abl protooncogenes. J Clin Invest 76:365–369, 1985

124. Haines ME, Goldman JM, Worsley AM, et al: Chemotherapy and autografting for chronic granulocytic leukemia in transformation: probable prolongation of survival for some patients. Br J Haematol 58:711–721, 1984

125. Buckner CD, Stewart P, Clift RA et al: Treatment of blastic transformation of chronic granulocytic leukemia by chemotherapy, total body irradiation and infusion of cryopreserved autologous marrow. Exp Hematol 6:96–109, 1978

126. Coulombel L, Kalousek DK, Eaves CJ, et al: Long-term marrow culture reveals chromosmally normal hematopoietic progenitor cells in patients with Philadelphia chromosome-positive chronic myelogenous leukemia. N Engl J Med 308:1493–1498, 1983

127. Dube ID, Gupta CM, Kolousek DK et al: Cytogenetic studies of early myeloid progenitor compartments in Ph^1-positive chronic myeloid leukaemia (CML). I. Persistence of Ph^1-negative committed progenitors that are suppressed from differentiating in vivo. Br J Haematol 56:633–644, 1984

128. Thomas DE, Clift RA, Fefer A et al: Marrow transplantation for the treatment of chronic myelogenous leukemia. Ann Intern Med 104:155–163, 1986

129. Champlin R: Bone marrow transplantation for chronic leukemias. In Champlin R (moderator): Chronic leukemias: oncogenes, chromosomes, and advances in therapy. Ann Intern Med 104:671–688, 1986

130. Champlin RE, Gale RP: The early complications of bone marrow transplantation. Semin Hematol 21:101–108, 1984

131. Sullivan KM, Deeg HJ, Sanders JE et al: Late complications after marrow transplantation. Semin Hematol 21:53–63, 1984

132. Talpaz M, Kantarjian HM McCredie K et al: Hematologic remission and cytogenetic improvement induced by recombinant human inteferon alpha in chronic myelogenous leukemia. N Engl J Med 314:1065–1069, 1986

133. Aglietta M, Piacibello W, Stacchini A et al: Effect of interferon gamma (IFN) on HLA class II antigens and on sensitivity to prostaglandin E by normal and chronic myeloid leukemia progenitors (abstr). Exp Hematol 14:462, 1986

134. Brodsky I: Speculations on the treatment and pathophysiology of polycythemia vera and chronic myelogenous leukemia. Cancer Invest 4:281–285, 1986

135. Yoffe G, Blick M, Gutterman J et al: Molecular and cytogentic evidence for complete suppression of Philadelphia chromosome in a patient treated with alpha interferon (abstr). Exp Hematol 14:462, 1986

136. Silver RT, Reich SD, Coleman M et al: Gamma interferon (IFN) has activity in treating chronic myeloid leukemia (CML) (abstr). Blood 68 (Suppl 1):808, 1986

137. Arlin ZA, Mertelsmann R, Berman E et al: 13 cis-retinoic acid does not

increase the true remission rate and the duration of true remission (induced by cytotoxic chemotherapy) in patients with chronic phase chronic myelogenous leukemia. J Clin Oncol 3:473–476, 1985

138. Hardisty RM, Speed DE, Till M: Granulocytic leukaemia in childhood. Br J Haematol 10:551–566, 1964

139. Smith KL, Johnson W: Classification of chronic myelocytic leukemia in children. Cancer 34:670–679, 1974

140. Altman AJ, Palmer CG, Baehner RL: Juvenile "chronic granulocytic" leukemia: A panmyelopathy with prominent monocyte involvement and circulating monocyte colony-forming cells. Blood 43:341–350, 1974

141. Bader JL, Miller RM: Neurofibromatosis and childhood leukemia. J Pediatr 92:925–929, 1978

142. Mays JA, Neerhout RC, Bagby GC, Koler RD: Juvenile chronic granulocytic leukemia. Emphasis on cutaneous manifestation and underlying neurofibromatosis. Am J Dis Child 134:654–658, 1980

143. Palmer CG, Provisor AJ, Weaver DD et al: Juvenile chronic granulocytic leukemia in a patient with trisomy 8, neurofibromatosis, and prolonged Epstein-Barr virus infection. J Pediatr 102:888–892, 1983

144. Herrod HG, Dow LW, Sullivan JL: Persistent Epstein-Barr infection mimicking juvenile chronic myelogenous leukemia: Immunologic and hematologic studies. Blood 61:1098–1104, 1983

145. Shannon K, Nunez G, Dow LW et al: Juvenile chronic myelogenous leukemia: surface antigen phenotyping by monoclonal antibodies and cytogenetic studies. Pediatrics 77:330–335, 1986

146. Estrov Z, Grunberger T, Chan HSL, Freedman MH: Juvenile chronic myelogenous leukemia: Characteristics of the disease using cell cultures. Blood 67:1382–1387, 1986

147. Suda T, Miura Y, Mizoguchi H et al: Characterization of hemopoietic precursor cells in juvenile-type chronic myelocytic leukemia. Leuk Res 6:43–53, 1982

148. Maurer HC, Vida LN, Honig GR: Similarities of the erythrocytes in juvenile chronic myelogenous leukemia to fetal erythrocytes. Blood 39:778–784, 1972

149. Travis SF: Fetal erythropoiesis in juvenile chronic myelocytic leukemia. Blood 62:602–605, 1983

150. Cannat A, Seligmann M: Immunological abnormalities in juvenile myelomonocytic leukaemia. Br Med J 1:71–74, 1973

151. Ghione F, Merucci C, Symann M: Cytogenetic investigation in childhood chronic myelocytic leukemia. Cancer Genet Cytogenet 20:317–323, 1986

152. Hoffman R, Zanjani ED: Erythropoietin dependent erythropoiesis during the erythroblastic phase of juvenile chronic granulocytic leukaemia. Br J Haematol 38:511–516, 1978

153. Lilleyman JS, Harrison JF, Black JA: Treatment of juvenile chronic myeloid leukemia with sequential subcutaneous cytarabine and oral mercaptopurine. Blood 49:559–562, 1977

154. Chan HS, Estrov Z, Weitzman SS, Freedman MH: The value of intensive combination chemotherapy for juvenile chronic myelogenous leukemia. J Clin Oncol 5:1960–1967, 1987

155. Sanders JE, Buckner CD, Stewart P, Thomas ED: Successful treatment of juvenile chronic granulocytic leukemia with marrow transplantation. Pediatrics 63:44–46, 1979

156. Holton CP, Johnson WW: Chronic myelocytic leukemia in infant siblings. J Pediatr 72:377–383, 1968

157. Castro-Malaspina H, Schaison G, Passe S et al: Subacute and chronic myelomonocytic leukemia in children (juvenile CML). Clinical and hematologic observations, and identification of prognostic factors. Cancer 54:675–686, 1984

158. Thomas WJ, North RB, Poplack DG et al: Chronic myelomonocytic leukemia in childhood. Am J Hematol 10:181–194, 1981

159. Stockley RJ, Eden OB: Chronic myelomonocytic leukaemia in infancy: A case report. Med Pediatr Oncol 11:284–286, 1983

160. Weisgerber G, Schaison G, Chavelet F et al: Les leucemies myelo-monocytaires de l'enfant. Arch Fr Pediatr 29:11–30, 1972

161. Solal-Celigny P, Desaint B, Herrara A et al: Chronic myelomonocytic leukemia according to FAB classification; analysis of 35 cases. Blood 63:634–638, 1984

162. Pearson HA, Diamond LK: Chronic monocytic leukemia in childhood. J Pediatr 53:259–270, 1958

163. Orchard NP: Letterer-Siwe's syndrome: Report of a case with unusual peripheral blood changes. Arch Dis Child 25:151, 1950

164. Sonnier JA, Buchanan GR, Howard-Peebles PN et al: Chromosomal translocation involving the immunoglobulin kappa-chain and heavy-chain loci in a child with chronic lymphocytic leukemia. N Engl J Med 309:590–594, 1983

165. Rewald R, Estevez ME, Sen L: Monoclonal B-cell lymphocytosis in early childhood. A case report. Am J Pediatr Hematol Oncol 7:331–335, 1985

166. Sardemann H: Chronic lymphocytic leukemia in an infant. Acta Paediat Scand 61:213–216, 1972

167. Behm FL, McWilliams NB, Westin EH, Trench G: Chronic lymphocytic leukemia in a child (abstr 883). Proc APS/SPR 19:258A, 1985

168. Casey TP: Chronic lymphocytic leukaemia in a child presenting at the age of two years and eight months. Aust Ann Med 17:70–74, 1968

169. Darte JMM, McClure PD, Saunders EF et al: Congenital lymphoid hyperplasia with persistent hyperlymphocytosis. N Engl J Med 284:431–432, 1971

170. Holowach J: Chronic lymphoid leukemia in children. J Pediatr 32:84–86, 1948

171. Gahrton G, Robert K-H: Chromosomal aberrations in chronic B-cell lymphocytic leukemia. Cancer Genet Cytogenet 6:171–181, 1982

172. Han T, Ozer H, Sadamori H et al: Cytogenetic abnormalities in chronic lymphocytic leukemia (CLL): A clinical correlation (abstr). Blood 60 (Suppl 1):127a, 1982

nineteen

Myeloproliferative and Myelodysplastic Syndromes

Cindy L. Schwartz and
Harvey J. Cohen

BASIC BIOLOGICAL CONSIDERATIONS

The myeloproliferative and myelodysplastic syndromes are hematologic disorders of the myeloid cells. Their hallmarks are excessive proliferation or abnormal maturation, respectively, with a variable tendency for evolution to acute nonlymphocytic leukemia. These disorders, while uncommon in children, may be of prime importance in unraveling the mechanisms by which hematopoietic disturbances can result in leukemia. Proliferation and differentiation are the essential mechanisms by which multipotential hematopoietic stem cells produce mature functional blood cells. In this section, hematopoiesis and leukemogenesis are reviewed with an emphasis on biological mechanisms that result in proliferation and differentiation, myeloproliferative syndromes (MPS) and myelodysplastic syndromes (MDS).

Normal Hematopoiesis

There are several models of hematopoiesis. All agree that multipotential hematologic stem cells carry the genetic information of all possible hematologic progeny. Stem cells can either self-renew or become committed multipotent stem cells (myeloid or lymphoid), which then undergo progressive restriction of lineage potential from oligopotent (two or three lineages) to unilineage and finally to mature blood cells (Fig. 19-1).[1] Erythrocytes, platelets, granulocytes, eosinophils, basophils, and monocytes are considered myeloid cells, produced by a myeloid stem cell. Proliferation (expansion of a population) must be coupled with differentiation (progressive maturation of cells), resulting in appropriate numbers of all hematopoietic cells with maintenance of a stem cell pool.

The likelihood that a cell will develop along a particular genetic program may be determined by stochastic processes[2] or by environmental stimuli.[3,4] The stochastic model assumes that division of hematopoietic cells is an entirely random event that may result in self-replication or in maturation in any of a variety of differentiation pathways. The environmental model suggests that growth factors and cell–cell interactions affect the differentiation pathway of a given cell. A theory encompassing the stochastic model of hematopoiesis and the apparent effect of regulatory factors has been suggested.[5] In this model, differentiation occurs as in the stochastic model. Environmental stimuli affect the proliferation of specific multilineage or unilineage cells. Thus, an erythroid stimulus would result in preferential proliferation of those cells that, by random events, had become erythroid. A growth factor affecting multilineage progenitors would cause proliferation of a multipotent stem cell and thereby increase the entire hematopoietic pool.

Protein growth factors have been identified that appear to be stimuli for hematopoietic cells. Interleukin-3 (IL-3) is a multilineage hematopoietic growth factor that stimulates proliferation of erythroid cells, megakaryocytes, neutrophils, macrophages, and mast cells.[6] Granulocyte-macrophage, macrophage, and granulocyte colony-stimulating factors (GM-CSF, M-CSF, and G-CSF) support the growth of their respective committed progenitors.[7,8] G-CSF has also been called a differentiation-inducing factor because it appears to induce terminal differentiation of myeloid leukemia cells.[8] It is unclear whether differentiation-inducing factors exist in normal hematopoiesis.

Stromal cells are known to produce growth factors such as GM-CSF, erythroid burst-promoting activity (BPA), and megakaryocyte-CSF (Mg-CSF) when stimulated by monocytes.[9,10] Extramedullary hormones such as erythropoietin (renal production)[11] add to the regulatory control of hematopoiesis (see also Chap. 14).

Evidence is mounting that growth factors initiate a cascade of cellular events that result in regulatory control of the hematopoietic cell.[12,13] Proteins encoded for by a variety of cellular oncogenes enable this cascade to proceed (Table 19-1). Four classes of such oncogene products have been described (see also Chap. 3). The first class codes for the growth factors themselves. For example, the peptides of platelet-derived growth factor (PDGF), which causes fibroblasts to proliferate,[14] have a protein sequence similar to P28^{sis}, the gene product of the transformed simian sarcoma virus (SSV) oncogene, v-sis.[15,16] The comparable cellular oncogene is c-sis. A second class codes for protein kinases, most of which have specificity for tyrosine residues and serve as intracellular signals. These oncogene products are located in the plasma membrane or cytoplasm. Some also appear to be growth factor receptors. For example, c-fms encodes the receptor for M-CSF.[17] It probably spans the plasma membrane, with an external receptor and an internal tyrosine kinase domain that functions as an intracellular signal to nuclear regulatory proteins. Another tyrosine kinase located in the cytoplasm is produced by the c-fes onco-

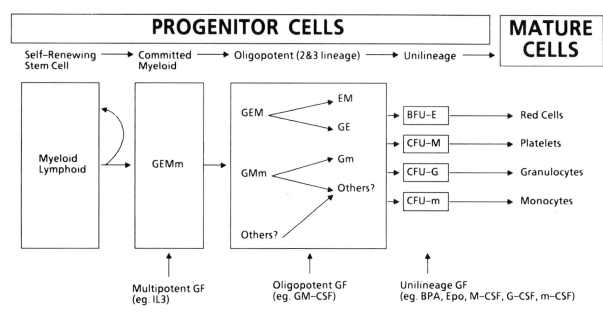

FIGURE 19-1. Schema of hematopoiesis showing progressive restriction of lineage potential, with progenitor cells replicating and producing more differentiated cells. Growth factors that affect proliferation of progenitors are shown. (Based on data from Refs. 1–11.) G = granulocyte; E = erythroid; M = megakaryocyte; m = monocyte; GF = growth factor; BFU-E = erythroid burst forming unit; CFU = colony forming unit.

Table 19-1
Oncogenic Proteins and the Regulation of Hematopoiesis

Class of Protein	Oncogene (Chromosome No.)	Location	Cascade Function*
I. Growth factors	c-sis (22)	Secreted	Growth factor (PDGF)
II. Protein kinase	c-fms (5)	Transmembrane	Receptor/IS† (M-CSF receptor)
	c-abl (9)	Plasma membrane	Receptor/IS
	c-fes (15)	Cytoplasm	IS† (cellular response to GM-CSF)
III. GTP binding protein	c-ras^H (11)	Inner plasma membrane	Intracellular signal
	c-ras^k (12)		Intracellular signal
IV. Nuclear proteins	c-fos (2)	Nucleus	Affect DNA (differentiation)
	c-myc (8)	Nucleus	Affect DNA (proliferation)
	c-myb (6)	Nucleus	Affect DNA (proliferation)

* Oncogenic cascade: growth factor → receptor → intracellular signal → affect DNA synthesis.
† IS = intracellular signal.

gene and appears to play a role in cellular responsiveness to GM-CSF.[18] The *ras* genes (H-*ras* and K-*ras*) code for GTP binding proteins that may also be intracellular signals affecting cell regulation. Expression of *ras* genes is increased in many hematopoietic malignancies.[12,19] Oncogene products of the fourth class are located in the nucleus and include c-*myc*, c-*myb*, and c-*fos*. c-*fos* increases transiently before differentiation of cells, followed by increased n-*myc* expression. It has been proposed that c-*fos* is associated with differentiation, particularly of monocytes and macrophages, whereas n-*myc* is associated with proliferation and increased DNA synthesis.[20,21] Thus, several proteins produced by normal cellular oncogenes appear to function in hematopoietic control. Abnormalities in any of these oncogenes may result in abnormal hematopoiesis.

Abnormal Hematopoiesis

If hematopoietic regulation is under genetic control, aberrant hematopoiesis may occur with chromosomal disturbances. Aberrant growth factors or receptors for growth factors may be produced. An abnormal tyrosine kinase has been noted when c-*abl* translocates to chromosome 22 in chronic myelogenous leukemia (CML)(see Chap. 18).[22] This may cause an abnormal responsiveness to growth factors, thus affecting proliferation or differentiation. In patients with the 5q− syndrome who have refractory anemia, myeloid hyperplasia, abnormal thrombopoiesis, and thrombocytosis, the M-CSF receptor, c-*fms* (located on the deleted portion of chromosome 5), is hemizygous, probably accounting for the regulatory abnormality.

Abnormal proteins may also be excreted by abnormal hematopoietic or stromal cells, affecting adjacent karyotypically normal cells. When medium conditioned by the growth of a murine myelomonocytic cell line (WEHI-3) is added to long-term normal marrow cultures, phenotypic changes are seen in the karyotypically normal cells. These cells are then indistinguishable from WEHI-3 cells. This may be due to the effect of an abnormal differentiating factor.[23] Such factors may cause the dysmyelopoiesis of karyotypically normal cells in the myelodysplastic syndromes and may enhance the ability of an abnormal clone to establish predominance.

Abnormalities in growth factors and differentiating factors, or abnormalities of the receptors or intracellular signals, may play a major role in the development of the myeloproliferative and myelodysplastic syndromes and their evolution into acute nonlymphoblastic leukemia (ANLL).

Leukemogenesis

It appears likely that a two-step process results in malignancies such as retinoblastoma and Wilms' tumor.[24] Sachs has suggested that uncoupling of pathways of gene expression controlling growth and differentiation results in leukemia.[25] Myeloproliferative and myelodysplastic syndromes may represent a first step, in which either proliferation or differentiation of a myeloid stem cell becomes aberrant. Leukemia affecting myeloid cells arises when a second event results in aberrance of both pathways, such that an immature cell proliferates excessively. This may occur by an additional genetic change in an already abnormal cell, perhaps one that produces a change in proliferation in the myelodysplastic syndrome or a change in differentiation in myeloproliferative disorders. Genetic changes, such as amplification of c-*abl* in CML during blast crisis[26] with emergence of the new immature cell line, have been noted.

In susceptible mice, Friend leukemia virus (FLV) causes a hemolytic anemia followed by erythroleukemia. This two-step event has recently been shown to be under the influence of two separate genomic regions.[27] However, increased erythropoiesis does appear to set the stage, in that stimulation of erythropoiesis by a hemolytic agent results in a more rapid onset of erythroleukemia.[28] An initial hematologic abnormality may thus set up conditions that favor the emergence of an abnormal, leukemic clone.

An example of a disorder in which an abnormal cell may affect the environment, giving a proliferative advantage to the cell itself or to another abnormal clone, is juvenile chronic myelogenous leukemia, in which monocytic cells secrete an inhibitor of normal hematopoiesis.[29] Whether the leukemias that arise in the myeloproliferative and myelodysplastic syndromes are genetically "preprogrammed" at the time of onset of the hematologic disturbance (as in FLV), or arise as a random event, possibly influenced by the use of mutagenic therapies, is unclear.

The hematopoietic disturbances of the individual myeloproliferative and myelodysplastic syndromes can be considered in terms of these biological events. The unique characteristics of each disorder reflect the particular abnormality involved, whereas their similarities may result from more generalized effects of hematopoietic responses. The biology and clinical features of these disorders and the likelihood of their evolution to leukemia are described in the following sections.

MYELOPROLIFERATIVE SYNDROMES

In 1951, Dameshek suggested that CML, polycythemia vera, essential thrombocythemia, and agnogenic myeloid metaplasia/myelofibrosis were not "pure" proliferations of granulocytes, erythrocytes, platelets, and fibroblasts, respectively, but somewhat variable manifestations of the proliferative activity of bone marrow cells, "perhaps due to a hitherto undiscovered stimulus."[30] He labeled them the "myeloproliferative syndromes" collectively and noted that, to varying degrees, stimulation of all hematopoietic cells was seen in these disorders. He hypothesized that this might be due to a "myelostimulatory principle."[30]

Current knowledge, both clinical and laboratory, confirms the logic of examining these disease entities jointly. During the course of their illness, patients with one MPS may have symptoms classically associated with another.[31] This is particularly true for polycythemia vera, essential thrombocythemia, and agnogenic myeloid metaplasia/myelofibrosis, which have the greatest morphologic similarity,[32,33] reflected in hyperplasia of all lineage cells, particularly megakaryocytes.[34] Abnormality of a multipotent myeloid stem cell is etiologic in all of these syndromes, resulting in many common clinical and laboratory features (Fig. 19-2). These three syndromes are discussed here, as is the myeloproliferative syndrome of trisomy 21; CML is discussed in Chapter 18.

Polycythemia Vera

Definition and Epidemiology

Polycythemia vera (PV) is a primary MPS involving a pluripotential stem cell.[35] It is characterized by erythrocytosis with varying degrees of thrombocytosis, leukocytosis, and splenomegaly. The incidence has been reported to be 0.6 to 1.8 per 100,000.[36,37] The median age of affected patients is 60 years, with only 0.1% younger than 20.[38] Fewer than 20 pediatric

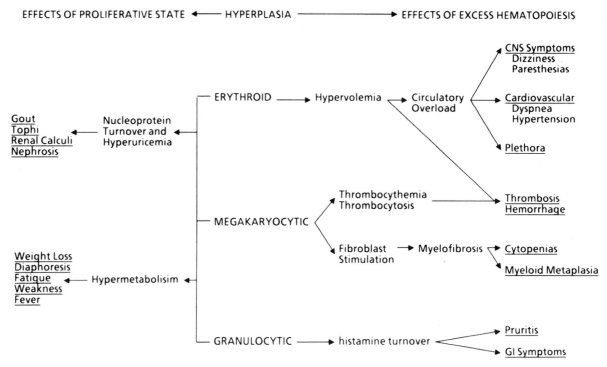

FIGURE 19-2. Schema of the pathophysiology of the myeloproliferative syndrome, showing clinical symptomatology that can be attributed to effects of the increased proliferation and hematopoiesis.

cases have been reported, and some are not clearly primary polycythemias.[39–46]

Biology and Genetics

The clonal nature of PV was demonstrated by Adamson and colleagues in a female heterozygons for glucose-6-phosphate dehydrogenase (G6PD) in whom multilineage hematopoietic cells expressed only one G6PD isoenzyme.[35] Clonal chromosomal abnormalities, including trisomies 8 and 9 or aberrations of chromosomes 1, 5, or 20, are seen in 10% to 25% of patients at diagnosis and 25% to 40% of previously treated patients. This may reflect either a natural progression of a clonal abnormality or a tendency for treatment to increase the chromosomal abnormality. Complex cytogenetic abnormalities are almost universal if leukemic transformation occurs and may be similar to those of chemotherapy-related acute myelogenous leukemia (particularly the deletions of all or parts of chromosomes 5 and 20).[47,48] Reports of a familial incidence of PV suggest that a genetic predisposition may exist.[49–52]

Marrow colony-forming assays have shown that multipotent myeloid progenitor cells (CFU-GEMM) and erythroid progenitor burst-forming units (BFU-E) in PV respond to erythropoietin with a greater proliferative response than that of normal controls. The use of antierythropoietin antibody prevents colony formation in normal controls and decreases but does not entirely prevent colony formation in patients with PV.[53–56] This increased proliferative response may allow the abnormal cells to become the dominant clone. The proportion of normal progenitors decreases over time in a given patient.[57]

Pathogenesis and Natural History

PV has many manifestations that can be attributed to the abnormal proliferation and function of erythrocytes, granulo-cytes, and platelets (see Fig. 19-2). Erythrocytosis with hypervolemia, thrombocytosis with abnormal platelet function, disturbed cerebral circulation, pruritis, hypermetabolic symptoms, hyperuricemia, myelofibrosis, extramedullary hematopoiesis, and hypersplenism occur.[58] The course of the disease can be divided into the proliferative, stable, and spent phases. Most patients are diagnosed in the proliferative phase, in which excessive erythrocytosis occurs, with varying degrees of thrombocytosis and granulocytosis. During this phase, thrombohemorrhagic events are of greatest concern. Serious complications noted in children include hypersplenism, splenic infarction, hypertension, strokes, hemorrhage, and coagulation abnormalities.[39] A significant minority progress to the stable phase, during which blood counts normalize without therapy. This is believed to result from some degree of marrow fibrosis. Many patients ultimately enter the spent phase, or postpolycythemic myeloid metaplasia (PPMM), characterized by extensive marrow fibrosis with hepatosplenomegaly. Peripheral cytopenias then become the major clinical problems.[59] Leukemia may develop at any time in the disease course but is most common in the spent phase.[60,61]

Clinical Presentation

The most common presenting symptoms of PV in adults are headache (48% of patients), weakness (47%), pruritis (43%), and dizziness (43%). Splenomegaly (70%), plethora (67%), conjunctival plethora (59%), engorged retinal veins (46%), and a palpable liver (40%) are common physical findings. (Table 19-2).[38] Manifestations of the disease are similar in children. In one review, 12 of 31 patients aged 13 to 40 at diagnosis of PV had severe thromboembolic episodes before beginning therapy.[62] Cerebral thrombosis, hepatic and portal vein thrombosis, and splenic infarction are most commonly noted.

Table 19-2
*Clinical Features of the Myeloproliferative Syndromes**

	Syndrome				
	PV	*ET*	*AMMM*	*AMF*	*C-AMF*
Symptoms					
Weight loss	+	−	+	++	++
Weakness/malaise	++	++	++	+++	+++
Fever	−	−	+	++	++
CNS (headache, dizziness, visual, paresthesia)	++	++	−	−	−
Thrombosis	+	+	−	−	−
Hemorrhage	+	++	+	++	++
Pruritis	++	+	−	−	−
Physical/Laboratory					
Circulatory overload					
Plethora	++	−	−	−	−
Hypertension	++	−	−	−	−
Hepatomegaly	++	+	++	+	+++
Splenomegaly	+++	++	+++	−	+++
Myelofibrosis	+§	−	+++	+++	+++
Osteosclerosis	−	−	++	−	−
Cytopenia	+§	−	+	+++	+++
Hypruricemia	++	++	+	−	−

* Symbols: + = 5%–35% of patients; ++ = 35%–70%; +++ = 70%–100%; − = not reported as a feature, or <5% of patients.
§ In spent phase.

Laboratory abnormalities include an elevated erythrocyte volume (>36 ml/kg in adult males; >32 ml/kg in females) in all patients (by definition), a leukocyte count > 12,000 in half, and a platelet count > 400,000 in two thirds. Leukocyte alkaline phosphatase (LAP) is increased in 70%, vitamin B_{12} in 30%, and uric acid in >50% of adult patients.[38] Laboratory findings in children are similar. The blood smear is notable for increased numbers of erythrocytes, and often for increased numbers of platelets and leukocytes (Fig. 19-3A). Bone marrow biopsy at diagnosis shows hyperplasia of erythroid, granulocytic, and megakaryocytic elements. Stainable iron is absent. A mild to moderate increase in reticulin fibers was found in 11% of pretreatment specimens of 226 Polycythemia Vera Study Group (PVSG) patients, but was not indicative of imminent PPMM.[61]

Differential Diagnosis

PV, in which erythopoietin is not increased, must be differentiated from secondary polycythemia, in which erythropoietin is increased either appropriately (when there is decreased tissue oxygenation) or inappropriately (when tissue oxygenation is normal). Also to be differentiated is relative polycythemia, in which the hematocrit is elevated because of decreased plasma volume, but erythrocyte mass is normal (Table 19-3). Splenomegaly is common only in PV. PV, secondary polycythemia, and relative polycythemia can be differentiated in most patients by history, physical examination, measurement of total erythrocyte mass with radioactively labeled erythrocytes, arterial blood oxygen saturation (Pao_2), measurement of oxygen pressure at which hemoglobin is 50% saturated, and an intravenous pyelogram or an ultrasonogram to rule out renal disease. The PVSG has required an abnormal erythrocyte volume (>36 ml/kg in males; >32 ml/kg in females), Pao_2 > 92%, and

splenomegaly or, in the absence of splenomegaly, two of the following: thrombocytosis (platelets > 400,000/mm³), leukocytosis (>12,000/mm³), elevated LAP, or elevated serum B_{12} or unbound B_{12} binding capacity. Urinary erythropoietin can be determined when the differential diagnosis remains unclear; it will be low in PV and high in secondary polycythemia.[38]

Prognosis and Treatment

Treatment with phlebotomy, myelosuppressive agents or both has produced median survivals of 9 to 14 years. During the proliferative phase, therapy attempts to decrease the incidence of thrombohemorrhagic phenomena. The PVSG performed a randomized study comparing phlebotomy versus radioactive phorphorus (^{32}P) versus chlorambucil.[63] Fatality rates were similar early in the study, although thrombosis-related events were more common in phlebotomy-treated patients. Chlorambucil-treated patients had the highest incidence of acute leukemia, lymphocytic lymphomas, and skin and gastrointestinal (GI) carcinoma, particularly after the fifth year. Phosphorus-32-treated patients were also at increased risk of developing leukemia, although onset was somewhat later. Overall, thrombosis accounted for 31% of deaths, acute leukemia for 19%, other neoplasms for 15%, and hemorrhage and the spent phase for 5% each. In another study, anticoagulation with aspirin or dipyrimadole increased the incidence of hemorrhage without decreasing the incidence of thrombosis.[64]

Hydroxyurea, a nonalkylating myelosuppressive agent, has recently been used because it may not induce cancer. Preliminary results suggest that control of thrombosis is better with hydroxyurea than with phlebotomy alone, but it is too early to assess the likelihood that patients will develop leukemia.[65] The incidence of acute leukemia is increased even in

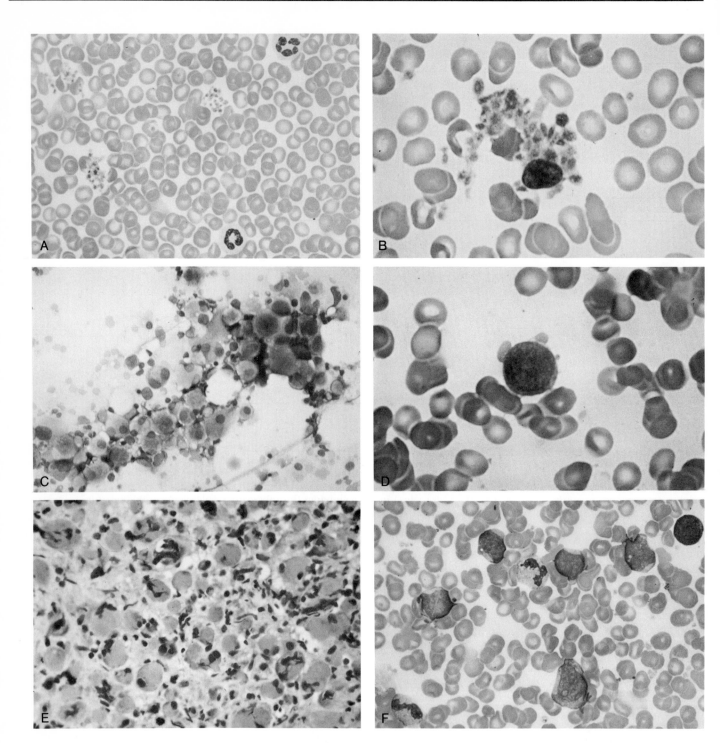

FIGURE 19-3. Myeloproliferative syndromes. (**A**) PV (blood)—increased numbers of erythrocytes (no thinner areas present) and increased numbers of platelets, forming clumps (×200). (**B**) ET (blood)—increased numbers of platelets resulting in platelet clumps; a megakaryocyte fragment is seen (×400). (**C**) ET (marrow aspirate)—increased numbers of small, hypolobulated megakaryocytes (×80). (**D**) C-AMF (marrow biopsy)—cellular specimen consisting of an abnormal megakaryocytic proliferation (×125). (**E**) C-AMF (marrow aspirate)—hypocellular specimen with an abnormal micromegakaryoblast with blue, budding cytoplasm (often confused with lymphoblasts) (×400) (**F**) neonatal myeloproliferative syndrome of trisomy 21 (blood)—leukocytosis with numerous myeloblasts (×200). (Photomicrographs of blood and marrow kindly provided by J. Schaffer, Division of Hematology, University of Rochester Medical Center.)

Table 19-3
Features of Primary and Secondary Polycythemia

Primary (normal erythropoietin)
    Polycythemia vera
Secondary (increased erythropoietin)
    Appropriate response to decreased tissue oxygenation
        High altitude
        Right-to-left cardiac shunt
        Pulmonary disease
        High oxygen affinity hemoglobinopathy
        Congenital decreased erythrocyte DPG
        Pickwickian syndrome
    Inappropriate response to normal tissue oxygenation
        Tumors
        Renal abnormalities
Relative (decreased plasma volume, normal erythrocyte
      mass)

patients treated by phlebotomy alone, so it is unlikely that hydroxyurea will entirely prevent this complication.

Current recommendations suggest phlebotomy alone for young patients because thrombotic events are less likely in the young, whereas the risk of leukemia over a long life span may be significant. If the phlebotomy requirement is high or there is a history of thrombotic events, hydroxyurea is recommended.[63]

Essential Thrombocythemia

Definition and Epidemiology

Essential thrombocythemia (ET) is a myeloproliferative syndrome characterized by persistent thrombocytosis for which no etiology can be determined. It is considered to be a disorder of adulthood (median age = 61; range, 21–84 in the PVSG),[66] with few well-documented and described cases in children.[67,68] However, a more recent study reviewing all patients in one hospital found that 13 of 94 patients with ET (14%) were younger than 20.[69] This group also found the distribution to be bimodal, with a major peak in older adults and a second one for younger women (approximately 30 years).

Biology and Genetics

Several studies of G6PD isoenzymes have suggested that ET is a clonal disorder with multilineage involvement.[70–72] Myeloid cells from approximately 5% of patients have detectable chromosomal abnormalities initially. Some have developed chromosomal abnormalities later, at the time of transformation to acute leukemia.[69,73] A 21q− abnormality in ET has been described.[74,75] The PVSG did not find this abnormality, but 21% of patients had aneuploidy in their myeloid cells and 1 of 37 had an abnormal myeloid clone.[66] A familial form of ET with an autosomal dominant mode of inheritance has also been reported.[76] The patients with this genetic disorder were asymptomatic despite laboratory evidence of platelet dysfunction. A genetically determined, nonclonal abnormality of regulation was hypothesized to be responsible for this form of ET.

Pathogenesis and Natural History

As long as ET remains a diagnosis of exclusion, it will be difficult to adequately describe its pathogenesis. Because thrombocytosis is the hallmark of the disease, platelet function has been studied most frequently. Results are often contradictory, perhaps because patients have been analyzed as a group, with no distinction based on presence or absence of thrombohemorrhagic events. Spontaneous platelet aggregation occurred in four of five patients with thrombosis but in none of eight without thrombosis.[77] Studies have shown that platelets from many, but not all, patients with ET demonstrate decreased platelet aggregability to epinephrine (19 of 32 patients), adenosine 5′-diphosphate (ADP) (21 of 69), collagen (7 of 73), or ADP + collagen (35 of 64).[69,78–80] Two patients with decreased aggregability to epinephrine were found to have a decreased number of adrenergic receptors.[79] Decreased activation of adenylate cyclase by prostaglandin D_2 (PGD_2) found in some patients suggests that PGD_2 receptors may be decreased.[81] This observation may explain the tendency for thrombosis, since adenylate cyclase activation normally inhibits platelet aggregation.

Many of these platelet studies were also performed in patients with PV and produced similar results. Morphologically, the megakaryocytes appear identical in PV and ET. Several patients with ET have later demonstrated an increased erythrocyte mass. This tendency for erythrocytosis may have been masked by hemorrhage or iron deficiency at diagnosis.[66] The cause of preferential megakaryopoiesis in ET is unclear.

The natural course of ET is highly variable. Some patients, particularly those who are younger, have been followed for long periods of time without complications.[82] Morbidity and mortality are primarily due to thrombosis or hemorrhage, with rare instances of leukemic conversion.

Clinical Presentation

Many patients are asymptomatic, and ET is found by blood counts obtained for an unrelated problem. Approximately one third of patients present with thrombohemorrhagic events.[69] Thrombotic events suggesting transient cerebral ischemia include weakness, headache, paresthesia, dizziness, and visual phenomena. Peripheral vascular ischemia may cause toe and fingertip thrombosis, sometimes requiring amputation. Venous thrombosis, manifested as deep vein thrombosis or priapism, may occur. Pruritis, splenomegaly, and hepatomegaly are less severe and less frequent in ET than in PV. Results of laboratory studies overlap with PV, with elevations seen in leukocyte counts, LAP scores, vitamin B_{12}, urate, and cholesterol.[66,69] The blood smear is remarkable only for the presence of clumps of platelets (Fig. 19-3B); megakaryocytic hyperplasia is found in the marrow (Fig. 19-3C).

The few well-described cases of ET in children tend to involve thromboembolic phenomena, mild to moderate splenomegaly, and mild hepatomegaly. These complications are similar to those in adults but occur more frequently. A significant bias may exist, such that only those children with severe complications of ET may be diagnosed and reported.

Differential Diagnosis

Many causes of thrombocytosis exist in childhood (Table 19-4).[83] Until unique biological features are determined, ET will be a diagnosis of exclusion. The other myeloproliferative disorders must be excluded by criteria such as those suggested by the PVSG. Criteria for the diagnosis of ET include platelet count > 600,000; normal erythrocyte mass; stainable iron in the marrow or failure of an iron trial to increase erythrocyte mass; absence of the Philadelphia chromosome; absence of marrow fibrosis or, in a patient without splenomegaly or leukoerythro-

Table 19-4
Thrombocytosis in Childhood

Primary
   Myeloproliferative syndromes
   Acute megakaryoblastic leukemia
Secondary
   Inflammatory/immune
      Infection: Acute—recovery phase
                    Chronic—osteomyelitis, tuberculosis
      Mucocutaneous lymph node syndrome
      Inflammatory bowel syndrome
      Collagen-vascular disorders
      Nephrotic syndrome
      Sarcoid
      Graft versus host disease
      Caffey's disease
   Asplenia
   Anemia
      Iron deficiency
      Vitamin E deficiency
      Megaloblastic anemia
      Hemolytic anemia
   Drugs
      Epinephrine
      Corticosteroids
      Vinka alkaloids
      Citrovorum factor
   Neoplasia
      Lymphomas
      Neuroblastoma
      Carcinoma
      Histiocytosis
   Miscellaneous
      Hemorrhage
      Surgery
      Trauma
      Thrombosis (pulmonary embolism, thrombophlebitis,
         cerebrovascular accident)
      Hyperadrenalism

(Modified from Addiego and coworkers[83])

blastosis, less than one third of biopsy area showing fibrosis; and no known cause of reactive thrombocytosis.[66]

Prognosis and Treatment

In both adults and children, ET appears to have a better prognosis than the other myeloproliferative syndromes. Of the ten children noted earlier, only one, who had been treated with ^{32}P, died after a leukemic conversion[67,84]; one child developed idiopathic myelofibrosis.[85] In adults, the probability of surviving longer than 100 months has been calculated to be 0.8.[69] Five of 94 patients in one study had a leukemic conversion 32 to 192 months after diagnosis.[69] All five had received therapy for their disease (two with hydroxyurea only, and three with melphalan or ^{32}P).

A variety of myelosuppressive agents have been used to treat ET. The PVSG patients with platelet counts > 1 million were treated with melphalan or [32]P. Response rates were greater and response was more rapid with melphalan. Because of the high incidence of leukemia in PV patients receiving ^{32}P or chlorambucil, clinical trials using hydroxyurea are now being performed.[66] Prostaglandin inhibitors have been used but may cause a higher incidence of hemorrhage.[86]

Children with ET appear to have a more benign course than adults,[82] perhaps because they tolerate thrombocytosis of any etiology better. Since alkylating agents and radiation may increase the likelihood of leukemic transformation, these treatments are not recommended for asymptomatic children. Hydroxyurea should be considered for children who have had thrombotic episodes or hemorrhage.

Idiopathic Myelofibrosis

Definition and Epidemiology

Idiopathic myelofibrosis (IMF; fibrosis of the marrow) was originally thought by Dameshek to be a manifestation of marrow proliferation, primarily involving fibroblasts.[30] He considered the possibility that this actually represented a peculiar leukemia, perhaps of megakaryoblastic origin. The clinical similarity to phases of PV and CML was noted, resulting in classification of IMF as a myeloproliferative syndrome.

Since that time, two forms of IMF have been described in adults: agnogenic myeloid metaplasia and myelofibrosis (AMMM) and acute myelofibrosis (AMF). AMMM was described in detail by Ward and Block as a syndrome of myelofibrosis and extramedullary hematopoiesis (myeloid metaplasia) that occurs in patients who are symptomatic for approximately 5½ years before diagnosis at an average age of 61 years.[32] The peripheral blood smears show poikilocytosis, teardrops, nucleated erythrocytes, and blasts. Osteosclerosis is common (40%). The onset is insidious and survival is prolonged in many patients (median = 10.6 years from onset).[32] AMF, as first described by Lewis and Szur, has a rapidly fatal course with the following features: marrow fibrosis with bizarre megakaryocytes and frequently unclassifiable blast cells, absence of myeloid metaplasia, and a rapidly progressive course with nonspecific symptoms of fatigue, weight loss, and dyspnea. Pancytopenia is common, and the morphology of the peripheral smear is unremarkable.[87]

IMF in children is usually different from both AMMM and AMF. Only one child has been described who appears to have had AMMM,[88] and another has been found to fit the criteria for AMF.[89] A number of children described in the literature have had a rapid course similar to AMF, but a leukoerythroblastic blood picture, myeloid metaplasia, or both were seen. This childhood form of AMF (C-AMF) has most frequently been described in young children (under 4 years), particularly in those with trisomy 21.[90-97]

Genetics

C-AMF is seen with increased frequency in Down's syndrome. Two children with Down's syndrome and C-AMF had chromosomal abnormalities in addition to their trisomy,[96] suggesting the possibility that genomic instability is a predisposing factor. It has been noted that patients with trisomy 21 have an inherent abnormality of thrombopoiesis.[98] Perhaps those oncogenes that regulate megakaryocytic differentiation and proliferation are affected by the extra chromosomal material and are more likely to undergo leukemic transformation. Megakaryoblastic leukemia and myelofibrosis have also been reported in a patient with Fanconi's anemia, another disorder with chromosomal instability.[99]

Myelofibrosis and myeloid metaplasia was diagnosed by Sieff and Malleson in two siblings with normal chromosomes at the ages of 7 and 8 weeks.[100] This may represent a constitutional genetic abnormality causing abnormal regulation of fibroblast or megakaryocyte proliferation.

Biology

Myelofibrosis is defined by the presence of reticulin, the silver-staining precollagen produced by fibroblasts. AMMM has been shown in a G6PD heterozygote to be a clonal disorder involving the granulocytes, erythrocytes, and platelets but not the marrow fibroblasts.[101] The fibroblastic proliferation thus appears to be a secondary phenomenon. A predominance of megakaryocytes, usually atypical, has been noted in the hematopoietic areas of fibrotic marrow.[32] The alpha granules of platelets and megakaryocytes contain PDGF, platelet factor 4 (PF4), and beta-thromboglobulin (BTG).[12,102,103] It has been proposed that PDGF, which is known to stimulate fibroblast growth, is released from the abnormal megakaryocytes or platelets, causing myelofibrosis. Sacchi and colleagues reported elevated plasma and decreased intraplatelet content of PF4 and BTG in AMMM, findings suggestive of excessive release of alpha granular proteins.[104]

AMMM does, on occasion, transform to acute myelocytic or myelomonocytic leukemia.[105-108] A man with a 17-year history of AMMM whose disease evolved into acute megakaryoblastic leukemia (AMgL) was recently reported.[109] The patient's blast cells showed a marked increase in expression of c-sis mRNA, which is known to code for one of the polypeptides of PDGF.[16] The authors proposed that activation of the c-sis gene may play a central role in the malignant evolution of myelofibrosis. Thus, AMMM may have been the first step in a two-step process of leukemogenesis.

Patients with AMF also have an increased number of abnormal megakaryocytes. Often, blasts are present that, by light microscopic appearance and ultrastructural demonstration of alpha granules and platelet peroxidase, appear to be megakaryoblasts. These findings suggest that AMF is actually AMgL.[90,110-112] The clinical courses of cases described as AMF and AMgL are similar. Both are characterized by pancytopenia associated with bone marrow fibrosis, absence of organomegaly, and a rapid course.

AMgL in children differs from that in adults in that both organomegaly and leukocytosis commonly occur.[113] These are the same features by which C-AMF usually differs from AMF Both AMgL and C-AMF are characterized by a proliferation of bizarre megakaryoblasts in the marrow, which is accompanied by myelofibrosis in C-AMF and some cases of AMgL. As shown in Table 19-5, many children with C-AMF, particularly those younger than 4 years, have Down's syndrome. Four of the 20 children with AMgL found in a recent literature review also had trisomy 21; they too were younger than 4 years.[113] Other reports of an association between AMgL and Down's syndrome exist.[114] The overlap of clinical symptomatology, marrow findings, and population at risk suggests that C-AMF may also be AMgL. In some instances, other myeloid cells may be involved in the leukemic proliferation. Chan and coworkers reviewed several cases of IMF in childhood and noted that many had courses consistent with AMgL.[115]

AMF and C-AMF appear to represent true leukemias rather than myeloproliferative syndromes. However the possibility of leukemic transformation of AMMM and the similarities in pathogenesis of these forms of IMF (AMMM, AMF, C-AMF) confirm the benefits of studying these disorders jointly in an attempt to better understand the leukemogenic process.

Table 19-5
*Children Described in the Literature as Having Idiopathic Myelofibrosis**

Reference (Case)	Age	Trisomy 21	↑L/S	LEB	Blasts	↑MKC	Comments	Probable Diagnosis
88	10 mo–10 yr	−	+	+	+	+	Alive at 120+ mo; blasts 105 mo	AMMM
89	4 yr	−	−	−	−	+		AMF
92 (1)	18 mo	+	+	+	+	+		C-AMF
92 (2)	22 mo	+	+	+	+	+		C-AMF
93 (1)	23 mo	+	+	?	+	+	Undifferentiated mononuclear cells	C-AMF
94	24 mo	+	+	+	+	+	Undifferentiated myeloblasts	C-AMF
95	12 mo	+	+	+	+	+	Myeloblasts	C-AMF
96 (1)	26 mo	+	+	+	+	+		C-AMF
96 (2)	27 mo	+	+	+	+	+	Peroxidase−; not lymphoblasts	C-AMF
93 (2)	13 mo	−	+	?	−	+	Varicella → death	C-AMF
97 (1)	16 yr	−	+	+	+	+	? Lymphs versus myeloblasts	C-AMF
123	8 yr	+	−	+	+	−		ALL
124 (2)	5 mo	−	−	+	+	−		ALL
125 (1)	5 yr	−	−	?	+	−		ALL
125 (2)	8 yr	−	+	?	+	−		ALL
125 (4)	5 yr	−	+	?	+	−		ALL
125 (5)	3 yr	−	+	?	+	−		ALL
131	3–8 yr	−	+	+	+	−	? Course similar to monosomy 7	AML
130	7½ mo	−	+	?	−	−		Rickets
132	9½ mo	+	+	+	−	−	Slight hypocalcemia, lamellar periostitis and sclerosis	? Metabolic bone disease
133	10 yr	−	−	+	−	−	Osteosclerosis	? Bone disease

* ↑L/S = increased liver or spleen; LEB = leukoerythroblastosis; ↑MKC = megakaryocyte proliferation; + = present; − = absent.

Pathology

Three histologic patterns have been described in the bone marrow of patients with AMMM: [1] panhyperplasia with megakaryocytic and erythroid predominance and a slight increase in reticulum; [2] myeloid atrophy and fibrosis, with only 30% of the marrow space showing hyperplastic hematopoietic tissue (megakaryocytic predominance); and [3] myelofibrosis and osteosclerosis, with 30% bone trabeculae and minimal amounts of hematopoietic tissue (occasional clumpy megakaryocytes).[32] It has been hypothesized that alterations in the marrow stroma increase the access of hematopoietic cells to the circulation. Trapping of these cells in splenic sinusoids results in intrasinusoidal hematopoiesis and splenomegaly, which increases with duration of disease.[116] In C-AMF, bone marrow biopsies usually show marked fibrosis with a few islands of cellularity composed of fibroblasts and large multinucleated cells, which appear to be megakaryocytes (Fig. 19-3D). Poorly differentiated mononuclear cells are sometimes seen, particularly in the liver and spleen. Hepatosplenomegaly thus may be due to leukemic infiltration as well as fibrosis.

Natural History and Clinical Presentation

Adults with AMMM are often well-nourished and asymptomatic at presentation, despite splenomegaly and a leukoerythroblastic blood picture. Years later, malaise, weight loss, dyspnea, splenic pain, and hyperuricemia occur. Patients ultimately develop anemia, and many die of heart failure (and artherosclerosis) or pneumonia. Transition to leukemia may be seen.[32]

Adults with AMF are usually severely ill, with fatigue, weight loss, and pancytopenia, but have minimal abnormalities of erythrocyte morphology and no organomegaly.[117] C-AMF patients also have cytopenias and an acute course, but organomegaly and a leukoerythroblastic blood picture may be present. Blasts may also be seen in the peripheral blood and are sometimes increased in the marrow (Fig. 19-3E). Untreated patients die of bleeding or infection.

Differential Diagnosis

Myelofibrosis may occur as a secondary phenomenon in several situations, including granulomatous disease, autoimmune illness, Hodgkin's disease, metastatic tumor, ALL, exposure to toxins (e.g., fluoride, benzene) or estrogenic substances, renal osteodystrophy, and rickets.[97,118–130] Other myeloproliferative disorders, such as PV and CML, may have associated myelofibrosis.

The presence of increased numbers of abnormal megakaryocytes (often bizarre in appearance) can be used to differentiate patients with a proliferative abnormality of megakaryoblastic or combined megakaryoblastic–myeloblastic origin (AMMM, AMF, C-AMF) from those with other disorders. Increased, but normal appearing, megakaryocytes were present in a patient with systemic lupus erythematosus and myelofibrosis, but autoimmune thrombocytopenia may have played a role.[119] A review of children reported as having IMF (Table 19-5) shows how well those with C-AMF can be differentiated by the presence of abnormal megakaryocytes[92–97] from patients with probable ALL,[123–125] ANLL without megakaryoblastic involvement,[131] renal osteodystrophy,[126,127] or rickets,[128–130] and from atypical patients with some bone abnormalities.[132,133] All patients with increased megakaryocytes had blasts noted, except one child who died of overwhelming varicella and may have had a spontaneous remission of leukemia.[93]

The evaluation of myelofibrosis must include tests for granulomatous disorders, autoimmune disorders, renal dysfunction, and rickets. ALL may be confused morphologically with AMgL. Ultrastructural, cytochemical (platelet peroxidase), or monoclonal antibody techniques may be helpful in distinguishing these possibilities. If possible, chromosomal analysis should be performed in children with IMF.

Prognosis and Treatment

AMMM in adults is a slowly progressive disease that usually requires only supportive care until the terminal stages, when splenectomy or chemotherapy may be considered. Most patients become anemic and pancytopenic.

IMF of childhood must be evaluated fully to determine the true etiology. Those children who have metabolic disorders or ALL can be differentiated by the lack of megakaryocytic proliferation and should respond to appropriate therapy.[123,125,128–130]

Children with C-AMF treated with the newer chemotherapeutic regimens for ANLL have had prolonged remissions,[114] as has a child treated with allogeneic bone marrow transplantation.[89]

Myeloproliferative Syndrome Associated with Trisomy 21

Infants with Down's syndrome may be born with an MPS that appears identical to ANLL. The leukocyte count may be elevated (5000 to 400,000/mm^3) and myeloblasts (up to 95%) may be seen in the periphery. Erythroid and myeloid hyperplasia are common marrow findings, with up to 60% myeloblasts present (Fig. 19-3F).[134] Hepatosplenomegaly, skin infiltrates, anemia, and thrombocytopenia may occur.[135] Many of these children undergo spontaneous remission within 1 to 2 months, while others have a persistent leukemia. Controversy exists as to whether those with a transient course have a transient acute leukemia[136] or ineffective regulation of granulopoiesis masquerading as congenital leukemia.[137] Also problematic is our inability to predict which children will have a spontaneous remission and which will develop a persistent leukemia.

Chromosomal studies have been performed on the bone marrow cells of several patients. Some revealed only trisomy 21, but other patients had additional chromosomal abnormalities that disappeared as the MPS resolved.[138,139] This is suggestive of a clonal leukemic or preleukemic disorder that remits, possibly as hormonal or other regulatory influences allow the normal trisomic hematopoietic cells to gain dominance over the abnormal clone. Of interest is a patient reported by Honda and colleagues who had an extra C chromosome in 6% of the trisomy 21 cells during neonatal MPS.[140] The MPS resolved, although the minor cell line could still be demonstrated at age 6 months. Leukemia arose at 26 months, at which time 93% of the cells had the extra chromosome. This cell line could simply have been more unstable than the normal trisomic cells, or it may have been a leukemic line that was suppressed initially but then proliferated.

In vitro assays of CFU-GM are normal in many of these children in whom the MPS is transient.[141–144] No colonies grew for one patient who did not go into remission.[144] More studies are needed to see if colony assays are truly predictive of outcome. Patients with detectable chromosomal abnormalities in addition to trisomy need to be studied to determine if the normal colony growth is due to evolving dominance of the normal trisomic cells, or if cells that form these normal appearing colonies include those of the aberrant line. The latter finding would suggest that the abnormal clone is not leukemic and that the MPS is probably due to ineffective regulation of hematopoiesis.

Until this MPS is better understood, these children should be supported as long as possible without the use of chemotherapy to determine whether the disorder is transient.

MYELODYSPLASTIC SYNDROMES

Definition and Epidemiology

An MDS is a syndrome of hematopoietic dysfunction that may precede the development of ANLL. Hematopoiesis is ineffective, as shown by the presence of progressive peripheral blood cytopenias with a hypercellular (or at least normocellular) marrow. Morphologic abnormalities occur in at least one and often multiple hematopoietic cells, particularly erythrocytes. The spectrum of abnormalities has resulted in a confusing array of terminology. In 1978, Linman and Bagby devised criteria for the "preleukemic syndrome or hematopoietic dysplasia" that included [1] anemia and oval macrocytosis in the peripheral blood; [2] megaloblastoid erythropoiesis or ringed sideroblasts, abnormal megakaryocytes or disorderly granulopoiesis, and the absence of overt leukemia in the marrow; and [3] absence of vitamin B_{12} or folate deficiency, and no cytotoxic therapy in the previous 6 months.[145] In 1982 the French–American–British (FAB) group devised a more inclusive classification based on the number of blasts in the periphery and marrow, peripheral blood monocytes, and ringed sideroblasts. Patients are classified as having refractory anemia, (RA), RA with ringed sideroblasts (RARS), chronic myelomonocytic leukemia (CMML), RA with an excess of blasts (RAEB), or RAEB in transition (RAEBt) (Table 19-6).[146] This classification has introduced a degree of uniformity in patient grouping that permits evaluation of clinical and biological studies.[147] More basic biological classifications may follow.

Pre-ANLL is commonly considered a disorder of the elderly (median age = 60). Childhood cases do exist, and, based on the observation of MDS in 6 of 37 children with ANLL, it has been suggested that a myelodysplastic syndrome precedes ANLL in children as often as it does in adults.[148] Childhood MDS is very similar to MDS in adults, although the incidence of monosomy 7 is considerably higher. An increased incidence of MDS occurs in all patients treated with alkylating agents.[149,150]

Biology and Genetics

The MDS involve cells of multiple hematopoietic lineage. *In vitro* colony assays have been used to evaluate patterns of cell growth, maturation, and regulation. Granulocyte and macrophage colonies formed by the committed progenitors CFU-GM may be normal (particularly in patients with RA who do not have clinical granulocyte-monocyte involvement) or may be decreased. In the latter instance, increased numbers of abortive myeloid clusters are found that exhibit defective maturation similar to that seen in leukemia.[151-153] This pattern is common in RAEB and RAEBt, which progress inexorably to ANLL. CMML, characterized by monocytosis, has increased numbers of CFU-GM. Anemia is present in 90% of all MDS patients. BFU-E (erythroid progenitors) are often unable to proliferate *in vitro*.[152,154,155] Megakaryocyte colony formation may also be reduced in MDS.[153,156] It is unclear whether the abnormal hematopoiesis reflects the growth pattern of the abnormal clone itself or the effect of the abnormal clone on normal progenitor cells, perhaps mediated by inhibitors of hematopoiesis.

Table 19-6
FAB Classification of Myelodysplastic Syndromes

| MDS | Peripheral | | Marrow | |
	Blasts	Other	Blasts	Other
Refractory anemia (RA)	<1%	Reticulocytopenia Oval macrocytes Rarely, platelets and PMN decreased or dysplastic	<5%	Erythroid hyperplasia Dyserythropoiesis
RA with ringed sideroblasts	<1%	As in RA, plus Basophilic stippling Dimorphic erythrocytes (hypo- and normochromic)	<5%	Erythroid hyperplasia Dyserythropoiesis 15% ringed sideroblasts
Chronic myelomonocytic leukemia	<5%	As in RA, plus Monocytes ↑Mature granulocytes Thrombocytopenia Pelger–Huet PMN Hypogranular PMN	≤20%	Monocytic hyperplasia Erythroid hyperplasia
RA with excess blasts (RAEB)	<5%	As in RA, plus Dysplasia and cytopenia of at least 2 cell lines Pelger–Huet PMN Hypogranular PMN Hypogranular and abnormal sized platelets	5%–20%	Granulocytic hyperplasia Erythroid hyperplasia Dyserythropoiesis Dysgranulocytopoiesis Dysmegakaryopoiesis
RAEB in transition	>5%		20%–30%	Auer rods

(Data from Bennett and coworkers.[146])

Chromosomal abnormalities,[157] particularly deletions of part or all of chromosomes 5 or 7 or trisomy 8, are reported in 50% to 60% of patients with MDS. Monosomy 7 occurred in 4 of 10 children with MDS in one study[158] and 25 of 51 children described in the literature.[159] Of the other 26, 16 had chromosome studies performed; 7 of these had abnormalities.

Natural History and Pathogenesis

Leukemia has been defined as an uncoupling of differentiation and proliferation.[25] Differentiation is certainly aberrant in MDS, as seen by the morphologic myelodysplasia *in vivo* and delayed maturation *in vitro*.[160] A mixture of normal and abnormal cells may coexist for a prolonged period.[161] A proliferative abnormality that in true leukemia, results in the expansion of an abnormal clone at the expense of normal cells, may occur after a variable time period. It is not known whether the cells apparent at the time of leukemic proliferation result from an acute karyotypic change of the dysplastic cells or from abnormal cells that slowly gain predominance over the normal ones.

Abnormal hematopoietic cells are likely to occur in patients exposed to mutagenic agents. Thus, MDS, particularly with deletions of chromosomes 5 or 7, occurs more frequently in patients treated with cytotoxic chemotherapy or radiation, as well as in people who have been exposed to chemicals, petroleum solvents, pesticides, and industrial metal.[149,162] Loss of part or all of a chromosome may result in loss of genetic material that regulates cell growth or, as proposed in retinoblastoma and Wilms' tumor, may allow for the expression of a mutant gene.[24] The c-*fms* proto-oncogene product, which appears related to be the receptor for mononuclear phagocytic growth factor M-CSF[18], is lost in the 5q deletion of RA.[163]

Monosomy 7, as it occurs in children, is characterized by disease onset at a young age, with recurrent bacterial infections that are probably due to granulocyte dysfunction.[164,165] The genes responsible for this regulatory dysfunction are not known. This disorder has a very aggressive course, with 19 of 25 children described in the literature progressing to ANLL and 5 dying during a preleukemic phase. The natural history of other MDS in children is similar: 23 of 26 developed overt leukemia, and the other 3 died in the preleukemic stage.[159]

Clinical Presentation

Weakness due to anemia, bleeding due to platelet dysfunction, and infection due to granulocyte dysfunction are common presenting symptoms. Although half of adults are said to be asymptomatic,[147] a study of preleukemia in 28 children (16 pre-ANLL, 12 pre-ALL) found only 1 asymptomatic child. Fever (12 of 28), pallor (8 of 28), hemorrhage (14 of 28), and infection (11 of 28) were seen most commonly.[166] Of six children with pre-ANLL in one report, all had pallor, adenopathy, and unusual infections.[148] Hepatosplenomegaly is common, particularly in children with monosomy 7.[159]

Laboratory studies in adults with MDS reveal anemia in 90% and pancytopenia in 50%. Fewer than 5% of patients have isolated involvement of platelets, granulocytes, or monocytes. Oval macrocytosis and basophilic stippling of erythrocytes, circulating megaloblastoid nucleated erythrocytes, Pelger–Huet abnormalities, hypersegmentation and hypogranularity of neutrophils, and hypogranulation of platelets are seen (Fig. 19-4A, 19-4B). Five of six children with MDS initially had normocytic and normochromic anemia, with macrocytosis and ovalocytosis occurring later, followed by poikilocytosis and anisocytosis. Leukocyte abnormalities occurred but were more subtle than erythrocyte abnormalities.[148] Children with monosomy 7 often have monocytosis and occasionally have granulocytosis.[164]

The bone marrow is usually hypercellular, reflecting ineffective hematopoiesis (Fig. 19-4C, 19-4D). Ringed sideroblasts are seen in about 20% of adults, but are not a feature of childhood MDS. Dyserythropoiesis occurs, with megaloblastoid and multinucleated erythroid precursors that are similar in appearance to those of folate or vitamin B_{12} deficiency. Megakaryocytes are reported to be increased in adult studies,[147] although Kobrinsky and colleagues report decreased megakaryocytes in children.[167] Megaloblastic changes in myeloid precursors are seen, often with hypogranulation. Blasts seen in five of six pediatric patients were monocytoid or myelomonocytic, with Auer rods seen in two.

Other laboratory abnormalities reported, primarily in adults, include abnormal iron metabolism, altered erythrocyte enzyme activity (decreased pyruvate kinase and 2,3-diphosphoglyceromutase), increased fetal hemaglobin, increased expression of erythrocyte i antigen, and decreased A and H substances.[145,168,169] Paroxysmal nocturnal hemoglobinuria may be an associated finding.[170] Decreased LAP, myeloperoxidase, chemotaxis, phagocytosis, and bactericidal function have been reported in neutrophils.[171,172] Six pediatric patients all had elevated vitamin B_{12} levels.[148]

Differential Diagnosis

Preleukemia can be diagnosed unequivocally only when a transformation to leukemia occurs. Clues to the diagnosis of preleukemia from peripheral blood findings include anemia, cytopenias, and peripheral blasts. Marrow clues are hypercellularity, progressive megaloblastosis, >5% blasts, dyserythropoiesis, abnormal megakaryocytes, chromosome abnormalities, and reduced colony-to-cluster ratio in *in vitro* colony assays.[148] Cytopenias with nonrandom chromosome abnormalities have been found to terminate in ANLL in 70% of adults.[173] Such studies are not available in children.

The differential diagnosis in children is complicated by the occurrence of two types of preleukemia—pre-ANLL and pre-ALL (Table 19-7). Presenting symptoms are not specific. Peripheral cytopenia with marrow hypoplasia is more common in pre-ALL than pre-ANLL. Ineffective hematopoiesis of erythroid and myeloid lineage occurs in both, but ineffective megakaryopoiesis occurs only in pre-ANLL. Granulocytic hyperplasia also occurs only in pre-ANLL. Morphologic abnormalities of all cell lines are seen primarily in pre-ANLL. Pre-ANLL is seen throughout childhood, while pre-ALL occurs more often in children aged 1 to 6. Males predominate in pre-ANLL, whereas females predominate in pre-ALL. Karyotypic abnormalities, particularly monosomy 7, are frequent in pre-ANLL and rare in pre-ALL.[166]

Seven pediatric patients with hematopoietic dysplasia and features similar to preleukemia were found by Kobrinsky and colleagues by review of all pediatric marrow examinations over a 10-year period (7 of 760).[167] Six had constitutional abnormalities, which included coarse or unusual facies (4 patients), short stature (4 patients), mental retardation (3 patients), skin abnormalities (5 patients), and endocrine abnormalities (2 patients). One otherwise normal patient had a hydrocele. Four of these six children developed ANLL and another died of hemorrhage. Two of the four children with ANLL had family histories of childhood leukemia. Another appeared to have Schwachman syndrome, which has previously been associated with hematopoietic dysplasia and progression to ANLL.[174] Hematopoietic dysplasia, monosomy 7, and cerebellar atrophy have been

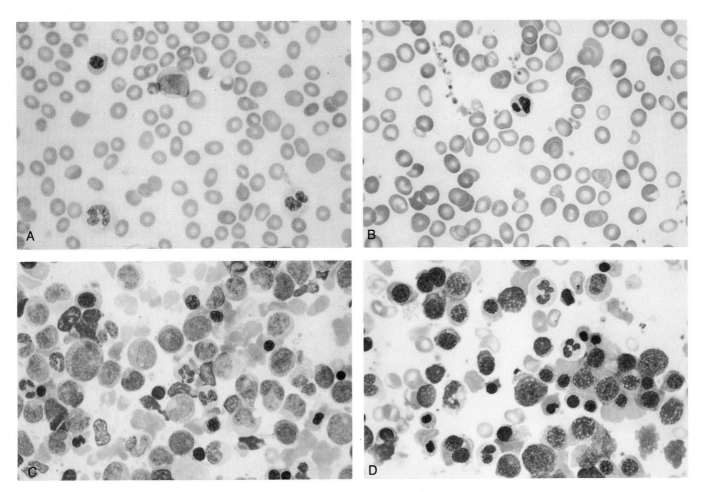

FIGURE 19-4. Myelodysplastic syndromes. (**A**) Blood smear showing a nucleated erythrocyte, myeloblast, hypogranulated neutrophil, ovalocytes, and teardrops (×200). (**B**) Blood smear showing the Pelger–Huet abnormality and poikilocytosis (×200). (**C**) Marrow aspirate showing dysgranulopoiesis with hypogranularity and abnormal segmentation, erythropoiesis with dyssynchronous cytoplasmic maturation, megaloblastoid changes, irregular nuclear budding, (×22). (**D**) Marrow aspirate showing dyserythropoiesis with dyssynchronous cytoplasmic maturation, megaloblastoid changes, multinucleated forms (×200). (Photomicrographs of blood and marrow kindly provided by J. Schaffer, Division of Hemotology, University of Rochester Medical Center.)

described in one kindred.[175] Pediatric MDS may thus include a group of patients with constitutional hematopoietic dysplasia.

Several other constitutional disorders are associated with an increased incidence of acute leukemia but do not have a preleukemic phase with myelodysplasia and are therefore not included in the MDS. These include Kostmann's agranulocytosis, Down's syndrome, Bloom's syndrome, and Diamond–Blackfan syndrome. Patients with Fanconi's anemia and idiopathic aplastic anemia also have an increased incidence of leukemia.[145,176]

Prognosis and Treatment

Significant variability exists in the time of evolution of MDS to ANLL. Adults with CMML, RAEB, and RAEBt usually die as a direct consequence of the disorder. RA and RARS are more indolent, and patients die of other disorders.[177] The presence of an abnormal karyotype increases the likelihood of transformation to ANLL.[178] Evidence of leukemic evolution by *in vitro*

assays of cell growth (decreased colony:cluster ratio) or by karyotypic evolution is a poor prognostic sign.[147]

Children have rarely been classified by the FAB system, but do not appear to have RARS, RA, or CMML. Most probably have RAEB or RAEBt. Chromosomal abnormalities are common (32 of 41 patients). The preleukemic phase in children has been calculated to last 1 to 60 months (median = 12–18 months).[159] Because the evolution to leukemia is often rapid in childhood, the likelihood of death from unrelated causes, as is seen in the elderly patients, is low.

Supportive care with antibiotics and blood products is necessary in most patients. Curative therapy, if it existed, would of course be ideal. Treatment with aggressive chemotherapy has been disappointing. Responses in adult MDS have been less frequent than in *de novo* ANLL, and periods of aplasia have been prolonged.[179] Reports of successful chemotherapy in childhood MDS do not exist, although improved treatment of ANLL in general may improve the outcome in these patients.[180] Children and young adults have been treated successfully with cyclophosphamide and total body irradiation followed by allo-

Table 19-7
Comparison of Pre-ANLL and Pre-ALL in Children

Variable	Pre-ANLL	Pre-ALL
Age	Throughout childhood	Peak 1–6 years
Sex (M:F)	2:1	1:2
Duration (median/mean)	12 mo/18 mo	4 mo/6 mo
Symptoms	*Same for pre-ANLL and pre-ALL:* fever, infection, hemorrhage, fatigue, malaise, joint symptoms	
Physical examination	*Same for pre-ANLL and pre-ALL:* pallor, splenomegaly, hepatomegaly, lymphadenopathy, skin lesions	
Blood smear	Myelodysplastic changes Cytopenias	Normal morphology Cytopenias
Marrow	Ineffective erythropoiesis (60%) Ineffective thrombopoiesis Increased myelopoiesis	Ineffective erythropoiesis (40%) Hypoplasia of all cell lines, particularly myelopoiesis
Chromosomes	50% monosomy 7 75% abnormal clone	No specific abnormalities Usually normal

geneic bone marrow transplantation.[181] Seven of nine patients were alive and well 478 to 1080 days after transplantation. For children with an available allogeneic donor, this is currently the preferred therapy.

Experience with the use of maturational agents has accumulated in adults, particularly those considered unable to withstand aggressive chemotherapy. Low-dose cytosine arabinoside (ara-C) was initially used as a maturational agent, although it is currently thought to work by cytotoxic suppression of the abnormal clone. Review of several studies suggests that approximately 50% of patients had improved hematopoiesis for 3 to 27 months, but hospital admissions for myelosuppression were significant.[147] The difference in duration of survival of the responders and nonresponders (12 months versus 9 months) is not impressive.[182] Swanson and colleagues studied MDS marrow cells treated with 13-cis retinoic acid, another maturational agent, and noted enhanced CFU-GM differentiation and increased BFU-E growth in the majority.[183] A preliminary study of patients treated with retinoic acid for MDS suggested some improvement in granulocyte count in some patients, but there was no change in transfusion requirement.[184]

A new approach has been suggested by Francis and co-workers, who have found *in vitro* evidence of synergy when inducers of maturation (retinoic acid or N-methylformamide) are used with agents that slow proliferation by inhibition of DNA synthesis (6-mercaptopurine, ara-C, or aphidicolin).[185] Myelotoxic effects *in vitro* were not synergistic. Slowing of proliferation does not seem likely to change the overall distribution of mature and immature cells. Francis and colleagues proposed that cells may be responsive to differentiation inducers in only one phase of the cell cycle, and that this phase may be lengthened by slowing DNA synthesis.[185] Alternatively, those agents that slow proliferation may act preferentially on multipotent progenitor cells while proliferation of mature cells continues normally. The presence of a differentiation inducer thus results in significantly increased numbers of mature cells that can respond to normal proliferative signals.

As we begin to understand more about the abnormalities of proliferation and differentiation that occur in myeloproliferative and myelodysplastic syndromes, we will hopefully be able to treat the consequences of the diseases and prevent their transformation into leukemia.

REFERENCES

1. Korn AP, Henkelman RM, Ottensmeyer FP, Till JE: Investigations of a stochastic model of haemopoiesis. Exp Hematol 1:362, 1973
2. Till JE, McCulloch EA, Siminovitch L: A stochastic model of stem cell proliferation, based on the growth of spleen colony-forming cells. Proc Natl Acad Sci USA 51:29–36, 1964
3. Dexter TM, Allen TD: The regulation of growth and development of normal and leukemic cells. J Pathol 141:415–433, 1983
4. Van Zandt G, Goldwasser E: Simultaneous effects of erythropoietin and colony-stimulating factor on bone marrow cells. Science 198:733–735, 1977
5. Bender JG, Van Epps DE, Stewart CC: A model for the regulation of myelopoiesis by specific factors. J Leuk Biol 39:101–111, 1986
6. Ihle NJ, Keller J, Henderson L, Palaszynski E: Procedures for the purification of interleuken 3 to homogeneity. J Immunol 129:2431–2435, 1982
7. Burgess AW, Camakaris J, Metcalf D: Purification and properties of colony-stimulation factor from mouse lung-conditioned medium. J Biol Chem 652:1998–2003, 1977
8. Nicola NA, Metcalf D, Matsumoto M, Johnson GR: Purification of a factor inducing differentiation in murine myelomonocytic leukemia cells. J Biol Chem 258:9017–9023, 1983
9. Gualtieri RJ, Shadduck RK, Baker DG, Quesenberry PJ: Hematopoietic regulatory factors produced in long-term murine bone marrow cultures and the effect of *in vitro* irradiation. Blood 64:516–525, 1984
10. Broudy VC, Zuckerman KS, Jetmalani S, Fitchen JH, Bagby GC: Monocytes stimulate fibroblastoid bone marrow stromal cells to produce multilineage hematopoietic growth factors. Blood 68:530–534, 1986
11. Jacobsen LO, Goldwasser E, Fried W, Plzak L: Role of the kidney in erythropoiesis. Nature 179:633–634, 1957
12. Pierce JH, Eva A, Aaronson SA: Interactions of oncogenes with haematopoietic cells. Clin Haematol 15:573–596, 1986
13. Hunter T: The proteins of oncogenes. Sci Am 251:70–79, 1985
14. Castro-Malaspina H, Rabellino EM, Yen A, Nachman RL, Moore ASM: Human megakaryocyte stimulation of proliferation of bone marrow fibroblasts. Blood 57:781–787, 1981
15. Doolittle RF, Hunkapiller MW, Hood LE, Devare SG, Robbins KC, Aaronson SA, Antoiades HN: Simian sarcoma virus oncogene, v-sis is derived from the gene (or genes) encoding a platelet-derived growth factor. Science 221:275–276, 1983
16. Waterfield MD, Scrace GT, Whittle N, Stroobant P, Johnsson A, Wasteson A, Westermark B, Heldin CH, Huang JS, Deuel TF: Platelet-derived growth factor is structurally related to the putative transforming protein p28^{sis} of simian sarcoma virus. Nature 304:35–39, 1983
17. Sherr CJ, Rettenmier CW, Sacca R, Roussel MF, Look AT, Stanley ER: The c-fms proto-oncogene product is related to the receptor for the mononuclear phagocyte growth factor, CSF-1. Cell 41:665–676, 1985
18. Feldman RA, Gabrilove JL, Tam JP, Moore MAS, Hanafusa H: Specific

expression of the human cellular fps/fes-encoded protein NCP92 in normal and leukemic myeloid cells. Proc Natl Acad Sci USA 82:2379–2383, 1985

19. Murray MJ, Cunningham JM, Parada LF, et al: The HL-60 transforming sequence: A ras oncongene coexisting with altered myc genes in hematopoietic tumors. Cell 33:749–757, 1983
20. Kelly K, Cochran BH, Stiles CD, Leder P: Cell-specific regulation of the c-myc gene by lymphocyte mitogens and platelet-derived growth factor. Cell 37:603–610, 1983
21. Muller R, Bravo R, Burckhardt J: Induction of c-fos gene and protein by growth factors precedes activation of c-myc. Nature 312:716–720, 1984
22. Konopka JB, Watanabe SM, Witte ON: An alteration of the human c-abl protein in K562 leukemia cells unmasking associated tyrosine kinase activity. Cell 37:1035–1042, 1984
23. Dexter TM, Garland J, Scott D, Scolnick E, Metcalf D: Growth of factor-dependent hemopoietic precursor cell lines. J Exp Med 152:1036–1047, 1980
24. Knudson FG: Mutation and cancer: Statistical study of retinoblastoma. Proc Natl Acad Sci USA 68:820–823, 1971
25. Sachs L: Constitutive uncoupling of pathways of gene expression that control growth and differentiation in myeloid leukemia: A model for the origin and progression of malignancy. Proc Natl Acad Sci USA 77:6152–6156, 1980
26. Collins SJ: Breakpoints on chromosomes 9 and 22 in Philadelphia chromosome positive chronic myelogenous leukemia (CML). J Clin Invest 78:1392–1396, 1986
27. Sitbon M, Sola B, Evans L, Nishio J, Hayes SF, Nathanson K, Garon CF, Cheseboro B: Hemolytic anemia and erythroleukemia, two distinct pathogenic effects of Friend MuLV: Mapping of the effects to different regions of the viral genome. Cell 47:851–859, 1986
28. Ruscetti S, Feild J, Davis L, Oliff A: Factors determining the susceptibility of NIH Swiss mice to erythroleukemia induced by Friend murine leukemia virus. Virology 117:357–365, 1982
29. Estrov Z, Grunberger T, Chan HSL, Freedman MH: Juvenile chronic myelogenous leukemia: Characterization of the disease using cell cultures. Blood 67:1382–1387, 1986
30. Dameshek W: Editorial: Some speculations on the myeloproliferative syndromes. Blood 6:372–375, 1951
31. Editorial: Myelofibrosis. Lancet 1:127–129, 1980
32. Ward HP, Block MH: The natural history of agnogenic myeloid metaplasia (AMM) and a critical evaluation of its relationship with the myeloproliferative syndrome. Medicine 50:357–419, 1971
33. Duhamel G, Najman A, Andre R: L'Histologie de la moelle osseuse dans la maladie de vaquez et le probleme de la myelosclerose. Nouv Rev Fr Hematol 10:209–222, 1970
34. Weinfeld A, Branehog I, Kutti S: Platelets in the myeloproliferative syndrome. Clin Haematol 4:373–392, 1975
35. Adamson JW, Fialkow PJ, Murphy S, Prchal JF, Steinmann L: Polycythemia vera: Stem-cell and probable clonal origin of the disease. N Engl J Med 295:913–915, 1976
36. Modan B: An epidemiological study of polycythemia vera. Blood 26:657–667, 1965
37. Silverstein MN, Lanier AP: Polycythemia vera 1935–1969. Mayo Clin Proc 46:751–753, 1971
38. Berlin NI: Diagnosis and classification of the polycythemias. Semin Hematol 12:339–351, 1975
39. Danish EH, Rasch CA, Harris JW: Polycythemia vera in childhood: Case report and review of the literature. Am J Hematol 9:421–428, 1980
40. Natelson EA, Lynch EC, Britton HA, Alfrey CP: Polycythemia vera in childhood. Am J Dis Child 122:241–244, 1971
41. Hann HWL, Festa RS, Rosenstock JS, Cifuentes E: Polycythemia vera in a child with acute lymphocytic leukemia. Cancer 43:1962–1965, 1979
42. Marlow AA, Fairbanks VF: Polycythemia vera in an eleven-year-old girl. N Engl J Med 263:950–952, 1960
43. Dykstra OH, Halbertsma T: Polycythemia vera in childhood. Am J Dis Child 60:907–916, 1940
44. Wick H: Polycythemia vera mit neurologischen Komplikationen bein enem 12 jahrigen Kind. Schweiz Med Wochenschr 99:186–189, 1969
45. Aggeler PM, Pollycove M, Hoag S, Donald WG, Lawrence HJ: Polycythemia vera in childhood. Studies of ion kinetics with Fe59 and blood clotting factors. Blood 17:345–349, 1961
46. Heilmann E, Klein CE, Beck JD: Primary polycythaemia in childhood and adolescence. Folia Haematol (Leipz) 110:935–941, 1983
47. Testa JR, Kanofsky JR, Rowley JD, Baron JM, Vardiman JW: Karyotypic patterns and their clinical significance in polycythemia vera. Am J Hematol 11:29–45, 1981
48. Berger R, Bernheim A, Le Coniat M, Vecchione D, Flandrin G, Dresch C, Najean Y: Chromosome studies in polycythemia vera patients. Cancer Genet Cytogenet 12:217–223, 1984
49. Friedland ML, Wittels EG, Robinson RJ: Polycythemia vera in identical twins. Am J Hematol 10:101–103, 1981
50. Brubaker LH, Wasserman LR, Goldberg JD, Pisciotta AV, McIntyre OR, Kaplan ME, Modan B, Flannery J, Harp R: Increased prevalence of polycythemia vera in parents of patients on Polycythemia Vera Study Group protocols. Am J Hematol 16:367–373, 1984
51. Burnside P, Salmon DC, Humphrey CA, Robertson JH, Morris TCM: Polycythemia rubra vera in monzygotic twins. Br Med J 283:56–561, 1981
52. Fairrie G, Black AJ, McKenzie AW: Polycythaemia rubra vera and congenital deafness in monozygotic twins. Br Med J 283:194–195, 1981
53. Golde DW, Cline MJ: Erythropoietin responsiveness in polycythaemia vera. Br J Haematol 29:567–573, 1975
54. Golde DW, Bersch N, Cline MJ: Polycythemia vera: Hormonal modulation of erythropoiesis in vitro. Blood 49:399–405, 1977
55. Zanjani ED, Lutton JD, Hoffman R, Wasserman LR: Erythroid colony formation by polycythemia vera bone marrow in vitro. J Clin Invest 59:841–848, 1977
56. Fauser AA, Massner HA: Pluripotent hematopoietic progenitors (CFU-GEMM) in polycythemia vera: Analysis of erythropoietin requirement and proliferative activity. Blood 58:1224–1227, 1981
57. Adamson JW, Singer JW, Catalano P, Murphy S, Lin N, Steinmann L, Ernst C, Fialkow PJ: Polycythemia vera: Further in vitro studies of hematopoietic regulation. J Clin Invest 66:1363–1368, 1980
58. Gilbert HS: The spectrum of myeloproliferative disorder. Med Clin North Am 57:355–393, 1973
59. Silverstein MN: The evolution into and the treatment of late stage polycythemia vera. Semin Hematol 13:79–84, 1976
60. Silverstein MN: Postpolycythemia myeloid metaplasia. Arch Intern Med 134:113–115, 1974
61. Ellis JT, Peterson P, Geller SA, Rappaport H: Studies of the bone marrow in polycythemia vera and the evolution of myelofibrosis and second hematologic malignancies. Semin Hematol 23:144–155, 1986
62. Le Mercier N, Najean Y: Polyglobulie des sujets jeunes. Nouv Presse Med 8:93–97, 1979
63. Berk PD, Goldberg JC, Donovan PB, Fruchtman SM, Berlin NI, Wasserman LR: Therapeutic recommendations in polycythemia vera based on polycythemia vera study group protocols. Semin Hematol 23:132–143, 1986
64. Tartaglia AP, Goldberg JD, Berk PD, Wasserman LR: Adverse effects of anti-aggregating platelet therapy in the treatment of polycythemia vera. Semin Hematol 23:172–176, 1986
65. Kaplan ME, Mack K, Goldberg JD, Donovan PB, Berk PD, Wasserman LR: Long term management of polycythemia vera with hydroxyurea in a progress report. Semin Hematol 23:167–171, 1986
66. Murphy S, Iland H, Rosenthal D, Laszlo J: Essential thrombocythemia: An interim report from the Polycythemia Vera Study Group. Semin Hematol 23:177–182, 1986
67. Sceats DJ, Baitlon D: Primary thrombocythemia in a child. Clin Pediatr 19:298–300, 1980
68. Linch DC, Hutton R, Cowan D, Moore AR, Richards JDM, Wilkinson LS: Primary thrombocythaemia in childhood. Scand J Haematol 28:72–76, 1982
69. Bellucci S, Janvier M, Tobelem G, Flandrin G, Charpak Y, Berger R, Boiron M: Essential thrombocythemias. Cancer 58:2440–2447, 1986
70. Fialkow PJ, Faguet GB, Jacobsen RJ, Vaidya K, Murphy S: Evidence that essential thrombocythemia is a clonal disorder with origin in a multipotent stem cell. Blood 58:916–919, 1981
71. Gaetani GF, Ferraris AN, Galiano S, Giuntini P, Canepa L, d'Urso M: Primary thrombocythemia: Clonal origin of platelets, erythrocytes, and granulocytes in a GdB/GdMediterranean subject. Blood 59:76–79, 1982
72. Singal U, Prasad AS, Halton DM, Bishop C: Essential thrombocythemia: A clonal disorder of hematopoietic stem cell. Am J Hematol 14:193–196, 1983
73. Third International Workshop on Chromosomes in Leukemia: Report on essential thrombocythemia. Cancer Genet Cytogenet 4:138–142, 1979
74. Zaccaria A, Tura S: A chromosomal abnormality in primary thrombocythemia. N Engl J Med 298:1422–1423, 1978
75. Fuscaldo KE, Erlick BJ, Fuscaldo AA, Brodsky I: Correlation of a specific

chromosomal marker, 21q–, and retroviral indicators in patients with thrombocythemia. Cancer Lett 6:51–56, 1979

76. Eyster ME, Saletan SL, Rabellino EM, Karanas A, McDonald TP, Locke LA, Luderer JR: Familial essential thrombocythemia. Am J Med 80:497–502, 1986

77. Wu KK: Platelet hyperaggregability and thrombosis in patients with thrombocythemia. Ann Intern Med 88:7–11, 1978

78. Boneu B, Nouvel C, Sie P, Carnaobe C, Combes D, Laurent G, Pris J, Bierme R: Platelets in myeloproliferative disorders. Scand J Haematol 25:214–220, 1980

79. Kaywin P, Mcdonough M, Insel PA, Shattil SJ: Platelet function in essential thrombocythemia. N Engl J Med 299:505–509, 1978

80. Cortelazzo S, Barbui T, Bassan R, Dini E: Abnormal aggregation and increased size of platelets in myeloproliferative disorders. Thromb Haemost 43:127–130, 1980

81. Cooper B, Schafer AI, Puchalsky D, Handin RI: Platelet resistance to prostaglandin D_2 in patients with myeloproliferative disorders. Blood 52:618–625, 1978

82. Hoagland HC, Silverstein MN: Primary thrombocythemia in the young patient. Mayo Clin Proc 53:578–580, 1978

83. Addiego JE, Mentzer WC, Dallman PR: Thrombocytosis in infants and children. J Pediatr 805–807, 1974

84. Ozer FL, Truax WE, Miesch DC, Levin WC: Primary hemorrhagic thrombocythemia. Am J Med 807–823, 1960

85. Amato D, Freedman MH: Editorial correspondence: Eleven-year follow-up of "primary thrombocythemia" in a child. J Pediatr 107:650, 1985

86. Kessler CM, Klein HG, Havlik RJ: Uncontrolled thrombocytosis in chronic myeloproliferative disorders. Br J Haematol 50:157–167, 1982

87. Lewis SM, Szur L: Malignant myelosclerosis. Br Med J 2:472–477, 1963

88. Boxer LA, Camitta BM, Berenberg W, Fanning JP: Myelofibrosis-myeloid metaplasia in childhood. Pediatrics 55:861–865, 1975

89. Brovall C, Mitchell M, Saral R, Santos GW, Civin CI: Acute myelofibrosis in a child. J Pediatr 103:91–93, 1983

90. Weisenburger DD: Acute myelofibrosis terminating as acute myeloblastic leukemia. Am J Clin Pathol 73:128–132, 1980

91. Bain BJ, Catovsky D, O'Brien M, Prentice HG, Lawlor E, Kumaran TO, McCann SR, Matutes E, Galton DA: Megakaryoblastic leukemia presenting as acute myelofibrosis—A study of four cases with the platelet-peroxidase reaction. Blood 58:206–213, 1981

92. Evans DIK: Acute myelofibrosis in children with Down's syndrome. Arch Dis Child 50:458–462, 1975

93. Rosenberg HS, Tayler FM: The myeloproliferative syndrome in children. J Pediatr 52:407–415, 1958

94. Hillman F, Forrester RM: Myelofibrosis simulating acute leukemia in a female infant with Down's syndrome. Irish J Med Sci 1:167–173, 1968

95. Okada H, Liu PI, Hoshino T, Yamamato T, Yamaoka H, Murakami M: Down's syndrome associated with a myeloproliferative disorder. Am J Dis Child 124:107–110, 1972

96. Ueda K, Kawaguchi Y, Kodama M, Tanaka Y, Usui T, Kamada N: Primary myelofibrosis with myeloid metaplasia and cytogenetically abnormal clones in 2 children with Down's syndrome. Scand J Haematol 27:152–158, 1981

97. Wood EE, Andrews CT: Subacute myelosclerosis. Lancet 2:739–743, 1949

98. Lewis DS, Thompson M, Hudson E, Liberman MM, Samson D: Down's syndrome and acute megakaryoblastic leukaemia. Acta Haematol 70:236–242, 1983

99. Dharmasena F, Catchpole M, Erber W, Mason D, Gordon-Smith EC: Megakaryoblastic leukaemia and myelofibrosis complicating Fanconi anaemia. Scand J Haematol 36:309–313, 1986

100. Sieff CA, Malleson P: Familial myelofibrosis. Arch Dis Child 55:888–893, 1980

101. Jacobsen RJ, Salo A, Fialkow PJ: Agonogenic myeloid metaplasia: A clonal proliferation of hematopoietic stem cells with secondary myelofibrosis. Blood 51:189–193, 1978

102. Groopman JE: The pathogenesis of myelofibrosis in myeloproliferative disorders. Ann Intern Med 92:857–858, 1980

103. Kaplan DR, Chao FC, Stiles CD, Antoniades HN, Scher CD: Platelet granules contain a growth factor for fibroblasts. Blood 53:1043–1052, 1979

104. Sacchi S, Curci G, Piccinini L, Messerotti A, Cucci F, Bursi R, Zaniol P, Torelli U: Platelet alpha-granule release in chronic myeloproliferative disorders with thrombocytosis. Scand J Clin Lab Invest 46:163–166, 1986

105. Silverstein MN, Brown AL, Linman JW: Idiopathic myeloid metaplasia. Arch Intern Med 132:709–712, 1973

106. Rosenthal DS, Moloney WC: Occurrence of acute leukaemia in myeloproliferative disorders. Br J Haematol 36:373–382, 1977

107. Bearman RM, Pangalis GA, Rappaport H: Acute "malignant" myelosclerosis. Cancer 43:279–293, 1979

108. Ragni MV, Shreiner DP: Spontaneous "remission" of agnogenic myeloid metaplasia and termination in acute myeloid leukemia. Arch Intern Med 141:1481–1484, 1981

109. Marcus RE, Hibbin JA, Matutes E, Whittle N, Waterfield MD, Goldman JM: Megakaryoblastic transformation of myelofibrosis with expression of the c-sis oncogene. Scand J Haematol 36:186–193, 1986

110. Breton-Gorius J, Reyes F, Duhamel G, Nagman A, Gorin NC: Megakaryoblastic acute leukemia: Identification by the ultrastructural demonstration of platelet peroxidase. Blood 51:45–60, 1978

111. Den Ottolander GJ, Te Velde J, Brederoo P, Geraedts JPM, Slee PHT, Willemze R, Zwaan FE, Haak HL, Muller HP, Bieger R: Megakaryoblastic leukaemia (acute myelofibrosis): A report of three cases. Br J Haematol 42:9–20, 1979

112. Bevan D, Rose M, Greaves M: Leukemia of platelet precursors; diverse features in four cases. Br J Haematol 52:147–164, 1982

113. Cairney AEL, McKenna R, Arthur DC, Nesbit ME, Woods WG: Acute megakaryoblastic leukaemia in children. Br J Haematol 63:541–554, 1986

114. Lewis DS: Association between megakaryoblastic leukemia and Down's syndrome. Lancet 2:691, 1981

115. Chan WC, Brynes RK, Kim TH, Verras A, Schick C, Green RJ, Ragab AH: Acute megakaryoblastic leukemia in early childhood. Blood 62:92–98, 1983

116. Wolf BC, Neiman RS: Myelofibrosis with myeloid metaplasia: Pathophysiologic implications of the correlation between bone marrow changes and progression of splenomegaly. Blood 65:803–809, 1985

117. Truong LD, Saleem A, Schwartz MR: Acute myelofibrosis. Medicine 63:182–187, 1984

118. Erf LA, Herbut PR: Primary and secondary myelofibrosis (A clinical and pathological study of thirteen cases of fibrosis of the bone marrow). Ann Intern Med 21:863–869, 1944

119. Daly HM, Scott GL: Myelofibrosis as a cause of pancytopenia in systemic lupus erythematosus. J Clin Pathol 36:1219–1222, 1983

120. Myers CE, Chabner BA, DeVita VT, Gralnick HR: Bone marrow involvement in Hodgkin's disease: Pathology and response to MOPP chemotherapy. Blood 44:197–204, 1974

121. Carroll WL, Berberich R, Glader BE: Pancytopenia with myelofibrosis. Clin Pediatr 25:106–108, 1986

122. Kiang DT, McKenna RW, Kennedy BJ: Reversal of myelofibrosis in advanced breast cancer. Am J Med 64:173–176, 1978

123. Nordan UZ, Humbert JR: Myelofibrosis and acute lymphoblastic leukemia in a child with Down syndrome. J Pediatr 94:253–255, 1979

124. Marino R, Altshuler G, Humphrey GB: Idiopathic myelofibrosis followed by acute lymphoblastic leukemia. Am J Dis Child 133:1194–1195, 1979

125. Tobin MS, Tan C, Argano SAP: Myelofibrosis in pediatric age group. NY State J Med 1:1080–1083, 1969

126. Schlackman N, Green AA, Naiman JL: Myelofibrosis in children with chronic renal insufficiency. J Pediatr 87:720–724, 1975

127. Weinberg SG, Lubin A, Wiener SN, Deoras MP, Ghose MK, Kopelman RC: Myelofibrosis and renal osteodystrophy. Am J Med 63:755–764, 1977

128. Cooperberg AA, Singer OP: Reversible myelofibrosis due to vitamin D deficiency rickets. Can Med Assoc J 94:392–395, 1966

129. Yetgin S, Ozsoylu S: Myeloid metaplasia in vitamin D deficiency rickets. Scand J Haematol 28:180–185, 1982

130. Say B, Berkel I: Idiopathic myelofibrosis in an infant. J Pediatr 4:580–585, 1964

131. Krasilnikoff PA: Myelofibrosis and myeloid leukaemia. Acta Paed Scand 56:424–429, 1967

132. Lau SO, Ramsay NKC, Smith CM, McKenna R, Kersey JH: Spontaneous resolution of severe childhood myelofibrosis. J Pediatr 98:585–588, 1981

133. Tebbi K, Zarkowsky HS, Siegel BA, McAlister WH: Childhood myelofibrosis and osteosclerosis without myeloid metaplasia. J Pediatr 84:860–862, 1974

134. Weinstein HJ: Congenital leukaemia and the neonatal myeloproliferative disorders associated with Down's syndrome. Clin Haematol 7:147–154, 1978

135. Ganick DJ: Hematological changes in down's syndrome. CRC Crit Rev Oncol Haematol 6:55–69, 1986

136. Engel RR, Hammond D, Eitzman DV, Pearson H, Krvit W: Transient congenital leukemia in seven infants with mongolism. J Pediatr 64:303, 1964

137. Ross JD, Moloney WC, Desforges JF: Ineffective regulation of granulopoiesis masquerading as congenital leukemia in a mongoloid child. J Pediatr 63:1–10, 1963

138. Lazarus KH, Heerema NA, Palmer CG, Baehner RL: The myeloproliferative reaction in a child with Down syndrome: Cytological and chromosomal evidence for a transient leukemia. Am J Hematol 11:417–423, 1981

139. Morgan R, Hecht F, Cleary ML, Sklar J, Link MP: Leukemia with Down's syndrome: Translocation between chromosomes 1 and 19 in acute myelomonocytic leukemia following transient congenital myeloproliferative syndrome. Blood 66:1466–1468, 1985

140. Honda F, Punnett HH, Charney E, Miller G, Thiede HA: Serial cytogenetic and hematologic studies on a mongol with trisomy-21 and acute congenital leukemia. J Pediatr 65:880–887, 1964

141. Denegri JF, Rogers PCJ, Chan KW, Sadoway J, Thomas JW: In vitro cell growth in neonates with Down's syndrome and transient myeloproliferative disorders. Blood 58:675–677, 1981

142. Barak Y, Mogilner BM, Karov Y, Nir E, Schlesinger M, Levin S: Transient acute leukaemia in a newborn with Down's syndrome. Acta Paediatr Scand 71:699–701, 1982

143. Inoue S, Ottenbreit MJ, Ravindrath Y, Lusher JM: Leukemoid reaction in Down's syndrome in vitro maturation of circulating stem cells. Pediatr Res 15:579, 1981

144. deAlarcon PA, Goldberg J, Allen J: Leukemia in trisomy 21: Progressive or transient? Pediatr Res 16:202A, 1982

145. Linman JW, Bagby GC: The preleukemic syndrome (hemopoietic dysplasia. Cancer 42:854–864, 1978

146. Bennett JM, Catovsky D, Daniel MT, Flandrin G, Galton DAG, Gralnick HR, Sultan C: Proposals for the classification of the myelodysplastic syndromes. Br J Haematol 51:189–199, 1982

147. Koeffler HP: Myelodysplastic syndromes (preleukemia). Semin Hematol 23:284–299, 1986

148. Blank J, Lange B: Preleukemia in children. J Pediatr 98:565–568, 1981

149. Rowley JD, Golomb HM, Vardiman JW: Nonrandom chromosome abnormalities in acute leukemia and dysmyelopoietic syndromes in patients with previously treated malignant disease. Blood 58:759–767, 1981

150. Kantarjian HM, Keating MJ, Walters RS, Smith RL, Cork A, McCredie KB, Freireich RJ: Therapy-related leukemia and myelodysplastic syndrome: Clinical, cytogenetic, and prognostic features. J Clin Oncol 4:1748–1757, 1986

151. Greenberg PI, Mara B: The preleukemic syndrome. Am J Med 66:951–958, 1979

152. Ruutu T, Partanen S, Lintula R, Teerenhovi L, Knuutila S: Erythroid and granulocyte-macrophage colony formation in myelodysplastic syndromes. Scand J Haematol 32:395–402, 1984

153. Partanen S, Juvonen E, Ruutu T: In vitro culture haematopoietic progenitors in myelodysplastic syndromes. Scand J Haematol 36:98–101, 1986

154. Carbonell F, Heimpel H, Kubanek B, Fliedner TM: Growth and cytogenetic characterizations of bone marrow colonies from patients with 5q– syndrome. Blood 66:463–465, 1985

155. Chui DH, Clarke BJ: Abnormal erythroid progenitor cells in human preleukemia. Blood 60:362–367, 1982

156. Juvonen E, Partanen S, Knuutila S, Ruutu T: Megakaryocyte colony formation by bone marrow progenitors in myelodysplastic syndrome. Br J Haematol 63:331–334, 1986

157. Nowell PC: Cytogenetics of preleukemia. Cancer Genet Cytogenet 5:265–278, 1982

158. Nowell P, Wilmoth D, Lange B: Cytogenetics of childhood preleukemia. Cancer Genet Cytogenet 10:261–266, 1983

159. Wegelius R: Preleukaemic states in children. Scand J Haematol 36:133–139, 1986

160. Golde DW, Cline MJ: Human preleukemia. N Engl J Med 88:1083–1086, 1973

161. Streuli RA, Testa JR, Vardiman JW, Mintz U, Golomb HM, Rowley JD: Dysmyelopoietic syndrome: Sequential clinical and cytogenetic studies. Blood 55:636–644, 1980

162. Golomb HM, Alimena G, Rowley JC, Vardiman JW, Testa JR, Sovik C: Correlation of occupation and karyotype in adults with acute nonlymphocytic leukemia. Blood 60:404–411, 1982

163. Neinhuis AW, Bunn HF, Turner PH, Gopal TV, Nash WG, O'Brien ST, Sherr CJ: Expression of the human c-fms proto-oncogene in hematopoietic cells and its deletion in the 5q– syndrome. Cell 42:421–428, 1985

164. Sieff CA, Chessellis JM, Harvey BAM, Pickthall VJ, Lawler SD: Monosomy 7 in childhood: A myeloproliferative disorder. Am J Hematol 49:235–249, 1981

165. Ruutu P, Ruutu T, Repo H, Vuopio R, Timonen T, Kosunen TU, de la Chapelle A: Defective neutrophil migration in monosomy-7. Blood 58:739–745, 1981

166. Saarinen UM, Wegelius R: Preleukemic syndrome in children. Am J Pediatr Hematol Oncol 6:137–143, 1984

167. Kobrinsky NL, Nexbit ME, Ramsay NKC, Arthur DC, Krivit W, Brunning RD: Hematopoietic dysplasia and marrow hypocellularity in children: A preleukemic condition. J Pediatr 100:907–913, 1982

168. Valentine WN, Konrad PN, Paglia DE: Dyserythropoiesis, refractory anemia, and "preleukemia": Metabolic features of the erythrocytes. Blood 41:857–873, 1973

169. Dreyfus B, Sultan C, Rochant H, Salmon Ch, Mannoni P, Cartron JP, Boivin P, Galand C: Anomalies of blood group antigens and erythrocyte enzymes in two types of chronic refractory anaemia. Br J Haematol 16:303–312, 1969

170. Jenkins DE, Hartmann RC: Paroxysmal nocturnal hemoglobinuria terminating in acute myeloblastic leukemia. Blood 33:274–291, 1969

171. Breton-Gorius J, Houssay D, Vilde JL, Dreyfus B: Partial muramidase deficiency in a case of preleukemia. Br J Haematol 30:279–288, 1979

172. Ruutu P, Ruutu T, Vuopio P, Kosunen TU, de la Chapelle A: Function of neutrophils in preleukaemia. Scand J Haematol 18:317–325, 1977

173. Nowell P, Finan J: Chromosome studies in preleukemic states. Cancer 42:2254–2261, 1978

174. Woods WG, Roloff JS, Lukens JN, Krivit W: The occurrence of leukemia in patients with the Shwachman syndrome. J Pediatr 99:425–428, 1981

175. Li FP, Hecht F, Kaiser-McCaw B, Barbanko PV, Upp Potter N: Ataxia-pancytopenia: Syndrome of cerebellar ataxia, hypoplastic anemia, monosomy 7, and acute myelogenous leukemia. Cancer Genet Cytogen 4:189–196, 1981

176. Kleihauer E: The preleukemic syndromes (hematopoietic dysplasia) in childhood. Eur J Pediatr 133:5–10, 1980

177. Foucar K, Langdon RM, Armitage JO, Oldson DB, Carroll TJ: Myelodysplastic syndromes. Cancer 56:553–561, 1985

178. Jacobs RH, Cornbleet MA, Vardiman JW, Larson RA, Le Beau MM, Rowley JD: Prognostic implications of morphology and karyotype in primary myelodysplastic syndromes. Blood 67:1765–1772, 1986

179. Murray C, Cooper B, Kitchens LW: Remission of acute myelogenous leukemia in elderly patients with prior refractory dysmyelopoietic anemia. Cancer 52:967–970, 1983

180. Weinstein HJ, Maryer RJ, Rosenthal DS, Coral FS, Camitta BM, Gelber RD: Chemotherapy for acute myelogenous leukemia in children and adults: VAPA Update. Blood 62:315–319, 1983

181. Deeg HJ: Marrow transplantation in preleukemia. JNCI 76:1329–1332, 1986

182. Griffin JC, Spriggs D, Wisch JS, Kufe DW: Treatment of preleukemic syndromes with continuous intravenous infusion of low-dose cytosine arabinoside. J Clin Oncol 3:982–991, 1985

183. Swanson G, Picozzi V, Morgan R, Hecht F, Greenberg P: Responses of hemopoietic precursors to 13-cis retinoic acid and 1,25 dihydroxyvitamin D$_3$ in the myelodysplastic syndromes. Blood 67:1154–1161, 1986

184. Picozzi VJ, Swanson GF, Morgan R, Hecht F, Greenberg PL: 13-cis retinoic acid treatment for myelodysplastic syndromes. J Clin Oncol 4:589–595, 1986

185. Francis GE, Guimaraes JETE, Berney JJ, Wing MA: Synergistic interaction between differentiation inducers and DNA synthesis inhibitors: A new approach to differentiation induction in myelodysplasia and acute myeloid leukaemia. Leuk Res 9:573–581, 1985

twenty

Malignant Non-Hodgkin's Lymphomas

Ian T. Magrath

OVERVIEW

Most cancers are neoplastic proliferations of an organ or tissue, and therefore originate in a circumscribed anatomic location and spread from the point of origin either by local invasion or by the process of metastasis. Malignant lymphomas differ radically from this pattern in that they are neoplasms of the constituent cells of the immune system—cells that normally circulate throughout the body in order to subserve their functions. Consequently, almost all lymphomas in children are generalized diseases from the outset (there are some exceptions) and have patterns of spread that mimic the migration patterns of their normal counterpart lymphoid cells.[1] The complex process whereby foreign substances or microorganisms are contained or eliminated is executed and regulated by a variety of cell types, each of which is generated by a process of differentiation or activation from precursor cells. These precursor cells range from multipotential stem cells that can generate progeny belonging to different cell lineages (*e.g.,* lymphoid and myeloid) to resting lymphocytes capable only of being activated into a single type of executive cell with a highly specific function (*e.g.,* production of an antibody molecule or stimulation of the function of another specific cell type). Malignant transformation can occur in any of the functionally different subpopulations of lymphoid cells, and the resultant neoplasm may be expressed at any of the levels of differentiation or activation of the particular subpopulation.[1,2] Clearly, an understanding of the pathology and clinical features of malignant lymphomas must derive from knowledge of the cellular composition and interactions of the normal lymphoid system. It should be recognized that the study of the latter has been considerably enhanced by the availability of large numbers of monoclonal antibodies (see Chap. 4). Many of the monoclonal antibodies have been raised against neoplastic lymphoid cells, which have also been used for biochemical studies of relevant genes and their products (*e.g.,* the immunoglobulin and T-cell antigen receptor genes) as well as for the preparation of reagents of immense value in both the study of the normal immune system and its neoplasms (*e.g.,* monoclonal antibodies directed against lineage or differentiation specific cell surface antigens).[3] As increasingly precise tools for the study of intracellular and intercellular molecular interactions have been developed, the limitations of cell and tissue morphology as a diagnostic modality have become increasingly apparent, although at present, histopathology remains the primary and most widely used means of classifying the lymphoid neoplasms.

A detailed knowledge of the normal immune system is not, of course, sufficient in itself to comprehend the diversity of lymphoid neoplasia. It is essential to understand the deviations in the malignant cell from its normal counterpart. Such information not only can provide additional approaches to the diagnosis and classification of lymphomas, but also should lead, ultimately, to the development of much more specific therapy, directed toward the unique features of the malignant clone. Recent advances in molecular biology have provided the means to examine the origins of neoplastic behavior at the level of gene expression. As a result it has become increasingly clear that lymphoid neoplasms occur as a consequence of a genetic change in a lymphoid cell, frequently a chromosomal translocation. As such, the genetic changes must surely provide the ultimate definition of the disease entity, although caution is needed in developing new taxonomies since a number of different genetic lesions (*e.g.*, translocation, mutation, deletion) can have the same end result on the level of expression or the regulation of the expression of a particular gene product. Moreover, it is necessary to differentiate between pathogenetically relevant genetic changes and secondary changes that may occur as a consequence of the neoplastic state. An additional complication is brought about by the current assumption, based on experimental systems, that more than one genetic change is necessary for the induction of a true neoplastic state.[4] In some cases virus infection may provide one or more of these necessary (or facilitating) steps in oncogenesis, since viruses manipulate the expression of cellular genes, whether from necessity for replication of the viral genome, or by chance, such as when virally derived gene activating factors that regulate the expression of viral genes also alter the expression of cellular genes. A good example of this is the several transactivating factors synthesized by the human T-cell tropic retroviruses. The products of HTLV I and HTLV II transactivating genes stimulate the expression of both cellular interleukin-2 and its receptor, providing the potential for polyclonal activation of the infected T cells and a setting in which the likelihood of further genetic changes relevant to the induction of a malignant T-cell tumor is increased (see Chap. 3).[5-7]

In this chapter, the biology and treatment of the malignant non-Hodgkin's lymphomas will be discussed, emphasizing recent advances in our comprehension of these diseases and indicating, where possible, the impact that this new understanding will have on their diagnosis and management.

HISTORICAL PERSPECTIVE

To the new student of the non-Hodgkin's lymphomas the existence of several histologic classification schemes and the superimposition of immunologic, cytogenetic, or molecular genetic categories can be overwhelming. One of the major causes for confusion is the plethora of terms, originating from many different disciplines and perspectives (witness Ki-1 lymphoma versus lymphoblastic lymphoma versus Burkitt's lymphoma) and the not infrequent application in different classification schemes of the same term to different tumors (*e.g.*, lymphoblastic lymphoma). This apparent semantic mire can be negotiated only by a consideration of the origins of our current concepts of the pathology of lymphoid neoplasms. Similarly, modern treatment approaches have evolved empirically over many years, with the consequence that an understanding of current practice is more readily gained by a historical rather than a rational perspective. In this section, therefore, an outline of the chronological development of present concepts of pathology and management will be presented not only to provide an explanation for and guide to modern terminology and practice, but also to indicate that the basis for currently accepted definitions and treatment approaches is sometimes tenuous, while our understanding of lymphoid neoplasia and our therapeutic stategems are continually evolving.

Origins of Modern Concepts of the Pathology of Malignant Lymphomas

Lymphomas were originally recognized as swellings of lymph nodes (hence Virchow's use of the word "lymphoma") unrelated to a recognized disease entity such as tuberculosis or to obvious pathology in the drainage area of a group of lymph nodes. Thus they were not perceived as neoplasms in the modern sense of the word. Sporadic descriptions of generalized lymph node swelling of unknown cause, often associated with splenic enlargement, occur in the literature in the latter part of the 18th century and the first half of the 19th century, including those of Cruickshank, Hodgkin, Wunderlich, Wilkes, and Trousseau.[8-12] Not surprisingly, these observations in different countries led to the coining of numerous appellations: in England, Hodgkin's disease (an eponym first used by Wilkes); in Germany, Pseudoleukämie (to distingush this entity from the recently described "Leukämie" of Virchow, in which a high white cell count was associated with lymph node and splenic enlargement); and in France, l'adenie, to name but a few. Since the clinical features and the gross pathologic appearance were the only available diagnostic criteria until the value of the histologic features came to be recognized in the late 19th and early 20th centuries, these diseases must have included the whole range of malignant lymphomas (both Hodgkin's and non-Hodgkin's lymphomas) as we know them today, and doubtless some non-neoplastic lymphadenopathies as well as leukemias with low white cell counts.

Undergoing a separate evolution in Germany was the disease known as Lymphosarkoma, characterised by localized swelling of a lymph node or lymph node region. This disease, according to Kundrat, was classified with the other sarcomata —that is, cellular growths arising in connective tissue—and separated from "lymphatic growths."[13] In Kundrat's experience, this disease was confined to lymph nodes or lymphatic tissue in mucus membranes and could spread from its local origin to other lymph node groups. He referred to this progressive form as "Lymphosarkomatosis" and distinguished it on clinical grounds from Pseudoleukämia, although his categories would clearly not correspond to any modern subdivisions, except perhaps clinical stages.

By the early 20th century the histologic appearance subsequently equated with what we now know as Hodgkin's disease had been recognized, permitting the separation between Hodgkin's disease and lymphosarcoma to be based on histologic grounds (see Chap. 21).[14] This also led to a change in the meaning of these terms, which were originally based primarily on clinical subdivisions. The diagnosis of "Pseudoleukämia" gradually fell into disuse, although other terms used to describe lymph node swelling such as "lymphadenoma" persisted as synonyms for Hodgkin's disease. The description of "reticulum cell sarcoma" by Oberling in 1928[15] and "giant follicular lymphoma" by Brill in 1925[16] and Symmers in 1927[17] provided sufficient major categories for the classification scheme published by Gall and Mallory in 1942,[18] one of the first to be based on histology alone. Since that time, and until very recently, histology has been the primary basis for classification, although the distinctive clinical features of more recently recognized pathologic entities such as Burkitt's lymphoma[19] and lymphoblastic lymphoma (using the term as defined by Nathwani and Rappaport[20]) have been important in leading to their acceptance as separate diseases. Not surprisingly, a purely morphologic schema untempered by any real knowledge of the functional nature of the cells that had become neoplastic was less than satisfactory, as indicated by the subsequent proliferation of alternative classification schemes.[21-28] In recent years, the introduction of immunophenotyping and genetic analysis of malignant lymphomas has greatly enhanced our knowledge of the biology of these tumors and is already having an impact on therapy, since diagnosis is more precise and prognostic categories can therefore be more clearly defined (see Chap. 6). However, no classification scheme has yet been designed in which the immunologic phenotype or karyotype, to say nothing of specific molecular genetic changes, is required to be measured for purposes of diagnostic classification.

Pediatric Lymphomas and the Evolution of Present Treatment Approaches

Although the occurrence of lymphomas in childhood had been reported since the 19th century, only recently was the difference in their histologic spectrum from the adult lymphomas recognized. Burkitt's lymphoma was first brought to prominence as a clinical entity in 1958 by Burkitt in Uganda[19] and was recognized as a malignant lymphoma in 1962 by O'Conor.[29] Subsequently, O'Conor, Dorfman, Wright, and others realized that a proportion of childhood lymphomas in Europe and the United States was histologically indistinguishable from Burkitt's lymphoma described in Africa.[30-32] Nonetheless, at this time, perhaps because of a surviving remnant of the concept of a clinical rather than a histologic classification, a diagnosis of Burkitt's lymphoma was made only in the absence of bone marrow involvement and was more likely to be made in the presence of jaw involvement. Rappaport differentiated between undifferentiated lymphomas of Burkitt's and non-Burkitt's types,[33] and Lukes and Collins believed that they could identify similar cells in normal germinal centers in lymphoid tissue and proposed the descriptive term "malignant lymphoma of small non-cleaved follicular center cells" for this entity.[26] By now, the division of the immune system into humoral (B) and cellular (T) components was established, and also the recognition that lymphomas could be classified on that basis. Because of their presumptive germinal center origin, Lukes and Collins considered Burkitt's lymphoma to be a tumor of B cells. This was confirmed by the finding of surface IgM.

Sixteen years after the early descriptions of Burkitt's lymphoma, Lukes and Collins described a malignant lymphoma of convoluted lymphocytes.[26] They suggested that this entity was likely to be of T-cell origin and commented on the frequent involvement of the thymus and the higher frequency of the tumor in children and adolescents. Shortly afterward, Nathwani and colleagues distinguished "lymphoblastic lymphoma" from the Rappaport category of diffuse poorly differentiated lymphocytic lymphoma and identified it with Lukes and Collins' convoluted T-cell lymphoma, although they also realized that many otherwise morphologically identical tumors lacked nuclear convolutions.[20] This was an important distinction because other diffuse poorly differentiated lymphocytic lymphomas are of quite different origin, the term being applied now to a rather uncommon B-cell tumor that occurs in adults. It soon became apparent, in part from the examination of retrospective series of patients with mediastinal or "non-Burkitt's lymphoma," that lymphoblastic lymphomas had a predilection for the bone marrow and central nervous system and that most patients developed recurrent disease at these sites.[2,34,35] These two entities—small noncleaved (undifferentiated or Burkitt's lymphoma) and lymphoblastic lymphoma (convoluted T-cell lymphoma)—account for the bulk of pediatric malignant lymphomas (70–80%), the remainder being large cell lymphomas, half of which are immunoblastic and half of which fulfill the criteria for lymphomas of large follicle center cells, as described by Lukes and Collins.[26]

The results of treatment of pediatric lymphomas before the 1970s were extremely poor, with 5-year survival ranging from 5% to 33% in various series.[2] The only therapy that could lead to cure in, at best, half of patients with localized disease (Stage I) was radiation.[2,36] The use of single cytotoxic agents only slightly enhanced the results with radiation alone except in the case of Burkitt's lymphoma, in which some remarkable cures were observed by Burkitt and others with single doses of cyclophosphamide or other agents.[37,38] Some North American patients with limited disease also achieved long-term survival following treatment with cyclophosphamide as a single agent.[39] The success of the MOPP combination drug regimen in Hodgkin's disease,[40] however, heralded the modern era of combination chemotherapy, and application of a combination of cyclophosphamide, methotrexate, and vincristine in African Burkitt's lymphoma initially, and in American patients subsequently, demonstrated the advantages of combinations of drugs over single-agent chemotherapy.[41] Meanwhile, the clinical and morphologic similarity of lymphoblastic lymphoma to acute lymphoblastic leukemia, as well as the high frequency of bone marrow relapses in nonlymphoblastic lymphomas, was instrumental in developing the concept that malignant lymphomas in children represent variants of acute leukemia. This led to the application of regimens designed for acute lymphoblastic leukemia to the treatment of children with malignant non-Hodgkin's lymphomas, even in the absence of bone marrow involvement. The most successful of the leukemia regimens was the LSA_2-L_2 regimen used at the Memorial Sloan–Kettering Center in New York,[42] and the success of this regimen led to the need to determine which of the two main approaches—"lymphoma" therapy, derived primarily from the combination used in Burkitt's lymphoma, or "leukemia" therapy, based on the LSA_2-L_2 protocol—was more appropriate for the treatment of childhood lymphomas (see below).

Of interest is the fact that the treatment regimens in Africa did not include radiation therapy, since this was not available in Uganda, and because, in Nairobi, Swedish radiation therapists reported very poor local control of Burkitt's lymphoma with gamma rays.[43] Although the cure of a proportion of patients with localized non-Hodgkins lymphoma by radiation therapy in the United States and Europe[36,44] led to the use of radiation therapy directed at sites of bulk disease in patients with more extensive disease (in whom chemotherapy was clearly the major treatment modality), the precise role of radiation therapy in the treatment of childhood lymphomas has, even now, not been finally agreed upon. There is increasing evidence, however, that with modern drug combinations, radiation adds little except toxicity to primary therapy.[45,46] Surgery, on the other hand, as shown originally in African Burkitt's lymphoma patients,[47] can convert patients from a poor to a good prognostic group when essentially complete resection is accomplished.

The modern era, in the context of childhood malignant lymphomas, stems from the early 1970s. Since then, alongside major improvements in the results of treatment, rapid progress in the disciplines of immunology, cytogenetics, and molecular biology has led to dramatic advances in the understanding of the origins of non-Hodgkin's lymphomas from the cells of the immune system and of the genetic abnormalities relevant to their pathogenesis.[1,48,49] These areas will be discussed further in the relevant sections of this chapter.

EPIDEMIOLOGY AND PATHOGENESIS

Lymphomas constitute about 10% of all childhood cancers in the more developed countries, being third in relative frequency after acute leukemias and brain tumors. In the United States between the years 1973 and 1982, according to the SEER surveillance/epidemiology program of the National Cancer Institute, lymphomas constituted 12.6% of all cancers in white children younger than 15 years of age, non-Hodgkin's lymphomas accounting for 7% and Hodgkin's disease the remainder.[50] The average annual incidence of non-Hodgkin's lymphomas was 9.1 per million white children. In black children lymphomas constituted 9% of all neoplasms, non-Hodgkin's lymphomas accounting for 4%, with an average annual incidence of 4.6 per million. Thus in this age group as a whole, non-Hodgkin's lymphomas have a slightly higher incidence than does Hodgkin's disease, but the incidence of Hodgkin's disease in children increases with age, thus accounting for a greater proportion of the lymphomas in older children (Table 20-1). Unlike Hodgkin's disease, which has a bimodal incidence curve, the incidence of non-Hodgkin's lymphomas increases steadily with age throughout life, and children younger than 16 years of age account only for about 3% of all patients with non-Hodgkin's lymphomas (Fig. 20-1).[51] Non-Hodgkin's lymphomas have a higher incidence in males than females, the male to female ratio being 2 or 3 to 1.

Not only are lymphomas relatively less common in children than in adults, but also the range of histologic appearances in childhood lymphomas is considerably narrower than that of adult lymphomas. The clinical features also differ inasmuch as adult lymphomas are predominantly nodal, whereas childhood lymphomas are predominantly extranodal. It is highly probable that these differences between childhood and adult non-Hodgkin's lymphomas reflect age-related differences in the cellular composition of the immune system, with resultant differences in the lymphoid cell population at greatest risk for malignant transformation (see below).

Geographical Differences in the Incidence of Lymphoid Neoplasms in Children

Childhood lymphomas occur throughout the world, although the relative frequency of non-Hodgkin's lymphoma varies quite markedly from country to country (see Chap. 1).[52] In equatorial Africa, for example, approximately 50% of childhood cancers are lymphomas. This markedly increased frequency is the consequence of the very high incidence of Burkitt's lymphoma in this region (Table 20-2). Both lymphoblastic and large cell lymphomas also occur in equatorial Africa, probably with a similar incidence to that in the more developed countries, although accurate figures are not available and little is known of their biology. In Europe and the United States about 33% of childhood lymphomas are lymphoblastic lymphomas, about 50% small noncleaved cell lymphomas (including Burkitt's lymphoma), about 15% large cell lymphomas, and the remainder unclassified (the designations used here are from the National Formulation; see below).

Interestingly, there are a number of differences between equatorial, African Burkitt's lymphoma (endemic) and Burkitt's lymphoma in other parts of the world (sporadic) (Table 20-3), and it seems probable that these are distinct, though

closely related, disease entities.[48,52,53] African Burkitt's lymphoma was originally recognized because of the high incidence of jaw tumors, but this is not a site of predilection in patients outside Africa, although abdominal involvement is frequent in both endemic and sporadic varieties. One of Burkitt's major contributions was to demonstrate the remarkable geographic distribution of the endemic tumor in equatorial Africa and subsequently to show that the apparent limits of its distribution were climatically determined.[54] This observation led to the hypothesis that a vectored virus could be of pathogenetic importance and prompted a search for tumor-associated viruses that resulted in the discovery of Epstein–Barr Virus (EBV).[55] However, although 95% of all equatorial African tumors carry EBV genomes in their cells, this is true for only about 10% to 20% of North American tumors.[56] Moreover, this difference does not simply reflect exposure to EBV, since most patients with endemic tumors, and therefore predominantly EBV negative tumors, have antibodies to EBV regardless of their country of origin.[53,57] It is still not clear whether EBV infection simply predisposes to the development of African Burkitt's lymphoma (and presumably those sporadic tumors that contain EBV sequences) or whether EBV is, in such cases, an essential component of pathogenesis. It has been shown, however, that EBV infection occurs at an early age in equatorial Africans (almost the entire population has been infected by the age of 3) compared to individuals in more developed countries, where primary infection frequently occurs in late adolescence or early adulthood.[58] It seems probable that the B-cell mitogenic effect of EBV increases the size of certain B- or pre-B-cell populations and also causes individual cell clones to remain in a proliferative state, both of which may increase the likelihood of genetic changes developing and the subsequent selection of a clone with the specific genetic abnormalities that result in neoplastic behavior. An alternative hypothesis—that EBV immortalizes cells that already contain a specific translocation—has been proposed,[59] although direct evidence supporting either of these hypotheses is lacking. Although the dependence of Burkitt's lymphoma on climatic factors led to the discovery of EBV, this virus is ubiquitous and its presence in African Burkitt's lymphoma is therefore unlikely to explain the geographical distribution of Burkitt's lymphoma.[58] The areas of high incidence do correspond, however, to regions of holoendemic malaria, which may also predispose to the development of the tumor, since, like EBV, malaria is a B-cell mitogen and also causes a defect in T-cell suppression, both effects of which combine to produce a marked B-cell hyperplasia.[60,61] Early infection by EBV and malaria probably work in concert to increase markedly the risk of developing Burkitt's lymphoma in holoendemic malarial regions such as Africa and New Guinea (Fig. 20-2).

Another difference between endemic and sporadic Burkitt's lymphoma lies in the precise locations of the breakpoints that result in the characteristic 8:14 chromosomal translocation (also see Chaps. 2 and 3). These findings are described in detail below and presumably indicate that the cell of origin of the endemic and sporadic tumors differs.[52,53] It should be pointed out that the differences in EBV association and chromosomal breakpoint location are not absolute. The small proportion of EBV negative tumors in equatorial Africa may represent sporadic tumors that happen to occur in the endemic region. Considerably more work in this area needs to be done. Burkitt's lymphoma in North Africa, for example, is associated with EBV in more than 85% of cases,[56] but detailed information on breakpoint location has not yet been published. The EBV association and chromosomal breakpoint locations of Burkitt's lymphoma in other parts of the world are also largely unstudied.

Table 20-1
Actual Number of Lymphoma Cases Diagnosed Between 1973 and 1977 (White Males and Females, United States)

Age Group	Hodgkin's (%)	Non-Hodgkin's (%)
<5	6 (0.2)	39 (0.5)
5–9	30 (1.1)	63 (0.8)
10–14	119 (4.3)	86 (1.0)
15–19	300 (11)	79 (1.0)
>20	2301 (83)	7828 (97)
All ages	2756	8095

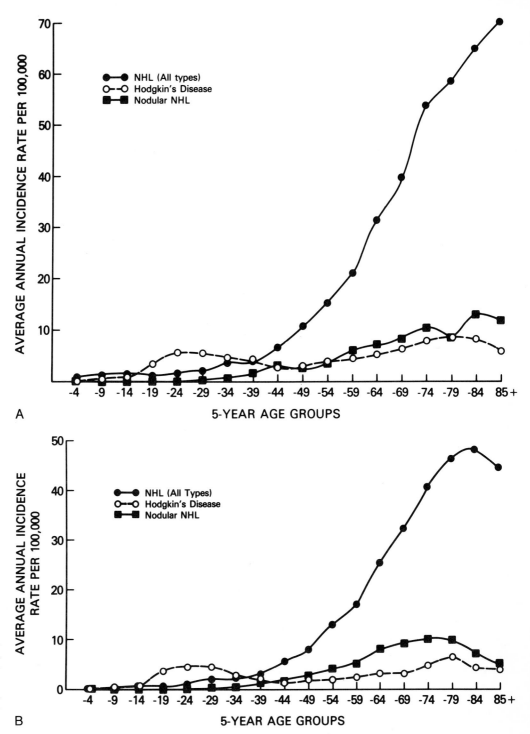

FIGURE 20-1. Average annual incidence of non-Hodgkin's and Hodgkin's lymphomas in the United States according to age. **A.** Males. **B.** Females. These data have been obtained from the SEER program, NCI.

Little epidemiologic information is available with regard to the other varieties of childhood non-Hodgkin's lymphoma, although both lymphoblastic and large cell lymphomas clearly occur throughout the world. Preliminary information indicates that lymphoblastic lymphomas are considerably more common than undifferentiated tumors in some countries (*e.g.,* India), although caution must be exercised in interpreting the scanty data available because the distinction from acute lymphoblastic leukemia is not always made in the same way (also see Chap. 1). No virus association has been yet observed, nor is there a single nonrandom chromosomal abnormality asso-

ciated with lymphoblastic lymphomas. Even though lymphoblastic lymphomas are predominantly of T-cell origin, this is not invariably so,[62] and it seems likely that this histologic entity encompasses several etiologically distinct diseases. It remains possible that in some areas, tumors not seen, or rarely seen in the more developed countries, represent a significant proportion of childhood malignant lymphomas.

Large cell lymphomas in childhood have been poorly characterized but clearly represent a heterogeneous group. Some, at least, appear to have the same chromosomal translocations as undifferentiated lymphomas, although whether the

Table 20-2

Comparison of Frequencies of Childhood Cancer Among Four Population Groups

	Frequency (%)			
Tumor Type	American Blacks (162)†	Manchester* (994)†	Uganda* (766)†	Nigeria (1325)†
Leukemia, all types	27.8	29.5	7.1	4.5
Lymphomas (including Burkitt's and Hodgkin's)	9.8	8.7	49.2	59.0
Gliomas and intracranial tumors	11.2	17.0	1.3	2.2
Sympathetic nervous system tumors	15.5	7.5	2.2	2.6
Retinoblastoma	4.9	3.1	7.4	7.4
Nephroblastoma	10.5	5.4	7.3	5.8
Soft tissue tumors	9.2	11.7	14.75	6.3
Bone tumors	1.2	4.4	—	2.5
Liver tumors	6.2	0.4	—	1.3
Germ cell tumors	3.1	4.1	—	1.6

(Reprinted with permission from Olisa EG, Chandra R, Jackson MA et al: J Natl Cancer Inst 55:281–284, 1975)
* See Davies JN: Some variations in childhood cancers throughout the world. In Marsden HB, Steward JK (eds): Tumours in Children, pp 13–36. New York, Springer-Verlag, 1968.
† Values in parentheses indicate number of children.

breakpoint locations in such cases conform to one or another of the patterns seen in Burkitt's lymphoma is not known. Others, usually designated as immunoblastic lymphomas, may express few surface markers or minimal evidence of a T-cell or B-cell origin. Some of these tumors react with monoclonal antibodies raised against Hodgkin's lymphoma cell lines and designated as Ki-1 or Heffe-1.[63,64] The occurrence of the various subtypes of large cell lymphomas on a world-wide basis is quite unknown at present.

A recognized predisposing factor to malignant non-Hodgkin's lymphoma is immunodeficiency, usually inherited in children, but rarely due to the acquired immune deficiency syndrome (AIDS). The majority of the lymphomas occurring in such individuals are histologically classified as large cell or immunoblastic lymphomas that are predominantly of B-cell origin.[65] Some of these tumors, however, have been diagnosed histologically as Burkitt's lymphoma, and EBV appears to play an important role in pathogenesis.[66] The frequency of AIDS-related non-Hodgkin's lymphomas in Africa, where HIV infection is particularly common, is unknown but likely to come under increasing scrutiny. Whether human immunodeficiency virus (HIV) infection (see Chap. 36) in equatorial African children will further increase the incidence of Burkitt's lymphoma is currently unknown but seems a likely possibility.

Prelymphomatous States

Since lymphomas arise from the constituent cells of the immune system, it is not surprising that disorders associated with abnormal regulation of lymphocytes are associated with an increased incidence of non-Hodgkin's lymphomas (see Chap. 4). This is probably a consequence of alterations in the size and proliferative or self-renewal potential of selected lymphoid subpopulations. EBV also appears to be important in the pathogenesis of lymphomas in immunodeficiency states, since most of these lymphomas contain EBV genomes.[66,67] One possible explanation of this is that defective T-cell regulation permits the expansion of EBV-infected clones of B cells that would normally be tightly controlled but which, due to the influence of viral genes, have a selective advantage over unin-

Table 20-3

Differences Between Endemic and Sporadic Burkitt's Lymphoma

Variable	Endemic	Sporadic
Average annual incidence (children below 16 years)	10 per 100,000	0.2 per 100,000
Occurrence	Climatically determined	Not climatically determined
Association with EBV*	95%	15%
Chromosome 8 breakpoints	Upstream of c-*myc*	Within c-*myc*
Immunologic features	"Blast" Ags CALLA−, Tül+, B2+ No IgM secretion	Few "blast" Ags CALLA+, Tül−, B2− Secretion of IgM
Common sites of tumor	Jaw Abdomen Orbit Paraspinal	Abdomen Bone marrow Nasopharynx Lymph nodes
Response of recurrent tumor (incl. CNS)	Poor	Good

* Presence of Epstein–Barr viral DNA in tumor cells.

fected cells. Such cell clones would then be at increased but not exclusive risk to develop a genetic change capable of causing neoplastic behavior. In such patients, however, the boundary between lymphoproliferation that is not neoplastic and true neoplasia is not easy to discern and is, perhaps, to some extent a semantic debate. Some families, for example, carry a sex-linked disorder known as X-linked lymphoproliferative syn-

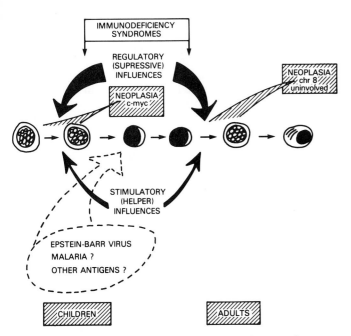

FIGURE 20-2. Diagrammatic depiction of the influence of environmental factors (*e.g.,* malaria, EBV, HIV, or iatrogenic immunosuppression) and inherited immunodeficiency disease on the genesis of B-cell lymphomas. Such factors probably increase the probability of a lymphoma developing by increasing the size of the cell pool that provides a "target" for the lymphomagenic event—possibly the random occurrence of a relevant chromosomal translocation. The differentiation pathway from committed B cells through resting lymphocytes to plasma cells is shown from left to right.

drome (XLP), which is characterized by the occurrence of aplastic anemia, fatal infectious mononucleosis, and malignant non-Hodgkin's lymphomas (see Chaps. 4 and 22).[67] Whether or not patients die of infectious mononucleosis or lymphoma presumably reflects the degree to which immune reactivity against EBV infection is impaired. Individuals with essentially no ability to regulate the proliferation of EBV infected cells die as a consequence of primary EBV infection, whereas those with some ability to control EBV infected cells may simply be at increased risk for a B-cell lymphoma because of an enlarged pool of EBV-infected B cells and consequent increased risk of developing a genetic abnormality that leads to a clonal lymphoma. As already mentioned in patients with AIDS (see Chap. 36) some of the lymphomas that develop have the histologic features of Burkitt's lymphoma and also carry the same chromosomal abnormalities (with breakpoint locations similar to those in sporadic Burkitt's lymphoma).[68-70] Before these lymphomas develop, there is B-cell hyperplasia in which expansion of a small number of clones occurs but in which the genetic changes associated with Burkitt's lymphoma are not present,[70] strongly supporting the above interpretation. HIV is not present in the tumor cells themselves, although it may be present in interspersed lymphocytes.

In children the genetically determined immune deficiency syndromes with the greatest risk of lymphoma development are ataxia telangiectasia, Wiscott–Aldrich syndrome, common variable immune deficiency disease, severe combined immune deficiency syndrome (SCID), and XLP (see Chap. 4). The estimated risk of non-Hodgkin's lymphoma in these syndromes is between 1% (SCID) and 35% (XLP). About 12% to 14% of patients with Wiskott–Aldrich syndrome develop non-Hodgkin's lymphomas. Other genetically deter-

mined immune deficiency syndromes are associated with a much lower risk of lymphoma development. In some of these syndromes the decreased ability to repair DNA and predisposition to chromosomal abnormalities (*e.g.,* ataxia telangiectasia, Bloom's syndrome, and xeroderma pigmentosum) may also play a role in inducing lymphomas.[65]

Transplant recipients are also at risk of developing non-Hodgkin's lymphomas as a consequence of iatrogenic immunosuppression. Lymphomas have been described in kidney, heart, and bone marrow recipients (see Chaps. 22 and 48).[65,71] In some series as many as 25% of renal or cardiac allograft recipients have developed non-Hodgkin's lymphomas after 1 year. Patients treated with the monoclonal antibody T3 also have developed EBV-associated lymphomas,[72] most likely from the consequent reduction in regulatory subsets of T lymphocytes.

Prelymphomatous states of adults such as alpha-heavy-chain disease[73] and angioimmunoblastic lymphadenopathy[74] are very rare in children, and, although a retrovirus (HTLV I) has been implicated in the pathogenesis of a mature T-cell malignancy of adults occurring particularly in Japan, the Caribbean, and Africa, retroviruses to date have not been implicated in childhood lymphomas. The possibility that an as-yet-unknown virus is causally implicated in the pathogenesis of one or more of the childhood lymphomas cannot be excluded.

Drugs and Radiation as Predisposing Factors

Evidence that radiation induces lymphoma is scanty. Unlike leukemia, there was no early lymphoma peak in exposed young persons among atomic bomb survivors in Nagasaki and Hiroshima, and, although there appeared to be an increased incidence in persons who received 200 rad or more in Nagasaki and those exposed to more than 100 rad in Hiroshima, there was no significant trend for increased incidence with increased dose.[75] The possible "lymphomagenic" effects of thymus gland irradiation in children are doubtful.

Patients with Hodgkin's disease treated with combined modality therapy are at increased risk of developing non-Hodgkin's lymphoma—perhaps 4% to 5% will develop non-Hodgkin's lymphoma within 10 years. The precise risk for children with Hodgkin's disease treated with either chemotherapy alone or combined modality therapy has not been determined.

Apart from immunosuppressive drugs used in transplant recipients, information on the capacity of other drugs to induce lymphoma is limited. Hydantoin derivatives are known to cause pseudolymphomas that regress with cessation of therapy, but there are reports of the development of lymphomas in recipients taking these drugs long-term.[75] Unfortunately, no accurate figures are available on the size of this risk, but in view of the widespread use of these compounds it is likely to be very low. Various organic solvents, including dioxins and benzene, have been incriminated in the etiology of non-Hodgkin's lymphomas, but there is no evidence that they represent significant factors in the occurrence of childhood lymphomas.[75]

BIOLOGY

The differences in the characteristic features of childhood and adult lymphomas are presumably a consequence of age-related differences in the immune system. In essence, the child must develop an immunologic repertoire that can respond to a very high number of environmental antigens and, self-evidently, has a much greater number of *primary* encounters with antigen than does the adult. Moreover, since the generation of a specific immune response ultimately involves the selection of a clone of lymphocytes in which rearrangement of the antigen receptor genes (whether immunoglobulin genes or T-cell antigen receptor genes) has produced molecules with the appropriate reactivity, and since the "memory" compartment is relatively small in children, it is likely that the immune system in children contains a much higher proportion of lymphocyte precursor cells, namely, cells undergoing the molecular rearrangements necessary to generate specific immunologic reactivity or cells that have rearranged their immunoglobulin genes but have not yet encountered antigen (see Chap. 4). This is substantiated in the case of the T-cell system by the large size of the thymus during childhood—the anatomic site at which T-cell differentiation occurs. Indeed, lymphoblastic lymphoma, the major T-cell lymphoma of childhood, involves the thymus in a high proportion of cases. Detailed phenotypic studies, predictably, have identified this tumor as a neoplasm of the precursors of functional T cells.[76,77] This, coupled with the recognition that acute lymphoblastic leukemia is a group of neoplasms arising in pre-B cells or T-cell precursors which, in general, are even more immature than those from which thymic lymphoblastic lymphomas arise,[76-78] is consistent with the concept that the lymphoid tumors of childhood arise predominantly in lymphocyte precursors in the bone marrow and thymus rather than in immunocompetent lymphoid cells capable of, or even currently participating in, an immune response (see also Chap. 16). In other words, childhood lymphoid tumors occur mainly (but not exclusively) in the primary rather than in the secondary lymphoid organs and are the neoplastic counterparts of cells that have not yet encountered antigen. In contrast, most adult non-Hodgkin's lymphomas have characteristics consistent with their origins in cells taking part in an immune response, that is, cells activated by antigen. This is particularly obvious in tumors arising from follicular center cells.

Despite the fact that the small noncleaved tumors of childhood, including Burkitt's lymphoma, occur predominantly in the first two decades of life and that in the United States a high proportion of these patients have bone marrow involvement sometime during their clinical course,[53] it has not been clearly demonstrated that these cells are of virgin lymphocyte origin (i.e., unexposed to antigen). Indeed, some investigators favor an origin from memory B cells.

It is clear from these remarks that an understanding of cell biology of the neoplasms of the immune system can be gained only by relating them to their normal counterpart cells. Similarly, an understanding, even if incomplete, of their pathogenesis requires a knowledge of the processes that occur during normal lymphocyte differentiation. The following sections of this chapter will therefore provide sufficient information about normal lymphocyte differentiation to permit a general understanding of the biology of lymphoid neoplasia.

Differentiation Pathways of Normal B Cells

In mammals, cells committed to lymphoid differentiation arise in the bone marrow from multipotential stem cells. Whereas T cells undergo further differentiation in a circumscribed location—the thymus—there is no similar organ that serves exclusively as a site for the early phases of B-cell differentiation (i.e., antigen independent differentiation). This is not the case in birds, in which the bursa of Fabricius subserves this function. Because of this, the characteristics of immature B cells in mammals are less well known than are the characteristics of immature T cells. The bone marrow, the site at which primary

B-cell differentiation occurs in mammals, is both a primary and secondary lymphoid organ because it contains both the most mature (plasma cells) and the most immature cells of the B-cell series (committed B cells not yet synthesizing immunoglobulins) as well as a large number of other cell lineages. Consequently it has not proved possible to obtain pure populations of immature B cells readily and investigate the stages of early differentiation as has been done so elegantly for T cells. Currently existing information on the sequence of events in the early phases of B cell differentiation in humans has been derived predominantly from the analysis of acute lymphoblastic leukemia of pre-B-cell origin.[78] It must be remembered that this information is derived from neoplastic cells and may not reflect normal processes in every respect. It remains, however, the only information available in humans at present, at least with regard to the sequence of antigen expression and immunoglobulin gene rearrangements.

Molecular Events Occurring in B Cell Precursors

The molecular events occurring in B cells during differentiation are directed toward the generation of an immunoglobulin molecule with reactivity to an antigen, or rather to a specific epitope of an antigen. The diversity of the immune response, that is the synthesis of a large number of discrete antigen receptor molecules capable of reacting to a broad range of epitopes, is brought about by the rearrangement (i.e., approximation) of the initially separate component parts of the genes to permit the formation of whole immunoglobulin molecules in cells destined to become B cells, and T-cell antigen receptor molecules in cells destined to become T cells.[79] The immunoglobulin heavy chain genes are situated on chromosome 14 (q24) and arranged in tandem sequence, whereas lambda light chain genes are on chromosome 22 (q11) and kappa chain genes on chromosome 2 (p11) (Fig. 20-3). The ability to clone immunoglobulin genes and study their structure by the methods of recombinant DNA technology has led to the recognition that the parts of the gene coding for the variable (antigen binding) region of immunoglobulin molecules are spacially separated on the chromosome from the constant regions. Moreover, the generation of a gene coding for a functional immunoglobulin molecule requires the approximation of one of the multiple variable (V) regions with the constant region via one each of the other multiple discontinuous segments called D (for diversity region) and J (for joining region). In the heavy chain locus, one of the 5D segments first joins to one of the 6J segments that lie immediately upstream of the first heavy chain constant region expressed during development, namely, $C\mu$. Subsequently, one of the 100 or so variable regions is approximated to the DJ region, bringing with it the promoter and leader sequences of the immunoglobulin gene that now come under the influence of the enhancer region of the immunoglobulin locus (see Fig. 20-4), a region of DNA situated downstream of J, which acts on the promoter to initiate transcription. In the light chain loci similar events occur, except that there is no D region, and one of the 200 or so variable regions is directly approximated to one of the J regions. Based on studies in acute lymphoblastic leukemia,[80] there appears to be an ordered sequence of immunoglobulin gene rearrangements, the first being VDJ joining of one of the two μ alleles. If the recombination is precise (errors may occur) and a functional immunoglobulin gene is created, the second μ gene on the allelic chromosome remains unrearranged so that only one antibody specificity is generated per cell (allelic exclusion). The gene product itself (i.e., μ chains) appears to be responsible for inhibiting the joining of V to D on the allelic chromosome.[79] If a functional gene is not created, the second allele is

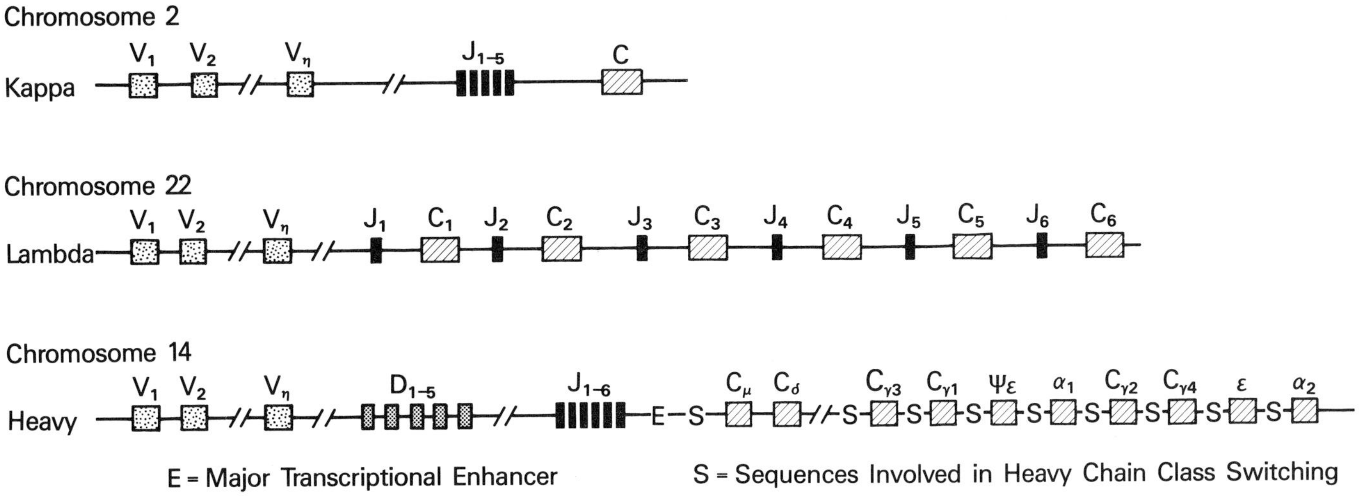

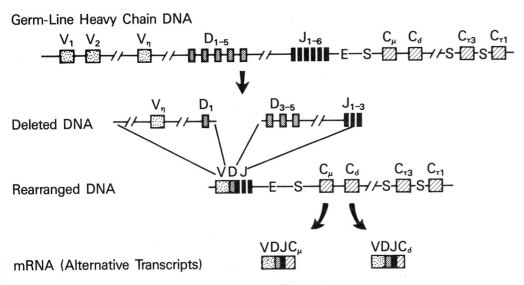

FIGURE 20-3. Molecular organization of the immunoglobulin genes on chromosomes 2 (kappa chains) 22 (lambda chains), and 14 (heavy chains).

FIGURE 20-4. Diagrammatic depiction of the process of VDJ joining.

rearranged. If the resultant gene is still not functional, the cell presumably cannot become a B cell. Based on the occurrence of rearranged μ genes in a small proportion (about 10%) of T-cell acute lymphoblastic leukemias,[81,82] such cells may sometimes go on to rearrange their T-cell receptor genes and become T cells (see Chap. 16). If a functional μ gene is produced, signaled by the synthesis of μ chains, VJ joining of one kappa allele occurs, with allelic exclusion or rearrangement of the second allele depending on the functional consequence of the rearrangement of the first allele, as in the heavy chain locus. If no functional kappa rearrangement is produced, the lambda genes undergo sequential rearrangements in similar fashion to the kappa genes.

The recombinational processes that result in the approximation of variable regions to constant regions is one of the mechanisms for generating antibody diversity. Because this process occurs in both heavy and light chain loci, and because both heavy and light chain variable regions make up the final antigen combining region of the immunoglobulin molecule, a considerable amount of diversity of immunoglobulin molecules is generated at this level alone. However, another important mechanism for generating diversity is the random replacement of nucleotides (so-called N [nucleotide] regions) at the join sites (which are imprecise) between variable and D region domains and D and J domains during the process of VDJ joining. This is accomplished by an enzyme expressed in immature lymphoid cells called terminal deoxyribonucleotide transferase (TdT), which inserts nucleotides without the need of a DNA template.[83] Interestingly, the insertion of N regions appears not to occur at VJ junctions in light chains. Additional somatic mutations occur at random in the variable region during the process of recombination and possibly also during the process of heavy chain class switching described below. It is probable that these modifications of the variable region after VDJ joining are primarily responsible for the acquisition of increasing affinity of the antibodies produced during the course of an immune response, a process that is presumably dependent on selection of those mutations that increase affinity for the epitope in question, probably by a process involving competition for antigen.

Once the cell is committed to the B-cell lineage, that is, there is a successful recombination of one μ allele, the cell is referred to as a pre-B cell. Such cells express cytoplasmic μ chains, HLA-DR antigens, and a B-cell-specific surface antigen known as B4. This has also been referred to as cluster of differentiation antigen (CD19). After the appearance of B4, other B-cell-specific or -associated (*i.e.*, not confined to B cells) antigens are expressed, including the common ALL antigen (CD10), BA-1 (CD24), B1, (CD20) and B2 (the C3d complement component receptor, CD21). Although μ chains are initially confined to the cytoplasm, once the light chain is also synthesized it combines with the heavy chain to form a complete immunoglobulin molecule. The resultant IgM is expressed at the cell surface, and the cell is by definition a B cell. These molecular events occur in a large, dividing cell, but once the cell has successfully synthesized a complete immunoglobulin molecule (always IgM initially) it ceases to divide and becomes a small resting cell competent to respond to antigen by virtue of its expression of surface immunoglobulin, which is, of course, the B-cell antigen receptor. Recently generated virgin B cells that have never encountered antigen leave the bone marrow and circulate for a short time through the perifollicular lymphoid tissue in lymph nodes and the marginal zone of the spleen.[84] Although there is still controversy as to the phenotypic differences between these virgin B cells and memory B cells that have previously encountered antigen, there is evidence that virgin cells, or at least a proportion of them, belong to the leu 1 (CD5) positive population of B cells.[85] These cells synthesize a special subclass of low affinity antibodies capable of broad reactivity (including antibodies against single-stranded DNA and rheumatoid factors). At least some of the leu-1-positive B cells, which include the normal counterpart cells of chronic lymphocytic leukemia, also express surface IgD.

Molecular Events Following Antigenic Stimulation

Under normal circumstances virgin B cells appear to be short lived, being converted to long-lived lymphocytes only if they encounter antigen. It seems likely that circulating lymphocytes that express both IgM and IgD, a phenomenon that involves differential splicing of a long RNA transcript that reads through both μ and δ constant regions, are long-lived lymphocytes and presumably, therefore, memory B cells. These cells recirculate through the primary follicles of lymphoid tissue and, if antigen is encountered, are activated and develop into or enter a germinal center of a secondary follicle. The cells surrounding the germinal center (*i.e.*, which make up the mantle zone) have the same characteristics as those of the primary follicles from which they are presumably derived, namely, surface IgM and IgD. The germinal follicle may be the predominant site for somatic mutation of V regions and of class switching, that is, the site at which the immune response is more precisely tailored with regard to the affinity of antibodies for antigen and where the reapproximation of the variable region to constant regions with different functional capacities takes place. In the latter process, the variable region is moved from its position adjacent to the μ constant region to a position adjacent to one of the other heavy chain constant regions.[79,86] This recombination occurs at specific sites in the immunoglobulin locus, called switch regions, which lie immediately in front (5') of the constant regions (Fig. 20-5). During heavy chain class switch recombination, the DNA sequences between two switch regions are deleted, the switch regions fuse, and a new transcript composed of the same variable sequences as before, coupled now to a new heavy chain constant region (*e.g.*, τ or α), is synthesized. Cells that secrete antibody also process the Ig messenger RNA differently in that the region coding for the membrane anchoring region—the lipophilic region at the carboxy terminal of the molecule—is spliced out of the RNA.[87] The resultant molecules are not inserted into the cell membrane but exported from the cell.

At a morphologic level, activated B cells develop nuclear clefting and undergo rapid enlargement. While still small in size, they are referred to as small cleaved cells. As they enlarge within a germinal center, they become large cleaved cells that may lose most of their surface immunoglobulin, including surface IgD. Eventually the nuclear clefts are lost and the cells develop large quantities of rough endoplasmic reticulum as they begin to synthesize large quantities of immunoglobulin, including surface immunoglobulin. Such cells are referred to as immunoblasts and are usually found in the medullary cords of the lymph node, having exited from the germinal follicle. Finally the cells take on the appearance of plasma cells, and many of them return to the bone marrow, which is the predominant site of antibody production in a secondary immune re-

FIGURE 20-5. Diagrammatic depiction of the process of heavy chain class switching.

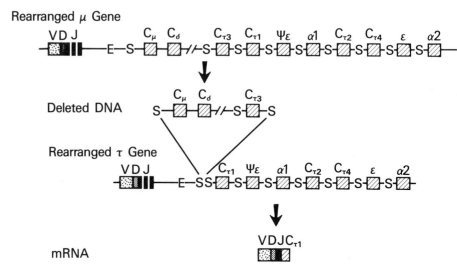

sponse. By now they have lost their surface immunoglobulin but possess large amounts of cytoplasmic immunoglobulin and express plasma-cell-associated antibodies such as T10 and PCA-1.[88]

Cellular Origins of B-Cell Lymphomas in Childhood

Small noncleaved and most large cell lymphomas of childhood are of B-cell phenotype. They express surface immunoglobulins, almost exclusively of the IgM class, associated with either kappa or lambda light chain, and the B-cell-specific antigens, including those detected by the monoclonal antibodies B4 and B1 (CD19, CD20) (see Chap. 4).[48,52,89] Some of these tumors also express a protein that can bind both complement subcomponents (Cd3) and EBV, these sites being detected, respectively, by the monoclonal antibodies B2 and HB5 (CD21). HLA-DR antigens are also invariably present,[89] and since the cells express surface immunoglobulin and therefore, by definition, are true B cells that have completed their immunoglobulin rearrangements, they do not contain the enzyme TdT. The protein detected by the monoclonal antibody leu 1 (CD5), which is expressed by most T cells but only a subclass of B cells (including those that produce IgM antibodies against the Fc region of IgG [*i.e.,* rheumatoid factors], and antibodies to single-stranded DNA), and the cells from which chronic lymphocytic leukemia arises, are not expressed on B-cell lymphomas of children. These tumors frequently express, however, the common ALL antigen, which is present on the surface of both pre-B cells and a fraction of the more mature follicle center cells. There are no reported phenotypic differences at the level of cell surface markers between large cell lymphomas of B-cell type and small noncleaved lymphomas, although it is likely that this is simply a consequence of the lack of sufficiently detailed studies. Differences at a phenotypic level, however, have been described between equatorial and North American small noncleaved lymphomas. North American tumors, for example, secrete IgM (often detectable as a serum monoclonal band on protein electrophoresis), whereas African Burkitt's lymphoma cells appear not to.[90,91] In addition, African Burkitt's lymphoma cells tend to express more of the antigens present on EBV-transformed normal lymphocytes and more EBV receptor than does the sporadic lymphoma.[92-94] There also seems to be a reciprocal relation between reactivity with the antibody against Tü1, which is present on mantle zone cells, and CALLA. Cell lines derived from African tumors express more Tü1 and less CALLA than do sporadic tumors, which usually lack detectable Tü1 expression but nearly always express CALLA.[94] Burkitt's tumor cells do not express receptors for the B-cell growth factor II (BCGF II), detected by the monoclonal antibody B1H5, whereas the expression of receptors for BCGF I appears to correlate directly with the presence or absence of the EBV genome.[95] These findings suggest that the equatorial African and North American forms of Burkitt's lymphoma have different cellular origins or pathogenesis, or both—a suggestion that is supported by data showing that there are differences in the precise locations, at a molecular level, of the breakpoints in the chromosomes involved in the specific translocations associated with these tumors[96] (see below).

Differentiation Pathways of Normal T Cells

Because T-cell differentiation occurs predominantly in a specific anatomic location (the thymus), it has been relatively easy to explore the stages through which T cells pass during their maturation (Fig. 20-6). Pre-T cells arise in the marrow and migrate to the thymus, during which time there is progressive rearrangement of T-cell antigen receptor genes (Ti, the i indicating that the antigen is idiotypic) and progressive alteration in the expression of surface receptors (see also Chap. 4). Three different Ti loci code for α, β, and τ chains (Fig. 20-7). The α locus is on chromosome 14 (q11), whereas the β and τ loci are on chromosome 7 (q35-6 and 7p15, respectively).[97-99] A complete antigen receptor molecule comprises two of these chains, most often α and β, which form a heterodimer similar to an immunoglobulin molecule comprising heavy and light chains. This heterodimer is associated with another molecule, T3 (CD3), on the cell surface to form the complete antigen detection complex.[100] The rearrangement of the T-cell antigen receptor genes is very similar to that of the immunoglobulin genes. Each allele has discontinuous variable (V), joining (J), and constant (C) regions in the germline (unrearranged state), and the β locus, at least, also has D regions as well as two C regions. When rearrangement of the β locus occurs, one of a small number of V regions, perhaps only 15 for this locus, joins to one of the 6 D regions and one of the 6 J regions (DJ joining precedes VD joining as in the immunoglobulin locus) which are located upstream of the $C_{\beta 1}$ or $C_{\beta 2}$ regions to form a functional gene.[101] A similar process of VJ joining occurs in the α and τ loci, although each varies with regard to the number of V, J, and C regions. During thymocyte differentiation it appears that the Tτ gene is the first to rearrange, followed by the T$_\beta$ gene, then the Tα gene. Tβ is present in the cytoplasm before the complete antigen receptor complex, which includes α and

FIGURE 20-6. Differentiation of T-cell precursors (TdT positive) in the thymus. Some of the antigens expressed at various stages are shown on the right. CD groups are as follows: 3A1, CD7; T6, CD1; T4, CD4; T8, CD8; T3, CD3.

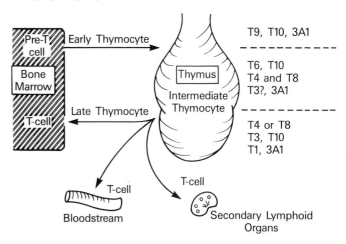

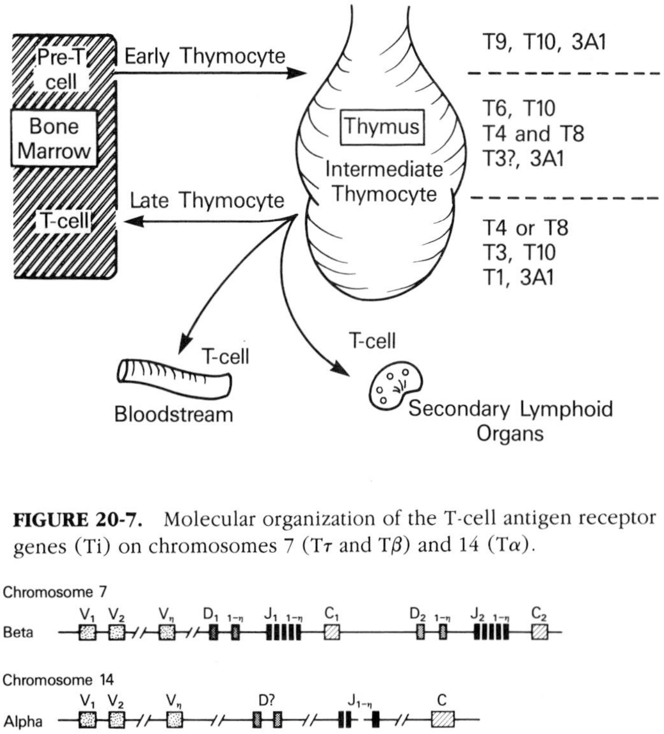

FIGURE 20-7. Molecular organization of the T-cell antigen receptor genes (Ti) on chromosomes 7 (Tτ and Tβ) and 14 (Tα).

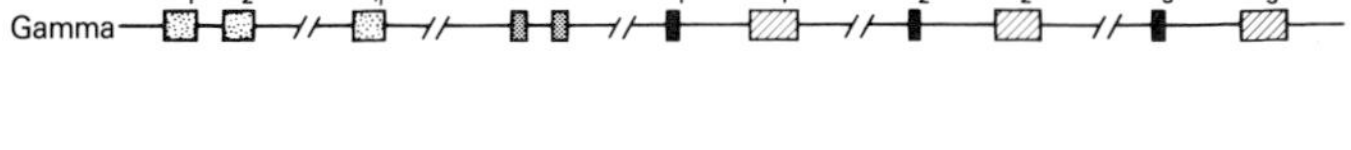

T3 (CD3) molecules expressed at the cell surface.[102,103] This is analogous to μ immunoglobulin expression before light chain rearrangement in pre-B cells. The Tτ gene is distinct from this complex (the τ chain of the T3 molecule should not be confused with Tτ), and its function is as yet unknown, although its rearrangement appears to be an early event in T-cell differentiation and it is rearranged in a variety of functionally different T-cell populations, including helper and cytotoxic/suppressor T cells.[104,105] As in B-cell tumors, the enzyme TdT has been shown to be involved in adding random nucleotides to either side of the D gene segment in the rearranging Ti genes,[105,106] although, unlike in B cells, somatic mutation does not appear to be a mechanism involved in the generation of antigen receptor diversity.[101] Early thymocytes express an antigen (of unknown function) recognized by the monoclonal antibodies 3A1, 4H9 (leu 9), and WT1 (CD7)[107-109] as well as the transferrin receptor (T9) and an antigen also present on activated T cells and plasma cells (T10).[110] Some, but not all, early T cells express the T11 antigen (CD2), which is the sheep red cell receptor, formerly detected by sheep red cell rosetting.[108,109] T cells can be activated by means of this receptor, which is expressed on most thymocytes and peripheral T cells.[111] Tτ but not Tβ receptor genes are rearranged at the earliest stage of intrathymic differentiation. At an intermediate level of differentiation, thymocytes express an antigen called T6 (CD1), as well as both T4 (CD4) and T8 (CD8), the antigens expressed by T cells that are activated in the presence of class II and class I HLA antigens, respectively.[110] Intermediate thymocytes have rearranged Tβ genes but do not express Ti molecules or the associated T3 antigen (CD3) at the cell surface.[102,103] As the cells mature further, they express at the cell surface either T4 or T8 antigens but not both, and also express the antigen receptor (Ti) in conjunction with T3.[102,103,110] T4-positive cells are helpers of other cell types, including cells responding to antigen and mitogen stimulation, suppressor and cytotoxic T cells, and antibody-producing cells. T8-positive cells include suppressor and cytotoxic cells of various kinds.[112,113] Self-HLA antigens appear to be necessary for the development of helper cells in the thymus.[114]

Activation of T cells is associated with the expression of a variety of "activation" antigens, including interleukin-2 receptor (CD25), transferrin receptor, HLA Class II antigens T10, Ki-1 (CD30), and others,[115] but since, with the exception of some large cell lymphomas, childhood lymphomas appear to arise only from immature T cells, such antigens will not be discussed here.

Cellular Origins of T-Cell Lymphomas in Childhood

Lymphoblastic lymphoma, in addition to its distinctive histologic appearance, differs from all other lymphomas by virtue of the almost invariable presence of TdT.[116] The relevance of this enzyme to the generation of both T- and B-cell receptor diversity has been discussed above, and its presence indicates that the cell type is immature and likely to be at the differentiation stage when rearrangement of its antigen receptor genes is occurring. This may be significant with regard to the role of translocations in pathogenesis, since some translocations may arise as a consequence of inappropriate interchromosomal recombination during the process of physiological intrachromosomal recombination between variable and constant region gene segments.[117] Differentiation beyond this stage and loss of TdT may take the place, however, even after the translocation has occurred. Regardless of its physiological role, TdT provides an objective means of dividing the childhood lymphomas into two broad categories, being present in all lymphoblastic

lymphomas (Rappaport terminology; see below) and acute lymphoblastic leukemia but no other morphologic category.

Most lymphoblastic lymphomas (and some large cell lymphomas) express T-cell markers, including the glycoprotein (gp 40) recognized by the monoclonal antibodies 4H9, 3A1, or WT1 (leu 9). Although absent from some more mature T-cell neoplasms, this antigen is present on essentially all immature T-cell malignancies, that is, lymphoblastic lymphomas and leukemias of T-cell type, and is therefore a particularly good marker of the T lineage when the cells are immature.[107-109] T1 (CD5) is frequently present, particularly on more mature thymocytes. Additional antigens expressed by T-cell lymphoblastic lymphomas predominantly reflect an intermediate (3A1, T11, T6, T4, and T8) or late (3A1, T11, T3, and either T4 or T8) thymocyte phenotype,[76,77] although atypical patterns are quite frequently observed.[76,77,118] It is of interest that, in contrast, a high proportion of T-cell acute lymphoblastic leukemias express early thymocyte markers and usually lack T6, T3, T4, and T8.[76,119]

One difficulty in concluding that lymphoblastic leukemia is generally the counterpart of an earlier precursor T cell than is lymphoblastic lymphoma is the indistinct borderline between these diseases.[120] Arbitrary separation on the basis of the percentage of blast cells in the bone marrow is unsatisfactory, and the numerical cutoff usually chosen (25%) appears to have little prognostic significance. It would appear more rational to conclude that although neoplasms with an "early" thymocyte phenotype almost always present as leukemia, neoplasms with a more mature phenotype can also involve the bone marrow (see also Chap. 16). A small proportion of T-cell lymphoblastic lymphomas express the common ALL antigen, but HLA-DR is seen uncommonly. Infrequently, lymphoblastic lymphomas express the phenotype of pre-B cells as seen in acute lymphoblastic leukemia (B4, HLA-DR, usually with common ALL antigen, and with or without other B-cell markers such as B1 or even less commonly B2, but without surface immunoglobulin).[62,121-123] Very recently, lymphoblastic lymphoma was described in which the phenotype was that of natural killer cells.[124] The significance of these findings to therapy remains uncertain at present.

Poorly Characterized Lymphomas

Some rare childhood lymphomas fall histologically into the large cell category and are sometimes further defined as immunoblastic lymphomas that do not conform to the more usual B- or T-cell phenotypes that occur in large cell lymphomas. Some of these tumors express an antigen first detected on cell lines derived from Hodgkin's lymphoma, which can be detected by a monoclonal antibody known as Ki-1(CD30).[63] This protein is not present on circulating lymphocytes, activated monocytes, or tissue macrophages but is expressed on activated lymphocytes. Such Ki-1 lymphomas often present with cutaneous lesions and peripheral adenopathy and arise from activated perifollicular T or B cells, the T-cell type being in the majority.[125] Ki-1 lymphomas may express few surface markers, and their lineage may be apparent only by examination of immunoglobulin or T-cell antigen receptor gene rearrangements.[63]

The cellular origins of other lymphomas that do not express T- or B-cell characteristics has not been determined with precision, although some may be of true histiocytic origin.[126] Frequently, lymphomas that occur in children with immune deficiency syndromes are designated as immunoblastic lymphomas. Although most such lymphomas are of B-cell origin, this is not always the case.[127] Detailed characterization remains to be performed.

Cytokinetics of Childhood Lymphomas

All childhood lymphomas are rapidly growing neoplasms with very high growth fractions (approaching 100% in some cases) and potential doubling times (*i.e.,* calculated doubling times that do not take into account spontaneous cell death in the neoplasm) ranging from 12 hours to a few days.[128] In practice, even small noncleaved cell lymphomas, one of the most rapidly growing of all neoplasms, has a measured (actual) doubling time of several days (the mean of 3 skin tumors was 66 hours), although there is considerable variation from patient to patient and between different tumor sites in the same patient, since the spontaneous cell death rate is dependent on tumor size (being greater in larger tumors) and, probably, the nature of the tissue in which it resides, although no studies have been done to examine this. The spontaneous cell death rate has been measured in African Burkitt's lymphoma to be about 70% of all progeny cells.[128] Among the childhood lymphoid neoplasms, B-cell tumors have the highest growth fractions, and up to 27% of the cells may be in S-phase (by flow cytometry).[130]

These observations have relevance to management. The high spontaneous cell turnover rate in untreated tumors is the immediate cause of pretreatment hyperuricemia, which, as expected from the cytokinetic parameters, occurs more frequently in the B-cell neoplasms. The short actual doubling times mean that patients should be worked up rapidly and treatment begun at the earliest possible time, particularly in B-cell neoplasms. Any delay will increase both the chance of complications and worsen the prognosis, since tumor burden is perhaps the single most important prognostic factor. The high growth fraction is also beneficial because it is likely that this is a critically important factor in the excellent response of childhood lymphomas to a wide range of chemotherapeutic agents and the fact that these neoplasms can be cured.

GENETICS AND MOLECULAR PATHOLOGY

The specific cytogenetic findings in undifferentiated lymphomas, including Burkitt's lymphoma, have been of paramount importance in the development of an understanding of the pathogenesis of these tumors and have led to the detection of a series of molecular markers that provide a new and substantially more precise means of characterization than any other available method (see also Chap. 3). Moreover, it has now become clear that even within an apparently homogeneous phenotype there may be more than one tumor, as defined at a molecular genetic level. The relevance to the clinician of this new ability to subcategorize at a molecular level remains to be determined, but particular genetic abnormalities may correlate with prognosis so that refinement of therapy may be possible. Some of the genetic changes may provide specific markers that could enhance our ability to detect residual tumor cells (*e.g.,* in patients with bone marrow involvement). Molecular markers may even increase our understanding of the reasons for failure, since they could be used to determine whether the malignant clone can persist in cell types that differ morphologically from the recognized tumor cells (*e.g.,* having the morphology of mature lymphocytes). Finally, improved understanding of pathogenesis could eventually lead to the development of new approaches to treatment that are directed toward the abnormal biochemistry of the neoplastic cell.[131]

The translocations of B- and T-cell neoplasms described below strongly suggest a general pattern for the translocations in which the involved chromosomal regions include the antigen receptor locus (Ig or Ti) and another region involved in cellular proliferation or differentiation. It seems likely that the genetic rearrangements of the antigen receptor are relevant to the genesis of the translocations, which may occur as a mistake during normal physiologic rearrangements of these genes, or at least take place at the stage of differentiation when these events are occurring, perhaps rendering specific regions of the T- and B-cell receptor loci more vulnerable to breaks.

Small Noncleaved Cell (Undifferentiated) Lymphomas

The discovery in 1976 of the characteristic chromosomal translocation involving chromosomes 8 and 14 in Burkitt's lymphoma (Fig. 20-8)[132] led to crucially important insights into the pathogenesis of this disease, for not only did the breakpoints in the involved chromosomes coincide with the location of, on the one hand, a proto-oncogene (c-*myc,* on chromosome 8, band q24) and, on the other, the immunoglobulin heavy chain genes (on chromosome 14, band q32), but also it was soon shown that the c-*myc* gene is translocated from chromosome 8 to the heavy chain locus on chromosome 14.[133,134] The involvement of the immunoglobulin heavy chain locus in a translocation present in a B-cell tumor suggested pathogenetic significance, and this was soon endorsed by the demonstration of additional chromosomal translocations occurring in a small proportion of Burkitt's lymphomas in which a breakpoint was still present on the q24 band of chromosome 8, but the other breakpoint was situated in either the kappa immunoglobulin light chain locus on chromosome 2 or the lambda light chain locus on chromosome 22 (Fig. 20-8).[135] In these so-called variant translocations, the c-*myc* gene remains on chromosome 8, but a part of the relevant light chain region is translocated onto this chromosome distal to the c-*myc* gene.[136] Thus, although at first sight rather different, there is a common feature to the 8:14 and variant translocations, for in all cases the c-*myc* gene comes to lie adjacent to immunoglobulin constant region sequences, whether of heavy or light chain origin (Fig. 20-9). Further confirmation that these chromosomal translocations are of pathogenetic significance, and not simply secondary changes, was obtained through experiments conducted with somatic cell hybrids between Burkitt's lymphoma cells and mouse plasmacytomas. In these hybrid cells, human chromosomes are selectively lost so that clones containing only some of the human chromosome content can be obtained. It was shown that the c-*myc* allele on the uninvolved chromosome 8 is silent, whereas the c-*myc* allele involved in the translocation is expressed (whether translocated to chromosome 14 or remaining on chromosome 8).[137] These findings led to the conclusion that the proto-oncogene c-*myc* is in some way "activated" (abnormally expressed) by its proximity to immunoglobulin sequences. However, since the level of c-*myc* messenger RNA in the cytoplasm is similar to that in other proliferating cells, including those of B-lymphocyte origin,[138] the abnormality is not simply one of quantity but is more likely to involve inappropriate expression. It has been proposed that there is no expression at all of c-*myc* in the normal counterpart cell of Burkitt's lymphoma.[48] The product of the c-*myc* oncogene is known to be necessary for cellular proliferation,[139] and it seems likely that the inappropriate expression of c-*myc,* occasioned by the translocation, maintains the cell in a proliferative state when, under normal circumstances, it should be a resting cell.

Because the immunoglobulin genes and the translocated c-*myc* gene are arranged in opposite transcriptional orientation in the more frequent 8;14 translocations, the activation mechanism cannot involve the immunoglobulin promotor. Nor is it possible that the recognized transcriptional enhancer situated in the heavy chain locus between the J and switch regions is

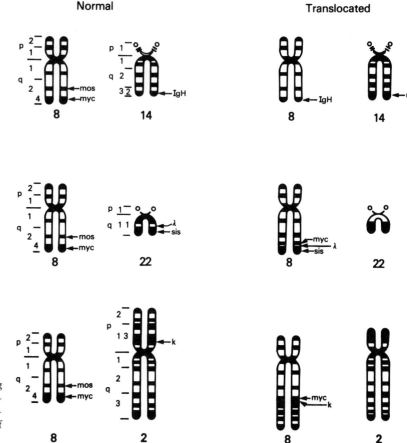

FIGURE 20-8. Chromosomal translocations occurring in small noncleaved cell lymphomas. The banding patterns and relevant gene locations are shown in the normal chromosomes on the left, and the consequences of the translocations are shown on the right.

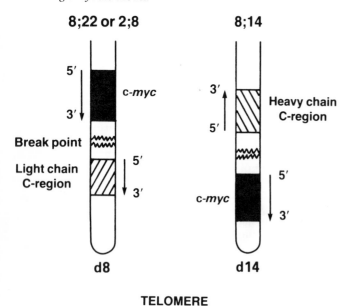

FIGURE 20-9. Juxtaposition of the c-*myc* and immunoglobulin genes brought about by the specific chromosomal translocations in Burkitt's lymphoma. Note the opposite transcriptional orientation of the genes in the 8;14 translocation (*arrows*). Only the derivative chromosomes containing c-*myc* are shown.

relevant to altered c-*myc* regulation because in many 8;14 translocations, depending on the precise location of the breakpoint in the heavy chain locus, this is a part of the reciprocal translocation product that comes to lie on chromosome 8 while at the same time the c-*myc* gene has been moved to chromosome 14 (Fig. 20-10). It seems likely that there are several different methods of activating the c-*myc* gene, one of the strongest pieces of evidence for this being the observation that the location of the breakpoint on chromosome 8 varies markedly (Fig. 20-11). In the 8;14 translocations it may be upstream of c-*myc*, within the gene (though not within the protein coding sequences, *i.e.,* exons II and III), or in the immediate 5′ flanking sequences. In the variant translocations, the breakpoint is downstream of the gene. Of interest is a correlation between the site of the breakpoint on chromosome 8 and the geographic origin of the tumor. In equatorial African Burkitt's lymphomas (endemic) the breakpoint is usually some distance upstream of the gene, but it appears that in this circumstance there are mutations in the first exon of the c-*myc* gene that probably influence the regulation of transcription. The protein coding sequences of the gene, however, appear to be normal in the majority of Burkitt's lymphomas[48] (Fig. 20-11). In North American tumors (sporadic) the breakpoint is usually within the gene or in its flanking sequences, which are almost certainly involved in the regulation of its expression.[96]

Thus in the endemic tumors there are mutations in the regulatory sequence, whereas in the sporadic tumors the regulatory sequences are partly or wholly lost. The distinction be-

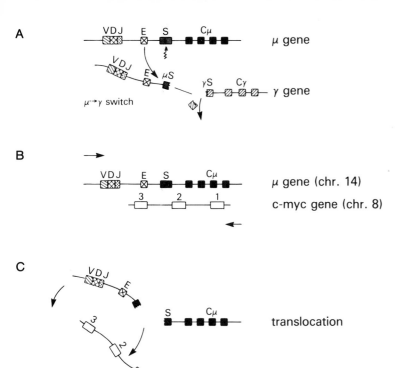

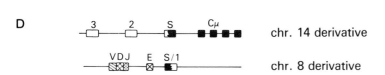

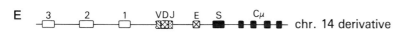

FIGURE 20-10. Diagrammatic depiction of the molecular rearrangements that occur as a consequence of the 8:14 translocation. **A.** A μ gene that has undergone VDJ joining undergoes normal heavy chain class switching from μ to τ. Note that the known enhancer region (*E*) moves with the variable region to the τ constant region. **B.** Normal μ and c-*myc* genes arranged side by side. Arrows show directions of transcription. **C.** Translocation occurring between μ and c-*myc* genes. The breakpoint on chromosome 14 is depicted as being in a switch region, and the breakpoint on chromosome 8 falls within the first exon of the c-*myc* gene. **D.** The derivative chromosomes after the translocation shown in c. The known enhancer is now on chromosome 8 in this example and hence could not influence transcription of the translocated c-*myc* gene. **E.** A derivative 14 chromosome in which the breakpoints were in different regions: 5′ of c-*myc* and in the V immunoglobulin region. In this case the enhancer is on the same chromosome as c-*myc*.

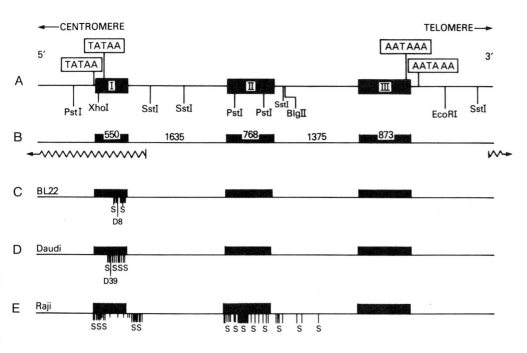

FIGURE 20-11. **A.** Structure of the normal c-*myc* gene, showing the three exons, the alternative promoters (TATAA boxes), poly A addition sites (AATAAA), and sites cut by various restriction endonucleases. **B.** Regions at which breakage can occur as a consequence of the chromosomal translocations (*wavy line*). The numbers indicate the number of base pairs in various regions of the gene. **C, D, E.** c-*myc* genes that were obtained from Burkitt's lymphoma cell lines and sequenced. Note the normality of the second and third (protein coding) exons in two of the genes and the mutations (substitutions and deletions) in the first exons (involved in regulation of transcription) of all three.

tween endemic and sporadic tumors is not, however, absolute, and about 10% to 25% of tumors do not conform to the more usual pattern for the region. Despite this, these observations are consistent with the probability that the cell in which the translocation occurs is at a different stage of differentiation in most endemic versus most sporadic tumors. The normal counterpart cell of Burkitt's lymphoma has not been definitively identified, although there is increasing evidence that it is a resting lymphocyte, either one that has recently exited the marrow (*i.e.*, a virgin B cell) or a memory B cell.[53,140] This does not necessarily mean that the chromosomal translocation occurs in this type of cell. It has been proposed that the translocation occurs as a mistake during physiological immunoglobulin gene rearrangement (*i.e.*, a more immature cell) and that the enzymes involved (recombinases) are those normally utilized during this process.[117] Figure 20-12 depicts a hypothetical scenario that brings these pieces of information together to provide a reasonable account of the pathogenesis of Burkitt's lymphoma, at least in the context of the 8;14 chromosomal translocation occurring around the time of VDJ recombination and the resultant abnormalities of c-*myc* gene expression. In tumors with either an 8;22 or a 2;8 translocation, the translocation presumably occurs in proximity to physiological light chain rearrangement rather than heavy chain rearrangement. The tumors with variant translocations are too infrequent for analysis of the clinical or prognostic implications of these translocations to have been performed so far, although such a study would be of considerable interest.

It remains unknown as to why the translocations occur and to what extent they are random events. Band q24 of chromosome 8 has been recognised as a "fragile site," that is, a chromosomal location which, for unknown reasons, though possibly related to the precise positioning of histones and other DNA binding proteins on the DNA strand, is particularly susceptible to breaks induced *in vitro* by agents such as caffeine.[141] Thus band q24 may simply be *more likely* to be a site of random DNA damage.

One final component of the genesis of translocations could be a relative deficiency in DNA repair, demonstrated to be present in mice susceptible to plasmocytoma development. Of interest, mouse plasmocytomas bear homologous translocations to Burkitt's lymphoma.[142] Whether patients with Burkitt's lymphoma have an inherited predisposition to such translocations because of relatively infficient DNA repair or whether an altered ability to repair DNA could be induced by an environmental factor are topics for further research.

Lymphoblastic Lymphomas

Although specific nonrandom chromosomal abnormalities occurring in a high proportion of lymphoblastic lymphomas have not been found to date,[143] several translocations have been described in small numbers of cases of T-cell lymphoblastic leukemias and lymphomas that involve chromosomal regions relevant to T-cell differentiation, including, in most cases, the Ti receptor genes (particularly Tα situated on chromosome 14q11). This is very reminiscent of the translocations involving immunoglobulin genes in B-cell tumors. In the translocations described to date, translocations between chromosomes 14(q11) and 11 (p13/15) have been most often observed (in

FIGURE 20-12. Hypothetical schema depicting the pathogenesis of Burkitt's lymphoma. On the left are shown the normal series of differentiation steps (including VDJ joining) for the earliest stages of B cells, resulting in cytoplasmic μ chains (*C*) and then surface IgM (*E*). The earliest cells expressing surface IgM (virgin B cells) are resting cells, unlike their more immature counterparts, and have switched off expression of c-*myc*. On the right, chromosomal translocation and deregulation of c-*myc* have occurred, with resultant indefinite proliferation of the cells containing the translocation.

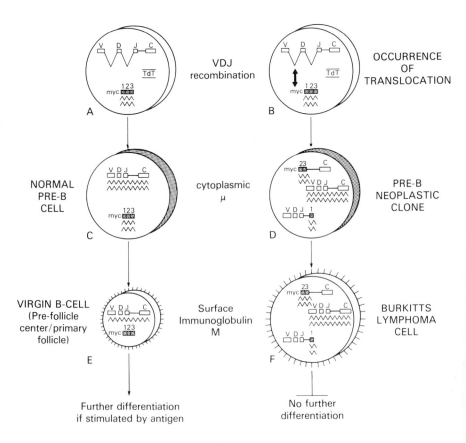

∿∿∿ gene expression

VDJC variable, diversity, joining and constant immunoglobulin gene regions.

both leukemia and lymphoma), but 1;14, 8;14, and 10;14 translocations have also been described.[144–151] In one tumor from which a cell line was derived, an inversion of the long arm of chromosome 14 was seen. Molecular studies in the cell line have demonstrated a remarkable rearrangement in which the variable region of the α chain of the T-cell receptor gene is juxtaposed to the J region of the heavy chain immunoglobulin locus, and *vice versa*.[145] Although RNA derived from the hybrid $V_{Ig}J_\alpha C_\alpha$ gene has been demonstrated, it is not known at present whether a hybrid protein is made or whether this rearrangement has pathogenetic significance. These findings strongly suggest that the rearrangement of genetic material occurred during the process of cell differentiation at a time when rearrangements of T-cell receptor gene subunits normally occur—at an early thymocyte stage. As could be the case with B-cell tumors, the enzymes that are involved in the pathologic recombinations may be responsible for physiological gene rearrangement. It is also likely, particularly in view of the inversion described above, that these enzymes are common to B- and T-cell antigen receptor gene recombinations.[152] Molecular cloning of the cell line (MOLT 16) containing an 8:14 (q24;q11) translocation has demonstrated the translocation of the Tα constant region from its location in chromosome 14 (the breakpoint being in the J region of the Tα gene) to chromosome 8 distal to c-*myc*. A second cell line with a similar rearrangement has been described. These translocations are analogous to the variant translocations observed in small noncleaved lymphomas. The breakpoint on chromosome 11 in the 11:14 (p15;q11) translocations is between the genes for insulin and the insulin-like growth factor.[149] The regulation of the latter could be disturbed by the translocation. The 10;14 translocation reported in four T-cell lymphoblastic neoplasms results from chromosomal breaks in the q11 band (Tα) on chromosome 14 and band q24 on chromosome 10, which includes the gene coding for TdT. To what extent these various translocations are associated with specific clinical presentations (*e.g.,* lymphoma versus leukemia) remains unclear at present. Specific nonrandom translocations in non-T-lymphoblastic lymphomas have not yet been described, although translocations have been described in acute lymphoblastic leukemia with the same phenotype (see Chap. 16).

Large Cell Lymphomas

Characteristic karyotypic abnormalities have also not yet been observed for large cell lymphomas in children.[153] This is not surprising because these tumors, as described above, are phenotypically heterogeneous. Some, at least, bear the same karyotype as small noncleaved lymphomas, namely, an 8:14 translocation,[154] but these tumors have not been sufficiently analyzed at a molecular level. The similarity or differences between small noncleaved and large cell lymphomas with 8;14 chromosomal translocations remain to be determined. The chromosomal translocation that occurs in follicular lymphomas and in some large cell lymphomas in adults, namely, the 14:18 translocation,[155,156] has not so far been described in children. In view of the absence of true follicular lymphomas in children, this is not surprising, but it also indicates that the spectrum of large cell lymphomas in children and adults differs in that the majority of those in adults, unlike those in children, are of follicular center cell origin.

HISTOPATHOLOGY

At a histologic level, pediatric non-Hodgkin's lymphomas can be divided, according to the NCI formulation (Table 20-4), into three major categories[1,2]: lymphoblastic (about 30% of childhood non-Hodgkin's lymphomas, depending on the way in which the distinction is made between leukemia and lymphoma); small noncleaved (about half of the childhood non-Hodgkin's lymphomas); and large cell lymphomas (about 20% of childhood non-Hodgkin's lymphomas). All are diffuse lymphomas of high grade (in the formulation nomenclature) except for some large cell lymphomas (large noncleaved or large cleaved), which are technically of intermediate grade according to the formulation. Such lymphomas, however, are uncommon in children and account for perhaps half of the large cells lymphomas, the other half comprising the immunoblastic lymphomas. Lymphoma cells tend to efface the architecture of lymphoid tissue, although in the early stages of involvement there may be preservation of the architecture in some areas of the lymph node. In nonlymphoid tissue, the neoplastic cells

Table 20-4
Comparison of Terminology in Different Classification Schemes

Classification Scheme	Indistinguishable from ALL	Indistinguishable or Similar to BL	Large Lymphoid Cells
Rappaport	Lymphoblastic lymphoma (convoluted or nonconvoluted)	Undifferentiated lymphoma, Burkitt or non-Burkitt	Histiocytic lymphoma
Lukes and Collins	ML of convoluted lymphocytes (T cell)	ML of small noncleaved follicle center cells	ML of large follicle center cells Immunoblastic sarcoma (T or B cell) Histiocytic
Kiel	ML lymphoblastic, convoluted and unclassified types	ML lymphoblastic, Burkitt type	ML centroblastic ML immunoblastic
British National Lymphoma	Lymphocytic poorly differentiated (lymphoblast)—convoluted cell mediastinal lymphoma	Lymphocytic poorly differentiated (lymphoblast)—Burkitt's tumor NonBurkitt's tumor	Undifferentiated large cell (large lymphoid cell) Histiocytic cell (Mononuclear phagocytic cell)
World Health Organization	Diffuse lymphosarcoma, lymphoblastic	Diffuse lymphosarcoma, Burkitt's tumor	Diffuse lymphosarcoma, immunoblastic Reticulosarcoma
Working Formulation	ML lymphoblastic, convoluted and nonconvoluted types	ML small noncleaved cell	ML large cells ML immunoblastic

infiltrate between the normal cells, collagen, or muscle fibers of involved tissues.

Lymphoblastic lymphomas are indistinguishable histologically and cytologically from the lymphoblasts of acute lymphoblastic leukemia. The cells are usually quite uniform in appearance, but a percentage of the cells may have irregular nuclear margins and linear markings in the nuclei caused by nuclear convolutions (sometimes likened to the imprint of a crow's foot). The nuclear convolutions are not always present, and there is variation in the quantity of cytoplasm from one tumor to another. The nuclear chromatin is finely stippled, and, although multiple nucleoli are present, they are difficult to see. There is usually a thin rim of pale cytoplasm (*i.e.,* a high nuclear:cytoplasmic ratio (Fig. 20-13). The distinction of lymphoblastic lymphoma from acute lymphoblastic leukemia is arbitrary at present and can be done only on the basis of clinical features. Some pediatric oncologists have advocated using the extent of bone marrow involvement as a means of making a separation: Leukemia is diagnosed if at least 25% of the nucleated cells are lymphoblasts, and lymphoma if the degree of infiltration is less than 25%. Such a distinction is of questionable biological significance, particularly because it depends on adequate sampling of the marrow. Further, with sufficient delay the percentage of marrow blasts may increase.

Small noncleaved cell lymphomas are either indistinguishable or differ only with regard to the degree of pleomorphism or the number of large, single nucleoli from African Burkitt's lymphoma. Thus the small noncleaved cell lymphomas can be subdivided into Burkitt's and non-Burkitt's lymphomas (Fig. 20-14), although there are no known clinical, phenotypic, karyotypic, or molecular features that correspond to this histologic subdivision. Small noncleaved cells also have a high nuclear:cytoplasmic ratio, although in cytologic preparations not quite as high as in the case of lymphoblastic lymphoma. The nucleus is round or oval and has a more "open" nuclear chromatin pattern, giving the appearance of being able to see through the network of chromatin, than does lymphoblastic lymphoma. There are multiple (usually 2–5), readily discernible nucleoli. Occasional cells may have only a single central nucleolus, but if such cells are frequent, many pathologists would diagnose non-Burkitt's lymphoma. The rim of cytoplasm is very basophilic (staining intensely with methyl green pyronine) and usually contains lipid vacuoles that stain with lipid stains such as oil red O. The cells are frequently

interspersed with macrophages in which nuclear debris is discernible and which give rise to the oft-quoted "starry sky" appearance. This pattern is not pathognomonic and may be seen in any rapidly proliferating tumor.

Large cell lymphomas differ from small noncleaved lymphomas mainly with regard to size and have a significantly greater quantity of cytoplasm. The term immunoblastic lymphoma is reserved for large cell lymphomas that do not meet the criteria for large cell lymphomas of germinal center origin. The latter are more commonly seen in adults and are designated as large cleaved or noncleaved cell lymphomas. As implied, the nuclei may or may not be cleaved and the nucleoli are frequently closely applied to the inner aspect of the nuclear membrane. The recently described Ki-1 lymphoma is usually classified as immunoblastic, but the frequent very large cells have led some to use the term "bizarre large cell lymphoma" (Fig. 20-15).[125] Ki-1 lymphomas characteristically involve the lymph node sinuses. A very small number of large cell lymphomas may be of true histiocytic origin.[126]

Although these categories are the primary determinants of

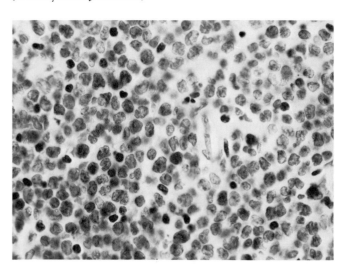

FIGURE 20-13. Histologic appearance of lymphoblastic lymphoma. (Courtesy of Dr. J. Cossman)

FIGURE 20-14. Histologic appearance of small noncleaved (undifferentiated) lymphomas. **A.** Burkitt's lymphoma. **B.** Non-Burkitt's lymphoma. This tumor was not diagnosed as Burkitt's lymphoma largely because of the frequent single large nucleoli. (Courtesy of Dr. J. Cossman)

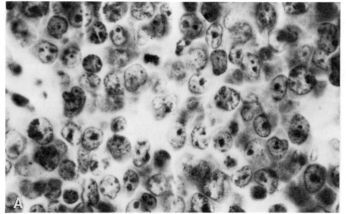

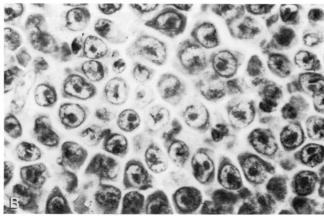

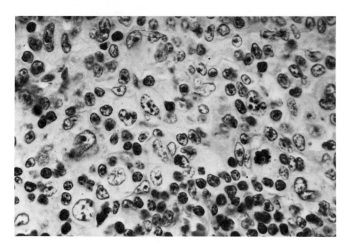

FIGURE 20-15. Histologic appearance of large cell lymphoma (immunoblastic, Ki-1). (Courtesy of Dr. J. Cossman)

Table 20-5
Correspondence Between Histology and Immunophenotype

Histology	Phenotype
Lymphoblastic	Immature T cell (thymocyte)
	Pre-B cell
Small noncleaved	B cell (surface IgM)
Large cell:	
Large follicle center cell	B cell
Immunoblastic	B cell
	T cell

treatment decisions at present, they are not homogeneous even when morphology alone is used as the discriminant. Each category can be subdivided on the basis of morphology (particularly small noncleaved and large cell) or phenotype (particularly lymphoblastic and large cell) and doubtless, as more information accumulates, karyotype and molecular genetics. One needs to be aware that there are several classification nomenclatures currently in widespread use that employ quite different terms derived from histogenetic or purely descriptive cytologic designations (Table 20-4).[20,22,23,25–28] Unfortunately, the same term is sometimes applied to quite different tumors in different classification systems. The term lymphoblastic lymphoma in the Kiel and British Lymphoma classification schemes, for example, includes small noncleaved lymphomas, which is a separate category in other classification schemes.

Reproducibility of a histologic diagnosis, particularly between pathologists, is often less than satisfactory. Perhaps the most reproducible histologic distinction is that between lymphoblastic lymphoma and all other tumors, often collectively referred to as nonlymphoblastic lymphomas.[158] There is difficulty, on occasion, in distinguishing between small noncleaved lymphomas and large cell lymphomas, and even more in subdividing the small noncleaved category into Burkitt's and non-Burkitt's lymphomas. The correspondence between histology and immunophenotype is shown in Table 20-5, which demonstrates that while the histologic classification of childhood lymphomas is initially much less confusing than that of adult lymphomas, it fails to distinguish between several distinct pathologic entities. The relevance of this to therapy may

take some time to elucidate because of the rarity of several of the subtypes. Nevertheless, unless phenotyping and cytogenetic analysis are routinely performed, it will never be possible to determine their significance as prognostic factors.

CLINICAL PRESENTATIONS

Clinical Presentations Related to Histology

Patients with non-Hodgkin's lymphoma present, for the most part, with a limited number of syndromes, most of which correlate well with cell type. Patients with lymphoblastic lymphomas most commonly manifest intrathoracic tumor, particularly a mediastinal mass (50–70%) and often pleural effusions. Symptoms may include pain, dysphagia, dyspnea, or swelling of the neck, face, and upper limbs from superior vena caval obstruction. If such patients have lymphadenopathy (which occurs in 50–80% of all patients), it is likely to be above the diaphragm, in the neck, the supraclavicular regions, or the axillae. Readily detectable abdominal involvement is singularly uncommon, although when it occurs it is more likely to involve only liver and spleen, a syndrome more often seen in patients with bone marrow involvement who are usually diagnosed as having acute lymphoblastic leukemia. Generalized peripheral lymphadenopathy may occur but should also raise suspicions of bone marrow involvement. These and other "peripheral" sites of disease, including bone and skin, are not usually associated with a large mediastinal mass and may be composed of cells of a more mature phenotype.

In contrast to lymphoblastic lymphoma, which presents commonly as a supradiaphragmatic tumor, patients with small noncleaved cell lymphomas (in the United States) present with abdominal tumor in all except a small number of cases.[53,159] This is manifested as abdominal pain or swelling, sometimes with a symptom complex caused by intussusception, a change in bowel habits, nausea and vomiting, evidence of gastrointestinal bleeding, or, rarely, intestinal perforation.[160] Presentation with a right iliac fossa mass is quite common and can be confused with an inflammatory appendiceal mass. Lymphadenopathy in such patients is more likely to be inguinal or iliac in distribution. In patients with Burkitt's lymphoma in equatorial Africa, jaw involvement, involving multiple jaw quadrants in a high proportion of cases, is the most frequent site of involvement, although it is very much age dependent, occurring particularly in young children. In an early series 70% of children younger than 5 years of age with Burkitt's lymphoma had jaw involvement, as compared to 25% of patients older than 14 years.[161] In very young children, orbital involvement is often present in patients who do not have jaw tumors, although at least some of these orbital tumors arise in the maxilla. Jaw involvement in sporadic Burkitt's lymphoma occurs in about 15% to 20% of patients at presentation and is not age related.[162] Abdominal involvement is also frequent in endemic Burkitt's lymphoma, being present in a little more than half the patients. There are still differences between endemic and sporadic Burkitt's lymphoma, however, since in the latter, involvement of the right iliac fossa (appendiceal/cecal region) is very common, occurring in almost half of all patients and being localized to that region in about 25% of patients.[163] Presentation with a resectable right iliac fossa mass is very uncommon in African patients. A comparison of sites of disease at presentation in equatorial African and North American Burkitt's lymphoma is shown in Table 20-6. Patients in North Africa appear to have a spectrum of organ involvement that more closely approximates that of the sporadic disease rather than the endemic form.[164]

Table 20-6
Disease Sites at Presentation in Burkitt's Lymphoma

	Percentage of Patients with Involvement*	
	Sporadic	*Endemic*
Abdomen (all)	58	91
Pleural effusion	3	19
Bone marrow	7	20
Peripheral nodes	9	13
Bone	8	9
CSF/CNS	19	14
Paraspinal	17	2
Testis	2	6
Pharynx	0	10
Jaw	58	7
Mediastinum	<1	3
Orbit	11	1
Miscellaneous†	17	15

* Many patients had multiple sites of disease.
† Includes thyroid, breast, skin, shoulder, and thigh.

Cervical adenopathy alone, marrow involvement, skin, bone, central nervous system disease, pharyngeal disease, or testicular involvement occur at low frequency in tumors of any histology, although unusual sites of involvement—for example, lung, face, intracerebral—usually prove to be of large cell histology. Large cell lymphomas of B-cell type may also involve the mediastinum, although this is very rare in the case of small noncleaved lymphomas.

Bone Marrow Involvement

One site of involvement worthy of more discussion is the bone marrow. In small noncleaved lymphomas this may occur in 20% of patients at presentation,[165] although there is evidence from the culture and karyotyping of microscopically uninvolved bone marrow that occult involvement occurs in approximately another 20% of patients.[166] Some patients present with a clinical syndrome consistent with leukemia without any solid lymphomatous masses, apart from lymphadenopathy and hepatosplenomegaly. This is usually referred to as "L3" (after the French-American-British classification) or Burkitt's cell leukemia, although it has become clear that not all leukemias that conform to the criteria of L3 morphology express surface immunoglobulin and have 8;14 translocations—both of which confirm the particular neoplasm to be a small noncleaved cell tumor.[165] The true B-cell acute leukemia of this type responds poorly to standard acute lymphoblastic leukemia therapy[165,168] and should be considered and treated as a small noncleaved cell lymphoma. Such neoplasms constitute 2% to 5% of most large series of patients with acute lymphoblastic leukemia and thus have a similar incidence (perhaps 1–2 per million children younger than 16 years old) to small noncleaved cell lymphomas that present with solid masses with or without bone marrow involvement. Viewed from this perspective, bone marrow involvement occurs at presentation in about two thirds of patients with small noncleaved cell neoplasms in the United States and Europe! This is not the case in African patients with Burkitt's lymphoma, in whom marrow involvement is uncommon, occurring in only about 8% of patients at presentation.

There are no estimates of the proportion of patients who have occult bone marrow involvement or the frequency of B-cell leukemia in Africa. The rarity of marrow involvement at relapse in African patients, even after multiple relapse, and the very high frequency of marrow involvement at relapse in North American patients (perhaps 90% of patients) also speak to the fact that the frequency of bone marrow involvement in these two geographic regions is very different.

In lymphoblastic lymphoma, marrow involvement is also common, but in view of the semantic debate over what constitutes leukemia and lymphoma it is difficult to obtain estimates. In the United States and Great Britain, T-cell acute lymphoblastic leukemia accounts for about 15% of all cases of acute lymphoblastic leukemia (see Chap. 16). This form of T-cell acute lymphoblastic neoplasia is significantly more common than lymphoblastic lymphoma diagnosed on the usual basis of having less than 25% of blasts in the bone marrow. In earlier series of patients with lymphoblastic lymphoma, treated inadequately by modern standards, bone marrow involvement occurred at some stage during the disease in more than 50% of cases.[34,35]

Central Nervous System Involvement

Involvement of the central nervous system can include meningeal infiltration, cranial nerve infiltration, intracerebral disease, paraspinal disease, or some combination of these, most often meningeal and cranial nerve.[169,170] At presentation, CNS involvement is uncommon, although it is distinctly more common in the presence of bone marrow disease.[159,165] Without CNS prophylactic therapy, however, CNS spread will occur in a high proportion of patients, particularly those with extensive disease or head and neck primary tumors. Intracerebral involvement is extremely uncommon at presentation, occurring rarely at any time, but is more frequent in patients with persistent meningeal involvement.[171] Any cranial nerve can be involved, but the ophthalmic nerves and the facial nerve are more often affected. Very rarely the optic nerve can be infiltrated, giving rise to blindness. CNS involvement, particularly paraspinal, is distinctly more common in patients with endemic Burkitt's lymphoma. Paraplegia occurs in some 15% of equatorial African patients at the time of presentation but rarely (1–2%) in patients outside this region.[55,159]

METHODS OF DIAGNOSIS

Histology remains the primary mode of diagnosis, but it is important to supplement this, whenever possible, with studies of phenotype and karyotype. Distinction between lymphomas and other "small round cell tumors," usually taken to include round cell sarcomas (*e.g.,* Ewings sarcoma and some rhabdomyosarcomas), and neuroblastoma, is usually not difficult on histologic grounds alone, but phenotyping or molecular studies, or both, will resolve any diagnostic problems. The distinction from a non-neoplastic lymphoproliferative process (see Chap. 22), particularly in a child with an underlying immunologic disorder that may include longstanding lymphadenopathy, is often more difficult on morphologic grounds alone. For this reason, at the time of biopsy of a suspected pediatric neoplasm, it is preferable that tissue is provided unfixed to the pathologist so that some can be frozen, some used for immunologic and molecular studies, and some provided for karyotyping. It is essential that material used for these special studies is known to contain minimal amounts of normal tissue unless molecular or combined morphologic/phenotyping studies are to be performed. Clonal populations can be detected by molecular techniques (Southern blot) even if representing only a small percentage (as little as 1%) of the normal cells. For purposes of demonstrating that a molecular abnormality is confined to the tumor tissue, it is important that some normal tissue (*e.g.*, peripheral leukocytes) be available for comparison. To date, no antigen expressed exclusively on a tumor cell (excepting idiotypes) has been identified, so that all surface markers utilized will also be present on at least some populations of normal cells. Thus, apart from the monoclonality of a lymphoid proliferative process, which in the B-cell system can be determined, for all practical purposes, on the basis of the expression of a single light chain type, phenotype alone cannot distinguish between a malignant and nonmalignant lymphoproliferation except when a specific phenotype is observed in an inappropriate anatomic location—for example, CD6 positive cells is a lymph node. Even monoclonality is by no means a guarantee of malignancy (witness benign monoclonal gammopathy), and some lymphoproliferative processes arising in allogeneic organ or tissue transplant recipients that have been diagnosed histologically as malignant lymphomas have been shown to be polyclonal.[173,174] This is, to an extent, a semantic debate, since absolute criteria for the diagnosis of a malignant non-Hodgkin's lymphoma have not been agreed on. In any event, at present, phenotyping should be considered as an extremely useful supplement to morphology which can provide confirmation that a malignant tumor is of lymphoid origin and can also assist greatly in further delineating the subtype of lymphoma (see above).

The presence of the leukocyte common antigen,[174] which is not present on nonhematologic neoplasms, provides sufficient confirmation of a lymphoid cell population, but it is rare that sufficient tumor tissue is not available for additional testing to be performed, particularly since immunophenotyping can be done on cytocentrifuge preparations, imprints, or smears of cells, which require very little material. Similar material can also be used for *in situ* hybridization using nucleic acid probes (DNA or RNA) for genes expressed only in lymphoid cells such as immunoglobulin or T-cell receptor genes. Confirmation of a T- or B-cell phenotype, with or without the presence of TdT, provides irrefutable evidence of a lymphoid origin. Some immunoblastic lymphomas may not express surface markers of this type, although in this case it is likely that the Ki-1 antigen will be present. A lymphoid origin in this case can be ascertained by demonstrating that the tumor tissue contains immunoglobulin or T-cell receptor gene rearrangements, which also provide evidence of clonality for both T and B lineages.[78,80–82] Such information at present can be obtained only from fresh or frozen tissue from which nucleic acids can be extracted. It has the additional potential of detecting small numbers of tumor cells (which may not be apparent morphologically) in bone marrow or peripheral blood.[175] Rarely, a true histiocytic tumor may be encountered. Such a tumor will have evidence of its lineage in the form of nonspecific esterases. Sometimes the presence of the CD6 (T6) antigen (expressed on Langerhans' cells) or other monocyte antigens, and phagocytosis may be demonstrable.

The presence of TdT is a very useful criterion, both for the identification of lymphoid cells and for further delineation of subtype, since only acute lymphoblastic leukemias and lymphoblastic lymphomas of both B- and T-cell phenotype express this enzyme,[116] and TdT positive cells under normal circumstances are found only in the bone marrow.[176] Electron microscopy will also provide definitive evidence of a lymphoid origin,[177] although phenotyping is considerably more convenient and provides lineage information not obtainable by electron microscopy. The latter may, however, provide definitive evidence of the tumor type when it is nonlymphoid (*e.g.*, evidence of neural differentiation or muscle differentiation). This is discussed in detail in Chapter 6.

Serum studies at present cannot provide diagnostic information for lymphomas but may provide evidence of a nonlymphoid origin when, for example, there are high levels of catechol amines or their metabolites or in the presence of other tumor markers such as α-fetoprotein or carcinoembryonic antigen. Lactate dehydrogenase elevations are nonspecific, and the presence of high serum levels of soluble interleukin-2 receptor (SIL-2-R) and other molecules associated with lymphoid cells, such as beta 2-microglobulin (β2-m), although they provide prognostic information and may prove to be of diagnostic value in the future, require more study before their usefulness in this regard can be ascertained.[178,179] The presence of weak but discrete monoclonal immunoglobulin bands has been reported in the serum of patients with small noncleaved lymphomas.[91] These bands can, however, be used only to help confirm a B-lymphoid origin, since a number of benign lymphoproliferative processes could produce a similar serum pattern. Despite these provisos, the value of the measurement of the serum levels of lymphocyte-associated molecules depends on the question being asked. If the problem is one of differentiation between a benign and malignant lymphoid proliferation, then IL-2R and β2-m, for example, may be of little or no value, since both types of lymphoproliferation result in increases in serum levels of these substances. They may, however, be of value in distinguishing lymphoid from nonlymphoid tumors. It seems probable that other markers of lymphoid neoplasia will be identified in serum. Because, however, some lymphoid antigens are also expressed on other tissues, including epithelial tissues,[3] considerable work will need to be done to clarify the role of such serum markers.

Karyotyping can provide specific information only when one of the specific translocations described above is detected. Normal cells are not known, under any circumstances, to contain these translocations. Even without karyotyping information, the presence of one of the specific chromosomal translocations associated with Burkitt's lymphoma, for example, can be inferred by the presence of a molecular rearrangement or specific mutation of the c-*myc* oncogene, which is often detectable by means of a simple Southern blot. One or another of these structural alterations in c-*myc* is present in almost all Burkitt's lymphomas.[96] Rearrangements of other presumptive oncogenes (BCL1 and BCL2) known to be involved in translocations associated with certain adult lymphomas such as follicular lymphomas, some large cell lymphomas, and well-differentiated lymphomas, namely, 11;14 (involving 14q32) and 14:18 translocations,[155,157,180] have not yet been detected in childhood lymphomas.

STAGING SYSTEMS AND STAGING PROCEDURES

Staging systems in childhood non-Hodgkin's lymphoma predominantly reflect the tumor volume. Several systems are in common use,[53] but only the most widely used—those of St. Jude Hospital and the National Cancer Institute—will be described here. The former system is modified from the system proposed at Ann Arbor for Hodgkin's disease. It is applicable to all histologic types of childhood lymphoma and separates patients with limited stage disease (one or two masses on one side of the diaphragm) from those with extensive intrathoracic or intra-abdominal disease. The meaning of the term "extensive" is not defined. Patients with bone marrow infiltration with fewer than 25% tumor cells seen on aspirate and patients with involvement of the CNS are separated into the worst

Table 20-7
Staging Systems for Childhood Non-Hodgkin's Lymphoma

Staging System	Stage	Definition
St Jude (NHL)	I	Single tumor (extranodal); single anatomic area (nodal); excluding mediastinum or abdomen
	II	Single tumor (extranodal) with regional node involvement; primary gastrointestinal tumor with or without involvement of associated mesenteric nodes only. On same side of diaphragm: a) two or more nodal areas; b) two single (extranodal) tumors with or without regional node involvement
	III	On both sides of the diaphragm: a) two single tumors (extranodal); b) two or more nodal areas. All primary intrathoracic tumors (mediastinal, pleural, thymic); all extensive primary intra-abdominal disease; all primary paraspinal or epidural tumors regardless of other sites
	IV	Any of the above with initial CNS or bone marrow involvement (<25%)
Uganda Cancer Institute (Burkitt's lymphoma)	A	Single extra-abdominal tumor
	AR	Completely resected intra-abdominal tumor without extra-abdominal tumor
	B	Multiple extra-abdominal tumors
	C	Intra-abdominal tumor with or without a single jaw tumor
	D	Intra-abdominal tumor with extra-abdominal sites other than a single jaw tumor
Proposed NCI (ML SNC/ undiff.)	I	Single extra-abdominal tumor
	IR	Resected (>90%) intra-abdominal tumor
	II	Multiple extra-abdominal sites excluding bone marrow and CNS
	III$_A$	Unresected intra-abdominal tumor; epidural tumor not otherwise in Stage IV
	III$_B$	Intra- and extra-abdominal tumor except bone marrow
	IV$_A$	Bone marrow involvement without abdominal or CNS tumor
	IV$_B$	Bone marrow and abdominal tumor*
	IV$_c$	CNS disease (malignant CSF pleiocytosis/cranial nerve palsies)
Proposed NCI (LL)	I	Single extrathoracic tumor
	II	Multiple extrathoracic tumors excluding bone marrow and CNS
	III A	Single mediastinal (thymic) tumor
	III B	Mediastinal tumor with pleural effusion; mediastinal tumor with extrathoracic tumor excluding bone marrow and CNS
	IV A	CNS disease (malignant CSF pleiocytosis/cranial nerve palsies) without bone marrow involvement
	IV B	Bone marrow and intrathoracic tumor (without CNS)
	IV C	Bone marrow and extrathoracic tumor (without CNS)
	IV D	Bone marrow and CNS disease
		[Stages IV B, C, and D are probably better diagnosed as ALL]

NHL = non-Hodgkin's lymphoma; ML SNC/undiff. = malignant lymphoma small noncleaved/undifferentiated; LL = lymphoblastic lymphoma.
* Does not include diffuse hepatosplenomegaly.

prognostic group (Table 20-7). The system used at the National Cancer Institute was originally devised as a staging system for African patients with Burkitt's lymphoma and reflects the rarity of marrow involvement and the high curability (50%) of patients with CNS disease in Africa. This scheme should not, therefore, be applied to patients with lymphoblastic lymphoma and has been recently modified to take into account the poor prognosis of patients with marrow and CNS disease in the United States (Table 20-7).[181] It differs from the St. Jude scheme in that it includes a stage that reflects the advantage of complete surgical resection of abdominal disease[53] and does not incorporate the use of the diaphragm as a determinant of disseminated disease, something that makes more sense in Hodgkin's disease, in which there is orderly progression of involvement of lymph node regions, than in the predominantly extranodal non-Hodgkin's lymphomas of childhood.

Staging laparotomy is not advocated in patients with non-Hodgkin's lymphoma because chemotherapy is the primary therapeutic modality. Moreover, in nonlymphoblastic lym-phomas, abdominal involvement is so frequently present (in more than 90%) that a high proportion of patients will have had a laparotomy in order to make the diagnosis. In contrast, abdominal involvement is so uncommon in lymphoblastic lymphomas that laparotomy would be unlikely to reveal tumor. Modern imaging methods, including ultrasonography and computed tomography (CT), provide adequate means of evaluating disease sites.[182,183] Ultrasonography has advantages over CT scanning when retroperitoneal fat is minimal (e.g., in small children) and when the liver is being scanned (see Chap. 7). Gallium scanning provides a useful whole body screen, particularly for small noncleaved cell lymphomas that avidly take up the isotope. Lymphangiogram is much less useful than in Hodgkin's disease because of the high frequency of extranodal tumor, and is thus performed infrequently. A bone scan is the most sensitive means of detecting bony involvement but may add nothing to a gallium scan in this regard. Radionuclide liver and spleen scans also appear to add little to CT and ultrasound images, and the role of magnetic resonance imaging

(MRI) and positron emission tomography is not sufficiently well defined for these imaging techniques to be used routinely, although MRI has been shown to be useful in detecting patchy bone marrow involvement in adult lymphomas. Bone marrow and CSF examination are an essential part of staging, although when prophylactic intrathecal drug administration is simultaneously initiated with systemic therapy, the initial CSF examination can be carried out at the same time. Bilateral bone marrow aspirates and biopsies are necessary if the rate of detection of marrow involvement is to be maximized. An acceptable list of investigations relevant to staging is given in Table 20-8.

Clinical staging and, when performed as part of the diagnostic evaluation, pathologic staging provide both an abbreviated designation for the approximate volume and extent (*i.e.,* distribution) of disease and an indicator of prognosis. Although clinical examination and imaging studies are essential for the determination of the sites of disease, quantitative biochemical or immunochemical measurements may provide simpler and more objective measurements of tumor volume. Such measurements should be included in the evaluation of the patient at initial presentation, and, with time, may become an accepted component of stage. Specific examples are discussed in the next section.

PROGNOSTIC FACTORS

There is substantial evidence that the main determinant of treatment outcome in childhood non-Hodgkin's lymphomas is the tumor burden at presentation.[184,185] This is reflected in the clinical stage (although not all staging systems reflect stepwise increments in tumor burden) and the presence of elevated serum levels of molecules either secreted or shed by the tumor cells or that accumulate as a consequence of tumor cell breakdown. These include lactic dehydrogenase, IL-2R, β2-m, uric acid, lactic acid, and polyamines.[178,179,184–187] In African Burkitt's lymphoma the titer of antibody against the early antigen of EBV has also been shown to be of prognostic significance. Although this antigen is not readily detectable in viable tumor

cells, it is probably expressed and subsequently released from dying cells.[184,188] It seems highly probable that numerous molecules expressed by tumor cells, as yet not studied, are present in greatly increased amounts in the serum of patients with malignant lymphomas, and it is quite likely that one or more of these molecules will provide even better correlates of prognosis than those observed to date. However, of the biochemical correlates of prognosis thus far examined, the best appears to be serum IL-2R (Fig. 20-16).[179] In a detailed multivariate analysis involving statistical modeling conducted on patients with non-Hodgkin's lymphoma treated at the NCI according to protocol 77-04 (see below), serum IL-2R was shown to be superior to all other prognostic variables examined. Interestingly, despite the original designation of IL-2 as T-cell growth factor and the high rate of production of IL-2R by cell lines derived from relatively mature T-cell neoplasms, IL-2R serum levels were of particular value in the B-cell lymphomas, in which levels of less than 1000 (arbitrary units) were associated with an excellent prognosis and levels above this value with a very poor prognosis. IL-2R is known to be expressed on B-cell lymphomas and is present in high amounts in malignant serous effusions containing small noncleaved lymphoma cells.[179] The value of IL-2R level as a predictor of relapse and IL-2R levels in CSF in the presence or absence of CNS disease has not been examined.

The importance of such biochemical correlates of prognosis is severalfold. The determination of serum levels provides a much more objective measure of tumor burden than any other available method, and this should allow more accurate categorization of patients into different risk groups and facilitate the comparison of different patient study groups (*e.g.,* patients treated in different treatment arms of randomized studies or in different centers). These molecules could also provide tumor markers of value in assessing the progress of therapy, in the same way that human chorionic gonadotropins,

Table 20-8
Investigations Required for Accurate Staging

Physical examination

Complete blood count
Liver and renal serum chemistries
Serum LDH
Serum uric acid
Serum lactate (optional)
Serum IL2-R (optional)

Chest x-ray
Chest CT scan (if chest x-ray findings are abnormal or suspiciously abnormal)
Abdominal ultrasound examination (include liver/spleen; kidneys; abdomen; pelvis)
Gallium-67 scan
Abdominal CT scan (can be waived if ultrasound and gallium scan are done)
Bone scan (optional or if gallium scan suggests bone involvement)
MRI (research)

Bone marrow examination
CSF examination

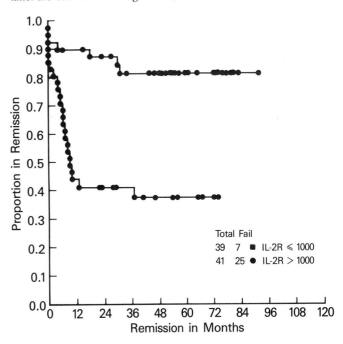

FIGURE 20-16. Disease-free interval (failure-free survival) of patients with non-Hodgkin's lymphomas according to serum IL-2R level. The patients were treated at the NCI with the 77-04 protocol. All patients, even those not achieving a complete response, are shown. The latter are counted as having a disease-free interval of zero.

catecholamines, α-fetoprotein, and carcinoembryonic antigen are currently used in various nonlymphoid malignancies. The advantages of serum analyses to supplement or in some cases substitute for immunologic analysis of tumor biopsies are apparent. Finally, these molecules have implications for therapeutic approaches involving biological response modification, which very often involve the use of molecules synthesized by lymphocytes (*e.g.*, τ-interferon, interleukin-2). Clearly many of these molecules or their receptors may also be secreted by lymphoid neoplasms. Inhibitory interactions of the therapeutic agent and the product of the lymphoma cells may occur either directly or because of opposing effects of the molecules on normal cell populations (usually lymphoid cells) involved in the therapeutic response.

TREATMENT

Choice of Treatment Modality

Although the extent of disease may govern, to a degree, the choice of treatment protocol, the primary therapeutic modality for all histologies and stages of childhood non-Hodgkin's lymphoma is chemotherapy. This is based not only on the belief that non-Hodgkin's lymphomas are generalized diseases, but also on empirical clinical experience. Children with limited disease have a markedly better prognosis when treated with chemotherapy than with radiation alone, and there is accumulating evidence that irradiation adds no therapeutic benefit in this situation but does increase both short-term and long-term toxicity.[36,46] In patients with extensive disease, radiotherapy can, at best, subserve only an ancillary role, that is, as emergency treatment for involvement of the nervous system, for testicular involvement, or when there is a severe mass effect, as in superior vena caval compression. When used as a component of primary therapy in conjunction with an effective chemotherapy regimen, as in the case of localized disease, radiation adds toxicity without overall therapeutic benefit.[45] This is not the case with surgery, for patients with bulky abdominal disease in whom tumor can be completely resected before chemotherapy have an excellent prognosis, which is better than that of patients with unresected abdominal disease.[47,163] A prospective randomized study designed to evaluate the role of surgery in patients in whom surgery is a feasible option has not been carried out. Such a study would be extremely difficult to design in an ethical fashion. The probable benefits of surgery, including prevention of gastrointestinal bleeding, bowel perforation, and the acute tumor lysis syndrome, with relatively minor disadvantages (many patients in this category require laparotomy, in any event, to establish the diagnosis), render such a trial a low priority.

At present, the differentiation between lymphoblastic lymphomas and all other lymphomas is widely used as a useful means of categorizing patients for therapeutic decisions. In many centers, all nonlymphoblastic lymphomas are treated with regimens used for the therapy of small noncleaved cell lymphomas. Large cell lymphomas have been treated effectively with protocols used for both lymphoblastic and nonlymphoblastic lymphomas.[189-191]

Principles of Chemotherapy of the Non-Hodgkin's Lymphomas

All the childhood non-Hodgkin's lymphomas respond to a wide range of chemotherapeutic agents, in part, no doubt, because of the high growth fraction (see Chap. 9). Response rates

in African Burkitt's lymphoma are shown in Table 20-9. Previous experience has clearly indicated that combination therapy is necessary in all these diseases if cures are to be obtained, but the optimal drug combination and sequence have yet to be determined. Issues that are frequently debated include, Which drugs should be used? How are they best combined? What should the dose intensity be? What is the optimum duration of therapy? What is the best form of prophylaxis against CNS disease? Unfortunately these questions can be answered only by empirical trial. In the B-cell tumors there has been a trend toward using intensive alkylating agent therapy for a short duration, whereas in the T-cell tumors the tendency has been to use therapy more akin to that for acute lymphoblastic leukemia, in which alkylating agent therapy has a minor role and therapy is prolonged. In view of the success of some salvage regimens of very high intensity, even when only a single therapy cycle is used (see below), it has been questioned as to whether such an approach might provide an effective stratagem for high-risk patients regardless of histology.

Despite the fact that there remains room for improvement, it is clear that a high proportion of patients can be cured with the use of present combination drug regimens combined with prophylactic therapy directed toward the CNS. CNS relapse is not a major problem in any of the protocols discussed below (it occurs only in a small percentage of patients) with the exception of B-cell tumors with bone marrow spread. However, even here, when CNS spread is present in almost a third of patients, it is likely that inadequate CNS prophylactic therapy is not the primary reason for ultimate failure—rather, it is the inability to control systemic tumor. It is also clear that the approach used in acute lymphoblastic leukemia is not appropriate for the small noncleaved lymphomas.[192,193] In the past, a proportion of such tumors have been cured with short duration, pulsed, alkylating agent therapy, even a single dose of cyclophosphamide,[41,195,196] so that the general strategy should be a small number of intensive cycles of therapy, the main bulwark of which is cyclophosphamide (although in the future this could be replaced). It would also appear that it is inappropriate to

Table 20-9
*Single-Agent Activity in African Burkitt's Lymphoma**

Drug	Number†	CR‡	R§	% R‖
Cyclophosphamide	163	43	132	81
Nitrogen mustard	61	10	44	72
Melphalan	26	8	16	61
Chlorambucil	12	3	10	83
Procarbazine	6	0	0	0
Orthomelphalan	14	?	14	100
BCNU	5	0	4	80
Vincristine	21	10	17	81
Vinblastine	2	0	0	—
Methotrexate	45	11	26	58
6-Mercaptopurine	3	0	0	—
Cytosine arabinoside (cytarabine)	3	2	2	—
Epipodophyllotoxin	2	2	2	—
Actinomycin D (dactinomycin)	4	1	4	—
Terephthalanilide	18	1	14	78

* See Reference 53.
† Number of patients tested.
‡ Complete response.
§ Complete and partial responses.
‖ Percentage of patients responding.

leave too long an interval between successive cycles of therapy unless the cycles are delivered at extremely high doses, since the possibility of regrowth of tumor prior to marrow recovery is significant. Extremely high-dose therapy, with or without bone marrow rescue, for primary treatment should be considered only in a research setting at present.

An approach used at the NCI to meet these requirements was to administer high-dose methotrexate 10 or 14 days after the initial cyclophosphamide-containing regiment for a period sufficiently long to allow all cycling cells to be exposed during S phase.[185] Similar approaches, sometimes with the addition of other agents, have been applied successfully by others,[189,192,193] and all successful protocols incorporate moderate or high-dose methotrexate as one component of CNS prophylactic therapy and for its systemic effect.

This approach may not be optimal for the treatment of lymphoblastic lymphomas. It has been applied successfully in patients with large mediastinal masses without bone marrow involvement but unsuccessfully in a small number of patients with marrow infiltration.[185] For the latter patients, optimal therapy at present should approximate that designed for intensive high-risk acute lymphoblastic leukemia. Such treatment protocols contain continuous or weekly therapy, with 2-week rest periods between phases (induction, consolidation, reinforcement, maintainance). Alkylating agents have a minor role.[189,197] The optimal therapy duration for lymphoblastic lymphoma has not been determined, although 18 months appears to provide effective treatment.[189]

Protocol strategies in the large cell lymphomas are not well defined largely because they represent a mixture of tumors. Optimal therapy for Ki-1 lymphomas is unknown since this subclass has been defined only recently, but the large cleaved and noncleaved lymphomas occurring in older adolescents or young adults have a good prognosis when treated with protocols designed for these tumors in adults.[198] In young children therapy is usually the same as that given for small noncleaved cell lymphomas. The basic tenets of this strategem are similar to those of the adult large cell lymphomas. Success has also been reported, however, from some centers using protocols based on treatment designed for acute lymphoblastic leukemia.[190,191] Clearly, it is imperative to fully characterize the large cell lymphomas in childhood if a rational and uniform approach to treatment is to be achieved.

Management of Lymphoblastic Lymphomas

Immediate Considerations

Patients with extensive lymphoblastic lymphomas may present with a number of complications that require urgent intervention (also see Chap. 37). Almost always, the most appropriate course of action is to initiate specific chemotherapy as soon as a diagnosis has been established. The most common complications result from a large mediastinal mass and include dyspnea, dysphagia, superior vena caval (SVC) obstruction, and rarely cardiac irregularities or tamponade. Uric acid nephropathy is sometimes encountered (see section on B-cell lymphomas). Patients with large mediastinal masses are also at increased risk for complications when undergoing anesthesia, and acute cardiac arrest and increased bleeding from engorged mediastinal veins in this circumstance have been described.[199] If tracheal intubation is performed, it may be difficult to extubate the patient until considerable reduction in the mediastinal mass has been achieved. The diagnosis in the patient with a large mediastinal mass is therefore best established, whenever possible, from a lymph node biopsy done under local anesthetic or by detailed characterization of cells present in a serous effusion. The bone marrow should also be examined before performing a surgical procedure, since this may reveal malignant cells. When tumor is limited to the mediastinum, biopsy is best performed by mediastinoscopy or biopsy via a small parasternal incision. Although dysphagia and dyspnea may result from the presence of a large mediastinal mass, they are not usually of severe degree, and the most frequently encountered serious complication resulting from the compression of surrounding structures in patients with lymphoblastic lymphomas is SVC obstruction. SVC obstruction from a wide range of tumors has been traditionally treated with radiation therapy, but in highly chemotherapy responsive tumors such as lymphoblastic lymphoma there is no advantage to this, and, indeed, irradiation can increase toxicity without therapeutic gain. Several studies have shown that very good overall results in the treatment of lymphoblastic lymphoma involving the mediastinum can be obtained without mediastinal irradiation.[181,185,191] In one trial in the United Kingdom in which a significant survival advantage to patients receiving mediastinal irradiation was demonstrated, survival without irradiation was extremely poor (18%), whereas survival in patients who received irradiation (more than 60%) was no better than in other trials in which radiation was not used.[200] There seems, therefore, to be no cogent reason to irradiate the mediastinum routinely, even in the presence of SVC obstruction, when effective chemotherapy is given. On the other hand, the potential for added toxicity such as esophagitis and pericarditis, especially if Adriamycin, which enhances radiation damage, is included in the treatment regimen, argues against the use of routine mediastinal irradiation for lymphoblastic lymphoma causing SVC obstruction. In the rare case in which no response to specific chemotherapy is observed within a few days in patients with large, symptomatic mediastinal masses, mediastinal irradiation should be given. Radiation therapy may also be administered in circumstances in which the patient is so compromised that immediate relief of symptoms is imperative and the added security of combined modality therapy is desirable. In all of these circumstances, relatively low-dose therapy—for example, to a total of 1200 cGy—is preferable, since irradiation represents emergency treatment only.

Rarely, patients with lymphoblastic lymphoma may manifest cardiac tamponade from pericardial tumor or pericardial effusion, and rapid institution of specific therapy coupled with pericardial paracentesis, when appropriate, may be life saving.

Other complications of lymphoblastic lymphoma that require urgent intervention are uncommon. Pleural effusions may be sufficiently massive to require paracentesis, but until a response to systemic chemotherapy has been achieved, reaccumulation is likely to be rapid, particularly when the patient is being hydrated. Initially, then, repeated aspirations will probably be necessary. Further measures, such as pleurodesis with a sclerosing agent, are not recommended as initial treatment. Such approaches may be useful as palliation in relapsed patients in whom systemic therapy is ineffective. Involvement of the pharynx, itself uncommon, usually responds rapidly to specific chemotherapy so that other measures such as tracheostomy or irradiation are rarely necessary. Involvement of the central nervous system is also unusual at presentation, and in this circumstance radiation should be considered in view of the more limited chemotherapeutic options and the serious long-term consequences of failure to achieve rapid control of tumor growth. Involvement of the facial or optic nerves, intracerebral extension of tumor, and paraplegia are therefore usually treated with full doses of irradiation (usually 3000 cGy). This practice in the case of paraplegia is, however, of questionable advantage.

Chemotherapy of Lymphoblastic Lymphoma

The most widely used chemotherapy regimens for lymphoblastic lymphoma are based upon protocols designed for acute lymphoblastic leukemia,[201-207] but one needs to be aware that not all such protocols are equally satisfactory. The St. Jude Study VIII protocol, for example, produced very poor results in lymphoblastic lymphoma, only 10% of patients surviving at 2 years.[203] Much more successful protocols are the German BFM protocol (Fig. 20-17),[204] an intensive protocol that has produced among the best results in the world for acute lymphoblastic leukemia and is equally successful regardless of the phenotype of the leukemic cells, and the LSA$_2$-L$_2$ protocol (Fig. 20-18), originated by the Memorial Sloan–Kettering Cancer Institute.[42,189] The latter protocol has been used with similar degrees of success in several centers, producing results in the region of 60% to 80% predicted long-term disease-free survival for patients with extensive disease (Fig. 20-19) and 90% or more for patients with limited disease.[205,206] Why these protocols are more effective than, for example, the St. Jude Study VIII is not known with certainty, but both are more intensive and contain additional drugs. It seems probable that anthracyclines are an important component of drug regimens designed for the treatment of lymphoblastic lymphoma, since almost all effective regimens to date have included either Adriamycin or daunorubicin. A recent report, however, described a simple acute lymphoblastic leukemia-like regimen containing cytosine arabinoside (cytarabine) and VM-26 in which no anthracycline was included. Although the number of evaluable patients was small (23) and further follow up will be required (median follow-up duration was 30 months), the results appeared to be very good, with predicted disease-free survival at 4 years of 73%.[207] These drugs are also included in the effective BFM regimen, although the latter protocol contains an anthracycline as well.

It has often been presumed that the therapy of children with lymphoblastic lymphomas (generally equated with T-cell lymphomas) should be different from that of children with all other kinds of lymphoma (generally equated with B-cell lymphomas). This is based on the results of the randomized trial conducted by the Children's Cancer Study Group in which it was shown that for extensive non-Hodgkin's lymphomas the COMP regimen (cyclophosphamide, vincristine, methotrexate, and prednisone) was less effective for lymphoblastic lymphoma than was the LSA$_2$-L$_2$ regimen, but that for B-cell lymphomas the reverse was true.[189] This is not so for the NCI Pediatric Branch 77-04 protocol,[185] which provides effective therapy for all childhood lymphomas without bone marrow involvement, although the number of patients with lymphoblastic lymphoma studied is small. The potential advantages of this protocol include simplicity and a shorter duration of therapy than some of the regimens based on leukemia therapy. Clearly more needs to be learned about the treatment of lymphoblastic lymphoma, and the determination of optimal therapy will depend on the identification of better prognostic indicators, with refinement of treatment approaches within prognostic subgroups.

LIMITED DISEASE. Patients with limited lymphoblastic lymphoma (Stage I or II in the St. Jude system) have an excellent long-term survival, being in the region of 90% in all recent protocols. In the CCSG study, early results seemed to indicate that the COMP and LSA$_2$-L$_2$ regimens were equally effective. More recent analysis suggests a survival advantage for LSA$_2$-L$_2$.[46] Radiation appears to add toxicity but has no survival advantage over chemotherapy alone in these patients.[46] The treatment approach to lymphoblastic lymphoma has so far not been varied according to stage, although patients with limited disease may require a shorter duration of treatment, a question currently under study.

MARROW INVOLVEMENT. The arbitrary distinction between leukemia and lymphoma, based on whether there is more or less than 25% involvement of the marrow, has not generally been found to be of prognostic significance,[201] although in the POG modified LSA$_2$-L$_2$ study patients with greater than 25% blast cells in the marrow and associated lymphomatous masses

FIGURE 20-17. A. BFM therapy schema (BFM NHL 1981/3) for patients with lymphoblastic (non-B) lymphomas. *V:* Cytoreductive phase with cyclophosphamide and prednisone. *I:* Protocol I. Subscripts designate protocol phase. CNS irradiation is given only during phase 2A). *III:* Protocol III. Reinduction therapy similar to protocol I. *Down arrows:* intrathecal methotrexate—under 1 year, 6 mg; 1 to 2 years 8 mg; 2 to 3 years 10 mg; above 3 years 12 mg. *Up arrows:* 24-hour infusion of MTX (500 mg/m^2) with leucovorin rescue after 48 hours. *Shaded area:* oral 6-MP and MTX. Thymic tumors were irradiated only in the presence of residual tumor after protocol I. **B.** Schema of protocol I. (Reproduced with permission from Müller–Weihrich S et al: BFM trials for childhood non-Hodgkin's lymphomas. In Cavalli F et al [eds]: Malignant Lymphomas and Hodgkin's Disease: Experimental and Therapeutic Advances, p 633. Boston, Martinus Nijhoff, 1985)

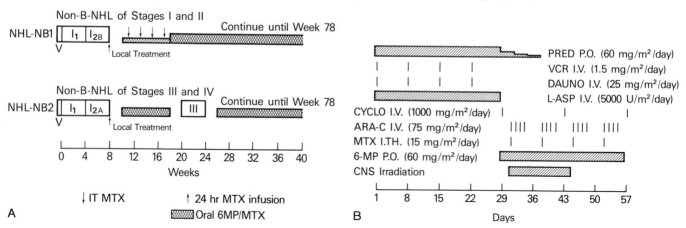

A

B

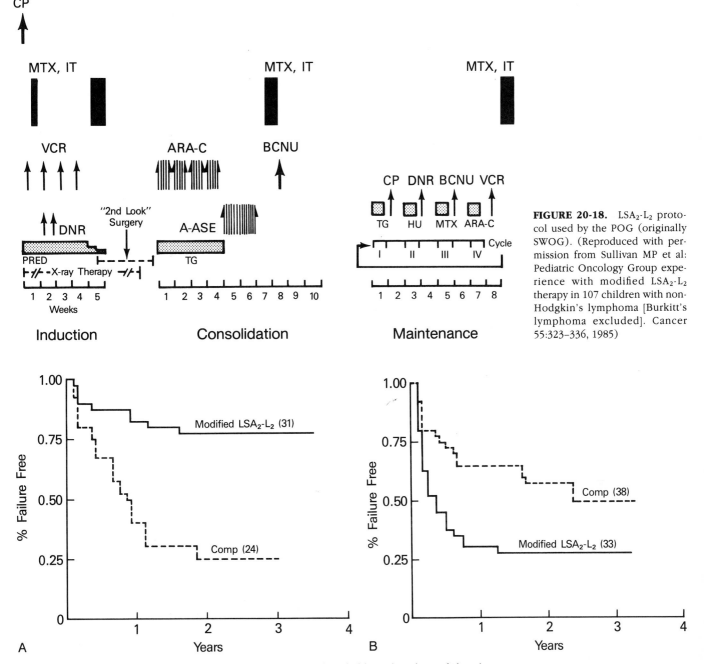

FIGURE 20-18. LSA$_2$-L$_2$ protocol used by the POG (originally SWOG). (Reproduced with permission from Sullivan MP et al: Pediatric Oncology Group experience with modified LSA$_2$-L$_2$ therapy in 107 children with non-Hodgkin's lymphoma [Burkitt's lymphoma excluded]. Cancer 55:323–336, 1985)

FIGURE 20-19. Failure-free survival of patients with extensive lymphoblastic lymphoma (**A**) and nonlymphoblastic lymphoma (**B**) treated according to the LSA$_2$-L$_2$ and COMP protocols. (Reproduced with permission from Anderson JR et al: The results of a randomized therapeutic trial comparing a 4-drug regimen [COMP] with a 10-drug regimen [LSA2-L2]. N Engl J Med 308:559, 1983)

did appear to have a worse prognosis.[191] However, this result should be interpreted with caution, since in patients with T-cell ALL (marrow blasts greater than 25%) treated with LSA$_2$-L$_2$ by the POG the results were similar to those in patients with lymphoblastic lymphoma.[208] Within the patients with T-cell ALL a higher white cell count correlated with a worse prognosis, so that it would appear that the most important prognostic factor is tumor burden rather than marrow involvement *per se*. In any event, the arbitrary choice of 25% marrow blasts as a dividing line between leukemia and lymphoma suffers from

practical difficulties arising from bone marrow sampling differences (both anatomic and chronologic). Some chemotherapy regimens, such as the APO protocol,[202] a protocol used in the treatment of acute lymphoblastic leukemia, and protocol 77-04 of the NCI,[185] are much less effective in patients with marrow disease.

MEDIASTINAL MASSES.   Patients who present with a mediastinal mass but no involvement of the bone marrow or central nervous system may represent a biologically separate subgroup of patients with lymphoblastic lymphoma, although unfortunately in most clinical trials they are not analyzed separately. In the POG LSA_2-L_2 study this group of patients had an actuarial disease-free survival of 40% at beyond 4 years—a poor result that raises the question as to whether LSA_2-L_2 represents appropriate therapy for these patients.

CENTRAL NERVOUS SYSTEM PROPHYLAXIS. Central nervous system involvement in patients with lymphoblastic lymphoma is uncommon at presentation, and although at one time it was a frequent site of relapse, occurring in 50% or more of all patients in various trials,[34,35] CNS recurrence is rarely encountered when effective CNS prophylaxis is given.[185,189,192,204] Because of the lower incidence of lymphomas compared to leukemias in children in the United States and Europe, controlled clinical trials comparing different methods of CNS prophylaxis in non-Hodgkin's lymphomas have not been carried out. In some protocols, cranial irradiation and intrathecal methotrexate are administered,[204] and in others, intrathecal methotrexate or cytosine arabinoside, or both, coupled with intermediate or high-dose methotrexate.[185,189] Optimal therapy has yet to be agreed on, but despite the absence of controlled studies, regimens that do not include cranial irradiation clearly prevent CNS spread. It would seem prudent, therefore, to avoid cranial irradiation with its known physical and psychological complications (see Chap. 16). Intrathecal therapy along with intermediate- or high-dose methotrexate infusions would appear to be the treatment of choice for CNS prophylactic therapy at present.

Management of Patients with Nonlymphoblastic Lymphomas

Immediate Considerations

HYPERURICEMIA AND THE ACUTE TUMOR LYSIS SYNDROME. It has been shown that the fraction of cells in S phase is higher in B-cell lymphomas and leukemias than in T-cell neoplasms.[130,209] The resultant higher cell turnover is probably the major reason for the more frequent occurrence of uric acid nephropathy in patients with nonlymphoblastic lymphomas, although another factor may be the tendency of the latter patients to have higher tumor burdens at the time of presentation. The extent to which these factors are interrelated is not known. There is no doubt, however, that the likelihood of uric acid nephropathy prior to the initiation of chemotherapy or of the development, immediately after chemotherapy, of the biochemical abnormalities leading ultimately to renal failure, which have collectively become known as the "acute tumor cell lysis syndrome" (Fig. 20-20), correlates directly with the tumor burden.[210,211] This syndrome does not occur, of course, in patients with completely resected disease. Because of the short doubling time of small noncleaved lymphomas, the initiation of therapy should be considered a medical emergency, and staging procedures should be completed as expeditiously as possible (see also Chap. 37). Nevertheless, when biochemical abnormalities are already present, their correction, or at least improvement, prior to the initiation of chemotherapy outweighs considerations of added increase in tumor bulk, because further tumor lysis caused by chemotherapy would cause severe biochemical abnormalities, including such rapid and profound hyperkalemia that even renal dialysis may prove inadequate to prevent fatal cardiac arrhythmia. Before therapy is begun it is essential to ensure that the serum uric acid level is not elevated and that the patient is not only well hydrated but also able to

maintain a high urine flow.[210,211] This period of biochemical correction should not exceed 24 to 48 hours at most. The reduction of serum uric acid to normal levels can usually be accomplished within this period by alkaline diuresis and allopurinol administration in all except those with additional renal compromise such as ureteric obstruction or, less commonly, massive involvement of the kidneys by tumor. In such circumstances there may be no other alternative than to institute hemodialysis prior to chemotherapy. In this case, chemotherapy should be begun after the completion of a period of hemodialysis when biochemical parameters are close to normal, since further dialysis is unlikely to be required for at least a few hours, thus minimizing the possibility of removing drugs (e.g., cyclophosphamide) by dialysis.

In all patients with a high tumor burden it is imperative to maintain a high urine flow (as much as 250 ml/m^2 per hour in the patients at highest risk) for the first few days after the initiation of chemotherapy to ensure that the high solute burden from tumor lysis is accommodated without the onset of hyperkalemia or acute renal failure from intratubular deposits of oxypurines and phosphates, a consequence of exceeding their solubility in urine. Because of relatively poor solubility of phosphate in an alkaline urine, it is preferable to maintain the urine pH at about 7, and not to administer bicarbonate during chemotherapy. At this pH, uric acid is some 10 to 12 times more soluble (solubility is about 150 mg/liter at pH 5 and 2000 mg/liter at pH 7) and xanthine more than twice as soluble (solubility at pH 5 is about 50 mg/liter and at pH 7 about 130 mg/liter) than at pH 5. The solubility of hypoxanthine differs little at either pH (1400–1500 mg/liter). Allopurinol should be given at high doses—for example, 10 mg/kg, a dose that will ensure that a significant proportion of purine metabolites is excreted as xanthine and hypoxanthine. It is not advisable to prevent uric acid production completely because it is over ten times more soluble in urine than xanthine and slightly more soluble than hypoxanthine. The objective of allopurinol therapy, therefore, is to increase the total amount of oxypurine that can be excreted in a given volume of urine rather than to prevent uric acid formation.

The acute tumor lysis syndrome was originally recognized because of sudden death occurring as a consequence of hyperkalemia, which may occur within hours of the initiation of therapy.[212] It is important, therefore, to avoid potassium supplements shortly before and during the first few days of therapy, except in exceptional circumstances. Ideally the patient should be mildly hypokalemic before the start of chemotherapy. Hyperkalemia is most unlikely to occur in the presence of a high urine output, and in fact urine flow is the key to the management of the tumor lysis syndrome. As long as a high urine flow can be maintained, other interventions are unlikely to be needed. If this is not the case, rapid progression of biochemical abnormalities will occur, necessitating urgent hemodialysis. Hypocalcemia, a consequence of hyperphosphatemia, should not be treated unless symptomatic, and intravenous calcium chloride should be given with great caution, if at all, because of the risk of extraosseous calcification. Systemic alkalinity increases the possibility of symptomatic hypocalcemia, including tetany. This is another reason why alkalinization of the urine is recommended only before chemotherapy, not during, and need be sufficient only to increase the urine pH to 7. Rarely, hemodialysis may be required for symptomatic hypocalcemia.

A problem that can considerably complicate the management of the tumor lysis syndrome is a tendency for fluids to collect in a third space, including serous effusions (more often ascites but frequently complicated by pleural effusions) or even limb edema from venous or lymphatic obstruction, or

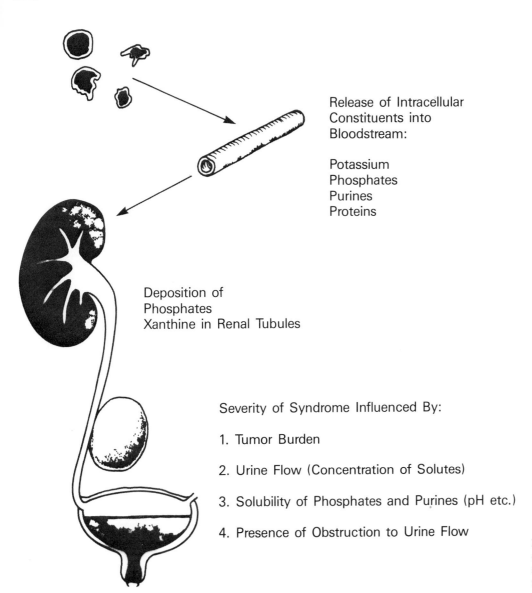

Release of Intracellular
Constituents into
Bloodstream:

Potassium
Phosphates
Purines
Proteins

Deposition of
Phosphates
Xanthine in Renal Tubules

Severity of Syndrome Influenced By:

1. Tumor Burden

2. Urine Flow (Concentration of Solutes)

3. Solubility of Phosphates and Purines (pH etc.)

4. Presence of Obstruction to Urine Flow

FIGURE 20-20. Diagrammatic depiction of the etiology of the acute (chemotherapy-induced) tumor lysis syndrome.

both. In such patients, vigorous hydration is complicated by weight gain and an inappropriate urine flow. This situation usually can be managed by the judicious use of diuretics. Some form of central pressure monitoring, such as central venous pressure or pulmonary wedge capillary pressure, is extremely helpful in this circumstance, and if an acceptable urine output cannot be maintained, there is no alternative but to hemodialyze. It is clear that patients at high risk for the acute tumor lysis syndrome are best managed in a critical care unit.

OTHER COMPLICATIONS ENCOUNTERED AT PRESENTATION. Less common complications encountered at presentation are airway obstruction from a large pharyngeal tumor, necessitating immediate initiation of therapy, or gastrointestinal hemorrhage as a consequence of tumor infiltration of the bowel. Intestinal obstruction may occur, most commonly due to intussusception resulting from the intraluminal projection of a small tumor mass. The latter is a relatively common presentation of non-Hodgkin's lymphoma in children and leads to laparotomy, which establishes the diagnosis and, in some patients, also leads to the removal of all apparent tumor, thus adding therapeutic advantage. In patients with gastrointestinal bleeding,

surgical intervention should be strongly considered before specific treatment, since tumor necrosis following chemotherapy is likely to considerably worsen the bleeding.

CNS complications are uncommon at presentation but should be managed in the same way as discussed for lymphoblastic lymphomas.

Chemotherapy of Nonlymphoblastic Lymphoma

Several different studies have demonstrated that treatment protocols based on the principles shown to be effective for acute lymphoblastic leukemia, such as the LSA$_2$-L$_2$, the BFM 1976-81, and the APO regimens, are suboptimal for the treatment of small noncleaved cell lymphomas.[189,190,204] Large cell lymphomas may respond adequately to these regimens, however, as exemplified by the good results obtained with the APO and LSA$_2$-L$_2$ regimens in the POG trial (but not in the CCG trial; see Table 20-10) in patients with large cell lymphomas.[190,204] These data are based on histologic diagnoses only, and in view of apparent discrepancies between the results in different trials (Table 20-10) and the heterogeneity of the large cell lymphomas,[191,213] it will be essential to further dissect prognostic

Table 20-10
Response Rates in Childhood NHL with Current Regimens

Protocol	Stage*	Number of Patients	FFS† (%)	Follow-Up‡ (mo)	Reference
Lymphoblastic Lymphoma					
LSA₂-L₂ (POG-7615)	I-III	29	55§	48	191
	IV <25%	12	58	48	
	IV >25%	8	13	48	
LSA₂-L₂ (CCG-551)	III	24	78‖	>18	213
	IV¶	7	71	>18	
BMF 75/81**	III/IV††	42	78	>48	204
NCI 7704	III	10	70	48	‡‡
	IV§§	6	16	48	
Nonlymphoblastic Lymphoma					
COMP (CCG-551)	III	32	62	>18	213
	IV	6	33	>18	
NCI 7704	III	38	60	48	‖‖
	IV	9	28	48	
BMF 81/83¶¶	III	75	73	21	214
	IV	15	57	21	214
LMB-0281	III	72	73	>20	216
	IV	42	48***	>20	
LMB-84†††	III	126	74	2–14	216
	IV‡‡‡	34	65	2–14	
Total B	III	17	81	24	217
	IV	12	17	24	

* St. Jude staging system except that Stage IV includes patients with any degree of bone marrow involvement unless otherwise stated.
† Failure-free survival. Includes all patients.
‡ Median follow-up.
§ At 24 months (actuarial estimate).
‖ At 24 months.
¶ <25% blasts in bone marrow.
** Non-B cell.
†† <25% blasts in the marrow.
‡‡ Recent unpublished update of the series reported in Reference 185.
§§ All except two patients had >25% blasts in the marrow. The surviving patient had CNS disease without marrow involvement.
‖‖ Recent unpublished update of the series reported in Reference 185.
¶¶ Two trials, 81/83 and 83/86, are combined here. The present protocol, B-NHL/ALL 86, is similar except for the substitution of ifosfamide for cyclophosphamide on alternate cycles and increased doses of ara-C, MTX, and VM-26.
*** No difference between patients with <25% or >25% blasts in the marrow.
††† This protocol includes a randomization between five and eight courses of therapy and does not include patients with CNS disease. Preliminary analysis shows no difference between the arms.
‡‡‡ Excluding patients with CNS disease.

groupings using additional diagnostic criteria as they become available. Several protocols using cyclical cyclophosphamide-containing combinations coupled with intermediate- or high-dose methotrexate (Figs. 20-21 through 20-25), have been shown to be highly effective for all patients with nonlymphoblastic lymphomas except those with bone marrow disease. With such protocols, overall survival rates of 50% to 75% have been reported (Table 20-10).[185,189,204,214–219] Because of differences in the patient populations (recognized and unrecognized) it is not clear that any one of these protocols is better than another. For comparative purposes, a more useful indicator than stage might be a more direct measure of tumor burden such as LDH or serum IL-2R. In Figure 20-26, a comparison of the results of the Total Therapy B and 77-04 protocols is shown by LDH. When compared in this way, the results are remarkably similar. The decision as to which of these protocols to use should therefore be based on familiarity with the drug regimen used, although it is appropriate to point out that all patients should be entered into a research protocol. There is a suggestion in some studies (*e.g.,* the NCI Pediatric Branch protocol 77-04(185)) that children younger than 10 years of age have a better prognosis, but this has not been substantiated. Nonetheless, when comparing the results of different protocols, the possible influence of age on prognosis should be considered. For example, the median age in protocol NCI 77-04 is 16 years, whereas that of the French LMB-01 protocol is 8 years. In addition, within each stage there may be significant differences in tumor burden, so that similarity of distribution by stage of study populations does not necessarily confirm similarity of tumor burden. The ability to compare the results of different trials would be considerably enhanced by the routine reporting of other measures of tumor burden, such as LDH or serum IL-2R.[179,184–186]

All reported successful protocols include cyclophosphamide in doses of at least 1 g/m² and either high- or intermediate-dose methotrexate. Most also include an anthracycline

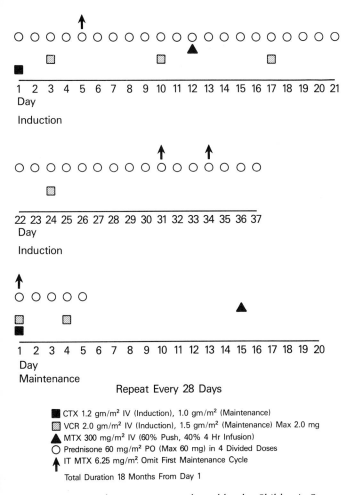

CTX 1.2 gm/m² IV (Induction), 1.0 gm/m² (Maintenance)
VCR 2.0 gm/m² IV (Induction), 1.5 gm/m² (Maintenance) Max 2.0 mg
MTX 300 mg/m² IV (60% Push, 40% 4 Hr Infusion)
Prednisone 60 mg/m² PO (Max 60 mg) in 4 Divided Doses
IT MTX 6.25 mg/m². Omit First Maintenance Cycle

Total Duration 18 Months From Day 1

FIGURE 20-21. The COMP protocol used by the Children's Cancer Study Group, which includes radiation to the sites of bulk disease. (Schema prepared according to information provided in Ref. 189)

(exceptions are the CCG COMP protocol[189] and a study carried out at the M. D. Anderson Hospital[217]), the role of which is being studied at present in a randomized study conducted by the CCG. Preliminary results do not demonstrate a difference between the two arms of this study.[218]

LIMITED DISEASE. Patients with limited disease, that is localized or completely resected intra-abdominal disease (Stages I and II, St. Jude, and A and AR, NCI), have an excellent prognosis (at least 90% cure rate) and require less intensive treatment than do patients with more extensive disease (all other stages). In the BFM protocols 81/83 and 83/86, these patients receive only 8 and 6 weeks of therapy, respectively, whereas six cycles are given in the NCI 77-04 protocol and 6 months in CCG-551 and 501 studies. In the CCSG trials, the results at 6 months were not inferior to those at 18 months.[218] The preliminary result of the POG study examining the role of radiation to local sites of disease does not support a role for this modality, a conclusion that is in concert with the similar results obtained in protocols in which such therapy was given, for example, in the CCSG COMP protocol,[189] to those obtained using other protocols that do not include irradiation.[185,215,219] The one exception to the limited value of local irradiation may be in the presence of testicular involvement, but no controlled studies have been done in B-cell lymphomas in childhood.

ABDOMINAL DISEASE. Patients with abdominal disease without bone marrow or CNS involvement (the majority of patients) have an expectancy of cure that is between 60% and 80% in all major protocols (Table 20-10). It is not clear that differences among these protocols reflect differences in efficacy rather than differences in the patient groups under study.

BONE MARROW AND CNS DISEASE. In contrast to patients with limited disease, patients with bone marrow involvement have a poor prognosis, ranging from 10% to 40% prolonged survival in most reported studies. An exception appears to be the French LMB-0281 protocol, in which 76% of 21 patients with bone marrow disease (but without CNS involvement)

FIGURE 20-22. The 77-04 protocol of the NCI.

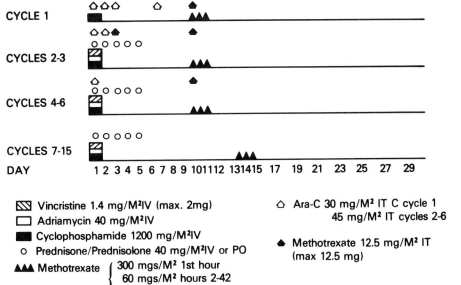

Vincristine 1.4 mg/M²IV (max. 2mg)
Adriamycin 40 mg/M²IV
Cyclophosphamide 1200 mg/M²IV
Prednisone/Prednisolone 40 mg/M²IV or PO
Methotrexate { 300 mgs/M² 1st hour
60 mgs/M² hours 2-42
Leukovorin rescue

Ara-C 30 mg/M² IT C cycle 1
45 mg/M² IT cycles 2-6

Methotrexate 12.5 mg/M² IT (max 12.5 mg)

Cycles commence as soon as granulocytes over 1500/cu. mm (or day 28 cycles 7-15)

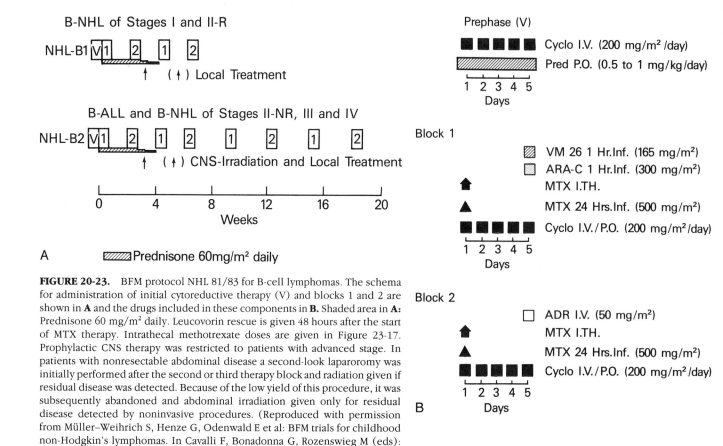

FIGURE 20-23. BFM protocol NHL 81/83 for B-cell lymphomas. The schema for administration of initial cytoreductive therapy (V) and blocks 1 and 2 are shown in **A** and the drugs included in these components in **B**. Shaded area in **A**: Prednisone 60 mg/m² daily. Leucovorin rescue is given 48 hours after the start of MTX therapy. Intrathecal methotrexate doses are given in Figure 23-17. Prophylactic CNS therapy was restricted to patients with advanced stage. In patients with nonresectable abdominal disease a second-look laparoromy was initially performed after the second or third therapy block and radiation given if residual disease was detected. Because of the low yield of this procedure, it was subsequently abandoned and abdominal irradiation given only for residual disease detected by noninvasive procedures. (Reproduced with permission from Müller–Weihrich S, Henze G, Odenwald E et al: BFM trials for childhood non-Hodgkin's lymphomas. In Cavalli F, Bonadonna G, Rozensweig M (eds): Malignant Lymphomas and Hodgkin's Disease: Experimental and Therapeutic Advances, p 633. Boston, Martinus Nijhoff, 1985)

achieved long-term survival.[215] No difference was apparent between patients with less than or more than 25% of tumor cells in the bone marrow. It is not certain at present whether the apparent advantage to the LMB-02 protocol reflects a true superiority in this subgroup of patients or differences in the patients themselves. In all protocols, even earlier protocols with only three cycles of therapy, some patients with bone marrow involvement survive.[41,194] Thus, such patients should not be considered to be a uniform group.

All patients with CNS disease at diagnosis, though representing only a small proportion of patients, have a poor prognosis, regardless of the protocol used.[70,71] Improved treatment approaches are clearly required in such patients. Some patients, however, particularly African children, have achieved long-term cure when treated only with intrathecal and systemic chemotherapy. It is therefore likely that it is only a matter of time before this problem is solved.[69,72]

CNS PROPHYLACTIC THERAPY. As with lymphoblastic lymphoma, CNS prophylaxis is indicated in patients with nonlymphoblastic lymphomas. Since effective prophylaxis has been achieved without the use of cranial irradiation,[56,70] a combination of intrathecal therapy with intermediate- or high-dose methotrexate represents appropriate treatment. It has been suggested that patients with completely resected abdominal disease do not require intrathecal prophylaxis. This is based on the observed low frequency of this complication in such patients. However, much depends on the type of patient subjected to debulking surgery, and the risk of CNS disease may depend on the bulk of tumor resected. If this is so, patients in

whom a large mass of tumor is resected may not be totally without risk. Because of the minimal increase in toxicity associated with the administration of intrathecal therapy but the very poor prognosis of patients who develop CNS recurrence, it seems appropriate, until more definitive information is available, to continue to treat such patients with a small number (*e.g.*, 4–6) of intrathecal injections of methotrexate and ara-C.

THERAPY DURATION. An issue that needs to be addressed is the optimal duration of therapy. Most protocols have given therapy for 12 to 18 months, but there is an increasing realization that a shorter therapy duration may be equally effective, since relapse occurs predominantly in the first 8 months and is almost unknown after 10 months. Moreover, there is no obvious difference between the results of treatment protocols with a short-duration therapy—for example, the BMF 83/86 protocol in which even high-risk patients received only 12 weeks of therapy[214]—and those with a long duration—for example, earlier CCSG, NCI, and SIOP protocols.[185,189,216] The attendant advantages with regard to toxicity, convenience, and cost of short duration protocols provide a strong incentive to routinely reduce treatment to a few months.

Treatment of Recurrent Non-Hodgkin's Lymphoma

In general, patients with recurrent disease after modern, intensive chemotherapy have a very low chance of survival if retreated with conventional therapy, and such patients should be considered candidates for massive chemotherapy with or

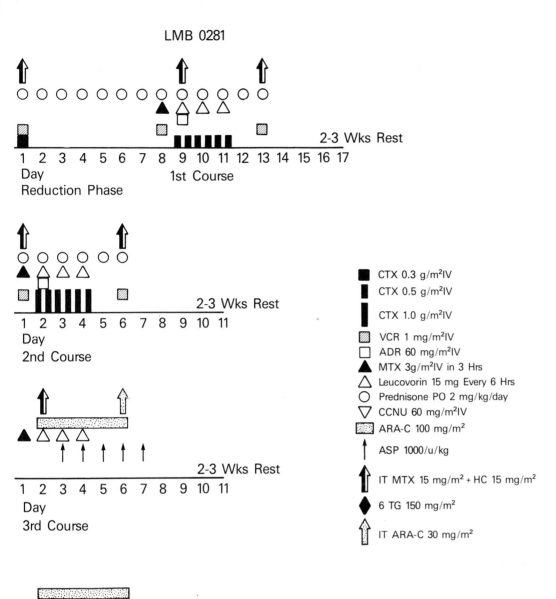

LMB 0281

2-3 Wks Rest

Day
Reduction Phase
1st Course

2-3 Wks Rest

Day
2nd Course

2-3 Wks Rest

Day
3rd Course

CTX 0.3 g/m²IV
CTX 0.5 g/m²IV
CTX 1.0 g/m²IV
VCR 1 mg/m²IV
ADR 60 mg/m²IV
MTX 3g/m²IV in 3 Hrs
Leucovorin 15 mg Every 6 Hrs
Prednisone PO 2 mg/kg/day
CCNU 60 mg/m²IV
ARA-C 100 mg/m²
ASP 1000/u/kg
IT MTX 15 mg/m² + HC 15 mg/m²
6 TG 150 mg/m²
IT ARA-C 30 mg/m²

2-3 Wks Rest

Day
4th Course

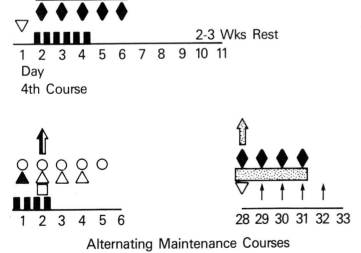

Alternating Maintenance Courses

FIGURE 20-24. LMB-02 protocol of the SIOP for B-cell lymphomas, other than stages I and II. (Large nasopharyngeal primaries in stage II are included.) Cyclophosphamide is given at the doses shown daily in two fractions. Maintenance courses are given monthly. During maintenance courses, ara-C is given as two SC fractions; otherwise it is given as a continuous IV infusion. (Schema prepared from information in Ref. 215)

A

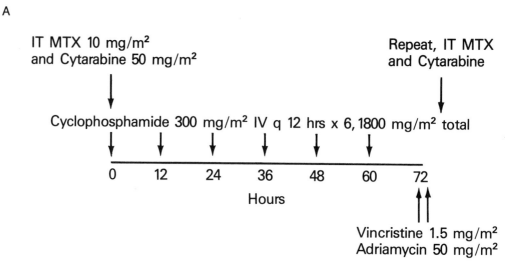

B

FIGURE 20-25. "Total therapy B" protocol used at St. Jude Hospital. Successive cycles (**A** followed by **B**) are given as soon as hemopoietic recovery has occurred (18–21 days) to a total of four cycles each of **A** and **B**. Five to 6 months are required for completion. In succeeding courses after the first, the second IT treatment in cycle **A** is omitted, and the infusion dose of ara-C in cycle **B** is escalated to a total of 3200 mg/m². (Reproduced with permission from Murphy S, Bowman WP, Abromowitch M et al: Results of treatment of advanced stage Burkitt's lymphoma and B-cell (SIg+) acute lymphoblastic leukemia with high-dose fractionated cyclophosphamide and coordinated high-dose methotrexate and cytarabine. J Clin Oncol 4:1732, 1986)

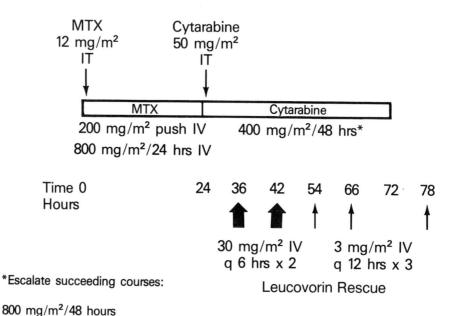

without bone marrow rescue from myelotoxicity. In addition to attempting to salvage relapsed patients, chemotherapy regimens used in this patient group should be considered as potential new approaches for the primary therapy of high-risk patients.

Some relapse protocols have met with a degree of success, notably the very intensive "BACT" protocol, consisting of a single cycle of BCNU (200 mg/m² on day 1), high-dose cyclophosphamide (1600 mg/m² daily for 4 days on days 2 to 5), 6-thioguanine and cytosine arabinoside (both 100 mg/m² every 12 hours for 8 doses on days 2 to 5). This drug combination has been used primarily in relapsed Burkitt's lymphoma, originally at the NCI[220] and subsequently at the Centre Léon Bérard in Lyon, France.[221] In the first study, half of the patients received autologous bone marrow that had previously been cryopreserved after intensive therapy. Without total body irradiation, however, the regimen is not totally marrow ablative,

and marrow recovery occurred in all patients who survived therapy regardless of bone marrow rescue. In this first series of patients, 4 of 19 patients achieved long-term survival (8–14 years disease-free). Similar results were obtained in France in which autologous bone marrow transplantation (ABMT) was used after the BACT regimen or a derivative protocol, BEAM, which incorporates VP-16 and melphalan.[222,223]

A successful outcome of these salvage therapies can be predicted according to the previous response to therapy (Fig. 20-27). Patients with relapse responsive to conventional approaches have a much better prognosis with high-dose therapy, with relapse-free survival that may approach 50%.[223] Patients with tumor totally resistant to conventional therapy have an extremely poor prognosis, with no survivors after 9 months.[223] Patients with a partial response to primary treatment (*i.e.*, with residual disease but not progressive disease) appear to have a good prognosis, although the definition of this group of pa-

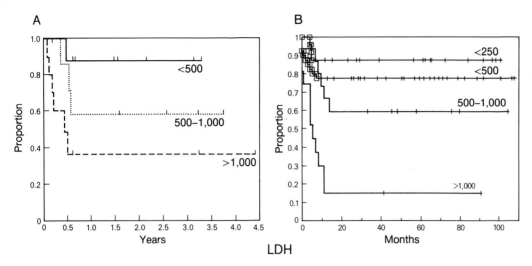

FIGURE 20-26. Comparison of total therapy B protocol from St. Jude Hospital with the 77-04 protocol (**A**) and when failure-free survival is plotted according to LDH level (**B**). (**A** reproduced with permission from Murphy S, Bowman WP, Abromowitch M et al: Results of treatment of advanced stage. Burkitt's lymphoma and B-cell (SIg+) acute lymphoblastic leukemia with high-dose fractionated cyclophosphamide and coordinated high-dose methotrexate and cytarabine. J Clin Oncol 4:1732, 1986)

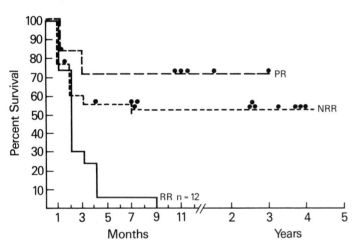

FIGURE 20-27. Results of ABMT obtained in selected patients with initial partial response (*i.e.,* residual, surgically documented disease after three cycles of therapy): PR, nonresistant relapse (NRR), and resistant relapse (RR). This series of patients with Burkitt's lymphoma was reported from the Centre Léon Bérard in Lyon, France. (Reproduced with permission from Cabanillas F, Jagannath S, Philip T: Management of refractory disease. In Magrath IT [ed]: The Non-Hodgkin's Lymphomas. London, Edward Arnold [in press])

tients is subjective. In interpreting these results it should be remembered that patients with marrow involvement at the time of relapse are not usually considered for ABMT, so that the above results have been obtained in a selected subgroup.

Another group of patients that appears to do well with high-dose salvage therapy including ABMT is that in which isolated CNS relapse occurs. In one series of 19 such patients 47% of patients were reported to achieve long-term survival.[223] The survival of some patients with isolated CNS recurrence when treated with conventional-dose systemic therapy, intrathecal therapy, and cranial irradiation[170] raises issues regarding the optimal form of therapy for this subgroup of patients, but it is most unlikely that, with present results, as many as 50% of patients with isolated CNS relapse would survive. In African patients, however, such a result has been reported in patients treated with systemic and intrathecal therapy but without radiation.[224] Fortunately, patients with isolated CNS relapse are now

few in number because prophylactic therapy directed toward the CNS is highly successful.

A question that may be legitimately asked is whether the ABMT and TBI are really necessary. ABMT always carries the risk of reinfusion of malignant cells, and although considerable effort has been put into purging bone marrow with drugs or monoclonal antibodies,[225] a definite advantage to such procedures has not been demonstrated. ABMT performed with and without TBI seems to give similar results except that there is slightly more toxicity with TBI.[223,226] This introduces the possibility of using massive therapy without the need for ABMT (as in the earliest NCI BACT protocol). Drugs such as high-dose ara-C and VP-16 may have an important role in such protocols in the future. High-dose cytosine arabinoside has been shown to be active in relapsed patients,[227,228] and a regimen of high-dose ara-C, VP-16, and ifosfamide for patients with relapsed nonlymphoblastic lymphomas is under study at the NCI.

Allogeneic bone marrow transplantation usually following high-dose cyclophosphamide and TBI has also been explored in relapsed patients with non-Hodgkin's lymphoma. Overall results are quite similar to those in the ABMT experience, with patients with progressive disease at the time of transplant doing poorly.[229]

The promising results of massive therapy in relapsed patients suggests that for selected subgroups of patients with a very high risk (*e.g.,* those with CNS involvement and possibly bone marrow disease at diagnosis), massive therapy during the first remission could provide such patients with an improved outlook. At present, the role of allogeneic marrow transplantation in Stage IV patients who achieve a first complete remission, and for whom a matched donor is available, is being explored by the Pediatric Oncology Group. In Switzerland, a small number of patients in first remission have been treated by intensive therapy followed by ABMT,[230] and a similar approach has been adopted in France in patients with initial CNS disease, since this patient group has a poor prognosis with the French LMB-02 protocol. Five of nine patients in the latter study remain free of disease in excess of 1 year after transplantation.[223] These approaches are clearly experimental, and interpretation of results at present is hindered by the small numbers and patient selection. Such approaches must also be viewed in the context of the markedly improved results of systemic therapy that are currently being obtained and the added toxic risks of massive therapy. In the Lyon series, 12% of patients died from toxicity.[223]

Long-Term Complications of Therapy

The long-term complications of the treatment of non-Hodgkin's lymphoma in children have become less of a problem as treatment has been refined (see also Chap. 50). The potentially serious consequences of radiation therapy have almost ceased to exist as this modality has played a smaller and smaller role in overall therapeutic strategies, including prophylactic therapy against CNS spread. The trend toward shorter therapy durations in the small noncleaved lymphomas will further reduce the likelihood or seriousness of long-term complications. Perhaps the three most serious potential problems common to all patients are impaired reproductive function, the risk of second malignancies, and the psychological consequences of life-threatening illness.

Reproductive function is normally severely impaired in males undergoing chemotherapy, particularly when alkylating agents are used, but the consequences of treatment appear to be much less in the prepubertal patient, although azoospermia may still occur.[231] In women treated before the age of 20 years who do not receive abdominal irradiation, reproductive function later in life appears to be normal.[232] Regimens based on acute leukemia therapy appear to be relatively benign with regard to reproductive function, even in males.[233]

In contrast to Hodgkin's disease and the solid tumors of children, malignancies have not been a significant problem in patients with non-Hodgkin's lymphomas.[234] Among the cytotoxic drugs, alkylating agents have the greatest tendency to induce second tumors, so that the potential for this problem exists. It is likely to be significantly less with short-duration therapy.

FUTURE CONSIDERATIONS

The treatment of non-Hodgkin's lymphomas in children has improved greatly over the past 15 years. Now perhaps two thirds of all such patients can be expected to be cured when treated with one of the major treatment protocols. This result has been achieved largely by the use of intensive combination drug therapy and prophylactic therapy directed against the development of CNS involvement. Yet many challenges remain. The first is to improve the results of treatment to the point that almost all patients are cured. The second is to minimize the morbidity of treatment.

Immediate Possibilities

At present, patients with small noncleaved cell lymphomas who have bone marrow involvement and particularly those with CNS disease at presentation have a poor prognosis, and special consideration should be given to these groups. The most promising avenues for exploration would appear to be incorporating intensive regimens, derived from the experience with patients who relapse, into primary regimens. Whether ABMT or allogeneic transplantation will also be necessary remains to be seen, but this seems unlikely in view of the apparent minimal value of TBI. Even outside these high-risk groups, there is room for improvement in results as well as reduction in toxicity. It is likely that this can be achieved by the "fine-tuning" of existing chemotherapy regimens with regard to dose, the utility of component drugs, and the precise drug combination. This will go hand-in-hand with further identification of risk factors, perhaps based on molecular genetics, biochemical features of the disease, or even the advent of improved imaging techniques, including the possible computerized combination

of the results obtained from CT scans, MRI, and radionuclide scans, the latter possibly targeted by means of specific monoclonal antibodies.[235] Improved ability to categorize patients will improve patient selection for different regimens, thus achieving the best outcome for the least morbidity. Perhaps these measures will be sufficient to improve cure rates to greater than 90%, but in view of the relative rarity of childhood lymphomas, such approaches, still based on empirical clinical trials, will require many years of study before their efficacy can be ascertained. Nonetheless, these are worthy goals and represent the most promising approaches at present.

Attempts to improve the results of treatment with existing drugs are likely to be supplemented by the development of new drugs with higher therapeutic indices.[236] A precedent for this has already been established with the development of analogues of established chemotherapeutic agents that appear to have less of one of the dose-limiting toxicities of the parent compound, including anthracyclines with less cardiac toxicity, and platinum coordination compounds with less renal toxicity. There is increasing sophistication with regard to drug design, such that agents which bind, for example, to specific enzymes can be developed. The possibility exists of overcoming, by such means, some types of drug resistance as well as developing new agents that could have synergistic effects with existing agents. This is particularly likely with the antimetabolites. Similarly, drugs with greater efficacy against tumor in the CNS are likely to be available soon, and in this regard promising new approaches have included the use of thiotepa and monoclonal-antibody-targeted immunotoxins.[237,238] Recent progress in the amelioration of regional toxicities, such as the prevention of oxazaphosphorine-induced hemorrhagic cystitis with the sulphydryl agent 2-mercaptoethanesulfonate (mesna), or the lessening of the renal toxicity of cisplatin by hyperchloremic diuresis is representative of another approach to the improvement of therapeutic index. The use of cloned hemopoietic growth factors such as specific colony-stimulating factors[239] could ameliorate myelosuppression—a particularly important consideration in tumors with a rapid doubling time, because the frequent problem of tumor regrowth (clinically or subclinically) prior to marrow recovery might be avoided by this means, with potentially marked improvement in the therapeutic outcome, to say nothing of lessened morbidity from infectious complications of neutropenia. Studies with such molecules are underway.[240]

More Distant Possibilities

With the dramatic increase of knowledge regarding the pathogenesis of lymphoid neoplasms, perhaps the most exciting possibility is the development of therapy directed toward the specific pathogenetic lesion in the tumor cells. There are few neoplasms in which this could be contemplated at present, but the large and increasing body of data on the molecular genetic abnormalities of the small noncleaved lymphomas resulting from the specific chromosomal translocations associated with these tumors provides one of the best opportunities to examine this approach. Targeting therapy toward, for example, the abnormal expression of the c-myc gene, possibly by an antisense oligonucleotide (i.e., a nucleic acid molecule with a sequence complementary to the c-myc messenger RNA), and causing down regulation of the c-myc gene by targeting the immediate cause of abnormal regulation (not yet identified) are real possibilities, although much work remains before such approaches can be realistically contemplated in the clinic. Other kinds of targeting, are less distant possibilities, such as use of anti-idiotypic or other monoclonal antibodies, perhaps coupled with drug, toxin, or radionuclide. One such immunotoxin relevant to T-cell neoplasia in children is currently under study.[238,241] The efficacy and the overall role in therapy of such immunotoxins will take years to define.

Finally, the use of biological response modifiers still has promise as a treatment approach, possibly combined with conventional therapy, but studies in this area with the childhood lymphomas have been few[242] and there is no clear lead to follow at present. Nonetheless, the major progress that has been made in understanding the regulation of growth in lymphoid cells in recent years provides promise that ultimately regulation of neoplastic growth may be possible by utilizing relevant growth factors or their analogues. (Modifications of the structure and function of cloned molecules by means of recombinant DNA technology are eminently feasible). These considerations justify increased effort directed toward understanding the pathogenesis of the childhood non-Hodgkin's lymphomas. If such studies also lead to the identification of specific individuals at high risk to develop lymphomas, the ultimate intervention—prevention—might also be entertained. At present, no one can predict that such a goal might ever be achieved.

REFERENCES

1. Magrath IT: Lymphocyte differentiation pathways—An essential basis for the comprehension of lymphoid neoplasia. J Natl Cancer Inst 67:501, 1981
2. Magrath IT: Malignant lymphomas. In Levine AS (ed): Cancer in the Young, p 473. New York, Masson, 1982
3. Foon KA, Todd RF: Immunologic classification of leukemia and lymphoma. Blood 68:1–31, 1986
4. Klein G, Klein E: Evolution of tumors and the impact of molecular oncology. Nature 315:190–195, 1985
5. Greene W, Leonard WJ, Wano Y et al: Trans-activator gene of HTLV-II induces IL-2 receptor and IL-2 cellular gene expression. Science 232:877–880, 1986
6. Cross SL, Feinberg MB, Wolf JB et al: Regulation of the human interleukin-2 receptor alpha chain promoter: Activation of a nonfunctional promoter by the transactivator gene of HTLV I. Cell 49:47–56, 1987
7. Gendelman HE, Phelps W, Fiegenbaum L et al: Transactivation of the human immunodeficiency virus long terminal repeat sequence by DNA viruses. Proc Natl Acad Sci USA 83:9759–9763, 1986
8. Cruickshank W: The anatomy of the absorbing vessels of the human body. London, G Nicol, 1786
9. Hodgkin T: On some morbid appearances of the absorbent glands and spleen. Med Chir Trans 17:68–114, 1832
10. Wunderlich CA: Zwei Fälle von progressiven multiplen Lymphdrüsenhypertrophien. Arch Physiol Heilk 12:122–131, 1858
11. Wilkes S: Cases of lardaceous disease and some allied affectations, with remarks. Guy's Hosp Rep 17:102–132, 1856
12. Trousseau A: De l'adenie. Clin Méd Hotel-Dieu Paris 3:555–581, 1865
13. Kundrat H: Ueber Lympho-sarkomatosis. Wien Klin Wochenschr 12:211, 1893
14. Reed DM: On the pathological changes in Hodgkin's disease, with especial reference to its relation to tuberculosis. Johns Hopkins Hosp Rep 10:133–196, 1902
15. Oberling C: Les réticulosarcomes et les reticulo-endothelio-sarcomes de la moelle ossuese (sarcomes de Ewing). Bull Assoc Franc Etude Cancer 17:259–296, 1928
16. Brill NE, Baehr G, Rosenthal N: Generalized giant lymph follicle hyperplasia of lymph nodes and spleen. A hitherto undescribed type. JAMA 84:668–671, 1925
17. Symmers D: Follicular lymphadenopathy with splenomegaly. A newly recognized disease of the lymphatic system. Arch Pathol Lab Med 3:816–820, 1927
18. Gall EA, Mallory TB: Malignant lymphoma. A clinicopathological survey of 618 cases. Am J Pathol 18:381–429, 1942
19. Burkitt D: A sarcoma involving the jaws in African children. Br J Surg 46:218–223, 1958
20. Nathwani BW, Kim H, Rappaport H: Malignant lymphoma, lymphoblastic. Cancer 38:964–983, 1976
21. Robb–Smith AHG: The lymph node biopsy. In Dyke SC (ed): Recent Advances in Clinical Pathology, pp 350–370. London, J & A Churchill, 1947
22. Rappaport H: Tumors of the hematopoietic system. In Atlas of Tumor Pathology, sect III, fasc 8. Washington, DC, Armed Forces Institute of Pathology, 1966
23. Bennett MH, Farrer–Brown G, Henry K, Jeliffe AM: Classification of non-Hodgkin's lymphomas. Lancet 1:1295, 1974
24. Dorfman RF: The non-Hodgkin's lymphomas. In Rebuck J, Berard CW, Abell MR (eds): The Reticuloendothelial System, p 262. Baltimore, Williams & Wilkins, 1975
25. Lennert K, Mohri N, Stein H, Kaiserling E: The histopathology of malignant lymphoma. Br J Haematol 31(suppl):193, 1975
26. Lukes RJ, Collins RD: New approaches to the classification of the lymphomata. Br J Cancer 31(suppl II):1–28, 1975
27. Mathé G, Rappaport H, O'Conor GT, Torloni H: Histological and Cytological Typing of Neoplastic Diseases of the Hemopoietic and Lymphoid Tissues. Geneva, World Health Organization, 1976
28. National Cancer Institute sponsored study of classifications of non-Hodgkin's lymphomas. Summary and description of a working formulation for clinical usage. Cancer 49:2112–2135, 1982
29. O'Conor G: Malignant lymphoma in African children: II. A pathological entity. Cancer 14:270–283, 1961
30. O'Conor G, Rappaport H, Smith EB: Childhood lymphoma resembling Burkitt's lymphoma in the United States. Cancer 18:411–417, 1965
31. Dorfman RF: Childhood lymphosarcoma in St Louis, Missouri, clinically and histologically resembling Burkitt's lymphoma. Cancer 18:418–430, 1965
32. Wright DH: Burkitt's tumor in England: A comparison with childhood lymphosarcoma. Int J Cancer 1:503–514, 1966
33. Rappaport H, Braylan RC: Changing concepts in the classification of malignant neoplasms of the hematopoietic system. Int Acad Pathol Monogr 16:1–19, 1975
34. Wanatabe A, Sullivan MP, Sutow WW, Wilbur JR: Undifferentiated lymphoma, non-Burkitt's type: Meningeal and bone marrow involvement in children. Am J Dis Child 125:57–61, 1973
35. Hutter JJ, Favara BE, Nelson M, Holton LP: Non-Hodgkin's lymphoma in children. Correlation of CNS disease with initial presentation. Cancer 36:2132–2137, 1975
36. Glatstein E, Kim H, Donaldson S et al: Non-Hodgkin's lymphoma: VI. Results of treatment in childhood. Cancer 34:204, 1974
37. Burkitt D: Long term remissions following one and two dose chemotherapy for African lymphoma. Cancer 20:756–759, 1967
38. Clifford P: Long term survival of patients with Burkitt's lymphoma. An assessment of treatment and other factors which may relate to survival. Cancer Res 27:2578–2615, 1967
39. Arseneau JC, Canellos GP, Banks PM, Berard CW, Gralnick HR, De Vita VT: American Burkitt's lymphoma—A clinicopathological study of 30 cases: I. Clinical factors relating to long term survival. Am J Med 58:314–321, 1975
40. De Vita VT Jr, Serpick A, Carbone PP: Combination therapy in the treatment of advanced Hodgkin's disease. Ann Intern Med. 73:881–895, 1970
41. Ziegler JL: Treatment results of 54 American patients with Burkitt's lymphoma are similar to the African experience. N Engl J Med 297:75–80, 1977
42. Wollner N, Burchenal JH, Liebermann PH et al: Non-Hodgkin's lymphoma in children: A comparative study of two modalities of therapy. Cancer 37:123, 1976
43. Norin T, Clifford P, Einhorn J et al: Radiotherapy in Burkitt's lymphoma. Conventional or superfractionated radiation therapy in Burkitt's lymphoma. Acta Radiol 10:545–557, 1971
44. Van der Werf–Messing: Radiotherapy of extranodal non-Hodgkin's lymphoma. In Mathé G, Seligmann M, Tubiana M (eds): Recent Results in Cancer Research. Lymphoid Neoplasias: II, pp 111–128. Berlin, Springer, 1978
45. Murphy SB, Hustu HO: A randomized trial of combined modality therapy of childhood non-Hodgkin's lymphoma. Cancer 45:630–637, 1980
46. Link MP, Donaldson S, Berard C et al: High cure rate with reduction in toxicity for children with localized non-Hodgkin's lymphoma: Results of the Pediatric Oncology Group. In Cavalli F, Bonnadonna G, Rosencweig M (eds): Proceedings of the Third International Conference on Malignant Lymphoma (in press)
47. Magrath IT, Lwanga S, Carswell W et al: Surgical reduction of tumour bulk in management of abdominal Burkitt's lymphoma. Br Med J 2:308, 1974
48. Magrath IT: Burkitt's lymphoma as a human tumor model: New concepts in etiology and pathogenesis. In Pochedly C (ed): Pediatric Hematology Oncology Reviews, pp 1–51. Westport, Praeger, 1985

49. Jaffe ES, Cossman J: Immunodiagnosis of lymphoid and mononuclear phagocytic neoplasms. Dev Oncol 34:83–115, 1985
50. Young JL, Ries LG, Silverberg E, Horm JW, Miller RW: Cancer incidence, survival and mortality for children younger than age 15 years. Cancer 58:598–602, 1986
51. West R: Childhood cancer mortality: International comparisons 1955–1974. World Health Statistics 37:98, 1984
52. Magrath IT: Biological features of pediatric non-Hodgkin's lymphomas in Hodgkin's disease and non-Hodgkin's lymphoma. In Ford RJ, Fuller L, Hagermeister (eds): New Perspectives in Immunotherapy, Diagnosis and Treatment, pp 201–212. New York, Raven Press, 1984
53. Magrath IT: Burkitt's lymphoma. In Mollander D (ed): Diseases of the Lymphatic System: Diagnosis and Therapy, pp 103–139. Heidelberg, Springer-Verlag, 1983
54. Burkitt DP: Geographical distribution. In Burkitt DP, Wright DH (eds): Burkitt's Lymphoma, pp 186–197. Edinburgh, Livingstone, 1970
55. Epstein MA, Achong BG, Barr YM: Virus particles in cultured lymphoblasts from Burkitt's lymphoma. Lancet 1:702–703, 1964
56. Lenoir G, Philip T, Sohier R: Burkitt-type lymphoma; EBV association and cytogenetic markers in cases from various geographical locations. In Magrath IT, O'Conor G, Ramot B (eds): Pathogenesis of Leukemias and Lymphomas: Environmental Influences, pp 283–295. New York, Raven Press, 1984
57. Levine PH, Kamaraja LS, Conelly RR et al: The American Burkitt's lymphoma registry; eight years experience. Cancer 49:1016–1022, 1982
58. Henle W, Henle G: Seroepidemiology of the virus. In Epstein MA, Achong BG (eds): The Epstein Barr virus, pp 61–78. New York, Springer, 1979
59. Lenoir GM, Bornkamm GW: Burkitt's lymphoma, a human cancer model for the study of the multistep development of cancer: Proposal of a new scenario. In Klein G (ed): Advances in Viral Oncology, vol 6 (in press)
60. Moss DJ, Burrows SR, Castelino DJ et al: A comparison of Epstein-Barr virus-specific T-cell immunity in malaria-endemic and -nonendemic regions of Papua New Guinea. Int J Cancer 31:727–732, 1983
61. Whittle HC, Brown J, Marsh K et al: T-cell control of Epstein-Barr virus infected B-cells is lost during P. falciparum malaria. Nature 312:449–450, 1984
62. Cossman J, Chused TM, Fisher RI et al: ES: Diversity of immunological phenotypes of lymphoblastic lymphoma: Cancer Res 43:4486, 1983
63. Kadin M, Sako K, Berliner N et al: Childhood Ki-1 lymphoma presenting with skin lesions and peripheral lymphadenopathy. Blood 68:1042–1049, 1986
64. Hsu SM, Yang K, Jaffe ES: Phenotypic expression of Hodgkin and Reed-Sternberg cells in Hodgkin's disease. Am J Pathol 118:209, 1985
65. Filipovitch AH: Lymphoproliferative disorders associated with immunodeficiency: In Magrath IT (ed): The Non-Hodgkin's Lymphomas. London, Edward Arnold (in press)
66. Saemundsen AK, Purtilo D, Sakamoto K et al: Documentation of Epstein-Barr virus infection in imunodeficnet patients with life-threatening lymphoproliferative diseases by Epstein-Barr virus complementary RNA/DNA and viral DNA/RNA hybridization. Cancer Res 41:4237–4242, 1981
67. Purtilo D: Immunoregulatory defects and Epstein Barr virus-associated lymphoid disorders. In Magrath IT, O'Conor G, Ramot B (eds): Pathogenesis of Leukemias and Lymphomas: Environmental Influences, pp 235–257. New York, Raven Press, 1984
68. Whang–Peng J, Lee EC, Sieverts H, Magrath IT: Burkitt's lymphoma in AIDS: A cytogenetic study. Blood 63:818–822, 1984
69. Chaganti RSK, Jhanwar S, Kozinar B et al: Specific translocations characterize Burkitt's-like lymphoma of homosexual men with the acquired immunodeficiency syndrome. Blood 61:1269–1272, 1983
70. Pelicci PG, Knowles DM, Arlin ZA et al: Multiple monoclonal B cell expansions and c-myc oncogene rearrangements in acquired immune deficiency syndrome-related lymphoproliferative disorders. Implications for lymphomagenesis. J Exp Med 164:2049–2060, 1986
71. Filipovitch AH, Zerbe D, Spector BD et al: Lymphomas in persons with naturally occurring immunodeficiency disorders. In Magrath IT, O'Conor G, Ramot B (eds): Pathogenesis of Leukemias and Lymphomas: Environmental Influences, pp 225–234. New York, Raven Press, 1984
72. Tosado G: Personal communication
73. Salem P, El-Hashimi L, Anaissi E et al: Immunoproliferative small intestinal disease. Dev Oncol 32:269–277, 1985
74. Watanabe S, Sato Y, Shimoyama M et al: Immunoblastic lymphadenopathy, angioimmunoblastic lymphadenopathy, and IBL-like T-cell lymphoma. A spectrum of T-cell neoplasia. Cancer 58:2224–2232, 1986
75. Finch S: Ionizing radiation and drugs in the pathogenesis of lymphoid neoplasia. In Magrath IT, O'Conor G, Ramot B (eds): Pathogenesis of Leukemias and Lymphomas: Environmental Influences, pp 207–223. New York, Raven Press, 1984
76. Bernard A, Boumsell L, Reinherz EL et al: Cell surface characterization of malignant T cells from lymphoblastic lymphoma using monoclonal antibodies: Evidence for a phenotypic difference between malignant T cells from patients with acute lymphoblastic leukemia and lymphoblastic lymphoma. Blood 57:1105, 1981
77. Roper M, Crist WM, Metzger R et al: Monoclonal antibody characterization of surface antigens in childhood T-cell malignancies. Blood 61:830, 1983
78. Nadler LM, Korsmeyer SJ, Anderson KC et al: B cell origin of non-T cell acute lymphoblastic leukemia. A model for discrete stages of neoplastic and normal pre-B cell differentiation. J Clin Invest 74:332, 1984
79. Alt FW, Blackwell TK, Depinho RA, Reith MG, Yancopoulos GD: Regulation of genome rearrangement events during lymphocyte differentiation. Immunol Rev 89:5–30, 1986
80. Korsmeyer SJ, Hieter PA, Ravetch JV et al: Developmental hierarchy of immunoglobulin gene rearrangements in human leukemic pre-B-cells. Proc Natl Acad Sci USA 78:7096–7100, 1981
81. Pellici P-G, Knowles DM, Dalla Favera R: Lymphoid tumors displaying rearrangements of both immunoglobulin and T cell receptor genes. J Exp Med 162:1015–1024, 1985
82. Bertness V, Kirsch I, Hollis G et al: T-cell receptor gene rearrangements as clinical markers of human T-cell lymphomas. N Engl J Med 313:534–538, 1985
83. Desiderio SV, Yancopoulos GD, Paskind M et al: Insertion of N regions into heavy-chain genes is correlated with expression of terminal deoxytransferase in B cells. Nature 311:752, 1984
84. MacLennan ICM, Gray D: Antigen-driven selection of virgin and memory B cells. Immunol Rev 91:61–82, 1986
85. Casali P, Burastero SE, Nakamura M, Inghirami G, Notkins AL: Human lymphocytes making rheumatoid factor and antibody to ssDNA belong to Leu-1+ B-cell subset. Science 236:77–81, 1987
86. Radbruch A, Burger C, Klein S, Muller W: Control of Immunoglobulin class switch recombination. Immunol Rev 89:69–83, 1986
87. Alt FW, Bothwell AKM, Knapp ALM et al: Synthesis of secreted and membrane-bound immunoglobulin mu heavy chains is directed by mRNAs that differ at their 3'-ends. Cell 20:293, 1980
88. Anderson KC, Bates MP, Slaughenhoupt B et al: A monoclonal antibody with reactivity restricted to normal and neoplastic plasma cells. J Immunol 132:3172–3179, 1984
89. Sandlund JT, Kiwanuka J, Marti GE, Goldschmidts G, Magrath IT: Characterization of Burkitt's lymphoma cell lines with monoclonal antibodies using an ELISA technique. In Reinherz EL, Hayes BF, Nadler LM, Bernstein ID (eds): Leukocyte Typing, vol 2. Proceedings of the 2nd International Congress of Human Leukocyte Antigens, pp 403–410. New York, Springer-Verlag, 1986
90. Benjamin D, Magrath IT, Maguire R et al: Immunoglobulin secretion by cell lines derived from African and American undifferentiated lymphomas of Burkitt's and non-Burkitt's type. J Immunol 129:1336, 1982
91. Magrath I, Benjamin D, Papadopoulos N: Serum monoclonal immunoglobulin bands in undifferentiated lymphomas of Burkitt's and non-Burkitt's types. Blood 61:726, 1983
92. Magrath IT, Freeman CB, Pizzo P, Gadek J, Jaffe E, Santaella M, Hammer C, Frank M, Reaman G, Novikovs L: Characterization of lymphoma derived cell lines: Comparison of cell lines positive and negative for Epstein-Barr virus nuclear antigen: II. Surface markers. J Natl Cancer Inst 64:477–483, 1980
93. Ehlin–Henriksson B, Manneborg-Sandlund A, Klein G: Expression of B-cell-specific markers in different Burkitt lymphoma subgroups. Int J Cancer 39:211–218, 1987
94. Favrot MC, Philip I, Philip T et al: Distinct reactivity of Burkitt's lymphoma cell lines with eight monoclonal antibodies correlated with the ethnic origin. JNCI 73:841–847, 1984
95. Favrot M, Philip I, Comparet V et al: Receptors of B cell activation and differentiation are variable expressed on EBV negative and positive cell lines. In Cavalli F, Bonnadonna G, Rosencweig M (eds): Proceedings of the Third International Conference on Malignant Lymphoma
96. Pellici P-G, Knowles D, Magrath I et al: Chromosomal breakpoints and tructural alterations of the c-myc locus differ in endemic sporadic forms of Burkitt lymphoma. Proc Natl Acad Sci USA 83:2984, 1986
97. Croce CM, Isobe M, Palumbo A et al: Gene for alpha-chain of human T-cell receptor: Location on chromosome 14 region involved in T-cell neoplasms. Science 227:1044–1047, 1985

98. Le Beau MM, Diaz MO, Rowley JD et al: Chromosomal localization of the human T cell receptor beta-chain genes (lett). Cell 41:335, 1985

99. Murre C, Waldmann RA, Morton CC et al: Human gamma-chain genes are rearranged in leukaemic T cells and map to the short arm of chromosome 7. Nature 316:549–552, 1985

100. Meuer SC, Acuto O, Hussey RE et al: Evidence for the T3-associated 90K heterodimer as the T cell antigen receptor. Nature 303:808–810, 1983

101. Hood L, Kronenberg M, Hunkapillar T: T cell antigen receptors and the immunoglobulin supergene family. Cell 40:225–229, 1985

102. Royer HD, Acuto O, Fabbi M et al: Genes encoding the Tiβ subunit of the antigen/MHC receptor undergo rearrangement during intrathymic ontogeny prior to surface T3-Ti expression. Cell 39:261–266, 1984

103. Royer HD, Ramarli D, Acuto O et al: Genes encoding the T-cell receptor alpha and beta subunits are transcribed in an ordered manner during intrathymic ontogeny. Proc Natl Acad Sci USA 82:5510–5514, 1985

104. Lefranc M-P, Rabbitts TH: Two tandemly organised human genes encoding the T cell τ constant-region sequences show multiple rearrangement in different T-cell types. Nature 316:464–466, 1985

105. Haars R, Kronenberg M, Gallatin WM, Weissman IL, Owen FL, Hood L: Rearrangement and expression of T cell antigen receptor and gamma genes during thymic development. J Exp Med 164:1–24, 1986

106. Siu G, Kronenberg M, Strauss E et al: The structure, rearrangement and expression of D beta gene segments of the murine T-cell antigen receptor. Nature 311:344–350, 1984

107. Haynes BF: Differentiation pathways of human lymphocytes: Use of monoclonal antibodies and malignant T cells as investigative probes. Immunobiology 159(1/2):14, 1981

108. Vodinelich L, Tax W, Bai Y, Pegram S, Capel P, Greaves MF: A monoclonal antibody (WT1) for detecting leukemias of T-cell precursors (T-ALL). Blood 62:1108–1113, 1983

109. Link M, Warnke R, Finlay J et al: A single monoclonal antibody identifies T-cell lineage of childhood lymphoid malignancies. Blood 62:722, 1983

110. Reinherz EL, Kung PC, Goldstein G, Levey RH, Schlossman SF: Discrete stages of human intrathymic differentiation: Analysis of normal thymocytes and leukemic lymphoblasts of T-cell lineage. Proc Natl Acad Sci USA 77:1588–1592, 1980

111. Casten LA, Lakey EK, Jelachich ML et al: Anti-immunoglobulin augments the B-cell antigen-presentation function independently of internalization of receptor-antigen complex. Proc Natl Acad Sci USA 82:5890–5894, 1985

112. Royer HD, Reinherz EL: T Lymphocytes: Ontogeny, function, and relevance to clinical disorders. N Engl J Med 317:1136–1142, 1987

113. Blue ML, Schlossman SF: Biology of the T cell. Prog Clin Biol Res 224:11–20, 1986

114. Blue ML, Schlossman SF: Ontogeny of human T cells: Acquisition of a functional program. Serono Symp Publ Raven Press 28:3–11, 1986

115. Reinherz EL, Schlossman SF: Human T-cell leukemias in the context of normal T-lineage ontogeny and function. In Murphy SB, Gilbert JR (eds): Leukemia Research: Advances in Cell Biology and Treatment, pp 85–95. New York, Elsevier Biomedical, 1983

116. Braziel RM, Keneklis T, Donlon JA et al: Terminal deoxynucleotidyl transferase in non-hodgkin's lymphoma. Am J Clin Pathol 80:655–659, 1983

117. Haluska FG, Finver S, Tsujimoto Y et al: The t(8;14) translocation occurring in B-cell malignancies results from mistakes in V-D-J joining. Nature 324:158, 1986

118. Bernard A, Boumsell L: Cell-surface heterogeneity of human T-cell malignancies. Prog Cancer Res Ther 21:93, 1982

119. Reinherz EL, Nadler LM, Sallan SE, Schlossman SF: Subset derivation of T-cell acute lymphoblastic leukemia in man. J Clin Invest 64:392–397, 1979

120. Haynes BF: Human T lymphocyte antigens as defined by monoclonal antibodies. Immunol Rev 57:127–161, 1981

121. Bernard A, Murphy SB, Melvin S et al: Non-T, non-B lymphomas are rare in childhood and associated with cutaneous tumor. Blood 59:549, 1982

122. Link MP, Hoper M, Dorfman RF et al: Cutaneous lymphoblastic lymphoma with pre-B markers. Blood 61:838, 1983

123. Grogan T, Spier C, Wirt D et al: Immunologic complexity of lymphoblastic lymphoma. Diagn Immunol 4:81–88, 1986

124. Sheibani K, Winberg CD, Burke JS: Lymphoblastic lymphoma expressing natural killer cell-associated antigens: A clinicopathologic study of six cases. Leuk Res 11:371–377, 1987

125. Stein H, Gerdes J, Tippelmann G et al: Ki-1 lymphoma: Experimental and clinical findings. In Cavalli F, Bonnadonna G, Rosencweig M (eds): Proceedings of the Third International Conference on Malignant Lymphoma (in press)

126. Van der Valk P, Meijer CJLM, Willemze R, Van Oosteruom AT, Spaander PJ, Te Velde J: Histiocytic sarcoma (true histiocytic lymphoma): A clinicopathological study of 20 cases. Histopathology; 8:105–123, 1984

127. Cotelingam JD, Witebsky FG, Hsu SM et al: Malignant lymphoma in patients with the Wiskott-Aldrich syndrome. Cancer Invest 3:515, 1985

128. Iverson U, Iverson OH, Ziegler JL et al: Cell kinetics of African cases of Burkitt's lymphoma. A preliminary report. Eur J Cancer 8:305–310, 1972

129. Braylan RC, Fowlkes BT, Jaffe ES et al: Cell volumes and DNA distributions of normal and neoplastic human lymphoid cells. Cancer 41:201–209, 1978

130. Murphy SB, Melvin SL, Mauer AM et al: Correlation of tumor cell kinetic studies with surface marker results in childhood non-Hodgkins lymphoma. Cancer Res 39:1534–1538, 1979

131. Magrath IT: Treatment approaches directed towards molecular lesions in neoplastic cells. In Magrath IT (ed): New Directions in Cancer Treatment. Heidelberg, Springer (in press)

132. Zech L, Haglund U, Nilsson K et al: Characteristic chromosomal abnormalities in biopsies and lymphoid-cell lines from patients with Burkitt and non-Burkitt lymphomas. Int J Cancer 17:47, 1976

133. Taub R, Kirsch I, Morton C et al: Translocation of the c-myc gene into the immunoglobulin heavy chain locus in human Burkitt lymphoma and murine plasmacytoma cells. Proc Natl Acad Sci USA 79:7837, 1982

134. Dalla-Favera R, Bregni M, Erikson J et al: Human c-myc onc gene is located on the region of chromosome 8 that is translocated in Burkitt lymphoma cells. Proc Natl Acad Sci USA 79:7824, 1982

135. Bernheim A, Berger R, Lenoir G: Cytogenetic studies on African Burkitt's lymphoma cell lines: t(8;14), t(2;8) and t(8;22) translocations. Cancer Genet Cytogenet 3:307, 1981

136. Rappold GA, Hameister H, Cremer T et al: c-myc and immunoglobulin kappa light chain constant genes are on the 8q+ chromosome of three Burkitt lymphoma lines with t(2;8) translocations. EMBO J 3:2951, 1984

137. ar-Rushdi A, Nishikura K, Erikson J et al: Differential expression of the translocated and the untranslocated c-myc oncogene in Burkitt lymphoma. Science 222:390, 1983

138. Maguire RT, Robins TS, Thorgeirsson SS et al: Expression of cellular myc and mos genes in undifferentiated B cell lymphomas of Burkitt and non-Burkitt types. Proc Natl Acad Sci USA 80:1947, 1983

139. Armelin HA, Armelin MC, Kelly K et al: Functional role for c-myc in mitogenic response to platelet-derived growth factor. Nature 310:655–660, 1984

140. Ehlin-Henriksson B, Manneborg-Sandlund A, Klein G: Expression of B-cell specific markers in different Burkitt lymphoma subgroups. Int J Cancer 39:211–218, 1987

141. Yunis JJ: Fragile sites and predisposition to leukemia and lymphoma. Cancer Genet Cytogenet 12:85, 1984

142. Sanford KK, Parshad R, Potter M et al: Chromosomal radiosensitivity during G2 phase and susceptibility to plasmacytoma induction in mice. Curr Top Microbiol Immunol 132:202, 1986

143. Kristoffersson U, Heim S, Heldrup J: Cytogenetic studies of childhood non-Hodgkin lymphomas. Hereditas 3:77, 1985

144. Smith SD, Morgan R, Link MP et al: Cytogenetic and immunophenotypic analysis of cell lines established from patients with T cell leukemia/lymphoma. Blood 67:650, 1986

145. Denny CT, Yoshikai Y, Mak TW et al: A chromosome 14 inversion in a T-cell lymphoma is caused by site-specific recombination between immunoglobulin and T-cell receptor loci. Nature 320:549–551, 1986

146. Levine EG, Arthur DC, Frizzera G et al: There are differences in cytogenetic abnormalities among histologic subtypes of the non-Hodgkin's lymphomas. Blood 66:1414, 1985

147. Dube ID, Raimondi SC, Pi D, Kalousek DK: A new translocation, t(10;14)(q24;q11), in T cell neoplasia. Blood 67:1181–1184, 1986

148. Mathieu-Mahul D, Sigaux F, Zhu C et al: A t(8;14)(q24;q11) translocation in a T-cell leukemia (L1-ALL) with c-myc and TCR-alpha chain locus rearrangements. Int J Cancer 38:835–840, 1986

149. Le Beau MM, McKeithan TW, Shima EA et al: T-cell receptor alpha-chain gene is split in a human T-cell leukemia cell line with a t(11;14) (p15;q11). Proc Natl Acad Sci USA 83:9744–9748, 1986

150. Smith SD, Morgan R, Link MP et al: Cytogenetic and immunophenotypic analysis of cell lines established from patients with T cell leukemia/lymphoma. Blood 67:650–656, 1986

151. McKeithan TW, Shima EA, Le Beau MM et al: Molecular cloning of the breakpoint junction of a human chromosomal 8;14 translocation involving the T cell receptor alpha-chain gene and sequences on the 3' side of MYC. Proc Natl Acad Sci USA 83:6636–6640, 1986

152. Finger LR, Harvey RC, Moore RCA et al: A common mechanism of chromosomal translocation in T and B cell neoplasia. Science 234:982–985, 1986

153. Le Beau MM, Rowley JD: Chromosomal abnormalities in leukemia and lymphoma: clinical and biological significance. Adv Hum Genet 15:1–54, 1986

154. Bloomfield CD, Arthur DC, Frizzera G, Levine EG, Peterson BA, Gaji–Peczalska KJ: Non-random chromosome abnormalities in cancer. Cancer Res 43:2975–2984, 1983

155. Tsujimoto Y, Finger LR, Yunis J, Nowell PC, Croce C: Cloning the chromosome breakpoint of neoplastic B cells with the t(14;18) chromosome translocation. Science 226:1097–1099, 1984

156. Bakhshi A, Jensen JP, Goldman P, Wright JJ, McBride OW, Epstein AL, Korsmeyer SJ: Cloning the chromosomal breakpoint of t(18;14) bearing human lymphomas clustering around JH on chromosome 14 and near a transcriptional unit on 18. Cell 41:899–906, 1985

157. Cossman J, Berard CW: Histopathology of childhood non-Hodgkin's mphomas. In Graham–Pole J (ed): Non-Hodgkin's Lymphomas in Children. Masson Monographs in Pediatric Hematology/Oncology, p 177. New York, Masson Publishing USA, 1980

158. Wilson JF, Jenkin RD, Anderson JR et al: Studies on the pathology of non-Hodgkin's lymphoma of childhood: I. The role of routine histopathology as a prognostic factor. A report from the children's cancer study group. Cancer 53:1695, 1984

159. Magrath IT, Sariban E: Clinical Features of Burkitt's Lymphoma in the USA. Proceedings. Burkitt's Lymphoma—A Human Cancer Model, pp 119–127. Lyon, France, IARC Publications, 1985

160. Meyers PA, Potter VP, Wollner N, Exelby P: Bowel perforation during initial treatment for childhood non-Hodgkin's lymphoma. Cancer 56:259–261, 1985

161. Burkitt DP: General features and facial tumours. In Burkitt DP, Wright DH (eds): Burkitt's Lymphoma. Edinburgh, Livingstone, 1970

162. Sariban E, Donahue A, Magrath IT: Jaw involvement in American Burkitt's lymphoma. Cancer 53:141–146, 1984

163. Janus C, Edwards BK, Sariban E, Magrath IT: Surgical resection and limited chemotherapy for abdominal undifferentiated lymphomas. Cancer Treat Rep 68:599–605, 1984

164. Ladjadj Y, Philip T, Lenoir GM et al: Abdominal Burkitt-type lymphomas in algeria. Br J Cancer 49:503–512, 1984

165. Magrath IT, Ziegler JL: Bone marrow involvement in Burkitt's lymphoma and its relationship to acute B-cell leukemia. Leukemia Res 4:33–59, 1980

166. Benjamin D, Magrath IT, Douglass EC, Corash LM: Derivation of lymphoma cell lines from microscopically normal bone arrow in patients with undifferentiated lymphomas: Evidence of occult bone marrow involvement. Blood 61:1017–1019, 1983

167. Mangan KF, Rauch AE, Bishop M et al: Acute lymphoblastic leukemia of Burkitt's type (L-3 ALL) lacking surface immunoglobulin and the 8;14 translocation. Am J Clin Pathol 83:121–126, 1985

168. Kersey JH, Lebien TW, Hurwitz R et al: Childhood leukemia-lymphoma. Heterogeneity of phenotypes and prognoses. Am J Clin Pathol 72:(suppl):746–752, 1979

169. Ziegler JL, Magrath IT: Burkitt's lymphoma. In Ioachim HL (ed): Pathobiology Annual, pp 129–142. New York, Appleton-Century-Croft, 1974

170. Sariban E, Janus C, Edwards B, Magrath IT: Central nervous system involvement in American Burkitt's lymphoma. J Clin Oncol 11:677–681, 1983

171. Magrath IT, Mugerwa J, Bailey I, Olweny C, Kiryabwire Y: Intracerebral Burkitt's lymphoma: Pathology clinical features and treatment. Q J Med 43:489–508, 1974

172. Hanto DW, Frizzera G, Purtilo DT et al: Clinical spectrum of lymphoproliferative disorders in renal transplant recipients and evidence for the role of Epstein-Barr virus. Cancer Res 41:4253–4261, 1981

173. Sklar J: Multiclonal lymphomas. In Cavalli F, Bonnadonna G, Rosencweig M (eds): Proceedings of the Third International Conference on Malignant Lymphoma, 1987

174. Battifora H, Trowbridge IS: A monoclonal antibody useful for the differential diagnosis between malignant lymphoma and nonhematopoietic neoplasms. Cancer 51:816–821, 1983

175. Hu E, Trela M, Thompson J et al: Detection of B-cell lymphoma in peripheral blood by DNA hybridisation. Lancet 2:1092–1095, 1985

176. Janossy G, Bollum F, Bradstock K et al: Terminal transferase positive human bone marrow cells exhibit the antigenic phenotype of common acute lymphoblastic leukemia. J Immunol 123:1525–1529, 1979

177. Vezzoni P, Giardini R, Lombardi L et al: Multienzymatic analyses of human malignant lymphomas. Correlation of enzymatic data with pathologic and ultrastructural findings in Burkitt's and lymphoblastic lymphomas. Cancer 54:489–499, 1984

178. Hagberg H, Killander A, Simonsson B: Serum β_2-microglobulin in malignant lymphoma. Cancer 51:2220–2225, 1983

179. Wagner DK, Kiwanuka J, Edwards BK et al: Soluble interleukin II receptor levels in patients with undifferentiated and lymphoblastic lymphomas. J Clin Oncol 5:1262–1274, 1987

180. Erikson J, Finan J, Tsujimoto Y, Nowell P, Croce C: The chromosome breakpoint in neoplastic B cells with the t(11;14) translocation involves the immunoglobulin heavy chain locus. Proc Natl Acad Sci USA 81:4144–4148, 1984

181. Magrath IT: Malignant non-Hodgkin's lymphomas in children. Hemat Oncol Clin North Am 1:577–602, 1987

182. Shawker TH, Dunnick NR, Head GL, Magrath IT: Ultrasound evaluation of American Burkitt's lymphoma. J Clin Ultrasound 7:279–283, 1979

183. Krudy AD, Dunnick NR, Magrath IT, Shawker TH, Doppman JL, Spiegel R: CT of American Burkitt's lymphoma. AJR 136:747–754, 1981

184. Magrath IT, Lee YJ, Anderson T, Henle W, Ziegler J, Simon R, Schein P: Prognostic factors in Burkitt's lymphoma: Importance of total tumor burden. Cancer 45:1507–1515, 1980

185. Magrath I, Janus C, Edwards B et al: An effective therapy for both undifferentiated (including Burkitt's) lymphomas and lymphoblastic lymphomas in children and young adults. Blood 63:1102, 1984

186. Csako G, Magrath IT, Elin R: Serum total and isoenzyme lactate dehydrogenase activity in American Burkitt's lymphoma. Am J Clin Pathol 78:712–717, 1982

187. Desser H, Waldner R, Klaring W, Lutz D: Polyamines and histamine in serum from patients with hematological diseases. Adv Polyamine Res 4:49–58, 1983

188. Magrath IT: Clinical and pathobiological features of Burkitt's lymphoma and their relevance to treatment. In Levine PH, Ablashi DV, Pearson GR, Kottaridis SD (eds): Epstein-Barr Virus and Associate Diseases. Proceedings of the First International Symposium on Epstein-Barr Virus and Associated Malignant Diseases, pp 631–643. Boston, Martinus Nijhoff Publishing, 1985

189. Anderson JR, Wilson JF, Jenkin RD et al: The results of a randomized therapeutic trial comparing a 4-drug regimen (COMP) with a 10-drug regimen (LSA2-L2). N Engl J Med 308:559, 1983

190. Weinstein HJ, Lack EE, Cassady JR: APO Therapy for malignant lymphoma of large cell ''histiocytic'' type of childhood: analysis of treatment results for 29 patients. Blood 64:422, 1984

191. Sullivan MP, Boyett J, Pullen J: Pediatric Oncology Group experience with modified LSA$_2$L$_2$ therapy in 107 children with non-Hodgkin's lymphoma (Burkitt's lymphoma excluded). Cancer 55:323–336, 1985

192. Gadner H, Muller–Weihrich S, Riehm H: Treatment strategies in malignant non-Hodgkin lymphomas in childhood. Onkologie 9:126, 1986

193. Muller–Weihrich S, Henze G, Langermann HJ et al: Childhood B-cell lymphomas and leukemias. Improvement of prognosis by a therapy developed for B-neoplasms by the BMF study group. Onkologie 7:205, 1984

194. Ziegler JL, Magrath IT, Deisseroth AB et al: Combined modality treatment of Burkitt's lymphoma. Cancer Treat Rep 62:2031–2034, 1978

195. Burkitt DP: Long-term remissions following one- and two-dose chemotherapy for African lymphoma. Cancer 20:756–759, 1967

196. Ziegler JL: Burkitt's lymphoma. N Engl J Med 305:734–745, 1981

197. Duque–Hammershaimb L, Wollner N, Miller D: LSA$_2$L$_2$ protocol treatment of stage IV non-Hodgkin's lymphoma in children with partial and extensive bone marrow involvement. Cancer 52:39–43, 1983

198. Glick JH: Non-Hodgkin's lymphomas: Current trials in the United States. In Cavalli F, Bonnadonna G, Rosencweig M (eds): Proceedings of the Third International Conference on Malignant Lymphoma (in press)

199. Carabell SC, Goodman RL: Oncologic emergencies: Superior vena cava syndrome. In DeVita VT Jr, Hellman S, Rosenberg SA (eds): Cancer: Principles and Practice of Oncology, 2nd ed, pp 1855–1860. Philadelphia, JB Lippincott, 1985

200. Mott MG, Chessells JM, Willoughby ML et al: Adjuvant low dose radiation in childhood T cell leukaemia/lymphoma (report from the United Kingdom childrens' cancer study group—UKCCSG). Br J Cancer 50:457, 1984

201. Bernard A, Boumsell L, Patte C et al: Leukemia versus lymphoma in children: a worthless question? Med Pediatr Oncol 14:148, 1986

202. Weinstein HJ, Cassady Jr, Levey R: Long-term results of the APO protocol (vincristine, doxorubicin [adriamycin] and prednisone) for treatment of mediastinal lymphoblastic lymphoma. J Clin Oncol 1:537, 1983

203. Murphy S: The management of childhood non-Hodgkin's lymphoma. Cancer Treat Rep 61:1161, 1977

204. Müller–Weihrich S, Henze G, Odenwald E et al: BFM trials for childhood non-Hodgkin's lymphomas. In Cavalli F, Bonadonna G, Rosenswieg M (eds): Malignant Lymphomas and Hodgkin's Disease: Experimental and Therapeutic Advances, p 633. Boston, Martinus Nijhoff, 1985

205. Pichler E, Jurgenssen OA, Radaszkiewicz T et al: Results of LSA2-L2 therapy in 26 children with non-Hodgkin's lymphoma. Cancer 50:2740, 1982

206. Bogusawska–Jaworska J, Koscielniak E, Sroczynska M et al: Evaluation of the LSA2L2 protocol for treatment of childhood non-hodgkin's lymphoma. A report from the polish children's leukemia/lymphoma study group. Am J Pediatr Hematol Oncol 6:363, 1984

207. Dahl GV, Rivera G, Pui CH et al: A novel treatment of childhood lymphoblastic non-Hodgkin's lymphoma: Early and intermittent use of teniposide plus cytarabine. Blood 66:1110, 1985

208. Pullen DJ, Sullivan MP, Falletta JM et al: Modified LSA$_2$L$_2$ treatment in 53 children with E-rosette positive T-cell leukemia: Results and prognostic factors (a Pediatric Oncology Group Study). Blood 60:1159–1168, 1982

209. Hirt A, Baumgartner C, Imbach P et al: Differentiation and cytokinetic analysis of normal and neoplastic lymphoid cells in B and T cell malignancies of childhood. Br J Haematol 58:241, 1984

210. Cohen LF, Balow JE, Magrath IT: Acute tumor lysis syndrome: A review of 37 patients with Burkitt's lymphoma. Am J Med 68:486, 1980

211. Tsokos GE, Balow JE, Spiegel RJ: Renal and metabolic complications of undifferentiated and lymphoblastic lymphomas. Medicine 60:218, 1981

212. Arseneau JC, Bagley CM, Anderson T, Canellos GP: Hyperkalemia, a sequel to chemotherapy of Burkitt's lymphoma. Lancet 1:10–14, 1973

213. Anderson JR, Jenkin RDT: Treatment of childhood non-Hodgkin's lymphoma (lett). N Engl J Med 309:311, 1983

214. Müller–Weihrich S, Ludwig R, Reiter A et al: B-Type non-Hodgkin's lymphomas and leukemia: The BFM study group experience. In Cavalli F, Bonnadonna G, Rosencweig M (eds): Proceedings of the Third International Conference on Malignant Lymphoma, 1987

215. Patte C, Philip T, Rodary C et al: Improved survival rate in children with stage III and IV B cell non-Hodgkin's lymphoma and leukemia using multi-agent chemotherapy: Results of a study of 114 children from the French Pediatric Oncology Society. J Clin Oncol 4:1219, 1986

216. Zucker JM, Patte C, Philip T et al: Update results of the protocols LMB of the French Pediatric Oncology Society (SFOP) for B-cell advanced stage non-Hodgkin's lymphoma (NHL). In Cavalli F, Bonnadonna G, Rosencweig M (eds): Proceedings of the Third International Conference on Malignant Lymphoma, 1987

217. Murphy S, Bowman WP, Abromowitch M et al: Results of treatment of advanced stage Burkitt's lymphoma and B-cell (SIg+) acute lymphoblastic leukemia with high-dose fractionated cyclophosphamide and coordinated high-dose methotrexate and cytarabine. J Clin Oncol 4:1732, 1986

218. Siegel S, Chilcote R, Coccia P et al: A decade of progress in childhood non-Hodgkin's lymphoma (NHL). The Childrens Cancer Study Group (CCSG) experience. In Cavalli F, Bonnadonna G, Rosencweig M (eds): Proceedings of the Third International Conference on Malignant Lymphoma

219. Sullivan M, Ramirez I: Curability of Burkitt's lymphoma with high-dose cyclophosphamide, high dose methotrexate therapy and intrathecal chemoprophylaxis. J Clin Oncol 3:627–636, 1985

220. Appelbaum FR, Deisseroth AB, Graw RG Jr et al: Prolonged complete remission following high dose chemotherapy of Burkitt's lymphoma in relapse. Cancer 41:1059, 1978

221. Philip T, Pinkerton R, Hartmann O et al: The role of massive therapy with autologous bone marrow transplantation in Burkitt's lymphoma. Clin Haematol 15:205, 1986

222. Philip T, Biron P, Philip I et al: Massive therapy and autologous bone marrow transplantation in pediatric and young adults Burkitt's lymphoma (30 courses on 28 patients: a 5-year experience). Eur J Cancer Clin Oncol 22:1015–1027, 1986

223. Philip T, Biron P, Philip I et al: ABMT in Burkitt's lymphoma (50 cases in the Lyon protocol). In Cavalli F, Bonnadonna G, Rosencweig M (eds): Proceedings of the Third International Conference on Malignant Lymphoma, 1987

224. Ziegler J, Magrath IT, Olweny CLM: Cure of Burkitt's lymphoma: 10 year follow-up of 157 Ugandan patients. Lancet 2:936–938, 1979

225. Favrot M, Philip T: Bone marrow purging. In Magrath IT (ed): New Directions in Cancer Treatment. Heidelberg Springer-Verlag (in press)

226. Philip T, Pinkerton R, Hartmann et al: The role of massive therapy with autologous bone marrow transplantation in Burkitt's lymphoma. Clin Haematol 15:205–217, 1986

227. Jones GR, Ettinger LJ: Continuous infusion of high-dose cytosine arabinoside for treatment of childhood acute leukemia and non-Hodgkin's lymphoma in relapse. Semin Oncol 12(suppl 3):150, 1985

228. Lie SO, Sirdahl S: High-dose cytosine arabinoside in the treatment of childhood malignancies. Semin Oncol 12(suppl 3):1605, 1985

229. Appelbaum F, Sullivan K, Thomas E et al: Treatment of malignant lymphoma in one hundred patients with chemotherapy, total body irradiation and marrow transplantation. J Clin Oncol 5:1340–1367, 1987

230. Baumgartner C, Bleher EA, Brun del Re G et al: Autologous bone marrow transplantation (ABMT) for childhood non-Hodgkin's lymphoma (NHL): Limitations by acute extramedullary toxicity. In Cavalli F, Bonadonna G, Rozenswieg M (eds): Malignant Lymphomas and Hodgkin's disease: Experimental and therapeutic advances, p 419. Boston, Martinus Nijhoff, 1985

231. Sullivan MP, Jaffe N, Boren H et al: Male reproductive functions in long-term survivors of childhood cancer: Assessment by sperm count analysis (sca) (abstr) Proc Annu Meet Am Assoc Cancer Res 26:182, 1985

232. Hall BH, Green DM: Sexual and reproductive function following treatment during childhood and adolescence for cancer (abstr). Proc Annu Meet Am Soc Clin Oncol 2:C-272, 1983

233. Pasqualini T, Chemes H, Domene H et al: Evaluation of testicular function following long-term treatment for acute lymphoblastic leukemia. Am J Pediatr Hematol Oncol 5:11–20, 1983

234. Meadows AT, Baum E, Fossati–Bellani F et al: Second malignant neoplasms in children: An update from the late effects study group. J Clin Oncol 3:532–538, 1985

235. Lichter AS, Fraass BA, McShan DL et al: Radiotherapy treatment planning: Past, present and future. In Magrath IT (ed): New Approaches to Cancer Treatment. Heidelberg, Springer-Verlag (in press)

236. Magrath IT: New directions in cancer treatment: An overview. In Magrath IT (ed): New Directions in Cancer Treatment. Heidelberg, Springer-Verlag (in press)

237. Arndt C, Colvin M, Balis F et al: Intrathecal administration of 4-hydroperoxycyclophosphamide (hpc) (abstr). Proc Annu Meet Am Assoc Cancer Res 28:439, 1987

238. Hertler A, Schlossman D, Lester C et al: Intrathecal administration of WT1-ricin, a chain immunotoxin (abstr). Proc Am Soc Clin Oncol 6:A989, 1987

239. Wong GG, Temple PA, Leary AC et al: Human CSF-1: Molecular cloning and expression of 4-Kb cDNA encoding the human urinary protein. Science 235:1504–1508, 1987

240. Giardyina SL, Fooy KA, Beatty SM, Morgan AC Jr: Evaluation of clinical application of partially purified human urinary colony-stimulating factor. Immunobiology 172:205–212, 1986

241. Myers CD, Thorpe PE, Ross WC et al: An immunotoxin with therapeutic potential in T cell leukemia: WT1-ricin A. Blood 63:1178–1185, 1984

242. Ochs J, Abromowitch M, Rudnick S et al: Phase I–II study of recombinant alpha-2 interferon against advanced leukemia and lymphoma in children. J Clin Oncol 4:883–887, 1986

twenty-one

Hodgkin's Disease

Brigid G. Leventhal and
Sarah S. Donaldson

The original paper by Hodgkin in 1832 was entitled "On some morbid appearances of the absorbent glands and spleen."[1] In that era of anatomic description of disease, investigators were concerned with differentiating inflammatory disease from infection or idiopathic hypertrophy of the lymphoid organs. It was not until the second half of the 19th century, as the criteria for making diagnoses came to depend more on microscopic morphology, that investigators recognized that there were abnormal giant cells in Hodgkin's material. Sternberg in 1898[2] and Reed in 1902[3] are generally credited with the first definitive and thorough descriptions of the histopathology of Hodgkin's disease. Reed, in particular, gave a precise description of the multinucleated giant cells in this disease, which led her finally to refute the idea that it was an unusual form of tuberculosis despite the not-infrequent association of the two diseases in the same individual. After the histologic definition of the disease was established, Fox, in 1926,[4] reexamined the histology from Hodgkin's original seven cases and concluded that three of them, one of whom was a pediatric patient,[5] met the new criteria for definition of the disease.

In the ensuing years, although it was recognized that Hodgkin's disease might well be a malignancy, the possibility of an infectious or autoimmune etiology was still considered.[6] The pleomorphic nature of the cellular infiltrate in Hodgkin's disease has left investigators uncomfortable with the idea that this is a clonal proliferation of a single malignant cell. However, the successful cultivation by Kaplan and Gartner[7] and by Long and associates[8] of Reed–Sternberg cells permitted the demonstration that they are aneuploid, heterotransplantable, mitotically active malignant cells and reinforced the idea that Hodgkin's disease was, indeed, a malignant disorder.

In 1902, Pusey[9] and in 1903, Senn[10] reported the first cases of Hodgkin's disease treated with radiotherapy. Dramatic regressions occurred, usually followed by recurrence, with the disease inevitably being fatal. With improvement in radiotherapeutic equipment and techniques, however, cure of early-stage disease with radiotherapy alone is now common. In 1940, as a byproduct of wartime work on compounds related to the mustard gases, it was discovered that the nitrogen mustards had powerful lymphocytolytic effects on normal and malignant lymphoid tissue.[11] Experimental studies indicating the desirability of using combinations of agents with nonoverlapping toxicities led to the introduction in 1964 of the four-drug MOPP regimen (mustard, Oncovin, procarbazine, prednisone)[12] (Table 21-1) and later of other four-drug combinations. Early in the reports of treatment of this disease, it was suggested that children had a less-favorable prognosis than young adults,[13] but with more extensive study, this has not proved to be the case.

Table 21-1
Chemotherapy Regimens for Hodgkin's Disease

Name	Drugs	Dose and Route*		Days of Administration
MOPP	Mechlorethamine (nitrogen *m*ustard)	6	mg/m² IV	1, 8
	Vincristine (*O*ncovin)	1.4 mg/m² IV		1, 8
	*P*rocarbazine	100 mg/m² PO		1–14
	*P*rednisone	40 mg/m² PO		1–14 (Prednisone in cycles 1 and 4 only)
	Repeat cycle every 4 weeks for six courses or two beyond complete response, whichever is longer.			
COPP	Cyclophosphamide OR	600 mg/m² IV 300 mg/m² IV		1 1, 8 } (substituted for mechlorethamine in MOPP)
CVPP	Lomustine (*CC*NU)	75	mg/m² IV	1 (substituted for mechlorethamine in MOPP)
	*V*inblastine (Velban)	6	mg/m² IV	1 (substituted for vincristine in MOPP)
MVOPP	Mechlorethamine			
	Vinblastine			
	Vincristine			
	Oncovin			
	Procarbazine			
	Prednisone			
ChlVPP	Chlorambucil			
	Vinblastine			
	Procarbazine			
	Prednisolone			
ABVD	Doxorubicin (*A*driamycin)	25	mg/m² IV	1, 15
	*B*leomycin	10	U/m² IV	1, 15
	*V*inblastine	6	mg/m² IV	1, 15
	*D*acarbazine	375	mg/m² IV	1, 15
	Repeat every 28 days.			

* IV = inravenous; PO = orally.

EPIDEMIOLOGY

There is a definite bimodal age peak in the incidence of Hodgkin's disease not seen for most other lymphomas (Fig. 21-1).[14] The second peak occurs in late adulthood. In developing countries, the early peak occurs before adolescence, whereas in industrialized countries, including the United States, the early peak occurs in the mid to late 20s. In these industrialized countries, there is an association of Hodgkin's disease in young patients with higher family socioeconomic status. This pattern, similar to that seen with paralytic poliomyelitis 50 years ago, has led some investigators to postulate that an infectious agent is responsible for Hodgkin's disease.

There is a slight overall male predominance in the incidence of Hodgkin's disease. In childhood cases, this is most marked in the very young patient. A summary of cases in the United States from the National Cancer Institute Surveillance, Epidemiology, and End Results (SEER) Program is shown in Table 21-2.[15] From these data, several generalizations can be made. First, Hodgkin's disease is rare before the age of 5 years. Second, in children older than 15 years, the disease is more common in the white race than in other races. Finally, in the child younger than 10 years, the incidence seems much higher in males than females, whereas in the teenager, the incidence is about equal.

The difference in incidence by race might suggest an environmental or a genetic etiology. Studies looking for specific associations with HLA types have not been convincing. However, there are numerous reports of Hodgkin's disease in first-degree relatives, including siblings, particularly those of the same gender,[14] as well as in parent–child concordant pairs. Concordance that might represent transplacental transmission of the disease[16] is extremely rare, as are reports of Hodgkin's disease in married couples.[17]

Hodgkin's disease does appear to be more common in individuals with an underlying immunodeficiency disease such as ataxia telangiectasia,[18] and this fact might account for the slight increase in familial incidence. There is an apparent increase in some families of other diseases of the lymphoreticular system. There is a definite increase in lymphoma including Hodgkin's disease in patients with iatrogenic or acquired immune deficiency syndromes such as AIDS.[19]

The possibility of a contagious component in the transmission of Hodgkin's disease has been the focus of a number of epidemiologic studies. There have been case clusters reported, such as among students and teachers in a particular school,[20] but later statistical analyses have generally cast doubt on the validity of these observations on the grounds that such apparent clustering could well occur by chance alone.[21] Many viruses and bacteria have been looked for as etiologic agents through the years. The one puzzling association that appears to be real is the increased incidence of Hodgkin's disease in patients with high titers of antiviral antibody after serologically diagnosed infectious mononucleosis, although Epstein-Barr viral DNA has not been isolated from the genome of tumor cells.[22]

BIOLOGY

There is general agreement that the malignant cell of Hodgkin's disease is the Reed–Sternberg cell, but its normal counterpart has not yet been identified. The availability of cultured cell lines derived from Reed–Sternberg cells and monoclonal

FIGURE 21-1. Bimodal peak of age incidence of Hodgkin's disease in the United States, with the early peak in young adults and the later peak in elderly individuals. (Grufferman SL, Delzell E: Epidemiology of Hodgkin's disease. Epidemiol Rev 6:76–106, 1984)

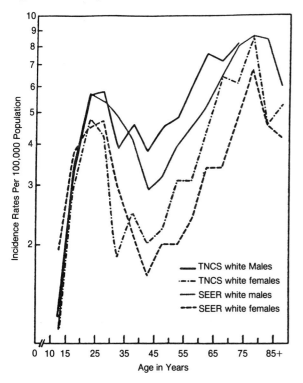

antibodies that identify tissue-specific and differentiation antigens has intensified research in this area but still has not allowed definite conclusions.

Popular theories have included origin from activated B or T lymphocytes or some form of antigen-presenting cells. Antigen-presenting cells are divided by immunologic and functional characteristics into two distinct types: monocyte/macrophages and interdigitating reticulum/dendritic cells (see Chap. 4).[23] The former category of "histiocyte" is rich in degradative lysosomal enzymes, including lysozyme; actively phagocytic; largely distributed in the sinusoids of the lymph nodes and spleen; and derived from the peripheral blood monocyte.[24] The latter category of "histiocyte," including the interdigitating reticulum cells of the lymph node paracortex, dendritic cells in the lymph node follicles, and the Langerhans' cells in the epidermis, is only weakly phagocytic, poor in degradative enzymes, a potent stimulator of the mixed lymphocyte response, and of unknown derivation.[25]

Reed Sternberg cells and their mononuclear variants have Fc and C_3 receptors and Ia antigen. They also have intracytoplasmic immunoglobulin, but this is polyclonal and therefore presumably ingested rather than synthesized by the cell itself. The cell lines also express Ia antigen and rosette with T lymphocytes but usually lack demonstrable Fc and C_3 receptors. All of these findings would be consistent with origin from an antigen-presenting cell. The cells are not phagocytic, and they lack diffuse activity of nonspecific esterase and acid phosphatase.[26] In addition, they do not react with a panel of antibodies to differentiation antigens of the monocyte/macrophage system,[23] which suggests that the cells arise from an interdigitating reticulum cell[27] rather than a cell of monocytic origin.

Knowles and coworkers studied the organization of the immunoglobulin and T-cell receptor β-chain (T-β) gene loci in 18 cases of Hodgkin's disease. They found that clonal immunoglobulin or T-β gene rearrangements were not detectable in cases containing more than 25% Reed–Sternberg cells, although minor clonal B- or T-cell populations unrelated to Reed–Sternberg cells were occasionally found. However, those authors thought that their data might be consistent with the interpretation that Reed–Sternberg cells represent polyclonal activated T cells, because the Reed–Sternberg cells express a variety of antigens associated with T-cell activation such as Ia, Leu M1, and Tac (interleukin-2 receptor), which are absent from resting peripheral T cells. Some of these markers are also characteristic of activated B cells.

The monoclonal antibodies KI-1[29] and HeFi-I[30] prepared against Hodgkin's disease cell lines, which preferentially react with Reed–Sternberg cells, also react with activated, but not with resting, T lymphocytes. KI-1 in normal tissues also stains a small mononuclear cell in the parafollicular zone, as well as cells in certain other lymphomas and inflammatory conditions. The interdigitating reticulum cell in man has not been isolated

Table 21-2
Incidence of Hodgkin's Disease per 100,000 (1973–1982)[14]

Age at Diagnosis	White M	White F	Black M	Black F	Puerto Rican M	Puerto Rican F	Mexican M	Mexican F
0–4	0.06	0.07	0.32	0.11	0.29	—	0.40	—
5–9	0.68	0.25	0.60	0.10	1.06	0.24	0.79	0.41
10–14	1.37	1.67	1.43	0.38	1.22	1.32	2.33	0.81
15–19	3.67	4.18	2.38	1.59	1.85	1.59	1.49	3.40

and purified, so its reactivity cannot be evaluated in the same way.

At the moment, the interdigitating reticulum cell is probably the leading candidate for the normal counterpart of the Reed–Sternberg cell; however, there are no specific positive markers that identify this cell in normal tissues. On the basis of marker studies, one could make a case for some form of polyclonal activated T or B lymphocyte as the Reed–Sternberg analogue, but this would complicate the interpretation of the malignant nature of this disease.

One of the most confusing histologic features of Hodgkin's disease has been the multicellular or "reactive" appearance of the infiltrate that accompanies the Reed–Sternberg cells. The established cell lines produce mediators of biological activity including E-rosette inhibition factor, interleukin 1 (IL-1)-like activity, fibroblast growth-promoting activity, colony-stimulating factor, macrophage-inhibiting factor (MIF), and inhibiting activity for pokeweed mitogen (PWM)-induced B-cell transformation.[31] Some of these activities have also been detected in the sera of patients with Hodgkin's disease. The liberation of factors with such activities could well explain the presence of multiple cell types at the site of the primary malignant lesions.

PATHOLOGY

Overview

Histologically, one sees an admixture of apparently normal reactive cells including lymphocytes, plasma cells, and eosinophils along with the cytologically abnormal Reed–Sternberg cells. The diagnosis of Hodgkin's disease rarely should be made in the absence of Reed–Sternberg cells, although the presence of such a cell, by itself, is not pathognomonic of the disease. Cells simulating Reed–Sternberg cells have been found in reactive lymphoid hyperplasias such as infectious mononucleosis, non-Hodgkin's lymphomas, and nonlymphoid malignancies including carcinomas and sarcomas.[26]

Reed–Sternberg cells are large (15–45 µm or more in diameter), with abundant cytoplasm and either multiple or multilobed nuclei. The nuclear membrane is usually intensely stained, and the delicate chromatin network within it typically gives way to a peculiar halo-like clear zone around the nucleolus. The nucleoli are also large and prominent (Fig. 21-2). Mononuclear cells (often called Hodgkin's cells) with identical nuclear and nucleolar features are also seen. Variants include the "lacunar" cells seen characteristically in nodular sclerosing disease (see below). In some patients, Hodgkin's cells are more bizarre and pleomorphic and may be difficult to distinguish from diffuse pleomorphic histiocytic lymphomas.[32]

Definition of Histologic Subtypes

The first clinically useful subclassification of Hodgkin's disease was developed by Jackson and Parker.[33] In this scheme, about 10% of patients had indolent disease classified as "paragranuloma," whereas another 10% had highly aggressive disease or "sarcoma." The other 80% of cases were called Hodgkin's granuloma. A later scheme, proposed by Lukes and Butler[32] and later simplified into the Rye classification, is the one currently used. In the Rye classification, Hodgkin's disease is divided into four categories: lymphocytic predominance (LP), mixed cellularity (MC), lymphocytic depletion (LD), and nodular sclerosis (NS). The prognosis in the first three

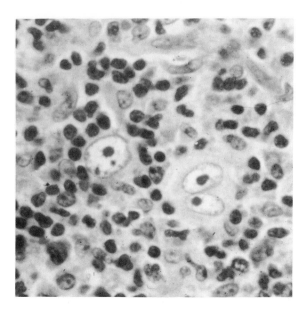

FIGURE 21-2. Characteristic Sternberg–Reed cell and mononuclear variant of Hodgkin's disease. (Hematoxylin and eosin; magnification ×400)

categories is generally proportional to the ratio of lymphocytes to abnormal cells.

In LP Hodgkin's disease, the lymph node architecture may be partially or completely destroyed. The cellular proliferation involves benign-appearing lymphocytes with or without benign histiocytes and may be misinterpreted as reactive hyperplasia. It is often necessary to examine multiple sections to identify a diagnostic Reed–Sternberg cell; fibrosis usually is not seen.

In MC Hodgkin's disease, Reed–Sternberg cells and their variants usually are quite plentiful (5 to 15 per high-power field). The lymph node is usually diffusely effaced. Fine interstitial fibrosis may be seen, and focal necrosis may be present but usually is not marked.

In LD Hodgkin's disease, there are principally abnormal cells with a relative paucity of lymphocytes. Fibrosis and necrosis are common but diffuse and not of the broad type seen in nodular sclerosis.

The NS type of Hodgkin's disease is morphologically distinctive. The lacunar variant of the Reed–Sternberg cell may be seen. In Formalin-fixed tissue, the abundant pale cytoplasm often artifactually retracts and gives the appearance of a cell in a space. The second feature, seen in most (but not all) cases, is a thickened capsule with a proliferation of orderly collagenous bands that divide the lymphoid tissue into circumscribed nodules (Fig. 21-3). This process has a striking propensity to involve the lower cervical, supraclavicular, and mediastinal lymph nodes.

Involvement of other organs, most notably the spleen, generally begins as small nodular infiltrates, which may be no more than a few millimeters in diameter. The size of the spleen and the degree of involvement do not necessarily correlate, since the spleen may be enlarged without being involved or involved without being enlarged. The entire spleen must be sectioned and examined at 1- to 3-mm intervals before it can be satisfactorily called tumor free. Figure 21-4 shows the focal nature of splenic involvement. Studies in adults have shown the number of nodules in the spleen to have prognostic significance; that is, a better prognosis with no more than five nod-

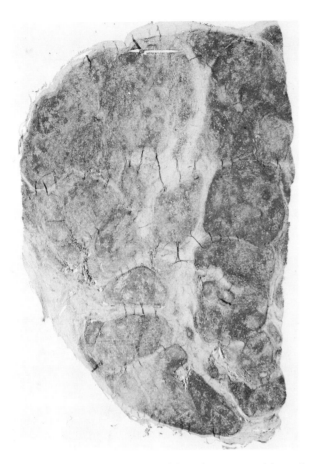

FIGURE 21-3. Lymph node, nodular sclerosing Hodgkin's disease. Cellular nodules are surrounded by dense fibrous bands. (Hematoxylin and eosin; magnification ×8)

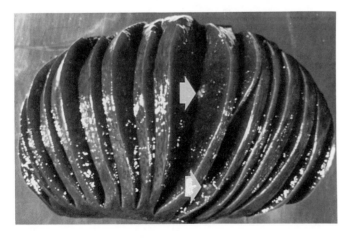

FIGURE 21-4. "Bread-loafed" spleen revealing two foci of disease (*arrows*). The spleen was of normal size and weight. The two areas of disease were not apparent by inspection or palpation and might not have been recognized if only a hemisplenectomy been performed or if the spleen had not been sectioned at 5-mm intervals.

ules.[34] For complete evaluation, wedge biopsies of the liver also must be performed, since infiltration of this organ is also usually focal.

At the time of relapse, it is usual to find the same histologic subtype of disease. However, progression from the more favorable LP type to a less favorable MC or LD type has been noted in sequential biopsies of untreated areas.[35]

About two-thirds of pediatric patients have NS disease at the time of presentation, although LP and MC disease are relatively more common in children 10 years or younger than in older children. Data from two institutions are shown in Table 21-3.

CLINICAL PRESENTATION

Lymphadenopathy

The usual clinical presentation is one of painless supraclavicular or cervical adenopathy. The lymph nodes often feel firmer than inflammatory nodes and have a rubbery texture. They may be tender if they have grown rapidly. At least two-thirds of the patients have mediastinal involvement of some degree at presentation. It is extremely important to obtain a chest film as soon as Hodgkin's disease becomes part of the differential diagnosis (Fig. 21-5). The competency of the airway should be thoughtfully assessed before any procedures such as node biopsies are undertaken. Axillary or inguinal adenopathy may also be presenting signs, although primary disease presenting in a subdiaphragmatic site is rare, occurring in only about 3% of cases.[37] Splenomegaly, hepatomegaly, or both often indicate advanced disease, although involvement of these organs must be surgically assessed. Intrathoracic structures such as pulmonary parenchyma, pleura, and pericardium are the most commonly involved extranodal sites of disease.

Systemic Symptoms

About one-third of patients with Hodgkin's disease have nonspecific systemic symptoms at the time of presentation that may include fatigue, anorexia, and weight loss. The specific symptoms of unexplained fever with temperatures above 38.0°C orally, unexplained weight loss of 10% in the previous 6 months, and drenching night sweats are thought to be of prognostic significance; if any of these is present, the patient is considered to have B disease as opposed to A disease (asymptomatic). Some patients suffer symptoms such as pruritus or pain that worsens with ingestion of alcohol, but this does not carry prognostic significance.

Hematologic Picture

Abnormal blood counts may indicate the presence of advanced disease. There are two known mechanisms of anemia in Hodgkin's disease. The first is hemolysis, which will be accompanied by reticulocytosis and normoblastic hyperplasia of the bone marrow. The Coombs' test is rarely positive. The second is impaired mobilization of iron stores, which occurs in the presence of excessive iron stores in the liver and spleen.[38] At the onset of disease, the absolute lymphocyte count is usually normal in children,[39] although adults with extensive disease not uncommonly have lymphopenia. Some patients develop an idiopathic thrombocytopenic purpura (ITP)-like picture. In addition, 11 of 17 patients studied during active disease, five of whom were thrombocytopenic, had platelet-associated IgG.[40] Thus thrombocytopenia or platelet-associated IgG may be a sign of active disease in patients who are otherwise asympto-

Table 21-3
Histologic Subtype at Presentation

| | | | Percentage of Patients | | | | |
Series	Age	Number of Patients	LP*	NS	MC	LD	Other
Donaldson and Link[36]	≤10	65	17	45	32	0	6
	11–15	126	10	72	13	2	3
Leventhal	≤10	17	18	41	35	0	6
	11–16	38	11	70	18	0	0

* LP = lymphocytic predominance; NS = nodular sclerosis; MC = mixed cellularity; LD = lymphocytic depletion; Other = interfollicular and unclassified.

matic. Rarely, patients develop symptomatic hypersplenism with anemia, leukopenia, and thrombocytopenia.

Immunologic Status

Anergy is a common concomitant of advanced Hodgkin's disease. These patients fail to respond to intradermal recall antigens, and their lymphocytes do not have a normal *in vitro* response to PHA stimulation.[39,41] Immunologic parameters usually return toward normal with successful therapy for the disease, although abnormalities of T-cell function may persist for years.[41] This deficiency has been postulated to be secondary to involvement of the antigen-presenting cells in this disease, which could render T cells unresponsive despite normal numbers.

DIFFERENTIAL DIAGNOSIS

Hodgkin's disease must be differentiated from other inflammatory causes of lymphadenopathy, particularly those with a relatively indolent course such as atypical mycobacterial infections and toxoplasmosis (see also Chap. 5). In addition, non-Hodgkin's lymphoma may present with similar signs and symptoms. The growth rate in non-Hodgkin's lymphoma will often be more rapid than in Hodgkin's disease, and signs of rapid tissue turnover such as elevated uric acid or lactic dehydrogenase will be more common (see also Chap. 20). Occasionally, lymphadenopathy for which it was thought there was an explanation, such as infectious mononucleosis or "reactive hyperplasia,"[42] will recur or persist beyond a reasonable period of time, and repeat biopsy will lead to the diagnosis of lymphoma. Metastatic cervical adenopathy can also be the presenting complaint in patients with other primary tumors, such as nasopharyngeal carcinoma or soft-tissue sarcoma (see Chaps. 30 and 35). Ultimately, the diagnosis of any of these conditions will have to be made by biopsy.

A somewhat more difficult problem is that of a mediastinal mass that must be differentiated from normal thymus in an otherwise asymptomatic patient. The thymus is maximal in size on computed tomography (CT) in patients at about the age of 10 and may be differentiated from tumor by its texture by an extremely experienced interpreter.[43] However, biopsy is required to establish a diagnosis. Interpretation of mediastinal CT scans and radiographs may be complicated after therapy. First, often the mediastinum does not return to normal even in patients who have been cured.[44] Second, a situation that is

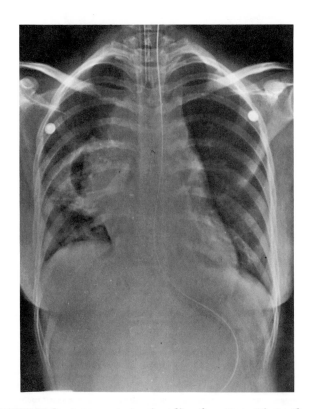

FIGURE 21-5. Anteroposterior chest film of a patient with significant tracheal compression below the distal endotracheal tube. Emergency radiotherapy may be required for such patients before laparotomy can be staged.

particularly vexing to interpret occurs in patients after therapy, where rebound growth of mediastinal tissue may mimic relapse.[45]

DIAGNOSTIC WORK-UP

Table 21-4 shows the steps in the diagnostic work-up of a child with Hodgkin's disease. A careful physical examination with assessment of all node-bearing areas including Waldeyer's ring is essential, with direct measurement of any enlarged nodes so that later changes can be quantitated. Chest radiography with anteroposterior and lateral projections is required. The ratio of

Table 21-4
Steps in Diagnostic Work-up of Patients with Hodgkin's Disease

Physical examination with measurement of enlarged nodal areas
Posteroanterior and lateral chest radiographs
Complete blood count, erythrocyte sedimentation rate, serum
    copper, liver- and renal-function tests, alkaline phosphatase
    assay. Baseline thyroid-stimulating hormone and free T4
Lymph node biopsy to establish diagnosis
Chest CT scan
Gallium scan (optional)
Abdominal and pelvic CT scan*
Lymphangiogram*
Staging laparotomy*
  Splenectomy
  Sampling of splenic hilar, celiac and porta hepatis, mesenteric,
    iliac, and para-aortic lymph nodes
  Wedge biopsies of both lobes of liver
Bone marrow biopsy
Bone scan (optional)

* For indications and details, see text.

the maximum diameter of mediastinal mass to the maximum intrathoracic diameter should be calculated, since masses more than one-third the thoracic diameter may carry a poor prognosis.[46,47] The adequacy of the airway must be assessed. The airway may be compressed by anterior structures so that the most marked abnormality is appreciated on the lateral film. Next, a biopsy of nodal tissue is performed to establish a histologic diagnosis before proceeding with the studies noted below.

Thoracic disease should be further assessed with a CT scan. Rostock and associates found that approximately 50% of previously untreated patients had disease discovered on CT that had been missed on plain films, including pericardial or chest-wall invasion, retrocardiac masses, and pulmonary parenchymal involvement.[48] If high cervical nodes are involved, CT of neck to include Waldeyer's ring should be performed, since nasopharynx mirror examination may be difficult in a small or uncooperative child. Magnetic resonance imaging (MRI) is also an effective tool for evaluating intrathoracic structures.

The CT scan can be used to assess the extent of abdominal and pelvic disease, although evaluation by this technique is complicated in children by the lack retroperitoneal fat. Furthermore, CT not ideal in imaging retroperitoneal lymph nodes, since enlargement is detected, but architecture is not well characterized.

The classic method of evaluating the extent of retroperitoneal adenopathy in patients with Hodgkin's disease is the lymphangiogram (LAG). This study is currently the most accurate way of evaluating pelvic and para-aortic lymph nodes in Hodgkin's disease, although it usually does not image the mesenteric nodes or upper abdominal celiac and porta hepatis nodes (see Chap. 7). The technique has the advantage that the nature of the nodes can be determined and that specific nodes can be identified for biopsy during a staging laparotomy. Moreover, because the retroperitoneal nodes remain opacified for months after the procedure, one can use a plain abdominal radiograph to determine the accuracy of operative sampling, to design radiotherapy treatment portals appropriately, and to monitor the residual abnormal nodes for response to therapy.

There are some drawbacks to the technique, however. The false-positive rate may be higher in children than in adults, perhaps because children are more likely to have reactive lymph nodes. Dudgeon and associates found that 16 of 47 pediatric patients had abnormal LAGs, but at staging laparotomy, only five had retroperitoneal lymph nodes that contained Hodgkin's disease.[49] Thirty-one patients had a normal LAG, and three of these had histologically positive retroperitoneal lymph nodes. Thus, those investigators found an overall accuracy of only 70%. Dunnick and coworkers, however, found a 95% accuracy in their radiographic–histologic correlation.[50] The LAG may carry with it some toxicity. Patients may develop a lipoid pneumonitis, with subsequent respiratory distress. Therefore, the test should not be performed in patients who have respiratory compromise. In addition, the LAG is time consuming and requires an expert team for performance and interpretation in a pediatric population. For these reasons, although there is no doubt that an LAG in good hands is a most effective diagnostic tool, in many pediatric institutions, there is reluctance to use it routinely.

Gallium-67 scanning may be a useful screen in patients with Hodgkin's disease.[51] Gallium citrate has shown a great affinity for lymphomas, particularly NS and LP Hodgkin's disease. A ^{67}Ga scan will have a true-positive rate of approximately 70%, although not all lesions even within the same patient will necessarily be equally gallium avid. The study can be particularly useful in patients for whom a LAG is contraindicated. It may indicate otherwise obscure sites of disease and may be very helpful in the detection of recurrent disease in patients with a normal physical examination but worrisome systemic symptoms or abnormal laboratory values. This test is nonspecific, however, and will not distinguish a lymphoma from an inflammatory lesion. It should be remembered that the contrast medium used for LAG will cause an inflammatory response in lungs and lymphoid tissue, so if both studies are to be done, the ^{67}Ga scan should be done first.

Bone marrow involvement at the time of initial presentation of Hodgkin's disease is rare. Nevertheless, the bone marrow should be evaluated. An aspirate is an inadequate sample, since involvement when present is spotty. A biopsy should be performed, although this can be deferred until the time of the staging laparotomy in patients in clinical stage I or IIA. If the patient has hematologic abnormalities suggesting bone marrow involvement, B symptoms, or clinical stage III–IV disease, then biopsy should be done prior to laparotomy, since it may obviate that particular staging procedure.

Since Hodgkin's is a disease of the reticuloendothelial system, tests that reflect activation of this system, such as the erythrocyte sedimentation rate and serum copper, will often have abnormal results in patients with active disease. These nonspecific tests, if abnormal at diagnosis, are useful during follow-up.[52]

Adequate evaluation of the spleen must be surgical, as must that of the liver. Hepatic and renal function should be assessed along with other metabolic measures such as serum uric acid prior to initiating therapy, but these studies will not show the extent of involvement with disease. Serum alkaline phosphatase, a nonspecific indicator of disease activity, may be elevated in children as a function of normal bone growth, so age-appropriate norms should be compared.

A ^{99}Tc bone scan is a reasonable initial screen at the time of diagnosis, particularly when the patient has bone complaints or has an elevated serum alkaline phosphatase concentration. However, since bone involvement is extremely rare, it is usually not necessary to repeat this test in the absence of specific symptoms.

STAGING

Overview

There is strong evidence that Hodgkin's disease generally spreads from one adjacent nodal area to another, at least until very late in the disease.[6] The staging classification for Hodgkin's disease currently in use is based on this assumption (Table 21-5). It was adopted in 1971 at a workshop in Ann Arbor, Michigan.[53] The lymph node chains that would be designated as "regions" for the purpose of staging[54] are shown in Figure 21-6.

The classification of extralymphatic disease is sometimes difficult. Extralymphatic disease may be widespread, in which case the patient is considered to have Stage IV disease. In an occasional patient, however, extralymphatic disease is small, in which case it is designated substage E. The designation "E" was originally intended for extralymphatic disease so limited in extent or location that it could be subjected to definitive treatment by radiotherapy.[6]

Another area to which a great deal of attention has recently been paid is the subdivision of Stage IIIA disease. Disease limited to the spleen or splenic hilar or porta hepatis nodes has been said to have a favorable prognosis relative to other Stage IIIA disease and designated $IIIA_1$[55] (Fig. 21-7). Disease represented by fewer than five nodules in the spleen is said to have a particularly favorable prognosis.[34] For some, this has represented the distinction between those patients who can be treated by definitive radiotherapy alone and those who are better treated with combined-modality therapy. This distinction may be less important for younger patients, who are all likely to receive combined-modality therapy.

There is an important distinction between clinical stage and pathologic stage. Pathologic staging involves surgical staging, often with a laparotomy and splenectomy. The importance of the staging laparotomy was emphasized after the discovery of an unusually high number of patients who had clinically unsuspected splenic involvement at presentation.[56] Of 133 children clinically staged prior to laparotomy, 10 were downstaged as a result of their surgery and 27 were upstaged, for an overall change in status of 28%.[57] When patients are to be treated by radiotherapy alone, a precise anatomic notation of the sites involved is critical to the design of the portals. When all patients receive chemotherapy, precise staging may be less

FIGURE 21-6. Anatomic definition of separate lymph node regions used for staging purposes. (Modified from Kaplan HS, Rosenberg SA: The treatment of Hodgkin's disease. Med Clin North Am 50:1591–1610, 1966)

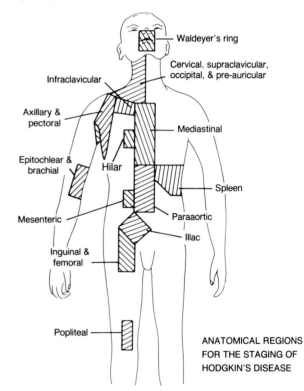

FIGURE 21-7. Diagram of lymph node regions in the abdomen showing the demarcation of stage $IIIA_1$ disease (nodal involvement limited to groups above the line) from stage $IIIA_2$ (nodal involvement including groups below the line). (Desser RK et al: Prognostic classification of Hodgkin's disease in pathologic stage III, based on anatomic considerations. Blood 49:883–893, 1977. Copyright © 1977 Grune & Stratton)

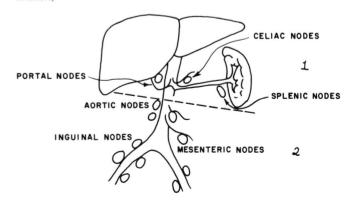

Table 21-5
Ann Arbor Staging Classification for Hodgkin's Disease

Stage	Definition
I	Involvement of a single lymph node region (I) or of a single extralymphatic organ or site (I_E)
II	Involvement of two or more lymph node regions on the same side of the diaphragm (II) or localized involvement of an extralymphatic organ or site and one or more lymph node regions on the same side of the diaphragm (II_E)
III	Involvement of lymph node regions on both sides of the diaphragm (III), which may be accompanied by involvement of the spleen (III_S) or by localized involvement of an extralymphatic organ or site (III_E) or both (III_{SE})
IV	Diffuse or disseminated involvement of one or more extralymphatic organs or tissues with or without associated lymph node involvement

The absence or presence of fever, night sweats, or unexplained loss of 10% or more of body weight in the 6 months preceding admission are to be denoted in all cases by the suffix letters A or B, respectively.

Table 21-6
Stage of Hodgkin's Disease at Presentation in Pediatric Patients

Number of Patients	Pathologic Stage								Reference
	1A	*1B*	*2A*	*2B*	*3A*	*3B*	*4A*	*4B*	
60	14	21	0	5	9	4	3	4	46
133	15	2	51	12	34	11	4	4	57
92	14	0	36	9	9	15	9		58
65	9	0	30	1	10	5	6	4	Authors' data
350	52	23	117	27	62	35	17	17	
Total (%)	(15)	(7)	(33)	(8)	(18)	(10)	(5)	(5)	

Table 21-7
Indications for Staging Laparotomy

Patients Who Require a Staging Laparotomy

All patients in stage I or II at the end of clinical staging.

All patients for whom localized radiation therapy to involved areas is contemplated as part of the management (even if chemotherapy is also given).

Patients Who Do Not Require a Staging Laparotomy

Patients who otherwise can be shown to have histologically proved stage III or IV disease and in whom only chemotherapy will be used for management, such as those with positive biopsies from lymph node groups both above and below the diaphragm.

N.B.: The presence or absence of splenic involvement cannot be determined by nonsurgical techniques at present.

important. It cannot be overemphasized, however, that therapeutic results in patients who have been clinically staged only cannot be compared with those of patients who have been pathologically staged. About two-thirds of pediatric patients will have pathologic Stage I or II disease at the time of presentation, and about one-quarter will have B symptoms. Data from several pediatric series are summarized in Table 21-6.

Staging Laparotomy

A staging laparotomy and splenectomy should be performed if management decisions depend on precise identification of the location of abdominal disease (Table 21-7).[59] Emergency radiotherapy to the mediastinum may be required prior to general anesthesia. Laparotomy should include detailed inspection of the abdomen and removal of the entire spleen and any accessory spleens. Partial splenectomy, which was previously suggested in order to leave functional splenic tissue *in situ,* is not adequate for evaluation of disease spread, since splenic involvement in Hodgkin's disease is commonly focal. Wedge and needle biopsies of both lobes of the liver should be performed at laparotomy, unless hepatic involvement can be proved by less-extensive biopsy of an abnormal area seen either directly or by another technique; for example, a filling defect on CT scan. For the liver, the question to be answered is *whether* there is involvement rather than the extent, since any degree of involvement represents stage IV disease.

After inspection and palpation of the nodal groups, a biopsy should be taken of the right and left para-aortic and iliac nodes regardless of their character on palpation with attention

to biopsy of nodes suspicious or abnormal on LAG. In addition, lymph nodes should be removed from the splenic hilar, celiac/porta hepatis, mesenteric, and iliac regions. In patients with a positive LAG, it is important to be certain that the suspicious nodes have actually been sampled; this can be checked with an intraoperative abdominal film.

Bone marrow biopsy may be performed as part of the laparotomy. If abdominal radiotherapy is anticipated as part of the management, then oophoropexy with transposition of the ovaries to a midline position posterior to the uterus should be performed.[60] This will minimize ovarian exposure during irradiation of pelvic nodal areas.

In general, the use of laparotomy as a second-look operation in patients with Hodgkin's disease has not been recommended. Rebiopsy to establish the persistence or recurrence of disease after therapy is recommended before second-line therapy is reinstituted.

Staging laparotomy is a major surgical procedure. Potential complications, including wound infections, wound dehiscence, retroperitoneal hematoma, subphrenic abscess, pancreatitis, and acute pulmonary complications of atalectasis and pneumonia, may occur, although they have been seen in no more than 1% of pediatric cases.[61] Late complications such as adhesions with intestinal obstruction may occur even in those patients who do not receive abdominal radiation and have been reported in 3%[61] to 12%[62] of children.

TREATMENT

Principles of Radiotherapy

The exquisite radiation responsiveness of Hodgkin's disease was recognized shortly after the discovery of x-rays. Even in the 1950s when only orthovoltage equipment was available, it was realized that one could effectively treat patients with Hodgkin's disease by irradiating all involved areas to high doses. With the development of megavoltage irradiation equipment, and specifically of the linear accelerator, Kaplan and colleagues at Stanford devised techniques allowing one to treat large fields to high doses, with resultant cures.[63] These pioneering efforts provide much of the basis for current standards of practice. In the early years, all patients, irrespective of age, were managed and treated alike. It was not until 1970 that the first protocol was devised specifically for the management of children.[61] This protocol proposed the combination of chemotherapy and low-dose radiation to preserve more-normal growth patterns.

The decisions regarding use of radiation therapy in the treatment program are a function of patient age, tumor burden, and concern about potential complications of therapy. All newly diagnosed Hodgkin's disease in children should be treated with curative intent. Good treatment planning with evaluation of sites of disease is an essential component of patient management.

Radiotherapy Techniques

Appropriate radiotherapy involves treatment with megavoltage irradiation, ideally using a 4- to 8-MeV linear accelerator. Cobalt-60 has significant limitations of scatter irradiation that should be minimized when irradiating children. Orthovoltage radiation is contraindicated. One must use an extended source-to-skin distance in order to achieve large treatment volumes. Distances of less than 80 cm should be avoided because of poor depth-dose characteristics. Each field should be treated each day, with treatment five times a week. Each field must be simulated. Attention must be given to calculating appropriate gaps when adjacent areas are treated. Field edges should be permanently marked with tattoos. In young patients in whom there may be movement or risk of daily variation in fields, immobilization devices such as casts may improve daily reproducibility.

Fields and Volumes

A preauricular (Waldeyer's) field is used prophylactically, when there is disease involving the high cervical lymph nodes and radiation is the sole therapeutic modality, or therapeutically, when there is actual involvement of the preauricular nodes or Waldeyer's lymphoid tissue.

The supradiaphragmatic mantle field is the most complex and important treatment field utilized in the management of Hodgkin's disease.[64] It is designed to treat the submandibular, submental, cervical, supraclavicular, infraclavicular, axillary, mediastinal, and pulmonary hilar lymph nodes[6,65] (Fig. 21-8). The treatment volume may be enlarged to encompass the entire cardiac silhouette or lungs, or these organs may be treated to a low dose by means of a partial transmission block.[66] Proper

design and localization of the mantle field requires a simulator to individualize the size and position of the lead or cerrobend blocks to protect vital structures. The mantle field involves treatment of a large volume; therefore, specific beam-shaping devices must be added. Both anterior and posterior field are used that in general are similar. However, the infraclavicular lymph nodes are generally treated from the anterior field only. Blocks should be used over the occipital area and the spinal cord from the posterior fields.

Because of the difference in thickness of various parts of the body, the daily dose to different portion of the mantle field may vary as much as 10%, requiring that multiple point doses be recorded and corrected for by individualized compensators in order to deliver a uniform dose to each area of disease. The use of a shrinking-field technique is important when treating a mantle field in a patient with large mediastinal adenopathy. A dramatic response may be seen after radiation doses of as little as 1000–1500 cGy. One may take advantage of this response and perform a repeat set-up, designing new and larger blocks to provide more protection of critical normal structures. An initial course of mantle irradiation in a symptomatic patient with extensive disease often will result in prompt relief of symptoms and enable continuation of work-up and laparotomy when the thoracic disease has begun to regress.

The subdiaphragmatic field covers the splenic pedicle or spleen and the para-aortic nodes (Fig. 21-9). The pelvic field includes the common iliac, external iliac, and inguinal–femoral lymph nodes (Fig. 21-10). These fields may be treated together as the "inverted-Y" field,[67] although they are usually treated sequentially, particularly in a patient who is receiving combined-modality therapy. They are treated both anteriorly and posteriorly. In patients with a negative staging laparotomy

FIGURE 21-9. Spleen–upper abdomen radiotherapy field, showing spleen–upper abdomen anterior set-up. Radiographic horizontal and vertical marks are placed on the skin for localization. Although the kidneys are opacified in an attempt to provide shielding, more of the superior pole of the kidney is included within the splenic volume than occurs when the patient has had a laparotomy with a surgically placed splenic hilar clip.

FIGURE 21-8. Mantle radiotherapy field; a mantle set-up, anterior field. Shaped lung blocks are used to contour the mediastinal–hilar silhouette. Humeral head, larynx, and axillary flash blocks are individualized.

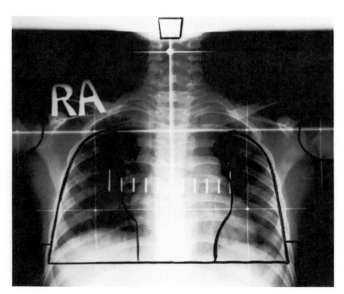

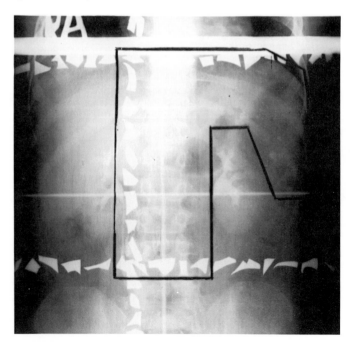

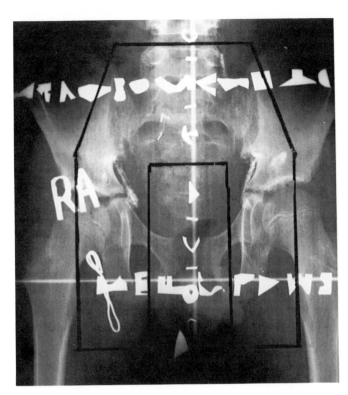

FIGURE 21-10. Pelvic radiotherapy field; an anterior pelvic set-up. The radiopaque horizontal and vertical marks are placed on the skin for localization. The right inguinal biopsy site is opacified with a wire marker.

who are treated by irradiation alone, a spade field may be used, which differs from the inverted-Y field in that the inferior extent is blocked below the common iliac lymph nodes, so that the true pelvis is not treated (Fig. 21-11).

For patients who have not undergone laparotomy and splenectomy but in whom subdiaphragmatic treatment is indicated; for example, those with positive lymph node biopsies above and below the diaphragm, the entire spleen must be treated along with the upper abdominal lymph nodes. In this situation, a significant volume of the left kidney often must be irradiated in order to encompass the entire splenic volume. In addition, irradiation of the spleen may result in the development of a pleural reaction at the left lung base.

In young women in whom pelvic irradiation is indicated, transposition of the ovaries to a central midline position allows the use of a midline pelvic block to protect ovarian function.[60] The translocated ovarian dose can be reduced to 8% of the adjacent pelvic lymph-node dose when pelvic radiation is given.[68] In males, a testicular shield is used, which minimizes the scatter irradiation dose to the testes to 0.75% of the pelvic lymph-node dose.[69] The testicular shield is easily employed for postpubertal males; individual shielding devices must be fabricated for prepubertal males.

When using radiotherapy alone in the management of patients with splenic disease, the liver is at risk for occult disease. Hepatic irradiation can be administered safely by using a partial hepatic transmission block.[70] With this technique, one can deliver a lower dose of radiation to the liver while the adjacent nodal areas are simultaneously treated to full dose. When radiation alone is used in the treatment program, extended-field radiotherapy with consideration of prophylactic organ irradiation is recommended.

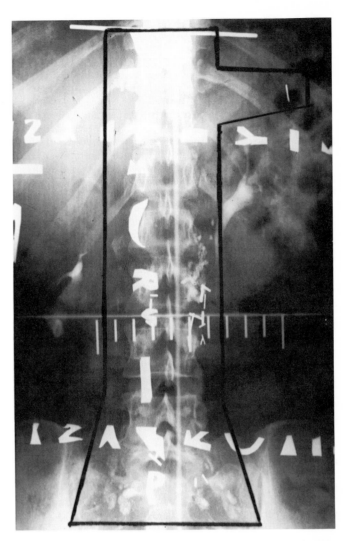

FIGURE 21-11. An anterior spade radiotherapy field; the fields encompass the surgically placed clips. Radiographic horizontal and vertical marks are placed on the skin for localization. A lymphangiogram clip on the splenic hilar region and renal contrast are helpful landmarks in the design of this field.

With planned combined-modality programs, the radiotherapy fields may be minimized to the use of an involved or extended field in conjunction with chemotherapy. The definition of fields is a function of the original site of disease, and no specific guidelines exist. In general, an involved field implies treatment of an entire region as defined by the Ann Arbor stage, with fields designed to minimize retreatment match-line problems in the event of subsequent regional recurrence. Table 21-8 provides useful functional definitions of involved radiation fields for various regions. It is unwise to treat smaller fields such as a unilateral axillary field without including the adjacent supraclavicular, infraclavicular, and low cervical areas because of the indistinct divisions between areas.

Dose and Time Factors

A well-defined radiation dose–response curve has demonstrated the risk of recurrence to be 10% or less if radiation doses of 3500 to 4400 cGy are used.[6] Thus, when radiotherapy

Table 21-8
Involved Field Regions

Mantle	Supradiaphragmatic disease involving mediastinum as well as one or both cervical, supraclavicular, infraclavicular, or axillary lymph nodes
Minimantle	Bilateral supramediastinal disease involving axillae, supraclavicular, infraclavicular, or cervical lymph node chains
Hemi-minimantle	Unilateral supramediastinal disease involving axilla, supraclavicular, infraclavicular, or cervical lymph node chains
Mediastinum	Disease in mediastinum, one or both hila
Para-aortic–Splenic hilar–Spleen	Subdiaphragmatic disease in spleen, splenic hilar, or para-aortic areas
Spade	Subdiaphragmatic disease in spleen, splenic hilar, para-aortic, and iliac areas
Pelvis	Disease in bilateral iliac and inguinal–femoral areas
Hemi-pelvis	Disease in unilateral iliac and inguinal–femoral areas
Inverted-Y	Subdiaphragmatic disease in spleen, splenic-hilar, para-aortic, and pelvic areas.

alone is used, a minimum recommended dose to clinically involved areas is 4000 to 4400 cGy, while subclinical disease appears to be controlled with 3000 to 4000 cGy.[71] The dose-time relationship is less well known. Because of normal tissue tolerance, patient acceptance, and tumor control, however, tumor doses of 150 to 200 cGy per day five times a week appear to be most appropriate. When large volumes are treated, doses of 150 cGy are best tolerated. There is no indication for large fraction sizes to be employed.

When combined-modality programs are planned, lower radiation doses have been successful, with a local-control rate of 97%.[72] On the basis of these data, many current protocols now employ 2500 cGy or less with a minimum of six cycles of chemotherapy. Data are not yet available detailing long-term local-control rates when low doses of radiation are used in a setting of fewer than six cycles of chemotherapy. In the planned combined-modality setting, if a child does not achieve an optimal response to chemotherapy, it is unwise to administer only a low dose of radiotherapy. High-dose radiotherapy should be used in this unfavorable setting.

General Principles of Chemotherapy

Early in the history of clinical chemotherapy, it became clear that the administration of single drugs only rarely produced durable complete remissions in any type of tumor. It is generally held now that effective drug regimens can be achieved when agents with the following properties are combined: (1) individually active against the tumor in question; (2) differing mechanisms of action, so that different biochemical events in the cell can be attacked simultaneously and so that the combi-

nation will be able to circumvent resistance that might exist to some but not all of the constituent agents; and (3) nonoverlapping toxicities, so that each agent can be given at or near its full single-agent dose. The combination of agents selected for the original combination therapy of Hodgkin's disease—MOPP—appears to fulfill these qualifications (see Table 21-1).

A long-term follow-up of the initial group of 188 patients treated at the National Cancer Institute has recently been published.[73] The mean age at diagnosis was 32 years, with a range from 12 to 69. Most (95%) of the patients had Stage III or IV disease, and 89% had B symptoms. The complete-remission rate was 84%, and 54% remain disease free at 10 years. This rate was not affected by whether the patients received maintenance therapy with additional MOPP courses or with carmustine (BCNU). Overall, 48% of the group are still alive after 10 years: 77 in their first remission, 8 in their second, 2 in their third, and 2 in their fourth and 1 undergoing a fourth course of induction therapy.

Several generalizations can be made from these data that probably apply to children as well as to adults. First, cure of about half the patients with advanced disease can be achieved with combination chemotherapy. Second, maintenance therapy beyond a certain point is not helpful in extending the remission. Third, doses of drug should be as high as possible within the combination. Fourth, even with 10-year follow-up, there may be further deaths due to disease, since those patients in their third or later remission may not be cured. Fifth, long-term follow-up with actual assessment of causes of severe morbidity and death in patients who may be cured of their disease is extremely important, since not all deaths are due to disease. Some deaths may be due to late effects of therapy and some to other causes. Of the 98 patients who died, 68 had progressive Hodgkin's disease, and 30 died free of Hodgkin's disease. Causes of death in the latter group include acute nonlymphocytic leukemia, non-Hodgkin's lymphoma, myocardial infarction, sepsis, and automobile accidents.

In 1974, about 10 years after the initial studies of MOPP, Bonadonna and associates developed a combination regimen of doxorubicin (Adriamycin), bleomycin, vinblastine, and dacarbazine (ABVD) that originally was intended for the treatment of MOPP-resistant disease (see Table 21-1).[74] This combination was developed with the same general principles in mind, namely that each agent had individual activity in the treatment of Hodgkin's disease and that the toxicities were nonoverlapping. In addition, each agent was thought to have a different mechanism of action from those included in the MOPP combination. The initial success in inducing complete remission in 54% of 70 patients with MOPP-resistant disease led to the proposal that an alternating MOPP/ABVD schedule might be more effective than either combination alone. The initial study, which compared MOPP/ABVD with MOPP alone, suggested that this was indeed true.[75] This observation was placed on a firmer mathematical footing by Goldie and Coldman, who adapted the somatic mutation theory to model the development of biochemical resistance to drugs as an acquired, heritable property of tumor cells.[76] Assuming that mutations to drug resistance are random events, the theory considers that the longer any tumor cell is in place, the greater its likelihood of undergoing a resistant mutation. This formulation predicts, then, that optimal therapy should consist of the maximum number of active drugs given as early after diagnosis as possible with the maximum dose intensity possible. The MOPP/ABVD hybrid was developed with this theory in mind.[77] Trials specifically comparing regimens in a prospective fashion that might test this hypothesis are currently under way in adult patients.

Combined-Modality Therapy

As noted above, radiation was the first definitive therapy for Hodgkin's disease. However, MOPP combination chemotherapy was also shown to be effective by 1970.[12] These findings, coupled with the then-emerging observation of substantial late effects on growth and development when children were irradiated, provided the impetus for combined-modality studies using lower doses of radiation in conjunction with chemotherapy for children. In 1970, a program was designed to ascertain whether multiple cycles of MOPP chemotherapy could replace a fraction of the radiation dose in children with Hodgkin's disease.[78] Although novel in concept at that time, the use of low-dose radiation combined with multiagent chemotherapy has been extremely effective, with long-term cure rates in the range of 90%.[72] This approach has now become standard therapy in the management of children with Hodgkin's disease.

The proper sequencing of radiotherapy and chemotherapy is not yet established. Concern over the inability to deliver full doses of chemotherapy following radiotherapy or, alternatively, the inability to deliver full doses of radiotherapy following chemotherapy, has led to the concept of alternating the two modalities.[79,80] There are theoretical reasons why this might result in increased tumor sensitivity to both modalities.[81] Alternation of courses of chemotherapy and radiotherapy is well tolerated and does enable maximal doses of both modalities to be given.

The benefit of combined-modality therapy is that the cure rate may be increased, presumably because chemotherapy and radiotherapy are each active treatments with different mechanisms of action. If they are given sequentially, then the second modality is administered in a setting of minimal residual disease, which not only is more likely to result in cure, but which also may allow lower doses to be effective.

The risks of combined-modality therapy are, first, that each modality may limit the amount of the other that can be given. For example, the total dose of doxorubicin that can be given safely without cardiotoxicity is less in the patients who have received mediastinal radiation than in those who have not. In addition, combined-modality therapy, although it may reduce the risk of radiation toxicity since lower doses are given, increases the spectrum of toxicity to which the patient is exposed. Chemotherapy carries with it the risk of sterility and damage to other organ systems such as the lungs and heart. There is some suggestion that combined-modality therapy will result in an increased incidence of second malignancies when compared with either therapy alone.[82]

There is an added complication in devising ideal therapy for Hodgkin's disease where either modality alone cures a significant percentage of patients. If the end-point being assessed is disease-free survival; that is, the time from which complete remission is achieved until the time that disease recurs, then there is no question that combined-modality therapy is more effective than radiation alone. However, because chemotherapy is effective in salvaging patients who have relapsed after radiotherapy, there is some question whether the best overall strategy would be to use radiotherapy alone in limited-stage disease and administer chemotherapy only to those patients who relapse, thereby sparing many patients the toxicity of chemotherapy. This question has as yet not been rigorously evaluated in children, and because the full answer depends on the rate of late relapses and late toxicity, extremely long follow-up (more than 10 years) may be required in order to compare the strategies.

Chemotherapy is considered the primary treatment for patients with advanced-stage disease. At the same time, there is some question whether those patients with bulky disease may not do better with the addition of radiotherapy. Thus, the therapeutic question in early-stage disease is whether chemotherapy should be given at presentation in addition to low-dose radiotherapy; the question in advanced disease is whether radiotherapy should be added to chemotherapy. An additional potential advantage of administering chemotherapy to all patients might be that clinical staging would be adequate and laparotomy no longer required.

TREATMENT RESULTS

The initial management decisions about a new patient must be made collaboratively by the radiation oncologist, pediatric oncologist, and pediatric surgeon working with the pathologist, diagnostic radiologist, and other medical and paramedical personnel who may affect the management of the child. Each member of the team should have a chance to examine the patient and review the diagnostic findings. It is not appropriate for a child to be managed primarily by the radiation oncologist and subsequently referred to the pediatric oncologist for salvage chemotherapy in the event of a relapse, nor is it appropriate for the pediatric oncologist to initiate chemotherapy and subsequently request radiation therapy for consolidation or treatment of residual disease. Optimal therapy today involves a multidisciplinary approach from the time of diagnosis.

Stages I and IIA Disease

Radiation therapy has been the cornerstone in the treatment of early-stage Hodgkin's disease. The 5-year disease-free survival (DFS) rate for children with pathologic Stage I or IIA Hodgkin's disease treated with full-dose (3600–4000 cGy) involved-field or extended-field radiation at single institutions has been relatively high (70% to 86%), although the rate falls to 30% to 40% when multiple institutions are engaged in a clinical trial (Table 21-9). This failure of the large multi-institution studies to duplicate single-institutional results is disappointing and makes it difficult to know what the true cure rate is for patients treated in the community with radiation alone. When three to six courses of MOPP are added to radiotherapy, the 5-year DFS rate rises to around 90% in both single-institution and group studies. When the dose of radiation given with the chemotherapy is lowered to 2000 cGy, the results remain excellent (Table 21-9). Only very small numbers of patients with limited-stage disease have been treated with chemotherapy alone, and therefore the long-term cure rate of this treatment is not known.

Current therapy of Stages I and IIA disease without unfavorable prognostic features generally would include chemotherapy with six courses of MOPP plus low-dose (2500 cGy) radiation to involved fields for the young child who is still growing, whereas definitive radiation alone at full dose (3500–4000 cGy) to extended fields is given to the fully grown teenager. If unfavorable features such as large mediastinal mass (greater than one-third of the thoracic diameter) or invasion of chest wall are present, then patients should receive chemotherapy plus irradiation regardless of age (Table 21-10).

Stage IIB Disease

The treatment of Stage IIB disease is controversial. Some groups of clinicians believe that the fully grown adolescent with Stage IIB disease fares as well as one with IIA disease and

Table 21-9
Treatment Results in Limited-Stage Hodgkin's Disease

Stage and Treatment*	Number of Patients	% Disease-Free (Total) Survival		Reference
		5 Years	10 Years	
Radiotherapy Alone (full-dose IF or EF)				
Single-institution studies				
PS IA, IIA	11	70 (100)	70 (100)	83
PS I, II A, B	40	76 (97)	— —	84
PS I	14	86 (93)	— —	58
PS IIA	36	81 (100)	— —	
Multiple-institution studies				
PS I, II IF	43	28 (96)		85
EF	53	40 (96)		
CS I, II†	35	33 (80)	33 (66)	86
Full-dose Radiotherapy plus 3 or 6 Courses of Chemotherapy				
CS I, II	41	88 (88)		87
CS I, II	52	94 (94)	88 (94)	86
PS I, II	119	95 (96)		85
Low-dose Radiation plus 6 Courses of Chemotherapy				
PS, I, II	27	96 (100)	96 (100)	80
CS II, III	27	88 (92)		88
CS I–IIIA	17	86 (100)		83
Chemotherapy Alone				
CS I–II	7	100 (100)		89
CS I–II (2-year follow-up)	10	90 (100)		90
CS I–II	11	100 (91)		91

* CS = clinical stage; PS = pathologic stage; full-dose radiotheapy = minimum dose to any nodal field ≥3000 cGy; low-dose radiotherapy = maximum dose to any nodal field ≤2550 cGy; IF = involved field; EF = extended field.
† Some patients also received single-agent chemotherapy.

can be managed with radiation alone,[92] whereas others believe that all children with this stage, regardless of age, should be treated with combined-modality therapy.

Stage IIIA Disease

The standard therapy for Stage IIIA disease is also controversial. Most investigators agree that patients with Stage IIIA$_2$ disease (*i.e.,* disease involving the para-aortic, iliac, or mesenteric nodes) should receive chemotherapy. The conflict arises over whether patients with involvement only of the spleen with or without the high abdominal nodes should be treated with radiation alone, and if so, what, if any, dose of radiation should be administered to the liver. In general, patients with Stage IIIA$_1$ disease are treated in similar fashion to those with Stage I or IIA disease; that is, definitive radiotherapy for those patients who have achieved their full growth and who have no unfavorable prognostic features such as large mediastinal mass, with chemotherapy plus low-dose radiation given to the younger patient or the patient with more aggressive disease.

Stages IIIB and IV Disease

There is general agreement that patients with Stage IIIB or IV disease should receive chemotherapy as their primary management. The questions are what chemotherapy, for how long, and should radiotherapy be given as well? The complete-remission rate in adult patients with Stage III or IV disease treated with MOPP or some variant of MOPP has ranged from 44% to 87% (median 72%)[73] and that for patients given multiagent chemotherapy plus MOPP from 77% to 92% (median 88%).[77] It has not as yet been proved in concurrent randomized studies that adding agents to MOPP provides a distinct advantage in terms of complete-remission, disease-free, or overall survival rates. The series reported to date for children generally have involved treatment with MOPP or some variant with or without radiotherapy. It can be seen in Table 21-11 that response rates in children are in the same range as those for adults. A description of standard treatment regimens is given in Table 21-10.

Most relapses in patients with Hodgkin's disease occur within the first 3 years, although there are patients who relapse as much as 10 years after their initial diagnosis. The DFS rate in

Table 21-10
Recommended Therapy for Patients with Hodgkin's Disease

	Patient Features	Recommended Therapy
Stages IA, IB, IIA	Attained full growth; no unfavorable signs	Full-dose radiotherapy*
	Still growing or large mediastinal mass or chest wall or pericardial invasion	Low-dose radiotherapy plus 6 courses of MOPP Other chemotherapy (experimental)
Stages IIB, IIIA₁	Attained full growth; no unfavorable signs	Full-dose radiotherapy; definitive hepatic radiotherapy for patients with splenic involvement treated with radiation alone
	Still growing or large mediastinal mass†	Low-dose radiotherapy plus 6 courses of MOPP; other chemotherapy (experimental)
Stages IIIA₂, IIIB, IVA, IVB		6 courses MOPP ± full dose IF radiotherapy; or 12 courses alternating MOPP/ABVD; or 6 courses MOPP + low-dose TNLI; or other chemotherapy (experimental)

* Full-dose radiotherapy = 3500–4400 cGy; low-dose = ≤2500 cGy.
† Some would treat these patients as though they had advanced (stage IIIA₂–IV) disease.

Table 21-11
Results in Patients with Advanced-Stage Disease (Pathologic Stages III and IV Unless Otherwise Noted)

				5-year Survival (%)		
Chemotherapy	Radiotherapy	Number Treated	Complete Remission Rate	DF	Total	Reference
MOPP (6–12)	None	8	88	80	92	90
MVOPP	None	16	70	45	91	91
MOPP Stage IV	None	6	86	66	66	58
MOPP Stage III	Full dose*	15	—	87	100	58
ChlVPP Stage III	Full dose	20	100	77	—	47
Stage IV		13	85	67	—	
MOPP	Low dose	28	90	84	78	
MOPP CS† IV	Low dose	15	—	65	85	88
MDP‡ Stage IV	Low dose	8	—	88	88	93
CCP‡ Stage IIB–IVB	Low dose	33	—	60	86	93

* Full dose = minimum dose to any treatment field ≥3000 cGy; low dose.= maximum dose to any treatment field ≤2550 cGy.
† Clinical stage.
‡ MDP = multidrug protocol chemotherapy with cyclophosphamide, procarbazine, Adriamycin, and vincristine; CCP = several different combinations used at this institution.

adults treated with MOPP alone at intervals from 1 to 15 years ranges from 47% to 60%.[73] In the studies using the additional chemotherapy, the range is from 73% to 92%.[77] The DFS rate in children with advanced-stage disease treated with MOPP with or without radiotherapy ranges from 40% to 100%, with the overall survival ranging from 40% to 92%. A number of the deaths that occurred in patients in remission from Hodgkin's disease were from sepsis or second malignancies.

Overall, then, with current treatment, one could expect at least 80% of children with advanced-stage disease to achieve complete remission and perhaps 70% of them to remain disease free at 5 years, which means that approximately half these patients will be cured with their initial therapy (0.80 × .70 = 0.56). It thus appears that there is room for more-aggressive

approaches to therapy to be investigated in these patients. Preliminary data suggest that alternating combinations similar to MOPP/ABVD is safe in children,[80,94,95] and larger trials are under way.

RELAPSED DISEASE

There is a significant salvage rate in patients who relapse after therapy.[96] In the Intergroup Hodgkin's Disease Study,[85] the overall survival in all groups of patients was 96% despite the recurrence of disease in 60% of the patients treated with radiation alone. However, the follow-up at the time of this report was less than 10 years. In a series of adult patients who were treated with different combination-chemotherapy regimens after relapse from prior treatment with radiation alone, complete-remission rates ranged from 70% to 82%, with a 5-year failure-free survival rate of 49%.[97] The salvage rate for patients who had initial multimodality therapy may be lower. In three pediatric series, the following data were seen. Jenkin and associates treated 110 patients initially with low-dose radiation and MOPP and had 25 relapses; 17 were retreated with MOPP, five with ABVD, and three with other chemotherapy regimens. The 5-year survival and disease-free survival rates of these patients measured from first day of relapse were 76% and 43%, respectively.[88] Mauch and coworkers observed 15 relapsed patients, of whom 11 were rendered disease-free following retreatment.[58] Bayle–Weisgerber and colleagues had 47 relapses in 212 children. Of the 43 who relapsed among those treated without MOPP, 24 remained in a second complete remission, two had a second relapse but were still alive, and 17 had died.[86] Of the four who relapsed after initial MOPP plus irradiation, none was still in a second complete remission, although all were still alive. Thus, it appears that, at best, 50% of those patients who relapse after combined-modality therapy will be cured.

Reinduction therapy with agents non-cross-resistant with MOPP and ABVD are being explored. The combination of cisplatin, cytosine arabinoside, and etoposide, for example, may be promising in children.[98] Experimental therapy is also being tried. A number of investigators are exploring the possibility of high-dose chemotherapy with a single agent, such as melphalan,[99] or with combinations of agents that have individual activity in the disease, followed by autologous bone-marrow reinfusion.[100,101]

Another new approach to therapy is based on the observation that in many cases Hodgkin's disease cells make a high titer of ferritin. Antiferritin antibody labeled with ^{131}I has been used to treat 38 adult patients who had failed at least two combination-chemotherapy regimens; objective partial remissions were seen in 40%.[102] The use of antibody prepared in rabbit, pig, and monkey allowed the administration of several courses without serious concerns about anaphylaxis. This type of experimental therapy is being explored further.

ACUTE TOXICITY

Acute Radiation Effects

Acute side-effects of irradiation are reversible and generally not serious (see also Chap. 11). They are a function of the total dose delivered and the volume irradiated, with the most acute toxicity seen when high-dose, large-volume therapy is administered. In general, one should anticipate erythema, hyperpigmentation, or both of irradiated skin. Mild gastrointestinal disturbance, and, possibly, thrombocytopenia and granulocytopenia can also occur. Lhermitte's syndrome, a sensation of "electric shock" radiating down the back and into the extremities upon flexion of the neck, may be observed occasionally. This is thought to be related to transient demyelination of nerve fibers in the spinal cord. It is self-limited and reversible and does not represent a prodrome of later neurologic dysfunction.

Immediate Effects of Chemotherapy

Both MOPP and ABVD will cause nausea and vomiting, the latter regimen more than the former. This can be severe enough, particularly in a teenager, that anticipatory nausea and vomiting may occur and lead to reluctance to complete therapy. This effect is almost never severe enough, however, to lead to interruption of therapy or to necessitate hyperalimentation.

Nitrogen mustard, vincristine, and Adriamycin all may cause severe local tissue damage if infiltrated outside the veins through which they are being administered, and vinblastine and dacarbazine can cause a local burning sensation as they are being given. Both combinations will cause reversible alopecia of some degree. The neurotoxicity of vincristine, the cardiac toxicity of Adriamycin, and the pulmonary toxicity of bleomycin as well as other side-effects are discussed in Chapter 9. A thorough review of the toxicities of individual agents should be made before one administers any of them either alone or in combination.

Infection

The most common dose-limiting acute toxicity of combination chemotherapy is myelosuppression. A number of courses of treatment may have to be delayed because of low blood counts, transfusions may be required for thrombocytopenia, and some patients may have to be admitted to the hospital for antibiotic therapy if they develop fever during a period of neutropenia.

The risk of serious bacterial infection among children is related to the intensity of the treatment given rather than to whether a splenectomy has been performed.[103,104] Serious infections, defined as bacteremia, meningitis, pneumonia, or pyelonephritis, occured in 1 of 71 splenectomized children (1.4%) and 2 of 71 nonsplenectomized children (2.8%) treated with irradiation alone.[103] However, when chemotherapy was added to the treatment program, the risk rose to 13 of 71 (18.3%) for splenectomized children and 6 of 26 (23.1%) for nonsplenectomized children ($p < 0.05$). The liberal use of prophylactic antibiotics such as penicillin (or erythromycin in the penicillin-allergic patient) has greatly reduced the incidence of infection. In addition, vaccines are now available against pneumococci, *H. influenzae,* and meningococci, which may further decrease the risk for these patients, although antibody titers are not sustained in patients receiving chemotherapy. The management of immunosuppressed patients with these and other infections is discussed in Chapter 39.

LATE EFFECTS*

Soft-Tissue and Bone Growth Alterations

Early reports described a disproportionate alteration in sitting height compared to standing height among a group of children who had received axial skeletal irradiation.[105] The growth impairment was greater in those patients receiving 3500 cGy or more to the axial skeleton than in those given no more than 2500 cGy and was particularly marked in those individuals 13 years of age or younger at the time of treatment. Boys appeared more severely affected than girls. Shortening of the clavicles with a decrease in intraclavicular distance is also characteristic of children given high-dose irradiation to a mantle field at a young age. Underdevelopment and fibrosis of the soft tissues of the neck have also been seen. Growth disturbance is not a significant complication of high-dose radiation for children

---

* This subject also is discussed in Chapter 50.

whose bone age is 14 to 15 years or greater at the time of radiotherapy.

A number of soft-tissue toxic effects are less common now that megavoltage radiotherapy is employed. A few patients will have relatively permanent thinning of the hair in the posterior cervical area of the mantle field if full-dose radiation is given, but total hair loss in this region is rare.

Avascular necrosis of bone has been reported in as many as 10% of long-term survivors who receive chemotherapy including prednisone in addition to irradiation and is a known complication of long-term steroid administration.

Pulmonary and Cardiac Sequelae

Significant pulmonary injury from irradiation is related to total radiation dose, daily fraction size, and the volume of lung included in the high-dose irradiated area. Symptomatic pulmonary injury occurred in 3.6% of children receiving high-dose mantle therapy.[61] A higher frequency would be expected in patients also receiving chemotherapy, particularly bleomycin. To date, significant pulmonary reactions have not been observed among the 55 children receiving low-dose radiotherapy and six cycles of MOPP. This lower incidence reflects both a reduction in radiation dose and volume, as well as shrinking radiation fields and the use of shaped and "thin" lung blocks.[72] In 118 adult patients receiving ABVD and radiation and 114 receiving MOPP plus radiation, fatal radiation pneumonitis was seen in 2.5% and 2.6%, respectively.[106] Formal pulmonary function tests showed no difference between the two groups; however, with systematic reevaluation of chest roentgenograms for a minimum of 2 years, only 41% of patients in the ABVD group showed *no* evidence of lung damage, compared to 70% of patients in the MOPP group ($p < 0.001$). In 4 of 57 ABVD-treated patients who showed radiologic signs of postirradiation paramediastinal fibrosis, there was persistent dyspnea on effort up to 3 years after completion of therapy.

Cardiac injury from radiation is also related to dose, volume, and fraction size. Both the pericardium and the myocardium may be affected. Disease may appear as asymptomatic and transient cardiac enlargement recognized only radiographically or with increasing severity ranging all the way to delayed constrictive pericarditis requiring pericardiectomy. The approximately 13% incidence of cardiac injury among children following high-dose mantle irradiation does not differ from that observed in adults. Arterial vascular injury, including underdevelopment of the great vessels, coronary artery disease with coronary fibrosis, and accelerated atherogenesis, has been observed in long-term survivors of Hodgkin's disease who underwent mantle irradiation.[61]

Doxorubicin is known to cause myocardial damage. The late effects of the use of this drug in combination with radiation are unknown. In addition, Raynaud's phenomenon is reported in patients receiving the combination of vinblastine and bleomycin and may be a significant form of morbidity for patients treated with combinations including these drugs.

Endocrine Sequelae

Using an elevated TSH level to define hypothyroidism, the incidence of thyroid dysfunction in irradiated patients has ranged from 4% to 79%. The sensitivity of the growing thyroid may be higher than that of the adult gland. The iodine load of a preradiotherapy LAG has been implicated as a factor in thyroid damage. The dose of radiation is important: only 17% of children who received neck-irradiation doses of less than 2600 cGy developed thyroid abnormalities, compared to 78% of children who received 2600 cGy or more. In this series, there was improvement in 36% of biochemically hypothyroid children with time.[107] Thyroid nodules, hyperthyroidism, and thyroid cancer have all been observed in patients treated for Hodgkin's disease. It is recommended that TSH and free T4 levels be checked annually in patients who have received radiotherapy to the neck and that children who have elevated TSH levels receive thyroid replacement therapy to reduce stimulation from prolonged TSH elevation.

Sterility, alterations in fertility, and potential gonadal injury following staging and treatment are important issues that must be addressed at the time of diagnosis and prior to therapy.[108] Pelvic irradiation carries the high likelihood of ablation of ovarian function. The technique of oophoropexy, with removal of the ovaries to a midline location, has allowed the preservation of ovarian function in young women with Hodgkin's disease.[68]

The younger the woman at the time of therapy, the higher the probability of maintenance of regular menses following therapy. In an assessment of menstrual status among girls with Hodgkin's disease 13 to 18 years of age at the time of treatment, it was shown that following oophoropexy, all 18 girls treated with radiation alone and 22 of 25 (88%) of those treated with combined-modality therapy maintained normal menses.[57] Pregnancies have occurred in girls treated for Hodgkin's disease with no increased risk of fetal wastage or spontaneous abortion.[61] Of the pregnancies that have been carried to term, no increase in birth defects has been observed when compared to the offspring of sibling controls. However, despite the fact that menses may be resumed or continued after therapy, it appears that a significant proportion of women treated with combination chemotherapy will undergo early menopause. In a recent study, very few treated women continued to menstruate beyond the age of 35 regardless of the age at first treatment.[109] Thus, the biological clock may be ticking faster for these women, and it may be unwise for them to delay having their families.

The sterility issue in males is of much greater severity. Primary gonadal dysfunction may exist at the time of diagnosis of Hodgkin's disease in 30% to 40% of patients,[110] but, despite this, pretreatment storage of sperm should be considered in the older patient. High-dose irradiation to the pelvis in a standard inverted-Y field may be associated with a transient oligospermia or azoospermia; however, recovery of function is common.[69] Six courses of MOPP chemotherapy has led to universal sterility in male patients, although there is a suggestion that fertility will be maintained in as many as 50% of patients after only three courses of MOPP.[111] In general, the hormone-producing cells of the testis are more resistant to the effects of treatment than are the spermatogonia, so the patients will continue to grow and develop normally; however, in one series, 9 of 13 Ugandan adolescent boys with Hodgkin's disease who were 10 to 16 years of age at the time of MOPP treatment developed gynecomastia, complete germinal aplasia, increased serum follicle-stimulating hormone and luteinizing hormone, and decreased serum testosterone.[112] In contrast, the prepubertal boys showed no change in gonadotropin levels and no clinical gynecomastia, although males treated in childhood still had azoospermia.[113] In 25 adults less than 45 years of age when treated with ABVD and radiotherapy, azoospermia was observed in 9 (36%) and oligospermia in 5 (20%). Full recovery of spermatogenesis was documented within 18 months in all 13 patients in whom the sperm count was repeated. Thus, ABVD appears to cause less permanent impairment of gonadal function than does MOPP.[106]

Second Malignant Tumors

The problem of second malignancies among patients surviving their initial cancer is well recognized. Acute nonlymphocytic leukemia (ANLL) and its precursor—a pancytopenic myelodysplastic syndrome—are the most common second cancers, and the risk of ANLL may be as high as 1% per year for the first 10 years after treatment. The incidence of secondary leukemia in patients treated with radiotherapy alone is low, less than 1% in most series. The incidence in patients treated with MOPP alone may be 5% to 7%[82] and increases to 10% as MOPP is given with radiotherapy. There have been no secondary ANLL cases reported in patients treated with ABVD either alone or in combination with radiation.[114] A 15% incidence of secondary leukemia has been reported when radiation is given initially and chemotherapy is used as salvage therapy. It appears that the risk of secondary leukemia is higher in adult patients, particularly in those older than 40 at the time of first treatment, than in pediatric patients and that the risk of secondary leukemia may decrease after 10 years.[115]

There is an increased risk of other solid tumors as well.[82] Non-Hodgkin's lymphoma has been reported in as many as 4% of patients after therapy. The solid tumors do not all appear within the radiation field, and the risk of solid tumors increases with increasing age. It is clear that long-term follow-up is essential in assessing the true risk of these second malignant tumors, as the risk increases with age and length of follow-up. There is some suggestion that the peak incidence for these other tumors will be later than the 10 years post-therapy suggested for ANLL.

In choosing definitive treatment, the efficacy and the risks should be balanced. It should be emphasized that cure with minimal morbidity and the highest quality of life is our goal in the management of children with Hodgkin's disease.

REFERENCES

1. Hodgkin T: On some morbid appearances of the absorbent glands and spleen. Med Chir Trans 17:68–114, 1832
2. Sternberg C: Uber eine Eigenartige unter dem Bilde der Pseudoleukämie verlaufende Tuberculose des lymphatischen Apparates. Z Heilk 19:21–90, 1898
3. Reed DM: On the pathological changes in Hodgkin's disease, with especial reference to its relation to tuberculosis. Johns Hopkins Hosp Rep 10:133–196, 1902
4. Fox H: Remarks on microscopical preparations made from some of the original tissue described by Thomas Hodgkin, 1832. Ann Med Hist 8:370–374, 1926
5. Sullivan MP, Fuller LM, Butler JJ: Hodgkin's disease. In Sutow WW, Fernbach DF, Vietti TJ (eds): Clinical Pediatric Oncology, pp 416–451. St Louis, CV Mosby, 1984
6. Kaplan HS: Hodgkin's Disease, 2nd Ed. Cambridge, Harvard University Press, 1980
7. Kaplan HS, Gartner S: "Sternberg–Reed" giant cells of Hodgkin's disease: Cultivation in vitro, heterotransplantation, and characterization as neoplastic macrophages. Int J Cancer 19:511–525, 1977
8. Long JC, Zamecnik PC, Aisenberg AC, Atkins L: Tissue culture studies in Hodgkin's disease: Morphologic, cytogenetic, cell surface, and enzymatic properties of cultures derived from splenic tumors. J Exp Med 145:1484–1500, 1977
9. Pusey WA: Cases of sarcoma and of Hodgkin's disease treated by exposures to X-rays: A preliminary report. JAMA 38:166–169, 1902
10. Senn N: Therapeutical value of roentgen ray in treatment of pseudoleukemia. New York Med J 77:665–668, 1903
11. Goodman LS, Wintrobe MM, Dameshek W, Goodman MJ, Gilman AZ, McLennan MT: Nitrogen mustard therapy: Use of methyl-bis-(-chloroethyl)amine hydrochloride for Hodgkin's disease, lymphosarcoma, leukemia and certain allied and miscellaneous disorders. JAMA 132:126–132, 1946
12. DeVita VT Jr, Serpick A, Carbone PP: Combination chemotherapy in the treatment of advanced Hodgkin's disease. Ann Intern Med 73:881–895, 1970
13. Young RC, DeVita VT Jr, Johnson RE: Hodgkin's disease in childhood. Blood 42:163–174, 1973
14. Grufferman SL, Delzell E: Epidemiology of Hodgkin's disease. Epidemiol Rev 6:76–106, 1984
15. Spitz MR, Sider JF, Johnson CC, Butler JJ, Pollack ES, Newell GR: Ethnic patterns of Hodgkin's disease incidence among children and adolescents in the United States, 1973–1982. JNCI 76:235–239, 1986
16. Priesel A, Winkelbauer A: Placentare Ubertragung des Lymphogranuloma. Virchows Arch Pathol Anat 262:749–765, 1926
17. Fogel TD, Peschel RE, Papac R: Hodgkin's disease in married couples. Cancer 55:2495–2497, 1985
18. Gatti RA, Good RA: Occurrence of malignancy in immunodeficiency disease: A literature review. Cancer 28:89–98, 1971
19. Ioachim HL, Cooper MC, Hellman GC: Lymphomas in men at high risk for acquired immune deficiency syndrome (AIDS): A study of 21 cases. Cancer 56:2831–2842, 1985
20. Vianna NJ, Greenwald P, Davies JNP: Extended epidemic of Hodgkin's disease in high school students. Lancet 1:1209–1211, 1971
21. Smith PG, Pike MC: Case clustering in Hodgkin's disease: A brief review of the present position and report of current work in Oxford. Cancer Res 34:1156–1160, 1974
22. Nonoyama M, Kawai Y, Huang CH et al: Epstein Barr virus DNA in Hodgkin's disease, American Burkitt's lymphoma and other human tumors. Cancer Res 34:1228–1231, 1974
23. Strauchen JA, Dimitriu–Bona A: Immunopathology of Hodgkin's disease: Characterization of Reed–Sternberg cells with monoclonal antibodies. Am J Pathol 123:293–300, 1986
24. Van Voorhis WC, Steinman RM, Hair L, Luban J, Witmer M, Koide S, Cohn Z: Specific antimononuclear phagocyte monoclonal antibodies: Application to purification of dendritic cells and the tissue localization of macrophages. J Exp Med 158:126–145, 1983
25. Van Voorhis WC, Witmer M, Steinman RM: The phenotype of dendritic cells and macrophages. Fed Proc 42:3114–3118, 1983
26. DeVita VT Jr, Jaffe ES, Hellman S: Hodgkin's disease and the non-Hodgkin's lymphomas. In DeVita VT Jr, Rosenberg SA, Hellman S (eds): Principles and Practice of Oncology, 2nd Ed, pp 1623–1709. Philadelphia, JB Lippincott, 1985
27. Kadin ME: Possible origin of the Reed–Sternberg cell from an interdigitating reticulum cell. Cancer Treat Rep 66:601–608, 1982
28. Knowles DM, Neri A, Pelicci PG et al: Immunoglobulin and T-cell receptor beta-chain gene rearrangement analysis of Hodgkin's disease: Implications for lineage determination and differential diagnosis. Proc Natl Acad Sci USA 83:7942–7946, 1986
29. Stein H, Mason DY, Gerdes J et al: The expression of the Hodgkin's disease associated antigen KI-1 in reactive and neoplastic lymphoid tissue: Evidence that Reed–Sternberg cells and histiocytic malignancies are derived from activated lymphoid cells. Blood 66:848–858, 1985
30. Hecht TT, Longo DL, Cossman J, Bolen JB, Hsu SM, Israel M, Fisher RI: Production and characterization of a monoclonal antibody that binds Reed-Sternberg cells. J Immunol 134:4231–4236, 1985
31. Diehl V, Pfreundschuh M, Fonatsch C, Stein H, Falk M, Burrichter H, Schaadt M: Phenotypic and genotypic analysis of Hodgkin's disease derived cell lines: Histopathological and clinical implications. Cancer Surv 4:399–419, 1985
32. Lukes RJ, Butler JJ: The pathology and nomenclature of Hodgkin's disease. Cancer Res 26:1063–1081, 1966
33. Jackson H, Parker F: Hodgkin's disease I: General considerations. N Engl J Med 230:1–8, 1944
34. Hoppe RT, Cox RS, Rosenberg SA, Kaplan HS: Prognostic factors in pathologic Stage III Hodgkin's disease. Cancer Treat Rep 66:743–749, 1982
35. Strum SB, Rappaport H: Interrelations of the histologic types of Hodgkin's disease. Arch Pathol 91:127–134, 1971
36. Donaldson SS, Link MP: Childhood lymphomas: Hodgkin's disease and non-Hodgkin's lymphoma. In Moosa AR, Robson MC, Schimpff SC (eds): Comprehensive Textbook of Oncology, pp 1161–1169. Baltimore, Williams & Wilkins, 1986
37. Krikorian JG, Portlock CS, Mauch PM: Hodgkin's disease presenting below the diaphragm: A review. J Clin Oncol 4:1551–1562, 1985
38. Cline MJ, Berlin N: Anemia in Hodgkin's disease. Cancer 16:526–532, 1963

39. Tan CT, DeSousa M, Good RA: Distinguishing features of the immunology of Hodgkin's disease in children. Cancer Treat Rep 66:969–975, 1982

40. Berkman AW, Kickler T, Braine H: Platelet-associated IgG in patients with lymphoma. Blood 63:944–948, 1984

41. Fisher RI: Implications of persistent T cell abnormalities for the etiology of Hodgkin's disease. Cancer Treat Rep 66:681–687, 1982

42. Butler JJ: Non neoplastic lesions of lymph nodes of man to be differentiated from lymphomas. Natl Cancer Inst Monogr 32:233–255, 1969

43. Heiberg E, Wolverson MK, Sundaram N, Nouri S: Normal thymus characteristics in subjects under 20. AJR 138:491–494, 1982

44. Jochelson M, Mauch P, Balikian J, Rosenthal D, Canellos G: The significance of the residual mediastinal mass in treated Hodgkin's disease. J Clin Oncol 3:637–640, 1985

45. Cohen M, Hill CA, Cangir A, Sullivan MP: Thymic rebound after treatment of childhood tumors. Am J Radiol 135:152–156, 1980

46. Roskos RR, Evans RC, Gilchrist GS, Burgert EO Jr, Ilstrup DM: Prognostic significance of mediastinal mass in childhood Hodgkin's disease. Cancer Treat Rep 66:961–968, 1982

47. Robinson B, Kingston J, Nogueira-Costa R, Malpas JS, Barrett A, McElwain TJ: Chemotherapy and irradiation in childhood Hodgkin's disease. Arch Dis Child 59:1162–1167, 1984

48. Rostock RA, Siegelman SS, Lenhard RE, Wharam MD, Order SE: Thoracic CT scanning for mediastinal Hodgkin's disease: Results and therapeutic implications. Int J Radiat Oncol Biol Phys 9:1451–1457, 1983

49. Dudgeon DL, Kelly M, Ghory MJ, Halden WJ, Kaufman SL, Wharam M: The efficacy of lymphangiography in the staging of pediatric Hodgkin's disease. J Pediatr Surg 21:233–235, 1986

50. Dunnick NR, Parker BR, Castellino RA: Pediatric lymphography: Performance, interpretation and accuracy in 193 consecutive children. Am J Roentgenol 129:639–645, 1977

51. Horn ML, Ray RC, Kriss JP: Gallium-67 citrate scanning in Hodgkin's disease and non-Hodgkin's lymphoma. Cancer 37:250–257, 1976

52. Hrgovic M, Tessmer CF, Minckler TM et al: Serum copper levels in lymphoma and leukemia: Special reference to Hodgkin's disease. Cancer 21:743–755, 1968

53. Carbone PP, Kaplan HS, Husshoff K et al: Report of the committee on Hodgkin's disease staging classification. Cancer Res 31:1860–1861, 1971

54. Kaplan HS, Rosenberg SA: The treatment of Hodgkin's disease. Med Clin North Am 50:1591–1610, 1966

55. Desser RK, Golomb HM, Ultmann JE et al: Prognostic classification of Hodgkin's disease in pathologic stage III, based on anatomic considerations. Blood 49:883–893, 1977

56. Glatstein E, Guernsey JM, Rosenberg SA, Kaplan HS: The value of laparotomy and splenectomy in the staging of Hodgkin's disease. Cancer 24:709–718, 1969

57. Russell KJ, Donaldson SS, Cox RS, Kaplan HS: Childhood Hodgkin's disease: Patterns of relapse. J Clin Oncol 2:80–87, 1984

58. Mauch PM, Weinstein H, Botnick L, Belli J, Cassady JR: An evaluation of long-term survival and treatment complications in children with Hodgkin's disease. Cancer 51:925–932, 1983

59. Cohen IT, Higgins GR, Powars DR, Hays DM: Staging laparotomy for Hodgkin's disease in children: Evaluation of the technique. Arch Surg 112:948–951, 1977

60. Ray GR, Trueblood HW, Enright LP, Kaplan HS, Nelsen TS: Oophoropexy: A means of preserving ovarian function following pelvic megavoltage radiotherapy for Hodgkin's disease. Radiology 96:175–180, 1970

61. Donaldson SS, Kaplan HS: Complications of treatment of Hodgkin's disease in children. Cancer Treat Rep 66:977–989, 1982

62. Jenkin RDT, Brown TC, Peters MV et al: Hodgkin's disease in children: A retrospective analysis, 1958–1973. Cancer 35:979–990, 1975

63. Kaplan HS: On the natural history, treatment and prognosis of Hodgkin's disease. In Harvey Lectures 1968–1969, pp 215–259. New York, Academic Press, 1970

64. Page V, Gardner A, Karzmark CJ: Physical and dosimetric aspects of the radiotherapy of malignant lymphomas I: The mantle technique. Radiology 96:609–618, 1970

65. Hoppe RT: Treatment planning in the radiation therapy of Hodgkin's disease. In Vaeth JM, Meyer J (eds): Front Radiat Ther Oncol 21:270–287, 1987

66. Palos B, Kaplan HS, Karzmark CJ: The use of thin lung shields to deliver limited whole-lung irradiation during mantle-field treatment of Hodgkin's disease. Radiology 101:441–442, 1971

67. Page V, Gardner A, Karzmark CJ: Physical and dosimetric aspects to the

68. le Floch O, Donaldson SS, Kaplan HS: Pregnancy following oophoropexy in total nodal irradiation in women with Hodgkin's disease. Cancer 38:2263–2268, 1976

69. Pedrick TJ, Hoppe RT: Recovery of spermatogenesis following pelvic irradiation for Hodgkin's disease. Int J Radiat Oncol Biol Phys 12:117–121, 1986

70. Schultz HP, Glatstein E, Kaplan HS: Management of presumptive or proven Hodgkin's disease of the liver: A new radiotherapy technique. Int J Radiat Oncol Biol Phys 1:1–8, 1975

71. Hanks GE, Kinzie JJ, Herring DR et al: Patterns of care outcome studies in Hodgkin's disease: Results of the national practice and implications for management. Cancer Treat Rep 66:805–808, 1982

72. Donaldson SS, Link MP: Combined modality treatment with low-dose radiation and MOPP chemotherapy for children with Hodgkin's disease. J Clin Oncol 5:742–749, 1987

73. Longo DL, Young RC, Wesley M, Hubbard SM, Duffey DL, Jaffe ES, DeVita VT Jr: Twenty years of MOPP therapy for Hodgkin's disease. J Clin Oncol 4:1295–1306, 1986

74. Bonadonna G, Zucali R, Monfardini S, DeLena M, Uslenghi C: Combination chemotherapy of Hodgkin's disease with Adriamcyin, bleomycin, vinblastine, and imidazole carboxamide versus MOPP. Cancer 36:252–259, 1975

75. Bonadonna G, Valagussa P, Santoro A: Alternating non-cross-resistant combination chemotherapy or MOPP in stage IV Hodgkin's disease. Ann Intern Med 104:739–746, 1986

76. Coldman AJ, Goldie JH: Role of mathematical modeling in protocol formulation in cancer chemotherapy. Cancer Treat Rep 69:1041–1046, 1985

77. Klimo P, Connors JM: MOPP/ABV hybrid program: Combination chemotherapy based on early introduction of seven effective drugs for advanced Hodgkin's disease. J Clin Oncol 3:1174–1182, 1985

78. Donaldson SS: Hodgkin's disease: Treatment with low dose radiation and chemotherapy. Front Radiat Ther Oncol 16:122–133, 1982

79. Hoppe RT, Portlock CS, Glatstein E, Rosenberg SA, Kaplan HS: Alternating chemotherapy and irradiation in the treatment of advanced Hodgkin's disease. Cancer 43:472–478, 1979

80. Donaldson SS, Link MP, McDougall IR, Parker BR, Shochat SJ: Clinical investigations of children with Hodgkin's disease at Stanford University Medical Center: A preliminary overview using low dose irradiation and alternating ABVD/MOPP chemotherapy. In Kamps WA, Poppema S, Humphrey B (eds): Pediatric Oncology: Current Status and Controversies in Hodgkin's Disease. Boston, Martinus Nijhoff (in press)

81. Looney WB, Hopkins HA: Alternation of chemotherapy and radiotherapy in cancer management III: Results in experimental solid tumor systems and their relationship to clinical studies. Cancer Treat Rep 70:141–162, 1986

82. Coleman CN: Secondary malignancy after treatment of Hodgkin's disease: An evolving picture. J Clin Oncol 4:821–824, 1986

83. Lange B, Littman P: Management of Hodgkin's disease in children and adolescents. Cancer 51:1371–1377, 1983

84. Tan C, Jereb B, Chan KW, Lesser M, Mondora A, Exelby P: Hodgkin's disease in children: Results of management between 1970–1981. Cancer 51:1720–1725, 1983

85. Sullivan MP, Fuller LM, Chen T et al: Intergroup Hodgkin's Disease in Children Study of stages I and II: A preliminary report. Cancer Treat Rep 66:937–947, 1982

86. Bayle-Weisgerber C, Lemercier N, Teillet F, Asselain B, Gout M, Schweisguth O: Hodgkin's disease in children: Results of therapy in a mixed group of 178 clinical and pathologically staged patients over 13 years. Cancer 54:215–222, 1984

87. Cramer P, Andrieu JM: Hodgkin's disease in childhood and adolescence: Results of chemotherapy-radiotherapy in clinical stages IA–IIB. J Clin Oncol 3:1495–1502, 1985

88. Jenkin D, Chan H, Freedman M et al: Hodgkin's disease in children: Treatment results with MOPP and low-dose, extended-field irradiation. Cancer Treat Rep 66:949–959, 1982

89. Olweny CLM, Katongole-Mbidde E, Kiire C, Lwange SK, Magrath I, Ziegler JL: Childhood Hodgkin's disease in Uganda. Cancer 42:787–792, 1978

90. Ekert H, Waters KD: Results of treatment of 18 children with Hodgkin disease with MOPP chemotherapy as the only treatment modality. Med Pediatr Oncol 11:322–326, 1983

91. Jacobs P, King HS, Karabus C, Hartley P, Werner D: Hodgkin's disease in

children: A ten-year experience in South Africa. Cancer 53:210–213, 1984

92. Crnkovich M, Hoppe R, Rosenberg S: Stage IIB Hodgkin's disease: The Stanford experience. J Clin Oncol 4:472–479, 1986

93. Jereb B, Tan C, Bretsky S, He SQ, Exelby P: Involved field (IF) irradiation with or without chemotherapy in the management of children with Hodgkin's disease. Med Pediatr Oncol 12:325–332, 1984

94. Willoughby MLN, Razak K, Keel A, Cameron FG: Alternating chemotherapy for childhood Hodgkin's disease. Lancet 2:763, 1982

95. Weiner M, Leventhal B, Falletta J, Brecher M: Treatment for advanced Hodgkin's disease (HD) in children (abstract). Proc Am Assoc Cancer Res 26:185, 1985

96. Bergsagel DE: Salvage treatment for Hodgkin's disease in relapse. J Clin Oncol 5:525–526, 1987

97. Vinciguerra V, Propert KJ, Coleman M et al: Alternating cycles of combination chemotherapy for patients with recurrent Hodgkin's disease following radiotherapy: A prospectively randomized study by the Cancer and Leukemia Group B. J Clin Oncol 4:838–846, 1986

98. Wimmer R, Weiner M, Strauss L, Leventhal B, Adair S, Kletzel M, Hartmann G: Treatment of pediatric patients for relapsed Hodgkin's disease (HD) with cytosine arabinoside, (A), cisplatin (P) and etoposide (E) (abstract). Proc Am Soc Clin Oncol 6:191, 1987

99. Selby PJ, Mbidde BK, Maitland J, McElwain TJ: High dose melphalan and autologous bone marrow transplant as treatment for refractory Hodgkin's disease. J Clin Oncol 4:612, 1986

100. Jagannath S, Dicke KA, Armitage JO et al: High-dose cyclophosphamide, carmustine and etoposide and autologous bone marrow transplantation for relapsed Hodgkin's disease. Ann Intern Med 104:163–168, 1986

101. O'Reilly S, Connors J, Voss N, Fiarey R, Herzig G, Klimo P, Phillips G: High dose cyclophosphamide, BCNU and etoposide (CBVB) and autologous bone marrow transplantation (ABMT) in progressive Hodgkin's disease (HD) (abstract). Proc Am Soc Clin Oncol 6:196, 1987

102. Lenhard RE Jr, Order SE, Spunberg JJ, Asbell SO, Leibel SA: Isotopic immunoglobulin: A new systemic therapy for advanced Hodgkin's disease. J Clin Oncol 3:1296–1300, 1985

103. Donaldson SS, Glatstein E, Vosti KL: Bacterial infections in pediatric Hodgkin's disease: Relationship to radiotherapy, chemotherapy and splenectomy. Cancer 41:1949–1958, 1978

104. Rosenstock JG, D'Angio GJ, Kiesewetter WB: The incidence of complications following staging laparotomy for Hodgkin's disease in children. Am J Roentgenol 120:531–535, 1974

105. Probert JC, Parker BR, Kaplan HS: Growth retardation in children after megavoltage irradiation of the spine. Cancer 32:634–639, 1973

106. Santoro A, Bonadonna G, Valagussa P et al: Long term results of combined chemotherapy–radiotherapy approach in Hodgkin's disease: Superiority of ABVD plus radiotherapy versus MOPP plus radiotherapy. J Clin Oncol 5:27–37, 1987

107. Constine LS, Donaldson SS, McDougall IR, Cox RS, Link MP, Kaplan HS: Thyroid dysfunction after radiotherapy in children with Hodgkin's Disease. Cancer 53:878–883, 1984

108. Damewood MD, Grochow LB: Prospects for fertility after chemotherapy or radiation for neoplastic disease. Fertil Steril 45:443–459, 1986

109. Horning SJ, Hoppe RT, Kaplan HS, Rosenberg SA: Female reproductive potential after treatment for Hodgkin's disease. N Engl J Med 304:1377–1382, 1981

110. Chapman RM, Sutcliffe SB, Malpas JS: Male gonadal dysfunction in Hodgkin's disease: A prospective study. JAMA 243:1323–1328, 1981

111. deCunha MF, Meistrich ML, Fuller LM et al: Recovery of spermatogenesis after treatment for Hodgkin's disease: Limiting dose of MOPP chemotherapy. J Clin Oncol 2:571–577, 1984

112. Sherins RJ, Olweny CLM, Ziegler JL: Gynecomastia and gonadal dysfunction in adolescent boys treated with combination chemotherapy for Hodgkin's disease. N Engl J Med 299:12–16, 1978

113. Whitehead E, Shalet SM, Morris–Jones P, Beardwell CG, Deakin DP: Gonadal function after combination chemotherapy for Hodgkin's disease in childhood. Arch Dis Child 47:287–291, 1982

114. Valagussa P, Santoro A, Fossati–Bellanti F, Banfi A, Bonadonna G: Second acute leukemia and other malignancies following treatment for Hodgkin's disease. J Clin Oncol 4:830–837, 1986

115. Blayney DW, Longo DL, Young RC et al: Decreasing risk of leukemia with prolonged follow-up after chemotherapy and radiotherapy for Hodgkin's disease. N Engl J Med 316:710–714, 1987

twenty-two

Lymphoproliferative Disorders

Nita L. Seibel,
Jeffrey Cossman, and
Ian T. Magrath

Lymphoproliferative disorders represent a heterogeneous array of diseases involving B-cell proliferations that range from reactive polyclonal hyperplasias to true monoclonal malignant lymphomas. This chapter focuses on those lymphoproliferative disorders in which an underlying condition leads to a defect in the host, thereby predisposing, or permitting, the expansion of lymphoid cell populations that would be more strictly regulated in the normal individual. These conditions are not usually self-limited disorders and may be inherited, iatrogenically induced, or acquired immunodeficiencies. Defects in immunoregulation and immune surveillance may be similar in these conditions. As a result of these defects, particularly in regulation, an increased pool of a subpopulation of lymphocytes may be present, an unchecked proliferation of this subpopulation may occur, and within this setting new irreversible cytogenetic aberrations may take place.[1]

In an extreme situation of immunosuppression, death may result from polyclonal proliferation (*e.g.,* fatal mononucleosis), but the lymphoproliferation in any event increases the risk of malignancy because of genetic aberrations. Additional factors may include defects in DNA repair, direct effects of viruses that have infected subpopulations of cells and that have themselves altered the proliferation characteristics of such subgroups, and that lymphocytes undergo recombinational events whereby their receptor genes are rearranged and made functional. These chromosomal regions may be preferential sites for chromosomal changes.[2]

EPIDEMIOLOGY AND PATHOGENESIS

Inherited Immunodeficiencies

Inherited abnormalities of the immune system encompass a heterogeneous group of genetically determined immunodeficiency diseases (also see Chap. 4). It has been estimated that patients with inherited immunodeficiencies are 100 to 10,000 times more likely to develop cancer, in particular neoplasia of the lymphoreticular system.[3] A recent review of the Immunodeficiency Cancer Registry (ICR) revealed that non-Hodgkin's lymphoma (NHL) constituted more than 50% of the reported tumors in patients with immunodeficiencies.[4] The largest number of cases of NHL were recorded in ataxia-telangiectasia (69 of 150 tumors), Wiskott–Aldrich syndrome (59 of 79), common variable immunodeficiency (55 of 120), and severe combined immunodeficiency (31 of 42). The median age at diagnosis of NHL in patients with primary immunodeficiencies is 7 years.[5]

Ataxia-telangiectasia

Ataxia-telangiectasia (AT) has provided insight into how chromosomal rearrangements can link immunodeficiency to cancer (see Chaps. 2 and 4). AT is a complex primary immunodeficiency syndrome inherited as an autosomal recessive trait with an incidence of about 1 in 40,000. Children with AT are known to be cancer prone; it has been estimated that 12% to 40% of patients develop malignancy.[6] Lymphoid malignancies (both B and T cell) predominate although other types occur.[4] Adults with AT have an increased predisposition to develop T-cell chronic lymphocytic leukemia (CLL).[7] Heterozygotes have a two to threefold overall risk of developing neoplasia, particularly breast cancer in females.[8]

Ataxia telangiectasia is associated with increased chromosomal breakage, the emergence of clones with characteristic chromosomal rearrangements, and, as noted, a predisposition to lymphoid malignancy. Lymphocytes from patients with AT frequently carry clonal populations of nonmalignant lymphoid cells identifiable by the presence of chromosome rearrangements involving breakpoints at sites 14q11, 7p14, 7q35, 2p12, 14q32, and 22q11. These chromosomal loci represent locations of the alpha chain of the T-cell receptor (TCR) (14q11), the gamma- and beta-chain genes of the TCR (7p14 and 7q35, respectively), and the immunoglobulin gene loci for the heavy chain (14q32), kappa light chain (2p12), and lambda light chain (22q11).[6] These breakpoints refer to the same regions involved in physiologic rearrangements. It has been proposed that the etiology of the high level of chromosomal rearrangements in lymphocytes of AT patients is due to either faulty rearrangement of T-cell antigen receptor and immunoglobulin genes or breakage at sites of high transcriptional activity.[2,9]

Cases have been described from AT patients in which a T-cell neoplasm developed from within clones carrying either a translocation or inversion involving chromosome 14.[10] These clones may exist for many years as a high proportion of the T cells before the neoplasm develops. This suggests that the rearrangement by itself is not sufficient to cause the evolution to a malignant state; however, in the presence of further chromosomal rearrangements, transformation from a benign to a malignant clone may occur.[11]

The underlying defect in the patient with AT has not been defined. In culture, AT fibroblasts exhibit increased sensitivity to chromosomal aberrations by ionizing radiation and radiomimetic chemicals.[12] One hypothesis based on this hypersensitivity is that they have a defect in DNA synthesis or repair.[13] A low molecular weight clastogenic peptide is thought to be responsible for the DNA repair defect.[14] Another theory has proposed a defect in tissue differentiation as evidenced by the immature appearance of the thymus and elevated levels of α_1-fetoprotein and carcinoembryonic antigen.[15–17] This defect could be responsible for the immunologic abnormalities.

In addition to the cytogenetic changes seen in AT cells, cellular and humoral immune responses are deficient. Modest reduction in lymphocyte numbers is seen, and T-cell specific cell-surface markers demonstrate an abnormal ratio of CD4:CD8 cells.[18] Other T-cell defects include blunting of delayed hypersensitivity reactions, failure to reject allografts normally, and reduced response of lymphocytes to phytohemagglutinin.[19]

Patients with AT exhibit abnormal antibody responses to Epstein–Barr virus (EBV).[20] Although EBV DNA has been detected in a B-cell lymphoma from a patient with AT, additional data will be required to prove an association between EBV and the pathogenesis of lymphoma.[21] The most consistent B-cell defect is a low level or absence of IgA in the serum, seen in 70% of affected persons.[19]

Wiskott–Aldrich

The Wiskott–Aldrich syndrome (WAS) is an X-linked recessive disorder characterized by immunodeficiency, thrombocyto-

penia, and eczema. Recurrent infection reflects involvement of both the humoral and cellular arms of the immune system. Immunologically there is poor antibody response to polysaccharide antigens, increased rate of serum immunoglobulin catabolism, and defective cytotoxic killer cell activity by T cells and monocytes.[22,23]

The risk of developing malignancy has increased proportionately to the sophistication of pediatric care and infection control. The incidence of malignant disease increases with age.[24] The typical NHL of childhood, Burkitt's lymphoma, and lymphoblastic lymphomas are the predominant tumor types, and the other common pediatric tumors (neuroblastoma, Wilms' tumor, Ewing's sarcoma, osteosarcoma, among others) are not increased in incidence.[25] The etiology of the malignancies in WAS remains obscure although chromosomal instability or latent viral activation has been postulated.[26,27] Papovavirus has been isolated from one brain tumor in a patient with WAS.[28]

Combined Immune Deficiencies

Severe combined immune deficiency (SCID) and common variable hypogammaglobulinemia (CVID) cover a broad classification of immunologic diseases involving both humoral and cellular systems (see Chap. 4). B-cell lymphoproliferative disorders have been reported after thymic epithelium transplants in children with SCID. Eleven patients have developed NHL in this setting.[29] Polyclonality was demonstrated in three cases (of six cases studied), and in one case in which EBV studies were performed, EBV was detected.[30,31] Immunoreconstitution (by thymic transplant) in these cases does not seem to alter the occurrence of lymphoproliferative disorders in SCID.[29] In contrast, no cases have been reported after successful bone marrow transplantation from a histocompatible donor.[32] Thirty percent of patients with CVID have T-cell lymphopenia and abnormal delayed hypersensitivity skin reactions.[33] Based on 220 patients with CVID observed in Great Britain, an estimated 30-fold increase in lymphoma was noted when compared to the incidence in the general population.[34]

X-linked Lymphoproliferative Syndrome

The initial descriptions in three families of a new X-linked lymphoproliferative syndrome (XLP) to EBV were made in 1974 and 1975 (see Chaps. 2, 4, and 20).[35–37] The syndrome is characterized by marked susceptibility to diseases induced by EBV, which is the only virus to which these males appear to have a heightened susceptibility. To date more than 161 affected males within 44 unrelated kindreds have been reported. Approximately 57% of XLP patients developed fatal infectious mononucleosis (IM), 29% had acquired hypogammaglobulinemia, and 24% developed malignant lymphoma. Median age of onset of fatal IM was 1.7 years, 4.9 years for lymphoma, and 6.9 years for hypogammaglobulinemia. The mortality rate in childhood is 80%; by the age of 10, 70% have died and all have died by age 40. Duration of survival was longest among patients with acquired hypogammaglobulinemia (70% long-term survival) and those with both hypogammaglobulinemia and malignant lymphoma in remission that occurred sequentially or concurrently (67% long-term survival). Sixty-five percent of the patients who died of IM had fulminant hepatitis concurrent with a hemophagocytic syndrome[38] (see Chap. 23).

The estimated risk of malignant lymphoma in patients with XLP is 200 times greater than that of the general population. Malignant lymphoma in the XLP syndrome has been described in 34 patients. Six of these cases were associated with hypogammaglobulinemia, and two patients had fatal IM and hypogammaglobulinemia as well as lymphoma. Two patients who had survived lymphoma later died of IM. All cases analyzed have been B-cell NHL (45% small noncleaved), and 78% of the lymphomas have occurred in the intestine, particularly the ileocecal region. Seventy-eight percent had localized disease (Stages I and II). Of 18 evaluated patients the median survival was 6 months. The patients with lymphoma in remission and hypogammaglobulinemia have survived the longest. Although the disease is clinically heterogeneous, an age relationship has emerged wherein younger patients have more fulminant disease.[38]

Immunologic studies of patients surviving the XLP syndrome reveal numerous humoral and cellular immunologic defects. They include inverted CD4:CD8 ratios, diminished lymphocyte transformation response to mitogens, hypogammaglobulinemia, failure of normal switching from IgM to IgG class responses after secondary challenge by bacteriophage φX174, defective natural killer cell activity, and diminished or absent regression of autologous lymphoblastoid cell lines in the presence of the patient's T cells, demonstrating decreased immunity toward EBV.[38] Only lymphocyte-mediated antibody-dependent cellular cytotoxicity was unchanged in survivors.[39]

Recently, the mutation responsible for the syndrome has been genetically linked to a restriction length polymorphism detected with the DNA probe DXS42 (from chromosome Xq24-q27). This now enables detection of female carriers of the XLP syndrome and can be used for prenatal diagnosis.[40]

The pathogenesis of the XLP syndrome may be attributed to a defect in regulation of the T-cell-mediated immune response (possibly controlled by an X-linked gene) triggered by EBV.[38] As a consequence of this defect, cytotoxic T cells, in response to invading EBV-infected B cells, also destroy adjacent hepatocytes and hematopoietic organs.[41] Because of this uncontrolled killer cell activity, either fatal IM or immune deficiency is seen if the male survives the EBV infection. These defects in immune surveillance potentially could predispose patients to opportunistic infections or sustained EBV polyclonal B-cell proliferations.[38]

Iatrogenically Induced Immunodeficiencies

The incidence of malignancy in renal allograft recipients is 6% which is 100 times greater than that of the general population when matched for age.[42] Skin and lip carcinomas are the most common, followed by lymphomas, which make up about 20% of the total. There is a 40 times greater risk of a recipient of a renal allograft developing lymphoma.[43] The incidence of malignancy in children undergoing renal transplants is reported to be 1.3%.[44]

Lymphoproliferative disorders have now been reported in patients undergoing liver, heart, heart–lung, and renal and bone marrow transplants. The risk of developing a lymphoproliferative disorder in transplant recipients ranges from 1% to 2.5% in renal patients, 2.3% in liver patients, and 5% in heart patients, when calculations are based on all patients transplanted.[45–47] Hodgkin's disease is rare in transplant patients, as compared to the general population.[48] Various hypotheses have been proposed to explain the increased incidence, including impaired T-cell regulation of B cells, particularly those infected by EBV, chronic antigenic stimulation from the allograft, and a direct oncogenic effect of immunosuppressive drugs.[48,49–51]

Bone marrow transplantation (BMT) (see Chap. 48) differs from other organ allografting in that the patient is essentially receiving a new immune system donated from an HLA-matched family member.[48] The pretransplantation regimen is designed to treat the tumor with ablative doses of radiation and chemotherapy and effectively immunosuppresses the host, resulting in marrow engraftment. After BMT, further im-munosuppression may be administered (in the form of methotrexate, prednisone, or cyclosporin A) to prevent graft-versus-host disease (GVHD).[52] Progressive development of the functional integrity of the immune system following BMT requires a period of 6 months to 2 years.[53] Development of acute or chronic GVHD or continued immunosuppression interferes with this maturation.

The frequency of lymphoproliferative disorders after allogeneic BMT has been estimated to be 0.6%.[54] From review of cases who developed lymphoproliferative disorders after BMT, certain risk factors have emerged. Severe GVHD combined with use of high-dose immunosuppressive treatment, HLA disparity between donor and recipient, and T-cell depletion of donor marrows appear to contribute to the development of lymphoproliferative disorders in these patients.[52,54] The use of anti-T-cell monoclonal antibodies for treatment of acute GVHD was the most identifiable risk factor. EBV genomic sequences have been demonstrated in most cases.[54]

Virally Induced Immunodeficiencies

Epstein–Barr Virus

Epstein–Barr virus, a ubiquitous lymphotrophic virus of the herpesvirus family, has attracted much attention since it was first described in 1964 by Epstein in cultured Burkitt's lymphoma cells.[55] As detailed in the previous sections, it has been associated with lymphoproliferative disorders in immunologically compromised individuals.

Primary infection with EBV occurs silently in young children. Children from lower-level socioeconomic backgrounds acquire EBV at a younger age than do middle-class children—perhaps reflective of more crowded living conditions. One-half to two-thirds of adolescents manifest IM at the time of primary infection.[56]

In humans, EBV is transmitted horizontally through the release of virus into oropharyngeal secretions, although cell-free virus has recently been demonstrated in female genital tract secretions, raising the possibility of sexual transmission.[57] The virus is replicated in the epithelial cells of the upper respiratory tract and in the salivary glands and then released into the oral cavity, thereby gaining access to the lymphoreticular system.[58]

Thirty to 50 days after initial contact with the virus, EBV-infected B cells will be found in the peripheral blood, although only a small percentage of the B cells (1–2%) contain EBV[59] (see Fig. 22-1). Once B cells are infected, activation occurs, resulting in B-cell proliferation and later immunoglobulin secretion. A prominent increase in peripheral blood T cells bearing the CD8 suppressor-cytotoxic phenotype is detectable, with a resultant diminution of T helper:suppressor ratios to below 1.0 that persists for weeks in primary IM. Recovery from the primary infection is associated with decreased virus shedding in the oral cavity and from virally infected lymphocytes in the peripheral blood. Suppressor-cytotoxic T cells return to normal levels during convalescence.[61]

Primary EBV infection (asymptomatic or IM-associated) is followed by a virus carrier state that usually lasts for the lifetime of the host. Virus persistence will be found at the same sites in the EBV carrier state as in primary infection and will produce the same type of infection (*i.e.,* productive in the oropharynx, latent in peripheral blood), although the virus burden is much lower after the acute phase has subsided.[62]

The humoral response to primary infection to EBV is defined serologically by the following: presence of antibodies directed to viral capsid antigen (VCA) (IgM initially, which

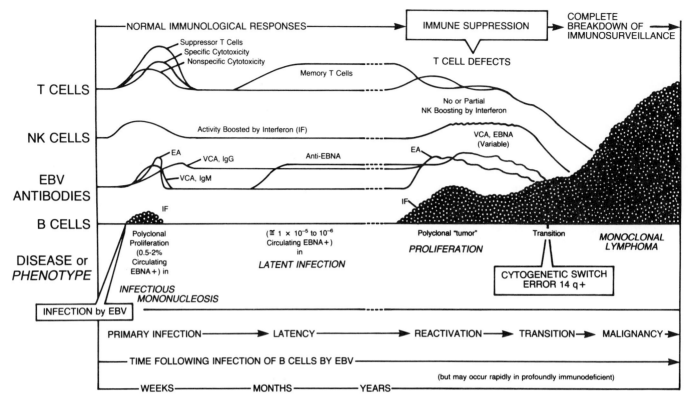

FIGURE 22-1. Normal immune responses to primary infection with EBV noted on the left. Events that may occur with an inherited immune deficiency or reactivation in individuals with acquired immune deficiency are depicted on the right. Conversion from polyclonal B-cell proliferation to monoclonal proliferation is postulated to occur through a specific cytogenetic event. EA = early antigen; VCA = viral capsid antigen; EBNA = Epstein–Barr nuclear-associated antigen; NK = natural killer cells. (Purtillo DP: Immunodeficiency predisposing to Epstein-Barr virus induced lymphoproliferative disease: The x-linked lymphoproliferative syndrome as a model. Adv Cancer Res 34:279–312, 1981. Published with permission of Academic Press)

later declines coincidentally with the appearance of IgG antibodies against VCA), increase in anti-early antigen (EA), increase in antimembrane antigen (MA), and absence of anti-Epstein–Barr nuclear-associated antigen (EBNA).[63] Antibodies against the MA complex are important because they include virus-neutralizing antibodies and are generally low during acute IM as compared to convalescence.[64] The anti-MA antibodies are the only antibodies that could play a role in control of primary EBV infection because the antigens they recognize are surface antigens. They influence the course of infection because of neutralization of the virus, which could prevent viremia, and subsequent infection of circulating lymphocytes.[65] Whether they can prevent passage of virus from infected epithelial cells to susceptible B lymphocytes or prevent infection of epithelial cells in the oropharnyx from the virus is unclear.[62]

In immunologically compromised individuals, the serologic responses may be abnormal. Although definitive patterns have not yet been established it appears that antibody titers to VCA and EA tend to increase, whereas antibodies to EBNA often decrease and disappear. This is likely a result of a decrease in or absence of T cells that are EBV specific and cytotoxic T cells that cause EBNA release of infected B cells.[66]

Cellular immunity is believed to play the most important role in immune surveillance against EBV. Primary control of active EBV infection in the normal host occurs through EBV-specific cytotoxic T cells that bear the suppressor-cytotoxic phenotype, with contributions by antibody-dependent cellular cytotoxicity, natural killer cell activity, and alpha interferon.[67] Specific T-cell immunity is responsible for the regulation of latent EBV-infected B cells as demonstrated by abrogation of outgrowth of infected B-cell lines when cocultured with autologous memory T cells.[68] Lymphocyte-determined membrane antigen (LYDMA), defined functionally, has not yet been defined biochemically.[69]

Because of the importance of T cells in the control of EBV, it is not surprising that patients with defects in certain T-cell functions may fail to regulate EBV-infected cells, leading to serious consequences. For example, as noted earlier, patients treated with high doses of anti-T-cell monoclonal antibody (CD3) or cyclosporin A as a form of treatment of severe GVHD following BMT may develop EBV-associated lymphoproliferative disorders. Cyclosporin A is a fungal product that has profound immunosuppressive effects and demonstrates a selective activity for T-cell functions, including the induction of gamma interferon by thymocytes and T lymphocytes. On the other hand, an exaggerated T-cell response to EBV infected cells is the probable cause of agammaglobulinemia reported after a primary infection with EBV. In these cases it has been suggested that abnormal persistence of suppressor T cells (which nonspecifically suppress immunoglobulin production) is responsible.[70] Normally these suppressor T cells disappear from the circulation within a few weeks to months after diagnosis.

Retroviruses

Human retroviruses represent a group of viruses that include human T-cell leukemia virus type I (HTLV-I) and human immunodeficiency virus type I (HIV), notable for their tropism for a subset of helper T lymphocytes possessing the CD4 antigen (see Chap. 36). Depending on the specific viral subgroup, the patient may exhibit proliferation of virus-infected T lymphocytes which, in some cases, are ultimately manifested as adult T-cell leukemia/lymphoma (ATL) or may become severely immunosuppressed as a consequence of depletion of helper T cells. This process results ultimately in the development of acquired immune deficiency syndrome (AIDS). These differences are not completely separate, for HTLV-I can cause immunosuppression and opportunistic infections[71] (see Chap. 36).

ATL, an aggressive lymphoproliferative disorder, was first recognized in patients born in southwestern Japan in 1977.[72] Subsequently the disease has been observed rarely in American-born blacks from the southeastern United States and among individuals who have emigrated from the West Indies to the United States and Britain.[73] HTLV-I has been implicated as the etiologic agent for this aggressive T-cell leukemia. Antibodies against HTLV-I have been found in the sera of these patients as well as in the sera of healthy individuals in endemic areas, where, as in the case of EBV, children have low levels of positivity and the likelihood of seropositivity increases with age.[74] Healthy HTLV-I carriers have demonstrated marked suppression of T-cell control of EBV-infected B cells. This finding suggests that persistent infection with HTLV-I may induce immune suppression and potentially development of ATL.[75] In the Japanese with ATL there is an insidious clinical onset characterized by abnormal T lymphocytosis often persisting for longer than a year. This lymphocytosis will either remit or develop into overt ATL. Chromosomal rearrangements involving 14q11.2 are characteristic of Japanese ATL. In the T-lymphocytosis phase, visible breaks in 14q11.2 have been observed. The transition to overt ATL occurs when these visible breaks give rise to rearrangements of 14q11.2.[6]

The relation of HTLV-I to lymphoproliferative disorders in children is unknown and is now beginning to be examined. Seropositive healthy individuals have persistent HTLV-I infection as demonstrated by cultured HTLV-I obtained from their infected T lymphocytes.[76] Individuals who acquire seropositivity through blood transfusions manifest persistent HTLV-I infection as demonstrated by viral antigen and proviral DNA of HTLV-I in the cloned lymphocytes of seropositive recipients.[77] Routes of transmission in children include blood transfusions and milk (mother-to-child). In a prospective study of children born of carrier mothers in Japan, antigen-positive mothers were found to be at higher risk of transferring virus to their children than were antigen-negative mothers. Approximately 50% of the children born to antigen-positive mothers become positive usually by 2 years of age.[74] HTLV-I antibodies have not been found in children with acute leukemia (including T-cell ALL), including those in the southeastern United States where HTLV-I may be endemic.[78]

PATHOLOGY

The histopathology of lymphoproliferative processes seen either in patients with primary immunodeficiency disorders or in those who have received immunosuppressive therapy shows a spectrum of morphologies ranging from atypical lymphoid hyperplasias to high-grade malignant lymphoma.

Congenital immunodeficiency syndromes are associated with localized histologic abnormalities in lymphoid tissues. For example, the paracortical T-cell zones of lymph nodes, periarteriolar T-cell lymphatic sheath of spleen, and germinal center B-cell areas are often diminished in their cellular content in disorders such as Wiskott–Aldrich syndrome, ataxia-telangiectasia, and variable immunodeficiency (Figs. 22-2 and 22-3). Occasionally one or both of these zones may be absent in these conditions, particularly in SCID.[79]

The lymphoproliferations are histologically similar regardless of the cause of immunosuppression, and the lymphomas are usually classified as large cell lymphomas, most commonly of the immunoblastic lymphoma subtype (Fig. 22-4). Hodgkin's disease is a less frequent complication of immunodeficiency disorders, and its relative incidence is approximately one-third that of non-Hodgkin's lymphomas in immunodeficient patients.[80]

FIGURE 22-2. Lymph node from a patient with Wiskott–Aldrich syndrome. The B-cell cortical areas are markedly reduced, and only a single primary follicle remains (*arrow*) with no evidence of germinal center development. The adjacent paracortex is moderately hypocellular.

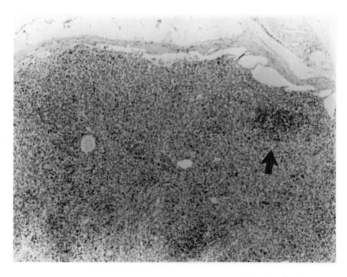

FIGURE 22-3. Spleen from a patient with Wiskott–Aldrich syndrome. The B-cell follicle is atrophic (***black arrow***) and shows no evidence of germinal center development. The periarteriolar T-cell lymphatic sheath is absent (*open arrow*).

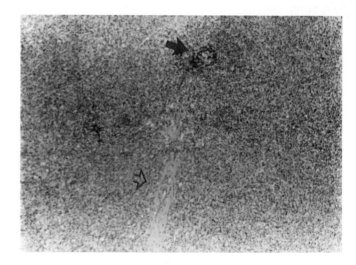

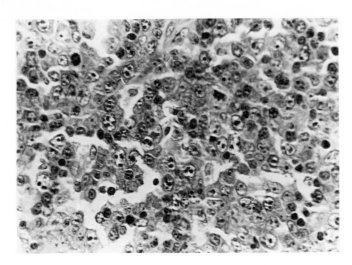

FIGURE 22-4. Large cell lymphoma, immunoblastic, arising in Wis-kott–Aldrich syndrome exemplifies one type of large cell immunoblastic lymphoma that may develop in this setting. A range of large cell lymphoma morphologies occurs in immune deficiency disorders that are not histologically distinguishable from large cell lymphomas and large cell immunoblastic lymphomas seen in other patients.

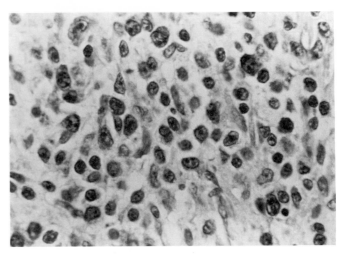

FIGURE 22-5. Infectious mononucleosis. The lymph node contains sheets of immunoblasts with multiple nucleoli, abundant amphophilic cytoplasm, and a background of lymphocytes, plasmacytoid lympho-cytes, and plasma cells. Although the large cells simulate the cells of a large cell lymphoma, the cellular environment is polymorphous, as expected in a reactive lymphoproliferative process.

Although the morphologic features of large cell lymphoma are well defined, a controversy exists concerning the malignant nature of lymphoproliferative processes in patients with either primary or secondary immunodeficiencies. Immunophenotypic analysis has suggested that some processes may be polyclonal by virtue of mixtures of cells expressing either kappa or lambda light chains together in the same tissue. Lack of restriction to a single light chain gene expression is suggestive of a polyclonal rather than a monoclonal disorder.[81]

Patients with X-linked lymphoproliferative syndrome show widespread immunoblastic infiltration of lymphoreticular organs.[82] The liver will show an intense periportal B-cell EBNA containing infiltrate surrounded by T cells (suppressive-lytic phenotype). In addition to lymphoreticular organ infiltration, lungs, heart, and CNS may be involved. Lymph nodes may actually show total effacement of normal architecture with necrosis and an immunoblastic proliferation; however, in other patients lymphoid depletion may be present. These changes may be present in the same patient in sporadic lymph node groups. The thymus will be hyperplastic in early stages of the disease but later becomes depleted of lymphocytes and Hassall's bodies.[38]

The morphology of lymphoid tissue in post-transplant lymphoproliferative processes may mimic the histologic features of lymph nodes in patients with IM (Fig. 22-5), a feature that is not unexpected because EBV DNA is frequently found in post-transplantation lymphoproliferative disorders. The marked immunoblastic proliferation seen in lymph nodes of patients with IM may be quite worrisome because sheets of cells bear a remarkable similarity to large cell immunoblastic lymphoma. However, IM lesions tend to be more polymorphous than large cell lymphoma and often contain admixed lymphocytes, plasma cells, and other inflammatory cells. The cytologic features of immunoblasts in lymph nodes of patients with IM may be confused with the Reed–Sternberg cells of Hodgkin's disease.[83] The nucleoli of the immunoblasts in IM can be distinguished from Reed–Sternberg cells by their baso-philia, irregular shapes, and perinuclear clear zone.[84] Moreover, the overall architecture of the lymph node is more likely to be intact in IM than in a malignant lymphoma. In view of the lymphoma-like histology of IM, it may be unwise to submit a patient with classic serologic and clinical features of IM to lymph node biopsy.[83]

MOLECULAR BIOLOGICAL ASPECTS OF LYMPHOPROLIFERATIVE DISORDERS

Many neoplastic processes have been shown to be clonal disorders that result from genetic changes within cells, leading to altered expression or function of normal cellular genes. However, cellular proliferation could also occur as a consequence of failure of the normal regulatory mechanisms. In the latter case, the proliferating cell is likely to be polyclonal at least initially. Thus the determination of clonality is relevant to an understanding of the pathogenesis of the lymphoproliferative syndromes arising in immunosuppressed individuals. The use of new genetic tools has opened a series of questions concerning the diagnosis of malignancy among lymphoproliferative processes. Clonality can be determined by either conventional cytogenetics or by DNA hybridization using Southern blot techniques (see Chap. 3). The Southern blot DNA hybridization technique is sensitive and can detect clonal populations, which represent as few as 1% of the total cells within a peripheral blood or lymphoid tissue sample. In certain settings clonal populations can be identified by their rearrangement of immunoglobulin or T-cell receptor genes, but these clones do not necessarily progress to malignant lymphoma or leukemia. Such clones, present in low frequency, have been identified in patients with altered immune function, such as in the WAS[85] or angioimmunoblastic lymphadenopathy with dysproteinemia (AILD).[86] Minor clonal populations can also be identified in iatrogenically immunosuppressed patients after organ or bone marrow transplantation.[87,88] Molecular genetic analysis of the lymphoid proliferations observed in a series of postcardiac transplant patients has indicated that lesions are clonal because immunoglobulin gene rearrangements may be detected.[89] In a subsequent study, Cleary and co-workers analyzed multiple samples from individuals after cardiac transplant and found that, although each lymphoid proliferation was clonal, the gene rearrangement patterns varied from site to site in the same patient. This finding suggested that each lesion was a separate clone and represented multiclonal lymphoma.[90]

A similar biological process may occur in some patients with primary immunodeficiency. One example is a patient with WAS who developed lymphadenopathy that histologically appeared to be an atypical follicular hyperplasia (Fig. 22-6). Although mantle zones were depleted, the germinal centers appeared polymorphous while staining for immunoglobulins revealed polyclonality. A diagnosis of malignant lymphoma could not be rendered on this tissue. However, immunoglobulin gene rearrangement analysis indicated the presence of a small but detectable B-cell clone that contained rearrangements of both heavy and kappa light chain genes.[85] Although this patient later died of opportunistic infection, no lymphoma was detected at autopsy. Thus the presence of a B-cell clone in lymphoid tissue is not necessarily diagnostic of a malignant lymphoma. The results of gene hybridization studies should be taken in context in view of the histologic picture and the usual clinical information that one must consider when developing a diagnosis of malignant lymphoma.

CLINICAL PRESENTATION

Inherited Immunodeficiencies

Lymphadenopathy is often a characteristic physical finding of the inherited immunodeficiency syndromes (*e.g.,* WAS, CVID). Detection of lymphoproliferative disorders within the context of chronic lymphadenopathy may be difficult. The lymph nodes are not usually the sites of occurrence of lymphoproliferative disorders in these patients. Locations more commonly associated with lymphoproliferative disorders include gastrointestinal tract, central nervous system, lung, and soft tissue of head and neck.[80] Patients with the most severe T-cell defects may present with wide systemic involvement (including CNS).[5] AT patients who develop CLL may present with nonspecific constitutional symptoms and leukocytosis without lymphadenopathy or organomegaly.[91]

FIGURE 22-6. Follicular hyperplasia in Wiskott–Aldrich syndrome. The lymph node contains numerous well-developed germinal centers, but lymphoid cuffs are absent. The cellular composition of the germinal centers is polymorphous and includes the range of cell types seen in reactive follicular hyperplasias.

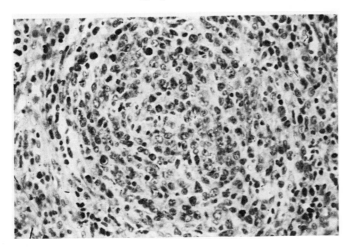

Other naturally occurring immunodeficiency diseases associated with lymphoproliferative disorders include Bloom's syndrome and Chédiak–Higashi syndrome. Patients with Bloom's syndrome exhibit chromosomal instability and increased susceptibility of cultured fibroblasts to gamma irradiations.[92] Chédiak–Higashi syndrome is a rare, autosomal recessive syndrome characterized by partial oculocutaneous albinism, photophobia, frequent pyogenic infections, and abnormally large lysosomal inclusions in cells throughout the body. Eighty-five percent of patients will enter an accelerated phase manifested by pancytopenia, fever, jaundice, hepatosplenomegaly, lymphadenopathy, neurologic changes, and a diffuse mononuclear cell infiltration. The infiltrate is usually considered neoplastic when the architecture of the lymphatic tissue is obscured and benign if the architecture is preserved.[93] Whether this accelerated phase is a reaction to a virus is unknown, although DNA from EBV has been detected in mononuclear cells of lymph node, blood, and bone marrow.[94] One patient in the accelerated phase demonstrated a T-cell infiltrate in the lymph node consistent with non-Hodgkin's T-cell lymphoma.[95] Patients with Chédiak–Higashi syndrome demonstrate *in vitro* abnormalities predisposing them to malignancy, including deficiency of natural killer cell activity and defects in DNA repair.[96,97]

Iatrogenically Induced Immunodeficiencies

Lymphoproliferative disorders occurring in renal transplants have been categorized into two groups. The first group manifests a nonspecific mononucleosis illness consisting of fever, pharyngitis, and lymphadenopathy. Individuals in this group are usually young (mean age, 21 years), and rapid development of illness after transplantation usually occurs around 9 months. The other group consists of older patients (mean age, 47 years) who develop localized extranodal tumor masses at a longer interval from transplantation (mean, 5.3 years).[98] Two other categories of lymphoproliferative disorders emerge when evaluating other solid organ transplants in addition to kidney: lymphomas confined to the brain and gastrointestinal lymphoproliferative diseases manifested by perforation, obstruction, or hemorrhage. The most important predisposing factor to the development of a lymphoproliferative disorder in organ transplant recipients is the degree of immunosuppression rather than a particular type.[66] Bone marrow transplant patients who develop lymphoproliferative disorders may present with significant deterioration of neuropsychological function in addition to fever, adenopathy, organomegaly (resembling IM), and necrotic, umbilicated skin lesions.[99]

Virally Induced Clinical Syndromes

Fatal Infectious Mononucleosis

Fatal IM refers to the disease seen in patients in whom uncontrolled proliferation of EBV-infected B cells occurs. Children in families with the X-linked lymphoproliferative (XLP) syndrome are at risk for fatal infectious mononucleosis. Fatal IM can also occur without a family history of XLP. Survivors have recovered completely, and they produce the normal pattern of antibodies to EBV over the usual time-course. The affected members have demonstrated a deficiency of natural killer cells as seen with XLP patients.[100]

The most common presentation of the XLP syndrome is fatal IM occurring at a median age of 2.7 years, with a median survival duration of 32 days. Clinically these patients present with a severe EBV infection, fever, pharyngitis, generalized lymphadenopathy with marked cervical lymphadenopathy, and hepatosplenomegaly. A faint maculopapular rash may be present. An atypical lymphocytosis is detected in the peripheral blood along with elevations in serum immunoglobulin and transaminase concentrations.[38,82]

A diagnosis of EBV infection can be made by detection of heterophil antibodies, anti-VCA (IgM), and anti-EA. In 10 of 33 patients infection could not be documented serologically. However, five of these patients had EBV DNA detected in postmortem tissues.[38]

HIV Infection

Babies and children with AIDS-related complex (ARC) commonly have nonspecific symptoms of candidiasis and lymphadenopathy (see Chap. 36). Patients at high risk for developing AIDS (such as seropositive hemophiliacs or recipients of blood products) will often develop a generalized lymphadenopathy that may represent a prodrome to AIDS.[101] These patients show fluctuations in their lymphadenopathy that is present for a minimum of 3 months, show immunologic abnormalities, but lack other constitutional symptoms.[102] Lymph node biopsies in these patients can be a dilemma because the majority will show benign hyperplasia. Findings demonstrating lymphocyte depletion may be predictive of impending AIDS. Lymph node biopsy is suggested in the setting of a rapidly enlarging single lymph node in order to determine whether malignancy has developed.[103,104]

Lymphocytic interstitial pneumonia (LIP) is more common in childhood AIDS than in adults and is not considered to be a neoplastic process. There is diffuse infiltration of the alveolar septa and peribronchiolar areas with plasmacytoid lymphocytes and immunoblasts. Lymphomatous transformation, which occurs rarely, is characterized by cellular atypia and involvement of the hilar or mediastinal lymph nodes or parietal pleura.[105] Patients have a restrictive defect with impaired carbon monoxide diffusing capacity. Clinical manifestations include cough and dyspnea with or without fever and can often be confused with pneumocystis or CMV pneumonia. Radiographic findings of a reticulonodular pattern can be pathognomonic.[106] Both HIV-I and EBV DNA have been identified from lung biopsies in patients with LIP.[105,107]

Infants have been reported to present with a lymphadenopathic form of Kaposi's sarcoma consisting of abnormally small nodes infiltrated by tumor.[108] Non-Hodgkin's lymphoma occurs in patients with AIDS (adults more than children), particularly in extranodal sites.[109]

HTLV-I Infection

One Sicilian child had a smoldering T-cell lymphoma that presented within the first year of life with lymphadenopathy, skin eruption, and atypical lymphocytes in the peripheral blood. Antibodies to HTLV-I were detected both in child and mother.[110]

LYMPHOPROLIFERATIVE DISORDERS INFREQUENTLY ENCOUNTERED IN PEDIATRICS

Angioimmunoblastic Lymphadenopathy with Dysproteinemia

Angioimmunoblastic lymphadenopathy with dysproteinemia is a potentially fatal disease of unknown etiology, more frequently seen in adults but which has been reported in children

as young as 5 years of age.[111] Manifestations include fever, generalized lymphadenopathy, hepatosplenomegaly, skin rash, polyclonal hypergammaglobulinemia, hemolytic anemia, and increased hypersensitivity reactions. Histologically the lymph node is effaced with infiltration of immunoblasts, plasma cells, eosinophils, histiocytes, and atypical lymphocytes. Arborizing small vessels often accompany the polymorphic infiltrate, and in some cases deposition of amorphous eosinophilic material is noted.[112] The clinical course covers a spectrum from regression without cytotoxic therapy to transformation to a more aggressive course, with a median survival of 30 months.[113] Fifty percent of the patients will develop an aggressive (immunoblastic) NHL, usually of T-cell type. Attempts have been made to define the malignant potential of AILD at onset. Clonal proliferations of B cells, T cells, or both have been identified in the peripheral blood and lymph nodes of patients with AILD.[86] Lymphomas in patients who have developed AILD have included B or T cell, either polyclonal or monoclonal.[114,115] Karotypic abnormalities have also been demonstrated in lymph nodes from patients with AILD and lymphoma.[116]

Lymphomatoid Granulomatosis

Lymphomatoid granulomatosis is a poorly understood form of angiitis and granulomatoses that can affect any organ system, however, pulmonary, neurologic, and cutaneous manifestations are most frequent. Pulmonary involvement, consisting of multiple bilateral nodules with a tendency to wax and wane, may resemble Wegener's granulomatosis. Characteristic histology includes a granulomatous process with a polymorphous lymphoreticular infiltration comprising atypical lymphocytes and plasmacytoid cells. Better prognosis correlates with the presence of a large number of small lymphocytes or plasma cells in the inflammatory infiltrate rather than atypical lymphocytes.[117] Most patients present with fever, cough, malaise, and weight loss. The disease is seen primarily in middle age; however, in the four reported lymphoblastic cases of the disease in childhood, two of the children were in remission for acute lymphoblastic leukemia.[118–121]

The disorder may be considered both premalignant and postmalignant because about 13% of reported cases progress to lymphoma or may occur within that setting.[118] Patients with lymphomatoid granulomatosis have had severe T-lymphocyte functional impairment.[122]

The relation of this disease to EBV is unknown. A case of lymphomatoid granulomatosis has been reported in a patient who initially presented with reactivated EBV infection, and another has been described in an immunodeficient patient with acute EBV infection.[82,123] The prognosis of lymphomatoid granulomatosis is extremely poor, with a mortality rate between 60% and 90%.[82,118]

Sinus Histiocytosis with Massive Lymphadenopathy

Sinus histiocytosis with massive lymphadenopathy refers to a clinical disorder consisting of massive bilateral, painless cervical lymphadenopathy. All lymph node groups of the neck can be involved as well as axillary and inguinal regions. A progression is seen from early stages in which the lymph nodes are mobile and discrete to later stages in which they adhere to each other, resulting in a multinodular mass. Extranodal sites such as skin, eyelid and orbit, salivary gland, bone, and respiratory tract have been reported. This disease occurs worldwide, usually, but not exclusively, presenting in blacks within the first decade of life without predilection for either sex.[124]

Fever, leukocytosis with neutrophilia, mild normochromic anemia, elevated erythrocyte sedimentation rate, and polyclonal hypergammaglobulinemia are commonly associated findings. The condition usually persists for 3 to 9 months. However, one case reportedly has lasted for 11 years. The course of the disease is not influenced by various treatments but usually resolves spontaneously. Evolution into amyloidosis or malignant lymphoma has been described in individual patients.[125] Histologically the disorder shows distinctive features, including capsular and pericapsular fibrosis and dilatation of the sinuses filled with large granular or vacuolated histocytes. Phagocytosis of lymphocytes, plasma cells, and erythrocytes by sinus histiocytes is the most striking feature. The etiologic agent for this disorder remains unknown although elevated titers to EBV and measles virus have been observed.[124]

Giant Lymph Node Hyperplasia

Giant lymph node hyperplasia (angiomatous lymphoid hamartoma, Castleman's disease) refers to an accumulation of nonneoplastic lymphoid tissue interspersed with plasma cells and blood vessels. Its etiology is unknown. The most frequent site is the mediastinum, but lesions may also be found in the abdomen, pelvis, and cervical and axillary regions. Ages of patients have ranged from 8 to 70 years. Solitary lesions have ranged in size from 1.5 to 16 cm.[126] Two histologic types exist: hyaline vascular and plasma cell. The hyaline vascular type is more common, is solitary, and is generally asymptomatic. In contrast, the plasma cell type makes up 10% to 20% of the lesions, involves multiple lymph nodes, and is usually associated with systemic symptoms. The latter is associated with a syndrome characterized by fever, anemia, and hypergammaglobulinemia.[127] Case reports in the pediatric literature have also been associated with growth retardation and bleeding tendencies.[128] Resolution of the symptoms occurs after surgical excision.

Heavy Chain Diseases

Alpha heavy chain disease is a lymphoproliferative disorder of B lymphocytes that can evolve into malignant lymphoma. In this disorder there is proliferation of plasma cells accompanied by secretion of an abnormal immunoglobulin molecule consisting of incomplete alpha chains devoid of light chains. People aged 10 to 30 years old are primarily affected by the disease.[129]

Two forms of the disease exist: a respiratory form and an intestinal form. The respiratory form is very rare and has occurred in patients in Europe and the United States. The intestinal form is seen in areas where bacterial, parasitic, and viral intestinal infections are common (Mediterranean region, Northern Africa, and Asia). Clinical features include chronic diarrhea and severe malabsorption syndrome, consisting of weight loss, steatorrhea, hypocalcemia, and excessive fecal fluid and electrolyte losses. Abdominal pain may often predominate the clinical picture along with palpable abdominal masses and finger clubbing. Detection of abnormal IgA molecules in the serum is necessary for diagnosis.

Three stages appear to exist in the intestinal form of alpha heavy chain disease. The initial stage is characterized histologically as having a diffuse and massive infiltration of lymphoid cells (predominantly plasma cells, with interspersed lymphoplasmacytic cells and occasional immunoblasts). These areas are located in the lamina propria without extension into the submucosa of the small intestines (duodenum and jejunum mainly) and mesenteric lymph nodes. Secondary villous atrophy and sparsity of crypts have also been detected. The late stage is characterized by large cell (usually immunoblastic) lymphoma. An intermediate stage shows deeper extension of the infiltrate into the submucosa accompanied by more atypical cells and immunoblasts.[130] It has been suggested that the entity known as Mediterranean lymphoma is analogous to the late stage of alpha chain disease but has either a subclinical or absent prodrome.[131]

The etiology of the transition from the initial stage to that of immunoblastic lymphoma is unknown. Complete and prolonged remissions have been obtained in early stage patients by treatment with oral antibiotics alone, which lends support to the benign nature of the early stage.[129] The large cells of the immunoblastic lymphoma are believed to be derived from the same B-cell clone as in the initial plasma cell proliferation based on the detection of immunoglobulin molecules devoid of light chains on the surface of the cells.[132] Environmental factors have been postulated to play a role in the pathogenesis of this disease because of the strong association between the intestinal form and geographical area. It is unlikely that environmental factors could trigger the clonal proliferation; rather, they could represent predisposing factors.[129]

Gamma heavy chain disease is another lymphoproliferative disorder that occurs more frequently in adults older than 40. However, cases have been reported in patients as young as 12 years of age.[133] The clinical manifestations include general lymphadenopathy, anemia, fever, malaise, weakness, and hepatosplenomegaly. Often the lymph nodes in Waldeyer's ring will be enlarged, leading to palatal edema and respiratory difficulties. The disease course varies between a few months to as long as 5 years and often occurs in the setting of other chronic diseases such as rheumatoid arthritis, lupus erythematosus, Sjögrens, and myasthenia gravis.[134]

Ocular Adnexal Lymphoid Proliferations

Ocular adnexal lymphoid proliferations represent 10% to 15% of orbital tumor masses. These occur both in the conjunctiva and in the orbit predominantly in adults. Benign lesions outnumber malignant lesions in the conjunctiva with the converse being true in the orbit. Ocular pseudolymphomas resemble benign reactive lymph nodes histologically, with polyclonal proliferations of lymphocytes, whereas the lymphomas show monoclonal B-cell proliferations with accompanying histologic features. Ocular pseudolymphomas have been reported rarely in children.[135,136]

Sjögren's Syndrome

Sjögren's syndrome is a chronic autoimmune disease consisting of features of lymphocytic infiltration of the lacrimal and salivary glands eventually progressing to keratoconjunctivitis sicca and xerostomia. The disease is seen frequently in middle-aged women and identified only rarely in children (36 cases reported, predominantly female, with the youngest 2 years old).[137,138] Adult patients with a history of parotid enlargement, lymphadenopathy, and splenomegaly have been documented to have an increased risk of developing NHL.[139] This has not been reported in the pediatric population, in which a fulminant autoimmune connective tissue disease (systemic lupus erythematosus or rheumatoid arthritis) is more likely to develop.[137]

DIFFERENTIAL DIAGNOSIS

Lymphadenopathy in children is a common finding and usually represents a transient proliferative response to localized infection (see Chap. 5). Consideration of all the causes of lymphadenopathy in pediatric patients and particularly of infectious origin is beyond the scope of this chapter (see Table 22-1). Only conditions that can resemble lymphoproliferative disorders in pediatric patients will be discussed.

Reactive hyperplasia, defined as a proliferation of one or more cell components, is the most common histologic diagnosis in children undergoing lymph node biopsy.[149,150] The stimulus for most of the hyperplasias is usually unknown, and appearance depends on the patient's age, immunologic capabilities, and previous exposure to the inciting agent, as well as the duration. Approximately 20% of the pediatric patients initially showing reactive hyperplasias later develop a specific pathologic process, emphasizing the need for careful follow-up of these patients.[149]

Infectious mononucleosis is a self-limited benign disorder characterized by fever, sore throat, lymphadenopathy, splenic enlargement, and lymphocytosis in the peripheral blood combined with the presence of atypical lymphocytes. Epstein–Barr virus is the most common cause of IM, however, other agents can cause mononucleosis syndromes, including cytomegalovirus, herpes simplex II, rubella, adenovirus, and Toxoplasma gondii.[151,152] Diagnosis of IM caused by EBV can usually be made by detection of heterophil antibodies or EBV-specific antibodies (VCA, EA, EBNA).[63]

Persistent lymphocytosis lasting months to years has been observed in a number of patients after EBV infection. One patient exhibited a CD8 T-cell lymphocytosis associated with neutropenia following acute EBV infection that lasted more than 5 years.[153] Epstein–Barr virus infection in infants is rare but has been reported in a clinical syndrome similar to juvenile chronic myelogeneous leukemia. Presenting signs of these infants included hepatosplenomegaly, leukocytosis, thrombocytopenia, and increased fetal hemoglobin. This syndrome can be distinguished from juvenile onset chronic myelogeneous leukemia by normal bone marrow and peripheral blood karyo-

type combined with serologic evidence of recent EBV infection. Clinical symptoms may persist for months to years but usually resolve spontaneously.[154]

An additional illness to be considered is an incompletely defined syndrome named chronic active EBV infection or chronic IM.[155] This disorder includes a symptom complex consisting of persistent fatigue and constitutional symptoms with a duration of at least 18 months following a primary infection with EBV. The sera of these patients characteristically contain antibodies to EBV-related antigens, the absence of antibodies to EBNA, and generally higher than normal titers of antibodies to VCA. Serum immunoglobulin levels are usually normal along with normal numbers of EBV-infected cells in the circulation.[70,156]

Another group of patients with extraordinarily high titers of EBV antibodies (IgG-VCA, EA) has pancytopenia, chronic lymphadenopathy, hepatosplenomegaly, interstitial pneumonitis, and chronic liver dysfunction in the face of chronic EBV infection. An abnormal humoral immune response to EBNA antigen or infection with a variant EBV strain is thought to be associated with this state. The relation between EBV and the clinical syndrome is suggested by the clinical response to acyclovir.[157] Interleukin-2 (IL-2) may also have a role in treatment.[158]

Generalized lymphadenopathy is seen in approximately 40% of children with juvenile rheumatoid arthritis often accompanied by splenomegaly and less commonly hepatomegaly. Lymphadenopathy frequently precedes joint involvement.[142] Systemic lupus erythematosus is associated with lymphadenopathy in 70% of the patients; in approximately 35% of cases it is generalized. An increased incidence of lymphomas has been seen in adults with rheumatoid arthritis and systemic lupus erythematosus.[142,159]

Sarcoidosis is a multisystem disease of unknown etiology occurring rarely in children. It is seen more frequently in blacks between the ages of 20 and 50 years of age. The average age of occurrence of childhood sarcoidosis is 13.[145,160] Presenting symptoms are nonspecific but include weight loss, cough, malaise, bone and joint pain, and peripheral lymphadenopathy. Nontender, movable, firm lymph nodes are the most common physical findings.[145] Eye and skin changes are seen frequently in the disease, more commonly in very young children.

Phenytoin therapy has been associated with a hypersensitivity response in children consisting of fever, rash, lymphadenopathy, hepatitis, and eosinophilia. The term pseudolymphoma has been applied to this condition because of the striking lymphadenopathy identified and the histologic similarities such as predominance of immunoblasts or presence of Reed–Sternberg-like cells.[161-163] Clinical manifestations usually disappear with drug withdrawal. Cases have been reported of both Hodgkin's disease and NHL developing in patients treated with phenytoin for prolonged periods.[161,164] Histiocytosis X is mentioned here because of the overlap in the clinical manifestations with lymphoproliferative disorders; it is discussed in Chapter 23.

DIAGNOSIS

The understanding of the relationship of specific underlying disease states with lymphoproliferative disorders has evolved over the past 20 years. Factors such as the patient's age, underlying disease, immunologic capabilities, and exposure to agents that interfere with these capabilities need to be considered when dealing with these groups. At the time of presentation a thorough history is essential. Patients need to be evalu-

---

Table 22-1
Causes of Lymphadenopathy in Children

Nonspecific reactive hyperplasia

Infections: bacterial, fungal, parasitic (toxoplasmosis), viral (EBV, HSII, HIV, adenovirus), spirochetes (secondary syphilis), cat scratch fever

Postvaccination including postvaccinial lymphadenitis[140,141]

Autoimmune: rheumatoid arthritis, systemic lupus erythematosus, serum sickness[142-144]

Sarcoidosis[145]

Drugs

Histiocytoses X

Reactive lymphohistiocytoses: XLP, lymphomatoid granulomatosis, sinus histiocytosis with massive lymphadenopathy

Angioimmunoblastic lymphadenopathy with dysproteinemia

Giant lymph node hyperplasia

Primary and metastatic malignancy

Mucocutaneous lymph node disease

Hyperthyroidism[146]

Storage diseases: Niemann–Pick, Gaucher's

Beryllium exposure[147]

Autoimmune hemolytic anemia[148]

ated for viral-specific immune defects by examining antibody titers. Both humoral and cellular defects need to be evaluated in relation to viral infection. Attempts to culture the virus (HIV, HTLV-I) should be made in the premalignant state and then serially. Lymph node biopsy may be necessary to establish a definitive diagnosis, particularly in patients with generalized lymphadenopathy or bulky or abdominal adenopathy.[103] Clonality and karyotyping should be determined on all tumors, and, when possible, virus-specific probes should be used.[1]

PREVENTION AND TREATMENT

Prevention is the best way to handle patients at risk for lymphoproliferative disorders. Bone marrow transplantation performed in an attempt to fully reconstitute the immune system in primary immunodeficiencies is the treatment of choice for patients with histocompatible donors. There is a much lower risk of developing lymphoproliferative disorder after full immune reconstitution.[32] Avoidance of EBV exposure or prophylaxis by using IV IgG or acyclovir has been suggested for patients at high risk (such as patients with XLP, bone marrow transplant recipients, and those with Chédiak–Higashi syndrome).[1]

Depending on the patient's underlying disease and the location of the lymphoproliferative disorder, treatment needs to be individualized. In some cases, such as in the inherited immunodeficiency syndromes, local therapy, biological response modifiers (*e.g.*, interferon, IL-2), or monoclonal antibodies might be chosen. If the patient's underlying immunodeficiency (whether inherited or acquired) is manifested only to a minor degree, then standard therapy should be instituted[165] (see Chap. 20). Patients who have been treated successfully for their lymphoproliferative disorders remain at high risk and can develop different lymphoproliferative syndromes.[166] Acyclovir (9-[2-hydroxyethoxy)-methyl] guanine) has been used in patients documented to have an EBV carrying polyclonal lymphoproliferation and serologic evidence of a primary reactivated infection. Acyclovir blocks the EBV-associated DNA polymerase therefore inhibiting the EBV DNA replication only in virus-producing cell lines.[167] In recipients of renal transplant, three patient groups have been identified in their responsiveness to acyclovir.[45,98,168] In patients with an EBV-induced IM-like illness characterized by a polyclonal B-cell proliferation without cytogenetic abnormalities treated with acyclovir, complete resolution of the disease was noted during therapy on standard doses of immunosuppressives.[98] The second group is similar to the first group, but with morphologic features of malignancy and clonal karyotypic abnormalities detected in a small percentage of cells. These patients respond to acyclovir, but immunosuppression needs to be decreased or stopped because of the risk of progression from a polyclonal to a monoclonal B-cell proliferation.[168] The third group consists of older patients with extranodal solid tumors that are morphologically malignant and monoclonal and may contain clonal karyotypic abnormalities. Latently infected EBV B cells make up these tumors; they are therefore insensitive to acyclovir, and treatment should consist of combination radiation therapy and chemotherapy and discontinuation of immunosuppressive therapy (see Chap. 20). This group has the highest mortality rate (greater than 80%).[66]

Treatments of other transplant recipients besides renal transplant recipients have varied but have included reduction of immunosuppressives or surgical resection (site-dependent) or both; however, it appears that reduction of immunosuppression is not sufficient for most patients.[66] Primary CNS disease has been treated with a combination of radiation therapy and a

reduction in immunosuppression, although this has usually resulted in a high recurrence rate and short survival.[45]

Treatment of the malignant lymphomas in the XLP have included surgery, radiation therapy, or chemotherapy, resulting in long-term survival. Patients with related hypogammaglobulinemia have survived with antibiotic therapy and gammaglobulin.[38] Patients with acute IM have had cessation of EBV shedding and more rapid return to a subjective feeling of well-being when treated with acyclovir. Two patients with chronic IM have responded to acyclovir therapy.[169] At present, studies are under way to evaluate the role of acyclovir in EBV infections.

FUTURE DIRECTIONS

The role of molecular genetics is central to the knowledge of lymphoproliferative disorders. Not only is molecular genetics being applied to define malignancy but also it is being applied to detect etiologic agents and predict those individuals at risk. New questions have arisen with regard to the criteria of malignancy and the relationship to clonality and histology. By continued application of viral and cellular molecular probes to lymphomas and tissue from lymphoproliferative disorders, coupled with histology and cytogenetics, further insight and understanding of the process of lymphomagenesis will be gained. Prevention of lymphoproliferative disorders may be possible in the future through genetic engineering, genetic counseling, and selective application of antiviral therapy (including vaccines) and immunotherapy.[170]

REFERENCES

 1. Purtillo DT, Linder J: Oncological consequences of impaired immune surveillance against ubiquitous viruses. J Clin Immunol 3:197–206, 1983
 2. Kirsch IR, Brown JA, Lawrence J et al: Translocations that highlight chromosomal regions of differentiated activity. Cancer Genet Cytogenet 18:159–171, 1985
 3. Gatti RA, Good RA: Occurrences of malignancy in immunodeficiency diseases. A literature review. Cancer 28:89–98, 1971
 4. Filipovich AH, Heinitz KJ, Robison L et al: The immunodeficiency cancer registry, a research resource. Pediatr Hematol Oncol 9:183, 1987
 5. Filipovich AH, Shapiro R, Robison L et al: Lymphoproliferative disorders associated with immunodeficiency. In Magrath I (ed): Non-Hodgkins Lymphoma. London, Arnold (in press)
 6. Hecht F, Hecht BK: Chromosome changes connect immunodeficiency and cancer in ataxia-telangiectasia. Am J Pediatr Hematol Oncol 9:185–188, 1987
 7. Spector BD, Filipovich AH, Perry GS III et al: Epidemiology of cancer in ataxia-telangiectasia. In Bridges BA, Harnden DG (eds): Ataxia-telangiectasia: A cellular and molecular link between cancer, neuropathology, and immune deficiency, pp 103–138. Chichester, England, John Wiley, 1982
 8. Swift M, Reitnauer PJ, Merrell D et al: Breast and other cancers in families with ataxia-telangiectasia. N Engl J Med 316:1289–1294, 1987
 9. Fiorilli M, Carbonari M, Crescenzi M et al: T cell receptor genes and ataxia-telangiectasia. Nature 313:186, 1985
10. McCaw BK, Hecht F, Harnden DG et al: Somatic rearrangement of chromosome 14 in human lymphocytes. Proc Natl Acad Sci USA 72:2071–2075, 1975
11. Taylor AMR, Butterworth SV: Clonal evolution of T cell chronic lymphocytic leukemia in a patient with ataxia-telangiectasia. Int J Cancer 37:511–516, 1986
12. Taylor AMR, Harnden DG, Arlett CF et al: Ataxia-telangiectasia: A human mutation with abnormal radiation sensitivity. Nature 258:427–429, 1975
13. Waldmann TA, Misiti J, Nelson DL et al: Ataxia-telangiectasia: A multi-system hereditary disease with immunodeficiency, impaired organ maturation, x-ray hypersensitivity, and a high incidence of neoplasia. Ann Intern Med 99:367–379, 1983
14. Shaham M, Becker Y: The ataxia-telangiectasia clastogenic factor in a low molecular weight peptide. Hum Genet 58:422–424, 1981

15. Waldmann TA, McIntire KR: Serum alpha-fetoprotein levels in patients with ataxia-telangiectasia. Lancet 2:1112, 1972

16. Sugimoto T, Swada T, Tozawa M et al: Plasma levels of carcinoembryonic antigen in patients with ataxia-telangiectasia. J Pediatr 92:436–439, 1978

17. Peterson RD, Kelly WD, Good RA: Ataxia-telangiectasia: Its association with a defective thymus, immunological-deficiency disease, and malignancy. Lancet 1:1189–1193, 1964

18. Fiorilli M, Businco L, Pandolfi F et al: Heterogeneity of immunological abnormalities in ataxia-telangiectasia. J Clin Immunol 3:135–141, 1983

19. McFarlin DD, Strober W, Waldmann TA: Ataxia-telangiectasia. Medicine (Baltimore) 51:281–314, 1972

20. Berkel AI, Henle W, Henle G et al: Epstein-Barr virus-related antibody patterns in ataxia-telangiectasia. Clin Exp Immunol 35:196, 1979

21. Saemundsen AK, Berkel A, Henle W et al: Epstein-Barr virus carrying lymphoma in a patient with ataxia-telangiectasia. Br Med J 282:425–427, 1981

22. Blaese RM, Strober W, Levy AL et al: Hypercatabolism of IG, IgA, IgM, and albumin in the Wiskott-Aldrich syndrome, a unique disorder of serum protein metabolism. J Clin Invest 50:2331–2338, 1971

23. Poplack DG, Bonnard GD, Holiman BJ et al: Monocyte mediated antibody dependent cellular cytotoxicity: A clinical test of monocyte function. Blood 48:809–816, 1976

24. Perry GS, Spector BD, Shuman LM et al: The Wiskott-Aldrich syndrome in the US and Canada (1892–1979). J Pediatr 97:72–78, 1980

25. Cotelingam JD, Witebsky FG, Hsu SM et al: Malignant lymphoma in patients with the Wiskott-Aldrich Syndrome. Cancer Invest 3:515–522, 1985

26. Chaganti RSK, Weigensberg M, Smithwick EM et al: Wiskott-Aldrich syndrome. Chromosomal instability in phytohemagglutinin-stimulated blood lymphocytes. Am J Human Genet 31:90(a), 1979

27. Schwartz RS: Immunoregulation, oncogenic viruses and malignant lymphomas. Lancet 1:1266–1269, 1972

28. Takemoto KK, Rabson AS, Mullarkey MF et al: Isolation of papovavirus from brain tumor and urine of a patient with Wiskott-Aldrich syndrome. J Natl Cancer Inst 53:1205–1207, 1974

29. Filipovich AH: Personal communication based on the updated Immunodeficiency Cancer Registry.

30. Borzy MS, Hong R, Horowitz SD: Fatal lymphoma after transplantation of cultured thymus in children with combined immunodeficiency disease. N Engl J Med 301:565–568, 1979

31. Reece ER, Gartner JG, Seemayer TA et al: Epstein-Barr virus in a malignant lymphoproliferative disorder of B-cells occurring after thymic epithelial transplantation for combined immunodeficiency. Cancer Res 41:4243–4247, 1981

32. Neudorf SM, Filipovich AH, Kersey JH: Immunoreconstruction by bone marrow transplantation decreases lymphoproliferative malignancies in Wiskott-Aldrich and severe combined immune deficiency syndromes. In Purtillo DT (ed): Immune deficiency and cancer: Epstein-Barr virus and lymphoproliferative malignancies, pp 471–480. New York, Plenum Press, 1984

33. Webster AO, Malkovsky M, Patterson S et al: Isolation of retroviruses from two patients with common variable hypogammaglobulinemia. Lancet 1:581–583, 1986

34. Cunningham–Rundles C, Siegal FP, Cunningham–Rundles S et al: Incidence of cancer in 98 patients with common varied immunodeficiency. J Clin Immunol 7:294–299, 1987

35. Bar RS, Delor CJ, Clausen KP et al: Fatal infectious mononucleosis in a family. N Engl J Med 290:363–367, 1974

36. Provisor AJ, Iacuone JJ, Chilcote RR et al: Acquired agammaglobulinemia after a life-threatening illness with clinical and laboratory features of infectious mononucleosis in three related male children. N Engl J Med 293:62–65, 1975

37. Purtillo DT, Yang JP, Cassel CK et al: X-linked recessive progressive combined variable immunodeficiency (Duncan's disease). Lancet 1:935–941, 1975

38. Grierson HL, Purtillo DT: Epstein-Barr virus infections in males with the x-linked lymphoproliferative syndrome. Ann Intern Med 106:538–545, 1987

39. Argov S, Johnson DR, Collins M et al: Defective natural killing activity but retention of lymphocyte-mediated antibody-dependent cellular cytotoxicity in patients with x-linked lymphoproliferative syndrome. Cell Immunol 100:1–9, 1986

40. Skare JC, Milunsky A, Byron KS et al: Mapping the x-linked lymphoproliferative syndrome. Proc Natl Acad Sci USA 84:2015–2018, 1987

41. Sullivan JL, Byron KS, Brewster FE et al: X-linked lymphoproliferative syndrome. J Clin Invest 71:1765, 1983

42. Penn I: The price of immunotherapy. Curr Probl Surg 18:681, 1981

43. Hoover R, Fraumeni JF: Risk of cancer in renal transplant recipients. Lancet 2:55, 1973

44. Kaskel FJ, Feld LG, Schoeneman MJ: Renal replacement therapy in infants and children. Adv Pediatr 31:197–267, 1985

45. Hanto DW, Gajl-Peczalska KJ, Frizzera G et al: Epstein-Barr virus induced polyclonal and monoclonal B-cell lymphoproliferative diseases occurring after renal transplantation. Ann Surg 198:356, 1983

46. Starzl TE, Nalesnick MA, Porter KA et al: Reversibility of lymphomas and lymphoproliferative lesions developing under cyclosporin-steroid therapy. Lancet 1:583, 1984

47. Bieber CP, Herberling RL, Jamieson SW et al: Lymphoma in the cardiac transplant recipients associated with cyclosporin A, prednisone and antithymocyte globulin (ATG). In Purtillo DT (ed): Immune Deficiency and Cancer, p 309. New York, Plenum Press, 1984

48. Penn I: Lymphomas complicating organ transplantation. Transplantation Proc 15:2790, 1983

49. Klein G, Klein E: Immune surveillance against virus-induced tumors and nonrejectability of spontaneous tumors: contrasting consequences of host versus tumor evolution. Proc Natl Acad Sci USA 74:2121, 1977

50. Louie S, Schwartz RS: Immunodeficiency and the pathogenesis of lymphoma and leukemia. Semin Hematol 15:117, 1978

51. Matos AJ, Simmons RL, Najarian JS: Chronic antigenic stimulation, herpesvirus infection, and cancer in transplant recipients. Lancet 1:1277, 1975

52. Forman SJ, Sullivan JL, Wright C et al: Epstein-Barr virus-related malignant B cell lymphoplasmacytic lymphoma following allogeneic bone marrow transplantation for aplastic anemia. Transplantation 44:244–249, 1987

53. Forman SJ, Gallagher MT: Reconstitution of the immune system. In Blume KG, Petz LD (eds): Clinical Bone Marrow Transplantation, p 65. New York, Churchill Livingstone, 1983

54. Zutter MM, Martin PJ, Sale GE et al: Epstein-Barr virus lymphoproliferation after bone marrow transplantation. Blood (in press)

55. Epstein MA, Achong BG, Barr YN: Virus particles in cultures lymphoblasts from Burkitt's malignant lymphoma. Lancet 1:702–703, 1964

56. Henle W, Henle G, Lennette EL: The Epstein-Barr virus. Sci Am 241:48, 1979

57. Sixby JW, Lemon SM, Pagano JS: A second site for Epstein-Barr virus shedding: The uterine cervix. Lancet 2:1122, 1986

58. Sixby JW, Nedrud JG, Raab–Traub N et al: Epstein-Barr virus replication in oropharyngeal epithelial cells. N Engl J Med 310:1225, 1984

59. Svedmyr E, Ernberg I, Seeley J et al: Virologic, immunologic and clinical observations on a patient during the incubation, acute and convalescent phases of infectious mononucleosis. Clin Immunol Immunopathol 30:437, 1984

60. Purtillo DP: Immunodeficiency predisposing to Epstein-Barr virus induced lymphoproliferative diseases: The x-linked lymphoproliferative syndrome as a model. Adv Cancer Res 34:279–312, 1981

61. De Waile M, Theilemans C, Van Camp BKG: Characterization of immunoregulatory T cells in Epstein-Barr virus-induced infectious mononucleosis by monoclonal antibodies. N Engl J Med 304:460, 1981

62. Tosato G: Epstein-Barr virus and the immune system. Adv Cancer Res 49:75–125, 1987

63. Henle W, Henle G, Horowitz CA: Epstein-Barr virus specific diagnostic tests in infectious mononucleosis. Hum Pathol 5:551, 1974

64. Rocchi G, de Felici AP, Rogona G et al: Quantitative evaluation of Epstein-Barr virus infected mononuclear peripheral blood leukocytes in infectious mononucleosis. N Engl J Med 296:132–134, 1977

65. Thorley–Lawson DA, Geilinger K: Monoclonal antibodies against the major glycoprotein (gp 350/220) of Epstein-Barr virus neutralize infectivity. Proc Natl Acad Sci USA 77:5307–5311, 1980

66. Hanto DW, Frizzera G, Gajl–Peczalska KJ: Epstein-Barr virus, immunodeficiency, and B cell lymphoproliferation. Transplantation 39:461–472, 1985

67. Royston I, Sullivan JL, Periman PO et al: Cell-mediated immunity to Epstein-Barr-virus-transformed lymphoblastoid cells in acute infectious mononucleosis. N Engl J Med 293:1159–1163, 1975

68. Moss DJ, Rickinson AB, Pope JH: Long term T-cell mediated immunity to Epstein-Barr virus in man. Complete regression of virus-induced transformation in cultures of seropositive donor leukocytes. Int J Cancer 22:662–668, 1978

69. Klein E, Klein G, Levine PH: Immunological control of human lymphoma: Discussion. Cancer Res 36:724–727, 1976

70. Tosato G, Blaese RM: Epstein-Barr virus infection and immunoregulation in man. Adv Immunol 37:99–149, 1985

71. Wong–Staal F, Gallo RC: Human T-lymphotropic retroviruses. Nature 317:395–403, 1985

72. Takatsuki K, Uchiyama J, Sagawa K et al: Adult T-cell leukemia in Japan. In Seno S, Takaku K, Irino S (eds): Topics in Hematology, pp 73–77. Amsterdam, Excerpta Medica, 1977

73. Bunn PA, Schechter GP, Jaffe E et al: Clinical source of retrovirus-associated adult T-cell lymphoma in the United States. N Engl J Med 309:257–264, 1983

74. Sugiyama H, Doi H, Yamaguchi K et al: Significance of postnatal mother-to-child transmission of human T lymphotropic virus type I on the development of adult T-cell leukemia/lymphoma. J Med Virol 20:253–260, 1986

75. Katsuki T, Katsuki K, Imai J et al: Immune suppression in healthy carriers of adult T-cell leukemia retrovirus (HTLV-I): Impairment of T cell control of Epstein-Barr virus-infected B cells. Jpn J Cancer Res 78:639–642, 1987

76. Popovic M, Sarin PS, Robert–Gierroff M et al: Isolation and transmission of human retrovirus. Science 219:856–859, 1983

77. Hara T, Takahashi Y, Sonoda S et al: Human T-cell lymphotropic virus Type I infection in neonates. Am J Dis Child 141:764–765, 1987

78. Williams DL, Ragab A, McDougal JS et al: HTLV-I antibodies in childhood leukemia. JAMA 253:2496, 1985

79. Snover DC, Frizzera G, Spector BD et al: Wiskott-Aldrich syndrome: Histopathologic findings in the lymph nodes and spleens of 15 patients. Hum Pathol 12:821–831, 1981

80. Frizzera G, Rosai J, Dehner LP et al: Lymphoreticular disorders in primary immunodeficiencies. New findings based on an up-to-date histologic classification of 35 cases. Cancer 46:692–699, 1980

81. Levy R, Warnke R, Dorfman RF et al: The monoclonality of human B-cell lymphomas. J Exp Med 145:1014–1028, 1977

82. Sullivan JL: Hematologic consequences of Epstein-Barr virus infection. Hematol Oncol Clin North Am 1:397–417, 1987

83. Schnitzer B: Reactive lymphoid hyperplasia. In Jaffe ES (ed): Surgical Pathology of the Lymph Nodes and Related Organs, pp 22–56. Philadelphia, WB Saunders, 1985

84. Tindle BH, Parker JW, Lukes RJ: "Reed-Sternberg cells" in infectious mononucleosis. Am J Clin Pathol 58:607–617, 1972

85. Arnold A, Cossman J, Bakhshi A et al: Immunoglobulin gene rearrangements as unique clonal markers in human lymphoid neoplasms. N Engl J Med 309:1593–1599, 1983

86. Lipford EH, Smith HR, Pittaluga S et al: Clonality of angioimmunoblastic lymphadenopathy and implications for its evolution to malignant lymphoma. J Clin Invest 79:637–642, 1987

87. Hecht F, Hecht BK: Ataxia telangiectasia breakpoints in chromosome rearrangement reflect genes important to T and B lymphocytes. KROC Found Ser 19:189–195, 1985

88. Cleary ML, Chao J, Warnke R et al: Immunoglobulin gene rearrangement as a diagnostic criterion of B cell lymphoma. Proc Natl Acad Sci USA 81:593–597, 1984

89. Cleary M, Warnke R, Sklar J: Monoclonality of B-lymphocyte proliferations in cardiac transplant recipients: Clonal analysis based on immunoglobulin gene rearrangement. N Engl J Med 310:477–482, 1984

90. Cleary ML, Sklar J: Lymphoproliferative disorders in cardiac transplant recipients are multiclonal lymphomas. Lancet 2:489–493, 1984

91. Kaiser–McCaw B, Hecht F: Ataxia-telangiectasia; chromosomes and cancer. In Bridges BA, Harnden DG (eds): Ataxia-telangiectasia: A Cellular and Molecular Link Between Cancer, Neuropathology, and Immune Deficiency, pp 243–257. New York, John Wiley & Sons, 1982

92. Gianelli F, Benson PF, Pawsey SA et al: Ultraviolet light sensitivity and delayed DNA-chain maturation in Bloom's syndrome fibroblast. Nature 265:466, 1977

93. Barak Y, Nir E: Chediak Higashi Syndrome. Am J Pediatr Hematol Oncol 9:42–55, 1987

94. Rubin CM, Burke BA, McKenna RW et al: The accelerated phase of Chediak–Higashi syndrome: An expression of the virus-associated hemophagocytic syndrome? Cancer 56:524–530, 1985

95. Argyle JC, Kjeldsberg CR, Marty J et al: T-cell lymphoma and the Chediak-Higashi syndrome. Blood 60:672–676, 1982

96. Roder JC, Haliotis T, Klein M et al: A new immunodeficiency disorder in human involving NK cells. Nature 284:553, 1980

97. Tanaka H, Ito T, Orii T: DNA repair mechanism in Chediak-Higashi cells. J Inherited Metab Dis 5:65–66, 1982

98. Hanto DW, Frizzera G, Gajl–Peczalska KJ et al: Acyclovir therapy of Epstein-Barr virus (EBV)-induced posttransplant lymphoproliferative. Transplant Proc 17:89, 1985

99. Tate MN, Henslee PJ, Cibull M et al: Clinico-pathologic manifestations of Epstein-Barr virus (EBV) related lymphoproliferative disorder following bone marrow transplantation. Blood 70:315a, 1987

100. Fleisher G, Starr, S, Koven N et al: A non-x-linked syndrome with susceptibility to severe Epstein-Barr virus infections. J Pediatr 100:727–730, 1982

101. Gill JC, Menitove JE, Wheeler D et al: Generalized lymphadenopathy and T cell abnormalities in hemophilia. J Pediatr 103:18–22, 1983

102. Kohn DB, Trigg ME, Borcherding W et al: Immunologic studies of lymph node lymphocytes in the generalized lymphadenopathy syndrome. Am J Pediatr Hematol Oncol 9:1–7, 1987

103. Abrams DI: AIDS-related lymphadenopathy: The role of biopsy. J Clin Oncol 4:126–127, 1986

104. Meyer PR, Yanagihara ET, Parker JW et al: A distinctive follicular hyperplasia in the acquired immune deficiency syndrome (AIDS) and the AIDS related complex. Hematol Oncol 2:319–347, 1984

105. Ryan B, Connor E, Minnefor A et al: Human immunodeficiency virus infection in children. Hematol Oncol Clin North Am 1:381–395, 1987

106. Bernstein LJ, Rubinstein A: Acquired immunodeficiency syndrome in infants and children. Prog Allergy 37:194–206, 1986

107. Andiman WA, Martin K, Rubinstein A et al: Opportunistic lymphoproliferations associated with Epstein-Barr viral DNA in infants and children with AIDS. Lancet 2:1390–1393, 1985

108. Buck BE, Scott GB, Valdes–Dopena M et al: Kaposi sarcoma in two infants with acquired immune deficiency syndrome. J Pediatr 103:911–913, 1983

109. Fahey JL, Ojo–Amaize E: Acquired immune deficiency syndrome and neoplasia. Am J Pediatr Hematol Oncol 9:193–195, 1987

110. Vilmer E, Le Deist F, Fischer A et al: Smouldering T lymphoma related to HTLV-I in a Sicilian child. Lancet 2:1301, 1985

111. Stensvold K, Brandtggzaeg P, Kvaly S et al: Immunoblastic lymphadenopathy with early onset in 2 boys: Immunohistochemical study and indication of decreased proportion of circulating T helper cells. Br J Haematol 56:417, 1984

112. Lukes RJ, Tindle BH: Immunoblastic lymphadenopathy: A hyperimmune entity resembling Hodgkin's disease. N Engl J Med 292:1, 1975

113. Pangalis GA, Moran EM, Nathwani BW et al: Angioimmunoblastic lymphadenopathy: Long term follow-up study. Cancer 52:318–321, 1983

114. Boros L, Bhaskar AG, D'Souza JP: Monoclonal evolution of angioimmunoblastic lymphadenopathy. Am J Clin Pathol 75:856–860, 1981

115. Grier JJ, York JC, Cousar JB et al: Peripheral T cell lymphoma: A clinicopathologic study of 42 cases. J Clin Oncol 2:788–798, 1984

116. Ganesan TS, Dhaliwal HS, Dorreen MS et al: Angioimmunoblastic lymphadenopathy: A clinical, immunological and molecular study. Br J Cancer 55:437, 1987

117. Patton WF, Lynch JP: Lymphomatoid granulomatosis. Medicine 61:1–12, 1982

118. Liebow AA, Carrington CRB, Friedman PJ: Lymphomatoid granulomatosis. Hum Pathol 3:457–549, 1972

119. Shen SC, Heuser ET, Landing BH et al: Lymphomatoid granulomatosis-like lesions in a child with leukemia in remission. Hum Pathol 12:276–280, 1981

120. Bekassy AN, Cameron R, Garwicz S et al: Lymphomatoid granulomatosis during treatment of acute lymphoblastic leukemia in a 6 year old girl. Am J Hemat Oncol 7:377–380, 1985

121. Pearson AD, Kirpalani H, Ashcraft T et al: Lymphomatoid granulomatosis in a 10 year old boy. Br Med J 286:1313–1314, 1983

122. Sordillo PP, Epremian B, Koziner B et al: Lymphomatoid granulomatosis: An analysis of clinical and immunologic characteristics. Cancer 49:2070–2076, 1982

123. Veltri RW, Raich PC, McClung JE et al: Lymphomatoid granulomatosis and Epstein-Barr virus. Cancer 50:1513–1517, 1982

124. Foucer E, Rosai J, Dorfman RF: Sinus histiocytosis with massive lymphadenopathy. Cancer 54:1834–1840, 1984

125. Rosai J, Dorfman RF: Sinus histiocytosis with massive lymphadenopathy: A pseudolymphomatous benign disorder. Cancer 30:1174–1188, 1972

126. Keller AR, Hochholzer L, Castleman B: Hyaline-vascular and plasma-cell types of giant lymph node hyperplasia of the mediastinum and other locations. Cancer 29:670–683, 1972

127. Miller FS, Miller JJ: Benign giant lymph node hyperplasia presenting as fever of unknown origin. J Pediatr 87:237–239, 1975

128. Buchanan GR, Chipman JJ, Hamilton BL et al: Angiomatous lymphoid hamartoma: Inhibitory effects on erythropoiesis, growth and primary hemostasis. J Pediatr 99:382–388, 1981

129. Seligmann M, Rambaud JC: Alpha-chain disease: An immunoproliferative

disease of the secretory immune system. Ann NY Acad Sci 190:478–485, 1983

130. Galian AM, Lecestre J, Scotto C et al: Pathological study of alpha-chain disease, with special emphasis on evolution. Cancer 39:2081–2101, 1977

131. Rambaud JC, Matuchansky C: Alpha-chain disease: Pathogenesis and relation to Mediterranean lymphoma. Lancet 1:1430–1432, 1973

132. Ramot B, Levanon M, Hahn Y et al: The mutual clonal origin of the lymphoplasmocytic and lymphoma cell in alpha heavy chain disease. Clin Exp Immunol 27:440–445, 1977

133. Franklin EC: Gamma and mu heavy chain diseases and related disorders. J Clin Pathol 27:65–71, 1974

134. Frangioni B, Franklin EC: Heavy chain diseases: Clinical features and molecular significance of the disordered immunoglobulin structure. Semin Hematol 10:53–63, 1973

135. Knowles DM, Halpen JP, Jakobiec FA: The immunologic characterization of 40 extranodal lymphoid filtrates. Cancer 49:2321–2335, 1982

136. Knowles DM, Jakobiec FA: Ocular adnexal lymphoid neoplasms: Clinical, histopathologic, electron microscopic, and immunologic characteristics. Hum Pathol 13:148–162, 1982

137. Franklin DJ, Smith RJ, Person DA et al: Sjogren's Syndrome in children. Otolaryngol Head Neck Surg 94:230–235, 1986

138. Vermylen C, Meurant A, Noel H et al: Sjogren's Syndrome in a child. Eur J Pediatr 144:266–269, 1985

139. Kassan SS, Thomas TL, Moutsopoulos HM et al: Increased risk of lymphoma in Sicca syndrome. Ann Intern Med 89:888–892, 1978

140. Hartsock RJ: Postvaccinial lymphadenitis. Cancer 21:632–649, 1968

141. Lapin JH, Tuason J: Immunization adenitis. JAMA 158:472, 1955

142. Calabro JJ, Holgerson WB, Conpal GM et al: Juvenile rheumatoid arthritis: A general review and report on 100 patients observed for 15 years. Semin Arthritis Rheum 5:257, 1976

143. Fox RA, Rosahn PD: The lymph nodes in disseminated lupus erythematosis. Am J Pathol 19:73, 1943

144. Kojis FG: Serum sickness and anaphylaxis. Am J Dis Child 64:133, 1942

145. Pattishall EN, Strope GL, Spinola SM et al: Childhood sarcoidosis. J Pediatr 108:169–177, 1986

146. Zeulzer WW, Kaplan J: The child with lymphadenopathy. Semin Hematol 12:323, 1975

147. Constantinidis K: Acute and chronic berylliosis disease. Br J Clin Pract 32:127, 1978

148. Canale VC, Smith CH: Chronic lymphadenopathy simulating malignant lymphoma. J Pediatr 70:891, 1967

149. Lake AM, Oski FA: Peripheral lymphadenopathy in childhood. Am J Dis Child 132:357–359, 1978

150. Knight PJ, Mulne AF, Vassy LE: When is a lymph node biopsy indicated in children with enlarged peripheral nodes? Pediatrics 69:391–396, 1982

151. Horowitz CA, Henle W, Henle G et al: Heterophil-negative infectious mononucleosis and mononucleosis-like illnesses. Am J Med 63:947, 1977

152. Klemola E, Kaariainen L: Cytomegaloviruses as a possible cause of a disease resembling infectious mononucleosis. Br Med J 2:1099, 1965

153. Herrod HG, Wang WC, Sullivan JL: Chronic T cell lymphocytosis with neutropenia associated with Epstein-Barr virus infection. Am J Dis Child 139:405, 1985

154. Herrod HG, Dow LW, Sullivan JL: Persistent Epstein-Barr virus infection in two children with a syndrome mimicking juvenile chronic myelogenous leukemia. Blood 61:1098, 1983

155. Straus SE, Tosato G, Armstrong G et al: Persisting illness and fatigue in adults with evidence of Epstein-Barr virus infection. Ann Intern Med 102:7–16, 1985

156. Tobi M, Ravid Z, Feldman–Weiss V et al: Prolonged atypical illness associated with serological evidence of persistent Epstein-Barr virus infection. Lancet 1:61–64, 1982

157. Schooley RT, Carey RW, Miller G et al: Chronic Epstein-Barr virus infection associated with fever and interstitial pneumonitis. Ann Intern Med 104:636, 1986

158. Kawa–Ha K, Franco E, Doi S et al: Successful treatment of chronic active Epstein-Barr virus infection with recombinant interleukin-2. Lancet 1:154, 1987

159. Miller DG: The association of immune disease and malignant lymphoma. Ann Intern Med 66:507–521, 1967

160. Cohen DL: Sicca Syndrome: An unusual manifestation of sarcoidosis in childhood. Am J Dis Child 137:289–290, 1983

161. Li FP, Willard DR, Goodman R et al: Malignant lymphoma after diphenylhydantoin (Dilantin) therapy. Cancer 36:1359–1362, 1975

162. Choovivathanavanich P, Wallace EM, Scaglione PR: Pseudolymphoma induced by diphenylhydantoin. J Pediatr 76:621–623, 1970

163. Powers NG, Carsen SH: Idiosyncratic reactions to phenytoin. Clin Pediatr 26:120–124, 1987

164. Hyman GA, Sommers SC: Development of Hodgkin's disease and lymphoma during anticonvulsant therapy. Blood 28:416–427, 1966

165. Ziegler JA, Magrath M: Lymphoma in HIV positive individuals. In Magrath I (ed): Non-Hodgkins Lymphoma. London, Arnold (in press)

166. Barriga F, Whang–Peng J, Lee E et al: Development of a second clonally discrete Burkitt's lymphoma in a human immunodeficiency virus (HIV) positive patient. Blood (in press)

167. Colby BM, Shaw JE, Elion GB et al: Effect of acyclovir on Epstein-Barr virus DNA replication. J Virol 34:560–568, 1980

168. Hanto DW, Frizzera G, Gajl–Peczalska KJ et al: Epstein-Barr virus-induced B cell lymphoma after renal transplantation. N Engl J Med 306:913–918, 1982

169. Sullivan JL, Byron KS, Brewster FE et al: Treatment of life-threatening Epstein-Barr virus infections with acyclovir. Am J Med 73:262, 1962

170. Thorley–Lawson DA: A virus-free immunogen effective against Epstein-Barr virus. Nature 281:486, 1979

twenty-three

The Histiocytoses

Stephan Ladisch and Elaine S. Jaffe

The childhood histiocytoses are a very rare and diverse group of disorders that have presented great difficulties in diagnosis and treatment to pediatricians. This has been true for nearly a century, since the first clear description of a childhood histiocytosis, Hand-Schuller-Christian disease.[1] The confusion surrounding the childhood histiocytoses is exemplified by the term coined for one group of these disorders, histiocytosis X. This term, with "X" standing for unknown, was proposed by Lichtenstein in 1953 to underscore the lack of understanding of these disorders.[2] Likewise, the rarity of the histiocytoses has prevented adequate epidemiologic studies to date. The only form of histiocytosis that has a definite genetic component is familial erythrophagocytic lymphohistiocytosis.

The forms of histiocytosis are frequently difficult to distinguish on a clinical basis. Yet they must be unequivocally differentiated from one another, as they require very different treatment approaches. Correct and complete pathological diagnosis is essential. Paradoxically, although the diagnosis and treatment of these disorders is frequently relegated to the pediatric oncologist, the majority of the histiocytoses are not malignancies. The actual distinction between malignant and nonmalignant forms of childhood histiocytosis has been difficult in the past. This confusion undoubtedly has led to suboptimal treatment in some cases. In fact, the prognosis of many of the childhood histiocytoses has been considered with more pessimism than is justified. Formulation of an appropriate treatment plan rests on the ability to distinguish among the various severe forms of childhood histiocytosis and establish an accurate diagnosis. This requires an understanding of the biological features of this group of diseases and their relationship to the normal histiocytic subsets of the reticuloendothelial system.

BIOLOGY

The historical association of several childhood diseases and syndromes into the single category of histiocytosis resulted from histopathologic findings that at least at a superficial level appeared to be common to all of these diseases. The term histiocytosis literally signifies an increase in the number of histiocytes, or mononuclear phagocytic cells of bone marrow origin. The diseases and syndromes included under histiocytosis are characterized by an infiltration and accumulation of cells of the monocyte/macrophage series in the involved tissues. However, not all diseases in which histiocytic infiltrations are prominent are classified as histiocytoses. In some instances, histiocytic infiltration represents a secondary rather than a primary process. Some examples include graft-versus-host disease, the X-linked lymphoproliferative syndrome, and certain of the inherited lipidoses. This implies that in the future, diseases currently classified as histiocytoses of unknown etiology may be found to have an etiology which establishes the histiocytic infiltration as a secondary process, not a primary process. An understanding of the histiocytoses requires understanding of the normal histiocyte.

The origin of normal histiocytes is the bone marrow, and the differentiation of these cells occurs according to the following sequence: The most primitive precursor of the tissue macrophage is the uncommitted stem cell, found in the bone marrow. Current theory suggests that this stem cell undergoes one differentiation step to become a stem cell committed to further development in the granulocyte/macrophage series. Upon exposure to colony stimulating factors, soluble factors promoting bone marrow proliferation and differentiation, the committed stem cell further differentiates into a colony forming cell or myeloblast/monoblast. As the next step, this precursor cell matures into the monocyte which is found in the peripheral blood. This circulating monocyte then undergoes terminal differentiation into cells that are found in essentially every organ of the body. These cells are known by various names according to their tissue location, for example, bone marrow macrophages, Kupffer cells in the liver, and Langerhans cells in the skin.

The cells of the histiocytic system can be classified into two major subsets thought to be derived from the same bone marrow precursor: antigen processing or phagocytic cells and antigen presenting or dendritic cells (Table 23-1).[3-7] Dendritic cells are generally not phagocytic and have as their major function the presentation of antigen to both T and B lymphocytes. Dendritic reticulum cells (DRCs) are found in lymph node follicles and present antigen to B lymphocytes. The interdigitating reticulum cells (IRCs) and Langerhans cells (LCs) are functionally related and both present antigen to T lymphocytes. LCs are found primarily in the skin but are also present in other organs. LCs are relatively rare in unstimulated lymph nodes, but their numbers increase in certain reactive conditions. IRCs are found throughout the paracortex of normal and reactive lymph nodes.

Phenotypically, dendritic cells lack the abundant lysosomal enzymes characteristic of phagocytic macrophages (Table 23-2).[8] Both IRCs and LCs have small amounts of lysosomal enzyme activity for acid phosphatase and nonspecific esterase. The reactivity generally has a punctate perinuclear distinction and is localized to the golgi region. DRCs lack lysosomal enzyme activity. All three dendritic cell types, however, manifest enzyme activity for ATPase.

The dendritic cell types have strong reactivity for HLA-DR or Class II antigens on their cell surface membranes.[9] Class II antigens play an important role in the presentation of antigen to T and B lymphocytes (see also Chap. 4). It is the CD4-positive subpopulation of T cells that recognizes antigen in the context of Class II antigens.[10] In contrast the CD8-positive T-cell subset recognizes antigen in the context of Class I.

All three dendritic cell subpopulations manifest IgG Fc receptors and under some conditions will manifest complement receptors.[11] DRCs have strong receptors for the C3d receptor, recognized by antibodies of the CD21 class (B2, BL10).[12] DRC is a specific monoclonal antibody that reacts exclusively with DRCs in frozen sections and is very useful in their identification in normal and neoplastic lymph nodes (Table 23-3). IRCs and LCs are characterized by strong reactivity for S100 protein, which is totally lacking on DRCs. Lesser amounts of S100 immunoreactivity can be identified in activated monocytes and macrophages.[13]

LCs demonstrate immunoreactivity for the CD1 antigen as identified by T6 monoclonal antibodies (see Table 23-3).[14] This antigen is also expressed on cortical thymocytes. IRCs generally lack the CD1 antigen, but it is controversial as to whether T6 immunoreactivity can be induced on IRCs in certain reactive conditions. The T6 immunoreactive cells that appear in dermatopathic lymphadenitis may represent infiltrating LC, derived from outside the lymph node, or CD1 immunoreactivity induced on resident IRCs. LCs have characteristic ultra-

---

Table 23-1
Histiocytic and Reticulum Cell Subsets

Antigen Processing Cells (Phagocytic)	Antigen Presenting Cells (Dendritic)
Tissue macrophages	Dendritic reticulum cell (lymph node follicle)
Monocytes	Interdigitating reticulum cell (lymph node paracortex)
Tingible body macrophages (lymph node follicle)	Langerhans cell (skin, *etc.*)
Sinusoidal histiocytes	
Epithelioid histiocytes	

Table 23-2
Features of Macrophage and Reticulum Cell Subsets

	FcIgG	CD21 CR	HLA-DR	AP/NSE	Phg	ATPase	S100	Lyso	AT
Monocyte	+	+	+	+	+	−	−	+	+
Macrophage	+	+	+	++	+	−	+/−	+/−	+
DRC	+	+	+	−	−	+	−	−	−
IRC	+	−	+	+/−	−	+	+	−	−
LC	+	−	+	+/−	−	+	+	−	−

FcIgG, receptor for the Fc fragment of IgG; CR, complement receptor (C3d); AP/NSE, acid phosophatase/nonspecific esterase; Phg, phagocytic activity; S100, reactivity with S100 proteins; lyso, lysozyme; AT, alpha 1-anti-trypsin activity; DRC, dendritic reticulum cell; IRC, interdigitating reticulum cell; LC, Langerhans cell.

Table 23-3
Immunoreactivity of Macrophage and Reticulum Cell Subsets

	CD11c LEUM5	CD25 TAC	T9	CD4 T4	CD14 MY4	CD13/CD33 MY7/9	DRC	CD1 T6	CD45 LCA
Monocyte	+	+	+	+	+	+	−	−	+
Macrophage	+	+	+	+	+	−	−	−	+
DRC	−	−	−	−	−	−	+	−	+
IRC	−	−	+/−	+/−	−	−	−	−	+
LC	−	−	−	+/−	−	−	−	+	+

structural organelles known as Birbeck granules.[15] They are rod-shaped structures of variable length that contain a central striation and a vesicular expansion and produce a racket shape. The function of the Birbeck granule is unknown. The dendritic cell populations in general lack many of the antigens expressed on monocytes and macrophages described below.

Tissue histiocytes or macrophages are found in all the major compartments of the normal lymph node. Sinus histiocytes are the principal cells involved in the phagocytosis of foreign particulate matter and are located predominantly within lymph node sinuses. Tingible body macrophages are phagocytic cells found in normal germinal centers. In the presence of a florid follicular hyperplasia, these cells become more numerous. They frequently contain karyorrhectic nuclear debris, presumably derived from spontaneous necrosis and karyorrhexis of proliferating germinal center cells. Tingible body macrophages are also conspicuous in high-grade malignant lymphomas and are especially prominent in Burkitt's lymphoma, where they have been described as demonstrating a starry-sky pattern (see Chap. 20). Their role in these tumors is the same as in the normal lymph node, and they contain karyorrhectic debris derived from necrotic lymphoid cells.

Tissue macrophages or histiocytes are also prominent in the paracortex of lymph nodes. In paracortical lymphoid hyperplasias, such as viral lymphadenitis, these histiocytes become prominent and produce a mottled pattern. Epithelioid histiocytes and multinucleated giant cells are associated with granulomatous lesions involving lymph nodes.

The macrophages of the reticuloendothelial system share many enzyme histochemical and immunophenotypic characteristics. They have abundant and diffuse activity for lysosomal enzymes including acid phosphatase and nonspecific esterase.[16,17] As stated above, all of these cells can also demonstrate phagocytosis under appropriate conditions. HLA-DR antigens, complement receptors, and receptors for the Fc fragment of IgG are common to all macrophages in lymph nodes. Activity for lysozyme and alpha 1 antitrypsin can be seen in all of the above subtypes as well but is most prominent in epithelioid histiocytes.[18] Activity for lysozyme decreases abruptly with phagocytosis, presumably because of its loss into lysosomal vacuoles.

A variety of monoclonal antibodies have been derived that react with monocytes and macrophages.[19-21] Unfortunately, none of these reagents is specific for the mononuclear phagocytic system, and all have been shown to react with other hematopoietic cells as well: myeloid cells, T cells, or B cells (see Chap. 4). The CD11c antigen detected by LeuM5 is present on monocytes and macrophages, and is absent on normal T and B lymphocytes. However, this antigen is found on the cells of hairy cell leukemia (a B-cell lymphoproliferative disorder) and in some cases of B-cell chronic lymphocytic leukemia.[22] Similarly, the CD14 antigen detected by MY4 is present on mono-

cytes and macrophages as well as on most normal and neoplastic B lymphocytes. Within normal lymph nodes, CD14 expression is strong on mantle zone B and weak on germinal center B cells.

Cross-reactivities with T cells are present as well. For example, the CD4 antigen characteristic of the so-called helper T-cell subset is found in normal monocytes and macrophages.[23] Receptors for interleukin-2 (CD25), formerly known as T-cell growth factor, in addition to being found on activated T lymphocytes, are found on normal monocytes and macrophages.[24,25] Transferrin receptors, normally a feature of activated or proliferating hematopoietic and nonhematopoietic cells, are strongly expressed on monocytes and macrophages, even if these cells do not appear to be undergoing cellular proliferation.[26]

The MY7 (CD13) and MY9 (CD33) antigens that are characteristic of cells of the granulocytic series are also expressed on normal peripheral blood monocytes but to a lesser extent in tissue macrophages.[27]

All of the macrophage and reticulum cell subsets express the leukocyte common antigen detected by CD45 antibodies, attesting to their common hematopoietic origin.

Pathophysiology of the Histiocytoses

Several theories have been advanced to explain the pathophysiology of the four major severe childhood histiocytoses. In the case of histiocytosis X (now more correctly called Langerhans cell histiocytosis [LCH]; see subsequent discussion) it is suspected that immunologic stimulation of a normal antigen-processing cell, the LC, continues in an uncontrolled manner, resulting in the proliferation and accumulation of these cells. That this results in disordered immunoregulation that may be central to the disease process is suggested by recent findings of defective immunologic function in patients with LCH.[28] These patients showed autocytotoxicity, or destruction of their own fibroblasts and antibody-coated erythrocytes by their own effector cells *in vitro*. These immunologic findings were associated with abnormal thymic histology.[28,29] Furthermore, the administration of thymic extract was associated with clinical improvement and reversal of the defective immunologic responses *in vitro*. Although it has been suggested that LCH is a malignancy, there has been no experimental support for this concept by demonstration of a clonal origin of these cells, although the cells may show some cytologic atypia.

Histiocytic reactions that are secondary to known causes would be expected to disappear upon resolution of the underlying disease process. As will be discussed in detail later in this chapter, this is the case in infection-associated hemophagocytic syndrome. Thus, it is possible that in this syndrome, the macrophage is reacting to a foreign antigen adsorbed onto the formed blood elements, including erythrocytes.

An alternate explanation is that the hemophagocytic syndrome might be secondary to excessive lymphokine production by normal or neoplastic T lymphocytes.[30] Such a lymphokine has been isolated from CD4-positive T lymphocytes.[31,32] The lymphokine, termed phagocytosis inducing factor (PIF), was isolated from normal T cells, cloned T-cell lines, and mononuclear cells from patients with angiocentric immunoproliferative diseases.[31] The lymphokine can stimulate the cells of the U937 histiocytic cell line to undergo histiocytic differentiation and phagocytosis of IgG-coated red blood cells. Thus, it is hypothesized that in certain clinical situations, in particular in association with defective T-cell function, there exists a state of abnormal immune regulation. A precipitating event such as an infection results in marked stimulation of the immune system. T cells become activated and elaborate lymphokines, including PIF. However, lymphokine production fails to be shut off, possibly because of abnormal feedback regulation. The excessive lymphokine production continues unchecked with marked stimulation of mononuclear phagocytes and the development of a hemophagocytic syndrome.

In the case of familial erythrophagocytic lymphohistiocytosis (FEL), the pathophysiology of the disease clearly includes an element of immunodeficiency associated with plasma inhibitory activity.[33] The cell-mediated immune defects may be responsible for the opportunistic infections frequently suffered as terminal events in patients with FEL. The immune defects are secondary, however, because treatment (e.g., plasmapheresis) can remove plasma immunosuppressive activity and result in complete recovery of cellular immunodeficiency *in vivo*.[34] How this secondary immunodeficiency relates to the underlying genetic (autosomal recessive) disease, and to the unknown trigger of the clinical exacerbations of FEL, is not known at this time.

Finally, only in the case of neoplastic proliferation of cells of the monocyte/macrophage series (e.g., malignant histiocytosis) is the pathophysiology clearly one of a clonal proliferation of histologically malignant cells, as is the case in other diseases discussed in this book.

PATHOLOGY

A recently formed international group, The Histiocyte Society, has proposed a system for the classification of the childhood histiocytoses.[35] The basis for classification is to relate these lesions to the normal histiocytic and reticulum cell subsets. This classification system is a pathologic one, as the ultimate diagnosis of all the childhood histiocytoses rests upon the findings of pathologic examination. While this schema does not include all proliferative histiocytic lesions of children or adults, it provides a conceptual approach to the diagnosis and classification of these disorders. The major forms of childhood histiocytosis are grouped into three classes, as presented in Table 23-4.

Class I Histiocytoses

Class I includes those histiocytoses in which the central cell has the histopathologic features of the LC. LCH, formerly known as histiocytosis X, is the principal disease in this class, and also the main proliferative lesion of the LC. LCH replaces the term histiocytosis X as well as the syndromes eosinophilic granuloma, Hand-Schuller-Christian disease, and Letterer-Siwe disease, which had been included under the terms histiocytosis X.[28,36-43] LCH is not considered a neoplasm but a proliferative lesion, possibly secondary to a defect in immunoregulation.[29,44] The cells of LCH demonstrate the phenotypic

Table 23-4
Classification of Childhood Histiocytoses

Class I	Class II	Class III
	Diseases Included	
Langerhans cells histiocytosis*	Infection-associated hemophagocytic syndrome (IAHS); familial erythrophagocytic lymphohistiocytosis (FEL)	Malignant histiocytosis; acute monocytic leukemia; true histiocytic lymphoma
	Cellular Characteristics of the Lesions	
Langerhans cells with cleaved nuclei and Birbeck granules seen by electron microscopy, cell surface antigens include S-100 and CD-1; cells mixed with varying proporations of eosinophils; multinucleated giant cells sometimes seen	Morphologically normal, reactive macrophages with prominent erythrophagocytosis; process involves entire reticuloendothelial system	Neoplastic cellular proliferation of cells exhibiting characteristics of macrophages or their precursors; localized or systemic
	Proposed Pathophysiologic Mechanisms of the Histiocytosis	
Immunologic stimulation of a normal antigen-processing cell—the Langerhans cell—in a somehow uncontrolled manner	Secondary histiocytic reaction an unknown antigenic stimulation (FEL) or an infectious agent (IAHS), with erythrophagocytosis possibly reflecting foreign antigens adsorbed on erythrocytes or activation of macrophages by excess lymphokine production because of abnormal immunoregulation	Neoplasm; clonal autonomous uncontrolled proliferative process

* Previously known as histiocytosis X and its related syndromes of eosiniophilic granuloma, Hand-Schuller-Christian disease and Letterer-Siwe disease.

characteristics of normal LCs including S-100-positivity, CD1 (OKT6) expression, and Birbeck granules (Fig. 23-1).[45-48] In contrast to normal LCs, the cells of LCH also express antigens associated with phagocytic histiocytes such as CD11 and CD14 (Table 23-5).[49,50]

Grossly, the lesions of LCH are granulomatous and, when visible, appear yellow-brown in color. As such, they are easily seen in the skin. The hallmark of these lesions is the presence of LCs by light microscopy. These cells have deeply indented nuclei and low nuclear:cytoplasmic ratios (Fig. 23-2). The lesions in LCH may consist of either pure histiocytic infiltrates or mixed histiocytic/eosinophilic lesions, as are commonly seen in lytic bone lesions of this disease.[51-53] In addition to the varying proportion of eosinophils present, multinucleated giant cells are also sometimes present. Necrosis may be evident. In partially involved lymph nodes, the process involves

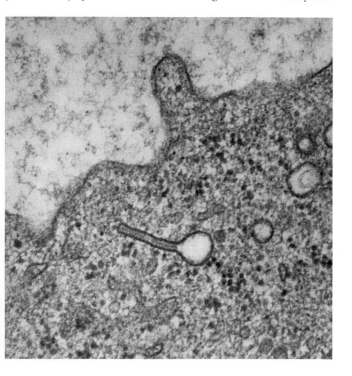

FIGURE 23-1. Electron micrograph of a Langerhans cell showing Birbeck granules. This cell was obtained by needle aspiration from a patient with lymph node involvement of Langerhans cell histiocytosis.

the paracortex. Although cytologic atypia may be observed in the LC, cytologic atypia is said not to be a significant prognostic factor.[54]

The key pathologic finding in LCH is the presence of Birbeck granules[10] in cells of the lesions detected by electron microscopy (see Fig. 23-1). The significance of this diagnostic structure is not known,[11] although it is also found in the normal LC of the skin, a cell whose role is to process antigens. It has therefore been suggested that LCH might represent an uncontrolled immunologic reaction to an unknown foreign antigen.[55] In support of this possibility are the findings of autocytotoxicity previously discussed. The presence of Birbeck granules in cells of the lesions is the diagnostic finding in LCH.

As noted earlier, although it had been suggested that LCH might be a malignancy there has been no experimental support for this concept by demonstration of a clonal origin of these cells, although the cells may show some cytologic atypia. LCs have been described in lymph nodes in association with a variety of malignant lymphomas, most often Hodgkin's disease.[56-58] In this situation LCH appears to be an incidental finding to a localized process and does not have any independent prognostic importance. Malignant proliferations of LCs have not been recognized.[46]

Class II Histiocytoses

The Class II histiocytoses represent the largest group of disorders and include the nonmalignant histiocytoses in which the accumulating mononuclear cell is of the phagocytic (antigen-processing) cell type (see Table 23-1). This contrasts them with the Class I diseases, also reactive histiocytoses but of antigen-presenting or dendritic cell type. In the Class II histiocytoses, the normal monocyte/macrophage is the predominant cell, frequently in a mixed lymphohistiocytic infiltrate. The characteristic findings on lymph node biopsy include infiltration of the node, especially of the sinusoids, cortex, and paracortex, without effacement of nodal architecture. Involved nodes may later evidence lymphocytic depletion with increased numbers of histiocytes.

The striking major histopathologic finding in the Class II histiocytoses (FEL and infection-associated hemophagocytic syndrome [IAHS]) is the morphologically normal appearance of the involved cells; there is no cytologic atypia (Fig. 23-3). The marked histiocytic proliferation is observed throughout the reticuloendothelial system. Sites most markedly affected include the bone marrow, splenic red pulp, hepatic sinusoids, and lymph node sinuses.[30,59] Cytologically, the histiocytes ap-

Table 23-5
Phenotypes of Proliferative Histiocytic Lesions

	CD11C LeuM5	CD21 TAC	T9	CD4 T4	CD14 MY4	CD13/CD33 MY7/9	DRC	CD1 T6	S100	CD30 Ki-1
THL	+	−	+	+/−	+	−	−	−	+/−	−
AMOL	+	+	+	+/−	+	+	−	−	nd	−
SHML	+	+	+	+	+	−	−	−	+	−
LCH	+	+	+/−	+	+	+/−	−	+	+	−
SLCL	−	+	+	+/−	−	−	−	−	nd	+

(Adapted from Wood GS, Warner NL, Warnke RA: Anti-Leu-3/T4 antibodies react with cells of monocyte/macrophage and Langerhans lineage. J Immunol 131:212–216, 1983)

THL, true histiocytic lymphoma; AMOL, acute monocytic leukemia; SHML, sinus histiocytosis with massive lymphadenopathy; LCH, Langerhans cell histiocytosis; SLCL, sinusoidal large cell lymphoma.

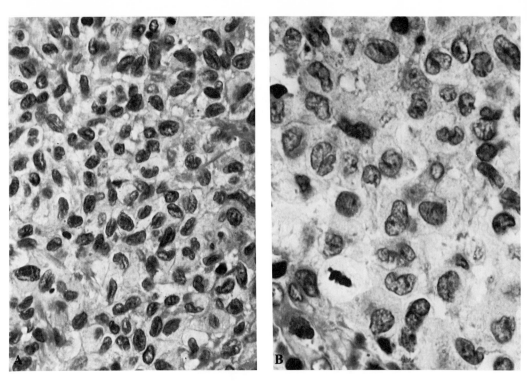

FIGURE 23-2.   Histopathologic features of Langerhans cell histiocytosis. **A.** Langerhans cells exhibit delicate nuclear chromatin with fine nuclear grooves. **B.** Cytologic atypia in Langerhans cells may be seen in some cases but is said not to be a significant prognostic feature.

pear activated, with abundant cytoplasm and prominent phago-cytosis of the formed elements of the blood, including erythro-cytes, leukocytes, and platelets. These reactive histiocytes have low nuclear:cytoplasmic ratios, mature nuclear chromatin, in-conspicuous nucleoli, and abundant cytoplasm.[12] Striking erythrophagocytosis (and in fact phagocytosis of all cellular blood elements) is characteristic of both IAHS and FEL. On histopathologic criteria alone, FEL and IAHS may be indistin-guishable from each other but should be clearly distinguish-able from both Class I and Class III histiocytoses.

With respect to the evolution of the lesions, resolution of the infection in the case of IAHS results in complete resolution of the histiocytic infiltration and the erythrophagocytosis. Simi-larly, apparent clinical remission in FEL is associated with dis-appearance of the pathologic infiltrates. Thus, the Class II syn-dromes are characterized by a clearly secondary accumulation of histiocytes. The mechanisms causing these accumulations, however, remain unknown. In both cases, electron microscopy is negative for the Birbeck granules that characterize the cells of LCH. The mixed lymphohistiocytic infiltrates further help to distinguish the disseminated Class II histiocytoses from Class I disease, in which either mixed histiocytic/eosinophilic or pure histiocytic infiltrates are seen.

Several other rare Class II histiocytoses are mentioned, primarily because they enter into the differential diagnosis of lymphadenopathy or skin lesions in which histiocytic infiltra-tion is prominent.

In sinus histiocytosis with massive lymphadenopathy (SHML), affected lymph nodes demonstrate a marked fibrous thickening of the capsule. Residual follicles are usually present and demonstrate a florid follicular hyperplasia. In keeping with the polyclonal hypergammaglobulinemia seen in these patients, a prominent plasmacytosis is present as well. The sinuses and interfollicular regions are expanded by a marked histiocytic proliferation. The histiocytes have abundant clear

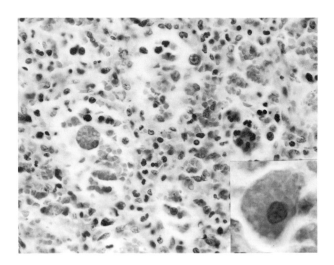

FIGURE 23-3.   Infection-associated hemophagocytic syndrome. His-tiocytic infiltrates with prominent erythrophagocytosis (*inset*) are characteristic of both this syndrome and familial erythrophagocytic lymphohistiocytosis. Histiocytes are cytologically normal.

cytoplasm and distinct cytoplasmic membranes. A characteris-tic feature is the phenomenon of emperipolesis in which ap-parently viable lymphocytes and plasma cells are identified within vacuoles within the cytoplasm of the histiocytic cells.

The nuclei of the proliferating histiocytes appear activated and may contain small but distinct nucleoli. However, cyto-logic anaplasia indicative of malignancy has not been de-scribed.

Phenotypically, the cells of SHML demonstrate many of the properties of phagocytic macrophages.[51] The cells contain abundant activity of lysosomal enzymes. They also demonstrate weak reactivity for S100 protein.[52] Although S100 protein is more characteristic of IRCs, weak activity may be seen in normal and reactive sinus histiocytes. The cells of SHML are negative with the DRC and T6 monoclonal antibodies but do demonstrate reactivity for CD4, CD11, CD14, CD25, and transferring receptors. Of course, all of the above are present on normal histiocytes and macrophages.

In histiocytic necrotizing lymphadenitis (Kikuchi's disease), histiocytes constitute a significant component of the inflammatory lesion that characterizes this disease.[60–62] The cause of this reactive lymphadenopathy is unknown. Kikuchi's disease is characterized by a focal necrotizing lesion within lymph nodes, usually located in the paracortex. Although karyorrhexis is conspicuous, neutrophils are absent. The proliferating cells are predominantly histiocytes and immunoblasts. The process is often misdiagnosed as a large cell or histiocytic lymphoma because of the prominent immunoblastic component and partial obliteration of lymph node architecture that may be seen.[62]

Two pediatric benign histiocytic proliferative disorders are characterized primarily by skin involvement with multiple cutaneous nodules. In juvenile xanthogranuloma (multiple cutaneous nodules), lesions are composed of a monotonous cellular infiltrate of histiocytes with frequent multinucleated Touton giant cells in the subcutaneous tissue. The cytoplasm is abundant and eosinophilic. Cytologically the cells appear benign. The cells cytochemically and ultrastructurally have the features of macrophages.[63] They are strongly positive for lysozyme.

In self-healing reticulohistyocytosis, the cutaneous nodules are composed of large histiocytic cells that may demonstrate cytologic atypia. This feature distinguishes this disease from juvenile xanthogranuloma, in which cytologic atypia is less prominent. Multinucleated forms may be present and mitotic figures are observed. The cells contain either foamy or eosinophilic ground glass-like cytoplasm. Erythrophagocytosis is not a conspicuous feature.

Class III Histiocytoses

Class III comprises the malignant disorders of mononuclear phagocytes, including acute monocytic leukemia, malignant histiocytosis, and true histiocytic sarcoma. These three malignancies represent a spectrum in terms of their degree of dissemination and can be conceptually related to different stages of maturation and differentiation in the mononuclear phagocytic series.[64] Acute monocytic leukemia relates to a bone marrow–derived monoblast. This malignancy arises in the bone marrow compartment with secondary involvement of the peripheral blood and usually a markedly elevated white blood cell count. In contrast to acute myeloid leukemia, there is a somewhat higher incidence of involvement of nonhematopoietic sites, with frequent involvement of skin and gingiva. Hepatosplenomegaly and lymphadenopathy are relatively common (25% and 50%, respectively).[65] Acute monocytic leukemia is discussed further in Chapter 17.

Malignant histiocytosis represents a malignancy of mononuclear phagocytes that are intermediate in differentiation between monocytes and monoblasts and fixed tissue histiocytes. In many instances the syndromes of acute monocytic leukemia and malignant histiocytosis may merge, and the distinction may be arbitrary and somewhat semantic.[66,67] Malignant histiocytosis is a systemic malignancy involving the entire reticuloendothelial system.[68–71] Within the lymphoreticular system there is preferential involvement of sites normally populated by histiocytes, such as lymph node sinuses, splenic red pulp, and hepatic sinusoids. Bone marrow involvement is common, and although abnormal cells can be seen in the peripheral blood, if peripheral blood involvement is extensive a diagnosis of acute monocytic leukemia should be considered. Other frequent sites of involvement include skin and bone.[72]

The cells in malignant histiocytosis have atypical characteristics (Fig. 23-4). The nucleus is large with a reticular chromatin pattern and prominent nucleolus. Cells exhibit a basophilic cytoplasm and stain positively for acid phosphatase and nonspecific esterase.[5,13] Erythrophagocytosis may be present but is not prominent, as it is in the Class II histiocytoses. Even if phagocytosis is observed, it is virtually always clinically insignificant. The clinical syndrome of histiocytic medullary reticulosis, characterized by hepatosplenomegaly, pancytopenia, and jaundice, once thought to be a variant of malignant histiocytosis, is recognized now as a manifestation of the Class II histiocytoses, most often IAHS.

The end point of the spectrum is the most rare form, histiocytic sarcoma or "true histiocytic lymphoma." This is a malignancy of the mononuclear phagocytic series at the stage of fixed tissue histiocytes. As such, the lesions in histiocytic sarcoma are localized and relatively discrete. In addition to the

FIGURE 23-4. Malignant histiocytosis. **A.** Neoplastic cells preferentially invade lymph nodes sinuses and, as seen in **B**, exhibit cytologically malignant features.

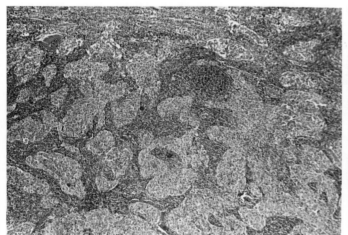
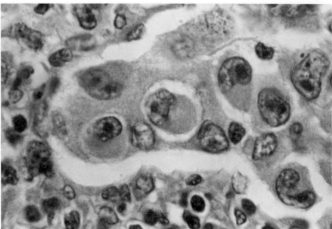

reticuloendothelial system, common sites of involvement include skin and bone.[64] Cytologically, the cells are unquestionably malignant. Without the benefit of specialized diagnostic tools, these lesions would fall into the category of large cell, immunoblastic lymphomas in the working formulation.[64,74]

Enzyme cytochemistry and histochemistry remain a reliable adjunct to morphology in the diagnosis of malignancies of the mononuclear phagocytic system. The cells have diffuse activity for nonspecific esterase, which is usually at least partially fluoride sensitive.[75] Preferable methods for detection of esterase activity include the alpha naphthyl butyrate esterase reaction because activity will not be observed in myeloid cells.[16] Myeloid cells also contain minimal, if any, activity for alpha naphthyl acetate esterase. The use of the naphthol ASD acetate esterase reaction requires the use of fluoride to distinguish myeloid and mononuclear phagocytic cells. Activity for acid phosphatase and B-glucuronidase is usually present as well. In all cases the activity should be relatively diffuse throughout the cytoplasm and not punctate. Punctate reactivity localized to the Golgi region is more characteristic of lymphoid than mononuclear phagocytic cells. Caution should be exercised in the use of enzyme cytochemistry because these enzymes are not specific for mononuclear phagocytes and can be seen in certain carcinomas and sarcomas.[76]

Note should be taken of one form of immunoblastic lymphoma that in some ways mimics a true histiocytic lymphoma. True histiocytic lymphomas preferentially involve lymph node sinuses. However, this feature is not specific and can be seen in certain T-cell immunoblastic lymphomas.[77,78] Indeed, most instances of so-called malignant histiocytosis appear to represent this variant of Ki-1-positive immunoblastic lymphoma. In this tumor the malignant cells have a propensity to invade lymphoid sinuses. Because of the sinusoidal location of the tumor cells, misdiagnosis as malignant histiocytosis or metastatic carcinoma has been common.[77] In most cases studied, the malignant cells express some T-cell antigens, although the cells have a markedly aberrant phenotype. T-cell gene rearrangement has also been shown in some instances.[79] A consistent feature is the expression of the Hodgkin's disease associated antigen CD30, detected by Ki-1 and Hefi-1. This antigen, although present on the malignant cells of Hodgkin's disease, is also found in activated T and B lymphocytes (but not in macrophages).

This tumor can present in all age groups but appears relatively common in children and young adults.[78] A high incidence of cutaneous disease has been reported. The skin lesions are deep dermal, but ulceration of the overlying epidermis may be seen in larger tumors. The process should be approached clinically as a large cell or aggressive non-Hodgkin's lymphoma (discussed further in Chap. 20).

To summarize, the new pathologic classification of the childhood histiocytoses includes LCH in Class I, the Class II histiocytoses that result from the accumulation of benign histiocytes as a secondary response to disease processes of unknown pathogenic mechanisms, and the Class III malignant histiocytic disorders. Histopathologic diagnostic criteria are summarized in Table 23-1. Accurate diagnosis of the childhood histiocytoses is vital. The presence of those pathologic features of definitive value in classifying these disorders must be identified: Birbeck granules uniformly and only in Class I histiocytoses, malignant characteristics uniformly and only in Class III histiocytoses, and benign reactive histiocytes comprising Class II histiocytoses. Attempting to make a clinical diagnosis without these histopathologic findings is not appropriate.

CLINICAL PRESENTATION AND TREATMENT

Class I Histiocytoses

Langerhans Cell Histiocytosis

The clinical presentation of LCH is extremely variable and may range from mild discomfort and irritability to specific lytic bone lesions (Fig. 23-5) that may have been diagnosed only incidentally on a radiograph obtained for another reason.[80-83] Other symptoms may include chronic otitis, diabetes insipidus, or generalized symptoms such as fever and weight loss. This varied clinical presentation may make the diagnosis of LCH difficult. As noted previously, the definitive diagnosis (see Table 23-6) rests on confirmation of the presence of the Birbeck granule–positive cells in the lesions of the disease as determined by electron microscopy. Other findings include positive immunostaining for S100 protein and the CD1 antigen (formerly known as the OKT6 antigen), neither of which is present on normal histiocytes.[9] It is important that the biopsy be obtained from a clearly involved tissue because normal LCs containing Birbeck granules are present in the skin as well. Multiple organ systems may be involved in this disorder (Table 23-7).

The clinical hallmark of LCH is the presence of lytic bone lesions (see Fig. 23-3) in the majority of cases.[81,84] When either single or multiple bone lesions alone were present, the disease was referred to as eosinophilic granuloma.[42,43] When granulomas were more widespread, causing bone lesions, diabetes insipidus (by involvement of the pituitary), and exophthalmos (by the presence of retroorbital granulomas), the disease was termed Hand-Schuller-Christian disease.[37-39] Finally, the disseminated form of LCH was previously called Letterer-Siwe disease.[28,40,41] This latter presentation is more commonly seen in infants and very young children (under the age of 2) and is characterized by wasting, hepatosplenomegaly, generalized

FIGURE 23-5. Langerhans cell histiocytosis. Radiograph of the characteristic lytic bone lesion, as seen in the skull of a patient whose other findings included exophthalmos and diabetes insipidus.

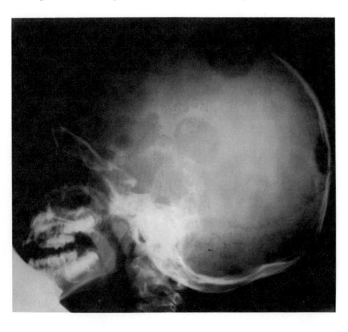

Table 23-6
Clinical, Prognostic, and Therapeutic Aspects of the Major Childhood Histiocytoses

Class I (LHC)	Class II (IAHS)	Class II (FEL)	Class III
Clinical Presentation			
Wide spectrum, from mild discomfort related to lesions (lytic bone lesions, chronic otitis, diabetes insipidus) to generalized symptoms including fever and weight loss	Pancytopenia, hepatosplenomegaly, fever, coagulopathy	Irritability, fever, wasting, sometimes with a coagulopathy, and hepatosplenomegaly	Variable, from systemic disease in acute monocytic leukemia to localized mass in true histiocytic lymphoma
Diagnostic Findings			
Birbeck granules and CD-1 expression in lesional cells	Morphologically normal macrophages; often documented infection and negative family history	Morphologically normal lymphocytes and macrophages; lack of specific infectious etiology; sometimes positive family history	Malignant macrophages
Prognosis			
Variable, but a self-resolving disease process in most cases	Excellent, providing underlying infection is controlled and immunosuppression can be reversed	Extremely poor; uniformly rapidly fatal	Poor for acute monocytic leukemia. Improving for MH and THL; up to 75% survival at 40 months reported with appropriate therapy
Recommended			
None to mild radiation or chemotherapy (vinblastine and steroids) for certain lesions	Avoidance of all immunosuppressive therapy	Experimental	Adriamycin in a combination chemotherapy regimen for MH and THL; appropriate treatment for acute monocytic leukemia

Table 23-7
Organ System Involvement in Langerhans Cell Histiocytosis

Site	Percentage of Cases Involved
Bone	80
Skin	60
Liver, spleen, lymph nodes	33
Bone marrow	30
Lungs	25
Orbit	25
Orodental	20
Otological	20
Central nervous system	
Diabetes insipidus	15
Hydrocephalus, nerve palsies	<5
Gastrointestinal tract	<5

(Callihan TR: The surgical pathology of the differentiated histiocyses. In Jaffe ES [ed]: Surgical Pathology of the Lymph Nodes and Related Organs, pp 357–380. Philadelphia, WB Saunders, 1985)

lymphadenopathy, anemia, and sometimes pancytopenia. The milder forms of LCH are seen primarily in older children and less commonly in adults. The clinical finding of seborrheic dermatitis deserves special mention. It is often present on the scalp, and in infants may easily be confused with a nonspecific dermatitis. However, as with the other lesions of LCH, biopsy and examination by electron microscopy or immunohisto-chemistry, or both, is diagnostic. In addition to the clinical findings discussed above, virtually every tissue may be involved in LCH, including the lung, gastrointestinal tract (colon), and central nervous system (the cerebellum as well as the pituitary gland and hypothalamus). How the sometimes protean manifestations of the disease process are linked to one another remains to be determined. Therefore, clinical classification of the forms of LCH remains to be further developed.

The outcome of LCH is extremely variable, but in most cases the disease is a self-resolving process. The two prognostic factors appear to be age at the time of diagnosis and degree of organ involvement.[80,83,85] Children younger than 2 years of age at the time of diagnosis have a higher mortality rate than do older children. Likewise, the presence of organ dysfunction (*e.g.,* liver, lungs, bone marrow) has been found to be a poor prognostic sign, with the involvement of multiple organ systems having an additive negative effect on survival. Fortunately, children with these poor prognostic features constitute fewer than 15% of LCH cases. Other than these two factors and the knowledge that the disease usually resolves completely and spontaneously, little is known about the natural evolution of the disease process and the effects of intervention.

The approaches to treatment of LCH over the last century have been as varied as the clinical presentation of the disease.[28,85–91] Thus, treatment has ranged from antimicrobial therapy, based on the assumption that LCH is an infectious disease, to chemotherapy, based on the belief that this disorder is an aggressive malignancy. Although a number of reports in the literature have supported a role for chemotherapy by demonstrating improvement in the overall survival rate compared to historical controls, careful diagnosis and stratification for severity of disease were not always been applied in these studies. When such analyses were performed on a large number of patients, all uniformly classified, it was concluded that disseminated LCH, with multiple organ involvement, has a relatively poor prognosis that has not been changed substantially by various treatments.[55] In contrast, mild disease has an excellent prognosis that also has not changed by the administration of any particular therapy.[55,92] These findings suggest that very little progress has been made in the development of definitive therapy for LCH. As this concept is now relatively widely accepted by pediatric oncologists, current treatment approaches tend to employ less intensive therapy, when it is indicated. Specifically, this includes use of vinblastine, with or without the addition of prednisone, and low dose radiation therapy.

In the absence of a specific, definitive treatment, the therapeutic approach to the child with LCH should be directed toward preventing permanent, that is, irreversible damage to normal tissues by LCH lesions which eventually will spontaneously resolve. Thus, treatment should be directed toward halting or reversing the progression of lesions. This approach has been widely applied to cases of isolated bone involvement in LCH, and may also be applicable to more disseminated disease. However, even the use of mild therapy remains controversial because of the absence of definitive prospective studies evaluating various treatment approaches to this entity. A sufficiently large, prospective, randomized treatment study is necessary if we are to improve our knowledge of the evolution of the childhood histiocytoses and reach firm conclusions regarding the indications for and the optimal mode of therapy. In the interim, the use of low-dose radiation therapy to specific lesions that threaten permanent damage is recommended. Doses in the range of 500 to 1000 cGy have been administered to such single lesions. Systemic therapy, vinblastine (0.4 mg/kg weekly) with or without corticosteroids, has been used similarly in the case of more widespread disease. Newer approaches such as treatment with thymic hormone are being studied. These trials are based on findings that suggest a role for autoimmunity in this disease.[28,86]

Dendritic and Interdigitating Reticulum Cell Tumors

Although LCH is the major form of histiocytosis included in Class I, at least two additional very rare lesions have recently been described that have a proposed derivation from DRCs and IRCs, respectively.[93,94,95] These disorders tend to present as localized lymph node disease. Although local recurrence may occur, systemic spread does not. These tumors are often associated with an inflammatory background or necrosis, or both. Whether these proliferations represent benign or malignant neoplasms, or even possibly atypical reactive processes, has not been determined. Only limited phenotypic studies have been performed in such cases. Those lesions derived from DRC have been characterized by prominent desnosomal attachments, which are also seen ultrastructurally on normal DRCs.

Class II Histiocytoses

Diseases falling into this category consist of those in which reactive cells of the mononuclear phagocytic cell series, excluding LCs, are found in the lesions. The histiocytic reaction is presumed secondary to a primary underlying disease process. Since the histiocytic proliferation may result from different pathogenetic mechanisms, it could be predicted that both the prognosis and treatment of the individual diseases in this class may be widely different. This is in fact the case. The two major diseases in this category are FEL and IAHS.

Familial Erythrophagocytic Lymphohistiocytosis (FEL)

FEL is characterized by the presence of hemophagocytosis and a positive family history.[96–99] Early in the disease, biopsy of lymph nodes demonstrates lymphoid proliferation. Later, however, lymphoid depletion occurs. Patients exhibit multiple defects in cellular and humoral immunity; a plasma inhibitor of lymphocyte blastogenesis has been demonstrated.[33]

FEL is a rare and almost always rapidly fatal disease. An autosomal recessive pattern of inheritance has been recognized since the initial studies of Farquar and Claireaux,[97] but a genetic marker for this disease has not yet been identified. The pathogenesis of FEL is not understood. The clinical presentation is that of a generalized disease. Affected children, usually under 3 or 4 years of age at the time of diagnosis, most often present with a fever of unknown origin and weight loss. They may have the overall clinical appearance of failure to thrive. Physical examination may reveal hepatosplenomegaly and sometimes a maculopapular skin eruption. The latter is distinguished from the yellow brown eruption of LCH by its color, which is frequently red to purple. The central nervous system may be involved, with symptoms including disorientation, seizures, and sometimes coma.[100] Laboratory findings may include marked hyperlipidemia, hypofibrinogenemia, and the cellular immunologic dysfunction mentioned earlier. Although it was initially thought that some or all of these laboratory findings were related to the underlying primary disease process, this is apparently not the case because the onset of temporary clinical remission results in normalization of all laboratory parameters.[34] It now appears more likely that these abnormalities are a secondary phenomenon, as is the histiocytic reaction, in this genetic disease of undefined pathogenesis. Chromosomal abnormalities of a nonspecific nature have been reported.[101] Erythrophagocytosis in FEL is very marked, particularly late in the course of the disease, and the terminal phase, which resembles the hemophagocytic syndromes, is frequently characterized by pancytopenia and jaundice.[102]

The diagnosis of FEL rests on identification of a lymphohistiocytic infiltrate, often with conspicuous erythrophagocytosis, together with an appropriate clinical and family history. The diagnosis may be made from examination of lymph nodes, spleen, liver, bone marrow, or lungs. The presence of a positive family history is obviously very helpful. However, since it is inherited in an autosomal recessive fashion, frequently this history will not be available. Often the correct diagnosis is not reached until a second family member is affected.

The rapid and fulminant course of FEL, coupled with findings of marked lymphohistiocytic organ infiltration, has resulted in the erroneous consideration of this disease as a malignancy. Consequently, cytotoxic chemotherapy has been employed in the treatment of FEL.[103] Agents that have been used include vinblastine, VP-16, and other more convenient antileukemic drugs. In general, however, treatment has been unsuccessful, with the usual rapidly fatal course of the disease only slightly prolonged by the administration of therapy. The lack of benefit from chemotherapy is not surprising given that the disease is histopathologically benign. Because of the relative lack of success of these treatments, other more experimental therapeutic approaches have been employed. Plasma exchange therapy, consisting of a series of plasmaphereses or plasma exchange transfusions, was based on the findings of circulating immunosuppressive activity in this disease.[34] Following exchange therapy, reduction in plasma inhibitory activity and reversal of the depressed cellular immune responses have been observed. Although clinical improvement was noted in an early trial of this approach, the disease subsequently relapsed. Another experimental approach applied to the treatment of FEL is bone marrow transplantation. This strategy is based on the hypothesis that the disease represents either an autonomous or uncontrolled proliferation of lymphocytes and histiocytes. One patient has been treated, apparently successfully, by this approach. In general, however, the treatment approaches for FEL are unsatisfactory. Further understanding of the disease process is essential before effective treatment for FEL is likely to be identified.

Infection-Associated Hemophagocytic Syndrome (IAHS)

IAHS was first described as a response to a viral infection in an immunocompromised host.[59] Subsequently, IAHS has been reported in association with a variety of infections, including viral, bacterial, fungal, and parasitic infections.[104,105] This hemophagocytic syndrome usually occurs in a setting of immunodeficiency. The immunodeficiency may be iatrogenic, as in organ transplant recipients receiving immunosuppression, or congenital. IAHS has also been seen in association with lymphoid malignancies, most often of a the T-cell type, such as acute lymphocytic leukemia and the angiocentric immunoproliferative disorders.[30,106–110] The clinical features of IAHS are similar to those of FEL, and include fever and other constitutional symptoms, liver function and coagulation abnormalities, and anemia. The coagulopathy appears to be multifactorial. Clotting factors are markedly diminished, presumable secondary to liver disease, and a component of consumption coagulopathy is also seen.[59] It should be stressed that although the overwhelming nature of the histiocytic proliferation has resulted in this syndrome being confused with malignant histiocytosis, histopathologic analysis can clearly distinguish these two forms of childhood histiocytosis. Moreover, the clinical features associated with IAHS are not characteristic of true histiocytic malignancies, malignant histiocytosis and true histiocytic lymphoma.[49] It is important to distinguish IAHS from a true histiocytic malignancy because cytotoxic chemotherapy is contraindicated for IAHS.

The diagnosis of IAHS is most readily made on bone marrow aspirate where frequent benign-appearing histiocytes containing platelets and red cells are seen. Lymph nodes usually demonstrate lymphoid depletion and marked infiltration by benign histiocytes. As the histiocytes are normal and reactive, they demonstrate all of the phenotypic and enzyme cytochemical characteristics of normal activated macrophages.[30]

As mentioned above, IAHS usually occurs in a clinical setting characterized by immunodeficiency. If the diagnosis is made, immunosuppression should be withdrawn and supportive care instituted. Treatment for the underlying infection should be instituted. Acyclovir administration has been useful in some patients with Epstein-Barr viral infections and IAHS.[111]

Other Class II Histiocytoses

Sinus histiocytosis with massive lymphadenopathy (SHML) (Rosai-Dorfman disease) presents primarily in the first two decades of life.[112] It affects boys and girls equally and is seen more often in blacks than in other races. Patients generally present with massive cervical lymphadenopathy, although many other sites can be involved, including skin, orbit, bone, salivary gland, and the upper respiratory tract. Patients usually exhibit some systemic symptoms, including fever, increased erythrocyte sedimentation rate, polyclonal hypergammaglobulinema, and neutrophilic leukocytosis.[113] The etiology of SHML remains obscure. A relation to an underlying immunodeficiency has been postulated. Although SHML is not considered a malignant disorder, considerable morbidity and mortality can result.[114,115] The lesions are locally destructive and can involve almost every organ system. Both radiotherapy and chemotherapy have been used with some success, and in some cases the lesions spontaneously regress.[116,117]

Histiocytic necrotizing lymphadenitis (HNL) is a reactive lymphadenopathy, the cause of which is unknown. The disorder usually presents in cervical or axillary lymph nodes. It affects women much more often than men and is more common in Orientals than in whites or blacks. The peak incidence is in the third decade of life, but it may be seen in children and adolescents. Clinically, patients exhibit mild constitutional symptoms, fever, fatigue, and localized adenopathy. An infectious etiology is suspected but has not been confirmed. No bacteria or fungi are seen on special stains, and serologic evaluations for toxoplasmosis or Epstein-Barr viral infection have been negative. Because HNL is entirely benign and has a self-limited clinical course, correct diagnosis is critical. No treatment is indicated.

Juvenile xanthogranuloma is a benign histiocytic lesion of the skin first described by Helwig and Hackney.[118] It occurs predominantly in neonates and young children. The process is characterized by one or more cutaneous nodules, often restricted to the head, neck, trunk, and proximal portions of the extremities. Extracutaneous involvement has also been reported. The lesions usually persist for 1 to 2 years and then spontaneously resolve.[118]

Self healing reticulohistiocytosis presents in the perineonatal period.[119] Patients present with multiple firm cutaneous nodules that range in color from dark red to dark blue. The nodules resolve spontaneously within 2 or 3 months. In some patients, hematologic abnormalities such as neutropenia or lymphocytosis, or both, have been reported. The process is distinguished from juvenile xanthogranuloma in that more cytologic atypia of the histiocytic cells is evident. The clinical course is benign, and no therapy other than supportive care is indicated.

Class III Histiocytoses

The histiocytoses that are true neoplasms constitute a minority of the childhood histiocytoses. As noted previously, three major forms are known (acute monocytic leukemia, malignant histiocytosis, and true histiocytic lymphoma). Acute monocytic leukemia, included in this class because of its cell origin, is discussed in Chapter 17.

True malignant histiocytosis is a very rare disease. When it occurs it is usually seen in older children and adults but has been described in young children. Affected children present with symptoms of a generalized illness. Clinical symptoms and findings include fever, wasting, lymphadenopathy, and hepatosplenomegaly. Raised skin lesions, peripheral lymphadenopathy, and subcutaneous inflammatory infiltrates also may be seen. Each of these findings represents infiltration by tumor cells. Thus, the clinical presentation may be very similar to that of FEL or IAHS. Indeed, some cases diagnosed as malignant histiocytosis in the past may have actually belonged to one of the hemophagocytic syndromes in Class II.[120,121]

As discussed earlier in the section on pathology, the diagnosis may best be made on a lymph node biopsy. Circulating tumor cells are rarely observed in these patients, who nevertheless almost always exhibit some degree of peripheral pancytopenia. Malignant histiocytosis must be distinguished from the other histiocytoses and from disseminated (Stage IV) Hodgkin's disease, immunoblastic non-Hodgkin's lymphoma, and immunoblastic lymphadenopathy. In these latter disorders, immunophenotypic characterization may be a helpful diagnostic tool.

True histiocytic lymphomas may involve lymph nodes, the reticuloendothelial system, and skin and bone. When initially confined to the skin, this disease has been reported to pursue an indolent clinical course with spontaneous regression of lesions observed in some cases.[122] The entity initially described as regressing atypical histiocytosis may represent histiocytic sarcoma with this characteristic presentation.[123] Alternatively, the clinical and pathologic features of the cutaneous lesions are remarkably similar to lymphomatoid papulosis, a chronic self-remitting T-cell lesion of the skin.[124] Therefore, the nature of regressing atypical histiocytosis and isolated histiocytic sarcomas of the skin need to be reassessed.[125,126] Indeed, clonal rearrangements of the T-cell antigen receptor genes have been demonstrated in one case of regressing atypical histiocytosis.[127]

The appropriate treatment of the Class III malignant histiocytic disorders of childhood is based on accurate diagnosis. Acute monocytic leukemia should be approached with treatment appropriate for that disorder. Because the diagnosis and classification of malignant histiocytic disorders have undergone such dramatic change in recent years, critical evaluation of previous clinical series is problematic and conclusions regarding therapeutic efficacy are difficult. As noted earlier, many cases previously diagnosed as malignant histiocytosis represented either hemophagocytic syndromes (a benign disorder) or Ki-1 positive large cell immunoblastic lymphoma (an aggressive non-Hodgkin's lymphoma) (see Chap. 20).[77,79,128,129]

However, malignant histiocytosis is one childhood histiocytosis in which a marked change in prognosis has occurred over the last years. Formerly, this disease was considered to be almost uniformly fatal. However, survival has now improved markedly, apparently because of the addition of Adriamycin to the combination chemotherapy treatment regimens for malignant histiocytosis.[129] With the addition of this agent, a median survival of less than 6 months has been increased to one of approximately 40 months. It has been recommended that children with malignant histiocytosis receive induction therapy with vincristine, prednisone, cyclophosphamide, and Adriamycin, and subsquent maintenance therapy consisting of vincristine, cyclophosphamide, and Adriamycin.[68] The use of intensive, aggressive, Adriamycin-containing regimens also appears to be effective in the treatment of true histiocytic lymphomas.[49]

CONCLUSION

Most of the childhood histiocytoses have historically been discussed in pediatric oncology textbooks only because of their traditional assignment to this subspecialty of pediatrics. Since most of these disorders are not true malignancies, the use of antineoplastic agents in their treatment should be carefully limited (with the exception of the treatment of Class III histiocytoses). Careful documentation of the natural history of the childhood histiocytoses, and use of the new system of pathologic classification discussed in this chapter, may help provide a framework for the eventual development of optimal therapeutic approaches. Ultimately, improvement in the outcome for children with the histiocytoses will depend on further elucidation of the etiology and pathogenesis of these diseases.

REFERENCES

1. Hand A Jr: Polyruia and tuberculosis. Arch Pediatr 10:673–675, 1893
2. Lichtenstein L: Histiocytosis X: Integration of eosinophilic granuloma of bone, 'Letterer-Siwe' and 'Schuller-Christian disease' as related manifestations of a single nosologic entity. Arch Pathol 56:84–102, 1953
3. Lasser A: The mononuclear phagocytic system: A review. Hum Pathol 14:108–126, 1983
4. Weiss L: The Cells and Tissues of the Immune System. Structure, Functions, Interactions. Englewood Cliffs, NJ, Prentice-Hall, 1972
5. VanFurth R, Taeburn JA, van Zwet TL: Characteristics of human mononuclear phagocytes. Blood 54:485–500, 1979
6. Steinman RM, Nussenzweig MC: Dendritic cells: Features and functions. Immunol Rev 53:125–147, 1980
7. Tew JG, Thorbecke GJ, Steinman RM: Dendritic cells in the immune response: Characteristics and recommended nomenclature. J Reticuloendothel Soc 31:371–380, 1982
8. Beckstead JH, Wood GS, Turner RR: Histiocytosis X cells and Langerhans cells: Enzyme histochemical and immunologic similarities. Hum Pathol 15:826–833, 1984
9. Stingl G, Katz SI, Clement L, et al: Immunological functions of Ia-bearing epidermal Langerhans' cells. J Immunol 121:2005–2010, 1978
10. Royer HD, Reinherz EL: T lymphocytes: Ontogeny, function, and relevance to clinical disorders. N Engl J Med 317:1136–1142, 1987
11. Stingl G, Wolff-Schreiner EC, Pichler WJ, et al: Epidermal Langerhans' cells bear Fc and C3 receptors. Nature 268:245–246, 1977
12. Stein H, Gerdes J, Mason DY: The normal and malignant germinal center. Clin Haematol 11:531–559, 1982
13. Wood GS, Turner PR, Shiurba RA, et al: Human dendritic cells and macrophages: In situ immunophenotypic definition of subsets that exhibit specific morphologic and microenvironmental characteristics. Am J Pathol 119:73–82, 1985
14. Murphy GF, Bhan AK, Harrist TJ, et al: In situ identification of T6-positive cells in normal human dermis by immunoelectron microscopy. Br J Dermatol 108:423–431, 1983
15. Birbeck MD, Breathnach AJ, Everall JD: An electron microscopic study of basal melanocytes and high level clear cells (Langerhans cells) in vitiligo. J Invest Dermatol 37:51–64, 1961
16. Shibata A, Bennett JM, Castoldi GL, et al: Recommended methods for cytochemical procedures in haematology. Clin Lab Haematol 7:55–74, 1985
17. Braziel RM, Hsu S-M, Jaffe ES: Lymph nodes, spleen, and thymus. In Spicer SS, Garvin AJ, Hennigar GR (eds): Application of Histochemistry to Pathologic Diagnosis, pp 203–256. New York, Marcel Dekker, 1986
18. Mason DY, Taylor CR: The distribution of muramidase (lysozyme) in human tissues. J Clin Pathol 28:124–132, 1975
19. Todd RF, Nadler LM, Schlossman SF: Antigens on human monocytes by monoclonal antibodies. J Immunol 126:1435–1438, 1981
20. Hanjan SNS, Kearney JF, Cooper MD: A monoclonal (MMA) that identifies a differentiation antigen on human myelomonocytic cells. Clin Immunol Immunopathol 23:172–176, 1982
21. Reinherz EL, Haynes BF, Nadler LM, et al: Leukocyte Typing II. Human Myeloid and Hematopoietic Cells, vol 3. New York, Springer-Verlag, 1988
22. Schwarting R, Stein H, Wang CY: The monoclonal antibodies S-HCL 1 (Leu-14) and S-HCL 3 (Leu-M5) allow the diagnosis of hairy cell leukemia. Blood 65:974–983, 1985
23. Wood GS, Warner NL, Warnke RA: Anti-Leu-3/T4 antibodies react with cells of monocyte/macrophage and Langerhans lineage. J Immunol 131:212–216, 1983
24. Robb RJ, Greene WC: Direct demonstration of the identity of T cell growth factor binding protein and the Tac antigen. J Exp Med 158:1332–1340, 1983
25. Lando Z, Sarin P, Megson M, et al: Association of human T-cell leukemia/lymphoma virus with the Tac antigen marker for the human T-cell growth factor receptor. Nature 305:733–735, 1983
26. Hsu S-M, Yang K, Jaffe ES: Phenotypic expression of Hodgkin's and Reed-Sternberg cells in Hodgkin's disease. Am J Pathol 118:209–217, 1985
27. Abt AF, Denenholz EJ: Letterer-Siwe's disease: Splenomegaly associated with widespread hyperplasia for non-lipid storing macrophages Discussion of the so-called reticuloendothelioses. Am J Dis Child 51:499, 196
28. Osband ME, Lipton JM, Lavin O, et al: Histiocytosis X: Demonstration of abnormal immunity, T-cell histamine H2-receptor deficiency, and successful treatment with thymic extract. New Engl J Med 304:146–153, 1981

29. Hamoudi AB, Newton WA Jr, Mancer K, et al: Thymic changes in histiocytosis. Am J Clin Pathol 77:169, 1982

30. Jaffe ES, Costa J, Fauci AS, et al: Malignant lymphoma and erythrophagocytosis simulating malignant histiocytosis. Am J Med 75:741–1749, 1983

31. Simrell CR, Margolick JB, Crabtree GR, et al: Lymphokine-induced phagocytosis in angiocentric immunoproliferative lesions (AIL) and malignant lymphoma arising in AIL. Blood 65:1469–1476, 1985

32. Margolick JB, Ambrus JL Jr, Volkman DJ, et al: Human T4+ lymphocytes produce a phagocytosis-inducing factor (PIF) distinct from interferon— and interferon. J Immunol 136:546–554, 1986

33. Ladisch S, Poplack D, Holliman B, et al: Immunodeficiency in familial erythrophagocytic lymphohistiocytosis. Lancet 1:581–583, 1978

34. Ladisch S, Ho W, Matheson E, et al: Immunological and clinical efforts of repeated blood exchange in familial erythrophagocytic lymphohistiocytosis. Blood 60:814–821, 1982

35. Writing group of the histiocyte society: Histiocytosis syndromes in children. Lancet 1:208–209, 1987

36. Aver ME, MacAffe JG: The course and prognosis of reticuloendotheliosis (eosinophilic granuloma, Schuller-Christian disease and Letterer-Siwe disease): A study of forty cases. Am J Med 22:636–652, 1957

37. Schuller A: Uber eigenartige Schadeldefekte in Jugendalter, Fortschr Roentgenstr 23:12, 1916

38. Christian HA: Defects in membranous bones, exophthalmos and diabetes insipidus: An unusual syndrome of dyspituitarism. Med Clin North Am 3:849, 1920

39. Letterer E: Aleukamische Retikulase: Ein Betrag zu den proliferativen Erkrankungen des Retikuloendothelial apparates. Z Pathol 30:377, 1924

40. Siwe SA: Die Reticuloendotheliase—ein neues Krankheitsbild unter den Hepatosplenomegalien. Z Kinderheilk 55:212, 1933

41. Lichtenstein L, Jaffe HL: Eosinophilic granuloma of bone, with report of a case. Am J Pathol 16:479, 1940

42. Farber S: The nature of "solitary or eosinophilic granuloma" of bone. Am J Pathol 17:625, 1941

43. Enriquez P, Dahlin DC, Hayles AB, et al: Histiocytosis X: A clinical study. Mayo Clin Proc 42:88, 1967

44. Tomooka Y, Torisu M, Miyazaki S, et al: Immunological studies on histiocytosis X. I. Special reference to the chemotactic defect and the HLA antigen. J Clin Immunol 6:355–362, 1986

45. Favara BE, McCarthy RC, Mierau GW: Histiocytosis X. In Finegold M (ed): Pathology of Neoplasia in Children and Adolescents, pp 126–144. Philadelphia, WB Saunders, 1986

46. Harrist TJ, Bhan AK, Murphy GF, et al: Histiocytosis-X: In situ characterization of cutaneous infiltrates with monoclonal antibodies. Am J Clin Pathol 3:294–300, 1983

47. Mierau GW, Favara BE: S-100 protein immunohistochemistry and electron microscopy in the diagnosis of Langerhans cell proliferative disorders: A comparative assessment. Ultrastruct Pathol 10:303–309, 1986

48. Rowden G, Connelly EM, Winkelman RK: Cutaneous histiocytosis X. The presence of S-100 protein and its use in diagnosis. Arch rmatol 119:553–559, 1983

49. Schwab GM, Bookman M, Braziel R, et al: True histiocytic neoplasia: An immunophenotypic, morphologic, and clinical study. Am J Clin Pathol (in press)

50. McMillan EM, Humphrey GB, Stoneking L, et al: Analysis of histiocytosis X infiltrates with monoclonal antibodies directed against cells of histiocytic, lymphoid, and myeloid lineage. Clin Immunol Immunopathol 3:295–301, 1986

51. Nezelof C: Histiocytosis X: A histological and histogenetic study. Perspect Pediatr Pathol 5:153–178, 1979

52. Favara BE, McCarthy RC, Mierau GW: Histiocytosis X. Hum Pathol 14:663–676, 1983

53. Jaffe R: Pathology of histiocytosis X. Perspect Pediatr Pathol 9:4–47, 1987

54. Risdall RJ, Dehner LP, Duray P, et al: Histiocytosis X (Langerhans' cell histiocytosis). Prognostic role of histopathology. Arch Pathol Lab Med 107:59–63, 1983

55. Ladisch S: Histiocytosis. In Willoughby MLN, Seigal SE (eds): Butterworths' International Medical Reviews. Pediatrics, vol 1, pp 95–109. London, Butterworth Scientific, 1982

56. Kjeldsberg CR, Kim H: Eosinophilic granuloma as an incidetal finding in malignant lymphoma. Arch Pathol Lab Med 104:173, 1980

57. Burns BF, Colby TV, Dorfman RF: Langerhans' cell granulomatosis (histiocytosis X) associated with malignant lymphomas. Am J Surg Pathol 6:529–533, 1983

58. Almanaseer IY, Kosova L, Pellettiere EV: Composite lymphoma with immuno-

59. Risdall RJ, McKenna RW, Nesbit ME, et al: Virus-associated hemophagocytic syndrome—A benign histiocytic proliferation distinct from malignant histiocytosis. Cancer 44:993–1002, 1979

60. Kikuchi M: Lymphadenitis showing focal reticulum cell hyperplasia with nuclear debris and phagocytes: A clinicopathological study (in Japanese). Nippon Ketsueki Gakkai Zasshi 35:379–380, 1972

61. Pileri S, Kikuchi M, Helbron D, et al: Histiocytic necrotizing lymphadenitis without granulocytic infiltration. Virchows Arch 340:257–270, 1982

62. Turner RR, Martin J, Dorfman RF: Necrotizing lymphadenitis: A study of 30 cases. Am J Surg Pathol 7:115–123, 1983

63. Seo S, Min KW, Mirkin LD: Juvenile xanthogranuloma: Ultrastructural and immunocytochemical studies. Arch Pathol Lab Med 110:911–915, 1986

64. Jaffe ES: Malignant histiocytosis and true histiocytic lymphomas. In Jaffe ES (ed): Surgical Pathology of Lymph Nodes and Related Organs, pp 381–411. Philadelphia, WB Saunders, 1985

65. Sultan C, Imbert M, Richard MF, et al: Pure acute monocytic leukemia. A study of 12 cases. Am J Clin Pathol 68:752–757, 1977

66. Lampert IA, Catovsky D, Bergier N: Malignant histiocytosis: A clinicopathological study of 12 cases. Br J Haematol 40:65–77, 1978

67. DiSant'Agnese PA, Ettinger LJ, Ryan CK, et al: Histomonocytic malignancy—A spectrum of disease in an 11-month-old infant. Cancer 52:1417–1422, 1983

68. Ducaman BS, Wick MR, Morgan TW, et al: Malignant histiocytosis: A clinical, histologic, and immunohistochemical study of 20 cases. Hum Pathol 15:368–377, 1984

69. Esseltine DW, Leeuw NKM, Berry GR: Malignant histiocytosis. Cancer 52:1904–1910, 1983

70. Vardiman JW, Byrne GE, Rappaport H: Malignant histiocytosis with massive splenomegaly in asymptomatic patients. A possible chronic form of the disease. Cancer 36:419–427, 1975

71. Huhn D, Meister R: Malignant histiocytosis: Morphologic and cytochemical findings. Cancer 42:1341–1349, 1978

72. Jaffe ES: Histiocytosis of lymph nodes: Biology and differential diagnosis. Semin Diagnostic Pathol (in press)

73. Koeffler HP, Munday GR, Golde DW, et al: Production of bone resorbing activity in poorly differentiated monocytic malignancy. Cancer 41:2438–2443, 1978

74. Writing Committee of the National Cancer Institute study of classification of non-Hodgkin's lymphomas. Summary and description of a working formulation for clinical usage. Cancer 49:2112, 1982

75. Azar HA, Jaffe ES, Berard CW, et al: Diffuse large cell lymphomas (reticulum cell sarcomas, histiocytic lymphomas). Correlation of morphologic features with functional markers. Cancer 46:1428–1441, 1980

76. Jeffree GM: Enzymes of round cell tumours in bone and soft tissue: A histochemical survey. J Pathol 113:101–115, 1974

77. Stein H, Mason DY, Gerdes J, et al: The expression of Hodgkin's disease associated antigen Ki-1 in reactive and neoplastic lymphoid tissue: Evidence that the Reed-Sternberg cells and histiocytic malignancies are derived from activated lymphoid cells. Blood 66:848–858, 1985

78. Kadin ME, Sako D, Berliner N, et al: Childhood Ki-1 lymphoma presenting with skin lesions and peripheral lymphadenopathy. Blood 68:1042–1049, 1986

79. O'Connor NTJ, Stein H, Gatter KC, et al: Genotypic analysis of large cell lymphomas which express the Ki-1 antigen. Histopathology 11:733–740, 1987

80. Nezelof C, Frileux-Herbet F, Cronier-Sachot J: Disseminated histiocytosis X: Analysis of prognostic factors based on a retrospective study of 50 cases. Cancer 44:1824–1838, 1979

81. Kaufman A, Bukberg PR, Werlin S, et al: Multifocal eosinophilic granuloma ("Hand-Schuller-Christian Disease"). Am J Med 60:541–548, 1976

82. Williams JW, Dorfman RF: Lymphadenopathy as the initial manifestation of histiocytosis X. Am J Surg Pathol 3:405–421, 1979

83. Lahey ME: Prognostic factors in histiocytosis X. Am J Pediatr Hematol Oncol 3:57–65, 1981

84. Callihan TR: The surgical pathology of the differentiated histiocytoses. In Jaffe ES: Surgical Pathology of the Lymph Nodes and Related Organs, pp 357–380. Philadelphia, WB Saunders, 1985

85. Broadbent V: Fabourable prognostic features in histiocytosis X: Bone involvement and absence of skin disease. Arch Dis Child 61:1219–1221, 1986

86. Consolini R, Cini P, Cei B, et al: Thymic dysfunction in histiocytosis-X. Am J Pediatr Hematol Oncol 9:146–148, 1987

87. Monk BE, McKee PH, duVivier A: Histiocytosis X of the scalp and face responding to topical nitrogen mustard. J R Soc Med 11:6–7, 1985

88. Anonsen CK, Donaldson SS: Langerhans' cell histiocytosis of the head and neck. Laryngoscope 97:537–542, 1987

89. Iwatsuki K, Tsugiki M, Yoshizawa N, et al: The effect of phototherapies on cutaneous lesions of histiocytosis X in the elderly. Cancer 57:1931–1936, 1986

90. Dehner LP: Allogenic bone marrow transplantation in a patient with chemotherapy-resistant progressive histiocytosis X. N Engl J Med 317:773–774, 1987

91. Matus-Ridley M, Raney RB Jr, Thawerani H, et al: Histiocytosis X in children: Patterns of disease and results of treatment. Med Pediatr Oncol 11:99–105, 1983

92. Berry DH, Gresik MV, Humphrey GB, et al: Natural history of histiocytosis X: A pediatric oncology group study. Med Pediatr Oncol 14:1–5, 1986

93. Monda L, Warnke R, Rosai J: A primary lymph node malignancy with features suggestive of dendritic reticulum cell differentiation. A report of 4 cases. Am J Pathol 122:562–572, 1986

94. Feltkamp CA, van Heerde P, Feltkamp-Vroom TM, et al: A malignant tumor arising from interdigitating cells; light microscopical, ultrastructural, immuno- and enzyme-histochemical characteristics. Virchows Arch [A] 393:183–192, 1981

95. Chan W, Zaatari G: Lymph node interdigitating reticulum cell sarcoma. Am J Clin Pathol 85:739–744, 1986

96. Chan JK, Ng CS, Law CK, et al: Reactive hemophagocytic syndrome: A study of 7 fatal cases. Pathology 19:43–50, 1987

97. Farquhar JW, Claireaux AE: Familial hemophagocytic reticulosis. Arch Dis Child 27:519–525, 1952

98. Soffer D, Okon E, Rosen N, et al: Familial hemophagocytic lymphohistiocytosis in Israel. Cancer 54:2423–2431, 1984

99. Perry MC, Harrison EG, Burgert EO, et al: Familial erythrophagocytic lymphohistiocytosis. Cancer 38:209–218, 1976

100. Rettwitz W, Sauer O, Burow HM, et al: Neurological and neuropathological findings in familial erythrophagocytic lymphohistiocytosis. Brain Dev 5:322–327, 1983

101. Kletzel M, Gollin SM, Gloster ES, et al: Chromosome abnormalities in familial hemophagocytic lymphohistiocytosis. Cancer 57:2153–2157, 1986

102. Wieczorek R, Greco MA, McCarthy K, et al: Familial erythrophagocytic lymphohistiocytosis: Immunophenotypic, immunohistochemical, and ultrastructural demonstration of the relation to sinus histiocytes. Hum Pathol 17:55–63, 1986

103. Fischer A, Virelizier JL, Arenzana-Seisdedos F, et al: Treatment of four patients with erythrophagocytic lymphohistiocytosis by a combination of epipodophyllotoxin, steroids, intrathecal methotrexate, and cranial irradiation. Pediatrics 76:263–268, 1985

104. Risdall RJ, Brunning RD, Hernandez JI: Bacteria-associated hemophagocytic syndrome. Cancer 54:2968–2972

105. Campo E, Condom E, Miro MJ, et al: Tuberculosis-associated hemophagocytic syndrome. A systemic process. Cancer 58:2640–2645, 1986

106. Yin JAL, Kumaran TO, Marsh GW, et al: Complete recovery of histiocytic medullary reticulosis-like syndrome in a child with acute lymphoblastic leukemia. Cancer 51:200–202, 1983

107. Chen T, Nesbit M, McKenna R, et al: Histiocytic medullary reticulosis in acute lymphocytic leukemia of T-cell origin. Am J Dis Child 130:1262–1264, 1976

108. Rubin M, Rothenberg SP, Panchacharam P: A histiocytic medually reticulo-sis-like syndrome as the terminal event in lymphocytic lymphoma. Am J Med Sci 287:60–62, 1984

109. Theodorakis ME, Zamkoff KW, Davey FR, et al: Acute nonlymphocytic leukemia complicated by severe cytophagocytosis of formed blood elements by nonmalignant histiocytes: Cause of significant clinical morbidity. Med Pediatr Oncol 11:20–26, 1983

110. Liang DC, Chu ML, Shih CC: Reactive histiocytosis in acute lymphoblastic leukemia and non-Hodgkin's lymphoma. Cancer 58:1289–1294, 1986

111. Sullivan JL, Woda BA, Herrod HG, et al: Epstein-Barr virus-associated hemophagocytic syndrome: Virological and immunopathological studies. Blood 65:1097–1104, 1985

112. Rosai J, Dorfman RF: Sinus histiocytosis with massive lymphadenopathy: A pseudolymphomatous benign disorder. Analysis of 34 cases. Cancer 30:1174–1188, 1972

113. Foucar E, Rosai J, Dorfman RF, et al: Immunologic abnormalities and their significance in sinus histiocytosis with massive lymphadenopathy. Am J Clin Pathol 5:515–525, 1984

114. Foucar E, Rosai J, Dorfman RF: Sinus histiocytosis with massive lymphadenopathy. An analysis of 14 deaths occurring in a patient registry. Cancer 9:1834–1840, 1984

115. Marsh WL, McCarrick JP, Harlan DM: Sinus histiocytosis with massive lymphadenopathy. Arch Pathol Lab Med 112:298–301, 1988

116. Suarez CR, Zeller WP, Silberman S, et al: Sinus histiocytosis with massive lymphadenopathy: Remission with chemotherapy. Am J Pediatr Hematol 5:235–241, 1983

117. Newman SP, Sweet DL, Vardiman JW: Sinus histiocytosis with massive lymphadenopathy: Response to cyclophosphamide therapy. Cancer Treat Rep 68:901–902, 1984

118. Helwig EB, Hackney VC: Juvenile xanthogranuloma (nevoxanthoendothelioma). Am J Pathol 30:625, 1954

119. Hashimoto K, Griffin D, Kohsbaki M: Self-healing reticulohistiocytis: A clinical histologic, and ultrastructural study of the fourth case in the literature. Cancer 49:331–337, 1982

120. Karcher DS, Head DR, Mullins JD: Malignant histiocytosis occurring in patients with acute lymphocytic leukemia. Cancer 41:1967–1973, 1978

121. Starkie CM, Kenny MW, Mann JR, et al: Histiocytic medullary reticulosis following acute lymphoblastic leukemia. Cancer 47:537–544, 1981

122. Willemze R, Rinter DJ, Willem A, et al: Reticulum cell sarcomas (large cell lymphomas) presenting in the skin. High frequency of true histiocytic lymphoma. Cancer 50:1367–1379, 1982

123. Flynn KJ, Dehner LP, Gajl-Peczalska KJ, et al: Regressing atypical histiocytosis: A cutaneous proliferation of atypical neoplastic histiocytes with unexpectedly indolent biologic behavior. Cancer 49:959–970, 1982

124. Valentino LA, Helwig EG: Lymphomatoid papulosis. Arch Pathol 96:409–416, 1973

125. Kadin M, Nasu K, Sako D, et al: Lymphomatoid papulosis, a cutaneous proliferation of activated helper T cells expressing Hodgkin's disease-associated antigens. Am J Pathol 119:315–325, 1985

126. Weiss LM, Wood GS, Trela M, et al: Clonal T-cell populations in lymphomatoid papulosis. N Engl J Med 315:475–479, 1986

127. Headington JT, Roth MS, Ginsburg D, et al: T-cell receptor gene rearrangement in regressing atypical histiocytosis. Arch Dermatol 123:1183–1187, 1987

128. Ishii E, Hara T, Okamura J, et al: Malignant histiocytosis in infants: Surface marker analysis of malignant cells in two cases. Med Pediatr Oncol 15:102–108, 1987

129. Zucker JM, Cailaux JM, Vanel D, et al: Malignant histiocytosis in childhood: Clinical study and therapeutic results in 22 cases. Cancer 45:2821–2829, 1980

twenty-four

Tumors of the Central Nervous System

Richard L. Heideman,
Roger J. Packer,
Leland A. Albright,
Carolyn R. Freeman, and
Lucy B. Rorke

At the beginning of the 20th century, parasitic or tuberculous cysts accounted for half of the intracranial masses that occurred in children.[1] With the advent of effective microbial therapy, brain tumors are now the most common intracranial mass in children, particularly in the developed world. The central nervous system (CNS) tumors of children form a broad spectrum of diseases whose unifying features are their common intracranial location and the therapeutic dilemmas posed by their development in this site in patients with relatively immature nervous systems. Primary CNS neoplasms account for 20% of all pediatric malignancies and are the most common solid tumors in children (Fig. 24-1). They are exceeded only by leukemia and lymphoma as a cause of malignant disease in this population. With a rate of 2.4 new cases per 100,000 children per year, more than 1200 new cases are estimated to occur.[2] Surprisingly, only half of these patients are identified and treated in universities, cancer centers, or tertiary-care locations, and experience with these tumors in any single institution is often limited.[3]

This chapter discusses the epidemiology, biology, classification, and diagnosis of these tumors and reviews the neurologic, surgical, radiotherapeutic, and chemotherapeutic approaches to treatment. Those tumors most frequently encountered are then addressed, with the purpose of providing current relevant information on their diagnosis and management.

EPIDEMIOLOGY

There are limited data in the literature regarding the epidemiology of CNS tumors. Two peaks in the incidence have been described. A small but consistently noted peak of 2.2 to 2.5 cases per 100,000 children per year with a slight male predominance (1.1:1) occurs in the first decade of life. A much larger peak begins in the third to fourth decade and has its zenith beyond age 60.[7,8] Within the first peak there is a predominance of embryonal CNS neoplasms and a relative absence of the adult gliomas. This persists into early adolescence, at which time a sudden increase in the incidence of typically adult CNS (supratentorial) tumors appears. Such distinct patterns of incidence and histology suggest that the occurrence of these tumors is not random and that in children, CNS tumors may have a distinctly different etiology than in adults.

Familial and Heritable-Disease Associations

Recognizable associations between the occurrence of primary CNS tumors and several heritable syndromes have been observed, the most frequently noted being that with the phacomatoses.[9,10] The association between neurofibromatosis and visual-pathway gliomas, other glial tumors, and meningiomas is well known.

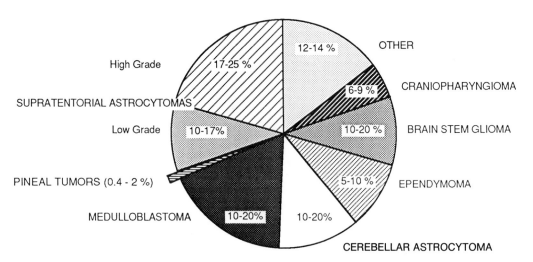

FIGURE 24-1. Approximate incidence of common CNS tumors. "Other" category includes ganglioglioma, meningioma, choroid plexus tumors, and teratomas of unspecified site (all with incidence less than 1%). Also included are unclassified tumors. Data have been compiled from References 3–6.

In tuberous sclerosis, glial tumors and occasionally ependymomas have been reported. In patients with von Hippel–Lindau syndrome, cerebellar hemangioblastoma, pheochromocytoma, and retinal tumors have been observed.

A number of families without any identifiable heritable or genetic abnormalities have been described in which often-identical CNS tumors have aggregated in siblings and other close relatives.[9,11,12] In most instances, these events have been limited to one or two interfacing generations and have not occurred in prior or subsequent generations.

Hereditary associations are somewhat more apparent in the astrocytic tumors, especially glioblastoma multiforme. In addition to the well-established association of astrocytomas with phacomatoses, family clusters have been described that appear to fit a pattern of polygenic or autosomal dominant inheritance.[12] Such mechanisms account for no more than 5% of astrocytic tumors, however.

Although no recognizable pattern of inheritance is observed in medulloblastoma, rare congenital occurrences have been reported. Additionally, instances of temporally concordant and nonconcordant tumors in monozygotic twins and non-twin siblings have been reported, but familial concordance beyond one generation has not been observed. The numbers of patients are insufficient to demonstrate other than a rare familial susceptibility in which hereditary factors do not appear to be prominant.[12] Medulloblastoma has also been described in patients with the autosomal dominant nevoid basal-cell carcinoma syndrome and the recessive Turcot and ataxia telangiectasia syndromes.

A smaller number of patients with familial clustering of pinealoma (which may be histologically indistinguishable from medulloblastoma) and of choroid plexus papilloma have been reported.[12]

Associations with Other Malignancies

Pituitary tumors occur in patients with various forms of the multiple endocrine adenomatosis syndromes. Pineoblastoma has been documented in association with retinoblastoma in the trilateral retinoblastoma syndrome.[13]

An association between embryonal CNS and renal neoplasms has recently been demonstrated. In six unrelated infants with malignant rhabdoid tumors of the kidney and a seventh with Wilms' tumor, close temporal associations with medulloblastoma, pineoblastoma, medulloepithelioma, astrocytoma, or primitive neuroepithelial tumor occurred. This curi-

ous and enigmatic association had no other recognizable heritable etiology.[14]

Cytogenetic Associations

A few well-defined cytogenetic abnormalities repeatedly have been associated with CNS tumors. An acquired monosomy 22 has been noted in the cells of meningiomas and acoustic neuromas,[15,16] and the presence of double minutes and extra chromosomes in the 6–12 and 4–5 group occur frequently in medulloblastoma cells.[12] In retinoblastoma, both constitutional and tumor-cell deletions in the long arm of chromosome 13 have been noted.

Associations with Ionizing Radiation

Various types of radiation exposure, including both preconception radiation and *in utero* diagnostic radiation, have been related to the occurrence of CNS tumors in childhood.[17] An increased occurrence of meningiomas, as well as other benign and malignant intracranial tumors, has been observed in children treated with radiation for tinea capitis.[18] Of interest, a similar association with meningiomas has been noted with low-dose medical and dental x-ray use in adults.[19]

A recent report describing primary adult-onset CNS gliomas in four patients who received radiation therapy to the head for prior childhood malignancies is of interest.[20] The doses to which these patients were initially exposed were between 1800 and 5900 cGy, and the latency between treatment and CNS tumors was 5 to 25 years. Two additional patients who received craniofacial radiation almost two decades prior to developing brain-stem glioma have also been documented.[21] The obvious implications of these reports for the survivors of pediatric malignancies who have received cranial radiation are troubling.

Immunologic Associations

Exogenous immunosuppression in transplant recipients has been reported to be associated with an increased risk of both peripheral and CNS neoplasms. However, virtually all of these CNS tumors were lymphoid neoplasms; no true primary CNS tumors were observed.[22,23] Similarly, endogenous immunosuppression, as in the Wiskott–Aldrich syndrome and ataxia telangiectasia, has been associated with lymphoid malignancies and only sporadically with a true primary CNS tumor.[9]

Environmental and Chemical Exposure Associations

Increases in the incidence of primary CNS neoplasms have been demonstrated in a number of industrial settings. Although individual reports may not attain statistical significance, the association appears repeatedly.[22] A number of organic compounds, particularly the nitrosamines, nitrosureas, hydrazines, triazines, and polycyclic hydrocarbons, are effective CNS carcinogens in experimental animals, where exposures *in utero* or soon after birth are regularly associated with the development of CNS tumors.[24,25] The recent observation of an increased incidence of CNS tumors in the children of parents who work where exposures to such agents may be frequent is of particular interest.[26,27]

Associations between CNS tumors and exposure to other exogenous agents such as barbiturates and insecticides and contact with sick animals also have been suggested. However, the data appear weak and unconvincing.

BIOLOGY

Tumor Genetics and Cytogenetics

Fluorescence-activated cell sorting (FACS) and direct chromosomal preparations from biopsy specimens have demonstrated that the low-grade gliomas, meningiomas, and pituitary adenomas almost universally possess a unimodal diploid DNA content.[28] In contrast, direct-biopsy preparations from the more aggressive and malignant tumors such as anaplastic glioma and glioblastoma multiforme frequently show bizarre chromosomal and histologic aberrations as well as many cells with obvious deviations from diploidy. Similarly, in cultured cell lines from these tumors, triploid and tetraploid cells dominate. It is surprising, then, that when FACS and karyotyping are done on freshly prepared tumor-cell populations, the majority of the cells are near-diploid. Thus, the expected relation between increased DNA content and more aggressive clinical behavior suggested by *in vitro* results does not appear to hold for fresh tumor.[28–31] Additionally, recent evidence suggests that the substrate of malignant behavior in these aggressive gliomas lies in the population of small, diploid, undifferentiated cells rather than the dramatically abnormal cells that are so often characteristic of these tumors. It is these small diploid or near-diploid anaplastic cells that appear to harbor drug resistance and which also appear to be involved in the repopulation of previously treated tumors and the rare instances of rapid anaplastic transformation in initially less-aggressive tumors.[32–34]

Several qualitative karyotypic abnormalities have been described in the malignant gliomas and glioblastoma multiforme. The most frequent of these are the presence of double minutes and the loss or displacement of the distal portions of 9p.[28] The significance of these abnormalities is unclear, but the presence of double minutes has been associated with amplifications of genes that code for cellular drug resistance in some non-CNS tumors.[35,36]

Discrete deviations in chromosome number have also been described. The most common of these are gains of chromosome 7 and losses of chromosomes 10 and 22 and of the sex chromosomes.[28] Losses of part or all of chromosome 22 appear regularly in meningiomas and acoustic neuromas.[15,16] As abnormalities in the control of gene expression have been proposed as contributors to the presence and maintenance of the transformed (malignant) state, these abnormalities and their

persistence in fresh tumor tissue as well as glioma-derived cell lines is intriguing, all the more because of the presence of human cellular proto-oncogenes on some of these abnormal chromosomes.

Oncogenes

Although associations suggesting a role for various oncogenes in the genesis of human tumors continue to be reported (see Chap. 3), in most instances, the evidence remains only circumstantial.

Epidermal growth factor (EGF) is a product of the *erb*-B oncogene located on the terminal portion of the long arm of human chromosome 7. The fact that EGF is a potent stimulator of neuroectodermal-derived cells and that both amplified *erb*-B sequences and gains of chromosome 7 have been found in some human gliomas suggests that this locus may be involved in the malignant behavior of these tumors.[37,38] Additionally, the *neu* oncogene, which is closely homologous with *erb*-B, has been found to be amplified in chemically induced murine neurogenic tumors, and transforming activity has been demonstrated in DNA preparations from some of these tumors.[39,40]

A potential role for platelet-derived growth factor (PDGF), another oncogene-derived protein and a potent glial mitogen, may exist in human glial tumors. This potential link results from the observation that the simian sarcoma virus is a very efficient inducer of glial tumors in several animals including primates and that the histologic features of these tumors are remarkably similar to those of humans. The transforming protein of this virus is a product of the v-*sis* oncogene and appears identical to the β chain of human PDGF, which is coded for by the c-*sis* locus on chromosome 22. In addition, PDGF or a closely homologous protein that is at least partly encoded by c-*sis* has been found to be synthesized and secreted by some human glial cell lines.[38,41] It seems unusual, however, that increased PDGF has been demonstrated despite the fact that amplified c-*sis* sequences have not been detected and that losses rather than gains of chromosome 22 are frequent in these tumors. This may imply alternative mechanisms of oncogene participation in malignant transformation, different from the usual amplification of these loci. Such a mechanism has been hypothesized in familial and sporadic acoustic neuroma, where loss of all or a part of chromosome 22 is a frequent finding. A proposal for a mechanism similar to that strongly implicated in the embryonal neoplasms, Wilms' tumor and retinoblastoma, and involving some perturbation at a recessive cellular allele has been advanced (see Chaps. 3 and 25).[15] Such a mechanism would be important in light of the frequency of chromosome 22 deletions in meningiomas and gliomas. Broader investigation of this possibility in the embryonal CNS tumors of children would also be of interest.

Tumor-Cell Kinetics

Tumor labeling indexes obtained both before and after biopsy provide a measure of cellular DNA synthesis, which generally reflects a tumor's growth fraction and degree of clinical aggressiveness. For example, within the glial tumors, the mean labeling index is relatively high (9.3%) for glioblastoma multiforme, intermediate (4%) in the less-aggressive anaplastic and moderately anaplastic gliomas, and low (1%) in the well-differentiated and clinically unaggressive astrocytomas.[42]

It is apparent that more fundamental and intrinsic kinetic measures, such as those relating to the cell cycle and cell renewal, are also important in assessing tumor proliferation.

For example, juvenile pilocytic astrocytomas have been described that possess unusually high labeling indices (5%–8%) but which display typically unaggressive clinical behavior.[42,43] In such cases, long cell cycles and long tumor-cell doubling times account for the slow growth and less aggressive clinical features despite the high labeling index.[43] Differences in self-renewal capabilities also may help explain differences in the clinical behavior of aggressive and nonaggressive tumors. For example, it has been suggested that a continued full renewal capacity exists in all or most of the progeny of malignant gliomas. In contrast, the more "benign" gliomas have limited proliferative capacity in which many cells appear to follow a path toward terminal differentiation and nonrenewal.[44] This hypothesis correlates well with the slow linear growth and long-term persistence of injected radiolabel in cells of the "benign" glial tumors compared with the near-exponential growth and rapid dilution and loss of label in the malignant and aggressive tumors.[42,44] Observations such as these suggest that even histologically similar tumors (*e.g.,* the gliomas), are individually distinct, with different biological properties. They do not, as suggested by some classification systems, belong to a biological continuum.

Biological characteristics other than tumor-cell kinetics significantly affect tumor growth and clinical behavior. For example, medulloblastoma and the malignant gliomas show similar kinetic characteristics, yet their prognoses differ. This difference reflects intrinsic differences in their responses to radiation and chemotherapy.[42,43,45]

CLASSIFICATION

Classification schemes are arbitrary, hypothetical statements that do not necessarily reflect the natural order of the things being classified and which may change significantly with time and knowledge. In medicine, such schemes should be clinically relevant and provide a structure within which a subject may be arranged for study. In reality, however, both goals have rarely been achieved by the same scheme. Disagreement among neuropathologists regarding which structure or scheme best reflected the biological paradigms of the time have led to a variety of classifications. Elaboration and detailed evaluation of brain tumor classification is beyond the scope of this chapter but has been elegantly reviewed.[46,47] A synopsis of the evolution and status of classification is presented here.

Classification systems for brain tumors are of relatively recent origin. In 1926, Bailey and Cushing advanced their classification of CNS tumors, which was based on the concepts of Ribbert, who had earlier suggested that tumors developed from cells that had been arrested at various stages of their anatomic and functional development. Thus, for each developmental stage of a glial cell, Bailey and Cushing suggested that a corresponding tumor could be identified. Although their classification includes CNS neoplasms that are not strictly gliomas, such as pineal tumors, it gained popularity because it reflected some aspects of clinical behavior and prognosis, accumulated from Cushing's experience.[47,48] Figure 24-2 outlines the relations among the five different cell types (choroidal epithelium, pineal proparenchyma, spongioblast, medulloblast, and neuroblast) these authors suggested as emanating from the primitive neural substrate or medullary epithelium, as well as the 14 individual tumors that were presumed to develop from these cell lineages. Modifications of this seminal work have continued to be the basis for most morphologically and histogenetically based classifications.[46,49,50]

Methods of Classification

Morphologic and Histogenetic Classification

PROPOSED SYSTEMS.   Bailey and Cushing recognized that tumors were composed of a heterogeneous cell population and classified them on the basis of the morphology of the

FIGURE 24-2.   Bailey and Cushing schema of normal developing cells and neuroepithelial tumors derived from them.

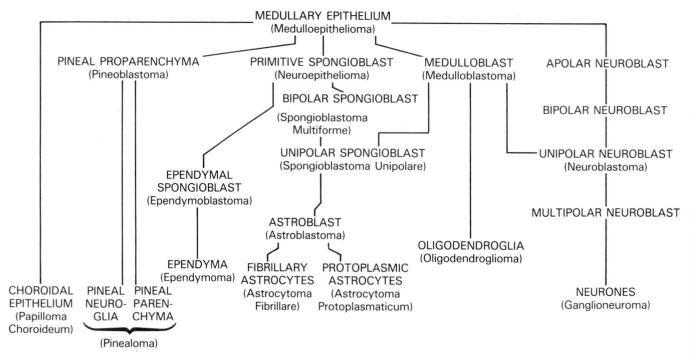

predominant cell type. Most currently used classifications; for example, that of Russell and Rubinstein[49] and that advanced by the World Health Organization (WHO),[50] are based to various degrees on the morphologic and histogenetic concepts of Bailey and Cushing. Other classifications, such as that of Kernohan and associates,[51] are based on the concept that glial tumor cells become progressively more anaplastic rather than on the idea of neoplastic transformation of cells at various stages of development. This concept led to a proposal to simplify CNS tumor classification by grading tumors I to IV to reflect the degree of anaplasia. At present, only that portion of this system relating to the astrocytomas remains in (limited) use.

Table 24-1 provides a comparison of the above four morphologic classification systems. The Russell and Rubinstein classification is a reorganization of that proposed by Bailey and Cushing along lines that reflect modern concepts of histogenesis. The WHO system is an amalgamation of classifications that recognizes both traditional morphologic entities and degree of anaplasia. Additionally, this classification provides for the designation of a tumor's location within the CNS.

PITFALLS OF MORPHOLOGIC AND HISTOGENETIC CLASSIFICATION. Even though these systems are generally adequate for the description and diagnosis of most CNS tumors, in light of present knowledge, their underlying concepts are no longer tenable. The diversity of histologic features within a tumor is amplified by the changes resulting from divergent differentiation and genotypic instability of neoplastic cells.[52,53] Moreover, cell populations displaying similar, even identical, patterns of differentiation may not have a common embryogenesis.[54]

Table 24-1
Comparison of Classification Systems for CNS Tumors

WHO (Modified for Pediatrics)	Russell and Rubinstein	Kernohan and Associates	Bailey and Cushing
Glial Tumors	**Tumors of the Glial Series**		
1. Astrocytic astrocytoma Anaplastic astrocytoma Subependymal giant-cell tumor Giagnatocellular glioma	I. Astrocytic astrocytoma Astroblastoma Polar spongioblastoma	1. Astrocytoma grades I–IV	1. Astrocytoma 2. Astroblastoma
2. Oligodendroglial tumors Oligodendroglioma Anaplastic oligodendroglioma	II. Oligodendroglial tumors Oligodendroglioma	2. Oligdendroglioma grades I–IV	3. Oligodendroglioma
3. Ependymal tumors Ependymoma Anaplastic ependymoma Myxopapillary ependymoma	III. Tumors of the ependyma and its homologues Ependymoma	3. Ependymoma grades I–IV	4. Ependymoma 5. Ependymoblastoma
4. Choroid plexus tumors Choroid plexus papilloma Anaplastic choroid plexus tumor	Colloid cyst Choroid plexus papilloma		6. Choroid plexus papillomas
5. Mixed gliomas 6. Glioblastoma multiforme	IV. Glioblastoma multiforme	(Astrocytoma IV)	7. Glioblastoma multiforme
Neuronal Tumors	**Tumors of the Neurone Series**	4. Neuroastrocytoma grades I–IV	
1. Gangliocytoma 2. Ganglioglioma 3. Anaplastic ganglioglioma	1. Ganglioneuroma 2. Ganglioglioma 3. Neuroblastoma		8. Ganglioglioma 9. Neuroblastoma
Primitive Neuroectodermal Tumors			
1. PNET not otherwise specified 2. PNET with differentiation (astrocytic, ependymal, neuronal); oligodendroglial, mixed	4. Medulloblastoma	5. Medulloblastoma	10. Medulloblastoma
3. Medulloepithelioma	5. Medulloepithelioma	(Ependymoma IV)	11. Medulloepithelioma
Pineal Cell Tumors	**Pineal Parenchymal Tumors**		
1. Pineocytoma 2. PNET (pineoblastoma)	1. Pineocytoma 2. Pineoblastoma		12. Pinealoma

Thus, classifications based on the predominant cell type in a tumor cannot be presumed to reflect its ancestry, future identity, or behavior.

Although classification of tumors according to the degree of anaplasia is not difficult for grade I (histologically benign and clinically unaggressive) and grade IV (histologically and clinically malignant) tumors and generally provides accurate prognostic correlations, objective criteria for identification of less-discrete prognostic correlations is a problem in the intermediate-grade (II and III) tumors. Further, the assumption that one or a few histologic features adequately reflect the clinical behavior of tumors regardless of other pathologic and clinical features is unsupportable. For example, a recent comparison of three cerebellar tumor types (medulloblastoma, astrocytoma, and ependymoma) with different prognoses revealed a disturbingly broad overlap in multiple discretely identifiable histologic features.[55]

Phenotypic Classification

An alternative to classification based exclusively on morphologic and histogenetic concepts is the phenotypic approach. Here, immunohistochemistry and molecular biology are utilized to allow more precise identification of cells than was previously possible.[56-58] The general application of many of these techniques is discussed elsewhere in Chapter 6. Utilization of these techniques to complement standard light and electron microscopy has the potential to provide a more objective identification and classification for CNS tumors.[55,59] For example, the identification of nervous system marker antigens such as cytoskeletal and membrane proteins, hormonal polypeptides, and neurotransmitter substances with the use of monoclonal and polyclonal antibodies and the immunofluorescent and immunoperoxidase techniques has contributed significantly to the accurate identification of CNS tumors. Table 24-2 summarizes the most commonly used and widely available markers, which include glial fibrillary acidic protein (GFAP), neuron-specific enolase (NSE), neurofilament protein (NFP), and S100 protein.[56-58] A few non-neural markers such as cytokeratins, vimentin, desmin, and alpha-fetoprotein, as well as a variety of immunoglobulins and pituitary hormones, also are available for identification of cellular elements.

As in all other aspects of diagnostic tumor pathology, critical interpretation of findings is necessary. For example, what percentage of cells must demonstrate the antigen for the test to be interpreted as positive? Distinction must also be made between reactive and neoplastic astrocytes when using GFAP. Moreover, cells other than astrocytes may stain positively for GFAP, and some cells with undeniable light microscopic features of astrocytes may not stain at all.

Recent application of molecular genetics and the use of cytogenetic markers to investigate specific chromosomal features of retinoblastoma[60] and peripheral neuroblastomas[61,62] holds promise that these techniques may eventually be applicable to the classification of CNS tumors (see Chaps. 3, 6, and 25).

Status of Pediatric Brain-Tumor Classification

Pediatric CNS tumors differ markedly from those of the adult. There is a predominance of supratentorial tumors in the adult, nearly all of which are astrocytomas. In contrast, the majority of pediatric tumors are infratentorial, and as many as 40% of these are undifferentiated embryonal neoplasms.

The two most popular CNS tumor classifications, those of Russell and Rubinstein and the WHO, are inadequate to address the differences between adult and pediatric CNS tumors.[47,63,64] Site of origin, a significant factor in prognosis, is not adequately emphasized in any current classification except that proposed by Rorke and associates as a modification of the WHO.[64] Further, similar-appearing tumors in different locations may have different prognoses because of variances in surgical accessibility or biology.[47] Another major problem in the classification of childhood CNS tumors is the approach to the embryonal, undifferentiated, or primitive neuroectodermal tumors (PNET).[63,64]

The Problem of the Primitive Neuroectodermal Tumor

Of the many different histologic types of CNS tumors, none have excited more misunderstanding, discussion, and controversy than this broad group of embryonal tumors that appear to be formed by poorly differentiated neuroepithelial cells. Justi-

Table 24-2
Common Markers for Diagnosis of CNS Tumors

Marker	Tumor Types Containing Positive Cells
Glial fibrillary acidic protein (GFAP)	Astrocytoma, ependymoma, mixed glioma, gliosarcoma, ganglioglioma, glioblastoma multiforme
	Some positive cells may be found in oligodendroglioma, capillary hemangioblastoma, choroid plexus papilloma, primitive neuroectodermal tumor
S100 protein	Variety of normal and neoplastic cells of neural and non-neural origin; of questionable utility for diagnostic purposes
Neuron-specific enolase (NSE)	Variety of normal and neoplastic cells of neural and non-neural origin; of questionable utility for diagnostic purposes
Neurofilament proteins	Ganglioglioma, gangliocytoma, primitive neuroectodermal tumors with differentiation
Vimentin	Mesenchymal tumors, meningioma, sarcoma; also melanoma, lymphoma, ependymoma, astrocytoma, chordoma
Desmin	Tumors containing muscle (rhabdomyosarcoma, teratoma, etc.)
Cytokeratin	Chordoma
Epithelial membrane antigen	Meningioma, rosettes of ependymomas
Alpha-fetoprotein	Embryonal carcinoma, endodermal sinus (yolk sac) tumor
Human chorionic gonadotropin	Choriocarcinoma, mixed germ-cell tumors

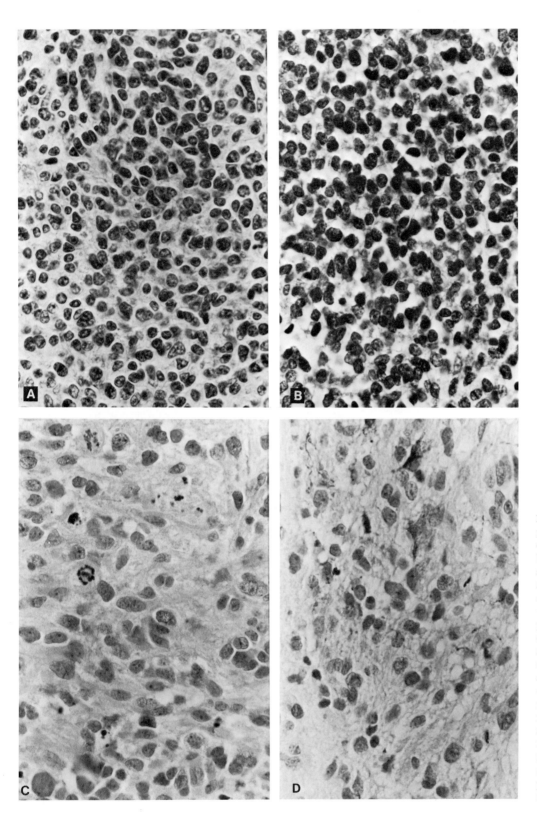

FIGURE 24-3 **A.** Typical field of primitive neuroectodermal tumor of the posterior fossa (medulloblastoma). Tumor is formed by apparently undifferentiated, basophilic round to oval nuclei with minimal perceptible cytoplasm. (H & E ×400) **B.** Typical field of primitive neuroectodermal tumor of pineal (pineoblastoma). Note similarity to the photomicrograph in **A.** (H & E ×400) **C.** One of several nests of malignant astrocytes in primitive neuroectodermal tumor of cerebrum displaying mild pleomorphism and several mitotic figures. (H & E ×400) **D.** Another similar field from same tumor shown in *C* stained with glial fibrillary acidic protein showing a few cells staining for GFAP. (GFAP × 400)

fication for a classification of these primitive neuroectodermal tumors is based on several observations. First, these tumors occur almost exclusively in childhood. Second, they display a common clinical behavior characterized by a strong propensity for widespread lepto-meningeal dissemination that generally mandates prophylactic craniospinal irradiation as part of the therapeutic approach. Third, they are composed primarily of primitive or undifferentiated neuroepithelial cells, although they may also contain cells that morphologically resemble neoplastic astrocytes, oligodendrocytes, ependymal cells, neurones, or melanocytes. Some may even contain smooth or striated muscle or fibrocollagenous tissue, although there is disagreement as to whether the latter is reactive or neo-plastic.[57,65]

Tumors with the above features are most common in the cerebellum and are identified as medulloblastoma in most current classifications. However, histologically identical tumors may also occur in the cerebrum, pineal gland, brain stem, and spinal cord and include entities with labels such as ependymoblastoma, pineoblastoma, retinoblastoma, and cerebral neuroblastoma (Fig. 24-3).[66] Thus, the concept emerges that a number of neoplasms currently named on the basis of morphology and location, but which have similar clinical and pathologic characteristics, should perhaps be considered variants of a single tumor type, the PNET.[59]

The antithesis of this idea is that these tumors, despite their apparent similarity, are independent entities recognizable by distinctive patterns of differentiation from a unique presumed cell of origin. Differentiation is thought to result from ill-defined effects of the local environment or area of the CNS in which the tumor arises.[65]

In reaction to a growing body of contradictory concepts and diagnostic terms applied to this group of tumors, a classification based on the phenotypic characteristics of the tumor has been proposed (Table 24-3).[59] This classification rejects the multitude of names and assumptions regarding origins and differentiation potential implied in other systems and is included in the proposed modification of the WHO for pediatric CNS tumors.[64] It addresses only the "small round-cell" or primitive neuroepithelial cell tumors of the CNS and specifically excludes medulloepithelioma, retinoblastoma, and olfactory neuroblastoma.

Although this proposal has been criticized as simplistic and a semantic convenience reflecting failure to achieve a specific cytologic diagnosis,[67] several authors have adopted some of its terminology and concepts.[63,68,69] Reviews of the origin and status of this controversy may be found in several recent publications.[59,66,69]

These classifications continue to generate much controversy, and it seems clear that new proposals and revisions will appear until these tumors are defined at the phenotypic and genotypic levels.

CLINICAL PRESENTATION: THE NEUROLOGY OF CNS TUMORS

The signs and symptoms of neurologic dysfunction in a child with a brain tumor are varied and depend more on the site of origin than the histology of the neoplasm. Age and the pre-morbid developmental level of the child also affect the clinical presentation.

Increased Intracranial Pressure

Brain tumors may cause neurologic compromise directly, by infiltrating or compressing normal CNS structures, or indirectly, by causing obstruction of cerebrospinal fluid (CSF) flow and increased intracranial pressure. The latter is responsible for some of the earliest clinical manifestations of CNS tumors. Although acute onset and rapid progression of these symptoms is not frequent, when they are present, they strongly suggest a rapidly growing midline or posterior fossa tumor and the need for immediate evaluation. In most patients, however, the classic triad of raised intracranial pressure—morning headaches, vomiting without nausea, and diplopia or other visual disturbances—is absent until considerable tumor growth has occurred.

More commonly, the initial signs of increased intracranial pressure are subacute, nonspecific, and nonlocalizing. In school-age children, declining academic performance, fatigue, personality changes, and complaints of vague intermittent headaches are common. Much emphasis has been placed on the "classic" headache of increased intracranial pressure; head pain present on arising that is relieved by vomiting and lessens during the day. However, vague and nonspecific complaints of head pain are probably more common. When headaches are present, their duration prior to diagnosis is generally less than 4 to 6 months, and additional tumor-related symptoms have usually become apparent within this time. The clinical suspicion of tumor should be greatest in those children with recent and continuing complaints of headache and should prompt a careful history and evaluation for related symptoms.[70,71]

In the first few years of life, irritability, anorexia, developmental delay, and, later, regression of intellectual and motor abilities are frequent early signs of increased intracranial pressure. Thus, mentation, as well as developmental reflex patterns in younger children, should always be evaluated. Likewise, head circumference should be measured, as the cranial sutures remain unfused through the first few years of life, and chronically increased pressure thus will result in macrocephaly. Funduscopic evaluation of these patients may reveal only optic pallor and no evidence of papilledema. The setting-sun sign, manifest by an impaired upgaze and a seemingly forced downward deviation of the eyes, may be seen in infants with increased pressure.

Table 24-3
Proposed Terminology for Undifferentiated Neuroepithelial Round-Cell Tumors Based on Best Available Light Microscopic, Immunocytochemical, and Ultrastructural Evidence

Operational Definition of Neoplasm	Proposed Terminology
Undifferentiated neuroepithelial cells	Primitive neuroectodermal tumor, nos*†
Undifferentiated neuroepithelial cells plus glial differentiation	Primitive neuroectodermal tumor with glial differentiation*†
Undifferentiated neuroepithelial cells plus ependymal differentiation	Primitive neuroectodermal tumor with ependymal differentiation
Undifferentiated neuroepithelial cells plus neuronal differentiation	Primitive neuroectodermal tumor with neuronal differentiation*†
Undifferentiated neuroepithelial cells plus glial and neuronal differentiation	Primitive neuroectodermal tumor with multipotential or biopotential differentiation*†

* Add (medulloblastoma) if tumor is located on cerebellum.
† Add (pineal parenchymal tumor) if tumor is located in pineal body.

Common Signs and Symptoms of Infratentorial (Brain Stem and Cerebellar) Tumors

Deficits of balance or brain-stem function (truncal steadiness, upper-extremity coordination and gait, cranial nerve function) strongly suggest an infratentorial tumor. Early in the course of tumors that fill the posterior fossa but do not erode into brain tissue, localized deficits may be absent or limited to truncal unsteadiness, with the nonlocalizing symptoms of increased intracranial pressure dominating the clinical picture. In contrast, tumors arising in the cerebellar hemispheres (cerebellar astrocytomas) more commonly cause lateralizing signs such as appendicular dysmetria early in their courses, predating signs and symptoms of increased intracranial pressure.

Inability to abduct one or both eyes (VIth-nerve palsy) may be a false localizing sign, which does not necessarily imply a posterior fossa lesion, as it may result from increased intracranial pressure from any source. However, inability to deviate both eyes conjugately (gaze palsy) or the inability to adduct an eye properly on attempted lateral gaze implies intrinsic brainstem pathology.[72] These latter findings alone or, more likely, in combination with deficits of the Vth, VIIth, and IXth cranial nerves strongly suggest invasion of the brain stem. Head tilt and vertical or diagonal diplopia may suggest trochlear nerve palsy but may also be a sign of cerebellar tonsil herniation. A partial Horner's syndrome with ipsilateral ptosis and miosis is frequently missed in patients with hypothalamic, brain stem, or upper cervical-cord disease, where the descending sympathetic tracts may be compromised.

Common Signs and Symptoms of Supratentorial Tumors

Children with supratentorial tumors may demonstrate a variety of deficits, depending on the size and location of the tumor, that generally precede the signs of increased intracranial pressure by considerable periods of time. Nonspecific headaches may be associated with early cortical symptoms, seizures being particularly common. Grand mal seizures, as well as more subtle episodes with incomplete loss of consciousness (complex partial seizures) or transient focal events without loss of consciousness (partial seizures) may also occur. Hemiparesis, hemisensory loss, and visual field defects also may be present. In some patients with lesions involving "silent" areas of the cortex such as the frontal or parietal–occipital lobes, or in those with third-ventricular lesions, increased intracranial pressure may occur largely in isolation.

In any child with visual symptomatology, there should be a careful search for optic nerve or chiasmatic dysfunction. A relative afferent pupillary defect (the "Marcus–Gunn" pupil) should be looked for by evaluating the direct and consensual pupillary responses to a bright light. Absence or a significant delay in the direct reflex in the tested eye and no consensual response in the companion eye indicates an optic pathway lesion on the tested side. In addition, visual field testing is mandatory to map and follow any disruption of the visual pathway.

A specific quartet of symptoms, "Parinaud's syndrome," should be looked for in any child with hydrocephalus or symptoms of increased intracranial pressure. This syndrome is caused by compression of the caudal midbrain and is frequent in patients with pineal area tumors. It is manifested by poor upward gaze, slightly dilated pupils that react on accommodation but not to light, retraction or convergence nystagmus, and lid retraction.[72] Similar symptoms are sometimes caused by third-ventricular dilatation due to shunt malfunction.[73]

As many as 15% of primary CNS tumors, particularly primitive neuroectodermal varieties and germ cell tumors, will have disseminated to other CNS sites by the time of diagnosis.[74] Although such dissemination is often asymptomatic, neurologic dysfunction from such lesions sometimes overshadows the symptoms of the primary tumor. For example, spinal cord and cauda equina involvement may cause back or radicular pain, bowel or bladder dysfunction, or long-tract symptoms. Thus, examination at the time of diagnosis should include a search for local (percussion) tenderness of the spine, focal extremity weakness, or sensory loss (especially a sensory level).

After treatment, careful and focused neurologic examinations are integral to the detection of early recurrence and to the recognition of treatment-related sequelae. Although neurologic examination may not be as objective as MRI or CT, being more dependent on the cooperation of the child, it does play a role in evaluating the response of a lesion to treatment. Indeed, in some cases, such as infiltrating gliomas and leptomeningeal disease, neurologic evaluation may be more sensitive to changes in tumor size than are available imaging techniques.

METHODS OF DIAGNOSIS: NEUROIMAGING

Initial Evaluation

The advent of CT has greatly facilitated the evaluation of children with brain tumors (also see Chap. 7). When performed with and without contrast medium, CT can detect the lesions in at least 95% of cases.[75,76] Skull radiography and pneumoencephalography infrequently add new or useful information and have little utility in the routine evaluation of these patients. Occasionally, angiography may be used preoperatively to determine the vascularity and surrounding vascular anatomy of cortical, pineal, or suprasellar lesions as well as to rule out the presence of vascular malformations.

MRI has recently been added to the neuroimaging armamentarium (see also Chap. 7). MRI has obvious advantages when compared with CT: there is no radiation exposure, it does not require intravenous contrast agents, images can be obtained in multiple planes, and bone artifacts are avoided.[77] The spatial resolution of current MRI equipment is similar to that of CT, and the method may be more sensitive than CT in detecting some brain tumors. For example, MRI may detect early infiltrating (primarily low-grade glial) lesions that are missed by CT.[78] MRI is also the procedure of choice for evaluating and designing radiation portals for brain-stem lesions and infiltrating glial tumors, as the extent of disease is much better defined than on CT. Figure 24-4 contrasts CT and MRI scans of the same large cystic and exophytic brain-stem tumor. The superiority of MRI is obvious. However, for detection of other posterior fossa mass lesions, MRI does not appear to be superior to CT.

The sensitivity of MRI has generated some interesting biological questions about CNS tumors. For example, the presence of abnormal signal intensity in clinically unaffected areas of the brain in children with CNS tumors (especially those with neurofibromatosis) leads to the question of whether these areas represent tumor or abnormal but non-neoplastic tissue.[79] Additionally, MRI may be capable of demonstrating areas of treatment-related white-matter damage not appreciable on CT. The location and degree of such abnormality may correlate with the severity of neurologic abnormality noted clinically and suggests a role for MRI in the evaluation and follow-up of the adverse sequelae of CNS tumor therapy.[80]

MRI also has some disadvantages. It is more sensitive to

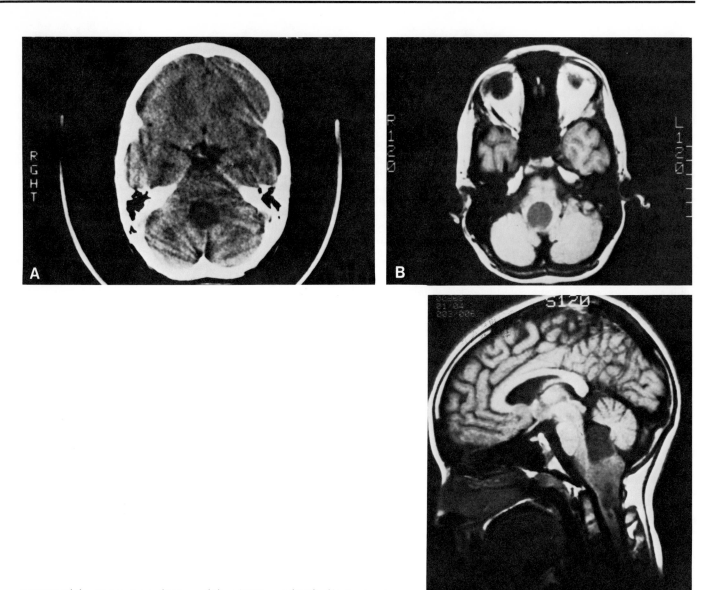

FIGURE 24-4. Comparison of CT scan (**A**) and MRI scan (**B, C**) of brain-stem tumor in same patient. Note greater resolution and detail in MRI.

movement artifacts and at present requires longer scanning times than CT. Also, although MRI is extremely sensitive in detecting abnormal tissues, it is not very specific, and differentiation of residual disease from postoperative changes may be difficult or impossible, thus limiting MRI utility in follow-up and early detection of tumor recurrence.[77] Additionally, MRI has so far not been useful in detecting leptomeningeal disease.[81] Although it was originally hoped that MRI could obviate myelography in children, this goal has not yet been realized.

At the current level of sophistication, a child with a presumed CNS tumor can be evaluated initially by either CT or MRI. In the medically stable, cooperative child, MRI is the procedure of choice because of its safety and the detail it provides. For infiltrating glial tumors, MRI is probably the only neuroimaging technique needed prior to treatment. For extra-axial lesions, especially those in the posterior fossa, additional information concerning the most likely type of tumor and the extent of meningeal disease may be gained by CT. For a medically unstable child or one difficult to sedate, CT with or without contrast will provide much of the information needed for initial treatment planning.

Leptomeningeal disease spread may occur, both before and after diagnosis, in a significant number of children with primitive neuroectodermal tumors, anaplastic gliomas, and germinomas.[74] Finding of such spread impacts greatly on the prognosis and affects management; thus, myelography and CSF cytology evaluations have a significant role.[74] CSF cytologic examination alone is inadequate to assess subarachnoid tumor spread, particularly in patients with primitive neuroectodermal tumors and germ cell neoplasms. As many as 50% of patients with these diseases have evidence of subarachnoid disease on myelography despite normal CSF analysis, and both procedures are necessary to evaluate and treat these patients properly. Although lumbar puncture and myelography are not without theoretical risks, especially in posterior fossa tumors, such procedures can be performed safely in almost all patients 10 to 21 days after their initial operation and intracranial decompression.[74]

Positron emission tomography (PET) is another potentially useful technique for evaluation of CNS tumors. PET is performed using various agents that measure brain metabolism (2-^{11}C-deoxy-D-glucose for glucose metabolism and ^{11}C-L-methionine for protein metabolism) and provides the first truly metabolic images of the brain.[82] Preliminary work in adults suggests that PET may demonstrate metabolic abnormalities in areas outside those demonstrated by CT or MRI. PET can also distinguish recurrent or residual tumor from radionecrosis and may be useful in suggesting a tumor's degree of malignancy by means of its overall metabolic activity.

Follow-up Evaluation

Both CT and MRI simplify the follow-up of children with brain tumors. Although the optimal timing of post-treatment scans in the evaluation of patients for both response to therapy and recurrence has yet to be determined, most observers would agree that routine surveillance should be performed every 3 to 6 months during the first 2 years and every 6 to 12 months for the following 2 to 3 years after diagnosis and treatment.[83]

SURGICAL APPROACH AND TREATMENT

The neurosurgical care of children with brain tumors has changed significantly during the past decade. Tumors are detected earlier and are localized more accurately with the ad-

vent of CT and MRI. Additionally, children are more often operated on by pediatric neurosurgeons, and tumors are removed more thoroughly with less morbidity and lower mortality rates. An outline of the neurosurgical approach and considerations in patients with primary CNS tumors is presented here (Table 24-4).

Preoperative and Perioperative Considerations

Preoperatively, anticonvulsants are begun if the child has had seizures, has a tumor in an epileptogenic area, or the operative approach to the tumor is likely to evoke seizures. Sodium phenytoin (4–8 mg/kg per day) is the anticonvulsant of choice as it can be initiated rapidly without significantly altering the level of consciousness and can be given intravenously if necessary. Corticosteroids, usually dexamethasone (0.5–1 mg/kg initially, then 0.25–0.5 mg/kg divided into four daily doses), are begun to diminish the preoperative and postoperative peritumoral edema and to reduce the likelihood of surgically related aseptic meningitis. Preoperative medications, especially narcotics and sedatives, should be used with great caution in patients with already increased intracranial pressure, altered consciousness, or decreased respirations, as they may exacerbate

Table 24-4
Surgical Approaches and Problems in CNS Tumors

Site	Tumor	Operation Attempted		Approach	Percent and Types of Morbidity		Comments
		Biopsy	*Resection*				
Infratentorial	Medulloblastoma Ependymoma	–	Yes	Post. fossa craniotomy	20	Dysmetria, cranial nerve palsy, paresis	Resection may improve survival
	Cerebellar astrocytoma	–	Yes	Post. fossa craniotomy	10–20	Dysmetria, ataxia	Resection usually curative
	Pontine glioma	Debated	–	Stereotactic or retromastoid craniotomy	10–20	Cranial nerve palsies, paresis	Resection attempted only in the 15%–20% with focal enhancing tumors
Supratentorial	Craniopharyngioma	–	Yes	Subfrontal craniotomy	70–100	Increased neuroendocrine deficits	Morbidity increased by aggressive attempt at total resection
					10–20	Occasional visual and psychological	
	Optic glioma	Debated	Rarely	Subfrontal craniotomy		Variable visual decline up to 70% with biopsy alone and 100% with resection of optic nerve	Partial removals in infants may delay radiotherapy and its effects on immature CNS
	Nuclear/ diencephalic	Yes	Occasionally	Stereotactic or transcallosal craniotomy	20–30	Hemiparesis, hemisensory loss	More frequently biopsied and resected now
	Pineal region	Often	Often	Craniotomy	20–30	Diplopia, abnormal eye movements	Because histology differs considerably, open biopsies are increasingly common
Supratentorial lateral	Gliomas	–	Yes	Craniotomy		Varies with site	Outcome varies widely according to histologic type

these problems. Although vagolytic agents such as atropine or scopolamine are not generally contraindicated, they should be used as close to the time of the operation as possible and be documented in the patient record to prevent the sedation and pupillary dilatation they cause from being confused with uncal herniation.

In patients with increased intracranial pressure, anesthesia is induced with thiopental if intravenous access can be obtained easily with a minimum of struggling and crying, which may increase the pressure. Inhalation agents such as halothane may be used to induce anesthesia in other circumstances, after which intravenous access may be established with fewer problems.

Hydrocephalus is present to various degrees in many patients with CNS tumors. The need to treat it depends on its clinical severity and the likelihood that surgery can reopen the obstructed CSF pathways. For some patients, corticosteroids may lower the intracranial pressure and allow preoperative shunts or ventricular drains to be avoided. However, if depressed consciousness persists despite steroids, a CSF diversion procedure should be strongly considered. Hydrocephalus from most midline posterior fossa tumors can be temporarily treated with an external ventricular drain, as tumor removal is likely to reestablish CSF flow in most of these patients.[84,85] These devices can often be removed within a week of the operation. However, recurrence of hydrocephalus usually indicates the need for a permanent shunt. In patients with deep midline intra-axial and thalamic tumors, surgery infrequently reestablishes normal CSF flow, and placing a permanent shunt during the initial operation should be strongly considered.

Whether a pretreatment biopsy is always necessary is a matter of controversy. For example, tumors of the optic nerve and chiasm can be accurately diagnosed by CT or MRI and have a relatively uniform histology, and biopsy of these tumors rarely influences treatment. In contrast, with tumors of the diencephalon and brainstem, histology is variable, and biopsy findings may influence treatment decisions, especially as new treatment protocols and therapeutic options evolve. As biopsy of these areas has historically been attended by considerable risks, it should be attempted only by neurosurgeons experienced in this procedure. It is suggested that biopsy be done whenever possible to improve clinicopathologic correlations and understanding of tumor biology.

Direct open biopsy is generally the preferred approach for most pediatric brain tumors. Although stereotactic biopsies can obtain diagnostic material from within 1 mm of the desired target in as many as 95% of patients, these procedures are more difficult in the very young, as their heads are often too small for the stereotactic frames (Fig. 24-5) and their skulls may be perforated by the pins used to position and hold the head. In older children, however, stereotactic biopsies both provide tissue

with which to make therapeutic decisions and obviate extensive and often riskier open procedures. Despite the potential problems posed by deep vascular structures, the stereotactic approach is gaining popularity for the biopsy of brain stem, diencephalon, and recurrent tumors as well as for the instillation of radiocolloids such as ^{32}P and ^{90}Y into cystic lesions. It may also aid in distinguishing radionecrosis from recurrent tumor. The mortality rate from stereotactic biopsy is less than 1%; morbidity is less than 5% and is characterized predominantly by an increased neurologic deficit or development of postbiopsy hematomas that require removal.[86-88]

Intraoperative Considerations and Surgical Technique

Most pediatric brain tumors are operated on via craniotomies, often with the aid of mannitol and CSF drainage to lower the intracranial pressure, and by routes designed to minimize cortical damage and brain retraction. Tumors on the cortical surface are approached via a local craniotomy. Deep tumors are often approached through the anterior corpus callosum, a route that causes minimal if any deficit. Choroid plexus and other ventricular neoplasms are approached through the dilated ventricles. If the location of deep tumors is in question, intraoperative ultrasound can be used to locate them accurately.

For supratentorial craniotomies, children are generally placed in the supine or lateral position. For infratentorial craniotomies, the prone or lateral position is used more often than the upright position because of concern over potential venous air embolism. Intraoperatively, the heads of young children are positioned on soft rings rather than held by pins, which can perforate an infant's skull or cause a depressed fracture. Intraoperative monitoring of evoked potentials from the visual, auditory, somatosensory, or motor areas appears to enhance the safety of resection of tumors located near the monitored pathways.

The operating microscope is an invaluable adjunct. Its illumination and magnification permit surgeons to distinguish tumor margins from adjacent structures. It is nearly always used in operations where exposure is limited: deep hemispheric tumors and tumors near the skull base. Microsurgical forceps, scissors, and dissectors are narrow, elongated instruments that permit delicate manipulations at a depth of several centimeters. However, their fine movement makes them ill-suited for the intratumoral decompression of medium or large tumors. Such decompressions are accomplished by the ultrasonic surgical aspirator or the laser, both of which remove tumors with far less trauma to surrounding brain than conventional forceps and scissors. The ultrasonic aspirator has a 1 × 5-mm tip that vibrates at 22,000 Hz, breaking off microfrag-

FIGURE 24-5. **Left.** Leksell stereotactic frame, arc, and biopsy guide. **Middle.** Frame applied to a child's head in CT scanner. **Right.** Stereotactic biopsy being obtained.

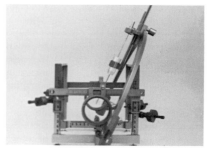
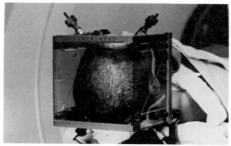
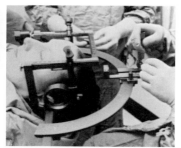

ments of tumor. The tip is surrounded by two concentric channels, one dispensing saline to solubilize the fragments and another suctioning away that suspension. The most commonly used laser is the CO_2 variety, which emits a narrow beam of light that vaporizes tissue (tumor) at its focal point.

Circumscribed, well-encapsulated tumors may be removed *in toto,* although few brain tumors have discrete enough margins for this to occur regularly. For example, most low-grade gliomas have margins that blend imperceptibly into normal white matter, precluding complete resection. In such cases, resection may begin within the core of the tumor and proceed outward toward the margins, ceasing when neoplasm cannot be distinguished from normal tissue.

There is debate over whether the extent of resection correlates with the survival rate in pediatric CNS tumors. In medulloblastoma and malignant astrocytomas, there does appear to be an association between total or near-total resection and longer survival.[89] However, this relation is less certain in the low-grade gliomas, which make up the largest proportion of pediatric tumors. This issue is important because of the obvious risks of overly aggressive resections. At present, the operative mortality rate in pediatric craniotomies is less than 1%. Morbidity is dependent on the tumor site, the preoperative neurologic condition, and the extent of removal. The current morbidity rate in polar gliomas and cerebellar astrocytomas is 10% to 20% and that in nuclear tumors, 20% to 30%. The likelihood of neurologic recovery depends on the severity of the deficits and whether they result from tumor infiltration and destruction of tissues or from tumor compression.

Although recurrent brain tumors are not frequently reoperated on, such procedures may be indicated in certain patients. For individuals with recurrent juvenile pilocytic astrocytomas in the posterior fossa, and occasionally in other recurrent gliomas, papillomas, and craniopharyngiomas, reoperation may be considered if the child is in good preoperative condition and if surgery with or without adjunctive therapy has the potential for producing a reasonable quantity and quality of life.[90] The risks of such operations are generally similar to those of the initial operation.

RADIATION THERAPY

The general principles of radiotherapy are reviewed in Chapter 11, and only those issues that are unique to the treatment of pediatric brain tumors will be discussed here.

Radiotherapy plays a major role in the management of children with brain tumors. Accurate assessment of tumor volume and precise, reproducible treatment techniques are essential. Custom-made casts may be useful in achieving this goal. Sedation is rarely needed except in very young children.

General Considerations

Volume

With an emphasis on sparing uninvolved tissues, the optimal treatment volume and field arrangement will depend on the size and location of the tumor, as well as on the expected pattern of tumor spread. Table 24-5 outlines this interaction. Although there is controversy over the most appropriate volume in individual situations, some general principles exist to guide that choice. Volumes of less than the whole brain are used for tumors that tend to remain relatively localized. Whole-brain fields are used for tumors that involve the brain

Table 24-5
Radiotherapy Treatment Volumes for CNS Tumors

Volume	Tumor
Local (less than whole brain)	Low-grade astrocytoma (cerebellar and cerebral, optic gliomas) Midbrain and brain-stem gliomas Supratentorial ependymoma Craniopharyngioma Pituitary adenoma Meningioma
Whole brain (with boost to primary tumor)	Grades III and IV astrocytoma Lymphoma
Whole CNS (with boost to primary tumor and other macroscopic disease)	Medulloblastoma Infratentorial and/or high-grade ependymoma Primitive neuroectodermal tumor Pineoblastoma Germ cell tumor

extensively and whole-CNS fields for tumors with a significant propensity for seeding along CSF pathways.

Treatment of the whole CNS poses unique technical problems and in most medical centers is accomplished by the use of lateral opposed fields covering the whole brain along with a direct posterior field covering the spinal axis. Field matching over the cervical cord is optimized by angling the brain fields parallel with the divergent edge of the spinal field (Fig. 24-6). In order to avoid underdosage or overdosage at the junction, the latter field will usually be moved weekly during the course of treatment.

Because the penetration depth of electrons can be controlled, they may be used to treat the spinal axis so that irradiation of underlying structures (especially the thyroid) can be reduced. However, field matching over the cervical cord is more difficult with this technique than with photons.

Dose, Fractionation, and Time

For most tumors, the dose of radiotherapy is influenced by both the need for tumor control and the tolerance of normal brain. This tolerance, in turn, depends on a number of factors including the anatomic location (the brain stem and hypothalamus are more sensitive than other areas), the volume irradiated, and, perhaps most important, the age of the child.[91] Doses of 5400 cGy, 4500 cGy, and 3500 cGy, given at a rate of 160 to 180 cGy daily 5 days per week, for local fields, whole brain, and spinal axis, respectively, are considered within tolerance for a child older than 3 years in whom brain development is largely complete (Table 24-6). However, such doses may cause unacceptable damage in a younger child, in whom some radiotherapists consider dose reductions of 20% to be necessary.[92,93]

The fractionation schedule and total treatment time are also of considerable importance. Late effects on normal tissue seem to depend largely on the size of the dose per fraction. Thus, there may be a theoretical advantage to the use of a larger number of smaller fractions ("hyperfractionation") to reduce late damage. With "accelerated hyperfractionation," a higher total radiation dose is given in a similar or shorter time than in conventional therapy. This technique is postulated to increase tumor control. Several studies have tested the feasibility of these approaches, and some show promising early results.[94–97]

Newer Approaches

Hyperbaric oxygen and the hypoxic cell sensitizers metronidazole and misonidazole have been used in an attempt to overcome the problem of reduced radiation sensitivity of poorly oxygenated tissues, which make up a significant portion of many solid tumors.[96,98–100] Other attempts at overcoming this problem, such as the use of neutrons, which have less dependence on an ionizing interaction with oxygen for their biological effects, have been accompanied by unacceptable brain damage in spite of good local tumor control.[101]

Retreatment

For the most part, failure in patients with brain tumors occurs at the site of original disease. Additional radiotherapy may provide excellent palliation for some patients.[92,102,103] In general, the radiotherapy volume should be limited to the area of recurrence and the dose to that which is adequate for symptom control. Retreatment doses of 1500 to 2000 cGy given in 180-cGy daily fractions are generally tolerated and when given 1 year or more after initial radiotherapy may not substantially increase the risk of serious brain damage. Higher doses, approaching those used in the initial treatment, have also been used with tolerable effects.[102,103] In any event, prior fields and doses to particularly radiosensitive areas such as the cervical cord must be considered in choosing dose and fields.

Complications of Radiotherapy

Early (During the First Month After Therapy)

Worsening of the neurologic status is rarely seen during radiotherapy. Although radiation-induced cerebral edema may occur during the first week of treatment, it is unusual unless larger-than-conventional treatment fractions are used. Patients are generally given steroids (dexamethasone, 0.5 mg/kg divided into three or four daily doses with a maximum of 4 mg/dose) during the early part of their treatment; the dose usually can be tapered after the first week or two.

Temporary alopecia within the radiotherapy field is universal. If the dose to the skin is excessive, as may be the case over the frontal region, vertex, and occiput, where the radiation beam enters tangentially and so loses the skin-sparing properties of a perpendicular beam, permanent partial or even total alopecia may occur. A mild erythema of the skin may be seen in the first week of treatment. A brisker reaction occurring after the fourth week is usually limited to no more than a moderate erythema and dry desquamation, but moist desquamation may occur behind the ears where skin sparing is lost. Such reactions usually subside within 1 to 2 weeks following completion of treatment. Topical steroid creams are generally

adequate if treatment is necessary. Otitis externa and secretory otitis media may be a problem in the later part of treatment. Fullness in the ear, earache, tinnitus, and mild hearing loss usually resolve spontaneously, although surgical drainage may be necessary. Transient hematologic suppression may be observed with whole-CNS radiotherapy.

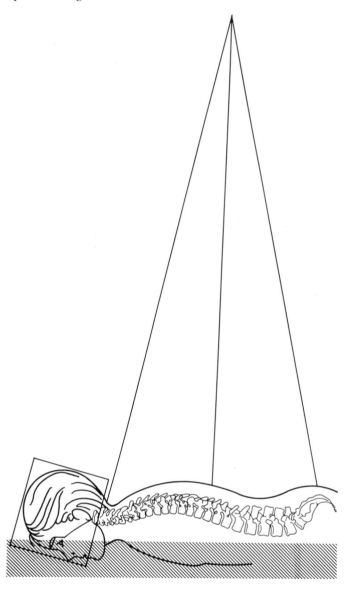

FIGURE 24-6. Diagram of radiation field matching over the cervical cord with craniospinal treatment. Note parallel meeting of cranial and spinal field edges.

Table 24-6
Radiation Dose (cGy), Fractionation, and Overall Treatment Time in Children

Age (Years)	Local Fields	Whole Brain	Spinal Cord
<3	5040 in 28 fx in 6 wk	3960 in 22 fx in 4.5 wk	3040 in 19 fx in 4 wk
≥3	5400 in 30 fx in 6 wk	4500 in 25 fx in 5 wk	3520 in 22 fx in 4.5 wk

Early–Delayed (Up to 6 Months After Therapy)

Transient symptoms attributed to temporary demyelination have been seen 6 to 8 weeks after completion of radiotherapy to the brain and spinal cord. The "somnolence syndrome" has been best described after radiotherapy for CNS prophylaxis in acute lymphoblastic leukemia[104] and consists of lethargy, anorexia, and headache that usually last about 2 weeks. Although no consistent CT abnormalities or CSF cytology changes are noted, electroencephalographic changes of slow-wave activity consistent with diffuse cerebral disturbance have been described. Whereas this syndrome has been reported to some degree in as many as 79% of leukemia patients, it appears to be less frequent after the higher doses of radiotherapy used for the treatment of brain tumors, although this observation has not been documented.

Lhermitte's sign, the sensation of electric discharge down the spine and limbs upon neck flexion, is thought to be an indicator of a temporary demyelination in the spinal cord.[105,106] Like the somnolence syndrome, symptoms usually appear 8 weeks after the completion of radiotherapy, although they may persist longer (up to 3 months). Again, this finding has been described more commonly after moderate rather than higher radiotherapy doses (Hodgkin's disease versus primary head and neck cancer) and treatment of tumors other than those of the CNS.

Late (6 Months to Many Years After Therapy)

Late or delayed radiation-induced damage to the CNS is likely due to a combination of direct injury of glial cells, especially oligodendroglia, and damage to the vasculature. Cell injury appears to predominate in the first months and years after treatment, whereas vascular damage becomes apparent in the late (several months to years) post-treatment phase.[91,107] The risk of such changes increases with the dose of radiation, and most cases of frank brain necrosis have occurred at much higher doses than are commonly used,[108,109] with larger-than-conventional daily fraction sizes, or with the use of experimental modalities such as neutrons and combined radiotherapy–chemotherapy programs. Concomitant use of systemic high-dose methotrexate is also associated with late CNS injury as manifested by necrotizing leukoencephalopathy. Symptoms are variable, ranging from mild intellectual impairment to headache, focal neurologic problems, progressive dementia, seizures, and even death.

The principal difficulty with such late injury lies in distinguishing it from progressive tumor. The electroencephalographic and CT abnormalities do not appear to correlate well with the clinical findings, although MRI may be more useful in this regard.[80] The analogous process in the spinal cord, radiation myelopathy, is distinctly unusual unless larger-than-conventional radiation doses are delivered, as for example in an area of field overlap. Classically, this syndrome is characterized by progressive sensory changes in the lower extremities followed by motor weakness and bowel and bladder dysfunction occurring in a patient with a normal myelogram.[106]

PRINCIPLES OF CHEMOTHERAPY

Recently published reviews of ongoing clinical trials and currently useful individual chemotherapeutic agents in CNS tumors continue to demonstrate that the utility of chemotherapy for CNS tumors lags considerably behind that for solid tumors found elsewhere in the body.[110–112] Some of the reasons for this are highlighted below.

Blood–Brain Barrier and Factors Influencing Drug Penetration

The presence of the blood–brain barrier (BBB) profoundly influences the CNS penetration of most substances. For some time, it was thought that the tight endothelial cell junctions of this structure limit penetration to all but small-molecular-weight (200 Daltons), highly lipophilic, un-ionized (at physiologic pH) compounds.[113] However, current evidence shows that the BBB is not uniformly intact, and various degrees of disruption have been described repeatedly. An understanding of the relative contribution of these individual changes to increased permeability is not yet available.[114,115] It is clear, however, that the frequency and distribution of such changes vary considerably, both and among CNS tumors and within an individual tumor.

In general, it appears that small tumor foci as well as the peripheral portions of larger tumors behave as if the BBB were relatively intact, whereas the central portions of most tumors and very large individual tumors tend to have absent BBB characteristics. This latter feature appears to be independent of central necrosis.[116] These findings may be partly explainable by the tendency of advancing margins of tumor initially to parasitize normal CNS capillaries possessing an intact BBB and for abnormal tumor-induced vascularity to arise in and dominate more-established areas of tumor.[117]

Other independent factors, among them capillary permeability and surface area, blood flow (F) across the tumor, and those physiochemical properties of a drug that are largely related to liposolubility, also influence drug penetration. These influences are summarized in the term E, which represents the fractional extraction of drug across the tumor capillaries.[116,118]

Another operational expression, K, reflects the blood–tissue transfer constant or "driving force" behind drug penetration. This parameter is directly related to F and E and is expressed in a simplified way as

$$K = FE.$$

With the appropriate considerations for concentration of drug (C) and time of exposure (T), K can be used to model tumor drug penetration (P). An elementary illustration of this concept is

$$P = K (CT).$$

In most clinical instances, where the chosen drug does not lie at the extremes of lipid or aqueous solubility, the degree of its penetration is described by more complex equations that also consider drug metabolism, protein binding, half-life, and other pharmacokinetic parameters.[116,118] It is instructive, however, to examine the extremes of drug solubility under "ideal" circumstances, where the complexity of drug penetration reduces to only a few factors.

For drugs that are highly lipophilic and whose E is high (~100%), the amount of BBB disruption and capillary surface area available for exchange is less important than the rate of drug delivery (F) and the amount (C) of drug available locally. A similar situation applies when T is small (use of a drug with a short *in vivo* half-life). Conversely, for poorly lipophilic agents whose E is low, the available surface area for exchange and the degree of capillary permeability or BBB disruption become the dominant influences behind penetration.[116,118] Table 24-7 lists some commonly used drugs in order of liposolubility and other important parameters related to their CNS penetration as discussed above.

Table 24-7
Physiochemical Properties of Some Common CNS Antitumor Agents

Drug	Molecular Weight (daltons)	Solubility (log P)*	K†
Nitrosoureas		Lipid	
CCNU	234	2.85	—
BCNU	214	1.54	0.588
PCNU	263	0.37	—
		Lipid	
AZQ‡	364	0.5	0.145
Procarbazine	258	Water	—
5-fluorouracil	130	Water	0.0096
Methotrexate	454	Water	0.0014
		−2.52	
Cisplatin	300	Water	—

* Preferential solubility (lipid versus water); log P = 1-octanol/water partition coefficient; liposoluble drugs partition more in octanol.
† K = blood-to-tissue transfer constant.[116]
‡ AZQ = aziridinylbenzoquinone.

In all animal and human tumors so far studied, K varies broadly. Regional variability in K as great as 100-fold can be seen within the same tumor as well as across individual tumors.[116,119] This variability leads to significant intratumor and intertumor differences in drug penetration that partly underlie the poor response of CNS tumors to chemotherapy. Such penetration differences reflect the great heterogeneity in the integrity of the BBB in CNS tumors, a factor that is an intrinsic property of these tumors and independent of their histologic identity or classification.[116,118]

Drug Delivery Strategies

High-Dose Systemic Therapy

In attempts to improve the response rate of CNS tumors to chemotherapy, several recent trials have increased the systemic drug concentration by high-dose therapy, often with autologous bone-marrow reinfusion to rescue the resultant hematologic toxicity. However, such trials (BCNU in doses of 600–2850 mg/m^2) have been unable to avoid other systemic toxicity and have resulted in several instances of severe hepatic, pulmonary, and CNS toxicity without clearly improving patient survival rates.[120–122]

Regional Therapy

Other attempts to enhance drug penetration have employed regional (carotid artery) infusions. The rationale here is to increae the drug concentration in the tumor without increasing the systemic concentration and toxicity. Drugs that have a high systemic clearance but which otherwise penetrate tumor well are the best candidates for such use. One group of such drugs is the nitrosoureas, which have been used for regional therapy of CNS tumors.

Although such treatment does provide better local drug delivery, penetration is increased in surrounding normal brain tissue as well as in the tumor. Thus, in spite of decreased systemic toxicity, diffuse and focal CNS toxicity, particularly retinal damage, has followed intracarotid infusions.[123,124] Nonuniform local mixing of drug and blood at the infusion site can lead to a separate stream of even higher drug concentration within the flow of the vessel. This "streaming" during arterial delivery and the possible effects of alcohol-containing diluents have been suggested as being partly responsible for increased CNS toxicity of regional therapy.[124,125]

Blood–Brain Barrier Disruption

Reversible opening of the BBB with hyperosmolar infusions of mannitol or arabinose can enhance the penetration of a variety of compounds of various sizes, molecular weights, and liposolubility.[126] The principal advantage of this approach lies in the feasibility of administering water-soluble and large-molecular-weight substances where limited penetration relative to blood flow and rate of delivery is dominant. Increases in CNS and CSF drug levels have been documented and can be correlated with improved clinical response in some instances.[126–128] However, enhanced CNS toxicity, similar to that in regional therapy, can occur.[129] The possibility of longer-term, less-intense BBB opening with continuous dehydrocholate infusions has theoretical appeal but is as yet untried.[130] The application of other approaches for BBB disruption, including the use of dimethylsulfoxide, hypercapnia, and ionizing or microwave radiation, have been unsuccessful.[110]

Self-contained implantable devices for continuous intraventricular and local tumor therapy may also play a role in the treatment of CNS tumors. Applications for the treatment of malignant meningitis and intra-axial prophylaxis in primitive neuroectodermal neoplasms such as medulloblastoma are possible.[131,132]

Immunotherapy

Although attempts at immunotherapy in CNS tumors are in their infancy, the potential applications are possible. Osmotic BBB disruption in animals allows significant penetration of high-molecular-weight substances such as monoclonal antibody into both the brain parenchyma and the CSF, where 24% of the concomitant plasma levels may be obtained. The potential of this technique for diagnosis and treatment requires further investigation.[133,134]

Interleukin-2 and lymphokine-activated killer cells have been suggested as having a role in the treatment of CNS tumors similar to that reported in systemic malignancies.[135] *In vitro* activity has been demonstrated against gliomas, and phase I trials of direct intracerebral administration have not demonstrated any specific toxicity.

In Vivo and In Vitro Drug Testing

Skipper has pointed out that no individual animal or human tumor can be thought of as a good model for another tumor, yet a number of murine and canine tumors of various origins have, of necessity, been used to model human CNS tumors. These systems have been useful in demonstrating and studying the unique physiology of these tumors and the effects of the BBB. Although they are frequently used to screen for active tumor agents, they are not particularly good predictors of human response. Recent development of murine–human xenograft brain-tumor models may overcome some of these problems.[136–140]

In vitro chemosensitivity testing of CNS tumors may have utility in predicting the therapeutic profile of a tumor, although it may better predict clinical failure than response. In spite of multiple problems in the choice of exposure times and drug concentrations representative of the *in vivo* situation, this model is frequently used,[141,142] and recent experiences with it and comparisons with simultaneous *in vivo* test results in medulloblastoma show that clinically useful information may be obtained.[142]

MEDULLOBLASTOMA (PRIMITIVE NEUROECTODERMAL TUMOR ARISING IN THE CEREBELLUM)

Epidemiology

Medulloblastoma is a predominantly midline cerebellar tumor that arises in the area of the cerebellar vermis adjacent to the roof of the fourth ventricle. It accounts for between 10% and 20% of primary CNS neoplasms in children and about 40% of all posterior fossa tumors. The peak age of incidence is 5 years, and most tumors occur within the first decade of life with a 1.3–2:1 male-to-female ratio.[5,143,144]

Pathology and Patterns of Spread

The term "medulloblastoma" was first used by Bailey and Cushing in 1925. Although the term was meant to imply that the tumor arose from the medulloblast, a putative CNS germinal cell with the ability to differentiate along neuronal or glial lines, no such cell has ever been identified. Most current literature proposes the cells of the external granular layer of the cerebellum as the origin of this tumor.[60,145] Recently, however, the primitive neuroepithelial cell present in subependymal regions throughout the nervous system has been suggested as the more probable cell of origin.[60] This concept provides an explanation for the occurrence of other histologically identical embryonal neoplasms elsewhere in the CNS and makes the term "primitive neuroectodermal tumor (PNET) arising in the cerebellum" more appropriate than "medulloblastoma."

Medulloblastomas are highly cellular, soft, and friable tumors composed of small, round, undifferentiated cells with hyperchromatic nuclei and generally abundant mitoses (Fig. 24-7). Homer–Wright rosettes and pseudorosettes are variably present, and a generally inconspicuous stromal component is confined to the vasculature. Various degrees of glial or neuroblastic differentiation may be seen, and in rare circumstances, muscle or pigmented cells or both may also be found. A histologic variant, the desmoplastic medulloblastoma (Fig. 24-8), occurs dominantly in the lateral cerebellar areas of adolescents and adults and has a more abundant stromal component than the classic tumor.[60,145,146]

Medulloblastomas often grow to several centimeters in size and may fill the posterior fossa, invading surrounding CNS structures as they grow into the regional subarachnoid and ventricular spaces. As with other CNS tumors of presumed primitive neuroepithelial origin, widespread seeding of the subarachnoid space may occur (Fig. 24-9). The frequency of CNS spread outside the area of the primary tumor at diagnosis has been reported as 11% to 43% and has been as high as 92% in some autopsy series.[93,147–149]

Of all pediatric CNS neoplasms, medulloblastoma has the greatest propensity for extraneural spread. Although rare at diagnosis, extraneural dissemination is eventually observed in 5% to 35% of patients. Bone is the most common site, accounting for more than 80% of metastases. Bone marrow, lymph nodes, liver, and lung are other common sites.[150–152]

Clinical Presentation

The earliest and most persistent signs and symptoms are the nonspecific, nonlocalizing findings of increased intracranial pressure resulting from obstruction of the fourth ventricle.

FIGURE 24-7. Typical histology of medulloblastoma (PNET). Tumor formed by apparently undifferentiated basophilic round to oval nuclei with minimal perceptible cytoplasm. (H & E × 400)

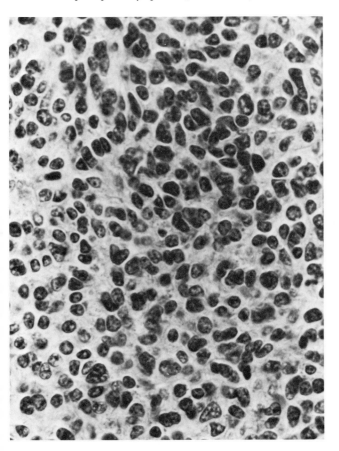

FIGURE 24-8. Primitive neuroectodermal tumor of cerebellum showing linear arrangement of cells along delicate background fibers characteristic of what has been called "desmoplastic medulloblastoma." (H & E × 400)

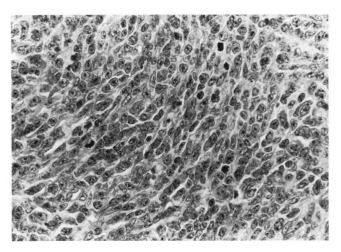

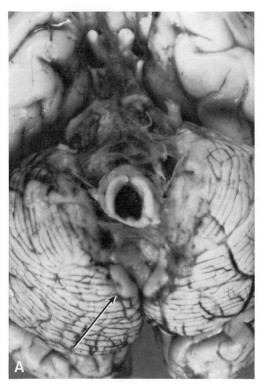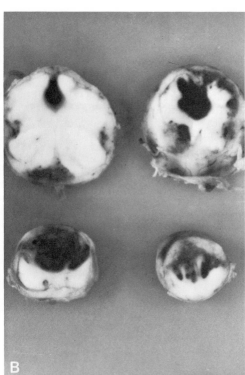

FIGURE 24-9. A. Nodules of primitive neuroectodermal tumor (medulloblastoma) in cisterna magna (*arrow*). There is a hemorrhage in the medulla. **B.** Transverse sections of medulla and spinal cord showing metastatic primitive neuroectodermal tumor (medulloblastoma) in subarachnoid space. Tumor is partially hemorrhagic and has invaded the neural tissue to a variable extent at the different levels.

Papilledema, headache, emesis, and lethargy are present in more than 80% of patients at diagnosis.[148,153,154] Because many of these symptoms are intermittent and subtle, they are often overlooked, and delays in diagnosis of 3 months or more may result.[146,153,154]

With increasing tumor size and compromise of the surrounding brain tissue, more characteristic signs appear. A progressively worsening ataxia involves the lower extremities, often with relative sparing of the upper extremities and trunk. Diplopia and abnormalities of the Vth, VIIth, and other cranial nerves may become apparent due to tumor compromise of the brain stem. Hyporeflexia or hyperreflexia, hypotonia, and other motor signs may become apparent with medullary and cervical tract involvement.[153] With further extension toward the foramen magnum, complete obstruction of the fourth ventricle may occur, which in turn may increase hydrocephalus and intracranial pressure, leading to herniation of the cerebellar tonsils. Although the development of a stiff neck and head tilt may be due to an oculomotor paresis, they should be considered ominous signs that suggest impending herniation and the need for immediate neurosurgical intervention.

Differential Diagnosis and Evaluation

The differential diagnosis of medulloblastoma includes other posterior fossa tumors such as cerebellar astrocytoma, ependymoma, and, less frequently, brainstem gliomas. Additionally, infectious encephalitis may lead to an acute syndrome of vomiting, lethargy, and ataxia. Although this syndrome has a more acute onset and a more prominent component of truncal ataxia than is seen in most patients with medulloblastoma or other posterior fossa tumors, these characteristics alone are not sufficiently reliable to rule out tumor.

On CT, prominent hydrocephalus and a solid, homogenous, isodense to hyperdense, contrast-enhancing midline

mass is characteristic.[155,156] Similar-appearing midline cerebellar astrocytomas and brain-stem gliomas may occasionally give rise to diagnostic confusion. MRI may be useful in such instances by better demonstrating the anatomic origin and extent of tumor.

Evaluation of the spinal axis for evidence of leptomeningeal dissemination is an essential part of the pretherapeutic investigation of patients with medulloblastoma. However, neither clinical symptomatology nor negative CSF cytology findings can be relied on to indicate the presence of nodular spinal cord disease (Fig. 24-10), as a high proportion of such patients are asymptomatic and have negative cytology results. Thus, metrizamide myelography is necessary to evaluate the spinal axis fully in all patients prior to therapy.[93,147,149,157] The lumbar puncture for this procedure and for simultaneous CSF cytology can be safely done in the majority of patients within 2 to 4 weeks of surgery. It should never be attempted prior to surgical decompression of hydrocephalus (by either tumor resection or placement of a shunt device) for fear of precipitating tonsillar herniation.

The measurement of CSF polyamines has been suggested as a method of monitoring for recurrent disease. Elevations of putrescine and spermidine concentrations are associated with increased DNA turnover and cell proliferation, and CSF elevations of these substances can be seen in patients who harbor rapidly growing tumors near the ventricular system. The finding of such elevations has predicted tumor regrowth several weeks in advance of cytology or CT.[158]

Prognostic Considerations

Prognostic significance has been reported for several histologic and clinical features (Table 24-8).

In a proposed clinical staging system that evaluated extent of disease as well as size, tumors greater than 3 cm in diameter

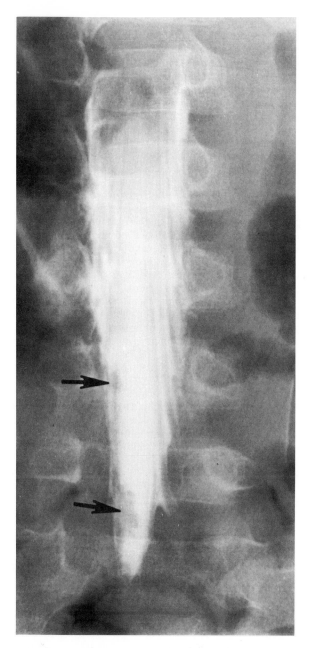

FIGURE 24-10. Metrizamide myelogram showing gross nodular tumor (medulloblastoma).

and extending beyond the cerebellar vermis were associated with a poor prognosis.[159] In attempts to confirm the utility of this system, size, disease extent, and other clinical features were evaluated as a part of two large cooperative-group therapeutic trials in medulloblastoma.

Tumor Size

Tumors localized to the midline and smaller than the volume of the fourth ventricle are reported by the International Society of Pediatric Oncology (SIOP) Multi-Institutional Study Group as having a 54% compared with a 23% disease-free survival rate at 54 months. However, a similarly conducted Children's Cancer Study Group (CCSG) trial and other institutional series

Table 24-8
Putative Prognostic Factors in Medulloblastoma*

Factor	Comment
Tumor size	Uncertain significance; larger tumors associated with poor prognosis only in some studies
Tumor extent	Brain stem, intra-axial subarachnoid, and extraneural disease associated with poorer prognosis
CSF cytology	Positive cytology alone generally without prognostic significance
Histology	Classic versus desmoplastic histology generally of no significance; tumor-cell differentiation of conflicting significance
Age at diagnosis	Less than 5 years of age associated with poorer short-term survival independent of tumor extent and treatment
Extent of resection	Generally improved short-term survival with greater extent of resection

* See text for details.

have found no significant or independent prognostic association with size alone.[89,144,150,160,161]

Disease Extent

The extent of disease has been the most consistently useful prognostic factor. Patients with localized disease have a significantly better prognosis than those with disseminated disease. A 58% versus 32% disease-free survival advantage in favor of patients with localized disease was present at 54 months in a recent CCSG study.[89]

CSF Cytology

The prognostic meaning of an isolated positive CSF cytology result in the absence of myelographic evidence of subarachnoid disease is unclear. Although intraoperative and early postoperative CSF samples frequently show tumor cells, their presence at this time does not appear to correlate with the eventual occurrence of widespread intra-axial disease.[150,162] Similarly, the persistence of positive cytology, or its first discovery 2 to 4 weeks postoperatively (*e.g.,* at the time of myelography), although sometimes associated with interaxial diseases,[93] is not a reliable indicator of the presence of myelographically demonstrable subarachnoid disease. Ongoing studies are attempting to evaluate the significance of isolated positive CSF cytology.

Age at Diagnosis

Young patients, especially those under age 5 at diagnosis, are consistently reported to have a poorer prognosis than older patients, although the magnitude of this difference is often no greater than 10% and it largely disappears beyond 5 years from diagnosis in some studies. This difference may be partly due to the often larger and more extensive tumors in these younger patients and the common practice of giving reduced doses of radiation to this group, although poorer survival persists even when these factors are taken into consideration.[89,93,144,146,150,159,161,163]

Histology

Although patients with classic histology have been reported to have a 10% to 15% better survival rate at 5 and 10 years compared with patients with desmoplastic histology,[25] most authors find little prognostic significance to these features.[144,146] It has also been suggested that the degree of cellular differentiation influences prognosis. For example, a recent report noted a 70% versus 32% survival advantage at 4 years for patients with undifferentiated tumors as compared to those with neuronal or ependymal differentiation.[164] Astrocytic differentiation has also been associated with improved survival.[165] However, other reports have found no correlation between the degree of differentiation and survival.[166]

Shunts

It has been suggested that shunts placed to relieve hydrocephalus are associated with a greater incidence and earlier onset of systemic metastases.[85,150,151,161,167] However, more than 80% of patients with systemic metastases have never had a shunt.[151] Further, the presence of other poor prognostic features, retrospective case selection, and the absence of a survival difference between shunted and nonshunted patients in other recent series cast doubt on the idea that shunts might accelerate metastases.[84,93,144,151,152,161,168,169]

Treatment

Surgery

Although the goal of complete tumor resection is achievable in about 50% of patients, the ultimate impact of radical resection appears limited. Complete resection produces a 30% to 50% survival advantage at 1 year compared with biopsy or partial resection, but only small differences (*e.g.,* 10% at 5 years) or a "trend" toward improvement are present thereafter in most recent series.[89,150,153,167]

Medulloblastomas are approached surgically through a suboccipital craniotomy. After removal of a roughly quadrangular portion of the inferior occipital bone, the dura and cisterna magna are opened to reveal the posterior fossa and the tumor. As the tumor is often quite friable, gentle suction may be used to remove much of it. With the aid of the operating microscope, forceps or an ultrasonic surgical aspirator can be used to remove more-adherent portions. Because modern neurosurgical techniques permit complete or nearly complete resection with little or no significant increase in morbidity and mortality rates over those of more conservative surgery,[154] and at least short-term the survival rate is enhanced, attempts at complete resection are encouraged in current treatment protocols. Even with vigorous attempts at complete removal, surgical mortality rates are now 0 to 8% compared with 30% in earlier reports.[90,150,153,161,167] As surgical estimates of the extent of resection may not be reliable, CT validation has been recommended[170] and is required in the new cooperative group trials.

Radiation

Medulloblastoma is one of the most radiosensitive primary CNS tumors of childhood. Total neuraxis therapy is standard in all patients, and survival is seriously compromised in patients who do not receive such treatment.[90,170] Many authors have demonstrated the need for doses of at least 5000 cGy to the posterior fossa, showing that local control of the primary tumor and survival decline at doses below this.[150,160,170,171] However, the most appropriate dose for craniospinal therapy remains a subject of debate. A general trend toward increasing the dose delivered to these fields is apparent over the past several years, paralleling the increases given to the posterior fossa. Although most current treatment protocols utilize 3500 to 4000 cGy, doses of as little as 1900 cGy do not appear to differ in their ability to prevent isolated spinal recurrence.[89,170-172]

Attempts to reduce the dose of craniospinal radiation are important because of the significant intellectual and endocrinologic morbidity associated with such therapy in young children. In reported series with adequately detailed relapse information, the incidence of isolated spinal or supratentorial relapse is less than 10%. This figure is significantly less than the incidence of metachronous neuraxis and posterior fossa recurrences that comprise the majority of such events.[147,149,150,159,160,161,171,173] In view of these results and the fact that 60% to 80% of treatment failures occur in the posterior fossa alone, it may be possible to reduce the craniospinal radiation doses safely (preserving current posterior fossa dose recommendations) in well-staged patients with negative CSF cytology and myelography without substantially increasing the risk of failure outside the primary site. Early but encouraging results of such an approach have been reported recently,[174] and a similar intergroup study is currently being conducted by the CCSG and the Pediatric Oncology Group (POG).

The most appropriate treatment for the patient who is younger than 3 years is debatable. In spite of the recognition that children of this age have a poorer prognosis, dose reductions of 20% to 30% are recommended because of the significant neurologic and intellectual morbidity that may occur with full-dose therapy.[92,93] However, in view of the data presented above, it is likely that such dose reductions will be associated with a greater incidence of posterior fossa relapse. In an attempt to circumvent this problem, both the CCSG and POG are beginning to evaluate the use of chemotherapy alone in such patients and are delaying radiation for 1 to 2 years, that is, until age 3 or older.

The survival rates of representative groups of patients treated with postoperative radiation therapy alone are presented in Table 24-9.

Chemotherapy

Several single-agent and multiagent chemotherapy trials over the last decade have shown little more than transient responses and marginal or no overall survival advantage.[111,144,177] Table

Table 24-9

Actuarial Survival (%) in Medulloblastoma with Postoperative Radiation Therapy

Number of Patients	Survival in Years				Reference
	1	*3*	*5*	*10*	
39	71	45	35	35	153
58		60	40	31	159
57		61	54		175
20	90	56	45		176
32	80	47	41	22	173
22	77	50			174

24-10 outlines the results of some recent adjuvant chemotherapy trials, and the results of three recent phase III chemotherapy trials are presented in Table 24-11. In the large trials conducted by the CCSG and SIOP, only a 10% survival advantage was observed for patients treated with a similar postradiation chemotherapy program over those given postoperative radiation alone. Despite these disappointing results, both studies showed that chemotherapy was more beneficial for patients with the greatest extents of disease, a group in whom a beneficial effect would be the easiest to detect because of their poorer prognosis. In contrast, no effect was observed on the survival of patients with apparently completely resected disease.[89]

Preradiation chemotherapy has been employed in the hope of attaining additional tumor kill at a time (postoperatively) when the tumor burden is theoretically the smallest. However, in a recent European trial, intrathecal methotrexate in addition to intravenous vincristine and procarbazine followed by postradiation maintenance chemotherapy with CCNU did not produced survival rates any better than those obtained with postoperative radiation alone.[185,186]

A unique preradiation and postradiation chemotherapy program, "eight drugs in 1 day," has recently produced a 56% response rate in a CCSG phase II trial.[187] This program employs eight individual drugs—CCNU, vincristine, procarbazine cisplatin, cyclophosphamide, methylprednisolone, hydroxy-

urea, and cytosine arabinoside—all of which have individual utility in CNS tumors. The underlying rationale is that multiple noncross-resistant single agents are necessary to overcome the innate occurrence of drug resistance. This aggressive treatment should be undertaken only by institutions familiar with its use and equipped to deal with its potential toxicities. Similar responses were noted in a small European study, and the CCSG is currently comparing this regimen with their prior nitrosourea-containing combination.[188]

Human medulloblastoma cell lines have been used *in vitro* and in murine xenograft models to explore the sensitivity of this tumor to different chemotherapeutic agents. Although this approach is still experimental, useful, clinically applicable information appears feasible.[177]

EPENDYMOMAS

Epidemiology

Ependymomas usually arise within or adjacent to the ependymal lining of the ventricular system or the central canal of the spinal cord and constitute 5% to 10% of all primary childhood CNS tumors. Sixty to seventy-five per cent of intracranial ependymomas occur in the posterior fossa and the remainder in the supratentorial area. Although the mean age of occurrence is 5 to 6 years, the peak age of incidence appears to be at 1 to 2 years. There is no gender predilection.[189-192] Ependymomas constitute as many as 25% of spinal cord tumors and rarely occur before the age of 12 years. These are considered separately in another section of this chapter.

Pathology and Patterns of Spread

Ependymomas tend to be well demarcated, partially encapsulated tumors that are frequently hemorrhagic and cystic. The most consistently used classification scheme is a numerical grading system that classifies tumors from I to IV on the basis of increasing anaplasia, cellular pleomorphism, cellularity, and mitosis. The grades I and II (low-grade) tumors are often referred to as "benign," although they can behave aggressively despite their well-differentiated appearance. Grades III and IV tumors are referred to as anaplastic, malignant, or high-grade.[189-193] Some investigators prefer not to use such grading systems, pointing out that they do not possess reliable prognostic value. Indeed, grading is not a part of the proposed pediatric revision of the WHO CNS tumor classification.[64]

The low-grade tumors are composed of polygonal or fusiform cells with round to ovoid nuclei. The most characteristic and diagnostic feature of these tumors is the ependymal rosette, which is composed of cells radially aligned about a central lumen. Perivascular pseudorosettes are more commonly seen than are the characteristic ependymal rosette (Fig. 24-11). Mitoses are, uncommon. In addition to these features, high-grade tumors demonstrate increased cellularity, frequent mitoses, necrosis, and bizzare multinucleated cells.[194] The overall appearance of these tumors may be similar to that of the high-grade astrocytomas.

There is disagreement over the inclusion of ependymoblastoma in the ependymoma tumor category. This largely undifferentiated, primitive-appearing tumor is probably best considered part of the primitive neuroectodermal tumor group, with which it shares a high proclivity for neuraxis dissemination. For the purposes of this review, it is not considered an ependymoma.[52,60]

Table 24-10
Actuarial Survival (%) in Medulloblastoma with Adjuvant* Chemotherapy

Agents†	Number of Patients	Survival in Years			Reference
		1	*3*	*5*	
CCNU	47	67	43	27	178
CCNU, VCR, It MTX	37		75	71	179
VCR, PCB, P	20		44	–	180
BCNU, MTX	40	68‡		56	181
VCR, CTX, It MTX	29		55	20	182
CCNU, VCR, It Mtx	34	95	82	71	162

* Postsurgical and postradiation.
† P = prednisone; It = intrathecal; MTX = methotrexate; VCR = vincristine; PCB = procarbazine; CTX = cyclophosphamide.
‡ Two-year survival.

Table 24-11
Results of Recent Randomized Chemotherapy Trials for Medulloblastoma

Agents*	Number of Patients	Actuarial Survival at 5 Years (%)		Reference
		RAD*	*RAD + CHEMO*	
VCR, It MTX, It HC	34	62	18	183
CCNU, VCR, P (CCSG)	237	49†	60†	89
		56	64	184
CCNU, VCR (SIOP)	232	42†	52†	89

* VCR = vincristine; It = intrathecal; P = prednisone; MTX = methotrexate; HC = hydrocortisone; RAD = radiation; RAD + CHEMO = radiation plus chemotherapy.
† Disease-free survival rate.

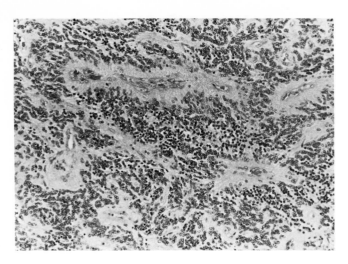

FIGURE 24-11. Section from fourth ventricular ependymoma displaying typical perivascular pseudorosettes. (H & E × 250)

Table 24-12
Spinal Subarachnoid Seeding (%) in Ependymomas by Tumor Grade and Location[195,196]

Location	Low Grade	High Grade	Total
Supratentorial	0–7	4–18	0–18
Infratentorial	12–15	52–63	12–63
Total	0–15	4–63	

The subependymoma histologically resembles a low-grade ependymoma but behaves differently. In most instances, this tumor is silent, being noted incidentally at autopsy, although it occasionally causes obstructive hydrocephalus *ante mortem.*

Ependymomas are locally invasive tumors with an incidence of spinal subarachnoid dissemination averaging 11% to 12% in combined patient series.[183,195,196] An interplay between tumor location and histologic grade is apparent in many series. Supratentorial tumors have a 3.5% to 8% overall incidence of such spread, whereas infratentorially located tumors have a rate of 20% to 33%.[74,195,196] When evaluated by histology alone, a 23% incidence of dissemination occurs in the high-grade tumors, in contrast to an 8% incidence in the low-grade tumors.[196] Table 24-12 integrates site and grade to demonstrate the relative risk of spinal subarachnoid dissemination for the various combinations of these features.

Tumors may also extend contiguously to produce intraspinal disease in the absence of subarachnoid spread.[9] Systemic metastases are rare and when present show a preference for liver, lung, lymph node, and bone.[4]

Clinical Presentation

The initial signs and symptoms of ependymomas are usually nonspecific and nonlocalizing and related to increased intracranial pressure. Posterior fossa tumors may lead to cerebellar dysfunction with ataxia and dysmetria. Cranial nerve findings and vomiting are more common with ependymomas than with the medulloblastoma because of tumor adherence and invasion of the fourth-ventricular floor.

In patients with supratentorial lesions, seizures and focal cerebral deficits similar to those accompanying other tumors in this location are frequent.

The duration of symptoms before diagnosis may range from a few weeks to well over a year and is inversely related to the grade of the tumor.[189,190]

Differential Diagnosis and Evaluation

The posterior fossa ependymomas may mimic brain-stem tumors, medulloblastomas, and astrocytomas as well as the nonmalignant conditions included in the differential diagnosis of these entities. In the lateral and third ventricles, ependymomas may produce a clinical picture similar to that seen in choroid plexus and midline astrocytic tumors.

As with other CNS tumors, the CT scan is the most reliable tool for demonstrating the tumor mass. Although there is great variability in the CT appearance of these tumors, they are generally hyperdense and homogeneously contrast-enhancing lesions. Hydrocephalus is present in almost all patients, and both cystic areas and calcification are frequent, occasionally leading to confusion between posterior fossa ependymomas and cerebellar astrocytomas.[197,198] Although experience with MRI in ependymomas is limited, it is likely to delineate the extent and degree of infiltration better than does CT.

Because of the significant incidence of subarachnoid seeding (Table 24-12), especially from posterior fossa tumors, myelography and CSF cytology should be included in the postoperative evaluation of these patients. Such a procedure can be safely done within 2 to 4 weeks postoperatively.

Prognostic Considerations

It has been suggested that children with ependymomas have a poorer prognosis than adults. However, study results are frequently contradictory on this point.[189,192,195] The discrepancy may be partly due to the inclusion of ependymoblastomas and the greater surgical mortality rate in earlier series of pediatric patients.

The effects of tumor site and grade on outcome are outlined in Table 24-13. With the exception of the markedly better survival in spinal tumors, which probably reflects the dominance of low-grade tumors, no consistent relation between location and outcome is evident. The most reliable prognostic factor is the grade of the tumor.[189,195–199,200] A 30% to 40% 5-year survival advantage in favor of low-grade tumors is regularly noted in recent series. Most other histologically based classifications have no consistent relation to outcome.[191]

Treatment

Surgery

Although surgery is important in establishing the diagnosis and helping to reestablish normal CSF flow, the impact of total versus subtotal resection on survival is unclear. Although gross macroscopic resections may be possible in two-thirds of supratentorial ependymomas, similar resections are much less frequent in the posterior fossa, where tumor adherence to the floor of the fourth ventricle is common and operative morbidity and mortality rates are high.[195,201] This concern, together with the lack of data indicating a significantly improved long-

Table 24-13
Ependymoma 5-Year Survival Rates (%) by Tumor Grade and Location

All Locations and Grades	Grade Only		Location Only		Reference
	High	Low	Supratentorial	Infratentorial	
18*	15	28	29	17	190
40*			33	46	202
17†			0	25	
47†‡	40				179
41 (10-year)	21	47			
37*	11	71			199
50‡					199
69 (10-year)*	67	75	35	33	192
44 (10-year)‡					192
39‡					195
51†‡	34	62			
60*	42 (III)§	78			200
	23 (IV)§				
54 (10-year)					
29‡					200
28‡					201

* Combined adult and child cases.
† Operative deaths excluded.
‡ Children only.
§ Histologic grade (Kernohan).

term outcome for patients with total versus subtotal resections, has led most clinicians to attempt the resection of gross tumor and to stop their resection when the tumor enters the brain stem.[191,192,195,201,202]

The perioperative mortality rates in ependymomas, which were as high as 50% in early series, are 0 to 11% in recent series, reflecting better operative techniques and supportive care.[191,195,201]

Radiation

Postoperative radiation therapy increases the overall survival of patients with ependymoma at 5 years from 15%–25% to 40%–50%.[12] Local failure remains the greatest cause of relapse and occurs in more than 50% of patients.[74,179,192] Local radiation doses of at least 4500 cGy are needed to establish reliable local control. The effect of greater doses has not been concurrently or prospectively evaluated even though most radiotherapists strongly encourage doses of 5000 to 5500 cGy.

Dose reductions of 20% have been recommended for children younger than 3 years.[179,192] The impact of this reduction on the survival rate of these patients has not been evaluated, however. One recent study demonstrated that younger (less than age 6) and older children have the same long-term survival rate (45% at 5 years), implying that dose reductions do not adversely affect ultimate survival.[192] However, the number of children younger than 3 years in this study is not stated.

The volume of radiation necessary for adequate prophylaxis against spinal subarachnoid disease is a matter of controversy. Even though it is apparent from Table 24-13 that both tumor site and grade affect such spread, most reported treatment series do not permit independent evaluation of these factors with respect to treatment volume and subarachnoid spread, and no prospective evaluation has been done, although the POG currently is attempting to address this issue.

At present, most radiotherapists recommend craniospinal coverage for high-grade tumors in any location because of their substantial incidence of subarachnoid dissemination. This approach has produced 5-year survival rates of 47% or better compared to 0 to 15% for local therapy only or no irradiation.[190,192,202]

For the low-grade ependymomas, therapy recommendations depend largely on the tumor site. In the supratentorial lesions, where the frequency of spinal disease is less than 7%, routine spinal prophylaxis may not be justified, and most therapists suggest local fields alone or with wide local margins.[196] Although whole-brain therapy has also been suggested,[192] the 5-year survival rate for this therapy (67%) is not significantly better than the 60% to 75% survival rates reported for local fields alone in older series.[190,199,203] In infratentorial low-grade ependymomas, most radiotherapists recommend wide local fields.[196] These fields usually encompass an upper cervical cord segment in addition to the posterior fossa and exclude the cerebrum, as spread to this area from the posterior fossa is rare.[195]

Chemotherapy

Several nitrosourea-containing drug combinations with and without intrathecal therapy with other agents have been used in newly diagnosed and recurrent disease. The number of patients treated has been small in any single series, and no consistent evidence of more than transient stabilization of disease has been shown.[200,204,205] Cisplatin has produced the best overall response rate in phase II trials.[206] A phase III trial of adjuvant CCNU and vincristine in 14 patients demonstrated an increase in the 5-year survival rate to 70% from 44% for historical controls, but the groups had identical survival rates (44%) at 7 years.[179] Aside from the lack of concurrent controls, a greater radiation volume was used in the chemotherapy-treated patients. Thus, any improvement in 5-year survival rates cannot be attributed independently to chemotherapy.

CEREBELLAR ASTROCYTOMA

Epidemiology

Cerebellar astrocytomas account for between 10% and 20% of childhood CNS tumors and occur throughout the first decade of life without a discrete incidence peak.[5,207–211] The male-to-female ratio is 1.3:1.

Pathology and Patterns of Spread

Two principal histologic variants of the cerebellar astrocytoma have been described.[145] The classic, or pilocytic, astrocytoma accounts for 80% to 85% of these tumors (Fig. 24-12). This tumor is characterized by firm, compact areas merging with looser, poorly cellular areas of spongy texture. The modestly cellular areas are composed of fusiform cells interwoven with a fine fibrillary background. A prominent microcystic component is generally visible. Rosenthal fibers, which are thought to represent benign degenerative changes, as well as focal areas of calcification and oligodendroglial cells are also seen frequently. The second variety, the diffuse astrocytoma, accounts for 15% of these tumors and differs from the classic piloid variety in being a more solid and densely cellular tumor that generally lacks microcysts. This tumor is said to closely resemble Russell and Rubinstein's fibrillary astrocytoma, which is most frequent in the cerebral hemispheres and has a poorer prognosis than piloid tumors.

Although mitoses are rare, focal leptomeningeal invasion, endothelial hyperplasia, and pleomorphic and hyperchromic nuclei are frequently seen in cerebellar astrocytomas. Although such features are associated with malignant behavior in other astrocytomas, the cerebellar astrocytoma generally follow an indolent clinical course.

A mural nodule surrounded by a large cyst that contains a thick proteinaceous fluid often dominates the gross appearance of cerebellar astrocytomas, particularly the piloid tumors. Such macrocystic tumors may constitute half or more of all cerebellar astrocytomas.[211] The walls of these cysts are often highly vascular, and spontaneous hemorrhages may occur.

Rarely, glioblastoma multiforme occurs in the cerebellum.

FIGURE 24-12. Typical biphasic pattern of piloid astrocytoma. Note dense, relatively anuclear fibrillar areas alternating with looser honeycombed fields. (H & E × 250)

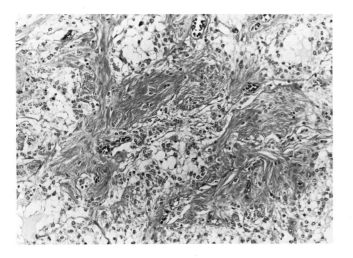

The clinical course is identical to that of tumors in the more common cerebral location.[216]

Although cerebellar astrocytomas are considered to be well-circumscribed, noninvasive tumors, recent observations demonstrate that one-third of newly diagnosed patients may have clinically silent involvement of noncontiguous posterior fossa and more-distant sites.[208] Additionally, extensive neuraxis involvement by well-differentiated piloid tumor in the absence of positive CSF cytology has been reported.[216] Some authors have suggested that these instances of noncontiguous well-differentiated disease may evidence a multifocal neoplastic process.[208]

Clinical Presentation

Because of their common location, the signs and symptoms of cerebellar astrocytomas may resemble those of medulloblastoma. However, cerebellar astrocytomas grow more slowly and have a less acute clinical onset.[207,211,217] As with medulloblastoma, more than 90% of patients present with nonspecific and nonlocalizing symptoms of increased intracranial pressure. Midline cerebellar signs are present in 70% of patients, even though the tumor is more frequently located in the lateral cerebellar hemispheres.[207,211,217] Such signs may be secondary to pressure on the midline areas rather than to direct tumor involvement. When there is invasion of the cerebellar peduncles and brain stem, cranial nerve signs, hyperreflexia, and Babinski signs also appear.

Prognostic Considerations

A poor prognostic influence has been suggested for the diffuse histologic subgroup of cerebellar astrocytomas. This pattern has been associated with a 38% 25-year survival rate in contrast to a 94% survival rate in patients with the classic piloid tumor.[212] However, others have been unable to confirm these results although their follow-up times are often much shorter.[213,214]

Winston and associates retrospectively described a number of discretely identifiable histologic and clinical features that strongly correlate with survival.[209] The histologic features were described without reference to the nomenclature and assumptions embedded in more-conventional classifications such as those of Russell and Rubinstein and of the WHO. A statistical analysis revealed clusters of phenotypic features that describe two major tumor types with differing prognoses (see classification section). The type A tumor has a 94% 10-year survival rate and any or all of the following histologic features: Rosenthal fibers, oligodendroglial foci, microcysts, and leptomeningeal deposits. At the clinical level, headaches, dysmetria, and gait disturbances are noted. The second tumor, type B, has a 29% 10-year survival rate. Its histologic features include perivascular pseudorosettes, foci of necrosis, high cell density, mitoses, and foci of calcification. Lethargy and altered consciousness are the important clinical features. Whereas 70% of type A tumors have a macrocyst, only 23% of type B tumors have this feature. The above conclusions and the tumor definitions are undergoing a prospective evaluation by the multi-institutional Childhood Brain Tumor Consortium.

Perhaps the most consistently observed clinically relevant variable predictive of outcome is the presence of brain-stem involvement which carries a poor prognosis regardless of tumor histology or size.[213,217,221]

Differential Diagnosis and Evaluation

The differential diagnosis of these tumors includes vascular malformations, the rare cerebellar degenerative diseases, and other primary posterior fossa tumors such as medulloblastoma and ependymoma.

The CT appearance of cerebellar astrocytoma may be similar to that of medulloblastoma in some instances; both generally demonstrate hydrocephalus, good contrast enhancement, and a cerebellar location. However, the cerebellar astrocytoma is generally a less dense tumor and often has a prominant cystic component in which the cyst wall and mural nodule may also enhance with contrast medium. Contrast enhancement in the cerebellar astrocytoma does not imply the same aggressive clinical behavior it typically does for the cerebral astrocytomas.[218,219]

Treatment

Surgery

The surgical approach to cerebellar astrocytomas is via a suboccipital craniotomy, similar to that used for medulloblastoma. As complete tumor excision improves survival and large portions of the cerebellar hemispheres can be removed without significant permanent neurologic or cerebellar dysfunction, aggressive attempts at resection of tumor located in these areas is warranted. However, tumor located in the cerebellar midline or peduncles is much more difficult to resect totally, as significant cerebellar dysfunction may result from damage to or interuption of the cerebellar nuclei and pathways.[211,212,214,217,222] In the current era, 80% to 90% of patients have complete resections, compared with 65% in earlier series, and the operative mortality rate is less than 1%.[209,211,212,217,222] Preoperative shunting may be necessary, and as many as one-third of patients may require permanent shunting.[228]

The relapse-free survival rate for patients with complete resections is at least 80%, and more than 90% of these patients will survive disease free for periods of up to 30 years. Further therapy is unnecessary after complete resection.[209,211,221,223,225]

The survival rates of patients with subtotally resected tumors are deceptive. Whereas actuarial survival rates may initially be similar to those after total resection, relapse-free survival rates are considerably poorer. Despite occasional reports of 15- and 30-year relapse-free survivors, recent data suggest that as few as 36% of patients with subtotal resections are relapse-free survivors at 6 years.[211,217,223]

Radiation

The role of radiation therapy in incompletely resected tumors is unclear. Table 24-14 outlines the results of radiation therapy after partial and complete resection. Although many authors have suggested that postoperative radiation therapy improves the survival of patients with incomplete resections,[223,225,229] similar results are reported in unirradiated patients.[211,217,221] Additionally, radiation has had no effect on the survival of patients with poor prognostic features, a group in which the benefits of effective therapy should be the easiest to observe.[209,212,216,226–228] Although radiation has been reported to improve the relapse-free survival rate in newly diagnosed disease and the freedom from subsequent relapse in patients with initially recurrent tumor, the numbers of patients studied are small.[223] As there are no substantive data to indicate otherwise, radiation may reasonably be withheld until there is evidence of disease progression or relapse.

Intracavity ^{32}P appeared to be useful in patients with recurrent macrocystic disease.[224]

Chemotherapy

Chemotherapy has been given only to a few patients, and no reliable judgments can be made about its effectiveness.[224]

SUPRATENTORIAL ASTROCYTOMAS

Epidemiology

Supratentorial astrocytic tumors comprise about 35% of childhood CNS tumors. One-third to one-half of them are located in the cerebral hemispheres, and the remainder occur in the ventricles or in other midline diencephalic or nuclear structures (thalamus, hypothalamus, and basal ganglia). The peak incidence is bimodal, with an early peak between ages 2 and 4 and another in early adolescence. The overall male-to-female ratio is somewhat higher than in other CNS tumors and approaches 2:1.[3,5,230]

Pathology and Patterns of Spread

The classification of astrocytic tumors is confusing because of the variety of terms that have been applied to them (see Table 24-1). Astrocytomas are a heterogeneous group of tumors that includes a number of well-differentiated subtypes (protoplasmic, fibrillary, pilocytic, gemistocytic) that have a rather uniform microscopic appearance. The presence of anaplastic changes (increased cellularity, mitoses, cellular pleomorphism) is associated with the appearance of progressively less-differentiated astrocytic tumors, the anaplastic astrocytoma, and glioblastoma multiforme. In an attempt to simplify the

Table 24-14
Survival Rate (%) with and Without Radiation in Complete and Incompletely Resected Cerebellar Astrocytomas

Treatment	5 Years	10 Years	Reference
Complete resection	76–100	79–100	211, 217, 223–225
Incomplete resection			
Without radiation	79, 36,* 74*	66; 68	217, 223, 224, 228
With radiation	56–92	40–70; 83*	211, 217, 223–225, 228

* Relapse-free survival rate.

classification of astrocytomas, Kernohan proposed grading these tumors I to IV on the basis of increasing anaplasia.[51] Despite its subjective nature and conceptual drawbacks, this system has remained popular because it has some correlation with prognosis and is intuitively easy to apply and understand (see classification). Its use is not recommended in the revised WHO classification of CNS tumors, however.

The histologic subtypes common in children include the fibrillary and pilocytic tumors, and the malignant anaplastic astrocytoma and glioblastoma multiforme.[145] The pilocytic tumors tend to occur more frequently in the diencephalic structures and ventricles and have microscopic features identical to those of the classic pilocytic cerebellar astrocytomas (Fig. 24-12). The fibrillary astrocytomas are more densely cellular and less cystic than the pilocytic tumors and have a more diffuse and microscopically uniform appearance. Cellular pleomorphism may be seen, and mitoses are rare.[145] These tumors are more common in the cerebral hemispheres.

The anaplastic astrocytoma (Fig. 24-13) is distinguished by the presence of anaplastic changes interspersed with areas of better-differentiated and typical astrocytic cells. In the glioblastoma multiforme (Fig. 24-14), anaplastic change dominates the microscopic picture. Giant and bizarre multinucleated cells and aberrant mitoses as well as grossly visible areas of degenerative changes (hemorrhage, necrosis) are also present in this latter tumor.

The Kernohan grade I and II (low-grade) tumors are well-differentiated, bland-appearing neoplasms without mitoses. These tumors comprise 50% to 75% of supratentorial astrocytomas, have an indolent clinical course, and remain locally infiltrative.[3,5,51,145,230,231] Because of their well-differentiated appearance and slow growth, these tumors blend into the surrounding normal brain tissue without a clear demarcation.

The grade III and IV (high-grade) tumors are best exemplified by the anaplastic astrocytoma and glioblastoma multiforme: highly cellular, undifferentiated tumors with frequent mitoses, cellular pleomorphism, and areas of necrosis and hemorrhage. These are clinically aggressive tumors that are widely invasive. Because of their rapid growth, effacement of local tissues often produces a grossly clear demarcation from normal brain. However, extensive microscopic extension beyond this margin is the rule. About 25% to 50% of all supratentorial astrocytomas are high grade, and most occur in hemispheric rather than diencephalic locations. Glioblastoma multiforme, in particular, has the potential for both neuraxis and systemic dissemination, although this is more frequent in adults than in children. Lung, lymph nodes, liver, and bone are the favored metastatic sites.[3,5,51,145,230–233]

FIGURE 24-13. Highly cellular tumor composed of anaplastic astrocytes. A few vessels with compressed lumina are formed by swollen epithelial cells. (H & E × 250)

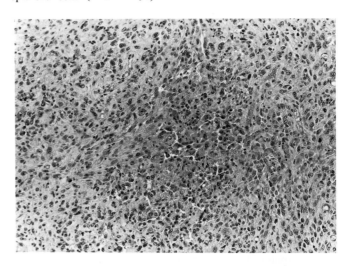

FIGURE 24-14. A. Typical field in glioblastoma multiforme showing pseudopalisading (*upper left*), neovascularity, nuclear anaplasia, and multinucleated giant cells (*lower right*). (H & E × 250) **B.** Higher magnification of different field from same tumor showing cellular anaplasia, multinucleated cells, and bizarre mitosis (*upper left corner*). (H & E × 400)

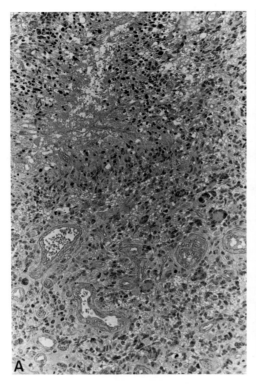

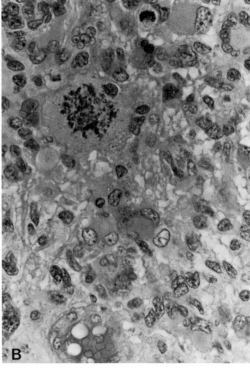

Clinical Presentation

The major clinical signs at diagnosis are nonspecific and non-localizing features related to increased intracranial pressure; these occur in 50% to 75% of patients regardless of tumor location. Papilledema occurs in 80% of patients, and other visual disturbances, weakness, hemiplegia, and cranial nerve findings are present in 25% to 50%.[230,232,236–238]

Seizures, most frequently grand mal, are present at diagnosis in at least 25% of patients with supratentorial astrocytomas overall and in as many as 55% of those with hemispheric tumors. Although as many as one-third of patients with high-grade tumors have seizures, the frequency is actually higher in the more slowly evolving low-grade tumors, where they may precede diagnosis by several months to as much as 1 or 2 years. In contrast, seizures in patients with high-grade tumors have an onset closer to diagnosis.[230,232,234,235,238,239]

Diencephalic astrocytomas present with a spectrum and frequency of nonspecific findings similar to that in patients with hemispheric tumors, although earlier CSF obstruction causes a more acute and earlier onset of symptoms.

The more specific signs of supratentorial tumors relate to tumor location and the compromise of surrounding structures and neural pathways.[230,232,233,236–238] Focal motor deficits and pyramidal tract findings such weakness and monoplegias or hemiplegias are particularly common with lateral hemispheric and central diencephalic tumors, occurring in 40% or more of these patients.[239] In some patients with diencephalic tumors, weakness, dysmetria, tremor, and ataxia may occur, mimicking the findings in posterior fossa tumors.[239] Similar features may be seen in some individuals with frontal lobe involvement.[240] Dysmetria and chorea are seen in many patients with basal ganglia tumors. Hypothalamic tumors are often associated with growth and endocrine abnormalities, and weight loss occurs in as many as 50% of these patients. Optic atrophy and diabetes insipidus are also frequent.[239] The classic diencephalic syndrome (emesis, emaciation, and unusual euphoria in infants with diencephalic tumors) is uncommon, however, and is rare beyond age 3 years.

Differential Diagnosis and Evaluation

The differential diagnosis of supratentorial tumors includes abscess, vascular malformations, the uncommon demyelinating diseases, and cerebritis. The acuteness of onset and the constellation of clinical features and the CT findings are generally able to differentiate these possibilities. Cerebral angiography may help to rule out a vascular malformation and aid in operative planning by demonstrating the blood supply of the tumor and its proximity to major vascular structures.

Germ cell tumors and teratomas must be considered in the differential diagnosis of diencephalic tumors, particularly those in the hypothalamic and pineal areas. These tumors are discussed later in this chapter.

Both the density and contrast enhancement noted on the CT scan correlate with the degree of malignancy. In low-grade tumors, a homogenous low-density pattern with contrast enhancement is present in as many as 50% of patients. The high-grade tumors show a more heterogeneous and mixed density pattern with generally diffuse contrast enhancement. A mass effect is almost universal in the high-grade, but infrequent in the low-grade, tumors.[241,242] MRI generally reveals a greater extent of tumor than does CT and more clearly distinguishes peritumoral edema from hypodense surrounding tumor.

Prognostic Considerations

Several prognostically significant features can be identified in the supratentorial astrocytomas, including tumor grade and histology, patient age, and tumor location.

Survival is inversely correlated with the Kernohan grade of the tumor. In adult patients with glioblastoma multiforme, a giant-cell or "monstrocellular" histology is associated with longer survival in hemispheric tumors, but this has not been evaluated in the pediatric population.[3,243–245] The presence of tumor cysts is associated with a more favorable outcome in hemispheric locations, although this feature is probably not an independent variable and is often found in the more favorable low-grade tumors. A long duration of symptoms prior to diagnosis and the presence of seizures have a similar prognostic significance and association with low-grade tumors.[232,237,244,246,247]

With hemispheric tumors, younger age is generally associated with a better prognosis. Children consistently have longer survivals than adults, and within the pediatric population, younger patients appear to do better than older ones with the exception of those less than 2 years old. The reasons for this latter observation are unclear but may partly reflect the greater surgical mortality rates and the higher-grade tumors in the very young patients described in earlier series. The shift from the better prognosis of childhood appears to occur by age 10 and is clearly established in the adolescent.[3,230,236,243,248,249] No clear age influence is noted in the diencephalic tumors.

Diencephalic and ventricular tumors appear to have survival rates similar to those of other supratentorial tumors of the same grade.[88,225,241,250–252] Thalamic tumors may be an exception to this generalization in that a greater incidence of high-grade tumors has been reported in this location by some[253] although not all[88] observers.

Treatment

Much of the literature on the treatment of supratentorial astrocytomas does not allow clear and independent evaluations of tumor site, histology, degree of resection, and effects of subsequent radiation or chemotherapy. Moreover, adult and pediatric patients are frequently reported together. Nevertheless, definable response patterns do exist and are summarized below and in Tables 24-15 and 24-16. Although hemispheric and diencephalic sites are not separated in most articles, response and survival patterns appear similar in these sites when tumor grade is considered.

Surgery

Although complete excision favorably influences survival regardless of site or histology, it is often precluded because of unfavorable tumor location and the unacceptable morbidity of an aggressive approach. Gross total excisions are possible in 40% to 80% of hemispheric tumors; however, less than 40% of diencephalic tumors have been similarly resectable.[230,231,254] In a recently reported institutional series, a 90% resection rate for thalamic tumors was possible with microsurgical techniques.[88]

The beneficial effects of resection are most evident in the low-grade tumors, where complete removal may lead to 80% survival rates at 7 years compared with 15% to 50% in patients with subtotal resections.[231] Removal of the mural nodule alone in macrocystic piloid tumors has led to mean survivals of at least 70% for periods of 13 to 17 years, and in some instances of these low-grade and cystic tumors, surgery appears to be curative.[225,232,236,237,247,252,255,259] In the high-grade tumors, a recent report shows patients with at least partial resection have better survival rates than those undergoing biopsy alone. However, no difference between the effects of complete and partial resection was evident in this adjuvant chemotherapy trial.[259]

The current operative mortality rate is less than 3%, although figures as high as 14% to 27% were common in earlier literature, particularly for the deep midline tumors and in younger children.[225,231,236,247] Morbidity depends on tumor location and is highest in the diencephalic tumors, where a 10% to 20% incidence of hemiparesis or visual field cut may occur.

Radiation

In high-grade gliomas, only a modest increase in short-term survival is apparent with radiation therapy. The effect appears little influenced by the tumor site or the extent of resection and is generally short lived.[241,248,255] In grade III tumors, postoperative radiation influences early survival, but by 5 years, there is no difference in the survival of irradiated and unirradiated patients. In grade IV tumors, the benefit of radiation is even more limited, and it rarely prolongs survival beyond 1 to 2 years.[238,243,255]

Radiation has no apparent effect in patients with completely resected low-grade tumors, where 5-year survival rates are as high as 90%.[232,237,246,254] In patients with incomplete resection, a positive effect on survival appears limited to the first 5 to 10 years after therapy.[230,237,243,244,254,255] Although tumor doses of 5000 to 5500 cGy are recommended, little change in survival rates with doses between 3500 and 5000 cGy has been reported by others.[225,242,248,256] In contrast, the use of higher-dose therapy (conventionally fractionated doses of 6000–7500 cGy) may modestly prolong survival in high-grade tumors, although it does not alter the 3 to 5-year survival.[260]

There is little or no evidence to suggest that whole-brain therapy is needed, and radiation to the tumor bed with generous margins appears adequate, as 90% of recurrences are local.[225,248,254,261] Interstitial irradiation (see Chap. 11) may have a role in some well-localized midline tumors.

Chemotherapy

Chemotherapy has no established role in the adjuvant treatment of low-grade tumors. Reports of its use in a few relapsed patients with low-grade tumors suggest that objective tumor response and improved survival may be obtained with nitrosourea-containing regimens or high-dose methotrexate.[179,262–264]

With one exception, chemotherapy has demonstrated little effect on high-grade tumors. A recent pediatric phase III chemotherapy trial in high-grade gliomas produced a 45%

Table 24-15
Survival Rate (%) in Low-Grade Supratentorial Astrocytomas According to Therapy

Treatment	Survival in Years					References
	3	5	7	10	20	
Complete resection		90	60 (d)*	86	25	231, 254
Incomplete resection		13–62		15–48	0–48	225, 230, 250
		25 (I), 0 (II)				255
Incomplete resection		41–81		28–81	40	88, 225, 254, 256
plus radiation	58 (d)	58–72 (d)		67 (d), 17 (t)		252, 257, 258
		58 (I), 25 (II)				225

* d = diencephalic tumors; t = thalamic tumors; I = grade I; II = grade II (all other figures are for grades I and II combined).

Table 24-16
Survival Rate (%) in High-Grade Astrocytomas According to Therapy

Treatment	Survival in Years						References
	1	2	3	5	7	10	
Incomplete resection	8 (IV)*		0 (IV)	0 (IV)			255
				2 (III/IV)			255
Incomplete resection	33–67 (IV)	15–17 (IV)	7 (IV)	0–26 (IV)			225, 238, 255, 256
and radiation	30 (d)			0–18 (III)			225, 255, 256
				10–28 (III/IV)	22 (d)		88, 231
						23 (III/IV)‡	250, 259
Incomplete resection	24 (IV)		6 (IV)	0 (IV)			255
and radiation	80 (III/IV)			45 (III/IV)			249, 255
plus							
chemotherapy							

* Grade of tumor; d = diencephalic tumors.
† 10-year survival.

versus a 13% 5-year disease-free survival rate with adjuvant CCNU, vincristine, and prednisone.[259] The effect was most apparent in glioblastoma multiforme and appeared to be related to the degree of surgical resection, with the best survival occurring in those patients who had at least a partial resection.

The "8 in 1" chemotherapy regimen has recently produced a 36% response rate (complete and partial) in a phase II trial in malignant gliomas.[187] This treatment program is similar to the "8 in 1" program outlined in the medulloblastoma section of this chapter, except that DTIC is substituted for cyclophosphamide. A phase III trial of preradiation and postradiation chemotherapy comparing this combination with the CCNU, vincristine, and prednisone program referred to above is currently being conducted by the CCSG.

High-dose methotrexate with citrovorum rescue appears to have some limited utility in patients with recurrent tumor without prior chemotherapy.[264]

BRAIN-STEM GLIOMAS

Epidemiology

Brain-stem gliomas comprise between 10% and 20% of all childhood CNS tumors. The peak age of incidence lies between 5 and 8 years, and as many as 77% of patients are less than age 20 at diagnosis. The male-to-female ratio is near unity.[265-269]

Pathology and Patterns of Spread

Nearly half of these tumors arise in the pons, with the medulla and midbrain being the next most frequent sites.[265-269] In recent series, 53% of patients had low-grade (Kernohan I and II) astrocytomas, which are generally of the diffuse fibrillary pattern similar to that noted in the cerebral hemispheres; only a minority had tumors with the more favorable characteristics of pilocytic astrocytomas.[51,145] Higher-grade (III and IV) tumors, anaplastic astrocytoma and glioblastoma multiforme, respectively, account for about 38% of brain-stem tumors. However, in autopsy series, a greater proportion of high-grade tumors is noted, suggesting either "malignant progression" of tumor or, more likely, an initially inadequate biopsy.[265,270] In combined patient series, as many as 10% of brain-stem tumors are ependymomas or primitive neuroectodermal tumors.[269,271-293]

Direct intra-axial extension of tumor into contiguous CNS sites is the dominant mode of growth and often results in symmetric and asymmetric enlargement of the brain stem. Exophytic growth into the posterior fossa may also occur.[270,273] Although distant neuraxis dissemination has been considered uncommon, an incidence as high as 20% has been reported in recent combined patient series. Patients harboring the most anaplastic tumors show the most extensive local invasion and are also the most likely to have distant disease.[265,274,275]

Clinical Presentation

As tumors encroach on the fourth ventricle, obstruction of CSF flow occurs, which may result in hydrocephalus. Although some evidence of hydrocephalus may occur in many patients at diagnosis, papilledema is an uncommon finding at this time, suggesting that increased intracranial pressure and hydrocephalus develop slowly.[268,276] The initial nonlocalizing and nonspecific clinical features of these tumors such as headache, nausea, and emesis result from direct tumor involvement of

vagal nuclei and meningeal traction rather than overtly increased pressure.

Cranial nerve palsies are particularly frequent and most often involve the IIIrd, Vth, VIth, VIIth, IXth, and Xth nerves. Tumor involvement of the cerebellar peduncles and brainstem cerebellar tracts may lead to ataxia and other cerebellar signs. Likewise, compromise of motor and sensory tracts may produce contralateral anesthesia, spastic hemiparesis, and hemiplegia.[277] Personality changes characterized by apathy, withdrawal, and emotional lability are particularly frequent in patients with pontine tumors.[278,279]

Differential Diagnosis and Evaluation

The most common differential diagnoses of brain-stem tumors include vascular malformations and brain-stem encephalitis. Demyelinating processes such as multiple sclerosis and subacute necrotizing encephalomyelopathy should also be considered. Although rare, an epidermoid cyst, hematoma, or tuberculoma may also mimic a brain-stem tumor.[269] An evaluation of the CSF for inflammatory findings such as pleocytosis, increased protein, myelin basic proteins, and oligoclonal bands may help to distinguish among the above possibilities. However, a lumbar puncture should not be undertaken until clinical evaluation and CT scan confirm the absence of hydrocephalus and fourth-ventricular obstruction.

CT and MRI are the most useful diagnostic procedures. The CT appearance of most tumors is that of an isodense or hypodense, often poorly contrast-enhancing, mass (Fig. 24-4A).[280,281] Contrast-enhancing exophytic tumors filling the fourth ventricle can be confused with medulloblastoma on CT scan. MRI is helpful in such situations, as it can better demonstrate the anatomic origins and extent of the tumor (Fig. 24-4B,C).[282,283] This capability is of considerable importance in defining the radiotherapy fields in tumors such as these, where the dominant mode of failure is local recurrence.

Brain-stem evoked potentials may be useful both in helping to make the diagnosis and in intraoperative monitoring, which can increase the safety of direct surgical intervention.[284,285]

Prognostic Considerations

The principal prognostic factors in brain-stem gliomas relate to the location and histology of the tumor.[265,267,274,276] In general, the more superiorly located tumors, particularly those of the diencephalon and, to a lesser extent, the midbrain, tend to have lower-grade histology and longer survival times. Pontine tumors are said to be intermediate, and medullary tumors appear to have the most malignant histologies and the worst survival. Although a recent report has described several cervicomedullary tumors with low-grade histology and good survival, these tumors may have been medullary extensions of the more favorable spinal cord glioma.[274]

The Kernohan tumor grade is inversely correlated with survival: patients with low-grade (I or II) lesions survive longer than those with high-grade (III or IV) lesions. Even so, more than half of those with low-grade lesions eventually die of their disease. The presence of Rosenthal fibers and calcification and the absence of mitotic figures have recently been said to indicate improved survival and presumably reflect a low-grade favorable histology, as in cerebellar astrocytomas.[209,286,287] However, unlike the cerebellar tumors, the presence of a gross or microscopic cystic component appears to have no impact on survival.[270,286]

Cranial nerve palsies are strongly correlated with high-grade or malignant histology. Patients with these findings usually have a rapidly worsening clinical course and early demise.[286]

The CT appearance also has prognostic significance[286,288]; 60% to 100% of patients with hypodense (prior to contrast injection) diffusely intrinsic brain-stem tumors die of recurrence within 1 year of diagnosis, whereas only 10% to 60% of patients with local or focally intrinsic isodense (prior to contrast) tumors—some of which may show contrast enhancement—die within 2 years. The longest survivals occur in patients with dorsally exophytic tumors that fill the fourth ventricle. These patients are remarkable in that their survival rate at 4.5 years may be greater than 90%.[288] In small institutional series, these individuals make up as many as 22% of patients and tend to be young, often less than 2 years, and to have low-grade tumors.[269,273,288] Exophytic growth alone, however, does not appear to have any consistent independent relation to histology or survival in other series.[271,276,286]

Treatment

The overall prognosis for patients with brain-stem tumors is poor, and recent reports demonstrate virtually no improvement in the median survival time of these patients over several decades.[266,271]

Surgery

The surgical approach to brain-stem tumors is hazardous and the degree of resectability extremely limited. For these reasons and the potential problems posed by small biopsy specimens from nonhomogeneous tumors, the morbidity, and the lack of substantially effective therapy, histology has not been relied on for diagnosis or management.[274] Thus, in most instances, clinical and radiographic diagnosis alone has been regarded as satisfactory. However, in several recent reports, either direct or stereotactic biopsy was done safely, and good clinicopathologic correlations were obtained with little morbidity.[272,276,288–291]

The recent ability to resect some focal low-grade tumors subtotally[274] and the improved survival in three of four patients with partial tumor resections as compared with the larger number of unselected patients in a recent CCSG study[268] suggest an increasingly valuable role for surgery in this disease. Additionally, it should be noted that the good prognosis associated with the exophytic tumors described by Hoffman and associates involved unusually large tumor resections, a factor that may partly account for their good results.[273] All the above suggest that biopsy and attempted resection of brain-stem gliomas by an experienced neurosurgeon can aid in patient management.

Radiation

Radiation remains the only routinely used therapeutic modality. Although most investigators show increases in the median survival of patients given at least 5000 cGy to the tumor and a surrounding margin, improvement is generally transient. Although occasional reports have described survival rates of better than 40% to 50% at 5 years, these results appear skewed by significant numbers of diencephalic tumors, which have a better prognosis than brain-stem lesions.[265,292–294] A survival rate of 20% to 30% at 3 years is more consistent with the results of recent large studies.[266–269,271]

Radiation therapy appears to be most beneficial for patients with low-grade tumors. Little benefit is apparent for patients with high-grade tumors, their survivals being the same as

or less than the approximately 15 months reported for some untreated patients.[145,268,269,276] Radiation sensitizers have not improved the response in either group of patients. Hyperfractionated radiation therapy with 120 cGy twice daily to a total dose of 6480 to 6600 cGy has had no effect on survival.[295] However, longer survival is appearing with total hyperfractionated doses of 7200 cGy delivered in 100-cGy fractions twice daily.[97] The long-term toxicity and ultimate utility of this experimental approach remain to be determined.

Chemotherapy

Although reports of response to several single agents and drug combinations have been published, the numbers of patients are generally small and the responses short lived.[111]

Adjuvant multiagent chemotherapy has also been disappointing. In a recently conducted CCSG trial, 74 children with brain-stem gliomas were randomized to radiation alone versus postradiation CCNU, vincristine, and prednisone. No statistical difference in the 5-year survival rate was apparent (17% versus 23%).[268] Similarly, results with a variety of other nitrosourea-containing programs, with and without the use of radiosensitizers, have shown no benefit.[267,296,297]

INTRAMEDULLARY SPINAL CORD TUMORS

Epidemiology

Four percent to 6% of primary CNS tumors in children occur in the spinal cord. These tumors occur sporadically throughout childhood, with a median age of 10 years and a male-to-female ratio of 1.3:1. A limited association (5%) with neurofibromatosis is present.[5,298,299]

Pathology and Patterns of Spread

About two-thirds of intramedullary tumors are astrocytomas, and one-fourth to one-third are ependymomas. In general, the intramedullary astrocytomas and ependymomas are well-differentiated low-grade tumors with histology identical to that of their counterparts in other CNS locations. High-grade or anaplastic features occur in 11% of astrocytomas and less frequently in ependymomas. Large cysts, both within the tumor and at the superior and inferior margins, are common. In as many as 60% of cases, extensive and often holocord involvement by tumor and cysts may be present. In the remainder, the location in the spinal cord appears to be random, with an incidence in any anatomic region being roughly proportional to the length of that region: thoracic greater than cervical greater than lumbar. Slow and contiguous extension across an average of six vertebral segments with compression and effacement of normal tissues is the usual mode of growth.[5,298–300] Rare instances of leptomeningeal dissemination are confined to the high-grade tumors, and the presence of multiple discrete tumors is associated with neurofibromatosis.

Clinical Presentation

Because of their slow growth, the symptoms of these tumors develop insidiously and may be present for up to 24 months or longer prior to diagnosis.[299,301,302] The most frequent clinical findings are weakness (85%), pain and other sensory changes (60%–70%), gait disturbance (40%–50%), and sphincter dysfunction (20%). Weakness is of variable extent and severity, ranging from that confined to an extremity to quadriparesis. Likewise, pain is variable and may suggest spinal, nerve root, or neural tract involvement. In 70% of patients, the pain is localized to the vertebral segments adjacent to the tumor and is described as dull and aching, worse at night and increased by coughing or sneezing. This pain probably is due to tumor distention of the dura, which is temporarily increased with Valsalva-maneuver-induced venous and CSF pressure. In another 10% to 20% of patients, pain typical of nerve root involvement and encompassing one or two dermatomes is present. A vague burning pain and paresthesias occur in other patients, suggesting lateral spinothalamic-tract compromise. This latter pain often bears no anatomic relation to the site of the tumor, perhaps reflecting the significant longitudinal dispersion of pain and touch fibers along the cord prior to their crossing into the contralateral spinothalamic tracts.[299,301] Gait disturbance may result from both motor-tract and posterior-column involvement.[299,301]

Papilledema and other signs and symptoms of increased intracranial pressure are present in 12% of patients. These findings are generally attributed to increased CSF viscosity from an elevated protein content, which is frequently 250 mg/dl or more, with levels as high as 1500 to 2000 mg/dl below the level of obstruction. Arachnoiditis or fourth-ventricular obstruction in high cervical tumors may also contribute to elevated intracranial pressure.[299,301]

Differential Diagnosis and Evaluation

The differential diagnosis of intramedullary tumors must include syringomyelia and hydromyelia, which can generally be distinguished with neuroradiographic studies or MRI. Extramedullary tumors such as schwannomas and meningiomas, as well as the rare spinal demyelinating diseases, may produce similar clinical findings.[3,6] Spinal metastases from other systemic malignancies are generally distinguishable by their acute onset and the other systemic findings.

Plain radiographs are abnormal in 50% of patients with intramedullary tumors. A widened spinal canal with medial erosion of the pedicles, posterior scalloping of the vertebral bodies, and kyphoscoliosis are common. Metrizamide myelography shows a block at the inferior tumor margin in 50% to 90% of cases. If such a block is found, a second myelogram via a C1–2 puncture should be done to define the tumor's upper limit and to help plan the extent of surgery. Repeat CT scans 12 to 24 hours later after water-soluble myelography dyes have diffused into these spaces may be helpful in demonstrating cysts and ruling out a syrinx.[298,299–301]

MRI is probably the best modality for demonstrating clearly the extent and components of intramedullary tumors (Fig. 24-15) and may obviate for myelography.[299,302]

Treatment

Surgery

Surgical exploration for diagnosis and potential resection is mandatory. In earlier series of patients, complete tumor resections were associated with longer survivals, although such resections were frequently not possible except perhaps in the well-demarcated ependymomas. Although a cleavage plane is much less evident in astrocytomas, recent series indicate that complete, near-complete (99%), and gross total resections are possible in most patients using the ultrasonic surgical aspirator

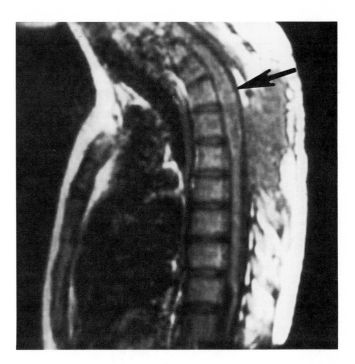

FIGURE 24-15. T-1 weighted MRI of an anaplastic astrocytoma of the upper thoracic cord. Note presence of cystic change.

and the laser. Intraoperatively monitored somatosensory evoked potentials may further improve safety. These tumors are best approached by osteoplastic laminectomies, removing as a single unit all lamina covering the solid portion of the tumor. Replacement after surgery not only helps protect the cord but may lessen the risk of subsequent spinal deformity. Operative mortality is low; morbidity and the amount of neurologic recovery are proportional to the degree of preoperative dysfunction.

Postoperative orthopedic follow-up and monitoring for spinal deformity is important. In 25% to 40% of children, the development or progression of such deformity occurs within a mean of 3 years. In earlier series, deaths from pulmonary complications related to these deformities were more common than deaths from tumor.[298–303]

Radiation

No controlled trial of radiation has been done in the intramedullary tumors, and evidence for its utility is inferred from the treatment of similar tumors in other CNS locations. Radiation is thought to be unnecessary if the tumor appears to have been resected completely. With incomplete resections, 4500 to 5000 cGy is recommended to the area of involvement. These doses are lower than those usually given for gliomas and ependymal tumors in other locations because of concern that the radiation tolerance of the spinal cord may be decreased by surgery and the presence of tumor.[298–301]

The overall survival rates for low-grade astrocytomas with various degrees of resection and postoperative radiation therapy are 70% at 5 years and 55% at 10 years. With apparently complete resection, patients may have survival rates as high as 100% at 5 years. In small series of ependymomas, survival rates of 70% to 80% at 5 years and 50% to 70% at 10 years are reported. Patients with anaplastic or high-grade tumors die from their disease within several months of diagnosis.[299,300,303]

Chemotherapy

No role for chemotherapy has been demonstrated in these tumors.

VISUAL-PATHWAY GLIOMAS

Epidemiology

Gliomas of the visual pathway (VPGs), including the optic nerves, chiasm, and optic tracts, comprise up to 5% of primary CNS tumors in children. More than 75% of isolated optic-nerve gliomas occur in the first decade of life, with the peak in the first 5 years, and 90% by age 20. Patients with chiasmal involvement tend, as a group, to be older. The male-to-female ratio is near unity. An association with neurofibromatosis is present in 50% to 70% of patients with isolated optic-nerve tumors and in 16% to 20% of those with chiasmal or deeper optic-tract tumors (also see Chap. 2).[304–310]

Pathology and Patterns of Spread

Histologically, these tumors are usually low-grade fibrillary or pilocytic astrocytomas whose microscopic features are virtually identical to those of the classic cerebellar astrocytoma and other midline pilocytic tumors. Malignant degeneration is rare.[309]

Although these tumors are usually confined to the structures of the visual pathways and extend in contiguity along them (Fig. 24-16), they also may extend into the frontal lobes, hypothalamus, thalamus, and other midline structures. Such events are more frequent in chiasmal tumors. Overall, tumor growth is slow, although alternating periods of clinical progression and stability suggest an erratic growth pattern.[304–310]

Clinical Presentation

The signs and symptoms of VPGs depend on their location and the age of the patient. Young children rarely complain of the slow and progressive visual loss characteristic of these tumors. More commonly, children under age 3 are brought to medical attention because of strabismus, nystagmus, or developmental difficulties. Children with neurofibromatosis are often visually asymptomatic at the time of diagnosis, the tumor being identified during the course of screening examinations. Mild proptosis is usually present with primary intraorbital tumors, whereas less than 20% of patients with intracranial disease have proptosis. Although funduscopic examination discloses optic pallor and atrophy in the involved eye, papilledema and other signs of increased intracranial pressure are rare except in large chiasmal or hypothalamic tumors that impinge on the anterior third ventricle.[304–310]

Visual acuity is frequently reduced to less than 20/200. The pattern of visual loss in patients with intraorbital tumors is most commonly that of a decrease in central vision. In patients with chiasmatic tumors, bitemporal hemianoptic field loss is often noted, although its absence does not preclude such involvement.[309,311] A fine, rapid, unilateral or bilateral nystagmus is often present in the involved eye, and amblyopia is frequent in blind or severely compromised eyes.[312]

Growth and endocrine disturbances, as well as precocious puberty and the diencephalic syndrome (failure to thrive in spite of adequate calories, euphoria, and overactivity in association with a diencephalic tumor in infants) have been reported

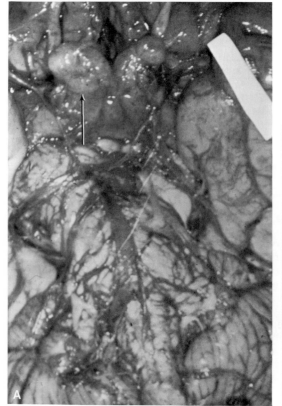

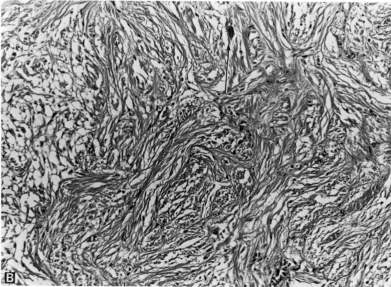

FIGURE 24-16. A. Diffuse infiltrating glioma of right optic nerve (*left, arrow*). Note diffuse enlargement of nerve and absence of a separate mass lesion. **B.** Optic nerve glioma formed by elongated, swirling piloid processes of astrocytes, the nuclei of which are inconspicuous. Note plump Rosenthal fiber (*upper center, arrow*). (H & E × 250)

with intracranial tumors of the chiasmatic–hypothalamic area.[306,307]

Differential Diagnosis and Evaluation

The differential diagnosis of an intraorbital mass must include rhabdomyosarcoma of the orbit and metastases from systemic solid tumors such as neuroblastoma. Orbital angiomas and lymphangiomas may produce a similar clinical picture. The rare meningiomas of the optic nerve sheath, midline gliomas originating in the hypothalamus or ventricles, craniopharyngioma, and other suprasellar tumors should also be considered. In infants, spasmus nutans, a disorder of eye movement producing pendular nystagmus, has also caused diagnostic confusion.[304–309,313]

Although plain radiographs of the orbital foramina often show enlargement on the involved side, CT and MRI have all but replaced this and other diagnostic tools in the primary evaluation of VPGs. The CT scan generally shows an isodense mass lesion. Contrast enhancement is generally present in optic nerve lesions, and it may be more pronounced in the chiasmal tumors and their extensions. Contiguous involvement of other visual-pathway structures and surrounding tissue may also be visible. Hydrocephalus is frequent with intracranial tumors. The MRI scan often shows a larger and more infiltrative lesion than does the CT scan.[77,310,314]

The utility of CT as a follow-up tool for VPGs is less certain. Declines in vision or responses to therapy may not be associated with changes in tumor size, and stable vision does not exclude tumor growth.[310] Thus, both detailed ophthalmologic evaluations, including visual-fields and acuity testing, and CT evaluations are important. Visual evoked responses may aid in follow-up, particularly in young children, where clinical and CT evaluations are the most difficult.[315,316]

Prognostic Considerations

Individuals with intracranial tumors (chiasm or deeper) generally have a more aggressive clinical course and greater mortality rates. Whether this is a reflection of tumor biology or partly due to tumor proximity to, and the ease of involvement of, other midline structures is unknown. The 10-year survival rate for patients with chiasmal tumors approximates 50%, in con-

trast to the 90% to 100% survival rate for patients with intraorbital tumors.[308,309,317]

Although the location of chiasmal tumors (anterior or posterior) has been suggested as having prognostic significance, recent reviews demonstrate that such divisions are rather arbitrary and have little or no prognostic importance.[304,308]

The behavior and survival of patients with optic gliomas is similar with or without associated neurofibromatosis. There is some suggestion, however, that chiasmal tumors in individuals with neurofibromatosis have a more favorable outcome than those in other patients.[309]

Treatment

The natural history of VPGs is extremely erratic. Some patients without treatment will experience long-term stabilization, whereas others will develop progressive disease with increasing visual loss and neurologic deterioration culminating in death.[308,311,318,319] Because of this erratic behavior, no consensus on the most appropriate management of these tumors has developed.

In the absence of severe proptosis, rapidly progressive visual decline, or extensive chiasmal tumors with gross distortion or invasion of the optic tracts, hypothalamus, or third-ventricular area, a period of observation without treatment is the most prudent approach, as there is no evidence that early surgery or radiation improves the eventual survival or visual status of the clinically nonacute and nonprogressive patient. The initial election to resect the tumor ignores the fact that the course of these pathologic processes is generally measured in decades and the well-documented and frequent occurrence of stable disease. A similar case can be made for withholding radiation therapy. This point is well demonstrated by comparing the effects of observation alone or radiation therapy in 195 cases taken from the literature (Table 24-17). The efficacy of any form of therapy is difficult to document.

Surgery

Although biopsy is the only way to confirm the diagnosis of VPG, this procedure may further compromise vision in as many as 75% of patients.[311,320,321] The CT or MRI scan is highly reliable for making a clinical diagnosis of many VPGs, and biopsy

Table 24-17
*Visual Status and Survival of 195 Patients with Visual-Pathway Gliomas Treated by Observation Only (O) or Radiation (R) at Diagnosis**

| Tumor Location | Treatment (No.) | Visual Status | | | |
		Deteriorated	Stable	Improved	Died
Optic nerve alone	O (6)	3	3	0	0
	R (12)	2	9	1	0
Chiasm alone ± optic nerve	O (27)	5	17	2	3
	R (79)	23	27	15	14
Chiasm and hypothalamus ± optic nerve	O (21)	7	10	2	2
	R (38)	10	8	6	14
Unspecified	R (?)		10	2	–

* Data from References 304–306, 308, 318–320, 322.

can be reserved for unusual clinical or radiographic circumstances.

The principal indications for neurosurgical intervention in patients with isolated intraorbital tumors are cosmesis in a severely proptotic blind or seeing eye and pain or jeopardy to the health of the globe and the cornea caused by severe proptosis.[307] Some also suggest that resection is wise in the very young, where evaluation of tumor progression is difficult.[306] In many instances, the tumor can be removed with preservation of the globe. However, if complete resection is to be done, the resected segment of the optic nerve should be as long as possible (preferably to the chiasm) to diminish the risk of local recurrence.[307] A transcranial approach across the orbital roof or a lateral orbitotomy may be used, depending on the surgical goals and the extent of the tumor.

In patients with chiasmal or deeper intracranial involvement, biopsy may be necessary to distinguish VPG unequivocally from craniopharyngioma or hypothalamic glioma. Although complete resection is usually impossible and is associated with significant neurologic and neuroendocrine morbidity, limited debulking of a large of cystic lesion through a transcranial or transcollosal route may relieve obstructive hydrocephalus.[307,308]

Radiation

The potential benefit of radiation therapy for VPGs is controversial. Although there are reports of diminished tumor growth and improved vision in isolated optic-nerve tumors as well as improved survival rates in patients with intracranial tumors,[305,320] the value of such therapy has not been unequivocally established.[308,309,311,319] Nevertheless, radiotherapy has been recommended as the best initial treatment for patients with seeing eyes in whom there is a need to treat proptosis or to attempt to arrest the decline of vision. Similarly, radiation may be useful in the treatment of large or growing chiasmatic lesions, as it can reduce tumor size, although this effect is observed in less than 50% of patients.[77,305] Its ability to stabilize vision in these patients is less certain, although this outcome has been reported in more than 70% in some series.[305] If an effect on growth and vision does occur, it is often limited.[305–308]

The disadvantages of radiotherapy are that it may take several weeks or months for its effect to become apparent and that it is associated with significant intellectual and neuroendocrine sequelae in young children with chiasmal lesions. In this latter instance, especially when there is rapid deterioration, a limited surgical resection and immediate or delayed radiation therapy may be a good alternative with less overall morbidity.[323,324]

Current recommendations for the use of radiotherapy are local doses of between 4500 and 5500 cGy over 5 to 6 weeks.[305,320]

Chemotherapy

Although chemotherapy is not routinely used for these tumors, in a recent series 15 patients younger than 5 years with newly diagnosed or recurrent VPGs were treated with dactinomycin and vincristine, and disease stabilization or regression occurred in 80%.[325] Further, these patients retained normal endocrinologic function, and the majority had normal intellectual function with follow-up periods of as long as 5 years for newly diagnosed tumors and 8 years for recurrent tumors. It is unclear how long such control will last, but chemotherapy may at least delay the need for radiotherapy in very young patients, in whom its morbidity is the highest.

PINEAL-AREA TUMORS

Epidemiology

Tumors of the pineal area account for 0.4% to 2% of all primary CNS neoplasms in children. Two principal groups, the pineal parenchymal tumors and the germ cell tumors, account for majority of neoplasms in this area. Pineal parenchymal tumors are more frequent in the first decade of life and in females. The intracranial germ cell tumors have a male-to-female ratio of 2–3:1 and are more frequent in the second decade of life, with a peak incidence at ages 12 to 14 years.[326–328]

Pathology and Patterns of Spread

Pineal Parenchymal Tumors

The pineal parenchymal tumors—pineoblastoma and pineocytoma—comprise 20% to 40% of pineal-area tumors. Pineoblastoma is a primitive undifferentiated tumor that accounts for about 50% of these tumors (Fig. 24-3). Except for its location, this tumor may be histologically indistinguishable from medulloblastoma and is probably best considered a variant of the primitive neuroectodermal tumors. It is a highly cellular tumor in which mitoses and areas of focal necrosis are frequent. The occasional presence of Flexner–Wintersteiner rosettes indicates differentiation toward retinoblastoma.[327]

Although the histologic appearance of the pineocytoma (Fig. 24-17) may overlap that of the pineoblastoma, the cells are generally larger and have a recognizable relation with blood vessels, and true rosettes are rarely seen. Occasional evidence of astrocytic, neuronal, or ganglion-cell differentiation is noted.[327]

Germ Cell Tumors

The germ cell tumors include a spectrum of embryonal neoplasms and teratomas that are believed to be derived from totipotent germ cells that aberrantly migrated to the cranial midline during embryogenesis. Overall, these tumors account for about 50% of pineal area tumors. The germinoma (Fig. 24-18) comprises 50% to 65% of tumors in this spectrum and is

FIGURE 24-17. Primary pineal tumor displaying prominent perivascular growth of neoplastic cells characteristic of pineocytoma. Note papillary pattern. (H & E × 250)

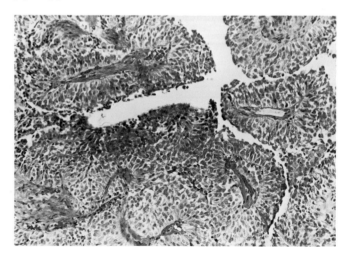

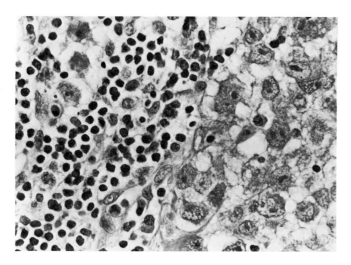

FIGURE 24-18. Typical field of germinoma displaying large cells with large nucleoli and focus of lymphocytes (on *right* half of field). (H & E × 400)

a histologically primitive tumor indistinguishable from gonadal germinomas.[326-329]

Teratomas and mixed germ-cell tumors harboring a variety of mature and immature elements comprise 18% to 25% of germ cell tumors. The less-frequent embryonal carcinoma, choriocarcinoma, and endodermal sinus tumors collectively account for only 5% to 15% of the intracranial germ cell tumors.[327-330]

Both contiguous regional extension and distant intra-axial dissemination are common in pineal-area tumors. The overall incidence of leptomeningeal dissemination in larger series of patients is approximately 10%, with pineoblastomas and germinomas demonstrating the greatest frequency of such spread.[326-330] A recent report suggests that the pineocytoma, often considered a slow-growing, locally infiltrative tumor, may also have a high incidence of leptomeningeal seeding.[331]

Teratomas generally remain local, well encapsulated, and noninvasive. However, areas with more-primitive germ-cell features may be present and are associated with a more aggressive clinical course and neuraxis dissemination.[327,329]

Systemic metastases, although uncommon, may occur in pineoblastoma and germinoma as well as in embryonal carcinoma and choriocarcinoma. Bone, lung, and lymph nodes are the most common sites of such dissemination.[329]

Clinical Presentation

The dominant signs and symptoms of pineal-area tumors are the nonspecific and nonlocalizing features of increased intracranial pressure secondary to tumor extension and compression of third-ventricular outflow.[326,328] Other signs and symptoms depend on the location and amount of tumor extension.[326,328] Masses extending anteriorly and caudally may involve the posterior portion of the midbrain (the midbrain tegmentum) and cause various degrees of vertical gaze paresis such as Parinaud's syndrome (see section on neurology), an often-characteristic finding. Tumors that compress or infiltrate the overlying thalamus may result in hemiparesis, incoordination, visual difficulties, or movement disorders. The primary germ-cell tumors are somewhat more likely to cause upper-midbrain or tegmental dysfunction, whereas focal motor deficits are more common with infiltrating glial tumors. Although

technically outside the pineal region, the suprasellar area also frequently harbors germ cell tumors (so-called ectopic pinealomas), which may produce pituitary and hypothalamic dysfunction. Visual loss and neuroendocrine abnormalities are the most frequent of these, followed by precocious puberty and emotional and thermoregulatory dysfunction.[326,328]

Differential Diagnosis and Evaluation

Pineal masses are uncommon in children. In addition to the above tumors, the differential diagnosis includes glioma, meningioma, nonmalignant epidermal or arachnoid cysts, and vascular malformations. Encephalitis and demyelinating diseases may produce similar clinical features.[326-328]

Although the CT scan reliably demonstrates the mass in the pineal region, it is unreliable for specific diagnosis, as there is significant overlap in the CT characteristics of the pineal-area tumors. The CT appearance of germ cell tumors is generally that of an irregular lesion of mixed density and homogeneous contrast enhancement; calcium may be present. The pineal parenchymal tumors are calcified to various extents and show a similar pattern of density and contrast enhancement. Teratomas usually have a mosaic pattern with mixed areas of density and contrast enhancement as well as irregular calcification.[326,332] Periventricular contrast enhancement implies diffuse ventricular seeding. Although calcification is said to be frequent in patients with pineal-area tumors, this finding is less common in preadolescent patients.[332]

In patients with pineoblastoma or germ cell tumor, both CSF cytology and myelography should be performed, as cytology alone is inadequate, much as in medulloblastoma. In all other tumors, CSF cytology is, at a minimum, strongly encouraged.[147,326,329,333,334] These studies can be safely done within 2 to 4 weeks of surgery.

Alpha-fetoprotein (AFP) and human chorionic gonadotropin (hCG) may be secreted by any of the germ cell tumors, and elevated levels may be found in the serum or CSF. Although not reliable for diagnosis, serial measurements of these markers may be useful in following the response to treatment and in detecting relapse.[326,329,335]

Prognostic Considerations

Tumor histology has general prognostic significance, with the germinomas having the best overall survival rate and response to therapy followed by the teratomas and the pineal parenchymal tumors. The remaining germ cell neoplasms have a generally rapid clinical course, with death within a year of diagnosis. Leptomeningeal, wide regional, or hypothalamic involvement also implies a poor prognosis.[326,328,329,333] The age at diagnosis has conflicting significance in various series and probably has no great overall prognostic influence.[326,328,329,333]

Treatment

Surgery

Because of the variable natural history and response to treatment of the various pineal-area tumors, biopsy is recommended whenever possible.[326,329] Current neurosurgical technique allows biopsy in most patients with morbidity that is generally limited to transient worsening of prior visual symptoms, although new or permanent losses may occur. The mortality rate is generally below 1%. Direct visually guided biopsy is usually the preferred and safest route in the pediatric patient, as prominent vascular structures often preclude a stereotactic approach.

Except for well-encapsulated teratomas, extensive local or regional disease usually precludes complete tumor resection. Because there is no evidence that wide resection improves the outcome, and because significant morbidity and mortality rates are associated with aggressive resection, biopsy only or limited debulking to relieve hydrocephalus may be the most prudent approach.[328,329,334]

An alternative approach to diagnosis and therapy has been to treat all patients who have enhancing pineal-region lesions with 2000 to 3000 cGy of radiotherapy prior to pathologic confirmation. Although the response is said to suggest the presence of a radiocurable germinoma and to obviate biopsy, this approach is not reliable and not advocated, as pineoblastoma or mixed germ-cell tumors may respond similarly.[326,328,334]

Radiotherapy

Radiotherapy is the primary treatment modality for pineal-area tumors. There is a consensus that whole-brain radiation is indicated, with usual doses of 3500 to 4500 cGy and an additional 1000 to 1500 cGy to the area of the tumor for germ cell tumors and pineoblastomas. The extent of radiotherapy needed to control pineocytomas is unclear, and the need for routine spinal irradiation in pineal parenchymal and germ cell tumors is a matter of debate. Some therapists think that the 10% incidence of spinal dissemination is too low to justify routine spinal prophylaxis. However, patients with positive CSF cytology or myelography are candidates for spinal irradiation, and those with pineoblastomas, germinomas, embryonal carcinomas, and possibly pineocytomas, which tend to have a greater incidence of spinal dissemination, should also be strongly considered for such therapy.[326–328,331,333,336,337]

Local recurrence, generally within 2 to 3 years of diagnosis, is the dominant mode of failure.[326,329]

Chemotherapy

The absence of a blood–brain barrier in the pineal area and the success of chemotherapy in many germ cell tumors outside the CNS has led to chemotherapy use in the pineal germ-cell tumors. No current evidence of efficacy is available for pineal parenchymal tumors. Significant responses have been documented with vinblastine, bleomycin, and cisplatin-containing regimens in the germinomas, and methotrexate may be similarly useful in choriocarcinomas.[326,329,338,339] The potential benefit of such therapy is further reason to require biopsy.

Results

Survival rates for most individual tumor types are difficult or impossible to state with any accuracy because of the infrequency of biopsy in most series. Germinomas clearly have the best prognosis, with 60% to 85% 5-year disease-free survival rates being reported. This probably reflects the radiosensitivity of these tumors. With the exception of teratomas, some of which may have a 50% 5-year survival rate, the other germ cell tumors have very poor prognoses, with at least half the patients expiring within 1 year of diagnosis.

On the basis of the combined results of small series of patients, it appears likely that no more than one-third of patients with pineal parenchymal tumors, the majority of these being pineocytomas, survive 5 years.[326–330,333,336,337]

CRANIOPHARYNGIOMAS

Epidemiology

Craniopharyngiomas account for between 6% and 9% of all primary CNS tumors in children. Two-thirds occur before age 20, but occurrence is unusual before age 2 years.[5,145,340] The median age at diagnosis is 8. There is no apparent male or female predilection. Although predominantly suprasellar tumors, which occur in the pituitary stalk and hypothalamus, these tumors also arise within the sella turcica. Except for location, the craniopharyngioma may appear similar or identical to epidermal cysts that occur in parasellar and other CNS locations; tumors described as craniopharyngiomas have been found within the chiasm and cerebellopontine angle (also see Chap. 34).

Pathology and Patterns of Spread

Tumors in suprasellar and intrasellar locations are presumed to arise from epithelial cell rests along the involuted hypophyseal–pharyngeal duct, although it has also been suggested that they represent metaplasia in the epithelial portions of the pituitary.[145] Grossly, these tumors are smooth, lobulated, solid, cystic, or mixed solid–cystic masses. The cyst contents may range from gelatinous to a viscous, oily fluid rich in cholesterol crystals. Rupture of a cyst into the CSF may cause an intense sterile meningitis. Calcification is frequently seen on cut section. Both the cystic lining and the solid portions of the tumor are characterized by squamous epithelium, usually with some evidence of keratinization and various amounts of connective tissue.

Although craniopharyngioma is a histologically benign tumor composed of well-differentiated tissue, it is malignant by virtue of its location and its ability to efface surrounding normal structures. A thick glial layer encasing the tumor is tightly adherent to surrounding tissue. Small islands of epithelial tumor arising within this gliotic scar can extend into adjacent tissues.[341]

Clinical Presentation

The nonspecific signs and symptoms of increased intracranial pressure, particularly headache, occur in 50% to 90% of patients.[145,340–343] Obstruction of the third ventricle and foramen of Monro by superior tumor extension causes hydrocephalus in half of the patients.[343] Because of slow tumor growth, papilledema is less common than optic pallor.[341,342,344] More localizing signs are related to tumor site and impingement on the adjacent optic chiasm, hypothalamus, and pituitary. Visual-field defects of various degrees of severity occur in 50% to 90% of patients, with homonomous hemianopsia and bitemporal hemianopsia being the most frequent.[341,342,344] Various neuroendocrine deficits, including abnormalities of growth hormone, adrenocorticotropin, thyroid-stimulating hormone, thyroid-releasing hormone, antidiuretic hormone, and the gonadotropins, are present in as many as 83% of patients at diagnosis.[345,346] Although diabetes insipidus and short stature are frequent findings, the signs and symptoms of increased intracranial pressure more commonly bring the patient to clinical attention.

Differential Diagnosis and Evaluation

Intrinsic hypothalamic gliomas, large chiasmal gliomas, and suprasellar germ cell tumors or teratomas are the most frequent entities in the differential diagnosis of craniopharyngiomas. Other diencephalic tumors and large epidermoid cysts in the hypothalamic/third-ventricle region may also mimic craniopharyngiomas.

Plain skull radiographs are a valuable screening tool. An enlarged or distorted sella is present in 45% of patients, and visible tumor calcifications may be present in 50% to 80%.[340,341] The CT scan characteristically demonstrates a cystic, low-density, contrast-enhancing lesion with calcification. In most instances, the hypophyseal–hypothalamic origin of the tumor is clear, but large low-density chiasmal gliomas and supratentorial teratomas may cause some diagnostic confusion. Preoperative angiography and metrizamide cisternography to define the local vascular anatomy, rule out an aneurysm, and delineate tumor extent may be helpful. MRI scans define the solid and cystic nature of the tumor, its extent, and its relation to adjacent structures better than any other procedure (Fig. 24-19).

Because of the high incidence of clinical and subclinical neuroendocrinologic deficits at diagnosis, a thorouvaluation of the hypothalamic–pituitary axis should be done prior to surgery. Abnormalities of adrenal function and of the regulation of fluid and electrolytes balance, in particular, can lead to serious perioperative problems if not anticipated. Neuroendocrine evaluations should be repeated postoperatively and periodically thereafter for at least a year, as hormonal deficits, which routinely increase after surgery, may take several months to become fully apparent.

Prognostic Considerations

The extent of tumor resection is the overriding prognostic factor; patients with totally excised tumors have vastly better survival rates than those managed by biopsy alone or by subtotal resection.[323,340,347] The purported prognostic significance of tumor size[358] is probably not an independent variable but rather is related to the extent of resection.

Although the data show only a trend, patients with purely cystic lesions appear to survive longer than those with solid or mixed solid and cystic lesions.[349] Gender has no prognostic significance. There also is a trend toward poorer survival for patients less than age 5 at diagnosis.[323,349]

Treatment

The optimal therapy for craniopharyngioma is a matter of intense debate, with some authors strongly recommending radical surgery[340,342,350] and others partial resection followed by local radiation.[323,340,347-349] Survival alone is an inadequate measure of therapeutic efficacy in this tumor: the multitude of neuroendocrinologic, visual, and neuropsychologic problems related to the location and treatment of this tumor must also be considered carefully.

Surgery

Surgery has been the primary therapeutic mode for most patients with craniopharyngioma, although debate over its extent continues. There is clear evidence, in several series of patients, that survival times are longer and recurrences fewer in patients who have complete tumor excisions.[351] In the current era, with the use of microsurgical technique, postsurgical CT scans show no evidence of tumor postoperatively in 74% to 88% of patients.[341,342]

In combined series of patients, the recurrence rate after total excision is 23%, although rates as high as 50% have been reported.[340,344,347,351-353] Half of all relapses occur within 2 years and 75% within 5 years.[347,354] Although the surgical mortality rate is now less than 5%,[145,340,347,353] significant nonendocrine-related surgical morbidity (*i.e.,* hematoma) and neurologic or visual–motor problems occur in 18% to 22% of patients.[324,344,347,353] Additionally, there is an inevitable increase in the number and severity of neuroendocrine deficits following surgery, and post surgical decline in the neuropsychologic and functional status is seen in many patients.[324,343,349,355]

Preoperative corticosteroids are strongly recommended in all patients not already receiving dexamethasone for control of increased intracranial pressure. Hydrocortisone, 100 mg intravenously followed by 25 mg every 6 hours for four more doses, is generally adequate until maintenance steroids can be resumed in a postoperatively stable patient. Preoperative vasopressin is not needed unless the patient is symptomatic.

A right frontal or frontotemporal craniotomy is generally used to expose the tumor, although other approaches may be used depending on tumor extent and location. For example, tumors located primarily in the sella can be removed transphenoidally, and large cystic tumors extending to the roof of the third ventricle can be approached through the corpus callosum. A lumbar drain may be inserted to remove CSF intraop-

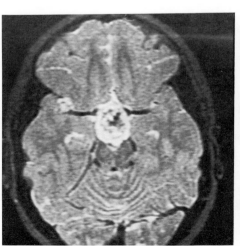
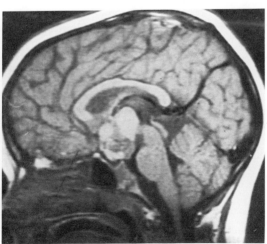

FIGURE 24-19. Axial and sagittal T-2 weighted MRI of mixed density craniopharyngioma with foci of calcification (black).

eratively to minimize brain retraction, and if significant hydrocephalus is present, shunting may be necessary.

Postoperative CT scans are necessary to confirm the extent of resection. If no visible calcification or tumor is present, the risk of recurrent disease is low, and 10-year disease-free survival rates of greater than 70% are frequent. The primary cause of demise in these patients is either recurrent tumor or chronic or late-occurring neuroendocrine problems.[355]

If residual disease is noted, recurrence is likely.[354,356] Without postoperative radiotherapy, fewer than half of such patients survive 10 years, and as many as 50% to 75% have recurrent disease within 2 to 5 years.[347,354]

Radiation

Table 24-18 shows the actuarial survival ranges for patients with different degrees of resection and postoperative radiotherapy. It is apparent that radiation can significantly decrease the recurrence rate and enhance the survival of patients with incomplete tumor resections.[323,347-349,357-359] Even with minimal surgery (biopsy and cyst drainage) and in patients with recurrent disease, radiation is capable of prolonging survival.[323,347,349,354,357]

When morbidity is considered, patients with incomplete resection followed by irradiation have less neuroendocrine dysfunction and fewer serious neurologic (sensory, motor, visual) deficits. They are likely to have an improved level of function and better quality of life than patients treated with radical surgery alone.[323,343,347,340,354] Additionally, neuropsychologic function is reported to be preserved better in the combined-therapy group despite the known detrimental effect of radiation on these abilities.[324] However, these conclusions are based on relatively few patients treated over many years, and direct comparisons may not yet be reliable. Recommended doses of radiation are 5000 to 5500 cGy to local fields only.

Local radiation using intracystic ^{90}Y, ^{128}Au, or ^{32}P in recurrent disease has been tried. Although this therapy has been effective, its use is limited to tumors with a relatively large cyst. It is not useful in solid tumors. This approach must be used with caution, because of the potential for radiation-induced visual problems.[360]

At present, most observers recommend that the patient with a suspected craniopharyngioma have surgery with cyst decompression and debulking of easily accessible tumor. Total resection may be attempted provided the size and extent of tumor and its adhesiveness to surrounding structures permit relatively easy dissection. Radical attempts at resection are not warranted in view of the results achievable with radiation therapy of subtotally resected tumors.

Table 24-18
Actuarial Survival Rates (%) in Craniopharyngioma with Surgery and Radiation

Treatment	5 Years	10 Years	References
Total resection	58–100 77*	24–100 47*–74	323, 347, 349, 350, 354, 356–359
Subtotal resection	37–71 14*	31–52 7*	323, 347, 354, 359
Subtotal resection and radiation	69–95 85*	62–84 79*	323, 343, 347, 349, 354, 356, 359

* Disease-free survival.

Chemotherapy

There is no established role for chemotherapy in craniopharyngiomas. A response to a vincristine, BCNU, and procarbazine combination has been described in a patient with a cystic tumor that had recurred after surgery alone.[361] This result suggests that chemotherapy might be capable of postponing or even augmenting irradiation in some patients.

CHOROID PLEXUS NEOPLASMS

Epidemiology

Choroid plexus neoplasms comprise 3% of brain tumors in children younger than 17 years and 10% to 20% of CNS tumors occurring during the first year of life, with a few congenital tumors having been reported. As many as 85% of these tumors arise in the lateral ventricles, 10% to 50% in the fourth ventricle, and only 5% to 10% in the third ventricle.[362,363] The male-to-female ratio is near unity in combined series.[364]

Pathology and Patterns of Spread

Choroid plexus neoplasms generally arise as functioning intraventricular papillomas capable of secreting CSF. Grossly, the choroid plexus papillomas (CPPs) resemble coral; fronds of tumor attached to a pedicle float in the CSF. Microscopically, these tumors are similar to normal choroid plexus and have cuboidal or columnar epithelium and a well-preserved epithelial–stromal border overlying fibrovascular septa. Their neoplastic nature is reflected in the heaping and redundancy of the epithelial component.

A more aggressive and anaplastic tumor, the choroid plexus carcinoma (CPC), accounts for 10% to 20% of choroid plexus tumors. This tumor has lost the well-differentiated papillary structure and the epithelial–stromal border of the CPP. It is a hypercellular tumor with pleomorphic cells, frequent mitoses, and foci of necrosis.[362]

CPPs tend to be slow growing and often reach a size of 60 to 70 g before coming to clinical attention. Both papillomas and carcinomas are capable of leptomeningeal dissemination. In the former, the clinical behavior and histology of the isolated and frequently noted deposits is benign, and symptoms are uncommon. Conversely, diffuse and aggressive leptomeningeal spread occurs in CPCs.

Clinical Presentation

In more than 90% of cases, hydrocephalus and the symptoms of increased intracranial pressure are the presenting and dominant features of either CPP or CPC. These signs and symptoms may develop on the basis of increased CSF production by the tumor (rates of four times normal have been documented), overt ventricular obstruction, and basilar arachnoiditis secondary to repeated small tumor hemorrhages into the CSF. The onset and progression of these features may be rapid.

Midline tumors may cause hydrocephalus and intracranial hypertension without any other localizing findings. However, tumors in the fourth ventricle frequently produce associated cerebellar findings such as ataxia. Ocular palsies, seizures, hemiparesis, and hemianopsia may also occur, depending on the patient's age, the acuteness and degree of increased pressure, and the degree to which accommodation to increased CSF pressure is possible.[362,365]

Differential Diagnosis and Evaluation

The differential diagnosis of choroid plexus tumors includes ependymomas and midline astrocytomas, which may have similar clinical and radiographic features. Plain skull radiographs reveal sutural widening in 70% of patients, and skull asymmetry as a result of asymmetric hydrocephalus may be present in one-third of patients. On CT scan, hydrocephalus along with an isodense to hyperdense and brightly contrast-enhancing intraventricular tumor is characteristic. MRI scans clearly show the fronds of tumor and may be diagnostic (Fig. 24-20).

Cerebral angiography is routinely performed to identify the vascular pedicle so that it may be clipped during surgery. An irregular vascular stain at the trigone and hypertrophy of one or more of the choroidal arteries is generally seen in midline tumors. Fourth-ventricular tumors may produce enlargement of the superior or posteroinferior cerebellar artery.

Treatment

Surgery

Surgical excision is the primary mode of therapy for CPPs. The commonest of these tumors, those in the trigone, are approached via a temporoparietal craniotomy. Tumors of the anterior third ventricle or foramen of Monro may be approached transcallosally and fourth-ventricular tumors by the suboccipital route. Intraventricular tumors outside the posterior fossa may be more easily removed if the ventricles are large, and for this reason, preoperative shunting may not be done in otherwise stable patients. Although a surgical morbidity of 40% to 50% and a mortality rate of 15% to 45% occurred in earlier series, current neurosurgical practice has reduced these figures to less than 20% and 5%, respectively. Complete resections are possible in 75% to 100% of patients and are generally curative. Long-term survival is the rule, but no recent series reflecting current surgical techniques have been published. Older 1- and 5-year survival rates were 67% and probably reflect the greater surgical risks of the time.[5,366] Even after complete tumor removal, persistent hydrocephalus and the need for a postcraniotomy shunt may be present in 60% of patients. Adjunctive radiation or chemotherapy is not recommended, as neither has established utility in the treatment of CPPs.

In the CPCs, occasional long-term survivals after surgery alone have been reported. However, 80% or more of reported patients have died either from the tumor itself or from surgical complications. The mean survival time in children is less than 7 years.

Radiation

Although postoperative radiation therapy has frequently been used to treat CPC and the survival times of some irradiated patients may be marginally better than those of unirradiated patients, such results are not entirely separable from those of surgery alone. The utility of radiotherapy beyond that of slowing disease progression is uncertain.[362]

Chemotherapy

Chemotherapy may have a role in these tumors, as the blood–brain barrier is absent in the vessels of the choroid plexus (although a blood–CSF barrier is present along the choroid epithelium), and drug penetration thus should be relatively easy. However, there are no reports of chemotherapy use.

SUPRATENTORIAL PRIMITIVE NEUROECTODERMAL TUMORS

The supratentorial primitive neuroectodermal tumors (SPNET) comprise 2% to 3% of primary CNS tumors in children. These tumors have been referred to by variety of terms including cerebral or central neuroblastoma, PNET of the cerebrum, cerebral medulloblastoma, and others.[59,367] A review of the nosologic controversy surrounding these tumors is provided in an earlier section of this chapter. A total of 122 patients with these diagnoses has been abstracted from recent literature and form the basis for this discussion.[68,368,376–382]

Epidemiology

Although a broad age range, from neonate through adult (age 35), is noted, these tumors occur predominantly in the first decade of life, with a median age of 8 years and a peak inci-

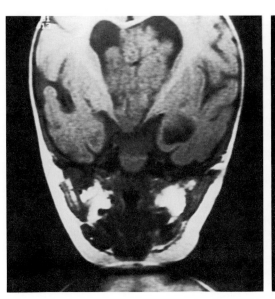
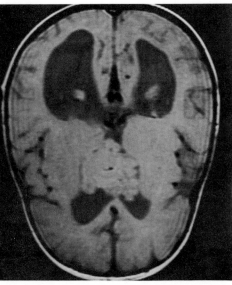

FIGURE 24-20. Axial and coronal MRI showing third ventricular choroid plexus papilloma with extension into the lateral ventricles.

dence distributed evenly between birth and age 5. Equal numbers of males and females are effected. The SPNET have a predilection for the cerebral hemispheres; 90% of reported cases have occurred in this location, with the frontal, parietal, temporal, and occipital lobes involved in order of increasing frequency. Less than 10% of these tumors occur in the midline structures, including the ventricular areas, corpus callosum, thalamus, and basal ganglia. Spinal cord PNET make up less than 5% of reported cases.

Pathology and Patterns of Spread

Despite the presence of considerable microscopic extension, these tumors generally appear as well-circumscribed masses. Grossly, they are lobulated, soft, hemorrhagic, often cystic, masses. Microscopically, sheets of uniform embryonal-appearing small round cells with hyperchromatic oval nuclei and frequent mitoses are noted (see Fig. 24-3 A–C). Both Homer–Wright rosettes and perivascular pseudorosettes, as well as areas of necrosis, are common. Although foci with various degrees of glial, neuronal, or ependymal differentiation are seen in 70% of tumors, light microscopy and ultrastructural evaluation generally reveal the majority of individual cells to be primitive and undifferentiated.

Wide local and regional tumor extension is common, and instances of transcollosal extension into the opposite hemisphere have been reported. Diffuse leptomeningeal or spinal subarachnoid disease occurred eventually in 31% of 74 evaluable patients.[368–370,372–374,377–379] Four of these 74 patients had systemic metastases, with bone and lung being the favored sites.

Clinical Presentation

The nonspecific, nonlocalizing signs and symptoms of increased intracranial pressure, headache, vomiting, and papilledema are the predominant presenting features. Because of the hemispheric location of these tumors, seizures and motor signs such as weakness and hemiplegia are frequent, being observed in 20% and 40% of these patients, respectively. The period from the onset of symptoms to diagnosis is variable but generally is between 3 and 10 months.

Prognostic Considerations

Age, gender, and tumor site appear to have no prognostic significance. The degree of differentiation may have some prognostic significance, however; a recent article reported increased survival in a small group of patients with less than 90% of their tumor composed of undifferentiated cells.[68] A similar finding has been described for medulloblastoma.[382]

Differential Diagnosis and Evaluation

The differential diagnosis of the SPNETs is the same as that for other supratentorial tumors, consisting of the common tumors and nonmalignant vascular abnormalities of the hemispheres and midline structures.

CT scans demonstrate hydrocephalus in many cases as well as the presence of a mass lesion, which may be partially calcified and show cystic changes.[164,376,379] Various degrees of contrast enhancement are noted.

Like medulloblastoma, leptomeningeal dissemination is common with SPNETs, and postoperative CSF cytology study and myelography should be part of the evaluation in all patients. In most instances, this can be safely accomplished within 14 to 21 days of surgery.

Treatment

Surgery

Although complete tumor resection is frequently not possible because of the size, location, and extent of tumor, it appears to be associated with improved prognosis and should be attempted when possible. Gross total resection in four newly diagnosed cases in one small series[374] and in one patient with recurrent disease[373] has been associated with long-term survival. However, similar survivals have occurred in small numbers of patients given radiation therapy after subtotal resection.[68,373–375,377]

Radiation

Most of the reported patients received postoperative radiotherapy. The dose and volume of such treatment are often unspecified; where such information is available, doses to the tumor bed of 4000 to 6000 cGy and prophylactic craniospinal doses of 3000 to 4000 cGy have been used. Tumor doses less than 4500 cGy appear to be associated with poorer outcomes.[378] Both whole-brain and wide local fields have been used for treating the primary tumor.[68,369,373] Although radiation does appear to lengthen survival, most patients still succumb to locally or regionally recurrent disease within 1 to 2 years.

Chemotherapy

A variety of single agents and combination programs based on the use of a nitrosourea have been reported. Temporary responses have been documented with oral procarbazine alone (two patients) and with BCNU, cyclophosphamide, and vincristine combination (one patient).[371,378] The use of similar combination chemotherapy as an adjuvant has not been independently evaluated; the evidence overall suggests that it does not materially influence outcome or survival.[164]

Results

The overall survival in these tumors is poor. Recent results show a 64% 1-year survival followed by 36% and 25% 2- and 5-year survival rates,[68] which appears no better than the 8- to 24-month mean survival of older series.[376]

SEQUELAE OF TREATMENT IN THE YOUNG CHILD

As many as 10% of all childhood brain tumors occur in patients under the age of 2, and it is these children who are the most likely to suffer the severest sequelae of therapy.[5,383,384] Most long-term survivors seem free of crippling neurologic deficits and lead active lives apparently without disability.[385] However, on close inspection, impairment of neurocognitive functions and endocrinologic deficits are frequently present[92,175,386] (see also Chap. 50).

Damage to the CNS from several sources may play a role in these deficits. Direct distortion and destruction of normal brain tissue by tumor as well as by increased intracranial pressure

Table 24-19
Syndromes of Postradiation CNS Damage in Childhood

Syndrome	Etiology	Incidence	Onset	Clinical Manifestation	Outcome
Somnolence syndrome	Whole-brain RT*	Increases with increasing doses of RT; ? >50% after 2400 cGy	4–8 weeks after RT	7–14 days of lethargy, malaise, nausea, vomiting; psychological alterations	Usually resolution; ? later neurologic deficits
Radionecrosis	Idiosyncratic; increased with higher total dose or increased dose per fraction; usually after >5500 cGy	0.1%–1% with conventional RT range 1–2 months to ?	Usually 6 months to 3 years after RT; obtundation; coma	Focal neurologic dysfunction; seizures	May lead to death
Necrotizing leukoencephalopathy	Higher total dose or dose per fraction, usually >240 cGy; potentiated by use of It MTX or HDMTX; occurs rarely after HDMTX alone	0.5%–2.0% of children receiving 2400 cGy RT alone; up to 55% with concomitant IV HDMTX or It MTX	Usually 4–12 months after RT; range 3 months to ?	Spasticity, ataxia, lethargy, dementia, pseudobulbar paresis	Variable; may be progressive or stabilize
Mineralizing microangiopathy with dystrophic calcification	≥2000 cGy RT; ? potentiated by It MTX or It ARAC	? 25%–30%+ of treated patients; 17% of children with ALL (autopsy)	Unknown; 9 months after RT to ?	None; possible headaches, seizures	Unclear (often an autopsy finding)
Neuropsychological damage	Primarily whole-brain RT; ? with local RT; increases with increasing total dose or It or IV MTX	Common; ? >50% after >2400 cGy; increased with younger age at treatment	Increases with time after treatment; ? peaks 3 years after treatment	Cognitive deficits, learning deficits, behavioral abnormalities	Static or may progress
Endocrinologic dysfunction	RT to hypothalamus (? pituitary); usually 2400 cGy	Common; ? 80%–100% after 3600 cGy	Biphasic; early dysfunction; fixed damage 1–5 years after RT	Growth failure, less common thyroid or gonadotropin deficiency	Static; requires hormonal replacement

* RT = radiotherapy; It = intrathecal; MTX = methotrexate; HDMTX = high-dose methotrexate; ARAC = cystosine arabinoside; ALL = acute lymphocytic leukemia.

and surgical trauma may cause some degree of irreversible neurologic damage.[387] Likewise, chemotherapy, especially in combination with radiation, appears capable of inducing encephalopathy. However, it is radiation therapy that has been implicated as the chief cause of these and many other adverse long-term sequelae, which are listed in Table 24-19.[175,383,386,388–392]

Intellectual impairment is among the most frequent problems of the young child treated with radiotherapy.[92,383,393–395]

Some reports suggest that most children receiving whole-brain radiation have moderate to severe intellectual compromise as judged by IQ test scores.[153,175,386,396] More recent studies have identified deficits in specific neurocognitive functions such as memory and fine-motor and visual–perceptive behavior that may contribute to significant learning disabilities and underlie the poor intellectual performance.[153,175,386,387,396]

The impact of the volume of radiation on such deficits is not entirely clear. Although whole-brain radiation is believed to be the most detrimental, even radiation fields not encompassing the cerebral hemispheres may produce intellectual declines.[385,386] The dose of radiation also influences the development of these deficits, with more severe sequelae occurring with higher doses. Although the slope of the dose–effect curve is not well defined, variable intellectual deficits and CT abnormalities of the brain occur regularly in young children with leukemia given doses of 2400 cGy or more to the whole brain, and such abnormalities have been demonstrated even with whole-brain doses as low as 850 to 1800 cGy.[396] Because the majority of patients with neurocognitive deficits do not have observable histopathologic changes, the location and pathogenesis of their problems are not identifiable. Thus, the effects of radiation and other forms of CNS treatment on axonal growth, dendritic arborization, and synaptogenesis, all of which occur at an increased rate in early childhood and alteration of which is presumably critical to the development of these problems, are unknown.[153,175]

Neuroendocrinologic damage frequently occurs in children who have received radiotherapy to the hypothalamic–pituitary region.[385] Both whole-brain irradiation and the inclusion of the posterior hypothalamus in most radiation portals used to treat posterior fossa tumors have been incriminated in the genesis of these problems. Impaired growth-hormone secretion, the most commonly observed abnormality, is both more frequent and more severe in younger children. Abnormal responses to provocative growth-hormone testing and diminished growth velocity may become apparent after as little as 2400 cGy of cranial irradiation.[385,396–399] Replacement therapy should be considered in patients who grow less than 4 cm per year and in whom there is no response to provocative growth-hormone testing or abnormally blunted basal pulsatile growth hormone output.[385]

Other, less frequent, hormonal deficits also are seen. Hypothyroidism secondary to inclusion of this organ in the portals for craniospinal radiation may occur in some patients.[175,385,398] In addition, delayed puberty, abnormalities of gonadotropin secretion, Addison's disease, and panhypopituitism have occasionally been documented.[398]

Management of these sequelae of treatment is suboptimal. The first step is the recognition that they may not occur or become fully manifest for 3 years or more after therapy. Because of this, yearly psychological and endocrine evaluations should be done for at least the first 3 years after therapy.[385,396] Children who demonstrate intellectual impairment require further evaluation so that proper educational remediation can begin. Those with endocrine deficits may be candidates for hormone replacement.

Although prevention of these deleterious sequelae is beginning to receive attention, the efficacy of current interventions remains difficult to judge. Attempts to obviate or to delay radiotherapy have been made. Dactinomycin and vincristine have postponed the need for radiation in some young children with chiasmatic gliomas.[325] Similar results may be obtained using MOPP and cisplatin-containing regimens in other young children.[400–402] However, chemotherapy itself may have deleterious effects on the developing nervous system.[175,385,386,396]

Another potential means of reducing radiation sequelae has been use of hyperfractionated therapy, in which the total daily dose is divided into two or more fractions given several hours apart. Such treatment is postulated to be at least as effective as conventional fractionation and to have less-deleterious effects on normal tissue. Although experience with this modality in young children is limited, some evidence for a reduced incidence of growth hormone impairment has come from leukemic patients treated with smaller fractions of prophylactic CNS radiation.[403]

Reduction in the dose and volume of cranial irradiation has also been advocated in young children.[92,404] However, such doses have yet to be proved as effective in tumor control or significantly less damaging than conventional therapy.

Although attempts such as these to postpone the need for or to reduce the dose of radiation may be useful, the age beyond which significant neurologic maturation is present and radiation can be more safely delivered is unclear. Age 3 years, the time by which myelinization is thought to be complete, has been suggested as the point beyond which full or only marginally reduced radiation could be delivered. However, even patients as old as 8 years appear to have a greater incidence of both abnormal CT scans and neuropsychologic evidence of radiation-induced neurologic sequelae.[387,396]

MRI may offer a means of locating and following areas of CNS damage. A recent report suggests that this tool is capable of demonstrating areas of treatment-related white-matter abnormalities not visible on CT that may correlate with the degree of clinical neurologic compromise.[80] A prospective evaluation of the use of MRI in children with CNS malignancy may improve understanding of the location and dynamics of CNS damage associated with various therapeutic interventions.

Because the numbers of patients are relatively small and there is usually a time lag between therapy and the onset of these sequelae, it is unlikely that the many questions regarding risk, detection, and control of these problems will be answered outside of multi-institutional studies.

REFERENCES

1. Holt LM: The Diseases of Infancy and Childhood, pp 728–734. New York, Appleton, 1897
2. Young J, Miller R: Incidence of malignant tumors in U.S. children. J Pediatr 86:254–258, 1975
3. Duffner PK, Cohen ME, Meyers MH et al: Survival of children with brain tumors: SEER program 1973–1980. Neurology 36:597–601, 1986
4. Ertel IJ: Brain tumors in children. Cancer 30:306–321, 1980
5. Farwell JR, Dohrman GJ, Flannery JT: Central nervous system tumors in children. Cancer 40:3123–3132, 1977
6. Yates AJ, Decker LE, Sachs LA: Brain tumors in childhood. Childs Brain 5:31–39, 1979
7. Schoenberg B, Christine B, Wishnant J: The descriptive epidemiology of primary intracranial neoplasms—the Connecticut experience. Am J Epidemiol 104:499–510, 1976
8. Schoenberg B, Schoenberg D, Christine B et al: The epidemiology of primary intracranial neoplasms of childhood: A population study. Mayo Clin Proc 51:51–56, 1976
9. Schoenberg B, Glista G, Reagan T: The familial occurrence of glioma. Surg Neurol 3:139–145, 1975
10. Schoenberg B: Multiple primary neoplasms and the nervous system. Cancer 40:1961–1967, 1977
11. Lesnick J, Chayt K, Bruce D et al: Familial pineoblastoma: Report of two cases. J Neurosurg 62:930–932, 1985
12. Tijssen CC, Halprin MR, Endtz LJ (eds): Familial brain tumors. In Developments in Oncology, vol 9. The Hague, Martinus Nijhoff, 1982
13. Bader J, Meadows A, Zimmerman L et al: Bilateral retinoblastoma with ectopic intracranial retinoblastoma: Trilateral retinoblastoma. Cancer Genet Cytogenet 5:203–213, 1982
14. Bonnin J, Rubinstein L, Palmer N et al: An association of embryonal tumors originating in the kidney and in the brain. Cancer 54:2137–2146, 1984
15. Seizinger BR, Martuza RL, Gusella JF: Loss of genes on chromosome 22 in tumourigenesis of human acoustic neuroma. Nature 322:644–647, 1986
16. Zang KD: Cytological and cytogenetical studies on human meningioma. Cancer Genet Cytogenet 6:249–274, 1982
17. Shioro P, Chung C, Myrianthopouios N: Preconception radiation, intrauterine diagnostic radiation and childhood neoplasia. JNCI 65:681–686, 1980
18. Shore R, Albert R, Pasternack B: Followup study of patients treated by x-ray epilation for tinea capitis. Arch Environ Health 31:21–28, 1976
19. Spallone A, Gagliardi F, Vagnozzi R: Intracranial meningiomas related to external cranial radiation. Surg Neurol 12:153–159, 1979

20. Liwnicz B, Berger T, Liwnicz R et al: Radiation-associated gliomas: A report of four cases and analysis of postradiation tumors of the central nervous system. Neurosurgery 17:436–445, 1985

21. Hood T, Gerbarski S, McKeever P et al: Stereotaxic biopsy of intrinsic lesions of the brain stem. J Neurosurg 65:172–176, 1986

22. Hoover R, Fraumeri J: Risk of cancer in renal transplant recipients. Lancet 2:55–57, 1973

23. Schneck S, Penn I: De novo brain tumours in renal transplant recipients. Lancet 1:983–986, 1971

24. Zeller WJ, Ivankovic S, Habs M et al: Experimental chemical production of brain tumors. Ann NY Acad Sci 381:250–263, 1982

25. Rice J, Ward J: Age dependence of susceptibility to carcinogenesis in the nervous system. Ann NY Acad Sci 381:274–289, 1982

26. Kwa S, Fine L: The association between parental occupation and childhood malignancy. J Occup Med 22:792–794, 1980

27. Peters J, Preston–Martin S, Yu M: Brain tumors in children and occupational exposure of parents. Science 213:235–237, 1981

28. Bigner SH, Bjerkvig R, Laerum OD: DNA content and chromosomal composition of malignant human gliomas. Neurol Clin 3:769–784, 1985

29. Mark SJ, Laerum OD: Modal DNA content of human intracranial neoplasms studied by flow cytometry. J Neurosurg 53:198–204, 1982

30. Christov R, Zapryanov Z: Flow cytometry in brain tumors I: Ploidy abnormalities. Neoplasma 33:49–55, 1986

31. Cravioto H: Human and experimental gliomas in tissue culture. In Zimmerman H (ed): Progress in Neuropathology, vol 6, pp 165–188. New York, Raven Press, 1986

32. Shapiro JR: Cellular characterization and BCNU resistance of freshly resected and early passage human glioma cells. In Zimmerman H (ed): Progress in Neuropathology, vol 6. New York, Raven Press, 1986

33. Giangospero F, Burger P: Correlations between cytologic composition and biologic behavior in the glioblastoma multiforme: A postmortem study of 50 cases. Cancer 52:2320–2333, 1983

34. Schmitt HP: Rapid anaplastic transformation in gliomas of adulthood: "Selection" in neuro-oncogenesis. Pathol Res Pract 176:313–323, 1983

35. Gebhart E, Brederlein S, Tulsan AH et al: Incidence of double minutes, cytogenetic equivalents of gene amplification in human carcinoma cells. Int J Cancer 34:369–373, 1984

36. Baker PE: Double minutes in human tumor cells. Cancer Genet Cytogenet 5:81–94, 1982

37. Liberman PA, Nusbaum HR, Razon N et al: Amplification, enhanced expression and possible rearrangement of EGF receptor gene in primary human brain tumours of glial origin. Nature 313:144–147, 1985

38. Westermark B, Ninster M, Heldin C: Growth factors and oncogenes in "human malignant glioma." Neurol Clin 3:785–799, 1985

39. Schecheter AL, Stern DF, Vaidyanathan L et al: The neu oncogene: An erb-B-related gene encoding a 185,000-M, tumour antigen. Nature 312:513–515, 1984

40. Perantoni A, Reed CD, Watatani M et al: Tissue-specific activation of ERB B-related oncogene sequences in nitrosoethylurea (ENU)-induced rat neurogenic tumors (abstract). Proc Annu Meet Am Assoc Cancer Res 27:75, 1986

41. Pantazis P, Pelicci P, Dalla–Favaro R et al: Synthesis and secretion of proteins resembling platelet-derived growth factor by human glioblastoma and fibrosarcoma cells in culture. Proc Natl Acad Sci USA 82:2404–2408, 1985

42. Hoshino T, Nagashima T, Murovic J et al: In situ cell kinetics studies on human neuroectodermal tumors with bromodeoxyuridine labeling. J Neurosurg 64:453–459, 1986

43. Pertuiset B, Dougherty D, Cromeyer C et al: Stem cell studies of human malignant brain tumors 2: Proliferation kinetics of brain-tumor cells in vitro in early-passage cultures. J Neurosurg 63:426–432, 1985

44. Hoshino T: A commentary on the biology and growth kinetics of low-grade and high-grade gliomas. J Neurosurg 61:895–900, 1984

45. Hoshino T, Kobayashi S, Townsend J et al: A cell kinetic study on medulloblastomas. Cancer 55:1711–1713, 1985

46. Zulch KJ: Brain Tumors: Their Biology and Pathology, 3rd Ed., pp 1–26. Berlin, Springer-Verlag, 1986

47. Gilles FH: Classifications of childhood brain tumors. Cancer 56:1850–1857, 1985

48. Bailey P, Cushing H: A Classification of Tumors of the Glioma Group. Philadelphia, JB Lippincott, 1926

49. Russell DS, Rubinstein LJ: Pathology of Tumours of the Nervous System. London, Arnold, 1977

50. Zulch KJ: Histologic Typing of Tumours of the Central Nervous System. Geneva, World Health Organization, 1979

51. Kernohan JW, Mabon RF, Swien JH et al: A simplified classification of the gliomas. Proc Staff Meet Mayo Clin 24:71–75, 1949

52. Schnipper LE: Clinical implications of tumor cell heterogeneity. N Engl J Med 314:1423–1431, 1986

53. Kobayashi H: The biological modification of tumor cells as a means of inducing their regression: An overview. J Biol Response Mod 5:1–11, 1986

54. Gould VE: Histogenesis and differentiation: A re-evaluation of these concepts as criteria for the classification of tumors. Hum Pathol 17:212–215, 1986

55. Gilles FH, Leviton A, Hedley–Whyte TE et al: Perspectives in pathology: Childhood brain tumor update. Hum Pathol 14:834–843, 1983

56. Clark HB: Immunohistochemistry of nervous system antigens: Diagnostic application in surgical neuropathology. Semin Diagn Pathol 1:309–316, 1984

57. Bonnin JM, Rubinstein JL: Immunohistochemistry of central nervous system tumors. J Neurosurg 60:1121–1133, 1984

58. Coakham HB, Brownell B: Monoclonal antibodies in the diagnosis of cerebral tumors and cerebrospinal fluid neoplasia. In Cavanaugh JB (ed): Recent Advances in Neuropathology, Vol 3, pp 25–53. Edinburgh, Churchill-Livingstone, 1986

59. Rorke LB: The cerebellar medulloblastoma and its relationship to primitive neuroectodermal tumors. J Neuropathol Exp Neurol 42:1–15, 1983

60. Vogel F: Genetics of retinoblastoma. Hum Genet 52:1–54, 1979

61. Brodeur GM, Green AA, Hayes FA et al: Cytogenetic features of human neuroblastomas and cell lines. Cancer Res 41:4678–4686, 1984

62. Gilbert F, Feder M, Balaban G et al: Human neuroblastomas and abnormalities of chromosomes 1 and 17. Cancer Res 44:5444–5449, 1984

63. Becker LE: An appraisal of the World Health Organization classification of tumors of the central nervous system. Cancer 56:1858–1864, 1985

64. Rorke LB, Gilles FH, Davis RL et al: Revision of the World Health Organization classification of brain tumors for childhood brain tumors. Cancer 56:1869–1886, 1985

65. Rubinstein LJ: The cerebellar medulloblastoma: Its origin, differentiation, morphological variants, and clinical behavior. In Vincken PJ, Bruyn GW (eds): Tumors of the Brain and Skull, part III, pp 167–194. New York, Elsevier, 1975

66. Becker LE, Hinton D: Primitive neuroectodermal tumors of the central nervous system. Hum Pathol 14:538–550, 1983

67. Rubinstein LJ: Embryonal central neuroepithelial tumors and their differentiating potential: A cytogenetic view of a complex neuro-oncological problem. J Neurosurg 62:795–805, 1985

68. Gaffney CC, Sloane JP, Bradley NJ et al: Primitive neuroectodermal tumors of the cerebrum. J Neuro-oncol 3:23–33, 1985

69. Dehner LP: Peripheral and central primitive neuroectodermal tumors. Arch Pathol Lab Med 110:997–1005, 1986

70. Honig PJ, Charney EB: Children with brain tumor headaches. Am J Dis Child 136:121–124, 1982

71. Leurssen TC, Siegel KR, Packer RJ et al: Long prodromal presentation of pediatric brain tumors (abstract). Proceedings of American Association of Neurological Surgeons, Section of Pediatric Neurology, 1984

72. Burde RM, Savino PJ, Trobe JD: Clinical decisions in neuroophthalmology, pp 132–146. St Louis, CV Mosby, 1985

73. Barrer SJ, Schut L, Bruce DA: Global rostral midbrain dysfunction secondary to shunt malfunction in hydrocephalus. Neurosurgery 7:322–325, 1980

74. Packer RJ, Siegel KR, Sutton LN et al: Leptomeningeal dissemination of primary central nervous system tumors of childhood. Ann Neurol 18:217–227, 1985

75. Segall MD, Batnizky S, Zee CS et al: Computed tomography in the diagnosis of intracranial neoplasm in children. Cancer 56:1748–1755, 1985

76. Batnizky S, Segall MD, Cohen ME: Radiologic guidelines in assessing children with intracranial tumors. Cancer 56:1756–1762, 1985

77. Packer RJ, Batnizky S, Cohen ME: Magnetic resonance imaging in the evaluation of intracranial tumors of childhood. Cancer 56:1767–1772, 1985

78. Packer RJ, Zimmerman RA, Leurrson T: Nuclear magnetic resonance in the evaluation of brain stem gliomas of childhood. Neurology 35:397–401, 1985

79. Cohen ME, Duffner PK, Kuhn JP et al: Neuroimaging and neurofibromatosis (abstract). Ann Neurol 20:444, 1986

80. Packer RJ, Zimmerman RA, Bilaniuk LT: Magnetic resonance imaging in the evaluation of treatment related central nervous system damage. Cancer 58:635–640, 1986

81. Packer RJ, Zimmerman RA, Sutton LN et al: Magnetic resonance imaging (MRI) of spinal disease of childhood. Pediatrics 78:251–256, 1986

82. Phelps ME, Mazziotta JC, Huang SC: Study of cerebral function with positron computed tomography. J Cerebral Blood Flow Metab 2:113–162, 1982

83. Kun LE, D'Souza B, Tefft M: The value of surveillance testing in childhood brain tumors. Cancer 56:1818–1823, 1984

84. Albright AL: The value of precraniotomy shunts in children with posterior fossa tumors. Clin Neurosurg 30:278–285, 1983

85. McLaurin RL: Disadvantages of the preoperative shunt in posterior fossa tumors. Clin Neurosurg 30:286–292, 1983

86. Lunsford LD: Diagnosis of mass lesions using the Leksell system. In Lunsford LD (ed): Modern Stereotactic Surgery. Boston, Martinus Nijhoff, 1987

87. Broggi G, Franzini A, Migliavacca F et al: Stereotactic biopsy of deep brain tumors in infancy and childhood. Childs Brain 10:92–98, 1983

88. Albright AL, Price RA, Guthkelch AN: Diencephalic gliomas of children: A clinico-pathologic study. Cancer 55:2789–2793, 1985

89. Allen JC: Childhood brain tumors: Current status of clinical trials in newly diagnosed and recurrent disease. Pediatr Clin North Am 32:633–651, 1985

90. Barrer SJ, Schut L, Sutton LN et al: Re-operation for recurrent brain tumors in children. Childs Brain 11:375–386, 1984

91. Rubin P, Casaret GW (eds): Clinical Radiation Pathology. Philadelphia, WB Saunders, 1968

92. Bloom HJG, Wallace ENK, Henk JM: The treatment and prognosis of medulloblastoma in children: A study of 82 verified cases. Am J Roentgenol 105:43–62, 1969

93. Allen J, Epstein F: Medulloblastoma and other primary malignant tumors of the CNS. J Neurosurg 57:446–451, 1982

94. Douglas BG, Worth AJ: Superfractionation in glioblastoma multiforme: Results of a phase II study. Int J Radiat Oncol Biol Phys 8:1787–1794, 1982

95. Shin KH, Muller PJ, Geggie PH: Superfractionated radiation therapy in the treatment of malignant astrocytoma. Cancer 52:2040–2043, 1983

96. Shin KH, Urtasun RC et al: Multiple daily fractionated radiotherapy and misonidazole in the management of malignant astrocytoma: Phase III prospective clinical trial: Preliminary report. Ann Roy Coll Physicians Surgeons Can 16:362, 1983

97. Wara WM, Edward MSB, Levin VA et al: A new treatment regimen for brain stem glioma: A pilot study of the Brain Tumor Research Center and Children's Cancer Study Group. Int J Radiat Oncol Biol Phys 12(Suppl 1):143, 1986

98. Chang CH: Hyperbaric oxygen and radiation therapy in the management of glioblastoma. Natl Cancer Inst Monogr 46:163–169, 1977

99. Urtasan R, Band P, Chapman JD et al: Radiation and high-dose metronidazole in supratentorial glioblastomas. N Engl J Med 294:1364–1367, 1976

100. Phillips TL, Wasserman TH, Johnson RJ et al: Final report on the United States Phase I clinical trial of the hypoxic cell sensitizer, misonidazole (RO-07-0582: NSC #261037). Cancer 48:1697–1704, 1981

101. Laramore GE, Griffin TW, Gerdes AJ et al: Fast neutron and mixed (neutron/photon) beam teletherapy for grades III and IV astrocytomas. Cancer 42:96–103, 1978

102. Bouchard J (ed): Radiation Therapy of Tumors and Diseases of the Nervous System. Philadelphia, Lea & Febiger, 1966

103. Kim TH, Chin HW, Pollan S, Hazel JH, Webster JH: Radiotherapy of primary brain stem tumors. Int J Radiat Oncol Biol Phys 6:51–57, 1980

104. Freeman JE, Johnston PG, Voke JM: Somnolence after prophylactic cranial irradiation in children with acute lymphoblastic laeukemia. Br Med J 4:523–525, 1973

105. Jones A: Transient radiation myelopathy (with reference to Lhermitte's sign of electrical paresthesia). Br J Radiol 37:727–744, 1964

106. Reagan TJ, Thomas JE, Colby MY: Chronic progressive radiation myelopathy: Its clinical aspects and differential diagnosis. JAMA 203:128–132, 1968

107. deRenck J, van der Eechen H: The anatomy of late radiation encephalopathy. Eur Neurol 13:481–494, 1975

108. Kramer S, Lee KF: Complications of radiation therapy: The central nervous system. Semin Roentgenol 9:75–83, 1974

109. Martins AN, Johnston JS, Henry JM et al: Delayed radionecrosis of the brain. J Neurosurg 47:336–345, 1977

110. Greig NH: Chemotherapy of brain metastases: Current status. Cancer Treat Rev 11:157–186, 1984

111. Levin V: Chemotherapy of primary brain tumors. Neurol Clin 3:855–866, 1985

112. Allen J, Bloom J, Ertel J: Brain tumors in children: Current cooperative and institutional chemotherapy trials in newly diagnosed and recurrent disease. Semin Oncol 13:110–122, 1986

113. Rall D, Zubrod C: Mechanisms of drug absorption and excretion: Passage of drugs in and out of the central nervous system. Annu Rev Pharmacol 2:109–128, 1962

114. Vick N, Khandekar J, Bigner D: Chemotherapy of brain tumors: The "blood brain barrier" is not a factor. Arch Neurol 34:523–526, 1977

115. Waggener J, Beggs J: Vasculature of neural neoplasms. Adv Neurol 15:27–49, 1976

116. Blasberg R, Groothuis D: Chemotherapy of brain tumors: Physiological and pharmacokinetic considerations. Semin Oncol 13:70–82, 1986

117. Levin V, Freeman–Dove M, Landahl H: Permeability characteristics of brain adjacent to tumors in rats. Arch Neurol 32:785–791, 1975

118. Molnar P, Blasberg R, Horowitz M et al: Regional blood-to-tissue transport in RT-9 brain tumors. J Neurosurg 58:874–884, 1983

119. Blasberg R, Molnar P, Horowitz M: Regional blood flow in RT-9 brain tumors. J Neurosurg 58:863–873, 1983

120. Hochberg F, Parker L, Takvorian T et al: High-dose BCNU with autologous bone marrow rescue for recurrent glioblastoma multiforme. J Neurosurg 54:455–460, 1981

121. Burger P, Komenar E, Schold S et al: Encephalomyelopathy following high-dose BCNU therapy. Cancer 48:1318–1327, 1981

122. Mortimer J, Hewlett J, Bay J et al: High dose BCNU with autologous bone marrow rescue in the treatment of recurrent malignant gliomas. J Neuro Oncol 1:269–273, 1983

123. Kapp J, Vance R, Parka J et al: Limitations of high dose intra-arterial BCNU chemotherapy for malignant gliomas. Neurosurgery 10:715–719, 1982

124. Blacklock J, Wright D, Dedrick R et al: Drug streaming during intra-arterial chemotherapy. J Neurosurg 64:284–291, 1986

125. Ross R, Kapp J, Hochberg F et al: Solvent systems for intracarotid BCNU infusion. Neurosurgery 12:512–514, 1983

126. Neuwelt E, Frenkel E: Is there a therapeutic role for blood–brain barrier disruption? Ann Intern Med 93:137–139, 1980

127. Neuwelt E, Diehl J, Vu L et al: Monitoring methotrexate delivery in patients with malignant brain tumors after osmotic barrier disruption. Ann Intern Med 94:449–454, 1981

128. Neuwelt E, Balaban D, Diehl J et al: Successful treatment of primary central nervous system lymphomas with chemotherapy after osmotic blood–brain barrier opening. Neurosurgery 12:662–671, 1983

129. Neuwelt E, Glasberg M, Frenkel E et al: Neurotoxicity of chemotherapeutic agents after blood–brain barrier modification: Neuropathological studies. Ann Neurol 14:316–324, 1983

130. Spigelman M, Zappalla R, Malis L et al: Intracarotid dehydrocholate infusion: A new method for prolonged reversible blood–brain barrier disruption. Neurosurgery 12:606–612, 1983

131. Dakhil S, Ensminger W, Kindt G: Implanted system for intraventricular drug infusion in central nervous system tumors. Cancer Treat Rep 65:401–411, 1981

132. Ommaya A: Implantable devices for chronic access and drug delivery to the central nervous system. Cancer Drug Deliv 1:169–177, 1984

133. Neuwelt EA, Barnett PA, McCormick CI et al: Osmotic blood–brain barrier modification: Monoclonal antibody, albumin and methotrexate delivery to cerebrospinal fluid and brain. Neurosurgery 17:419–423, 1985

134. Neuwelt EA, Specht HD, Hill SA: Permeability of human brain tumor to 99 mTc-glucoheptonate and 99 mTc albumin. J Neurosurg 65:194–198, 1986

135. Jacobs SK, Wilson DJ, Kornblith PL: Interleukin-2 and autologous lymphokine-activated killer cells in the treatment of malignant glioma. J Neurosurg 64:743–749, 1986

136. Kaye A, Morstyn G, Gardner I et al: Development of a xenograft glioma model in mouse brain. Cancer Res 46:1367–1373, 1986

137. Saris S, Bigner S, Bigner D: Intracerebral transplantation of a human glioma line in immunosuppressed rats. J Neurosurg 60:582–588, 1984

138. Friedman H, Colvin O, Ludeman S et al: Experimental chemotherapy of human medulloblastoma with classical alkylators. Cancer Res 46:2827–2833, 1986

139. Friedman H, Schold S, Bigner D: Chemotherapy of subcutaneous and intracranial human medulloblastoma xenografts in athymic nude mice. Cancer Res 46:224–228, 1986

140. Weizsacker M, Nagamune R, Rathmer K et al: Brain tumor growth and response to chemotherapy in the subrenal capsule assay. J Cancer Res Clin Oncol 106:229–233, 1983

141. Kimmel DW, Shapiro JR, Shapiro WR: In vitro drug sensitivity testing in human gliomas. J Neurosurg 66:161–171, 1987

142. Friedman H, Schold S, Muhlbaier L et al: In vitro versus in vivo correlations of chemosensitivity of human medulloblastoma. Cancer Res 44:5145–5149, 1984

143. McFarland DR, Horwitz H, Saenger EL: Medulloblastoma—A review of prognosis and survival. Br J Radiol 42:198–214, 1969

144. Choix M, Lena G, Hassoun J: Prognosis and long term followup in patients with medulloblastoma. Clin Neurosurg 30:246–277, 1983

145. Russell DR, Rubinstein LJ: Pathology of Tumors of the Nervous System, 4th Ed., pp 32–38, 135–183, 244–255. Baltimore, Williams & Wilkins, 1977

146. Muller W, Afra D, Schroder R et al: Medulloblastoma: Survey of factors possibly influencing the prognosis. Acta Neurochir 64:215–224, 1982

147. Deutsch M, Reigel D: The value of myelography in the management of childhood medulloblastoma. Cancer 45:2194–2197, 1980

148. Liebner E, Pretto J, Hochhauser M et al: Tumors of the posterior fossa in childhood and adolescence: Their diagnostic and radiotherapeutic patterns. Radiology 82:193–201, 1964

149. Dorwart R, Ward W, Norman D et al: Complete myelographic evaluation of spinal metastases from medulloblastoma. Radiology 139:403–408, 1981

150. Berry M, Jenkin D, Keen C et al: Radiation treatment for medulloblastoma: A 21 year review. J Neurosurg 55:43–51, 1981

151. Kleinman G, Hochberg F, Richardson E: Systemic metastases from medulloblastoma: Report of two cases and review of the literature. Cancer 48:2296–2309, 1984

152. Campbell A, Chan H, Becker L et al: Extracranial metastasis in childhood primary tumors. Cancer 53:974–981, 1984

153. Raimondi A, Tomita T: Medulloblastoma in childhood: Comparative results of partial and total resection. Childs Brain 5:310–328, 1979

154. Hoffman HJ, Hendrick EB, Humphreys RP: Management of medulloblastoma. Clin Neurosurg 30:226–245, 1983

155. Zimmerman R, Bilaniuk L, Pahlajani H: Spectrum of medulloblastomas demonstrated by computed tomography. Radiology 126:137–141, 1978

156. Tsuchida T, Tanaka R, Fukuda M et al: CT findings of medulloblastoma. Childs Brain 11:60–68, 1984

157. Packer RJ, Segal KR, Schut L et al: Central nervous system spread of childhood brain tumors at diagnosis and recurrence. Concepts Pediatr Neurosurg 6:16–24, 1985

158. Seidenfield J, Marton LJ: Biological markers of CNS tumors. In Humphrey GB, Dehner LJ, Grindey GB et al (eds): Pediatric Oncology 1, pp 117–163. The Hague, Martinus Nijhoff, 1981

159. Harisiadis L, Chang CH: Medulloblastoma in children: A correlation between staging and results of treatment. Int J Radiat Oncol Biol Phys 2:833–841, 1977

160. Silverman C, Simpson J: Cerebellar medulloblastoma: The importance of posterior fossa dose to survival and patterns of failure. Int J Radiat Oncol Biol Phys 8:1869–1876, 1982

161. Gerosa M, diStefano E, Olivi A et al: Multidisciplinary treatment of medulloblastoma: A 5 year experience with the SIOP trial. Childs Brain 8:107–118, 1981

162. Fossati F, Gasparini M, Lombardi F et al: Medulloblastoma: Results of sequential combined treatment. Cancer 54:1956–1961, 1984

163. Park TS, Hoffman HJ, Hendrick BE et al: Medulloblastoma: Clinical presentation and management: Experience at the Hospital for Sick Children, Toronto 1950–1980. J Neurosurg 58:543–552, 1983

164. Packer RJ, Sutton LN, Rorke LB et al: Prognostic importance of cellular differentiation in medulloblastoma of childhood. J Neurosurg 61:296–301, 1984

165. Chatty EM, Earle KM: Medulloblastoma: A report of 201 cases with emphasis on the relationship of histologic variants to survival. Cancer 28:977–983, 1971

166. Camins MB, Cravioto HM, Epstein F et al: Medulloblastoma: An ultrastructural study: Evidence for astrocytic and neuronal differentiation. Neurosurgery 6:398–411, 1980

167. Norris D, Bruce D, Byrd R et al: Improved relapse free survival in medulloblastoma utilizing modern techniques. Neurosurgery 9:661–664, 1981

168. Hoffman H, Hendrick E, Humphreys R: Metastasis via ventriculoperitoneal shunt in patients with medulloblastoma. J Neurosurg 44:562–566, 1976

169. McComb J, Davis R, Isaacs H: Extraneural metastatic medulloblastoma during childhood. Neurosurgery 9:548–551, 1981

170. Brown R, Gunderson L, Plenk H: Medulloblastoma: A review of the LDS Hospital experience. Cancer 40:56–60, 1977

171. Cumberlin R, Luk K, Ward W: Medulloblastoma treatment results and effect on normal tissues. Cancer 43:1014–1020, 1979

172. Landberg T, Lindgre M, Cavallin–Stohl E et al: Improvements in the radiotherapy of medulloblastoma, 1946–1975. Cancer 45:670–678, 1980

173. Mealy J, Hall P: Medulloblastoma in children—Survival and treatment. J Neurosurg 46:56–63, 1977

174. Tomita T, McClone DG: Medulloblastoma in childhood: Results of radical resection and low-dose neuraxis radiation therapy. J Neurosurg 64:238–242, 1986

175. Hirsch DR, Czernichow P, Benveniste L et al: Medulloblastoma in children: Survival and functional results. Acta Neurochir 48:1–15, 1979

176. Chin HW, Maruyama Y: Results of radiation treatment of cerebellar medulloblastoma. Int J Radiat Oncol Biol Phys 7:737–742, 1981

177. Friedman HS, Schold SC: Rational approaches to the chemotherapy of medulloblastoma. Neurol Clin 3:843–853, 1985

178. Mazza C, Pasqualin A, Da Pian R et al: Treatment of medulloblastoma in children: Long term results following surgery, radiotherapy and chemotherapy. Acta Neurochir 46:163–175, 1981

179. Bloom HJG: Intracranial tumors: Response and resistance to therapeutic endeavors 1970–1980. Int J Radiat Oncol Biol Phys 8:1083–1113, 1982

180. Seiler RW, Bernasconi S, Berchtold W et al: Adjuvant chemotherapy with procarbazene, vincristine and prednisone for medulloblastoma: A preliminary report. Helv Paediatr Acta 36:249–253, 1981

181. Woo SY, Sinks LF, Sackmann–Muriel F et al: Update of adjuvant methotrexate and BCNU in treatment of medulloblastoma (abstract). Am Soc Clin Oncol 2:66, 1983

182. Gerosa M, Di Stefano E, Carli M et al: Combined treatment of pediatric medulloblastoma: A review of an integrated program. Childs Brain 6:263–273, 1980

183. Van Eys J, Chen T, Moore T et al: Adjuvant chemotherapy for medulloblastoma and ependymoma using IV vincristine, intrathecal methotrexate, and intrathecal hydrocortisone: A Southwest Oncology Group study. Cancer Treat Rep 65:681–684, 1981

184. Zeltzer PM: Chemotherapy for medulloblastoma: A review of treatment in de novo tumors. In Zeltzer PM, Pochedly C (eds): Medulloblastomas in Children: New Concepts in Biology, Diagnosis and Treatment, pp 164–199. New York, Praeger, 1986

185. Riehm HJ, Niedhardt MK, Janka G: Postoperative combination chemotherapy before neuraxis irradiation in childhood medulloblastoma. Neuropediatrics 2:80–85, 1981

186. Neidhardt MK, Havefield F, Henze G et al: Treatment of medulloblastoma with post operative chemotherapy before neuraxis irratiation: An interim progress report on the Berlin pilot study and the West German cooperative trial (abstract). Proceedings of the International Society of Pediatric Oncology XIII Annual Meeting, p 39, 1983

187. Pendergrass TW, Milstein JM, Geyer RJ et al: Eight drugs in one-day chemotherapy for brain tumors: Experience in 107 children and rationale for preradiation chemotherapy. J Clin Oncol 5:1221–1231, 1987

188. Olive P, Phillip T, Zucker J et al: Efficacy of 8 drug combination regimen in the treatment of brain tumors (abstract). Am Soc Clin Oncol 3:80, 1984

189. Coulon RA, Till K: Intracranial ependymomas in children: A review of 43 cases. Childs Brain 3:154–168, 1977

190. Dohrmann GJ, Farwell JR, Flannery JT: Ependymomas and ependymoblastomas in children. J Neurosurg 45:273–283, 1976

191. Liu HM, Boggs J, Kidd J: Ependymomas of childhood I: Histological survey and clinicopathological correlation. Childs Brain 2:92–110, 1976

192. Salazar OM, Casto–Vita M, Van Houtte D et al: Improved survival in cases of intracranial ependymoma after radiation therapy: Late report and recommendations. J Neurosurg 59:652–659, 1983

193. Mabon RF, Svien NJ, Kernohan JW et al: Symposium on new and simplified concept of gliomas: Ependymomas. Proc Staff Meet Mayo Clin 24:65–71, 1949

194. Rubinstein LJ: The definition of the ependymoblastoma. Arch Pathol 90:35–45, 1970

195. Pierre–Kahn A, Hirsch JF, Roux FX, Renier D, Sainte-Rose C: Intracranial ependymomas in childhood: Survival and function results of 47 cases. Childs Brain 10:145–156, 1983

196. Cohen ME, Duffner PK: Ependymomas. In Cohen ME, Duffner PK (eds): Brain Tumors in Childhood: Principles of Diagnosis and Treatment, pp 136–155. New York, Raven Press, 1984

197. Enzmann DR, Norman D, Levin V, Wilson C, Newton TH: Computed tomography in the follow-up of medulloblastoma and ependymomas. Radiology 128:57–63, 1978

198. Kingsley DPE, Kendall BE: The CT scanner in posterior fossa tumors of childhood. Br J Radiol 52:769–776, 1979

199. Chin HW, Maruyama Y, Markesberry W et al: Intracranial ependymoma: Results of radiotherapy at the University of Kentucky. Cancer 49:2276–2280, 1982

200. Garret PG, Simpson WJ: Ependymomas: Results of radiation treatment. Int J Radiat Oncol Biol Phys 9:1121–1124, 1983

201. Oi S, Raimondi A: Ependymoma. In Pediatric Neurosurgery: Surgery of the Developing Nervous System, pp 419–427. New York, Grune and Stratton, 1982

202. Mørk SJ, Loken AC: Ependymoma: A follow-up study of 101 cases. Cancer 40:907–915, 1977

203. Sheline GE: Conventional radiation therapy of gliomas. Recent Results Cancer Res 51:125–138, 1975

204. Gutin PH, Wilson CB, Kumar AR et al: Phase II study of procarbazine, CCNU, and vincristine in the treatment of metastatic brain tumors. Cancer 35:1398–1404, 1975

205. Wilson CB, Gutin P, Boldrey EB et al: Single agent chemotherapy of brain tumors. Arch Neurol 33:739–744, 1976

206. Khan AB, D'Souza BJ, Wharan MD et al: Cis-platinum therapy in recurrent childhood brain tumors. Cancer Treat Rep 66:2013–2020, 1982

207. Matson D: Cerebellar astrocytoma in childhood. Pediatrics 18:150–158, 1956

208. Gilles F: Cerebellar tumors in children: Clin Neurosurg 30:181–188, 1983

209. Winston K, Gilles F, Leviton A et al: Cerebellar gliomas in children. JNCI 58:833–838, 1977

210. Koos W, Miller M: Intracranial tumors of infants and children. St Louis, CV Mosby, 1971

211. Gol A, McKissock W: The cerebellar astrocytomas: A report on 98 verified cases. J Neurosurg 16:287–296, 1959

212. Gjerris F, Klinken L: Long-term prognosis in children with benign cerebellar astrocytoma. J Neurosurg 49:179–184, 1978

213. Szenasy J, Slowik F: Prognosis of benign cerebellar astrocytomas in children. Childs Brain 10:39–47, 1983

214. Palma L, Russo A, Celli P: Prognosis of the so-called "diffuse" cerebellar astrocytoma. Neurosurgery 15:315–317, 1984

215. Chin H, Maruyama Y, Tibbs P et al: Cerebellar glioblastoma in children. J Neuro-oncol 2:79–84, 1984

216. Auer R, Rice G, Hinton G et al: Cerebellar astrocytoma with benign histology and malignant clinical course. J Neurosurg 54:128–132, 1981

217. Geissinger J, Bucy P: Astrocytomas of the cerebellum in children: Long term study. Arch Neurol 29:125–135, 1971

218. Butler A, Horii S, Kricheff I et al: Computed tomography of astrocytomas. Radiology 129:433–439, 1978

219. Zimmerman R, Bilaniuk L, Bruno L et al: Computed tomography of cerebellar astrocytoma. AJR 130:929–933, 1978

220. Klein D, McCullough D: Surgical staging of cerebellar astrocytomas in childhood. Cancer 56:1810–1811, 1985

221. Ferbert A, Gullotta F: Remarks on the followup of cerebellar astrocytomas. J Neurol 232:134–136, 1985

222. Bucy P, Thieman P: Astrocytomas of the cerebellum: A study of a series of patients operated upon over 28 years ago. Arch Neurol 18:14–19, 1968

223. Griffin TW, Beaufait D, Blasko JC: Cystic cerebellar astrocytoma in childhood. Cancer 44:276–280, 1979

224. Edwards MS, Levin VA, Wilson CB: Chemotherapy of pediatric posterior fossa tumors. Childs Brain 7:252–260, 1980

225. Leibel SA, Sheline GE, Wara WM et al: The role of radiation therapy in the treatment of astrocytomas. Cancer 35:1551–1557, 1975

226. Salazar OM, Rubin P: The spread of glioblastoma multiforme as a determining factor in the radiation treated volume. Int J Radiat Oncol Biol Phys 1:627–637, 1976

227. Kopelson G: Cerebellar glioblastoma. Cancer 50:308–311, 1982

228. Bruno L, Schut L, Bruce D: Cerebellar astrocytoma. In Pediatric Neurosurgery: Surgery of the Developing Nervous System, pp 367–374. New York, Grune and Stratton, 1982

229. Herbst M: Radiation therapy in the treatment of the astrocytomas and midline tumors of childhood. In Voth D, Gutjahr P, Laingmaid C (eds): Tumors of the Central Nervous System in Infants and Children, pp 325–332. Berlin, Springer-Verlag, 1982

230. Gjerris F: Clinical aspects and long-term prognosis in supratentorial tumors of infancy and childhood. Acta Neurol Scand 57:445–470, 1978

231. Tiyaworabun S, Kazkaz S, Nicola N et al: Supratentorial tumors in infants and children. In Voth D, Gutjahr P, Langmaid C (eds): Tumors of the Nervous System in Infancy and Childhood, pp 420–425. New York, Springer-Verlag, 1981

232. Mercuri S, Russo A, Palma L: Hemispheric supratentorial astrocytomas in children: Long term results in 29 cases. J Neurosurg 55:170–173, 1981

233. Cohen ME, Duffner PK: Brain Tumors in Children: Principles of Diagnosis and Treatment, p 185. New York, Raven Press, 1984

234. Backus RE, Millichap JG: The seizure as a manifestation of intracranial tumor in childhood. Pediatrics 29:978–984, 1962

235. Page LK, Lombroso CT, Matson DD: Childhood epilepsy with late detection of cerebral glioma. J Neurosurg 31:253–261, 1969

236. Gol A: Cerebral astrocytomas in childhood: A clinical study. J Neurosurg 19:577–582, 1962

237. Palma L, Guidetti B: Cystic pilocytic astrocytomas of the cerebral hemispheres. J Neurosurg 62:811–815, 1985

238. Dohrmann GJ, Farwell JR, Flannery JT: Glioblastoma multiforme in children. J Neurosurg 62:811–815, 1985

239. Menenzes AH, Bell WE, Perret GE: Hypothalamic tumors in children. Childs Brain 3:265–280, 1977

240. Low NL, Correll JW, Hammill JW: Tumors of the cerebral hemispheres in children. Arch Neurol 13:547–554, 1965

241. Weisberg LA: Cerebral computed tomography in the diagnosis of supratentorial astrocytoma. Comput Tomogr 4:87–105, 1980

242. Tars JT, Jongh IE: Computed tomography of supratentorial astrocytomas. Clin Neurol Neurosurg 80:157–168, 1979

243. Stage WS, Stein JJ: Treatment of malignant astrocytomas. Am J Roentgenol Radium Ther Nucl Med 120:7–18, 1974

244. Weir B, Grace M: The reactive significance of factors affecting postoperative survival astrocytomas grades one and two. Can J Neurol Sci 3:47–50, 1976

245. Burger PC, Vollmer RT: Histologic factors of prognostic significance in the glioblastoma multiforme. Cancer 46:1179–1186, 1980

246. Loftus CM, Copeland BR, Carmel PW: Cystic supratentorial gliomas: Natural history and evaluation of modes of surgical therapy. Neurosurgery 17:19–24, 1985

247. Gol A: The relatively benign astrocytomas of the cerebrum. J Neurosurg 28:501–506, 1961

248. Scanlon PW, Taylor WF: Radiotherapy of intracranial astrocytomas: Analysis of 417 cases treated from 1960 through 1969. Neurosurgery 5:301–308, 1979

249. Phuphanich S, Edwards M, Levin V et al: Supratentorial malignant gliomas of childhood. J Neurosurg 60:495–499, 1984

250. Bloom HJ: Treatment of brain gliomas in children. In Bleehen NM (ed): Tumors of the Brain, pp 121–125. New York, Springer-Verlag, 1986

251. Bloom HJ: Recent concepts in the conservative management of intracranial tumors in children. Acta Neurochir 50:103–116, 1979

252. Marsa GW, Probert JC, Rubinstein LJ et al: Radiation therapy in the treatment of childhood astrocytic gliomas. Cancer 32:646–655, 1973

253. Wald SL, Fogelson H, McLaurin RL: Cystic thalamic gliomas. Childs Brain 9:381–393, 1981

254. Fazekas JT: Treatment of grades I and II brain astrocytomas: The role of radiotherapy. Int J Radiat Oncol Biol Phys 2:661–666, 1977

255. Sheline GE: Radiation therapy of brain tumors. Cancer 39:873–881, 1977

256. Rutter EH, Kazam I, Joop L: Post operative radiation therapy in the management of brain astrocytoma—Retrospective study of 142 patients. Int J Radiat Oncol Biol Phys 7:191–195, 1981

257. Sheline GE: Radiation therapy of tumors of the central nervous system in childhood. Cancer 35:957–964, 1975

258. Greenburger JS, Cassady JR, Martin B et al: Radiation therapy of thalamic, midline, and brain stem gliomas. Radiology 122:463–468, 1977

259. Sposto R, Ertel IJ, Jenkin RD et al: Results of the CCSG 943 protocol: Adjuvant chemotherapy with CCNU, vincristine, and prednisone in high-grade astrocytomas: Update of results as of January 1987 (submitted for publication)

260. Salazar OM, Rubin P, Feldstein ML et al: High dose radiation therapy in the treatment of malignant gliomas: Final report. Int J Radiat Oncol Biol Phys 5:1733–1740, 1979

261. Choucair AK, Levin VA, Gutin PH et al: Development of multiple lesions during radiation therapy and chemotherapy in patients with gliomas. J Neurosurg 65:654–658, 1986

262. Bloom HJ: Intracranial tumors: Response and resistance to therapeutic endeavors, 1970–1980. Int J Radiat Oncol Biol Phys 8:1083–1113, 1982

263. Sumer T, Freeman AI, Cohen ME et al: Chemotherapy in recurrent noncystic low grade astrocytomas of the cerebrum in children. J Surg Oncol 10:45–54, 1978

264. Djerassi I, Kim JS, Regger A: Response of astrocytoma to high-dose methotrexate with citrvorum factor rescue. Cancer 55:2741–2747, 1985

265. Mantravadi R, Phatak R, Bellur S et al: Brain stem gliomas: An autopsy study of 25 cases. Cancer 49:1294–1296, 1982

266. Shin K, Fisher G, Webster J: Brain stem tumors in children: A review of 26 cases 1960–1976. J Can Assoc Radiol 30:77–78, 1979

267. Fulton DS, Levin VA, Wara WM et al: Chemotherapy of pediatric brain-stem tumors. J Neurosurg 54:721–715, 1981

268. Jenkin RD, Bosel C, Ertel I et al: Brain stem tumors in childhood: A prospective randomized trial of irradiation with and without adjuvant CCNU, VCR and prednisone: A report from the Children's Cancer Study Group. J Neurosurg 66:227–233, 1987

269. Littman P, Jarrett P, Bilaniuk L et al: Pediatric brain stem gliomas. Cancer 45:2787–2792, 1980

270. Berger MS, Edwards MSB, LaMasters D et al: Pediatric brain stem tumors: Radiographic, pathological, and clinical correlations. Neurosurgery 12:298–302, 1983

271. Kim TH, Chin HW, Pollan S et al: Radiotherapy of primary brain stem tumors. Int J Radiat Oncol Biol Phys 6:51–57, 1980

272. Albright L, Price R, Guthkelch N: Brain stem gliomas of children: A clinico-pathological study. Cancer 52:2313–2319, 1983

273. Hoffman HJ, Becker L, Craven MA: A clinically and pathologically distinct group of benign brain stem gliomas. Neurosurgery 7:243–248, 1980

274. Epstein F, McCleary E: Intrinsic brain stem tumors of childhood: Surgical indications. J Neurosurg 64:11–15, 1986

275. Packer R, Allen J, Nielson S et al: Brainstem glioma: Clinical manifestations of meningeal gliomatosis. Ann Neurol 14:177–182, 1983

276. Reigel D, Scarff T, Woodford J: Biopsy of pediatric brain stem tumors. Childs Brain 5:329–340, 1979

277. Rothman S, Olanow C: Brain stem glioma of childhood: Acute hemiplegic onset. J Can Sci Neurol 8:263–264, 1981

278. Lassman L, Long M, Anjona V: Pontine gliomas of childhood. Lancet 1:913–915, 1967

279. Panitch E, Berg B: Brain stem tumors in childhood and adolescence. Am J Dis Child 119:465–472, 1970

280. Bilaniuk L, Zimmerman R, Littman P et al: Computed tomography of brain stem gliomas in children. Neuroradiology 134:89–95, 1980

281. Weisberg L: Computed tomography in the diagnosis of brain stem gliomas. Comput Tomogr 3:145–153, 1979

282. Packer R, Zimmerman R, Luerssen T et al: Brainstem gliomas of childhood: Magnetic resonance imaging. Neurology 35:397–401, 1985

283. Lee B, Kneeland J, Walker R et al: MR imaging of brainstem tumors. AJNR 6:159–163, 1985

284. Nodar R, Hahn J, Levine H: Brain stem auditory evoked potentials in determining site of lesion of brain stem gliomas in children. Laryngoscope 90:258–266, 1980

285. Davis S, Aminoff M, Berg B: Brainstem auditory evoked potentials in children with brain stem or cerebellar dysfunction. Arch Neurol 42:156–160, 1985

286. Albright A, Guthkelch A, Packer R et al: Diagnosis and management of pediatric brain stem gliomas. J Neurosurg 65:745–750, 1986

287. Cohen M, Duffner P, Heffner R et al: Prognostic factors in brain stem gliomas. Neurology 36:602–605, 1986

288. Stroink AR, Hoffman HJ, Hendrick EB et al: Diagnosis and management of pediatric brain stem gliomas. J Neurosurg 65:745–750, 1986

289. Hood T, Gerbarski S, McKeever P et al: Stereotaxic biopsy of intrinsic lesions of the brain stem. J Neurosurg 65:172–176, 1986

290. Albright A, Scalabassi R: Use of the Cavitron ultrasonic surgical aspirator and evoked potentials for the treatment of thalamic and brain stem tumors in children. Neurosurgery 17:564–568, 1985

291. Coffey R, Lunsford L: Stereotactic surgery for mass lesions of the midbrain and pons. Neurosurgery 17:12–18, 1985

292. Whyte T, Colby M, Layton D: Radiation therapy of brain stem tumors. Radiology 93:413–416, 1969

293. Lee F: Radiation of infratentorial and supratentorial brain stem tumors. J Neurosurg 43:65–68, 1975

294. Ryan M, King G, Chung C et al: Irradiation of primary brain stem tumors. Radiology 131:503–507, 1979

295. Packer RJ, Littman P, De Angio P et al: Results of hyperfractionated radiation therapy in children with brain stem glioma. Proceedings of the International Society for Pediatric Oncology 18th Annual Meeting, pp 127–128, 1986

296. Levin J, Edwards M, Ward W et al: 5-Fluorouracil and CCNU followed by hydroxyurea, misonidazole and irradiation for brain stem gliomas: A pilot study of the Brain Tumor Research Center and the Children's Cancer Group. Neurosurgery 14:679–681, 1984

297. Pompili A, Riccio A, Jandolo B et al: CCNU chemotherapy in adult patients with tumors of the basal ganglia and brain stem. J Neurosurg 53:361–363, 1980

298. Epstein F, Epstein N: Surgical treatment of spinal cord astrocytomas of childhood: A series of 19 patients. J Neurosurg 57:685–689, 1982

299. Reimer R, Onofrio BM: Astrocytomas of the spinal cord in children and adolescents. J Neurosurg 63:669–675, 1985

300. Peschel RE, Kapp DS, Cardinale F et al: Ependymomas of the spinal cord. Int J Radiat Oncol Biol Phys 9:1093–1096, 1983

301. Epstein F, Epstein N: Intramedullary tumors of the spinal cord. In Pediatric Neurosurgery: Surgery of the Developing Nervous System, pp 529–540. New York, Grune & Stratton, 1982

302. Cooper PR, Epstein F: Radical resections of intramedullary spinal cord tumors in adults: Recent experience in 29 patients. J. Neurosurg 63:492–499, 1985

303. Epstein F: Spinal cord astrocytomas of childhood. Adv Tech Stand Neurosurg 13:136–169, 1985

304. Miller NR, Iliff WJ, Green WR: Evaluation and management of gliomas of the anterior visual pathway. Brain 97:743–754, 1975

305. Danoff BF, Kramer S, Thompson N: The radiotherapeutic management of optic gliomas of children. Int J Radiat Oncol Biol Phys 6:45–50, 1980

306. Oxenhandler DC, Sayers MP: The dilemma of childhood optic gliomas. J Neurosurg 48:34–41, 1978

307. Tenny RT, Laws ER, Younge BR et al: The neurosurgical management of optic glioma. J Neurosurg 57:452–458, 1982

308. Packer RJ, Savino PJ, Bilaniuk K et al: Chiasmatic gliomas of childhood: A reappraisal of natural history and effectiveness of cranial irradiation. Childs Brain 10:393–403, 1983

309. Rush JA, Young BR, Campbell RJ, MacCarthy CS: Optic glioma: Long-term follow-up of 85 histopathologically verified cases. Ophthalmology 89:1213–1219, 1982

310. Fletcher WA, Imes RK, Hoyt WF: Chiasmatic gliomas: Appearance and long-term changes demonstrated by computed tomography. J Neurosurg 65:154–159, 1986

311. Glaser JS, Hoyt WF, Corbett J: Visual morbidity with chiasmal glioma. Arch Ophthalmol 85:3–12, 1971

312. Farmer J, Hoyt CS: Monocular nystagmus in infancy and early childhood. Am J Ophthalmol 98:504–509, 1984

313. Albright AL, Sclabassi RJ, Slamovits TL, Bergman I: Spasm nutans associated with optic gliomas in childhood. J Pediatr 105:778–780, 1984

314. Savoiardo M, Harwood–Nash DC, Tadmor R et al: Gliomas of the intracranial anterior optic pathways in children. Radiology 138:610–614, 1981

315. Wenze D, Harms D, Brandl U et al: Electrophysiological diagnosis and followup controls in cases of tumors of the optic chiasm. In Voth D, Gutjahi P, Langmaid C (eds): Tumors of the Central Nervous System in Infancy and Childhood. New York, Springer-Verlag, 1982

316. Cohen ME, Duffner PK: Visual evoked responses in children with optic gliomas with and without neurofibromatosis. Childs Brain 10:99–111, 1983

317. Eggers H, Jokobiec FA, Jones IS: Optic nerve gliomas. In Duane TD, Jaeger EA (eds): Clinical Ophthalmology, pp 1–17. New York, Harper & Row, 1985

318. Chutorian AM, Schwartz JF, Evans RA, Carter S: Optic gliomas in children. Neurology 14:83–95, 1964

319. Hoyt WF, Baghdassarian SA: Optic glioma of childhood. Br J Ophthalmol 53:793–798, 1969

320. Montgomery AB, Griffin T, Parker RG et al: Optic nerve glioma: The role of radiation therapy. Cancer 40:2079–2080, 1977

321. Dosoetz DE, Blitzer PH, Wang CL: Management of gliomas of the optic nerve and/or chiasm. Cancer 45:1467–1471, 1980

322. MacCarty CS, Boyd AS, Childs DS: Tumors of the optic nerve and optic chiasm. J Neurosurg 33:439–444, 1970

323. Richmond IL, Wara WM, Wilson CB: Role of radiation therapy in the management of craniopharyngioma in children. Neurosurgery 33:439–444, 1980

324. Cavazzuti V, Fischer E, Welch K et al: Neurological and psychosocial sequelae following different treatments of craniopharyngioma in children. J Neurosurg 59:409–417, 1983

325. Rosenstock JG, Packer RJ, Bilaniuk LT et al: Chiasmatic optic glioma treated with chemotherapy: A preliminary report. J Neurosurg 63:862–866, 1985

326. Packer RJ, Sutton LN, Rosenstock JG et al: Pineal region tumors of childhood. Pediatrics 74:97–103, 1984

327. Herrick MK: Pathology of pineal tumors. In Neuwelt EA (ed): Diagnosis and Treatment of Pineal Region Tumors, pp 31–60. Baltimore, Williams & Wilkins, 1984

328. Abay EO III, Laws ER Jr, Grado GL et al: Pineal tumors in children and adolescents: Treatment by CSF shunting and radiotherapy. J Neurosurg 55:889–895, 1981

329. Jennings MA, Gelman R, Mochberg F: Intracranial germ-cell tumors: Natural history and pathogenesis. J Neurosurg 63:155–167, 1985

330. Wara WM, Jenkins RDT, Evans A et al: Tumors of the pineal and suprasellar region: Children's Cancer Study Group treatment results 1960–1975. Cancer 43:698–701, 1979

331. D'Andrea AD, Packer RJ, Rorke LB et al: Pineocytoma of childhood: A

reappraisal of natural history and response to therapy. Cancer 59:1353–1357, 1987

332. Zimmerman RA, Bilaniuk LT, Dolinskas C: Computed tomography of pineal, peripineal and histologically related tumors. Radiology 137:669–677, 1980

333. Rao YTR, Medini E, Haselow RE et al: Pineal and ectopic pineal tumors: The role of radiation therapy. Cancer 48:708–713, 1981

334. Chapman PH, Lingood RM: The management of pineal area tumors: A recent reappraisal. Cancer 46:1253–1257, 1980

335. Allen JC, Nisselbaum J, Epstein F et al: Alphafetoprotein and human chorionic gonadotropin determination in cerebrospinal fluid: An aid to the diagnosis and management of intracranial germ-cell tumors. J Neurosurg 51:368–374, 1979

336. Salazar OM, Castro-Vita H, Bakos RS: Radiation therapy for tumors of the pineal region. Int J Radiol Oncol Biol Phys 5:491–499, 1979

337. Onoyama K, Ono K, Nakajima T et al: Radiation therapy of pineal tumors. Radiology 130:757–760, 1979

338. Neuwelt EA, Frenkel EP: Germinomas and other pineal tumors: Chemotherapeutic responses. In Neuwelt EA (ed): Diagnosis and Treatment of Pineal Region Tumors, pp 332–343. Baltimore, Williams & Wilkins, 1984

339. Rustin GJ, Newland ES, Bagshawe KD et al: Successful management of metastatic and primary germ cell tumors of the brain. Cancer 57:2108–2113, 1986

340. Cohen ME, Duffner PK: Craniopharyngiomas. In Brain Tumors in Children, pp 193–210. New York, Raven Press, 1983

341. Bruce DA, Schut L, Rorke LB: Craniopharyngiomas in a capsule? In Concepts in Pediatric Neurosurgery, vol 1, pp 29–35. Basel, Karger, 1981

342. Hoffman HJ, Chuang S, Ehrlich R et al: The microsurgical removal of craniopharyngiomas in childhood. In Concepts in Pediatric Neurosurgery, vol 6, pp 52–62, Basel, Karger, 1985

343. Fischer EG, Welch K, Belli JA et al: Treatment of craniopharyngiomas in children: 1972–1981. J Neurosurg 62:496–501, 1985

344. Baskin DS, Wilson CB: Surgical management of craniopharyngiomas: A review of 74 cases. J Neurosurg 65:22–27, 1986

345. Thomsett MJ, Conte FA, Kaplan SL et al: Endocrine and neurologic outcome in children with craniopharyngioma: Review of effect of treatment in 42 patients. J Pediatr 97:728–738, 1980

346. Newman CB, Levin LS, New MI: Endocrine function in children with intrasellar and suprasellar neoplasms. Am J Dis Child 135:259–262, 1981

347. Sung DI, Chang CH, Harisiadis L et al: Treatment results of craniopharyngiomas. Cancer 47:847–852, 1981

348. Manaka S, Teramoto A, Takakura K: The efficacy of radiotherapy for craniopharyngiomas. J Neurosurg 62:648–656, 1985

349. Danoff BF, Cowchock FS, Kramer S: Childhood craniopharyngioma: Survival, local control, endocrine and neurologic function following radiotherapy. Int J Radiat Oncol Biol Phys 9:171–175, 1983

350. Hoffman HJ, Hendrick EB, Humphreys RP et al: Management of craniopharyngioma in children. J Neurosurg 47:218–227, 1977

351. Amacher AL: Craniopharyngioma: The controversy regarding radiotherapy. Child's Brain 6:57–64, 1980

352. Baskin DS, Wilson CB: Surgical management of craniopharyngioma. J Neurosurg 65:22–27, 1986

353. Symon L, Sprich W: Radical excision of craniopharyngioma. J Neurosurg 62:174–181, 1985

354. Carmel PW, Antunes JL, Chang CH: Craniopharyngiomas in children. Neurosurgery 11:382–389, 1982

355. Lyen KR, Grant DB: Endocrine function, morbidity and mortality after surgery for craniopharyngioma. Arch Dis Child 57:837–841, 1982

356. Shapiro K, Till K, Grant D: Craniopharyngiomas in childhood: A rational approach to treatment. J Neurosurg 50:617–673, 1979

357. Calvo FA, Hornedo J, Arellano A et al: Radiation therapy in craniopharyngiomas. Int J Radiat Oncol Biol Phys 9:493–496, 1983

358. Amendola BE, Gebarski SS, Bermudez AG: Analysis of treatment results in craniopharyngioma. J Clin Oncol 3:252–258, 1985

359. Chin HW, Maruyama Y, Young B: The role of radiation treatment in craniopharyngioma. Strahlentherapie 159:741–744, 1983

360. Kabayashi T, Kageyama N, Ohara K: Internal irradiation of cystic craniopharyngioma. J Neurosurg 55:896–903, 1981

361. Bremer AM, Nguyen TQ, Balsyo R: Therapeutic benefits of combination chemotherapy with vincristine, BCNU, and procarbazine on recurrent cystic craniopharyngioma. J Neuro-oncol 2:47–51, 1984

362. Carpenter DB, Michelsen WG, Hays AP: Carcinoma of the choroid plexus. J Neurosurg 56:722–727, 1982

363. Laurence KM: The biology of choroid plexus papilloma in infancy and childhood. Acta Neurochir 50:79–90, 1979

364. Velasco-Siles JM, Raimondi AJ: Choroid plexus papilloma. In Pediatric Neurosurgery: Surgery of the Developing Nervous System, pp 451–460. New York, Grune and Stratton, 1982

365. Milhorat TH, Hammock MK, Davis DA et al: Choroid plexus papilloma: Proof of cerebrospinal fluid overproduction. Childs Brain 2:273–289, 1976

366. Raimandi AJ, Gutierrez FA: Diagnosis and treatment of choroid plexus papillomas. Childs Brain 1:81–115, 1975

367. Dehner LP: Primitive neuroectodermal tumors of the central nervous system in childhood: Retrospective and overview. In Humphrey GB, Dehner LP, Grindey GB et al (eds): Pediatric Oncology 1, pp 277–288. The Hague, Martinus Nijhoff, 1981

368. Knapp J, Daisy F, Van Eys J et al: Primitive neuroectodermal tumors of brain in childhood: Literature review and the M.D. Anderson experience. Ibid., pp 215–224

369. Wara WM, Edwards MS, Surti NR et al: Primary cerebral neuroblastoma. Ibid., pp 225–228

370. Wald B, Siegel SE, Isaacs H et al: Cerebral primitive neuroectodermal tumor (primary cerebral neuroblastoma). Ibid., pp 229–234

371. Sexauer CP, Krous HF, Kaplan RJ et al: Supratentorial primitive neuroectodermal tumor: Clinical response to vincristine, cyclophosphamide, and BCNU. Ibid., pp 235–237

372. Baum ES, Morgan ER, Dal Canto MC et al: Review and experience with primitive neuroectodermal tumors of childhood. Ibid., pp 238–242

373. Jenkin D: Primitive neuroectodermal tumour. Ibid., pp 243–246

374. Priest J, Dehner LP, Sung JH et al: Primitive neuroectodermal tumors (embryonal gliomas) of childhood: A clinicopathologic study of 12 cases. Ibid., pp 247–264

375. Bruno LA, Rorke LB, Norris DG: Primitive neuroectodermal tumors of infancy and childhood. Ibid., pp 265–267

376. Cohen ME, Duffner PK: Primitive neuroepithelial tumors. In Cohen ME, Duffner PK (eds): Brain Tumors in Children, pp 274–279. New York, Raven Press, 1983

377. Parker JP, Mortara RH, McCloskey JJ: Biologic behavior of the primitive neuroectodermal tumors: Significant supratentorial childhood gliomas. Surg Neurol 4:383–388, 1975

378. Humphrey GB, Dehner LP, Kaplan RJ et al: Overview on the management of primitive neuroectodermal tumors. In Humphrey GB, Dehner LP, Grindey LP et al (eds): Pediatric Oncology 1, pp 289–294. The Hague, Martinus Nijhoff, 1981

379. Duffner PK, Cohen ME, Heffner RR: Primitive neuroectodermal tumors of childhood: An approach to therapy. J Neurosurg 55:376–381, 1981

380. Kosnik EJ, Boesel CP, Bay J et al: Primitive neuroectodermal tumors of the central nervous system in children. J Neurosurg 48:741–746, 1978

381. Hart MN, Earle KM: Primitive neuroectodermal tumors of the brain in children. Cancer 32:890–897, 1973

382. Markesbery WR, Challa VR: Electron microscopic findings in primitive neuroectodermal tumors of the cerebrum. Cancer 44:141–147, 1979

383. Danoff BF, Cowchock S, Marquette C et al: Assessment of the long-term effects of primary radiation therapy for brain tumors in children. Cancer 49:1580–1586, 1982

384. Raimondi AJ, Tomita T: Brain tumors during the first year of life. Childs Brain 10:193–207, 1983

385. Duffner PK, Cohen ME, Thomas PRM, Lansky SB: The long-term effects of cranial irradiation on the central nervous system. Cancer 56:1841–1847, 1985

386. Duffner PK, Cohen ME, Thomas PRM: Late effects of treatment on the intelligence of children with posterior fossa tumors. Cancer 51:233–237, 1983

387. Packer RJ, Bruce DA, Atkin TA et al: Factors impacting on neurocognitive outcome in long-term survivors of primitive neuroectodermal tumors/medulloblastoma (PNET-MB). Ann Neurol 20:396–397, 1986

388. Bleyer WA, Griffin TW: White matter necrosis, microangiopathy, and intellectual abilities in survivors of childhood leukemia, association with central nervous system irradiation and methotrexate therapy. In Gilbert HA, Kagan AR (eds): Radiation Damage to the Nervous System, pp 155–174. New York, Raven Press, 1980

389. Crosley CJ, Rorke LB, Evans AE, Nigro M: Central nervous system lesions in childhood leukemia. Neurology 28:678–685, 1978

390. Price RA, Birdwell DA: The central nervous system in childhood leukemia III: Mineralizing microangiopathy and dystrophic calcification. Cancer 42:717–728, 1978

391. Price RA, Jamieson PA: The central nervous system in childhood leukemia II: Subacute leukoencephalopathy. Cancer 35:306–318, 1975

392. Rottenberg DA, Chernik NL, Deck MDF et al: Cerebral necrosis following radiotherapy of extracranial neoplasms. Ann Neurol 1:339–357, 1977

393. Spunberg JJ, Chang CH, Goldman M et al: Quality of long-term survival following irradiation for intracranial tumors under the age of two. Int J Radiat Oncol Biol Phys 7:727–736, 1981

394. Kun LE, Malhern RK, Crisco JJ: Quality of life in children treated for brain tumors: Intellectual, emotional and academic function. J Neurosurg 58:1–6, 1983

395. Li FP, Winston KR, Gimbrene K: Followup of children with brain tumors. Cancer 54:135–138, 1984

396. Poplack DG, Brouwers P: Adverse sequelae of central nervous system therapy. Clin Oncol 4:263–285, 1985

397. Shalet SM, Beardwell CG, Pearson D, Morris–Jones PH: The effect of varying doses of cerebral irradiation on growth hormone production in childhood. Clin Endocrinol 5:287–290, 1976

398. Duffner PK, Cohen ME, Andersen SW et al: Long-term effects of treatment on endocrine function in children with brain tumors. Ann Neurol 14:528–532, 1983

399. Oberfield SE, Allen JC, Pollack J et al: Long-term endocrine sequelae after treatment of medulloblastoma: Prospective study of growth and thyroid function. J Pediatr 105:219–223, 1986

400. Van Eys J, Cangir A, Coady D, Smith B: MOPP regimen as primary chemotherapy for brain tumors in infants. J Neuro-oncol 3:237–244, 1984

401. Packer RJ, Siegel KR, Sutton LN et al: Efficacy of combination chemotherapy with cis-platinum (CPDD), lomustine (CCNU) and vincristine (VCR) in children with primitive neuroectodermal tumors—medulloblastoma (PNET-MB) of childhood. Ann Neurol 18:394, 1985

402. Duffner PK, Cohen ME, Horowitz M et al: Postoperative chemotherapy and delayed irradiation in children less than 36 months of age with malignant brain tumors. Ann Neurol 20:424, 1986

403. Shalet SM, Beardwell LA, Morris–Jones PH et al: Normal growth despite abnormalities of growth hormone secretion in children treated for acute leukemia. J Pediatr 94:719–722, 1979

404. Raimondi AJ, Tadanori T: The disadvantage of prophylactic whole CNS postoperative radiation therapy for medulloblastoma. In Paroletti P, Walker M, Butti G et al (eds): Multidisciplinary Aspects of Brain Tumor Therapy, pp 209–218. Amsterdam, Elsevier North-Holland Biomedical Press, 1979

twenty-five

Retinoblastoma

Sarah S. Donaldson and
Peter R. Egbert

Retinoblastoma is a malignant tumor of the embryonic neural retina. It is congenital, although usually not recognized at birth, and affects predominantly young children. It may have a variable growth rate, originating from single or multiple foci in one or both eyes, and may be manifest in one eye many months before the other. Retinoblastoma is the most common intraocular tumor of childhood and is extremely interesting in several respects. It may occur sporadically or may be inherited; patients with the hereditary type have a particular susceptibility to other malignant tumors. Retinoblastoma serves as the prototype and model for understanding of the heredity and genetics of childhood cancer.

EPIDEMIOLOGY

The Third National Cancer Survey indicates an average incidence in the United States of 11.0 new cases of retinoblastoma per million population less than 5 years of age, or 1 in 18,000 live births.[1] The estimated frequency of bilaterality ranges from 20% to 30%.[2] Thus, an estimated 200 children per year will develop retinoblastoma, of which at least 40 to 60 cases will be bilateral. There is no racial or gender predilection.

Retinoblastoma is often present at birth and is almost entirely restricted to early childhood. About 80% of cases are diagnosed before age 3 to 4 years, with a median age at diagnosis of 2 years.[3] The discovery of retinoblastoma beyond the age of 6 is decidedly rare. Bilateral cases are diagnosed earlier than unilateral cases. Sporadic bilateral retinoblastoma has been associated with advanced parental age.[4,5]

The occurrence of multiple congenital anomalies in association with retinoblastoma has been reported, but this is rare, being found in only approximately 0.05% of U.S. cases.[6] The reported anomalies are congenital cardiovascular defects, cleft palate, Bloch–Sulzberger syndrome, infantile cortical hyperostosis, dentinogenesis imperfecta, incontinentia pigmenti, and familial congenital cataracts.[3] An association with mental retardation has been suggested in children with the D-deletion syndrome. However, most patients with retinoblastoma have no intellectual impairment.

GENETICS

Etiology

The etiology of retinoblastoma is not known, but it is known to arise in hereditary, nonhereditary, and chromosomal deletion forms.[7] The retinoblastoma gene may be transmitted by a parent, giving rise to the hereditary (familial) form of the disease. Alternatively, the gene may be acquired by a new mutation and be expressed as a sporadic case of the tumor. Approximately 90% of newly diagnosed cases are sporadic; that is, there is no family history of retinoblastoma.[4]

There are important differences between the hereditary and nonhereditary types (Table 25-1). The nonhereditary type accounts for approximately 60% of all retinoblastomas.[8] The other 40% are inherited from an affected survivor parent or from a nonaffected nonmanifesting gene carrier parent or are the result of a new germinal mutation in a healthy parent. In most of the sporadic hereditary cases, the affected individuals are the product of new germinal mutations. Hereditary retinoblastoma is present in those clinical situations in which there is a positive family history of the tumor or, in the case of sporadic disease, where the individual is affected bilaterally. Patients with nonhereditary retinoblastoma have unilateral disease and no family history. However, approximately 10% to 12% of patients with sporadic unilateral disease actually have the hereditary form. In the chromosomal deletion form of the tumor, the peripheral lymphocytes have a deletion of chromosomal region 13q14.[7] The terms "hereditable," "familial," and "germinal" may be used interchangeably.

On the basis of experimental carcinogenesis data as well as the clinical characteristics of sporadic familial retinoblastoma, Knudson proposed a two-mutation hypothesis to explain retinoblastoma tumorigenesis.[8,9] He proposed that two independent events are necessary for a cell to acquire the potential to develop into retinoblastoma. In the dominantly inherited form, the first mutation, a germinal one, occurs prezygotically and is present in every retinal cell, whereas the second mutation occurs in a somatic retinal cell. In nonhereditary retinoblastoma, the two (or more) consecutive events are presumed to be somatic mutations in the same retinal cell. Therefore, although the second event is always a somatic mutation, the first event varies: it may be a new mutation in the ovum or sperm precursor cells (germinal mutation) of an unaffected parent, a germinal mutation from an affected parent, or a somatic mutation. Patients who have inherited a germinal mutation develop multiple tumors in one or both eyes and develop them earlier than do noncarriers. On the other hand, in the noncarrier, the two events must take place in a single retinal cell before malignant growth is initiated, accounting for the later age at diagnosis in these patients. Retinoblastoma gene carriers acquire chiefly bilateral tumors. Approximately 5% do not develop the tumor.[10] Some patients with the retinoblastoma gene develop multiple tumors in both eyes. The number of tumors acquired by a gene carrier follows a Poisson distribution.[8,9]

Cytogenetic Studies

Karyotyping does not routinely show abnormalities in patients with retinoblastoma. However, bilateral retinoblastoma is sometimes associated with a special syndrome in which there is a deletion or translocation on chromosome 13[11] (see also Chap. 2). This syndrome includes microcephaly, malformed ears, eye defects, high arched and cleft palate, multiple skeletal abnormalities including absent or hypoplastic thumbs, and psychomotor retardation.[11,12]

Genetic and physical mapping has located the retinoblastoma gene (Rb) on chromosome 13 in the region 13q14, which is common to all cases of the 13-deletion syndrome that include retinoblastoma (see also Chap. 3).[13–16] The Rb gene is closely linked to the genetic locus for esterase D, a gene-dose-dependent human polymorphic enzyme assigned to 13q14.[16,17]

There is substantial evidence that the two independent genetic events proposed by Knudson consist of loss or inactivation of wild-type Rb alleles. The data suggest that the Rb

Table 25-1
Features of Hereditary and Nonhereditary Types of Retinoblastoma

Hereditary	Nonhereditary
Diagnosed earlier	Diagnosed later
Bilateral or unilateral	Unilateral
Chromosomal abnormality from germinal mutation or inherited	Chromosomal abnormality from somatic mutation
Offspring affected	Offspring normal
Risk of other malignancies	No increased risk of other malignancies

gene is recessive and that the loss of one Rb allele is insufficient for tumor development, whereas the loss of both alleles is associated with tumor formation.[7] Thus, homozygosity for a mutated Rb locus is associated with tumorigenesis, and this can be produced in transformed cells by several mechanisms including nondisjunction (chromosome loss) with or without reduplication of the chromosome carrying the "first hit," a mitotic recombination event, or gene conversion, as well as by point mutation.[18]

Investigators using recombinant DNA technology have isolated a human complementary DNA segment that detects a chromosomal segment having properties of the retinoblastoma gene that maps to chromosome 13q14. The data strongly suggest that this segment is the carrier of the Rb DNA sequence.[19,20] This sequence is deleted in some patients with retinoblastoma and some with osteosarcoma, thus providing an explanation for the association of these malignancies (see Chap. 32).

The cytogenetic data now available support the two-mutation theory of Knudson. Retinoblastoma patients carry the first mutation, an abnormality of chromosome 13, which is closely linked to the esterase D locus. The second mutational event is the development of homozygosity for the abnormal segment of chromosome 13. The availability of two markers for the abnormal chromosomal segment, polymorphism for esterase D and DNA restriction length fragments, will aid in the identification of high-risk offspring of successfully treated patients.[3,21]

Genetic Counseling

Retinoblastoma may be a nonheritable type or a heritable type that shows an autosomal dominant inheritance pattern with high penetrance (80% to almost 100%).[22,23] If there is a positive family history, genetic counseling is straightforward, because one is clearly dealing with a heritable disease. The difficulty arises in the sporadic cases that constitute the majority of new patients, because these may be either nonheritable or heritable.

It is useful to separate the unilateral and bilateral sporadic cases. The bilateral sporadic cases are always heritable, and it follows that each child of those patients who survive will have a 50% risk of having retinoblastoma. The unilateral sporadic cases may be heritable or nonheritable, and empiric risk studies tell us that 10% to 12% of these patients have the heritable type and that the first child of a survivor has a 5% to 6% chance of having the disease (Fig. 25-1).[22]

A sporadic case is usually a spontaneous mutation, but there is a small chance that the parents are unaffected carriers or have an undiagnosed retinocytoma, so the parents should

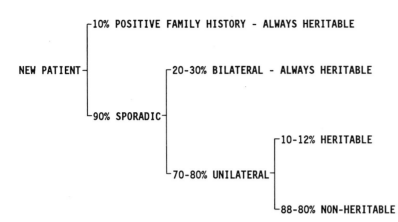

NEW PATIENT ┬ 10% POSITIVE FAMILY HISTORY - ALWAYS HERITABLE

└ 90% SPORADIC ┬ 20-30% BILATERAL - ALWAYS HERITABLE

└ 70-80% UNILATERAL ┬ 10-12% HERITABLE

└ 88-80% NON-HERITABLE

FIGURE 25-1. Flow diagram of statistical probabilities for a newly diagnosed patient with retinoblastoma.

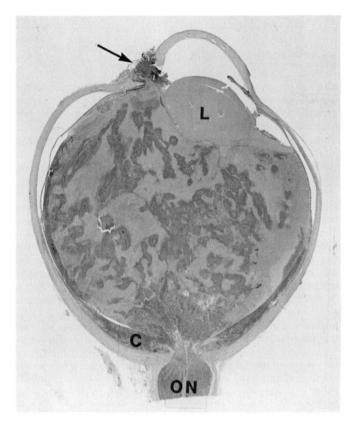

FIGURE 25-2. An eye filled with retinoblastoma. Numerous light staining lakes of necrosis are interspersed between the darker areas of viable tumor cells. The retina is totally destroyed and cannot be seen. The lens (*L*) is compressed. The choroid (*C*) and optic nerve (*ON*) are massively invaded by tumor. Extraocular extension is present through the limbus (*arrow*).

Until recently, it has been impossible to distinguish an asymptomatic carrier from a normal person unless an affected child was produced. However, recent use of recombinant DNA probes for sequences along chromosome 13q has recognized differences in the size of fragments ("restriction fragment-length polymorphism"), which have been used to identify disease among families predisposed to retinoblastoma.[24] Thus, prenatal and postnatal prediction of susceptibility using recombinant DNA markers may make genetic counseling more accurate and, one hopes, lead to earlier tumor detection.

PATHOGENESIS

Natural History

Retinoblastoma is characterized by rapid growth. The tumor enlarges over weeks to destroy increasing amounts of the retina where it arose, filling the eye either by direct enlargement or by growth of tumor seeds (Fig. 25-2). After the globe is largely filled, the tumor grows into the orbit.

Retinoblastoma has been said to have a spontaneous regression rate of 1%,[25] but this figure has confused two separate processes. First, there is true regression in large intraocular tumors, which become totally necrotic; subsequently, the tumor and the eye atrophy, resulting in a small, disorganized, blind eye. The second process is the occurrence in functional eyes of a benign variant of retinoblastoma that has been termed either retinocytoma[26,27] or retinoma.[25] These rare tumors are composed entirely of viable, benign-appearing tumor cells showing a high degree of photoreceptor differentiation. Ophthalmoscopically, these retinomas resemble retinoblastomas that have regressed after radiotherapy, which explains the confusion. Eyes containing retinomas often have normal vision, and the genetic implications are the same as for a retinoblastoma, which makes it important to search for them in the relatives of a new retinoblastoma patient.

Associated Malignancies

Patients with heritable retinoblastoma have a substantial risk of developing a second malignant tumor. The chromosomal abnormality that accounts for this risk has been discussed in the genetics section. Of 688 bilaterally and unilaterally irradiated children with hereditary retinoblastoma, 89 developed second tumors: 62 (70%) in the field of irradiation and 27 (30%) outside the irradiation field.[28,29] Of 23 additional patients who had never received radiotherapy, five developed second malignant tumors, one in what would have been an irradiated field and

always have an ophthalmoscopic examination. If normal parents have one affected child, the risk of their next child having retinoblastoma is about 1% if the first child has a unilateral tumor and 6% if that child has bilateral tumors.[22,23] Nussbaum and Puck have useful mathematical treatments of more complicated counseling situations.[23] For example, the risk of retinoblastoma in the first child of a survivor of sporadic retinoblastoma is 5% to 6%. But if that survivor has had one normal child, what is the occurrence risk in the next child? It can be calculated as about 3%, and if there are two normal children, the risk is 2%.

the others outside the head and neck area. The latent period was 10.4 years. These tumors were predominantly sarcomas, with osteosarcoma being the most frequently seen.[28,29]

The incidence of second malignant tumors increases with time. In the New York series, for irradiated patients, the incidence after 10 years was 20%; at 20 years, it was 50%, and at 30 years, it approached 90%.[28] For non-irradiated patients, the incidence of second malignant tumors was 10% at 10 years, 30% at 20 years, and 68% at 32 years.[28] Others have confirmed an increased risk of second malignant tumors but with lower incidence rates. From a series of 882 patients, Draper and associates reported a cumulative incidence of 2% in all patients by 12 years after diagnosis and 4.2% after 18 years. Among those with the genetic form of retinoblastoma, the cumulative incidence rate after 18 years was 8%, with 6% for osteosarcoma alone.[30] The use of chemotherapy, particularly cyclophosphamide, may also increase the risk of a second malignant tumor among those with retinoblastoma.[30] In addition, there is some suggestion that patients with genetic retinoblastoma are particularly sensitive to the carcinogenic effects of radiation, as fibroblasts from such patients have an increased radiation sensitivity and defective DNA repair.[31-33] However, the newer molecular genetic observations strongly suggest a genetic basis for the second malignant tumors, specifically osteosarcoma, in the long-term survivors of hereditary retinoblastoma (see Chap. 3).[34] To what degree treatment with ionizing radiation or chemotherapy increases this risk is not known.

A second form of malignancy associated with retinoblastoma is ectopic intracranial retinoblastoma, thought to arise in cells of photoreceptor origin in the pineal gland and suprasellar region.[35] These tumors, which are histologically consistent with retinoblastoma, often show a high degree of photoreceptor differentiation, which is not seen in metastatic retinoblastoma. Because the ectopic retinoblastoma almost invariably occurs in subjects with bilateral retinoblastoma, it has been termed "trilateral retinoblastoma."[36]

PATHOLOGY

Histologic Features

Retinoblastomas are malignant neuroblastic tumors that may arise in any of the nucleated retinal layers.[27] The predominant cells have hyperchromatic nuclei of various sizes and scanty cytoplasm; mitotic figures are numerous. The tumor has a ten-

dency to outgrow its blood supply, with resulting necrosis, so that one regularly sees a sleeve of viable cells around a blood vessel, whereas 90 to 100 μm away, the cells undergo ischemic coagulative necrosis (Fig. 25-2). Calcification appears in necrotic areas, especially in large tumors.

Retinoblastomas exhibit various degrees of differentiation. A feature that is highly characteristic, although not necessary for the diagnosis, is the formation of Flexner–Wintersteiner rosettes (Fig. 25-3). Electron-microscopy of these rosettes reveals that the cells have many features of normal retinal photoreceptors, including terminal bars of the luminal limiting membrane analogous to those that form the outer limiting membrane of the retina, cytoplasmic microtubules, cilia, and acid mucopolysaccharide in the lumina.[37] Additional signs of well-differentiated areas are groups of cells with more abundant eosinophilic cytoplasm and bouquet-like clusters of cells termed "fleurettes."[37]

Intraocular Spread and Its Consequences

The pattern of tumor growth and the resulting changes in the normal structures of the eye are important in understanding certain clinical variations of retinoblastoma. Endophytic retinoblastomas grow mainly from the inner surface of the retina toward the vitreous. Exophytic tumors grow from the outer layers of the retina toward the subretinal space, elevating the retina. Most tumors have a combination of these two growth patterns.

Retinal detachments are common with large tumors, particularly of the exophytic type, and first occur because of the tumor mass and then enlarge with accumulation of subretinal fluid. The detachment is often extensive, so that the retina is pushed anteriorly against the posterior surface of the lens and the retinoblastoma becomes visible through the retina (Fig. 25-4). A detachment will usually disappear after successful treatment of the tumor.

Retinoblastoma cells often break off from the main mass and grow independently in a new position as spheroidal aggregates, a process known as seeding. When seeding occurs in the vitreous, the cells may be confused clinically with an inflammatory disease. These cells frequently settle on the retina, causing new retinal masses, and they rarely accumulate in the anterior chamber or on the iris. When seeding occurs into the subretinal space, these cells can also attach to the retina and multiply into a mass. It is often difficult to determine whether multiple retinal masses represent multifocal tumor origin or seeding. Subretinal seeds may also invade the retinal pigment epithelium and from there can cross Bruch's membrane into the choroid. Tumor in the choroid is exposed to the rich vascularity of this tissue, and hematogenous spread may become more likely.

A visually disastrous consequence of certain retinoblastomas is glaucoma, which has one of two causes. First, either massive tumor growth or total retinal detachment may push the iris forward sufficiently to occlude the trabecular meshwork. Second, a neovascular membrane may grow on the iris and over the trabecular meshwork so that aqueous fluid egress is blocked, and the intraocular pressure rises (Fig. 25-5). Walton and Grant found iris neovascularization in 44% of eyes removed for retinoblastoma, the incidence being greater with larger tumors.[38] Folkman has demonstrated an angiogenic factor produced by retinoblastoma.[39] Iris neovascularization and neovascular glaucoma may be exacerbated by radiotherapy; therefore, patients presenting with these findings are not good candidates for radiotherapy.

FIGURE 25-3. Flexner–Wintersteiner rosettes in retinoblastoma.

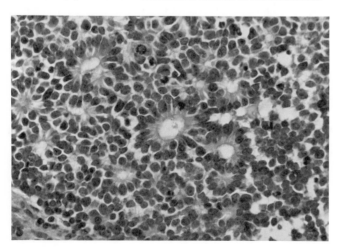

Patterns of Spread

Retinoblastoma spreads by direct extension into the orbit along scleral emissary vessels, by invasion of the optic nerve, by the hematogenous route, or by lymphatic extension.[27] All retinoblastomas have a tendency to invade the optic nerve. Once there, the tumor may spread directly along the axons toward the brain or may cross the pia into the subarachnoid space of the nerve sheath and be carried by the circulating cerebrospinal fluid to the brain. In addition, the tumor may exit the optic nerve to reach the orbit where the central retinal vessels perforate the sheath, about 15 mm behind the eye. Lymphatic spread occurs less often because the eye and orbit are generally considered not to have a lymphatic drainage; however, the conjunctiva and lid do have lymphatic drainage to the preauricular and submandibular nodes, and these nodes may be involved with large retinoblastomas that have anterior extraocular extension. Hematogenous dissemination leads to widespread metastases to bone, brain, and other organs. The pattern of metastases has been described in a review of metastatic retinoblastoma, whose authors found that one-third of their patients had metastases to the cranial vault whereas two-thirds had cranial-vault plus distant metastases.[40] The first symptoms of metastases included anorexia, weight loss, vomiting, and headache. Metastatic disease was recognized an average of 12 months after the diagnosis of the ocular primary. Laboratory tests that most often were positive included the bone-marrow aspirate, lumbar puncture, skull radiography, and computed tomography (CT) scan. However, it was unusual for the disease to be diagnosed by laboratory tests prior to the appearance signs or symptoms; at present, there is no good screening test for metastatic retinoblastoma. Death from metastatic disease occurred after an average of 5 to 6 months despite treatment.

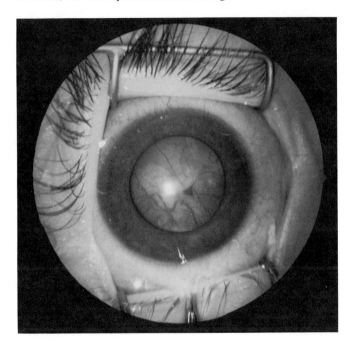

FIGURE 25-4. Exophytic group 5 retinoblastoma filling the vitreous cavity and pushing the retina forward. The retina is actually touching the posterior surface of the lens, and the retinal blood vessels as well as tumor vessels are visible. The dark triangle is blood on the surface of the tumor; the white spot is a reflection of light.

CLINICAL PRESENTATION

Most cases of retinoblastoma in the United States are diagnosed while the tumor remains intraocular. For example, among 60 consecutive new cases seen from 1974 to 1978 at the Wills Eye Hospital in Philadelphia, there were no examples of extraocular extension or metastases at the time of diagnosis, and four tumors were found by routine examination.[41] In contrast, in developing countries, late diagnosis is the rule, with the diagnosis being made only after an enlarged eye or gross orbital extension is apparent.

The signs and symptoms of an intraocular tumor depend on its size and position. The most common sign is leukocoria

FIGURE 25-5. Iris neovascularization (rubeosis iridis). **Left.** Clinical photograph in which the vessels of a fibrovascular membrane (*arrowheads*) are apparent on the surface of the iris. The membrane has also grown over the lens to form a pupillary membrane (*M*), leaving only a small open portion of the pupil (*P*). **Right.** Fibrovascular membrane (*arrows*) on the surface of the iris (*I*). This membrane has drawn the iris up to the cornea (*C*), resulting in occlusion of the trabecular meshwork (*TM*).

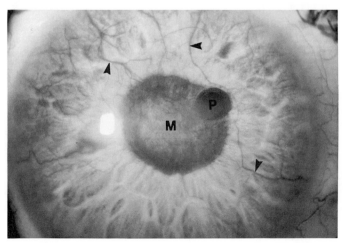

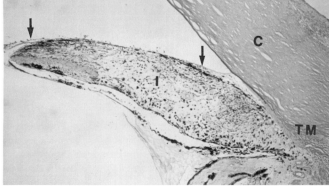

of one or both eyes, which has been termed the cat's eye reflex but which parents describe as an unusual appearance of the eye (Fig. 25-6). Leukocoria is manifest when the tumor is fairly large or has caused a total retinal detachment, leading to a retrolental mass that is visible through the pupil. The next most common presenting sign is strabismus, which occurs when a tumor arises in the macula causing loss of central vision and thereafter loss of the fusional reflex so that the eye may drift, resulting in esotropia or exotropia. Other occasional presenting signs are orbital inflammation, hyphema, fixed pupil, and heterochromia iridis.[41] Vision loss is not a symptom because young children do not complain of unilaterally decreased vision. Intraocular tumors are not painful unless there is secondary glaucoma or inflammation.

Newly diagnosed cases are bilateral 20% to 30% of the time.[2] Bilateral disease is multifocal, with several tumors in each eye. When the tumor is in an advanced stage, it is difficult to distinguish seeding from multifocal origin, so the exact number of independent tumors cannot be determined.

Diagnosis

Most commonly, parents of a child with retinoblastoma note an abnormality of the eye that prompts physician evaluation (also see Chap. 5). The diagnosis is established clinically via ophthalmoscopic examination. Whereas the gross appearance of a

FIGURE 25-6. Child exhibiting leukokoria in the left eye, the most common presenting sign of retinoblastoma.

mass, creamy pink to snow white in color, projecting into the vitreous (Fig. 25-7) is suggestive of retinoblastoma, associated findings of retinal detachment, vitreous hemorrhage, or opaque media may make inspection difficult. Pupillary dilatation and examination under anesthesia is essential to evaluate the retina fully. Characteristically, the diagnosis must be made by the ophthalmoscopic and radiographic appearance without pathologic confirmation.

Two-dimensional B-scan ultrasonography is of particular value in demonstrating the presence or absence of a mass in the posterior segment in cases where the fundus may be obscured by detachment or hemorrhage. Retinoblastoma exhibits high internal acoustic reflectivity due to calcium and the many interfaces between viable and necrotic areas.[42-45] In addition, ultrasound is a useful tool for the radiotherapy set-up procedure and as a guide to the response to treatment. CT (Fig. 25-8) is useful in demonstrating intraocular extent as well as possible extraocular extension.[46] More recently, magnetic resonance imaging (MRI) (Fig. 25-9) has been employed as an adjunct in determining the extent of orbital and central nervous system disease[47] and in the differential diagnosis of leukocoria.[47,48] MRI is complementary to CT in evaluating the intracanalicular and cisternal portions of the optic nerve, subarachnoid seeding, and brain involvement. No comparative studies of CT versus MRI for retinoblastoma are available (see Chap. 7). Plain films of the skull may show tumor calcification, which is pathognomonic of retinoblastoma, and a CT scan is even more sensitive.

In the course of an ophthalmological examination under anesthesia for suspected retinoblastoma, bone marrow aspiration and biopsy and lumbar puncture for cytologic examination of the cerebral spinal fluid should be performed. An elevated lactic acid dehydrogenase (LDH) concentration in the aqueous humor may be useful, as it often is elevated in patients with

FIGURE 25-7. Group 2 retinoblastoma arising from the macula. The normal optic nerve head is at the left. The tumor is hemispherical, translucent white, and incorporates the retinal blood vessels. A characteristic focus of calcium is present in the edge of the tumor nearest the nerve head.

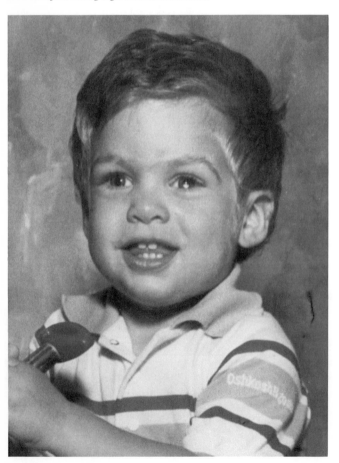

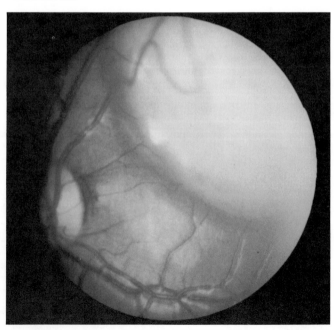

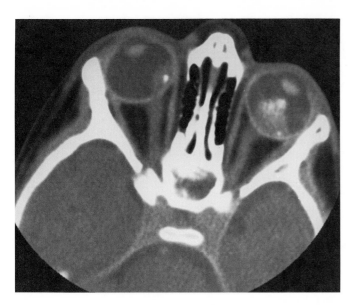

FIGURE 25-8. Computed tomographic (CT) scan through the mid-section of the globes reveals bilateral retinoblastoma, retinal detachment, and calcifications typical of retinoblastoma. No optic nerve, orbital involvement, or brain involvement is present.

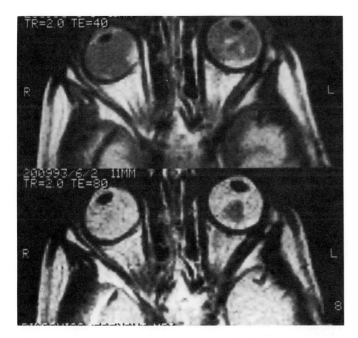

FIGURE 25-9. Magnetic resonance imaging (MRI) through the midsection of the globe in the same child as shown in Figure 25-8 reveals the same extent of bilateral retinoblastoma, retinal detachment, and calcifications as demonstrated by CT. No extension beyond the globe is present.

retinoblastoma,[49,40] but this test is not performed routinely because of the potential risk of extraocular seeding via the needle tract.

The differential diagnosis includes Coats' disease, retrolental fibroplasia, persistent hyperplastic primary vitreous, *Toxocara canis,* toxoplasmosis, and other types of severe uveitis.[51] The clinical diagnosis is usually straightforward and accurate. Nevertheless, in one review of eyes removed because of clinical suspicion of retinoblastoma, one-fourth had non-neoplastic lesions.[52] Institutions experienced in ocular oncology have greater accuracy rates, however, and ultrasonic examination, which is of considerable help, has become widely available only in the last few years.

A more serious, though fortunately less frequent, problem is delayed diagnosis caused by failure to suspect retinoblastoma when it is present. Stafford and associates found that 14% of patients with histologically proved retinoblastomas had their treatment delayed by an initially mistaken diagnosis of other conditions, particularly endophthalmitis or uveitis.[53]

Traditionally, patients with retinoblastoma have been referred to an oncologist after the diagnosis has been made by an ophthalmologist. Ideally, the radiation oncologist and pediatric oncologist participate in the initial examination and assist in the staging, work-up evaluation, and treatment planning. Efficient diagnosis and evaluation is important, since retinoblastoma has a rapid growth rate. Because the prognosis for visual acuity is related to tumor size at the initiation of treatment, an early diagnosis is extremely important.

STAGING

Because the management of retinoblastoma depends on the size of the tumor and the extent of disease, staging is important, and the classification of Reese and Ellsworth has become generally adopted as the standard for intraocular disease (Table 25-2).[2] This schema predicts the likelihood of tumor control and preservation of vision but does not predict survival.[54] It divides patients according to favorable, doubtful, or unfavorable likelihood of preservation of vision following radiotherapy on the basis of tumor size, number and location of lesions, and presence of vitreous seeding. Tumor size is conveniently expressed in comparison to the optic disk, which has a diameter of 1.5 mm. Each eye should be evaluated separately in selecting the treatment and deciding whether there is any potential for preserving or restoring useful vision.

There is no standard staging system for disease that has extended beyond the globe. One system proposed by investigators at St. Jude Children's Research Hospital distinguishes disease as follows: stage I = tumor confined to the retina; stage II = tumor confined to the globe; stage III = extraocular (regional) extension; stage IV = distant metastases.[55] However, for purposes of evaluating treatment programs, it suffices to subdivide stage with respect to intraocular tumor, optic nerve involvement, orbital extension, or distant metastases.

CONSIDERATIONS AFFECTING THERAPEUTIC DECISIONS AND PROGNOSIS

When disease is limited to the globe (Reese–Ellsworth groups I–V), where there is a high probability of cure, the therapeutic decision rests on the potential for vision. The choice of therapy depends on the size, location, and number of lesions; the treatment facilities and the experience gained at that medical center; and whether the entire retina must be considered as being at risk.

Most children with unilateral tumors have far-advanced disease when it is detected, often with little or no potential for vision in the affected eye. Thus, enucleation is the treatment of choice. When a diagnosis of a unilateral lesion is made at an

Table 25-2
Reese-Ellsworth Staging[2] Classification of Retinoblastoma

Group I. Very Favorable
  A. Solitary tumor, smaller than 4 disk diameters*, at or behind the equator
  B. Multiple tumors, none larger than 4 disk diameters, all at or behind the equator

Group II. Favorable
  A. Solitary tumor, 4 to 10 disk diameters in size, at or behind the equator
  B. Multiple tumors, 4 to 10 disk diameters in size, behind the equator

Group III. Doubtful
  A. Any lesion anterior to the equator
  B. Solitary tumors larger than 10 disk diameters behind the equator

Group IV. Unfavorable
  A. Multiple tumors, some larger than 10 disk diameters
  B. Any lesion extending anteriorly to the ora serrata

Group V. Very Unfavorable
  A. Tumors involving more than half the retina
  B. Vitreous seeding

* 1 disk diameter = 1.5 mm.

---

early stage, alternative treatment can be justified in an attempt to save vision. Such alternatives may include photocoagulation, cryotherapy, or radiation.

The management of bilateral disease depends largely on the extent and group of disease in each eye independently. Seldom is bilateral enucleation recommended as a treatment of choice; such a procedure is justified only when the disease is so extensive that no vision can be saved in either eye by any means. No longer is it appropriate to enucleate the more severely affected eye automatically in bilateral cases. If some vision is present in both eyes, then neither eye should be enucleated, and both should be irradiated. In cases of advanced bilateral disease, the potential for preservation of vision is difficult to ascertain. In such cases, an initial course of radiotherapy may result in tumor regression such that vision may be preserved. Rather than enucleate all eyes with unilateral disease or the worse eye in bilaterally affected cases, with modern radiotherapy, one may achieve a gratifying response, thus sparing vision and avoiding an unnecessary enucleation.[56,57] Nothing is lost by this approach as long as close follow-up with examinations under anesthesia is routine.

Optic nerve invasion by retinoblastoma carries a poor prognosis. When no optic nerve invasion is present, survival approaches 100% in many series,[58-61] and if there is optic nerve invasion to the lamina cribrosa, survival is still excellent (85%–95%).[3,58] However, when optic nerve invasion extends beyond the lamina cribrosa, survival drops to approximately 40%.[3,58]

Choroidal invasion can be diagnosed only after enucleation. It occurs most commonly with large tumors, and only massive invasion appears to affect prognosis.[62] When there is extension into the sclera, ciliary body, iris, or anterior chamber, survival drops to 20% to 40%.[58,59,61] The identification of such local extension predicts local recurrence as well.[58] Other poor prognostic signs are orbital invasion, central nervous extension, or hematogenous metastases at the time of presentation. Less than 10% of patients with orbital extension live longer than 2 years after diagnosis.[63]

Table 25-3
Indications for Surgical Procedures in Retinoblastoma

Enucleation	No potential for useful vision
	Neovascular glaucoma
	Failure to control tumor by conservative treatment
	Inability to examine retina following conservative therapy
Cryotherapy	Small (<4 disk diameters) primary tumors in anterior part of retina
	Small recurrences after radiotherapy
Photocoagulation	Small (<4 disk diameters) primary tumors in posterior part of retina
	Retinal neovascularization due to radiation retinopathy

TREATMENT

General Principles

The principal considerations in treatment planning include whether involvement is unilateral or bilateral, whether there is vision or any potential for vision, whether the tumor is confined to the globe or there is extension to the optic nerve, and whether there is orbital, central nervous system, or hematogenous extension. Treatment must be individualized; general recommendations for management are a function of each group or stage and must be considered guidelines only.

Surgery

Table 25-3 summarizes the indications for surgical treatment. Enucleation of the eye is indicated when there is no chance for useful vision even if the tumor is destroyed. For example, if the retinoblastoma has replaced most of the retina, then no useful vision is possible because the retina has no ability to repair itself. Glaucoma before treatment inevitably gets worse after conservative treatment and is also a reason for enucleation.[64] Other indications for enucleation are failure of conservative treatment and inability to examine an eye for resolution of the tumor after conservative treatment because of vitreous hemorrhage or cataract.

The operation itself is relatively simple and not painful. An important technical point is to remove a long section of the optic nerve with the globe in case retinoblastoma has begun to grow down the nerve. An artificial eye can be fitted about 6 weeks after surgery with a generally satisfactory appearance. Enucleation is simpler and has less morbidity than conservative treatment in many ways, inasmuch as the treatment is finished quickly and repeated examinations under anesthesia are not needed. A cosmetic disadvantage in children under 3 years of age is that the orbit ceases to grow normally after an eye is removed, and as the face of an infant grows, the orbit looks increasingly sunken. External-beam radiotherapy produces the same appearance due to inhibition of bone growth.

The indications for cryotherapy and photocoagulation are similar. Both techniques can successfully treat small (less than 4 disk diameters) primary tumors or new tumors appearing after radiotherapy. The advantage of these treatments compared to external-beam irradiation is the relative lack of ocular complications and the ability to repeat the treatment several times when necessary. The disadvantages are that large tumors or vitreous seeds cannot be treated adequately and that the therapy always leaves a nonseeing retinal scar that is larger than that resulting from radiation. This is particularly important for tumors involving the macula, where even a slightly larger scar may considerably worsen vision.

Cryotherapy is applied by a small probe placed directly on the conjunctiva or on the sclera through a small incision in the conjunctiva. The position of the probe under the tumor is observed by ophthalmoscopy, and a whitening of the tumor is seen as it freezes. Abramson and associates reported on 200 eyes treated with cryotherapy;[65] 95% of new tumors were cured, and 90% of tumors that showed a poor response to external irradiation were cured. The average size of the tumors in both cases was 1.5 (range 0.25–5) disk diameters.

Whereas cryotherapy is easier to apply to tumors in the anterior retina, photocoagulation is easier to apply to posteriorly situated tumors. Light from either an argon laser or a xenon arc photocoagulator is used to ring the tumor, occluding the feeding retinal blood vessels. An ischemic necrosis of the tumor ensues. The results with photocoagulation are similar to those obtained with cryotherapy for tumors less than 4 disk diameters in size.[66] Photocoagulation cannot be used for large tumors.

Photocoagulation may also be used to treat the neovascularization of radiation retinopathy that could lead to vitreous hemorrhage.

Radiotherapy

The introduction of megavoltage radiation has contributed greatly to the treatment of retinoblastoma. High-voltage, well-collimated x-rays, as produced by a linear accelerator, have distinct advantages over conventional kilovoltage (orthovoltage) x-rays, and there is no indication today for orthovoltage treatment to be given to a child with retinoblastoma (also see Chap. 11).

The purpose of radiotherapy for retinoblastoma is control of local disease while preserving vision. However, the advantages of this approach must be weighed against the potential short- and long-term complications. Since the majority of patients have multiple tumors in one or both eyes and these tumors may be multifocal in origin, radiation fields must include the entire geographic extent of the retina, the anterior border of which is the ora serrata. In an attempt to preserve vision, radiotherapy has become the treatment of choice in the treatment of the majority of children with retinoblastoma. Any eye that has a chance for useful vision should be considered for irradiation rather than enucleation.

Several techniques for external-beam radiotherapy have been employed. Some radiotherapists prefer an anterior field with a divergent lens block, together with a lateral field.[67] However, most radiotherapists utilize a D-shaped lateral field (for unilateral treatment) or opposed lateral fields (for bilateral treatment) (Fig. 25-10).[56,68–70] The large-institutional treatment series have almost universally utilized the lateral technique. The D-shaped field is contoured to include the entire retinal surface and vitreous plus 10 mm of anterior optic nerve while protecting the radiosensitive structures of the eye.

The radiation doses have differed but in general have been high. At the Ophthalmologic Center in New York and the M. D. Anderson Hospital, doses of 3500 cGy in 3 weeks for groups I to III tumors and 4500 cGy in 4 weeks for groups IV and V, given in three fractions per week, have been used.[71,72] At Utrecht, 4500 cGy in 5 weeks, three fractions per week at 300 cGy per fraction, are used independent of the stage of the

FIGURE 25-10. An anesthetized, immobilized infant in the treatment position with the lateral D-shaped treatment field as shown. The anterior border of the field lies at the fleshy canthus, which is located at the ora serrata in this child with bilateral group V retinoblastoma.

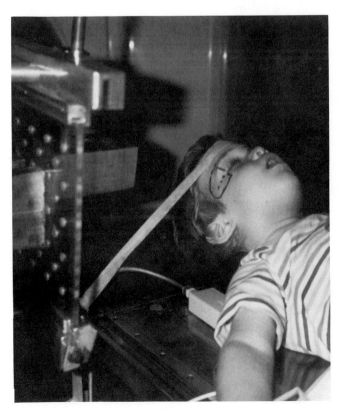

tumor.[69] At Stanford, higher doses have been used with smaller daily fractions in an attempt to maintain local control rates but minimize the complications of large-fraction radiotherapy; routinely, doses of 5000 to 5600 cGy in 5 to 5½ weeks using 200-cGy fractions have been administered using a 4 to 6 mV linear accelerator.[73] Each series has included supplemental photocoagulation or cryotherapy as needed.

Retinoblastomas are considered radiosensitive. However, because of the use of supplemental therapy and the variations in technique, fraction size, tumor group/stage, etc., dose–response data in the various series are difficult to obtain. Abramson has shown that 75% of intraocular tumors treated by radiation alone are cured and that when supplemental cryotherapy is added to radiotherapy, 90% are cured.[64]

Regression patterns following radiotherapy have been categorized into three types: (1) a "cottage-cheese" pattern due to calcium deposition; (2) partial shrinkage to a homogeneous, gray, nonvascular mass with an annulus of atrophic pigment around the base; and (3) a combination of types 1 and 2.[74] Interpretation of these regression patterns requires great experience. When the interpretation is unclear, there is the question of whether the tumor is sterilized. In such a situation, a patient should be monitored closely, even if the disease is stable; histologic examination of a persistent mass may show completely necrotic tumor without apparently viable tumor cells.

For optimal radiotherapy treatments, an infant must be anesthetized, immobilized in a reproducible fashion using a 3-point set-up, and treated by a consistent team of technical staff with fields checked by a physician daily (Fig. 25-10). The initial set-up should be done with the ophthalmologist and radiotherapist working together to establish the borders of the treatment field, as well as the posterior border of the lens, the ora serrata, and other key landmarks, to ensure adequate tumor coverage while avoiding the radiosensitive structures of the eye. Investigators at the Utrecht Retinoblastoma Center have developed a highly precise technique of positioning the field by magnetic fixation of the eye in the central position using a low-vacuum contact lens placed on the cornea.[68,70] The contact lens is attached to a soft iron pin, which is magnetically coupled to a millimeter scale on the collimator holder attached to the head of the linear accelerator. The anterior edge of the treatment field can easily be adjusted by measuring from the anterior extent of the cornea. Alternatively, the Comberg lens can be used for the set-up. This is a thin contact lens with a radiopaque marker that lies on the anterior surface of the cornea. In the infant, there is approximately a 1-mm separation between the posterior lens capsule and the temporal extent of the ora serrata. An examination under anesthesia in the treatment position when the pupils are dilated will help localize the anterior extent of the ora serrata in each individual case. In general, it is at or very near the fleshy canthus in a baby; 6 to 7 mm from the limbus when the pupils are in the central position. These measurements should be checked routinely during the radiotherapy procedures.

Figure 25-11 shows the isodose curves from a 4-mV linear accelerator using a 3.5 × 7-cm field blocked to 3.5 × 3.5 cm using a beam-splitting technique for opposing lateral fields and a single lateral field designed to cover the entire retina to the ora serrata. With this technique, theoretically, the dose at the ora serrata is approximately 50% of the given dose, while within 2 to 3 mm, the dose is 90% of the given dose. The lens and pituitary doses are less than 10% of the given dose. If one is concerned about the anterior extent of the tumor, the beam can be brought anteriorly 1 to 2 mm to increase the dose to the ora while simultaneously increasing the lens dose slightly.

Some authors have criticized the lateral fields on the basis of the potential for recurrence at the anterior margin of the beam. In practice, it is rare to see recurrence at the margin. However, for any suspicious area, cryotherapy may be used as a supplement to external-beam radiotherapy. Most radiotherapists believe it is optimal to use a lateral field in an attempt to prevent a radiation-induced cataract, which is universal if an anterior field is used without a lens block.

Because retinoblastoma is a rare neoplasm and optimal radiotherapy requires precise, tedious, and laborious treatment planning and execution, these children should be referred to a medical center with sufficient technical expertise and experience to ensure optimal therapy.

Radioactive plaques have been used in the treatment of solitary retinoblastoma and for localized recurrences following external-beam therapy. However, they have limited usefulness as primary initial therapy when one desires treatment of the entire retina; the isodose distribution is nonhomogenous, with an extremely high dose delivered to the immediate area where the applicator is sutured, the outer scleral surface of the globe, but with rapid dose fall-off within 1 mm. Such high doses may cause vascular injury and possible late hemorrhage, and therefore this modality is suitable only for accessible lesions, small lesions, and those tumors out of range of the optic disc.[75] Likewise, radioactive plaques should not be used in most patients with hereditary or bilateral disease who have multifocal multicentric disease.[76] Patients with residual optic nerve involvement or orbital tumor following surgery should be given orbital and optic nerve irradiation in doses of 5000 to 5600 cGy over 5 to 6 weeks. Cranial–spinal irradiation is indicated for patients with brain or meningeal extension, in an attempt to control central nervous system disease. However, few if any patients with regional spread or metastatic disease are likely to survive.

Chemotherapy

The role of chemotherapy for retinoblastoma remains undefined. In the past, chemotherapy was used in conjunction with radiotherapy to enhance the response of advanced intraocular disease. However, when triethylenemelamine (TEM), administered by intracarotid injection, was used in conjunction with radiotherapy, no clear advantage was seen over radiotherapy alone in local control rate or survival.[77] Adjuvant chemotherapy has also been tested in children with group V disease after enucleation, with no survival advantage shown over enucleation alone.[64] Because effective local control and survival is achieved in 90% of patients given local treatment (surgery or radiotherapy), chemotherapy is best restricted to patients with extraocular disease: regional or distant metastases.[67]

Even in extraocular retinoblastoma, however, the responses are unsatisfactory and of short duration. Single-agent chemotherapeutics that have been used include cyclophosphamide (with a response rate of 47%), Adriamycin (doxorubicin) (33%), and vincristine (16%).[3,78] Recently, ifosfamide produced a short-term partial response in a patient with extraocular retinoblastoma.[79] Combination chemotherapy using vincristine–cyclophosphamide–dactinomycin, cyclophosphamide–doxorubicin, and cisplatin-VM26 has achieved mixed or partial responses of only 1 to 5 months. Apparently complete responses have been observed in a few patients receiving vincristine–cyclophosphamide prior to high-dose radiotherapy.[79] Finally, cyclophosphamide and vincristine have been used prior to radiation in children with advanced intraocular tumors in an attempt to induce tumor regression, thus potentially permitting a smaller volume of radiation.[80] New agents are needed, and their value must be demonstrated in prospective

A   OPPOSED PAIR, NORMALIZED TO d1/2 OF OPEN AREA

CENTERED AT ORA SERRATA

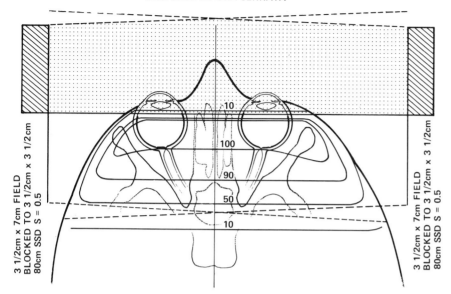

B   SINGLE FIELD NORMALIZED TO d3 OF OPEN AREA

CENTERED AT ORA SERRATA

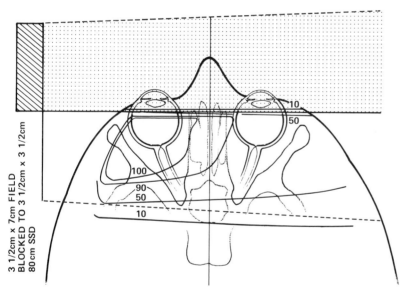

FIGURE 25-11. Isodose curves from a 4-MV linear accelerator for a 3½ × 7 cm field blocked to an effective field of 3½ × 3½ cm, with the anterior border of the treatment field located at the ora serrata. Using the beam splitting technique, the lens and pituitary receive less than 10% of the given dose. **A.** For bilateral treatment, using equally weighted opposed lateral fields, the dose is calculated at the midplane with the retina lying within the 90% isodose curve. **B.** For unilateral treatment the dose is calculated to a depth of 3 cm. The retina lies within the 90% isodose curve, whereas the opposite eye receives 50% to 70% of the given dose.

randomized trials before chemotherapy is used routinely in the treatment of retinoblastoma.

Nearly all patients present with disease confined to the globe, which can be controlled locally 90% of the time. Reserving chemotherapy for those patients with extraocular disease will subject only a small proportion of children with retinoblastoma to this treatment.

Results

Survival among patients with retinoblastoma is excellent; survival rates of better than 90% have been reported by several centers specializing in the treatment.[73,77,81] Among 1531 pa-

tients with retinoblastoma from the Ophthalmic Oncology Center in New York seen between 1914 and 1983, there has been modest improvement in survival from approximately 79% in the years 1914 to 1958 to approximately 87% in the period 1958 to 1983.[82] Among those with unilateral disease, no deaths from metastases have occurred later than 4 years after diagnosis, whereas among those with bilateral disease, deaths from metastases occur within 8 years of diagnosis.[82]

However, survival of the patient with bilateral retinoblastoma is dramatically worse than that of the patient with unilateral disease because of the high incidence of second malignant tumors among the former. Beginning 5 years after diagnosis, more patients die of second tumors than die of retinoblastoma.

Table 25-4
Results of Megavoltage Irradiation for Retinoblastoma

Group	Stanford 1956–1974[73] Eyes Saved/Total (%)*	Utrecht 1971–1981[69] Eyes Saved/Total (%)†	Total % Cured
I	7/8 (88)	14/14 (100)	95
II	3/5 (60)	9/9 (100)	86
III	7/8 (88)	10/12 (83)	85
IV	0/2 –	11/14 (79)	69
V	5/15 (33)	0/5 –	25
Total	22/38 (58)	44/54 (81)	80

* Median follow-up of 10 years.
† Median follow-up of 6 years.

These deaths continue for as long as follow-up is available. Patients with second malignant tumors should be treated aggressively using surgical resection with consideration of postoperative radiotherapy and possibly chemotherapy. Such aggressive treatment will salvage some of these unfortunate patients. In the Stanford series, of five children with bilateral retinoblastoma who have developed a second malignant tumor, all survive following aggressive salvage therapy, four without apparent evidence of disease with follow-up of 12 to 60 months (median 30 months). Thus long-term follow-up is essential, particularly in patients with hereditary disease, to assess the true impact on survival.

Because survival of retinoblastoma is excellent, successful treatment is now measured in terms of eradication of disease with preservation of useful vision. Comparison of results from two medical centers using definitive megavoltage radiation by a laterally placed field is shown in Table 25-4.[69,73] In both series, complementary photocoagulation or cryotherapy was used in addition to external-beam radiotherapy when necessary. The prognosis for vision depends largely on the size and location of the tumor. The ability to maintain vision is a function of the stage of disease. The percentage cure while maintaining vision is excellent among those with groups I to IV disease; however, even those with advanced disease have some potential for vision. The group V patients in the Stanford series presented with bilateral advanced disease such that it was not possible to predict which eye was the more advanced or which eye might have salvage of vision.[83] Tumor location is also important. Macular tumors involving the fovea always lead to poor central acuity, and in the Stanford series, this was the most common cause of a visual acuity less than 20/40. Table 25-5 shows the quality of vision among 22 of 38 patients subjected to irradiation who did not undergo a secondary enucleation. Five patients had a visual acuity better than 20/40, five had 20/50 to 20/100, nine had 20/200 to hand motion, and three had light perception only or no light perception with a follow-up of 4 to 19 years.[73]

Complications of Therapy

As the survival from retinoblastoma is excellent following conservative treatment, it is important to evaluate not only tumor control but also complications from treatment. The most frequent reason for secondary enucleation following radiotherapy is residual tumor, which is seen in approximately 16% of cases. In the Stanford radiotherapy series, the local control rate following radiotherapy; that is, the sterilization of the tumor, was 84%.[73] For those cases not controlled by radiotherapy, secondary therapy including enucleation is effective as salvage treatment and cure. Eyes removed for reasons other than persistent or recurrent tumor are usually in patients who had advanced disease at presentation. These cases include blind eyes enucleated because of pain, neovascular glaucoma, or difficulty in evaluating tumor status through opaque media or retinal detachment. Recurrent vitreous hemorrhage may occur from blood vessels in or at the edge of a previous tumor scar, but it often clears spontaneously. A diffuse radiation pigmentary epithelial change consisting of pigment mottling and occasional microaneurysms typically follows radiotherapy.

Table 25-5
Quality of Vision After Irradiation[73]

Group	Number of Eyes	Visual Acuity*
I	7	20/20, 20/20, 20/50, 20/100, 20/200, 20/400, HM
II	3	20/20, 20/100, 20/200
III	7	20/30, 20/100, 20/200, 20/200, 20/300, HM, NLP
IV	0	
V	5	20/30, 20/70, 20/200, LP, LP

* HM = hand motion; LP = light perception; NLP = no light perception.

The risk of cataract development is related to the radiotherapy technique. Recent studies with accurate reproducible radiation set-up techniques suggest that the threshold dose for a detectable opacity in the human lens is probably in the neighborhood of 1000 to 2000 cGy fractionated over 5 weeks, a higher dose than indicated in earlier reports.[70,84] The time to development of a radiation-induced cataract is variable and dose dependent. Some retinoblastoma survivors develop posterior lenticular densities detectable only by slit-lamp evaluation that do not interfere with vision. If a radiation-induced cataract does interfere with vision, it may be safely removed.

Retinal vascular injury is a more serious late radiation complication, the risk of which increases with the radiation dose. Doses of 4500 cGy carry a small risk of injury, but with 5000 to 6000 cGy, the risk of retinopathy and vitreous hemorrhage increases, and with doses greater than 6500 cGy in 6 weeks, the risk of retinal damage and optic atrophy leading to blindness is substantial.[85] Retinal artery occlusion may occur at lower doses.[85] When chemotherapy is added to radiotherapy, visual complications, including loss of vision, have been more frequent than when radiotherapy is given alone.[86]

Bone growth abnormalities may occur after surgery or radiotherapy. There is a significant decrease in the growth of the orbit following enucleation of the eye in children.[87] An orbital implant does not greatly affect subsequent orbital growth.

An increase in second malignant tumors, mainly osteosarcoma, is observed with heritable retinoblastoma and those with bilateral disease but not in the majority of survivors of unilateral retinoblastoma. Until recently, this increase was thought to be related to the fact that many of these children received orthovoltage radiation many years ago. The recent discovery of the coding sequence in the q14 region of chromosome 13 suggests that these findings have a genetic basis rather than one related to treatment.[19,20] As discussed earlier, there now is molecular genetic evidence that both retinoblastoma and osteosarcoma involve specific somatic loss of constitutional heterozygosity for the region of chromosome 13 that includes the Rb/1 locus.[34,88]

Treatment of Recurrent Disease

Recurrent or metastatic disease portends a very poor prognosis. Radiotherapy is useful for palliation of enlarging masses, central nervous system disease, or distant metastases. Long-term palliation can be achieved with 3500 to 4000 cGy. Systemic chemotherapy may provide palliation; however, most responses are partial and brief.

Follow-up

Patients with retinoblastoma should be monitored indefinitely for control of their primary tumor as well as second malignant tumors. The majority of recurrences occur within the first 3 years after diagnosis. Examinations under anesthesia should be performed every 4 to 6 weeks following radiotherapy, then every 2 to 3 months for the first year, every 3 to 4 months the second year, and every 6 months to age 6 years, assuming satisfactory regression of tumor. If there is any question of an inadequate regression or reactivation of tumor, patients must be examined more frequently. Until the patients are old enough to permit adequate fundus examination with scleral depression, examination must be done under general anesthesia with the pupils widely dilated. In addition to routine visual acuity and ophthalmologic testing, retinoblastoma patients require careful follow-up throughout their lifetimes because of their increased risk of second malignant tumors.

FUTURE CONSIDERATIONS

Current therapy for patients with retinoblastoma confined to the globe is excellent, with actuarial survival in excess of 85%. Results of treatment using survival as an end-point have not changed dramatically over the past 50 years. Great advances have been made, however, in treatment techniques, particularly with the use of the linear accelerator, allowing curative doses of radiation to the tumor without sacrificing normal surrounding tissues including the radiosensitive lens. Further efforts must be made to refer children to radiotherapy centers with the expertise to carry out this highly specialized form of treatment so that vision can be preserved while the tumor is controlled. However, deaths from second malignant tumors among patients with hereditary disease are increasing: analysis indicates that 50% of these patients will be dead 25 years after the initial diagnosis.[82]

Significant advances have been made in molecular genetic research over the past 5 years, which now make retinoblastoma the prototype tumor in our understanding of the genetic implications of childhood neoplasia. Further treatment-related research may be directed toward continuous refinement of radiotherapy techniques and perhaps exploration of new modalities such as hyperthermia or heavy-particle radiation. Recognition of the gene for retinoblastoma may make antenatal diagnosis of gene inheritance possible. Furthermore, these genetic advances may help determine if a particular retinoblastoma stems from an inherited lesion or a new mutation of somatic or germinal origin. Investigation in these areas will certainly improve our understanding of the factors responsible for tumorigenesis in retinoblastoma as well as in other childhood malignancies.

REFERENCES

1. Devesa SS: The incidence of retinoblastoma. Am J Ophthalmol 80:263–265, 1975
2. Ellsworth RM: The practical management of retinoblastoma. Trans Am Ophthalmol Soc 67:462–534, 1969
3. Greene DM: Retinoblastoma. In Diagnosis and Management of Malignant Solid Tumors in Infants and Children, pp 90–128. Boston, Martinus Nijhoff, 1985
4. Francois J, Matton MTh, deBie S et al: Genesis and gentics of retinoblastoma. Ophthalmologica 170:405–425, 1975
5. Pellie C, Briard ML, Feingold J et al: Parental age in retinoblastoma. Humangenetik 20:63–69, 1973
6. Jensen RD, Miller RW: Retinoblastoma: Epidemiologic characteristics. N Engl J Med 285:307–311, 1971
7. Murphree A, Benedict WF: Retinoblastoma: Clues to human oncogenesis. Science 223:1028–1033, 1984
8. Knudson AG: Mutation and cancer: Statistical study of retinoblastoma. Proc Natl Acad Sci USA 68:620–623, 1971
9. Knudson AG, Hethcote HW, Brown BW: Mutation and childhood cancer: A probabilistic model for the incidence of retinoblastoma. Proc Natl Acad Sci USA 72:5116–5120, 1975
10. Knudson AG: Retinoblastoma: A prototypic hereditary neoplasm. Semin Oncol 5:57–60, 1978
11. Cross HE, Hansen RC, Morrow G et al: Retinoblastoma in a patient with a 13q X p translocation. Am J Ophthalmol 84:548–554, 1977
12. Allerdice PW, Davis JG, Miller OJ et al: The 13q⁻ deletion syndrome. Am J Hum Genet 21:499–512, 1969
13. Knudson AG, Meadows AT, Nichols WW et al: Chromosomal deletion and retinoblastoma. N Engl J Med 295:1120–1123, 1976
14. Francke V, Kung F: Sporadic bilateral retinoblastoma in 13q⁻ chromosomal deletion. Med Pediatr Oncol 2:379–385, 1976
15. Cavenee W, Hansen M, Nordenskjold M: Genetic origin of mutations predisposing to retinoblastoma. Science 228:501–503, 1985
16. Sparkes RS, Murphree AL, Lingua RW et al: Gene for hereditary retinoblastoma assigned to human chromosome 13 by linkage to esterase D. Science 219:971–973, 1983
17. Squire J, Dryja TP, Dunn J et al: Cloning of the esterase D gene: A polymorphic gene probe closely linked to the retinoblastoma locus on chromosome 13. Proc Natl Acad Sci USA 83:6573–6577, 1986
18. Potluri VR, Helson L, Ellsworth RM et al: Chromosomal abnormalities in human retinoblastoma: A review. Cancer 58:663–671, 1986
19. Friend SH, Bernards R, Rogelj S et al: A human DNA segment with properties of the gene that predisposes to retinoblastoma and osteosarcoma. Nature 232:643–646, 1986
20. Harris H: Malignant tumours generated by recessive mutations. Nature 323:582–583, 1986
21. Junien C, Despoisse S, Turleau C et al: Retinoblastoma, deletion 13q14, and esterase D: Application of gene dosage effect to prenatal diagnosis. Cancer Genet Cytogenet 6:281–287, 1982
22. Vogel F: Genetics of retinoblastoma. Hum Genet 52:1–54, 1979
23. Nussbaum R, Puck J: Recurrence risks for retinoblastoma: A model for autosomal dominant disorders with complex inheritance. J Pediatr Ophthalmol 13:89–98, 1976
24. Wiggs J, Nordenskjold M, Yandell D et al: Prediction of the risk of hereditary retinoblastoma using DNA polymorphisms within the retinoblastoma gene. N Engl J Med 318:151–157, 1988
25. Gallie BL, Ellsworth RM, Abramson KH et al: Retinoma: Spontaneous regression of retinoblastoma or benign manifestation of the mutation? Br J Cancer 45:513–521, 1982

26. Margo CE, Hidayat A, Kopelman J et al: Retinocytoma: A benign variant of retinoblastoma. Arch Ophthalmol 101:1519–1531, 1983

27. Zimmerman LE: Retinoblastoma and retinocytoma. In Spencer WH (ed): Ophthalmic Pathology: An Atlas and Textbook, 3rd Ed., vol 2, pp 1292–1351. Philadelphia, WB Saunders, 1985

28. Abramson DH, Ellsworth RM, Kitchin FD et al: Second nonocular tumors in retinoblastoma survivors: Are they radiation induced? Ophthalmology 91:1351–1355, 1984

29. Kitchin FD, Ellsworth RM: Pleiotropic effects of the gene for retinoblastoma. J Med Genet 11:244–246, 1974

30. Draper GJ, Sanders BM, Kingston JE: Second primary neoplasms in patients with retinoblastoma. Br J Cancer 53:661–671, 1986

31. Weichselbaum RR, Nove J, Little JB: X-ray sensitivity of diploid fibroblasts from patients with hereditary or sporadic retinoblastoma. Proc Natl Acad Sci USA 75:3962–3964, 1978

32. Weichselbaum RR, Nichols WW, Albert DM et al: In vitro radiosensitivity of fibroblasts from patients with retinoblastoma and abnormalities of chromosome 13. Retina 3:126–130, 1983

33. Albert DM, Walton DS, Weichselbaum RR et al: Fibroblast radiosensitivity and intraocular fibrovascular proliferation following radiotherapy for bilateral retinoblastoma. Br J Ophthalmol 70:336–342, 1986

34. Dryja TP, Rapaport JM, Epstein J et al: Chromosome 13 homozygosity in osteosarcoma without retinoblastoma. Am J Hum Genet 38:59–66, 1986

35. Kingston JE, Plowman PN, Hungerford JL: Ectopic intracranial retinoblastoma in childhood. Br J Ophthalmol 69:742–748, 1985

36. Bader JL, Meadows AT, Zimmerman LE et al: Bilateral retinoblastoma with ectopic intracranial retinoblastoma: Trilateral retinoblastoma. Cancer Genet Cytogenet 5:203–213, 1982

37. Tso MOM, Zimmerman LE, Fine BS: The nature of retinoblastoma II: Photoreceptor differentiation: An electron microscopic study. Am J Ophthalmol 69:350–359, 1970

38. Walton D, Grant W: Retinoblastoma and iris neovascularization. Am J Ophthalmol 65:598–599, 1968

39. Folkman J: Tumor angiogenesis factor. Cancer Res 34:2109–2113, 1974

40. MacKay CJ, Abramson DH, Ellsworth RM: Metastatic patterns of retinoblastoma. Arch Ophthalmol 102:391–396, 1984

41. Shields JA: Diagnosis and Management of Intraocular Tumors, pp 437–533. St Louis, CV Mosby, 1983

42. Sterns JK, Coleman DJ, Ellsworth RM: The ultrasonographic characteristics of retinoblastoma. Am J Ophthalmol 78:606–611, 1974

43. Shields JA, Leonard BC, Michelson JB et al: B-scan ultrasonography in the diagnosis of atypical retinoblastomas. Can J Ophthalmol 11:42–51, 1976

44. Poujol J, Varene B: Contribution of echography to the diagnosis of retinoblastoma: A homogeneous B-scan study. Ultrasound Med Biol 11:171–175, 1985

45. Hermsen VM: Echographic diagnosis. In Blodi FC (ed): Contempory Issues in Ophthalmology, vol 2: Retinoblastoma, pp 111–127. New York, Churchill Livingstone, 1985

46. Arrigg PG, Hedges TR, Char DH: Computed tomography in the diagnosis of retinoblastoma. Br J Ophthalmol 67:588–591, 1983

47. Schulman JA, Peyman JA, Mafee MF: The use of magnetic resonance imaging in the evaluation of retinoblastoma. J Pediatr Ophthalmol Strabismus 23:144–147, 1986

48. Haik BG, Saint Louis L, Smith ME et al: Magnetic resonance imaging in the evaluation of leukocoria. Ophthalmology 92:1143–1152, 1985

49. Piro PA, Abramson DH, Ellsworth RM et al: Aqueous humor lactate dehydrogenase in retinoblastoma patients. Arch Ophthalmol 96:1823–1825, 1978

50. Dias PLR: Correlation of aqueous humour lactic acid dehydrogenase activity with intraocular pathology. Br J Ophthalmol 63:574–577, 1979

51. Searl SS, Moazed K, Albert DM et al: Ocular toxocariasis presenting as leukocoria in a patient with low ELISA titre to Toxocara canis. Ophthalmology 88:1302–1306, 1981

52. Margo CE, Zimmerman LE: Retinoblastoma: The accuracy of clinical diagnosis in children treated by enucleation. J Pediatr Ophthalmol Strabismus 20:227–229, 1983

53. Stafford WR, Yanoff M, Parnell B: Retinoblastoma initially misdiagnosed as primary ocular inflammations. Arch Ophthalmol 82:771–773, 1969

54. Ellsworth RM: The management of retinoblastoma. Jpn J Ophthalmol 22:389–395, 1978

55. Pratt CB: Management of malignant solid tumors in children. Pediatr Clin North Am 19:1141–1155, 1972

56. Bagshaw MA, Kaplan HS: Supervoltage linear accelerator radiation therapy VIII: Retinoblastoma. Radiology 86:242–246, 1966

57. Henderson JW: Orbital Tumors, pp 495–526. Philadelphia, WB Saunders, 1973.

58. Stannard C, Lipper S, Sealy R et al: Retinoblastoma: Correlation of invasion of the optic nerve and choroid with prognosis and metastasis. Br J Ophthalmol 63:560–570, 1979

59. Zimmerman LE: The registry of ophthalmic pathology: Past, present and future. Trans Am Acad Ophthalmol Otolaryngol 65:51–113, 1961

60. Carbajal UM: Observations in retinoblastoma. Am J Ophthalmol 45:391–402, 1958

61. Brown DH: The clinicopathology of retinoblastoma. Am J Ophthalmol 61:508–514, 1966

62. Sang D, Albert DM: Retinoblastoma: Clinical and histopathologic features. Hum Pathol 13:133–147, 1982

63. Rootman J, Ellsworth RM, Hofbauer J et al: Orbital extension of retinoblastoma: A clinicopathological study. Can J Ophthalmol 13:72–80, 1978

64. Abramson DH: Treatment of retinoblastoma. In Blodi FC (ed): Contemporary Issues in Ophthalmology, vol 2: Retinoblastoma, pp 63–93, New York, Churchill Livingstone, 1985

65. Abramson DH, Ellsworth RM, Rozakis GW: Cryotherapy for retinoblastoma. Arch Ophthalmol 100:1253–1256, 1982

66. Hopping W, Bunke-Schmidt A: Light coagulation and cryotherapy. In Blodi FC (ed): Contempory Issues in Ophthalmology, vol 2: Retinoblastoma, pp 95–110. New York, Churchill Livingstone, 1985

67. Pizzo PA, Miser JS, Cassady JR et al: Solid tumors of childhood. In Devita VT, Hellman S, Rosenberg SA (eds): Cancer: Principles and Practice of Oncology, 2nd Ed. pp 1536–1540. Philadelphia, JB Lippincott, 1985

68. Schipper J: An accurate and simple method for megavoltage radiation therapy of retinoblastoma. Radiother Oncol 1:31–41, 1983

69. Schipper J, Tan K, van Peperzeel H: Treatment of retinoblastoma by precision megavoltage radiation therapy. Radiother Oncol 3:117–132, 1985

70. Schipper J: Retinoblastoma: A Medical and Experimental Study. Thesis, University of Utrecht, The Netherlands, 1980

71. Tapley N, Strong L, Sutow WW: Retinoblastoma. In Sutow WW, Fernbach DJ, Vietti TJ (eds): Clinical Pediatric Oncology, 3rd Ed. pp 539–558, St Louis, CV Mosby, 1984

72. Tretter P: Radiotherapy of ocular and orbital tumors. In Reese AB (ed): Tumors of the Eye, pp 373–377. New York, Harper & Row, 1976

73. Egbert PR, Donaldson SS, Moazed K et al: Visual results and ocular complications following radiotherapy for retinoblastoma. Arch Ophthalmol 97:1826–1830, 1978

74. Ellsworth RM: Retinoblastoma. Mod Probl Ophthalmol 18:94–100, 1977

75. Rosengren B, Tengroth B: Retinoblastoma treated with a ^{60}Co applicator. Acta Radiol Ther Phys Biol 16:110–116, 1977

76. Kock E, Rosengren B, Tengroth B et al: Retinoblastoma treated with a ^{60}Co applicator. Radiother Oncol 7:19–26, 1986

77. Cassady JR, Sagerman RH, Tretter P et al: Radiation therapy in retinoblastoma. Radiology 93:405–409, 1969

78. Lonsdale P, Berry DH, Holcomb TM et al: Chemotherapeutic trials in patients with metastatic retinoblastoma. Cancer Chemother Rep 52:631–634, 1968

79. Pratt CB, Crom DB, Howarth C: The use of chemotherapy for extraocular retinoblastoma. Med Pediatr Oncol 13:330–333, 1985

80. Lemerle J, Bloch-Michel E: Chemotherapy in retinoblastoma: Preliminary report and warning. In Lommatzsch PK, Blodi FC (eds): Intraocular Tumors, pp 541–542. New York, Springer-Verlag, 1983

81. Bedford MA, Bedotto C, Macfaul PA: Retinoblastoma: A study of 139 cases. Br J Ophthalmol 55:19–27, 1971

82. Abramson DH, Ellsworth RM, Grumbach N et al: Retinoblastoma: Survival, age at detection and comparison 1914–1958, 1958–1983. J Pediatr Ophthalmol Strabismus 22:246–250, 1985

83. Donaldson SS: Retinoblastoma. In Levine A (ed): Cancer in the Young, pp 683–694. New York, Masson, 1982

84. Merriam GR, Focht EF: A clinical study of radiation cataracts and the relationship to dose. Am J Roentgenol 77:759–785, 1957

85. Shukovsky LJ, Fletcher GH: Retinal and optic nerve complications in a high dose irradiation technique of ethmoid sinus and nasal cavity. Radiology 104:629–634, 1972

86. Chan RC, Shukovsky LJ: Effects of irradiation on the eye. Radiology 120:673–675, 1976

87. Osborne D, Hadden OB, Deeming LW: Orbital growth after childhood enucleation. Am J Ophthalmol 77:756–759, 1974

88. Hansen MF, Koufos A, Gallie BL et al: Osteosarcoma and retinoblastoma: A shared chromosomal mechanism revealing recessive predisposition. Proc Natl Acad Sci USA 82:6216–6220, 1985

twenty-six

Hepatic Tumors

Mark Greenberg and Robert M. Filler

Tumors of the liver, although relatively infrequent in childhood, pose a considerable therapeutic and diagnostic challenge. Primary neoplasms of the liver comprise between 0.5% and 2.0% of pediatric tumors[1] and are the tenth most frequent tumor in children. The annual incidence of malignant hepatic tumors in the United States is 1.6 per million children, with hepatoblastoma accounting for 0.9 and hepatocellular carcinoma for 0.7.[2,3] Like Wilms' tumor, hepatic tumors most often present as an asymptomatic abdominal mass that is found on a routine physical examination or discovered incidentally by parents. In a child with a suspected liver tumor, one must distinguish hepatic malignancy from a benign hepatic tumor, nonneoplastic hepatomegaly, and other abdominal masses (particularly Wilms' tumor and neuroblastoma).[4]

A compilation of published series of hepatic tumors in children indicates that 57% are malignant (Table 26-1).[4-7] Approximately 60% of the benign liver tumors are hemangiomas or hamartomas. Most of these lesions present during the first 6 months of life. Benign vascular tumors can reach considerable size in infancy and may have an alarming clinical presentation, including high-output congestive heart failure (due to arteriovenous shunting), hemorrhage and bleeding with evidence of platelet consumption (the Kasabach–Merritt syndrome), and shock due to rupture of a vascular tumor mass. Cavernous hemangioma and hemangioendothelioma are the two most important benign lesions that must be distinguished from malignant hepatic tumors.

EPIDEMIOLOGY

No clear-cut geographic clustering is demonstrable for either hepatoblastoma or hepatocellular carcinoma. Both tumor types demonstrate a male predominance in North America, with male:female ratios of 1.7:1 and 1.4:1 for hepatoblastoma and hepatocellular carcinoma, respectively (Table 26-2).[3]

The median age at diagnosis of hepatoblastoma is 1 year,[9,10] and the bulk of patients are diagnosed within the first 18 months of life. In one series of 129 patients, there were 3 newborns and 11 children under 6 weeks of age.[4] The tumor occasionally presents in adolescence.

Hepatocellular carcinoma in the pediatric population has a median age of onset of 12 years.[5,11] The age range is wide, however, and may be influenced by associated underlying disease. The mean age of onset in the fibrolamellar subgroup is 20 years, with few cases seen before age 10.[12]

GENETICS AND BIOLOGY

Hepatoblastoma occurs in association with Beckwith–Wiedemann syndrome[13] and with its incomplete variants (see Chap. 2). Hemihypertrophy is seen in about 2% of children with hepatoblastoma. Whether this is an incomplete variant of

Table 26-1

*Frequency of Benign and Malignant Hepatic Tumors in Children:
Selected North American Series*

Tumor Type	Number	Percentage of Total
Malignant		
Hepatoblastoma	227	34.6
Hepatocellular carcinoma	148	22.5
Sarcoma*	45	6.8
Benign		
Adenoma	13	2
Focal nodular hyperplasia	12	2
Vascular tumors	118	18
Mesenchymal hamartoma	53	8
Other	40	6

(Data derived from References 3–6)
* Sarcomas often arose from extrahepatic biliary tree.

Table 26-2

*Incidence of Malignant Hepatic Tumors in Children Younger than 15 Years**

Race/Sex	Hepatoblastoma	Hepatocellular Carcinoma
White	0.97	0.7
Black	0.4	0.0

* Rate per 1 million children per year.

Beckwith–Wiedemann syndrome or a separate entity is unclear.[2,14] The synchronous occurrence of Wilms' tumor and hepatoblastoma,[2] both embryonal tumors, is compatible with gestational oncogenic events. It has been proposed that in embryonal tumors, a developmental disturbance occurs during organogenesis that permits inappropriate continuation of proliferation, resulting in a mass of immature tissue recognized as an embryonal tumor. In the case of Wilms' tumor, the homozygous expression of a recessive mutant allele at a locus on chromosome 11 band p13 can be found in tumor cell-derived DNA but not in DNA derived from surrounding normal kidney (see Chap. 27).[15] This locus has been designated the WAGR locus (for Wilms' tumor, aniridia, genital malformations, and mental retardation) because alleles coding for other developmental anomalies associated with Wilms' tumor also map to this locus. Similarly, in retinoblastoma, homozygosity for a mutant allele on chromosome 13 band q14 has been shown in tumor cells but not normal cells.[16,17] Homozygosity for a mutant recessive allele at the 11p locus corresponding to the WAGR locus has recently been shown in both biopsy tissue and explants in nude mice from two hepatoblastomas.[18] Both patients were constitutionally heterozygous for this locus. DNA hybridization and probing show the presence of normal copy numbers of chromosome 11, suggesting that the mitotic event responsible for the loss of heterozygosity of the mutant allele is a nondisjunctional loss of the wild-type chromosome with reduplication of the mutant chromosome.

Similar evidence for the loss of heterozygosity has been shown in rhabdomyosarcoma but not in Ewing's sarcoma or osteogenic sarcoma.[18] Thus, Wilms' tumor, rhabdomyosar-

coma, and hepatoblastoma appear to share a common chromosomal pathogenetic abnormality (see Chap. 3). The absence of a gene product necessary for the orderly maturation of these three specific tissues may result in the development of embryonal tumors.

Hepatoblastoma has been reported in association with maternal ingestion of both contraceptives[19,20] and gonadotropins[21] and in the fetal alcohol syndrome.[22]

Two families have been described in which two siblings had hepatoblastoma.[23,24] One of these sibling pairs had associated anomalies of the central nervous system.[24]

Hepatocellular carcinoma (HCC) in children younger than 15 shares the strong association with hepatitis B virus (HBV) seen in the adult population. Hepatitis B surface antigen (HBsAg) has been found in pediatric HCC, both in the presence of coexisting cirrhosis and in its absence.[25–27] Initial evidence for this association derived from the clustering in similar geographic sites of HCC and high HBV carrier rates.[28] Case-control studies demonstrate a much higher rate of serologically diagnosed active HBV infection in patients with HCC than in controls.[29] In a prospective study of a large cohort of Taiwanese men, the relative risk of developing hepatocellular carcinoma was increased 223-fold for HbsAg carriers compared to seronegative controls.[30] Studies using molecular hybridization with a ^{32}P HBV-DNA probe and restriction fragment length polymorphism analysis have shown that viral DNA is integrated into the DNA of cell lines derived from human HCC and from biopsy and autopsy tumor specimens.[31,32] However, the viral genome was also integrated into morphologically nonmalignant adjacent liver cells. Thus, the exact role of HBV in the oncogenic process remains undefined.

Clear cases have been documented of perinatal transmission of HbsAg, with the development of HCC 6 to 7 years later.[33–35] Although it is generally held that the latent period for HCC development is in excess of 20 years, the childhood cases demonstrating HBV involvement suggest a considerably shorter latency.

Children with the chronic form of hereditary tyrosinemia who survive beyond age 2 years have a strikingly high incidence of HCC. In a series of 43 cases, 16 children who survived beyond 2 years of age developed HCC.[36] All had concomitant cirrhosis, but this frequency of HCC in cirrhotic livers is considerably higher than that seen in adult patients with cirrhosis from all causes, suggesting oncogenic factors beyond the presence of cirrhosis.

Biliary cirrhosis secondary to extrahepatic biliary atresia has been associated with HCC in ten patients who survived longer than 3 years.[37,38] The syndrome of progressive familial cholestatic cirrhosis of childhood, another cause of biliary cirrhosis, has been associated with HCC in two sibships (four patients).[39,40] Hepatocellular carcinoma has also been reported in a 26-month-old boy with biliary cirrhosis secondary to prolonged parenteral nutrition.[41] Thus, childhood biliary cirrhosis caused by several different diseases has been associated with malignant transformation. Chronic cholestasis without cirrhosis does not predispose to HCC, nor does biliary cirrhosis in the adult have a significant association with HCC. Thus, there may be specific metabolic contributions to oncogenesis in childhood hepatic tumors that develop in biliary cirrhosis.

α_1-Antitrypsin is the main protease inhibitor in human serum. Its biosynthesis is controlled by a pair of genes at the Pi locus, for which more than 25 alleles exist. The PiZ variant is an electrophoretically slow variant; when inherited homozygously, it is designated PiZZ and reduces serum concentrations of α_1-antitrypsin to 10% to 15% of normal. The heterozygous form is designated PiMZ and reduces α_1-antitrypsin to 50% to 60% of normal. The homozygous ZZ phenotype is associated with a high incidence of hepatocellular and cholangiocellular carcinoma.[42] The MZ heterozygous phenotype has more recently been associated with HCC, and the retrospective finding of periodic acid-Schiff (PAS)-positive globules within the tumor in 10% of reviewed HCCs may imply a larger role of the heterozygote MZ phenotype in oncogenesis.[43] Nonetheless, the role of the heterozygote MZ phenotype in oncogenesis remains controversial.

Glucose-6-phosphatase deficiency (Type 1 glycogen storage disease) has been associated with the development of liver tumors, most of which are benign.[44,45] However, reports of HCC developing in longer-term survivors exist.[46]

Prolonged use of androgenic anabolic steroids, particularly the C17 alkylated forms (oxymethalone, methyltestosterone, testosterone enanthate, and methandienone), has produced hepatocellular neoplasms.[47,48] These tumors are multicentric in origin, well-differentiated, and nonmetastatic. They occur most frequently in patients with Fanconi's anemia but are also seen in patients taking these drugs for other reasons. Fanconi's anemia is characterized by a DNA repair defect and is associated with leukemia and squamous carcinomas but not with liver tumors in the absence of androgen administration. Metastatic spread and vascular invasion are rare in this androgen-induced tumor, and regression is seen in some instances on withdrawal of the androgen. These features have caused some to question whether this is a true hepatocellular carcinoma, but it is probably best regarded as such.

Hepatocellular carcinoma has been reported in children with lymphoblastic leukemia treated with daily oral methotrexate.[49,50] Methotrexate is hepatotoxic and causes portal fibrosis. Daily use of this drug is now unusual, and data from long-term follow-up studies suggest that HCC is a rare event in these patients. Other described associations with HCC include neurofibromatosis,[51] ataxia-telangiectasia, and familial polyposis.[52]

PATHOLOGY

Hepatoblastoma

Hepatoblastoma is most often unifocal, and the right lobe is more commonly affected.[53] Microscopic vascular spread may be found beyond an apparently encapsulated tumor. The gross appearance is that of a lobulated, bulging, tan mass, often punctuated by geographic areas of necrosis and surrounded by a pseudocapsule (Fig. 26-1). The tumor has no association with cirrhosis.

Most workers recognize two morphologic types of hepatoblastoma.[10] The pure epithelial type contains either fetal or embryonal cells, or admixtures of the two. The mixed hepatoblastoma contains mesenchymal tissue in addition to the epithelial elements (Fig. 26-2).

Fetal cells are slightly smaller than normal hepatocytes and have a relatively low nucleocytoplasmic ratio. Mitoses are infrequent (fewer than 2 per 10 high-power fields). The cells form slender cords that often contain canaliculi, with or without bile. There are no portal tracts or biliary ducts.

Embryonal cells have a much higher nucleocytoplasmic ratio, and mitoses are more frequent than in fetal cells. They assume acinar and tubular configurations that resemble early ducts of the embryonal liver. Ultrastructural studies also have been used to differentiate fetal from embryonic types. For example, embryonal cells contain fewer organelles than fetal cells.[54,55] Other ultrastructural differences have been described by Phillips and coworkers[56] and may be useful for differentiation in unusual cases.

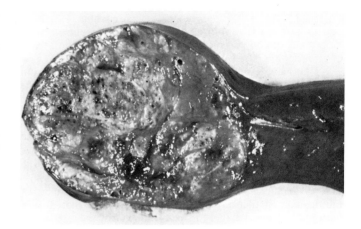

FIGURE 26-1. Gross specimen showing hepatoblastoma. The large tumor mass expands the liver. The cut surface is slightly variegated in appearance; one area is hemorrhagic.

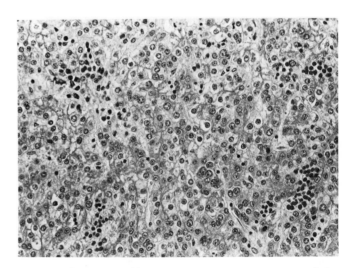

FIGURE 26-2. Hepatoblastoma. Microscopic appearance of the tumor shown in Figure 26-1. This is a fetal type of epithelial hepatoblastoma. The tumor cells are round or polygonal and much smaller than those seen in hepatocellular carcinoma (compare with Fig. 26-4). The dark staining cells in clusters are hematopoietic cells; they are a common finding in hepatoblastoma. (Hematoxylin and eosin × 400)

When a neoplastic mesenchymal component accompanies the epithelial elements, the tumor has been characterized as a mixed hepatoblastoma. The mesenchymal component usually consists of foci of small immature spindle cells that lie within or encompass neoplastic hepatocellular epithelium of either the embryonal or fetal type (see Fig. 26-2). Osteoid is frequently observed in these tumors. Extramedullary hematopoiesis is frequently present. Approximately 30% of hepatoblastomas are mixed tumors.[53]

Available data indicate that the epithelial component of hepatoblastoma is the most important histologic determinant of prognosis. The designation of hepatoblastoma as "mixed" has not been helpful in predicting behavior.[53] Watanabe[57] noted a 30% (9 of 31) 5-year survival for resectable tumors of the fetal type as compared to 5% (1 of 21) for the embryonal type. Sixty-two percent of the embryonal tumors and 78% of fetal tumors were resected. Similar trends have been noted by Foster and Berman,[58] Lack and colleagues,[6] and Weinberg and

Finegold.[53] These data suggest that the malignant potential of a hepatoblastoma is more dependent on the presence of *any* embryonal or undifferentiated cells than on the predominance of either epithelial cell type.

Metastatic spread most commonly affects the lungs and porta hepatis. Bone metastases are rare.

Hepatocellular Carcinoma

Hepatocellular carcinoma in childhood is similar in gross and microscopic features to its adult counterpart, except for the lack of underlying cirrhosis in most pediatric cases.[11,59] At the time of diagnosis, the tumor is often extensively invasive or multicentric, so that resection is possible in fewer than 30% of patients.[4,5] Hemorrhage and necrosis within the tumor are found more often than in hepatoblastoma, and pseudoencapsulation is less notable. The tumor is often bile-stained. Hepatocellular carcinoma is distinguished from hepatoblastoma microscopically by the presence of cells larger than normal hepatocytes, broad trabeculae, considerable nuclear pleomorphism, nucleolar prominence, tumor giant cells, and the absence of hematopoiesis. These distinctions may be difficult to apply to some tumors, especially when examination is limited to a biopsy (Figs. 26-3 and 26-4).[55,60–62]

A distinctive variant of HCC occurs in the noncirrhotic livers of older children and young adults.[63] This tumor, termed fibrolamellar carcinoma, has a more favorable prognosis than does the usual hepatocarcinoma.[64] It is characterized by plump, deeply eosinophilic hepatocytes encompassed by an abundant fibrous stroma composed of thin parallel fibrous bands that separate the epithelial cells into trabeculae or large nodules. Fibroblasts separate hepatocytes from the encompassing collagen.[65] The abundant fibrous tissue, which is unusual for hepatocellular carcinoma, may impart a gross appearance similar to focal nodular hyperplasia (Figs. 26-5 and 26-6).[66]

Hepatocellular carcinoma often has distinctive ultrastructural features that distinguish it from other tumors. Especially characteristic are large, round, centrally placed nuclei, prominent nucleoli, the abundance of large mitochondria, and the frequent occurrence of microvilli on the plasma membrane.[56] Other procedures that help prove the hepatocellular nature of

the tumor cells are the demonstration of alpha-fetoprotein (AFP) and α_1-antitrypsin by light or electron immunohistochemistry.

Metastatic spread is to lungs, regional lymph glands, and rarely, to bone.

Other Tumors

Rhabdomyosarcoma is the most common sarcoma seen in the liver. Its histologic appearance and clinical characteristics are similar to rhabdomyosarcoma at other sites (see also Chap. 30).

Although most vascular neoplasms (cavernous hemangioma and hemangioendothelioma) are benign, some observers believe that the presence of hemangioendothelioma at multiple sites indicates that this tumor can metastasize. Six cases of

FIGURE 26-4. Hepatocellular carcinoma. Microscopic appearance of the tumor shown in Figure 26-3. This is a well-differentiated hepatocellular carcinoma. Note large polygonal hepatic cells with central nuclei. A number of mitoses can be seen. (Hematoxylin and eosin × 400)

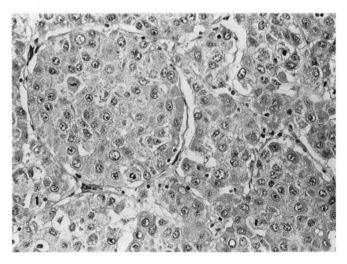

FIGURE 26-3. Gross specimen showing hepatocellular carcinoma. Large primary liver cell carcinoma in a noncirrhotic liver.

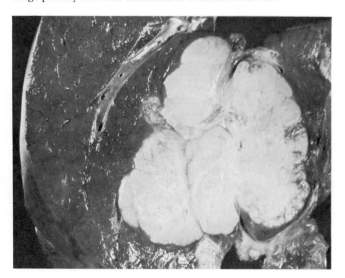

FIGURE 26-5. Gross specimen showing fibrolamellar carcinoma. Large tumor mass is multilobulated and extensively scarred.

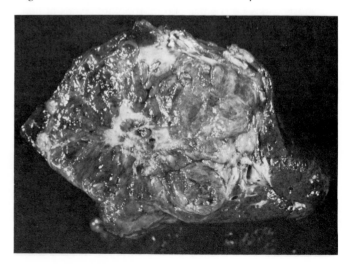

angiosarcoma developing in patients with hemangioendothelioma have been described.[53,67]

Excellent reviews of the characteristics of the less common benign and malignant hepatic neoplasms can be found in publications by Weinberg and Finegold[53] and Ishak and Rabin.[68] Table 26-3 lists the less common malignant tumors of the liver.

PRESENTING FEATURES

Hepatoblastoma

Hepatoblastoma most frequently presents as an asymptomatic abdominal mass in a child younger than 2 years. Anorexia, weight loss, vomiting, and abdominal pain are associated with advanced disease and are seen less frequently than in hepatocellular carcinoma. Rarely, the first presentation is one of acute abdominal crisis secondary to rupture of the tumor.

Approximately 10% of cases are first noted on routine physical examination. Physical examination is remarkable for the abdominal distention and associated hepatic enlargement. A discrete mass is not usually palpable. Pallor and evidence of weight loss are present in a minority of patients. Jaundice is rare, occurring in only 5% of published cases. Clubbing of the digits is seen rarely. Splenomegaly is occasionally present.

Other infrequent features include hemihypertrophy and

FIGURE 26-6. Fibrolamellar carcinoma. Note that the large polygonal hepatic cells that make up this tumor are separated by almost acellular collagen. This is the classic appearance of the fibrolamellar variant of hepatocellular carcinoma. (Hematoxylin and eosin × 400)

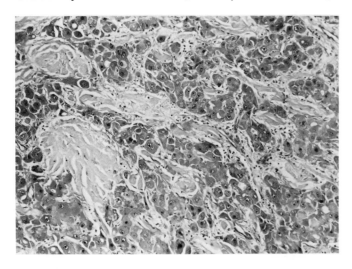

Table 26-3
Less Common Hepatic Malignancies

> Angiosarcoma
> Primary endocrine (APUD) or carcinoid
> Undifferentrated sarcoma
> Rhabdomyosarcoma
> Leiomyosarcoma
> Malignant teratoma
> Primary lymphoma

isosexual precocity, with penile and testicular enlargement in males and the presence of pubic hair. This latter syndrome occurs in the 3% of patients who secrete β-HCG (human chorionic gonadatropin).[69,70] The late features of the Beckwith–Wiedemann syndrome, including midface hypoplasia and slit-like indentations of the ear lobe, may also occur, although this syndrome is rare.

Severe osteopenia, with back pain, refusal to walk, and pathologic fractures of weight-bearing bones, may be a presenting clinical syndrome. Multiple vertebral compression fractures may be present on radiographs. Severe osteopenia is present in 20% to 30% of cases; some degree of osteopenia is present in the majority of cases and regresses with tumor resection.[71]

Hepatocellular Carcinoma

Abdominal distention and right upper quadrant mass are the most common presentations of HCC. These may be superimposed on the symptomatology of preexisting underlying disease such as tyrosinemia or cirrhosis. Abdominal pain occurs in approximately half of the patients, and nausea and vomiting are common. Systemic manifestations, including fever, weight loss, and anorexia, are more common than in hepatoblastoma, and the duration of symptoms is relatively short (mean = 1–2 months).[11] The mean duration of symptoms is considerably longer in the fibrolamellar type (mean = 11 months).[12,64]

Hemoperitoneum with an acute abdominal crisis is a well-recognized first presentation. Jaundice is more frequent in HCC than in hepatoblastoma, occurring in approximately 25% of cases. Splenomegaly may be present when there is coexisting cirrhosis, as may other features of chronic liver disease, such as spider angiomata. Polycythemia, with hemoglobin levels greater than 16 g/100 ml and increased erythrocyte mass, is occasionally present due to the extrarenal production of erythropoietin.[72,73]

DIAGNOSTIC WORKUP

Laboratory Tests

Mild normochromic normocytic anemia is usual, although polycythemia is occasionally seen in hepatocellular carcinoma (Tables 26-4 and 26-5). Thrombocytosis in excess of $1 \times 10^6/$ mm may be seen in both HCC and hepatoblastoma.[74] Modest elevations of liver enzymes and alkaline phosphatase can occur and are more frequent in HCC. Bilirubin is infrequently elevated.

The most valuable laboratory test for both diagnosis and monitoring of hepatic tumors, is AFP. This fetal antigen is a single-chain sialated glycoprotein with a molecular weight of 67,500 daltons (see also Chap. 8). Its synthesis, which begins at 28 days of fetal life, occurs initially in the yolk sac and the liver and by 11 weeks exclusively in the liver. By 14 weeks, peak levels are reached and it is the dominant serum protein. Thereafter, a rapid decline in concentration occurs until term, when levels are at concentrations of 20 to 120 μg/ml. In premature infants, levels at birth are higher.[75] In the first 2 months of life, the levels are in the 30 to 400 ng/ml range; by 6 months, they fall below 30 ng/ml. At 1 year, adult levels of 3 to 15 ng/ml are reached.[76]

The biological half-life of AFP is 5 to 7 days. Levels are elevated in two thirds of patients with hepatoblastoma (see also Chap. 8). Embryonal tumors produce AFP less frequently than do fetal ones. Levels are elevated in up to 50% of childhood HCC.[76] Elevated levels provide an excellent marker for following the course of disease. After complete resection, an exponential fall to the normal range can be expected. Failure to achieve normal levels implies residual disease, whereas secondary elevation suggests disease recurrence. Occasionally, non-AFP-producing metastases may follow resection of an AFP-secreting tumor.[77]

A specific abnormality of the vitamin B_{12} binding protein occurs in the fibrolamellar variant of HCC.[78] The level of unsaturated vitamin B_{12} binding protein is significantly elevated and rises with disease progression. This vitamin B_{12} binding protein differs from normal transcobalamin I by virtue of containing more sialic acid residues.[79]

Other diagnostic tests include serologic evaluation of previous exposure to HBV in the older child and β-HCG levels in children with precocious puberty. Although urinary cystathionine is significantly elevated in 40% to 70% of hepatoblastoma patients,[14,80] it is not a useful diagnostic test. Bone marrow aspirates are not necessary.

Table 26-4
Diagnostic Workup for Children with Suspected Liver Tumor

Child Younger Than 5 Years
Complete blood count
Liver function tests
AFP
β-HCG if precocious puberty present

Child Older Than 5 Years
Complete blood count
Liver function tests
AFP
Hepatitis B serology
Vitamin B_{12} binding protein

All Patients
Plain film of abdomen
Ultrasound
CT
Angiography if anatomic details unclear from CT

Diagnostic Imaging

Plain radiographs of the abdomen invariably demonstrate the presence of a right upper quadrant mass. Calcification is seen in approximately 6% of hepatic malignant tumors; hemangiomas demonstrate calcification in 12% of cases.[81]

Radionuclide imaging using ^{99m}Tc-labeled sulfur colloid is often carried out but yields little information beyond that derived from ultrasonography and computed tomographic (CT) scanning. Although it is a very sensitive technique, it is of low specificity.[82]

Ultrasonography is particularly useful in establishing the presence of a mass within an enlarged liver and in differentiating solid from cystic masses. Both hepatoblastoma and HCC demonstrate diffuse hyperechoic patterns on ultrasonography. By contrast, benign lesions are poorly echogenic, with scattered internal echoes. Hemangiomata and other vascular lesions contain areas with varying degrees of echogenicity. Ultrasound may reveal involvement of the inferior vena cava, hepatic veins, and portal veins.[82,83] Serial examination during preoperative chemotherapy reveals the development of echofree areas that reflect tumor necrosis.

CT scanning of the liver is particularly important for defining the extent of tumor involvement, the anatomic landmarks, and the tumor's operability.[84,85] Because of its blood supply, the portion of the left lobe of the liver lateral to the falciform ligament (*i.e.,* the lateral segment of the left lobe) can be regarded as a distinct "lobe." The presence or absence of tumor in the anatomic lobes of the liver usually can be determined by CT scan. Occasionally, this is difficult in the young child because of the paucity of fat in the ligamentum teres. CT scanning is of particular value in identifying the anatomy of left lobe tumors, in which angiography is often inconclusive.[82,86] The mass of hepatoblastoma and HCC characteristically is of lower attenuation than the surrounding normal hepatic tissue. Rarely, the tumor may be isodense and difficult to visualize. Contrast injection results in patchy enhancement throughout the tumor mass. Vascular tumors may be difficult to differentiate on unenhanced scans. With contrast, a specific pattern of enhancement may be seen, with initial dense peripheral enhancement and central low density and a gradual centripetal filling in of the central low-density area from the periphery. Regional lymph nodes are almost never involved;

Table 26-5
Useful Distinctive Features of Hepatic Tumors

Feature	Hepatoblastoma	HCC	Fibrolamellar Variant
Usual age at presentation	0–3 yr	5–18 yr	10–20 yr
Associated congenital anomalies	Dysmorphic features Hemihypertrophy Beckwith–Wiedemann	Metabolic	None
Advanced disease at presentation	40%	70%	10%
Usual site of origin	Right lobe	Right lobe–multifocal	Right lobe
Abnormal liver function tests	15%–30%	30%–50%	Rare
Jaundice	5%	25%	Absent
Elevated AFP	60%–70%	50%	10%
Positive hepatitis B serology	Absent	Present in some	Absent
Abnormal B_{12} binding protein	Absent	Absent	Present
Distinctive radiographic appearance	None	None	None
Pathology	Fetal and/or embryonal cells ± mesenchymal component	Large pleomorphic tumor cells and tumor giant cells	Eosinophilic hepatocytes with dense fibrous stroma

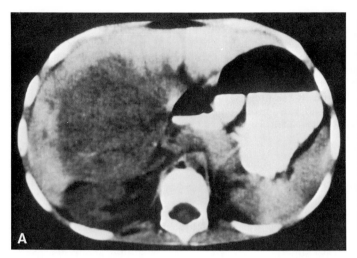

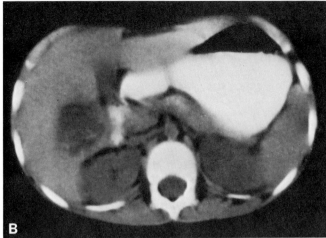

FIGURE 26-7. CT scans in 3-year-old boy with hepatoblastoma. **A.** At diagnosis a large tumor is noted in the right lobe of the liver. **B.** After four cycles of chemotherapy the mass is markedly reduced in size. Successful resection was performed. The child is alive and well 13 months later.

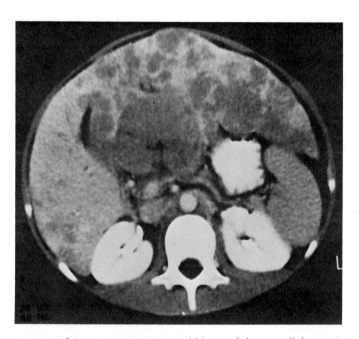

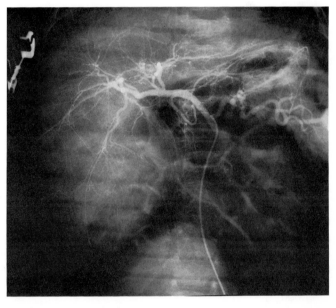

FIGURE 26-8. CT scan in 10-year-old boy with hepatocellular carcinoma. Tumor appears to be multicentric in origin and involves both right and left lobes and porta hepatis.

FIGURE 26-9. Angiogram in a 3-month-old infant with hepatoblastoma arising in the right lobe of the liver. Note the large size of the tumor and tumor vessels arising from the right hepatic artery. The left hepatic artery is visible and free of tumor.

if there is involvement, it may be detected on CT (Figs. 26-7 and 26-8).

The role of angiography in the era of rapid-imaging CT scanners is limited. Extra information was obtained from angiography in only 5 cases in a series of 45 children with hepatic masses,[82] and this series used early CT scanners with less resolution capacity than current scanners. The place of angiography may be limited to better defining the vascular anatomy in cases in which the tumor is centrally located, or in which the margins of the tumor are not clear on CT scanning (Fig. 26-9).

Experience to date with the use of magnetic resonance imaging (MRI) has been limited. The definition of anatomy and borders appears to be equivalent to but no better than that

of CT scanning. Whether this technology will prove a superior imaging modality awaits further study.

Investigation for metastatic spread should include CT scanning of the chest and bone scan.

DISEASE STAGING

A clinical grouping schema is essential for formulating prognoses and interpreting data from clinical trials. Although there is no universally accepted system, the most widely used approach is that of the Children's Cancer Study Group and the Southwest Oncology Group.[87] It is based on the extent of the tumor and of the surgical resection (Table 26-6). A study using this classification found good correlation between prognosis and clinical groups in a patient population comprising both hepatoblastoma and HCC (Fig. 26-10).

The Japanese Society for Pediatric Surgery attempted a classification based on the TNM (tumor, node, metastasis) system, using tumor size, number of lobes involved, regional node involvement, and presence of metastatic spread as criteria.[88] In 115 hepatoblastoma patients, positive regional nodes were noted in only 5 cases. The two determinants with prognostic significance were the number of liver segments involved with tumor and the presence of metastatic disease.

Thus, both staging systems demonstrate good correlation only between number of lobes involved and the presence of metastatic disease. Since both of these staging systems depend on operative findings, they are of little value in identifying those patients who would benefit from presurgical chemotherapy.

Table 26-6
Clinical Grouping of Malignant Hepatic Tumors

Designation	Criteria
Group I	Complete resection of tumor by wedge resection lobectomy, or by extended lobectomy as initial treatment
Group IIA	Tumors rendered completely resectable by initial irradiation and/or chemotherapy
Group IIB	Residual disease confined to one lobe
Group III	Disease involving both lobes of the liver
Group IIIB	Regional node involvement
Group IV	Distant metastases, irrespective of the extent of liver involvement

FIGURE 26-10. Life table analysis of survival in mixed population of children with hepatoblastoma and hepatocellular carcinoma showing correlation between survival probability and clinical grouping 0 to 60 months after diagnosis and treatment. (Evans EA et al: Combination chemotherapy in the treatment of children with malignant hepatoma. Cancer 50:821–826, 1982)

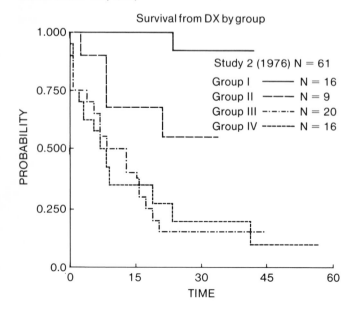

TREATMENT

Current data indicate that cure of malignant liver tumors in children is not possible without complete resection of the primary tumor; anatomic hepatic lobectomy is usually necessary. Recent studies indicate that preoperative chemotherapy may convert a nonresectable tumor to a resectable one. A summary of our current recommendations for the treatment of hepatoblastoma and HCC is given in Table 26-7.

Surgery

Anatomy

The anatomy of the liver is depicted in Figure 26-11. The division between right and left lobes is the plane that runs from the gall bladder fossa inferiorly to the suprahepatic inferior vena cava superiorly. The right lobe constitutes about 70% of the hepatic cell mass and is the site of most hepatic neoplasms. The left lobe is divided into a medial and lateral segment by the midline falciform ligament. Each segment represents about 15% of the liver mass. Because of the liver's remarkable ability to regenerate, as much as 85% of the liver can be removed safely, with complete regeneration of liver cell mass within 1 to 3 months following surgery. Thus, tumors that are contained in one lobe of the liver and those that arise in the right lobe but do not extend beyond the medial segment of the left lobe are amenable to surgical resection. Mortality from hepatic lobectomy ranges from 10% to 25% in various series. Current surgical techniques, as well as careful management before, during, and after surgery, minimize the hazards of hepatic resection.[89,90]

Biopsy

Some tumors may be judged unresectable because of their very large size or because they extend beyond the limits of a standard lobar resection (see Chap. 10). In these cases, preoperative chemotherapy, with or without radiation therapy, may render the tumor resectable. However, before instituting such therapy, a precise histologic diagnosis is required. Traditionally, tissue has been obtained by a wedge liver biopsy through a small laparotomy incision. The advantages of this "open" approach are that the liver and surrounding areas can be inspected for tumor involvement, a site likely to yield a definitive diagnosis can be biopsied, and hemostasis ensured. However, after trials in a large number of children, we now prefer to use needle biopsy, which avoids the need for general anesthesia and an incision. Bleeding and significant tumor spill appear to be less than with the open technique. The site to be biopsied is usually quite obvious, and one can ensure that the biopsy will be diagnostic by obtaining two or three specimens. Because CT scanning is now used routinely to determine the extent of tumor involvement, little additional useful information is obtained at laparotomy in the child whose tumor requires delayed resection.

Resection

PROCEDURE. The recommended procedure for hepatic resection in children is similar to that used in adults.[91,92] A thoracoabdominal approach is preferred because it offers excellent exposure and precludes the development of negative intrathoracic pressure, which may cause the aspiration of air into an open venous system (Fig. 26-12). This approach also provides excellent visualization of the entire supradiaphrag-

Table 26-7
Current Recommendations for Management of Hepatoblastoma and Hepatocellular Carcinoma

Tumor Extent	Surgery	Chemotherapy	Radiation
Small—confined to one lobe	Primary excision	Adjuvant	
Large—confined to one lobe or requires trisegmentectomy	Biopsy and delayed excision	Preoperative plus adjuvant	Rarely*
Any tumor with pulmonary metastases	Biopsy and delayed excision	Preoperative plus adjuvant	Rarely*

* If unresponsive to chemotherapy, or for pulmonary metastases.

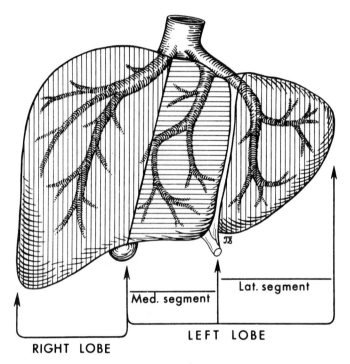

FIGURE 26-11. Lobar anatomy of the liver. The imaginary line between the bed of the gallbladder and the inferior vena cava divides the liver into right and left lobes. The falciform ligament divides the left lobe into medial and lateral segments. Only hepatic venous drainage is shown.

matic inferior vena cava, into which an internal venous shunt can be placed to isolate liver blood flow in the event of catastrophic hemorrhage.[93]

Once the porta hepatis is dissected, the vessels and bile ducts to the lobe to be excised are ligated and divided. The liver is mobilized by dividing its diaphragmatic attachments, and the diaphragm is divided radially to the vena cava. Tapes are passed around the vena cava above and below the liver to ensure control of any excessive bleeding. Before the hepatic veins are isolated, the liver capsule is incised along a lobar or segmental division and the liver substance is divided bluntly. Bridging vessels and bile ducts are ligated as they are encountered. Because of the very short extrahepatic length of the hepatic veins in children, these vessels are better approached by dissection through the liver substance rather

than at their exit from the liver. This technique minimizes inadvertent venous injury. After resection has been completed, hemostasis and bile drainage are controlled by compressing the raw surface of the liver with mattress sutures. Sump and Penrose drains are placed in the liver bed and the incision is closed. T-tube drainage of the common duct is not used because there is no conclusive evidence that it decreases postoperative bile leak, and stricture in the small bile duct of an infant is a potential risk.

Profound hypothermia with circulatory arrest has been used as an adjunct to surgery and may be employed in a difficult hepatectomy.[94] Before division of the liver, cardiopulmonary bypass is instituted and hypothermia induced. With the child's body temperature at 20°C, the circulation can be stopped for as long as 60 minutes and resection and repair of vascular structures can be performed in a bloodless operative field. Others have isolated and interrupted the hepatic circulation for periods as long as an hour to control massive bleeding by clamping the lower thoracic aorta, porta hepatis, and the vena cava above or below the liver, without any untoward effect on the liver remnant.[95]

INTRAOPERATIVE MANAGEMENT. The most frequent and serious intraoperative problem is hemorrhage. Even in the absence of uncontrolled bleeding, the loss of one blood volume (up to 800 ml in a 10 kg child) is not unusual. As a guide to proper replacement, precise measurement of blood loss and accurate assessment of intra-arterial blood pressure, central venous pressure, and urine output are necessary (see also Chap. 10). Since hypothermia tends to cause cardiac irritability, metabolic acidosis, and abnormal blood clotting, blood administered during surgery should be warmed to 37°C. Unless the procedure is performed with induced hypothermia, the child's normal body temperature should be maintained by providing a warm operating room temperature and by the use of a warming blanket. Adjusting the pH of banked blood (pH 7.0) to pH 7.4 also decreases the incidence of cardiac arrest, which can be triggered by the rapid infusion of large volumes of cold, acid blood.

Chemotherapy

Hepatoblastoma

As noted above, cure of hepatoblastoma appears possible only when complete surgical excision has been achieved. Complete excision is possible in 50% to 60% of cases, and there is a perioperative mortality of 11%.[3] Chemotherapy is used as an

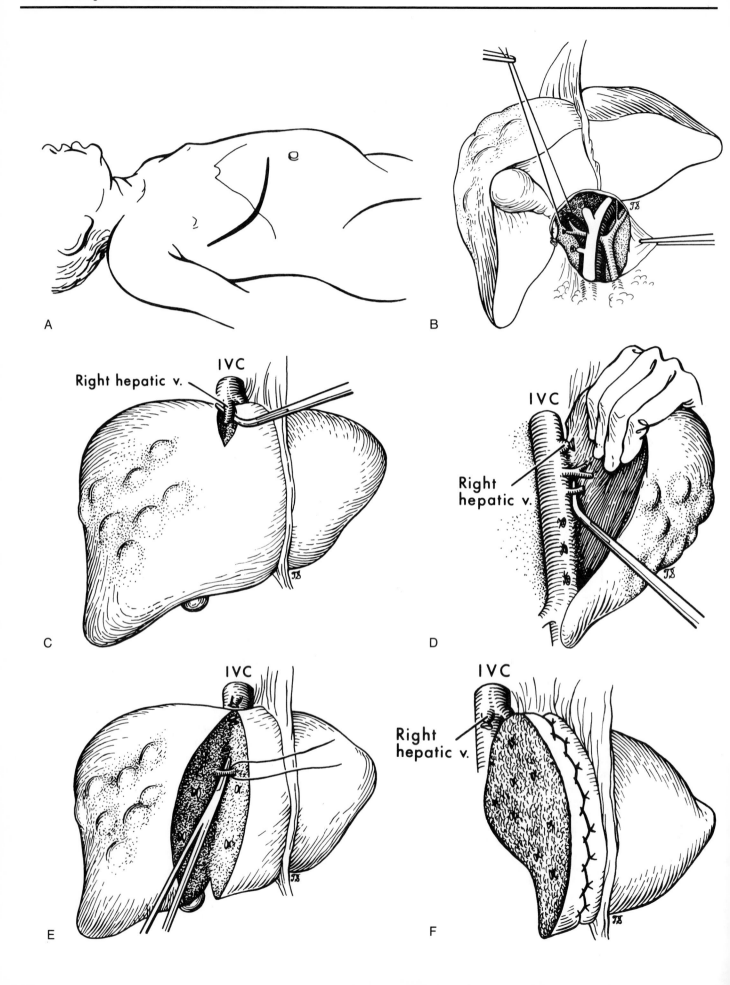

A

B

C

Right hepatic v.

IVC

D

IVC

Right hepatic v.

E

IVC

F

IVC

Right hepatic v.

Table 26-8
Preoperative Chemotherapy Regimens for Hepatoblastoma

Primary Agent and Dose	Other Agents	Number of Patients*	Number of Responders	References
Adriamycin 25 mg/m²/d × 3 every 3 wk or 30 mg × 1 d every 3 wk	Vincristine Cyclophosphamide Dactinomycin 5-FU DTIC	8	7	101
Adriamycin 60 mg/m² over 4 days or 75 mg/m² over 3 days	Cyclophosphamide 5-FU Vincristine Dactinomycin	6	4	102
CDDP 90 mg/m² × 1	Vincristine 5-FU	5 RD 6 PD	4 6	103
CDDP 100 mg/m² day 23 Adriamycin 40 mg/m² × 2, d 1, d 2	Vincristine Cyclophosphamide	9	8	104
CDDP 20 mg/m² d 1–5 Adriamycin 25 mg/m² d d 1–3		7	6	—†

* RD = resistant disease; PD = primary disease.
† Unpublished data, Hospital for Sick Children, Toronto.

adjuvant in tumors that are completely excised, and both pre-operatively and as an adjuvant in those tumors considered to be initially nonresectable or when primary resection would be hazardous.

ADJUVANT CHEMOTHERAPY. The first systematic multi-institutional study of adjuvant chemotherapy demonstrated clear benefit for the treated group. Only 1 of 16 patients who underwent complete resection followed by adjuvant chemotherapy developed distant metastases, compared to 7 of 11 historical controls who did not receive adjuvant chemotherapy.[87] Other studies have demonstrated excellent chemotherapeutic effects of cisplatin and Adriamycin.[96,97] We currently recommend cisplatin 20 mg/m²/day by continuous infusion for 5 days, given with Adriamycin 25 mg/m²/day for the first 3 days. Treatment is started approximately 4 weeks after hepatic resection to allow adequate regeneration of liver tissue, which can be evaluated by ultrasound or liver scan. Treatment cycles are administered 3 to 4 weeks apart for a total of six cycles. Other drugs with therapeutic effect in this tumor include vincristine, cyclophosphamide, and 5-fluorouracil (5-FU).[98–100]

PREOPERATIVE CHEMOTHERAPY. The various regimens used for preoperative chemotherapy and their results are listed in Table 26-8.[101–104] These regimens are either primarily Adriamycin based or primarily cisplatin based. Dose-limiting toxicity from Adriamycin has been mainly hematopoietic and cardiac. Preliminary evidence suggests Adriamycin administration by continuous infusion appears less toxic than and as effective as bolus administration.

Using continuous infusion Adriamycin and cisplatin, we have achieved a mean reduction in tumor size by CT scan in excess of 75% in five of six patients treated preoperatively (see Chaps. 9 and 10). Resectability was achieved in all five of these patients. We thus recommend that unless initial complete resection is clearly possible and safe, Adriamycin and cisplatin be used before resection (see Table 26-7). Three cycles are given approximately 3 weeks apart, and if CT scan confirms significant reduction in tumor size, resection is carried out when blood counts recover. Chemotherapy is resumed 4 weeks after resection, and another three cycles are given.

Although the presence of metastases considerably reduces the chances of long-term survival, we have seen complete regression of metastatic disease. Complete remissions, and possibly cures, have been recorded with the combined use of chemotherapy, surgery, and radiotherapy.[106]

Hepatocellular Carcinoma

Only one third of cases of hepatocellular carcinoma are amenable to complete resection.[4] Among patients who do undergo complete excision, only one third are long-term survivors. Adriamycin, etoposide (VP-16), and 5-FU have all been reported to produce partial remissions in 18% to 28% of cases.[107,108] However, remissions have been short-lived, with mean durations of a few months. Newer analogues, such as 4′ epidoxorubicin, may cause fewer side-effects but have not shown improved response rates.[109] Because of the multicentric origin of this tumor, it is less likely that preoperative chemotherapy will contribute significantly to operability. However,

◄**FIGURE 26-12.** Steps in performance of right hepatic lobectomy for tumor in right lobe. **A.** Thoracoabdominal skin incision. **B.** Division of right hepatic artery, right hepatic duct, right portal vein, and cystic duct in porta hepatis. **C.** The right hepatic vein is located in the substance of the liver and divided. **D.** Accessory right hepatic veins are divided as they enter the inferior vena cava. **E.** Vessels and bile ducts communicating between right and left lobes are ligated and divided. **F.** Mattress sutures are placed across the cut edge of the remaining left lobe for hemostases.

this has not been formally studied because of the limited experience in children.

Patients with the fibrolamellar variant apparently have a somewhat better prognosis. Of five children studied by Craig and colleagues,[64] resection was possible in four, and two were alive 5 to 15 years after resection. In 12 patients, Berman and colleagues[12] found 2- and 5-year survival rates of 82% and 62%, respectively. However, Lack and colleagues[11] found only a 20% long-term survival in five patients with the fibrolamellar variant. Three of four patients with fibrolamellar HCC treated at Toronto's Hospital for Sick Children were long-term survivors; two required resection of pulmonary metastases.[5]

Radiation Therapy

Dosages of radiation used to treat hepatic tumors have ranged from 1200 to 2000 cGy. Occasionally, higher doses to localized areas of tumor have resulted in tumor regression. However, even in combination with chemotherapy, such treatment has not been curative.[4,110]

As with chemotherapy, radiation to the liver immediately following resection will limit regeneration. Similarly, preoperative radiation to the primary tumor that includes uninvolved liver may also limit postresection regeneration. Radiation therapy therefore has a limited role in the treatment of hepatic malignancies. It is used only in the rare child with unresectable tumor in whom chemotherapy alone has failed to produce resectability. In this context, attempts should be made to exclude the uninvolved lobe from the radiation field. The use of limited localized field irradiation for microscopic residual disease at resection margins may have some merit.

FUTURE DIRECTIONS

Research directions that merit exploration in an attempt to improve outcome in hepatoblastoma and hepatocellular carcinoma include the following:

The development of methodologies to increase local concentrations of effective drug at tumor sites in the liver. Increasing concentration-over-time exposure of tumor cells without increasing systemic toxicity may be achieved by employing intra-arterial delivery of existing effective drugs bonded to slow-releasing inert compounds.

Delivering high concentrations of effective drug to malignant cells by using tumor-specific monoclonal antibodies as vectors. These antibodies may be membrane-determinant specific or may be directed at an intracellular component, but they must effect drug penetration of tumor cell membrane to ensure generation of lethal intracellular concentrations.

Definition, characterization, and synthesis of factors responsible for the differentiation of immature fetal and embryonal hepatocytes into their mature forms.

Determination of the role of liver transplant in tumors confined to the liver. This procedure would have to be combined with effective chemotherapy to eliminate the development of metastatic disease, as seen in the prechemotherapy-era patients treated with resection alone.

REFERENCES

1. Alagille D, Odievre M: Liver and Biliary Tract Disease in Children, p 311. New York, John Wiley & Sons, 1979
2. Fraumeni JF, Jr, Miller RW, Hill JA: Primary carcinoma of the liver in childhood: An epidemiologic study. J Natl Cancer Inst 40:1087–1099, 1968
3. Young JL Jr, Miller RW: Incidence of malignant tumors in U.S. children. J Pediatr 86:254–258, 1975
4. Exelby PR, Filler RM, Grosfeld JL: Liver tumors in children in the particular reference to hepatoblastoma in hepatocellular carcinoma. American Academy of Pediatric Surgical Section Survey 1974. J Pediatr Surg 10:329–337, 1975
5. Giacomantonio M, Ein SH, Mancer K, Stephens CA: Thirty years of experience with pediatric primary malignant liver tumors. J Pediatr Surg 19:523–526, 1984
6. Lack EE, Neave C, Vawter GF: Hepatoblastoma. A clinical and pathologic study of 54 Cases. Am J Surg Pathol 6:693–705, 1982
7. Weinberg AG, Finegold MJ: Primary hepatic tumors of childhood. Hum Pathol 14:512–537, 1983
8. Shafer AD, Selinkoff PM: Preoperative irradiation and chemotherapy for initially unresectable hepatoblastoma. J Pediatr Surg 12:1001–1007, 1977
9. Mahour GH, Wogu GU, Siegel SE, Isaacs H: Improved survival in infants and children with primary malignant liver tumors. Am J Surg 146:236–240, 1983
10. Ishak KG, Glunz PR: Hepatoblastoma and hepatocarcinoma in infancy and childhood. Report of 47 cases. Cancer 20:396–422, 1967
11. Lack EE, Neave C, Vawter GF: Hepatocellular carcinoma. Review of 32 cases of childhood and adolescence. Cancer 52:1510–1515, 1983
12. Berman MM, Libbey NP, Foster JH: Hepatocellular carcinoma. Polygonal cell type with fibrous stroma—An atypical variant with a favorable prognosis. Cancer 46:1448–1455, 1980
13. Sotelo-Avila C, Gonzalez-Crussi F, Fowler JW: Complete and incomplete forms of Beckwith-Wiedemann syndrome: Their oncogenic potential. J Pediatr 96:47–50, 1980
14. Geiser CF, Baez A, Schindler AM, Shih VE: Epithelial hepatoblastoma associated with congenital hemihypertrophy and cystathioninuria: Presentation of a case. Pediatrics 46:66–73, 1970
15. Koufos A, Hansen MF, Lampkin BC, Workman ML, Copeland NG, Jenkins NA, Cavenee WK: Loss of alleles at loci on human chromosome 11 during genesis of Wilm's tumor. Nature 309:170–174, 1984
16. Cavenee WK, Hansen MF, Nordenskjold M, Kock E, Maumenee I, Squire JA, Phillips RA, Gallie BL: Genetic origin of mutations predisposing to retinoblastoma. Science 228:501–503, 1985
17. Cavenee WK, Dryja TP, Phillips RA, Benedict WF, Godbout R, Gallie BL, Murphree AL, Strong LC, White RL: Expression of recessive alleles by chromosomal mechanisms in retinoblastoma. Nature 305:779–784, 1983
18. Koufos A, Hansen MF, Copeland NG, Jenkins NA, Lampkin BC, Cavenee WK: Loss of heterozygosity in three embryonal tumours suggests a common pathogenetic mechanism. Nature 316:330–334, 1985
19. Meyer P, LiVolse V, Cornog J: Hepatoblastoma associated with an oral contraceptive. Lancet 2:1387, 1974
20. Otten J, Smets R, der Jager R et al: Hepatoblastoma in an infant after contraceptive intake during pregnancy. N Engl J Med 297:222, 1977
21. Melamed I, Bujanover Y, Hammer J, Spirer Z: Hepatoblastoma in an infant born to a mother after hormonal treatment for sterility. N Engl J Med 307:820, 1982
22. Khan A, Bader JL, Hoy GR et al: Hepatoblastoma in child with fetal alcohol syndrome. Lancet 1:1403, 1979
23. Fraumeni JF Jr, Rosen PJ, Hull EW, Barth RF, Shapiro SR, O'Connor JF: Hepatoblastoma in infant sisters. Cancer 24:1086–1090, 1969
24. Napoli VM, Campbell WG Jr: Hepatoblastoma in infant sister and brother. Cancer 39:2647–2650, 1977
25. Ohaki Y, Misugi K, Sasaki Y, Tsunoda A: Hepatitis B surface antigen positive hepatocellular carcinoma in children. Report of a case and review of the literature. Cancer 51:822–828, 1983
26. Kew MC, Hodkinson J, Paterson AC, Song E: Hepatitis-B virus infection in black children with hepatocellular carcinoma. J Med Virol 9:201–207, 1982
27. Gasser RW, Judamier G, Nedden DZ, Aufschnatier M, Hofstaedter F: Primary hepatocellular carcinoma with hepatitis B virus infection in a 16-Year-Old noncirrhotic patient. Am J Gastroenterol 78:305–308, 1983
28. Szmuness W: Hepatocellular carcinoma and the hepatitis B virus: Evidence for a causal association. Progr Med Virol 24:40–69, 1978
29. Tabor E, Gerety RJ, Vogel CL et al: Hepatitis B viral infection and hepatocellular carcinoma. J Natl Cancer Inst 58:1197–2000, 1977
30. Beasley RP, Lin CC, Hwang LL, Chien CS: Hepatocellular carcinoma and

hepatitis B virus. A prospective Study of 22707 men in Taiwan. Lancet 2:1129–1132, 1981

31. Shafritz DA, Shouval D, Sherman HI, Hadziyannis SJ, Kew MC: Integration of hepatitis B virus DNA into the genome of liver cells in chronic liver disease and hepatocellular carcinoma. Studies in percutaneous liver biopsies and post-mortem tissue specimens. N Engl J Med 305:1067–1083, 1981

32. Brechot C, Pourcel C, Louise A, Rain B, Tiollais P: Presence of integrated grated hepatitis virus DNA sequences in cellular DNA of human hepatocellular carcinoma. Nature 286:533–535, 1980

33. Harvey VJ, Woodfield DG, Probert JC: Maternal transmission of hepatocellular carcinoma. Cancer 54:1360–1363, 1984

34. Beasley RP, Shiao I, Wu T, Hwang L: Hepatoma in an HBsAg carrier—Seven years after perinatal infection. J Pediatr 101:83–84, 1982

35. Shimoda T, Uchida T, Miyata H, Abe K, Ariga H, Shikata T, Fujii Y: A 6-year-old boy having hepatocellular carcinoma associated with hepatitis B surface antigenemia. Am Soc Clin Pathol 74:827–831, 1980

36. Weinberg AG, Mize CE, Worthen HG: The occurrence of hepatoma in the chronic form of herediatry tyrosinemia. J Pediatr 88:434–438, 1976

37. Deoras MP, Dicus W: Hepatocarcinoma associated with biliary cirrhosis. A case due to congenital bile duct atresia. Arch Pathol 86:338–341, 1968

38. Van Wyk J, Halgrimson CG, Giles G, Lily J, Martineau G, Starzl TE: Liver transplantation in biliary atresia with concomitant hepatoma. S Afr Med J 46:886–880, 1972

39. Ugarte N, Gonzalez-Crussi F: Hepatoma in siblings with progressive familial cholestatic cirrhosis of childhood. Am Soc Clin Pathol 76:172–177, 1981

40. Dahms B: Hepatoma in familial cholestatic cirrhosis of childhood. Its occurrence in twin brothers. Arch Pathol Lab Med 103:30–33, 1979

41. Vileisis RA, Sorensen K, Gonzalez-Crussi F, Hunt CE: Liver malignancy after parenteral nutrition. J Pediatr 88–90, 1982

42. Eriksson S, Carlson J, Velez R: Risk of cirrhosis and primary liver cancer in α_1-antitrypsin deficiency. N Engl J Med 314:736–739, 1986

43. Lieberman J, Silton RM, Agliozzo CM, McMahon J: Hepatocellular carcinoma and intermediate α_1-antitrypsin deficiency (MZ phenotype). Am J Clin Pathol 64:304–310, 1975

44. Howell R, Stevenson RE, Ben-Menachem Y, Phyliky RL, Berry DH: Hepatic adenomata with type 1 glycogen storage disease. JAMA 236:1481–1484, 1976

45. Mason HH, Andersen DH: Glycogen disease of the liver (von Gierke's disease) with hepatomata. Case report with metabolic studies. Pediatrics 16:785–799, 1955

46. Zangeneh F, Limbeck GA, Brown BI, Emch JR, Arcasoy MM, Goldenberg VE, Kelley VC: Hepatorenal glycogenosis (type I glycogenosis) and carcinoma of the liver. J Pediatr 74:73–83, 1969

47. Shapiro P, Ikeda RM, Ruebner BH, Connors MH, Halsted CC, Abildgaard CF: Multiple hepatic tumors and peliosis hepatis in fanconi's anemia treated with androgens. Am J Dis Child 131:1104–1106, 1977

48. Johnson FL, Lerner KG, Siegel M, Feagler JR, Majerus PW, Hartmann JR, Thomas ED: Association of androgenic-anabolic steroid therapy with development of hepatocellular carcinoma. Lancet 2:1273–1276, 1972

49. Ruymann FB, Mosijczuk AD, Sayers RJ: Hepatoma in a child with methotrexate-induced hepatic fibrosis. JAMA 238:2631–2633, 1977

50. Delbruck H, Schaison G, Chelloul N, Bernard J: Leberkarzinom bei einem Kind nach siebenjahriger kompletter Remission einer akuten Lymphoblastenleukamie. Dtsch Med Wochenschr 100:1792–1797, 1975

51. Ettinger LJ, Freeman AI: Hepatoma in a child with neurofibromatosis. Am J Dis Child 133:528–531, 1979

52. Kingston JE, Herbert A, Draper GJ, Mann JF: Association between hepatoblastoma and polyposis coli. Arch Dis Child 58:959–962, 1983

53. Weinberg AG, Finegold MJ: Primary hepatic tumors in childhood. In Finegold MJ (ed): Pathology of Neoplasia in Children and Adolescents, pp 333–372. Philadelphia, WB Saunders, 1986

54. Misugi K, Okajima H, Misugi N et al: Classification of primary malignant tumors of the liver in infancy and childhood. Cancer 20:1760, 1967

55. Ito J, Johnson WW: Hepatoblastoma and hepatoma in infancy and childhood. Light and electron microscopic studies. Arch Pathol 87:259, 1969

56. Phillips MJ, Poucell S, Patterson J, Valencia P: An Ultrastructural Atlas and Text of Liver Disease, pp 447–517. New York, Raven Press, 1986

57. Watanabe I: Histopathologic features of liver cell carcinoma in infancy in childhood and their relations to surgical prognosis. Jpn J Cancer Clin 23:691, 1977

58. Foster JH, Berman MM: Solid Liver Tumors. Philadelphia, WB Saunders, 1977

59. Jones E: Primary carcinoma of the liver with associated cirrhosis in infants and children. Arch Pathol 70:19, 1960

60. Bloustein PA: Association of carcinoma with congenital cystic conditions of the liver and bile ducts. Am J Gastroenterol 67:40, 1977

61. Randolph J, Chandra R, Leiken S: Malignant liver tumors in infants and children. World J Surg 4:71, 1980

62. Schiodt T: Hepatoblastoma and hepatocarcinoma in infancy and childhood. Acta Pathol Microbiol Scand 21(Suppl):181, 1970

63. Peters RL: Pathology of hepatocellular carcinoma. In Okuda K, Peters R (eds): Hepatocellular Carcinoma, p 107. New York, John Wiley & Sons, 1975

64. Craig JR, Peters RL, Edmondson HA, Omata M: Fibrolamellar carcinoma of the liver: A tumor of adolescents and young adults with distinctive clinicopathologic features. Cancer 46:372–379, 1980

65. Farhi DG, Shikes RH, Silverberg SG: Ultrastructure of fibrolamellar oncocytic hepatoma. Cancer 50:702, 1982

66. Vecchio FM, Fabiano A, Ghirlanda G et al: Fibrolamellar carcinoma of the liver: The malignant counterpart of focal nodular hyperplasia with oncoytic change. Am J Clin Pathol 81:521, 1984

67. Kirchner SG, Heller RM, Kasselberg AG et al: Infantile hepatic hemangioendothelioma with subsequent malignant degeneration. Pediatr Radiol 11:42, 1981

68. Ishak KG, Rabin L: Benign tumors of the liver. Med Clin North Am 59:995–1013, 1975

69. Murthy ASK, Vawter GF, Lee ABH, Jockin H, Filler RM: Hormonal bioassay of gonadotropin-producing hepatoblastoma. Arch Pathol Lab Med 104:513–517, 1980

70. McArthur JW, Toll GD, Russfield AB, Reiss AM, Quinby WC, Baker WH: Sexual precocity attributable to ectopic gonadotropin secretion by hepatoblastoma. Am J Med 54:390–403, 1973

71. Teng CT, Daeschner CW Jr, Singleton EB, Rosenberg HS, Cole VW, Hill LL, Brennan JC: Liver diseases and osteoporosis in children: I. Clinical observations. J Pediatr 59:684–702, 1961

72. Brownstein MH, Ballard HS: Hepatoma associated with erythrocytosis. report of eleven new cases. Am J Med 40:204–210, 1966

73. Kew MC, Fisher JW: Serum erythropoietin concentrations in patients with hepatocellular carcinoma. Cancer 58:2485–2488, 1986

74. Nickerson HJ, Silberman TI, McDonald TP: Hepatoblastoma, thrombocytosis, and increased thrombopoietin. Cancer 45:315–317, 1980

75. Goraya SS, Smythe PJ, Walker V: Plasma alpha-fetoprotein concentrations in pre-term neonates. Ann Clin Biochem 22:650–652, 1985

76. Yachnin S: The clinical significance of human alpha-fetoprotein. Ann Clin Lab Sci 8:84–90, 1978

77. Pritchard J, da Cunha A, Cornbleet NA et al: Alpha fetoprotein (AFP) monitoring of response to adriamycin in hepatoblastoma. J Pediatr Surg 17:429, 1982

78. Paradinas FJ, Melia WM, Wilkinson ML, Portmann B, Johnson PJ, Murray-Lyon IM, Williams R: High serum vitamin B_{12} binding capacity as a marker of the fibrolamellar variant of hepatocellular carcinoma. Br Med J 285:840–842, 1982

79. Waxman S, Gilbert HS: A tumor-related vitamin B_{12} binding protein in adolescent hepatoma. N Engl J Med 289:1053–1056, 1973

80. Geiser CF, Shih VE: Cystathioninuria and its origin in children with hepatoblastoma. J Pediatr 96:72–75, 1980

81. Miller JH, Gates GH, Stanley P: The radiologic investigation of hepatic tumors in childhood. Radiology 124:451–458, 1977

82. Liu P, Daneman A, Stringer DA: Diagnostic imaging of liver masses in children. J Can Assoc Radiol 36:296, 1985

83. Kaude JV, Felman AH, Hawkins IF Jr: Ultrasonography in primary hepatic tumors in early childhood. Pediatr Radiol 9:77–83, 1980

84. Korobkin M, Kirks DR, Sullivan DC, Mills SR, Bowie JD: Computed tomography of primary liver tumors in children. Radiology 139:431–435, 1981

85. Berger PE, Kuhn JP: Computed tomography of the hepatobiliary system in infancy and childhood. Radiol Clin North Am 19(3):431–444, 1981

86. Miller JH, Greenspan BS: Integrated imaging of hepatic tumors in childhood. Part 1: Malignant lesions (primary and metastatic). Radiology 154:83–90, 1985

87. Evans AE, Land VJ, Newton WA, Randolph JG, Sather HN, Tefft M: Combination chemotherapy in the treatment of children with malignant hepatoma. Cancer 50:821–826, 1982

88. Morita K, Okabe I, Uchino J, Watanabe I, Iwabuchi M, Matsuyama M, Takahashi H, Nakajo T, Hirai Y, Tsuchida Y, Katsumata K, Hasegawa H, Nishi T, Okamoto E, Ikeda K: The proposed Japanese TNM classification of primary liver carcinoma in infants and children. Jpn J Clin Oncol 13:361–370, 1983

89. Taylor PH, Filler RM, Nebesar RA et al: Experience with hepatic resection in childhood. Am J Surg 117:435–441, 1969

90. Clatworthy HW Jr, Schiller M, Grosfeld JL: Primary liver tumors in infancy and childhood: 41 cases variously treated. Arch Surg 109:143–147, 1974

91. Pack GR, Islami AH: Surgical treatment of hepatic tumors. In Popper H, Schaffner F (eds): Progress in Liver Diseases, vol 2, pp 499–511. New York, Grune & Stratton, 1965

92. Wilson H, Wolf RY: Hepatic lobectomy: Indications, technique and results. Surgery 59:472–482, 1966

93. Blaisdell FW, Lim RC: Liver resection. In Madding GF, Kennedy PA (eds): Major Problems in Clinical Surgery, pp 131–145. Philadelphia, WB Saunders, 1971

94. Theman T, Williams WG, Simpson JS et al: Tumor invasion of the upper inferior vena cava: The use of profound hypothermia and circulation arrest as a surgical adjunct. J Pediatr Surg 13:331–334, 1978

95. Offenstadt G, Huguet C, Gallot D et al: Hemodynamic monitoring during complete vascular exclusion for extensive hepatectomy. Surg Gynecol Obstet 146:709–713, 1978

96. Ragab AH, Sutow WW, Komp DM, Starling KA, Lyon GM, George S: Adriamycin in the treatment of childhood solid tumors. Cancer 36:1567–1571, 1975

97. Tan C, Rosen G, Ghavimi F, Haghbin M, Helson L, Wolner N, Murphy ML: Adriamycin (NSC-123127) in pediatric malignancies. Cancer Chemother Rep 6(Part 3):259–266, 1975

98. Selawry OS, Holland JF, Wolman IJ: Effect of veracristine on malignant solid tumors in children. Cancer Chemother Rep 52:497–500, 1968

99. Jacobs EM, Luce JK, Wood DA: Treatment of cancer with weekly intravenous 5 fluorouracil. Cancer 22:1233, 1968

100. Ikeda K, Suita S, Makagawaren A, Takabayasin K: Pre-operative chemotherapy for initially unresectable hepatoblastoma in children. Arch Surg 114:203–207, 1979

101. Weinblatt ME, Siegel SE, Siegel MM, Stanley P, Weitzman JJ: Preoperative chemotherapy for unresectable primary hepatic malignancies in children. Cancer 50:1061–1064, 1982

102. Andrassy RJ, Brennan LP, Siegel MM, Weitzmann JJ, Siegel SE, Stanley P, Mahour GH: Preopoperative chemotherapy for hepatoblastoma in children: Report of six cases. J Pediatr Surg 15:517–522, 1980

103. Douglas EC, Green AA, Wrenn E, Champion J, Shipp M, Pratt CB: Effective cisplatin (DDP) based chemotherapy in the treatment of hepatoblastoma. Med Pediatr Oncol 13:187–190, 1985

104. Kalifa C, Lemerle J, Caillaud MM, Valayer J: Respectability of childhood hepatoblastoma (HB) is improved by primary chemotherapy (CT) (abstr). Proc Am Soc Clin Oncol 3:C-308, 1984

105. Ortega JA, Woods W, Feusner J, Reaman G, Large B, Hammond D: Adriamycin continuous IV infusion for the treatment of childhood hepatic malignancies. In Proceedings of the First Symposium on Continuous Infusion Chemotherapy, p. 25, New York, 1985

106. Feusner J, Beach B, O'Leary M, Free E, Johnson LM, Betts J: Pulmonary metastatic disease does not preclude survival in children with hepatoblastoma. Proc Am Soc Clin Oncol 5:833, 1986

107. Chlebowski RT, Brzechwa-Adjukiewcz A, Cowden A, Block JB, Tong M, Chan KK: Doxorubicin (75 mg/m^2) for hepatocellular carcinoma: Clinical and pharmacokinetic results. Cancer Treatment Rep 68:487–491, 1984

108. Melia WM, Johnson PJ, Williams R: Induction of remission in hepatocellular carcinoma. A comparison of VP 16 with adriamycin. Cancer 51:206–210, 1983

109. Hochster HS, Green MD, Speyer J, Fazzini E, Blum R, Muggia FM: 4-Epidoxorubicin (Epirubicin): Activity in hepatocellular carcinoma. J Clin Oncol 3:1535–1540, 1985

110. Phillips R, Murikami K: Primary neoplasms of the liver: Results of radiation therapy. Cancer 13:714–720, 1960

twenty-seven

Wilms' Tumor (Nephroblastoma, Renal Embryoma)

Giulio J. D'Angio,
J. B. Beckwith, N. Breslow,
J. Finklestein, D. M. Green,
and P. Kelalis

The growth in understanding over the past 150 years of what has come to be termed Wilms' tumor and of its management traces the development of modern cancer clinical science.[1] The early advances were made by surgeons. This malignant childhood kidney tumor, first identified as a neoplasm by Rance in 1814,[2] was definitively described by a surgeon, Max Wilms.[3] Also known as the renal embryoma or nephroblastoma, this neoplasm remained a killer of children until other surgeons developed the necessary preoperative, operative, and postoperative techniques and management methods to permit the removal of these huge tumors from small patients. The tumor then was found to be radioresponsive, and postoperative irradiation became routine in many centers. The next stride forward came from the laboratory, where anticancer drugs were developed, and a third important modality—chemotherapy—was added to multimodality treatment. Later, major steps were taken by the cooperative group mechanism. Better and more refined treatments were developed and evaluated, and tumor characteristics were studied in detail for the accurate delineation of prognostic factors. Today, treatment can be limited to the bare essentials needed for the cure of most children predicted to be at low risk, thus lessening acute and late morbidity. The search goes on for better treatments for those at high risk.

EPIDEMIOLOGY

The incidence of Wilms' tumor is 7 per million children under age 16 per year.[4] Thus, approximately 1 child in 10,000 develops a Wilms' tumor. There is relatively little geographic variation in incidence, although rates appear to be slightly lower in Japan and Singapore and slightly higher in Scandinavia and some parts of Africa than they are in the United States, the United Kingdom, and Western Europe.[5] In 1978 Wilms' tumor represented 5% to 6% of childhood cancers in the United States, where the total incidence was estimated at 350 cases per year (see Chap. 1).[6]

Worldwide, the sex ratio is 1:1; however, there is some evidence that the frequency of Wilms' tumor may be slightly higher among females in the United States.[5,7] The distribution of age at diagnosis peaks at 2 to 3 years (Fig. 27-1). For 3442 National Wilms' Tumor Study (NWTS) cases found between 1969 and 1985, the median age was 36 months for males and 43 months for females with unilateral disease, and 23 months for males and 30 months for females with bilateral disease.

Reporting for all present and past members of the National Wilms' Tumor Study Committee, for whose help the authors are deeply grateful.

Supported in part by U.S. Public Health Service Grant CA-11722. Principal investigators at participating institutions also receive independent support from the National Cancer Institute.

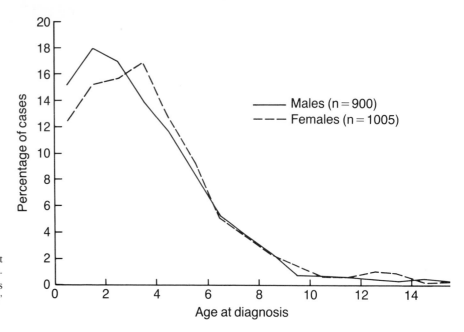

FIGURE 27-1. Frequency distribution of age at diagnosis for NWTS patients: 1969–1981. (Breslow NE, Beckwith JB: Epidemiological features of Wilms' tumor. Results of the National Wilms' Tumor Study. JNCI 68:427–436, 1982)

Wilms' tumor shows a strong association with certain congenital anomalies, notably aniridia, hemihypertrophy, and malformations of the genitalia (cryptorchidism, hypospadias, psuedohermaphroditism, and gonadal dysgenesis), especially in males.[7,8] Table 27-1 shows the numbers of cases and rates of occurrence of these anomalies observed in the NWTS. Aniridia and hemihypertrophy are extremely rare in the general population, and infants with either of these conditions should be screened carefully for Wilms' tumor. Wilms' tumor patients also have elevated rates of neurofibromatosis,[9] and the disease occurs in conjunction with the Beckwith–Wiedemann, Drash, and Perlman malformation syndromes.[10–12]

Several studies have compared parental occupations in Wilms' tumor patients to those of other childhood cancer patients or unaffected children, most with negative results.[13–15] Other research has indicated an increased risk for children whose fathers are occupationally exposed to hydrocarbons or lead[16] or work as mechanics or machinists.[17]

MOLECULAR BIOLOGY AND GENETICS

Significant advances have recently been made in understanding the molecular biology of Wilms' tumor. Although most patients with Wilms' tumor are karyotypically normal,[18] those with congenital aniridia frequently have a constitutional deletion at the 11p13 locus or have half-normal levels of the enzyme catalase, the gene for which has been mapped to this same region of the chromosome.[19,20] The deletion has also been reported in karyotypically normal Wilms' tumors by more sensitive analyses in patients without aniridia and with a normal constitutional karyotype (see Chaps. 2 and 3).[21,22] In most patients with this deletion in tumor cells, the uninvolved kidney and other somatic cells are not similarly affected. This suggests that genetic determinants on chromosome 11p can lead to the expression of Wilms' tumor when present in a hemizygous or homozygous state. Several workers have postulated that insulin-like growth factor II (ILGF II), the genetic locus for which is near the distal end of chromosome 11p, may be important in the pathogenesis of Wilms' tumor.[23–25] An 11p deletion was recently reported in a small nodule thought to be a precursor of Wilms' tumor.[26] Other cytogenetic abnormalities have been seen in occasional cases. There have been two re-

Table 27-1

Congenital Anomalies in 3442 NWTS Patients Registered During 1969–1985

Anomaly	Number of Cases	Prevalance (per 1000)
Aniridia	26	7.6
Hemihypertrophy	112	32.6
Cryptorchidism	53	32.7*
Hypospadias	37	22.8*
Other genital	24	7.0

* Rates for males only.

ported patients with Wilms' tumor and trisomy 18,[27,28] a condition known to be associated with an increased prevalence of precursor lesions of Wilms' tumor.[29]

Molecular analysis using DNA probes has suggested that expression of a recessive mutant allele at the 11p13 locus is involved in the development of Wilms' tumor; the same mechanism may play a role in hepatoblastoma and rhabdomyosarcoma.[22,28] Evidently, an abnormal somatic segregation event results in production of a cell that is homozygous or hemizygous for the mutant allele.

Case reports of the familial occurrence of Wilms' tumor are not uncommon.[30,31] Approximately 1% of NWTS cases have one or more family members with the disease (Table 27-2).[7] In view of the absence of parental consanguinity in such families, the mode of inheritance is generally thought to be autosomal dominant, with variable penetrance and expressivity.[32] Few of the kindreds reported in the literature involve affected parents; more often, the disease occurs in siblings, cousins, or other relatives. The NWTS experience is similar. The rate of synchronous and metachronous bilaterality among NWTS familial cases is no different from that for the NWTS population as a whole, and the mean age at diagnosis is intermediate between, although not statistically distinguishable from, the mean ages for unilateral and bilateral cases.[33] By contrast, familial cases reported in the literature have an increased occurrence of bilaterality and younger age at diagnosis compared to sporadic

Table 27-2
Occurrence of Familial Wilms' Tumor in 3442 NWTS Patients Registered During 1969–1985

Closest Affected Relative	Number of Cases*
Sibling	15 (8)
First cousin	11 (8)
Parent	5
Aunt/uncle	5
First cousin, once removed	3
Second cousin, once removed	2 (2)
Second cousin	1
Total	42

* Numbers in parentheses are numbers of cases where *both* the index case and the affected relative are NWTS patients.

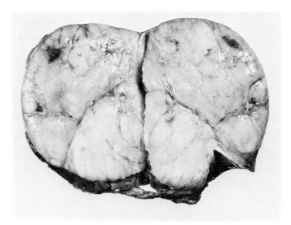

FIGURE 27-2. Typical Wilms' tumor, showing the uniform, pale, bulging cut surface and the sharp border between tumor and renal parenchyma.

cases.[32,34] The concepts of delayed mutation and host resistance have been advanced to explain the occurrence of pedigrees in which distant cousins with Wilms' tumor are related by unaffected family members.[32]

Recent molecular and cytogenetic findings lend support to a two-stage mutational model for the origin of Wilms' tumor that was developed earlier from epidemiologic data on the age distributions in different patient categories.[34] According to this model, a tumor may arise from two (or more) events. The first is either a germ cell or somatic cell mutation (*e.g.,* a recessive deletion at the 11p13 locus). The second event (or events) is always postzygotic (somatic); for instance, chromosomal nondisjunction or somatic recombination. Hereditary cases—those in which the initial mutation is germinal—are likely to be multicentric or bilateral and to be diagnosed at a younger age than sporadic cases. Nodular renal blastema, which is found in roughly 15% to 30% of patients with Wilms' tumor and is especially frequent in bilateral cases,[7,35] has been suggested as a precursor lesion in individuals who carry the "Wilms' " gene (see Chap. 3).[36]

The fraction of Wilms' tumor cases that are of hereditary origin was originally estimated to be 38%, but this has since been revised downward to 15% to 20%.[37] If the two-stage model is correct, one would expect to see increasing numbers of Wilms' tumors in the offspring of survivors of the disease, especially if they had the familial, bilateral, or other "hereditary" form. However, a survey of 59 children of 36 patients with unilateral Wilms' tumor did not identify a single case of cancer.[38] Thus, direct confirmation of the autosomal dominant inheritance pattern predicted by the two-stage model awaits systematic follow-up of offspring from survivors of the NWTS and other large series.

PATHOLOGY

The earliest known specimen of Wilms' tumor is on display in the Hunterian Museum of the Royal College of Surgeons in London, England.[39] This specimen of bilateral renal tumors from a young infant was prepared by John Hunter, who died in 1793, and is in an excellent state of preservation.

Wilms' tumor is characterized by tremendous histologic diversity, displaying a wide variety of cell and tissue types (see Chap. 6). It is in part because of this diversity that many terms have been used to describe this tumor. By 1975, at least 85 synonyms for the lesion had appeared in the literature.[40] The

terms nephroblastoma and Wilms' tumor now have achieved almost universal usage. Although the former is preferable for a number of reasons, the latter is in more general use.

Wilms' tumor is thought to be composed of, or derived from, primitive metanephric blastema. In addition to expressing a variety of cell types and aggregation patterns seen in the normally developing kidney, these neoplasms often contain tissues not found in the normal metanephros, such as skeletal muscle, cartilage, and squamous epithelium. It is thought that these heterotopic cell types reflect primitive developmental potentials of metanephric blastema that are not expressed in normal nephrogenesis.

This discussion emphasizes aspects of the gross and microscopic anatomy of Wilms' tumor that have clinical relevance in the context of modern therapy. Most of what follows is derived from the experience of the NWTS Pathology Center.[41,42] The center's collection of thousands of cases has enabled clinicopathologic correlative studies on a scale that was not formerly possible. Other childhood renal tumors are not discussed in detail unless they are related to, or frequently confused with, Wilms' tumor.

Gross Appearances and Patterns of Extension

Although most Wilms' tumors are unicentric lesions, a substantial number of specimens arise multifocally in the kidney. Of 1905 NWTS cases, 103 (5.4%) involved both kidneys either at presentation or subsequently, and an additional 133 (7%) were multicentric unilateral tumors.[7] There is no predilection for one side, and the tumor apparently may arise anywhere within the organ, which is usually markedly distorted by the neoplasm. Extrarenal Wilms' tumors are rare and generally occur in the retroperitoneum adjacent to, but unconnected with, the kidney. Others have occurred in the pelvis or inguinal region. The origins of extrarenal Wilms' tumor are diverse and are thought to include displaced metanephric elements, mesonephric remnants, and teratomas.

Most Wilms' tumors have a uniform pale gray or tan color on section (Fig. 27-2). Calcification is not often present, but hemorrhage and necrosis may impart a variegated appearance. Cysts are commonly encountered and may be a dominant feature. Not uncommonly, especially in infants, a polypoid extension into the pyelocalyceal lumen may resemble botryoid rhabdomyosarcoma growth patterns.[43] Tumors with a predominance of differentiating stromal elements may have a relatively firmer texture, but most specimens are notably soft and friable. This may contribute to the local spread of tumor cells when a tumor is ruptured either before or during operation.

Wilms' tumor usually appears as a sharply demarcated, relatively spherical mass. The border with the adjacent renal parenchyma is of the "pushing" type, and the tumor is usually enclosed by a distinct intrarenal pseudocapsule composed of compressed, atrophic renal tissues. This feature may help to distinguish Wilms' tumor from mesoblastic nephroma, clear cell sarcoma, rhabdoid tumors, and renal lymphomas. Exceptions to the pushing type of border are often seen when the tumor is composed of poorly cohesive blastemal cells, which may exhibit an infiltrative pattern at the periphery of the lesion.

Histology

The most distinctive microscopic feature of Wilms' tumor is its structural diversity. The classic pattern is triphasic, including blastemal, epithelial, and stromal cells (Fig. 27-3). Usually, these elements seem to recapitulate various stages of normal renal embryogenesis, but heterotopic cell types are commonly observed.[40,41] However, not all specimens are triphasic. Biphasic patterns (e.g., blastemal and stromal cells) are commonly encountered, and some specimens consisting predominantly or exclusively of one cell type are commonly included in the Wilms' tumor category if the cell type in question is one that is commonly seen in more conventional Wilms' tumor.[40] The interested reader is referred elsewhere for a more exhaustive histologic description of Wilms' tumor.[40,44,45]

Despite its diversity, childhood Wilms' tumor rarely presents a diagnostic problem. The primitive blastemal cells usually show distinctive patterns of aggregation into sharply outlined nodules or serpentine cords that are not likely to be confused with the other "small round blue cell" tumors of childhood.[42,44] Occasionally, there may be difficulty distinguishing a monophasic epithelial Wilms' tumor with papillary or tubular differentiation from a relatively undifferentiated specimen of renal cell carcinoma.[42] This problem is rarely encountered in childhood renal tumors, although in the adolescent or adult patient, it occasionally poses a challenge to the

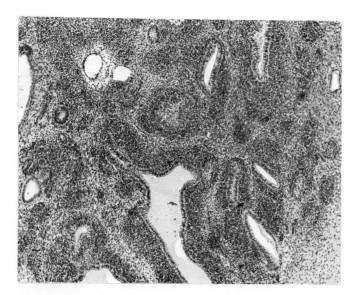

FIGURE 27-3. Triphasic Wilms' tumor, with well-defined tubules surrounded by dense clusters of blastemal cells and zones of pale-staining stromal differentiation. (H & E × 60)

surgical pathologist. It has been suggested that such tumors provide a conceptual link between two neoplastic entities that are usually, but not always, quite distinct from one another.[42] The histologic distinction between Wilms' tumor and the "sarcomatous" renal tumors of unfavorable histologic type is discussed later.

Special Studies

Because Wilms' tumor infrequently presents difficulties in recognition, the role of ultrastructural, immunohistochemical, and other special diagnostic studies is restricted. When a very small biopsy specimen is obtained, however, or the lesion is extremely undifferentiated, such studies may be helpful. Wilms' tumor is usually characterized ultrastructurally by numerous well-developed desmosomes, prominent cilia, and distinctive flocculent densities surrounding the tumor cells.[46,47] Immunohistochemistry is primarily of use in ruling out other primitive childhood tumors, such as neuroblastoma.[48–50]

Histopathology and Prognosis

The structural diversity of Wilms' tumor presents a potentially fertile field for exploring relationships between histopathology and the natural history of the tumor. Several workers have suggested that prominent tubular differentiation in a Wilms' tumor is associated with an improved outcome.[51–53] It is difficult to evaluate this hypothesis because of the very high relapse-free survival rates obtained in recent years. As cure rates increase, one becomes progressively less able to discriminate the most favorable variants of a tumor system, and only the most unfavorable variants remain as a distinctive subgroup.[54] It is therefore not surprising that analyses in the NWTS Pathology Center have identified markers associated with poor outcome but none associated with exceptionally favorable outcome. The outlook for children with Wilms' tumor with the histologic patterns so far described is good with modern therapies; they have therefore been termed tumors of "favorable histology."

The analysis of NWTS-1 showed that Wilms' tumors in which the tumor cells had extreme nuclear atypia (anaplasia), were associated with a high rate of relapse and death.[41] Monomorphous, apparently sarcomatous, tumors previously confused with Wilms' tumor were also identified as distinct and highly unfavorable clinicopathologic entities. Although these latter lesions have continued to be studied on the NWTS, they are currently viewed as tumor categories distinct from Wilms' tumor. These sarcomatous tumors (clear cell sarcoma of kidney and rhabdoid tumor) are discussed below.

ANAPLASIA. This cytologic change is a major indicator of poor outcome. Relapses and deaths with tumor present in 49 NWTS-1 and NWTS-2 Stage I, II, and III children with anaplastic tumors were 27 (55%) and 23 (47%), respectively. In contrast, these figures for 720 cohort patients without anaplastic neoplasms were 101 (14%) and 39 (5%), respectively.[55] The only exception is that Stage I anaplastic Wilms' tumor is associated with relapse and cure rates similar to those for nonanaplastic, "favorable histology" (FH) Stage I Wilms' tumor.[55] This finding suggests that Stage I anaplastic Wilms' tumor is not likely to be associated with occult micrometastases early in its course.

Anaplasia is recognized by the presence of three cytologic abnormalities, categorized by the NWTS as [1] obvious hyperdiploid mitotic figures, [2] threefold or greater nuclear enlargement, and [3] hyperchromasia of enlarged nuclei (Fig. 27-4A,B). These abnormalities are markers of extreme hyper-

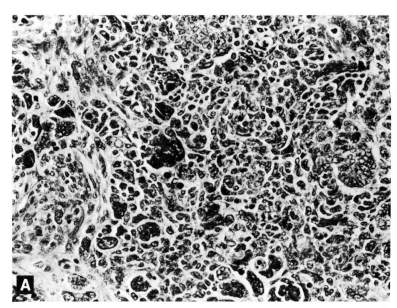
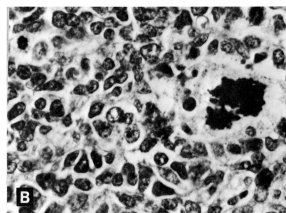

FIGURE 27-4. A. Anaplastic Wilms' tumor with several enlarged, hyperchromatic, bizarre nuclei. (H & E × 125) **B.** Anaplastic Wilms' tumor, showing markedly enlarged, hyperploid mitotic figure. (H & E × 400)

ploidy. Newer, more sensitive measures of ploidy, notably flow cytometry, promise to enhance the detection of prognostically significant changes in nuclear DNA content.[56,57]

Anaplasia was present in 4.5% of cases entered on NWTS-3 (unpublished data) and was related to patient age. It is rare in the first 2 years of life (8 of 362, or 2% of such patients), and then increases to a relatively stable rate of about 13% in those age 5 or older.[55] It is significantly more frequent in black than in white patients.[55]

Anaplasia in only one or a few small foci of a Wilms' tumor is sufficient to impart a markedly worse prognosis, and Stage II, III, and IV Wilms' tumor specimens must therefore be sampled thoroughly. The NWTS Pathology Center recommends that a minimum of one generous section be obtained for each centimeter of tumor diameter, and that each individual tumor be sampled in multicentric or bilateral cases. Meticulous attention to details of tissue preservation and slide preparation is necessary. Poor fixation, sectioning, or staining can easily lead to false-positive or false-negative interpretations.

CLEAR CELL SARCOMA OF THE KIDNEY (CCSK). Although not currently thought to be a Wilms' tumor variant, CCSK is an important entity to consider. Its site of origin and age distribution are identical to Wilms' tumor, yet it is associated with a significantly higher rate of relapse and death than FH Wilms' tumor. CCSK also displays a distinctively high rate of skeletal metastases. This variant was first recognized in the literature by Kidd in 1970,[58] and in 1978 was independently identified by pathologists of the NWTS and the U.K. Medical Research Council Nephroblastoma trial.[41,59] The descriptive term CCSK was used by the NWTS, whereas the British workers referred to "bone-metastasizing renal tumour of childhood" (BMRTC). Several points concerning CCSK deserve emphasis.

In contrast to Stage I anaplastic Wilms' tumor, Stage I CCSK is associated with a very high rate of tumor relapse, suggesting that micrometastases occur early with this tumor. For example, in NWTS-2, five of seven Stage I CCSK children relapsed and died with tumor.

The use of Adriamycin seems to be associated with a significantly improved outcome for CCSK.[60] This underscores the importance of correctly identifying CCSK and places a significant responsibility on pathologists.

CCSK has been found to be associated with brain as well as bone metastases.[60]

Most CCSK specimens have a distinct and easily recognized histologic appearance, but a number of variant patterns, such as epithelioid, spindling, myxoid, and cystic patterns, invite confusion with Wilms' tumor or other tumor types.[61-64] The reader is referred elsewhere for detailed descriptions and illustrations of both the classic and variant patterns.[42,59] An example of the former is shown in Figure 27-5.

RHABDOID TUMOR OF KIDNEY (RTK). A distinctive and highly malignant tumor type, RTK was identified for the first time in 1978 by NWTS pathologists.[41] The neoplasm, previously confused with Wilms' tumor, is a monomorphous tumor like CCSK. RTK tumor cells, unlike those of CCSK, characteristically have prominent acidophilic cytoplasm that often resembles that of myoblasts but is negative for ultrastructural or other markers of skeletal muscle. The term "rhabdomyosarcomatoid," used in the original description, was shortened to "rhabdoid" in a subsequent paper.[65] Figure 27-6 illustrates its typical histologic appearances. The cell of origin for this distinctive tumor remains unknown. It is not a variant of Wilms' tumor and will not be encountered as a focal change in a conventional Wilms' tumor. Several points regarding this important entity deserve emphasis.

RTK is characteristically seen in the infant or very young child. The median age of cases seen in the NWTS Pathology Center is 13 months, with a range from 2 months to 5 years.

It is associated with relapse and death rates of over 80%, and thus is one of the most malignant neoplasms in the pediatric population. The more aggressive therapeutic protocols

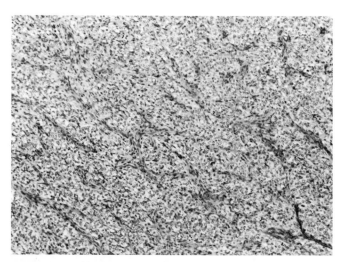

FIGURE 27-5. "Classic" clear cell sarcoma of the kidney. Cords and nests of pale-stained tumor cells are separated by an evenly spaced network of small vessels. (H & E × 60).

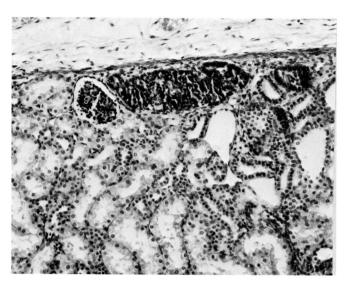

FIGURE 27-7. Persistent blastemal tissue beneath renal capsule of an infant. This is one of the forms of perilobar nephroblastomatosis. (H & E × 123)

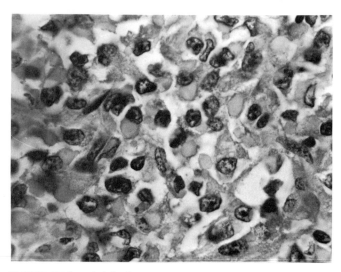

FIGURE 27-6. Rhabdoid tumor. Note prominent nucleoli in many cells and conspicuous globular hyaline inclusions in cytoplasm. Ultrastructurally, the inclusions are composed of whorled masses of intermediate filaments. (H & E × 625)

used in NWTS-3 did not significantly improve the outlook for patients with this tumor. Stage I tumors, as for CCSK, are associated with a high rate of relapse and death from advancing tumor, and, unlike CCSK, this pattern has not been altered by more aggressive therapies.[66]

Several cases have been reported in which apparently separate primary neuroectodermal tumors of the brain have developed in children with the rhabdoid tumor (RT).[67]

A few clear cases of RT do occur in extrarenal sites, but the majority of extrarenal RT and RTK in patients older than 5 years represent other neoplasms. They may mimic RTK closely, both at the light microscopic and ultrastructural level. Many of these "pseudorhabdoid" entities can, however, be identified by immunohistochemistry or other techniques to be carcinomas, melanomas, histiocytic tumors, or myosarcomas. Immunohistochemical studies of RT have not to date clarified the cell of origin.[68]

NEPHROBLASTOMATOSIS. The existence of precursor lesions to Wilms' tumor has been recognized for many years.[27,40] They take the form of small, usually microscopic clusters of blastemal cells, tubules, or stromal cells that are generally situated at the periphery of the renal lobe (Fig. 27-7). The nephroblastomatosis issue is an increasingly complex one. For example, a variant that occurs within the deeper cortex or medulla has been termed "intralobar nephroblastomatosis," to contrast with the more commonly encountered "perilobar" form. One or both of these variants are encountered in the renal parenchyma of approximately 25% of Wilms' tumor cases, and are present in about 1% of random perinatal postmortem examinations.[40] The neoplastic activation of these precursor lesions may affect a solitary focus, presumably in a single cell, giving rise to multicentric or bilateral Wilms' tumor. Diffuse overgrowth of these lesions may produce a thick "rind" of blastemal or tubular cells that enlarge the kidney but preserve its original shape.

Nephroblastomatosis is of great theoretical interest in the pathogenesis of Wilms' tumor and is also of practical importance. When multifocal precursor lesions are found in both kidneys at initial exploration or in a kidney removed for Wilms' tumor, there is an increased likelihood of subsequent tumor formation in the remaining parenchyma. This finding should be considered an indication for particularly close follow-up of the remaining kidney substance by physical examinations and appropriate imaging techniques (see Imaging Studies).

CONGENITAL MESOBLASTIC NEPHROMA (CMN). This term was applied by Bolande and colleagues in 1969 to a distinctive renal neoplasm of infancy.[69] It was characterized predominantly by bundles of spindle cells resembling fibroblasts or smooth muscle cells, with an interdigitating margin at the periphery that often extended a considerable distance into the renal parenchyma or the perirenal soft tissues. The frequent presence of tubules lined by basophilic cells in the lesion raised the possibility that this was a "cytodifferentiated variant of Wilms' tumor."[69] The most important aspect of these findings was the recognition that CMN was usually curable by nephrectomy alone. The appearance of a typical neonatal CMN is illustrated in Figure 27-8.

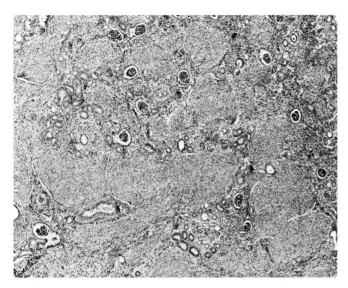

FIGURE 27-8. Congenital mesoblastic nephroma, showing typical pattern of extension into surrounding kidney tissue. (H & E × 30)

The subject of CMN was soon complicated by the recognition that a few such lesions could recur or even metastasize, and by the observation that a considerable proportion of specimens showed either focal or diffuse increases in cellularity, with high mitotic rates.[70] Some authors have suggested that the so-called cellular or atypical CMN should be treated as a potentially malignant tumor.[71] However, a review of all known cases of recurrent or metastatic CMN demonstrated that the cellular CMN is not associated with adverse outcome in infants younger than 3 months, with the exception of one instance in which incomplete removal of tumor was documented.[72] These considerations suggest the following conclusions:

Because of its characteristic tendency to extend into perirenal tissues, CMN deserves a radical surgical approach, with efforts to secure a wide margin of uninvolved tissue on all aspects of the specimen. Pathologists should carefully document the state of all resection margins.

Cellular CMN apparently is not of adverse prognostic significance in infants younger than 3 months. In older infants, the demonstration of dense cellularity and high mitotic rate is of some concern, because a few patients with such lesions have experienced local recurrence or distant metastases.

RENAL CELL CARCINOMA. In children, this tumor has a histologic appearance entirely similar to that seen in adults (see Chap. 35).[73]

PATTERNS OF SPREAD

Local

The first signs of spread beyond the tumor pseudocapsule are usually found in the renal sinus or intrarenal blood and lymphatic vessels. Tumors exhibiting these features are currently eligible for Stage I on the NWTS if the sinus infiltration does not extend beyond the hilar plane of the kidney and the vascular extension is limited to the renal parenchyma or small vessels of the renal sinus. Unless tumor cells are incorporated into a thrombus, are attached to vessel walls, or distend the vessel

lumen, one cannot be certain that they were not artifactually displaced into vessels during specimen manipulation.

Penetration through the renal capsule is the next most common site of extrarenal spread of Wilms' tumor. Here, one may see either tissue or vascular invasion, or both. The presence of tumor cells in perirenal fat is a criterion for up-staging the lesion. Not uncommonly, there is an inflammatory or granulation tissue response in perirenal connective tissues, yet penetration of the renal capsule by tumor cells cannot be demonstrated. This "inflammatory pseudocapsule" is most often associated with either hemorrhage into perirenal tissues or extensive necrosis of tumor just beneath the capsule. The presence of an inflammatory pseudocapsule is currently acceptable for Stage I tumors in the NWTS, as long as capsular penetration by tumor cells is not demonstrated. This finding is the usual explanation for cases in which the surgeon encounters adhesions of Wilms' tumor to adjacent organs but the pathologist, finding the specimen to be enclosed in fibrous connective tissue, correctly assigns a Stage I designation.

A recent study demonstrated that four features related to the degree of extension of tumor within the kidney were associated with relapses in Stage I FH Wilms' tumor.[74] These included the presence of an inflammatory pseudocapsule, extensive infiltration of the renal capsule, involvement of the renal sinus, and tumor in intrarenal vessels. When all four of these features were absent, there were no relapses attributable to the primary tumor in NWTS-3. The authors suggested that this subgroup of Stage I Wilms' tumor might be an appropriate study population for evaluating the efficacy of nephrectomy alone.

Distant

The most common sites of metastases of Wilms' tumor are the lungs, the regional nodes, and the liver. Of NWTS patients presenting with hematogenous metastases at diagnosis (Stage IV), the lungs were the only site of such metastases in approximately 85%. The liver was involved in perhaps 15% of these cases.[75] Other metastatic sites are distinctly uncommon in Wilms' tumor.

CLINICAL PRESENTATION

Typically, the child is found to have an asymptomatic mass (Fig. 27-9A). It is common for the tumor to be discovered by a visiting relative who feels it while bathing the child or notices an abdominal protuberance. Because the growth is insidious, the parents often fail to detect the gradual enlargement or are gratified to think their child is well-fed (see Chap. 5).

Associated signs and symptoms, each found in 20% to 30% of cases, include malaise, pain, and either microscopic or gross hematuria.[76] Sir William Osler provided the first description from North America of the signs and symptoms of the tumor that Wilms described 20 years later.[77] Hypertension, present in about 25% of cases, has been attributed to an increase in renin activity.[78]

A characteristic presentation for a subset of Wilms' tumor patients was described by Ramsey and coworkers.[79] Distinguishing features are rapid abdominal enlargement, anemia, hypertension, and sometimes fever. These may be associated with egg-shell-type calcification visible on plain radiographs of the abdomen. The syndrome appears to be related to sudden subcapsular hemorrhage, with the consequences described above.

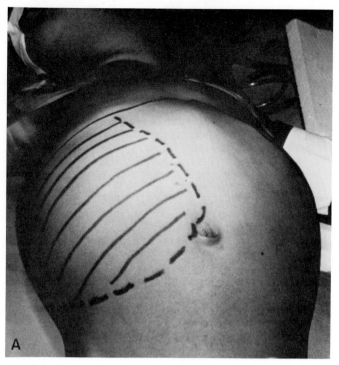

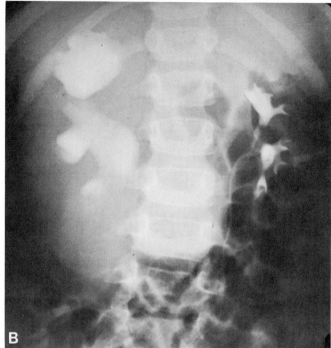

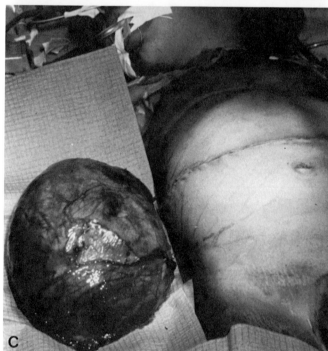

FIGURE 27-9 **A.** Obvious flank mass in a 7-year-old boy. **B.** Excretory urogram, showing distortion of intrinsic urinary pathways caused by an intrarenal mass. **C.** Tumor after removal, showing massive size relative to abdomen.

METHODS OF DIAGNOSIS

Differential Diagnosis

The chief differential diagnosis lies in distinguishing Wilms' tumor from neuroblastoma (see Chaps. 6 and 28). The distinction is usually relatively easy: Wilms' tumors, being intrarenal, show characteristic intrinsic displacement of the urinary collecting systems (Fig. 27-9B). Neuroblastoma, arising in the adrenal gland or the paravertebral sympathetic ganglia, displaces rather than distorts the kidney (Fig. 27-10). Neuroblas-

toma can, however, arise within the kidney substance, and preoperative distinction is then difficult if not impossible.[80] This remains the most common cause of error in preoperative diagnoses, accounting for 11 of the 32 such instances recorded in NWTS-3.[66]

Benign processes, such as multicystic kidneys, renal carbuncles, and hematomas, can lead to confusion.[80] Multilocular cysts can be strongly suspected on the basis of ultrasonagraphic findings. The so-called cystic, partially differentiated, nephroblastoma cannot be distinguished by any means other than pathologic examination.[81] This entity is characterized by

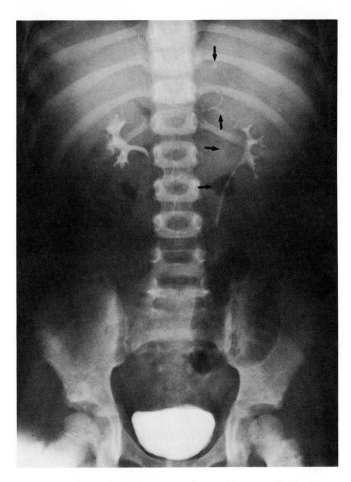

FIGURE 27-10. Left-sided suprarenal neuroblastoma. Unlike Figure 27-9B, the excretory urogram here shows displacement of renal collecting system by an extrinsic mass (*arrows,* which also indicate characteristic punctate ["pepper and salt"] calcifications).

small nests of Wilms' tumor within the walls of what otherwise seem to be typical cysts. Hematomas and carbuncles usually do not cause diagnostic problems, having characteristic clinical signs, symptoms, and history.

Less common intrarenal neoplasms include the mesoblastic nephroma, renal cell carcinoma, clear cell sarcoma, and rhabdoid tumor. Other entities that have been infrequently confused with Wilms' tumor include fibrosarcoma, rhabdomyosarcoma, adrenal carcinoma, hemangiopericytoma, malignant neurogenic tumor, hepatoblastoma, and non-Hodgkin's lymphoma.[66,76] Mesoblastic nephromas occur predominantly in males and in infants (median age = 2 months).[82] Rhabdoid tumors also tend to occur in male infants; 10 of 21 patients reported by Palmer and Sutow were in the first year of life and an additional 6 were younger than 2 years.[83] Renal cell carcinomas can occur at any age. A recent review of patients younger than 21 years with this diagnosis found an age range of 14 months to 19 years (median = 12 years); males were affected more often.[73]

Workup

Careful physical examination should take note of hemihypertrophy, aniridia, or the elements of the Beckwith–Wiedemann syndrome. Distended anterior abdominal veins may indicate

occlusion of the inferior vena cava by tumor thrombus. The mass itself is felt in the flank and must not be confused with the spleen in left-sided cases. Fixed tumors arising in or crossing the midline are more likely to be neuroblastomas; a displaceable mass crossing the midline may well be Wilms' tumor. A painful site beyond the abdomen (*e.g.,* a long bone) may indicate the presence of metastases and suggests the diagnosis of CCSK. Cerebral signs could be the result of brain metastases, which are seldom seen initially with favorable histology tumors but can develop in children with rhabdoid tumor or CCSK. Laboratory evaluation includes a complete peripheral blood cell count and urinalysis for evidence of hematuria.

Imaging Studies

Imaging studies preoperatively and in follow-up should be designed to assist the clinicians managing the child (see also Chap. 7). They must therefore take into account the known characteristics of the tumors at presentation and of metastatic patterns based on the tumor type. This discussion encompasses the following entities: FH Wilms' tumor, anaplastic Wilms' tumor, CCSK, RTK, mesoblastic nephroma, and renal cell carcinoma.

Renal Studies at Diagnosis

Imaging studies initially should be restricted to those necessary to establish the presence of an intrarenal space-occupying lesion. They should also provide information known to be of value to the surgeon and to the radiation therapist should postoperative radiation therapy be indicated. Data of importance to the surgeon include the presence and function of the opposite kidney, whether it is involved with tumor, and the presence and extent of intravascular tumor propagation (tumor thrombus). Excretory urography and careful real-time ultrasonography usually suffice for these purposes.

EXCRETORY UROGRAM. This study identifies the size and location of the tumor on the affected side and relates these findings to normal anatomic landmarks such as the vertebral bodies (see Fig. 27-9B). It also delineates the opposite kidney: whether it is present, whether it functions, and whether it is normal in configuration and outline. All of these findings are of value to radiation therapists, some of whom believe they can define their fields with greater accuracy by using this information rather than relying on the single reconstructed frontal view obtained by contrast-enhanced computed tomography (CT).

INFRADIAPHRAGMATIC ULTRASONOGRAPHY. This study gives the additional needed information.[84] Meticulously performed ultrasonography permits the examiner to establish whether there is a tumor thrombus in the ipsilateral or both renal veins and the inferior vena cava and, if so, whether it extends into the right atrium of the heart (Fig. 27-11A–E). Real-time ultrasonography also indicates whether the thrombus is attached to the walls. The stage of the primary lesion is immediately changed from Stage II if the thrombus is free-floating to Stage III if it is attached to the vessel wall. This information may influence subsequent management, especially in tumors considered inoperable at outset. Ultrasonography also again outlines the kidneys, their shapes and configurations, and indicates whether tumor is present on one or on both sides.

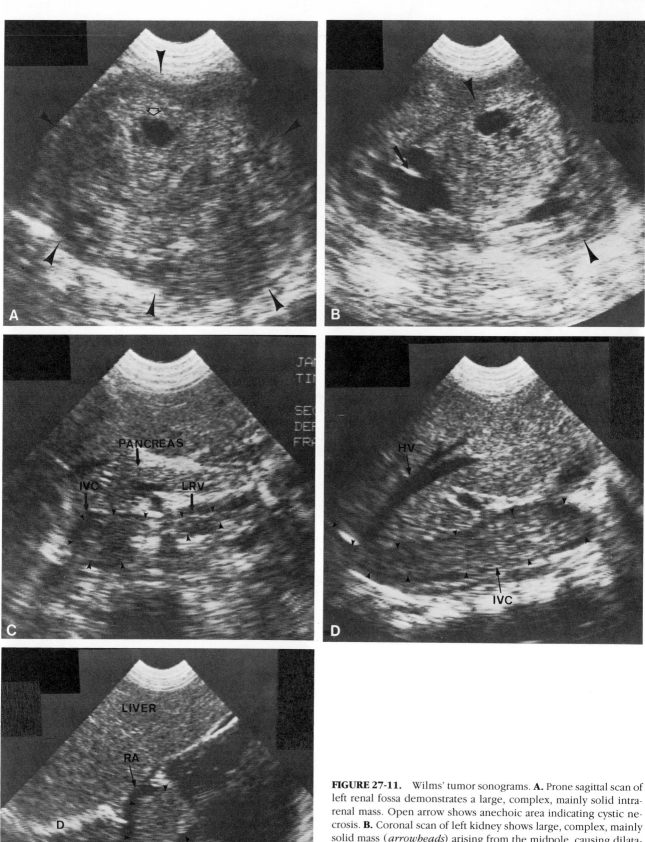

FIGURE 27-11. Wilms' tumor sonograms. **A.** Prone sagittal scan of left renal fossa demonstrates a large, complex, mainly solid intrarenal mass. Open arrow shows anechoic area indicating cystic necrosis. **B.** Coronal scan of left kidney shows large, complex, mainly solid mass (*arrowheads*) arising from the midpole, causing dilatation and splaying of the intrarenal collecting system (*arrow*). **C.** Transverse scan of inferior vena cava (*IVC*) and left renal vein (*LRV*) shows vessels almost entirely filled with echogenic tumor thrombus (*small arrowheads*). **D.** Sagittal view of inferior vena cava (*IVC*) demonstrates large intracaval thrombus extending superiorly to above the diaphragm. HV = hepatic vein (*arrowheads*). **E.** Subxyphoid transverse view of right atrium (RA) demonstrates extension of tumor thrombus into the heart. D = diaphragm (*arrowheads*).

INFRADIAPHRAGMATIC CT SCAN. The information added by this examination is not generally considered essential for patient management (see also Chap. 7). Like Ultrasonography, it can provide considerable detailed information regarding the existence of tumor thrombi, enlarged lymph nodes, the presence of cystic or necrotic spaces within the tumor, and the tumor's relation to adjoining structures.[84] Opacified CT also establishes function in the opposite kidney. The NWTS Committee concludes that this information can be derived from the excretory urogram and careful ultrasonography and that CT scanning of the kidney does not add information of sufficient value at diagnosis to make its routine use worthwhile. CT adds expense, is invasive, often requires sedation of the patient, and can delay definitive management when scheduling is a problem in busy radiology departments. This is not to deny the undisputed value of CT in problem cases where radiographic or ultrasonographic evidence is equivocal.[84]

MAGNETIC RESONANCE IMAGING (MRI). A relatively new method, MRI has unknown potential in Wilms' tumor. It may prove to be the single most valuable study, avoiding the need for excretory urography and ultrasonography.[85,86] MRI can delineate the anatomy and provide the needed relationships; it is also noninvasive. However, it is costly, usually requires sedation, does not provide evidence of function, and is not yet generally available. Additional study is needed before accurate conclusions can be drawn.[86]

Other Investigations at Diagnosis

LUNGS. Radiographic examination of the chest in four projections (posteroanterior, lateral, and both obliques) provides the necessary information. Small lesions are usually detectable on such studies, which suffice to establish whether the disease is Stage IV for practical purposes. CT scans can detect small nodules that are not visible on the standard radiographic views, but this can be a mixed blessing. A recent review of the NWTS files has been updated by Fernbach and colleagues,[87] who found that two of six biopsied NWTS-3 patients with nodules visible only on CT scanning had non-neoplastic lesions such as focal atalectasis. The physician is therefore faced with decisions concerning the need for biopsy proof of densities present on CT in one or both lungs. A positive result on one side is sufficient, but a negative result in the face of scattered unilateral or bilateral lesions poses difficult management decisions. For example, in Stage IV patients with tumors of any histology, irradiation of the entire thorax is given in the NWTS, and Adriamycin is added to dactinomycin (formerly actinomycin-D) and vincristine.[87,88] There is thus the potential for late complications in the heart and lungs.[88-90] The NWTS Committee therefore does not advocate routine CT scans of the chest at diagnosis in low-risk children. The survival for Stage I and II patients was excellent before CT scanners became generally available, and remains so.[66,91,92]

LIVER. There is no doubt that small, deeply placed metastases not detectable at surgery can be found by CT scanning.[84] However, the images can be confusing and, even when ultrasonography is added, it may not be possible to distinguish between cystic and solid lesions.[93] NWTS data suggest that the yield will be small and does not warrant routine CT scanning.

SKELETON AND BRAIN. Imaging studies of bone and brain are not advocated as part of the routine initial workup in the absence of signs or symptoms.

Immediate Postoperative Imaging Studies

The appropriate investigations after operation depend on the final histologic evaluation. If the neoplasm is found to be a renal cell carcinoma, a mesoblastic nephroma, or a Wilms' tumor of either favorable histology or anaplastic type, no additional imaging studies are needed beyond those listed above. Additional examinations are indicated for children with either CCSK or RTK.

CCSK. Clear cell sarcoma tends to metastasize to the skeleton and the brain.[59,60] Therefore, bone scans, radiographic skeletal surveys, or both are indicated, along with CT or MRI of the brain.

RTK. Rhabdoid tumor of the kidney is associated with brain metastases and with independent, second brain tumors of the primitive neuroectodermal type. Brain CT scans, MRI, or both are therefore indicated in the child with RTK.[67,94]

STAGING

The extent of disease at diagnosis and at surgery has long been known to be an important prognostic criterion, and various staging systems have been proposed that incorporate clinicopathologic elements considered to be important indicators.[95,96] The grouping method used by the NWTS in its first and second clinical trials evolved to the staging system used thereafter, when a retrospective validation indicated that the staging criteria provided better risk estimates.[97] The two systems are shown in Table 27-3.

PROGNOSTIC CONSIDERATIONS

Prognostic factors change as treatments become more effective.[54] For example, age at diagnosis, found to be important in NWTS-1, is no longer a factor.[98] Unfavorable histology, distant metastases (chiefly to the lung), and lymph node involvement remain adverse discriminants, the last mentioned as first documented by Jereb and Eklund years ago.[75,99]

GENERAL SURGICAL PRINCIPLES

Surgical extirpation remains the cornerstone of Wilms' tumor therapy.[100] The surgeon's responsibility is to assess the tumor spread precisely so that accurate staging and proper treatment will follow. Appropriate operative techniques must be used to remove the tumor without causing spread or spill by inadvertently rending the tumor capsule (see Chap. 10).

Technique

It is important to make a generous incision to afford maximal exposure. A transverse-transperitoneal incision with division of the ipsilateral rectus muscle is adequate in most cases. A formal thoracoabdominal incision is rarely needed, the exceptions being when very large tumors involve the upper pole and when excision of concurrent ipsilateral pulmonary metastatic lesions is planned.[101] Once the peritoneal cavity is entered, the extent of tumor should be assessed and the liver, periaortic area, and vena cava palpated to determine whether primary excision is advisable. The flank approach should never be used because adequate staging cannot be performed and, most im-

Table 27-3
*Clinicopathologic Staging**

Group	Stage*
I. Tumor limited to the kidney and completely resected. The surface of the renal capsule is intact. The tumor was not ruptured before or during removal. There is no residual tumor apparent beyond the margins of resection.	I. Tumor limited to the kidney and completely excised. The surface of the renal capsule is intact. The tumor was not ruptured before or during removal. There is no residual tumor apparent beyond the margins of excision.
II. Tumor extends beyond the kidney but is completely resected. There is local extension of the tumor (*i.e.,* penetration beyond the pseudocapsule into the perirenal soft tissues, or periaortic lymph node involvement). The renal vessel outside the kidney substance is infiltrated or contains tumor thrombus. There is no residual tumor apparent beyond the margins of resection.	II. Tumor extends beyond the kidney, but is completely excised. There is regional extension of the tumor (*i.e.,* penetration through the outer surface of the renal capsule into the perirenal soft tissues). Vessels outside the kidney substance are infiltrated or contain tumor thrombus. The tumor may have been biopsied or there has been local spillage of tumor confined to the flank. There is no residual tumor apparent at or beyond the margins of excision.
III. Residual nonhematogenous tumor confined to the abdomen. Any of the following may occur: a. The tumor has ruptured before or during surgery, or a biopsy has been performed. b. Implants are found on peritoneal surfaces. c. Lymph nodes are involved beyond the abdominal periaortic chains. d. The tumor is not completely resectable because of local infiltration into vital structures.	III. Residual nonhematogenous tumor confined to the abdomen. Any of the following may occur: a. Lymph nodes on biopsy are found to be involved in the hilus, the periaortic chains, or beyond. b. There has been diffuse peritoneal contamination by the tumor, such as by spillage of tumor beyond the flank before or during surgery, or by tumor growth that has penetrated through the peritoneal surface. c. Implants are found on the peritoneal surfaces. d. The tumor extends beyond the surgical margins either microscopically or grossly. e. The tumor is not completely resectable because of local infiltration into vital structures.
IV. Hematogenous metastases. Deposits beyond Group III (*e.g.,* lung, liver, bone, and brain).	IV. Hematogenous metastases. Deposits beyond Stage III (*e.g.,* lung, liver, bone, and brain).
V. Bilateral renal involvement either initially or subsequently.	V. Bilateral renal involvement at diagnosis. An attempt should be made to stage each side according to the above criteria on the basis of extent of disease prior to biopsy.

* The clinical stage is decided by the surgeon in the operating room and is confirmed by the pathologist who also evaluates the histology. Staging is the same for tumors with favorable and with unfavorable histologic features. The patient should be characterized, however, by a statement of both criteria (*e.g.,* Stage II/favorable histology or Stage II/unfavorable histology).

portant, the contralateral kidney cannot be examined.[102–104] It is axiomatic that the contralateral kidney should be explored before one proceeds with dissection of the tumor. Gerota's fascia of the contralateral kidney is opened and the kidney mobilized from its perirenal fat and fascia to allow thorough inspection and palpation of both anterior and posterior surfaces. The presence of bilateral Wilms' tumor alters the surgical approach significantly (see below); thus the status of the contralateral kidney must be determined *before* nephrectomy.

The colon is mobilized and reflected medially, with care taken to preserve the colonic blood supply. The renal vein, often splayed over the tumor, must be handled with extreme caution. Although early ligation of the renal vein does not appear to have an appreciable effect on survival, it is preferable (although not always possible) to ligate the renal artery and vein separately before tumor manipulation.

Complete surgical extirpation implies removal of the perirenal fascia and adrenal gland (with upper pole tumors) without opening Gerota's fascia. Recent evidence, however, suggests that simple nephrectomy is associated with similarly good survival rates. Excision of all tumor is desirable, but heroic surgical efforts to accomplish this are not necessary, because small amounts of residual tumor have not been associated with major decreases in survival rates. A subtotal ureterectomy is also performed. Nonresectable tumors should

be outlined with titanium clips for possible postoperative radiation therapy. These clips are radiopaque but scatter the beam less than other metal clips during postoperative CT scanning.

Wilms' tumor extends into the inferior vena cava in approximately 6% of cases and may be clinically asymptomatic in more than 50%.[100,105] Involvement of the renal vein or inferior vena cava by tumor does not adversely affect the prognosis if treatment is appropriate.

Preoperative ultrasonography usually identifies the types of tumor thrombus encountered within the cava. These are [1] free-floating tumor thrombus, extracted by cavotomy; [2] tumor thrombus adherent to the wall of the inferior vena cava, which can be dealt with by use of the Fogarty balloon catheter; [3] infiltration of the wall of the inferior vena cava by tumor thrombus, often requiring resection; and [4] extension of tumor thrombus into the right atrium. Free-floating thrombi (*i.e.,* those not attached to the intima of the extrarenal vessels), no matter how long, are classified as Stage II. Adherent or infiltrating tumors are Stage III.

Intracardiac Tumor

In patients with intracardiac extension of tumor, a median sternotomy and midline abdominal incision provide excellent exposure of the right atrium and the intrapericardial portion of the inferior vena cava.[106,107] Extracorporeal circulation is necessary in these situations. A recent review by Nakayama and colleagues shows that this finding does not adversely affect life expectancy.[107] Eleven of 14 (79%) NWTS children with intracardiac tumors of favorable histology survived. In extreme cases, preoperative shrinkage of the tumor can be achieved by chemotherapy, with or without irradiation. This approach is not preferred because it alters evaluation of the histology and extent of the infradiaphragmatic tumor, and also because the tumors are sometimes refractory to therapy. The primary tumors in patients given preoperative chemotherapy should be considered Stage III and managed accordingly.

The presence or absence of lymph node metastases is of major importance in determining relapse-free survival.[7,97,99] Thus, selective sampling of suspicious nodes is necessary for accurate staging. There is no evidence, however, that extensive lymph node removal alters the outcome in patients with Wilms' tumor. Therefore, the NWTS Committee does not advocate formal and aggressive lymph node dissections.

Second-Look Operations

Situations sometimes arise that require elective reexplorations (see Chap. 10). In patients in whom flank incisions were initially used for nephrectomy, second-look procedures by a transperitoneal approach have resulted in up-staging of the disease by identification of positive lymph nodes. The change in stage requires alterations of therapy. Further, Wilms' tumor deemed unresectable can be totally extirpated after appropriate cytoreductive chemotherapy. Indications for second-look procedures therefore include previous flank incision, abdominal recurrence, initially unresectable tumor, and bilateral Wilms' tumors.[102]

Preoperative Therapy

Preoperative therapy is used more or less routinely by many management teams, particularly in Europe.[108–110] It is not preferred in most North American centers, where its use is restricted to tumors so large that the surgical risk is considered too great or to cases in which other medically cogent reasons are present.[109] Preoperative irradiation or chemotherapy reduces the size of large tumors and makes excision less hazardous.[108–111] A thick capsule is produced around the tumor, which reduces the possibility of intraoperative spillage and in some cases makes even simple enucleation possible. This is the approach taken by the International Society of Pediatric Oncology in their successive clinical trials.[110,111] Their studies have been based on clinical diagnoses and have not included pretreatment biopsies. Because there continues to be an error rate of about 5% in reaching the correct preoperative diagnosis, pretreatment open biopsy is advised by some under these circumstances.[80,91] Primary cytoreductive chemotherapy can then be instituted before exploratory celiotomy. Percutaneous fine-needle aspiration biopsy may be a suitable alternative. Early experience with this technique indicates that it is a safe, reproducible, and relatively reliable method of establishing the pathologic diagnosis of the primary tumor in children with presumed neoplastic disease.[112,113] Some believe that formal exploration is needed for accurate staging to avoid the possibility of overtreatment or undertreatment due to either inaccurate assessment of nodal status or failure to recognize the histologic type.[114,115] Thus, the needle biopsy cannot provide all the relevant information.

Another method, preoperative embolization, avoids some but not all of the problems listed above. It has been reported to allow easier removal of large tumors.[116,117]

Bilateral Disease

Various reports record the incidence of synchronous bilateral Wilms' tumor as ranging from 4.4% to 7.0% and that of metachronous bilateral Wilms' tumor from 1.0% to 1.9% of affected children.[7,104,118–121] In about one third of patients, the bilaterality is missed in preoperative evaluation.[104] This emphasizes the need for visual inspection and palpation of both kidneys intraoperatively.

The traditional surgical approach to bilateral Wilms' tumors includes nephrectomy of the more involved side, combined with excisional biopsy or partial nephrectomy of the presumably smaller lesion in the remaining kidney. Patients are then treated with chemotherapy, radiation therapy, or both, followed by second-look procedures. With these methods, 75% of children with bilateral lesions had residual tumor in the remaining kidney, despite repeated surgical procedures. However, the survival rate was extremely high (87%).[119] This may be the result of several factors, including the earlier age at which bilateral lesions occur, the generally favorable histologic types (nearly 90% of cases), the preponderance of Stage I tumors in this group, and the excellent protection provided by chemotherapeutic agents.

A new method of management, designed to preserve as much renal parenchyma as possible, is under investigation. In brief, bilateral biopsies are followed by courses of chemotherapy, and second-look surgery is delayed until the full effects of chemotherapy are obtained. The guidelines of this investigational NWTS surgical project have been detailed by Blute and colleagues.[104]

GENERAL RADIOTHERAPEUTIC CONSIDERATIONS

Pioneering radiation therapists noted that Wilms' tumors were responsive to radiation therapy, and this modality then became routine postoperative treatment at the Boston Children's Hospital, where many of the initial observations concerning the management of these children were made.[122] Two methods were used at that institution to define the field. First, the field was extended across the midline to include the entire circumference of the implicated vertebral bodies.[123] This was done to equalize the growth suppression; irradiation of only one side of a vertebra had been shown to lead to an obligatory scoliosis convex away from the irradiated side. Concern for late treatment complications obviously was much in the minds of the early workers, notably M.H. Wittenborg. Second, the preoperative excretory urogram was used to define the location and size of the kidney and its associated mass, considered to be the tissues of the original tumor bed. The upper, lateral, and lower limits of the field were thus defined. The dosage was age-adjusted: babies received lower doses than 3- or 4-year-olds, not because it was assumed that tumors in younger children were more radioresponsive but because their normal tissues would suffer more. This was another early example of weighing risks versus benefits and trying to reach an appropriate compromise.

These radiation therapy (RT) precepts are still in use today, except for the age-adjusted dosages, which were shown to be unnecessary in subsequent trials (see Chap. 11). It must be emphasized that the Boston methods were developed in children who did not receive effective adjuvant chemotherapy. The advent of effective drugs has clearly had a profound impact not only on the general management of these children but also on the use of RT. There is evidence to suggest that chemotherapy can "substitute" for irradiation in achieving local control by ablating microscopic residual disease in the tumor bed. Perhaps the most definitive data along these lines have been accrued in the NWTS. NWTS-1 results suggested that younger Group I patients (under age 2) had equally good outcomes regardless of whether they received RT.[91,124] Children 2 years of age or older had a significantly worse 4-year survival experience without RT, however.[124] NWTS-2 and NWTS-3 explored these issues further. It had been shown that double-agent chemotherapy using actinomycin D plus vincristine gave much better results than actinomycin D alone.[91] It was therefore reasoned that these two drugs given postoperatively might substitute for RT. Therefore, in NWTS-2, postoperative RT was eliminated from the management of all Group I patients.[98] The results indicated that the overall relapse-free survival rate in all patients, regardless of age, was similar to that in the irradiated sample in NWTS-1 who had received only actinomycin D for maintenance, and was numerically superior in children aged 2 years or older. These data are shown in Table 27-4, which also includes figures demonstrating excellent survival expectancy.

Meanwhile, retrospective analyses of the data accumulated in NWTS-1 and NWTS-2 were under way. Patterns of relapse and evidence for a dose–response relationship were sought.[125-127] It was concluded that patients at low risk, defined as those with Group II/FH tumors as well as Group I/FH patients, derived doubtful benefit from postoperative irradiation. Also, the data did not indicate that doses in excess of 2000 cGy improved results; indeed, it appeared that 1000 cGy might provide adequate local protection.[126] These conclusions were always predicated on the fact that children would receive actinomycin D plus vincristine, with or without Adriamycin, in the maintenance period.

NWTS-3 was designed to test these hypotheses in a factorial design (see Chemotherapy section). The nonirradiated Stage II/FH patients fared no worse than their irradiated counterparts; the results were similar in Stage III children who received nominal doses of 1000 versus 2000 cGy (Table 27-5). It should be kept in mind that supplemental doses of 1000 cGy to areas of gross residual disease were permissible although not often administered. Meanwhile, excellent results continue to be recorded for Stage I/FH patients, none of whom received RT.[92]

It was concluded that Stage I and II patients with FH tumors did not require postoperative irradiation, and that doses of 1000 cGy should suffice for local control in Stage III/FH patients, with the provisos noted.

The analyses were refined and the results in each of the four arms of the factorial design for Stages II and III were considered. Examination of the infradiaphragmatic relapse rates suggested a slightly increased frequency among Stage III/FH children receiving 1000 cGy and only actinomycin D and vincristine. The remaining three arms had very low relapse rates. The differences were not statistically significant. With samples of approximately 70 patients each, the maximum number of abdominal relapses in any of the four treatment arms was only five.[66] It nonetheless seemed prudent to minimize the

Table 27-4
*NWTS Outcomes in Group I Patients**

		NWTS-1			NWTS-2		
Age	RT	N	RFS (%)	TYS (%)	N	RFS (%)	TYS (%)
<2 yr	Yes	38	90	97	—	—	—
	No	36	88	94	117	88	95
≥2 yr	Yes	39	77	97	—	—	—
	No	41	58	91	77	89	97

* RT = postoperative irradiation; RFS = 2-year relapse-free survival; TYS = overall 2-year survival.

Table 27-5
*Results in Randomized NWTS-3 Patients**

Stage/Histology	Regimen	N	2-Year Survival (%)	
			Relapse Free	Overall
I/FH	AMD+VCR, 10 wk vs. 6 mo	469	90 vs. 93	98
II/FH	15 mo. AMD+VCR vs. AMD+VCR+ADR* (±RT)	262	91 vs. 90	99 vs. 93
II/FH	AMD+VCR±ADR No RT vs. 2000 cGy*	262	90 vs. 91	95 vs. 96
III/FH	AMD+VCR vs. AMD+VCR+ADR* (15 mo; +RT)	264	77 vs. 88	88 vs. 95
III/FH	AMD+VCR±ADR 1000 vs. 2000 cGy*	264	82 vs. 83	92 vs. 91
Any IV, any UH	AMD+VCR+ADR vs. AMD+VCR+ADR+CPM (15 mo; +RT)	291	63 vs. 69	78 vs. 80

* Comparisons denoted by asterisks are collapsed regimens from the factorial design; persistent disease at last follow-up in Stage IV was scored as relapse. Data indicate that, in general, FH Stages II and III patients can be treated successfully with the less intensive regimens and that better treatment is needed for patients with UH and/or metastases, especially those with rhabdoid tumors. Stage I/FH children present particular problems for analysis. These results show the less intensive 10-week regimen to be no worse than 6 months, but other analyses suggest that 6 months of treatment may be better. Of the four possible treatment combinations for Stage III/FH, AMD+VCR+1000 cGy appears to produce inferior results when both relapse-free survival and infradiaphragmatic relapse are considered.

chances for intra-abdominal recurrences, given their grave implications. The question therefore was whether fewer late treatment-related effects could be expected after 2000 cGy (versus 1000 cGy) or after Adriamycin, if added to the other two drugs. The files of the Late Follow-up Study (LFUS), an integral part of the NWTS for several years, were examined.[128] No excess in cardiovascular sequelae had been recorded in children receiving Adriamycin. In contrast, musculoskeletal abnormalities and some second tumors at least appear to be related to radiation dose.[129,130] Deformities seen after kilovoltage irradiation are not avoided by the use of megavoltage machines or [60]Co (see Chaps. 11 and 50). The frequency remains about the same, although the severity appears to be less.[131,132] It was concluded that it would be preferable to add Adriamycin to actinomycin D and vincristine for Stage III/FH children, maintaining the postoperative radiation dose at 1000 cGy. This conclusion was strengthened by the fact that the relapse-free survival for the Adriamycin-containing arms seemed superior in Stage III children to those arms in which only actinomycin D and vincristine were given, even though the differences were not statistically significant.[66]

Similar analyses for Stage II/FH tumors yielded less compelling results in favor of either 2000 cGy or the three-drug regimen in terms of abdominal relapse rate. The relapse-free survival for all four arms was about 90%. The simplest of the four regimens was therefore selected for these patients; that is, two drugs and no postoperative irradiation.

These results were the basis for the design of NWTS-4 (described below), which does not address radiation therapy issues. Also, the observations regarding radiation were extended to the other categories of patients, including those with Stage IV/FH tumors and those with anaplastic lesions or with CCSK.

GENERAL CHEMOTHERAPY PRINCIPLES

Wilms' tumor was the first pediatric malignant solid tumor found to be responsive to a systemic chemotherapeutic agent, actinomycin D (AMD). The use of AMD for the adjuvant treatment of children with Wilms' tumor was pioneered by Farber and colleagues.[133] Other active agents were soon added to the list.[76] Chief among them were vincristine (VCR), with a reported 63% complete and partial response rate (17 of 27 pa-

tients) and, later, doxorubicin (Adriamycin, ADR), with a 60% response rate (31 of 52 patients). By contrast, the complete and partial response rate for cyclophosphamide was 27% (10 of 37 patients), whereas only 3 of 19 patients (16%) had partial responses to cisplatin. Too few patients have been tested with other drugs to draw valid conclusions.

The initial observations with AMD led to other single-institution studies and cooperative group randomized trials to evaluate the use of adjuvant single-agent chemotherapy in the treatment of these children.[91,110,134–138] The relative merits of AMD and VCR were studied in NWTS-1, and the two drugs were found to produce equal relapse-free survival rates of about 55% as they were used in that trial (Figs. 27-12 and 27-13).[91] The United Kingdom Medical Research Council (MRC) used VCR more intensively and reported a better relapse-free survival rate (78% versus 54% for AMD).[126] It should be noted that the MRC children treated in the VCR arm also received AMD immediately postoperatively and thus actually received two-drug chemotherapy.

Single-agent clinical investigations were soon superseded by trials of more complex regimens.[124] Those conducted by the NWTS and the International Society of Pediatric Oncology (SIOP) have taken different approaches. The NWTS has emphasized early surgery; the SIOP investigators have explored the value of preoperative therapies. Their efforts will therefore be discussed separately.

NWTS Trials

Since its inception, the NWTS has focused on identifying low- and high-risk groups so that treatment intensity and duration can be modulated. The designs of the successive NWTS studies reflect this concern, and the results are epitomized by NWTS-3, because each study built on the outcomes of the preceding one.

NWTS-3 stratified patients according to stage and histology (FH versus UH) and sought to minimize therapy for low-risk patients while intensifying treatment for the high-risk group. A shorter maintenance course for Stage I/FH patients was tested. In NWTS-2, patients with Group II, III, or IV tumors were randomly assigned to receive chemotherapy with VCR and AMD or these two drugs plus ADR. All received postoperative irradiation. The overall results showed statistically

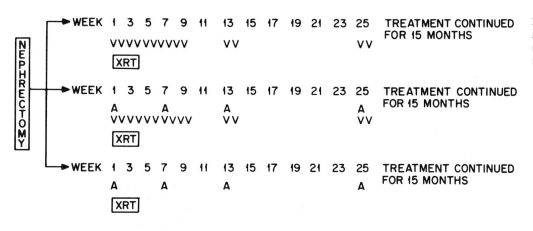

FIGURE 27-12. Randomization scheme for groups II and III in the first National Wilms' Tumor Study (NWTS-1).

A = ACTINOMYCIN D (15 MICROGRAMS/KG/DAY x 5 DAYS, IV)

V = VINCRISTINE (1.5 MG/M^2/DOSE, IV)

XRT = ABDOMINAL RADIATION THERAPY

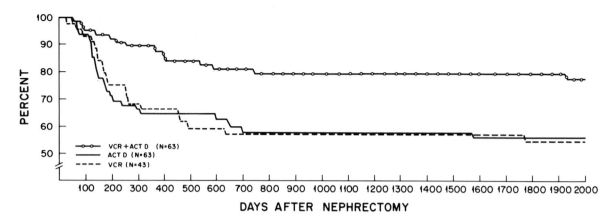

FIGURE 27-13.   Relapse-free survival rates for NWTS-1 groups II and III according to chemotherapy regimen.

NATIONAL WILMS' TUMOR STUDY-3
TREATMENT-STAGE II (FAVORABLE HISTOLOGY)

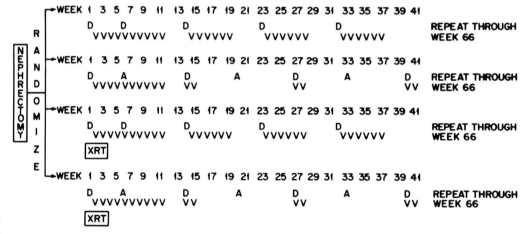

FIGURE 27-14. Randomization and treatments were the same for stage III favorable-histology patients except that postoperative radiation therapy was given to all in doses of either 1000 or 2000 cGy (rad).

significantly better 2-year relapse-free rates for the three-drug regimen (77%, compared to 63% for the two-drug scheme).[98] However, there was concern regarding the unknown potential for late cardiotoxicity of ADR, especially among the Stage II/FH and Stage III/FH children.[90,98] ADR was therefore excluded from one of the NWTS-3 study arms and a more intensive use of VCR was introduced as a possible substitute, on the bases of the MRC results (Fig. 27-14).[138] Finally, cyclophosphamide (Cytoxan, CTX) was added to the other three drugs in one of the two study regimens for the high-risk groups. Radiation therapy questions for Stage II/FH and Stage III/FH children were also addressed.

The results are shown in Table 27-5, which also reflects the randomized factorial scheme of NWTS-3.[92] These data, together with those derived from NWTS-1 and NWTS-2, are the bases for the following conclusions:

1. Postoperative radiation therapy is not needed for children with Stage I and II tumors of favorable histology.[91,92,98]

2. Combination chemotherapy with AMD + VCR is superior to either agent alone (Figs. 27-12 and 27-13) and is adequate for children with tumors of the following categories: Stage I/FH, Stage I/anaplasia, and Stage II/FH.[91,92,98]

3. ADR added to AMD + VCR gives better results in patients with Stage III/FH and Stage IV/FH tumors and those with CCSK.[60,66,91]

4. CTX added to AMD + VCR + ADR does not appear to improve results for children with Stage IV/FH tumors or RTK of any stage. The trial for anaplastic Stage II, III, and IV tumors is continuing, with AMD + VCR + ADR being tested against those three drugs plus CTX because the comparison data are inconclusive as yet.[60]

Previous success in treatment strategies has allowed the design of a unique study with the primary aims of continuing to improve treatment results while decreasing the cost of therapy through modification of the schedule of drug administration.

Table 27-6
Hematologic Toxicity After the 6-Week Course of Chemotherapy in NWTS-2

Group/Regimen	N	Leukocytes < 1000/mm³	Platelets < 50,000/mm³	Hgb < 8 g/dl
I/AMD+VCR, no RT	168	0.0%*	4.2%†	7.1%‡
II–IV/AMD+VCR+RT	158	1.9%	7.2%	16.4%
II–IV/AMD+VCR+ADR+RT	140	17.1%	7.6%	30.9%

* Percentage of patients who had a leukocyte count less than 1000/mm³.
† Percentage of patients who had a platelet count less than 50,000/mm³.
‡ Percentage of patients who had a hemoglobin count less than 8 g/dl.

Table 27-7
Relation Between Severe Neutropenia and Treatment Regimen for Irradiated NWTS-3 Patients*

Regimen	First	6 Week	12 Week
AMD+VCR	26.2%	29.6%	9.9%
AMD+VCR+ADR	31.2%	58.4%	18.1%
AMD+VCR+ADR+CPM	37.6%	75.0%	50.5%

* Percentages of patients who had leukocyte counts <2000/mm³ after that course of chemotherapy.

Table 27-8
Relation Between Severe Thrombocytopenia and the Administration of Actinomycin D ± Adriamycin Following Similar Radiation Doses in NWTS-3*

Regimen	First	6 Week
AMD+VCR	5.5%	27.0%
AMD+VCR+ADR	6.0%	7.2%

* Percentages of patients who had platelet counts <50,000/mm³ following that course of chemotherapy.

This study, NWTS-4, is based on experimental[139] and clinical[140–143] data demonstrating the safety and efficacy of AMD when administered in a single, moderately high dose.

The design of NWTS-4 will allow the results of intensive chemotherapy regimens employing single doses of AMD and ADR to be compared with current treatment regimens using divided-dose regimens of each drug. In addition, treatment durations of 6 and 15 months will be compared in patients with Stages II–IV/FH tumors.

Toxicity

A major objective of the NWTS has been to develop treatment regimens that cause less acute and long-term morbidity. Thus, evaluations of hematologic, hepatic, pulmonary, cardiac and skeletal toxicity have been performed, both during active treatment and as part of the NWTS long-term follow-up study.

Hematologic

Hematologic toxicity has been more profound in patients treated with regimens containing three or four agents, and following chemotherapy courses administered immediately after the completion of radiation therapy (Tables 27-6 and 27-7).[66,144]

The relation between the completion of radiation therapy and the occurrence of thrombocytopenia following the administration of actinomycin D was demonstrated clearly in NWTS-3.[66] The percentage of irradiated patients who experienced severe thrombocytopenia after the 6-week course of AMD in one regimen was 27.0%, compared with 7.2% among those treated with a regimen in which ADR was substituted for AMD at 6 weeks (Table 27-8).

The relation between patient age and the frequency and severity of hematologic toxicity was investigated by Morgan and colleagues.[144] They reported severe hematologic toxicity among 47% of infants younger than 12 months following treatment with full doses of chemotherapeutic agents, compared with 13% of similar patients treated with 50% of the protocol drug doses (see also Chap. 12). The use of lower drug doses did not increase the frequency of relapse among patients younger than 12 months.[144] These data confirmed the results of Jones and colleagues,[145] as well as anecdotal impressions that young infants tolerated treatment with several chemotherapeutic agents poorly, and led to the recommendation that all infants receive only 50% of the usual childhood dose of any chemotherapeutic agent.[145]

Hepatic

Radiation therapy and chemotherapy produced hepatic toxicity, manifested by hepatomegaly, liver enzyme elevations, and thrombocytopenia, in 5.8% of NWTS-1 patients[91] and 6.2% of NWTS-2 patients.[98] The type of toxicity is identical to that originally reported by Tefft and his colleagues.[146]

Cardiac

Cardiac toxicity causing death in the NWTS was infrequent. One NWTS-2 patient among the 27 with Group IV disease treated with the ADR-containing regimen died of cardiac toxicity. There were no such deaths among patients treated with only AMD and VCR.[98] The risk of cardiac toxicity following ADR administration is greater when the myocardium has also been irradiated in the course of either whole-lung or abdominal irradiation (see Chaps. 9, 11, 37, 50).[147,148]

International Society of Pediatric Oncology (SIOP) Studies

SIOP has placed its major emphasis on the role of preoperative therapies. This approach to the management of children with large abdominal tumors has long been championed by some and was originally based on preoperative irradiation,[149] because preoperative treatment reduces the bulk of the mass, thus facilitating the surgical removal.

SIOP evaluated preoperative irradiation in its first study.[110] Patients were randomized to receive or not receive preoperative RT. All received AMD. Although relapse-free and overall survival were not different between the two groups, the frequency of tumor rupture was less in the preoperative RT group (Table 27-9). The authors point out that the decreased frequency of intraoperative rupture meant that fewer patients required total abdominal irradiation postoperatively. Thus, the dose to the gonads was reduced, indubitably a major benefit.

Like the NWTS Committee, SIOP investigators sought to decrease the proportion of patients requiring RT of any sort. They therefore mounted a trial comparing the efficacy of preoperative chemotherapy with that of preoperative RT.[111] The advantages already noted for preoperative RT were also seen in the children receiving drugs before surgery. A subsequent trial (SIOP-6) divided patients without metastases at diagnosis to receive or not to receive postoperative irradiation according to their clinicopathologic findings.[150] Those children who after preoperative therapy did not have Stage III criteria (normal-risk group) did not receive RT; those still qualifying as Stage III (high risk) were given RT. The overall results in the entire sample were similar to those obtained in the NWTS with Stages I–III children. Excellent survival rates were obtained in the normal-risk group, whereas an understandably lower survival rate was reported in the SIOP Stage III patients with residual regional disease after treatment. Clearly, these children had more aggressive tumors and would be expected to fare worse than those qualifying as Stage III at the time of initial surgery without pretreatment.

Subsequent reports indicate that the normal-risk nonirradiated children in SIOP-6 have shown a disproportionate frequency of infradiaphragmatic relapses.[150] Careful statistical analyses are currently under way to determine whether artifacts, patient selection, or other factors might have influenced this result. The alternate explanation is that some patients with occult Stage III disease were down-staged by the treatment. It is known that a proportion of primary tumors are not only smaller but also totally necrotic after chemotherapy.[111] In this light, it is possible that preoperative chemotherapy destroys evidence of local extension, such as peritoneal seeding or lymph node involvement, but the risk of infradiaphragmatic relapse nonetheless remains unless postoperative RT is given. The results of the continuing SIOP analyses must be awaited before conclusions can be drawn.

COMMENT. The different approaches taken by the NWTS and SIOP investigators both yield excellent results for Wilms' tumor patients in the aggregate. The advantages and disadvan-

tages insofar as individual patients are concerned have been discussed elsewhere and are underscored by the tentative SIOP-6 results noted above.[114] In North America at least, most specialists who treat Wilms' tumor patients prefer initial surgery.

COMBINED MODALITY THERAPY

These recommendations are based on the results of the NWTS, which advocates early surgery without preoperative therapy, and modulates therapy according to stage and histology. It must be recognized that other points of view have been expressed.[110,111,149]

Chemotherapy

There are many chemotherapy regimens in use that appear to produce good results.[110,111,137,138] Those used by the NWTS Group will be detailed here because they have been tested in large numbers of patients.[92] The treatments are modulated in intensity according to risk, based on stage and histology considerations, as identified at surgery and at the pathology bench in non-pretreated patients.

The first course of chemotherapy is the same for all patients. This allows changes in treatment to be made thereafter should the initial stage, histology, or both require modification after more careful review.

In the following scheme, actinomycin D (AMD) is given in five daily intravenous doses of 15 μg/kg each, for a total of 75 μg/kg per course. Vincristine (VCR) is administered in single intravenous doses of 1.5 mg/m² each, and Adriamycin (ADR) in doses of 20 mg/m²/day IV for 3 consecutive days, for a total dose of 60 mg/m² per course.

Favorable Histology (FH) Tumors

Stage I, Regimen EE—AMD before postoperative day 6 and at weeks 5, 13, and 24. VCR once a week starting on day 7; then on days 1 and 5 of the AMD courses. No radiation therapy is given.

Stage II, Regimen K—As in Stage I for the first 10 weeks; then AMD at weeks 13, 22, 31, 40, 49, and 58, plus VCR once weekly for six injections at weeks 15, 24, 33, 42, 51, and 60. No radiation therapy is given.

Stage III and IV, Regimen DD—AMD before day 6 and at weeks 13, 26, 39, 52, and 65. VCR once a week starting on day 7 and continuing on days 1 and 5 of the AMD courses. ADR at weeks 6, 19, 22, 45, and 58. Postoperative irradia-

Table 27-9
*SIOP Preoperative Therapy Clinical Trials**

Preoperative Therapy	SIOP-1				SIOP-5			
	N	2-Year RFS	2-Year OS	Spill	N	4-Year RFS	4-Year OS	Spill
2000 cGy RT	63	52%	83%	4%	76	77%	83%	9%
None	64	44%	71%	33%	—	—	—	—
AMD+VCR, no RT	—	—	—	—	88	67%	89%	6%

* RFS = relapse-free survival; OS = overall survival. The original papers should be consulted for details of the trials.[110,111] None of the differences are statistically significant except the intraoperative tumor rupture rates in SIOP-1. Twelve of the 20 instances of tumor spillage ("spill") in the nonpretreated patients were major, compared with none of the 3 spills noted in the preoperatively irradiated children. Major spills required whole abdominal irradiation postoperatively (see text).

tion is added according to the relevant guidelines (see below).

Anaplastic Tumors

Stage I, Regimen EE—As in Stage I/FH.

Stages II–IV, Regimens DD and J—No really satisfactory regimen has yet been identified. Data from NWTS-3 suggest that more frequent VCR and cyclophosphamide (CPM) added to AMD and ADR (Regimen J) may be of benefit. That clinical trial is still under way. AMD, VCR, and ADR in Regimen J are given as in Regimen DD except that VCR is also added on days 1 and 3 of each ADR course, and CPM is given for 3 daily doses of 10 mg/kg during each ADR and each AMD course except the postoperative AMD course. Postoperative irradiation is added (see below).

Clear Cell Sarcoma

Stages I–IV, Regimen DD—As in Stages III/FH and IV/FH.

Rhabdoid Tumors

All stages—No satisfactory treatment has been developed for these children. Combinations of etoposide and cisplatin and of etoposide and ifosfamide are being tested.

Radiation Therapy

Megavoltage teletherapy apparatus or the equivalent is used, and daily doses of 180 cGy are delivered. The daily dose is reduced to 150 cGy when large volumes, such as the whole abdomen or the whole thorax, are included in the fields. Doses are specified as midplane values without correction for air transmission or bone absorption. The use of simulation and portal films is essential to ensure accurate beam direction (see Chap. 11).

Radiation therapy, when applicable, is initiated when the patient is stable postoperatively, free of ileus or diarrhea, and has a satisfactory absolute neutrophil cell count ($\geq 1000/mm^3$) and hemoglobin levels of at least 10 g/dl.

Favorable Histology

PRIMARY SITE—STAGES I AND II.   No postoperative RT is recommended in children receiving AMD plus VCR according to regimens similar to those reported in the NWTS.

STAGE III.   In children with tumors coming to the margin of the surgical specimen, doses of 1080 cGy are delivered to the tumor bed (Table 27-10). The tumor bed is defined as the kidney and its associated lesion as they are visualized on preoperative imaging studies. The portal is extended medially to include the entire vertebral column at the implicated levels (*i.e.,* across the midline medially). The lateral limit of the field is the properitoneal line. The field is extended as needed to include areas of known residual disease. The whole abdomen is treated in patients with gross peritoneal soilage by tumor rupture before or during surgery, or with diffuse peritoneal seeding. In these cases, the portal includes all the peritoneal surfaces and extends from the domes of the diaphragm to the inferior margins of the obturator foramina. External beam blocks are introduced to shield the femoral heads. Supplemental doses of 1080 cGy are recommended for areas of gross residual disease. These are defined as residual tumor masses ≥ 3 cm in maximum diameter. The fields are designed to encompass the residual disease, as visualized on imaging studies,

Table 27-10
Volume of Abdominal RT in Stages III and IV Disease

Extent of Disease	Volume of RT Required
Hilar nodes Gross* or microscopic residuum confined to flank Para-aortic nodes	Tumor bed crossing midline to include bilateral para-aortic nodes at implicated levels
Peritoneal seeding Gross residual abdominal disease* Diffuse spillage at surgery Preoperative intraperitoneal rupture	Whole abdomen

* Local 1080 cGy supplements to be given.

and a surrounding margin of at least 1 cm. Doses to more than one third of the remaining kidney should not exceed 1440 cGy.

STAGE IV.   No postoperative radiation is given to the flank in children with primary tumors that would qualify as Stage I or II. Postoperative irradiation is given to patients with more advanced lesions according to the guidelines described under Stage III above.

METASTATIC SITES.   Lung.   The entire thoracic cavity is irradiated without shields, except those protecting the humeral heads. The field extends from the apex of the lung to the posterior inferior recesses of the costophrenic sulci. The latter come to the bottom of T12 or lower in most children. Daily doses of 150 cGy are given to a total of 1200 cGy.

Shielding of mediastinal structures for fear of the effects on the heart of combined radiation plus Adriamycin is not recommended. Marginal recurrences in mediastinal lymph nodes have developed in patients managed in this way. Very few episodes of cardiotoxicity have been recorded in the NWTS in children given whole-thorax RT.[66,128]

Liver.   Nonresectable metastases present at diagnosis are irradiated. The treatment portal includes that portion of the liver known to be involved, as visualized on CT or MRI studies. Daily doses of 180 cGy are given to a total of 1980 cGy. The whole liver is treated in children with diffuse metastases. It is recognized that liver tolerance is approached by these recommendations, especially in view of the radiation-enhancing and radiation-reactivating drugs (AMD and ADR) used in the management of these children. Extreme caution is therefore recommended, with careful monitoring of liver function tests and blood counts during treatment. A selective thrombocytopenia can appear in these patients, who have a surprisingly good outlook after aggressive therapy. Breslow and coworkers reported 72% survival at 4 years in children with FH tumors and liver lesions, with or without lung metastases.[151] The NWTS Committee therefore considers the risks justified. Supplemental doses of 540 cGy to 1080 cGy can be given to small portions of the liver containing bulk lesions at the completion of the recommended 1980 cGy.

Other Sites.   Metastases to bulky lymph nodes, brain, bone, or other areas are treated like the liver, with supplemental doses reaching 3060 cGy for the brain and bone. The whole brain is treated in daily doses of 180 cGy, but the entire bone need not be irradiated for skeletal metastases. The field includes the lesion as seen on the best imaging study, with margins ≥ 3 cm in any direction.

Anaplastic Tumors

STAGE I. NWTS analyses have shown that children with Stage I anaplastic tumors have the same outlook as those with Stage I/FH lesions.[55] Therefore, no postoperative RT is advocated for this group of patients.

STAGES II–IV. The general outlook for these patients continues to be precarious, and postoperative radiation to control infradiaphragmatic relapse is still recommended. The daily doses and the field arrangements are the same as for the FH lesions; that is, the beam is directed to the flank as described under Stage III/FH above. The doses used in NWTS-3 are age-adjusted as follows: birth to 12 months—1200 to 1800 cGy; 13 to 18 months—1801 to 2400 cGy; 19 to 30 months—2401 to 3000 cGy; 31 to 40 months—3001 to 3500 cGy; 41 months or more—3501 to 4000 cGy.

METASTASES. These are treated like their FH counterparts except for those in the liver. Dosages for liver metastases are 3000 cGy in 3½ to 4 weeks, with 500 to 1000 cGy supplements permissible to small residual volumes. These doses are precarious, and careful monitoring during therapy is needed. The poor outlook for these patients justifies an increase in the level of acceptable risks, in the opinion of the NWTS Committee.

Clear Cell Sarcoma of the Kidney

Disease control for these patients has been improved dramatically through the addition of ADR to AMD and VCR.[60] These are, nonetheless, aggressive lesions; complacency is not warranted, and postoperative RT is recommended in NWTS-4 to patients with CCSK, regardless of the stage.

PRIMARY SITE. Stages I and II fields are like those for localized Stage III/FH as described above, and the dose is 1080 cGy. Irradiation for Stage III patients is as described for their FH counterparts. Stage IV patients undergo irradiation of infradiaphragmatic sites according to the local findings there. For example, tumors qualifying as Stage I or II receive 1080 cGy to the flank, and the fields are arranged according to those criteria that would qualify the child as Stage III if the disease were found to be more extensive.

METASTASES. Sites of metastatic disease are irradiated according to the criteria given for Stage IV/FH. NWTS-4 is exploring the tolerance of and response to higher doses, but in the absence of this evidence the recommendations for Stage IV/FH seem appropriate although aggressive in view of the poor prognosis for these children.

SPECIAL CONSIDERATIONS

Neonates and Infants

Wilms' tumor is rarely found in neonates (see Chaps. 10 and 12).[151] Neonates and all infants under 13 months of age require reduction of chemotherapy doses to 50% of those used in older children, after conversion of amounts cited per square meter of surface area to the dose/kilogram method.[145] Babies with pulmonary metastases pose particular problems. The NWTS Com-

mittee recommends that thoracic irradiation be given only to those children under 18 months of age who do not have complete resolution of metastases within 4 weeks of the AMD + VCR course. Patients who have total disappearance of metastases can then be observed. Children with residual nodules receive 900 cGy in 150 cGy daily doses with a single 150 cGy supplement to nodules that do not disappear after 900 cGy. Irradiation is recommended as the mainstay of treatment because of evidence from NWTS-3 suggesting that the best relapse-free survival is obtained in children who have thoracic irradiation added to chemotherapy.[153] An alternative to RT is surgical excision of lesion(s) that remain after the first cycle of AMD, VCR, and ADR (all such children should be on three-agent chemotherapy). Another alternative is to reserve surgical excision for those children who have residual masses after the delivery of 900 cGy to the whole chest. These operative approaches have not been tested systematically, although Green has recorded better results in NWTS-1 and NWTS-2 children who had surgical removal of metastases.[154]

Extrarenal Wilms' Tumor

This rare, extrarenal Wilms' tumor can be found in the pelvis and even the thorax as well as the retroperitoneal space.[155] The same general therapy precepts can be followed as when the kidney is affected, although it may be prudent to use the Stage III guidelines for chemotherapy and radiotherapy under these unusual circumstances.

Horseshoe Kidneys

Thirteen cases were found among 2961 (0.4%) NWTS patients reviewed by Mesrobian and associates.[156] Seven of the 13 had Stage I or II disease. Treatment was according to the guidelines for comparable stage unilateral disease, with an overall survival of 85% (mean follow-up = 3½ years). These findings indicate that the tumors are no more aggressive than unilateral tumors. By extension, patients with tumors in discoid kidneys can be managed successfully using preservative approaches.

FOLLOW-UP DURING AND AFTER MAINTENANCE CHEMOTHERAPY

Physical Examinations and Laboratory Studies

Examinations are conducted before each course of chemotherapy and include blood pressure recordings, urinalyses, and palpation of the abdomen for evidence of recurrent tumor at the primary site, in the liver, or in the remaining kidney. It is not enough that an imaging study a few weeks before showed no evidence of tumor in the contralateral kidney. A recent review of aniridic patients showed that tumor growth was first detected by the examining physician.[157] After the completion of chemotherapy, clinic visits for physical and laboratory checks coincide with the schedule for imaging studies given below. All children who received lung irradiation should have thyroid function tests performed at yearly intervals for 5 years to detect possible hypothyroidism, and the gland should be palpated yearly for life because of the known association between even low-dose irradiation and the subsequent appearance of thyroid adenomas and carcinomas.[158] Routine blood chemistries and peripheral blood cell counts are not needed once stable values have been reached.

Imaging Studies

The frequency of imaging studies is governed by the stage but not by the histology, with the exception of patients with mesoblastic nephroma (MN) who need no further studies because distant metastases are rare.[82] An exception is the child with MN who has sustained intraoperative tumor rupture, a not infrequent complication with neoplasms of this histology. Infradiaphragmatic recurrences can occur in that setting, and ultrasonographic studies at the intervals indicated below for Stages I and II Wilms' tumor are therefore advised.[46]

STAGES I AND II.   Four radiographic views of the chest are recommended at the following times after surgery: 6 weeks, 3 months, and a minimum of every 3 months for the first 18 months; then every 6 months to 3 years; then yearly through the fifth postoperative year and thereafter only as indicated clinically.

STAGE III.   Ultrasound examination of the abdomen is performed at the same time as the chest films described above.

STAGE IV, PULMONARY METASTASES.   Four-view radiographs are repeated at 6-week intervals until the metastases have not been visible for a minimum of 9 months. Thereafter, films are obtained every 3 months for an additional 15 months, after which the schedule for Stages I–III applies.

STAGE IV, METASTASES TO OTHER SITES.   Children with bone, liver, or brain metastases should have the relevant imaging examinations once every 3 months for 1 year; then every 6 months for 2 years; and then yearly to the fifth year. After this point, imaging studies can be dictated by clinical signs and symptoms.

PATIENTS WITH PREDISPOSING CHARACTERISTICS.   Children with sporadic aniridia, hemihypertrophy, the Beckwith–Wiedemann syndrome, or evidence of nephroblastomatosis in one or both kidneys require careful surveillance (see Chap. 5).[25,44,45] In those with excised unilateral Wilms' tumors, ultrasonography of the remaining kidney is performed every 3 months during the first 2 postoperative years, and then once every 6 months through the fifth postoperative year. Annual studies for an additional 5 years thereafter would seem prudent because the opposite kidney continues to be at risk for years, although with a decreasing likelihood of metachronous involvement.

Long-Term Follow-Up

A major objective of the NWTS has been to develop treatment regimens that cause less acute and long-term morbidity.[128] Therefore, evaluations of hematologic, hepatic, pulmonary, cardiac, and skeletal treatment-related complications have been performed during active treatment and as part of the NWTS long-term follow-up study.

The late effects of trunk irradiation—scoliosis and soft tissue underdevelopment—are still being seen since the advent of megavoltage irradiation.[131,132] One would expect the least deformity, of course, when RT is omitted entirely. That expectation has been documented by the NWTS, which recorded 66 instances of "musculoskeletal" difficulties (not otherwise defined) among 88 irradiated Stage I children followed

for 5 or more years versus 7 in 93 nonirradiated cohorts.*[144] By contrast, no difference in "cardiovascular" problems was found in cohorts of patients who did and did not receive ADR as part of primary therapy.[128]

Second malignant neoplasms (SMNs) can develop in Wilms' tumor survivors (see Chap. 50).[159] Most of these occur in irradiated areas. It is therefore not too surprising that thyroid and breast cancers have been recorded in some long-term Wilms' tumor survivors who were given thoracic bath radiation therapy for pulmonary metastases. There were four thyroid and two breast cancers among 36 Wilms' tumor survivors bearing SMNs recorded by the Late Effects Study Group (LESG).[159] As in other reports, sarcomas predominated (9 soft tissue and 6 bone); leukemia and lymphoma (7 cases) were next most common, despite prior evidence from the LESG that actinomycin D appeared to protect against radiation-associated SMNs.[160]

It is obvious that Wilms' tumor survivors must be followed carefully for life so that late adverse effects of therapy can be detected early, should they occur, and not vitiate what has been gained from so many years of successful clinical research.

FUTURE CONSIDERATIONS

Major progress has been made in the management of children with Wilms' tumor. More than 85% can be cured by current therapies. Future treatment research will follow both well-trodden paths and directions that can scarcely be glimpsed. Further refinements of surgery, radiation therapy, and chemotherapy remain to be made, with the aim of preserving as much normal tissue as possible. Partial nephrectomy, reduction of radiation doses (to zero in most cases) and elimination of as much chemotherapy as possible are visible and achievable goals. These will also have their rewards in reductions of both the immediate and future impact of the disease in the psychological, social, and economic spheres.

Research in epidemiology and molecular biology will without doubt lead to clinical applications. What these might be will become clear in the not too distant future. The horizon is bright with promise.

The authors thank the many physicians associated with the National Wilms' Tumor Study; Dr. Howard Snyder, Department of Surgery, Children's Hospital of Philadelphia, for permission to use Figure 27-9, and Dr. Spencer Borden and other staff members of the Department of Radiology, Children's Hospital of Philadelphia, especially Dr. Henrietta Rosenberg for permission to use Figure 27-11; we are also grateful to Martinus Nijhoff Publishing for permission to cite data contained in Chapter 4 of *Diagnosis and Management of Malignant Solid Tumors in Infants and Children*, pp 187–256, 1985.

* Some patients had more than one abnormality; for example, scoliosis and muscle hypoplasia, in which case two events were tallied in the numerator.

REFERENCES

1. D'Angio GJ: Oncology seen through the prism of Wilms' tumor. Med Pediatr Oncol 13:53–58, 1985
2. Rance TF: Cause of fungus haematodes of the kidneys. Med Phys J 32:19, 1814
3. Wilms M: Die Mischgeschwuelste der Niere. Leipzig, A Georgi, 1899
4. Young JL, Miller RW: Incidence of malignant tumors in U.S. children. J Pediatr 86:254–258, 1975

5. Breslow NE, Langholz B: Childhood cancer incidence: Geographical and temporal variations. Int J Cancer 32:703–716, 1983
6. Li FP: Cancers in children. In Schottenfeld D, Fraumeni JF Jr (eds): Cancer Epidemiology and Prevention, pp 1012–1024. Philadelphia, WB Saunders, 1982
7. Breslow NE, Beckwith JB: Epidemiological features of Wilms' tumor: Results of the National Wilms' Tumor Study. J Natl Cancer Inst 68:429–436, 1982
8. Miller RW, Fraumeni JF Jr, Manning MD: Association of Wilms' tumor with aniridia, hemihypertrophy and other congenital malformations. N Engl J Med 270:922–927, 1964
9. Stay EJ, Vawter G: The relationship between nephroblastoma and neurofibromatosis (von Recklinghausen's disease). Cancer 39:2550–2555, 1977
10. Beckwith JB: Macroglossia, omphalocele, adrenal cytomegaly, gigantism and hyperplastic visceromegaly. In Bergsma D, McKusick VA, Hall JG, Scott CI (eds): Birth Defects: Original Article Series, Vol 5, pp 188–196. New York, Stratton Intercontinental, 1969
11. Eddy MA, Mauer SM: Pseudohermophroditism, glomerulopathy and Wilms' tumor (Drash syndrome). Frequency in end-stage renal failure. J Pediatr 106:584–587, 1985
12. Greenberg F, Stein F, Cresick MV et al: The Perlman familial nephroblastomatosis syndrome. Am J Med Genet 24:101–110, 1986
13. Fabia J, Thuy TD: Occupation of father at time of birth of children dying of malignant diseases. Br J Prev Soc Med 28:98–100, 1974
14. Zack M, Cannon S, Lyod D et al: Cancer in children of parents exposed to hydrocarbon-related industries and occupations. Am J Epidemiol 111:329–336, 1980
15. Hakulinen T, Salonen T, Teppo L: Cancer in the offspring in hydrocarbon-related occupations. Br J Prev Soc Med 30:138–140, 1976
16. Kantor AF, McCrea Curren MG, Meigs JW et al: Occupations of fathers of patients with Wilms' tumor. J Epidemiol Community Health 33:253–256, 1979
17. Dwa SL, Fine LJ: The association between parental occupation and childhood malignancy. J Occup Med 24:792–794, 1980
18. Ferrell RE, Strong LC, Riccardi VM et al: A clinical cytogenetic and gene marker survey of 106 patients with Wilms' tumor (WT) and/or aniridia (AN). Am J Hum Genet 32:104A, 1980
19. Francke U, Holmes LB, Atkins L et al: Aniridia-Wilms' tumor association: Evidence for specific deletion of 11p13. Cytogenet Cell Genet 24:185–192, 1979
20. Junien C, Turleau C, de Grouchy J et al: Regional assignment of catalase (CAT) gene to band 11p13. Association with the aniridia-Wilms' tumor gonadoblastoma (WAGR) complex. Ann Genet 23:165–166, 1980
21. Kaneko Y, Eguel MC, Rowley JD: Interstitial deletion of short arm of chromosome-11 limited to Wilms' tumor patient cells in a patient without aniridia. Cancer Res 41:4577–4578, 1981
22. Koufos A, Hansen MF, Lamplin BC et al: Loss of alleles at loci on human chromosome 11 during genesis of Wilms' tumor. Nature 309:170–172, 1984
23. Scott J, Cowell J, Robertson ME et al: Insulin-like growth factor II gene expression in Wilms' tumor and embryonic tissues. Nature 317:260–262, 1985
24. Reeve AE, Eccles MR, Wilkins RJ et al: Expression of insulin-like growth factor II transcripts in Wilms' tumor. Nature 317:258–262, 1985
25. Olshan AF: Wilms' tumor, overgrowth factors: A hypothesis. Cancer Genet Cytogenet 21:303–307, 1986
26. Heideman R, MacGavran L, Walstein G: Nephroblastomatosis and 11p. The potential etiologic relationship to subsequent Wilms' tumor. Am J Pediatr Hematol Oncol 8:231–234, 1986
27. Karayalcin G, Shanske A, Honigman R: Wilms' tumor in a 13 year-old girl with trisomy 18. Am J Dis Child 135:665–667, 1981
28. Koufos A, Hansen MF, Copeland N et al: Loss of heterozygosity in three common embryonal tumors suggests common pathogenetic mechanism. Nature 316:330–334, 1985
29. Bove K, Koffler H, McAdams AJ: Nodular renal blastema. Definition and possible significance. Cancer 24:323–332, 1969
30. Meadows AT, Lichtenfeld JL, Koop CE: Wilms' tumor in three children of a woman with congenital hemihypertrophy. N Engl J Med 291:23–24, 1974
31. Kantor AF, Li FP, Fraumeni JF Jr et al: Childhood cancer in offspring of two Wilms' tumor survivors. Med Pediatr Oncol 10:85–89, 1982
32. Matsunaga E: Genetics of Wilms' tumor: Hum Genet 57:231–246, 1981
33. Breslow NB, Beckwith JB, Ciol M, Sharples K: The age distribution of Wilms' tumor. Cancer Res (in press)

34. Knudson AG, Strong LC: Mutation and cancer. A model for Wilms' tumor of the kidney. J Natl Cancer Inst 48:313–324, 1978
35. Machin GA: Persistent renal blastema (nephroblastomatosis) as a frequent precursor of Wilms' tumor: A pathological and clinical review. Am J Pediatr Hematol Oncol 2:165–172, 253–261, 353–362, 1980
36. Bove KE, McAdams AJ: The nephroblastomatosis complex and its relationship to Wilms' tumor: A clinicopathologic treatise. Perspect Pediatr Pathol 3:185–223, 1976
37. Knudson AG: Genetics and the child cured of cancer. In van Eys J, Sullivan MD (eds): Status of the Curability of Childhood Cancers, pp 295–305. New York, Raven Press, 1980
38. Green DM, Fine NE, Li FP: Offspring of patients treated for unilateral Wilms' tumor in childhood. Cancer 49:2285–2288, 1982
39. Beckwith JB: Wilms' tumor and other renal tumors of childhood: An update. J Urol 136:320–324, 1986
40. Bennington JL, Beckwith JB: Tumors of the kidney, renal pelvis and ureter. Atlas of Tumor Pathology, 2nd Series, Fascicle 12. Armed Forces Institute of Pathology, Washington, DC, 1975
41. Beckwith JB, Palmer NF: Histopathology and prognosis of Wilms' tumor. Results from the National Wilms' Tumor Study. Cancer 41:1937–1948, 1978
42. Beckwith JB: Wilms' tumor and other renal tumors of childhood: A selective review from the National Wilms' Tumor Study Pathology Center. Hum Pathol 14:481–492, 1983
43. Mahoney JP, Saffos RO: Fetal rhabdomyomatous nephroblastoma with a renal pelvic mass simulating sarcoma botryoides. Am J Surg Pathol 5:297–306, 1981
44. Gonzalez-Crussi F: Wilms' tumor (nephroblastoma) and related renal neoplasms of childhood. Boca Raton, FL, CRC Press, 1984
45. Pochedly C, Baum ES (eds): Wilms' tumor. Clinical and Biological Manifestations. New York, Elsevier, 1984
46. Schmidt D, Dickersin G, Vawter G et al: Wilms' tumor: Review of ultrastructure and histogenesis. Pathobiol Annu 12:281–300, 1982
47. Mierau GW, Weeks DA, Beckwith JB: Ultrastructure and histogenesis of the renal tumors of childhood: An overview. Ultrastruct Pathol 11:313–333, 1987
48. Kumar S, Carr T, Marsden HB: Study of childhood renal tumours using antisera to fibronectin, laminin, and epithelial membrane antigen. J Clin Pathol 39:5157, 1986
49. Altmannsberger M, Osborn M, Schaefer H et al: Distinction of neophroblastomas from other childhood tumors using antibodies to intermediate filaments. Virchows Arch [Cell Pathol] 45:113–124, 1984
50. Triche TJ, Askin FB, Kissane JM: Neuroblastoma, Ewing's sarcoma, and the differential diagnosis of the small-, round-, blue-cell tumors. Mod Probl Pathol 18:145–195, 1986
51. Chambers CH, Camitta BM, Tang TT, McCreadie SR: Nephroblastoma (Wilms' tumor): Tubule density and prognosis. Med Pediatr Oncol 5:127–135, 1978
52. Chatten J: Epithelial differentiation in Wilms' tumor—A clinicopathologic appraisal. Perspect Pediatr Pathol 3:225–254, 1976
53. Lawler W, Marsden HB, Palmer MK: Wilms' tumor—Histologic variation and prognosis. Cancer 36:1122–1126, 1975
54. Beckwith JB: Grading of pediatric tumors. In Care of the Child with Cancer, pp 39–44. New York, American Cancer Society, 1979
55. Bonadio JF, Storer B, Norkool P et al: Anaplastic Wilms' tumor: Clinical and pathological studies. J Clin Oncol 3:513–520, 1985
56. Douglass EC, Look AT, Webber B et al: Hyperdiploidy and chromosomal rearrangements define the anaplastic variant of Wilms' tumor. J Clin Oncol 4:975–981, 1986
57. Schmidt D, Wiedemann B, Keil W et al: Flow cytometric analysis of nephroblastomas and related neoplasms. Cancer 58:2494–2500, 1986
58. Kidd JM: Exclusion of certain renal neoplasms from the category of Wilms' tumor (abstr). Am J Pathol 59:16a, 1970
59. Marsden HB, Lawler W, Kumar PM: Bone metastazing renal tumor of childhood. Morphological and clinical features, and differences from Wilms' tumor. Cancer 42:1922–1928, 1978
60. Beckwith JB, Norkool P, Breslow N, D'Angio GJ: Clinical observations in children with clear-cell sarcoma (CCS) of the kidney (abstr). Proc Am Assoc Cancer Res 27:200, 1986
61. Haas JE, Bonadio JF, Beckwith JB: Clear cell sarcoma of kidney with emphasis on ultrastructural studies. Cancer 54:2978–2987, 1984
62. Schmidt D, Harms D, Evers KG et al: Bone metastasizing renal tumor (clear cell sarcoma) of childhood with epithelioid elements. Cancer 56:609–613, 1985

63. Lamego CMB, Zerbini MCH: Bone-metastasizing primary renal tumors in children. Radiology 147:449–454, 1983

64. Marsden HB, Lawler W: Bone metastasizing renal tumour of childhood. Histopathological and clinical review of 38 cases. Virchows Arch [A] 387:341–351, 1980

65. Haas JE, Palmer NF, Weinberg AG, Beckwith JB: Ultrastructure of malignant rhabdoid tumor of the kidney—A distinctive renal tumor of children. Hum Pathol 12:646–657, 1981

66. Statistical Report, Third National Wilms' Tumor Study, July 1986

67. Bonnin JM, Rubinstein LJ, Palmer NF, Beckwith JB: The association of embryonal tumors originating in the kidney and in the brain. Cancer 54:2137–2146, 1984

68. Vogel AM, Gown AM, Caughlan J et al: Rhabdoid tumors of the kidney contain mesenchymal specific and epithelial specific intermediate filament proteins. Lab Invest 50:232–238, 1984

69. Bolande RP, Brough AJ, Izant RJ: Congenital mesoblastic nephroma of infancy. Pediatrics 40:272–278, 1967

70. Beckwith JB: Mesenchymal renal neoplasms of infancy revisited. J Pediatr Surg 9:803–805, 1974

71. Joshi VV, Kasznicka J, Walters TR: Atypical congenital mesoblastic nephroma: Pathologic characterization of a potentially aggressive variant of conventional congenital mesoblastic nephroma. Arch Pathol Lab Med 110:100–106, 1986

72. Beckwith JB, Weeks DA: Congenital mesoblastic nephroma. When should we worry? Arch Pathol Lab Med 110:98–99, 1986

73. Raney RB Jr, Palmer N, Sutow WW et al: Renal cell carcinoma in children. Med Pediatr Oncol 11:91–98, 1983

74. Weeks DA, Beckwith JB, Luckey DW: Relapse-associated variables in Stage I favorable histology Wilms' tumor. A report of the National Wilms' Tumor Study. Cancer 60:1204–1212, 1987

75. Breslow NE, Churchill G, Nesmith B et al: Clinicopathologic features and prognosis for Wilms' tumor patients with metastases at diagnosis. Cancer 58:2501–2511, 1986

76. Green DM: Diagnosis and Management of Malignant Solid Tumors in Infants and Children. Boston, Martinus Nijhoff Publishing, 1985

77. Osler W: Two cases of striated-myosarcoma of the kidney. J Anat Physiol London 14:229–233, 1880

78. Ganguly A, Gribble J, Tune B et al: Renin-secreting Wilms' tumor with severe hypertension; report of a case and brief review of renin-secreting tumors. Ann Intern Med 79:835–837, 1973

79. Ramsay N, Dehner L, Coccia P et al: Acute hemorrhage into Wilms' tumor. J Pediatr 91:763–765, 1977

80. Ehrlich RM, Bloomberg SD, Gyepes MT et al: Wilms' tumor, misdiagnosed preoperatively. A review of nineteen National Wilms' Tumor Study-1 cases. J Urol 122:790–792, 1979

81. Joshi VV: Cystic partially differentiated nephroblastoma: An entity in the spectrum of infantile renal neoplasia. J Pathol 5:217–235, 1979

82. Howell CG, Othersen HB, Kiviat NE et al: Therapy and outcome in 51 children with mesoblastic nephroma: A report of the National Wilms' Tumor Study. J Pediatr Surg 17:826–831, 1982

83. Palmer NF, Sutow W: Clinical aspects of the rhabdoid tumor of the kidney: report of the National Wilms' Tumor Study Group. Med Pediatr Oncol 11:242–245, 1983

84. Miller JH: Imaging in Pediatric Oncology. Baltimore, Williams & Wilkins, 1985

85. Kangarloo H, Dietrich RB, Ehrlich RM et al: Magnetic resonance imaging of Wilms' tumor. Urology 28:203–207, 1986

86. Belt TG, Cohen MD, Smith JA et al: MRI of Wilms' tumor: Promise as the primary imaging method. AJR 146:955–961, 1986

87. Fernbach D, Pick T, Green D, Norkool P: The role of computerized tomograph in the clinical staging of Wilms' tumor. A report from the National Wilms' Tumor Study (NWTS) (abstr). Proc SIOP 16:5, 1984

88. Billingham ME, Bristow M, Glatstein E et al: Doxorubicin cardiotoxicity: Endomyocardial biopsy evidence of enhancement by irradiation. Am J Surg Pathol 1:17, 1977

89. Littman P, Meadows AT, Polgar G et al: Pulmonary function in survivors of Wilms' tumor. Cancer 37:2773–2776, 1976

90. Pratt CB, Ransom JL, Evans WE: Age-related doxorubicin cardiotoxicity in children. Cancer Treat Rep 62:1381–1385, 1978

91. D'Angio GJ, Evans AE, Breslow N et al: The treatment of Wilms' tumor. Results of the National Wilms' Tumor Study. Cancer 38:633–646, 1976

92. D'Angio GJ, Evans AE, Breslow N et al: Results of the third National Wilms' Tumor Study (NWTS-3): A preliminary report (abstr). Proc Am Assoc Cancer Res 25:183, 1984

93. Brick SH, Hill MC, Lande IM: The mistaken or indeterminate CT diagnosis of hepatic metastases: The value of sonography. AJR 148:723–726, 1987

94. Palmer NF, Sutow W: Clinical aspects of the rhabdoid tumor of the kidney: A report of the National Wilms' Tumor Study Group. Med Pediatr Oncol 11:242–245, 1983

95. Garcia M, Douglass C, Schlosser JV: Classification and prognosis in Wilms' tumor. Radiology 80:574–580, 1963

96. Cassady JR, Jaffe N, Filler RM: The increasing importance of radiation therapy in the improved prognosis of children with Wilms' tumor. Cancer 39:825–829, 1977

97. Farewell VT, D'Angio GJ, Breslow N, Norkool P: Retrospective validation of a new staging system for Wilms' tumor. Cancer Clin Trials 4:167–171, 1981

98. D'Angio GJ, Evans A, Breslow N et al: The treatment of Wilms' tumor: Results of the second National Wilms' Tumor Study. Cancer 47:2302–2311, 1981

99. Jereb B, Eklund G: Factors influencing the cure rate in nephroblastoma. Acta Radiol Ther 12:84–106, 1973

100. Leape LL, Breslow NE, Bishop HC: The surgical treatment of Wilms' tumor: Results of the National Wilms' Tumor Study. Ann Surg 187:351–356, 1978

101. Cole AT, Fried FA, Bissada NK: The supine subcostal modification of the thoraco-abdominal incision. J Urol 112:168–171, 1974

102. Grosfeld JL, Ballantine TVN, Baehner RL: Experience with "second-look" operations in pediatric solid tumors. J Pediatr Surg 13:275–280, 1978

103. Ehrlich RM: Complications of Wilms' tumor surgery. Urol Clin North Am 10:399–406, 1983

104. Blute ML, Kelalis PP, Breslow N et al: Bilateral Wilms' tumor. J Urol 128:968–973, 1987

105. Gonzalez R, Clayman RV, Sheldon CA: Management of intravascular nephroblastoma to avoid complications. Urol Clin North Am 10:407–415, 1983

106. Luck SR, De Leon S, Shkolnik A et al: Intracardiac Wilms' tumor: Diagnosis and management. J Pediatr Surg 17:551–554, 1982

107. Nakayama DK, deLorimier AA, O'Neill JA Jr et al: Intracardiac extension of Wilms' tumor. A report of the National Wilms' Tumor Study. Ann Surg 204:693–697, 1986

108. Bracken BR, Sutow WW, Jaffe N et al: Preoperative chemotherapy for Wilms' tumor. Urology 19:55–60, 1982

109. Broecker BH, Perlmutter AD: Management of unresectable Wilms' tumor. Urology 24:170–174, 1984

110. Lemerle J, Voute PA, Tournade MF et al: Preoperative versus post-operative radiotherapy, single versus multiple courses of actinomycin D in the treatment of Wilms' tumor. Cancer 38:647–654, 1976

111. Lemerle J, Voute PA, Tournande MF et al: Effectiveness of preoperative chemotherapy in Wilms' tumor: Results of an International Society of Paediatric Oncology (SIOP) clinical trial. J Clin Oncol 1:604–609, 1983

112. vanSonnenberg E, Wittich GR, Edwards DK et al: Percutaneous diagnostic and therapeutic interventional radiologic procedures in children: Experience in 100 patients. Radiology 162:601–605, 1987

113. Bray GL, Pendergrass TW, Schaller RT Jr et al: Preoperative chemotherapy in the treatment of Wilms' tumor diagnosed with the aid of fine needle aspiration biopsy. Am J Pediatr Hematol Oncol 8:75–78, 1986

114. D'Angio GJ: Editorial: SIOP and the management of Wilms' tumor. J Clin Oncol 1:595–596, 1983

115. Othersen HB Jr: Wilms' tumor (nephroblastoma). In Welch KJ, Randolph JG, Ravitch MM, O'Neill JA, Rowe MI (eds): Pediatric Surgery, 4th ed, pp 293–302. Chicago: Year Book Medical Publishers, 1986

116. Harrison MR, de Lorimier AA, Boswell WO: Preoperative angiographic embolization for large hemorrhagic Wilms' tumor. J Pediatr Surg 13:757–758, 1978

117. Danis RK, Wolverson MK, Graviss ER et al: Preoperative embolization of Wilms' tumors. Am J Dis Child 133:503–506, 1979

118. Bishop HC, Tefft M, Evans AE et al: Bilateral Wilms' tumor: Review of 30 National Wilms' Tumor Study cases. J Pediatr Surg 12:631–638, 1977

119. Malcom AW, Jaffe N, Folkman MJ, Cassady JR: Bilateral Wilms' tumor. Int J Radiat Oncol Biol Phys 6:167–174, 1980

120. Jones B, Hrabovsky E, Kiviat N et al: Metachronous bilateral Wilms' tumor. Cancer Clin Trials 5:545–550, 1982

121. Wasiljew BK, Besser A, Roffensperger J: Treatment of bilateral Wilms' tumors—A 22 year experience. J Pediatr Surg 17:265–268, 1982

122. Gross RE, Neuhauser EBD: Treatment of mixed tumors of the kidney in childhood. Pediatrics 6:843–852, 1950

123. Neuhauser EBD, Wittenborg MH, Berman CZ et al: Irradiation effects of roentgen therapy on the growing spine. Radiology 59:637, 1952

124. D'Angio GJ, Beckwith JB, Breslow NE et al: Wilms' tumor: An update. Cancer 45:1791–1798, 1980

125. Tefft M, D'Angio GJ, Grant W: Postoperative radiation therapy for residual Wilms' tumor. Review of Group III patients in National Wilms' Tumor Study. Cancer 37:2768–2772, 1976

126. D'Angio GJ, Tefft M, Breslow N et al: Radiation therapy of Wilms' tumor: Results according to dose, field, post-operative timing and histology. Int J Radiat Oncol Biol Phys 4:769–780, 1978

127. Thomas PRM, Tefft M, Farewell VT et al: Abdominal relapses in irradiated second National Wilms' Tumor Study patients. J Clin Oncol 2:1098–1101, 1984

128. Evans AE, Breslow N, Norkool P et al: Complications in long-term survivors of Wilms' tumor (abstr 808). Proc Am Assoc Cancer Res 27:204, 1986

129. Probert JC, Parker BR, Kaplan HS: Growth retardation in children after megavoltage irradiation of the spine. Cancer 32:634, 1973

130. Tucker MA, Meadows AT, Boice JD et al: Bone cancer (BC) linked to radiotherapy and chemotherapy in children (abstr C-932). Proc Am Soc Clin Oncol 4:239, 1985

131. Oliver JH, Gluck G, Gledhill RB et al: Musculoskeletal deformities following treatment of Wilms' tumor. CMA J 119:459–464, 1978

132. Heaston DK, Libshitz HI, Chan RC: Skeletal effects of megavoltage irradiation in survivors of Wilms' tumor. Am J Roentgenol 133:389–395, 1979

133. Farber S: Chemotherapy in the treatment of leukemia and Wilms' tumor. JAMA 198:826–836, 1966

134. Sutow WW, Thurman WG, Windmiller J: Vincristine (leurocristine) sulfate in the treatment of children with metastatic Wilms' tumor. Pediatrics 12:880–887, 1963

135. Wolff JA, D'Angio G, Hartmann J et al: Long-term evaluation of single versus multiple courses of actinomycin D therapy of Wilms' tumor. N Engl J Med 290:84–86, 1974

136. Wolff JA, Krivit W, Newton WA Jr et al: Single versus multiple dose dactinomycin therapy of Wilms' tumor. N Engl J Med 279:290–294, 1968

137. Green DM, Jaffe N: The role of chemotherapy in the treatment of Wilms' tumor. Cancer 49:2285–2288, 1979

138. Medical Research Council's Working Party on Embryonal Tumours in Childhood: Management of nephroblastoma in childhood. Arch Dis Child 53:112–119, 1978

139. Response of Ridgway Osteogenic Sarcoma (ROS) at Different Stages to a Variety of Drugs Given According to Different Schedules, Birmingham, AL, Southern Research Institute, 49:32–33, 1977

140. Green DM, Sallan SE, Krishan A: Actinomycin D in childhood acute lymphocytic leukemia. Cancer Treat Rep 62:829–831, 1978

141. Carli M, Pastore G, Paolucci G et al: High single doses versus 5 day divided doses of dactinomycin (AMD) in childhood rhabdomyosarcoma. Preliminary results (abstr). Proc Am Soc Clin Oncol 2:76, 1983

142. Blatt J, Trigg ME, Pizzo PA et al: Tolerance to single-dose dactinomycin in combination chemotherapy for solid tumors. Cancer Treat Rep 65:145–147, 1981

143. Benjamin RS, Hall SW, Burgess MA et al: A pharmacokinetically based phase I-II study of single dose actinomycin (NSC-3053). Cancer Treat Rep 60:289–291, 1976

144. Morgan E, Baum E, Breslow N et al: Chemotherapy-related toxicity in infants treated according to the second National Wilms' Tumor Study. J Clin Oncol 6:51–55, 1988

145. Jones B, Breslow N, Takashima J: Toxic deaths in the Second National Wilms' Tumor Study. J Clin Oncol 2:1028–1033, 1984

146. Tefft M, Mitus A, Das L et al: Irradiation of the liver in children: Review of experience in the acute and chronic phases, and in the intact normal and partially resected. Am J Roentgenol 108:365–385, 1970

147. Bhanot P, Cushing B, Phillipart A et al: Hepatic irradiation and Adriamycin cardiotoxicity. J Pediatr 95:561–563, 1979

148. Pinkel D, Camitta B, Kun L et al: Doxorubicin cardiomyopathy in children with left-sided Wilms' tumor. Med Pediatr Oncol 10:483–488, 1982

149. Silver HK: Wilms' tumor (embryoma of kidney). J Pediatr 31:643, 1947

150. Zucker JM, Tournade MF, Voute PA et al: Report on SIOP 6 nephroblastoma trials. Proc SIOP 18:31–34, 1986

151. Breslow NE, Churchill G, Nesmith B et al: Clinicopathologic features and prognosis for Wilms' tumor patients with metastases at diagnosis. Cancer 58:2501–2511, 1986

152. Hrabovsky E, Othersen HB, de Lorimier A et al: Wilms' tumor in the neonate: A report from the National Wilms' Tumor Study. J Pediatr Surg 385–387, 1986

153. Grundy P, Takashima J, Evans AE et al: Results of salvage therapy for relapsed third National Wilms' Tumor Study (NWTS-3) patients. Proc Am Soc Clin Oncol 4:245, 1985

154. Green DM: The treatment of advanced or recurrent malignant genitourinary urinary tumors in children. Cancer (in press)

155. Madanat F, Osborne B, Cangir A et al: Extrarenal Wilms' tumor. J Pediatr 93:439–443, 1978

156. Mesrobian H-GJ, Kelalis PP, Hrabovsky E et al: Wilms' tumor in horseshoe kidneys: A report of the National Wilms' Tumor Study group. J Urol 133:1002–1003, 1985

157. Palmer N, Evans AE: The association of aniridia and Wilms' tumor: Methods of surveillance and diagnosis. Med Pediatr Oncol 11:73–75, 1983

158. Mike V, Meadows AT, D'Angio GJ: Incidence of second malignant neoplasms in children: Results of an international study. Lancet 2:1326–1331, 1982

159. Meadows AT, Baum E, Fossati-Bellani F et al: Second malignant neoplasms in children: an update from the Late Effects Study Group. J Clin Oncol 3:532–538, 1985

160. D'Angio GJ, Meadows A, Mike V et al: Decreased risk of radiation associated second malignant neoplasms in actinomycin-D treated patients. Cancer 37(Suppl):1177–1185, 1976

twenty-eight

Neuroblastoma

Frances Ann Hayes and Edwin Ide Smith

Neuroblastoma was first described by Virchow in 1864.[1] The cellular similarities of this tumor to embryonic adrenal medulla were noted in 1910 by Wright,[2] and Robertson described its numerous histologic patterns, which ranged from highly anaplastic to well-differentiated, benign-looking cellular elements.[3] The neural character of the fibrils within these tumors was described and confirmed by several authors.[4-6]

Neuroblastoma is one of several tumors that originate in the neural crest cells, occurring in those cells that give rise to the sympathetic nervous system. This is one of the most biologically remarkable tumors of childhood. Not only does spontaneous regression occur,[7] but both spontaneous[8] and induced[9,10] maturation to benign ganglioneuroma are seen. In no other tumor is age such an important factor in prognosis, with significantly superior survival among infants younger than 1 year, regardless of extent of tumor at diagnosis.[11,12]

EPIDEMIOLOGY AND GENETICS

In the United States, the incidence of neuroblastoma is 9.6 per million white children per year and 7.0 per million black children.[13] It is the commonest extracranial solid tumor of childhood and comprises up to 50% of malignancies among infants[14] (median age at diagnosis = 2 years[15]). Neuroblastoma occurs slightly more frequently in males.[15]

The incidence of neuroblastoma is much lower in certain geographic areas. For example, in areas of Africa where Burkitt's lymphoma comprises up to 50% of childhood malignancies, neuroblastoma is rarely seen (see Chap. 1).[16] This may indicate that genetic or environmental factors affect the distribution of this tumor. Alternatively, lower incidences may reflect a low level of detection and reporting in these areas.

An interesting observation has been made in infants younger than 3 months dying of nonmalignant causes. Microscopic nodules of neuroblasts have been found in the adrenal glands of from 1 in 259 to 1 in 39 cases.[17,18] This "neuroblastoma in situ" is histologically indistinguishable from neuroblastoma. In fetuses, particularly between 17 and 20 weeks of gestation, these lesions have been found consistently. Whether these nodules represent malignancy that spontaneously regresses or are a normal embryonic stage of adrenal development unrelated to neuroblastoma is not known. The latter explanation seems reasonable and leads to the speculation that in those children who are genetically predisposed or who are exposed to relevant environmental factors, the normal regression or maturation of these embryonic nodules does not occur, and malignant neuroblastoma results.

Genetic predisposition is a possibility in neuroblastoma. The presence of neuroblastoma in siblings and in identical twins has been well documented.[19-21] Four of five siblings in one family had neuroblastoma, and their mother had elevated catecholamine excretion and a mediastinal mass. In another family, the parents of a child with neuroblastoma both had had children with the disease in previous marriages. Kushner and colleagues reviewed 23 familial aggregations of neuroblastoma, with 55 involved individuals.[22] They noted an increased incidence of multiple primary tumors (23% versus 5%) and a young age at diagnosis (60% versus 25% < 12 months) compared to unselected cases. However, from the available data the risk for siblings or offspring of neuroblastoma patients to develop the disease was calculated to be less than 6%. Knudson and Strong proposed that 20% to 25% of neuroblastomas are heritable and, as such, have a prezygotic (germinal) mutation and then a ''second hit'' or postzygotic (somatic) event. In the other 75% to 80% of cases, both ''hits'' or events are postzygotic.[23] The carriers of the germinal mutation may or may not develop tumors, and more than one tumor (multiple primaries) may be present. In nonheritable cases, only one primary tumor is present (see also Chap. 2).

Neuroblastoma has been observed with increased frequency in patients with neurofibromatosis, the Beckwith–Wiedemann syndrome, and nisidiroblastosis. However, no specific constellation of congenital anomalies has been associated with this tumor.[24–26] Neuroblastoma has been associated in several cases with the fetal hydantoin syndrome.[27]

BIOLOGY

Neuroblastoma is an important tumor biologically in that spontaneous regression and spontaneous and induced maturation occur with significant frequency. Spontaneous regression, seen most often in infants younger than 1 year, occurs in about 1% of children with neuroblastoma with gross residual disease after surgical excision. Unlike many malignancies, microscopic residual tumor in the tumor bed of localized neuroblastoma following gross surgical excision rarely results in recurrence (see Staging section). The role of host immunity in this phenomenon is unclear.

FIGURE 28-1. Induced conversion to ganglioneuroma. A 14-month-old child presented with biopsy-proven neuroblastoma in abdomen and liver metastases. The neuroblastoma treated with chemotherapy, and at repeat surgery biopsies showed ganglioneuroma only. Therapy was discontinued 4½ years ago. There has been no recurrence of neuroblastoma nor progression of residual unresectable ganglioneuroma.

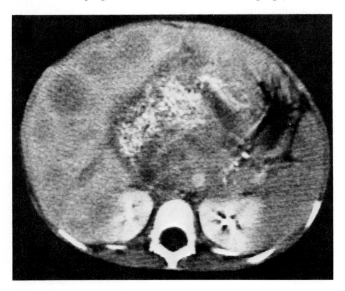

Differentiation of a malignant cohort of neuroblasts into benign ganglion cells occurs both spontaneously and following therapy. *In vitro* maturation of neuroblasts can be induced by a variety of substances that presumably act through cyclic adenosine monophosphate (cAMP), and by cAMP itself.[28,29] Two agents that increase cellular cAMP, 5-trifuoromethyl-2-deoxyuridine and papavarine, have been used in clinical trials to induce maturation.[30,31] However, because chemotherapeutic drugs were also used, the effects of these agents on maturation cannot be assessed.[32,33] Maturation to ganglioneuroma is not infrequently observed at surgery following induction chemotherapy (Fig. 28-1). Spontaneous maturation is thought to have occurred in patients presenting with benign ganglioneuromas, which are usually localized masses. Spontaneous maturation of disseminated disease does occur (Fig. 28-2).

FIGURE 28-2. Spontaneous conversion to ganglioneuroma. A 3½-year-old child presented with a thoracic mass and bone lesions. The resected mass and a biopsy of the maxillary lesion showed only ganglioneuroma. Follow-up without treatment has been 5½ years.

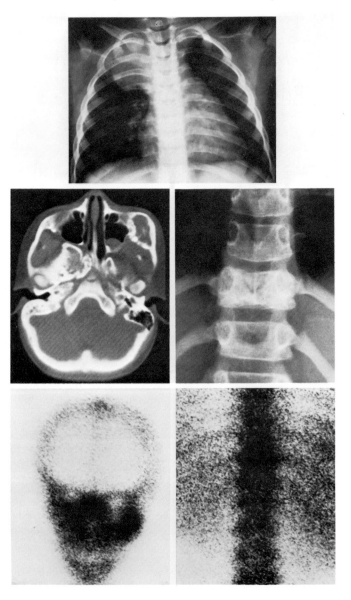

Immunology

Both cell-mediated and antibody-mediated cytotoxicity against neuroblastoma cells have been demonstrated in patients with neuroblastoma, in the mothers of these patients, and occasionally in other close relatives.[34,35] "Blocking antibodies," which interfere with cell-mediated cytotoxicity, have also been demonstrated in the sera of patients with active or progressive disease.[36] However, clinical immunotherapy trials using methanol-extracted residue of bacillus Calmette-Guerin (BCG), BCG- and neuraminidase-treated tumor cells, or viable tumor cells have not convincingly demonstrated therapeutic benefit.[37,38]

Multiple monoclonal antibodies have been developed that react with antigens on neuroblastoma cells.[39] None of these have been shown to react only with neuroblastoma, to react with all neuroblastoma cells (fresh tumor or cell lines), or to kill 100% of tumor cells *in vitro*. The antigen targets for most of these antibodies are probably glycoprotein differentiation antigens. At least one, however, is to the glycolipid G_{D2}, an antigen known to be present on the surface of neuroblastoma cells.[40] When these antibodies are injected into animals or humans, nonspecific localization in the reticuloendothelial system occurs, posing a significant limitation to their use for diagnostic scanning or targeted therapy.[39] The continued development of monoclonal antibodies of increased specificity, however, is an exciting and important area of research.

Genetics and Molecular Biology

Cytogenetic studies of neuroblastoma cells have demonstrated abnormalities in approximately 80% of cases.[41,42] The most consistent abnormality is a deletion or rearrangement of the short arm of chromosome 1. This finding is not specific for neuroblastoma—the same deletion is seen in many other tumors. The second most often involved chromosome is chromosome 17.

Recent studies indicate that the DNA content of tumor cells compared to normal cells (DNA index) is of prognostic importance in neuroblastoma. A DNA index can be obtained rapidly using flow cytometry to designate a tumor as pseudodiploid, diploid, or hyperdiploid. Look and coworkers have shown that in infants a DNA index of 1 rarely occurs in low-stage disease; in disseminated disease an index of 1 is associated with a poor response to cyclophosphamide and Adria-

mycin chemotherapy.[43] Gansler and associates reported similar findings.[44] Kaneko and colleagues found that pseudodiploidy was associated with higher stage disease and a poor prognosis.[45] It has been postulated that Evans Stage IV-S disease may not be a true malignancy. However, in the above studies[43,44] such patients have been shown to have aneupolid tumors, indicating that these neoplasms are composed of malignant cells.

Other nonspecific karyotypic abnormalities that occur with high frequency in neuroblastoma cell lines are double minute spheres (dms) and homogeneous staining regions (HSRs).[46,47] It has been suggested that the dms result from the breakdown of the HSRs. HSRs and dms have also been demonstrated in fresh neuroblastoma tissue. Current evidence would indicate that HSRs represent amplified cellular genes. The oncogenes N-*myc* and N-*ras* are amplified in neuroblastoma cells.[48] The cellular proto-oncogene N-*myc* is normally found in single copy on the short arm of chromosome 2.[49] In approximately 50% of tumors from patients with disseminated neuroblastoma, N-*myc* is amplified and multiple copies can be detected. However, amplification is rare in tumors from patients with localized neuroblastoma.[50,51] Studies of cell lines show that HSRs contain amplified N-*myc* sequences. N-*myc* is also amplified in retinoblastoma and malignant schwannoma.

N-*myc* DNA amplification and RNA expression have been reported to increase with tumor progression.[52] More recent findings indicate that N-*myc* copy number is homogeneous in a given tumor, and amplification generally does not increase with progressive disease but instead appears to be an intrinsic biological property present at the time of diagnosis.[53] The significance of this amplification in relation to prognosis or response to therapy has not been established.[50] (For a more in-depth review of oncogenes, see Chap. 3.)

Biological Markers

Urinary excretion of abnormally high levels of catecholamine metabolites occurs in 85% to 90% of patients with neuroblastoma (also see Chap. 8).[54,55] The metabolites most often measured are vanillylmandelic acid (VMA) and homovanillic acid (HVA) (Fig. 28-3). The absolute values of VMA and HVA are not of prognostic significance, but the VMA:HVA ratio in patients with disseminated disease correlates with outcome (the higher the value, the better the prognosis). The presence of vanillacetic acid (VLA) in the urine correlates with a poor prognosis.

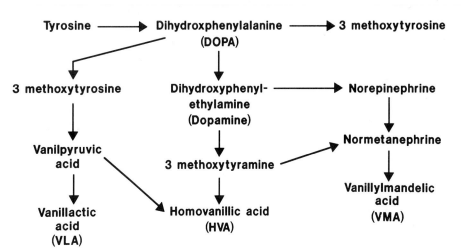

FIGURE 28-3. Schema of catecholamine metabolism.

In Japan, screening of urine for abnormal catecholamine excretion in 6-month-old infants to detect preclinical neuroblastoma has shown encouraging results.[56,57] Because the incidence of neuroblastoma is about equal to that of neonatal hypothyroidism and higher than either phenylketonuria or galactosemia, mass screening should be seriously considered in this disease.[58-60]

Plasma dopamine levels are elevated above normal levels (0.9–5.3 mg/ml) in approximately 90% of patients with neuroblastoma. The presence of elevated urinary levels of the amino acid cystathionine correlates with poor prognosis.[61]

Neuron-specific enolase (NSE) is elevated in the serum of 95% of patients with widespread neuroblastoma, whereas patients with localized or regional disease rarely have significantly elevated levels.[62] NSE is not specific for neuroblastoma, in that elevated levels can be found in normal children and in children and adults with other tumors. A value ≥ 100 mg/ml at diagnosis is of prognostic significance in infants younger than 365 days but is of only marginal prognostic value in older children.

Ferritin is produced by neuroblastoma cells *in vitro* and can be detected in the sera of nude mice bearing human neuroblastomas. Ferritin is rarely elevated in sera from patients with localized neuroblastoma but is elevated in approximately 40% to 50% of patients with Evans Stage III or IV disease at diagnosis. Patients with Stage III disease and normal ferritin levels have a significantly better prognosis than those with elevated levels (76% versus 23% disease-free at 2 years). For Stage IV patients, the difference is not as marked (27% versus 3%).[63]

Gangliosides (sialic acid-containing glycosphingolipids) occur primarily on the membrane of cells.[64] Several studies have shown that G_{D2} ganglioside is present in high concentrations on the surface of essentially all neuroblastoma cells and is shed into the circulation in amounts that are measurable in the serum of patients. G_{D2} is not present or is present in only small amounts on the surface of more differentiated ganglioneuroblastoma or ganglioneuroma. This ganglioside is the antigen target for one monoclonal antibody developed for scanning in neuroblastoma, and its level in serum may prove to be an important prognostic marker.[40]

PATHOLOGY

Neural crest cells give rise to the adrenal medulla, sympathetic ganglia, thyroid medullary C cells, meninges, Schwann cells, melanocytes, and membranous bone. The neural crest contains primitive stem cells that differentiate into sympathoblasts. It is from these cells that neuroblastoma is derived. The primitive cells may also differentiate into paraganglionic cells from which pheochromocytomas and paragangliomas are derived.

Neuroblastoma is one of the "small blue round cell" tumors of childhood. In its primitive form, it consists of dense nests of cells separated by fibrillar bundles and frequently demonstrates hemorrhage, necrosis, and calcification. A characteristic finding is the presence of rosettes in which tumor cells surround a pink fibrillar center. As maturation occurs, cells begin to differentiate toward ganglion cells, and increasing amounts of fibrillar material are present. Uniform maturation may occur, or there may be areas of maturation interspersed with areas of undifferentiated cells (composite ganglioneuroblastoma). At the completely differentiated end of the spectrum is ganglioneuroma, which is composed of well-differentiated ganglion cells, Schwann cells, and nerve bundles (Figs. 28-4–28-6). The same tumor may contain differentiated and undifferentiated areas, so that multiple sec-

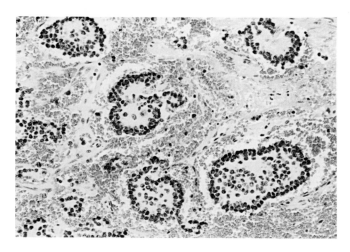

FIGURE 28-4.   Neuroblastoma.

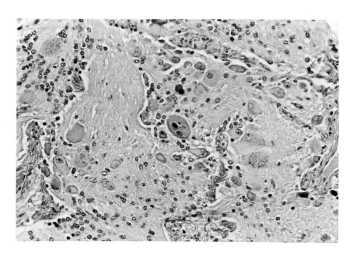

FIGURE 28-5.   Ganglioneuroblastoma.

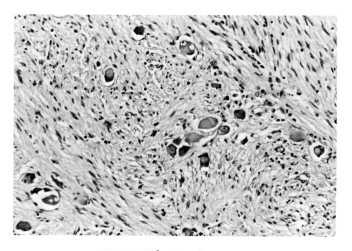

FIGURE 28-6.   Ganglioneuroma.

tions from all areas of a tumor mass must be sampled before a diagnosis of benign ganglioneuroma is made.

It may be very difficult to differentiate neuroblastoma from lymphoma, Ewing's sarcoma, rhabdomyosarcoma, and primitive neuroectodermal tumors by light microscopy. The pathologist must take into account the clinical and radiographic findings. Other aids to diagnosis include electron microscopy, immunodiagnosis, special stains, characteristic chromosomal abnormalities, and specific biochemical markers in urine or serum. (For a detailed discussion of the differential diagnosis of small round cell tumors, including neuroblastoma, see Chap. 6.)

Electron microscopy of neuroblastoma reveals neurosecretory dense core granules in the peripheral cytoplasm and neural processes containing microtubules. Immunodiagnosis using an antibody to NSE is helpful in differentiating neuroblastoma from the other common small round cell tumors (although NSE may also be present in primitive neuroectodermal tumors and, rarely, in rhabdomyosarcoma). Periodic acid-Schiff (PAS) stain is positive in Ewing's sarcoma and rhabdomyosarcoma but is typically negative in neuroblastoma. Lymphoid markers can be used to rule out lymphoma. Elevation of urinary catecholamines in patients with neuroblastoma is useful for diagnosis, but normal excretion does not rule out neuroblastoma (Table 28-1) (also see Chap. 8).

CLINICAL PRESENTATION AND PATTERNS OF SPREAD

Neuroblastoma may originate anywhere along the sympathetic nervous system chain. The most common site of primary tumor is within the abdomen, either in an adrenal gland (40%) or in a paraspinal ganglion (25%). Other sites are the paraspinal area of the thorax (15%), the neck (5%), and the pelvis (5%). A small proportion of patients do not have a discernible primary tumor at diagnosis. Age does affect the site of primary tumor, with infants (defined in this chapter as <365 days) having a higher proportion of thoracic primary tumors and a lower proportion of abdominal tumors compared with older children (Table 28-2).

Approximately 50% of infants and 70% of older children present with evidence of tumor spread beyond the primary site. The most common sites of metastases are lymph nodes (regional and disseminated), bone marrow, bone, liver, and subcutaneous tissue (Figs. 28-7–28-11).

Presenting signs and symptoms differ depending on the primary site and site of metastases. The presence of an abdominal mass is frequently the first sign of disease (see also Chap. 5). These masses are usually firm and irregular and often cross the midline. Thoracic masses are usually found coincidentally when a chest radiograph is obtained for another reason. Occasionally, the masses may be large enough to cause respiratory symptoms (see Chaps. 7 and 37). Cervical masses are often misdiagnosed as infection, even though the child is usually otherwise well. The presence of Horner's syndrome or heterochromia iridis should prompt one to rule out cervicothoracic neuroblastoma. Pelvic masses arising from the organ of Zuckerkandl may manifest as a palpable mass or may present with bladder and bowel symptoms resulting from compression by tumor. The liver may be markedly enlarged, especially in infants, which can result in respiratory embarrassment.

Large retroperitoneal abdominal or pelvic masses can

Table 28-1
Maximum Normal Urinary Excretion of VMA and HVA
(milligrams per gram of urinary creatinine)

Age (yr)	VMA	HVA
<0.5	12	16
0.5	10	14.5
1.0	8	13
1.5	6	11.5
2.0	4	10
>2.0	3.5	9

(Data compiled from Reference 55)

Table 28-2
Distribution of Primary Site by Age at Diagnosis

Site	Age	
	<1 year	>1 year
Neck	3 (5.2%)	4 (3%)
Chest	20 (33%)	23 (15.8%)
Abdomen		
Adrenal	22 (36.7%)	81 (55%)
Nonadrenal	11 (18.3%)	29 (19.9%)
Pelvic	3 (5.2%)	7 (4.8%)
Unknown	1 (1.6%)	2 (1.5%)
Total	60	146

FIGURE 28-7. Metastatic neuroblastoma in the mandible.

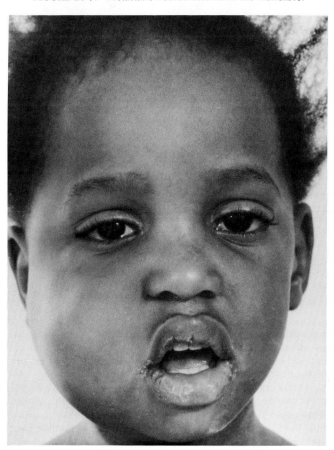

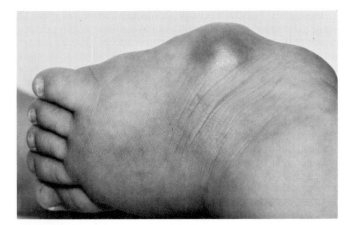

FIGURE 28-8. Subcutaneous metastasis of neuroblastoma.

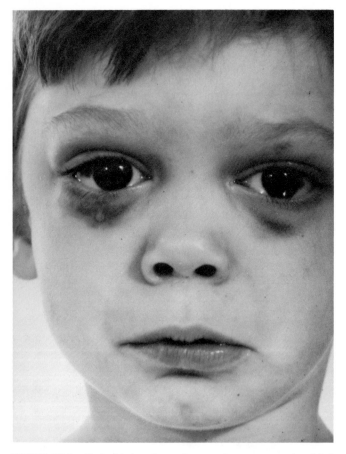

FIGURE 28-9. Periorbital ecchymosis secondary to metastatic orbital neuroblastoma.

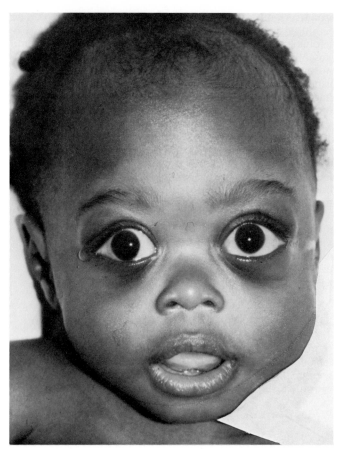

FIGURE 28-10. Cervical neuroblastoma with orbital metastases and proptosis.

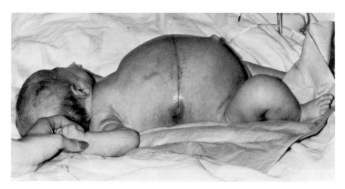

FIGURE 28-11. Massive liver enlargement caused by metastatic neuroblastoma.

cause vascular compression with edema of the lower extremities. Abdominal masses that produce stretching or compression of the renal vasculature can result in severe hypertension. Hypertension is rarely due to elevated catecholamines.

Paraspinal tumors in any site, but most frequently in the thorax and neck, may extend through the spinal foramina, with subsequent cord compression. Such patients may present with paresis, paralysis, or bladder or bowel dysfunction (see Chap. 37).

Skin or subcutaneous nodules are almost exclusively seen

in infants. They appear as nontender, bluish, mobile nodules, and there may be only a few or dozens present. Bone marrow and bone disease usually manifest in the child as pain that often results in limping or, in the younger child, refusal to walk. Sphenoid bone and retrobulbar tissue involvement is frequent and causes orbital ecchymosis with swelling and proptosis. Compression fractures of the vertebrae occur and in the older child can result in severe back pain.

Older children with neuroblastoma often present with rather nonspecific symptoms, such as intermittent fever, weight loss or failure to gain weight, refusal to play, or vague complaints of generalized pain.

An unusual presentation of this tumor is the syndrome of opsoclonus-myoclonus.[65,66] These patients have acute cerebellar and truncal ataxia and rapid, random eye movements ("dancing eyes, dancing feet"). The pathophysiology of this syndrome and its association with neuroblastoma is unknown; the favored view is that it is an autoimmune disorder. Jones and coworkers reviewed the experience at the Mayo Clinic and reported that half of the patients presenting with acute cerebellar ataxia were found to have neuroblastoma.[67] These patients tend to have localized disease and thus a good prognosis for cure of their tumor. However, 70% to 80% have permanent neurologic sequelae, with recurrences of ataxia, mental retardation, and extrapyramidal deficits.[68]

A syndrome of chronic watery diarrhea may also occur in patients with abdominal ganglioneuroblastoma.[69] The tumors and plasma of these patients contain a substance called vasoactive intestinal peptide (VIP), which causes increased intestinal motility and secretions. Removal of the tumor results in resolution of the diarrhea.

METHODS OF DIAGNOSIS

The history and physical examination usually lead to a high degree of suspicion of neuroblastoma. The workup should include a complete blood count, liver and kidney function studies, a coagulation screen, urinalysis, and urine assay for catecholamine metabolites. Diagnostic imaging studies should include a chest radiograph, computed tomography (CT) scan of the primary site and liver, bone scan, and skeletal survey with orbital views. A bone marrow aspirate with or without a biopsy should be obtained (Table 28-3). In patients with extensive orbital or cranial lesions, a CT scan of the head and orbits will define intracranial extension. CT scans of paraspinal primary sites should include views of the spine to evaluate cord compression. Magnetic resonance imaging (MRI) in neuroblastoma has not been studied prospectively to compare its utility to CT scans. The anatomic detail provided by MRI, especially in tumors impinging on the spinal cord, would indicate that this modality may replace CT scans in delineating the extent of mass disease (see Chap. 7). These studies are not only essential for staging of the tumor, but can often lead to a definite diagnosis without surgical intervention (*e.g.,* elevated catecholamines with classic bone marrow tumor and a clinical picture of neuroblastoma).

Newer diagnostic scanning materials may make many of the above studies obsolete.[40,70-72] ^{131}I-meta-iodobenzylguanidine (MIBG) is taken up by adrenergic secretory vesicles and competes with and is handled by the cells in the same manner as norepinepherine. Originally developed to visualize the adrenal medulla and pheochromocytoma, it has undergone extensive trials in neuroblastoma. In most patients, ^{131}I-MIBG is taken up both in the primary tumor and in metastatic deposits. Initial studies indicated that MIBG was only accumulated in tumors of patients with increased excretion of catecholamines. More current data, however, indicate that the majority of tumors accumulate MIBG, regardless of urinary catecholamine levels. Monoclonal antibodies are also undergoing evaluation as a scanning material attached to ^{131}I or [123]I. These antibodies are investigational and are not currently available for general *in vivo* use.[40,72,73]

At diagnosis, the hemoglobin is usually normal except in patients who have had hemorrhage into large tumors and, rarely, in patients with bone marrow tumor. Platelet counts are more often high than low. Coagulation studies may be abnormal, with evidence of disseminated intravascular coagulation present before therapy or developing during the initial days of chemotherapy. Elevations of lactate dehydrogenase (LDH) are common in patients with large tumors or in widely disseminated disease. It is unusual, even with extensive liver metastases, to find any abnormality of transaminases.

Radiographic findings depend on the site of the primary tumor and metastases. The chest radiograph may show a primary posterior mediastinal mass, paraspinal lymph node enlargement, or bone lesions of the ribs and vertebrae. Skeletal metastases are usually lytic in nature and are most often seen in the skull, orbits, and proximal long bones. Periosteal elevation may be evident, and occasionally pathologic fractures occur. The bone scan not only demonstrates most bone lesions, but in neuroblastoma, the ^{99m}Tc is taken up by the primary tumor. Symmetric bone lesions, especially in infants, may make interpretation of the bone scan very difficult. It is in these situations that ^{131}I-MIBG scans may be very useful.

With abdominal primaries, an abdominal film may reveal speckled calcifications in the mass lesion. Most centers now use contrast-enhanced CT scanning to assess mass lesions and hepatic metastases. Characteristically, abdominal neuroblastomas displace the kidneys and liver but do not invade them (Fig. 28-12). However, there are cases where clinical or radiographic differentiation from Wilms' tumor or hepatoblastoma

FIGURE 28-12. CT scan of an abdominal neuroblastoma at diagnosis.

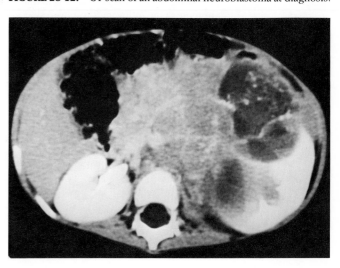

Table 28-3
Minimal Evaluation for Clinical Staging of Neuroblastoma

History and Physical Examination
Laboratory Studies
    Complete blood count, differential, platelets
    Liver and kidney function studies
    Urinary catecholamine excretion
Diagnostic Imaging
    Chest radiograph
    Skeletal survey with orbital views
    Bone scan
    CT scan of abdomen and pelvis
        (neck or thorax if primary in these areas)
Bone Marrow Aspirate ± Biopsy

is impossible (see Chaps. 26 and 27). Liver metastases may manifest as discrete nodules or may be diffusely scattered through the liver parenchyma. In the latter case, the CT scan or a liver scan with a radionucleotide may appear normal.

Bone marrow aspirates are most easily obtained from the posterior iliac spine. Tumor in marrow may be so extensive that a leukemic picture is present. However, careful evaluation reveals syncitia of cells, with fibrillar material more characteristic of neuroblastoma. Some patients have only occasional clusters of tumor cells. In all patients, it is essential that multiple slides be carefully studied before declaring the marrow uninvolved. If 1 or 2 cc of heparinized marrow is obtained, buffy coat smears can be made to search for tumor. In many centers, evaluation of marrow with monoclonal antibodies is now routine, whereas other centers use bone marrow biopsies.[74,75] Bone lesions are rarely present in the absence of marrow involvement. If bone lesions are detected on bone scan or radiograph and the initial bone marrow aspirate or biopsy is negative, multiple sites should be sampled to confirm the presence or absence of tumor.

STAGING

The classic staging system used in neuroblastoma is that proposed by Evans and colleagues in 1971 (Table 28-4).[76] This scheme was based on extent of disease as determined by physical examination, radiographic evaluation, and bone marrow examination. Tumor resectability of clinically localized disease was not incorporated into the original staging scheme.

Table 28-4
Evans Staging System for Neuroblastoma

Stage I	Tumor confined to the organ or structure of origin.
Stage II	Tumor extending in continuity beyond the organ or structure of origin but not crossing the midline. Regional lymph nodes on the homolateral side may be involved.
Stage III	Tumors extending in continuity beyond the midline. Regional lymph nodes bilaterally may be involved.
Stage IV	Remote disease involving bone, parenchymatous organs, soft tissues or distant lymph node groups, or bone marrow.
Stage IV-S	Patients who would otherwise be Stage I or II but who have remote disease confined to one or more of the following sites: liver, skin, or bone marrow (without evidence of bone metastases).

If the Evans staging system is used, more than half of children older than 1 year with Stages I through III disease will not survive, so that factors not included in this staging system must be considered.[77] One of these factors is spread of tumor cells to regional lymph nodes. Ninane and colleagues evaluated 33 children with Evans Stage II disease and found that of the 20 children with negative nodes, none died of tumor.[78] In contrast, 6 of the 13 with positive regional nodes died of tumor. In a review of Stages II and III patients, Hayes and coworkers found an 83% survival in patients without nodal disease compared to 31% in those with nodal disease.[79] Surgical resectability of the primary tumor, regardless of its size, is an important prognostic factor. If lymph nodes are negative for tumor, more than 90% of patients (regardless of age) with Pediatric Oncology Group (POG) Stage A disease will survive. Those with negative nodes and unresectable primaries also have an excellent prognosis with current therapy.[79] These studies have resulted in the POG staging system, which is based on the St. Jude Children's Research Hospital (SJCRH) surgical-pathologic staging of patients with clinically localized disease (Evans Stages I–III; Table 28-5).[79] A comparison of the Evans and POG staging systems is illustrated in Figure 28-13. Of the Evans Stage I patients, 85% will be POG Stage A and 15% Stage B. For Evans Stage II, 45% will be POG A, 45% POG B, and 10% POG C. Evans Stage III disease patients will in 10% of cases be POG Stage A, in 35% of cases POG Stage B, and in 55% POG Stage C.[79] The distribution of stage by age shows that there is a higher proportion of Stages A, B, and C disease in infants (Table 28-6).

Variable prognoses between and within stages have also been correlated with other factors, such as LDH, histologic grading of tumor,[80] serum ferritin,[63] serum NSE,[62] ploidy by flow cytometry,[43,44] and VMA:HVA ratio in the urine (see also Chap. 8).[55] In the future, these factors, combined with clinical-surgical-pathologic staging, may better define groups of patients requiring different treatment approaches. They will probably have their greatest impact in infants and in lower stage disease.

THERAPY

There are three main modalities for the treatment of neuroblastoma: surgery, radiation therapy, and chemotherapy.

Surgery

The role of surgery in neuroblastoma is both diagnostic and therapeutic (see also Chap. 10). Operations are classified as primary (prior to any chemotherapy or radiotherapy) and delayed or secondary (following therapy). The goals of a primary

Table 28-5
Pediatric Oncology Group (POG) Staging for Neuroblastoma

Stage A	Complete gross excision of primary tumor, margins histologically negative or positive. Intracavitary lymph nodes not intimately adhered to and removed with resected tumor are histologically free of tumor. If primary is in abdomen (including pelvis), liver is histologically free of tumor.
Stage B	Incomplete gross resection of primary. Lymph nodes and liver histologically free of tumor as in Stage A.
Stage C	Complete or incomplete gross resection of primary. Intracavitary nodes histologically positive for tumor. Liver histologically free of tumor.
Stage D	Disseminated disease beyond intracavitary nodes (*i.e.,* bone marrow, bone, liver, skin, or lymph nodes beyond cavity containing primary tumor).

Evans & D'Angio   POG*

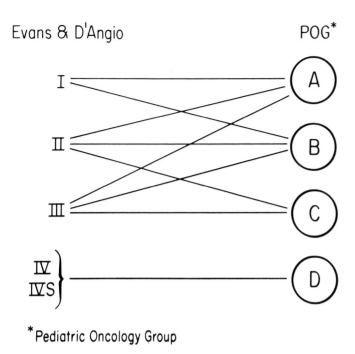

*Pediatric Oncology Group

FIGURE 28-13. POG versus Evans staging (clinical and surgical) of neuroblastoma.

Table 28-6
Pediatric Oncology Group (POG) Stage Distribution by Age at Diagnosis

	Age		
POG Stage	<1 Year	>1 Year	Total
A	16 (18.4%)	13 (8.7%)	29 (12.2%)
B	10 (11.5%)	10 (6.6%)	20 (8.4%)
C	19 (21.8%)	20 (13.4%)	39 (16.5%)
D	42 (48.3%)	107 (71.3%)	149 (62.9%)
Total	87 (36.7%)	150 (63.3%)	237 (100%)

procedure are to establish the diagnosis, to surgically stage the disease, and to excise the tumor or reduce its size by significant partial excision. Delayed or secondary operations assess the results of therapy and excise any residual primary disease.

The surgeon's approach to neuroblastoma must always be in the context of multidisciplinary therapy. Complete removal of the tumor affords the best chance of cure for localized disease, but where complete gross excision is not possible or distant disease is present, control by chemotherapy or radiotherapy is mandatory for cure.

It must be established preoperatively whether the disease is clinically localized or disseminated. This is critical, because in the presence of disseminated disease the diagnosis can frequently be made without surgical intervention. Where metastatic disease is present, primary operations should be limited to the least procedure necessary to establish the diagnosis—removal of a peripheral lymph node or simple abdominal or thoracic biopsy. In some cases, needle biopsy provides adequate tissue. In clinically localized disease, radiologic evaluation, including CT scan, or angiography, helps to delineate the

possibility of complete excision.[81,82] Boech and associates stress that tumors which cross the midline may be resectable, whereas unilateral tumors that distort major vessels or organs may not.[83] To establish disease stage in these patients, the surgeon must not only consider the resectability of the primary tumor, but must biopsy lymph nodes and, if the tumor is in the abdominal cavity, biopsy the liver.

Operative Technique

When the tumor is localized, a serious attempt should be made to remove it completely, although sacrifice of a major organ or vital structure should be avoided if at all possible. Because neuroblastoma does respond to chemotherapy, delayed resection is an alternative. The location of the tumor is an important consideration. Tumors that are located laterally, in the adrenal, thorax, and neck, are more amenable to excision than those located medially about the celiac axis or the superior mesenteric vessels, as has been stressed by Pellerin and colleagues.[84] It would appear that the inferior mesenteric artery can be sacrificed to gain tumor excision. In large pelvic primary tumors, where attempts at excision may result in neurologic deficits, preoperative chemotherapy appears to be beneficial.

Exploration of the abdomen is carried out through a generous transverse transperitoneal incision. The colon on the right or left is elevated to gain exposure to the retroperitoneal space. On the left the spleen and pancreas are elevated and reflected medially. Filler and colleagues have described an extraperitoneal approach, which is performed through a lateral thoracoabdominal incision with detachment of the diaphragm.[85] They suggest that this permits a safer and more complete dissection of the upper abdominal aorta when it is surrounded by tumor. This approach has been recommended for secondary operations as well.[85]

The surgeon can usually gain an idea of the resectability of the tumor by its mobility once the retroperitoneal space is entered. Although initial control of the blood supply is desirable, in practice this is often difficult to achieve without prior mobilization. Grosfeld has pointed out that while adrenal tumors are fed by multiple small vessels, the venous drainage is usually directly to the inferior vena cava on the right and into the left renal vein and subdiaphragmatic veins on the left.[86] Large tumors on both sides tend to distort the major aortic branches, and particular care must be taken to avoid injury to the superior mesenteric artery and the contralateral renal artery. Primary tumors tend to be quite friable and vascular and must be handled very carefully.

Excision of adjacent organs such as the spleen, pancreas, stomach, and colon is not indicated. The kidney typically is not invaded by the neuroblastoma and can usually be separated away. Involvement of the renal vessels by para-aortic primaries necessitates nephrectomy.

Thoracic tumors are approached through a standard posterolateral thoracotomy incision at an appropriate level. After the pleural cavity is entered, the endothoracic fascia is incised and a plane of dissection can usually be established. Thoracic neuroblastomas are almost always attached to the intervertebral foramina by gross or microscopic extensions. The tumor can usually be dissected free by sharp and blunt dissection. Involvement of major vessels and structures, particularly in the superior-most part of the thorax, may dictate biopsy or partial removal without sacrifice of a major vessel or vital organ. Attention must be paid to the feeding intercostal vessels, which are short and prone to retract.

Partial resection may be indicated if removal of more than 50% of the tumor—preferably 90% to 95%—is possible. There appears to be little advantage to lesser complete removal over simple biopsy.

Lymph node sampling is carried out in all cases unless precluded by the size and extent of the tumor. Nodal sampling in the abdomen should include ipsilateral and contralateral nodes along the major vessels superior and inferior to the tumor. It should be stressed that this is a sampling and not an *en bloc* nodal dissection. In the thorax, nodes are sought along the superior vena cava or the aorta and along the intercostal vessels. Nodes along the jugular and supraclavicular chains are sought in the neck. In the pelvis, bilateral iliac, mesenteric, paracaval, and para-aortic nodes are sampled. A needle biopsy of both lobes of the liver is performed for abdominal tumors.

The gross appearance of the node does not correlate predictably with the microscopic presence of tumor. Occult disease has also been found in the liver. The involvement of ganglia with tumor can be difficult to differentiate from a lymph node.

In delayed or secondary operations, the goal is to excise any residual tumor completely or to remove a major portion of residual tumor to reduce the tumor burden and to evaluate the results of chemotherapy (see also Chap. 10). Complete excision of the primary tumor enhances prognosis, so that additional risks are warranted, particularly in localized disease.[87] Exelby has estimated that 50% of secondary operations afford an opportunity for complete resection.[88] Treated tumors tend to be contracted, less vascular, and have some scarring to adjacent structures.[89] Grosfeld has reported that a very high percentage of patients judged to be in complete remission clinically will prove to have viable tumor in the primary site on exploration.[87]

The incidence of complications in surgery for neuroblastoma is acceptably low (<5%).[90] However, complications are reported to be most common in the younger age group, which has the best overall prognosis for tumor cure.[90] Since the response to chemotherapy in these infants is excellent, avoidance of surgical risk is of particular importance. The most common intraoperative complications are hemorrhage and hypertension. Postoperative complications include intestinal obstruction secondary to intussusception and later due to adhesions. Permanent and transient Horner's syndromes are seen after cervical and upper mediastinal operations.

Radiation Therapy

Although neuroblastoma is considered a radiosensitive tumor,[91] the tumoricidal dose of radiation in neuroblastoma *in vivo* is not known. The therapeutic doses usually delivered range from 15 Gy to 35 Gy, depending on the age of the child and the site being irradiated (see also Chap. 11). Several circumstances have resulted in the decreased use of radiation therapy (RT) as primary therapy for neuroblastoma. The high incidence of disseminated disease at diagnosis precludes this approach in the majority of patients. In lower stage disease, it is now known that surgery alone (POG Stage A) or surgery plus short-term chemotherapy (POG Stage B) is curative in most cases.[79] In more extensive regional disease (POG Stage C, Evans Stage III) there is controversy over whether RT increases cure rates over those attained with multidrug chemotherapy and surgery alone.

In more critical situations, such as spinal cord compression by tumor or loss of vision with orbital involvement, RT is an effective form of treatment. However, in newly diagnosed patients with epidural tumors, there is evidence that the prompt institution of effective chemotherapy will produce tumor resolution as rapidly as does RT.[92]

RT is very effective for pain control in patients who have symptomatic bone lesions and for the palliation of cosmetically disturbing skull lesions in patients with progressive disease. Doses of RT from 2 to 20 Gy can result in dramatic and relatively prolonged relief of symptoms.

Total body RT is part of preparative regimens for marrow transplant in some programs.[93,94] Whether the addition of total body RT to preparative chemotherapy regimens gives superior results is unknown. The usual dosages range from 9 Gy to 12 Gy over 3 to 5 days. Experimental delivery of targeted RT using MIBG or monoclonal antibodies as carriers is under evaluation (see also Chap. 14).[40,71,72] A current problem with this technique is estimating the dose of radiation delivered both to individual sites of tumor and to normal tissues such as the reticuloendothelial system.

The long-term consequences of RT include damage to normal organs, growth retardation, and the possibility of second malignancies (see Chap. 50).

Chemotherapy

Chemotherapy is the major modality of therapy for most patients with neuroblastoma. Complete plus partial response rates to effective single agents are as follows: cyclophosphamide, 59%; doxorubicin, 41%; cisplatin, 46%; epipodophyllotoxins, 30%; vincristine, 24%; dacarbazine, 14%; and peptichemio, 67%.[95]

Neuroblastoma is a chemotherapy-sensitive tumor, and chemotherapy is curative in the majority of patients with localized unresected disease and in infants with disseminated disease. For older children with disseminated disease, multiagent chemotherapy is effective in producing complete and partial responses in a significant proportion of patients but in most cases is not curative.[96-98]

The long-term consequences of chemotherapy in young children are largely unknown. Some effects, such as hearing loss from cisplatin, are irreversible. Careful follow-up of surviving children is needed to monitor for long-term effects of which we are currently unaware.

Therapy by Stage and Age

Treatment of neuroblastoma varies depending on the stage of disease and the age of the child (infants, defined as <365 days, and children >365 days). The treatment recommendations that follow are largely based on the POG staging system. For comparison, the respective distribution of patients staged by the Evans system (see Tables 24-4 to 24-6) are noted. The treatment of children with neuroblastoma categorized as POG Stage A or B is not modified for infants versus children. However, treatment recommendations are different for infants versus children with more advanced disease (*i.e.*, POG Stage C or D) and are noted accordingly.

POG Stage A

The majority of these patients have Evans Stage I or II disease; about 10% have Evans Stage III disease.

SURGERY. Surgical gross excision of the primary tumor mass will result in the cure of over 90% of these patients. Regardless of the patient's age, the presence of microscopic residual in the tumor bed does not affect outcome and is not an indication for therapy beyond surgery. As outlined in the previous discussion, regional lymph nodes and liver (if the tumor is in the abdomen) should be biopsied to delineate the stage correctly.

CHEMOTHERAPY AND RADIATION THERAPY.   These modalities are not indicated as primary therapy in this stage of disease. Careful follow-up and prompt treatment with chemotherapy, radiation therapy, or repeat surgery will salvage the majority of patients who relapse.

In a prospective POG study, 5 of 51 infants and 3 of 41 children have relapsed (median follow-up = 30 months). Only two older children have died of tumor.[99] At SJCRH, all 15 infants and children treated between 1976 and 1982 who received only surgical excision for Stage A disease are alive. One infant relapsed but is a long-term survivor following chemotherapy.[65]

POG Stage B

Approximately 40% of POG Stage B patients have Evans Stage II disease, and 60% have Evans Stage III.[79]

SURGERY.   Incomplete gross excision is accomplished at diagnosis. In these children, this is usually because of the size of the tumor or its intimate involvement with vital structures or organs. Following chemotherapy, the majority of these tumors will regress. If residual exists, a delayed surgical procedure can result in complete excision without sacrifice of major organs or vessels and nerves.

CHEMOTHERAPY AND RADIATION THERAPY.   In these previously untreated patients, RT would be expected in most cases to reduce tumor size so that delayed resection could be accomplished. However, the site of these tumors may necessitate relatively large ports. The inclusion in the port of portions of lung, kidney, liver, bladder, and growth centers in this young patient population may result in long-term complications. These can be avoided if short-term chemotherapy is used instead, with RT reserved for the small proportion of patients who do not respond well to current chemotherapy regimens or who have small residual masses remaining after second surgery. Current data indicate that more than 80% of patients with this stage of disease will have complete or very good partial responses to short-term chemotherapy. Sixteen prospectively staged patients were treated with cyclophosphamide (150 mg/m^2/day × 7) and Adriamycin (35 mg/m^2 day 8) every 21 days for 4 months, followed by postchemotherapy surgical excision of any residual tumor. Of these 16 patients, 15 were rendered disease-free and 14 remain disease-free at more than 5 years from diagnosis.[79] In a second study, 43 prospectively staged patients received cyclophosphamide and Adriamycin for 4 months, followed by surgery, with 32 rendered disease-free.[100] Of the 11 with residual tumor, 7 received cisplatin and VM-26, with 4 achieving complete responses.[101] Thus, of 39 patients receiving either two-drug[39] or four-drug[7] therapy, only 3 failed to achieve a disease-free status. Of the 36 who achieved complete remission, 4 have relapsed (median follow-up = 36 months).

In this group of patients with gross residual but localized disease, the use of other chemotherapy plus RT may result in cures. Before 1974, 17 children at SJCRH were treated with vincristine, cyclophosphamide, and RT. Although all 5 infants survived, only 5 of the 12 older children lived. In making a therapeutic decision, one must weigh the cure rate plus the acute and chronic side-effects of short-term chemotherapy against those of RT in these young patients.

POG Stage C or D in Infants

Age becomes a significant factor in outcome in POG Stages C and D and in decisions concerning the aggressiveness of therapy needed to effect cure.

SURGERY.   In Stage C disease the primary tumor may or may not be grossly excised at diagnosis. Regional lymph nodes separate from the primary tumor are biopsied and shown to contain tumor. In Stage D disease, an initial surgical approach to the primary tumor may not be indicated if the diagnosis can be made by other methods. Delayed or second surgery after chemotherapy induction serves two purposes: to remove any residual primary tumor and to document whether residual neuroblastoma is present in nodes and liver so that decisions can be made regarding the need for further therapy.

CHEMOTHERAPY AND RADIATION THERAPY.   Radiation therapy to the metastatic nodes and primary tumor site in Stage C disease may result in cure of some of these infants, but no prospective study has been done to evaluate RT as a single therapeutic modality. For Stage D disease, the presence of more disseminated tumor and the excellent response to chemotherapy argue against the use of RT except in selected cases where chemotherapy and surgery do not completely eradicate the primary tumor.

Chemotherapy is the primary modality in these infants. Finklestein and associates reported on 19 infants with Stage D disease treated with vincristine, cyclophosphamide, and DTIC ± Adriamycin for 24 months plus surgery, with or without RT. Ten of these infants were surviving at the time of publication.[96] Pritchard and coworkers delivered a median of six courses of cyclophosphamide, vincristine, cisplatin, and VM-26 to 8 infants with Stage D disease.[102] All 8 were alive and off therapy for 11 to 30 months (median = 21). One child received an autologous bone marrow transplant. Data from SJCRH indicate that short-term chemotherapy with 4 months of cyclophosphamide and Adriamycin plus delayed surgical excision of any residual primary will render approximately 65% of these patients disease-free. The availability of cisplatin and VM-26 combinations for those who fail increases the response rate to over 80%. From 1974 through 1985, 49 evaluable infants with Stage C ($N = 14$) or D ($N = 35$) disease were treated at SJCRH. Complete remission with 4 months of cyclophosphamide and Adriamycin and surgery was achieved in 33 patients. Of 4 who failed therapy before the standard use of cisplatin and VM-26 (1979), none achieved complete response with other therapies. Of 16 patients diagnosed before 1979, 7 died (2 in remission, 5 with tumor). In contrast, of 12 infants failing to achieve complete remission with cyclophosphamide and Adriamycin after the introduction of cisplatin and VM-26, 10 have achieved a disease-free status with the addition of these two agents. Thus, of 33 infants diagnosed from 1979 through 1985, 31 achieved complete remission and 28 survive (16 months–93 months, median = 59 months). Overall, 10 of 14 Stage C and 27 of 35 Stage D infants survive disease-free. These results indicate that the exposure of every infant with metastatic disease to multidrug chemotherapy with or without RT is not justified,[102,103] and more toxic therapy with drugs such as cisplatin should be reserved for those failing the two-drug chemotherapy.

Evans Stage IV-S

The therapeutic approach in infants with Evans Stage IV-S disease is controversial. That a certain proportion of these babies will have resolution of their disease without therapy beyond excision of the primary is not in question. The problem is in identifying which infants will do well without therapy and which will develop either mechanical problems due to tumor load or progressive or recurrent disease.

SURGERY. Surgery in this group remains somewhat controversial. There is general agreement that the primary tumor should be removed, either as an initial procedure or after chemotherapy, if given. A particular problem has been the infant with a massively enlarged liver. The use of a temporary Silastic silo has been proposed.[104] It certainly appears that avoidance of laparotomy in these infants is desirable. If liver biopsy is necessary, this can be done with a needle or with a very limited incision, and chemotherapy or RT can be used to control the liver metastases.

CHEMOTHERAPY AND RADIATION THERAPY. In a review by Evans and colleagues, 31 infants with Stage IV-S disease were reported.[104] The primary was removed in 19 patients and irradiated in 6. Three patients had no known primary, 1 died before treatment, and 2 were early in their courses. Only 9 patients had received no therapy other than removal of the primary tumor. Liver disease was present in 29 patients, with 11 receiving RT, 6 chemotherapy, and 6 both modalities. Of 16 patients with marrow disease, 8 received chemotherapy. The follow-up at the time of reporting ranged from 2 months to 40 months. Five patients had died, 8 were alive with disease, and 18 were alive and disease-free.

Late recurrences after spontaneous regressions are reported.[105] Currently, the decision to treat with short-term chemotherapy or low-dose radiation, or to not treat depends, on the individual investigators bias and the extent of disease.[104-106] If the decision is made to observe the child, frequent examinations are essential, as rapidly progressive disease can occur and can be life-threatening. Infants younger than 2 months with liver metastases have been reported to be at greatest risk for treatment failure.[107] Most investigators would elect to treat infants with massive liver enlargement and respiratory compromise and those with extensive bone marrow tumor.

POG Stage C in Children

These children have regional lymph nodes as their only site of tumor dissemination; 90% would be classified as having Evans Stage III disease.[79]

SURGERY. For these patients, a surgical procedure at diagnosis is necessary for a tissue diagnosis of neuroblastoma. The primary tumor may or may not be resected. The presence of tumor in regional lymph nodes defines these patients as having Stage C disease.

A second-look procedure following induction chemotherapy with or without RT serves the same purposes as for infants —removal of residual primary and documentation of response in lymph nodes.

CHEMOTHERAPY AND RADIATION THERAPY. Few studies have prospectively evaluated the effect of various therapeutic modalities in patients staged for the presence of lymph node disease as the only site of metastasis. One cannot make direct comparisons to treatment results for Evans Stage III disease because only 55% of those patients will have POG Stage C disease; the remainder, who have Stage A or B disease, would be expected to have excellent survival. For those with Stage C disease who have been prospectively staged, the outcome of therapy has been poor. Of 15 children treated with cyclophosphamide and Adriamycin or vincristine and cyclophosphamide ± RT, only 1 survives disease-free.[79]

This group of patients may respond better to more aggressive chemotherapy and radiotherapy, although this suggestion is controversial. Shafford and coworkers treated 7 Evans Stage III patients (nodal status unknown) with vincristine, cisplatin, VM-26, and cyclophosphamide ± Adriamycin ± RT, plus surgery and autologous marrow transplant; only 2 patients were disease-free survivors.[108] Rosen and colleagues reported on 8 Evans Stage III patients treated with four- or six-drug chemotherapy plus RT and surgery. All 8 survived disease-free for at least 1.5 years.[98] At SJCRH, 11 patients with prospectively staged Stage C disease have been treated with cyclophosphamide, Adriamycin, cisplatin, and VM-26 plus delayed surgery. Seven attained complete remission and 5 remain in first remission for 6, 6, 22, 82, and 87 months. The first three patients remain at high risk for relapse.

A POG study is currently in progress to evaluate the role of RT in the response to therapy and survival in a group of prospectively staged patients. In larger groups of patients, aggressive multidrug chemotherapy plus RT and surgery may be shown to improve survival in this stage of disease.

Available data would indicate that patients with regional node metastases have a prognosis that is not statistically different from those with more widely disseminated disease and that their therapy should be just as intensive as that of Stage D patients (Fig. 28-14).

POG Stage D in Children

Children with POG Stage D or Evans Stage IV disease are the largest group of patients with neuroblastoma. They also have been the group least responsive to curative treatment. As more chemotherapeutic agents have become available, duration of survival has been prolonged but ultimate outcome has not markedly changed (Fig. 28-15). Therapy for this disease stage is not standard, and multiple approaches are being used in both single-institution and cooperative group studies.

SURGERY. In the majority of children with Stage D disease, a diagnosis of neuroblastoma can be made on the basis of bone marrow tumor and catecholamine levels. Few patients require surgical intervention at the time of diagnosis. Delayed procedures to remove residual primary tumor following chemotherapeutic control of metastatic disease and to document remission status are incorporated into most current studies.

CHEMOTHERAPY AND RADIATION THERAPY. Chemotherapeutic control of metastatic disease is the primary treatment for this stage of disease. Current studies have moved beyond the previous use of combination chemotherapy with vincristine, cyclophosphamide, and DTIC[96] or cyclophosphamide and Adriamycin.[97] Almost all front-line studies now in progress include cisplatin and an epipodophyllotoxin in multiagent chemotherapy approaches. Dosages and schedules vary.

Several studies are evaluating the efficacy of autologous or allogeneic bone marrow transplant for remission consolidation and maintenance in children attaining good partial remission or complete remission with chemotherapy ± radiation therapy and surgery (see also Chap. 48).[94,108,109] Shaffard and colleagues treated 29 children with vincristine, cisplatin, VM-26, and cyclophosphamide ± Adriamycin ± RT and surgery fol-

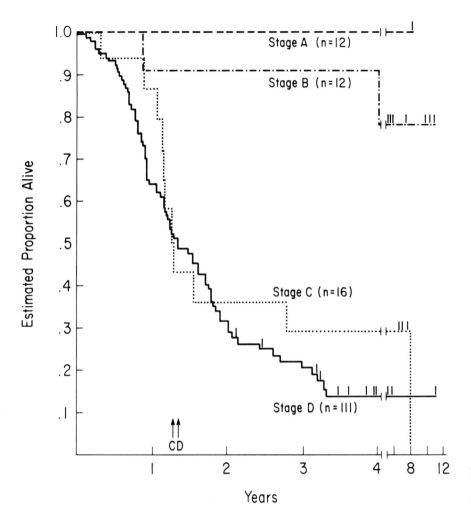

FIGURE 28-14. Survival of children older than 1 year of age with POG staged disease treated at SJCRH, 1974–1984.

lowed by high-dose melphalan and autologous marrow transplant. Twenty-two achieved good partial responses to induction therapy, and 7 survive disease-free 23 to 48 months from their last chemotherapy.[108]

Philip and coworkers reported on 45 patients who received chemotherapy for variable periods of time plus surgical resection of residual primaries.[94] At a median of 8 months postdiagnosis, 37 patients underwent total body irradiation, vincristine and melphalan chemotherapy, and bone marrow transplantation. Of 21 patients transplanted in partial remission, 10 survive free of disease 105 to 813 days after transplant (median = 180 days). Of 14 patients transplanted while in very good partial remission or complete remission, 5 survive disease-free at 90 to 1427 days posttransplant (median = 468 days). Nine of the 37 patients died of toxicity. Follow-up in this study is very short (median < 12 months posttransplant).

Comparable survival rates can be obtained without bone marrow transplant. At SJCRH 44 children with Stage D disease were treated with cyclophosphamide, Adriamycin, cisplatin, and VM-26 plus delayed surgery, with 35 attaining good partial response or complete response. Maintenance chemotherapy was given with the above agents for a total duration of therapy of 8 months. Six children are in first remission 41 to 81 months from diagnosis and 2 others survive at 58 months and 36 months.[110] In a study where these four agents were given in a more intensive fashion for 8 months, 28 of 28 Stage D patients had good partial responses or complete responses. Ten patients remain in first remission 9 to 30 months from diagnosis

(median = 17 months), and 19 survive. Two patients died in remission of causes other than neuroblastoma.[111] These regimens can result in significant toxicity, and treatment of these children is best provided in centers where full supportive care is available and where investigators are experienced in dealing with these problems.

These studies indicate that the major problem in treating children with Stage D disease is not attaining excellent responses but maintaining those responses.[108,111] Prospective studies are in progress using higher doses of chemotherapy,[112] autologous transplant with more intensive preparative regimens, tumor irradiation with ^{131}I-MIBG or radiolabeled monoclonal antibodies,[40,71,72] or biological response modifiers for patients who attain excellent responses to chemotherapy. With the rapid evolution of therapeutic protocols for this stage of disease, these children benefit most from being entered on organized prospective therapy trials. This also results in the most rapid evolution of clinical data on which new studies can be based.

Esthesioneuroblastoma

Esthesioneuroblastoma is an uncommon tumor of the olfactory region of the nasal cavity. The origin of this tumor is thought to be either neuroectodermal or neural crest, arising in the olfactory epithelium.[113] Peak ages of occurrence are 11 to 20 years

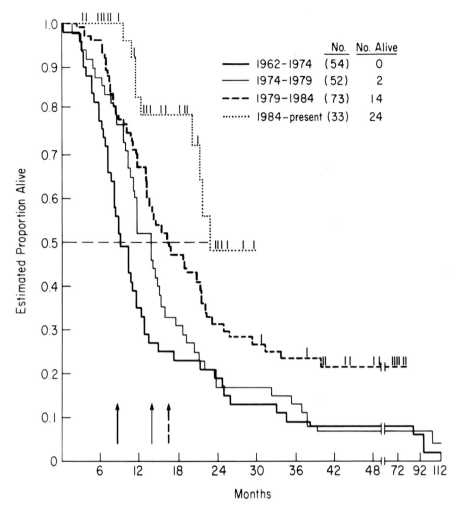

FIGURE 28-15. Survival of children older than 1 year of age with disseminated neuroblastoma treated at SJCRH 1962–1986. Treatment: 1962–1974, cyclophosphamide, vincristine ± Adriamycin and RT; 1974–1979, cyclophosphamide, Adriamycin; 1979–1984, cyclophosphamide, Adriamycin followed by cisplatin, VM-26; 1984–present, intensive cyclophosphamide, Adriamycin, cisplatin, and continuous infusion VM-26.

and 40 to 69 years, with 20% of cases occurring in childhood and adolescence. Management of these tumors has been largely with surgery and radiotherapy. Survival can be achieved in 85% to 90% of patients with disease localized to the nasal cavity and paranasal sinuses and in 50% of those with more extensive disease.[114]

FUTURE CONSIDERATIONS

The outcome for children with localized neuroblastoma and for infants with localized or disseminated neuroblastoma treated with currently available therapy is excellent. In these patients, biological markers may enable us to identify at diagnosis those infants who require more aggressive, multidrug therapy to survive their disease. Because the majority of these patients will survive, a major consideration must be the avoidance of long-term irreversible toxicities of therapy.

The majority of patients, however, present with disseminated disease and are older than 1 year. For these patients, therapy is far from satisfactory. Whether any of the approaches now under investigation will alter the cure rate for these children is unknown. Another approach must be to identify methods of earlier detection of disease, which might enable the diagnosis to be made at a time when disease is more localized or the child is younger.

REFERENCES

1. Virchow R: Hyperplasie der Zirbel und der Nebennieren. In Die krankhaften Geschwülste, vol 2. Berlin, A Hirschwald, 1864–1865
2. Wright JH: Neurocytoma or neuroblastoma, a kind of tumor not generally recognized. J Exp Med 12:556–561, 1910
3. Robertson HE: Virchows Arch 220:147, 1915. Cited by Willis RA: Pathology of Tumours, 4th ed, pp 857–885. New York, Appleton-Century-Crofts, 1967
4. Herxheimer G: Ueber Tumoren des Nebennierenmarkes, insbesondere das Neuroblastoma sympaticum. Beitr Pathol Anat 57:112, 1914
5. Rinscheid J: Virchows Arch 297:508, 1936. Cited by Willis RA: Pathology of Tumours, 4th ed, pp 857–885. New York, Appleton-Century-Crofts, 1967
6. Murray MR, Stout AP: Distinctive characteristics of the sympathicoblastoma cultivated in vitro. A method for prompt diagnosis. Am J Pathol 23:429–441, 1947
7. Everson TC, Cole WH: Spontaneous Regression of Cancer: A Study and Abstracts of Reports in the World Medical Literature and of Personal Communication Concerning Spontaneous Regression of Malignant Disease, pp 11–163. Philadelphia, WB Saunders, 1966
8. Evans AE: Natural history of neuroblastoma, In Evans AE (ed): Advances in Neuroblastoma Research. Raven Press, New York, 1980
9. Cushing H, Wolbach BB: The transformation of a malignant paravertebral sympathicoblastoma into a benign ganglioneuroma. Am J Pathol 3:203–215, 1927
10. MacMillan RW, Blanc WB, Santulli TV: Maturation of neuroblastoma to glioneuroma in lymph nodes. J Pediatr Surg 11:461–462, 1976
11. Breslow N, McCann B: Statistical estimation of prognosis for children with neuroblastoma. Cancer Res 31:2098–2103, 1971
12. Finkelsten JZ, Klemperer MR, Evans AE et al: Multiagent chemotherapy for

children with metastatic neuroblastoma: A report from Children's Cancer Study Group. Med Pediatr Oncol 6:179–188, 1979

13. Young JL, Miller RW: Incidence of malignant tumors in U.S. children. J Pediatr 86:254–258, 1975

14. Gale G, D'Angio G, Uri A, Chatten J, Koop CE: Cancer in neonates: The experience at the Children's Hospital of Philadelphia. Pediatrics 70:409–413, 1982

15. Kinnier-Wilson LM, Draper GJ: Neuroblastoma, its natural history and prognosis: A study of 487 cases. Br Med J 3:301–307, 1974

16. Miller RW: Ethnic differences in cancer occurrence: Genetic and environmental influences with particular reference to neuroblastoma. In Mulvihill JJ, Miller RW, Fraumeni JF Jr (eds): Genetics of Human Cancer, pp 1–14. New York, Raven Press, 1977

17. Beckwith JB, Perrin EV: In situ neuroblastoma: A contribution to the natural history of neural crest tumors. Am J Pathol 43:1089–1104, 1963

18. Guin GH, Gilbert EF, Jones B: Incidental neuroblastoma in infants. Am J Clin Pathol 51:126–136, 1968

19. Chatten J, Voorhees ML: Familial neuroblastoma. N Engl J Med 277:1230–1236, 1967

20. Hardy PC, Nesbit ME Jr: Familial neuroblastoma: Report of a kindred with a high incidence of infantile tumors. J Pediatr 80:74–77, 1972

21. Hecht F, Kaiser-McCaw B: Chromosomes in familial neuroblastoma (letter). J Pediatr 98:334, 1981

22. Kushner B, Gilbert F, Helson L: Familial neuroblastoma. Cancer 57:1887–1893, 1986

23. Knudson AG, Strong LC: Mutation and cancer. Neuroblastoma and pheochromocytoma. Am J Hum Genet 24:514–532, 1972

24. Bolande RP, Towler WF: Possible relationship of neuroblastoma in Von Recklinghausen's disease. Cancer 26:162–174, 1970

25. Grotting JC, Kassel C, Demner L: Nesidioblastosis and congenital neuroblastoma. Arch Pathol Lab Med 103:642–646, 1979

26. Emery LG, Shields M, Shah NR, Garbes A: Neuroblastoma associated with Beckwith Wiedemann syndrome. Cancer 52:176–179, 1983

27. Pendergrass TW, Hanson JW: Fetal hydantoin syndrome and neuroblastoma. Lancet 2:150, 1976

28. Haynes LW, Weller RO: Induction of some features of glial differentiation in primary cultures of human gliomas by treatment with dibutyryl cyclic AMP. Br J Exp Pathol 59:259–276, 1978

29. Prasad KN: Control mechanisms of malignancy and differentiation in cultures of nerve cells. In Evans AE (ed): Advances in Neuroblastoma Research. New York, Raven Press, 1980

30. Helson L, Helson C, Peterson RF, Das SK: A rationale for the treatment of metastatic neuroblastoma. J Natl Cancer Inst 57:727–729, 1976

31. Raaf JH, Congir A, Luna M: Induction of neuroblastoma maturation by a new chemotherapy protocol. Med Pediatr Oncol 10:275–282, 1982

32. Helson L: Chemotherapy of neuroblastoma. Clin Bull 5:47–50, 1975

33. Nitschke R, Cangir A, Crist W et al: Intensive chemotherapy for metastatic neuroblastoma: A SWOG study. Med Pediatr Oncol 8:281–288, 1980

34. Hellström IE, Hellström KE, Pierce GE, Bill AH: Demonstration of cell-bound and humoral immunity against neuroblastoma cells. Proc Natl Acad Sci USA 60:1231–1238, 1968

35. Hellström KE, Hellström IE, Bill AH, Pierce GE, Yang JPS: Studies on cellular immunity to human neuroblastoma cells. Int J Cancer 6:172–188, 1970

36. Hellström KE, Hellström I: Lymphocyte-mediated cytotoxicity and blocking serum activity to tumor antigens. Adv Immunol 18:209–277, 1974

37. Necheles TF, Rausen A, Kung F, Pochedly C: MER/BCG in the treatment of disseminated neuroblastoma (abstr). Proc Am Soc Clin Oncol 11:258, 1976

38. Nesbit ME, Kersey J, Finklestein J, Weiner J, Simmons R: Immunotherapy and chemotherapy in children with neuroblastoma. J Natl Cancer Inst 57:717–720, 1976

39. Seeger R, Siegel S, Sidell N: Neuroblastoma: Clinical prospectives, monoclonal antibodies, and retinoic acid. Ann Intern Med 97:873–884, 1982

40. Cheung NK, Saarinen U, Neely J, Landmeier B, Donovan D, Coccia P: Monoclonal antibodies to a glycolipid antigen on human neuroblastoma cells. Cancer Res 45:2642–2649, 1985

41. Brodeur GM, Sekhon GS, Goldstein MN: Chromosomal aberrations in human neuroblastomas. Cancer 40:2256–2263, 1977

42. Brodeur GM, Green AA, Hayes FA: Cytogenetic studies of primary human neuroblastomas. In Evans AE (ed): Advances in Neuroblastoma Research, pp 73–80. New York, Raven Press, 1980

43. Look AT, Hayes FA, Nitschke R, McWilliams NB, Green AA: Cellular DNA content as a predictor of response to chemotherapy in infants with unresectable neuroblastoma. N Engl J Med 311:231–235, 1984

44. Gansler T, Chatten J, Varello M, Bunin G, Atkinson B: Flow cytometric DNA analysis of neuroblastoma. Cancer 58:2453–2458, 1986

45. Kaneko Y, Kanda N, Maseki N, Sakurai M, Tsuchida Y, Takida T, Okabe I, Sakurai M: Different karyotypic patterns in early and advanced stage neuroblastoma. Cancer Res 47:311–318, 1987

46. Cowell JK, Rupniak HT: Chromosome analysis of human neuroblastoma cell with TR14 showing minutes and an aberration involving chromosome 1. Cancer Genet Cytogenet 9:273–280, 1983

47. Biedler JL, Ross RA, Shanske S, Spengler BA: Human neuroblastoma cytogenetics: Search for significance of homogeneously staining regions in double minute chromosomes. In Evans AE (ed): Advances in Neuroblastoma Research, pp 81–96. New York, Raven Press, 1980

48. Schwab M, Alitalo K, Klempnauer K-H, Varmus HE, Bishop JM, Gilbert F, Brodeur G, Goldstein M, Trent J: Amplified DNA with limited homology to myc cellular oncogene is shared by human neuroblastoma cell lines and a neuroblastoma tumour. Nature 305:245–248, 1983

49. Schwab M, Varmus H, Bishop J: Human N-myc gene contributes to neoplastic transformation of cells in culture. Nature 316:160–162, 1985

50. Brodeur GM, Seeger RC, Schwab M, Varmus HE, Bishop JM: Amplification of N-myc in untreated human neuroblastomas correlates with advanced disease stage. Science 224:1121–1124, 1984

51. Brodeur G, Seeger R: Gene amplification in human neuroblastomas: Basic mechanisms and clinical implications. Cancer Genet Cytogenet 19:101–111, 1986

52. Rosen N, Reynolds CP, Thiele C, Biedler J, Israel M: Increased N-myc expression following progressive growth of human neuroblastoma. Cancer Res 46:4139–4142, 1986

53. Brodeur G, Hayes FA, Green A, Casper J, Lee H, Seeger R: Consistent N-myc copy number in simultaneous or consecutive neuroblastoma samples from a given patients tumor. Proc Am Soc Clin Oncol 5:13, 1986

54. Gitlow SE, Bertani LM, Rausen A, Gribetz D, Dziedzic SW: Diagnosis of neuroblastoma by qualitative and quantitative determination of catecholamine metabolites in urine. Cancer 25:1377–1383, 1970

55. Laug W, Siegel S, Shaw K, Landing B, Baptista J, Gutenstein M: Initial urinary catecholamine metabolite concentrations and prognosis in neuroblastoma. Pediatrics 62:77–83, 1978

56. Sawada T, Nakata T, Takasugi N et al: Mass screening for neuroblastoma in infants in Japan. Lancet 2:271–273, 1984

57. Sawada T, Kidowaki T, Sakamoto I et al: Neuroblastoma, mass screening for early detection and its prognosis. Cancer 53:2731–2735, 1984

58. Levy HL, Kavolkewicz V, Houghton SA, MacCready RA: Screening the normal population in Massachusetts for phenylketonuria. N Engl J Med 282:1455, 1970

59. Levy HL: Screening for galactosemia. In Burman D, Holton JB, Pennock CA (eds): Inherited Disorders of Carbohydrate Metabolism, p 130. Lancaster, England, MTP Press Falcon House, 1980

60. Nyhan WL: Neonatal screening for inherited disease. N Engl J Med 313:43–44, 1985

61. Alvarado C, Faraj B, Kim T, Camp V, Bain R, Ragab A: Plasma dopa and catecholamines in the diagnosis and follow-up of children with neuroblastoma. Am J Pediatr Hematol/Oncol 7:221–227, 1985

62. Zeltzer P, Marganos P, Parma A et al: Raised neuron-specific enolase in serum of children with metastatic neuroblastoma. Lancet 2:361–363, 1983

63. Hann H, Evans A, Siegel S, Wong K, Sather H, Dalton A, Hammond D, Seeger R: Prognostic importance of serum ferritin in patients with stage III and IV neuroblastoma: The CCSG experience. Cancer Res 45:2843–2848, 1985

64. Wu ZL, Schwartz E, Seeger R, Ladisch S: Expression of G_{D2} ganglioside by untreated primary human neuroblastomas. Cancer Res 46:440–443, 1986

65. Moe PG, Nellhaus G: Infantile polymyoclonia-opsoclonus syndrome and neural crest tumors. Neurology 20:756–764, 1970

66. Bray PF, Ziter FA, Lahey ME, Myers GG: The coincidence of neuroblastoma and acute cerebellar encephalopathy. J Pediatr 75:983–990, 1969

67. Jones G, Groover R, Smithson W: Acute cerebellar encephalopathy (ACE): Its natural history and relationship to neuroblastoma. Proc Am Soc Clin Oncol 3:86, 1984

68. Senelick R, Bray P, Lakey ME, VanDyk H, Johnson D: Neuroblastoma and myoclonic encephalopathy: Two cases and a review of the literature. J Pediatr Surg 8:623–632, 1973

69. Kaplan S, Holbrook C, McDaniel H, Buntain W, Crist W: Vasoactive intestinal peptide secreting tumors of childhood. Am J Dis Child 134:21–24, 1980

70. Geatti O, Shapiro B, Sisson J, Hutchison R, Mallette S, Eyre P, Beierwaltes

WH: Iodine-131 metaiodobenzylguanidine scintigraphy for the location of neuroblastoma: Preliminary experience in ten cases. J Nucl Med 26:736–742, 1985

71. Haefnagel C, Voute P, DeKraker J, Marcuse H: Total body scintigraphy with ^{131}I-metaiodobenzylguanidine for detection of neuroblastoma. Diagn Imag Clin Med 54:21–27, 1985

72. Horne T, Granowska M, Dicks-Mireaux C, Hawkins L, Britton K, Mather S, Bomanji J, Kemshead J, Kingston J, Malpas J: Neuroblastoma imaged with ^{123}I-metaiodobenzylguanidine and with ^{123}I-labelled monoclonal antibody, UJ13A, against neural tissue. Br J Radiol 58:476–480, 1985

73. Kemshed J, Coakham H: The use of monoclonal antibodies for the diagnosis of intracranial tumors and the small round cell tumors of childhood. J Pathol 141:249–257, 1983

74. Reynolds CP, Moss T, Seeger R, Black A, Woody J: Sensitive detection of neuroblastoma cells in bone marrow for monitoring the efficacy of marrow purging procedures. In Evans AE (ed): Advances in Neuroblastoma Research, pp 425–441. New York, Alan R Liss, 1984

75. Frantz C, Duerst R, Ryan D, Gelsomino N, Constine L, Gregory P: Anti-neuroblastoma antibodies which do not bind to bone marrow cells. In Evans AE (ed): Advances in Neuroblastoma Research, pp 485–499. New York. Alan R Liss, 1984

76. Evans AE, D'Angio GJ, Randolph J: A proposed staging for children with neuroblastoma. Cancer 27:374–378, 1971

77. Breslow N, McCann B: Statistical estimation of prognosis for children with neuroblastoma. Cancer Res 31:2098–2103, 1971

78. Ninane J, Pritchard J, Morris-Jones PH et al: Stage II neuroblastoma: Adverse prognostic significance of lymph node involvement. Arch Dis Child 57:438–442, 1982

79. Hayes FA, Green A, Hustu HO, Kumar M: Surgicopathologic staging of neuroblastoma: Prognostic significance of regional lymph node metastases. J Pediatr 102:59–62, 1983

80. Shimada H, Chatten J, Newton J, Sachs W, Hamoudi N, Chiba T, Marsden H, Misugi K: Histopathologic prognostic factors in neuroblastic tumors: definition of subtypes of ganglioneuroblastoma and an age-linked classification of neuroblastomas. J Natl Cancer Inst 73:405–416, 1984

81. Ogita S, Tokiwa K, Majima S: Evaluation of aortography in assessing the resectability of retroperitoneal neuroblastoma in children. Jpn J Surg 15:312–317, 1985

82. Tsunoda A, Nishi T: Angiographic evaluation of neuroblastoma. J Pediatr Surg 16:712–716, 1981

83. Boechat MI, Ortega J, Hoffman AD, Cleveland RH, Kangarloo H, Gilsanz V: Computer tomography in stage III neuroblastoma. AJR 145:1283–1287, 1985

84. Pellerin D, Fekete CN, Revillon Y, Fernandes P: Place de la chirurgie dans le traitement du neuroblastome. Chir Pediatr 24:3–9, 1983

85. Pizzo PA, Cassady JR, Miser JS, Filler RM: Solid tumors of childhood. In DeVita VT Jr, Hellman S, Rosenberg SA (eds): Cancer. Principles and Practice of Oncology, 2nd ed, pp 1525–1536. Philadelphia, JB Lippincott, 1985

86. Grosfeld JL: Neuroblastoma in infancy and childhood. In Hays DM (ed): Pediatric Surgical Oncology, pp 63–85 Orlando, Grune & Stratton, 1986

87. Grosfeld JL: Neuroblastoma. In Welch KJ, Randolph JG, Ravitch MM, O'Neill JA Jr, Rowe MI (eds): Pediatric Surgery, 4th ed, pp 283–293. Chicago, Year Book Medical Publishers, 1986

88. Exelby PR: Pediatric oncologic surgery. In Sutow WW, Fernbach DJ, Vietti TJ (eds): Clinical Pediatric Oncology, 3rd ed, pp 154–166. St. Louis, CV Mosby, 1984

89. Smith EI, Krous HF, Tunell WP, Hitch DC: The impact of chemotherapy and radiation therapy on secondary operations for neuroblastoma. Ann Surg 191:561–568, 1980

90. Azizkhan RG, Shaw A, Chandler JG: Surgical complications of neuroblastoma resection. Surgery 97:514–517, 1985

91. Seaman WB, Eagleton MD: Radiation therapy of neuroblastoma. Radiology 68:1–8, 1957

92. Hayes FA, Thompson EI, Hvizdala E, O'Connor D, Green A: Chemotherapy as an alternative to laminectomy and radiation in the management of epidural tumor. J Pediatr 104:221–224, 1984

93. August C, Serata F, Koch P, Burkey E, Schlesinger H, Elkins, Evans A, D'Angio G: Treatment of advanced neuroblastoma with supralethal chemotherapy, radiation and allogeneic or autologous marrow reconstitution. J Clin Oncol 2:609–616, 1984

94. Philip T, Bernard J, Zucker J, Pinkerton R, Lutz P, Bordigoni P, Plouvier E, Robert A, Carton R, Philippe N, Philip I, Chauvin F, Favrot M: High dose chemoradiotherapy with bone marrow transplantation as consolidation treatment in neuroblastoma: An unselected group of stage IV patients over 1 year of age. J Clin Oncol 5:266–271, 1987

95. Carli M, Green A, Hayes FA, Rivera G, Pratt C: Therapeutic efficacy of single drugs for childhood neuroblastoma: A review. In Raybaud C, Clement R, LeBreuil G, Bernard J (eds): Pediatric Oncology, pp 141–150. Amsterdam, Excerpta Medica, 1982

96. Finklestein JZ, Klemperer MR, Evans A et al: Multiagent chemotherapy for children with metastatic neuroblastoma: A report from Children's Cancer Study Group. Med Pediatr Oncol 6:179–188, 1979

97. Green AA, Hayes FA, Hustu HO: Sequential cyclophosphamide and doxorubicin for induction of complete remission in children with disseminated neuroblastoma. Cancer 48:2310–2317, 1981

98. Rosen E, Cassady JR, Frantz C, Kretschmar C, Levey R, Sallan S: Neuroblastoma. The Joint Center for Radiation Therapy/Dana-Farber Cancer Institute/Children's Hospital experience. J Clin Oncol 2:719–732, 1984

99. Nitschke R, Smith EI, Altshuler G, Hayes FA, Shuster J: Localized neuroblastoma treated by surgery. A POG study. Proc Am Soc Clin Oncol 4:242, 1985

100. Green A, Casper J, Nitschke R, Smith EI, Hayes FA: The treatment of localized grossly unresectable (POG stage B) neuroblastoma. Proc Am Soc Clin Oncol 4:245, 1985

101. Hayes FA, Green A, Casper J et al: Clinical evaluation of sequentially scheduled cisplatin and VM-26 in neuroblastoma: Response and toxicity. Cancer 48:1715–1718, 1981

102. Pritchard J, Whelan R, Hill B: Sequential cis-platinum and VM26 in neuroblastoma: Laboratory and clinical (OPEC regimen) studies. In: Evans AE (ed): Advances in Neuroblastoma Research, pp 545–555. New York, Alan R Liss, 1984

103. Kretschmar C, Frantz C, Rosen E et al: Successful use of intensive chemotherapy for infants with stage IV neuroblastoma. Proc Am Soc Clin Oncol 2:78, 1983

104. Evans AE, Baum E, Chard R: Do infants with stage IV-S neuroblastoma need treatment? Arch Dis Child 56:271–274, 1981

105. Helson L: Death from progression following spontaneous regression of infantile neuroblastoma. Anticancer Research 3:313–316, 1983

106. McWilliams N: IV-S neuroblastoma—Treatment controversy revisited. Med Pediatr Oncol 14:41–44, 1986

107. Stephenson S, Cook B, Mease A, Ruymann F: The prognostic significance of age and pattern of metastases in Stage IV-S neuroblastoma. Cancer 58:372–375, 1986

108. Shafford E, Rogers D, Pritchard J: Advanced neuroblastoma: Improved response rate using a multiagent regimen (OPEC) including sequential cisplatin and VM26. J Clin Oncol 2:742–747, 1984

109. Hartmann O, Kalifa C, Benhamou E, Beaujean F, Patte C, Lemerle J: High-dose chemotherapy and ABMT as consolidation therapy in metastatic neuroblastoma. Proc Am Soc Clin Oncol 4:236, 1985

110. Green A, Hayes FA, Casper J, Sartain P, Abildgaard C: Extended disease-free survival for patients with disseminated neuroblastoma treated with cyclophosphamide, Adriamycin, cisplatin and VM-26. Proc Am Assoc Cancer Res 24:159, 1983

111. Green A, Hayes FA, Rao B: Disease control and toxicity of aggressive 4 drug therapy for children with disseminated neuroblastoma (DNb). Proc Am Soc Clin Oncol 5:210, 1986

112. Philip T, Ghalie R, Pinkerton R, Zucker J, Bernard J, Leverger G, Hartmann O: A Phase II study of high dose cisplatin and VP16 in neuroblastoma. J Clin Oncol (in press)

113. Chaudhry A, Haar J, Koul A, Nickerson P: Olfactory neuroblastoma. Cancer 44:564–579, 1979

114. Elkon D, Hightower S, Lim M, Cantrell R, Constable W: Esthesioneuroblastoma. Cancer 44:1087–1094, 1979

twenty-nine

Neuroepithelial Tumors

Mark A. Israel,
James S. Miser,
Timothy J. Triche, and
Timothy Kinsella

Peripheral neuroectodermal malignancies are a heterogeneous group of tumors that can occur either in supportive structures such as the nerve sheath (see Chap. 35) or in neuronal tissue itself. Among tumors of neuronal tissue, neuroendocrine malignancies, which occur very rarely during childhood, have a unique biology and have been considered separately (see Chaps. 3, 24, and 34). Tumors that have evidence of neuronal differentiation include neuroblastoma (see Chap. 28) and a variety of other tumors that occur outside recognized ganglia of the peripheral nervous system.

Peripheral neuroectodermal childhood tumors with histologic and cytologic neural features have been reported infrequently since 1918.[1] Historically, these tumors have been considered closely related to neuroblastoma, the best described and most extensively studied peripheral neural tumor of childhood. The recent identification of genetic, biochemical, and clinical characteristics of these tumors that distinguish them unambiguously from neuroblastoma, however, provides a basis on which they can be recognized as ontologically and biologically distinct entities (Table 29-1). The difficulty in identifying unique histopathologic features that distinguish neural tumors from neuroblastoma has confounded past attempts at their systematic classification. Although current diagnostic modalities cannot be retrospectively applied to previously reported tumors (*e.g.,* neuroepithelioma,[2-8] peripheral neuroectodermal tumor,[9] adult neuroblastoma,[10] primitive neuroectodermal tumor occurring outside the central nervous system,[11,12] malignant neuroepithelioma,[13] primitive neuroectodermal tumor of bone,[14-16] or malignant small cell tumor of the thoracopulmonary region[17-19]) review of the clinical and pathologic features of these and other tumors[20,21] and of ongoing studies (see below) strongly suggests that they are all a single nosologic entity. We will refer to this tumor as peripheral neuroepithelioma (PN), a term that reflects important features of this neuronal tumor that occurs outside the central nervous system (CNS).

EPIDEMIOLOGY

There have been no surveys or studies that indicate the incidence of PN. Many clinicians and pathologists have considered PN an uncommon presentation of neuroblastoma, and, in that context, this entity might be thought of as constituting a small fraction, perhaps 10%, of childhood neuroblastoma. On the other hand, it currently appears that PN is very closely related to Ewing's sarcoma, a tumor characterized by a chromosomal translocation indistinguishable from the t(11;22) (q24;q12) that occurs in PN (see below). Ongoing pathologic reviews at several major pediatric cancer centers suggest that as many as half of the tumors previously diagnosed as extraosseous Ewing's sarcoma may be PN,[22] and a similar proportion of Ewing's sarcoma of bone may have recognizable neural features.[23] If that observation can be generalized to all pediatric centers, the incidence of PN would clearly be increased.

Table 29-1
Comparison of Neuroepithelioma with Neuroblastoma and Ewing's Sarcoma

Variable	Neuroblastoma	Neuroepithelioma	Ewing's Sarcoma
Clinical Presentation			
Age	<4	Adolescence	Adolescence
Site	Abdominal	Thoracic, extremity, pelvis	Thoacic, extremity, pelvis
Biological Markers			
Cytologic features of neural differentiation	+	±	−
EM features of neural differentiation	+	±	−
Neurotransmitters	Adrenergic	Cholinergic	Cholinergic
Surface HLA expression	−	+	+
Cytogenetic Characteristics			
Chromosomal translocation	−	t(11;22) (q24;q11–12)	t(11;22) (q24;q11–12)
Gene amplification	+	−	−
Oncogene Expression			
N-*myc*	+	−	−
c-*myc*	−	+	+

There are few data on which to base a demographic characterization of PN. Two series reviewing 35 cases suggest that this tumor may be slightly more common in females than in males.[13,17] Although PN has been reported in very young children[17,24,25] and adults as old as 72 years,[10] the median ages of patients whose tumors were retrospectively identified in the two series cited above were 21 years[13] and 11 years[17] (the second review was limited to patients < 21 years). Clearly this is a tumor of older children, a finding compatible with the possibility that while adrenal neuroblastoma does rarely occur after age 5,[26] most such tumors occurring outside of known sympathetic ganglia are likely to be PN. Only one black child with PN has been reported, a finding reminiscent of the rarity of Ewing's sarcoma in black children.[24]

GENETICS

PN has not been reported to occur in familial clusters, and no predisposing genetic alterations have been identified. Only a small number of patients with this tumor have been evaluated for the presence of a constitutional cytogenetic abnormality; none has yet been identified. However, many cases of PN have been identified as having a t(11;22) (q24;q12) or a related, complex chromosomal rearrangement.[8,27] This translocation is cytogenetically indistinguishable from the rearrangement reported in Ewing's sarcoma.[28,29] In both Ewing's sarcoma and PN it has been possible to map the translocation breakpoint on chromosome 22 distal to 22q11 and distal to 11q23.3-24 on chromosome 11 (see Chaps. 3, 31).[30] An additional chromosomal rearrangement that seems to occur in PN more frequently than might be expected by chance alone is supernumerary 8. Interestingly, an extra copy of chromosome 8 is also a frequent finding in Ewing's sarcoma.[26]

An important feature of site-specific chromosome rearrangements that characterize human tumors is that they may lead to structural or regulatory changes in known proto-oncogenes.[31] The proto-oncogene c-*ets* 1 maps to 11q23.3-q24[32] at the breakpoint in PN, although with available molecular probes, it has not been possible to demonstrate either translo-

cation of a portion of this gene or alterations in its expression. In this regard, the presence of c-*myc* on chromosome 8 is of interest, since this proto-oncogene is expressed at high levels in PN.[33,34]

BIOLOGY, PATHOGENESIS, AND NATURAL HISTORY

The etiology of PN is unknown. Clinically, this tumor is an aggressive, rapidly growing malignancy that typically arises in the extremities, chest, or pelvis and metastasizes widely. The presence of neural features distinguishes PN from most other solid tumors of childhood (see below). When pathologic specimens of adrenal neuroblastoma do not reveal mature neuronal features, however, it is not possible to distinguish these two neural tumors histopathologically.

Nonetheless, as might be expected from the clinical differences between PN and childhood neuroblastoma, biological differences between these tumors can be identified (Table 29-1). Tumor cell lines from PN all have high levels of choline acetyltransferase, the rate-limiting enzyme for the synthesis of acetylcholine.[34] Cell lines from childhood neuroblastoma typically do not have detectable choline acetyltransferase but do have high levels of enzymes important for the synthesis of catecholamines, neurotransmitters in the sympathetic branch of the peripheral nervous system.[35] Choline acetyltransferase activity found outside the CNS is largely limited to postganglionic parasympathetic neurons, suggesting that PN may be a tumor of neurons in the parasympathetic nervous system. Such an interpretation is compatible with the broad distribution of sites at which PN can occur, since parasympathetic neurons are found in blood vessels throughout the body. The occurrence of PN in locations outside known sympathetic nervous system tissues would also explain the frequent, although not invariant, observation that patients with PN do not excrete high levels of urinary catecholamines, a reliable marker for childhood neuroblastoma.

CNS tissues and neuroblastoma do not express the major histocompatibility antigens on their surface,[36] although this is a characteristic of virtually all normal tissues and most tumors.

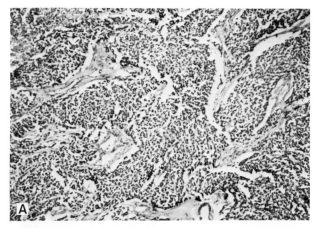

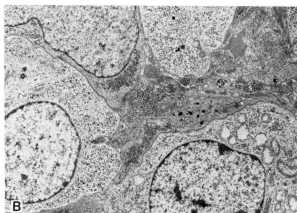

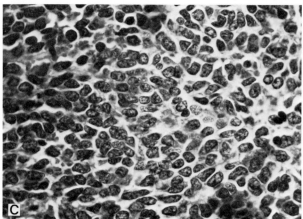

FIGURE 29-1. Peripheral neuroepithelioma (PN). **A.** Light microscopy. Fields of basophilic, small, blastic tumor cells sometimes arranged in lobules and (rarely) pseudorosettes are seen here. No ganglion cells, Schwann cells, or true rosettes with neuropil are seen in this tumor, in contrast to differentiating neuroblastoma. The light microscopic appearance is frequently nondiagnostic. (H & E; original magnification × 100) **B.** Electron microscopy. The ultrastructural appearance of PN is generally diagnostic. Specific neural features are found, including ill-formed neuritic processes, often with dense core granules (*center*). Individual granules (*upper right*) are also found in the perinuclear cytoplasm but are less reliable markers. Tumor cell cytoplasm is marked by abundant polyribosomes and occasional filaments or neurotubules (although the last two are more conspicuous and diagnostic when found in neuritic processes). (Uranyl acetate [UA] and lead citrate [PbCit]; original magnification × 4000) **C.** Immunocytochemistry. The single most useful marker for neural histogenesis is neuron specific enolase (NSE), illustrated here. Unfortunately, it alone is not sufficiently specific and reliable and must be interpreted in parallel with other neural antibodies or EM (as above). (Sternberger PAP technique, hematoxylin counterstain; original magnification × 400)

Cell lines from PN invariably express high levels of Class I histocompatibility antigens,[37] a feature that distinguishes them unequivocally from all neuroblastoma cell lines and tissues that have been reported. The evaluation of these surface antigens might provide a readily available approach for the pathologic characterization of these tumors, although no published data addressing this point are available.

PATHOLOGY

PN is a primitive round cell tumor with a largely undifferentiated light microscopic morphology, electron microscopic evidence of neural differentiation, and immunocytochemical evidence of neural antigen expression. We are unaware of any distinctive pathologic differences between PN, the malignant small cell tumor of the thoracopulmonary region in childhood ("Askin's tumor"), and primitive neuroectodermal tumors of bone. Although neural tumors arising in bone have not yet been evaluated for the presence of cytogenetic rearrangements, several thoracic wall tumors have been found to have a t(11;22) chromosomal rearrangement.[27] Further, cell lines from several such tumors are known to be cholinergic.[34] It seems likely that as more is learned about the biology of these tumors, they will be recognized as a single pathologic entity simply occurring at different sites throughout the body.

Histopathologic evaluation of PN reveals a tumor whose light microscopic appearance is similar to that seen in several other tumors of childhood—it is highly cellular and consists of a monotonous "blue pattern" of largely primitive round cells with scant cytoplasm. Although extensive light microscopic evaluation may reveal subtle neural features (Figure 29-1A) and a lobular growth pattern is sometimes evident, the overwhelming majority of these tumors lack conspicuous features of neural differentiation, such as obvious Homer–Wright rosettes or neuropil. Ganglion cell and Schwann cell differentiation is rarely if ever found.

The lack of distinctive light microscopic features that unambiguously define this tumor's cell of origin contrasts with electron microscopic and immunocytochemical evidence of neural differentiation. Usually these special studies are necessary to establish an accurate diagnosis. Electron microscopic evaluation of PN can reveal the presence of dense core granules, neurites, neurotubules, neurofilaments, and often prominent Golgi apparatus with associated neurosecretory vesicles (Fig. 29-1B). Unfortunately, in some cases, these features are infrequent or ambiguous and other methods of pathologic analysis are indicated. Immunocytochemical analysis is a particularly useful complement to electron microscopy in the evaluation of this tumor. The most useful antibody in establishing the diagnosis of a neural tumor is neuron specific enolase (NSE; see Fig. 29-1C). This enzyme can be detected in essentially all neural tissues and tumors, although it is not absolutely specific and can also be present in rhabdomyosarcoma (see Chap. 30). Other special stains are not particularly useful. Periodic acid-Schiff is positive in about two thirds of cases and therefore fails to distinguish this tumor from Ewing's sarcoma; even neuroblastoma can be positive in about 20% of cases. Silver staining for neurosecretory granules is virtually always negative.

The indistinguishable pathologic appearances of PN and the small round cell tumor of the thoracopulmonary region are highlighted in Figure 29-2. The lobular growth pattern of small, round, monomorphous tumor cells dominates the light microscopic appearance of this chest wall tumor, and only very rare rosettes can be identified (Figs. 29-2A,B). Ganglion cells, Schwann cells, or even distinct cell processes (manifest as refractile neuropil in the center of rosettes) providing firm evidence of neural differentiation cannot be detected. By electron microscopy, the ultrastructure of this tumor is characterized by such neural features as scant dense core granules that are usually somewhat pleomorphic and decidedly less uniform than the neurosecretory granules of neuroblastoma. Neurotubules and intermediate filaments (neurofilaments) are rarely if ever seen in these tumors. Similarly, electron microscopic evaluation of neuroectodermal tumors occurring in bone, which appear indistinguishable by light microscopy from other tumors of this group (Figure 29-3A), reveals similar neural features (Fig. 29-3B).

PN can be easily confused with Ewing's sarcoma when the pathologic evaluation is limited to light microscopic examination of tumor tissue. The presence of immunocytochemical and electron microscopic evidence of neuronal differentiation distinguishes this tumor from Ewing's sarcoma, in which these tissue-specific features are absent. What is the biological relationship of PN and Ewing's sarcoma? One possibility is that Ewing's sarcoma is simply the most undifferentiated form of a family of peripheral neuroectodermal tumors that occur outside the CNS. This interpretation is compatible with recent laboratory results demonstrating the expression of neural specific antigens[38] and the induction of neural differentiation in Ewing's sarcoma tumor cell lines.[39] However, it remains possible that the genetic alterations that give rise to tumors with the biological and pathologic features described here orchestrate the phenotype now recognized to characterize this "family" of tumors. If that is the case, the ontologic relationships between these tumors remain largely undefined.

CLINICAL PRESENTATION

The most commonly reported primary site of PN is the chest wall; other sites include the trunk, the abdomen and pelvis, and the extremities (occasionally, other sites are reported). Combining the results of two recently published series detailing the experience with a total of 47 patients with PN, 33 had tumors that arose in the chest wall.[24,25] The initial signs and symptoms caused by PN are related to the growth of the primary tumor and metastases, although there are usually no significant functional neurologic abnormalities at diagnosis. PN arising on the trunk and chest wall usually presents as an asymptomatic or locally painful palpable mass. The most common local complication of the chest wall lesion is an associated pleural effusion, which may or may not contain malignant cells. Tumor cells may spread throughout the pleural cavity, resulting in microscopic and macroscopic foci of tumor on the pleural surface. Because PN may arise in the paraspinal region as well as laterally or anteriorly on the chest wall, direct extension of the tumor into the spinal canal can occur. This possibility should always be considered and investigated if the primary

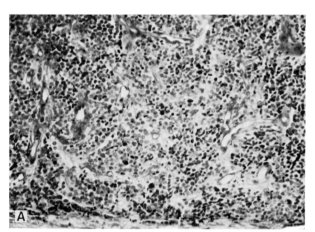
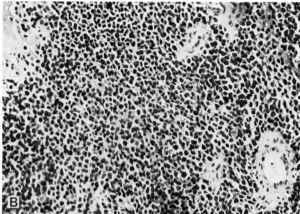
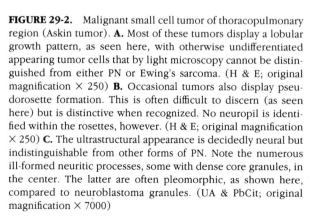
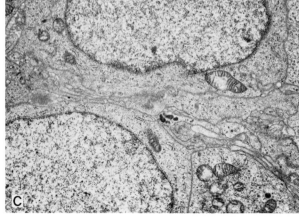

FIGURE 29-2. Malignant small cell tumor of thoracopulmonary region (Askin tumor). **A.** Most of these tumors display a lobular growth pattern, as seen here, with otherwise undifferentiated appearing tumor cells that by light microscopy cannot be distinguished from either PN or Ewing's sarcoma. (H & E; original magnification × 250) **B.** Occasional tumors also display pseudorosette formation. This is often difficult to discern (as seen here) but is distinctive when recognized. No neuropil is identified within the rosettes, however. (H & E; original magnification × 250) **C.** The ultrastructural appearance is decidedly neural but indistinguishable from other forms of PN. Note the numerous ill-formed neuritic processes, some with dense core granules, in the center. The latter are often pleomorphic, as shown here, compared to neuroblastoma granules. (UA & PbCit; original magnification × 7000)

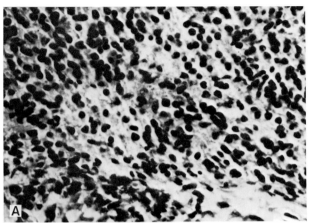

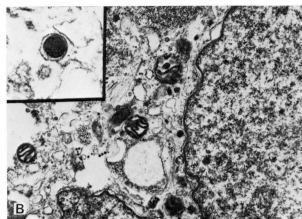

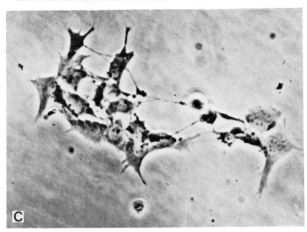

FIGURE 29-3. Primitive neuroectodermal tumor of bone (PNET of bone). **A.** This tumor is virtually indistinguishable from Ewing's sarcoma *or* PN by light microscopy, as is apparent here, compared with Figures 29-1A and 29-2A. Diffuse sheets of basophilic tumor cells are the rule. A tendency to develop a spindle cell component is also seen (but not illustrated here). (H & E; original magnification × 400) **B.** The ultrastructural appearance, as in other PNs, is generally diagnostic. Tumor cell cytoplasm contains abundant organelles, including filaments, rough endoplasmic reticulum, and granules. The last-mentioned is detailed in the inset (*upper left*); in this case (unlike many), it appears indistinguishable from neuroblastoma granules. (UA & PbCit; original magnification × 12,000) **C.** *In vitro,* the PNET of bone undergoes spontaneous neural differentiation, forming neurites visible by phase contrast microscopy. (Original magnification × 250)

or a metastatic tumor deposit involves the paraspinal region or a vertebra.

Tumors arising in bone may present as a painful tumor mass, in a fashion similar to Ewing's sarcoma. On physical examination, there is often a tender, swollen extremity indicative of the soft tissue mass commonly associated with the bone lesion. In many cases, it cannot be reliably determined whether the tumor arises in bone or soft tissue. PN arising in the pelvis is also very similar in presentation to Ewing's sarcoma: both are usually associated with a large soft tissue mass. Local pain is usually the only presenting symptom; however, there may be symptoms and signs of nerve and nerve root involvement, caused by direct extension of the tumor mass.

Metastases are often detectable at presentation. In the two largest series to date, 5 of 30 patients[24] and 8 of 17 patients[25] had metastatic disease at diagnosis. In the National Cancer Institute (NCI) series,[25] the most common sites of metastatic disease were bone (6 of 8), bone marrow (5 of 8), lung (3 of 8), and lymph node (2 of 8).

EVALUATION AND DIFFERENTIAL DIAGNOSIS

The initial evaluation of PN, like other malignancies of childhood, must include adequate tissue evaluation to allow precise diagnosis; determination of the extent of local disease; and definition of the extent of metastatic disease. Obtaining adequate tumor tissue is essential for pathologic and genetic studies to distinguish this tumor from other small round cell tumors such as neuroblastoma, rhabdomyosarcoma, and Ewing's sarcoma (see Chaps. 6 and 10). Evaluation of the local

tumor should include computed tomography (CT). Magnetic resonance imaging (MRI) is an effective method of defining the extent of soft tissue mass (see Chap. 7).

Metastatic evaluation should include a radionuclide bone scan, bone marrow biopsy and aspiration, chest radiograph, and CT scan of the chest to examine the three most likely sites of distant metastases at diagnosis. Because regional nodes are also frequently involved, a CT or MRI scan of the primary should include the locoregional lymph node basins. All lymph node groups should be examined. Although the optimal approach to identify nodal metastases has not yet been defined, biopsy of suspicious nodes must be considered. Autopsy studies have revealed liver and paraspinal metastases, but the incidence of such metastases at initial diagnosis is low. CT of the liver should be considered if hepatic involvement is suspected.

Both neural and non-neural tumors enter into the differential diagnosis of peripheral neural tumors. Some are almost certainly related tumors, although confirmatory data have not yet been published.

The major entities to consider in the differential diagnosis are both osseous and extraosseous Ewing's sarcoma. The former is illustrated and discussed in Chapter 31. The latter is illustrated in Figure 29-4. Because of a lack of distinguishing features, extraosseous Ewing's may represent a group of undifferentiated tumors, including primitive rhabdomyosarcoma. One such example is illustrated in Figure 29-5, both at presentation (where it was indistinguishable from extraosseous Ewing's) and at relapse following polychemotherapy (where frank myogenesis had occurred). Clearly, then, even undifferentiated rhabdomyosarcoma must be considered in the differential diagnosis.

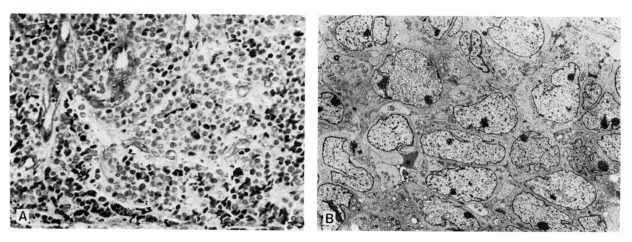

FIGURE 29-4. Extraosseous Ewing's sarcoma. **A.** The light microscopic appearance of extraosseous Ewing's sarcoma is indistinguishable from osseous Ewing's. No evidence of differentiation is detectable. Diffuse sheets of tumor cells with intervening vessels are seen. The tumor cell population is uniform. A light and dark cell dimorphic cellularity like that found in osseous Ewing's is often present, although not apparent here. (H & E; original magnification × 250) **B.** The electron microscopic appearance is also generally indistinguishable from osseous Ewing's sarcoma. Here, the tumor cells are somewhat more pleomorphic than usual, but still no evidence of differentiation is found. (UA & PbCit; original magnification × 1500)

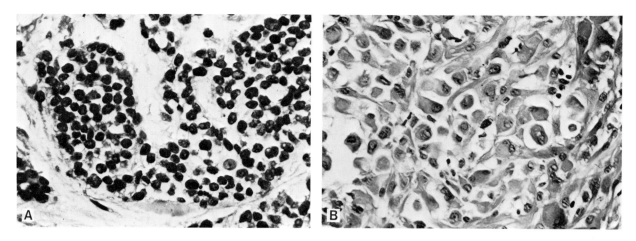

FIGURE 29-5. Primitive rhabdomyosarcoma. **A.** Initial biopsy. The appearance is indistinguishable from extraosseous Ewing's sarcoma as illustrated above. No differentiation of any type was detected by light microscopy. Immunocytochemistry for muscle markers was negative. (H & E; original magnification × 400) **B.** Post-treatment bone marrow relapse. Remarkable myogenesis affecting virtually every cell is obvious. Immunocytochemistry for skeletal muscle markers is now positive. (H & E; original magnification × 400) (Case courtesy of Dr. Vernon Pilon, Albany, NY)

Other tumors that must also be considered in the diagnosis of peripheral neural tumors include lymphoma, round cell tumors of bone (mesenchymal chondrosarcoma, small cell osteosarcoma), some densely cellular but otherwise undifferentiated spindle cell tumors of bone (termed primitive bone sarcomas at our institution), and certain primitive soft tissue sarcomas (vascular, synovial, and so forth). Other entities such as typical osteosarcoma, malignant fibrous histiocytoma, synovial cell sarcoma, and differentiated rhabdomyosarcoma are generally easily distinguished and are not included (see Chap. 31 for differential diagnosis and illustration).

Although the neural tumors discussed thus far appear to make up the majority of nonrhabdomyosarcomatous soft tissue tumors and nonosteosarcomatous bone tumors in children,

there are other less common neural tumors to consider. While a comprehensive discussion of all possibilities is beyond the scope of the present discussion, some such tumors are distinctive and warrant mention.

Perhaps the next most frequent and best delineated of the other neural tumors of children (and young adults) is esthesioneuroblastoma (or olfactory neuroblastoma, a synonomous term). This tumor appears to occur only in the nasal cavity, near the olfactory placode. It is generally just as undifferentiated in its appearance as the peripheral neuroepitheliomas discussed above. A typical example is illustrated in Figure 29-6A. When better differentiated, the neural character is more easily appreciated, both by light microscopy and immunocytochemistry (Fig. 29-6B). The ultrastructural appearance is diag-

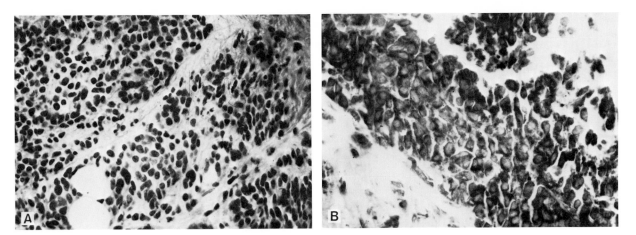

FIGURE 29-6. Esthesioneuroblastoma. **A.** Undifferentiated, light microscopy. The appearance is not diagnostic by light microscopy. Occurrence in the nasal cavity near the olfactory placode generally suggests the diagnosis, but confirmation requires other methods in tumors such as this. (H & E; original magnification × 400) **B.** Differentiated, immunocytochemistry. Tumors with larger, more eosinophilic tumor cells are typically more differentiated. Immunocytochemistry with antibodies such as neuron specific enolase (as here) confirms the impression of a neural phenotype. (Sternberger PAP, NSE; original magnification × 400)

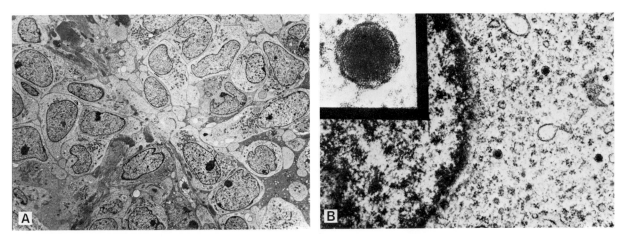

FIGURE 29-7. Esthesioneuroblastoma, ultrastructure. **A.** At low magnification, an undifferentiated tumor such as that in Figure 29-6A appears undifferentiated. No conspicuous neural features are seen at this magnification. (UA & PbCit; original magnification × 1000) **B.** At higher magnification, some undifferentiated tumors and all better-differentiated tumors can be seen to contain rather typical dense core neurosecretory granules. The inset details one such granule. (UA & PbCit; original magnification × 20,000; inset, original magnification × 100,000)

nostic, however (Fig. 29-7). The relationship of this tumor to neuroblastoma or other peripheral neural tumors is not known.

Another category of neural tumor that must be considered, albeit infrequently, is the central primitive neuroectodermal tumors (cPNETs). These tumors typically account for more than 25% of all childhood brain tumors and are second only to astrocytic tumors in frequency. The quintessential form is medulloblastoma, although numerous other entities are included in same group, including cerebral neuroblastoma, medulloepithelioma, and ependymoblastoma. Rarely, these tumors can occur outside the CNS and present as a primary, peripheral neuroectodermal tumor. In such cases, specific distinctive features allow these tumors to be distinguished from the more typical peripheral neuroepithelioma. A rare example is illustrated in Figure 29-8; this cPNET appeared vaguely epithelial,

even glandular by light microscopy, but by EM showed clearcut ependymal and possibly even neural tube differentiation (the latter typical of medulloepithelioma). Various other forms have been reported as well.

Finally, the possibility of mixed neural and non-neural tumors must be considered. The best described example of the latter among childhood tumors (although still quite rare) is the malignant ectomesenchymoma. Typically a tumor of the craniofacial region, where neural crest derived tissue gives rise to both neural and mesenchymal tissues of the head, malignant ectomesenchymoma has been clearly documented to display both classic neuroblastomatous and rhabdomyosarcomatous differentiation (Figure 29-9). The differential diagnosis of such tumors presents little problem when so clearly biphasic. It must be remembered, however, that the recurrent or persistent

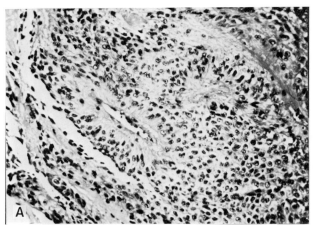

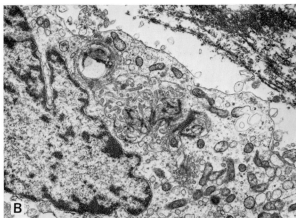

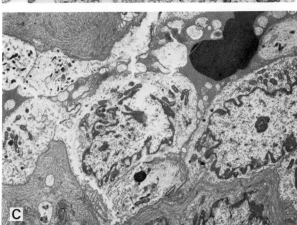

FIGURE 29-8. Central primitive neuroectodermal tumor (cPNET). **A.** This tumor is not completely undifferentiated, yet tissue-specific features are not immediately apparent by light microscopy. A vague suggestion of epithelial differentiation with a tendency to tube formation can be detected. Light microscopy alone, however, is insufficient to categorize this tumor. (H & E; original magnification × 250) **B.** By EM, frank epithelial differentiation with microvilli and junctional complexes is found in areas. Other cells showed abortive blepharoplasts, indicative of ependymal cell differentiation. **C.** Still other areas showed enormous oversynthesis of intact basal lamina, an absolute epithelial feature.

Taken together, these features are highly reminiscent of medulloepithelioma and ependymoma, normally a tumor of the central nervous system. This emphasizes the possibility that virtually any form of central PNET in the periphery could occur. (Case courtesy of Dr. Jonathan Finlay, Madison, WI)

tumor in several patients has been purely neuroblastic, presenting at least the theoretical possibility that some of these tumors might be confused with conventional peripheral neuroepithelioma.

Thoracic Neuroblastoma

The precise relationship of PN in the posterior chest wall and thoracic neuroblastoma, which usually occurs in patients younger than 5 years, is unknown. Thoracic neuroblastoma typically is not associated with elevations in the expression of urinary catecholamines and frequently has a more benign clinical course than that associated with abdominal neuroblastoma of comparable stage, suggesting that it is biologically different from typical adrenal neuroblastoma of childhood (see Chap. 28). Thoracic neuroblastoma also contrasts with PN in that it can usually be recognized as arising in the spinal ganglia and may be cured by surgery alone. It seems likely that thoracic neuroblastoma is a distinct pathologic entity, biologically distinct from both adrenal neuroblastoma and peripheral neuroblastoma.

STAGING AND PROGNOSTIC CONSIDERATIONS

The most appropriate clinical staging for PN is yet to be defined in a large prospective study. However, the staging definitions used in a recent NCI prospective trial were found to be clinically useful (Table 29-2).[25] It is clear, in the two largest studies reported to date, that small, resectable tumors have a more favorable outcome.[24,25] Whether surgical removal is a significant factor independent of tumor size or whether the extent of local spread is the important prognostic factor is not yet clear.

TREATMENT

The optimal treatment of PN has yet to be established. Although this tumor has only recently been recognized as a distinct clinical entity, it is known to be both radioresponsive and chemoresponsive.[24,25] A multimodality treatment approach including chemotherapy is both indicated and effective.

Surgery

The precise role of surgery in the treatment of PN requires further definition, but the complete removal of a small tumor, with pathologically confirmed negative margins, may avoid the need for radiation therapy and its potential toxicity.[25] There may also be some impact of complete resection on ultimate outcome; patients with completely resectable tumors in the two series reported to date have had a relatively good outcome.[24,25]

There are no data available to support the concept of debulking surgery (*i.e.,* surgery that does not completely remove the tumor) in patients with more extensive disease (see Chap. 10). In the NCI series of patients with advanced local and

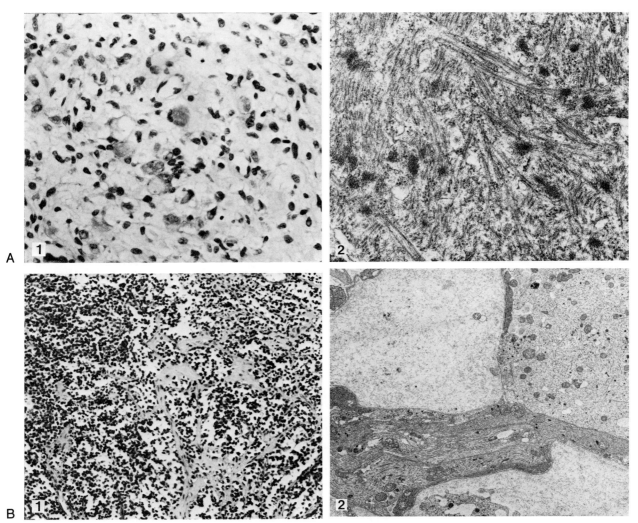

FIGURE 29-9. Malignant ectomesenchymoma. This complex tumor typically displays features of both mesenchymal and ectodermal tissues, usually rhabdomyosarcoma and neuroblastoma. **A.** Rhabdomyogenous component. [1] Numerous undifferentiated tumor cells are intermingled with occasional large, pink myoblasts. (H & E; original magnification × 250) [2] The myogenic character of the larger cells is confirmed by EM, where obvious thick and thin myofilaments plus Z-band material are easily identified. (UA & PbCit; original magnification × 60,000) **B.** Neuroblastic component. [1] Diffuse sheets of small, undifferentiated appearing tumor cells were present in other areas of this tumor. (H & E; original magnification × 200) [2] By EM, frank evidence of neuroblastic differentiation is found. Here, obvious bundles of neurites connect one cell to another. (UA & PbCit; original magnification × 10,000) (Courtesy of Dr. Dietmar Schmidt, Kiel, Germany)

systemic disease, no effect of surgery on outcome could be identified.[25]

Radiation Therapy

"Local" control of the primary tumor can be achieved by radiation therapy.[25] In the NCI series, with a follow-up of more than 2 years, there have been no local failures when radiation doses of 5000 to 5500 cGy were delivered in 180 cGy fractions with 2 to 5 cm margins five times a week to primary and metastatic lesions.[25] Unfortunately, the use of large radiation fields and high radiation doses in small children, especially on the chest wall, is associated with significant long-term deformities and toxicities. Future studies must address the dose and field size

required when radiation is given in conjunction with aggressive combination chemotherapy.

Careful attention to radiation therapy techniques is essential to minimize acute and late morbidities in children and adolescents with PN. Simulation with CT-assisted treatment planning should be done for all patients (see Chap. 11). For extremity lesions, immobilization during treatment by the use of casts is important and may avoid the need for complex field arrangements. For pelvic primaries, contrast should be used at simulation to identify the small bowel, bladder, kidneys, and rectum. Chest wall primaries can often be treated using tangential photon fields combined with an electron boost to minimize radiation injury to heart, lung, and upper abdominal viscera. Further discussion of the technical details and potential morbidities of radiation therapy is found in the discussion of

Ewing's sarcoma (Chap. 31)—the current approach to radiation therapy in these two tumors is identical.

Chemotherapy

Although no randomized study establishes the need for chemotherapy in the treatment of PN, the similarity of this disease to Ewing's sarcoma, its propensity to metastasize, and its recurrence at locations distant from the primary site of presentation all suggest the need for chemotherapy. A number of chemotherapeutic agents have documented activity in the treatment of PN. Although no single-agent response data are available, three drug combinations have proven to be active in the treatment of PN (Table 29-3): [1] vincristine, doxorubicin, and cyclophosphamide;[25] [2] ifosfamide and etoposide;[40] and [3] teniposide and cisplatin.[41] One report has suggested that actinomycin D also has efficacy in the treatment of PN;[24] however, response rates for this agent are not available, and limited experience with its use in combination with vincristine and cyclophosphamide in recurrent disease has not been rewarding.

In a Phase III trial where a measurable response to chemotherapy could be assessed in a group of newly diagnosed patients with Stage III and Stage IV PN, 14 of 15 patients (93%) had objective tumor responses (>50% reduction in tumor volume) when treated with an aggressive regimen of vincristine, doxorubicin, and cyclophosphamide.[25] Two additional previously treated patients also had partial responses to this regimen, yielding an overall response rate of 94%. In a second series, 11 of 16 patients had measurable partial or complete responses to several chemotherapy regimens, which included actinomycin D, vincristine, ifosfamide, and doxorubicin.[24]

In a Phase II evaluation of the efficacy of ifosfamide and etoposide in the treatment of recurrent PN, 5 of 8 children, but none of 2 adults, achieved a partial response, yielding an overall response rate of 50% for the group (see Table 29-3). Responses have been reported to the combination of teniposide and cisplatin, both alone and in combination with other agents.[15,41] Other information about response rates of PN to chemotherapy is anecdotal.

Combined Modality Therapy

There has been only one prospectively reported series of patients with PN treated with combined modality therapy;[25] however, a second, retrospectively evaluated group of patients also provides a basis for preliminary recommendations.[24] The combined results of these two series are given in Table 29-4. The prognosis is excellent when tumors are small and can be completely removed by surgery, and adjuvant chemotherapy is used.[24,25] In the retrospectively evaluated group of 30 patients (discovered to have PN on the basis of a histologic review of patients entered on trials for Ewing's sarcoma, soft tissue sarcoma, and neuroblastoma) 28 received chemotherapy in addition to local therapy. The disease-free survival of patients with complete removal of tumor was 100%, whereas four of five patients with metastatic disease relapsed.[24] Most patients with extensive local tumor or metastatic disease will achieve complete remission with chemotherapy regimens that include vincristine, doxorubicin, and an oxazaphosphorin,[25] although about half can be expected to relapse with prolonged follow-up (Table 29-4).[24,25] In a group of patients with more extensive disease treated in an NCI study, 8 of 15 patients with Stage III and IV disease have relapsed with a median follow-up of 2 years after being treated with intensive VADRIAC chemotherapy (vincristine, Adriamycin, and cyclophosphamide) and radiotherapy.[25]

Current recommendations for the chemotherapy of newly diagnosed PN are as follows: [1] for patients with Stage I or II lesions, adjuvant chemotherapy of moderate intensity and duration using vincristine, doxorubicin, and an oxazaphosphorin (either ifosfamide or cyclophosphamide); and [2] for patients with Stage III or IV lesions, similar chemotherapy using an intensive dose schedule. In the NCI trial for patients with extensive disease, intensive chemotherapy was delivered before

Table 29-2
Clinical Staging of Peripheral Neuroepithelioma

Stage I	Small tumor size (<5 cm diameter); complete resection performed; no metastases present
Stage II	Small tumor size (<5 cm diameter); gross tumor resection accomplished but microscopic disease remains; no metastases present
Stage III	Large tumor size (>5 cm diameter); gross tumor resection not usually possible; no metastases present
Stage IV	Primary tumor of any size; metastases present

Table 29-3
Response of Peripheral Neuroepithelioma to Chemotherapy Regimens*

Chemotherapy Regimen	Type of Patient	Number of Patients	Response CR	PR	Response Rate (%)	Reference
VCR+ADR+CTX	Recurrent	2	2	0	100	25
VCR+ADR+CTX	Newly diagnosed	15	14	0	93	25
IFOS+VP-16+MES	Recurrent	10	0	5	50	40
CPDD+VM-26	Newly diagnosed	6	0	4	67	41
VCR+CTX+CPDD+VM-26	Recurrent	1	1	0	100	†
VCR+AMD+CTX	Recurrent	2	0	0	0	†

* VCR = vincristine; ADR = Adriamycin; CTX = cyclophosphamide; IFOS = ifosfamide; MES = Mesna; CPDD = cisplatin; VM-26 = teniposide; VP-16 = etoposide; AMD = actinomycin D; CR = complete response; PR = partial response.
† Unpublished data.

Table 29-4
Outcome of Therapy for Peripheral Neuroepithelioma in Relation to Extent of Disease at Diagnosis

Extent of Disease	Retrospective Study*	Prospective Study†	Total Number
	(no. of relapses/no. of patients)		
Complete excision	0/13	0/1	0/14
Incomplete resection but no metastases	6/12	4/8	10/20
Metastases present at diagnosis	4/5	4/8	8/13

* Disease-free survival for patients with localized disease at 66 months is 52%.[25]
† Disease-free survival for the whole group at 2 years is 50%.[24]

radiation therapy to reduce the size and extent of the bulk disease, improve the local control rate, and avoid the toxicity of combined modality therapy in the initial 6 to 8 weeks of the regimen, when intensive systemic treatment of metastatic disease is crucial.[25] Preliminary data on disease-free survival suggest that with this approach, more than 50% of patients with limited resectable disease will remain in remission for extended periods of time, while 25% to 50% of patients with more extensive disease should remain in remission 2 to 3 years following achievement of complete remission.[24,25]

For the treatment of recurrent PN, the combination of ifosfamide and etoposide is the most effective regimen.[40] This further suggests that this combination may play an important role in the treatment of newly diagnosed patients with PN. Teniposide and cisplatin have also been used with some success in patients with recurrent PN.[15]

FUTURE CONSIDERATIONS

Recent research has provided a firm biological and clinical basis on which to determine the precise diagnosis of peripheral neuroepithelioma, whether presenting in bone or soft tissue. Continued laboratory research in this area should provide insight into the pathologic significance of the t(11;22) chromosomal rearrangement that characterizes this tumor and thereby provide additional information regarding its relationship to Ewing's sarcoma. The similarities in the natural histories of these two tumors, as well as the apparent similarities in their responsiveness to therapeutic intervention, suggest that such research may enhance our understanding of both tumors and of their relationship.

Several clinical studies have demonstrated the need for multiple modalities of therapy in the treatment of PN. Enhanced recognition of the natural history of this tumor and of the activity of agents such as ifosfamide and etoposide in patients who have relapsed suggests that continued improvement in disease-free survival rates can be anticipated. Toward this end, earlier intervention and improved chemotherapeutic regimens designed to capitalize on the high response rates of current approaches should be important focuses of future clinical research.

REFERENCES

1. Stout AP: A tumor of the ulnar nerve. Proc NY Pathol Soc 18:2–12, 1918
2. Stout AP, Murray MR: Neuroepithelioma of the radial nerve with a study of its behavior in vitro. Rev Can Biol 1:651–659, 1942
3. Penfield W: Tumors of the sheaths of the nervous system. In Cytology and Cellular Pathology of the Nervous System, pp 980–984, New York, Paul B Hoeber, 1932
4. Lagerkvist B, Ivemark B, Sylven B: Malignant neuroepithelioma in childhood. A report of three cases. Acta Chir Scand 135:641–645, 1969
5. Ishikawa S, Ohsima Y, Suzuki T, Oboshi S: Primitive neuroectodermal tumor (neuroepithelioma) of spinal nerve root. Report of an adult case and establishment of a cell line. Acta Pathol Jpn 29:289–301, 1979
6. Bolen JW, Thorning D: Peripheral neuroepithelioma: A light and electron microscopic study. Cancer 46:2456–2462, 1980
7. Harper PG, Pringle J, Souhami RI: Neuroepithelioma—A rare malignant peripheral nerve tumor of primitive origin. Report of two new cases and a review of the literature. Cancer 48:2282–2287, 1981
8. Whang-Peng J, Triche TJ, Knutsen T, Miser J, Douglass EC, Israel MA: Chromosome translocation in peripheral neuroepithelioma. N Engl J Med 311:584–585, 1984
9. Seemayer TA, Thelmo WL, Bolande RP, Wiglesworth FW: Peripheral neuroectodermal tumors. In Rosenberg HS, Boland RP (eds): Perspectives in Pediatric Pathology, pp 151–172. Chicago, Year Book Medical Publishers, 1979
10. Mackay B, Luna MA, Butler JJ: Adult neuroblastoma. Electron microscopic observations in nine cases. Cancer 37:1334–1351, 1976
11. Nesbitt KA, Vidone RA: Primitive neuroectodermal tumor (neuroblastoma) arising in the sciatic nerve of a child. Cancer 37:1562–1570, 1976
12. Samuel AW: Primitive neuroectodermal tumor arising in the ulnar nerve. A case report. Clin Orthop 167:236–238, 1982
13. Hashimoto H, Enjoji M, Nakajima T, Kyru H, Daimaru Y: Malignant neuroepithelioma (peripheral neuroblastoma): A clinicopathologic study of 15 cases. Am J Surg Pathol 7:309–318, 1983
14. Willis RA: Metastatic neuroblastoma in bone presenting the Ewing syndrome, with a discussion of "Ewing's sarcoma." Am J Pathol 16:317–332, 1940
15. Jaffe R, Santamaria M, Yunis EJ, Tannery NH, Agostini RM Jr, Medina J, Goodman M: The neuroectodermal tumor of bone. Am J Surg Pathol 8:885–898, 1984
16. Jaffe N et al: Bone Tumors in Children. Littleton, MA, PSG Publishing, 1979
17. Askin FB, Rosai J, Sibley RK, Dehner LP, McAlister WH: Malignant small cell tumor of the thoracopulmonary region in childhood. A distinctive clinicopathologic entity of uncertain histogenesis. Cancer 43:2438–2451, 1979
18. Scotta MS, DeGiacoma C, Maggiore G, Corbella F, Coci A, Castello A: Malignant small cell tumor of the thoracopulmonary region in childhood. A case report. Am J Pediatr Hematol Oncol 6:459–462, 1984
19. Linnoila I, Tsokos M, Triche TJ, Chandra R: Evidence for neural origin and periodic acid-Schiff-positive variants of the malignant small cell tumors of thoracopulmonary region ("Askin tumor") (abstr). Lab Invest 48:51A, 1983
20. Davidson KG, Walbaum PR, McCormack RJM: Intrathoracic neural tumours. Thorax 33:359–367, 1978
21. Abell MR, Hart WR, Olson VR: Tumors of the peripheral nervous system. Hum Pathol 1:503–551, 1970
22. Shimada H, Newton WA, Soul EA, Qualman SJ, Aoyama C, Mauer HM: Pathologic features of extraosseous Ewing's sarcoma: A report from the Intergroup Rhabdomyosarcoma Study (submitted for publication)
23. Perez-Atayde AR, Grier H, Weinstein H, Belarey M, Neslie N, Vawter G: Neuroectodermal differentiation in bone tumors presenting as Ewing's sarcoma. Proceedings of SIOP Meeting XIX, p 61, 1985
24. Gobel V, Jurgens H, Beck J, Brandeis W, Etspuler G, Gadner H, Harms D, Schmidt D, Sternschulte W, Treuner J, Gobel U: Malignant peripheral neuroectodermal tumors of childhood and adolescence: Retrospective analysis of treatment results in 30 patients. Proc Am Soc Clin Oncol 5:810, 1986
25. Miser JS, Kinsella TJ, Triche TJ, Steis R, Tsokos M, Wesley R, Horvath K, Belasco J, Longo DL, Glatstein E, Israel MA: Treatment of Peripheral neuroepithelioma in children and young adults. J Clin Oncol 5:1752–1758, 1987
26. Kaye JA, Warhol MJ, Kretschmar C, Landsberg L, Frei E: Neuroblastoma in adults. Three case reports and a review of the literature. Cancer 58:1149–1157, 1986
27. Whang-Peng J, Triche TJ, Knutsen T, Miser J, Kao-Shan S, Tsai S, Israel M: Cytogenetic characterization of selected small round cell tumors of childhood. Cancer Genet Cytogenet 21:185–208, 1986
28. Turc-Carel C, Philip I, Berger MP, Philip T, Lenoir GM: Chromosomal translocations in Ewing's sarcoma. N Engl J Med 390:496–497, 1983
29. Aurias A, Rimbaut C, Buffe D, Dubousset J, Mazabraud A: Chromosomal translocations in Ewing's sarcoma. N Engl J Med 309:496–497, 1983
30. Griffin CA, McKeon C, Israel MA, Gegonne A, Chysdael J, Stehelin D, Douglass EC, Green AE, Emanuel BS: Comparison of constitutional and

tumor-associated 11;22 translocations: Nonidentical breakpoints on chromosomes 11 and 22. Proc Natl Acad Sci USA 83:6122–6126, 1986

31. Bishop JM: The molecular genetics of cancer. Science 235:305–311, 1987

32. de Taisne C, Gregonne A, Stehelin D, Bernheim A, Berger R: Chromosomal localization of the human proto-oncogene c-ets. Nature 310:581–583, 1984

33. Thiele CJ, McKeon C, Triche TJ, Ross RA, Reynolds CP, Israel MA: Differential proto-oncogene expression characterizes histopathologically indistinguishable tumors of the peripheral nervous system. J Clin Invest 80:804–811, 1987

34. McKeon C, Thiele CJ, Ross RA, Kwan M, Triche TJ, Miser JS, Israel MA: Indistinguishable and predictable patterns of proto-oncogene expression in two histopathologically distinct tumors: Ewing's sarcoma and neuroepithelioma (submitted for publication)

35. Ross RA, Biedler JL, Spengler BA, Reis DJ: Neurotransmitter-synthesizing enzymes in 14 human neuroblastoma cell lines. Cell Molec Neurobiol 1:301–311, 1981

36. Lampson LA, Fisher CA, Whelan VP: Striking paucity of HLA-A, B, and B2-microglobulin on human neuroblastoma cell lines. J Immunol 130:2471–2478, 1983

37. Donner L, Triche TJ, Israel MA, Seeger RC, Reynolds CP: A panel of monoclonal antibodies which discriminate neuroblastoma from Ewing's sarcoma, rhabdomyosarcoma, neuroepithelioma, and hematopoietic malignancies. Prog Clin Biol Res 175:347–366, 1985

38. Lipinski M, Braham K, Philip I, Wiels J, Philip T, Goridis C, Lenoir GM, Tursz T: Neuroectoderm-associated antigens on Ewing's sarcoma cell lines. Cancer Res 47:183–187, 1987

39. Cavazzana AO, Miser J, Jefferson J, Triche TJ: Experimental evidence for a neural origin of Ewing's sarcoma of bone. Am J Pathol 127:507–518, 1987

40. Miser JS, Kinella TJ, Tsokos M, Jarosinski P, Forquer R, Wesley R, Magrath IT: Ifosfamide with mesna uroprotection and etoposide: An effective regimen in the treatment of recurrent sarcomas and other tumors of children and young adults. J Clin Oncol 5:1191–1198, 1987

41. Fink IJ, Kurtz DW, Cazenave L, Lieber MR, Miser JS, Chandra R, Triche TJ: Malignant thoracopulmonary small-cell ("Askin") tumor. Am J Radiol 145:517–520, 1985

thirty

Rhabdomyosarcoma and the Undifferentiated Sarcomas

R. Beverly Raney, Jr.,
Daniel M. Hays,
Melvin Tefft, and
Timothy J. Triche

A sarcoma is a malignant solid tumor arising from primitive mesenchymal cells, which are scattered throughout the body. Normally, mesenchymal cells develop into supportive tissues, such as fibrous tissue, muscle, cartilage, and bone. In the development of sarcomas, however, complete differentiation into mature structures is not achieved, although the pathologist can often find evidence of some maturation. For example, malignant tumors of cartilage may be designated as chondrosarcoma and those of fibrous tissue as fibrosarcoma, depending on the mature normal counterpart the tumor simulates most closely. Following this pattern, the term *rhabdomyosarcoma* connotes a tumor arising from tissue that imitates normal striated muscle.[1-3] Despite its name, rhabdomyosarcoma often arises from mesenchymal tissue in sites where striated muscle is not ordinarily found, such as the bladder. The undifferentiated sarcoma is a tumor whose cell of origin appears to be mesodermal, as opposed to ectodermal or endodermal, but whose degree of maturity is so primitive as to give no indication of a specific tissue type.

Rhabdomyosarcoma (RMS) is the most common soft tissue sarcoma in persons under age 21, and accounts for 5% to 8% of all cases of childhood cancer. It is important because of both its frequency and the multiple anatomic sites in which it can arise. Thus, surgical aspects appropriate to each site must be considered in planning management for individual patients. In addition, RMS is moderately sensitive to treatment with radiation therapy and chemotherapy. Progress in the use of all three modalities has led to impressive improvements in survival and to some diminution in the untoward late sequelae of therapy. With improved survival has come realization of the importance of prognostic factors in designing clinical trials and of the extraordinary variety of histologic subtypes and patterns of disease spread among tumors categorized as rhabdomyosarcoma and undifferentiated sarcoma (UDS).

All sarcomas of soft tissue can spread to areas of the body contiguous with and beyond their site of origin. Regardless of histologic subtype, all forms of RMS and UDS can infiltrate local structures and eventually invade both lymphatic tissues and the bloodstream. RMS and UDS can arise at virtually any site in the body. Accordingly, the site of origin, the regional lymphatic tissues, and more distant locations such as lungs, bone marrow, and bones must all be considered in the assessment of each patient with RMS or UDS.

HISTORICAL BACKGROUND

RMS and UDS can arise anywhere in the body and are divided into at least six conventional histologic types. A brief review of major contributions to our understanding of this extraordinarily complex group of cancers is presented here (see also Chap. 6).

Virchow (1821–1902) separated the sarcomas of soft tissue and bone from other forms of cancer, such as epithelial and hematologic malignancies.[4] Weber described rhabdomyosarcoma as a separate entity in 1854, in a report of a 21-year-old man with a recurrent growth in the tongue.[5] The first descriptive collection of cases appeared in 1946 with the landmark publication by A. P. Stout,[1] followed by Pack's report of the pathologic and clinical diversity of tumors arising in soft somatic tissues.[2,3] The pathologic descriptions of RMS were united by Horn and Enterline in 1958,[6] when they noted the presence of rhabdomyoblasts within malignant soft tissue tumors previously designated as embryonal rhabdomyosarcoma in young persons and as pleomorphic sarcomas in older persons.[7] Embryonal RMS, so called because the tissue simulates immature skeletal muscle, have since been divided into solid and botryoid (grape-like) forms. The distinction between the two varieties is related to the site of origin: solid embryonal RMS occurs within deep or superficial structures not covered with mucosa, whereas the more loosely arranged, relatively less common botryoid embryonal RMS arises in structures covered with mucosa and apposite to a body cavity, such as the bladder or nasopharynx.[8]

In 1956, Riopelle and Thériault used the term "alveolar" rhabdomyosarcoma, based on similarity of the tumor tissue pattern to that of normal lung parenchyma.[9] Enzinger and Shiraki summarized 110 patients with alveolar rhabdomyosarcomas in 1969.[10] More recently, a sarcoma arising in soft tissue but histologically similar to Ewing's sarcoma of bone has been described by several authors.[11,12]

The finding by Horn and Enterline in 1958 that RMS could be characterized by the presence of rhabdomyoblasts provided a uniform way to separate these tumors from fibroblastic, neurogenic, and other malignant proliferations of soft tissue.[6] Thereafter, cases of similar histologic appearance could be collected, and retrospective reports of experience with pediatric cases at large institutions began to appear over the next 20 years. Nevertheless, the total numbers of cases observed and treated over many years were often less than 100 per institution. Extensive lists of these publications can be found in review articles on rhabdomyosarcoma and other soft tissue sarcomas in childhood.[13–17]

EPIDEMIOLOGY

Soft tissue sarcomas are the sixth most common form of cancer in childhood, following acute leukemia, tumors of the central nervous system, lymphoma, neuroblastoma, and Wilms' tumor (see also Chap. 1).[18–20] Rhabdomyosarcoma is the most common soft tissue sarcoma in persons under age 15, and accounts for 5% to 8% of cases of childhood cancer.[18–20] Data from 1482 young people with cancer referred to the Children's Hospital of Philadelphia over a 10-year period revealed 122 cases of soft tissue sarcoma (8% of the total). RMS and UDS were the predominant forms of soft tissue sarcoma (72%) in children younger than 10 years; in the second decade of life, RMS and UDS comprised 57% of the cases.[21] Jenkin and Sonley reported that 71% of the young people referred to their institutions for treatment of soft tissue sarcoma had either RMS or UDS.[22]

The Third National Cancer Survey, conducted in two states and seven standard metropolitan areas of the United States from 1969 through 1971, found 130 cases of soft tissue sarcoma in white children and 9 in black children, taken from a total of approximately 5 million white and 700,000 black children. Of these, 69 cases in whites (53%) and 3 in blacks (33%) were classified as RMS. The overall rates were 8.4 cases of soft tissue sarcoma per million white children per year and 3.9 cases per million black children per year in these populations, which represented approximately 10% of the U.S. population at the time of the 1970 census.[18] These rates are similar to those for renal tumors (principally Wilms') in children. It has been estimated that approximately 500 new cases of Wilms' tumor are diagnosed in the United States annually,[23] and half of the soft tissue sarcomas are RMS, so one can estimate that approximately 250 new cases of RMS are diagnosed in this country each year.

Breslow and Langholz have recently summarized the world cancer registry experience and the SEER (surveillance, epidemiology, and end results) program of the National Cancer Institute (NCI) for childhood neoplasms.[19] RMS was somewhat less frequent than either neuroblastoma or Wilms' tumor, and somewhat more frequent in males than in females. There was no significant relationship with geographic location (among five continents) or change over the 20-year period (1958–1977) in the incidence of pediatric RMS.

The available information indicates that RMS and probably UDS occur throughout the world, that males are somewhat more likely than females to develop the disease, that RMS is predominantly a disease of persons younger than 21 years, and that there are no obvious differences among ethnic groups (in contrast to the distinctions seen for Burkitt's lymphoma in African as compared to American children; see Chap. 1).[24] There are some interesting and unexplained associations among age, site of the primary sarcoma, and tumor histology. Sarcomas of the bladder and vagina occur primarily in infants and nearly always have solid embryonal or botryoid histology, whereas sarcomas of the trunk and extremities occur in older persons and often have alveolar or undifferentiated histology. Tumors of the head and neck occur throughout childhood, but are more common in the first 8 years.[25] Further epidemiologic data are being collected prospectively under the auspices of the NCI and the Intergroup Rhabdomyosarcoma Study (IRS).

GENETICS

Reports of RMS arising within a congenital cyst of the lung in two children,[26,27] in two patients with Gorlin's nevoid basal cell carcinoma syndrome,[28,29] and in several children with fetal alcohol syndrome[30] or neurofibromatosis[31,32] have genetic implications (see also Chap. 2). The association with neurofibromatosis is particularly intriguing, because patients who develop neurogenic sarcoma may have evidence of rhabdomyosarcomatous differentiation within the mass. This pathologic entity, the malignant Triton tumor, may be found in patients with or without neurofibromatosis.[33,34]

Rarely, families with multiple tumors including RMS have been described. An association between maternal breast cancer and soft tissue sarcoma in offspring was first described in 1969 by Li and Fraumeni[35] and later amplified.[36] A similar association has been noted in England, where the risk of breast cancer in mothers of children with soft tissue sarcoma was as high as 13.5-fold increase.[37] Others have noted the excess occurrence in a kindred of RMS, glioblastoma, breast cancer, lung cancer, and adrenocortical carcinoma.[38] Knowledge of these associations and delineation of causal relationships await further investigations, but the implication is that genetic factors must have a role in the etiology of some soft tissue sarcomas in childhood.

The cytogenetics of soft tissue sarcomas themselves and of patients bearing these neoplasms have begun to be examined systematically in the last 10 to 15 years, coincident with the development of banding techniques that permit the detailed characterization of chromosomal abnormalities. The data are relatively limited, probably because of the low incidence of these tumors. Berger and coworkers examined peripheral blood lymphocytes of 45 consecutive adults (34 years and older) with soft tissue sarcomas admitted during the period 1980 to 1981.[39] Only one had RMS; three had unclassifiable sarcomas, and most were diagnosed with malignant fibrous histiocytoma, liposarcoma, or leiomyosarcoma. No significant differences in C-banding of chromosomes 1, 9, or 16 were found when compared to 78 randomly selected blood donors. Moriyama and associates have described a 2-year-old girl with embryonal RMS of the bladder whose peripheral blood lymphocytes showed a balanced reciprocal translocation between the long arms of chromosomes 2 and 5 in 20 prometaphase cells.[40]

Tumor specimens from two children with embryonal RMS[41,42] and two adults with alveolar RMS[43,44] have been studied for karyotypic abnormalities, as have two RMS tumors and five RMS cell lines,[45] plus one undifferentiated and one spindle cell sarcoma.[46] A variety of abnormalities have been found, as shown in Table 30-1 (see also Chap. 2). Whether one or more of these abnormalities will emerge as characteristic of RMS remains to be seen. The possible relationship between chromosomal abnormalities and alterations or expression of oncogenes is being studied (see Chap. 3). There is one case report of a 15-month-old with embryonal RMS who had N-*myc* amplification (by Southern blot analysis).[47] We are not aware of other similar cases involving RMS or UDS.

BIOLOGY

The biological behavior of RMS and UDS, which appear quite similar, has come under increasing scrutiny in the past 30 years as treatment techniques have improved. Until recently, knowledge of the evolution of these tumors was limited by their relative infrequency (even large institutions may accrue no more than 10 to 15 cases per year),[21] by the multiplicity of primary sites and histologic categories, and—before the discovery of effective chemotherapeutic agents—by the fact that most children with these tumors died within 2 years, usually of metastases in lung or marrow. Indeed, the experience with RMS and UDS was quite dismal as recently as 20 years ago. Soule and colleagues found only 19 survivors in a group of 102 children treated at the Mayo Clinic from 1950 through 1965 for RMS (15 of 75 alive) or UDS (4 of 27).[48] Kilman and colleagues reported an actuarial survival rate of only 14% at 5 years when children with RMS were treated by measures designed primarily to eradicate local tumor (surgical removal, radiation therapy, or both), without multiagent systemic chemotherapy after diagnosis.[49] A 5-year survival figure of 36% was reported by Myers and colleagues for 107 white children treated between

1965 and 1969 in various parts of the United States.[50] Other centers reported 5-year survival rates ranging from 10% to 30% before the introduction of standard multiagent chemotherapy.[51-55] A similar prechemotherapy era figure of 31% survival at 5 years has recently been reported by Flamant and associates from Villejuif, France.[56] These authors and others[57,58] noted that RMS had a high rate of eventual metastasis (approximately 65%–80%) and that often surgical measures alone could not eradicate local tumor, because many of the tumors occurred in the head and neck[57,59] or retroperitoneum and pelvis,[60] where surgical extirpation was not possible.

The etiology of primary RMS and UDS is still unknown. Radiation therapy can produce sarcomas in both soft tissue and bone, both primarily and secondarily (*i.e.*, after treatment for some other condition). Most current reports are concerned with secondary sarcomas in adults following radiation for breast cancer or other epithelial neoplasms.[61,62] There are also several reports of secondary sarcomas of bone and soft tissue in patients treated for pediatric cancer with radiation, with or without chemotherapy.[63,64] One child developed a pelvic RMS 3 years after treatment with chemotherapy and cranial irradiation for acute lymphocytic leukemia.[65] Perhaps by boosting the effect of radiation, the administration of actinomycin D has been associated with a lower rate of second malignancies in children.[66] A genetic predisposition to second malignancies, noted especially in children with the genetic form of retinoblastoma, can be associated with an increased rate of osteosarcoma, both in an irradiated area and in far-distant regions of the body (see Chaps. 3, 25, and 32).[67] Koufos et al. documented loss of heterozygosity in chromosome llp in RMS tissue of two patients compared to their normal tissue. This suggests that a mutant allele may cause RMS and two other embryonal tumors, Wilms' and hepatoblastoma.[68] In addition, the N-*ras* oncogene has been found in the RD human rhabdomyosarcoma cell line.[69] Interactions among genetic factors, environmental factors, the primary cancer itself, and treatments are still being defined (see Chap. 2).

Investigations of possible environmental causes of soft tissue sarcoma are of interest, although none is definitive. A relationship between exposure of adults to phenoxyacetic acids or chlorophenols has been postulated.[70,71] Even if confirmed, however, this finding will be less relevant to RMS or UDS in children, who are less likely to be so exposed. Preliminary information is available from a case-control study of 33 children with RMS in North Carolina, indicating a statistically significant association between RMS in children and cigarette smoking of fathers (but not mothers).[72] This suggests that carcinogens in cigarette smoke, which cause mutations in sperm cells, may be implicated. In addition, the RMS cases had more exposure to chemicals in the environment than did case-controls.[72] Further information is being collected to extend these observations.

There are several forms of soft tissue sarcoma that occur in animals after exposure to noxious agents such as chemicals and viruses. Methylcholanthrene, ethylnitrosourea, nickel sulfide, and other chemicals are capable of inducing soft tissue sarcomas in several species of animals.[73-78] Nickel sulfide injection has even produced testicular RMS, which is interesting because the testis does not normally contain striated muscle cells and because paratestis sarcoma occurs in male humans.[79]

Viruses can cause soft tissue sarcomas in mice and other rodents,[80] cats,[81] and woolly monkeys.[82] The existence of tumor viruses in animals, coupled with evidence implicating Epstein–Barr virus in Burkitt's lymphoma[83] and human T-lymphocyte viruses in some forms of leukemia,[84] suggests that viral causes of other forms of human cancer including RMS and UDS may be found.

Table 30-1

Chromosomal Abnormalities in Soft Tissue Sarcomas

Tumor Type	Patient Age	Chromosomal Abnormality	Reference
Embryonal RMS	7 yr	5q+, 9q+, 16p+, 17p+	41
Embryonal RMS	12 yr	Multiple nos. 2, 6, 8, 12, 13, 18, 20, 21; del(1)	42
Alveolar RMS	22 yr	t(2;13), three 2q+, del(13)	43
Alveolar RMS	32 yr	t(2;13) (q37;q14)	44
RMS	Child	t(1;3), 3p21 breakpoint	45
RMS	Child	t(1;?), 3p21 breakpoint	45
UDS	23 yr	t(X;18)	46
Spindle cell	59 yr	t(X;18)	46

Investigations of the cellular and molecular biology and growth kinetics of RMS and UDS are relatively limited, compared to those in leukemia and Burkitt's lymphoma (see also Chap. 4). Several long-term cell lines derived from human RMS were established 20 years ago.[85-87] In early immunologic studies, patients with RMS were found to have circulating peripheral blood lymphocytes that were cytotoxic to cultured tumor cells;[88] in one case, the lymphocytes of a healthy woman inhibited growth of cultured RMS cells taken from her identical twin sister.[89] Others have described inhibition of sarcoma-specific cellular immunity by sera from patients bearing progressive sarcomas.[90] Mice with methylcholanthrene-induced RMS produce serum factors that inhibit the mitogenic response of lymphoid cells, suggesting that tumor growth and immunosuppression are in some way related.[91,92] Cell kinetic studies have been conducted using both human- and rat-derived RMS cell lines.[93,94] RMS cell lines produce procollagen[95] and various kinds of cell surface glycoproteins involved in cell–cell interactions.[96] Cultured RMS cells also produce various growth-promoting and growth-inhibiting factors.[97-99] DNA extracted from human sarcoma cell lines can transform 3T3 cells and human fibroblasts.[100,101] In one study, evidence was presented suggesting that the transforming factor was an RNA type C virus.[102] Further investigations may shed more light on the ultimate causation of RMS in both animals and humans.

PATHOLOGY

General Concepts

The diagnosis of a soft tissue sarcoma in children can be reduced to two basic questions: [1] Is it rhabdomyosarcoma? [2] If so, what type is it, and how will it behave? These are actually quite separate issues. The first seeks to exclude all look-alike tumors, which account in aggregate for 17% of cases admitted to the IRS-I and IRS-II protocols. The second attempts to identify the two extremes of the vast spectrum of behavior inherent in this disease, where survival ranges from over 90% (in sarcoma botryoides) to less than 20% (in some series of alveolar RMS). Although the basic issues appear simple, consensus does not exist on either point.

Establishing the Diagnosis

Establishing a diagnosis of RMS, can be extremely difficult. Although RMS is the most common soft tissue sarcoma in children, it alone accounts for only about 50% of the total. The other possibilities (also discussed in Chaps. 6 and 31) include primitive tumors such as extraosseous Ewing's sarcoma and primitive neuroectodermal tumors (PNETs) of soft tissue, and usually highly characteristic entities such as synovial cell sarcoma, fibrosarcoma, alveolar soft part sarcoma, and hemangiopericytoma. Although the majority of these are straightforward diagnoses, sufficient uncertainty exists—especially in view of the propensity of RMS to be poorly differentiated—to warrant a thorough multimodality diagnostic evaluation in all but the most obvious cases.

The feature most often sought in the light microscopic diagnosis of rhabdomyosarcoma is also the least useful, that is, cross striations mimicking striated muscle, of which this tumor is thought to be a neoplastic analogue (Fig. 30-1A).[1-3,6,103] These cross striations are often inapparent on routine hematoxylin and eosin stained sections, but can be accentuated by special stains such as phosphotungstic acid (Fig. 30-1B). The past decade has witnessed the advent of immunocytochemical

diagnosis of many tumors, especially RMS; reliable antibodies directed against skeletal muscle and other myogenous proteins have been developed and widely used.[104,105] These include the muscle-specific proteins skeletal muscle myosin, myoglobin,[106,107] creatine kinase (MM isozyme),[108] skeletal muscle actin,[109] desmin,[110,111] and Z-band protein.[112] These antibodies can be extremely useful in establishing a diagnosis, since even a few cells in a field of hundreds can be diagnostic (Fig. 30-1C). Their relative value in diagnosis has been the source of some discussion, but most would agree that desmin is probably the single most useful antibody, although it must be substantiated by other markers because it is not specific for skeletal muscle, as opposed to all muscle. The IRS is currently evaluating these markers in the diagnosis of tumors from patients on the third IRS protocol; initial results substantiate the need for two or more markers, since no single marker is sufficiently reliable or free from false-positive results. It should also be noted that these same antibodies can be used in fluorescence-activated cell detection and sorting for diagnosis[113,114] and potentially for bone marrow purging.[115]

Finally, electron microscopy has been extremely useful in the diagnosis of RMS,[116] especially when the tumors are primitive, because distinction from other soft tissue sarcomas is mandatory.[117] The most characteristic feature (illustrated in Fig. 30-1D, E) is any indication of sarcomeric differentiation (e.g., actin-myosin bundles in register, or even convincing Z-band material). Even single filaments of 16 nm skeletal muscle myosin are diagnostic (Fig. 30-1F). Unfortunately, the actual situation is far more difficult; most cases of RMS are more easily differentiated by light microscopy augmented by immunocytochemistry. In some cases, addition of electron microscopy will clarify ambiguous results from these studies, both of which fail to detect all cases.[117,118] This caveat is especially true of primitive RMS and other soft tissue (and even bony) tumors, usually categorized as "small round cell tumors" (see Chap. 6). These tumors are a perennial source of diagnostic difficulty,[119-121] but the development of a host of new diagnostic techniques may resolve this problem. In some cases rebiopsy after chemotherapy may be diagnostic because of the tumor's propensity to undergo significant cytologic differentiation after treatment.[122]

Categorizing the Tumor

Once the diagnosis of RMS is established, the problem of precise categorization remains. This is a major problem, as noted earlier; failure to appreciate more or less aggressive forms of the disease necessarily results in over- or undertreatment on protocols that have high- versus low-risk arms, such as the current IRS and NCI protocols.

The history of RMS categorization is confusing. At first, only adult (pleomorphic) RMS was recognized.[1,2] Later, it was appreciated that the tumor was proportionally far more frequent in children than adults.[123] At present, the diagnosis of RMS has been virtually abandoned in adults[124]; they are now commonly diagnosed as pleomorphic malignant fibrous histiocytoma.[125] Juvenile rhabdomyosarcoma is a term that encompasses all forms of childhood RMS, including the two commonly recognized forms, embryonal and alveolar.[6]

The histologic appearance of most cases of RMS is characteristic enough to allow ready diagnosis by conventional schemes[103,126] as either embryonal (Fig. 30-2A) or alveolar (Fig. 30-2B). The more primitive cases (Fig. 30-2C) often require recourse to the techniques discussed above to establish the diagnosis of RMS. Botryoidal rhabdomyosarcoma, almost exclusively a tumor of young children, is histologically only a

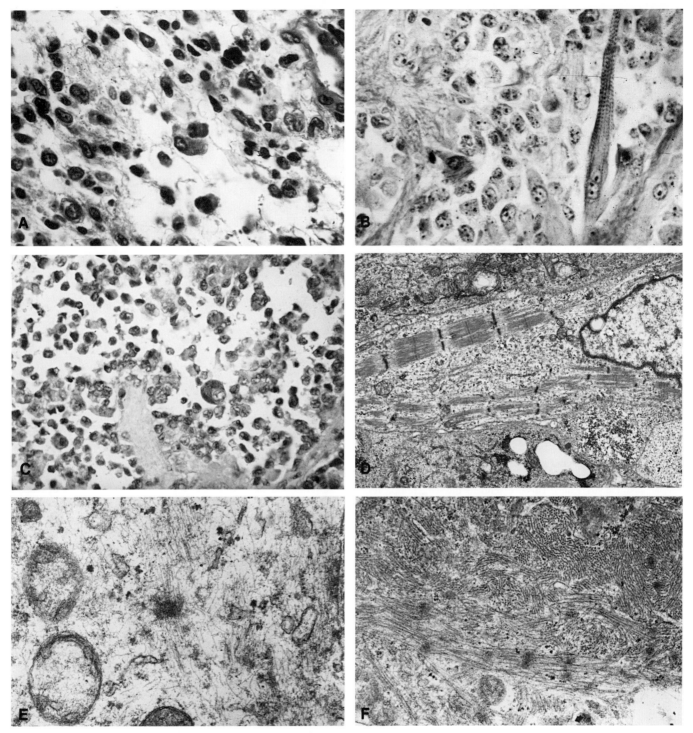

FIGURE 30-1. Diagnosis of rhabdomyosarcoma. **A.** Cross-striations, diagnostic of skeletal muscle differentiation, are visible even by hematoxylin and eosin (H & E) stained light microscopy in this field (*center*). This is a relatively uncommon event and will serve to detect only a few cases if this is the only criterion used for the diagnosis. **B.** Less apparent cross-striations are readily enhanced and made visible by special stains, especially phosphotungstic acid with hematoxylin counterstain (PTAH). The Z-band material found in benign and malignant striated muscle stains intensely by this method, as is readily apparent in the prominent strap cell (*right*). Even disoriented Z-band material will be detected by this method. Myofilaments, however, are not. **C.** By far the preferred method of unequivocal diagnosis, immunocytochemistry (ICC) with antibodies reactive with striated muscle specific proteins such as *skeletal muscle myosin, CK-MM, myoglobin,* or even myogenous proteins such as *desmin* are sufficient to detect even rather undifferentiated rhabdomyosarcomas, as here, where only one cell

stains intensely (*lower right center*). **D.** Historically, electron microscopy (EM) was the only alternative to special stains and H & E in the diagnosis of RMS. With the advent of immunocytochemistry, EM has assumed a complementary role. Questionable or negative results by ICC can be confirmed by EM, as here, where obvious sarcomeric differentiation, with Z bands and thick and thin filaments, is apparent. Tumors with this degree of differentiation, however, rarely require EM for diagnosis. **E.** This structure, invisible by light microscopy and usually undetectable by ICC, is clearly a fragmented version of the sarcomeres noted in D, above. It is therefore equally diagnostic and is, in fact, a more common finding in difficult cases than are the organized sarcomeres noted above. **F.** Because 14-nm myosin filaments are unique to striated muscle, the presence of these alone, as seen here, is diagnostic of striated muscle differentiation in a tumor. Because cardiac muscle (the only other striated muscle) tumors are virtually unreported, this equates with rhabdomyosarcoma.

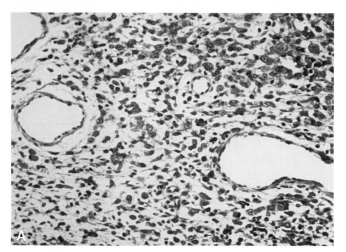

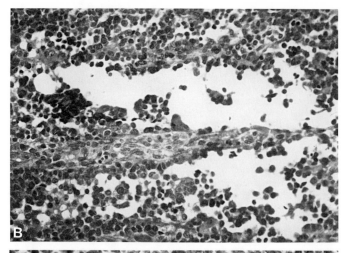

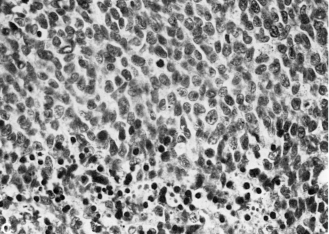

FIGURE 30-2. Classification of rhabdomyosarcoma. **A.** *Embryonal* rhabdomyosarcoma. The histologic appearance of this form of childhood rhabdomyosarcoma is highly characteristic, even in the closely related *botryoidal form.* These tumors have abundant myxoid stroma (in extreme amounts in botryoidal tumors) and a dominant spindle cell component among tumor cells. The tumor cells appear to "float" in this myxoid matrix. Even when sparse, the tumor cells are separated by it. This is a less densely cellular tumor than all forms of alveolar rhabdomyosarcoma. **B.** *Alveolar* rhabdomyosarcoma. The singular characteristic of this form of rhabdomyosarcoma is the presence of an obvious "alveolar" pattern, reminiscent of alveoli in lung, but lined by cytologically high-grade tumor cells. Tumor cells are *not* spindle shaped, as in embryonal, but are instead round and densely packed. A myxoid stroma is not characteristic of this tumor. **C.** *Solid variant* of alveolar rhabdomyosarcoma. This is essentially the same tumor illustrated in B, but here the alveolar pattern is absent. The cells are cytologically very similar or identical to those in B and distinctly different from those in C. This more primitive variant of conventional alveolar RMS is frequently misdiagnosed as another tumor, or embryonal RMS if found to be RMS. Both are incorrect diagnoses because the clinical behavior is at least as aggressive as that of alveolar RMS.

Table 30-2
Conventional Pathologic Subtypes and Sites of RMS and UDS

Pathologic Type	Predominant Primary Sites	Relative Frequency	Usual Age Range (yr)
Embryonal RMS	Head and neck, genitourinary tract	57%	3–12
Botryoid RMS	Bladder, vagina; nasopharynx	6%	0–3; 4–8
Alveolar RMS	Extremities, trunk	19%	6–21
UDS	Extremities, trunk	10%	6–21
Other	Extremities, trunk	8%	6–21

variation of embryonal rhabdomyosarcoma. Pleomorphic (adult type) rhabdomyosarcoma is vanishingly rare in children. In aggregate, however, these recognized entities account for no more than 80% of cases entered in the Intergroup Rhabdomyosarcoma Study (Ref. 126 and Newton and coworkers, unpublished observations); the other 20%, and even the placement of many of the first 80%, are the subject of considerable controversy, accentuated by the failure of the conventional histologic classification scheme outlined above to predict clinical behavior, despite previous publications to the contrary. The

conventional types of RMS and their relationship to patient age, primary site, and frequency of occurrence are shown in Table 30-2.

The lack of prognostic significance associated with conventional diagnoses of embryonal or alveolar RMS has prompted inquiry into the validity of the criteria used to make those distinctions. Bale and associates[127] require 70% of the tumor to possess an alveolar pattern for the diagnosis of alveolar RMS; the IRS-I and IRS-II criteria specified 50%. What if 1% were sufficient to impart the clinical behavior of a more aggressive tumor, which the alveolar form is presumed to be? Concern that this might be the case or, alternatively, that histology might be irrelevant, has prompted at least two independent studies of this question.

Palmer, in connection with the IRS, has proposed a cytologic (*i.e.,* cell nucleus) based classification scheme[128,129] that recognizes only anaplasia (Fig. 30-3A) and a particular cell type (monomorphous; Fig. 30-3B) as having poor prognostic features of childhood RMS. All other tumors, including alveolar RMS, are presumed to have a less clinically aggressive behavior, at least when treated on IRS-I or IRS-II protocols. This scheme was generated after an exhaustive multiparametric analysis of IRS-I cases. Unfortunately, it has not been so predictive in IRS-II cases. Widespread acceptance of the system also has been hampered by its failure to interface with conventional histologic criteria. A hybrid scheme, incorporating both cytologic and histologic features, is under study. Currently,

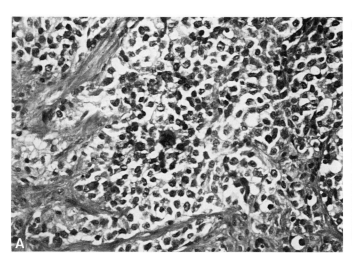

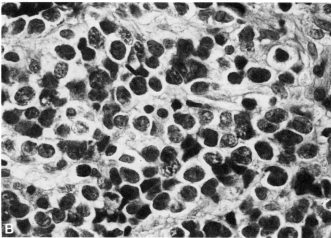

FIGURE 30-3. Palmer classification of rhabdomyosarcoma. **A.** *Anaplastic* RMS. The hallmark feature of this form of poor-prognosis RMS in the Palmer classification is the presence of cell mitoses similar to those seen in anaplastic Wilms' tumor. An example is seen in the center. The mitotic figure is at least three times the size of adjacent cell nuclei, is usually isolated in a field of bland appearing cells, and is easily identified even at low magnification. **B.** *Monomorphic* RMS. The other form of poor-prognosis RMS singled out in the Palmer classification method is composed of densely cellular fields of round tumor cells whose nuclei are rather basophilic and very similar in appearance to one another. Cytologically, this tumor would be termed *solid variant alveolar rhabdomyosarcoma* in the scheme used at the NCI.

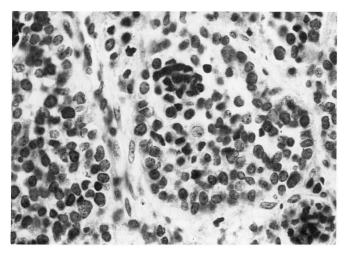

FIGURE 30-4. NCI "solid variant." The method used at the NCI recognizes all conventional forms of RMS, with the notable exception that tumors such as that illustrated here are grouped with alveolar rhabdomyosarcoma as so-called *solid variant ARMS.* As seen here, a nascent alveolar pattern, or at least a surrounding fibrous stroma, is evident. Other areas are composed of diffuse sheets of round tumor cells. Cytologically, these most resemble those seen in conventional alveolar rhabdomyosarcoma (and monomorphous, noted above) and are accordingly grouped therewith.

however, treatment decisions in the IRS are based on separating conventional alveolar RMS from the other types, including embryonal and botryoid RMS, undifferentiated sarcoma, and extraosseous Ewing's sarcoma.

A collaborative review of NCI and St. Jude Children's Research Hospital (SJCRH) cases, comparing three schemes (conventional, cytologic, and a variation of the conventional scheme), has been undertaken. Preliminary results with this case material were extremely promising,[130] but this approach

was less successful with a limited selection of IRS-II case material (Beltangady and colleagues, unpublished observations).

The essential point in both of the above schemes is the identification of a tumor type with extraordinary clinical aggressiveness, sufficient to distinguish it from all other types. In Palmer's scheme, anaplastic and monomorphous features are so identified. In the scheme used in the NCI/SJRCH series, a cytology similar to (and usually indistinguishable from) monomorphous (termed "solid variant of alveolar rhabdomyosarcoma"; Fig. 30-4) has been identified and associated with an aggressive clinical course, as has conventional alveolar RMS of any cytologic type. In this scheme, *any* evidence of an alveolar pattern, or even the cytology associated with alveolar RMS (*i.e.,* the solid variant thereof), is regarded as an ominous finding. This "0% standard" for alveolar histology in embryonal RMS is currently in use in IRS-III; the solid pattern is not recognized as alveolar at this point.

Thus, it is clear that there is no unanimously accepted classification scheme for RMS. Recognizing this, the principal proponents of all the above schemes, as well as their counterparts in another system used in Europe by the International Society of Pediatric Oncology (SIOP) pathologists, have agreed to a blinded review of 800 cases from the IRS-II archival pathology material, in an effort to determine which, if any, cytologic or histologic features are of prognostic utility. No results are yet available, but regardless of the outcome, for the first time, all major systems currently in use will be compared, analyzed, and evaluated in relationship to patient outcome on a standardized protocol. The goal of all participants is to develop a single, universal system for prognostic classification of childhood rhabdomyosarcoma.

PATHOGENESIS, CLINICAL PRESENTATION, AND PATTERNS OF SPREAD

Rhabdomyosarcoma and undifferentiated sarcoma produce clinically evident signs and symptoms in two main ways: the appearance of a mass lesion in a body region without history of temporally associated trauma and the disturbance of a normal body function by an otherwise unsuspected, critically located enlarging tumor. Typical signs, symptoms, and patterns of spread are discussed below by site of primary tumor involvement and are summarized in Table 30-3.

Head and Neck Region. RMS and UDS fall in three major subgroups.[131-133] Approximately one fourth of head and neck sarcomas arise in the orbit; one half arise in other parameningeal sites; and the remaining one fourth arise in nonorbital, nonparameningeal locations such as the scalp, face, buccal mucosa, oropharynx, larynx, and neck. The sex ratio is nearly equal and the median age at diagnosis is around 6 years.[132] The orbit–eyelid tumors produce proptosis and occasionally ophthalmoplegia.[134-136] Tumors in this site are nearly always diagnosed early, before distant dissemination has taken place; regional lymph node spread is also very unusual, probably because the orbit is only scantily supplied with lymphatic channels. Nonorbital parameningeal sarcomas arise most commonly in the nasopharynx and paranasal sinuses, the middle ear–mastoid region, and the pterygoid–infratemporal fossae. These tumors usually produce nasal, aural, or sinus obstruction, with or without a mucopurulent and sometimes sanguinous discharge. Cranial nerve palsy, sometimes multiple, may be present and indicates a high probability of direct extension toward the meninges.[137-143] Headache, vomiting, and systemic hypertension may result from intracranial growth of tumor following erosion of contiguous bone at the cranial base.[142,143] Autopsy studies of such patients show diffuse involvement of the cranial and spinal meninges[126] in a fashion reminiscent of CNS leukemia. These tumors can also spread distantly, primarily to lungs or bones.[144] Craniocervical sarcomas arising in areas other than the orbit and parameningeal sites usually present as a painless, progressively enlarging growth, and tend to remain localized.[145]

Genitourinary Tract. Sarcomas of this region are most frequently seen in the bladder and prostate. Bladder tumors tend to grow intraluminally, usually in or near the trigone, and present a polypoid appearance on gross examination. Hematuria, urinary obstruction, and occasionally the extrusion of mucosanguinous tissue can all occur, particularly when the tumor is botryoid. Usually, the affected children are under the age of 4 years. Prostate tumors usually produce large pelvic masses with or without urethral strangury; constipation may be present. These tumors can occur in infants or older children; even adults may be affected.[146] Bladder tumors tend to remain localized, whereas prostate tumors often disseminate early to lungs and sometimes to the bone marrow or bones.[146-152] Both the male and female genital tract can harbor sarcoma. Vaginal tumors are commonly botryoid in appearance and are almost exclusively found in very young children who may have a mucosanguinous discharge, reminiscent of that seen with a foreign body.[153] Cervical and uterine sarcomas are diagnosed more commonly in older girls than in infants, and present with a mass with or without vaginal discharge.[153-155] Paratesticular tumors usually produce painless unilateral scrotal or inguinal enlargement in either prepubertal or postpubertal males; regional retroperitoneal lymph nodes are often involved,[156] whereas regional lymphatics are less often found to harbor metastases in patients with bladder, prostate, and vaginal sarcoma.[157,158] Alveolar histology is distinctly unusual in sarcomas of both the head and neck and genitourinary tract.[126]

Sarcomas of the Extremity. These tumors are categorized by swelling in the affected body part. Nearly half have alveolar histology.[159-161] Sometimes the regional lymph nodes are enlarged by tumor deposits;[157] nodal spread may be more likely when the primary tumor is an alveolar RMS than an embryonal RMS or UDS.[162] The tumors may be quite extensive, owing to their propensity to spread along fascial planes. The fact that injuries are frequent in the extremities of school-aged children may lead to delay in diagnosis because of the tendency to expect bruises in that age group.

Tumors of the Trunk. These tumors are similar in evolution to those of extremities, both in exhibiting all histologic types (embryonal and alveolar RMS and UDS) and in their tendency for local recurrence despite wide local excision, and for distant spread. They are of relatively large diameter compared to head and neck and bladder tumors.[163] Contiguous involvement of the thoracolumbar spine may be present, depending on location of the primary lesion, but regional lymph node spread is unusual.

Intrathoracic[164] and Retroperitoneal-Pelvic Tumors[165-167]. These tumors can become quite large before the diagnosis is made, owing to their location deep within the body. As a result, they are often incompletely accessible to the surgeon, since vital

Table 30-3
Primary Site and Patterns of Spread of RMS and UDS

Primary Site	Relative Frequency (%)	Regional Sites	Distant Metastatic Sites
Head and Neck	40		
Orbit	10	Nodes infrequent	Lung—infrequent
Parameningeal	20	CNS $\approx$ 50%	Lung, bone
Other	10	Nodes infrequent	Lung
Genitourinary Tract	20		
Bladder-prostate	12	Nodes infrequent	Lung, marrow (mainly from prostate lesions)
Vagina-uterus	2	Nodes infrequent	Retroperitoneal nodes (mainly from uterus)
Paratesticular	6	Retroperitoneal lymph nodes $\approx$ 30%	Lung, bone
Extremities	20	Nodes $\approx$ 20%	Lung, marrow, bone, CNS
Trunk	10	Nodes infrequent	Lung, bone
Other	10	Nodes infrequent	Lung, bone, liver

vessels are usually surrounded. Wide infiltration is the rule, with an attendant high likelihood of local recurrence despite combined modality treatment.

Perineal-Perianal Tumors. Lesions in this region are unusual. They can mimic abscesses or polyps,[168] according to location, and are often of alveolar histologic type. A relatively high incidence of regional lymph node involvement was noted in the first series of these patients from the IRS.[169]

Biliary Tract Tumors. These tumors are even rarer than perineal-perianal tumors. They often produce obstructive jaundice and spread within the liver, and thence to the retroperitoneum or lungs.[170-172]

Other. Occasionally, the liver[173,174] or brain[175] may harbor a primary sarcoma.

METHODS OF DIAGNOSIS

The differential diagnosis of RMS and UDS includes other oncologic entities and an assortment of nononcologic conditions (see Chap. 5). Trauma may produce an enlarging soft tissue mass, especially over the extremities, face, or trunk. Generally, a history of an accident is available and an associated hematoma is tender and discolored. By contrast, sarcomas are nearly always nontender and impart no particular unusual hue to the overlying skin or subcutaneous tissue. Growth of a nontender mass, especially in the absence of a clear-cut history of trauma, should always lead to consideration of biopsy, especially when expansion is confirmed by repeated observations over 1 to 2 weeks. A mass within a body cavity can produce obstruction or discharge; both indicate the need for biopsy. Occasionally, a histologically benign lesion such as lipoma, rhabdomyoma, or neurofibroma may be diagnosed; if so, complete surgical removal should be performed, provided that mutilation can be avoided. Rarely, a very unusual condition such as myositis ossificans[176] or pyogenic myositis[177] may be discovered. Biopsy should also be considered when a young person has a mass and is failing to thrive, even if the affected region is tender and the patient is febrile (provided that appropriate studies for infection have been nonproductive) because a treatable neoplasm may be the underlying disorder.[177]

Other malignant neoplasms in childhood can mimic RMS or UDS. Non-Hodgkin's lymphoma, neuroblastoma, and Ewing's sarcoma can all simulate sarcoma at the light microscopic level, and special stains, electron microscopic ultrastructure, monoclonal antibodies, and collection of urine for catecholamine excretion studies may be necessary to distinguish among these entities (see Chap. 6). Occasionally, a leukemic chloroma[179] or collection of histiocytes (as in Langerhans' cell histiocytosis)[180] can produce unilateral proptosis or a mass in another body region, which should be biopsied to establish the correct diagnosis.

Once the diagnosis of RMS or UDS has been entertained, and even in the absence of confirmatory pathologic material, several clinical and radiographic studies may be in order to define the limits of the lesion and to look for evidence of spread. A careful, complete physical examination should be performed, with particular attention to regional lymphatic structures and to the surrounding tissues. Once RMS or UDS has been diagnosed by review of pathologic material, several laboratory studies should be obtained.[178] These include a complete blood count with liver and renal function tests, plus electrolytes, serum calcium and phosphorus, and a uric acid level, in anticipation of chemotherapy. Patients with bone

marrow metastases from a primary sarcoma may have altered peripheral blood values. Occasionally, a picture consistent with disseminated intravascular coagulation is present, and if so, other coagulation values should be determined.[181] Bone marrow aspiration and needle biopsy should be performed, even in the absence of altered blood counts or obvious metastases. When bone involvement is present, hypercalcemia may also be detected.[182]

Radiographic studies should include plain films of the affected part and a skeletal survey (see also Chap. 7). Nuclear medicine scans using ^{99m}Tc diphosphonate may be useful in assessing whether bones harbor metastatic tumor deposits; however one series suggests that bone survey may be the more sensitive procedure.[183] Gallium-67 has been used by some centers, but it can be concentrated in the bowel and in areas of inflammation, and therefore is not specific for sarcomatous tissue.[184]

Recently, considerable interest has been focused on the role of computed tomography (CT) in delineating the extent of soft tissue tumors. In areas such as the head and neck[185] and the pelvis,[186] CT scans without and with contrast enhancement are necessary for the radiation therapist to assess the volume at risk for subclinical tumor invasion and to plan treatment fields. Ultrasound examinations may be especially useful as an adjunct to CT in serial assessment of tumors of the pelvis (including the bladder and prostate and retroperitoneum) because the characteristic "water-density" of the urine-filled bladder helps in localization.[167] Ultrasonography has the advantage that no radiation is used, and dye injection is unnecessary. The types of investigations appropriate to the primary site are summarized in Table 30-4.

The newest technique, magnetic resonance imaging (MRI), has considerable promise as an adjunct to the more standard imaging studies.[187] As with ultrasonography, radiation is not used, nor are contrast dye injections needed. Another advantage of MRI lies in the ability of the imaging technologist to attenuate the bone artifact that can be so troublesome in lesions about the skull and spine.[188] The role of MRI in delineating the extent of pediatric sarcomas is unknown because of its newness, but we have been impressed with its utility in a few children with sarcomas of the head and neck (see also Chap. 7).

STAGING

Assessing the extent of the tumor in every patient is necessary, because therapy and prognosis depend upon the degree to which the mass has spread beyond the primary site (see Chap. 10). Patients with localized, surgically removable tumors have a better prognosis than do those whose disease has produced clinically detectable metastatic deposits. Because RMS and UDS can occur at any site in the body, and because complete surgical removal is not always possible, patients can be categorized in several ways. Several staging systems have been devised for clinical studies of pediatric sarcoma.[189-191] Many of these systems are surgical-pathologic in nature[189,191] because of the importance of operative removal (where feasible) as part of the treatment program. Although this approach is practical, it has the drawback that the surgical options are variable and not necessarily uniformly applied, thus hampering comparisons among groups of patients from different institutions. In addition, some systems categorize disseminated disease as Stage III and others as Stage IV, again leading to confusion.

Another approach is to categorize tumors without regard to the degree of surgical removal. The TNM (tumor, nodes, metastasis) system, which is based on pretreatment assessment

Table 30-4
Specific Diagnostic and Surgical Maneuvers for Various Primary Sites

Primary Site	Diagnostic Investigations*	Surgical Intervention
Head and neck	CT scan, to include cranial contents and any contiguous sinus or paraspinal region; LP for protein, cell count, and cytology; possibly MRI	Usually incisional biopsy for diagnosis; grossly complete removal of tumor often not feasible
Genitourinary	CT scan ± ultrasound of retroperitoneum	Incisional or cytoscopic biopsy for diagnosis; radical inguinal orchiectomy, retroperitoneal lymph node dissection or biopsy (paratestis only)
Extremity		
Upper	CT scan of primary	Biopsy of regional lymph nodes (axillary—upper,
Lower	CT scan of primary and retroperitoneum	inguinofemoral—lower); wide local excision if possible
Trunk	Consider myelogram if primary is paraspinal	Complete excision if possible
Gastrointestinal	Liver scan	Complete excision if possible

* *All* patients should have CT scans of chest and primary lesion, bone marrow aspirate ± biopsy, and bone survey ± scan, plus biopsy of any clinically suspicious regional lymph nodes.

Table 30-5
Intergroup Rhabdomyosarcoma Study Clinical Grouping System

Clinical Group	Definition
I	A. Localized, completely resected, confined to site of origin
	B. Localized, completely resected, infiltrated beyond site of origin
II	A. Localized, grossly resected, microscopic residual
	B. Regional disease, involved lymph nodes, completely resected
	C. Regional disease, involved lymph nodes, grossly resected with microscopic residual
III	A. Local or regional grossly visible disease after biopsy only
	B. Grossly visible disease after ≥50% resection of primary tumor
IV	Distant metastases present at diagnosis

of tumor extent, is used widely for adult tumor staging, and has also been applied to pediatric sarcomas in France[56] and the United States.[190,192] The IRS Committee developed a surgical-pathologic staging system[191] that has been used extensively since 1972. Currently, the IRS is attempting to compare this system, shown in Table 30-5, to a modified TNM system, shown in Table 30-6.[193] In the latter system, the size (widest diameter) and site of the primary tumor are noted, along with whether the tumor has invaded adjacent structures macroscopically. The size and consistency of regional lymph nodes are noted, and a clinical judgment is made as to whether the nodes have gross tumor involvement. Results of radiographic studies and bone marrow examination are used to ascertain whether distant metastases are present. Finally, the histologic subtype of the tumor is obtained on review of the pathologic specimen. In this way, tumors can be categorized without the variable of surgery. As the current IRS trials (IRS-III) continue, data will become available by which to judge the utility and validity of this modified TNM staging system for RMS and UDS.[194] The surgical-pathologic staging (clinical group) system has been retained because of its prognostic usefulness.[195]

The likelihood of infiltration of regional lymph nodes or adjacent structures varies with the site of the primary tumor.[157] Because regional nodal involvement is most likely with lesions arising in paratesticular structures or in an extremity, surgical staging should include sampling of the regional node-bearing areas. Radiation therapy is delivered to the region if tumor involvement of nodes is found on pathologic examination. Any enlarged regional lymph node at any site should also be removed and submitted for pathologic examination to ascertain whether radiation therapy may be advised as part of the patient's subsequent management.

PROGNOSTIC CONSIDERATIONS AND VARIABLES

The identification of prognostic variables is of major importance in understanding the behavior of sarcomas and developing careful clinical trials, the goals of which are to improve survival for all patients with RMS and UDS and to reduce morbidity.[195,196] Several prognostically significant variables have been identified. Thus far, the most important appears to be the clinical group, or extent of disease, at the time chemotherapy is initiated. Patients with no detectable metastases at diagnosis fare far better than those with widespread disease (Group IV).[58,195,197,198] Among patients with localized sarcoma, those whose tumors are completely excised surgically (Group I) have a better survival rate than those with microscopic residual tumor or with excised but regionally extensive lesions (Group II). Patients with gross residual sarcoma (Group III) fare less well, but have a superior survival rate compared to those with metastases at diagnosis.[58,195,197,198]

The histopathologic type of the tumor is also an important variable. It is clear that patients with alveolar RMS have a poorer survival than those with embryonal RMS or UDS.[199,200] There is ongoing discussion about the relative importance of primary site versus histology, especially in the case of alveolar lesions, because the IRS-I analysis[195,201,202] showed that patients with extremity tumors fared less well than did those with lesions arising elsewhere. The primary site is an important prognostic variable for several reasons. First, the location of a tumor determines the signs and symptoms that lead to diagnosis. Deeply situated tumors (*e.g.,* in the retroperitoneum or chest cavity) are often large, and have presumably been in place and possibly spreading over a longer period of time than have su-

Table 30-6
Intergroup Rhabdomyosarcoma Study TGNM System

Summary of pretreatment clinical staging based on clinical, radiographic and laboratory
      examination (plus histologic biopsy):
A. Localized tumor with favorable histology and clinically negative nodes
B. Locally extensive tumor with favorable histology and clinically negative lymph nodes
C. Any size tumor with clinically involved regional lymph nodes and/or unfavorable histology
D. Distant metastasis
Tumor: T_{site} 1—confined to anatomic site of origin; subscript indicates site*
        (a) <5 cm in size
        (b) ≥5 cm in size
      T_{site} 2—extension or fixation to surrounding tissues
        (a) <5 cm in size
        (b) ≥5 cm in size
Histology: G1—favorable histology (mixed, undifferentiated, embryonal, botryoid, other)
           G2—unfavorable histology (alveolar)
           GX—insufficient tumor for histologic classification
Regional lymph nodes: N-0—regional nodes not clinically involved
                     N-1—regional nodes *clinically* involved by neoplasm
                     N-X—clinical status of regional nodes unknown (especially sites that
                             preclude regional lymph node evaluation)
Metastases: M-0—no distant metastasis
              $M-1_{site}$—metastases present; subscript indicates site(s)†

* Subscripts for T_{site} hn = head and neck; or = orbit; ex = extremities; ex-lg = limb girdle; gu = pelvic GU; te
  = paratesticular; ot = other (includes trunk, retroperitoneal, and perineal).
† Subscripts for M_{site} dn = distant nodes; lu = lung or positive pleural effusion; li = liver; b = bone; m = marrow; n
  = CNS or positive CSF; s = soft tissue other than nodes; p = peritoneum or positive ascitic fluid.

perficial, readily visible tumors. Second, the likelihood of lymphatic spread (and hence hematogenous dissemination) varies with primary site.[157] Third, the location has implications for therapy: if a lesion cannot be removed *per primum,* the patient is placed in Clinical Group III, a prognostically unfavorable category compared to those whose sarcoma can be completely excised. There are also radiotherapeutic considerations based on the primary site with regard to the tolerance of adjacent normal structures to effective antisarcoma doses and volumes. Ongoing multivariate analyses are expected to provide answers as to the relative weight of these multiple prognostic variables. The most meaningful variable is the response to treatment.

TREATMENT

There are three currently recognized modalities of treating children with sarcomas: surgical removal (if feasible), radiation therapy (RT) for control of residual tumor, and systemic chemotherapy. Much of the information regarding current use of these modalities derives from therapeutic programs developed by the IRS.

Principles of Surgery

Primary operative management is the most rapid way to ablate the disease and should always be used when subsequent function or cosmesis will not be greatly impaired (see also Chap. 10). Operative management is related to location and extent of the tumor and is also influenced by the desire to preserve vital or functionally useful structures such as the eye or the urinary bladder. In those and nearby sites, and in most head and neck sites, incisional biopsy (for diagnosis) may be the only feasible surgical procedure, because of proximity to vital blood vessels

and nerves, cosmetic considerations, or both.[132] Tumors of the paratesticular region should be removed by radical inguinal orchiectomy to avoid scrotal contamination, which is likely if a transscrotal biopsy is performed. There is debate about the utility of subsequent retroperitoneal lymph node dissection, which is done to determine whether regional retroperitoneal lymph nodes harbor tumor deposits. The IRS Committee believes that retroperitoneal nodal RT should be given to patients with tumor-involved nodes, whereas RT can be deleted from the management program when nodal spread is not demonstrated.[156] Others believe that chemotherapy alone is adequate for patients with paratesticular sarcoma and no distant metastases.[203] The small number of patients with known nodal tumor makes execution of a controlled study difficult. The inguinal lymph nodes are not often involved, so dissection of that area is unnecessary unless scrotal contamination has occurred.

In lesions of an extremity, grossly complete surgical removal should be accomplished, provided that limb function is not greatly impaired, because the prognosis is considerably worse if grossly visible tumor is left behind.[161,195] As mentioned above, sampling of the regional lymph nodes is advisable. Amputation is usually not necessary, although it may be considered for patients with extensive lesions involving the bone or major neurovascular structures.

Surgical removal should also be attempted for lesions of the trunk. Tumors arising in the pelvis, retroperitoneum, or intrathoracic area often cannot be removed completely, either because of infiltration or encirclement of major blood vessels, nerves, or bones, or because of unwillingness to perform exenteration for pelvic-retroperitoneal tumors.[165–167]

When microscopic residual disease is found following an initial excision, or when the initial operation was carried out without knowledge of the type of neoplasm involved, reexcision of the area is indicated prior to nonsurgical management. In localized lesions of the trunk and extremities, improvement in survival duration can be produced by surgical removal of all residual tumor.

Occasionally, knowingly incomplete surgical removal (debulking surgery) is considered, in order to reduce the volume of residual tumor beyond that which would remain after incisional biopsy alone. Carefully reviewed data in support of this theoretically reasonable maneuver for children with RMS or UDS are not available. However, the IRS-III program is collecting such information and will ascertain whether there is a difference in the prognosis of Group III patients whose tumors have been <50% versus >50% excised. Data regarding secondary operations are also being collected in Group III patients enrolled in IRS-III, wherein a delayed resection of the residual primary tumor is recommended whenever possible after the first 20 weeks of treatment. Removal of metastatic deposits (e.g., pulmonary nodules) is another capability of surgical management that should be considered in selected cases, particularly when potentially active chemotherapeutic agents are still available.

When local or regional relapse occurs, retrieval therapy should include initial radical surgery where feasible, followed by radiotherapy when possible, and more intensive chemotherapy. For patients with lesions in certain sites, particularly vaginal and paratesticular locations, long-term survival can still be achieved.

Complications of operative management are related to the tumor site.[204] Any procedure involving the skin and subcutaneous tissue will produce a scar and loss of tissue in the region from which bulk tumor is removed, as in an extremity or on the trunk. Zealous, complete removal of large intramuscular masses in these areas can lead to unacceptable mutilation, loss of function, or both. The surgeon's experience is critical in executing the proper operation. Radical regional lymph node dissections are discouraged because of subsequent scarring and lymphedema. Skill is especially important in the surgical exploration of lesions arising in the head and neck, where major blood vessels and important nerves are so closely apposed. In the genitourinary region, total cystectomy for bladder or prostate tumors is currently deferred until it is clear that viable malignant cells have persisted despite chemotherapy and radiotherapy. In patients with paratesticular sarcoma,[156] bilateral retroperitoneal lymph dissection can produce retrograde ejaculation and is therefore discouraged.

Principles of Radiation Therapy

Radiation therapy is a major tool in the treatment of children with rhabdomyosarcoma and undifferentiated sarcoma (see also Chap. 11). RT is of particular utility in eradicating residual tumor cells from sites where surgical therapy alone cannot ablate the mass, especially in the head, neck, and pelvis. Soft tissue sarcomas infiltrate so widely that after simple excision or enucleation without wide excision, RT, or chemotherapy, local recurrence rates approximate 75%.[205]

Soft tissue sarcomas were generally considered insensitive to RT before 1960. Perry and Chu[206] and, later, McNeer and colleagues[207] were able to show that soft tissue sarcomas were sometimes sensitive to doses exceeding 3000 cGy. Suit and coworkers found that a tumor dose of 6300 to 7000 cGy produced local control (i.e., no detectable local tumor) in 50 of 57 patients, mainly adults, with various types of sarcomas.[205] Dritschilo and colleagues reported a local control rate of 96% in 27 children under age 16 years with RMS or UDS who received 5500 to 6500 cGy, delivered by a 4 MV or 8 MV accelerator.[208] Chemotherapy with VAC (vincristine, actinomycin D and cyclophosphamide) was also given over a 2-year

period. The precise contribution of surgical management was not clear, since some patients had radical operations, some had grossly complete removal of the primary tumor, and others underwent incisional biopsy only. Similarly high rates of local control with RT have been noted in other patients with RMS and UDS, with or without combination chemotherapy.[59,134,209–211]

As local control rates improved and the value of chemotherapy became established,[212] the need for RT following wide local excision of localized lesions with tumor-negative margins was questioned. The answer was obtained in Group I patients treated in IRS-I.[201] Of 47 patients treated with VAC but no RT, 6 developed recurrent sarcoma, 3 with local regrowth. Of 26 treated with VAC and 5000 cGy by random assignment, 4 developed recurrent sarcoma, 2 with local regrowth ($p = 0.38$). Thus, RT did not confer an advantage in disease-free survival or overall survival in these patients and was eliminated from the treatment program for patients in IRS-II.[213] Subsequent analyses of local control were reported by Tefft et al.[214] The IRS-I protocol called for a dose of 5000 to 6000 cGy to the tumor site in 6 weeks, delivered by supervoltage technique to all patients with any residual disease (children under age 5 received 4000 cGy in 4 weeks). Some patients in both age groups received less than 4000 cGy. Also, some children were treated to a smaller volume than the recommended entire muscle bundle from origin to insertion. The lower doses and volumes were selected on an individual basis and may have reflected concern about late deleterious effects on normal tissue in the treatment field, a well-established complication of high-dose RT when combined with multiagent chemotherapy.[215] The local control rates in IRS-I were as follows: 92% of patients in Clinical Groups I and II at doses of 3500 to 4000 cGy, and 95% at doses above 4000 cGy ($p = $ N.S.); 91% of children under age 6 years; and 68% in older children receiving doses less than 4000 cGy. In patients with adequately or inadequately treated volumes, respectively, local control rates were 92% and 84% in the <6-year group and 85% and 91% in the older children (all p values = N.S.). The authors concluded that a subsequent trial should consider changing the RT guidelines to include the following: [1] the minimum tumor dose for children with RMS and UDS should be 4000 cGy; [2] older children should receive a minimum dose of 4500 cGy; [3] tumors 5 cm wide or larger should be treated with 5000 to 5500 cGy; and [4] volumes could be reduced to a 5 cm margin beyond the evident gross tumor in all directions.[215]

These changes were implemented in the IRS-II protocol, initiated in 1978. A review of 362 patients entered in IRS-II showed that the locoregional recurrence rate was under 10% for all patients so treated, and doses in the range of 5000 to 5500 cGy were not more advantageous than 4000 to 4500 cGy doses. However, at doses less than 4000 cGy, the locoregional recurrence rate increased to 13% ($p = 0.02$). The nonirradiated Group I patients with unfavorable histology (primarily alveolar RMS) had a significantly higher rate of locoregional recurrence than did those with relatively favorable histology.[216] Thus far, the dosage and volume reductions have not led to impaired local control, except in the Group I patients with unfavorable histology. RT is currently given to these children as if they had microscopic residual tumor, but as in IRS-I and IRS-II, routine regional lymph node RT is not used.

Two subsets of children with RMS and UDS were analyzed subsequently. Local control was diminished to 72% in 40 infants (<1 year); 5 of the 10 receiving doses less than 4000 cGy failed to achieve local control, whereas 23 of the 30 remaining infants (80%) achieved local control after receiving 4000 cGy or more.[217] However, local control was achieved in 41 of 43 children with orbital sarcoma, including 6 patients whose dose

Table 30-7
Recommended Radiation Therapy Dosages for Primary RMS and UDS

Clinical Group (IRS), Histology, Site	Age (yr); Tumor Size (cm)	Radiation Dose (cGy)	Treatment Duration	Total Dose	Normal Tissue Margin
I, nonalveolar, any site	Any	None	—	—	—
II, any type; I, alveolar, any site	Any	180/day, 5 days/week	4–5 weeks	4140 cGy	5 cm
III + IV, any type, any site except special pelvic sites	<6 yr; <5 cm	180/day, 5 days/week	4–5 weeks	4140 cGy	5 cm
	<6 yr; ≥5 cm	180/day, 5 days/week	5 weeks	4500 cGy	5 cm
	≥6 yr; <5 cm	180/day, 5 days/week	5 weeks	4500 cGy	5 cm
	≥6 yr; ≥5 cm	180/day, 5 days/week	5–6 weeks	5040 cGy	5 cm
III, special pelvic sites—bladder, prostate; vagina, uterus*	As for III + IV (above)	180/day, 5 days/week	5–6 weeks	5040 cGy	2 cm

* Some patients may undergo limited resection with bladder preservation and avoid RT.

Table 30-8
Peak Radiation Therapy Dosages to Critical Areas (Normal Tissue Tolerance)

Organ	Dose (cGy)*	Timing (wk)
Kidney	1500	2–4
Liver		
Whole liver volume	2400	4
Two thirds liver volume	4000	5
Lungs		
Both lungs (entire)	1800	2
25% volume, both lungs	4500	5
Brain		
Whole brain	4500	5
One cerebral hemisphere	6000	7
Spinal cord		
Entire cord	4500	5
10 cm cord	5000	6
Gastrointestinal tract		
(*i.e.*, whole pelvis)	4500	5
Whole abdomen	1800	2–3

* Normal tissue tolerance.

was 3160 to 3960 cGy. Thus one must weigh the risk of local failure against the risk of untoward side-effects, especially in infants, because the majority of patients with local recurrence die of progressive sarcoma.[218]

RT is not now given to children with Group I (completely excised) nonalveolar RMS or UDS but is used for those with alveolar RMS, with the dosage adjusted according to age and size of the tumor, as above. Table 30-7 shows the current IRS recommendations. Patients in Group II receive doses adjusted according to age and tumor size, beginning at week 2 (nonalveolar RMS and UDS) or week 6 (alveolar RMS). Patients in Groups III and IV receive similarly adjusted doses beginning at week 6, except those patients with cranial parameningeal sarcoma with signs suggesting meningeal involvement, in whom RT is begun on the first day of chemotherapy. A 5-cm margin around the site of the primary tumor is recommended except for sarcomas arising in the bladder, prostate, vagina, or uterus (2 cm margin). Some children with pelvic tumors may have grossly and microscopically complete excision of tumor without cystectomy, in which case RT may not be necessary. Normal tissues are shielded at appropriate dosage levels, and areas of metastatic involvement are treated also. Specifics are given in great detail in the IRS-III protocol, which is available at institutions throughout North America and Europe that are members of the Children's Cancer Study Group, the Pediatric Oncology Group, or the United Kingdom Children's Cancer Study Group.

At times, an approach other than traditional external-beam megavoltage RT should be considered. One technique employs radiation implants, especially for children with small, critically located tumors of the head and neck, bladder or prostate, vagina, or extremity (see Chap. 11).[219–222] Because the dose is delivered to a carefully restricted volume, adjacent normal structures receive less scattered radiation and may be expected to have less fibrosis. Another, newer approach for large, deeply seated tumors is treatment of the tumor by the radiation therapist under direct vision while it is exposed in the operating room. More data are needed in pediatric patients to assess the utility of this method.[223]

In all cases, meticulous attention must be paid to normal tissue tolerance to minimize the risk of acute or late life-threatening damage to normal structures. Table 30-8 outlines the upper limits of normal tissue tolerance. Young age of the patient also calls for dosage reduction (*e.g.*, a limit of 1200 cGy to both lungs or of 2400 cGy to the brain). Also, large-field volumes such as the whole abdomen should receive lower daily doses (150 cGy) and total doses (1800 cGy). Details are given in the IRS-III protocol.

Sequelae of treatment are numerous. Radiation therapy can produce an acute reaction characterized by erythema and swelling of the irradiated volume, which can lead to desquamation if extreme. The later effects of radiation are loss of function or growth, chiefly due to fibrosis, which increases with increasing dose and volume and diminishes with increasing age of the patient.[215,224–227] Because certain chemotherapeutic agents contribute to the effect of RT, caution must be used in carrying out current recommendations for intensive therapy.

Principles of Chemotherapy

Chemotherapeutic agents with activity against RMS and UDS were first identified through single-drug trials, usually in children with recurrence or metastases. Several workers demonstrated objective tumor regression after the administration of actinomycin D,[228–230] cyclophosphamide,[231,232] vincristine,[233–235] and, later, doxorubicin (Adriamycin)[236–239] (Table 30-9). As agents became available, they were tested in combi-

Table 30-9

Responses in Single-Agent Trials in Children with RMS and UDS*

Reference	Drug	Number of Patients			Percentage of CR + PR
		Evaluable	CR	PR	
Pinkel[228]	Actinomycin D	4	0	2	50
Tan[229]	Actinomycin D	5	0	1	20
Shaw[230]	Actinomycin D	5	0	3	60
Haddy[231]	Cyclophosphamide	12	2	4	50
Sutow[232]	Cyclophosphamide	14	0	7	50
Sutow[233]	Vincristine	11	2	2	36
Sutow[234]	Vincristine	20	0	6	30
Selawry[235]	Vincristine	11	1	2	27
Bonadonna[236]	Doxorubicin	2	1	1	100
O'Bryan[237]	Doxorubicin	11	0	3	27
Sutow[239]	Doxorubicin	15	0	3	20
Tan[238]	Doxorubicin	12	0	4	33
Baum[255]	Cisplatin	19	1	3	21
Chard[256]	VP-16	5	0	1	20
Luce[257]	DTIC	2	0	1	50
Finkelstein[258]	DTIC	7	0	1	14
Bode[261]	Methotrexate	4	2	1	75
Horowitz[263]	Melphalan	4	0	3	75

* CR = complete response (100% tumor disappearance); PR = partial response (50%–99% disappearance).

nation, generally in patients with advanced inoperable sarcoma[240–242] (Table 30-10). It was then reasonable to consider using multiple agents after initial diagnosis for all patients with RMS or UDS, based on the generally poor outlook for survival at the time. Wilbur and colleagues pioneered in administering repetitive doses of vincristine, actinomycin D, and cyclophosphamide (VAC) to children with advanced RMS. Of 24 children with inoperable localized tumors (16 patients) or metastatic deposits at diagnosis (8 patients), 16 (67%) were alive and well at a median follow-up approaching 2 years.[243] Clinical trials in single institutions using varying combinations of these drugs, plus surgery and radiation therapy, made it clear that life was being prolonged and survival expectancy improved (Table 30-11).[49,52–56,244–252]

The next step was multicenter trials to recruit larger numbers of patients and thereby to ascertain better methods of treatment and to learn more about potential prognostic factors. The primary thrust of multi-institutional trials was to collect enough patients over a relatively short period of time (*e.g.,* 5 years) to ask such therapeutic and biological questions with a reasonable expectation of establishing statistically valid results. Controlled comparisons between two or more treatments could be made, provided that enough patients with similar extent of tumor could be found. The first relatively large-scale trial in pediatric RMS and UDS was initiated by the Children's Cancer Study Group (CCSG) in 1967, and eventually accrued 84 patients.[212] Later, 112 patients were entered by CCSG members into a successor study begun in 1970 and reported in 1977.[253] Subsequently, members of the CCSG and the Pediatric Divisions of the Southwest Oncology Group and the Cancer and Acute Leukemia Group B banded together to form the Intergroup Rhabdomyosarcoma Study in 1972.[192] The IRS investigations, still in progress, were designed to answer questions about the biology of RMS and UDS and to ascertain which of two or more alternative programs of treatment was preferable within various subgroups of patients. From November 1972

Table 30-10

Responses in Multiagent Trials in Children with RMS and UDS

Reference	Drugs*	Number of Patients			Percentage of CR + PR
		Evaluable	CR	PR	
Sitarz[240]	AMD, CMB, MTX	4	2	2	100
James[244]	AMD, VCR	6	1	5	100
Pratt[245]	VCR, AMD, CPM (VAC)	7	1	6	100
Green[241]	VAC	4	1	1	50
Gottlieb[242]	ADR, DTIC	18	2	7	50

* AMD = actinomycin D; CMB = chlorambucil; MTX = methotrexate; VCR = vincristine; CPM = cyclophosphamide; ADR = Adriamycin.

through November 1986, approximately 2000 patients with RMS, UDS, and extraosseous Ewing's sarcoma have been entered from over 60 institutions in the United States, Canada, and Western Europe on IRS protocols, constituting the largest collection of such patients in the world. As these studies have continued, the pathologic subtypes and primary sites of RMS and UDS have become better defined.

Once the major active drugs were identified in Phase II trials, combinations of these drugs were employed to achieve maximal antitumor effect without cumulative toxicity. Knowledge that patients who died of RMS or UDS usually had distant metastases provided the rationale for the use of combination chemotherapy after surgical intervention and along with radiation therapy. Even with such therapy, approximately 10% of Group I, 20% of Group II, 30% of Group III, and 70% of Group IV patients develop locoregional recurrence or distant metastases, and information from IRS-I indicates a 95% probability of

Table 30-11
Results of Single- and Limited-Institution Combined Modality Trials in RMS and UDS of All Sites, Histologic Subtypes, and Clinical Groups*

Reference	Number of Patients†	2-Year OS (%)	3-Year OS (%)	5-Year RFS (%)	5-Year OS (%)
Sutow,[58] 1970	78	47	40	—	28
Kilman,[49] 1973	38	—	—	—	71
Holton,[246] 1973	8	50	—	—	—
Ortega,[53] 1975	36	—	58	—	—
Ghavimi,[52] 1975	29	72	—	—	—
Pullen,[250] 1975	22	—	27	—	—
Jaffe,[54] 1977	20	80	—	—	—
Razek,[247] 1977	39	68	64	—	83‡
Jenkin,[22] 1980	25	—	—	52	43
Pratt,[249] 1981	90	36	—	—	41
Ghavimi,[189] 1981	53	83	—	—	—
Kingston,[251] 1983	73	—	—	45	58
Bale,[55] 1983	45	70	—	—	—
Flamant,[56] 1984	193	63	—	—	52
Pedrick,[193] 1986	74	—	—	43	47

* OS = overall survival; RFS = relapse-free survival; dash indicates data not available.
† Number of patients at risk at specified time-intervals.
‡ Five of six patients at risk.

death after recurrence despite further therapy given with curative intent.[218] Thus, new active agents are needed so that even more aggressive treatment can be given, with the goal of eliminating as many tumor cells as possible and preventing the development of drug resistance.[254]

Several newer drugs have been tested in the past decade. Rates of complete response (CR) plus partial response (PR) in children with recurrent RMS or UDS approximate 20% with cisplatin (CPDD)[255] and etoposide (VP-16),[256] and 15% with DTIC,[257,258] each given as single agents (see Table 30-9). It is important to incorporate as many active agents as possible to avoid the phenomenon of multiple drug resistance,[259] although increased toxicity is a likely result. Ifosfamide, an interesting congener of cyclophosphamide, is being used in combination with VP-16 for young people with recurrent sarcoma of soft tissue and bone, and a surprisingly favorable response rate of 69% has been reported for 9 of 13 patients with RMS from NCI.[260] One must be somewhat cautious in interpreting results from relatively small numbers of patients in Phase II trials, but the ifosfamide + VP-16 data will likely result in large-scale trials for previously untreated patients. Another candidate agent is methotrexate. Bode and associates recently reported that three of six children with recurrent RMS responded with CR or PR to methotrexate given intravenously over 42 hours.[261] Melphalan, an alkylating agent similar to cyclophosphamide, is very active against human RMS tumors transplanted into immune-deprived mice.[262] Although melphalan was of limited utility in a small group of children treated for recurrent soft tissue sarcomas at SJCRH, it was quite active in previously untreated patients with advanced RMS.[263] This finding supports the concept that active agents should be used before multiple drug resistance has occurred. Similar indirect evidence may be found in the possibly improved rates of response when CPDD with or without VP-16 is added to VAC + Adriamycin and RT for previously untreated patients with advanced RMS and UDS,[264] in contrast to a response rate of only 12% for CPDD + VP-16 in

relapsed patients with RMS or UDS.[265] Thus, optimal front-line therapy is still under development, as are strategies for patients whose disease escapes control.

Side-effects of chemotherapy (see Chaps. 9 and 50) can be divided into acute and later reactions. Most of the active agents cause temporary emesis, alopecia, and myelosuppression; mucositis can also occur. Repeated doses of vincristine can cause paralytic ileus and other forms of peripheral neuropathy; rarely, transient blindness may result.[266] Repeated doses of cisplatin can cause hearing loss and renal damage.[267] Later sequelae of cyclophosphamide include hemorrhagic cystitis and infertility;[268] cardiac failure can result from Adriamycin.[269]

Combined Modality Therapy

The general principle of complete surgical removal of tumor, where feasible, should be emphasized. Patients whose tumors are removed at the outset continue to fare better than those with gross residual sarcoma, especially with primary tumors of an extremity.[160,195] Operative removal should be considered after chemotherapy and radiation therapy for patients with initially unresectable tumors, with the goal of producing complete tumor regression surgically when the other modalities have failed to eradicate all detectable disease.[270] The timing of such secondary operative management is rather arbitrary; currently, IRS-III recommends repeat biopsy at week 20 for all patients with gross residual tumors (Group III) and those with lung metastases at diagnosis (Group IV).

Radiation therapy guidelines are summarized in Tables 30-7 and 30-8. The timing of RT in relation to chemotherapy has been somewhat variable. In the initial IRS programs, RT was begun at the same time as chemotherapy for patients with Group I or II sarcomas but was delayed until week 6 for those with Group III or IV tumors, in order to assess the response to chemotherapy and to minimize mucositis or other damage.[271] The "boost" effect of certain drugs, notably actinomycin D and Adriamycin, is well known.[272] However, there are data showing that delaying RT until week 6 for patients with cranial parameningeal sarcoma and evidence of meningeal involvement cranial nerve palsy, erosion of bone at the cranial base, or intracranial extension of tumor) may lead to diminished locoregional control and survival. In these patients, RT should be initiated as soon as possible after diagnosis, despite the increased risk of mucositis.[144,272]

Timing of RT may also be critical in another subset of patients. In IRS-II, children with localized tumors arising in the bladder or prostate were treated with repetitive courses of VAC every 4 weeks; if the tumor had shrunk by 50% or more after two cycles, two more cycles of VAC were administered and the response assessed by repeated biopsy. If persistent (but not recurrent) local tumor was found, RT (4000–4500 cGy for most patients) was initiated at week 16.[273] A preliminary analysis of 20 such patients undergoing repeat biopsy after completion of RT showed persistent local tumor in 14, suggesting a diminished response to RT. Therefore, in IRS-III, RT is begun at week 6, because local control rates in IRS-I patients with bladder or prostate sarcoma irradiated at week 6 were excellent.[148]

Chemotherapy is generally continued for 1 to 2 years after diagnosis because most relapses are seen in the first 2 years after initiation of therapy.[196,250] Drugs, doses, and schedules vary among institutions, and there are only a few randomized studies that provide guidelines. As a result, the approaches under investigation in IRS-III have been accepted for use by the major pediatric cooperative groups in the United States, Canada, and Great Britain. The IRS-III recommendations re-

Table 30-12
IRS-III Recommendations for Therapy of RMS and UDS in Childhood

Clinical Group, Histology, Site	Operative Management*	Radiation Therapy	Chemotherapy†
I, nonalveolar, any site	Complete excision, margins clear	None	AMD × 5, VCR × 6: Six 9-wk courses in 54 wk (*Reg. 31*)
I, alveolar, any site	As for Group I, nonalveolar	Begin day 14; follow guidelines in Tables 30-7 and 30-8	VCR, CPDD, ADR, CTX, AMD × 1 yr (*Reg. 38*)
II, nonalveolar, any site	Grossly complete excision with (A) microscopic residual, (B) regional extension-excised, or (C) both A and B	As for Group I, alveolar	Randomize: *Reg. 31* (see above) vs. AMD, VCR, and ADR (total of 360 mg/m²) × 1 year (*Reg. 33*)
II, alveolar, any site	As for Group II, nonalveolar	As for Group I, alveolar	*Reg. 38* (see above)
II + III, nonalveolar, cranial nonparameningeal	Grossly complete (II) or incomplete (III) excision	As for Group II or III	*Reg. 32* (see above)
II + III + IV, any histology, cranial parameningeal	As for nonparameningeal	Begin RT day 0 if meningeal signs present; otherwise begin day 14 (II) or 42 (III, IV)	Group II: Randomize: *Reg. 32* vs. *Reg. 33* Group III: *Reg. 34* vs. *Reg. 35* vs. *Reg. 36* (see below)
III, special pelvic (bladder, prostate, vagina, cervix, uterus)	Incisional or cystoscopic biopsy	See Tables 30-7 and 30-8; start wk 6 for bladder trigone and prostate lesions; start wk 20 if tumor present after excisional biopsy of lesion arising in vagina-uterus or bladder dome	VCR, CPDD, ADR, CTX, AMD × 2 yr, with RT at wk 6 (*Reg. 37-B*) or with optional RT at wk 20 (*Reg. 37-A*)
III, any histology, all other sites	Incomplete excision or incisional biopsy only	See Tables 30-7 and 30-8	Randomize: repetitive pulse VAC × 2 yr (*Reg. 34*) vs *Reg. 38* drugs × 2 yr (*Reg. 35*) vs *Reg. 35* + VP-16 for 2 yr (*Reg. 36*)
IV, any histology, any site except cranial parameningeal	Excise if possible	See Tables 30-7 and 30-8	Randomize: repetitive pulse VAC × 2 yr (*Reg. 34*) vs *Reg. 38* drugs × 2 yr (*Reg. 35*) vs *Reg. 35* + VP-16 for 2 yr (*Reg. 36*)

* See detailed guidelines in Table 30-4.
† Reg. = regimen; AMD = actinomycin D; VCR = vincristine; CPDD = cisplatin; ADR = Adriamycin; CTX = cyclophosphamide; VP-16 = etoposide.

Table 30-13
Results of Combined Modality Trials in RMS and UDS of the Head and Neck

Reference	Number of Patients	Site of Primary*	Survival (%)†			
			2 Years	3 Years	4 Years	5 Years
Donaldson,[59] 1973	19	All head/neck	74 OS	—	—	—
Pratt,[131] 1978	15	All head/neck	—	—	53 OS	—
Sutow,[132] 1982	103	All head/neck	—	66 RFS	—	—
Month,[133] 1986	30	All head/neck	73 RFS	—	—	—
Sagerman,[134] 1972	14	Orbit	64 OS	—	—	—
Flamant,[135] 1978	8	Orbit	—	88 OS	—	—
Wharam,[136] 1985	132	Orbit	—	—	—	88 RFS
Berry,[140] 1981	40	Orbit + PM	—	—	—	34 RFS; 35 OS
Raney,[144] 1987	68	PM (after 12/77)	—	57 RFS; 68 OS	—	—
Wharam,[145] 1984	63 in CR	Nonorbital, non-PM head/neck	—	—	—	78 RFS

* PM = cranial parameningeal.
† RFS = relapse-free survival; OS = overall survival.

Table 30-14
Results of Combined Modality Trials in RMS and UDS of the Pelvis

Reference	Number of Patients	Site of Primary*	Survival (%) 2 Years	Survival (%) 3 Years
Mahesh Kumar,[154] 1976	3	V, U	100 RFS and OS	—
Flamant,[221] 1979	7	V	—	86 RFS and OS
Hays,[155] 1985	19	V	—	89 OS
Hays,[155] 1985	9	U	—	44 OS
Ortega,[149] 1979	13	B, P, V, U	62 RFS	—
Voute,[150] 1981	6	B, P, V, U	67 RFS; 83 OS	—
Ghavimi,[151] 1984	25	B, P, V, U	72 RFS; 80 OS	—
Raney,[152] 1987	74—IRS-I	B, P, V, U	70 RFS; 82 OS	70 RFS; 78 OS
Raney,[152] 1987	128—IRS-II	B, P, V, U	48 RFS; 79 OS	46 RFS; 71 OS
Ransom,[165] 1980	16	R-P	13 OS	—
Crist,[166] 1985	70	R-P	44 RFS	42 RFS
Raney,[167] 1986	7	R-P	29 RFS; 43 OS	—

* V = vagina; U = uterus; B = bladder; P = prostate; R-P = retroperitoneum-pelvis.

Table 30-15
Results of Combined Modality Trials in RMS and UDS at Other Sites

Reference	Number of Patients	Site of Primary	Survival (%) 2 Years	Survival (%) 3 Years
Ransom,[159] 1977	13	Extremity	31 RFS and OS	—
Gehan,[195] 1981	19—Group I*	Extremity	62 RFS; 73 OS	—
	30—Group II	Extremity	63 RFS; 75 OS	—
	21—Group III	Extremity	24 RFS; 50 OS	—
	27—Group IV	Extremity	3 RFS; 25 OS	—
Raney,[163] 1982	28	Trunk	54 RFS and OS	—
Crist,[164] 1982	13	Intrathoracic	31 RFS and OS	—
Raney,[274] 1986	29	Perineum	—	31 RFS; 45 OS
Ruymann,[170] 1985	9	Biliary	22 RFS	—

* IRS clinical group (from IRS-I analysis).

Table 30-16
*Percentage of Patients Surviving at 3 Years, by Clinical Group**

Clinical Group	Heyn et al.,[212] 1974 (N = 84)	Heyn et al.,[253] 1977 (N = 112)	IRS-I (N = 686)	IRS-II (N = 956)
I	65 (− chemo) 87 (+ chemo)	Not studied	87	88
II	90	71	74	77
III	65	44	57	68
IV	22	28	23	32

* From the minutes of the IRS Meeting, November 1985.

garding surgery, radiation therapy, and chemotherapy for children with RMS and UDS of various histologic types and at various sites are outlined in Table 30-12. Many of the treatment schedules are toxic, especially those using cisplatin and Adria-mycin, and management of such patients requires skill, experience, and often supportive care in the form of intravenous antibiotics, blood component transfusions, hyperalimentation, and meticulous attention to fluid and electrolyte disturbances. Treatment programs for RMS and UDS are still evolving; the suggestions in Table 30-12 therefore should not be considered definitive.

Treatment Results

Results of single and limited institutional trials of multimodality management of young persons with RMS and UDS are listed in Table 30-11. The 3-year survival figure is probably most useful for comparisons, because of the readily distinguished endpoint and because most series show very little drop-off in survival curves beyond that time. Tables 30-13, 30-14, and 30-15 show the outcome data by primary site, both from single institutions and from the IRS. Table 30-16 presents 3-year survival rates from the prospective multi-institutional trials conducted in the combined modality era. These comparisons may be more valid because staging and clinical grouping were conducted in a planned manner and both pathologic review and statistical support were provided uniformly. Where series have employed staging systems other than that developed by the IRS, an attempt has been made to categorize the patients by equivalent IRS clinical groups. It can be seen in Table 30-16 that there is a rank order of survival by clinical group, with completely resected patients (Group I) faring the best and patients with metastases (Group IV) the worst. Data on histologic type and primary site are relatively limited in most series; findings from IRS-II are given in Tables 30-17 (primary site) and 30-18 (histology). As in smaller series, the alveolar RMS group fared less well than those with nonalveolar RMS and UDS, and patients with tumors of the extremity, retroperitoneum or pelvis, and perineum[274] have a worse outlook than those with tumors arising in the head and neck and the genitourinary tract.

Complications of the Therapy

Complications of therapy include residual effects of operative management, radiation therapy, and chemotherapy (see also Chap. 50). Clearly, the extent of surgical treatment has a bearing on the functional outcome. Extremity amputations and extensive formal lymph node dissections (other than, perhaps, in patients with paratesticular sarcoma) are rarely performed.

Infection, anemia, and bleeding can result from intensive drug combinations.[275] Infants develop more toxicity than older children.[276] Leukoencephalopathy, which is fortunately very uncommon, can be seen in patients with cranial parameningeal sarcoma given intensive chemotherapy and radiation ther-

apy, including repeated doses of intrathecal methotrexate, hydrocortisone, and cytosine arabinoside.[277] Fibrosis, diminished growth of underlying or surrounding structures, cataracts, disturbed dentition, and growth hormone deficiency have all been reported in children receiving multimodality therapy for tumors arising in the head and neck.[278-282] Combined therapy with drugs and radiation can produce severe fibrosis and limitation of function in irradiated sites (see Chap. 11).[215] The incidence of hematuria after cyclophosphamide therapy is increased as much as fourfold when pelvic irradiation has also been used.[283] Infertility can result from gonadal effects of cyclophosphamide[268] or radiation therapy, or from surgical interruption of nerves conveying impulses for antegrade ejaculation, as in boys with pelvic or paratesticular sarcoma.[156] Acute myeloid leukemia has now been reported in several children who have survived treatment for RMS,[278,279,284] as have several types of second solid tumors (see Chap. 50).[63]

Further information is needed for other large populations of survivors, especially those with primary genitourinary and extremity lesions. Nevertheless, it is clear that major advances have been made in the successful management of RMS and UDS in childhood over the past 20 years. Ongoing investigations should lead to the identification of better treatments with less long-term morbidity.

FUTURE CONSIDERATIONS

It is evident that improvements in disease control and survival are still much needed, particularly for the majority of patients (approximately 65%) who have gross residual or metastatic sarcoma at the time of diagnosis. Better ways of preserving the bladder and of lessening the late adverse effects on structures in the head and neck are other areas where progress is needed. As new agents with antisarcoma activity become available, it is possible that radiation therapy can be reduced still further (e.g., in patients with orbital lesions). Future research efforts should also concentrate on studies of etiology and epidemiology to increase our basic understanding of rhabdomyosarcoma and undifferentiated sarcoma.

Table 30-17
*Percentage of Patients Surviving at 3 Years in IRS-II**

Primary Site	Number Studied	Percentage Alive
Orbit	80	93
Genitourinary (other than Group III SP)†	98	80
Cranial parameningeal	155	71
Other head/neck	96	69
Genitourinary (mainly Group III SP)	116	64
Trunk	92	57
Extremity	159	56
Retroperitoneum-pelvis	110	46

* From the minutes of the IRS Meeting, November 1985; all clinical groups are combined.
† SP = special pelvic sites (bladder, prostate, vagina, cervix, uterus).

Table 30-18
*Percentage of Patients Surviving at 3 Years in IRS-II**

Histologic Type	Number Studied	Percentage Alive
Embryonal	506	69
Alveolar	198	56
Other	249	66

* From the minutes of the IRS Meeting, November 1985; all clinical groups are combined.

REFERENCES

1. Stout AP: Rhabdomyosarcoma of the skeletal muscles. Ann Surg 123:447–472, 1946
2. Pack GT, Eberhart WF: Rhabdomyosarcoma of skeletal muscle: Report of 100 cases. Surgery 32:1023–1064, 1952
3. Pack GT, Ariel IM: Sarcomas of the soft somatic tissues in infants and children. Surg Gynecol Obstet 98:675–686, 1954
4. Peltier LF: Historical note on bone and soft tissue sarcoma. J Surg Oncol 30:201–205, 1985
5. Weber CO: Anatomische Untersuchung einer hypertrophische Zunge nebst Bemerkungen ueber die Neubildung quergestreifter Muskelfasern. Virchows Arch Pathol Anat 7:115–138, 1854
6. Horn RC Jr, Enterline HT: Rhabdomyosarcoma: A clinicopathologic study and classification of 39 cases. Cancer 11:181–199, 1958
7. Stobbe GD, Dargeon HW: Embryonal rhabdomyosarcoma of the head and neck in children and adolescents. Cancer 3:826–836, 1950
8. Mackenzie AR, Whitmore WF Jr, Melamed MR: Myosarcomas of the bladder and prostate. Cancer 22:833–844, 1968
9. Riopelle JL, Thériault JP: Sur une forme méconnue de sarcome des parties molles: Le rhabdomyosarcome alvéolaire. Ann Anat Pathol 1:88–111, 1956
10. Enzinger FM, Shiraki M: Alveolar rhabdomyosarcoma: An analysis of 110 cases. Cancer 24:18–31, 1969
11. Angervall L, Enzinger FM: Extraskeletal neoplasm resembling Ewing's sarcoma. Cancer 36:240–251, 1975
12. Soule EH, Newton W Jr, Moon TE, Tefft M: Extraskeletal Ewing's sarcoma: A preliminary review of 26 cases encountered in the Intergroup Rhabdomyosarcoma Study. Cancer 42:259–264, 1978

13. Green DM, Jaffe N: Progress and controversy in the treatment of childhood rhabdomyosarcoma. Cancer Treat Rev 5:7–27, 1978

14. Pizzo PA: Rhabdomyosarcoma and the soft tissue sarcomas. In Levine AS: Cancer in the Young, pp 615–632. New York, Masson Publishing, 1982

15. Maurer HM, Ragab AH: Rhabdomyosarcoma. In Sutow WW, Fernbach DJ, Vietti TJ (eds): Clinical Pediatric Oncology, 3rd ed, pp 622–651. St Louis, CV Mosby, 1984

16. Miser JS, Pizzo PA: Soft tissue sarcomas in childhood. Pediatr Clin North Am 32:779–800, 1985

17. D'Angio GJ, Evans AE: Overview: Soft-tissue sarcomas in childhood. In D'Angio GJ, Evans AE: Bone Tumors and Soft-Tissue Sarcomas, pp 47–56. London, Edward Arnold, 1983

18. Young JL, Miller RW: Incidence of malignant tumors in U.S. children. J Pediatr 86:254–258, 1975

19. Breslow NE, Langholz B: Childhood cancer incidence: Geographical and temporal variations. Int J Cancer 32:703–716, 1983

20. Kramer S, Meadows AT, Jarrett P, Evans AE: Incidence of childhood cancer: Experience of a decade in a population-based registry. J Natl Cancer Inst 70:49–55, 1983

21. Raney B Jr: Soft-tissue sarcoma in adolescents. In Tebbi CK: Adolescent Oncology, pp 221–240. Mt Kisco, NY, Futura Publishing Co, 1987

22. Jenkin D, Sonley M: Soft-tissue sarcomas in the young: Medical treatment advances in perspective. Cancer 46:621–629, 1980

23. Miller RW: Deaths from childhood cancer in sibs. N Engl J Med 279:122–126, 1968

24. Mann RB, Jaffe ES, Braylan RC, Nanba K, Frank MM, Ziegler JL, Berard CW: Non-endemic Burkitt's lymphoma. N Engl J Med 295:685–691, 1976

25. Miller RW, Dalager NA: Fatal rhabdomyosarcoma among children in the United States, 1960–1969. Cancer 34:1897–1900, 1974

26. Ueda K, Gruppo R, Unger F, Martin L, Bove K: Rhabdomyosarcoma of lung arising in congenital cystic adenomatoid malformation. Cancer 40:383–388, 1977

27. Krous HF, Sexauer CL: Embryonal rhabdomyosarcoma arising within a congenital bronchogenic cyst in a child. J Pediatr Surg 16:506–508, 1981

28. Beddis IR, Mott MG, Bullimore J: Case report: Nasopharyngeal rhabdomyosarcoma and Gorlin's naevoid basal cell carcinoma syndrome. Med Pediatr Oncol 11:178–179, 1983

29. Schweisguth O, Gerard-Marchant R, Lemerle J: Naevomatose basocellulaire association a un rhabdomyosarcome congenital. Arch Fr Pediatr 25:1083–1093, 1968

30. Becker H, Zaunschirm A, Muntean W, Domej W: Alkoholembryopathie und maligner Tumor. Wien Klin Wochenschr 94:364–365, 1982

31. McKeen EA, Bodurtha J, Meadows AT, Douglass EC, Mulvihill JJ: Rhabdomyosarcoma complicating multiple neurofibromatosis. J Pediatr 93:992–993, 1978

32. Warrier RP, Kini KR, Shumaker B, Schwartz G, Raju U, Raman BS: Neurofibromatosis, factor IX deficiency, and rhabdomyosarcoma. Urology 28:295–296, 1986

33. Woodruff JM, Chernik NL, Smith MC, Millett WB, Foote FW Jr: Peripheral nerve tumors with rhabdomyosarcomatous differentiation (malignant "Triton" tumors). Cancer 32:426–439, 1973

34. Buck BE, Mahboubi S, Raney RB Jr: Congenital neurogenous sarcoma with rhabdomyosarcomatous differentiation. J Pediatr Surg 12:581–582, 1977

35. Li FP, Fraumeni JF Jr: Rhabdomyosarcoma in children: Epidemiologic study and identification of a familial cancer syndrome. J Natl Cancer Inst 43:1365–1373, 1969

36. Li FP, Fraumeni JF Jr: Prospective study of a family cancer syndrome. JAMA 247:2692–2694, 1982

37. Birch JM, Hartley AL, Marsden HB, Harris M, Swindell R: Excess risk of breast cancer in the mothers of children with soft tissue sarcomas. Br J Cancer 49:325–331, 1984

38. Lynch HT, Katz DA, Bogard PJ, Lynch JF: The sarcoma, breast cancer, lung cancer, and adrenocortical carcinoma syndrome revisited. Am J Dis Child 139:134–136, 1985

39. Berger R, Bernheim A, Mitelman F, Rydholm A: C-band pattern in lymphocytes of patients with soft-tissue sarcomas. Cancer Genet Cytogenet 9:145–150, 1983

40. Moriyama M, Shuin T, Kubota Y, Satomi Y, Sugio Y, Kuroki Y: A case of rhabdomyosarcoma of the bladder with a (2;5) chromosomal translocation in peripheral lymphocytes. Cancer Genet Cytogenet 22:177–181, 1986

41. Nelson-Rees WA, Flandermeyer RR, Hawthorne PK: Distinctive banded marker chromosomes of human tumor cell lines. Int J Cancer 16:74–82, 1975

42. Potluri VR, Gilbert F: A cytogenetic study of embryonal rhabdomyosarcoma. Cancer Genet Cytogenet 14:169–173, 1985

43. Seidal T, Mark J, Hagmar B, Angervall L: Alveolar rhabdomyosarcoma: A cytogenetic and correlated cytological and histological study. Acta Pathol Microbiol Immunol Scand [A] 90:345–354, 1982

44. Turc-Carel C, Lizard-Nacol S, Justrabo E, Favrot M, Philip T, Tabone E: Consistent chromosome translocation in alveolar rhabdomyosarcoma. Cancer Genet Cytogenet 19:361–362, 1986

45. Trent J, Casper J, Meltzer P, Thompson F, Fogh J: Nonrandom chromosome alterations in rhabdomyosarcoma. Cancer Genet Cytogenet 16:189–197, 1985

46. Limon J, Dal Cin P, Sandberg AA: Translocations involving the X chromosome in solid tumors: Presentation of two sarcomas with t(X;18) (q13;p11). Cancer Genet Cytogenet 23:87–91, 1986

47. Garson JA, Clayton J, McIntyre P, Kemshead JT: N-*myc* oncogene amplification in rhabdomyosarcoma at release. Lancet 1:1496, 1986

48. Soule EH, Mahour GH, Mills SD, Lynn HB: Soft-tissue sarcomas of infants and children: A clinicopathologic study of 135 cases. Mayo Clin Proc 43:313–326, 1968

49. Kilman JW, Clatworthy HW Jr, Newton WA Jr, Grosfeld JL: Reasonable surgery for rhabdomyosarcoma: A study of 67 cases. Ann Surg 178:346–351, 1973

50. Myers MH, Heise HW, Li FP, Miller RW: Trends in cancer survival among U.S. white children, 1955–1971. J Pediatr 87:815–818, 1975

51. Ehrlich FE, Haas JE, Kiesewetter WB: Rhabdomyosarcoma in infants and children: Factors affecting long-term survival. J Pediatr Surg 6:571–577, 1971

52. Ghavimi F, Exelby PR, D'Angio GJ, Cham W, Lieberman PH, Tan C, Miké V, Murphy ML: Multidisciplinary treatment of embryonal rhabdomyosarcoma in children. Cancer 35:677–686, 1975

53. Ortega JA, Rivard GE, Isaacs H, Hittle RE, Hays DM, Pike MC, Karon MR: The influence of chemotherapy on the prognosis of rhabdomyosarcoma. Med Pediatr Oncol 1:227–234, 1975

54. Jaffe N, Murray J, Traggis D, Cassady JR, Filler RM, Watts H, Weichselbaum R, Weinstein H: Multidisciplinary treatment for childhood sarcoma. Am J Surg 133:405–413, 1977

55. Bale PM, Parsons RE, Stevens MM: Diagnosis and behavior of juvenile rhabdomyosarcoma. Hum Pathol 14:596–611, 1983

56. Flamant F, Hill C: The improvement in survival associated with combined chemotherapy in childhood rhabdomyosarcoma: A historical comparison of 345 patients in the same center. Cancer 53:2417–2421, 1984

57. Sutow WW: Chemotherapeutic management of childhood rhabdomyosarcoma. In Neoplasia in Childhood, pp 201–208. Chicago, Year Book Medical Publishers, 1969

58. Sutow WW, Sullivan MP, Ried HL, Taylor HG, Griffith KM: Prognosis in childhood rhabdomyosarcoma. Cancer 25:1384–1390, 1970

59. Donaldson SS, Castro JR, Wilbur JR, Jesse RH Jr: Rhabdomyosarcoma of head and neck in children. Cancer 31:26–35, 1973

60. Lawrence W Jr, Jegge G, Foote FW Jr: Embryonal rhabdomyosarcoma: A clinicopathologic study. Cancer 17:361–376, 1964

61. Souba WW, McKenna RJ, Meis J, Benjamin R, Raymond AK, Mountain CF: Radiation-induced sarcomas of the chest wall. Cancer 57:610–615, 1986

62. Davidson T, Westbury G, Harmer CL: Radiation-induced soft-tissue sarcoma. Br J Surg 73:308–309, 1986

63. Meadows AT, D'Angio GJ, Miké V, Banfi A, Harris C, Jenkin RDT, Schwartz A: Patterns of second malignant neoplasms in children. Cancer 40:1903–1911, 1977

64. Strong LC, Herson J, Osborne BM, Sutow WW: Risk of radiation-related subsequent malignant tumors in survivors of Ewing's sarcoma. J Natl Cancer Inst 62:1401–1406, 1979

65. Crist WM, Edwards RH, Pereira F: Rhabdomyosarcoma diagnosed by electron microscopy in a child with acute lymphocytic leukemia. J Pediatr 93:893–894, 1978

66. D'Angio GJ, Meadows A, Miké V, Harris C, Evans A, Jaffe N, Newton W, Schweisguth O, Sutow W, Morris-Jones P: Decreased risk of radiation-associated second malignant neoplasms in actinomycin-D treated patients. Cancer 37:1177–1185, 1976

67. Abramson DH, Ellsworth RM, Kitchin FD, Tung G: Second non-ocular tumors in retinoblastoma survivors: Are they radiation-induced? Ophthalmology 91:1351–1355, 1984

68. Koufos A, Hansen MF, Copeland NG, Jenkins NA, Lampkin BC, Cavenee WK: Loss of heterozygosity in three embryonal tumours suggests a common pathogenetic mechanism. Nature 316:330–334, 1985

69. Chardin P, Yeramian P, Madaule P, Tavitian A: N-ras gene activation in the RD human rhabdomyosarcoma cell line. Int J Cancer 35:647–652, 1985

70. Hardell L, Sandstrom A: Case-control study: Soft-tissue sarcomas and exposure to phenoxyacetic acids or chlorophenols. Br J Cancer 39:711–717, 1979

71. Eriksson M, Hardell L, Berg NO, Moller T, Axelson O: Soft-tissue sarcomas and exposure to chemical substances: A case-referent study. Br J Industr Med 38:27–33, 1981

72. Grufferman S, Wang HH, DeLong ER, Kimm SYS, Delzell ES, Falletta JM: Environmental factors in the etiology of rhabdomyosarcoma in childhood. J Natl Cancer Inst 68:107–113, 1982

73. Kouri RE, Ratrie H, Whitmire CE: Evidence of a genetic relationship between susceptibility to 3-methylcholanthrene-induced subcutaneous tumors and inducibility of arylhydrocarbon hydroxylase. J Natl Cancer Inst 51:197–200, 1973

74. Jurgelski W, Hudson PM, Dunn RL, Falk HL: A new animal model for the direct induction of neoplasms during embryonic and fetal development. Proceedings of the Third International Symposium on the Detection and Prevention of Cancer 1, Part 1, Chap. 11, 1978

75. Allen JR, Hsu I-C, Carstens LA: Dehydroretronecine-induced rhabdomyosarcomas in rats. Cancer Res 35:997–1002, 1975

76. Grice HC, Mannell WA: Rhabdomyosarcomas induced in rats by intramuscular injections of Blue VRS. J Natl Cancer Inst 37:845–857, 1966

77. Bruni C, Rust JN: Fine structure of dividing cells and of nondividing, differentiating cells of nickel sulfide-induced rhabdomyosarcomas. J Natl Cancer Inst 54:687–696, 1975

78. Pot-Debrun J, Poupon M-F, Sweeney FL, Chouroulinkov I: Growth, metastasis, immunogenicity, and chromosomal content of a nickel-induced rhabdomyosarcoma and subsequent cloned cell lines in rats. J Natl Cancer Inst 71:1241–1245, 1983

79. Damjanov I, Sunderman FW, Mitchell JM, Allpass PR: Induction of testicular sarcomas in Fischer rats by intratesticular injection of nickel subsulfide. Cancer Res 38:268–276, 1978

80. Moloney JB: A virus-induced rhabdomyosarcoma of mice. Natl Cancer Inst Monogr 22:139–142, 1960

81. Gardner MB, Rongey RW, Arnstein P, Estes JD, Sarma P, Huebner RJ, Rickard CG: Experimental transmission of feline fibrosarcoma to cats and dogs. Nature 226:807–809, 1970

82. Theilen GH, Gould D, Fowler M, Dungworth DL: C-type virus in tumor tissue of a woolly monkey (Lagothrix spp.) with fibrosarcoma. J Natl Cancer Inst 47:881–889, 1971

83. Klein G: The Epstein-Barr virus and neoplasia. N Engl J Med 293:1353–1357, 1975

84. Shaw GM, Broder S, Essex M, Gallo RC: Human T-cell leukemia virus: Its discovery and role in leukemogenesis and immune suppression. Adv Intern Med 30:1–27, 1984

85. McAllister RM, Melnyk J, Finklestein JZ, Adams EC Jr, Gardner MB: Cultivation in vitro of cells derived from human rhabdomyosarcoma. Cancer 24:520–526, 1969

86. Chapman AL, Bogner P, Behbehani AM: A study of a new human tumor cell line (Rhabdomyosarcoma) (38250). Proc Soc Exp Biol Med 146:1087–1092, 1974

87. Sethi J, Hirshaut Y, Hajdu SI, Clements LG: Growing human sarcomas in culture. Cancer 40:744–755, 1977

88. Sinkovics JG, Shirato E, Cabiness JR, Martin RG: Rhabdomyosarcoma after puberty: Clinical, tissue culture and immunological studies. J Med 1:313–326, 1970

89. Sinkovics JG, Cabiness JR, Shullenberger CC: In vitro cytotoxicity of lymphocytes to human sarcoma cells. Bibl Haematol 39:846–851, 1973

90. Cohen AM, Ketcham AS, Morton DL: Specific inhibition of sarcoma-specific cellular immunity by sera from patients with growing sarcomas. Int J Cancer 11:273–279, 1973

91. Whitney RB, Levy JG: Effects of sera from tumor-bearing mice on mitogen and allogeneic stimulation of normal lymphoid cells. J Natl Cancer Inst 54:733–741, 1975

92. Levy JG, McMaster R, Kelly B, Whitney RB, Kilburn DG: Identity of a T-lymphocyte inhibitor with mouse immunoglobulin in the serum of tumour-bearing mice. Immunology 32:475–481, 1977

93. Kucheria K: Autoradiographic analysis of the cell cycle of five solid human tumours in vitro. Br J Cancer 24:283–289, 1970

94. Nusso M, Afzal J, Carr B, Kavanau K: Cell cycle kinetic measurements in an irradiated rat rhabdomyosarcoma using a monoclonal antibody to bromodeoxyuridine. Cytometry 6:611–619, 1985

95. Alitalo K, Myllyla R, Sage H, Pritzl P, Vaheri A, Bornstein P: Biosynthesis of type V procollagen by A-204, a human rhabdomyosarcoma cell line. J Biol Chem 257:9016–9024, 1982

96. Redini F, Moczar E, Poupon MF: Cell surface glycosaminoglycans of rat rhabdomyosarcoma lines with different metastatic potentials and of non-malignant rat myoblasts. Biochim Biophys Acta 883:98–105, 1986

97. Todaro GJ, Fryling C, DeLarco JE: Transforming growth factors produced by certain human tumor cells: Polypeptides that interact with epidermal growth factor receptors. Proc Natl Acad Sci USA 77:5258–5262, 1980

98. Lobb RR, Rybak SM, St. Clair DK, Fett JW: Lysates of two established human tumor lines contain heparin-binding growth factors related to bovine acidic brain fibroblast growth factor. Biochem Biophys Res Commun 139:861–867, 1986

99. Iwata KK, Fryling CM, Knott WB, Todaro GJ: Isolation of tumor cell growth-inhibiting factors from a human rhabdomyosarcoma cell line. Cancer Res 45:2689–2694, 1985

100. Marshall CJ, Hall A, Weiss RA: A transforming gene present in human sarcoma cell lines. Nature 299:171–173, 1982

101. Karpas A, Tuckerman E: Transformation of human fibroblasts with D.N.A. of cultured human rhabdomyosarcoma cells. Lancet 1:1138–1141, 1974

102. Cook B, O'Sullivan F, Leung J, Morse P, Graham B, Chapman AL: Transformation of human embryo cells with the use of cell-free extracts of a human rhabdomyosarcoma cell line (HUS-2): Brief communication. J Natl Cancer Inst 60:979–984, 1978

103. Patton RB, Horn RC Jr: Rhabdomyosarcoma: Clinical and pathological features and comparison with human fetal and embryonal skeletal muscle. Surgery 52:572–584, 1962

104. Roholl PJM, De Jong ASH, Ramaekers FCS: Application of markers in the diagnosis of soft tissue tumors. Histopathology 9:1019–1035, 1985

105. Eusebi V, Ceccarelli C, Gorza L, Schiaffino S, Bussolati G: Immunocytochemistry of rhabdomyosarcoma: The use of four different markers. Am J Surg Pathol 10:293–299, 1986

106. Corson JM, Pinkus GS: Intracellular myoglobin—A specific marker for skeletal muscle differentiation in soft sarcomas: An immunoperoxidase study. Am J Pathol 103:384–389, 1981

107. Brooks JJ: Immunohistochemistry of soft tissue tumors: Myoglobin as a tumor marker for rhabdomyosarcoma. Cancer 50:1757–1763, 1982

108. Tsokos M, Howard R, Costa J: Immunohistochemical study of alveolar and embryonal rhabdomyosarcoma. Lab Invest 48:148–155, 1983

109. De Jong ASH, van Kessel-van Vark M, Albus-Lutter Ch E, van Raamsdonk W, Voute PA: Skeletal muscle actin as tumor marker in the diagnosis of rhabdomyosarcoma in childhood. Am J Surg Pathol 9:467–474, 1985

110. Molenaar WM, Oosterhuis JW, Oosterhuis AM, Ramaekers FCS: Mesenchymal and muscle-specific intermediate filaments (vimentin and desmin) in relation to differentiation in childhood rhabdomyosarcomas. Hum Pathol 16:838–843, 1985

111. Altmannsberger M, Weber K, Droste R, Osborn M: Desmin is a specific marker for rhabdomyosarcomas of human and rat origin. Am J Pathol 118:85–95, 1985

112. Dickman PS: Electron microscopy for diagnosis of tumors in children. Perspect Pediatr Pathol 9:171–213, 1987

113. Barlogie B, Raber MN, Schumann J, Johnson TS, Drewinko B, Swartzendruber DE, Goehde W, Andreef M, Freireich EJ: Flow cytometry in clinical cancer research. Cancer Res 43:3982–3997, 1983

114. Allsbrook WC, Stead NW, Pantazis CG, Houston JH, Crosby JH: Embryonal rhabdomyosarcoma in ascitic fluid. Arch Pathol Lab Med 110:847–849, 1986

115. Kemshead JT, Treleaven JG, Gibson FM, Ugelstad J, Rembaum A, Philip T: Removal of malignant cells from bone marrow using magnetic microspheres and monoclonal antibodies. Prog Exp Tumor Res 29:249–255, 1985

116. Henderson DW, Raven JL, Pollard JAA et al: Bone marrow metastases in disseminated alveolar rhabdomyosarcoma: Case report with ultrastructural study and review. Pathology 8:329–341, 1976

117. Dickman PS, Triche TJ: Extraosseous Ewing's sarcoma versus primitive rhabdomyosarcoma: Diagnostic criteria and clinical correlation. Hum Pathol 17:881–893, 1986

118. Kahn HJ, Yeger H, Kassim O, Jorgensen AO, MacLennan DH, Baumal R, Smith CR, Phillips MJ: Immunohistochemical and electron microscopic assessment of childhood rhabdomyosarcoma: Increased frequency of diagnosis over routine histologic methods. Cancer 51:1897–1903, 1983

119. Dehner LP: Soft tissue sarcomas of childhood: The differential diagnostic dilemma of the small blue cell. Natl Cancer Inst Monogr 56:43–59, 1981

120. Triche TJ, Askin FB, Kissane JM: Neuroblastoma, Ewing's sarcoma, and the

differential diagnosis of small-, round-, blue-cell tumors. In Finegold M (ed): Pathology of neoplasia in children and adolescents, pp 145–195. Philadelphia, WB Saunders, 1986

121. Variend S: Small cell tumors in childhood: A review. J Pathol 145:1–25, 1985

122. Molenaar WM, Oosterhuis JW, Kamps WA: Cytologic "differentiation" in childhood rhabdomyosarcomas following polychemotherapy. Hum Pathol 15:973–979, 1984

123. Stout AP: Tumors of the soft tissues. In Atlas of Tumor Pathology, First Series, Sect II, Fasc 5. Washington, DC, Armed Forces Institute of Pathology, 1953

124. Stout AP, Lattes R: Tumors of the Soft Tissues. In Atlas of Tumor Pathology, Second Series, Fasc 1. Washington, DC, Armed Forces Institute of Pathology, 1967

125. Reddick RL, Michelitch H, Triche TJ: Malignant soft tissue tumors (malignant fibrous histiocytoma, pleomorphic liposarcoma, and pleomorphic rhabdomyosarcoma): An electron microscopic study. Hum Pathol 10:327–343, 1979

126. Gaiger AM, Soule EH, Newton WA Jr: Pathology of rhabdomyosarcoma: Experience of the Intergroup Rhabdomyosarcoma Study, 1972–78. Natl Cancer Inst Monogr 56:19–27, 1981

127. Bale PM, Parsons RE, Stevens MM: Pathology and behavior of juvenile rhabdomyosarcoma. In Finegold M (ed): Pathology of Neoplasia in Children and Adolescents, pp 196–222. Philadelphia, W B Saunders, 1986

128. Palmer N, Sachs N, Foulkes M: Histopathology and prognosis in rhabdomyosarcoma (IRS I) (abstr C-660). Proc Am Soc Clin Oncol 1:170, 1982

129. Palmer N, Foulkes M: Histopathology and prognosis in the second Intergroup Rhabdomyosarcoma Study (IRS-II) (abstr C-897). Proc Am Soc Clin Oncol 2:229, 1983

130. Tsokos M, Miser A, Pizzo P, Triche TJ: Histologic and cytologic characteristics of poor prognosis childhood rhabdomyosarcoma. Lab Invest 50:61A, 1984

131. Pratt CB, Smith JW, Woerner S, Mauer AM, Hustu HO, Johnson WW, Shanks EC: Factors leading to delay in the diagnosis and affecting survival of children with head and neck rhabdomyosarcoma. Pediatrics 61:30–34, 1978

132. Sutow WW, Lindberg RD, Gehan EA, Ragab AH, Raney RB Jr, Ruymann F, Soule EH: Three-year relapse-free survival rates in childhood rhabdomyosarcoma of the head and neck: Report from the Intergroup Rhabdomyosarcoma Study. Cancer 49:2217–2221, 1982.

133. Month SR, Raney RB: Rhabdomyosarcoma of the head and neck in children: The experience at the Children's Hospital of Philadelphia. Med Pediatr Oncol 14:288–292, 1986

134. Sagerman RH, Tretter P, Ellsworth RM: The treatment of orbital rhabdomyosarcoma of children with primary radiation therapy. Am J Roentgenol Rad Ther Nucl Med 114:31–34, 1972

135. Flamant F, Bloch-Michel E, Lemaistre O, Gerard-Marchant R, Schweisguth O, Campinchi R: Les possibilités actuelles de traitement du rhabdomyosarcome de l'orbite chez l'enfant: A propos de 20 cas observés à l'Institut Gustave Roussy (1960–1975). J Fr Ophtalmol 1:451–456, 1978

136. Wharam M, Beltangady M, Heyn R, Lawrence W, Newton W, Raney R, Ruymann F, Tefft M, Maurer H: Localized orbital rhabdomyosarcoma: A report of the Intergroup Rhabdomyosarcoma Study (abstr C-514). Proc Am Soc Clin Oncol 4:132, 1985

137. Tefft M, Fernandez C, Donaldson M, Newton W, Moon TE: Incidence of meningeal involvement by rhabdomyosarcoma of the head and neck in children. Cancer 42:253–258, 1978

138. Leviton A, Davidson R, Gilles F: Neurological manifestations of embryonal rhabdomyosarcoma of the middle ear cleft. J Pediatr 80:596–602, 1972

139. Chan RC, Sutow WW, Lindberg RD: Parameningeal rhabdomyosarcoma. Radiology 131:211–214, 1979

140. Berry MP, Jenkin RDT: Parameningeal rhabdomyosarcoma in the young. Cancer 48:281–288, 1981

141. Gasparini M, Lombardi F, Gianni C, Lovati C, Fossati-Bellani F: Childhood rhabdomyosarcoma with meningeal extension: Results of combined therapy including central nervous system prophylaxis. Am J Clin Oncol (CCT) 6:393–398, 1983

142. Prat J, Gray GF: Massive neuraxial spread of aural rhabdomyosarcoma. Arch Otolaryngol 103:301–303, 1977

143. Raney RB: Spinal cord "drop metastases" from head and neck rhabdomyosarcoma: Proceedings of the Tumor Board of the Children's Hospital of Philadelphia. Med Pediatr Oncol 4:3–9, 1978

144. Raney RB Jr, Tefft M, Newton WA, Ragab AH, Lawrence W Jr, Gehan EA, Maurer HM: Improved prognosis with intensive treatment of children with cranial soft tissue sarcomas arising in nonorbital parameningeal sites: A report from the Intergroup Rhabdomyosarcoma Study. Cancer 59:147–155, 1987

145. Wharam MD, Foulkes MA, Lawrence W Jr, Lindberg RD, Maurer HM, Newton WA Jr, Ragab AH, Raney RB Jr, Tefft M: Soft tissue sarcoma of the head and neck in childhood: Non-orbital and non-parameningeal sites: A report of the Intergroup Rhabdomyosarcoma Study (IRS)-I. Cancer 53:1016–1019, 1984

146. Hays DM: Pelvic rhabdomyosarcomas in childhood: Diagnosis and concepts of management reviewed. Cancer 45:1810–1814, 1980

147. Hays DM, Raney RB Jr, Lawrence W Jr, Soule EH, Gehan EA, Tefft M: Bladder and prostatic tumors in the Intergroup Rhabdomyosarcoma Study (IRS)-I. Cancer 50:1472–1482, 1982

148. Tefft M, Jaffe N: Sarcoma of the bladder and prostate in children: Rationale for the role of radiation therapy based on a review of the literature and a report of fourteen additional patients. Cancer 32:1161–1177, 1973

149. Ortega JA: A therapeutic approach to childhood pelvic rhabdomyosarcoma without pelvic exenteration. J Pediatr 94:205–209, 1979

150. Voute PA, Vos A, de Kraker J, Behrendt H: Rhabdomyosarcomas: Chemotherapy and limited supplementary treatment program to avoid mutilation. Natl Cancer Inst Monogr 56:121–125, 1981

151. Ghavimi F, Herr H, Jereb B, Exelby PR: Treatment of genitourinary rhabdomyosarcoma in children. J Urol 132:313–319, 1984

152. Raney RB Jr, Gehan EA, Hays DM, Tefft M, Newton WA Jr, Maurer HM: Primary chemotherapy with or without radiation therapy, surgery, or both for children with localized sarcoma of special pelvic sites (bladder, prostate, vagina, uterus, cervix) in Intergroup Rhabdomyosarcoma Study (IRS)-II: Comparison of results with IRS-I. Cancer (submitted)

153. Hays DM, Raney RB Jr, Lawrence W Jr, Gehan EA, Soule EH, Tefft M, Maurer HM: Rhabdomyosarcoma of the female genital tract. J Pediatr Surg 16:828–834, 1981

154. Mahesh Kumar AP, Wrenn EL Jr, Fleming ID, Hustu HO, Pratt CB: Combined therapy to prevent complete pelvic exenteration for rhabdomyosarcoma of the vagina or uterus. Cancer 37:118–122, 1976

155. Hays DM, Shimada H, Raney RB Jr, Tefft M, Newton W, Crist WM, Lawrence W Jr, Ragab A, Maurer HM: Sarcomas of the vagina and uterus: The Intergroup Rhabdomyosarcoma Study. J Pediatr Surg 20:718–724, 1985

156. Raney RB Jr, Tefft M, Lawrence W Jr, Ragab AH, Soule EH, Beltangady M, Gehan EA: Paratesticular sarcoma in childhood and adolescence: A report from the Intergroup Rhabdomyosarcoma Studies I and II, 1973–1983. Cancer 60:2337–2343, 1987

157. Lawrence W Jr, Hays DM, Moon TE: Lymphatic metastasis with childhood rhabdomyosarcoma. Cancer 39:556–559, 1977

158. Tefft M, Hays D, Raney RB Jr, Lawrence W, Soule E, Donaldson MH, Sutow WW, Gehan E: Radiation to regional nodes for rhabdomyosarcoma of the genitourinary tract in children: Is it necessary? A report from the Intergroup Rhabdomyosarcoma Study #1 (IRS-I). Cancer 45:3065–3068, 1980

159. Ransom JL, Pratt CB, Shanks E: Childhood rhabdomyosarcoma of the extremity: Results of combined modality therapy. Cancer 40:2810–2816, 1977

160. Hays DM, Sutow WW, Lawrence W Jr, Moon TE, Tefft M: Rhabdomyosarcoma: Surgical therapy in extremity lesions in children. Orthop Clin North Am 8:883–902, 1977

161. Hays DM, Soule EH, Lawrence W Jr, Gehan EA, Maurer HM, Donaldson M, Raney RB, Tefft M: Extremity lesions in the Intergroup Rhabdomyosarcoma Study (IRS-I): A preliminary report. Cancer 49:1–8, 1982

162. Heyn R, Hays D, Lawrence W, Newton W, Crist W, Tefft M, Foulkes M, Maurer H: Extremity alveolar rhabdomyosarcoma and lymph node spread: A preliminary report from the Intergroup Rhabdomyosarcoma Study (IRS)-II (abstr C-311). Proc Am Soc Clin Oncol 3:80, 1984

163. Raney RB Jr, Ragab AH, Ruymann FB, Lindberg RD, Hays DM, Gehan EA, Soule EH: Soft-tissue sarcoma of the trunk in childhood: Results of the Intergroup Rhabdomyosarcoma Study. Cancer 49:2612–2616, 1982

164. Crist WM, Raney RB Jr, Newton W, Lawrence W Jr, Tefft M, Foulkes MA: Intrathoracic soft tissue sarcomas in children. Cancer 50:598–604, 1982

165. Ransom JL, Pratt CB, Hustu HO, Mahesh Kumar AP, Howarth CB, Bowles D: Retroperitoneal rhabdomyosarcoma in children: Results of multimodality therapy. Cancer 45:845–850, 1980

166. Crist WM, Raney RB, Tefft M, Heyn R, Hays DM, Newton W, Beltangady M, Maurer HM: Soft tissue sarcomas arising in the retroperitoneal space in children: A report from the Intergroup Rhabdomyosarcoma Study (IRS) Committee. Cancer 56:2125–2132, 1985

167. Raney B, Carey A, Snyder H McC, Duckett JW, Schnaufer L, Rosenberg

HK, Mahboubi S, Chatten J, Littman P: Primary site as a prognostic variable for children with pelvic soft tissue sarcomas. J Urol 136:874–878, 1986

168. Srouji MN, Donaldson MH, Chatten J, Koblenzer CS: Perianal rhabdomyosarcoma in childhood. Cancer 38:1008–1012, 1976

169. Raney RB Jr, Donaldson MH, Sutow WW, Lindberg RD, Maurer HM, Tefft M: Special considerations related to primary site in rhabdomyosarcoma: Experience of the Intergroup Rhabdomyosarcoma Study, 1972–76. Natl Cancer Inst Monogr 56:69–74, 1981

170. Ruymann FB, Raney RB Jr, Crist WM, Lawrence W Jr, Lindberg RD, Soule EH: Rhabdomyosarcoma of the biliary tree in childhood: A report from the Intergroup Rhabdomyosarcoma Study. Cancer 56:575–581, 1985

171. Isaacson C: Embryonal rhabdomyosarcoma of the ampulla of Vater. Cancer 41:365–368, 1978

172. Mihara S, Matsumoto H, Tokunaga F, Yano H, Ota M, Yamashita S: Botryoid rhabdomyosarcoma of the gallbladder in a child. Cancer 49:812–818, 1982

173. Stanley RJ, Dehner LP, Hesker AE: Primary malignant mesenchymal tumors (mesenchymoma) of the liver in childhood: An angiographic-pathologic study of three cases. Cancer 32:973–984, 1973

174. Harris MB, Shen S, Weiner MA, Buckner H, Dasgupta I, Bleicher M, Fortner JG, Leleiko NS, Becker N, Rose J, Kasen L: Treatment of primary undifferentiated sarcoma of the liver with surgery and chemotherapy. Cancer 54:2859–2862, 1984

175. Olson JJ, Menezes AH, Godersky JC, Lobosky JM, Hart M: Primary intracranial rhabdomyosarcoma. Neurosurgery 17:25–34, 1985

176. Ferlito A, Barion U, Nicolai P: Myositis ossificans of the head and neck: Review of the literature and report of a case. Arch Otorhinolaryngol 237:103–113, 1983

177. Reid SE, Nambisan R, Karakousis CP: Pyomyositis: A differential diagnosis from sarcoma. J Surg Oncol 29:143–146, 1985

178. Wolff JA: Diagnostic procedures for evaluation of sarcomas of soft tissue and bone in childhood. Natl Cancer Inst Monogr 56:3–7, 1981

179. Lusher JM: Chloroma as a presenting feature of acute leukemia. A report of two cases in children. Am J Dis Child 108:62–66, 1964

180. Matus-Ridley M, Raney RB Jr, Thawerani H, Meadows AT: Histiocytosis X in children: Patterns of disease and results of treatment. Med Pediatr Oncol 11:99–105, 1983

181. Ruymann FB, Newton WA Jr, Ragab AH, Donaldson MH, Foulkes M: Bone marrow metastases at diagnosis in children and adolescents with rhabdomyosarcoma: A report from the Intergroup Rhabdomyosarcoma Study. Cancer 53:368–373, 1984

182. Hutchinson RJ, Shapiro SA, Raney RB Jr: Elevated parathyroid hormone levels in association with rhabdomyosarcoma. J Pediatr 92:780–781, 1978

183. Quddus FF, Espinola D, Kramer SS, Leventhal BG: Comparison between x-ray and bone scan detection of bone metastases in patients with rhabdomyosarcoma. Med Pediatr Oncol 11:125–129, 1983

184. Weinblatt ME, Miller JH: Radionuclide scanning in children with rhabdomyosarcoma. Med Pediatr Oncol 9:293–301, 1981

185. Raney RB Jr, Zimmerman RA, Bilaniuk LT, Littman P, Mandell G, Potsic W: Management of craniofacial sarcoma in childhood assisted by computed tomography. Int J Radiat Oncol Biol Phys 5:529–534, 1979

186. Baker ME, Silverman PM, Korobkin M: Computer tomography of prostatic and bladder rhabdomyosarcomas. J Comput Assist Tomogr 9:780–783, 1985

187. Kneeland JB, Lee BCP, Whalen JP, Knowles RJR, Cahill PT: NMR: The new frontier in diagnostic radiology. Adv Surg 18:37–65, 1984

188. Packer RJ, Zimmerman RA, Bilaniuk LT, Leurssen TG, Sutton LN, Bruce DA, Schut L: Magnetic resonance imaging of lesions of the posterior fossa and upper cervical cord in childhood. Pediatrics 76:84–90, 1985

189. Ghavimi F, Exelby PR, Lieberman PH, Scott BF, Kosloff C: Multidisciplinary treatment of embryonal rhabdomyosarcoma in children: A progress report. Natl Cancer Inst Monogr 56:111–120, 1981

190. Donaldson SS, Belli JA: A rational clinical staging system for childhood rhabdomyosarcoma. J Clin Oncol 2:135–139, 1984

191. Maurer HM: The Intergroup Rhabdomyosarcoma Study (N.I.H.): Objectives and clinical staging classification. J Pediatr Surg 10:977–978, 1975

192. Pedrick TJ, Donaldson SS, Cox RS: Rhabdomyosarcoma: The Stanford experience using a TNM staging system. J Clin Oncol 4:370–378, 1986

193. Lawrence W Jr, Gehan EA, Hays DM, Beltangady M, Maurer HM: Prognostic significance of staging factors of the UICC staging system in childhood rhabdomyosarcoma: A report from the Intergroup Rhabdomyosarcoma Study (IRS-II). J Clin Oncol 5:46–54, 1987

194. Gehan EA: Minutes of the IRS Committee Meeting, November 6–7, 1986

195. Gehan EA, Glover FN, Maurer HM, Sutow WW, Hays DH, Lawrence W Jr, Newton WA Jr, Soule EH: Prognostic factors in children with rhabdomyosarcoma. Natl Cancer Inst Monogr 56:83–92, 1981

196. D'Angio GJ, Clatworthy HW, Evans AE, Newton WA Jr, Tefft M: Is the risk of morbidity and rare mortality worth the cure? Cancer 41:377–380, 1978

197. Okamura J, Sutow WW, Moon TE: Prognosis in children with metastatic sarcoma. Med Pediatr Oncol 3:243–251, 1977

198. Maurer H, Foulkes M, Gehan E: Intergroup Rhabdomyosarcoma Study (IRS) II: Preliminary report (abstr C-274). Proc Am Soc Clin Oncol 2:70, 1983

199. Hays DM, Newton W Jr, Soule EH, Foulkes MA, Raney RB, Tefft M, Ragab A, Maurer HM: Mortality among children with rhabdomyosarcomas of the alveolar histologic subtype. J Pediatr Surg 18:412–417, 1983

200. Neifeld JP, Maurer HM, Godwin D, Berg JW, Salzberg AM: Prognostic variables in pediatric rhabdomyosarcoma before and after multimodal therapy. J Pediatr Surg 14:699–703, 1979

201. Maurer HM: The Intergroup Rhabdomyosarcoma Study: Update, November 1978. Natl Cancer Inst Monogr 56:61–68, 1981

202. Maurer HM, Moon T, Donaldson M, Fernandez C, Gehan EA, Hammond D, Hays DM, Lawrence W, Jr, Newton W, Ragab A, Raney B, Soule EH, Sutow WW, Tefft M: The Intergroup Rhabdomyosarcoma Study: A preliminary report. Cancer 40:2015–2026, 1977

203. Olive D, Flamant F, Zucker JM, Voute P, Brunat–Mentigny M, Otten J, Dutou L: Paraaortic lymphadenectomy is not necessary in the treatment of localized paratesticular rhabdomyosarcoma. Cancer 54:1283–1287, 1984

204. Hays DM: Rhabdomyosarcoma and other soft tissue sarcomas. In Hays DM: Pediatric Surgical Oncology, pp 87–122. New York, Grune & Stratton, 1986

205. Suit HD, Russell WO, Martin RG: Management of patients with sarcoma of soft tissue in an extremity. Cancer 31:1247–1255, 1973

206. Perry H, Chu FCH: Radiation therapy in the palliative management of soft tissue sarcomas. Cancer 15:179–183, 1962

207. McNeer GP, Cantin J, Chu F, Nickson JJ: Effectiveness of radiation therapy in the management of sarcoma of the soft somatic tissues. Cancer 22:391–397, 1968

208. Dritschilo A, Weichselbaum R, Cassady JR, Jaffe N, Green D, Friller RM: The role of radiation therapy in the treatment of soft tissue sarcomas of childhood. Cancer 42:1192–1203, 1978

209. Nelson AJ III: Embryonal rhabdomyosarcoma: Report of twenty-four cases and study of the effectiveness of radiation therapy upon the primary tumor. Cancer 22:64–68, 1968

210. Cassady JR, Sagerman RH, Tretter P, Ellsworth RM: Radiation therapy for rhabdomyosarcoma. Radiology 91:116–120, 1968

211. Jereb B, Cham W, Lattin P, Exelby P, Ghavimi F, D'Angio GJ, Tefft M: Local control of embryonal rhabdomyosarcoma in children by radiation therapy when combined with concomitant chemotherapy. Int J Radiat Oncol Biol Phys 1:217–225, 1976

212. Heyn RM, Holland R, Newton WA Jr, Tefft M, Breslow N, Hartmann JR: The role of combined chemotherapy in the treatment of rhabdomyosarcoma in children. Cancer 34:2128–2142, 1974

213. Maurer HM: The Intergroup Rhabdomyosarcoma Study II: Objectives and study design. J Pediatr Surg 15:371–372, 1980

214. Tefft M, Lindberg RD, Gehan EA: Radiation therapy combined with systemic chemotherapy of rhabdomyosarcoma in children: Local control in patients enrolled in the Intergroup Rhabdomyosarcoma Study. Natl Cancer Inst Monogr 56:75–81, 1981

215. Tefft M, Lattin PB, Jereb B, Cham W, Ghavimi F, Rosen G, Exelby P, Marcove R, Murphy ML, D'Angio GJ: Acute and late effects on normal tissues following combined chemo- and radiotherapy for childhood rhabdomyosarcoma and Ewing's sarcoma. Cancer 37:1201–1217, 1976

216. Tefft M, Wharam M, Ruymann F, Foulkes M, Gehan E: Radiotherapy (RT) for rhabdomyosarcoma in children: A report from the Intergroup Rhabdomyosarcoma Study #2 (IRS-2) (abstr C-909). Proc Am Soc Clin Oncol 4:234, 1985

217. Tefft M, Wharam M, Gehan E: Radiation therapy in embryonal rhabdomyosarcoma (ERS): Local control (LC) in children less than one year of age and in children with tumors of the orbit (abstr 803). Proc Am Soc Clin Oncol 5:205, 1986

218. Raney RB Jr, Crist WM, Maurer HM, Foulkes M: Prognosis of children with soft tissue sarcoma who relapse after achieving a complete response: A report from the Intergroup Rhabdomyosarcoma Study I. Cancer 52:44–50, 1983

219. Stowe SM, Littman P, Wara W, Raney RB, Tefft M: The use of implantation

in childhood tumors: The experience of the Children's Cancer Study Group member institutions (abstr 16). Am J Clin Oncol (CCT) 5:129, 1982

220. Novaes PERS: Interstitial therapy in the management of soft-tissue sarcomas in childhood. Med Pediatr Oncol 13:221–224, 1985

221. Flamant F, Chassagne D, Cosset J-M, Gerbaulet A, Lemerle J: Embryonal rhabdomyosarcoma of the vagina in children: Conservative treatment with curietherapy and chemotherapy. Eur J Cancer 15:527–532, 1979

222. Curran WJ, Littman P, Raney RB: Interstitial radiation therapy in the treatment of childhood soft tissue sarcomas. Int J Radiat Oncol Biol Phys 14:169–174, 1988

223. Kaufman BH, Gunderson LL, Evans RG, Burgert EO Jr, Gilchrist GS, Smithson WA: Intraoperative irradiation: A new technique in pediatric oncology. J Pediatr Surg 19:861–862, 1984

224. Tefft M: Radiation effect on growing bone and cartilage. In Vaeth JM: Frontiers of Radiation Therapy and Oncology, vol 6, pp 389–411. Basel, S Karger, 1972

225. Parker RG, Berry HC: Late effects of therapeutic irradiation on the skeleton and bone marrow. Cancer 37:1162–1171, 1976

226. Wohl MEB, Briscom NT, Traggis DG, Jaffe N: Effects of therapeutic irradiation delivered in early childhood upon subsequent lung function. Pediatrics 55:507–516, 1975

227. Probert JC, Parker BR, Kaplan HS: Growth retardation in children after megavoltage irradiation of the spine. Cancer 32:634–639, 1973

228. Pinkel D: Actinomycin D in childhood cancer: A preliminary report. Pediatrics 23:342–347, 1959

229. Tan CTC, Dargeon HW, Burchenal JH: The effect of actinomycin D on cancer in childhood. Pediatrics 24:544–561, 1959

230. Shaw RK, Moore EW, Mueller PS, Frei E III, Watkin DM: The effect of actinomycin D on childhood neoplasms. Am J Dis Child 99:628–635, 1960

231. Haddy TB, Nora AH, Sutow WW, Vietti TJ: Cyclophosphamide treatment for metastatic soft tissue sarcoma: Intermittent large doses in the treatment of children. Am J Dis Child 114:301–308, 1967

232. Sutow WW: Cyclophosphamide (NSC-26271) in Wilms' tumor and rhabdomyosarcoma. Cancer Chemother Rep 51:407–409, 1967

233. Sutow WW, Berry DH, Haddy TB, Sullivan MP, Watkins WL, Windmiller J: Vincristine sulfate therapy in children with metastatic soft tissue sarcoma. Pediatrics 38:465–472, 1966

234. Sutow WW: Vincristine (NSC-67574) therapy for malignant solid tumors in children (except Wilms' tumor). Cancer Chemother Rep 52:485–487, 1968

235. Selawry OS, Holland JR, Wolman IJ: Effect of vincristine (NSC-67574) on malignant solid tumors in children. Cancer Chemother Rep 52:497–500, 1968

236. Bonadonna G, Monfardini S, DeLena M, Fossati-Bellani F, Beretta G: Phase I and preliminary Phase II evaluation of Adriamycin (NSC-123127). Cancer Res 30:2572–2582, 1970

237. O'Bryan RM, Luce JK, Talley RW, Gottlieb JA, Baker LH, Bonadonna G: Phase II evaluation of Adriamycin in human neoplasia. Cancer 32:1–8, 1973

238. Tan C, Etcubanas E, Wollner N, Rosen G, Gilladoga A, Showel J, Murphy ML, Krakoff IH: Adriamycin—An antitumor antibiotic in the treatment of neoplastic diseases. Cancer 32:9–17, 1973

239. Sutow WW, Vietti TJ, Lonsdale D, Talley RW: Daunomycin in the treatment of metastatic soft tissue sarcoma in children. Cancer 29:1293–1297, 1972

240. Sitarz AL, Heyn R, Murphy ML, Origenes ML Jr, Severo NC: Triple drug therapy with actinomycin D (NSC-3053), chlorambucil (NSC-3088), and methotrexate (NSC-740) in metastatic solid tumors in children. Cancer Chemother Rep 45:45–51, 1965

241. Green DM: Evaluation of single-dose vincristine, actinomycin D, and cyclophosphamide in childhood solid tumors. Cancer Treat Rep 62:1517–1520, 1978

242. Gottlieb JA, Baker LH, Quagliana JM, Luce JK, Whitecar JP Jr, Sinkovics JG, Rivkin SE, Brownlee R, Frei E III: Chemotherapy of sarcomas with a combination of Adriamycin and dimethyl triazeno imidazole carboxamide. Cancer 30:1632–1638, 1972

243. Wilbur JR: Combination chemotherapy for embryonal rhabdomyosarcoma. Cancer Chemother Rep 58:281–284, 1974

244. James DH, Hustu O, Wrenn EL, Johnson WW: Childhood malignant tumors: Concurrent chemotherapy with dactinomycin and vincristine sulfate. JAMA 197:1043–1045, 1966

245. Pratt CB: Response of childhood rhabdomyosarcoma to combination chemotherapy. J Pediatr 74:791–794, 1969

246. Holton CP, Chapman KE, Lackey RW, Hatch EI, Baum ES, Favara BE: Extended combination therapy of childhood rhabdomyosarcoma. Cancer 32:1310–1316, 1973

247. Razek AA, Perez CA, Lee FA, Ragab AH, Askin F, Vietti T: Combined treatment modalities of rhabdomyosarcoma in children. Cancer 39:2415–2421, 1977

248. Gornall P, Mann JR, Corkery JJ, Cameron AH: Recent experience in the treatment of rhabdomyosarcoma. J Pediatr Surg 14:38–40, 1979

249. Pratt CB, Hustu HO, Mahesh Kumar AP, Johnson WW, Ransom JL, Howarth CB, George SL: Treatment of childhood rhabdomyosarcoma at St. Jude Children's Research Hospital, 1962–78. Natl Cancer Inst Monogr 56:93–101, 1981

250. Pullen DJ, Dyment PG, Humphrey GB, Lane DM, Ragab AH: Combined chemotherapy in childhood rhabdomyosarcoma. Cancer Chemother Rep 59:359–365, 1965

251. Kingston JE, McElwain TJ, Malpas JS: Childhood rhabdomyosarcoma: Experience of the Children's Solid Tumor Group. Br J Cancer 48:195–207, 1983

252. Ghavimi F, Exelby PR, Lieberman PH, Scott BF, Kosloff C: Multidisciplinary treatment of embryonal rhabdomyosarcoma in children: A progress report. Natl Cancer Inst Monogr 56:111–120, 1981

253. Heyn R, Holland R, Joo P, Johnson D, Newton W Jr, Tefft M, Breslow N, Hammond D: Treatment of rhabdomyosarcoma in children with surgery, radiotherapy and chemotherapy. Med Pediatr Oncol 3:21–32, 1977

254. Raney RB Jr: Combination chemotherapy for children with malignant solid tumors. In Hays DM: Pediatric Surgical Oncology, pp 21–36. New York, Grune & Stratton, 1986

255. Baum ES, Gaynon P, Greenberg L, Krivit W, Hammond D: Phase II trial of cisplatin in refractory childhood cancer: Children's Cancer Study Group Report. Cancer Treat Rep 65:815–822, 1981

256. Chard RL Jr, Krivit W, Bleyer WA, Hammond D: Phase II study of VP-16-213 in childhood malignant disease: A Children's Cancer Study Group report. Cancer Treat Rep 63:1755–1759, 1979

257. Luce JK, Thurman WG, Isaacs BL, Talley RW: Clinical trials with the antitumor agent 5-(3,3-dimethyl-l-triazene) imidazole-4-carboxamide (NSC-45388). Cancer Chemother Rep 54:119–124, 1970

258. Finkelstein JZ, Albo V, Ertel I, Hammond D: 5-(3,3-dimethyl-l-triazeno) imidazole-4-carboxamide (NSC-45388) in the treatment of solid tumors in children. Cancer Chemother Rep 59:351–357, 1975

259. Goldie JH, Coldman AJ: The genetic origin of drug resistance in neoplasms: Implications for systemic therapy. Cancer Res 44:3643–3653, 1984

260. Miser JS, Kinsella TJ, Triche TJ, Tsokos M, Jarosinski P, Foquer R, Wesley R, Magrath I: Ifosfamide with mesna uroprotection and etoposide: An effective regimen in the treatment of recurrent sarcomas and other tumors of children and young adults. J Clin Oncol 5:1191–1198, 1987

261. Bode U: Methotrexate as relapse therapy for rhabdomyosarcoma. Am J Pediatr Hematol Oncol 8:70–72, 1986

262. Houghton JA, Cook RL, Lutz PJ, Houghton PJ: Melphalan: A potential new agent in the treatment of childhood rhabdomyosarcoma. Cancer Treat Rep 69:91–96, 1985

263. Horowitz ME, Etcubanas E, Christensen ML, Houghton JA, George SL, Green AA, Houghton PJ: Phase II testing of melphalan in children with newly diagnosed rhabdomyosarcoma: A model for anticancer drug development. J Clin Oncol 6:308–314, 1988

264. Crist W, Raney RB, Ragab A, Heyn R, Wharam M, Webber B, Johnston J, Beltangady M: Intensive chemotherapy including cisplatin with or without etoposide for children with soft-tissue sarcomas. Med Pediatr Oncol 15:51–57, 1987

265. Raney RB Jr: Inefficacy of cisplatin and etoposide as salvage therapy for children with recurrent or unresponsive soft issue sarcoma. Cancer Treat Rep 71:407–408, 1987

266. Byrd RL, Rohrbaugh TM, Raney RB Jr, Norris DG: Transient cortical blindness secondary to vincristine therapy in childhood malignancies. Cancer 47:37–40, 1981

267. Blachley JD, Hill JB: Renal and electrolyte disturbances associated with cis-platinum. Ann Intern Med 95:628–632, 1981

268. Lentz RD, Bergstein J, Steffes MW, Brown DR, Prem K, Michael AF, Vernier RL: Postpubertal evaluation of gonadal function following cyclophosphamide therapy before and during puberty. J Pediatr 91:385–394, 1977

269. Goorin AM, Borow KM, Goldman A, Williams RG, Henderson IC, Sallan SE, Cohen H, Jaffe N: Congestive heart failure due to Adriamycin cardiotoxicity: Its natural history in children. Cancer 47:2810–2816, 1981

270. Etcubanas E, Rao B, Kumar M, Horowitz M, Pratt C, Hustu O, Vogel R:

Delayed surgery and local tumor control in childhood rhabdomyosarcoma (abstr C-302). Proc Am Soc Clin Oncol 3:78, 1984

271. Tefft M, Fernandez CH, Moon TE: Rhabdomyosarcoma: Response to chemotherapy prior to radiation in patients with gross residual disease. Cancer 39:665–670, 1977

272. Phillips T, Fu K: Quantification of combined radiation therapy and chemotherapy effects on critical normal tissues. Cancer 37:1186–1200, 1976

273. Raney RB Jr, Gehan EA, Hays DM, Tefft M, Newton WA Jr, Maurer HM: Primary chemotherapy with or without radiation therapy, surgery, or both for children with localized sarcoma of special pelvic sites (bladder, prostate, vagina, uterus, cervix) in Intergroup Rhabdomyosarcoma Study (IRS)-II: Comparison of results with IRS-I. Cancer (submitted)

274. Raney B, Crist W, Hays D, Newton W, Ruymann F, Tefft M: Soft tissue sarcoma of the perineal-anal region in childhood: A report from the Intergroup Rhabdomyosarcoma Study (IRS) Committee (abstr 822). Proc Am Soc Clin Oncol 5:209, 1986

275. Raney RB Jr, Gehan EA, Maurer HM, Newton WA Jr, Ragab AH, Ruymann RB, Sutow WW, Tefft M: Evaluation of intensified chemotherapy in children with advanced rhabdomyosarcoma. Cancer Clin Trials 2:19–28, 1979

276. Ragab AH, Heyn R, Tefft M, Hays DM, Newton WA Jr, Beltangady M: Infants younger than 1 year of age with rhabdomyosarcoma. Cancer 58:2606–2610, 1986

277. Fusner JE, Poplack DG, Pizzo PA, DiChiro G: Leukoencephalopathy following chemotherapy for rhabdomyosarcoma: Reversibility of cerebral changes demonstrated by computed tomography. J Pediatr 91:77–79, 1977

278. Heyn RM: Late effects of therapy in rhabdomyosarcoma. Clin Oncol 4:287–297, 1985

279. Fromm M, Littman P, Raney RB, Nelson L, Handler S, Diamond G, Stanley C: Late effects after treatment of twenty children with soft tissue sarcomas of the head and neck: Experience at a single institution with a review of the literature. Cancer 57:2070–2076, 1986

280. Hazra TA, Shipman B: Dental problems in pediatric patients with head and neck tumors undergoing multiple modality therapy. Med Pediatr Oncol 10:91–95, 1982

281. Heyn R, Ragab A, Raney RB Jr, Ruymann F, Tefft M, Lawrence W Jr, Soule E, Maurer HM: Late effects of therapy in orbital rhabdomyosarcoma in children: A report from the Intergroup Rhabdomyosarcoma Study. Cancer 57:1738–1743, 1986

282. Jaffe N: Non-oncogenic sequelae of cancer chemotherapy. Radiology 114:167–173, 1975

283. Jayalakshmamma B, Pinkel D: Urinary-bladder toxicity following pelvic irradiation and simultaneous cyclophosphamide therapy. Cancer 38:701–707, 1976

284. Meyers PA, Ghavimi F: Secondary acute non-lymphoblastic leukemia (ANLL) following treatment of childhood rhabdomyosarcoma (RMS) (abstr C-300). Proc Am Soc Clin Oncol 2:77, 1983

thirty-one

Ewing's Sarcoma and the Nonrhabdomyosarcoma Soft Tissue Sarcomas of Childhood

James S. Miser,
Timothy J. Triche,
Douglas J. Pritchard, and
Timothy Kinsella

Ewing's sarcoma is the second most common malignant bone tumor of children and young adults and accounts for about 1% of all childhood tumors.[1] The original report of this tumor described it to be of endothelial origin on the basis of the appearance of the tumor "in broad sheets of polyhedral cells without intervening stroma" and the close approximation of the tumor cells with primitive vascular channels.[2] Although the origin of Ewing's sarcoma has not yet been definitively determined, a recent report suggests that the tumor may not be of endothelial origin as initially thought but derived instead from primitive neural tissue.[3] Dr. Ewing's clinical description in 1921 was of a tumor that arose in the shaft of the long bones, often with sparing of the ends, that was not associated with bone production but rather with diffuse alteration of the bone structure, and that was radiosensitive.[2] All these features were in contrast to the more common bone tumor, osteogenic sarcoma. His pathologic description follows:

The growth was composed of broad sheets of small polyhedral cells with pale cytoplasm, small hyperchromatic nuclei, well-defined cell borders, and complete absence of intracellular material. Hydropic degeneration often affects large islands of cells, in which only nuclei and cell borders are visible. . . . In some sections the cells were of increased size, while in others they were smaller and more compact, and approached the morphology of plasma cells.[2]

Few additional criteria for the description of Ewing's sarcoma have been used over the past 65 years.

EPIDEMIOLOGY

Ewing's sarcoma occurs most frequently in the early portion to midportion of the second decade of life.[4,5] The tumor rarely occurs in children younger than 5 years of age and is equally uncommon in adults older than 30.[4,5] Although there is no difference in incidence related to sex in prepubertal individuals, in adolescence there is a slight preponderance of boys.[4] The most striking epidemiologic feature of this tumor is its very low incidence in blacks and Chinese (see Chaps. 1 and 2).[1,6–9] Its extreme rarity in these populations is in contrast to the incidence of Ewing's sarcoma in white children in the United States younger than 15 years of age: 1.7 cases per million individuals per year.

Unlike many of the pediatric tumors that occur in children younger than 5 years of age, Ewing's sarcoma has not been associated with any known congenital syndromes.[10] A recent preliminary review, however, has suggested an association with skeletal anomalies (*i.e.,* enchondroma, aneurysmal bone cyst) and genitourinary anomalies (*i.e.,* hypospadias, reduplication of the renal collecting system).[10] Others have reported the association of Ewing's sarcoma with the hereditary retinoblastoma syndrome.[11]

GENETICS

Although three pairs of siblings with Ewing's sarcoma have been described, there is no known pattern of hereditary transmission and no known constitutional karyotypic abnormality in patients with Ewing's sarcoma. Recently, a t(11:22) chromosomal translocation was discovered in tumor cells from both short-term tissue culture of Ewing's sarcoma and tumor cell lines derived from Ewing's sarcoma (see Chap. 3).[12,13] This chromosomal translocation has also been found in association with peripheral neuroepithelioma (PN), another small round cell tumor of children and young adults that is clearly of neural origin (see Chap. 29).[14] This common finding suggests that these tumors may be related both in cell of origin and mechanism of oncogenesis. Although this translocation has been a virtually constant feature of Ewing's cells evaluated in culture, there has as yet been no clear evidence that a particular oncogene is involved in the pathogenesis of this tumor. The pattern of oncogene expression, however, is indistinguishable from that seen with peripheral neuroepithelioma and very different from other tumors studied: c-*myc*, c-*myb*, c-*mil/raf*, and c-*src* are all expressed in similar levels in these tumors; c-*sis* is translocated from chromosome 22 to chromosome 11 but is not expressed; c-*ets*, located near the breakpoint on chromosome 11, is variably expressed.[16,17] These findings further suggest that a common cell of origin or mechanism of oncogenesis exists for these two tumors (see Chaps. 3 and 6).[15] High levels of choline acetyltransferase in both PN and Ewing's sarcoma suggests that this origin is neural.[15]

In contrast to the findings in Wilms' tumor and retinoblastoma,[16,17] the lack of a constitutional karyotypic abnormality in patients with Ewing's sarcoma suggests that the oncogenesis of this tumor is not likely to be due to the deletion of an antioncogene resulting in the homozygous recessive expression of specific genetic locus. Rather, it seems more likely that the specific t(11:22) or perhaps another cytogenetic finding will be associated with a dominantly expressed oncogene that is responsible for the oncogenesis of this tumor.

BIOLOGICAL STUDIES

The cell of origin of Ewing's sarcoma has not as yet been established. Early ultrastructural studies have been interpreted as providing evidence of a mesenchymal, an osteoblastic, an endothelial, and even a myelogenous origin.[18–21] In a detailed study of three established Ewing's cell lines in tissue culture, production of types I, III, and IV collagen was demonstrated. In contrast to osteosarcomas that produce principally type I collagen, chondrosarcomas that produce type II collagen, and fibrosarcomas that produce predominantly type III collagen, the Ewing's cells produced these three types of collagen simultaneously. This ability of the cells of Ewing's sarcoma to produce small amounts of three types of collagen supported the conclusion that Ewing's sarcoma was a tumor derived from primitive mesenchymal cells that are not yet committed to fibroblastic, osteoblastic, chondroblastic, endothelial, or myogenous differentiation.[21]

In contrast, because the t(11:22) translocation is shared by Ewing's sarcoma and peripheral neuroepithelioma, a tumor with clear ultrastructural and immunocytochemical evidence of a neural phenotype, it has been hypothesized that Ewing's sarcoma may, in fact, be of neural origin as well. A recent study of Ewing's sarcoma cell lines treated with differentiating agents under controlled conditions *in vitro* demonstrated that the cells exhibit a neural phenotype.[3] These *in vitro* data supported by the finding of choline acetyltransferase within the cells[15] provide biological data that these tumors may actually be neural in origin.

PATHOGENESIS AND NATURAL HISTORY

Except for the possible association with skeletal and genitourinary anomalies, there is no clearly predisposing process that underlies the development of Ewing's sarcoma.[10] Specifically, previous ionizing irradiation is not associated with the development of Ewing's sarcoma.[10] Although there is frequently a history of trauma in patients with Ewing's sarcoma, the role bone injury plays is not clear. It most likely represents just the event that brings attention to the malignant lesion.

The natural history of Ewing's sarcoma when treated only with local management, either radiation or surgery alone, has been clearly described: the 5- and 10-year survival rates for patients treated in this fashion were 12% and 9%, respectively, in one large retrospective series.[22] Further, the mortality rate 2 years after the diagnosis was greater than 70% for patients so treated.[22] Thus Ewing's sarcoma is a highly malignant lesion associated with systemic disease in most patients.

FIGURE 31-1. Schematic diagram of the differential diagnosis of Ewing's sarcoma. Although virtually any undifferentiated tumor could be considered, careful adherence to certain light microscopic criteria—such as whether the tumor is truly a round cell tumor, arises in bone, has nondescript ultrastructure, and is negative for all common immunocytochemical markers other than vimentin (by conventional Sternberger PAP immunocytochemistry)—will exclude these others. Unfortunately, at this time, the diagnosis of Ewing's sarcoma is a diagnosis of exclusion. No specific pathologic features are known.

Differential Diagnosis of Ewing's Sarcoma

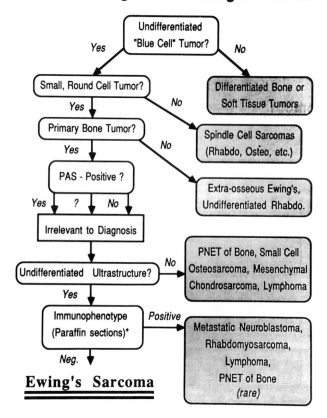

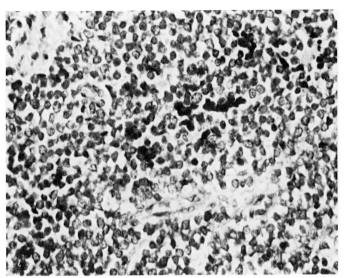
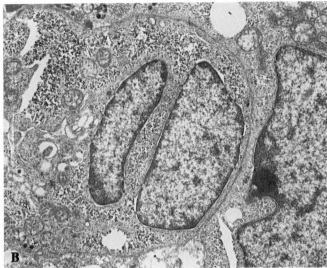

FIGURE 31-2. **Typical Ewing's sarcoma. A.** Light microscopy. The tumor is truly a round cell tumor with a dichotomous cell population of larger, clearer cells and smaller, darker cells. The nuclei are generally round to oval with a bland appearance that belies the strikingly malignant behavior of the tumor. No stroma (other than normal fibrovascular stroma) is present in this tumor. The histology is generally diffuse and unstructured. (H & E; original magnification × 250) **B.** Electron microscopy. The dominant feature by EM is the presence of cytoplasmic pools of glycogen, often admixed with scattered cytoplasmic organelles. The cytoplasm is otherwise nondescript and devoid of organelles other than polyribosomes. The nuclei often appear more convoluted by EM than LM, as here, where a nuclear groove creates the illusion of a binucleate cell. (UA/Pb Cit; original magnification × 12,000)

PATHOLOGY

Differential Diagnosis

The differential diagnosis of Ewing's sarcoma includes all the common solid tumors of childhood when they present in their primitive or undifferentiated form. These so-called small round blue cell tumors of childhood (see also Chap. 6) include Ewing's sarcoma; primary bone sarcomas (including small cell osteosarcoma and mesenchymal chondrosarcoma); rhabdomyosarcoma; lymphoma; metastatic neuroblastoma; and primitive neuroectodermal tumors (including the so-called Askin tumor of chest wall).

Ewing's sarcoma is a diagnosis of exclusion. The tumor possesses no unique morphologic markers that would allow reliable distinction from the other small round cell tumors. In contrast, each of the other diagnostic considerations possesses specific features that generally allow ready diagnosis, especially when specialized diagnostic techniques such as electron microscopy or immunocytochemistry are used. Thus the diagnosis of Ewing's sarcoma depends on the absence of any specific features that would exclude Ewing's from consideration. For convenience, these features can be categorized as light microscopic, ultrastructural, and immunocytochemical. For practical purposes, the diagnosis is approached in the sequence shown by the decision-tree in Figure 31-1.

Light Microscopic Criteria

By definition, Ewing's sarcoma, as described by James Ewing,[2] is an undifferentiated round cell tumor. This is manifest at the light microscopic level as a diffuse mass of tumor cells of similar appearance. The tumor may often present a biphasic population of larger, clear cells and smaller, dark cells (Fig. 31-2). In either case, the tumor generally infiltrates bone mar-

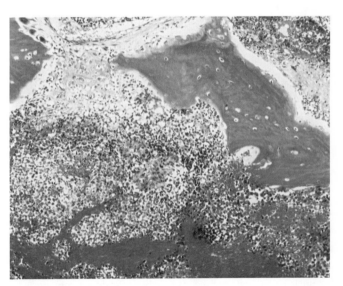

FIGURE 31-3. Light microscopy of typical Ewing's sarcoma in bone. The tumor generally replaces marrow elements but generally does not disturb bony trabeculae or cortex. Despite this, cortical permeation leads to rapid development of an extraosseous tumor component (see Fig. 31-4). (H & E; original magnification × 100)

row with surprisingly little destruction (Fig. 31-3) and in almost all cases secondarily involves adjacent soft tissues by diffuse infiltration (Fig. 31-4). Usually, the borders of tumor infiltration are infiltrative or "pushing"; however, in some cases, finger-like processes of compact, basophilic, tumor cell masses are seen to intertwine and form a lace-like or "filigree" pattern (Fig. 31-5). This particular pattern has been associated

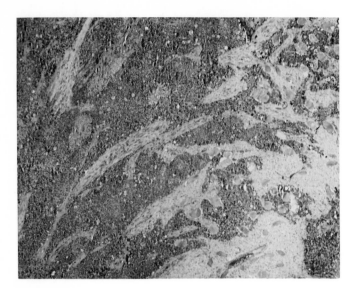

FIGURE 31-4. Light microscopy of soft tissue component of Ewing's sarcoma. The cytology is the same, but the pattern of infiltration is different. The architecture is diffuse, tending to lobular with (often) finger-like projections of infiltrating tumor, especially along fascial or periosteal planes. Entrapment of skeletal muscle is common, as here (*upper right*), and invasion of myotubes has been reported. (H & E; original magnification × 40)

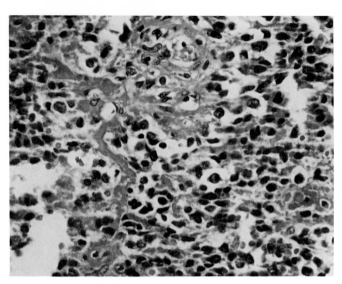

FIGURE 31-6. Small cell osteosarcoma. Although cytologically similar to Ewing's sarcoma, this tumor is distinguished by its production of osteoid stroma (seen here as homogeneous extracellular deposits). The amount is always scanty, focal, and sometimes absent in metastases or limited biopsies, thereby complicating this tumor's separation from Ewing's sarcoma. Ultrastructural analysis is definitive when available (see text). (H & E; original magnification × 250)

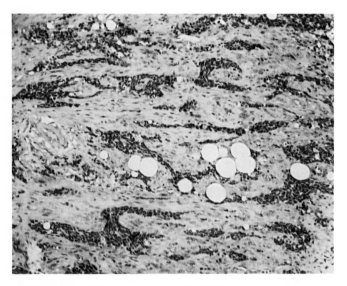

FIGURE 31-5. Filigree pattern in Ewing's sarcoma. Although no histologic or cytologic parameters have been linked with prognosis in Ewing's sarcoma in the past, recent publications have associated the pattern of soft tissue infiltration seen here (termed the *filigree* pattern) with poor prognosis. The tumor cells seen here, although condensed and hyperchromatic, are not effete or crushed when examined by EM. (H & E; original magnification × 100)

with a poorer prognosis by both the Intergroup Ewing's Sarcoma Study[23] and a group from the Institut Gustav Roussy and the University d' Valencia. This latter group also found that the presence of widespread tumor cell necrosis also predicted a poor-prognosis tumor.[24]

The most common clue to an incorrect diagnosis of Ewing's sarcoma is detection of atypical features by light mi-

croscopy. Many cases of poorly differentiated or undifferentiated variants of common entities are inadvertently diagnosed as Ewing's sarcoma. Some of the common entities that must be distinguished from Ewing's sarcoma follow (see also Chap. 6).

SMALL CELL OSTEOSARCOMA. Although an uncommon form of osteosarcoma, small cell osteosarcoma can appear identical to Ewing's sarcoma on superficial examination (Fig. 31-6) (see also Chap. 32).[25,26] A second entity, mesenchymal chondrosarcoma, is a closely related entity that presents as a small round cell tumor in association with malignant cartilage.[27-29] The most important distinguishing feature of these tumors is the presence of extracellular matrix, malignant osteoid in the case of small cell osteosarcoma and malignant chondroid in the case of mesenchymal chondrosarcoma. Ewing's sarcoma has none. This becomes apparent when conventional light microscopic special stains are used: reticulin and PAS with diastase (see Chap. 6). Neither stain reveals evidence of collagenous stroma (*i.e.,* positive extracellular staining) between Ewing's sarcoma tumor cells (Fig. 31-7). Virtually all other sarcomas (and occasional cases of lymphoma) will show some degree of extracellular matrix. In Ewing's sarcoma some such material will be present around blood vessels or adjacent to fibrous septae, for example, but will not extend beyond these areas.

UNDIFFERENTIATED PRIMARY SARCOMA OF BONE. In some cases, diagnostic osteoid or cartilage cannot be identified in a tumor that is otherwise too pleomorphic, contains some spindle cells, displays prominent fibrous matrix, or otherwise deviates too far from the usual descriptions of Ewing's sarcoma of bone as described and illustrated above. One such example is illustrated in Figure 31-8. Such tumors are virtually impossible to more precisely categorize by light microscopy alone. We have described these tumors as primary sarcomas of bone, recognizing that they may represent a heterogeneous group of tumors. Some will certainly prove to be small cell osteosarcoma or mesenchymal chondrosarcoma if osteoid or cartilage,

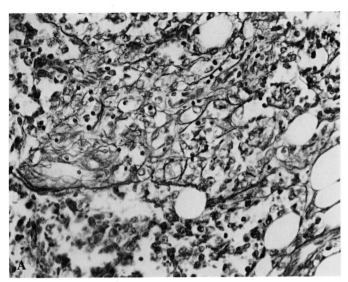
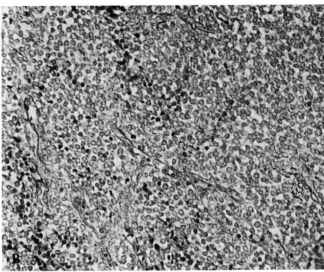

FIGURE 31-7. Comparison of small cell osteosarcoma and Ewing's sarcoma by reticulin stain. **A.** Small cell osteosarcoma. The scant stroma produced by this tumor is more easily detected by reticulin stain, as seen here. Individual tumor cells are enveloped by a halo of fine reticulin fibers that presumably represent beginning osteoid formation, since both are composed of type I collagen fibers. Other areas (*bottom*) are devoid of stroma, emphasizing the focal nature of the process. (Reticulin; original magnification × 250) **B.** Ewing's sarcoma. Stroma in this tumor is limited to vascular septae or occasional fascial planes. No extracellular matrix is deposited by Ewing's tumor cells, and therefore only preexisting stroma is identified. Individual tumor cells are never enveloped by reticulin fibers. (Reticulin; original magnification × 250)

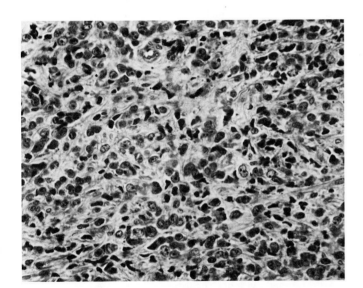

FIGURE 31-8. Primary sarcoma of bone. These primitive, primary bone tumors superficially resemble Ewing's sarcoma, but closer examination reveals a more pleomorphic tumor cell population, often with easily identified fibrous stroma, as here. However, no osteoid or cartilage is found, and these tumors cannot be precisely categorized as osteosarcoma, chondrosarcoma, or the like. At present, it is not clear whether these tumors are nascent true bone sarcomas related to small cell osteosarcoma and mesenchymal chondrosarcoma or are, instead, a heterogeneous group of tumors of unknown origin. (H & E; original magnification × 250)

respectively, are eventually identified; others may represent malignant fibrous histiocytoma of bone.[30] Others may be sarcomas that uncommonly arise in bone: rhabdomyosarcoma,

angiosarcoma, leiomyosarcoma, neurofibrosarcoma, and other soft tissue sarcomas.

RHABDOMYOSARCOMA. Virtually all cases of rhabdomyosarcoma of bone are metastatic; however, this tumor may also secondarily involve bone by direct extension (see Chap. 30). Most cases are readily identifiable by simple light microscopic examination alone (Fig. 31-9); nonetheless, certain undifferentiated tumors can represent serious diagnostic problems (Fig. 31-10). In such cases, confusion with Ewing's sarcoma is likely if no other diagnostic methods beyond light microscopy are employed.

SYNOVIOSARCOMA. Monophasic (especially stromal monophasic) synoviosarcoma is often composed of round and spindle cells that superficially resemble Ewing's sarcoma. This is especially true when there is no obvious osseous primary tumor. It must be recognized that even scattered spindle cells in areas of uncompressed tumor cell masses is strong evidence that the tumor in question is not Ewing's sarcoma (Fig. 31-11). Distinction between synoviosarcoma and other spindle cell sarcomas in children and young adults requires further diagnostic methods, as discussed below.

PRIMARY LYMPHOMA OF BONE. Lymphoma of bone, though not a common disease, is nonetheless sufficiently frequent to warrant consideration in the differential diagnosis of Ewing's sarcoma. Involvement may be solitary or multifocal at presentation (see also Chap. 20). In either case, the tumorous mass appears to be a solid tumor infiltrating marrow, quite similar to Ewing's sarcoma (Fig. 31-12A). At higher magnification, however (Fig. 31-12B), the cytology, especially the deeply basophilic nuclear staining with peripherally condensed heterochromatin, is inappropriate for Ewing's sarcoma. Further, periodic acid-Schiff (PAS) staining, virtually always positive in

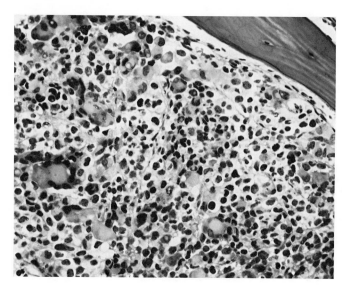

FIGURE 31-9.   Metastatic rhabdomyosarcoma in bone. Here, easily identified myoblasts intermingle with primitive round tumor cells, also part of this tumor. The presence of eosinophilic cells in a tumor otherwise similar to Ewing's sarcoma should always provoke consideration of a primary soft tissue sarcoma (particularly rhabdomyosarcoma) metastatic to bone. Apparent primary rhabdomyosarcoma of bone has also been reported, albeit rarely. (H & E; original magnification × 250)

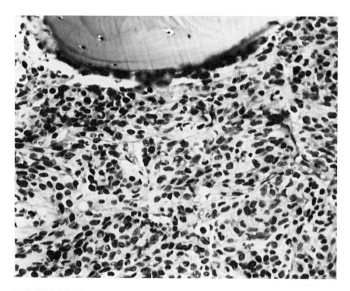

FIGURE 31-10. Primitive, metastatic rhabdomyosarcoma in bone. This round cell tumor is easily confused with Ewing's sarcoma. The diagnostic myoblasts are absent, and light microscopic appearance is not sufficient to distinguish the two. Immunocytochemistry and EM are necessary to distinguish them in this case. We have also seen cases with negative EM and ICC that have later shown myogenesis, thereby further complicating the distinction. (H & E; original magnification × 250)

Ewing's sarcoma, is almost always negative in lymphoma. It should also be noted, though, that the variable cytology of different types of lymphoma, including lymphoblastic and diffuse histiocytic or large cell, as well as the presence of punctate PAS positivity in lymphoblastic lymphoma, may make differentiation from Ewing's sarcoma by light microscopy difficult.

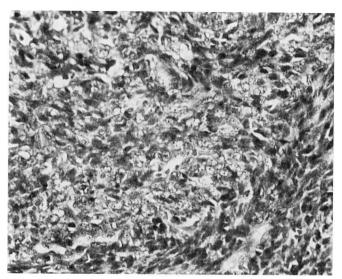

FIGURE 31-11.   Monophasic synoviosarcoma in bone. Although primarily a soft tissue sarcoma, this tumor not infrequently arises adjacent to and involves bone. The biphasic form is easily distinguished from round cell tumors of bone. The monophasic form, seen here, is virtually indistinguishable from a variety of spindle cell sarcomas of bone and soft tissue but is *not* readily confused with Ewing's sarcoma. There is often a tendency for a biphasic tumor cell population, with spindle cells resembling fibrosarcoma cells and larger, clearer, more rounded, or epithelioid cells, seen here diagonally across the center of the field. The latter offer a clue to the correct diagnosis, also easily confirmed by ICC with epithelial markers. (H & E; original magnification × 250)

For this reason, immunocytochemistry for common leukocyte antigen is imperative to distinguish hematopoietic malignancies from Ewing's sarcoma.

NEUROBLASTOMA.   When neuroblastoma metastasizes to bone, it generally diffusely infiltrates the marrow and involves multiple bones (see also Chap. 28). Confusion with a unifocal primary bone tumor is not a serious problem, but in rare cases an apparent single site may be present. In these cases, distinction from a primary neuroectodermal tumor of bone becomes imperative. Utilizing light microscopic criteria alone, this is not always possible; however, some useful morphologic guidelines include:

1. Neural tumors in general display some evidence of clustering if not overt rosette formation. Ewing's sarcoma may do so also, but this is not surprising in view of recent experimental evidence regarding its presumed neural origin.[3] Nonetheless, true rosettes are rare in neuroectodermal tumors in general, but common in neuroblastoma (Figs. 31-13A and B).
2. The development of neuropil, or tangled eosinophilic masses of cell processes (Fig. 31-13B), is tantamount to a diagnosis of metastatic neuroblastoma.

Because no single feature is sufficient to distinguish neuroblastoma from Ewing's sarcoma and neuroectodermal tumors in every case, immunocytochemistry and electron microscopy should be utilized to make this distinction.

PRIMITIVE NEUROECTODERMAL TUMORS.   These tumors, only recently separated as a distinct entity from Ewing's sarcoma and metastatic neuroblastoma,[31] are discussed in detail in

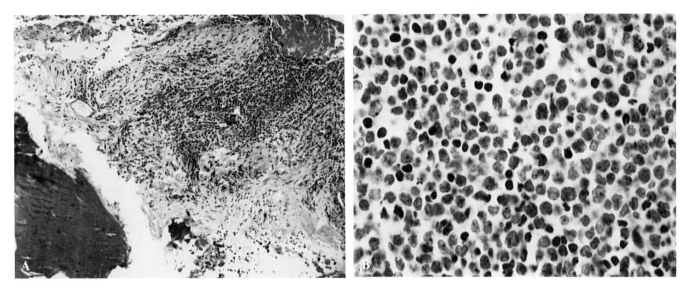

FIGURE 31-12.   Lymphoma of bone. A. Overview. Leukemic infiltrates, although more common, are distinguished from lymphoma of bone by the latter's destructive character mimicking a bone sarcoma. Like Ewing's, lymphoma is generally infiltrative of marrow and spares trabeculae, at least initially. Soft tissue extension is common, also like Ewing's. Unlike Ewing's, variable fibrosis (as seen here) may be present, a clue that the tumor is not Ewing's. (H & E; original magnification × 100) **B.** Cytology. Closer scrutiny of the cells in lymphoma of bone reveals typical lymphoid-type nuclear convolutions and chromatin pattern and a heterogeneity from cell to cell that is absent in Ewing's sarcoma. Although any childhood lymphoma can be found in bone, lymphoblastic has been the most common in our experience, as illustrated here. (H & E; original magnification × 630)

Chapters 6 and 29. Generally, they are exceedingly primitive and virtually impossible to distinguish from Ewing's sarcoma by light microscopy alone (Fig. 31-14).[32] For this reason, immunocytochemistry or electron microscopy must be used to distinguish clearly these two entities.

An unusual round cell tumor of chest wall, occurring predominantly in adolescents, has recently been shown to be yet another form of neuroectodermal tumor. This tumor, described by Askin and colleagues,[33] was virtually indistinguishable from Ewing's sarcoma. Recent immunocytochemical studies, among others, have clearly demonstrated that this tumor is yet another form of primitive neuroectodermal tumor.[34] These and other studies are discussed in detail in Chapters 6 and 29.

Specialized Diagnostic Procedures

In view of the utterly bland and featureless appearance of most cases of Ewing's sarcoma and its look-alikes, routine pathologic examination must be supplemented by other diagnostic procedures if a diagnosis of Ewing's sarcoma is to be substantiated. Although many possibilities exist (and are discussed in some detail in Chapters 3 and 6), two in particular are invaluable in the routine evaluation of tumor material: light microscopic immunocytochemistry of paraffin embedded tissue and electron microscopy (EM) of epoxy resin embedded tissue. The first is readily performed on routinely handled tissue; EM optimally requires glutaraldehyde fixation of very small fragments (<0.2 mm in at least one dimension). Sampling is thus a major concern in EM, and samples submitted therefore should be drawn from identical areas submitted for light microscopic study.

IMMUNOCYTOCHEMISTRY. Immunocytochemistry has become invaluable for distinguishing Ewing's sarcoma (for which no unique antigenic determinants have yet been identi-

fied) from other similar appearing tumors (for which many tumor specific antibodies often exist). Commonly available antibodies of value in the diagnosis of Ewing's sarcoma are summarized in Table 31-1, which compares each tumor and its pattern of antibody reactivity (see also Chaps. 4, 6, and 8).

ELECTRON MICROSCOPY. The other major practical approach to the diagnosis of Ewing's sarcoma and similar appearing round cell tumors is electron microscopy. EM complements immunocytochemistry, as it relies on categorically different findings for diagnosis. EM can identify intermediate filaments of unknown composition; immunocytochemistry can fail to identify a neural marker while EM documents unequivocal dense core (neural) granules. Thus, both procedures can be employed to benefit, and may be required in certain tumors. A detailed discussion of ultrastructural findings in context with other modalities can be found in Chapter 6. Certain unique features of typical and atypical Ewing's sarcoma and the tumors with which it is often confused are tabulated in Table 31-2.

PATTERNS OF SPREAD

If Ewing's sarcoma is treated without systemic therapy, over 90% of the patients will develop metastases.[22] The most common site of metastatic disease at diagnosis and at first relapse is the lung; other common sites of metastatic disease include the bones and bone marrow. Approximately 14% to 50% of patients in most series have evidence of overt metastases at diagnosis.[35,36] Interestingly, metastatic spread of Ewing's sarcoma to lymph nodes is very rare and usually occurs only after the disease has become very far advanced. This is in contrast to rhabdomyosarcoma, osteosarcoma, and peripheral neuroepithelioma (the closely related tumor) in which lymph node metastases occur more commonly. Retroperitoneal and me-

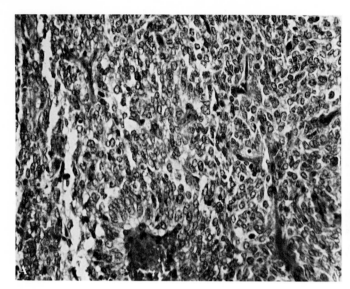

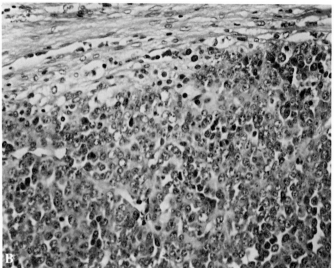

FIGURE 31-13.   Neural bone tumors. A. PNET of bone. This tumor varies in appearance from sarcomatous (as here) to epithelioid. The neural histogenesis is generally not detectable without the aid of EM or ICC. Often, they are histologically indistinguishable from Ewing's. The example illustrated here was originally diagnosed as Ewing's, but a spindle cell character is detectable on close examination; this precludes a diagnosis of Ewing's sarcoma. **B.** Metastatic neuroblastoma. Much has been written about the confusion between Ewing's sarcoma and neuroblastoma, most of it incorrect. Clinical considerations will identify almost all metastatic neuroblastomas (HVA/VMA alone is positive in >95% of cases), but when that fails, scrutiny of the cytologic appearance will virtually always disclose the characteristic "salt and pepper" chromatin pattern of neuroblastoma as well as heterogeneous tumor cells with variably abundant pink cytoplasm, absent in Ewing's. Both features are illustrated here. (H & E; original magnification × 250)

diastinal spread also rarely occurs at diagnosis but is not infrequent in far advanced cases. Preliminary evaluation of the early National Cancer Institute (NCI) series suggested that there was a significant incidence of central nervous system (CNS) involvement by Ewing's sarcoma at diagnosis and at first relapse. This led some therapists to treat the CNS with prophylactic irradiation. Further analysis has revealed that the incidence of CNS disease was only 2.2% with no patients presenting with CNS disease at diagnosis, with an actuarial incidence of 10% at 2 years with no effect of prophylactic CNS therapy on the incidence of subsequent CNS disease. Further, involvement of the CNS almost always occurred in the setting of widespread disseminated disease, frequently as a terminal event.[37–41]

Metastases to the spine and paraspinal region are relatively common in patients with Ewing's sarcoma. The occurrence of back pain with or without neurologic changes in the lower extremities or changes in bowel and bladder control in patients with Ewing's sarcoma must be considered strong evidence for metastatic involvement of the spinal cord due to direct extension of the tumor from a bony or paraspinal soft tissue metastasis.

CLINICAL PRESENTATION

The most common presenting symptoms of Ewing's sarcoma are pain and swelling of the affected bone or region. Patients with localized disease usually do not have systemic symptoms; however, fatigue, anorexia, weight loss, intermittent fever, and malaise are often present in patients with metastatic disease. These symptoms may lead to the diagnosis of chronic osteomy-

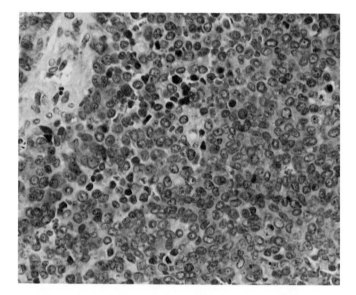

FIGURE 31-14.   Primitive neuroectodermal tumor (PNET). This group of tumors is frequently indistinguishable by light microscopy from Ewing's sarcoma. Subtle differences are generally noticeable, however, as here: nuclei are more heterogeneous in appearance (in contrast to the bland, "light and dark" pattern seen in Ewing's; see Fig. 31-2A); cytoplasm is more conspicuous; and stroma is evident (in striking contrast to Ewing's, where there is none). PAS stains are often positive, and therefore irrelevant. Confirmation of a diagnosis of PNET almost always requires recourse to EM and immunocytochemistry (see Tables 31-1 and 31-2 and Chap. 6).

Table 31-1
Immunocytochemistry of Ewing's Sarcoma and Related Tumors of Childhood*

Tumor	Antibodies													
	Neural								Myogenous					
	NSE	S100	Leu7	NFTP	Chromogranin	Synaptophysin	HSAN 1.2	HLA-1	Desmin	CK-MM	Myoglobin	Myosin	Vimentin	LCA
Ewing's sarcoma	–	–	–	–	–	–	–	+	–	–	–	–	+	–
Atypical Ewing's sarcoma	–	–	–	–	–	–	–	+	–	–	–	–	+	–
Small cell osteosarcoma	–	–	–	–	–	–	–	+	–	–	–	–	+	–
Mesenchymal chondrosarcoma	–	+	–	–	–	–	–	+	–	–	–	–	+	–
Primary bone sarcoma, NOS	–	–	–	–	–	–	–	+	–	–	–	–	+	–
Rhabdomyosarcoma	+	–	–	–	–	–	–	+	+	+	+	+	+	–
Lymphoma	–	–/+	–/+	–	–	–	–	+	–	–	–	–	+	+
Metastatic neuroblastoma	+	+	+	+	+	–	+	–	–	–	–	–	+	–
Primitive neuroectodermal tumor (PN, PNET, Askin tumor, PNET of bone)	+	+	–	+	–	+	+	+	–	–	–	–	+	–

* These are typical results, using the conventional Sternberger technique with no protease digestion of sections before application of the antibody. Exceptions occur, and results obtained with more sensitive techniques such as the avidin/biotin technique after protease predigestion are noticeably different. This information is intended only as a guide; results should always be evaluated in context with other data, including clinical information, routine light microscopy, and ulrastructure (noted in Table 31-2). See Chapter 6 for details.

Table 31-2
Ultrastructure of Ewing's Sarcoma and Related Tumors of Childhood*

EM Feature	Tumor								
	Ewing's Sarcoma	Atypical ESB	Small Cell Osteosarcoma	Mesenchymal Chondrosarcoma	Primary Bone Sarcoma	Rhabdomyo-sarcoma	Lymphoma	Neuroblastoma	PNET
Nuclei									
Irregular	No	Maybe	Variable	Variable	Yes	Yes	Usually	No	No
Dense chromatin	No	No	Yes	Yes	Variable	Yes	Always	Variable	No
Glycogen	Yes	Maybe	Usual	Always	Usually absent	Yes	Rare		
Intermediate filaments	Scant	Common	The rule	Also prominent	Common	Always	Absent	Variable	Rare
Rough endoplasmic reticulum	No	Some	Abundant	Abundant	Variable	Common	Uncommon	Some	Little
Dense core granules	Never	Possible	Never	Never	Never	Never	Never	Common	Some
Lysosomes	Variable	Common	Usual	Less common	Variable	Uncommon	Uncommon	Absent	Rare
Cell–cell attachments	Rare	Variable	Some	Some	Some	Common	Never	Usual	Some
Cell processes (neurites)	None	None	None	None	None	None	None	Usual	Rare
Fibrillar collagen Stroma									
Type I	Never	Rare	Always	Usual	Variable	Always	Never	Sometimes	Maybe
Type II	Never	Never	Never	Always	Never	Never	Never	Never	Never

* See Chapter 6 for details.

elitis and result in a significant delay in the diagnosis of Ewing's sarcoma (see also Chap. 5). The hemorrhage and necrosis commonly seen within the Ewing's tumor may result in an increase in the local temperature and in erythema, signs that mimic infection and may further obscure the diagnosis.

The most common bones affected by Ewing's sarcoma are the bones of the pelvis, the humerus, and the femur; however, Ewing's sarcoma may arise in any bone. Unlike osteosarcoma, which most commonly arises in the long bones of the extremities, Ewing's sarcoma most frequently involves the axial skeleton.

In the original description of the tumor, Ewing noted that a number of the patients had had symptoms for a prolonged period.[2] This is still the case; the duration of symptoms is often several months and may be even longer in patients with disease arising in the axial skeleton.

Although Ewing's sarcoma arises in the bone, there often is a significant soft tissue mass associated with the bony primary,[42] especially for primaries of the axial skeleton. The extent of this mass may not be initially appreciated without appropriate imaging. Often the viable enlarging soft tissue mass may be larger than the intraosseous component of the tumor, which is frequently necrotic.[42]

Less commonly appreciated modes of presentation of Ewing's sarcoma are related to the primary disease site: a primary tumor of the ribs may present with respiratory symptoms due to a massive pleural effusion; a neurogenic bladder may be the presenting sign of a tumor arising in the sacrum; nerve root symptoms may be the initial findings of a patient with a vertebral bone primary.

METHODS OF DIAGNOSIS

Differential Diagnosis

The most common nonmalignant entity confused with Ewing's sarcoma is osteomyelitis, because the tumor may frequently present with signs and symptoms of inflammation (see also Chap. 5). Other noninfectious causes of arthritides may also mimic Ewing's sarcoma. Trauma and structural nonmalignant bone lesions are also occasionally confused with Ewing's sarcoma. Malignant bone lesions that must be distinguished from Ewing's sarcoma are osteosarcoma, neuroblastoma, primitive neuroepithelioma, primary lymphoma of bone, leukemia, small cell osteosarcoma, and mesenchymal chondrosarcoma. Osteosarcoma usually, but not always, presents with an osteoblastic lesion and most commonly arises in the ends of the long bones in contrast with the metaphyseal and diaphyseal sites most commonly seen with Ewing's sarcoma (see Chap. 32). Neuroblastoma usually presents with multiple lesions and a primary tumor mass in the abdomen; however, urinary catecholamines, electron microscopy, immunocytochemistry, or oncogene expression may be required to make the distinction between these two tumors (see Chap. 28). Primitive neuroepithelioma of bone presents indistinguishably from Ewing's sarcoma. Pathologic differentiation between these two tumors may require immunocytochemical localization of fluorescent antibodies to neural antigens and ultrastructural evaluation (see Chap. 29). Leukemia and lymphoma may be distinguished by morphology, but immunocytochemistry, immunophenotyping, and gene rearrangement studies (immunoglobulin gene and T cell receptor gene rearrangement) may be required (see Chaps. 16 and 20). Small cell osteosarcoma and mesenchymal chondrosarcoma are distinguished by the presence of malignant osteoid or malignant chondroid in the setting of a small cell tumor. This malignant matrix must be differentiated from metaplastic bone and cartilage.

Evaluation

The most important aspect of the evaluation of Ewing's sarcoma is the initial diagnostic biopsy. The most common errors made here are obtaining inadequate tissue for light microscopy (frequently, the intramedullary portion is almost completely necrotic, whereas the associated soft tissue mass is usually viable); not obtaining or processing the tissue for electron microscopy and immunocytochemistry; not obtaining tissue for biological and cytogenetic studies; and creating a large bony defect in a weight-bearing bone when obtaining diag-

nostic material. An appropriate clinical evaluation of a patient with Ewing's sarcoma of bone includes adequate imaging of the primary tumor to adequately determine the extent of disease within the medullary cavity and size of the soft tissue component of the tumor. Recent studies suggest that the best technique for this evaluation is magnetic resonance imaging (see Chap. 7). Evaluation for metastatic disease should include imaging of the lung parenchyma with posteroanterior (PA) and lateral chest radiographs and with computed tomography (CT), imaging of the bones with a radionuclide bone scan, and microscopic assessment of the bone marrow with a bone marrow biopsy. Although there is no serum marker for Ewing's sarcoma, elevation of the serum lactate dehydrogenase (LDH) has been associated with the presence of metastatic disease and poor prognosis (see Chap. 8).[43,44]

PROGNOSTIC CONSIDERATIONS

The most important prognostic factor in the assessment of a patient with Ewing's sarcoma is the extent of disease. Evidence of metastatic disease at diagnosis dramatically reduces the projected survival of patients with this disease. Further, the type of metastatic disease also correlates with survival: most patients with metastatic disease to the bone marrow or bone can be expected to have a very poor prognosis. Patients with metastatic disease limited to the lung, especially those with only a small amount of disease, appear to fare better than those with metastatic disease in other sites.

A number of studies have attempted to determine what factors are of prognostic significance in the assessment of patients with Ewing's sarcoma.[43,45] Analysis of the NCI series revealed that the most favorable prognostic factors were a distal site of disease, a normal serum LDH at presentation, and the absence of metastatic disease at diagnosis. Pelvic disease and an elevated LDH were associated with a poor prognosis.[43] Analysis of the results of the first Intergroup Ewing's Sarcoma Study (IESS 1) confirmed that the site of primary disease was the most important prognostic variable in patients without metastases at diagnosis. Pelvic and sacral sites had the least favorable outcome, whereas the most favorable sites were the bones of the distal extremities and other sites (all other bones except the humerus, femur, and rib, which were intermediate in prognosis).[45]

The extent of the soft tissue extension of the primary tumor is now believed to be an important prognostic factor for patients with Ewing's sarcoma,[42,46] although a large prospective study of this factor will be required to establish this. In one small retrospective study, 87% of the patients with tumors confined to the bone were alive in 5 years. When extraosseous extension of the tumor was present, only 20% survived 5 years.[42] In a second study of 60 patients with Ewing's sarcoma, patients with tumor volumes <100 ml had a 3-year disease-free survival rate of 78% compared to a 17% disease-free survival rate for those with tumor volumes ≥ 100 ml.[46] This fact alone may account for the poor prognosis of patients with pelvic and sacral primaries.

Retrospective evaluation of the pathologic features of the IESS series and a European series has suggested that certain pathologic patterns may be associated with a poorer prognosis.[23,24] Specifically, the filigree pattern appeared to be associated with an increased risk of subsequent relapse. Detailed pathologic analysis of the NCI series has also suggested that the primary sarcomas of bone (distinguished from Ewing's sarcoma on the basis of electron microscopy) may have a poorer prognosis. Another pathologic entity, peripheral neuroepithelioma, which may be confused with Ewing's sarcoma on light microscopy alone, does not now imply a different prognosis with present therapy; however, prognostic differences may emerge as therapy changes.

Finally, it will be important to continue biological studies of Ewing's sarcoma. One can anticipate that, as with neuroblastoma, oncogene expression may have important prognostic implications.

STAGING

At present, there is no universally accepted staging system for Ewing's sarcoma. Most therapeutic studies have been stratified for the presence of metastatic disease or have actually had different therapies for patients with and without metastatic disease. Although the primary site has appeared to have prognostic significance in most studies, only a few studies have used primary site to determine therapy. Similarly, size of tumor has not been used to determine therapy despite data suggesting that it too has prognostic importance.[42,46]

As the prognosis for many of the subsets of patients with Ewing's sarcoma varies significantly, it will be important for the next generation of studies of Ewing's sarcoma to establish and subsequently apply a more detailed and accurate staging system. The most important factors now appear to be the size of the primary tumor and extent of metastatic disease; however, LDH, site of primary disease, and site(s) and extent of metastatic disease may also be important.

TREATMENT

The primary goals of treatment of Ewing's sarcoma include the preservation of as much function as possible, achievement of complete and permanent local control, and treatment and prevention of metastatic disease. Over the past 15 years the major thrust of therapeutic trials has been the improvement of survival. Although survival has significantly improved during this time for most patients, further advances need to be made, especially for those with large tumors and metastatic disease.[36,47–49] Moreover, future studies must begin to address optimum management of the primary tumor in order to maximize function, prevent second malignancies, and achieve permanent tumor control. Finally, the optimum dose-intensity of treatment regimens for patients with Ewing's sarcoma of differing prognoses must be determined to reduce both the short- and long-term morbidity of therapy while maximizing the survival of patients.

General Surgical Principles

The role of surgery in the management of Ewing's sarcoma is continuing to evolve. At one time, most Ewing's sarcomas were treated with surgery alone, but the results were poor. It was later found that radiation therapy could control most local lesions, and most patients were then treated with this modality.

When planning therapy to achieve local control of the primary lesion, the functional outcome of treatment plays an important role in deciding whether radiation or surgery is used (see Chaps. 10 and 11). When the treatment plan is being formulated, the risks, benefits, and functional outcome of both therapies should be carefully considered for every patient with newly diagnosed, primary, localized Ewing's sarcoma of bone. Although many patients are not suitable candidates for surgical treatment, when surgery is indicated the surgical philosophy is

to attempt removal of the entire tumor and obtain margins of normal tissue on all aspects of the tumor while preserving as much function as possible. It is best not to perform a surgical procedure until the patient has been treated with preoperative chemotherapy in order to judge the response of the tumor to chemotherapy. Some lesions that appear unresectable initially may become resectable after preoperative chemotherapy. Some lesions that fail to respond to chemotherapy may require amputation surgery. Those lesions that are located in surgically inaccessible sites or in sites that would require radical, mutilating surgical procedures in order to achieve margins histologically free of tumor are probably best treated by radiation therapy.

Biopsy

The proper planning and execution of the biopsy procedure is exceedingly important (see Chaps. 6 and 10). A poor biopsy procedure may lead to misdiagnosis, delay in diagnosis, and serious potential complications, including pathologic fracture and even the loss of an otherwise salvageable limb.

The first principle of the biopsy procedure is to obtain an adequate amount of a representative portion of the tumor to provide the pathologist with diagnostic tissue. When planning for the procedure, one should try to identify that portion of the suspected tumor that is accessible and yet has the expectation of providing adequate tissue. Most Ewing's tumors extend beyond the confines of the bone into the adjacent soft tissues. This is the area that should be approached for diagnostic tissue for several reasons: first, the tissue is likely to be soft and therefore easy to process in the pathology laboratory; second, the soft portion of the tumor is likely to be representative of the most malignant portion of the lesion while the intramedullary portion of the lesion is often necrotic; and third, if tissue can be obtained from the soft tissue, further violation of bony integrity can be avoided and the risk of pathologic fracture minimized. To obtain an adequate amount of tissue, it is usually necessary to perform an open biopsy; however, in certain clinical situations a needle biopsy may be satisfactory, particularly if the diagnosis is strongly suspected and the biopsy procedure is being used merely to confirm the diagnosis. In most situations, however, tissue obtained from needle biopsy is *not* adequate to allow the pathologist to formulate a diagnosis and to perform biologic studies that are now an important part of the pathologic evaluation of this tumor.

The biopsy needs to be planned in such a way as to provide direct access to the tumor and yet be placed so that the biopsy site itself can be excised at a later date if necessary. Moreover, it is always best to avoid transverse wounds on extremities because it is particularly difficult to perform subsequent limb salvage procedures in the presence of a transverse wound. When possible, the biopsy should be planned to avoid the tension side of the bone. This is particularly true for lesions that occur in the proximal femur. A lateral biopsy wound significantly increases the risk of subsequent pathologic fracture if the cortical bone is windowed to obtain tissue. Hence, it is better to approach such a lesion anteriorly, posteriorly, or medially rather than laterally.

The technique of the biopsy procedure is also important. The incision should be carried down to the tumor as directly as possible, avoiding unnecessary dissection around muscle planes. In general, it is better to go through a muscle than to dissect extensively around a muscle. Hemostasis needs to be maintained at all times during the procedure. Wound hematomas may be expected to disseminate tumor cells and should be avoided if at all possible. If a drain is used, it should be brought out either through the end of the wound or immediately adjacent to the wound, again realizing that the drain site is a potentially contaminated area.

There is another consideration in the biopsy of Ewing's tumors. Many patients present with a clinical course that is indistinguishable from osteomyelitis, that is, they may have pain, intermittent fever, an elevated sedimentation rate, and a radiographic appearance that does not distinguish between the two entities. At the time of biopsy, osteomyelitis and Ewing's sarcoma may be further confused because of the gross appearance of some Ewing's tumors. The tumor may be quite liquid and grossly indistinguishable from the purulence of infection. In such a situation the surgeon needs to be prepared to obtain material both for histology and for cultures. Some tumor material should be submitted for frozen section. If the immediate diagnosis is osteomyelitis, the surgeon should be prepared to treat the lesion accordingly. Hence, consideration needs to be made for this eventuality when one is planning a biopsy procedure.

Amputation: Indications and Procedures

Amputation offers the most definitive way of achieving control of the primary tumor (see Chap. 10). In practice, however, amputation is usually reserved for certain special clinical situations. Various clinical factors must be considered when one is contemplating an amputation to control local disease in a patient with Ewing's sarcoma, including the site and extent of the lesion and the age of the patient. In addition, the patient's response to primary or neoadjuvant chemotherapy may dictate whether an amputation is desirable. In general, amputations of the upper extremity are avoided. Further, most amputations are performed for lesions that are located in the distal portion of the lower extremity.

For those rare lesions that occur in the toes or small bones of the forefoot, ray amputations or hemiamputations of the foot may be preferable to radiation therapy at any age, but especially in younger patients. For lesions located in the distal fibula, tibia, talus, calcaneous, and hindfoot, below knee amputation has been used in patients of any age but, again, is more likely to be the treatment of choice in younger, growing patients. Very small lesions in these locations might be treated by either radiation therapy or resection surgery, but such situations are unusual. For tumors that arise in the region of the knee, either in the proximal tibia or distal femur, amputation may also be considered for young, growing children because radiation for tumors around the knee in this setting would probably produce an unacceptable leg length inequality. In addition to these specific situations, amputation should be considered whenever the tumor is huge or unresponsive to preoperative chemotherapy and when there is an otherwise unmanageable pathologic fracture.

Limb-Sparing Procedures

Limb-sparing procedures should be considered in certain surgically accessible sites, particularly if the lesion appears to be responding favorably to preoperative chemotherapy (see also Chaps. 10 and 32). Lesions of the proximal fibula, for example, can be resected if the tumor is reasonably small and there is little soft tissue involvement. The entire proximal four fifths of the fibula can be sacrificed without the need for reconstruction. If the peroneal nerve is sacrificed, the patients may need to wear a dropfoot brace or have a subsequent tenodesis procedure to prevent a dropfoot. If loss of the peroneal nerve is anticipated, radiation therapy may be an appropriate alternative with a better functional outcome. Tumors of the ribs can be treated by surgical excision. Resection should provide en bloc,

wide, tumor-free margins, which may include at least one normal rib above and one below the area of gross tumor, as well as the adjacent sternum and clavicle if necessary. The depth of resection should include at least full thickness of the chest wall, along with the adjacent pleura and wide resection of any areas of attachment to underlying lung parenchyma, pericardium, or diaphragm. Lesions that arise in the lateral four fifths of the clavicle can be excised if the extent of soft tissue involvement is not too great. Lesions involving the wing of the scapula may be resected if the chest wall itself does not seem to be invaded. Lesions of the forearm that involve only one of the two bones may be excised and the forearm reconstructed. These specific examples of resection for Ewing's sarcoma are probably the ones most commonly encountered; however, there may be other clinical situations, especially in young children, where resection surgery is worth consideration.

Management of Complications

One of the most difficult to manage complications of Ewing's sarcoma is the pathologic fracture, particularly if it involves a long bone and the patient has received prior irradiation. The situation is further compromised by ongoing chemotherapy, which may be responsible for delayed fracture healing. When pathologic fracture occurs in a major long bone, some form of surgical intervention is usually necessary. For example, if a pathologic fracture occurs in the subtrochanteric region of the proximal femur, open reduction and internal fixation using a Zickel nail or some other suitable device may be necessary to control the fracture. It may be desirable to evacuate tumor or necrotic debris in the region of the pathologic fracture and fill the resulting defect with methylmethacrylate. Pathologic fractures at the midshaft of the femur may require open reduction and internal fixation with an intramedullary rod, possibly supplemented with methylmethacrylate. Alternatively, one or more plates and multiple screws may be used for fixation. Similarly, fractures of the diaphysis of the humerus may necessitate open reduction and internal fixation either with intramedullary rods or with the use of plates and screws. On occasion, such fractures may be controlled using external casts or braces. This is an especially reasonable approach if the patient has widespread metastatic disease or other pathologic fractures. Some of the complications of radiation therapy can be managed by surgery. For example, the function of patients who develop severe joint contractures and marked leg length discrepancies may be improved by amputation.

Radiation Therapy

General Considerations

In his initial description, Ewing specifically remarked that this tumor was highly radioresponsive using the now antiquated treatment with radium molds.[2] Complete tumor regression following irradiation was observed, with gradual remodeling of bone matrix and return of normal limb function. Throughout the orthovoltage era and now in the megavoltage era of radiation therapy, the efficacy of local radiation therapy in Ewing's sarcoma has been repeatedly confirmed.[50–59]

Ewing's sarcoma is fundamentally a systemic disease: a significant number of patients have metastatic disease at presentation, and the predominant pattern of failure is systemic.[43,45,47] Given that Ewing's sarcoma is a systemic disease in most patients, it is important that local therapy not compromise delivery of effective systemic therapy. Before the use of chemotherapy, local control of Ewing's sarcoma was achieved in 50% to 85% of localized patients treated to >4000 cGy, although only 15% to 25% were long-term survivors.[50,51] The term "localized" is used advisedly because these patients were staged before the availability of routine lung tomography, CT scanning, and radionuclide bone scanning. Additionally, local irradiation was delivered with tumor volumes estimated by physical examination combined with conventional plain and contrast radiographic studies. Today, abnormalities and extent of disease defined by CT and magnetic resonance imaging (MRI) scanning have resulted in better radiation treatment planning, especially in delineating tumor volumes (see Chap. 11).

With the addition of adjuvant chemotherapy to local irradiation, it is apparent that local control and survival rates for patients with nonmetastatic Ewing's sarcoma are considerably better than those with radiation therapy alone.[50-59] Following combined modality therapy, fewer than 10% of patients with distal extremity lesions fail locally, compared to a 20% to 40% local failure rate in patients with primary lesions of the proximal extremity and pelvis.[47,55,56,58] An improvement in disease-free survival is most impressive in patients with a distal extremity primary tumor, where combined modality therapy may result in long-term (>3 years) disease-free survival in 60% to 70% of the patients. Unfortunately, fewer than 30% to 35% of patients with localized pelvic or proximal extremity disease are disease-free with 2 to 3 years of follow-up in published studies.[36,43,45,47,58] This latter localized patient group and patients who present with metastases represent poor prognosis groups in whom more aggressive combined modality therapy is indicated.

An analysis of local control in Ewing's sarcoma is particularly difficult for two reasons. First, the interpretation of follow-up diagnostic studies including plain radiographs, bone scans, CT scans, and MRI scans may be difficult following high-dose (>5000 cGy) irradiation and combination chemotherapy. Typically, there is significant tumor regression during the first 1 to 2 months of combined modality therapy, often associated with a decrease in pain, tenderness, and local erythema. In contrast, in patients with bulky (>10 cm) soft tissue masses, which usually arise in the pelvis, a significantly smaller but persistent soft tissue mass may be seen in follow-up CT and MRI scans during and for several months after treatment. Additionally, plain films and bone scans often continue to show abnormalities for months to years after treatment. These persistent abnormalities on follow-up diagnostic studies are a source of concern and frustration for oncologists, particularly in patients with no obvious metastatic disease. The differential diagnosis includes persistent tumor, radiation fibrosis of bone and soft tissue, a smoldering osteomyelitis, or, least likely, an evolving radiation-induced second tumor (see Chaps. 5 and 11). A routine bone or soft tissue biopsy in these patients is often not indicated based on the difficulty interpreting limited pathologic material obtained by needle biopsy or a small open biopsy, as well as the high risk of poor wound healing and infection following biopsy of heavily irradiated tissues. Obviously, close follow-up of these patients is indicated, with a planned, careful open biopsy if local symptoms and signs worsen or the persistent mass enlarges. An open biopsy should provide adequate material for light and electron microscopy and microbiological studies.

A second problem in assessing local control is that Ewing's sarcoma is a disease that commonly metastasizes to bone and there is the possibility of metastatic tumor reseeding a previously sterilized primary site. Although local tumor reseeding is speculative, it may, in part, explain the difference in clinical and pathologic local control rates. In the small autopsy series from the NCI, 13 of 20 evaluated patients with widespread disease showed histologic evidence of tumor at the primary site.[60] The clinical relevance of this limited autopsy data on local control after radiation therapy is unclear because most manifested no clinical evidence of local failure before death. Indeed, the most recent data from the NCI, using a very intensive combined modality treatment, show only a 10% local recurrence rate (as the initial site(s) of relapse), with a median follow-up of 2 years in patients with nonmetastatic disease in the proximal extremity or pelvis, or with metastatic disease at presentation.[59]

Based on results of combined modality therapy of Ewing's sarcoma in recent series, it appears that the combination of high-dose (>5000 cGy) local irradiation and multiagent chemotherapy is the treatment of choice for most patients. On the basis of retrospective reviews, an increased role for surgery has been advocated because of an observed apparent survival advantage for those undergoing surgery in the setting of combined modality therapy.[61-64] Unfortunately, the patient populations are by nature selected for either radiation or surgery, and thus direct comparisons of the efficacy and functional outcome of the two modalities in the treatment of similar tumor presentations are not possible. To date, there are no prospective controlled studies comparing surgery to radiation as local therapy of Ewing's sarcoma.

Technical Considerations

In general, the entire affected bone and the adjacent soft tissue extension are defined as the tumor volume for radiation therapy.[65] Since Ewing's sarcoma is known to infiltrate widely into surrounding normal tissues, a 3 to 5 cm margin is included, if possible, in the treatment fields around the gross tumor volume. Patients should be routinely simulated to optimize treatment planning. Additionally, CT scanning in the treatment position often results in further sparing of normal tissues by the use of customized blocks and isocentric oblique fields rather than opposing anteroposterior fields.

With extremity lesions, correct positioning of the extremity at simulation can sometimes obviate the need for complicated treatment plans (Fig. 31-15). The use of casts to immobilize the extremity during treatment is important, as the extremity's functional capabilities can change during treatment as a result of tumor response, normal tissue reaction to radiation therapy and chemotherapy, or the use of physical therapy. For distal extremity lesions, it is important to realize that the forearm and leg have two compartments with an interosseous membrane dividing the anterior and posterior muscle groups and sometimes serving as an effective barrier to tumor spread. In these situations, the uninvolved compartment may be excluded from the treatment fields to reduce the risk of late fibrosis and edema.

For the uncommon lesions arising in the hand and foot, a similar treatment philosophy is used.[66] Two recent series have documented that high-dose radiation therapy can be delivered with excellent local control (>90%) and with maintenance of normal to near-normal function.[67,68] Since the thickness of the hand or foot in the adolescent and young adult patient may be only a few centimeters, treatment of the lesion by immersion in a water bath or the generous use of bolus material for at least part of the treatment can improve radiation dose homogeneity (Fig. 31-16). Careful immobilization is still required, and the nail beds are usually excluded.

For the more common central axis primaries (primarily ribs and pelvis), CT-assisted treatment planning is necessary to adequately encompass the soft tissue extension, which is often bulky, and to limit irradiation of sensitive normal tissues (e.g., small and large intestine, kidney, liver, lung, heart). For pelvic primary tumors, contrast is used at simulation to identify small bowel, bladder, kidneys, and rectum. Additionally, treatment with a full bladder in the prone position may further displace small bowel from the radiation fields. Rib primaries can be

FIGURE 31-15. A technique for immobilizing the arm and forearm to treat a Ewing's sarcoma arising in the proximal radius with soft tissue extension to the antecubital fossa.

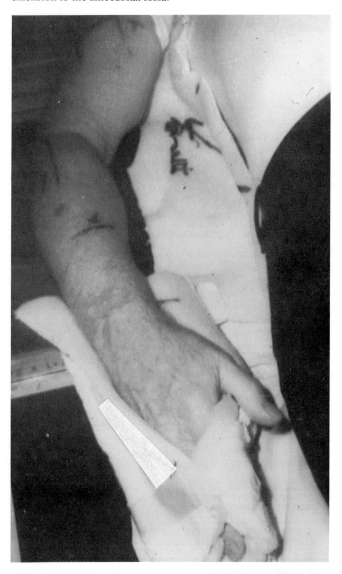

particularly difficult to simulate and treat because the tumor volume includes the entire rib and soft tissue extension. Rotating the treatment couch by 90° and angling the gantry are maneuvers that can be used to align the entire rib in one plane to minimize lung irradiation (Fig. 31-17). Additionally, the cone down "boost" irradiation may be delivered through matched or rotated electron fields.

Patients are usually treated using 175 to 200 cGy daily fractions to a total dose of 5000 cGy over 5 to 6 weeks. With bulky lesions (>10 cm), an additional 1000 cGy, usually at 200 cGy fractions, is used to "boost" any residual soft tissue mass, as well as the bone abnormality by plain radiograph and radionuclide scan. Higher doses of radiotherapy or unconventional radiation techniques may result in a higher incidence of treatment complications and are recommended for selected situations only.

Based on the pattern of failure in previously involved sites in patients with metastatic disease treated with chemotherapy alone,[43,44] it appears that gross metastatic disease is not usually controlled with chemotherapy alone. In many centers, high-dose local irradiation is used to treat sites of gross metastatic disease in addition to the primary tumor.

Both acute and late effects of irradiation can be reduced by the use of careful and proper irradiation technique (see Chaps. 11 and 50).[65] Acute effects occur during treatment or within a few weeks to months after treatment. These effects reflect a disruption of a normal homeostatic cell renewal system (*e.g.,* basal layer of skin, crypt cells of bowel) within a tissue and are both transient and reversible. Late effects occur from several months, usually more than 6 months, to several years after irradiation. The underlying mechanism of late injury to normal tissue is not completely understood, although it is believed to result probably from progressive, and often irreversible, damage to the supportive stroma of a normal tissue. It is important to note that the acute effects of radiation do not necessarily predict late effects. Also, both acute and late effects of normal tissues may be enhanced with the concomitant or sequential use of chemotherapy.

Acute radiation effects in treating extremity or chest wall lesions are primarily manifest as skin changes: erythema progressing to moist or dry desquamation during or shortly after therapy. Usually, these skin effects resolve within 1 to 2 weeks of stopping radiation therapy, although confluent moist desquamation may recur after chemotherapy with doxorubicin or dactinomycin. To minimize the risk of this drug–radiation toxicity, a planned radiation treatment break of 4 to 5 days at the time of chemotherapy administration may be helpful. In patients with pelvic primary tumors, acute radiation effects are usually manifested as diarrhea, proctitis, cramping, and, less commonly, dysuria. These symptoms are dependent on the extent of small bowel, large bowel, rectum, and bladder within

FIGURE 31-16. Radiation therapy setup for a Ewing's sarcoma of a metatarsal bone with soft tissue extension to the flexor surface of the foot (**A**). The soft tissue extension is outlined with solder wire on the x-ray (**B**). The foot is immersed in a water bath to improve radiation dose distribution and treated through opposed lateral fields using photons. A block to spare soft tissues on the plantar surface and nail beds is outlined with black lines on the x-ray (**B**).

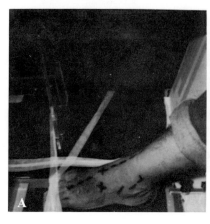

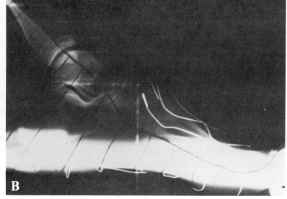

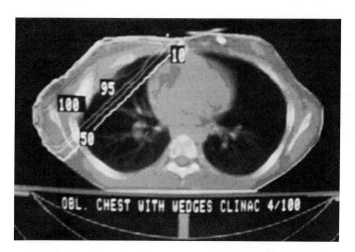

FIGURE 31-17. CT treatment plan for the boost field to a chest wall (rib primary) Ewing's sarcoma. The isodose curves for the opposed oblique fields are shown to illustrate the dose distribution to the tumor volume (95% isodose line) with sparing of underlying right lung and mediastinal structures.

the radiation treatment fields. Because cyclophosphamide is routinely used in these patients, attempts to limit the amount of bladder within the radiation fields may reduce the risk of acute cystitis. Finally, acute mucosal reactions of the upper digestive tract that vary from erythema to frank ulceration may occur in patients with upper chest wall and mandible primary tumors and can require temporary intravenous hyperalimentation. In general, these acute radiation effects are not a source of major morbidity, and most patients complete the planned radiation course to 5000 to 6000 cGy over 6 to 8 weeks.

On the other hand, late radiation effects are more worrisome.[65] In extremity lesions, late radiation effects range from minimal subcutaneous fibrosis to severe fibrosis with muscle contractures. Likewise, the irradiated bone can show long-term radiation effects ranging from mild osteopenia to marked cortical defects with a pathologic fracture. There is a considerable difference in the frequency of these late effects in the available literature. In a review of 29 patients with Ewing's sarcoma of the lower extremity treated at the NCI with high-dose irradiation (>5000 cGy) and combination chemotherapy, only 1 patient (<5%) had a functional deficit that was severe enough to warrant amputation. More than 50% of patients had essentially normal leg function, with a minimum follow-up of 2 years.[69] In a smaller series of 7 patients with Ewing's sarcoma of the hand or foot, 5 patients showed no functional limitation, whereas the other 2 patients had mild functional limitations but could perform routine activities.[68] The most recent experience with careful CT-assisted treatment planning at the NCI appears to be yielding further improvements in functional results with follow-up to 3 years.[59] These results are in direct contrast to an older series in which up to 50% of the patients had postirradiation functional deficits comparable to the deficit of an amputation.[70] The radiation techniques in this older series differed from present radiation approaches in volume, dose, and field arrangement.

In addition to radiation technique, lower extremity function following high-dose irradiation is also related to the age of the patient, the type of biopsy, and the routine use of physical rehabilitation. In the prepubertal patient, long bone irradiation results in growth arrest in the epiphyseal plate. It is often possible to exclude from the radiation field the epiphyseal plate at the opposite end of the bone primary to minimize the growth difference in the irradiated leg compared to the unirra-

diated leg in these prepubertal patients. Finally, a regular program of active and passive exercise of the lower extremity should be planned before treatment, implemented during irradiation, and continued after radiation therapy is completed. Skin care in the radiation fields should be stressed with avoidance of excessive physical or heat stress during and after treatment. For upper extremity lesions, similar treatment and follow-up recommendations are used.

For central axis primaries, late radiation injury can be manifested as vertebral body growth arrest, radiation enteritis varying from mild chronic diarrhea to intermittent partial bowel obstruction to life-threatening gastrointestinal bleeding or perforation, radiation cystitis, and radiation-induced hepatitis. Again, with careful attention to radiation treatment planning, it should be possible to avoid significant morbidity in treatment of these central axis primaries. Irradiation of the bones of the face and skull in prepubertal children will result in facial asymetry. Further, late radiation injury to the eye can result in cataract formation, decreased visual acuity, and chronic painful conjunctivitis.

Finally, the issue of second tumors as a late treatment complication needs to be discussed. Of 16 cases of second tumors reported in Ewing's sarcoma patients, 11 cases of bone sarcomas, primarily osteosarcoma, have been described as occurring within the radiation field.[71-73] These usually occurred after the use of orthovoltage irradiation. Nevertheless, although it appears that Ewing's sarcoma patients are at risk of developing bone sarcomas in the irradiated volume, the exact frequency cannot be accurately determined from the small patient groups analyzed to date.[71-73] Whether the combination of megavoltage radiation therapy and chemotherapy is potentially more or less carcinogenic is also not clear. Although the induction of second tumors is of major concern in these patients, the available data are by no means compelling enough to not recommend radiation therapy as the primary local treatment for many patients with Ewing's sarcoma. Hopefully, long-term follow-up of patients treated by the Intergroup Ewing's Sarcoma Studies and other large single institutions will provide in the near future a more complete analysis of the risk of second tumors.

Although most patients with Ewing's sarcoma can be adequately treated with definitive high-dose local irradiation to achieve local control and to maintain good function, it is important to realize that some cases may not be suitable for definitive radiation therapy. Occasional patients present with significant pretreatment functional deficits in an extremity related to infiltration of nerves and blood vessels who may be better treated with amputation. Further, in patients with extensive tumor destruction of a weight-bearing bone, which often is associated with a displaced pathologic fracture, the local treatment options include amputation or an attempt at limb salvage with a bone prosthesis. In the latter situation, preoperative local irradiation (up to 4500 cGy) and chemotherapy can be used to reduce soft tissue and bone tumor to facilitate resection and placement of the prosthesis. Following wound healing, additional local irradiation (1500 cGy) might be used for histologically positive margins along with continued chemotherapy. Finally, younger, prepubertal patients with Ewing's sarcoma will often have a significant reduction in growth of the irradiated bone and soft tissues leading to a poor functional outcome. Thus, the management of the primary tumor in young children is often limited to surgery and chemotherapy when possible.

Integration of Radiation Therapy and Chemotherapy

Any combined modality approach requires good communication between the radiation oncologist and pediatric oncologist to achieve the objective of tumor control with acceptable morbidity. Various sequences of radiation therapy and chemotherapy have been used to treat Ewing's sarcoma. The most common combined modality approach has been to initiate concomitant radiation and chemotherapy at the outset of therapy following staging. More recently, there has been a trend toward deferral of local treatment to assess the response of the primary to systemic chemotherapy. The rationale for this approach is as follows: Ewing's sarcoma is a systemic disease in most patients; combination chemotherapy including vincristine, cyclophosphamide, doxorubicin, and dactinomycin is usually quite effective, with most patients showing an objective response; and initial radiation therapy that includes a significant amount of bone marrow (*e.g.,* for pelvic primary tumors) may compromise delivery of initial full-dose chemotherapy because of prolonged myelosuppression or mucositis. In general, three to five cycles of chemotherapy are administered before radiation therapy except in certain clinical situations. These situations include patients with an initial significant neurologic deficit (*e.g.,* cord compression), patients with severe pain not responsive to the initial chemotherapy, and patients with obstruction of a hollow viscus such as the trachea or a main-stem bronchus.

Most patients will tolerate this aggressive combined modality treatment.[49,59,74] A reduced dose of doxorubicin of approximately 30% during the irradiation and a radiation treatment break of 3 to 5 days after the doxorubicin administration may reduce the drug–radiation interactions of normal tissues such as skin and gastrointestinal tract, which could result in prolonged radiation treatment breaks. As stressed previously, careful attention to the fine details of radiation treatment planning and delivery is of utmost importance to the successful use of combined modality therapy.

Total Body Irradiation

Total body irradiation (TBI) has been proposed as an experimental systemic adjuvant treatment in Ewing's sarcoma for three reasons. First, Ewing's sarcoma is considered to be a radioresponsive tumor. Based on the high response rate to gross, often bulky tumors, it is speculated that micrometastatic disease in high-risk patients with Ewing's sarcoma should respond to systemic irradiation, that is, TBI. Second, although recent combined modality trials have improved the complete response rates in high-risk patients, the predominant pattern of failure remains systemic.[36,47–49] In these patients, TBI is suggested as a non–cross-resistant agent. Third, some clinical data with a single 300 cGy fraction of TBI in patients with limited metastatic disease (isolated pulmonary metastases) suggest that TBI may be an effective systemic agent in the treatment of Ewing's sarcoma.[75] Although 3 of 11 patients treated with 300 cGy TBI remained disease-free for more than 10 years,[75,76] there has been no apparent benefit of sequential hemibody irradiation using the same 300 cGy fraction separated by 6 weeks.[77]

At the NCI, the use of adjuvant TBI in high-risk patients has evolved from a low-dose fractionated schedule (300 cGy/week for 5 weeks; total of 1500 cGy) to high-dose TBI consisting of two 400 cGy fractions on 2 consecutive days.[78,79] This latter high-dose schedule was based on the results of *in vitro* radiation survival and repair studies on tumor cell lines established from patients with recurrent disease.[80] It was argued that these cell lines might represent a resistant subpopulation of Ewing's cells that might persist as subclinical disease in patients treated with both chemotherapy and radiation therapy. The *in vitro* survival curve showed a surprisingly large "shoulder" on the radiation survival curve ($\bar{n}$ up to 6.0), im-

plying a substantial capacity for these cells to repair sublethal radiation damage with a single dose of less than 400 cGy. Additionally, experiments on plateau phase cells showed no repair of potentially lethal damage after 450 cGy.[80] Thus, the clinical study involved two 400 cGy fractions separated by 24 hours and delivered at 10 cGy to 15 cGy per minute.

This recent NCI regimen of TBI (400 cGy on days 1 and 2) combined with vincristine (1.5 mg/m^2 on day 3), doxorubicin (35 mg/m^2/day on days 3 and 4), and cyclophosphamide (1200 mg/m^2/day on days 3 and 4) followed by autologous bone marrow transplantation (day 6) was administered to patients who had achieved complete remission with an intensive induction and local irradiation.[74,79] Preliminary analysis of this consolidative regimen in patients with high-risk Ewing's sarcoma suggests an improvement in disease-free survival at 2 years in patients with both nonmetastatic and metastatic disease (predominantly to bone and bone marrow)—65% and 35% respectively. Although acute morbidity and mortality (5%) has been acceptable, further follow-up and investigation are needed before any definitive conclusions can be made.[79] In summary, TBI remains an interesting but clearly experimental approach in the treatment of Ewing's sarcoma.

Chemotherapy

Before the use of adjuvant chemotherapy in the treatment of Ewing's sarcoma, the survival of patients was very low. A number of retrospectively reported series documented a 5-year survival rate of 10% or less (Table 31-3).[22,50,81,82] As chemotherapeutic agents were developed in the early 1960s, significant activity was observed against Ewing's sarcoma with a number of the drugs (Table 31-4). Subsequently, many drugs have been found to have single agent activity in the treatment of Ewing's sarcoma (Table 31-4).[83–90] Initially, the most consistently effective agents were cyclophosphamide and doxorubicin; more recently, ifosfamide and etoposide have been a highly active combination even in patients who have failed previous chemotherapy.[91–93] Other agents found to have some activity in the disease are vincristine, dactinomycin, and 5-fluorouracil. Agents with reported activity, although little, are BCNU and cisplatin.[90,94] High-dose melphalan followed by autologous bone marrow transplantation has also had demonstrable activity.[95] Interpretation and comparison of single agent and phase II activity data such as that presented in Table 31-4 must be interpreted in light of the therapy to which the tumor has previously become resistant. For example, the single agent response rates for both ifosfamide and etoposide as well as the response rate for the combination of the two agents were determined in patients who had already failed at least one chemotherapeutic regimen, usually including both doxorubicin and cyclophosphamide.

Table 31-3

Five-Year Survival of Patients with Ewing's Sarcoma Treated Without Chemotherapy

Series	Number of Patients	Number Surviving at 5 Years
Nesbit [130]	374	36 (9.6%)
Bacci [102]	83	7 (8.4%)
Dahlin [22]	133	16 (12.0%)
Wang [50]	47	5 (10.6%)
Total	637	64 (10.0%)

Table 31-4
Single-Agent and Combination Activity in Ewing's Sarcoma in Phase II Studies

Agent (References)	Response (no. responding/total)	Response Rate (%) (CR or PR)
Cyclophosphamide (85–87, 103–106)	17/36	47
Doxorubicin (88, 107–112)	25/60	42
Ifosfamide (91, 122, 123)	12/37	32
Vincristine (83, 106, 113, 114)	4/10	40
Actinomycin D (84, 104, 115)	3/16	19
BCNU (90, 106)	6/18	33
5-fluorouracil (89, 116)	4/10	40
Etoposide (92, 117)	3/10	30
Cisplatin (94, 118–120)	2/27	7
Melphalan (high dose) (95, 121)	9/11	82
Ifosfamide/etoposide (93)	16/17	94

Despite the demonstrated single agent activity, the early studies of single chemotherapeutic agents used in an adjuvant fashion had only slight impact on the overall outcome of patients with Ewing's sarcoma. When effective agents were combined, however, the survival and disease-free survival rates of patients began to improve significantly.[35,47,48,49,52,96–102]

In 1973 a multi-institutional randomized trial was begun: the first Intergroup Ewing's Sarcoma Study (IESS 1) (see Tables 31-5 and 31-6).[47] One part of this study, designed for patients without metastatic disease, evaluated the addition of doxorubicin or pulmonary irradiation in the treatment of Ewing's sarcoma by adding these therapies to what was then considered to be standard therapy: vincristine, dactinomycin, and cyclophosphamide (VAC). The results of this study were important for several reasons. First, the overall survival rate (56% at 3 years) for the whole group was improved significantly over that for patients treated with no adjuvant therapy or with single agents. Second, the efficacy of pulmonary irradiation was established, providing further support for the role of systemic irradiation in this tumor. Third, the role of doxorubicin in the treatment of Ewing's sarcoma was clearly established. The 2-year disease-free survival rate was 74% for the patients receiving doxorubicin plus VAC compared to 35% for patients receiving VAC alone. Finally, the outcome was related to the site of disease, with the pelvic and proximal extremity sites faring worse than all other primary sites of disease.[47]

Also important in this initial study was the fact that of 44 patients who presented with advanced local disease in the chest wall or metastatic disease, 31 (70%) achieved a complete remission. At a median of 34 months, 41% of all of the patients and 33% of the patients with metastatic disease remained disease-free.[49] These results in patients with both localized and metastatic disease represented an important improvement in the results of therapy and formed the basis of future studies.[47,49]

The second Intergroup Ewing's Sarcoma Study (IESS 2), the results of which have not yet been published, evaluated the role of a more intensive regimen that relied heavily on the two most active agents at the time: cyclophosphamide and doxorubicin. The preliminary results of this study have demonstrated a benefit to this approach, especially in patients who had fared more poorly on the first study: those with pelvic primary sites.[100] Unfortunately, patients with metastatic disease continued to relapse at the same rate as those on the IESS 1.[100]

Several large single institutions or groups have also played important roles in the development of chemotherapy for Ewing's sarcoma. An important early report came from the Memorial Sloan-Kettering Cancer Center (MSKCC). Twelve children were treated with sequential doses of adjuvant chemotherapy with dactinomycin, doxorubicin, and the combination of vincristine and cyclophosphamide for 2 years (T2) (see Tables 31-5 and 31-6). All 12 children had localized disease at diagnosis, and all 12 continued disease-free for 10 to 37 months at the time of the first report.[96] In 1981, the 10-year experience with adjuvant chemotherapy at MSKCC was reviewed and detailed the results of the T2, T6, and T9 protocols for the treatment of patients with localized disease.[48] Sixty-seven patients were treated with combination chemotherapy regimens, 19 on the T2 protocol, 30 on the T6 protocol, and 18 on the T9 protocol. Fifty-three of the 67 patients with localized disease who were treated with aggressive chemotherapy in addition to local radiation or surgery were alive and disease-free at a median of 41 months from the beginning of therapy. Disease-free survival, as in IESS 1 and 2, appeared to be related to site of primary disease: 15 of 23 patients with axial disease (65%) were free of disease compared to 19 of 24 with proximal lesions (79%) and 19 of 20 (95%) with distal lesions. The chemotherapy regimens of these three successive studies evaluated, in single arm trials, the role of chemotherapy in general; however, the role played by both cyclophosphamide and doxorubicin in the protocols became more important with each study. The results confirmed the results of IESS 1 and 2: disease-free survival can be significantly improved with the use of an aggressive regimen including cyclophosphamide and doxorubicin.[48] The role of delayed therapy to the primary disease and the comparison of radiation and surgery in the control of the primary disease were also evaluated in these studies, although in a nonrandomized "selected" fashion. It was apparent from the T9 study that initial chemotherapy could significantly reduce tumor bulk. Further, the disease-free survival was similar for those treated with surgery (82%) and those treated with radiation (76%). However, 7 of the 34 patients treated with radiation but no surgery suffered local recurrences.[48]

In 1983, the first report of a different approach, one using sequential cyclophosphamide and doxorubicin, was published.[36] Twenty-two of 24 patients achieved a complete remission with this approach, and 4 of 10 patients with metastatic disease and 12 of 14 patients with localized disease remained disease-free from 9 to 41 months. This report again documented that cyclophosphamide and doxorubicin are very active in the treatment of Ewing's sarcoma and can be given with a moderately intense dosage and schedule with good result.[36]

A number of other studies have confirmed that therapy

Table 31-5
Results of Therapy for Nonmetastatic Ewing's Sarcoma

Institution or Author (Reference)	Regimen	Outcome
IESS 1 (47)	*Regimen 2:* Wkly VCR (1.5/m²)/CPM (500/m²) Dactino (15 μg/kg × 5) q 3 mo	Two-year relapse-free survival: 35%
	Regimen 1: Wkly VCR/CPM Dactino q 3 mo Doxo (60/m²) q 3 mo	Two-year relapse-free survival: 74%
	Regimen 3: Wkly VCR/CPM Dactino q 3 mo Bilateral pulmonary RT (1500–1800 cGY)	Two-year relapse-free survival: 58%
IESS 1 (58)	See above	N = 62 pelvic tumors: 34% disease-free survival at 5 years
IESS 1 (124)	See above	N = 21 rib primaries: 11 (52%) disease-free at 18–64 months
MSKCC (48, 96, 125)	T2	All 12 patients alive NED at 10–37+ months
	T6	23 of 28 patients alive NED at 12–46+ months

	T2–T9
	Wk 0: cyclo (1200/m²), doxo (20/m² × 3)
	    MTX (12/m² × 3), VCR (1.5/m²/wk × 5)
	Wk 3: bleo (10/m² × 3), cyclo (500/m² × 2), dactino
	    (500 μg/m² × 2)
	Wk 6: same as week 0. Cycle repeats at 9 weeks
		N = 67: 2-year disease-free survival: 79%

St Jude (36)	Sequential: Cyclo (150/m² × 7d) Doxo (35/m² day 8) Repeat q 2 weeks	14/14 achieved CR 12/14 disease-free at 9–41+ months
Istituto Ortopedico Rizzoli (101)	VCR (1.5/m²) Doxo (50/m²) CPM (300/m² × 2) Every 2 weeks	N = 80: 31 (39%) disease-free at mean of 45 months (21–96 months)
Istituto Ortopedico Rizzoli (102)		N = 124: 48% disease-free survival at a median of 65 months
Children's Solid Tumor Group (98)	VCR (1.5/m²) Doxo (40/m²) Cyclo (300/m²) Repeat q 2 weeks × 6, then q 3 weeks	N = 21: 14 disease-free at a median of 36 months
Adrani (126)	VCR Doxo Cyclo	N = 28: 55% disease-free survival at 3 years
Berry (77)	VCR Doxo Cyclo Hemibody radiation (500 upper, 600 lower)	N = 17: 49% survival at 3 years (no beneficial effect of hemibody irradiation)
Oberlin (127)	VCR Doxo Cyclo	N = 67 histologic responses: 41 good: 57% disease-free 26 bad: 9% disease-free

Table 31-5 (continued)

Institution or Author (Reference)	Regimen	Outcome
Zucker (128)	Vcr Doxo Cyclo Procarbazine	N = 30: 6 year disease-free survival: 49%
Gasparini (129)	VCR (1.4/m² × 2) Doxo (60/m²) Alt with VCR (1.4/m² × 2), Cyclo (1.0g/m²)	N = 34: 53% relapse-free survival at 4 years
NCI (78)	VCR, dactino, cyclo induction. Low-dose TBI. VCR, Doxo, Cyclo, DTIC maintenance	N = 24 high-risk patients (pelvis, chest wall; 4 with METS): 25% disease-free survival at 5 years
NCI (79)	VCR (1.5/m²) Doxo (60–90/m²) Cyclo (1.2–1.8 g/m²) Repeat q 3 weeks	N = 18: 70% disease-free survival at 18 months

Table 31-6
Results of Therapy for Metastatic Ewing's Sarcoma

Institution (Reference)	Regimen	Outcome
MSKCC (125)	T6	6/10 NED at 14–34 months
IESS (49)	*Regimen 1:* wkly VCR/CPM Dactino q 3 mo Doxo q 3 mo	31/44 achieved CR 17/44 disease-free at 75 weeks 5/7 with regional disease 12/37 with metastatic disease
St Jude (36)	*Sequential:* Cyclo (150/m² × 7) Doxo (35/m² × 8)	8/10 achieved CR 4/10 remained disease-free at 12–34 + months
NCI (79, 131)	S1–S4 therapy *High-risk protocol:* Induction VCR (2.0/m²), doxo (90/m²–>60/m²) Cyclo (1800/m² repeat q 3 weeks Consolidation VCR (2.0/m²), doxo (70/m²), cyclo (80/kg) Total body irradiation (400 cGY × 2) Autologous bone marrow transplant	N = 38: <5% survival at 5 years N = 13: 32% relapse-free survival at 2½ years

based on the use of these two agents produces good results when given as adjuvant therapy to localized patients.[98,101] Fourteen of 21 patients treated by the Children's Solid Tumor Group were disease-free at a median of 3 years from diagnosis, and 31 of 80 patients treated at the Istituto Ortopedico Rizzoli were disease-free at a median of 50 months of follow-up. Both studies used moderate doses of vincristine, doxorubicin, and cyclophosphamide administered every 2 weeks at modest dose intensity.[98,101]

Addressing a different problem, investigators at the NCI attempted to develop effective therapy for patients at high risk of relapsing, primarily those with widespread metastatic disease. The initial study, outlined previously in the radiation therapy section, used an induction with vincristine, dactinomycin, and cyclophosphamide followed by low dose total body irradiation and maintenance therapy, including doxorubicin.[79] Of these 24 high-risk patients, 4 of whom had metastatic disease, 20 (83%) achieved a complete remission. Six (25%) now remain in complete remission with more than 5 years of follow-up.[95] Building on this study and on the information available that the combination of cyclophosphamide and doxorubicin was effective adjuvant therapy, a second NCI study was developed for patients with disease with a poor prognosis on standard therapy. The induction consisted of vincristine, doxorubicin, and cyclophosphamide given at a higher dose than on previous studies. Once complete remission was achieved, an intensive consolidation was administered that included vincristine, doxorubicin, cyclophosphamide, and TBI, followed by autologous bone marrow transplantation. Of the 23 patients treated with this approach, 22 achieved a complete remission, and the actuarial disease-free survival at 18 months is 65% for the group with nonmetastatic disease and 32% for the group with metastatic disease.[79] In light of the fact that most patients with metastatic disease had either bone or bone marrow disease and most patients with localized disease had massive primary tumors, this approach seems worthy of further investigation. Unfortunately, it is also clear that much work needs to be done in the treatment of patients with metastatic disease.

To develop new approaches to the treatment of patients with metastatic Ewing's sarcoma, a phase II study evaluating the role of the combination of ifosfamide and etoposide in patients who had relapsed was begun at the NCI in 1985.[93] The study was based on the fact that ifosfamide is very similar in structure and mechanism of action to cyclophosphamide, an agent that is one of the most important in the treatment of Ewing's sarcoma (see Tables 31-5 and 31-6). It was also based on the fact that both ifosfamide and etoposide had significant single agent activity in patients who had failed primary therapy with regimens containing both cyclophosphamide and doxorubicin (see Table 31-5).[91,92,93] The rationale for the combination of these two agents administered sequentially on each of 5 successive days was based on the hypothesis that etoposide would significantly reduce the repair of ifosfamide-induced DNA damage if ifosfamide was administered when etoposide was present. Conversely, the ifosfamide might "fix" the reversible DNA damage caused by etoposide (see Chap. 9). The preliminary results of this phase II study have shown that most patients with Ewing's sarcoma will have significant responses to this combination even when resistant to a cyclophosphamide-based regimen.[93] This observation has led to the development of protocols at the NCI and elsewhere that will use this non–cross-resistant regimen in the treatment of newly diagnosed patients, alternating with the combination of vincristine, doxorubicin, and cyclophosphamide.

FUTURE DIRECTIONS

The current results of therapy are significantly better than those obtained with therapy available in the 1970s. Nevertheless, important progress must still be made if more patients are to survive with a better functional outcome. Local control has improved with the use of aggressive chemotherapy before radiation or surgery. The incidence of subsequent relapse has been reduced in patients by the use of adjuvant chemotherapy. The complete remission rate of patients with metastatic disease at diagnosis has improved. However, a number of questions remain. With the development of new techniques and reagents, it will become clear that all the small round cell tumors that are now included in the uniform diagnostic category of Ewing's sarcoma actually represent more than one diagnostic entity. These distinctions will likely have prognostic significance and important implications for treatment planning. Further evaluation and definition of important prognostic factors such as size of the primary lesion, pathologic subtype, and oncogene expression will be needed to optimize and individualize therapy. The role of a new chemotherapy regimen using ifosfamide and etoposide and the role of total body irradiation in high-risk patients must be further evaluated. The optimal duration of therapy must also be determined. Therapy varies from 6 months to 2 years in the presently published studies without apparent differences in outcome.

The response to preoperative chemotherapy, an important predictor of outcome in osteosarcoma, has not been evaluated extensively in Ewing's sarcoma. Nevertheless, initial studies suggest that this may be an important prognostic factor in this disease as well.[127] Because of the risk of second biopsies in patients with Ewing's sarcoma, an important aspect in the eval-

uation of the role of histologic response will be the development of new imaging modalities that correlate with histologic response to chemotherapy (*i.e.*, MRI and positron emision tomography).

Determination of the optimal local management of Ewing's sarcoma, that is, how to maximize local control while minimizing the occurrence of significant functional disabilities and of second malignancies in children of varying ages and stages of growth, remains a major goal for future studies. Retrospective review of single institution studies has suggested that surgery may also have a positive impact on outcome.[62–64,102] However, these reports have not prospectively analyzed and stratified the tumors for size, site, and pathologic characteristics of the lesions. Thus, a carefully controlled randomized study must be performed before it can be concluded that the use of surgery (as compared to radiation therapy) improves survival.

Most importantly, future therapeutic studies must be designed to encourage and allow the discovery and evaluation of the biology of Ewing's sarcoma using new molecular techniques.

OTHER NONRHABDOMYOSARCOMA SOFT TISSUE SARCOMAS OF CHILDHOOD AND ADOLESCENCE

The most common soft tissue sarcoma of children is rhabdomyosarcoma; however, 47% of all soft tissue sarcomas in children have a histology other than rhabdomyosarcoma (see also Chaps. 30 and 35).[1] Because these tumors make up 3% of all tumors in children, a better understanding of the biology and treatment of these rare and heterogeneous tumors is clearly needed. Although soft tissue sarcomas are more commonly seen in adults, the prognosis, in general, appears to be better for children with one of these tumors. This difference in prognosis is most pronounced for infants and younger children whose tumors often have a benign behavior and excellent prognosis with surgery alone. Soft tissue sarcomas that occur in adolescents often behave like the sarcomas that occur in adult patients. Thus, the management of soft tissue sarcomas in adolescents is similar to the management of these tumors in adults.

Soft tissue sarcomas may arise in any part of the body; however, the most common sites are the extremity and trunk, especially the retroperitoneum.[132,133] The standard approach to the management of these tumors in adults has undergone some change and significant debate over the past 10 years.[132,133] The optimal management may, indeed, be specific to anatomical site. Most therapeutic trials in adults have tested treatment strategies in groups of patients with heterogeneous histologies. This approach may or may not be correct in adults; however, it is unlikely to result in appropriate recommendations for the therapy of all children with nonrhabdomyosarcoma soft tissue sarcomas. For these reasons, treatment strategies have not yet been tested adequately in large groups of children in randomized trials.

The usual approach to the treatment of these tumors in adults is primarily surgical: the primary tumor is excised with wide margins.[132,133] Radiation therapy is added to the regimen when there is concern about the adequacy of the surgical margin or when limb-sparing procedures are performed.[132] The role of adjuvant chemotherapy in patients whose tumors have been completely excised is not yet generally agreed upon. Nevertheless, a small randomized study of adjuvant chemotherapy in 65 adults with soft tissue sarcomas of the extremities showed a disease-free survival difference for patients who received adjuvant chemotherapy with cyclophosphamide and doxorubicin.[133] In a larger report of 211 patients with resectable, high-grade soft tissue sarcomas of the extremities, adjuvant chemotherapy significantly prolonged disease-free sur-

Table 31-7
Features of the Common Childhood Soft Tissue Sarcomas

Tumor	Common Sites	Usual Age at Onset	Prognosis and Biological Features
Fibrosarcoma			
Congenital	Extremity (70%), trunk (30%)	Most < 2 years	Excellent with surgery alone
Adult form	Extremity (thigh, knee)	15 years	Outcome similar to adults
Neurofibrosarcoma	Extremity (40%), retroperitoneum (25%), trunk (20%)	—	Stage-related: I and II: good III and IV: poor Associated with von Recklinghausen's disease
Malignant fibrous histiocytoma	Extremity	Rare in children; usual age: 10–20 years	Stage-related: I and II: good III and IV: poor
Synovial sarcoma	Extremity (lower > upper)	31% of all cases occur <20 years	Stage-related: I and II: good (45–70% 5-year survival) III and IV: poor
Hemangiopericytoma			
Adult form	Extremity, retroperitoneum, head and neck	Most cases in children occur in 10–20 year age group	Stage-related: I and II: good (30–70% 5-year survival with adjuvant therapy) III and IV: poor
Infantile form	Extremity	Very rare	Excellent with surgery alone; rare metastases
Alveolar soft part sarcoma	Extremities (lower > upper) In children: head and neck	—	Short-term survival: very good Long-term survival: poor regardless of initial stage
Leiomyosarcoma	Retroperitoneum, GI tract, vascular tissue	—	Site-related: Non-GI tract—good GI tract—poor (high incidence of metastases)
Liposarcoma	Extremity, retroperitoneum	Two age peaks: 0–2 years; 2nd decade	Rarely metastasizes. Prognosis very good with complete excision

vival.[132] This study further suggested that patients who had undergone limb-sparing procedures plus postoperative radiotherapy had no difference in disease-free survival or overall survival from those patients who had had an amputation, although the local failure rate was higher for the limb-spared group. For patients who developed metastatic disease, the ability to surgically remove the metastases appeared to have important prognostic significance as measured by subsequent survival.[132]

Although the approach to children with these tumors may often be similar to that for adults, important differences exist. First, similar histologies may have very different biologies in children (Table 31-7). Second, the morbidity of radiation in a small and rapidly growing child may be much greater than that in an adult, depending on the site that requires irradiation. Third, it is more difficult to perform functionally successful limb-sparing procedures in young, growing children; however, newer techniques and expandable prostheses may allow a greater number of limbs of children to be salvaged. Finally, the long-term consequences of radiation and chemotherapy are of greater concern for children, whose potential survival after successful therapy will be much longer. Thus, in order to achieve the goal of maximum tumor control with minimum morbidity in both the short and long term, it will be important to carefully study these tumors in a prospective way and to be able ultimately to individualize therapy based on important prognostic factors.

Most of the information about the treatment of children with nonrhabdomyosarcomatous soft tissue sarcomas comes from retrospective analyses of the experiences of a single institution. Although these reports are valuable and provide an important basis upon which future studies can be developed, careful prospective multi-institutional studies are needed. The most important theme of most of these reports is that the ability to surgically extirpate the tumor is the most critical prognostic factor. In a retrospective review of 62 cases of childhood soft-tissue sarcomas other than rhabdomyosarcoma, 84% survived with no evidence of disease when the tumor could be completely removed, whereas only 1 of 26 patients survived when gross tumor remained after resection.[134] Factors besides the extent of disease that now appear to be important are age, histology, and primary site.

Fibrosarcoma

Epidemiology and Biology

Although rare, fibrosarcoma is one of the most common non-rhabdomyosarcomatous soft tissue sarcomas in children and adolescents.[135] Historical series of patients with congenital fibrosarcomas suggested that there was a predominance of boys[136,137]; however, a recent report and review of the literature reveals no significant sex predominance.[138] Fibrosarcomas occur most frequently on the extremity, often in the distal segments; 70% of the reported cases of congenital fibrosarcoma occur at this site. There appear to be two peaks in incidence of fibrosarcoma according to age: in infants and young children under 5 years of age and in patients 10 to 15 years of

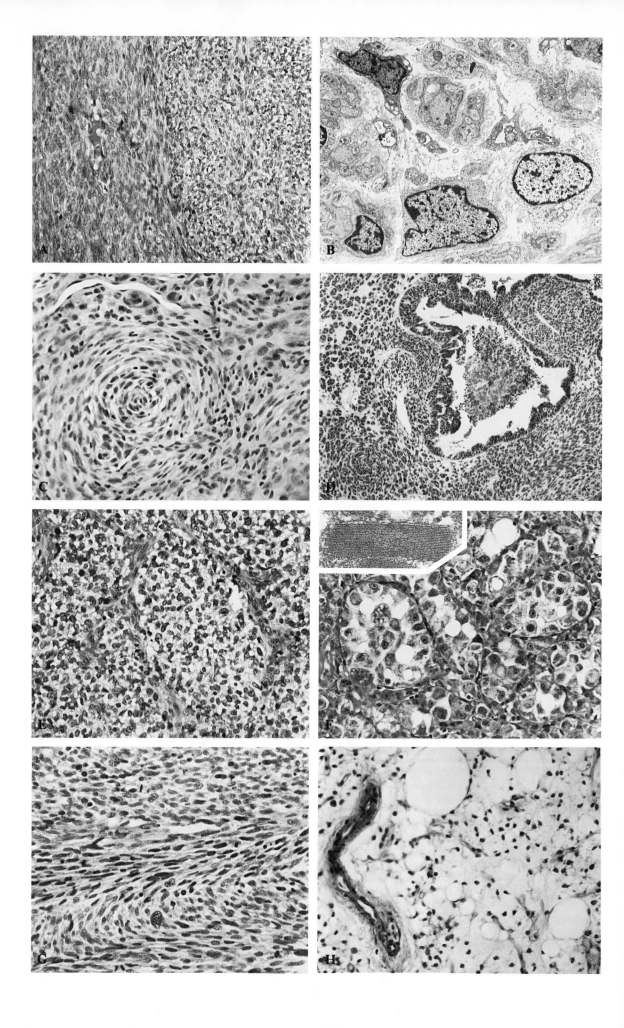

age. Although some authors believe that the biology of these tumors is similar in the two age groups, most think that the tumors in infants generally have a more benign course.[136,137,139]

Pathology

Fibrosarcoma is a spindle cell tumor with a characteristic herringbone pattern, or regularly interweaving fascicles of parallel arrays of tumor cells (Fig. 31-18A). Important features to look for are evidence of abnormal mitoses, nuclear pleomorphism, and increased basophilia of individual, sometimes anaplastic tumor cells. Cells are densely packed, but reticulin stain reveals a regular pattern of stromal collagen fibres not easily appreciated by light microscopy. The most important entities to distinguish are aggressive fibromatosis (which can be exceedingly aggressive locally, but which does not metastasize), nodular fasciitis, myositis ossificans, and inflammatory pseudotumor, among nonmalignant conditions, and neurofibrosarcoma and poorly differentiated embryonal rhabdomyosarcoma, among malignant tumors. Unfortunately, it is not always possible to distinguish congenital fibrosarcoma from fibromatosis, as noted by Stout[137] and others.[140,141] Individual tumors must be evaluated in light of clinical information such as age, site, history, and duration of the lesion. Serious mistakes have been made, especially with relation to myositis ossificans (a post-traumatic lesion) and nodular fasciitis.

Clinical Presentation

In a recent review of the literature detailing the experience with 52 cases of congenital fibrosarcoma, 37 occurred on an extremity and 15 on the trunk.[138] Of the patients with extremity primaries, 92% were free of metastatic disease and 95% were alive despite a 27% local recurrence rate. Thus, a local recurrence of a congenital fibrosarcoma arising on an extremity does not herald systemic spread of the tumor. This is in contrast to the usual clinical course in which a local recurrence appears after initial treatment of a small round cell sarcoma. In contrast, congenital fibrosarcomas of the trunk appear to be more aggressive, with 20% of patients developing metastases, 26% dying of their disease, and 13% suffering a local recurrence. Of the group of 52 reported congenital fibrosarcomas, only 6 patients have died (11.5%).[138] This is in contrast to fibrosarcoma in adolescents and young adults, which most commonly arises on the extremity, where the 5-year survival rate is approximately 60%.[142]

Principles and Recommendations for Treatment

Although a recent report details the benefit of preoperative chemotherapy in the treatment of fibrosarcoma in infants and young children,[143,144] the mainstay of treatment is surgical extirpation by wide local excision usually without additional therapy. Because late local recurrences do not appear to affect

◀ FIGURE 31-18. Differentiated soft tissue sarcomas other than rhabdomyosarcoma. **A.** Fibrosarcoma. This tumor is rare in adults and uncommon in older children but is one of the most common nonmyogenous soft tissue sarcomas in the first decade. Interlacing fascicles of spindle cells appear either elongate (*left*) or round (*right*) on section, depending on plane of section. The cells are closely packed, homogeneous, and resemble normal fibroblasts. Mitoses, pleomorphism, and nuclear hyperchromatism are rare. (H & E; original magnification × 250) **B.** Neurofibrosarcoma. The light microscopic appearance of this tumor may be indistinguishable from fibrosarcoma, yet the prognosis is very different. The former is a low-grade sarcoma, the latter high-grade. EM reveals evidence of nerve sheath differentiation, although not often as well developed as seen here, where some tumor cells envelop neurites (*upper center*), mimicking Schwann cells. More often, only fragmented basal lamina and slender cell processes are present. (EM; original magnification × 2000) **C.** Malignant fibrous histiocytoma. The most common soft tissue sarcoma of adults, MFH is uncommon in children. The angiomatoid variant, seen here, is the only type commonly seen in children. The propensity for tumor cells to form vascular-like structures (*center*) accounts for the name. (H & E; original magnification × 250) **D.** Synoviosarcoma. Classic biphasic synoviosarcoma is an unmistakable entity. Distinct epithelial, glandular differentiation (*center*) alternates with fibrosarcomatous stroma (*right*). Islands of tumor cells separated by hyaline stroma are sometimes seen (*left*), and staghorn vasculature (not illustrated) is often conspicuous. (H & E; original magnification × 100) **E.** Hemangiopericytoma. Thought to recapitulate normal pericytes, this tumor varies from Ewing-like (as here) to a spindle cell tumor resembling smooth muscle. In all cases, reticulin stains outline individual tumor cells and nests and EM demonstrates evidence of pericytic differentiation. Tumor cells do not form vascular spaces but surround them (*center*). (H & E; original magnification × 250) **F.** Alveolar soft part sarcoma. This problematic tumor is easily distinguished from all other sarcomas. The glandular or alveolar pattern is always prominent; tumor cells appear to rest on a basement membrane. Spaces within are variably present, as here. The tumor cells possess abundant pink cytoplasm that by light microscopy resembles muscle. However, PAS-positive, diastase-resistant cytoplasmic crystalloids (*center*) are present in tumor cells. By EM, these crystals are diagnostic (*inset*). Recent evidence, in fact, favors a myogenous origin of this tumor, although myogenous differentiation has never been identified by EM. (H & E; original magnification × 250) **G.** Leiomyosarcoma. Smooth muscle tumors in children are rare but do occur. Leiomyosarcoma in children and adults is characterized by spindle cells that resemble fibroblasts but stain intensely with eosin, due to their content of smooth muscle actin–myosin bundles. Some degree of pleomorphism (*bottom center*) and mitosis (*upper center*) are often found. (H & E; original magnification × 250) **H.** Liposarcoma. Of the four types of liposarcoma common in adults, only the myxoid type is common in children, and even then only rarely. This relatively low-grade sarcoma resembles fetal lipoblasts, often interspersed among more differentiated adipocytes (large clear cells). The vasculature (*left*) is routinely prominent in all liposarcomas and helps to distinguish the tumor from lipoblastoma and related benign fatty tumors. (H & E; original magnification × 400) overall survival of patients with congenital fibrosarcoma, conservative management aimed at maintaining as much function as possible and avoiding amputation is often the preferred approach. Because of the known long-term consequences of radiation therapy and the potential late effects of chemotherapy, the use of these modalities in the local management of congenital fibrosarcoma is generally not advised unless surgical removal is not possible. This is again in contrast to the treatment recommendations for older children and young adults. Here, an aggressive attempt to remove the tumor by wide local excision or amputation is the standard therapy. A recent report by Potter[132] suggests that if a limb-sparing procedure could be accomplished with close or microscopically positive margins, an excellent outcome could be expected with the addition of radiation therapy.

There is no evidence that adjuvant chemotherapy is indicated in the treatment of congenital fibrosarcoma and nonmetastatic fibrosarcoma of young children. This is in contrast to the experience in adults with high-grade spindle cell sarcomas in which chemotherapy appears to be of benefit in extremity lesions in both a randomized study and the overall experience at the surgery branch of the NCI.[132,133] Unfortunately, only four patients specifically with fibrosarcoma were treated in the randomized study, and thus the role of adjuvant chemotherapy has not yet been ascertained with certainty.[133]

Finally, although the role of chemotherapy in the adjuvant treatment of congenital fibrosarcoma has not been established, several recent reports clearly document that at least some of these tumors are sensitive to chemotherapy.[143,144] Thus, for patients who have unresectable metastatic or primary disease, chemotherapy is the initial treatment of choice. The following combinations of chemotherapy have been used successfully: vincristine, doxorubicin, and cyclophosphamide, and vincristine, dactinomycin, and cyclophosphamide. Further, use of the new combination of ifosfamide and etoposide has resulted in complete regressions of metastatic fibrosarcoma.[145]

Neurofibrosarcoma

Epidemiology, Genetics, and Biology

Neurofibrosarcomas, malignant tumors of nerve sheath origin, account for approximately 5% to 10% of all nonrhabdomyosarcomatous soft tissue sarcomas in children.[146–149] Although these tumors are not yet associated with a specific gene deletion or chromosome abnormality, it seems likely that such an abnormality will be discovered. Like retinoblastoma, which presents in association with the dominantly inherited retinoblastoma syndrome, neurofibrosarcoma also occurs in association with a dominantly inherited syndrome, neurofibromatosis (von Recklinghausen's disease) (see also Chaps. 2, 3 and 25).[150,151] With hereditary retinoblastoma, a primary mutation occurs in the germ line that is recessive at the cellular level to the normal allele.[152] The growth of a tumor ensues only after a second event occurs, resulting in loss of the normal allele and the unmasking of the altered allele. Unlike retinoblastoma in which the phenotypic expression of a retinal tumor occurs in 90% of patients, only 5% to 16% of patients with von Recklinghausen's disease, characterized by multiple neurofibromas and café au lait spots, develop neurofibrosarcomas.[150,151] Despite this lower penetrance, it has been hypothesized that these tumors may be associated with a specific gene deletion that results in the expression of a gene responsible for the development of the neurofibrosarcoma.[152,153] Recently, acoustic neuroma, a tumor associated with the neurofibromatosis II syndrome (bilateral acoustic neurofibromatosis), was found to have the loss of genes located on chromosome 22. Although the genetic abnormality producing the neurofibromatosis I

syndrome and neurofibrosarcomas is likely to be distinct from that producing neurofibromatosis II, a similar mechanism may be operative at a different genetic locus. Although only 20% of patients with neurofibrosarcoma presenting at all ages have von Recklinghausen's disease, neurofibrosarcoma in children is more commonly associated with this syndrome.[155] This further suggests that the neurofibrosarcoma in this setting is congenital in nature.

Pathology

Although superficially similar in appearance to fibrosarcoma, this is a vastly more aggressive lesion that must be distinguished from the less malignant fibrosarcoma. The cells are usually more variable in size and shape, a herringbone pattern is usually absent, and often typical features of adult neurofibrosarcomas can be found in some areas of the tumor: for example, a myxoid stroma, palisading of nuclei, and occasionally well-defined organoid arrays of nuclei (so-called Verocay bodies).[156] These features, common in benign schwannomas, are far less conspicuous in the malignant counterpart but can be diagnostic when present. EM is by far the most useful method of establishing the diagnosis; Schwann cell differentiation, lacking only neurites within cytoplasmic concavities (mesaxons), is usually conspicuous (Fig. 31-18B).

Clinical Presentation

In a recent report from the Children's Hospital of Philadelphia (CHOP), in which the experience with 24 patients is detailed, 16 children had the associated neurofibromatosis syndrome. The most common primary sites were extremity (42%), retroperitoneum (25%), and trunk (21%); 3 tumors occurred in other sites. Of the entire group only 2 patients had metastases at diagnosis.[155]

As with fibrosarcoma, surgery plays a key role in the management of children with neurofibrosarcoma. Of the 24 patients described above, 12 underwent gross total removal of the tumor, and 9 of these were tumor-free survivors at 3 years. In contrast, none of the 12 patients who could not have their tumors grossly removed were alive without disease at 3 years. In this small group of patients, it appeared that patients treated by complete removal with adequate margins and those treated by gross resection and radiation to microscopic residual disease had similar outcomes. This result is consistent with the experience in adult patients.[155]

The role of chemotherapy in the treatment of patients with neurofibrosarcoma is not yet clear. The experience with extremity sarcomas in adults at the NCI suggests that a regimen of doxorubicin and cyclophosphamide is effective in the adjuvant treatment of localized, grossly removed neurofibrosarcoma. However, only five patients with neurofibrosarcoma were entered onto the adjuvant trial: all survived, three treated with adjuvant chemotherapy and two without.[132,133] In the retrospective series from CHOP, there was no obvious difference in the outcome of patients whose tumors were grossly resected whether they were treated with or without chemotherapy; three of four treated with surgery alone survived disease-free, and five of eight treated with adjuvant chemotherapy were alive without disease.[155]

Although chemotherapy can produce tumor regressions in patients with gross local and metastatic disease, no chemotherapy regimen has emerged that can produce an adequate disease-free survival in patients with advanced disease. The most commonly used regimens include vincristine, cyclophosphamide, dactinomycin, and doxorubicin (VAC + ADR). None of the patients with gross residual disease after surgery in the above report survived disease-free despite the use of chemotherapy in 10 of the 12 cases (VAC ± ADR). Clearly, the optimum regimen has not been defined. Recently, the combination of ifosfamide and etoposide, a regimen highly active in the treatment of recurrent small round cell tumors of neural origin, has produced partial tumor regressions in 2 of the 4 patients with recurrent neurofibrosarcoma thus far evaluated.[145] Further investigation of this regimen is ongoing.

Malignant Fibrous Histiocytoma

Epidemiology

Although malignant fibrous histiocytoma (MFH) was the most common histologic diagnosis in the NCI series of adult patients with extremity sarcomas (accounting for 25% of the series, or 53 of 211 patients), it is much less common in children. In the St. Jude series in children, only 5 of the 62 cases (8%) of nonrhabdomyosarcomatous soft tissue sarcoma were diagnosed to have MFH.[134]

Pathology

Arthur Purdy Stout popularized the notion that many soft tissue sarcomas in adults were not simply fibrous lesions (i.e., fibrosarcoma), but rather possessed more than one tissue element (fat, fibrous tissue, tissue macrophages).[157] This concept has been widely adopted, and pathologists are now less likely to make a diagnosis of fibrosarcoma in adults. Not surprisingly, MFH is now recognized in children as well. The typical microscopic appearance resembles fibrosarcoma but is distinct therefrom by the presence of marked cellular pleomorphism, multiple cell types (especially lipid-laden tumor cells), and an overall more malignant appearance (Fig. 31-18C). A storiform pattern of tumor cells (described as radiating fascicles of tumor cells at right angles from one another) is virtually diagnostic of this tumor.[157-159]

Principles and Recommendations for Treatment

Because of the rarity of this tumor in childhood, the approach to treatment of this malignancy is based primarily on the experience with adults. The accepted initial management is wide local excision of the tumor. When the tumor arises in the extremity, limb-sparing operations with radiation to the tumor bed have been as successful as amputations; however, the tumor must be small and appropriately placed to allow such an approach. Although some experience in adults suggests that adjuvant chemotherapy is of benefit, the role of adjuvant chemotherapy has not yet been established in children with this tumor.[132,133] In a recent report of seven patients with MFH, two had their tumor completely removed; both were treated with adjuvant chemotherapy and were alive at 1.4 years and 9 years of follow-up, respectively.[160] In contrast, Tracy and colleagues reported six children treated with minimal chemotherapy (one patient) or no adjuvant chemotherapy (five patients) after complete removal of their tumors. All were alive without disease at a follow-up of 1 year for one patient and more than 3 years for the other five patients.[161]

Chemotherapy with vincristine, dactinomycin, and cyclophosphamide with or without doxorubicin has produced objective tumor regressions in patients with advanced disease; however, the optimal chemotherapy regimen has not yet been determined.[160,162-165] Four of the five patients treated by Raney and co-workers with group III or IV disease had complete (3 patients) or partial (1 patient) tumor regressions and two remained disease-free at 4.6 and 5.4 years, respectively. Responses to the combination of ifosfamide and etoposide have also been seen.[145] More information about the optimal treatment of children with MFH is needed.

Synovial Sarcoma

Epidemiology and Clinical Presentation

Synovial sarcoma is one of the most common soft tissue tumors in adults.[132] In the St. Jude series of nonrhabdomyosarcomatous soft tissue sarcomas in childhood, synovial sarcoma was the most common diagnosis, accounting for 29% of the patients.[134] The median age in most series of patients is in the third decade of life, with approximately 31% of cases occurring in patients younger than 20 years of age.[166-171] The male-to-female ratio is usually about 1.2:1 in most large series, suggesting a slight difference in incidence related to gender. The most common anatomical location in which the tumor arises is the lower extremity, often in the region of the thigh and the knee; the next most common site is the upper extremity. Approximately 15% to 20% occur on the head, neck, and trunk.[168-172]

Pathology

This peculiar soft tissue sarcoma of older children and young adults is unique for its propensity to differentiate into two distinct elements: a spindle cell fibrous stroma virtually indistinguishable from fibrosarcoma and a distinct glandular component with absolute epithelial differentiation (Fig. 31-18D). No other sarcoma does this, with the possible exception of rare nerve sheath tumors also containing glands. Epithelial differentiation can also be encountered in epithelioid sarcoma, a superficial soft tissue sarcoma with a granulomatous appearance.[172]

A major controversy in pathology concerns the existence of monophasic synoviosarcoma. The single phase is usually spindle cell stroma, although clusters of epithelial cells are sometimes found. Since the usual tumor is biphasic, and this is the unique characteristic of the tumor that sets it apart from other soft tissue sarcomas, especially fibrosarcoma, the absence of the glandular epithelial component renders the diagnosis extremely difficult unless immunocytochemistry with keratin antibodies is employed: the spindle cells are positive, unlike fibrosarcoma or any other soft tissue sarcoma except epithelioid sarcoma.[173]

Principles and Recommendations for Treatment

The factors reported to be of prognostic significance are small tumor size (less than 5 cm in diameter); a primary site around the hand, foot, or knee; a younger age; and a predominant epithelioid pattern.[170,171] The disease-free survival rate for adult patients with localized tumors of the extremity has been reported to be approximately 70% in a prospectively treated group.[132,133] Eight of the 18 patients treated at St. Jude were alive at follow-up.[134]

Because this tumor is relatively rare in children, the guidelines for its optimal treatment have not yet been established. Wide local excision is the treatment of choice to control the primary tumor. Analysis of the adult series suggests that limb-sparing procedures with limited surgical margins followed by radiation therapy to the tumor bed have an overall outcome that is similar to the outcome of patients treated with amputation.[132] Because most children are still growing rapidly, usually the optimal approach to these tumors in young patients is surgery alone in order to avoid the effects of ionizing irradiation of growing bones and soft tissues.[132] However, radiation therapy may be used to control microscopic disease if the treatment plan projects that normal function and normal growth can be maintained. The effectiveness of radiation in the control of large bulk disease has not yet been established.

Analysis of the retrospective series from St. Jude did not support the use of adjuvant chemotherapy in the treatment of synovial sarcoma in children and young adults[134]; however, the randomized adult trial evaluating cyclophosphamide and doxorubicin administered in an adjuvant fashion suggested a benefit of postoperative adjuvant therapy.[133] Tumor regressions in patients with advanced disease have been documented with a number of chemotherapy regimens.[167,174,175] Although these treatment plans have usually included cyclophosphamide and doxorubicin, a regimen of vincristine, dactinomycin, and cyclophosphamide has also been advocated.[164] Recently, objective tumor regressions have been seen with the combination regimen of ifosfamide and etoposide.[145] Because the lungs are often the only site of metastatic disease (metastases to lymph nodes occur in about 10% of the patients), aggressive attempts at resection of pulmonary metastatic disease have been of benefit.[132]

Hemangiopericytoma

Epidemiology

Hemangiopericytoma is rare in children and accounts for approximately 3% of all soft tissue sarcomas in this age group.[1] In the St. Jude series of nonrhabdomyosarcomatous soft tissue sarcomas, only 5 of the 62 patients had hemangiopericytoma.[134]

Pathology

This soft tissue neoplasm can be either benign or malignant. It is thought to be derived from vascular pericytes, the first layer of support cells adjacent to endothelial cells in normal vessels. The ultrastructural appearance of these tumors would seem to support this interpretation; pericyte differentiation of tumor cells is readily detected (Fig. 31-18E). Interestingly, malignant endothelial tumors of childhood are virtually unreported.

Clinical Presentation

The most common primary sites of disease are the extremities, especially the lower extremity; the retroperitoneum is the second most common site of disease, followed by the head and neck region and then the trunk. The most common sites of secondary disease are the lungs and bone.[176–179]

Principles and Recommendations for Treatment

The behavior of this tumor in older children is similar to that of hemangiopericytoma in adult patients.[176–180] The overall 5-year survival rate in most adult series varies from 30% to 70%.[176–180] The most widely accepted therapeutic approach is wide local excision followed by adjuvant chemotherapy.[176,177,179] As with other soft tissue sarcomas, radiotherapy is used when complete surgical removal of the tumor cannot be accomplished.[132] Local control has been achieved in this fashion with both microscopic and macroscopic disease remaining after surgery[181]; however, the experience with other soft tissue sarcomas suggests that the results of treatment of macroscopic residual disease will be significantly inferior to the results of treatment when all gross disease has been removed.

Responses to chemotherapy have been reported with the use of vincristine, cyclophosphamide, doxorubicin, dactinomycin, methotrexate, mitoxantrone, and other alkylating agents.[182,183] Although no randomized study has confirmed the role of adjuvant chemotherapy in this disease, the high incidence of metastatic disease and relative chemoresponsiveness of the tumor has led many investigators to treat these patients with chemotherapy after extirpation of the primary tumor.

Hemangiopericytoma may occur rarely in infants, and although similar in histologic appearance to the adult form, infantile hemangiopericytoma usually follows a more benign course.[180] These tumors usually arise in the subcutis; however, occasionally they may have extensive local infiltration and even metastases. The treatment of choice for infantile hemangiopericytoma is surgery alone when the tumor is localized; however, complete regression of metastatic disease in patients with this entity has been seen with chemotherapy.

Alveolar Soft Part Sarcoma

Epidemiology

Alveolar soft part sarcoma (ASPS) is a rare sarcoma that usually arises in individuals between the ages of 15 and 35 years.[184–186] In most adult series it accounts for less than 1% of the cases.[132,187] Although 6 of the 62 patients in the St. Jude series had ASPS,[134] the actual incidence in children and adolescents is probably lower. The tumor usually occurs in the skeletal muscle of the extremities in adults[184–187]; however, the head and neck region is a common site in children.[188]

Pathology

The noncommittal name of this sarcoma is a reflection of the uncertainty surrounding its histogenesis. Although ASPS was long thought to be a myogenous tumor,[189] current thinking is split over a myogenous versus neuroepithelial origin[190]; the authors favor the latter. By far the most distinctive feature of this sarcoma is the presence of PAS-positive, diastase-resistant inclusions in the cytoplasm by light microscopy (Fig. 31-18F). By EM, they show a regular crystalline structure (Fig. 31-18F, inset). Their biochemical nature is unknown despite a report of possible renin content and a similarity in appearance thereto.[191] Further, no biologically active secretory product has ever been detected in the tumor or patient. The finding that some inclusions closely resemble neurosecretory granules provokes suspicion that the tumor may be more neuroepithelial than not, but immunocytochemistry is inconclusive in this regard.

Clinical Presentation

Alveolar soft part sarcoma usually presents as a slow-growing, painless mass. The clinical course of patients with ASPS is often indolent. Despite the fact that more than 80% of children and young adults with ASPS are alive 2 years after the diagnosis, most patients die of this disease, sometimes as many as 20 years after the diagnosis has been made.[192,193] The most common sites of metastatic disease are lung, brain, bone, and lymph node.[192,193]

Principles and Recommendations for Treatment

Because of this indolent clinical course, the initial therapeutic approach is usually complete local excision alone with radiation and chemotherapy reserved for the treatment of recurrent disease.[193–195] With this standard approach, however, most patients eventually relapse and subsequently die of disease. This ominous fact strongly suggests that new approaches to the prevention of relapses are needed to treat this disorder. Because of the indolent nature of the disease, aggressive attempts to surgically remove metastatic disease should be made. Responses to chemotherapy have been reported.[192]

Leiomyosarcoma

Epidemiology and Clinical Presentation

Although leiomyosarcomas account for approximately 7% of all soft tissue sarcomas in adults, this tumor is rare in childhood, accounting for less than 2% of soft tissue sarcomas in children.[196-198] The most common primary sites of disease are the retroperitoneum, vascular tissue, peripheral soft tissue, and the gastrointestinal tract.[196-201]

Pathology

Leiomyosarcoma is an exceedingly uncommon soft tissue sarcoma in children and has been documented in a large series only recently.[202] Most smooth muscle-like tumors are in fact a variant of embryonal rhabdomyosarcoma (type A, or leioyomatous rhabdomyosarcoma) with an excellent prognosis. Nonetheless, occasional tumors with *bona fide* smooth muscle differentiation, indistinguishable from the adult counterpart, are encountered. The tumor cells are elongated with cigar-shaped nuclei and brightly eosinophilic cytoplasm (due to the content of myofilaments); they are closely packed in parallel arrays (Fig. 31-18*G*). The appearance is superficially similar to fibrosarcoma, but the eosinophilic cytoplasm, nuclei resembling smooth muscle in normal tissues, and usual monotonous regularity of tumor cells are clearly distinct therefrom.

Principles and Recommendations for Treatment

The most common approach to the treatment of these tumors has been wide local excision alone.[196-201] The role of chemotherapy and radiation therapy in the treatment of leiomyosarcoma in children is not yet known. If complete extirpation of the tumor can be achieved, the prognosis is usually good for tumors arising outside the gastrointestinal tract; however, tumors arising in this site generally have a poorer prognosis.[196-201,203] Leiomyosarcomas of the colorectal region in children, although extremely rare, appear to have a relatively good prognosis if the tumor can be successfully excised.[200]

Liposarcoma

Epidemiology and Clinical Presentation

Liposarcoma is one of the most common soft tissue sarcomas in adults; it usually accounts for approximately 5% to 18% of cases in most series.[132,204,205] Although it is primarily a disease of adults, with a peak age incidence of 40 to 60 years, this tumor may occur in children, most often in the early part of the second decade of life.[206-208] The tumor may rarely affect infants and young children, in whom its behavior is almost always benign if complete removal can be performed.[206] The two most common primary sites are the extremities and retroperitoneum.[206-208]

Pathology

To many, liposarcoma is not a tumor of childhood; most pathologists have been loathe to diagnose malignancy in a soft tissue neoplasm with lipoblastic differentiation, preferring instead to diagnose lipoblastomatosis or lipoma. This prejudice is unwarranted, in view of the documented examples of liposarcoma in children.[206] As in adults, the tumor may be well differentiated, myxoid, round cell, or pleomorphic, in increasing degree of malignancy and with decreasing rates of survival. A typical lipoblastic myxoid type is illustrated in Figure 31-18*H*. Most tumor cells are fibroblastic; only rare cells show conspicuous lipoblastic differentiation. The distinction from MFH can be difficult, but the presence of a myxoid stroma, conspicuous small blood vessels, and scant mitotic activity are all typical of liposarcoma, unlike MFH or even fibrosarcoma.

Principles and Recommendations for Treatment

Because these tumors rarely metastasize but can be locally invasive, the treatment of choice for localized liposarcoma is wide local excision alone.[206-208] Local recurrences may ultimately result in death of the patient by extension of the tumor into vital structures despite the absence of metastatic disease. The role of adjuvant chemotherapy in the treatment of liposarcomas of childhood has not yet been defined; however, the long-term prognosis for children with this rare tumor is very good with surgery alone as long as the tumor can be removed with adequate surgical margins.[206-208] Radiation appears to be effective in the control of microscopic disease in adult series[132]; however, its role in the treatment of children has not yet been determined. The effectiveness of radiation and chemotherapy in the treatment of gross residual disease has also not yet been established, but there are reports of responsiveness to chemotherapy.[145]

REFERENCES

1. Young JL, Miller RW: Incidence of malignant tumors in U.S. children. J Pediatr 86:245–258, 1975
2. Ewing J: Diffuse endothelioma of bone. Proc NY Pathol Soc 21:17–24, 1921
3. Cavazzana A, Triche TJ, Tsokos M et al: Experimental evidence for the neural origin of Ewing's sarcoma. Am J Pathol 127:507–518, 1987
4. Miller RW: Contrasting epidemiology of childhood osteosarcoma, Ewing's tumor and rhabdomyosarcoma. Natl Cancer Inst Monogr 56:9–14, 1981
5. Glass AG, Fraumeni JF: Epidemiology of bone cancer in children. J Natl Cancer Inst 44:187,199, 1970
6. Fraumeni JF, Glass AG: Rarity of Ewing's sarcoma among US negro children. Lancet 1:366–367, 1970
7. Jensen RD, Drake RM: Rarity of Ewing's tumor in negroes. Lancet 1:777, 1970
8. Lindin G, Dunn JE: Ewing's sarcoma in negroes. Lancet 1:1171, 1970
9. Li FP, Tu JT, Liu FS et al: Rarity of Ewing's sarcoma in China. Lancet 1:1255, 1980
10. Hanson MR, McKeen EA, Glaubiger DL et al: Ewing's sarcoma: A descriptive study of 154 patients. Proc ASCO 1:C-712, 1982
11. Schifter S, Vendelbo L, Jensen OM et al: Ewing's tumor following bilateral retinoblastoma. Cancer 51:1746–1749, 1983
12. Aurias A, Rimbaut C, Buffe D et al: Chromosomal translocation in Ewing's sarcoma. N Engl J Med 309:496–497, 1983
13. Turc-Carel C, Philip I, Berger MP et al: Chromosomal translocation in Ewing's sarcoma. N Engl J Med 309:497–498, 1983
14. Whang-Peng J, Triche TJ, Knutsen T et al: Chromosome translocation in peripheral neuroepithelioma. N Engl J Med 311:584–585, 1984
15. McKeon C, Thiele CJ, Ross RA et al: Indistinguishable and predictable patterns of proto-oncogene expression in two histopathologically distinct tumors: Ewing's sarcoma and neuroepithelioma (in press)
16. Knudson AG: Hereditary cancer, oncogenes, and antioncogenes. Cancer Res 45:1437–1443, 1985
17. Orkin SH: Reverse genetics and human disease. Cell 47:845–850, 1986
18. Roessner A, Voss B, Rauterberg J et al: Biologic characterization of human bone tumors: I. Ewing's sarcoma. J Cancer Res Clin Oncol 104:171–180, 1982
19. Miettinen M, Veli–Pekka L, Virtanen I: Histogenesis of Ewing's sarcoma. Virchows Arch 41:277–284, 1982
20. Harvey W, Squier MV, Duance VC et al: A biochemical and immunohistochemical study of collagen synthesis in Ewing's tumor. Br J Cancer 46:848–855, 1982
21. Dickman PS, Liotta LA, Triche TJ: Ewing's sarcoma: Characterization in established cultures and evidence of its histogenesis. Lab Invest 47:375–382, 1982
22. Dahlin DC, Coventy MD, Scanlon PW: Ewing's sarcoma: A critical analysis of 165 cases. J Bone Joint Surg [Am] 43:185–192, 1962
23. Kissane JM, Askin FB, Foulkes M et al: Ewing's sarcoma of bone: Clinicopathologic aspects of 303 cases from the Intergroup Ewing's Sarcoma Study. Hum Pathol 14:773–779, 1983
24. Llombart–Bosch A, Contesso G, Henry–Amar M et al: Histopathological predictive factors in Ewing's sarcoma of bone and clinicopathological correlations. A retrospective study of 261 cases. Virchows Arch 409:627–640, 1986

25. Martin SE, Dwyer A, Kissane JM et al: Small cell osteosarcoma. Cancer 50:990–996, 1982
26. Sim FH, Unni KK, Beabout JW et al: Osteosarcoma with small cells simulating Ewing's tumor. J Bone Joint Surg [Am] 61:207–215, 1979
27. Bertoni F, Picci P, Bacchini P et al: Mesenchymal chondrosarcoma of bone and soft tissues. Cancer :533–541, 1983
28. Huvos AG, Rosen G, Dabska M et al: Mesenchymal chondrosarcoma. Cancer 51:1230–1237, 1983
29. Dabska M, Huvos AG: Mesenchymal chondrosarcoma in the young. Virchows Arch 399:89–104, 1983
30. Huvos AG: Primary malignant fibrous histiocytoma of bone. Clinicopathologic study of 18 patients. NY State J Med 76:552–561, 1976
31. Hashimoto H, Kiryu H, Enjoji M et al: Malignant neuroepithelioma. A clinicopathologic study of 15 cases. Am J Surg Pathol 7:309–318, 1983
32. Jaffe R, Santamaria M, Yunis EJ et al: The neuroectodermal tumor of bone. Am J Surg Pathol 8:885–898, 1984
33. Askin FB, Rosai J, Sibley RK et al: Malignant small cell tumor of the thoracopulmonary region in childhood. Cancer 43:2438–2451, 1979
34. Linnoila RI, Tsokos M, Triche TJ et al: Evidence for neural origin and PAS-positive variants of the malignant small cell tumor of thoracopulmonary region. Am J Surg Pathol 10:124–133, 1986
35. Pilepich MV, Vietti TJ, Nesbit ME et al: Radiotherapy and combination chemotherapy in advanced Ewing's sarcoma: Intergroup Ewing's Sarcoma Study. Cancer 47:1930–1936, 1981
36. Hayes FA, Thompson EI, Hustu HO et al: The response of Ewing's sarcoma to sequential cyclophosphamide and Adriamycin induction therapy. J Clin Oncol 1:45–51, 1983
37. Marsa GW, Johnson RE: Altered metastases following treatment of Ewing's sarcoma with radiation and adjuvant chemotherapy. Cancer 27:1051–1054, 1971
38. Mehta Y, Hendrickson FR: CNS involvement in Ewing's sarcoma. Cancer 33:859–862, 1974
39. Kies MS, Kennedy PS: Central nervous system involvement in Ewing's sarcoma. Ann Intern Med 89:226–227, 1978
40. Trigg ME, Glaubiger D, Nesbit ME: The frequency of isolated CNS involvement in Ewing's sarcoma. Cancer 49:2404–2409, 1982
41. Trigg ME, Makuch R, Glaubiger D: Actuarial risk of isolated CNS involvement in Ewing's sarcoma following prophylactic cranial irradiation and intrathecal methotrexate. Int J Radiat Oncol Biol Phys 11:699–702, 1985
42. Mendenhall CM, Marcus RB, Enneking WF et al: The prognostic significance of soft tissue extension in Ewing's sarcoma. Cancer 51:913–917, 1983
43. Glaubiger DL, Makuch R, Schwarz J et al: Determination of prognostic factors and their influence on therapeutic results in patients with Ewing's sarcoma. Cancer 45:2213–2219, 1980
44. Bacci G, Capanna R, Orlandi M et al: Prognostic significance of serum lactic acid dehydrogenase in Ewing's tumor of bone. Ric Clin Lab 15:89–96, 1985
45. Gehan EA, Nesbit ME, Burgert EO et al: Prognostic factors in children with Ewing's sarcoma. Natl Cancer Inst Monogr 56:273–278, 1981
46. Gobel V, Jurgens H, Etspuler G et al: Prognostic significance of tumor volume in localized Ewing's sarcoma of bone in children and adolescents. J Cancer Res Clin Oncol 113:187–191, 1987
47. Nesbit ME, Perez CA, Tefft M et al: Multimodal therapy for the management of primary non-metastatic Ewing's sarcoma of bone: An Intergroup study. Natl Cancer Inst Monogr 56:255–262, 1981
48. Rosen G, Caparros B, Nirenburg A et al: Ewing's sarcoma: Ten-year experience with adjuvant chemotherapy. Cancer 47:2204–2213, 1981
49. Vietti TJ, Gehan EA, Nesbit ME et al: Multimodal therapy in metastatic Ewing's sarcoma: An intergroup study. Natl Cancer Inst Monogr 56:279–284, 1981
50. Wang CC, Schultz MD: Ewing's sarcoma. N Engl J Med 248:571–576, 1953
51. Phillips RF, Higinbotham NL: The curability of Ewing's endothelioma of bone in children. J Pediatr 70:391–397, 1967
52. Hustu HO, Pinkel D, Pratt CB: Treatment of clinically localized Ewing's sarcoma with radiotherapy and combination chemotherapy. Cancer 30:1522–1527, 1972
53. Johnson RE, Pomeroy TC: Evaluation of therapeutic results in Ewing's sarcoma. Am J Radiol 123:583–587, 1975
54. Zucker JM, Henry-Amar M: Therapeutic controlled trial in Ewing's sarcoma. Eur J Cancer 13:1019–1023, 1977
55. Tepper J, Glaubiger D, Lichter A: Local control of Ewing's sarcoma of bone with radiotherapy and combination chemotherapy. Cancer 46:1969–1973, 1980
56. Perez CA, Tefft M, Nesbit M et al: The role of radiation therapy in the

management of non-metastatic Ewing's sarcoma of bone. Report of the Intergroup Ewing's Sarcoma Study. Int J Radiat Oncol Biol Phys 7:141–149, 1980
57. Kinsella TJ, Triche TJ, Dickman PS et al: Extraskeletal Ewing's sarcoma: Results of combined modality treatment. J Clin Oncol 1:489–495, 1983
58. Evans R, Nesbit M, Askin FB et al: Local recurrence rate, sites of metastases, and time to relapse as a function of treatment regimen, size of primary, and surgical history in 62 patients presenting with non-metastatic Ewing's sarcoma of the pelvic bones. Int J Radiat Oncol Biol Phys 11:129–136, 1985
59. Kinsella TJ, Miser JS, Triche TJ et al: Treatment of ''high risk'' sarcomas in children and young adults: Analysis of local control using intensive combined modality therapy. Natl Cancer Inst Monogr (in press)
60. Telles NC, Rabson AS, Pomeroy TC: Ewing's sarcoma: An autopsy study. Cancer 41:2321–2329, 1978
61. Pritchard DJ: Indications for surgical treatment of localized Ewing's sarcoma of bone. Clin Orthop 153:39–43, 1980
62. Marcove RC, Rosen G: Radical en bloc excision of Ewing's sarcoma. Clin Orthop 153:86–91, 1980
63. Pritchard DJ, Dahlin DC, Dauphine RT et al: Ewing's sarcoma: A clinicopathological and statistical analysis of patients surviving 5 years or longer. J Bone Joint Surg [Am] 57:10–16, 1975
64. Wilkins RM, Pritchard, Burgert EO et al: Ewing's sarcoma of bone: Experience with 140 patients. Cancer 58:2551–2555, 1986
65. Kinsella TJ, Lichter AS, Miser JS et al: Local treatment of Ewing's sarcoma: Radiation therapy versus surgery. Cancer Treat Rep 68:695–701, 1984
66. Kinsella TJ: Limited surgery and radiation therapy for sarcomas of the hand and foot. Int J Radiat Oncol Biol Phys 12:2045–2046, 1986
67. Kliman M, Harwood AR, Jenkin RDT et al: Radical radiotherapy as primary treatment for Ewing's sarcoma distal to the elbow and knee. Clin Orthop 165:233–238, 1982
68. Kinsella TJ, Loeffler JS, Fraass BA et al: Extremity preservation by combined modality therapy in sarcomas of the hand and foot: An analysis of local control, disease-free survival, and functional result. Int J Radiat Oncol Biol Phys 9:1115–1119, 1983
69. Jentzsch K, Binder H, Cramer H et al: Leg function after radiotherapy for Ewing's sarcoma. Cancer 47:1267–1278, 1981
70. Lewis RJ, Marcove RC, Rosen G: Ewing's sarcoma: Functional effects of radiation therapy. J Bone Joint Surg [Am] 59:325–331, 1977
71. Li FP, Cassady JR, Jaffe N: Risk of second tumors in survivors of childhood cancer. Cancer 35:1230–1235, 1975
72. Strong LC, Herson J, Osborne BM et al: Risk of radiation-related subsequent malignant tumors in survivors of Ewing's sarcoma. J Natl Cancer Inst 62:1401–1406, 1979
73. Greene MH, Glaubiger DL, Mead GD et al: Subsequent cancer in patients with Ewing's sarcoma. Cancer Treatment Rep 63:2043–2046, 1979
74. Stea B, Kinsella TJ, Triche TJ et al: Treatment of pelvic sarcomas in adolescents and young adults with intensive combined modality therapy. Int J Radiat Oncol Biol Phys (in press)
75. Jenkin RDT, Rider WD, Sonley MJ: Ewing's sarcoma: A trial of adjuvant total body irradiation. Radiology 96:151–155, 1970
76. Jenkin RDT, Rider WD, Sonley MJ: Adjuvant total body irradiation, cyclophosphamide, and vincristine. Int J Radiat Oncol Biol Phys 1:407–413, 1976
77. Berry MP, Jenkin RDT, Harwood AR et al: Ewing's sarcoma: A trial of adjuvant chemotherapy and sequential half-body irradiation. Int J Radiat Oncol Biol Phys 1:407–413, 1976
78. Kinsella TJ, Glaubiger D, Deisseroth A et al: Intensive combined modality therapy including low dose TBI in high risk Ewing's sarcoma patients. Int J Radiat Oncol Biol Phys 9:1955–1960, 1983
79. Miser JS, Steis R, Longo DL et al: Treatment of newly diagnosed high risk sarcomas and primitive neuroectodermal tumors (PNET) in children and young adults. Proc ASCO 4:C-935, 1985
80. Kinsella TJ, Mitchell JB, McPherson S et al: In vitro radiation studies on Ewing's sarcoma cell lines and human bone marrow: Application to the clinical use of total body irradiation (TBI). Int J Radiat Oncol Biol Phys 10:1005–1011, 1984
81. MacIntosh DJ, Price CHG, Jeffree GM: Ewing's sarcoma: A study of behaviour and treatment in forty-seven cases. J Bone Joint Surg [Br] 57:331–340, 1975
82. Falk S, Alpert M: Five-year survival of patients with Ewing's sarcoma. Surg Gynecol Obstet 124:319–324, 1967
83. Sutow WW: Vincristine (NSC-67574) therapy for malignant solid tumors in children (except Wilm's tumor). Cancer Chemother Rep 52:485–487, 1968
84. Senyszyn JJ, Johnson RE, Curran RE: Treatment of metastatic Ewing's sar-

coma with actinomycin D (NSC-3053). Cancer Chemother Rep 54:103–107, 1970

85. Samuels ML, Howe CD: Cyclophosphamide in the management of Ewing's sarcoma. Cancer 20:961–966, 1967

86. Haggard ME: Cyclophosphamide (NSC-26271) in the treatment of children with malignant neoplasms. Cancer Chemother Rep 51:403–405, 1967

87. Sutow WW, Sullivan MP: Cyclophosphamide in children with Ewing's sarcoma. Cancer Chemother Rep 23:55–60, 1962

88. Oldham RK, Pomeroy TC: Treatment of Ewing's sarcoma with Adriamycin (NSC-123127). Cancer Chemother Rep 56:635–639, 1972

89. Krivit W, Bentley HP: Use of 5-fluorouracil in the management of advanced malignancies in childhood. Am J Dis Child 100:217–227, 1960

90. Palma J, Gakan S, Freeman A et al: Treatment of metastatic Ewing's sarcoma with BCNU. Cancer 30:909–913, 1972

91. Magrath IT, Sandlund JT, Raynor A et al: A phase II study of ifosfamide in the treatment of recurrent sarcomas in young people. Cancer Chemother Pharmacol 18(suppl):S25–S28, 1986

92. O'Dwyer PJ, Leyland–Jones B, Alonso MT et al: Etoposide (VP-16-213). Current status of an active anticancer drug. N Engl J Med 312:692–700, 1985

93. Miser JS, Kinsella TJ, Triche TJ et al: Ifosfamide with mesna uroprotection and etoposide: An effective regimen in the treatment of recurrent sarcomas and other tumors of children and young adults. J Clin Oncol 5:1191–1198, 1987

94. Baum ES, Gaynon P, Greenberg L et al: Phase II trial of cisplatin in refractory childhood cancer: Children's Cancer Study Group Report. Cancer Treat Rep 65:815–822, 1981

95. Cornbleet MA, Corringham RET, Prentice HG et al: Treatment of Ewing's sarcoma with high-dose melphalan and autologous bone marrow transplantation. Cancer Treat Rep 65:241–244, 1981

96. Rosen G, Wollner N, Tan C et al: Disease-free survival in children with Ewing's sarcoma treated with radiation therapy and adjuvant 4-drug sequential chemotherapy. Cancer 33:384–393, 1974

97. Rosen G: Primary Ewing's sarcoma: The multidisciplinary lesion. Int J Radiat Onc Biol Phys 4:527–532, 1978

98. Graham-Pole J: Ewing's sarcoma: Treatment with high dose radiation and adjuvant chemotherapy. Med Pediatr Oncol 7:1–8, 1979

99. Jaffe N, Traggis D, Sallan S et al: Improved outlook for Ewing's sarcoma with combination chemotherapy and radiation therapy. Cancer 38:1925–1930, 1976

100. Vietti TJ: Ewing's sarcoma. Presentation at the St Jude Symposium on the treatment of solid tumors, February 1985

101. Bacci G, Picci P, Gitelis et al: The treatment of localized Ewing's sarcoma. Cancer 49:1561–1570, 1982

102. Bacci G, Picci P, Gherlinzoni F et al: Localized Ewing's sarcoma of bone: Ten years' experience at the Istituto Ortopedico Rizzoli in 124 cases treated with multi-modal therapy. Eur J Cancer Clin Oncol 21:163–173, 1985

103. Finklestein JZ, Hittle RE, Hammond D: Evaluation of a high dose cyclophosphamide regimen in childhood tumors. Cancer 23:1239–1242, 1969

104. Goepfert H, Rochlin DB, Smart CR: Palliative treatment of Ewing's sarcoma. Am J Surg 113:246–250, 1967

105. Pinkel D: Cyclophosphamide in children with cancer. Cancer 15:42–49, 1962

106. Sutow WW, Vietti TJ, Fernbach DL et al: Evaluation of chemotherapy in children with metastatic Ewing's sarcoma and osteogenic sarcoma. Cancer Chemother Rep 55:67–78, 1971

107. Bonnadonna G, Beretta G, Tancici G et al: Adriamycin (NSC-123127) studies at the Istituto Nazionale Tumori, Milan. Cancer Chemother Rep 6:231–245, 1975

108. Evans AE, Baehner RL, Chard RL et al: Comparison of daunorubicin (NSC-83142) with Adriamycin (NSC-123127) in the treatment of late-stage childhood solid tumors. Cancer Chemother Rep 58:671–676, 1974

109. Pratt CB, Shanks EC: Doxorubicin in treatment of malignant solid tumors in children. Am J Dis Child 127:534–536, 1974

110. Ragab AH, Sutow WW, Komp DM et al: Adriamycin in the treatment of childhood solid tumors. Cancer 36:1567–1571, 1975

111. Tan CTC, Rosen G, Ghavimi F et al: Adriamycin (NSC-123127) in pediatric malignancies. Cancer Chemother Rep 6:259–266, 1975

112. Wang JJ, Holland JF, Sinks LF: Phase II study of Adriamycin (NSC-123127) in childhood solid tumors. Cancer Chemother Rep 6:267–270, 1975

113. James DH, George P: Vincristine in children with malignant solid tumors. J Pediatr 64:534–541, 1964

114. Selawry OS, Holland JF, Wolman IJ: Effect of vincristine (NSC-67574) on malignant solid tumors in children. Cancer Chemother Rep 52:497–500, 1968

115. Humphrey EW, Hymes AC, Ausman RK et al: An evaluation of actinomycin D and mitomycin C in patients with advanced cancer. Surgery 50:881–885, 1961

116. Haggard ME, Cangir A, Ragab AH et al: 5-Fluorouracil in childhood tumors. Cancer Treat Rep 61:69–71, 1977

117. Chard RL, Krivit W, Bleyer WA et al: Phase II study of VP-16-213 in childhood malignant disease: A Children's Cancer Study Group Report. Cancer Treat Rep 63:1755–1759, 1979

118. Kamalaker P, Freeman AI, Higby DJ et al: Clinical response and toxicity with cis-dichlorodiammineplatinum (II) in children. Cancer Treat Rep 61:835–839, 1977

119. Nitschke R, Fagundo R, Berry DH et al: Weekly administration of cisdichlorodiammineplatinum (II) in childhood solid tumors: A Southwest Oncology Group study. Cancer Treat Rep 63:497–499, 1979

120. Pratt CB, Hayes FA, Green AA et al: Pharmacokinetic evaluation of cisplatin in children with malignant solid tumors: A phase II study. Cancer Treat Rep 65:1021–1026, 1981

121. Graham-Pole J, Lazarus HM, Herzig RH et al: High dose melphalan for the treatment of children with refractory neuroblastoma and Ewing's sarcoma. Am J Pediatr Hematol Oncol 6:17–26, 1984

122. Antman KH, Montella D, Rosenbaum C et al: Phase II trial of ifosfamide with mesna in previously treated metastatic sarcoma. Cancer Treat Rep 69:499–504, 1985

123. Scheulen ME, Niederle N, Bremer K et al: Efficacy of ifosfamide in refractory malignant diseases and uroprotection by mesna: Results of a clinical phase II study with 151 patients. Cancer Treat Rev 10(suppl A):93–101, 1983

124. Thomas PR, Foulkes MA, Gilula LA et al: Primary Ewing's sarcoma of the ribs. A report from the Intergroup Ewing's sarcoma study. Cancer 51:1021–1027, 1983

125. Rosen G, Juergens H, Caparros B et al: Combination chemotherapy (T-6) in the multidisciplinary treatment of Ewing's sarcoma. Natl Cancer Inst Monogr 56:289–299, 1981

126. Advani SH, Rao DN, Dinshaw KA et al: Adjuvant chemotherapy in Ewing's sarcoma. J Surg Oncol 32:76–78, 1986

127. Oberlin O, Patte C, Demeocq F et al: The response to initial chemotherapy as a prognostic factor in localized Ewing's sarcoma. Eur J Cancer Clin Oncol 21:463–467, 1985

128. Zucker JM, Henry–Amar M, Sarrazin D et al: Intensive systemic chemotherapy in localized Ewing's sarcoma in childhood. A historical trial. Cancer 52:415–423, 1983

129. Gasparini M, Lombardi F, Gianni C et al: Localized Ewing sarcoma: Results of integrated therapy and analysis of failures. Eur J Cancer Clin Oncol 17:1205–1209, 1981

130. Nesbit ME: Bone tumors in infants and children. Paediatrician 1:273–287, 1972/1973

131. Glaubiger DL, Makuch RW, Schwarz J: Influence of prognostic factors on survival in Ewing's sarcoma. Natl Cancer Inst Monogr 56:285–288, 1981

132. Potter DA, Kinsella TJ, Glatstein E et al: High grade soft tissue sarcomas of the extremities. Cancer 58:190–205, 1986

133. Rosenberg SA, Tepper J, Glatstein E et al: Prospective randomized evaluation of adjuvant chemotherapy in adults with soft tissue sarcomas of the extremities. Cancer 52:424–434, 1983

134. Horowitz ME, Pratt CB, Webber BL et al: Therapy of childhood soft-tissue sarcomas other than rhabdomyosarcoma: A review of 62 cases treated at a single institution. J Clin Oncol 4:559–564, 1986

135. Anderson DH: Tumors of infancy and childhood. A survey of those seen in the pathology laboratory of the Babies Hospital during the years 1935–1950. Cancer 4:890–899, 1951

136. Soule EH, Pritchard DJ: Fibrosarcoma of infants and children. A review of 110 cases. Cancer 40:1711–1721, 1977

137. Stout AP: Fibrosarcoma in infants and children. Cancer 15:1028–1040, 1962

138. Blocker SH, Koenig J, Ternberg JL: Congenital fibrosarcoma. Presented at the American Academy of Pediatrics, Surgical Section, 1986

139. Exelby PR, Kuapper WH, Huvos AG et al: Soft tissue fibrosarcoma in children. J Pediatr Surg 8:415–420, 1973

140. Enzinger FM, Weiss SW: Fibrosarcoma. In Soft Tissue Tumors, pp 103–124. St Louis, CV Mosby, 1983

141. Cheung EB, Enzinger FM: Infantile fibrosarcoma. Cancer 38:729–739, 1976

142. Pritchard DJ, Soule EH, Taylor WF et al: Fibrosarcoma—a clinicopathologic and statistical study of 199 tumors of the soft tissues of the extremities and trunk. Cancer 33:888–897, 1974

143. Carli M, Perilongo G, Paolucci P et al: Role of primary chemotherapy in

childhood malignant mesenchymal tumors other than rhabdomyosarcoma. Preliminary results. Proc ASCO 5:816, 1986

144. Ninane J, Gosseye S, Pantion E et al: Congenital fibrosarcoma. Cancer 58:1400–1406, 1986

145. Miser JS, Kinsella TJ, Triche TJ et al: Treatment of recurrent childhood sarcomas and primitive neural tumors with ifosfamide, etoposide and mesna. J Clin Oncol (in press)

146. D'Agostino AN, Soule EH, Miller RH: Primary malignant neoplasms of nerves (malignant neurilemomas) in patients without manifestations of multiple neurofibromatosis (von Recklinghausen's disease). Cancer 16:1003–1014, 1963

147. D'Agostino AN, Soule EH, Miller RH: Sarcomas of the peripheral nerves and somatic soft tissues associated with multiple neurofibromatosis (von Recklinghausen's disease). Cancer 16:1015–1027, 1963

148. Storm FK, Eilber FR, Mira J et al: Neurofibrosarcoma. Cancer 45:126–129, 1980

149. Guccion JG, Enzinger FM: Malignant schwannoma associated with von Recklinghausen's neurofibromatosis. Virchows Arch Pathol Anat 383:43–56, 1979

150. Raney RB, Littman P, Jarrett P et al: Results of multimodal therapy for children with neurogenic sarcoma. Med Pediatr Oncol 7:229–236, 1979

151. Fienman NL, Yakovac WC: Neurofibromatosis in childhood. J Pediatr 76:339–346, 1970

152. Knudson AG: Hereditary cancer, oncogenes, and antioncogenes. Cancer Res 45:1437–1443, 1985

153. Orkin SH: Reverse genetics and human disease. Cell 47:845–850, 1986

154. Seizinger BR, Martuza RL, Gusella JF: Loss of genes on chromosome 22 in tumorigenesis of human acoustic neuroma. Nature 322:644–647, 1986

155. Raney RB, Schnaufer L, Zeigler M et al: Treatment of children with neurogenic sarcoma. Cancer 59:1–5, 1987

156. Enzinger FM, Weiss SW: Malignant schwannomas. In Soft Tissue Tumors, pp 625–639. St Louis, CV Mosby, 1983

157. Stout AP: Malignant fibrohistiocytic proliferations. In Armed Forces Institute of Pathology, Section 2, Fascicle 5. Washington, DC, Armed Forces Institute of Pathology, 1953

158. Weiss SW, Enzinger FM: Malignant fibrous histiocytoma: An analysis of 200 cases. Cancer 41:2250–2266, 1978

159. Kearney MM, Soule EH, Ivins JC: Malignant fibrous histiocytoma: A retrospective study of 167 cases. Cancer 45:167–178, 1980

160. Raney RB, Allen A, O'Neill J et al: Malignant fibrous histiocytoma of soft tissue in childhood. Cancer 57:2198–2201, 1986

161. Tracy T, Neifeild JP, DeMay RM et al: Malignant fibrous histiocytoma in children. J Pediatr Surg 19:81–81, 1984

162. Saiki JH, Baker LH, Rivkin SE et al: A useful high-dose intermittent schedule of Adriamycin and DTIC in the treatment of advanced sarcomas. Cancer 58:2196–2197, 1986

163. Leite C, Goodwin JW, Sinkovics JG et al: Chemotherapy of malignant fibrous histiocytoma: A Southwest Oncology Group report. Cancer 40:2010–2014, 1977

164. Bassett WB, Weiss RB: Prolonged complete remission in malignant fibrous histiocytoma treated with chemotherapy. Cancer Treat Rep 62:1405–1406, 1978

165. Clamon GH, Robinson RA, Olberding EB: Prolonged remission of metastatic malignant fibrous histiocytoma induced by combination chemotherapy. J Surg Oncol 26:113–114, 1984

166. Lee SM, Hajdu SI, Exelby PR: Synovial sarcoma in children. Surg Gynecol Obstet 138:701–704, 1974

167. Raney RB: Synovial sarcoma. Med Ped Oncol 9:41–45, 1981

168. Cameron HU, Kostvik JP: A long term follow-up of synovial sarcoma. J Bone Joint Surg (Br) 56:613–617, 1974

169. Cadman NL, Soule EH, Kelly PJ: Synovial sarcoma. Cancer 18:613–627, 1965

170. Hajdu SI, Shiu MH, Fortner JG: Tendosynovial sarcoma. Cancer 39:1201–1217, 1977

171. Wright PH, Sim FH, Soule EH et al: Synovial sarcoma. J Bone Joint Surg [Am] 64:112–133, 1982

172. Enzinger FM: Epithelioid sarcoma: A sarcoma simulating a granuloma or a carcinoma. Cancer 26:1026–1034, 1970

173. Krall RA, Kostianovsky M, Patchefsky AS: Synovial sarcoma. A clinical, pathological, and ultrastructural study of 26 cases supporting the recognition of a monophasic variant. Am J Surg Pathol 5:137–149, 1981

174. Gerner RE, Moore GE: Synovial sarcoma. Am Surg 81:22–25, 1975

175. Ryan JR, Baker LH, Benjamin RS: The natural history of metastatic synovial sarcoma. Clin Orthop Rel Res 164:257–260, 1982

176. Backwinkel KD, Diddams JA: Hemangiopericytoma. Report of a case and comprehensive review of the literature. Cancer 25:896–901, 1970

177. Enzinger FM, Smith BH: Hemangiopericytoma. An analysis of 106 cases. Hum Pathol 7:61–82, 1976

178. Wold LE, Unni KK, Cooper KL et al: Hemangiopericytoma of bone. Am J Surg Pathol 6:53–58, 1982

179. Auguste LJ, Razak MJ, Sako K: Hemangiopericytoma. J Surg Oncol 20:260–264, 1982

180. Kauffman SL, Stout AP: Hemangiopericytoma in children. Cancer 13:695–710, 1960

181. Mira JG, Chu FCH, Fortner JG: The role of radiotherapy in management of malignant hemangiopericytoma. Cancer 39:1254–1259, 1977

182. Ortega JA, Finkelstein JZ, Isaacs H et al: Chemotherapy of malignant hemangiopericytoma of childhood. Cancer 27:730–735, 1971

183. Wong PP, Yagoda A: Chemotherapy of malignant hemangiopericytoma. Cancer 41:1256–1260, 1978

184. Christopherson WM, Foote FW, Stewart FW: Alveolar soft-part sarcoma. Structurally characteristic tumors of uncertain histogenesis. Cancer 5:100–108, 1952

185. Lieberman PH, Foote FW, Stewart FW et al: Alveolar soft part sarcoma. JAMA 198:121–125, 1966

186. Ekfors TO, Kalimo H, Rantkokko V et al: Alveolar soft part sarcoma. Cancer 43:1672–1679, 1979

187. Balfour RS: The alveolar soft part sarcoma. Review of the literature and report of a case. J Oral Surg 32:214–220, 1974

188. Enzinger FM, Weiss SW: Alveolar soft part sarcoma. In Soft Tissue Tumors, pp 780–787. St Louis, CV Mosby, 1983

189. Fisher ER, Reidbord H: Electron microscopic evidence suggesting myogenous derivation on the so-called alveolar soft part sarcoma. Cancer 27:150–161, 1971

190. Mathew T: Evidence supporting neural crest origin of alveolar soft part sarcoma. Cancer 50:507–514, 1982

191. DeSchryver–Kecskemeti K, Kraus FT, Engelman BA: Alveolar soft part sarcoma—a malignant angioreninoma. Histochemical, immunocytochemical, and electron-microscopic study of four cases. Am J Surg Pathol 6:5–12, 1982

192. Unni K, Soule K: Alveolar soft part sarcoma. Mayo Clin Proc 50:591–598, 1975

193. Raney RB: Alveolar soft part sarcoma. Med Pediatr Oncol 6:367–370, 1979

194. Baum ES, Finkenstein L, Nachman JB: Pulmonary resection and chemotherapy of metastatic alveolar soft part sarcoma. Cancer 47:1946–1948, 1981

195. Roberfeld S: Radiation therapy in alveolar soft part sarcoma. Cancer 28:577–580, 1971

196. Botting AJ, Soule EH, Brown AL: Smooth muscle tumors of children. Cancer 18:711–720, 1965

197. Wile AG, Evans HL, Romsdahl MM: Leiomyosarcoma of soft tissue: A clinicopathologic study. Cancer 48:1022–1032, 1981

198. Yannopoulos K, Stout AP: Smooth muscle tumors in children. Cancer 15:958–971, 1962

199. Johnson H, Hutter JJ, Paplanus SH: Leiomyosarcoma of the stomach: Results of surgery and chemotherapy in an eleven-year old girl with metastases. Me Pediatr Oncol 8:137–142, 1980

200. Posen JA, Bar–Maor JA: Leiomyosarcoma of the colon in an infant. Cancer 52:1458–1461, 1983

201. Ranchod M, Kempson RL: Smooth muscle tumors of the gastrointestinal tract and retroperitoneum. A pathologic analysis of 100 cases. Cancer 39:255–262, 1977

202. Lack EE: Leiomyosarcoma in children. A clinicopathologic study of 10 cases. Pediatr Pathol 181–197, 1986

203. Angerpointer TA, Weitz H, Haas RJ: Intestinal leiomyosarcoma in childhood—case report and review of the literature. J Pediatr Surg 16:491–495, 1981

204. Enterline HT, Culberson JD, Rochlin DB et al: Liposarcoma. Cancer 13:932–950, 1960

205. Enzinger FM, Winslow DJ: Liposarcoma: A study of 103 cases. Virchows Arch Pathol Anat 335:367–388, 1962

206. Castleberry RP, Kelly DR, Wilson ER et al: Childhood liposarcoma. Report of a case and review of the literature. Cancer 54:579–584, 1984

207. Kauffman SL, Stout AP: Lipoblastic tumors of children. Cancer 12:912–925, 1959

208. Schmookler BM, Enzinger FM: Juvenile liposarcoma: An analysis of 15 cases. Am J Clin Pathol 133:245–246, 1982

thirty-two

Osteosarcoma

Michael P. Link and Frederick Eilber

In the 1920s, a celebrated surgeon of international repute summarized a scientific meeting on bone sarcomas by acknowledging, "If you do not operate, they die; if you do operate, they die just the same. Gentlemen, this meeting should be concluded with prayers." (quoted in Ref. 1). One might have drawn a similarly disheartening conclusion from meetings on osteosarcoma conducted in the 1960s and early 1970s—few therapeutic advances had occurred during the preceding half century, and the outlook for patients with osteosarcoma was indeed dismal. Despite aggressive surgery, more than 80% of children presenting without evidence of metastases developed tumor recurrences and died of their disease within 5 years of diagnosis.

Remarkable progress has been made in the treatment of osteosarcoma in the past two decades. As a result of the development of effective adjuvant therapy and advances in surgical and diagnostic imaging techniques, the majority of patients with limb primaries who present without metastases can now be cured. Advances in surgical techniques have also permitted improvement in the quality of life of survivors through the use of less radical surgery, particularly limb-sparing procedures, to control the primary tumor.

EPIDEMIOLOGY AND BIOLOGY

Osteosarcoma is a primary malignant tumor of bone, deriving from primitive bone-forming mesenchyme and characterized by the production of osteoid tissue or immature bone by the malignant proliferating spindle cell stroma.[2–4] Although primary bone tumors are rare in childhood (metastatic lesions to the skeleton are more common), they are the sixth most common group of malignant neoplasms in children;[5] in adolescents and young adults, they are the third most frequent neoplasms, exceeded in older children only by leukemias and lymphomas. Malignant bone tumors have been reported to occur in the United States at an annual rate of approximately 5.6 cases per million white children younger than 15 years[5] and at a slightly lower rate among black children. Only half of the bone tumors in childhood are malignant;[6] of these, osteosarcoma is the most frequent,[2,6] accounting for approximately 60% of malignant bone tumors in the first two decades of life.[6] (Ewing's sarcoma, the second most frequent primary bone cancer, is actually more common than osteosarcoma in children younger than 10 years.) Males are affected more frequently in most series.[2,7,8]

The peak incidence of osteosarcoma occurs in the second decade of life during the adolescent growth spurt (Fig. 32-1), a feature that suggests a relationship between rapid bone growth and the development of this malignancy. Several lines of evidence have been cited to support this relationship. First, patients with osteosarcoma are taller than their age peers.[9] Similarly, the risk of developing osteosarcoma in large breeds of dogs (e.g., the Great Dane and the St.

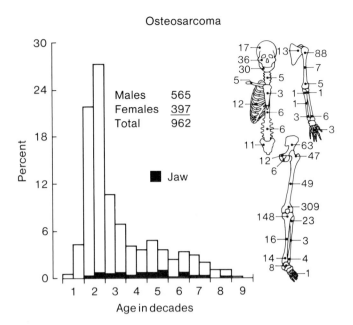

FIGURE 32-1. Age, sex, and skeletal site distribution of osteosarcomas in a large series of patients from the Mayo Clinic. (Reproduced with permission from Dahlin DC: Osteosarcoma of bone and a consideration of prognostic variables. Cancer Treat Rep 62:189–192, 1978)

Bernard) has been reported to be nearly 185 times that for small breeds.[10] Second, osteosarcomas occur at an earlier age in females than in males, corresponding to the more advanced skeletal age and earlier adolescent growth spurt of females,[11] while the increased risk for osteosarcoma among males may result from the larger volume of bone formed during a longer growth period in boys. Third, osteosarcoma has a predilection for the metaphyseal portions of the most rapidly growing bones in adolescents—the distal femur, proximal tibia, and proximal humerus—and tumors of the humerus tend to occur at a younger age than do tumors of the femur and tibia, corresponding to the earlier growth spurt of the humerus.[11] Thus, the tumor appears to occur most frequently at sites where the greatest increase in length and size of bone occurs. This has led to the speculation that bone tumors arise from an aberration of the normal process of bone growth in length and remodeling;[11,12] rapidly proliferating cells might be particularly susceptible to oncogenic agents, mitotic errors, or other events leading to neoplastic transformation.[9]

A viral etiology for osteosarcoma has been suggested based on older evidence in animals that bone sarcomas can be induced by viruses,[13,14] on the finding of C-type virus particles in thin sections of human and hamster osteosarcomas,[14,15] and on the development of osteosarcoma in hamsters injected with cell-free extracts of human osteosarcomas.[16] Moreover, in immunologic studies, antisarcoma-specific antibodies have been found in patients and also in high incidence in close relatives of patients with sarcomas.[17–19] In addition, lymphocytes cytotoxic to osteosarcoma cells have been found in the peripheral blood of patients with osteosarcoma and of their parents.[20] Data from these studies have been used to support the association of an infectious agent with osteosarcoma.[18] However, no time–space variations in the incidence of osteosarcoma have been detected that might suggest horizontal transmission,[21,22] nor have convincing data emerged from the laboratory to suggest a role for an infectious agent. Antecedent trauma has often been associated with the development of bone tumors, but

there is little evidence to support a causal relationship. Rather, injury (particularly pathologic fracture) often brings the patient to medical attention, and radiographs reveal the underlying neoplasm.

The only environmental agent known to produce bone sarcomas in humans is ionizing radiation. Radiation is implicated in approximately 3% of osteosarcomas,[7,8] although the incidence of postirradiation sarcoma is low in view of the extent to which therapeutic irradiation has been utilized.[2,23] An increased incidence is likely to be seen as more patients survive long enough after primary irradiation to develop this complication. Osteosarcomas resulting from therapeutic irradiation were initially seen following high orthovoltage radiation doses to bone (see Chap. 11).[24] More recently, osteosarcomas have also been reported as a complication of megavoltage radiation,[25] although the incidence after megavoltage irradiation may be lower because absorbed bone doses are considerably reduced with this technique.[25,26] The interval between irradiation and the appearance of osteosarcoma has ranged from 4 to more than 40 years (median, 12–16 years),[2,27] and bone sarcoma has occurred after irradiation for benign as well as malignant conditions. It is noteworthy that osteosarcomas have also been associated with the use of bone-seeking radioisotopes,[28] such as intravenous radium-224 for the treatment of ankylosing spondylitis and tuberculosis,[28,29] and Thorotrast used as a diagnostic radiocontrast agent.[30]

Osteosarcoma has been reported in patients with Paget's disease, and cases of osteosarcoma in patients older than 40 years are almost exclusively associated with this premalignant condition.[2] Approximately 2% of patients with Paget's disease develop osteosarcoma, and the occurrence of osteosarcoma is not necessarily related to the extent of involvement of the skeleton by Paget's disease.[2] Histologically, osteosarcomas in patients with Paget's disease are indistinguishable from conventional osteosarcoma, although multiple bone involvement is frequent[2] and the prognosis for such patients is poor.[8] Other benign bone lesions are also associated with an increased risk of the development of osteosarcoma. Lesions predisposed to such malignant degeneration include solitary or multiple osteochondroma, solitary enchondroma or enchondromatosis (Ollier's disease), multiple hereditary exostoses, fibrous dysplasia, and even chronic osteomyelitis and sites of bone infarcts.[2,8]

GENETICS

Several families have been described in which multiple members have developed osteosarcoma[2,31,32] suggesting that a genetic predisposition to this tumor exists (see also Chap. 2). Similar evidence for genetic predisposition has emerged from studies of dogs with osteosarcoma.[33] By far the strongest genetic predisposition to osteosarcoma is found in patients with hereditary retinoblastoma (see Chap. 25). The subsequent development of second nonocular tumors in patients who survive retinoblastoma has been reported in many case reports and series. The majority of second malignancies are sarcomas, and almost 50% are osteosarcomas.[34,35] Although the occurrence of secondary osteosarcoma in survivors of retinoblastoma was initially thought to represent a complication of radiotherapy,[34] it is now apparent that a relationship between osteosarcoma and hereditary (bilateral) retinoblastoma exists that is independent of therapy. Evidence for this relationship comes from several findings. First, more than 98% of patients with retinoblastoma who develop second nonocular tumors have bilateral (hereditary) disease, although the bilateral form of retinoblastoma is found in only 25% of cases.[36] Second, in hereditary retinoblastoma, osteosarcomas occur 2000 times more frequently in the skull after radiotherapy and 500 times more frequently in the extremities than would be expected in the general population.[36,37] Remarkably, the actuarial risk for development of second tumors among patients with bilateral retinoblastoma is 90% at 30 years.[38] Third, some patients with retinoblastoma have developed secondary osteosarcomas in the extremities at sites far distant from orbital radiation. Fourth, osteosarcoma has been reported in patients who did not receive radiotherapy to treat their primary ocular malignancy. A final observation relates to an obligate carrier for hereditary retinoblastoma who had two children with retinoblastoma by different wives, but who did not himself develop an ocular tumor; however, he developed osteosarcoma as an adult.[39]

The available evidence suggests that retinoblastoma is one of several tumors of childhood that arise as a result of recessive mutations (see Chaps. 3 and 25).[37,40,41] Recent data confirm that the specific locus involved in the generation of retinoblastoma (which has been mapped to chromosome 13) is also implicated in the generation of osteosarcoma,[42-44] even in patients without retinoblastoma. Tumor cells from osteosarcomas have been found to be homozygous at a variety of chromosome 13 loci tested,[42,43] although analysis of constitutional (nontumor) DNA from the same patients indicated heterozygosity at these same loci. Furthermore, part or all of the apparent retinoblastoma gene appears to be deleted in some osteosarcomas, and

RNA transcripts corresponding to the retinoblastoma locus are absent from the one osteosarcoma cell line tested, as they are in retinoblastoma cell lines.[44] Thus, homozygosity for the retinoblastoma allele occurring in an appropriate bone cell may lead to osteosarcoma, in much the same way that homozygosity for the allele in a retinoblast leads to the generation of retinoblastoma.[43] Rapidly proliferating regions of bone may be particularly susceptible to mitotic errors, which might result in homozygosity in the mutated retinoblastoma gene and in tumor formation. The genetic relationship between osteosarcoma and retinoblastoma may also explain the paucity of hereditary osteosarcoma families; such families are usually identified as hereditary retinoblastoma kindreds.[43]

PATHOLOGY

The diagnosis of osteosarcoma is based on histopathologic criteria and correlation with a confirmatory radiologic appearance. The histologic diagnosis of osteosarcoma depends on the presence of a frankly malignant sarcomatous stroma associated with the production of tumor osteoid and bone (Fig. 32-2). Great variability exists in the histologic patterns seen in this tumor and in the degree of osteoid production, so that extensive review of the pathologic material and, rarely, electron microscopy may be required to demonstrate tumor osteoid.

FIGURE 32-2.   A. Photomicrograph of a field of an osteosarcoma demonstrating extensive osteoid formation intimately associated with a sarcomatous stroma. (× 100) **B.** High-power view demonstrating cellular atypia and other features of the malignant cellular stroma. (× 400) (Reproduced with permission from Link MP: Osteosarcoma. In Schimpff SC, Robson MC, Moosa AR [eds]: Comprehensive Textbook of Oncology, pp 1179–1190. Baltimore, Williams & Wilkins, 1986)

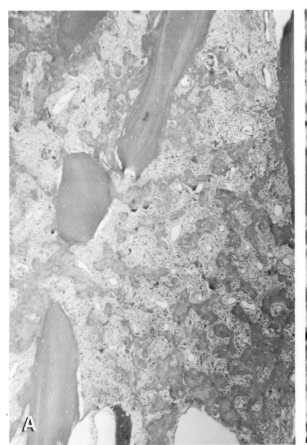
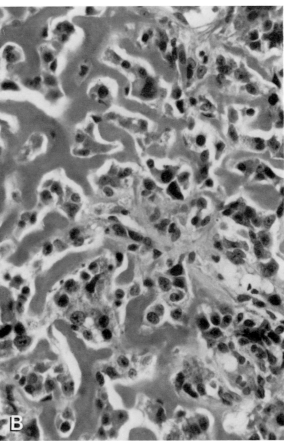

Since osteosarcomas are thought to arise from a stem mesenchymal cell capable of differentiating toward fibrous tissue, cartilage, or bone,[45] osteosarcoma shares many features with chondrosarcoma and fibrosarcoma—tumors of the same family (referred to generically as osteogenic sarcomas), with which osteosarcoma is easily confused (see Chaps. 6 and 31).[4] However, chondrosarcomas and fibrosarcomas are distinguished from osteosarcoma by their lack of production of osteoid substance, the *sine qua non* for the diagnosis of osteosarcoma. Features that distinguish chondrosarcoma and fibrosarcoma from osteosarcoma are summarized in Table 32-1.

A number of distinct clinicopathologic variants of osteosarcoma have been defined based on clinical, roentgenographic, and histologic features (Table 32-1). The largest group of osteosarcomas are the conventional osteosarcomas (Figs. 32-2 and 32-3), the variants of which are seen predominantly in children and adolescents. In conventional osteosarcoma, the connective tissue stroma variably appears as a mixture of large, atypical, spindle-shaped cells that are cytologically highly malignant, with large irregular nuclei and abnormal mitotic figures. The stroma may be largely anaplastic. Large numbers of benign appearing giant cells may be evident in up to 25% of cases. Interspersed in the pleomorphic stroma are areas of osteoid production and calcification intimately associated with the malignant cells.

Three categories of conventional osteosarcoma have been defined by Dahlin based on the predominant differentiation of the tumor cells.[6-8] Approximately 50% of cases of osteosarcoma are characterized by abundant production of osteoid and are classified as osteoblastic osteosarcoma. In about 25% of cases, the predominant differentiation is toward cartilage (chondroblastic osteosarcoma), and these tumors may be difficult to distinguish from pure chondrosarcoma when osteoid production is minimal. The remaining cases demonstrate a spindle cell stroma, with a herringbone pattern reminiscent of fibrosarcoma and minimal amounts of osteoid (fibroblastic osteosarcoma). The value of this subclassification of conventional osteosarcomas is not well established because the classification of an individual tumor is necessarily arbitrary and subject to errors of sampling,[8] and no significant differences in behavior or outcome can be determined among these subclasses.[7] Grading of osteosarcomas is difficult, but the majority are judged to be high grade.

Telangiectatic osteosarcoma[2,6] is an unusual variant (approximately 3% of all osteosarcomas) that characteristically appears as a purely lytic lesion on plain radiographs (Fig. 32-4), with little calcification or bone formation. Radiographically, telangiectatic osteosarcoma resembles aneurysmal bone cyst and giant cell tumor, with which it is easily confused. These tumors are grossly cystic, and they histologically demonstrate dilated spaces filled with blood and necrotic tissue, with viable tumor confined to the periphery of the lesion. The tumors are often anaplastic, with little evidence of osteoid formation. The telangiectatic variant of osteosarcoma has been reported to be associated with a particularly bleak outlook,[8,46] although other series have not confirmed this prognostic association.[47,48] Attempts to distinguish this entity from conventional osteosarcoma may be academic, because the natural his-

Table 32-1
The Family of Osteogenic Sarcomas

Tumor	Usual Age at Diagnosis	Common Primary Sites	Radiographic Appearance	Distinctive Features	Clinical Course
Fibrosarcoma	Second–sixth decade	Similar to osteosarcoma	Usually lytic	Spindle cells and collagen but no osteoid	Similar to osteosarcoma
Chondrosarcoma	Third–seventh decade; usually older adults	Most in trunk (especially pelvis) and proximal limbs	Bone destruction and fluffy calcification	Prolonged history of symptoms— proliferating tissue is fully developed cartilage without tumor osteoid	Metastases rare but may appear many years later
Osteosarcoma					
Conventional Osteoblastic Chondroblastic Fibroblastic	Second and third decade	Around knee joint and shoulder (see Fig. 32-1)	Variable, depending on degree of mineralization of osteoid (see text)	Tumor osteoid present; variable degrees of osteoblastic, chondroblastic, and fibroblastic differentiation (see text)	Early dissemination to lungs ± skeleton
Telangiectatic	Second and third decade	Similar to conventional osteosarcoma	Predominantly lytic lesion with little or no sclerosis	Cystic, cavity-like tumor; blood-filled spaces in tumor	Similar to conventional osteosarcoma
Multifocal		Synchronous involvement of multiple bones	Multiple skeletal sites showing densely sclerotic lesions	? Multiple primary tumors vs. metastatic primary tumor	Uniformly fatal
Parosteal (juxtacortical osteosarcoma)	Third decade or older	Posterior aspect of distal femur	Arises from cortex; encircles involved bone; pronounced ossification	Low-grade tumor with characteristic radiograph and pathology (see text)	Indolent clinical course with low propensity for metastases
Periosteal (juxtacortical chondrosarcoma)	First–seventh decade	Tibia and femur	Tumor located superficially in cortex	Tumor limited to periphery of cortex	Intermediate prognosis

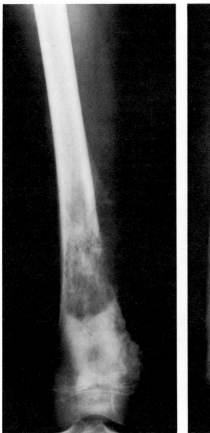
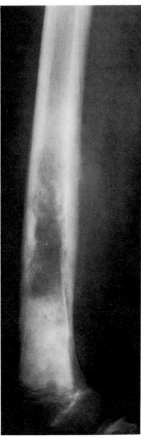
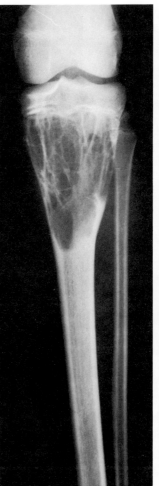
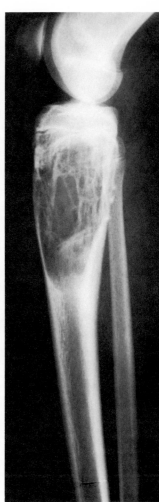

FIGURE 32-3. Radiographs (posteroanterior and lateral projections) of a conventional osteosarcoma involving the distal femur and extending up the shaft. The tumor demonstrates a mixed lytic and sclerotic appearance, a soft tissue mass with ossification apparent in the soft tissue, and periosteal reaction and the formation of Codman's triangle proximally. (Reproduced with permission from Link MP: Osteosarcoma. In Schimpff SC, Robson MC, Moosa AR [eds]: Comprehensive Textbook of Oncology, pp 1179–1190. Baltimore, Williams & Wilkins, 1986)

FIGURE 32-4. Radiographs (posteroanterior and lateral projections) of a telangiectatic osteosarcoma of the proximal tibia. The radiographic appearance is predominantly lytic with apparent expansion of the shaft. There is little evidence of ossification. The lesion is easily confused with benign entities, but erosion through the cortex posteriorly indicates the malignant nature of this lesion. (Radiograph courtesy of Thomas Slovis, M.D., Department of Radiology, Children's Hospital of Michigan.) (Reproduced with permission from Link MP: Osteosarcoma. In Schimpff SC, Robson MC, Moosa AR [eds]: Comprehensive Textbook of Oncology, pp 1179–1190. Baltimore, Williams & Wilkins, 1986)

tory and response to therapy appear to be the same as in conventional osteosarcoma. Similarly, malignant fibrous histiocytoma of bone may be difficult to distinguish from osteosarcoma, and the distinction may not be clinically significant.[8]

Certain variants of osteosarcoma have been distinguished from conventional osteosarcoma because of their unique clinicopathologic features and characteristic clinical behavior. The most important of these clinicopathologic variants is the parosteal osteosarcoma (juxtacortical osteosarcoma), which comprises less than 5% of all osteosarcomas.[4,8,49,50] The posterior aspect of the distal femur is the most commonly involved site, but other long bones may be affected. Clinically, these lesions occur in older patients with a relatively long history of symptoms (sometimes longer than 1 year). Parosteal osteosarcoma also presents a characteristic radiographic appearance (Fig. 32-5A, B); the tumor appears to arise from the cortex from a broad base without invasion of the medullary cavity (a finding that can be confirmed by tomography), and the lesion encircles the involved bone. Intense ossification is typical and, histologically, these lesions appear low grade. In contrast to classic osteosarcoma, parosteal osteosarcomas are clinically indolent and characterized by local recurrence after inade-

quate surgical excision rather than by distant metastatic spread. The outcome in patients who undergo radical excision of the primary tumor is usually favorable.[4,8,49,50] Rarely, lesions appearing to be parosteal osteosarcomas have been encountered that are high grade or that appear to invade the medullary cavity. Although such features may not be anticipated from the clinical or plain radiographic features, medullary invasion is sometimes demonstrable by tomography. Such lesions are much more ominous and behave aggressively, like classic high-grade osteosarcomas, with a high propensity for metastatic spread.

Another rare variant is the periosteal osteosarcoma,[51] which, like parosteal osteosarcoma, arises on the surface of bone without involvement of the marrow cavity. The lesion occurs frequently in the second decade of life and has a propensity for involvement of the upper tibial metaphysis, ap-

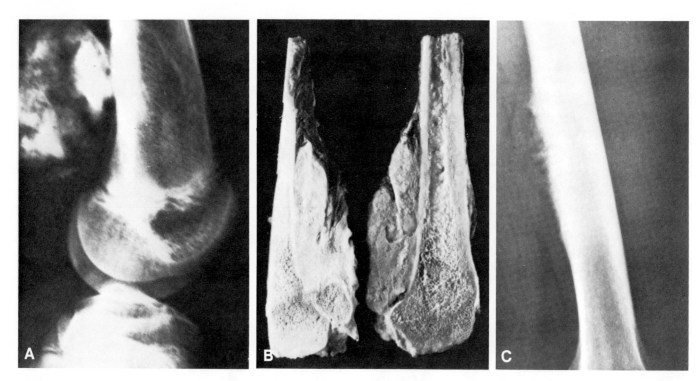

FIGURE 32-5. **A.** Radiograph of a typical parosteal osteosarcoma involving the posterior aspect of the distal femur. Intramedullary involvement is not evident. **B.** Sagittal section of gross specimen from a parosteal osteosarcoma (not the same case as in **A**). The bony mass is adherent to the underlying cortex and is situated entirely on the surface of the bone. **C.** Radiograph of a typical periosteal osteosarcoma. Tumor involving the midshaft of the femur is radiolucent, does not involve the marrow, and shows perpendicular spiculation. (Reproduced with permission from Dahlin DC, Unni KK. Osteosarcoma of bone and its important recognizable varieties. Am J Surg Pathol 1:61–71, 1977. Copyright © Raven Press, New York)

pearing as an ill-defined radiolucent lesion on the surface (Fig. 32-5C). Histologically, the tumors are relatively high-grade, predominantly chondroblastic osteosarcomas. The prognosis is worse than for parosteal osteosarcoma; the tumors tend to recur locally unless radical resection is performed, but only 25% of patients in one series died of metastatic disease.[8,51] It should be noted that conventional high-grade osteosarcomas may develop on the surface of bone and may be confused with parosteal or periosteal osteosarcoma. However, high-grade osteosarcoma of the surface of bone resembles conventional osteosarcoma histologically and in its clinical behavior. Low-grade intraosseous tumors[52] also occur, although they are rare. Intraosseous low-grade osteosarcomas are well differentiated, with minimal cytologic atypia, and can be mistaken for benign conditions, particularly fibrous dysplasia. A tendency to local recurrence, especially after inadequate surgery, is the rule, and distant metastases are unusual.[8,52]

Several additional variants of osteosarcoma are distinguished from classic osteosarcoma because of differences in biological behavior. Primary osteosarcoma of the jaw occurs most often in older patients, tends to demonstrate prominent chondroid differentiation, and is associated with a more indolent course, with a tendency to local recurrence rather than distant metastases.[53] By contrast, osteosarcoma occurring in patients with Paget's disease is associated with a very aggressive clinical course and there are few survivors.[8] Histologically, however, the tumors are identical to conventional osteosarcoma, as are osteosarcomas occurring in irradiated bones. Extraosseous osteosarcoma[54] is an uncommon variant that arises outside of bone and occurs most frequently in the soft tissues

of the lower extremity in middle-aged adults. Extraosseous osteosarcomas are seen (although not exclusively) as a late complication of radiotherapy. Local excision of these lesions is inadequate treatment because local recurrences and distant metastases invariably follow limited surgery.[54] Finally, multifocal osteosarcoma is a rare entity in which multiple synchronous skeletal tumors are present at diagnosis and each lesion resembles a primary tumor radiographically, suggesting a multicentric origin of the sarcoma. It is not clear whether such sarcomas arise in multiple sites, or whether one of the lesions is the true primary that has spread rapidly to other skeletal sites in the absence of lung metastases.[8,55]

CLINICAL PRESENTATION, NATURAL HISTORY, AND PATTERNS OF SPREAD

The majority of patients with osteosarcoma present with pain over the involved area, with or without an associated soft tissue mass. The average duration of symptoms is 3 months, although a history of 6 months or longer is not uncommon. Parosteal osteosarcomas, in particular, can be associated with painful symptoms of several years' duration, reflecting the relatively indolent behavior of this variant of osteosarcoma. Osteosarcoma characteristically involves the long tubular bones, especially adjacent to the knee joint. The distal femur and proximal tibia are the most frequently involved sites, followed by the proximal humerus and mid- and proximal femur (see Fig. 32-1).[2,6] Involvement of the flat bones of the axial skeleton, notably the pelvis, occurs in approximately 15% to 20% of cases but accounts for fewer than 10% of cases in the pediatric age group. Osteosarcoma of the jaw is a peculiar entity that accounts for less than 7% of all osteosarcomas and follows a more indolent course, as noted above.

Approximately 10% to 20% of patients with osteosarcoma present with visible macrometastatic disease. The majority of these metastatic lesions are found in the lungs, although a small fraction of patients present with bone metastases with or without concomitant pulmonary metastases. Presentations with multiple bone metastases may reflect multifocal primary tumors (multifocal sclerosing osteosarcoma) and carry an extremely grave prognosis.[8,55]

Since osteosarcoma has been demonstrated to be relatively unresponsive to radiation therapy, surgical removal of the primary tumor is necessary for durable local control (see below). Fortunately, the majority of patients with osteosarcoma present with primary tumors of the extremities, and local control can be readily achieved by amputation (see Chap. 10). In historical series (before 1970) the outlook for children with osteosarcoma was dismal, despite adequate surgical control of the primary tumor by amputation.[56-60] The overwhelming majority of patients presenting without evidence of metastases and treated only with surgery of the primary tumor ultimately developed distant metastases: 50% of patients developed metastases—virtually always in the lung—within 6 months of amputation and, overall, more than 80% ultimately developed recurrent disease. This discouraging natural history was documented at a number of centers and was summarized in a literature review in 1972.[60] Eleven studies conducted between 1946 and 1976 reporting data on 1337 patients were reviewed. Of 1286 patients with adequate follow-up treated with surgical ablation of the primary tumor (almost all amputations), only 253 (19.7%) survived 5 years. The 10-year survival dropped only slightly, to 16%, indicating that the majority of 5-year survivors were cured.

The appearance of metastatic disease was an ominous sign in historical series because few patients survived beyond 1 year after detection of tumor recurrence. The majority of patients developed multiple bilateral pulmonary metastases as the first evidence of recurrence,[4,61] and more than 95% of patients who died of metastatic disease had lung involvement at the time of death. Metastases to bones of the skeleton occur in 15% to 30% of patients. Less common sites of metastases occurring preterminally or discovered at autopsy include pleura, pericardium, kidney, adrenal gland, and brain.[59] Involvement of lymph nodes is unusual, but is a poor prognostic sign. Death from metastatic disease results from pulmonary failure due to widespread lung metastases, pulmonary hemorrhage, pneumothorax, and superior vena cava obstruction.

Although variability in overall outcome of patients with osteosarcoma was noted in historical series, the expectation that fewer than 20% of patients would survive beyond 5 years (based on data from multiple centers) served as the background for trials of adjuvant chemotherapy conducted in the 1970s and 1980s. The inescapable conclusion from historical studies was that 80% of patients presenting without overt metastatic disease in fact had microscopic subclinical metastases at the time of diagnosis, which were undetectable by techniques then available.

By the late 1970s it was clear that the prognosis for children with osteosarcoma was improving, an improvement largely attributed to the application of adjuvant therapies. However, data from the Mayo Clinic[62-64] suggested that the natural history of osteosarcoma had changed since the late 1960s, and that the prognosis for patients had improved independently of the administration of adjuvant therapy. Data from other small studies,[65-67] and particularly from a randomized controlled trial

of adjuvant chemotherapy conducted at the Mayo Clinic,[68] appeared to confirm this change in the natural history of osteosarcoma. Thus, at the beginning of the 1980s, the true natural history of osteosarcoma was controversial, and the efficacy of adjuvant therapy was difficult to assess. Trials of adjuvant chemotherapy for osteosarcoma undertaken in the 1970s were conducted without concurrent control groups, and benefits were inferred by comparison to historical controls and to the expectation that fewer than 20% of patients treated only with surgery would survive relapse-free. The controversy surrounding the apparent change in the natural history of osteosarcoma and its impact on the interpretation of results of trials of adjuvant therapy[69-71] cast doubt on the apparent benefits of adjuvant chemotherapy demonstrated in numerous uncontrolled trials of the 1970s.

Two trials conducted in the 1980s[72-74] were designed to address the natural history of surgically treated osteosarcoma of the extremity. The outcome of patients in these trials who were treated only with surgery of the primary tumor recapitulated the historical experience prior to 1970—more than half of these patients developed metastases within 6 months of diagnosis and, overall, more than 80% developed recurrent disease within 2 years of diagnosis. Thus, the natural history of osteosarcoma apparently has not changed over time, and fewer than 20% of patients treated only with surgery of the primary tumor can be expected to survive relapse-free. The bleak historical experience that had served as the background for numerous uncontrolled adjuvant trials of the 1970s appears to be an equally valid control for studies of the 1980s and beyond.

CLINICAL EVALUATION AND DIAGNOSTIC STUDIES

The evaluation of suspected osteosarcoma begins with history, physical examination, and plain radiographs. The duration of symptoms is variable and may have prognostic significance (see below). Pain in other bony sites may represent metastatic involvement, but metastases are most likely to occur in the lungs and do not produce respiratory symptoms in the absence of extensive lung involvement. Systemic symptoms, such as fever and weight loss, occur rarely in the absence of very advanced disease.[4,7] Physical examination is typically remarkable only for the soft tissue mass that is usually evident at the primary site; regional and distant lymph node metastases are rarely observed.

Laboratory evaluation is seldom revealing. Elevation of the serum alkaline phosphatase is observed in more than 40% of patients[4,75] but does not correlate reliably with disease extent, although the serum alkaline phosphatase may have prognostic significance (see below). The serum lactic dehydrogenase (LDH) may be elevated in approximately 30% of patients presenting without metastases.[76]

Radiologic Evaluation

Radiographic examination of the involved bone is extremely useful in the evaluation of the patient with a suspected malignant bone tumor (see Chap. 7). Plain films of malignant bone tumors usually reveal permeative destruction of the normal trabecular pattern, with indistinct margins and no endosteal bone response. Intense periosteal new bone formation and lifting of the cortex with formation of Codman's triangle is common (see Fig. 32-3).[77] A soft tissue mass is frequently observed as the tumor erodes from the medullary cavity through the cortex and into the adjacent soft tissue. Characteristic radiographic features, along with clinical information and tumor location, permit prediction of the histologic diagnosis from the plain radiographs in more than two thirds of cases of osteosarcoma.[77] The eccentric location of the tumor in the metaphyseal portion of the long bone is characteristic of osteosarcoma, whereas Ewing's sarcoma (the most frequent consideration in the differential diagnosis) tends to occur in the flat bones or in the diaphyseal portions of the long bones of the skeleton, and more frequently appears as a predominantly lytic lesion on plain radiographs. Ossification in the soft tissue in a radial or "sunburst" pattern is classic for osteosarcoma but is neither a reliable nor specific feature. None of the radiographic features is pathognomonic, however, and biopsy is always required to confirm the diagnosis. Radiographically, osteosarcomas may appear to be osteosclerotic in approximately 45% of cases, purely osteolytic in 30%, and mixed sclerotic and lytic in the remaining 25%.[77] Such radiographic findings reflect the degree of ossification and mineralization rather than the amount of osteoid found in the tumor, since uncalcified osteoid substance produces no radiopacity, even if present in large amounts.[8]

Although plain radiographs are extremely useful in evaluating malignant bone tumors, the extent of the primary lesion is often seriously underestimated by such studies. Further radiographic evaluation of the primary tumor is thus essential in planning the definitive surgery. Computerized tomography (CT scan) has been found to be particularly useful in evaluating the extent of the primary tumor in the medullary cavity and soft tissues, which is essential in planning the level of amputation or the proximal and distal resection margins when a limb-salvage procedure is an option. Magnetic resonance imaging (MRI) is apparently much more sensitive for detecting intramedullary extent of tumor[78] and may ultimately supplant the CT scan for this purpose.

The radionuclide bone scan is also indicated in the initial diagnostic evaluation to define the extent of the primary tumor. Because uptake of the radiopharmaceutical will extend slightly beyond the limits of tumor, it defines a safe margin to use in planning surgery of the primary lesion.[79,80] The sensitivity of radionuclide bone scanning is also useful in the detection of "skip lesions," which are seen infrequently in patients with osteosarcoma.[81] Increased uptake of radiopharmaceutical in a site separate from the primary but in the involved bone should alert the surgeon to the possible existence of skip lesions in planning the surgical approach to the tumor.

Arteriography may also be useful for evaluation of the primary tumor when limb-salvage procedures are a consideration, although some investigators find that angiograms are of limited value in determining local operability (see Chap. 7). Arteriograms performed in only the anteroposterior plane provide little definitive information on the relationship of the extramedullary tumor extent to the primary vascular structures. Arteriograms also provide poor visualization of veins, which may in fact be a more significant surgical problem than arteries.

The presence of metastases at diagnosis is an extremely important prognostic variable with a major impact on management, so appropriate surveillance must precede the definitive approach to the primary tumor. The lung is the first site of metastasis in 90% of children with osteosarcoma, and routine posteroanterior and lateral radiographs of the chest allow detection of metastases in the majority of cases. Linear tomography and CT of the chest are more sensitive in detecting pulmonary metastases—as many as 10% to 20% of patients have metastatic nodules found on linear or computed tomography of the chest that are undetectable on conventional chest radiographs.[82] Since CT is more sensitive than linear tomography, especially for the detection of pleural-based lesions,[77,83–85] the CT scan is probably the examination of choice for screening

patients with osteosarcoma for metastatic disease, although false-positive examinations have been a problem with this technique. If there is any doubt that a lesion on CT scan represents metastatic disease, histologic confirmation is indicated, especially if the lesion does not appear on plain radiographs.

Because metastases to other bones of the skeleton are seen in approximately 10% of patients with osteosarcoma, a radionuclide bone scan is also indicated in screening for metastatic disease. Scanning with methylene diphosphonate labeled with technetium-99m has been found to be very sensitive for the detection of metastatic bony sites, and in the majority of cases is more sensitive than plain radiographs.[79,86] Recently, radiolabeled monoclonal antibodies raised against human osteosarcoma have been used in scanning patients with a variety of tumors.[87,88] Although scanning with radiolabeled antibody successfully detected all five primary osteosarcomas tested in one report, the antibody scan failed to detect pulmonary metastases in two patients, reflecting the insensitivity of the technique. Moreover, the antibody used in that study is not specific for osteosarcoma, and scans of patients with other malignant tumors (notably Ewing's sarcoma and malignant fibrous histiocytoma) were also positive.[87] Nevertheless, better scanning techniques and the availability of more specific antibodies are likely to enhance the utility of such diagnostic studies, particularly for the detection of occult metastases.

Follow-Up Studies

Radiographic evaluations are also a critical component of follow-up. Patients with osteosarcoma should be followed frequently with radiographic studies for metastatic surveillance for at least 5 years from the completion of therapy. Because the overwhelming majority of first recurrences appear asymptomatically in the lungs, plain chest radiographs should be performed monthly for at least 2 years from diagnosis and with decreasing frequency thereafter. The importance of detecting metastases early cannot be overemphasized (see below). Thus, any abnormality detected on plain chest radiographs should be followed diligently. CT of the chest is a useful adjunct to plain radiographs for this purpose and should be performed routinely every 4 to 6 months for the first 2 years from diagnosis and whenever a persistent suspicious abnormality appears on plain films. Radionuclide bone scans should also be obtained every 4 to 6 months for the first 2 years. Although bone metastases are likely to produce symptoms, occasional asymptomatic metastases in the skeleton may be detected by bone scan, and any abnormality should be confirmed by plain radiographs. Evaluation of the stump after amputation and of the affected limb after tumor resection can be difficult because of bone scan and radiographic abnormalities resulting from unequal weight bearing and callus formation. However, evaluation of the primary site should not be overlooked because of the possibility of local recurrence, especially after limb-salvage procedures.

Biopsy

Although the radiographic findings in a patient with a suspected malignant bone tumor may be highly suggestive, a biopsy is always required to confirm the diagnosis. The timing of the biopsy in relation to the other diagnostic procedures has been debated; many investigators claim that interpretation of the bone scan, arteriogram, and CT scan (in terms of the extent of the primary tumor) may be unreliable if these investigations are undertaken after biopsy.[77,89] However, the tissue disturbance caused by the biopsy in most instances should be minimal and should not have a major impact on information from radiographic studies.

Several biopsy techniques have been proposed for the evaluation of malignant bone tumors. Fine needle aspiration, core needle biopsy, and open biopsy have been used successfully at different centers (see also Chap. 10). The majority of patients require an open biopsy. Previously, it was thought that a tourniquet should be placed proximal to the lesion at the time of biopsy to prevent the spread of tumor cells, but most investigators no longer consider this essential.

The location of the biopsy incision is a critical issue in planning the biopsy.[90] The incision should be made longitudinally in a fashion that disturbs as little of the normal anatomy as possible. In certain cases it is helpful to have available both plain radiographs and the CT scan to determine the shortest distance between the skin and the primary tumor. Dissection through the muscle directly down to the adjacent tumor through the shortest route disturbs the least amount of tissue. A frozen section performed at the time of biopsy ensures that adequate tissue has been obtained for diagnosis. Several studies have indicated that the frequency of tumor seeding of biopsy sites is high, and it is essential that the biopsy site be excised *en bloc* with the tumor during the definitive surgical procedure. Placement of the biopsy site with the view to the eventual definitive surgical procedure should thus be carefully planned (especially if limb-salvage surgery is a consideration), to allow excision of the biopsy tract in continuity with the definitive bony receptor. Meticulous hemostasis following the biopsy is also essential. Absorbable gelatin sponges or methylmethacrylate in the bone are useful to control bleeding, and efforts to control muscular vessels with external compression for 1 to 2 days may reduce the incidence of hematomas and subsequent wound infection in the biopsy site.

In the past, showering of tumor cells at the time of biopsy was felt to result from surgical manipulation and to account for the poor prognosis for patients with osteosarcoma. It was thought possible to reduce the dissemination of tumor cells by performing the definitive surgical procedure at the same time as the initial biopsy. A strategy was developed at the Mayo Clinic in which the biopsy was performed under tourniquet control, diagnosis was confirmed by frozen section, and immediate amputation was performed. The difficulty of rendering a definitive diagnosis in bone tumors based on frozen section alone has made this approach less popular. Moreover, the survival of patients treated in this manner has not been superior to that of patients undergoing biopsy and delayed definitive surgery.

Staging

Because of the unsuitability of standard staging systems when applied to skeletal tumors, Enneking and associates at the University of Florida established a staging system for malignant skeletal tumors based on a retrospective review of cases of primary malignant tumors of bone that were treated by primary surgical resection.[91] This system categorizes nonmetastatic malignant bone tumors by grade—low grade (Stage I) and high grade (Stage II)—and further subdivides by the local anatomic extent—intramedullary (A) or extramedullary (B). Patients with distant metastases are Stage III. The suitability of this staging system for high-grade skeletal lesions is not established, and its relevance to osteosarcomas, which are virtually all high-grade tumors, has been questioned. There are very few high-grade intramedullary lesions (*i.e.*, Stage II-A) because the majority of high-grade tumors (including osteosarcomas)

break through the cortex into the extramedullary tissues early in their natural history and most often present as Clinical Stage II-B lesions. It is also not clear that the size or extramedullary extent of the primary tumor in high-grade lesions is of major prognostic value. Nevertheless, the Enneking staging system remains the only one that is widely accepted for skeletal tumors, and its use facilitates comparison of outcomes of different therapy regimens.

PROGNOSTIC FACTORS

Several clinical characteristics are thought to be of prognostic significance for patients with osteosarcoma. Although treatment has an obvious impact on outcome, several factors appear to be prognostically important independent of therapy. Such factors may become less powerful prognostically as the outcome for patients with osteosarcoma continues to improve. The most important prognostic factor appears to be extent of disease at diagnosis, in that patients with overt metastatic disease have an unfavorable outcome. Although aggressive approaches to patients presenting with metastases have improved their prognosis somewhat (see below), the majority of such patients ultimately die of their disease.

As discussed above, histology exerts an important influence on outcome. Parosteal and intraosseous well-differentiated osteosarcomas, in particular, are associated with a favorable prognosis, and periosteal osteosarcomas have an intermediate outlook.[50–52] Among the variants of conventional osteosarcoma there appears to be no significant relationship between histologic subtype (osteoblastic, fibroblastic, and chondroblastic) and overall survival.[7] Telangiectatic osteosarcomas have been associated with a particularly poor prognosis in some series,[8,46] but not in others.[47,48] Osteosarcomas arising in preexistent lesions or from radiation exposure behave clinically like *de novo* lesions, except those in patients with Paget's disease, which are associated with an adverse prognosis.[8] Histologic grading has likewise not reliably correlated with outcome, in large part because the overwhelming majority of classic osteosarcomas are high-grade lesions. In preliminary studies, analysis of DNA content of bone tumors has been found to be a predictor of metastasis: tumors with a low percentage of diploid cells and an aneuploid peak were more likely to metastasize,[92] although several variables, especially histology and treatment, have confounded these results. Recently, lymphocytic infiltration of the primary tumor has been correlated with superior relapse-free survival in patients with osteosarcoma.[93] Such lymphocytic infiltration may represent the expression of specific host immunity to the tumor.

The primary site of disease is also an important variable. A review of survival figures from several large series[94,95] suggests that patients with axial skeleton primaries have a poor prognosis. Because complete surgical excision with clean margins is a prerequisite for long-term disease control, it is self-evident that tumors arising in certain axial skeleton sites (skull, vertebrae) are not amenable to curative surgery. There are now more innovative surgical strategies for tumors in certain axial skeleton sites (particularly primary tumors in the pelvis), and tumors once considered unresectable can be approached with curative intent. Less intuitive is the association of tibial primaries with a more favorable prognosis in most[76,94] but not all[4] series. Tumors of the proximal humerus have variably been associated with a favorable or unfavorable prognosis. In general, more distal primaries have been associated with a more favorable prognosis.

Tumor size has also been cited as a powerful prognostic factor—in the prechemotherapy era, small tumors (<5 cm) were associated with a favorable prognosis and large tumors (>15 cm) with a dismal prognosis.[4] This relationship has not been confirmed in all series, and the effect of tumor size may result from a correlation of size and primary site.[95] Duration of symptoms before treatment may be an indirect measure of tumor growth rate and has prognostic value—patients with longer durations of symptoms have a superior outcome.[4] In addition, patients with long intervals between the onset of symptoms and diagnosis are likely to have an indolent variant of osteosarcoma (particularly parosteal osteosarcoma).

Additional patient characteristics reported to be of prognostic value include age (children younger than 10 years fare worse; patients older than 20 years have a more favorable outlook), sex (females have a more favorable outcome),[96,97] and serum and tumor tissue alkaline phosphatase (elevated levels are associated with a greater risk of subsequent metastatic disease).[75,98] Results from the Multi-Institutional Osteosarcoma Study suggest that an elevated level of serum LDH is the most powerful single adverse prognostic factor for patients with nonmetastatic osteosarcoma of the extremity treated with adjuvant chemotherapy.[76] Thirty-one percent of the patients in that study were found to have elevated LDH at diagnosis. At 4 years, the projected event-free survival for patients with elevated LDH is 32% compared to 67% for patients with normal LDH at diagnosis ($p < 0.001$).

TREATMENT

Surgery of the Primary Tumor

Because osteosarcoma is generally unresponsive to conventional dose radiotherapy, the management of the primary tumor in extremity lesions is surgical. Removal of all gross and microscopic tumor is required to prevent local recurrence. Primary surgical procedures fall into two major categories—amputation and limb salvage procedures. Both approaches incorporate the basic principle of *en bloc* excision of the tumor and biopsy site through normal tissue planes. Other procedures, such as intralesional curettage or marginal resection, which are often successful for benign tumors of bone (giant cell tumor, chondroblastoma, and aneurysmal bone cysts), are inadequate for local control of osteosarcoma. Malignant tumors must be removed *en bloc* with a margin of normal uninvolved tissue. Local extension of malignant bone tumors occurs primarily by intramedullary and extramedullary extension. Once the tumors break through the cortex, they infiltrate normal muscle. However, direct invasion of adjacent arteries or nerves is rare, and involvement of veins is usually by tumor thrombus rather than direct invasion of the vein wall.

The selection of surgical procedure involves consideration of several interrelated factors, including tumor location, size or extramedullary extent, the presence or absence of distant metastatic disease, and patient factors such as age, skeletal development, and life-style preference that might dictate the suitability of limb salvage or amputation.

Amputation

The traditional surgical approach to local control of osteosarcoma of the extremity is amputation, which permits removal of all gross and microscopic tumor with clean margins and provides durable local control in the majority of cases. However, amputation, even with a wide margin of normal tissue, has not prevented stump recurrence in all cases. Stump recurrence has been attributed to the extensive intramedullary spread characteristic of osteosarcoma and to the existence of skip lesions—

tumor deposits in the affected bone that are separated from the primary tumor by several centimeters of normal bone—which have been reported to occur in up to 20% of cases of osteosarcoma.[81] This high incidence of skip lesions has led some surgeons to recommend the removal of the entire affected bone at the next proximal joint to ensure clean surgical margins and to avoid the problem of residual tumor in the stump. Such radical amputations result in considerable aesthetic and functional morbidity and seriously lessen the functional rehabilitation available with prostheses. The advent of more sensitive radionuclide bone scanning and, more recently, CT and MRI techniques to define the proximal intramedullary extent of tumor and to detect skip lesions has enabled orthopedic surgeons to proceed confidently with cross-bone amputations to treat the primary, allowing a safety margin of 6 to 7 cm above the most proximal medullary extent of tumor as defined by the bone scan and radiographs. The local recurrence rate has been acceptably low (<5%), indicating that skip lesions are indeed rare,[99] and the functional results are superior. Curettings from the medullary canal proximal to the amputation margin should be examined pathologically in any case to ensure the safety of the procedure. It has not been clearly shown that removal of the entire bone results in enhanced survival when compared to less radical procedures done with meticulous selection of surgical margins and with careful surgical techniques.

When amputation is performed, early rehabilitation and psychological preparation and support are important elements of the therapy (see Chaps. 46 and 47). Improvements in the prostheses available for amputees have enhanced the functional results for these patients. The functional ability of patients who have had below the knee amputations is excellent, with very little measurable functional disability. Low above the knee amputations also have successful functional outcome. More extensive amputations, such as high above the knee amputations, hip disarticulations, and hemipelvectomies, result in permanent functional problems because of mechanical disadvantage. There is currently no prosthesis available that adequately substitutes for a functional hand, so upper extremity amputations invariably result in severe loss of function. Thus, patients with tumors in more proximal segments of the extremity are likely to suffer more severe functional and cosmetic disability.

Limb-Salvage Surgery

With improvements in the survival of patients with osteosarcoma, investigators have attempted subamputative surgery in the hope of reducing functional and psychological morbidity (see Chap. 10). The selection of appropriate patients for limb-salvage surgery is essential. Certain tumors, including most distal tibial lesions and those proximal tibial lesions with a large extramedullary component, are poor candidates for limb-salvage surgical resections because an adequate soft tissue margin is difficult to achieve. Similarly, limb-salvage surgery in the lower extremity may be an inappropriate choice for young patients who have not achieved full growth potential and who would be left with a leg length discrepancy later in life, although creative endoprosthetic devices may circumvent this relative contraindication (see below). Advances in surgical techniques have increased the number of patients eligible for limb salvage surgery, and a variety of novel techniques have been used to repair the defect created by radical excision of tumor-bearing bones.

Tumors occurring in expendable bones, such as the ulna, patella, fibula, scapula, or ribs, although rare, provide a relatively straightforward opportunity for limb salvage. Surgical techniques for such tumors have been well described, and the

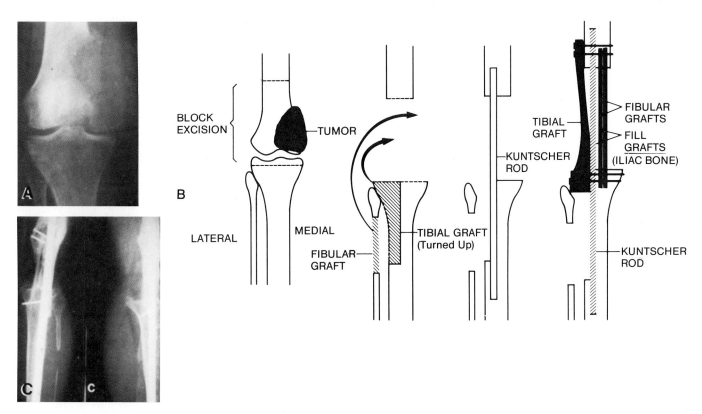

FIGURE 32-6. Sliding bone graft used in resection of distal femur osteosarcoma. **A.** Destructive lesion of distal femur. **B.** Stages of resection arthrodesis. **C.** Postoperative radiograph.

functional disability from excision of these areas is minimal. Bone grafting or endoprosthetic replacement is seldom necessary.

The majority of limb-salvage procedures for osteosarcoma require restoration of the structural integrity of the involved extremity, and clinical experience has centered around the use of biological materials and metallic endoprosthetic devices. Biological approaches to extremity, pelvic, or spinal reconstruction use cadaver allografts or grafts taken from the patient's own bone (autogenous graft or vascularized graft, *e.g.,* fibular or iliac). Once healed and incorporated, grafts provide an enduring solution to reconstruction problems of large bony structural defects by providing a structural lattice for the ingrowth of the patient's own bone elements; a stable anatomic setting of bone formation and remodeling is achieved that eventually is the same as that of nondiseased bones. Several options for limb reconstruction are available. The decision concerning the most appropriate procedure for an individual patient reflects consideration of the anatomy, the defect to be repaired, and the surgeon's personal preference.

AUTOLOGOUS GRAFTS.   The concept of autologous bone grafting is somewhat limited in tumor surgery because of the long segments of bone excised. Replacement then necessitates the use of an equal or almost equal length of normal uninvolved bone from another portion of the body, which often is not possible. Enneking and colleagues have described a sliding bone graft for replacement of the distal femur or proximal tibia that involves removal of approximately 180° of the circumference of the adjacent tibia or femur, which is then slid proximally to replace the distal femur or distally to replace the proximal tibia, and is supplemented with fibular grafts and fixed with a long intramedullary rod (Fig. 32-6).[100] Successful

knee arthrodesis can be achieved in 95% of patients, even when a long segment of bone has been excised. This procedure involves prolonged casting and bracing, and is complicated by a relatively high incidence of nonunion (35%), fatigue fracture (45%), and infection. However, in some instances the ultimate objective of incorporation with a solid bone union has been achieved. Although the operation successfully achieves tumor-free margins, the revascularization and rehabilitation processes are prolonged and complicated. Even when the outcome is successful, patients must readjust their lifestyles to accommodate the fused knee.

VASCULARIZED GRAFTS.   A relatively recent concept is the use of vascularized grafts (primarily using the fibula or iliac crest) with a nutrient blood supply. The vascularized segment is transposed to fill the defect created by excision of the primary tumor, and the nutrient vessels are reanastomosed by microvascular technique to adjacent vessels (Fig. 32-7).[101] The graft then remains viable throughout the entire course, and subsequent healing does not require the long periods of remodeling and regrowth of the tissue into the grafts. The major drawbacks of this procedure are the length of time required to perform the vascular dissection and reanastomosis, when added to a 4- to 5-hour *en bloc* excision procedure; and the transverse diameter discrepancy between the vascularized fibula and the excised segment of femur or humerus it replaces.

ALLOGRAFTS.   Allografts, whether obtained from surgical patients or cadaver donors, have been used to re-create structural integrity for many years. The success of allografts relates to the nonantigenic nature of bone, which permits the use of allografts without tissue typing. Freezing further decreases the rejection phenomenon. Glycerol preparations preserve the

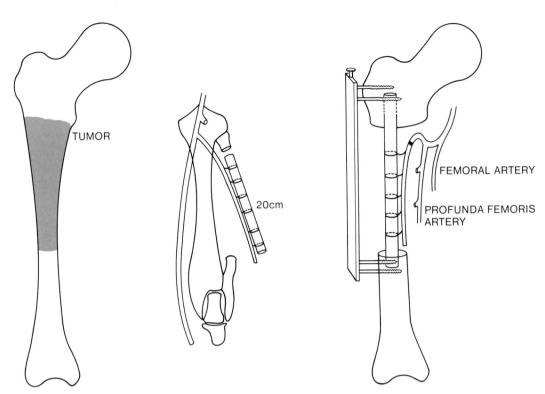

FIGURE 32-7. Schematic representation of tumor of midfemur. A vascularized fibular graft is used for intercalary replacement.

cartilage for invasive osteoarticular joint reconstructions, and adjacent tendons may be left attached to the donor bone to help stabilize the reconstruction.[102] Allografts are inexpensive, readily available, and are much more compatible in size to the excised segment than are vascularized or autologous grafts. It was hoped that these grafts would subsequently become incorporated by the host normal tissue, providing a structural lattice into which ingrowth of normal bone elements would occur. Short allograft segments are, in fact, incorporated without acute rejection, and, although they are probably eventually destroyed, this process occurs very slowly, retaining structural integrity. Clinical experience with larger segments of allografted bone has shown that subsequent incorporation is extremely unusual; fracture or dissolution of the allograft ultimately occurs in a high percentage of cases. Given that the bone removed for most primary bone tumors is 15 to 20 cm in length, the use of allogeneic materials is at present quite restricted.

ENDOPROSTHESIS. Endoprosthetic devices for bone and joint replacement have been developed as an offshoot of the experience with total joint arthroplasty. These devices are manufactured as casts of cobalt, chrome, or steel, or machined from titanium. They are custom-designed to reproduce accurately the structural dimensions of the excised bone, and clinically accomplish the goal of immediate attainment of structural integrity (Fig. 32-8). The long-term results and endurance of these prosthetic devices are not yet known. Three potential clinical problems have occurred: fatigue fracture, loosening, and infection. The fatigue fracture potential of the metal is a design and stress problem that can potentially be improved by changes in casting methods, use of stronger metals, or improvements in stress-relieving joint designs. Loosening of the endoprosthesis at the bone–cement–prosthesis interface is a

problem that is less easily resolved, but is minimized by using meticulous cement technique and stress-reducing total joint mechanics such as a rotating-hinge knee design. Infection is a difficult problem with the large endoprotheses because they act as a large foreign body. Management of this complication can be difficult and time-consuming, and, severe infection may result in a delayed amputation—although theoretically at a level no higher than if amputation had been used initially to approach the primary tumor.

Further improvements in endoprosthetic devices may result from active clinical and basic research. Porous ingrowth materials, such as woven meshes of titanium or metal alloys that are fixed to or coated on the surface of the metallic endoprosthesis, have been used. In animal experiments, these allow ingrowth of host tissue into the mesh and actual bone formation within these meshes. This encourages extramedullary ingrowth of the host's own bone along the metallic endoprosthesis shaft, thereby providing a biological fixation of the prosthesis.

Another fascinating biomechanical design advance is the expandable prosthesis, which uses the concept of a telescoping unit that can be expanded with a gear device (Fig. 32-9).[103] This permits gradual expansion of the overall length of the prosthesis and makes it possible to implant the endoprosthesis in skeletally immature patients, increasing the numbers of those eligible for limb-salvage surgery. The experience with this technique, although intriguing, is limited. It is also probable that when these prostheses reach their full length, they will have to be replaced because of the loss of structural strength with full extension.

EXCISIONS WITHOUT REPLACEMENT. Several surgical techniques have been used that involve resection of the tumor without replacement of the excised region. A procedure re-

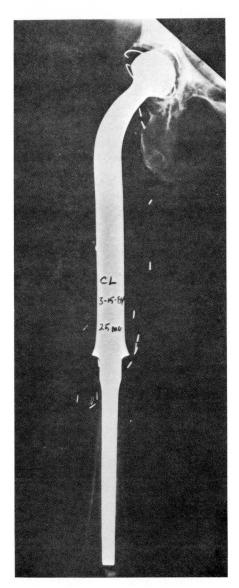

FIGURE 32-8. Anteroposterior radiograph depicting a proximal femoral replacement for extremity reconstruction following *en bloc* resection of an osteosarcoma of the proximal femur.

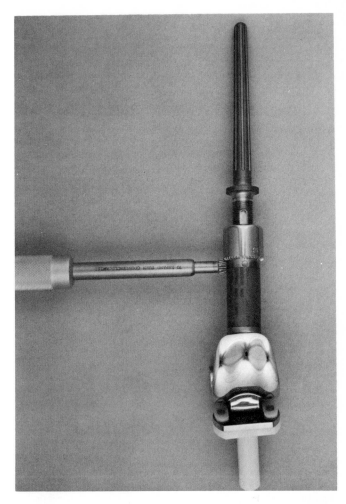

FIGURE 32-9. Expandable distal femoral endoprosthesis with kinematic rotating knee used for distal femur replacement in skeletally immature individuals (see text).

cently popularized by Saltzer is the tibial turnback, a variation of the Van Ness rotation.[104] This operation involves excision of the distal femur and adjacent musculature with preservation of the lower leg (tibia and foot) by maintenance of an intact neurovascular bundle. The defect created by the excision of the distal femur is replaced by 180° rotation of the distal extremity and fixation of the tibia to the proximal femur. This places the foot in an inverted position with the sole facing anteriorly, and the ankle functions as a knee joint (Fig. 32-10). The foot is retained, but an external prosthesis is still necessary—the patient is thus converted from a functional above the knee amputee to a functional below the knee amputee, with considerable improvement in function. This procedure permits the surgical excision of a great deal more tissue and achievement of a wider margin of resection than do operations that involve the use of an endoprosthesis or allograft. Its eventual acceptance remains to be seen; the appearance of the reconstructed limb presents cosmetic and psychological dif-

ficulties, but the functional results have thus far been encouraging.

In lesions of the proximal humerus, tumor excision without replacement has been extremely successful. The Tikhoff–Linberg resection is an alternative to interscapulothoracic amputation when the brachial plexus is not involved with tumor. The proximal humerus is excised in continuity with the scapula, without bony replacement,[105] preserving the distal arm and allowing normal elbow and hand function. The shoulder area is unstable, and telescoping of the intervening structures occurs if stresses are applied to the hand or forearm; stabilization is necessary in most instances. The recent development of endoprostheses for the scapula and humerus has permitted restoration of structural integrity in many of these cases (Fig. 32-11). The clinical and functional outcome is far superior to an amputation.

Although hemipelvectomy (hind-quarter amputations) were previously the only surgical option for malignant tumors of the pelvis, *en bloc* excision of the hemipelvis with preservation of the extremity can now be performed in most instances, with equal local tumor control. Reconstruction of the resultant defect has been difficult, and metallic endoprostheses have had limited success (80% failure) because of difficulties with the fixation of the prosthesis to the remaining pelvis. The large lever arms and forces applied to the fixation have resulted in

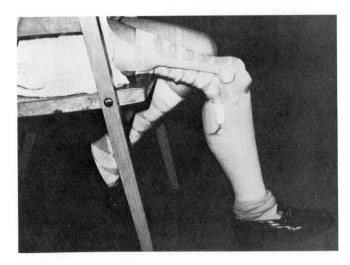

FIGURE 32-10. Tibial turnback operation with foot inverted and ankle functioning as a knee. A below-the-knee external prosthesis is in place.

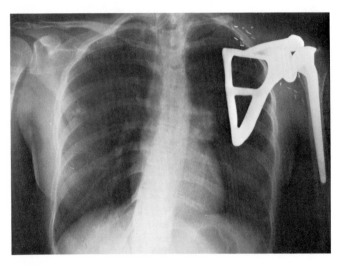

FIGURE 32-11. Postoperative radiograph of a patient who underwent resection of the entire scapula and proximal humerus with endoprosthetic replacement.

frequent loosening and migration of the endoprosthesis. Other methods of obtaining structural integrity have included fusion of the proximal femur to the ileum or sacrum and internal hemipelvectomy with no replacement at all (Fig. 32-12). When no replacement is used, a gap between the femur and pelvis is bridged by scar tissue from the adjacent soft tissue, and this fibrous union allows the patient to bear approximately 80% of his or her body weight.[106] There is approximately 2 to 4 inches of limb shortening, which requires additional shoe lifts, and most patients use a cane or crutch. However, even with these limitations, this procedure appears to be a useful alternative to amputative hemipelvectomy, with superior functional results.

UNRESOLVED ISSUES. Advances in techniques for limb salvage have increased the surgical options available, thus increasing the number of patients eligible for limb salvage and enhancing the results achieved. Although limb-salvage surgery is being used with increasing frequency and enthusiasm, several issues remain unresolved. The safety of limb salvage for

osteosarcoma has been questioned by investigators of the German Pediatric Oncology Group, who found a significantly higher distant failure rate for patients treated by *en bloc* resection than for those undergoing amputation.[107,108] In contrast, a retrospective review by the Musculoskeletal Tumor Society in the United States[108a] failed to show an increased risk of relapse for patients treated by limb salvage. In view of the close margins used in some limb-salvage procedures, one might anticipate higher rates of local recurrence compared to those associated with amputation, but this has not been the case. Follow-up from studies involving more patients treated by *en bloc* resection may help to resolve this issue. In addition, the long-term functional results of limb-salvage surgery have not been adequately assessed. The longevity of endoprosthetic devices remains problematic, and late infections and graft failure may result in delayed amputations for patients treated by limb resection. There is little doubt that limb salvage for upper extremity primaries results in a significant functional advantage; the advantage for patients with lower extremity primaries continues to be debated. Finally, the role of presurgical chemotherapy (see below) in facilitating limb salvage remains to be demonstrated, although it appears that centers which use preoperative therapy perform limb-salvage surgery on a higher proportion of patients than those centers which do not use presurgical therapy. Because few eligible patients who are given the opportunity will choose amputation rather than limb salvage, demonstration of the safety and efficacy of limb-salvage surgery in osteosarcoma is clearly an important priority for current studies.

Radiotherapy in the Management of the Primary Tumor

In the past, radiotherapy was recommended to treat the primary tumor in osteosarcoma. However, osteosarcoma has been found to be a highly radioresistant lesion. Radiation doses less than 6000 cGy have been associated with only transient tumor control,[109] and viable tumor has been observed in amputation specimens after doses of 8000 cGy or more.[110,111] The presence of a relatively high percentage of hypoxic tumor cells and *in vitro* evidence that osteosarcoma cells may have increased capacity to repair sublethal radiation injury[112] may explain the failure of conventional radiotherapeutic fractionation techniques to provide durable local control of osteosarcoma.

Before the 1970s, when osteosarcoma was almost uniformly fatal, a strategy of primary radiotherapy followed by delayed amputation evolved in an effort to avoid mutilating surgery in patients destined to die of their disease.[1,110] High-dose radiotherapy was administered initially and ablative surgery used only for those patients remaining free of disease 4 to 6 months after the completion of radiotherapy. However, in a subsequent assessment, primary radiotherapy was found to result in few responses; there were local recurrences in virtually all cases, and palliation (the ostensible goal of delayed surgery) was poor.[109]

With improvements in the control of micrometastatic disease by systemic chemotherapy in the 1970s and 1980s, the majority of patients should be approached with curative intent, which makes local recurrence intolerable. It appears that the overall control rate of the primary tumor with radiotherapy is significantly less than with ablative surgery, so radiotherapy has little role in the management of primary osteosarcomas that are controllable by surgery. The use of hypofractionated radiotherapy or other novel radiation fractionation techniques, with or without radiosensitizers to overcome the capacity of osteosarcoma cells to repair sublethal damage, may result in more durable control of primary osteosarcoma, although the

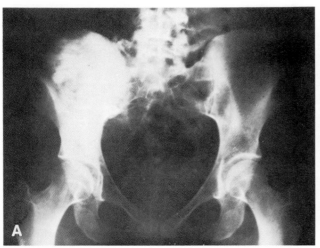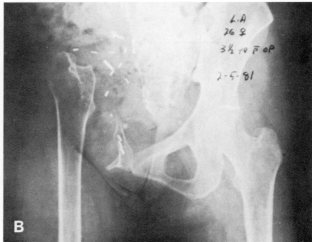

FIGURE 32-12. **A.** Anteroposterior radiograph of the pelvis of a patient with a large osteosarcoma of the ileum. **B.** Radiograph of the same patient 3½ years after internal hemipelvectomy.

Table 32-2
Representative Studies (Pooled Data) of Single-Agent Chemotherapy in Overt (Primary or Metastatic) Osteosarcoma

Agent	Number of Responders/ Number of Evaluable	Percentage of PR + CR*
Cyclophosphamide	4/28	15
Melphalan (L-PAM)	5/32	15
Mitomycin C	3/23	13
Vincristine/vinblastine	0/21	0
Uracil mustard	0/10	0
Hydroxyurea	0/10	0
Procarbazine	0/10	0
DTIC	2/14	14
Adriamycin	28/109	26
5-Fluorouracil	0/11	0
Cisplatin	8/24	33
Dactinomycin (actinomycin D)	4/26	15
Methotrexate (low dose)	0/14	0
High-dose methotrexate (plus vincristine and leucovorin)		
Every 3 weeks	11/26	42
Every week	9/11	82†
Ifosfamide	6/18	33

(Adapted from Bode U, Levine AS: The biology and management of osteosarcoma. In Levine AS [ed]: Cancer in the Young, pp 575–602. New York, Masson Publishing, 1982)
* PR = partial response; CR = complete response. CR is less than 10% of total response rate in all major trials.
† May include some patients who concurrently received surgery or coned-down radiation to metastases.

increased soft tissue injury that results may limit this approach.[112] However, such approaches may be especially useful as primary therapy or as an adjunct to debulking surgery for patients with unresectable lesions of the axial skeleton. In the past, such patients have fared poorly because local control has been difficult to achieve.

Adjuvant Treatment

Chemotherapy

Although control of the primary tumor is reliably accomplished by surgery, studies of osteosarcoma prior to 1970 indicated that more than 80% of patients with osteosarcoma treated only with surgery would develop metastatic disease and die. Microscopic subclinical metastatic disease was presumed to exist in the overwhelming majority of patients. Evidence from animal models supporting the notion that chemotherapy is more effective against microscopic than overt disease[113–116] had already been applied in a successful strategy of "prophylactic" or adjuvant systemic chemotherapy in other childhood tumors. Unfortunately, osteosarcoma is a relatively drug-resistant neoplasm. Studies of the activity of a variety of agents against macroscopic osteosarcoma (Table 32-2) have been extremely disappointing. Few drugs have produced responses in more than 15% of patients, and most responses are partial rather than complete. Notable exceptions have been seen in trials of Adriamycin,[118] cisplatin,[119–122] high-dose methotrexate (HDMTX),[123–125] and, more recently, ifosfamide.[126] Intuitively, the use of agents in the adjuvant setting that are not very active against macroscopic osteosarcoma would not be expected to exert a significant impact on the natural history of this disease. Nevertheless, the hopeless prognosis of patients with osteosarcoma led to the enthusiastic use of these agents, singly or in combination, as adjuvant therapy for patients with nonmetastatic osteosarcoma after amputation. Because of the expectation from historical data that 80% of patients not treated with adjuvant therapy were destined to relapse and die, none of the early adjuvant trials of the 1970s used concurrent non-adjuvantly treated control groups; the efficacy of adjuvant regimens was inferred by comparison to the historical experience, and results from two recent trials have confirmed the validity of this approach.[72–74] Reported results of some of the important adjuvant chemotherapy trials of the 1970s and early 1980s are summarized in Table 32-3.

Concerns have been raised that the favorable results achieved in patients treated with adjuvant chemotherapy may not hold with longer follow-up, as late relapses occur, and that adjuvant chemotherapy for osteosarcoma may delay but not prevent relapse. However, results of many of the adjuvant stud-

Table 32-3
Reported Results of Representative Trials of Adjuvant Chemotherapy for Osteosarcoma

Adjuvant Regimen*	Investigators	Number of Patients	Those Relapse-Free (%)
HDMTX, VCR	DFCI[127-130]	12	42
HDMTX, VCR ± BCG†	NCI[117,131]	39	38
ADR	CALGB[132-134]	88	39
ADR ± HDMTX†	CALGB[135]	62	50
ADR + VCR + HDMTX	DFCI[128-130]	22	59
ADR + VCR + HDMTX (weekly)	DFCI[93,128-130]	46	60
ADR + VCR + (HDMTX OR IDMTX)†	CCSG[136]	165	40
CONPADRI I (CTX, VCR, ADR, PAM)	SWOG[97,137,138]	43	49
COMPADRI II (CTX, VCR, ADR, PAM, HDMTX)	SWOG[97,138]	53	35
COMPADRI III (CTX, VCR, ADR, PAM, HDMTX)	SWOG[97,138]	84	38
ADR + HDMTX + CTX	Stanford[139]	29	47 (2 year)
			13 (4 year)
ADR + HDMTX + CTX (OSTEO 72)	SJCRH[140,141]	26	50
ADR + HDMTX + CTX (OSTEO 77)	SJCRH[141]	51	51
ADR + CDDP	Roswell Park[142,143]	22	64
HDMTX + VCR vs. no adjuvant therapy†	Mayo Clinic[68]	38	40 (chemo)
			44 (no chemo)
BCD + HDMTX + ADR + CDDP vs. no adjuvant therapy§	MIOS[72,73]	36 randomized, 77 nonrandomized	64 (chemo) 17 (no chemo)
BCD + HDMTX + VCR + ADR (+ intra-arterial ADR + RT) vs. no adjuvant therapy§	UCLA[74]	59	55 (chemo) 20 (no chemo)
HDMTX + VCR + ADR + CTX (T4 + T5 pooled)	MSKCC[144-146]	52 (<21 years)	48
HDMTX + VCR + ADR + BCD (T7)ǁ	MSKCC[145,146]	54 (<21 years)	80
HDMTX + VCR + ADR + BCD ± CDDP (depending on response) (T10)ǁ	MSKCC[146,147]	79 (<21 years)	92
ADR + HDMTX + (BCD or CDDP) ± interferon (COSS 80)†,ǁ	GPO[108,148]	116	68
HDMTX + ADR + CDDPǁ	Mount Sinai[149]	25	77

(Adapted from Link MP: Adjuvant therapy in the treatment of osteosarcoma. In DeVita VT Jr, Hellman S, Rosenberg SA (eds): Advances in Oncology 1986, pp 193–207. Philadelphia, JB Lippincott, 1986)
* HDMTX = high-dose methotrexate (5 g/m² or more) + leucovorin rescue; VCR = vincristine; BCG = bacillus Calmette-Guerin; ADR = Adriamycin; IDMTX = intermediate dose methotrexate (750 mg/m²) + leucovorin rescue; CTX = cyclophosphamide; PAM = phenylalanine mustard; CDDP = cisplatin; BCD = bleomycin, cyclophosphamide, actinomycin D combination; RT = radiotherapy; DFCI = Dana-Farber Cancer Institute; NCI = National Cancer Institute; CALGB = Cancer and Acute Leukemia Group B; CCSG = Children's Cancer Study Group; SWOG = Southwest Oncology Group; MIOS = Multi-Institutional Osteosarcoma Study; UCLA = University of California, Los Angeles; MSKCC = Memorial Sloan-Kettering Cancer Center; GPO = German Society for Pediatric Oncology; SJCRH = St. Jude Children's Research Hospital.
† Randomized study; no significant difference in relapse-free survival between treatment arms.
‡ Randomized study; no significant difference in relapse-free survival for patients receiving and not receiving adjuvant HDMTX (see text).
§ Randomized study; difference in results of treatments highly significant ($p < 0.01$) (see text).
ǁ Incorporates preoperative chemotherapy.

ies reported in Table 32-3 (some with follow-up beyond 10 years) suggest that life tables for relapse-free survival have stable plateaus beyond 4 years, and that relapses after 3 years are infrequent. The majority of patients surviving 3 years without evidence of recurrence are thus likely to be cured.

Examination of the results of adjuvant trials reveals a trend in the direction of improved outcome for patients treated on more recent protocols. This improvement in the adjuvant chemotherapy of osteosarcoma has been largely empiric. Regimens have evolved through the combination of agents with variable activity against macroscopic disease. The majority of regimens currently in use incorporate Adriamycin, high-dose methotrexate with leucovorin rescue, and cisplatin. The combination of bleomycin, cyclophosphamide, and actinomycin D (BCD)[150] is also used, although its activity is disputed. Although the activity of the available agents against macroscopic disease might be considered suboptimal, the empirically constructed adjuvant regimens have been surprisingly successful.

Approximately 60% of patients with osteosarcoma treated with modern adjuvant chemotherapy regimens will survive without recurrence. Thus, the favorable impact of postoperative chemotherapy on the natural history of osteosarcoma now appears incontrovertible, and adjuvant chemotherapy should be a component of treatment for all patients with this disease.

Whole-Lung Irradiation

Prophylactic irradiation of the lungs as an adjuvant to surgical treatment of the primary tumor was evaluated in several trials. Osteosarcoma is not considered to be a radioresponsive tumor; theoretic estimates of tumor burden in pulmonary micrometastases in patients with subclinical disease and radiobiological considerations of the "curability" by radiotherapy of patients presenting with fewer than 10⁵ tumor cells in micrometastases were used to justify these trials.[67,151] Results[66,67,151] have demonstrated only marginal (if any) benefit for irradiated patients, and the role of adjuvant whole-lung irradiation in the treatment of osteosarcoma remains to be defined.

Presurgical Chemotherapy

Presurgical ("neoadjuvant") chemotherapy has been used with increasing frequency in the past decade in the management of patients with osteosarcoma (see Chap. 10). This strategy has evolved along with the increasing enthusiasm among orthopedic surgeons for limb-sparing procedures. Initial attempts at limb salvage at the Memorial Sloan-Kettering Cancer Center in 1973 involved the fabrication of customized endoprostheses to be used after *en bloc* resection of the tumor in selected patients. During the presurgical delay necessary for production of the prosthesis—a process requiring up to 3 months—chemotherapy was administered to shrink the primary tumor and thus facilitate limited resection.[144] Patients treated with presurgical chemotherapy appeared to fare better than concurrent patients treated with immediate surgery and postoperative adjuvant therapy. The strategy of presurgical chemotherapy was explored further in several studies from Memorial Hospital.[145,146] Responsiveness of the primary tumor to preoperative chemotherapy (as assessed by histologic examination of the tumor at the time of resection) was found to be a powerful predictor of tumor recurrence: patients with a favorable response (Grade III or IV, indicating extensive to complete response in the primary tumor; Fig. 32-13) fared extremely well, whereas those with an unfavorable histologic response to preoperative chemotherapy (Grade I or II, indicating minimal tumor destruction) were likely to develop distant metastases despite continuation of chemotherapy after definitive surgery.[152] Thus, patients at high risk for the development of recurrent disease could apparently be identified early in treatment based on the poor response of the primary tumor to presurgical chemotherapy.

In addition to its value as a prognostic factor, preoperative chemotherapy is attractive because of other theoretic considerations.[145] Because chemotherapy is administered very soon after biopsy and diagnosis, treatment of micrometastases known to be present in the majority of patients can be insti-

FIGURE 32-13. Effect of preoperative chemotherapy. **A.** Section of tumor from biopsy prior to initiation of treatment demonstrating a cellular specimen with malignant cells intimately associated with osteoid characteristic of osteosarcoma. **B.** Section of tumor from specimen after 10 weeks of preoperative chemotherapy. This specimen is virtually acellular with residual lace-like osteoid. A grade IV response.

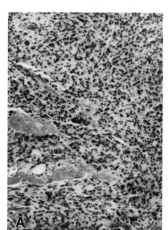
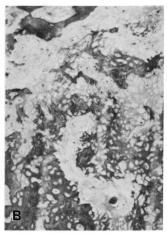

tuted early. This would represent a significant advantage over the traditional adjuvant approach, wherein the administration of systemic chemotherapy is delayed by a month (approximately one tumor doubling time for osteosarcoma) or more by surgery and the time necessary for wound healing.[153,154] In addition, the administration of preoperative chemotherapy provides a window of time for planning definitive therapy of the primary tumor, permitting the fabrication of customized internal prosthetic devices if required for limb salvage.

One of the most compelling rationales for presurgical chemotherapy is its use as an *in vivo* drug trial to determine the drug sensitivity of an individual tumor and to customize postoperative chemotherapy. Results of the Memorial Hospital studies suggest that patients whose tumors are responsive to presurgical therapy are destined to do well when the same therapy is continued postoperatively. Patients whose tumors are unresponsive to the presurgical regimen have a much less favorable outlook and might benefit from a change in chemotherapeutic agents. Although this is an attractive hypothesis, several objections can be raised on theoretic grounds. Considerations of cell kinetics predict that responsiveness (or lack thereof) of a bulky tumor may not predict responsiveness of micrometastases.[117] Data from leukemia trials indicate drugs active in the adjuvant (maintenance) setting may not be those that are most active against bulky macroscopic disease. Similarly, experimental data indicate that drugs with only modest activity against macroscopic tumor may still be active in the adjuvant setting. Finally, prolonged exposure to presurgical chemotherapy might select for drug-resistant tumor cells that might metastasize before definitive surgery.

The use of presurgical chemotherapy as an *in vivo* drug trial was tested at the Memorial Hospital in the T-10 protocol.[146,147] Patients were treated with HDMTX, the BCD combination, and Adriamycin preoperatively. Those with favorable histologic responses in the primary tumor continued to receive the same agents postoperatively, whereas those who had unfavorable histologic responses were treated with Adriamycin and cisplatin along with the BCD combination (without HDMTX) postoperatively. Only 39% of patients achieved a favorable (Grade III or IV) histologic response to presurgical chemotherapy, but almost all of these were projected to survive free of recurrence. Patients who demonstrated an unfavorable (Grade I or II) histologic response in the primary tumor were switched to the cisplatin-containing regimen, and nearly 85% were projected to remain relapse-free at 3 years. Overall, 90% of patients treated on the T-10 protocol with "custom-tailoring" of therapy based on response of the primary tumor were projected to remain disease-free at 3 years. Moreover, a significant difference in outcome was not detected between favorable and unfavorable responders to presurgical chemotherapy, supporting the contention that poor responders were "salvaged" by the selection of alternative postoperative chemotherapy. The outcome for patients on this protocol is the best yet reported in the treatment of osteosarcoma. Although these results have not yet been confirmed, data from other trials of presurgical chemotherapy[108,148,149] have at least confirmed the safety of this approach, have shown dramatic responses of primary tumors in 30% to 60% of patients, and have reaffirmed the predictive value of the histologic response of the primary tumor.

Presurgical chemotherapy has increasingly been administered via the intra-arterial route directly into the arterial supply of the tumor to maximize drug delivery to the tumor vasculature and drug extraction by the tumor.[155-157] Adriamycin and cisplatin, in particular, have been delivered by prolonged intra-arterial infusion into vessels of the extremity. High local drug concentrations have been documented by pharmacokinetic studies,[155] and dramatic responses in primary tumors have been observed. Whether the responses achieved are superior to those resulting from systemic intravenous administration of the same agents and whether systemic toxicity is ameliorated with intra-arterial administration has not been demonstrated convincingly. To date, the technique has appropriately been limited to centers with excellent angiographic support and facilities necessary to administer repeated courses of intra-arterial therapy preoperatively.

The enthusiasm with which the strategy of presurgical chemotherapy of osteosarcoma has been accepted is remarkable in view of the paucity of data supporting its use. Virtually every study of osteosarcoma initiated in the past 5 years has incorporated presurgical chemotherapy. However, a number of questions remain unanswered. Although the concept of presurgical chemotherapy is attractive from a theoretic standpoint, there are no data to suggest that presurgical chemotherapy leads to a superior overall outcome. Results from the COSS 80 study[108,148] of the German Pediatric Oncology Group (GPO), which used presurgical chemotherapy, are identical to results achieved with adjuvant chemotherapy (without presurgical chemotherapy) in the Multi-Institutional Osteosarcoma Study.[73] Thus, superior results achieved in recent studies of presurgical chemotherapy may reflect the use of more intensive multiagent therapy (incorporating cisplatin) and may be unrelated to the timing of chemotherapy relative to surgery. Further, the importance of custom-tailoring of therapy (*i.e.,* selecting postoperative treatment based on response of the primary tumor to presurgical chemotherapy) remains to be defined. This concept was tested in a follow-up study by the GPO (COSS 82). Preliminary results from this trial suggest that patients demonstrating poor response of the primary tumor are destined to do poorly, and that treatment of poor responders with "salvage regimens" (as in the T-10 protocol) is inadequate to improve their prognosis.[158] Investigators of the GPO conclude that active agents (*e.g.,* cisplatin) should not be withheld from the initial therapy of newly diagnosed patients. Thus, the value of presurgical chemotherapy (with or without tailoring of therapy based on tumor responsiveness) in the treatment of osteosarcoma remains to be demonstrated conclusively.

Use of Biological Response Modifiers

Therapeutic trials based on immunologic approaches to osteosarcoma have been stimulated by documentation of tumor-specific humoral[17,19] and cellular[20] immune responses in patients and animals with osteosarcoma. The presence in osteosarcoma patients of tumor-specific cytotoxic lymphocytes that are inhibited by a concomitant population of "inhibitor lymphocytes"[20] suggests a role for specific and nonspecific immune stimulation in the treatment of osteosarcoma. Early trials using the injection of inactivated osteosarcoma cells[159] or tumor cell lysates[160] induced evidence of cellular immune response in patients but produced no definitive therapeutic advantage. Similarly, cross-transplantation of biopsy specimens as a means of antitumor immunization resulted in no significant reduction in the incidence of metastatic disease.[159,161] Nonspecific immune stimulation with bacillus Calmette-Guerin (BCG) vaccine was not effective therapeutically,[159] even when administered in conjunction with adjuvant chemotherapy.[131] Interferon has been demonstrated to inhibit the growth of osteosarcoma cell lines *in vitro*[162] and was used as an adjuvant to surgery in an uncontrolled trial from the Karolinska Hospital in Sweden. A significant improvement over historical results was observed, but this improvement was less dramatic when compared to a concurrent group of patients treated only with surgery in other Swedish hospitals.[65,163] In the COSS 80 trial (see Table 32-3), patients were treated with presurgical and postsurgical adjuvant chemotherapy and were randomly assigned to receive or not to receive interferon in addition to chemotherapy. No benefit in relapse-free survival could be demonstrated for patients treated with interferon.[108]

Although trials of biological response modifiers have not yet yielded promising results, hybridoma technology and advances in the technology for cloning T-cells and expanding such clones for therapeutic purposes[164,165] provide interesting possibilities for future trials. Monoclonal antibodies raised against human osteosarcoma cell lines may prove useful in targeting drugs and toxins to tumor cells.[88,166,167] Similarly, T-cell clones have been isolated from the peripheral blood of patients with osteosarcoma[168] that are cytotoxic to autologous tumors and can be expanded *in vitro* for reinfusion into patients. It is possible that lymphocytes with enhanced antitumor reactivity may be cloned directly from tumor specimens[165] and provide a more potent source of immunoreactive cells for therapy of osteosarcoma.

Treatment of Metastases

Historically, patients with osteosarcoma who developed metastases had a poor prognosis and were treated palliatively. Most of these patients died within 1 year of developing metastatic disease. Although attempts at surgical resection of metastatic pulmonary nodules were undertaken as early as 1940,[169] the first systematic aggressive surgical approaches to these patients were initiated in the mid-1960s. There is little doubt that the development in the past 20 years of more effective salvage therapies for patients who develop metastases has contributed substantially to the improved survival of children with osteosarcoma.[169-180]

The biology of osteosarcoma offers the unique opportunity to cure patients who have developed metastases. More than 85% of recurrences are in the lung, where complete surgical resection of tumor nodules with wide margins can be accomplished relatively easily (and repeatedly). With the advent of CT of the chest, metastatic nodules can be detected when quite small and more easily resectable, although in most cases the surgeon will discover more lesions at thoracotomy than anticipated from the CT scan.[181] Moreover, in a significant proportion of patients, the lungs are likely to be the *only* site of metastases, especially when recurrences appear relatively late (*i.e.,* more than 1 year after diagnosis) and when the metastatic lesion is solitary. In such cases, the recurrent tumors are likely to have a more indolent behavior and may not themselves further metastasize. Such patients have been cured by thoracotomy alone (see below).

Complete surgical resection of all overt metastatic disease is a prerequisite for long-term salvage after relapse. Patients not treated by thoracotomy have little hope for cure.[175,176] The majority of pulmonary lesions can be resected successfully by wedge resection without risk of local recurrence,[171] while preserving the maximum lung tissue and allowing for the possibility of future pulmonary resections. Rarely, segmentectomy, lobectomy, or even pneumonectomy may be required to control more extensive lesions. Bilateral lung metastases can be approached by staged lateral thoracotomies done 1 to 2 weeks apart, a program that is well tolerated by otherwise healthy young adults and adolescents. Some surgeons have advocated an approach by median sternotomy. Although metastases can be removed from both lungs in one procedure using this approach, surgical exposure is not as complete (especially in the retrocardiac area and left lower lobe), and subsequent repeat thoracotomy is more difficult.

The completeness of surgical resection is an important determinant of outcome, in that patients left with measurable or microscopic disease at the resection margins are unlikely to be cured.[175] Evidence of disruption of the visceral pleura by tumor has been found to be associated with an adverse prognosis and is thought to carry the same implications as incomplete resection.[176,180] In one series, 9 of 11 (82%) patients who had complete resections without evidence of pleural disruption became long-term survivors, compared to only 2 of 15 (13%) who had incomplete resection or pleural disruption by tumor. More stringent criteria for complete resection, which include attention to the status of the pleura, are valuable prognostically, but even with an aggressive surgical approach only 42% of patients (11 of 26) could be rendered disease-free surgically in one series when these stringent criteria were applied.[176]

Several other prognostic factors have been examined in patients treated for metastases. Variables that appear to have significant prognostic value include the number of nodules detected on the prethoracotomy CT scan and the disease-free interval between initial diagnosis and the development of metastases. In general, patients with late-appearing (>1 year after surgery for the primary tumor) solitary pulmonary nodules are most likely to be cured, whereas those with more than three nodules that appear within 6 months of surgery have a less favorable outcome.[171,175,176] Although an initial disease-free interval of less than 6 months indicates a less favorable prognosis, this finding should not exclude the patient from consideration for salvage surgery;[175] the poor prognosis for patients who relapse within 1 year of initial diagnosis reported in some series may reflect the use of a less aggressive approach for such patients.[176] The number of nodules has also not been prognostically important in all series, although patients presenting with more than 16 nodules on preoperative tomography are unlikely to have successful complete resection.[175] Jaffe has reported that adjuvant chemotherapy for the primary tumor may reduce the number of metastatic nodules in patients destined to relapse, thus increasing the chance that these metastases will be resectable.[61]

Many investigators have advocated the use of postthoracotomy adjuvant chemotherapy (and even lung irradiation)[177-179] to destroy presumed residual microscopic deposits after surgical treatment of overt metastases. The contribution of such adjuvant therapy has not been examined in a controlled study. In small series, long-term survival has been reported without the use of further chemotherapy,[175,176,180] although survivors treated only with surgery were more likely to be those who had suffered late relapse with solitary pulmonary nodules.

Thus, when overt metastatic disease is discovered, a systematic approach is recommended. A careful search for all metastatic lesions, usually by thoracic CT scan and radionuclide bone scan, is essential; other investigations to search for metastases to other sites should be performed if clinically indicated. The discovery of unresectable extrathoracic metastases or of pulmonary disease that is obviously unresectable (because of hilar involvement, malignant pleural effusion, massive disease, or, perhaps, the presence of more than 16 nodules) is a contraindication to aggressive thoracotomy, and the patient should be treated palliatively. Radiotherapy may be particularly useful in palliative treatment. In selected patients with unresectable disease (especially those with no previous exposure to chemotherapy), an aggressive approach with curative intent may still be indicated. The use of chemotherapy (with or without radiotherapy) rarely produces complete response of all metastatic disease, but some patients with inoperable metastases may respond sufficiently to permit complete resection of disease at a later date, with a chance for long-term disease control. Rare patients with isolated bony metastases have also been cured by such an aggressive approach.

Patients with resectable lung disease should undergo thoracotomy to remove all evidence of disease. Bilateral disease is not a contraindication and can be approached by staged bilateral thoracotomies or median sternotomy. The role of adjuvant chemotherapy after thoracotomy remains to be defined, but such treatment is probably indicated at least for patients with multiple lesions (more than three) appearing within 6 months to 1 year of initial surgery and for patients who have incomplete resection of metastatic disease or evidence of pleural disruption by tumor. Repeat thoracotomies may be required for subsequent recurrence, and should be recommended so long as all evidence of disease can be resected.

Several approaches incorporating chemotherapy and radiotherapy administered before or after thoracotomy have been used to treat patients with metastases. There is no doubt that survival after relapse has been enhanced by approaches designed with curative intent that incorporate repeated aggressive surgery to remove overt disease. With such treatment, 30% to 40% of patients have been reported to survive beyond 5 years after relapse,[174-176,179,180,182] although not all of these patients will ultimately be cured. Such considerations emphasize the value of close follow-up, with frequent chest radiographs and thoracic CT scans to detect recurrent disease when it is still resectable. Thus, for the patient with osteosarcoma, presentation with or development of metastases is not a hopeless situation: aggressive systematic treatment of metastases offers prolonged survival for many patients and the possibility of cure for a significant fraction.

CONCLUSIONS AND FUTURE CONSIDERATIONS

In the past two decades, the prognosis for children with osteosarcoma has improved dramatically. The impact of adjuvant chemotherapy, which prevents recurrence in almost two thirds of patients with limb primaries, is now indisputable. Aggressive systematic approaches with thoracotomy have improved the outlook for patients presenting with or developing metastases after therapy. Nevertheless, refinements in therapy are needed. More than one third of children presenting without metastases will relapse after current therapy. Patients with axial skeleton primaries continue to fare poorly because local control cannot be achieved in the majority of cases. The morbidity related to therapy is considerable because the majority of patients are still treated with amputation to control the primary tumor, although newer approaches with limb-sparing surgery may provide durable local control with reduced morbidity for appropriate patients. The toxicity and expense of current chemotherapy regimens are substantial, and the late effects of such therapy have not yet been assessed.

The strategy of presurgical chemotherapy may well result in a further quantum improvement in prognosis for children with osteosarcoma. Although initial results of studies using presurgical chemotherapy are encouraging, longer follow-up is needed and comparative testing of preoperative chemotherapy against equally intensive adjuvant regimens must be performed to determine if the preoperative administration of chemotherapy is of value. Such a study is currently under way. Whether tailoring of therapy based on response of the primary tumor contributes substantially to patient management also awaits proof.

Limb salvage has been adopted enthusiastically by orthopedic surgeons, although questions persist regarding the safety of this approach, and it remains to be shown that the functional results in patients with lower extremity primaries are indeed superior to amputation. The psychological outcome for patients undergoing limb salvage is not clearly superior to that of amputees.[183] Prospective studies comparing the outcome and quality of life of patients undergoing limb salvage and amputation are now in progress. Approaches to sterilize the primary tumor site by administering intensive intra-arterial chemotherapy in the hope of avoiding surgery for the primary tumor altogether have been attempted, but results to date indicate an unacceptable local recurrence rate,[184] and this approach cannot yet be recommended.

New active drugs promise to add further to the armamentarium of chemotherapeutic agents available to use against osteosarcoma. Ifosfamide[126] has already been incorporated into front-line treatment regimens, and new platinum analogues may prove to be active agents with reduced toxicity (see Chap. 9).

Although immunotherapy of osteosarcoma has not yet proved successful, advances in technology have provided the immunotherapist with more active and more specific reagents. Monoclonal antibodies against osteosarcoma have already been used in scanning to detect metastases and may prove useful for delivering drugs or radiopharmaceuticals directly to tumor. Antibodies with exquisite specificity will be required for this purpose. Cloned cytotoxic T-cells may also provide more specific antitumor therapy and may prove most useful in the adjuvant setting.

The prospects for understanding the biology of osteosarcoma and improving therapy for affected children thus appear bright. Although numerous problems remain to be addressed, the current state of therapy—with more than two thirds of patients who have nonmetastatic osteosarcoma being cured of their disease—represents an exceptional advance, achieved in less than two decades. The celebrated surgeon of the 1920s who exhorted his colleagues to pray for children with osteosarcoma might well be gratified by the remarkable advances in treatment over the past 20 years.

REFERENCES

1. Cade S: Osteogenic sarcoma: A study based on 133 patients. J R Coll Surg Edinb 1:79–111, 1955
2. Huvos A: Bone Tumors: Diagnosis, Treatment and Prognosis. Philadelphia, WB Saunders, 1979
3. Sissons H: The WHO classification of bone tumors. Rec Results Cancer Res 54:104–108, 1976
4. McKenna R, Schwinn C, Soong K, Higinbotham N: Sarcomata of the osteogenic series (osteosarcoma, fibrosarcoma, chondrosarcoma, parosteal osteogenic sarcoma and sarcomata arising in abnormal bone): An analysis of 552 cases. J Bone Joint Surg [Am] 48:1–26, 1966
5. Young J, Miller R: Incidence of malignant tumors in U.S. children. J Pediatr 86:254–258, 1975
6. Dahlin D: Bone Tumors: General Aspects And Data On 6221 Cases, 3rd ed. Springfield, IL, Charles C Thomas, 1978
7. Dahlin D, Coventry M: Osteogenic sarcoma: A study of six hundred cases. J Bone Joint Surg [Am] 49:101–110, 1967
8. Dahlin D, Unni K: Osteosarcoma of bone and its important recognizable varieties. Am J Surg Pathol 1:61–72, 1977
9. Fraumeni J: Stature and malignant tumors of bone in childhood and adolescence. Cancer 20:967–973, 1967
10. Tjalma RA: Canine bone sarcoma: Estimation of relative risk as a function of body size. J Natl Cancer Inst 36:1137–1150, 1966
11. Price C: Primary bone-forming tumours and their relationship to skeletal growth. J Bone Joint Surg [Br] 40:574–593, 1958
12. Johnson L: A general theory of bone tumors. Bull NY Acad Med 29:164–171, 1953
13. Finkel M, Biskis B, Jinkins P: Virus induction of osteosarcoma in mice. Science 151:698–701, 1966
14. Friedlander G, Mitchell M: A virally induced osteosarcoma in rats: A model for immunological studies of human osteosarcoma. J Bone Joint Surg [Am] 58:295–302, 1976
15. Finkel M, Reilly C, Biskis B. Viral etiology of bone cancer. Front Radiat Ther Oncol 10:28–39, 1975
16. Finkel M, Biskis B, Farrell C: Osteosarcomas appearing in Syrian hamsters after treatment with extracts of human osteosarcomas. Proc Natl Acad Sci USA 60:1223–1230, 1968
17. Morton D, Malmgren R: Human osteosarcomas: Immunologic evidence suggesting an associated infectious agent. Science 162:1279–1281, 1968
18. Eilber F, Morton D: Immunologic studies of human sarcomas: Additional evidence suggesting an associated sarcoma virus. Cancer 26:588–596, 1970
19. Singh I, Tsang K, Blakemore W. Immunologic studies in contacts of osteosarcoma in humans and animals. Nature 265:541–542, 1977
20. Yu A, Watts H, Jaffe N, Parkman R: Concomitant presence of tumor-specific cytotoxic and inhibitor lymphocytes in patients with osteogenic sarcoma. N Engl J Med 297:121–127, 1977
21. Glass A, Fraumeni J: Epidemiology of bone cancer in children. J Natl Cancer Inst 44:187–199, 1970
22. Miller R: Etiology of childhood bone cancer: Epidemiologic observations. Rec Results Cancer Res 54:50–62, 1976
23. Phillips T, Sheline G: Bone sarcomas following radiation therapy. Radiology 81:992–996, 1963
24. Varela-Duran J, Dehner L: Post-irradiation osteosarcoma in childhood: A clinicopathologic study of three cases and review of the literature. Am J Pediatr Hematol Oncol 2:263–271, 1980
25. Freeman C, Gledhill R, Chevalier L, Whitehead V, Esseltine D: Osteogenic sarcoma following treatment with megavoltage radiation and chemotherapy for bone tumors in children. Med Pediatr Oncol 8:375–382, 1980
26. Haselow R, Nesbit M, Dehner L et al: Second neoplasms following megavoltage radiation in a pediatric population. Cancer 42:1185–1191, 1978
27. Sim F, Cupps R, Dahlin D, Ivins J: Postradiation sarcoma of bone. J Bone Joint Surg [Am] 54:1479–1489, 1972
28. Loutit J: Malignancy from radium. Br J Cancer 24:195–207, 1970
29. Spiess H, Mays C: Bone cancers induced by ^{224}Ra (Th X) in children and adults. Health Phys 19:713–729, 1970
30. Harrist T, Schiller A, Trelstad R, Mankin H, Mays C: Thorotrast-associated sarcoma of bone: A case report and review of the literature. Cancer 44:2049–2058, 1979
31. Colyer R: Osteogenic sarcoma in siblings. Johns Hopkins Med J 145:131–135, 1979
32. Swaney J: Familial osteogenic sarcoma. Clin Orthop 97:64–68, 1973
33. Bech-Nielsen S, Haskins M, Reif J et al: Frequency of osteosarcoma among first-degree relatives of St. Bernard dogs. J Natl Cancer Inst 60:349–353, 1978
34. Sagerman R, Cassady JR, Tretter P, Ellsworth R: Radiation induced neoplasia following external beam therapy for children with retinoblastoma. AJR 105:529–535, 1969
35. Schimke R, Lowman J, Cowan G: Retinoblastoma and osteogenic sarcoma in siblings. Cancer 34:2077–2079, 1974
36. Abramson D, Ellsworth R, Zimmerman L: Nonocular cancer in retinoblastoma survivors. Trans Am Acad Ophthal Otolaryngol 81:454–457, 1976
37. Murphee A, Benedict W: Retinoblastoma: Clues to human oncogenesis. Science 223:1028–1033, 1984
38. Abramson D, Ellsworth R, Kitchin F, Tung G: Second nonocular tumors in retinoblastoma survivors. Ophthalmology 91:1351–1355, 1984
39. Gordon H: Family studies in retinoblastoma. Birth Defects 10:185–190, 1974
40. Harris H: Malignant tumours generated by recessive mutations. Nature 323:582–583, 1986
41. Knudson A: Mutation and cancer: Statistical study of retinoblastoma. Proc Natl Acad Sci USA 68:820–823, 1971
42. Hansen M, Koufos A, Gallie B et al: Osteosarcoma and retinoblastoma: A shared chromosomal mechanism revealing recessive predisposition. Proc Natl Acad Sci USA 82:6216–6220, 1985
43. Dryja T, Rapaport J, Epstein J et al: Chromosome 13 homozygosity in osteosarcoma without retinoblastoma. Am J Hum Genet 38:59–66, 1986
44. Friend S, Bernards R, Rogelj S et al: A human DNA segment with properties of the gene that predisposes to retinoblastoma and osteosarcoma. Nature 323:643–646, 1986
45. Budd J, MacDonald I: A modified classification of bone tumors. Radiology 40:586–588, 1943

46. Matsuno T, Unni K, McLeod R, Dahlin D: Telangiectatic osteogenic sarcoma. Cancer 38:2538–2547, 1976

47. Farr G, Huvos A, Marcove R, Higinbotham N, Foote F: Telangiectatic osteogenic sarcoma: A review of twenty-eight cases. Cancer 34:1150–1158, 1974

48. Huvos A, Rosen G, Bretsky S, Butler A: Telengiectatic osteogenic sarcoma: A clinicopathologic study of 124 patients. Cancer 49:1679–1689, 1982

49. Ahuja S, Villacin A, Smith J et al: Juxtacortical (parosteal) osteogenic sarcoma. J Bone Joint Surg [Am] 59:632–647, 1977

50. Unni K, Dahlin D, Beabout J, Ivins J: Parosteal osteogenic sarcoma. Cancer 37:2466–2475, 1976

51. Unni K, Dahlin D, Beabout J: Periosteal osteogenic sarcoma. Cancer 37:2476–2485, 1976

52. Unni K, Dahlin D, McLeod R, Pritchard D: Intraosseous well-differentiated osteosarcoma. Cancer 40:1337–1347, 1977

53. Clark J, Unni K, Dahlin D, Devine K: Osteosarcoma of the jaw. Cancer 51:2311–2316, 1983

54. Wurlitzer F, Ayala A, Romsdahl M: Extraosseous osteogenic sarcoma. Arch Surg 105:691–695, 1972

55. Fitzgerald R, Dahlin D, Sim F: Multiple metachronous osteogenic sarcoma: report of twelve cases with two long-term survivors. J Bone Joint Surg [Am] 55:595–605, 1973

56. Marcove RC, Mike V, Hajek JV, Levin AG, Hutter RVP. Osteogenic sarcoma under the age of twenty-one. A review of 145 operative cases. J Bone Joint Surg [Am] 52:411–423, 1970

57. Mike V, Marcove RC: Osteogenic sarcoma under the age of 21: Experience at Memorial Sloan-Kettering Cancer Center. Prog Cancer Res Ther 6:283–292, 1978

58. Gehan EA, Sutow WW, Uribe-Botero G, Romsdahl M, Smith TL: Osteosarcoma: The M.D. Anderson experience, 1950–1974. Prog Cancer Res Ther 6:271–282, 1978

59. Uribe-Botero G, Russell W, Sutow W, Martin R: Primary osteosarcoma of bone: A clinicopathologic investigation of 243 cases, with necropsy studies in 54. Am J Clin Pathol 67:427–435, 1977

60. Friedman MA, Carter SK: The therapy of osteogenic sarcoma: Current status and thoughts for the future. J Surg Oncol 4:482–510, 1972

61. Jaffe N, Smith E, Abelson H, Frei E: Osteogenic sarcoma: Alterations in the pattern of pulmonary metastases with adjuvant chemotherapy. J Clin Oncol 1:251–254, 1983

62. Taylor WF, Ivins JC, Dahlin DC, Pritchard DJ: Osteogenic sarcoma experience at the Mayo Clinic, 1963–1974. Prog Cancer Res Ther 6:257–269, 1978

63. Taylor WF, Ivins JC, Dahlin DC, Edmonson JH, Pritchard DJ: Trends and variability in survival from osteosarcoma. Mayo Clinic Proc 53:695–700, 1978

64. Taylor WF, Ivins J, Pritchard D, Dahlin DC, Gilchrist GS, Edmonson JH: Trends and variability in survival among patients with osteosarcoma: a 7-year update. Mayo Clin Proc 60:91–104, 1985

65. Strander H, Adamson U, Aparisi T et al: Adjuvant interferon treatment of human osteosarcoma. Rec Results Cancer Res 68:40–44, 1979

66. Rab GT, Ivins JC, Childs DS, Cupps RE, Pritchard DJ: Elective whole lung irradiation in the treatment of osteogenic sarcoma. Cancer 38:939–942, 1976

67. Breur K, Cohen P, Schweisguth O, Hart A: Irradiation of the lungs as an adjuvant therapy in the treatment of osteosarcoma of the limbs: An EORTC randomized study. Eur J Cancer 14:461–471, 1978

68. Edmonson J, Green S, Ivins J et al: A controlled pilot study of high-dose methotrexate as post surgical adjuvant treatment for primary osteosarcoma. J Clin Oncol 2:152–156, 1984

69. Kolata GB: Dilemma in cancer treatment. Science 209:792–794, 1980

70. Lange B, Levine A: Is it ethical not to conduct a prospectively controlled trial of adjuvant chemotherapy in osteosarcoma? Cancer Treat Rep 66:1699–1704, 1982

71. Carter SK: Adjuvant chemotherapy in osteosarcoma: The triumph that isn't? J Clin Oncol 2:147–148, 1984

72. Link MP: Adjuvant therapy in the treatment of osteosarcoma. In DeVita VT Jr, Hellman S, Rosenberg SA (eds): Important Advances in Oncology 1986, pp 193–207. Philadelphia, JB Lippincott, 1986

73. Link MP, Goorin AM, Miser AW et al: The effect of adjuvant chemotherapy on relapse-free survival in patients with osteosarcoma of the extremity. N Engl J Med 314:1600–1606, 1986

74. Eilber F, Giuliano A, Eckardt J et al: Adjuvant chemotherapy for osteosarcoma: A randomized prospective trial. J Clin Oncol 5:21–26, 1987

75. Thorpe W, Reilly J, Rosenberg S: Prognostic significance of alkaline phos-

phatase measurements in patients with osteogenic sarcoma receiving chemotherapy. Cancer 43:2178–2181, 1979

76. Link MP, Shuster JJ, Goorin AM et al: Adjuvant chemotherapy in the treatment of osteosarcoma: Results of the Multi-Institutional Osteosarcoma Study. In Ryan JR, Baker LH (eds): Recent Concepts in Sarcoma Treatment. Proceedings of the International Symposium on Sarcomas, Tarpon Springs, Florida, October 8–10, 1987. Dordrecht, The Netherlands, Kluwer Academic Publishers, 1988

77. Kesselring F, Penn W: Radiological aspects of "classic" primary osteosarcoma: Value of some radiological investigations. Diagn Imaging 51:78–92, 1982

78. Aisen AM, Martel W, Braunstein EM et al: MRI and CT evaluation of primary bone and soft-tissue tumors. AJR 146:749–756, 1986

79. McKillop J, Etcubanas E, Goris M: The indications for and limitations of bone scintigraphy in osteogenic sarcoma. Cancer 48:1133–1138, 1981

80. Watts H: Surgical management of malignant bone tumors in children. In Jaffe N (ed): Bone Tumors in Children, pp 131–142. Littleton, MA, PSG Publishing, 1979

81. Enneking W, Kagan A: "Skip" metastases in osteosarcoma. Cancer 36:2192–2205, 1975

82. Neifeld J, Michaelis L, Doppman J: Suspected pulmonary metastases: Correlation of chest x-ray, whole lung tomograms and operative findings. Cancer 39:383–387, 1977

83. Muhm J, Brown L, Crowe J et al: Comparison of whole lung tomography and computed tomography for detecting pulmonary nodules. AJR 131:981–984, 1978

84. Schaner EG, Chang AE, Doppman JL, Conkle DM, Flye MW, Rosenberg SA: Comparison of computed and conventional whole lung tomography in detecting pulmonary nodules: A prospective radiologic-pathologic study. AJR 131:51–54, 1978

85. Vanel D, Henry-Amar M, Lumbroso J et al: Pulmonary evaluation of patients with osteosarcoma: Roles of standard radiography, tomography, CT, scintigraphy, and tomoscintigraphy. AJR 143:519–523, 1984

86. Kirchner PT, Simon MA: Current concepts review. Radioisotope evaluation of skeletal disease. J Bone Joint Surg [Am] 63:673–681, 1981

87. Armitage N, Perkins A, Pimm M et al: Imaging of bone tumors using a monoclonal antibody raised against human osteosarcoma. Cancer 58:37–42, 1986

88. Baldwin R, Pimm M, Embleton M et al: Monoclonal antibody 791T/36 for tumor detection and therapy of metastases. In Nicolson GL, Milas L (eds): Cancer Invasion and Metastases: Biologic and Therapeutic Aspects. pp 437–455. New York, Raven Press, 1984

89. Enneking W, Springfield D: Osteosarcoma. Orthop Clin North Am 8:785–803, 1977

90. Mankin HJ, Lange TA, Spanier SS: The hazards of biopsy in patients with malignant primary bone and soft-tissue tumors. J Bone Joint Surg [Am] 64:1121–1127, 1982

91. Enneking WF, Spanier SS, Goodman MA: Current Concepts Review: The surgical staging of musculoskeletal sarcoma. J Bone Joint Surg [Am] 62:1027–1030, 1980

92. Mankin H, Connor J, Schiller A, Perlmutter N, Alho A, McGuire M: Grading of bone tumors by analysis of nuclear DNA content using flow cytometry. J Bone Joint Surg [Am] 67:404–413, 1985

93. Goorin A, Perez-Atayde A, Gebhardt M et al: Weekly high dose methotrexate and doxorubicin for osteosarcoma: The Dana Farber Cancer Institute/The Children's Hospital Study III. J Clin Oncol 5:1178–1184, 1987

94. Lockshin M, Higgins I: Prognosis in osteogenic sarcoma. Clin Orthop 58:85–101, 1968

95. Simon R: Clinical prognostic factors in osteosarcoma. Cancer Treat Rep 62:193–197, 1978

96. Scranton P, DeCicco F, Totten R, Yunis E: Prognostic factors in osteosarcoma: A review of 20 years' experience at the University of Pittsburgh Health Center Hospitals. Cancer 36:2179–2191, 1975

97. Herson J, Sutow WW, Elder K et al: Adjuvant chemotherapy in nonmetastatic osteosarcoma: A Southwest Oncology Group Study. Med Pediatr Oncol 8:343–352, 1980

98. Levine A, Rosenberg S: Alkaline phosphatase levels in osteosarcoma tissue are related to prognosis. Cancer 44:2291–2293, 1979

99. Lewis R, Lotz M: Medullary extension of osteosarcoma: Implications for rational therapy. Cancer 33:371–375, 1974

100. Enneking WF, Shirley PD: Resection-arthrodesis for malignant and potentially malignant lesions about the knee using an intramedullary rod and local bone grafts. J Bone Joint Surg [Am] 59:223–236, 1977

101. Gross A, Langer F, McKee N et al: A biological approach to the restoration

of skeletal continuity following *en bloc* excision of bone tumors. Orthopedics 8:586–591, 1985

102. Mankin H, Doppelt S, Sullivan R, Tomford W: Osteoarticular and intercalary allograft transplantation in the management of malignant tumors of bone. Cancer 50:613–630, 1982

103. Lewis MM: The use of an expandable and adjustable prosthesis in the treatment of childhood malignant bone tumors of the extremity. Cancer 57:499–502, 1986

104. Kotz R, Salzer M: Rotation-plasty for childhood osteosarcoma of the distal part of the femur. J Bone Joint Surg [Am] 64:959–969, 1982

105. Linberg BE: Intrascapulo-thoracic resection for malignant tumors of the shoulder joint region. J Bone Joint Surg 10:344–349, 1928

106. Eilber FR, Grant TT, Sakai D et al: Internal hemipelvectomy—Excision of the hemipelvis with limb preservation: An alternative to hemipelvectomy. Cancer 43:806–809, 1979

107. Winkler K, Beron G, Kotz R et al: Einflus des localchirurgischen Vorgehens auf die Inzidenz von Metastasen nach neoadjuvanter Chemotherapie des Osteosarkoms. Z Orthop 124:22–29, 1986

108. Winkler K, Beron G, Kotz R et al: Neoadjuvant chemotherapy for osteogenic sarcoma: Results of a Cooperative German/Austrian Study. J Clin Oncol 2:617–624, 1984

108a. Simon MA, Aschliman MA, Thomas N, Mankin HJ: Limb-salvage treatment versus amputation for osteosarcoma of the distal end of the femur. J Bone Joint Surg (Am) 68:1331–1337, 1986

109. Jenkin R, Allt W, Fitzpatrick P: Osteosarcoma: An assessment of management with particular reference to primary irradiation and selective delayed amputation. Cancer 30:393–400, 1972

110. Lee S, MacKenzie D: Osteosarcoma: A study of the value of preoperative megavoltage radiotherapy. Br J Surg 51:252–274, 1964

111. Francis K, Phillips R, Nickson J et al: Massive preoperative irradiation in the treatment of osteogenic sarcoma in children. AJR 72:813–818, 1954

112. Martinez A, Goffinet D, Donaldson S et al: Intra-arterial infusion of radio-sensitizer (BUdR) combined with hypofractionated irradiation and chemotherapy for primary treatment of osteogenic sarcoma. Int J Radiat Oncol Biol Phys 11:123–128, 1985

113. Schabel FM: Rationale for adjuvant chemotherapy. Cancer 39:2875–2882, 1977

114. Schabel FM Jr: *In vivo* leukemic cell kill kinetics and "curability" in experimental systems. In The Proliferation and Spread of Neoplastic Cells, pp 379–408. Baltimore, Williams & Wilkins, 1968

115. Schabel FM Jr: The use of tumor growth kinetics in planning "curative" chemotherapy of advanced solid tumors. Cancer Res 29:2384–2389, 1969

116. Laster WR Jr, Mayo JG, Simpson-Herren L, Griswold DP et al: Success and failure in the treatment of solid tumors. II. Kinetic parameters and "cell cure" of moderately advanced carcinoma 755. Cancer Chemother Rep 53:169–188, 1969

117. Bode U, Levine AS: The biology and management of osteosarcoma. In Levine AS (ed): Cancer in the Young, pp 575–602. New York, Masson Publishing, 1982

118. Cortes EP, Holland JF, Wang JJ, Sinks LF: Doxorubicin in disseminated osteosarcoma. JAMA 221:1132–1138, 1972

119. Nitschke R, Starling KA, Vats T, Bryan H: Cis-diamminedichloroplatinum (NSC-119875) in childhood malignancies: A Southwest Oncology Group Study. Med Pediatr Oncol 4:127–132, 1978

120. Ochs JJ, Freeman AI, Douglass HO, Higby DS, Mindell ER, Sinks LF: Cis-Dichlorodiammineplatinum (II) in advanced osteogenic sarcoma. Cancer Treat Rep 62:239–245, 1978

121. Baum ES, Gaynon P, Greenberg L, Krivit W, Hammond D: Phase II study of cis-dichlorodiammineplatinum (II) in childhood osteosarcoma: Children's Cancer Study Group Report. Cancer Treat Rep 63:1621–1627, 1979

122. Gasparini M, Rouesse J, van Oosterom A et al: Phase II study of cisplatin in advanced osteogenic sarcoma. Cancer Treat Rep 69:211–213, 1985

123. Jaffe N, Farber S, Traggis D et al: Favorable response of metastatic osteogenic sarcoma to pulse high dose methotrexate with citrovorum rescue and radiation therapy. Cancer 31:1367–1373, 1973

124. Pratt C, Howarth C, Ransom J et al: High dose methotrexate used alone and in combination for measurable primary and metastatic osteosarcoma. Cancer Treat Rep 64:11–20, 1980

125. Jaffe N, Frei E, Traggis D, Watts H: Weekly high-dose methotrexate-citrovorum factor in osteogenic sarcoma. Cancer 39:45–50, 1977

126. Marti C, Kroner T, Remagen W et al: High-dose ifosfamide in advanced osteosarcoma. Cancer Treat Rep 69:115–117, 1985

127. Jaffe N, Frei E, Traggis D, Bishop Y: Adjuvant methotrexate and citrovorum-factor treatment of osteogenic sarcoma. N Engl J Med 291:994–997, 1974

128. Jaffe N, Frei E, Watts H, Traggis D: High dose methotrexate in osteogenic sarcoma: A 5-year experience. Cancer Treat Rep 62:259–264, 1978

129. Frei E, Jaffe N, Link M, Abelson N: Adjuvant chemotherapy of osteogenic sarcoma: Progress, problems and prospects. In Jones S, Salmon S (eds): Adjuvant Therapy of Cancer II, pp 355–363. New York, Grune & Stratton, 1979

130. Goorin A, Delorey M, Gelber R et al: The Dana-Farber Cancer Institute/The Children's Hospital adjuvant chemotherapy trials for Osteosarcoma: Three sequential studies. Cancer Treat Rep 3:155–159, 1986

131. Rosenberg SA, Chabner BA, Young RC et al: Treatment of osteogenic sarcoma. I. Effect of adjuvant high-dose methotrexate after amputation. Cancer Treat Rep 63:739–751, 1979

132. Cortes EP, Holland JF, Wang JJ et al: Amputation and adriamycin in primary osteosarcoma. N Engl J Med 291:998–1000, 1974

133. Cortes EP, Holland JF, Glidewell O: Amputation and adriamycin in primary osteosarcoma: a 5 year report. Cancer Treat Rep 62:271–277, 1978

134. Cortes EP, Holland JF, Glidewell O: Adjuvant therapy of operable primary osteosarcoma—Cancer and Leukemia Group B experience. Rec Results Cancer Res 68:16–24, 1979

135. Cortes E, Necheles TF, Holland JF et al: Adjuvant chemotherapy for primary osteosarcoma: A Cancer and Leukemia Group B Experience. In Salmon S, Jones S (eds): Adjuvant Therapy of Cancer, vol III, pp 201–210. New York, Grune & Stratton, 1981

136. Krailo M, Ertel I, Makley J et al: A randomized study comparing high-dose methotrexate with moderate dose methotrexate as components of adjuvant chemotherapy in childhood nonmetastatic osteosarcoma: A report from the Childrens Cancer Study Group. Med Pediatr Oncol 15:69–77, 1987

137. Sutow WW, Sullivan MP, Fernbach DJ, Cangir A, George SL: Adjuvant chemotherapy in primary treatment of osteogenic sarcoma. A Southwest Oncology Group Study. Cancer 36:1598–1602, 1975

138. Sutow WW, Gehan EA, Dyment PG, Vietti T, Miale T: Multidrug adjuvant chemotherapy for osteosarcoma: Interim report of the Southwest Oncology Group Studies. Cancer Treat Rep 62:265–269, 1978

139. Etcubanas E, Wilbur JR: Adjuvant chemotherapy for osteogenic sarcoma. Cancer Treat Rep 62:283–287, 1978

140. Pratt CB, Rivera G, Shanks E, Kumar APM, Green AA, George S: Combination chemotherapy for osteosarcoma. Cancer Treat Rep 62:251–257, 1978

141. Pratt CB: Personal communication

142. Ettinger LJ, Douglass HO, Higby DJ et al: Adjuvant adriamycin and Cis-diamminedichloroplatinum (Cis-platinum) in primary osteosarcoma. Cancer 47:248–254, 1981

143. Ettinger LJ, Douglass HO, Mindell ER et al: Adjuvant adriamycin and cisplatin in newly diagnosed, non-metastatic osteosarcoma of the extremity. J Clin Oncol 4:353–362, 1986

144. Rosen G, Murphy ML, Huvos AG, Gutierrez M, Marcove RC: Chemotherapy, *en bloc* resection, and prosthetic bone replacement in the treatment of osteogenic sarcoma. Cancer 37:1–11, 1976

145. Rosen G, Marcove RC, Caparros B, Nirenberg A, Kosloff C, Huvos AG: Primary osteogenic sarcoma. The rationale for preoperative chemotherapy and delayed surgery. Cancer 43:2163–2177, 1979

146. Rosen G, Marcove RC, Huvos AG, Caparros BI, Lane JM, Nirenberg A, Cacavio A, Groshen S: Primary osteogenic sarcoma: Eight-year experience with adjuvant chemotherapy. J Cancer Res Clin Oncol 106(Suppl):55–67, 1983

147. Rosen G, Caparros B, Huvos AG et al: Preoperative chemotherapy for osteogenic sarcoma: Selection of postoperative adjuvant chemotherapy based on the response of the primary tumor to preoperative chemotherapy. Cancer 49:1221–1230, 1982

148. Winkler K, Beron G, Kotz R et al: Adjuvant chemotherapy in osteosarcoma-effects of cisplatinum, BCD, and fibroblast interferon in sequential combination with HD-MTX and Adriamycin. Preliminary results of the COSS 80 study. J Cancer Res Clin Oncol 106(Suppl):1–7, 1983

149. Weiner M, Harris M, Lewis M et al: Neoadjuvant high-dose methotrexate, cisplatin, and doxorubicin for the management of patients with nonmetastatic osteosarcoma. Cancer Treat Rep 70:1431–1432, 1986

150. Mosende C, Gutierrez M, Caparros B, Rosen G: Combination chemotherapy with bleomycin, cyclophosphamide and dactinomycin for the treatment of osteogenic sarcoma. Cancer 40:2779–2786, 1977

151. van der Schueren E, Breur K: Role of lung irradiation in the adjuvant treatment of osteosarcoma. Rec Results Cancer Res 80:98–102, 1982

152. Huvos A, Rosen G, Marcove RC: Primary osteogenic sarcoma. Pathologic

aspects in 20 patients after treatment with chemotherapy, en bloc resection and prosthetic bone replacement. Arch Pathol Lab Med 101:14–18, 1977

153. Goldie JH, Coldman AJ: A mathematical model for relating the drug sensitivity of tumors to their spontaneous mutation rate. Cancer Treat Rep 63:1727–1733, 1979

154. DeVita VT: The relationship between tumor mass and resistance to chemotherapy. Cancer 51:1209–1220, 1983

155. Jaffe N, Knapp J, Chuang VP et al: Osteosarcoma: Intra-arterial treatment of the primary tumor with cis-Diammine-Dichloroplatinum II (CDP): Angiographic, pathologic and pharmacologic studies. Cancer 51:402–407, 1983

156. Jaffe N, Prudich J, Knapp J, Wang Y-M et al: Treatment of primary osteosarcoma with intra-arterial and intravenous high-dose methotrexate. J Clin Oncol 1:428–431, 1983

157. Jaffe N, Robertson R, Ayala A et al: Comparison of intra-arterial Cis-diamminedichloroplatinum II with high dose methotrexate and citrovorum factor rescue in the treatment of primary osteosarcoma. J Clin Oncol 3:1101–1104, 1985

158. Winkler K, Beron G, Delling G et al: Neoadjuvant chemotherapy of osteosarcoma: Results of a randomized cooperative trial (COSS-82) with salvage chemotherapy based on histological tumor response. J Clin Oncol 6:329–337, 1988

159. Eilber F, Townsend C, Morton D: Osteosarcoma: Results of treatment employing adjuvant immunotherapy. Clin Orthop 111:94–100, 1975

160. Green A, Pratt C, Webster R, Smith K: Immunotherapy of osteosarcoma patients with virus-modified tumor cells. Ann NY Acad Sci 277:396–411, 1976

161. Marsh B, Flynn L, Enneking W: Immunologic aspects of osteosarcoma and their application to therapy. J Bone Joint Surg [Am] 54:1367–1397, 1972

162. Strander H, Einhorn S: Effect of human leukocyte interferon on the growth of human osteosarcoma cells in tissue culture. Int J Cancer 19:468–473, 1977

163. Nilsonne U, Strander H: Traitement de l'osteosarcome par l'interferon et la chirugie differenciee. Rev Chir Orthop 67:193–197, 1981

164. Rosenberg S, Lotz M, Muul L et al: Special report: Observations on the systemic administration of autologous lymphokine-activated killer cells and recombinant interleukin-2 to patients with metastatic cancer. N Engl J Med 313:1485–1492, 1985

165. Rosenberg S, Spiess P, Lafreniere R: A new approach to the adoptive immunotherapy of cancer with tumor-infiltrating lymphocytes. Science 233:1318–1321, 1986

166. Garnett M, Embleton M, Jacobs E, Baldwin R: Preparation and properties of a drug-carrier antibody conjugate showing selective antibody-directed cytotoxicity in vitro. Int J Cancer 31:661–670, 1983

167. Embleton M, Byers V, Lee H et al: Sensitivity and selectivity of ricin toxin A chain-monoclonal antibody 791T/36 conjugates against human tumor cell lines. Cancer Res 46:5524–5528, 1986

168. Slovin S, Lackman R, Ferrone S, Kiely P, Mastrangelo M: Cellular immune response to human sarcomas: Cytotoxic T cell clones reactive with autologous sarcomas. I. Development, phenotype, and specificity. J Immunol 137:3042–3048, 1986

169. Martini N, Huvos A, Mike V, Marcove R, Beattie E: Multiple pulmonary resections in the treatment of osteogenic sarcoma. Ann Thorac Surg 12:271–280, 1971

170. Spanos P, Payne W, Ivins J, Pritchard D: Pulmonary resection for metastatic osteogenic sarcoma. J Bone Joint Surg [Am] 58:624–628, 1976

171. Telander R, Pairolero P, Pritchard D, Sim F, Gilchrist G: Resection of pulmonary metastatic osteogenic sarcoma in children. Surgery 84:335–341, 1978

172. Giritsky A, Etcubanas E, Mark J: Pulmonary resection in children with metastatic osteogenic sarcoma. J Thorac Cardiovasc Surg 73:354–362, 1978

173. Rosenberg S, Flye M, Conkle D, Seipp C, Levine A, Simon R: Treatment of osteogenic sarcoma II. Aggressive resection of pulmonary metastases. Cancer Treat Rep 63:753–756, 1979

174. Han M-T, Telander R, Pairolero P, Payne W et al: Aggressive thoracotomy for pulmonary metastatic osteogenic sarcoma in children and young adolescents. J Pediatr Surg 16:928–933, 1981

175. Putnam JB, Roth J, Wesley M, Johnson M, Rosenberg SA: Survival following aggressive resection of pulmonary metastases from osteogenic sarcoma: Analysis of prognostic factors. Ann Thorac Surg 36:516–523, 1983

176. Goorin A, Delorey M, Lack E, Gelber R et al: Prognostic significance of complete surgical resection of pulmonary metastases in patients with osteogenic sarcoma: Analysis of 32 patients. J Clin Oncol 2:425–431, 1984

177. Weichselbaum R, Cassady J, Jaffe N, Filler R: Preliminary results of aggressive multimodality therapy for metastatic osteosarcoma. Cancer 40:78–83, 1977

178. Beattie E, Martini N, Rosen G: The management of pulmonary metastases in children with osteogenic sarcoma with surgical resection combined with chemotherapy. Cancer 35:618–621, 1975

179. Rosen G, Huvos A, Mosende C, Beattie E, Exelby P et al: Chemotherapy and thoracotomy for metastatic osteogenic sarcoma. Cancer 41:841–849, 1978

180. Meyer WH, Schell MJ, Kumar APM, Rao BN, Green AA, Champion J, Pratt CB: Thoracotomy for pulmonary metastatic osteosarcoma. An analysis of prognostic indicators of survival. Cancer 59:374–379, 1987

181. Creagan E, Frytak S, Pairolero P et al: Surgically proven pulmonary metastases not demonstrated by computed chest tomography. Cancer Treat Rep 62:1404–1405, 1978

182. Marcove R, Martini N, Rosen G: The treatment of pulmonary metastasis in osteogenic sarcoma. Clin Orthop 111:65–70, 1975

183. Weddington W, Segraves K, Simon M: Psychological outcome of extremity sarcoma survivors undergoing amputation or limb salvage. J Clin Oncol 3:1393–1399, 1985

184. Jaffe N, Robertson R, Takaue Y: Osteosarcoma: Prolonged control of the primary tumor with chemotherapy. Proc Am Soc Clin Oncol 3:77, 1984

thirty-three

Germ Cell Tumors

Arthur Ablin and
Hart Isaacs, Jr.

Germ cell tumors are benign or malignant growths, presumably derived from primordial germ cells that can occur within the gonads or in extragonadal sites. When in the ovaries or testes, they must be distinguished from other gonadal tumors that are derived from sex cord–stromal or epithelial cells (discussed in Chap. 35).

EMBRYOGENESIS

The first germ cells can be recognized in the extraembryonic yolk sac of the 4-week-old human embryo. From this probable site of origin in the yolk sac endoderm, the cells migrate into the embryo through the midline dorsal mesentery and by the sixth week of fetal development can be identified in the germinal epithelium of the gonadal ridge, where they will populate either the developing testis or ovary (Fig. 33-1).[1] If during this migration, for reasons not yet understood, these cells miss their destination, they may multiply in sites foreign to their proper environment. At 6 to 8 weeks of fetal development, the gonadal ridge and the vertebral column, from the cervical to lower lumbar area, are in dorsal-ventral proximity. Mistakes in localization might cause these migrating cells to come to rest in some near-midline site, such as the sacrococcygeal area, the retroperitoneum, mediastinum, neck, or even the pineal area of the brain. If a malignant transformation takes place in those wandering cells, then a germ cell malignancy is produced that is either gonadal or extragonadal in location. The type of tumor depends on the degree of differentiation, with embryonal carcinoma at the malignant end of the spectrum and mature teratoma at the benign end.

EPIDEMIOLOGY

Germ cell tumors in all locations account for approximately 3% of malignant disease in children and adolescents (see also Chap. 1).[2] Because not all germ cell tumors are malignant, this percentage does not represent their true incidence. Approximately two thirds occur in extragonadal sites. The incidence of the most common germ cell tumor, sacrococcygeal teratomas (80% of which are benign), has been estimated to be 1 in 35,000 live births.[3] These tumors occur two to four times more frequently in girls than in boys.[4] Mortality from "teratoma" for children under age 15 was three times more frequent for girls than boys, reflecting both the higher incidence of sacrococcygeal teratomas in infancy and the younger age at which girls develop ovarian tumors compared to the development of testicular germinal tumors in males. After age 14, deaths from germ cell tumors are more frequent in boys than girls.[5]

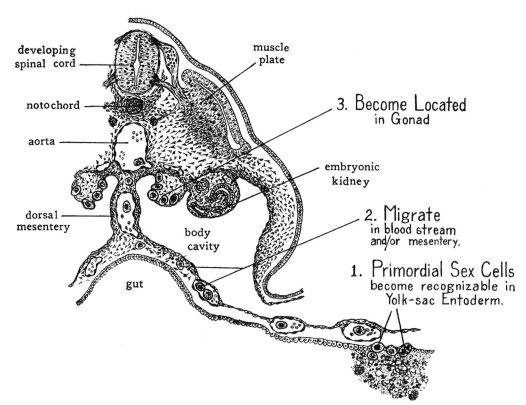

developing
spinal cord

muscle
plate

notochord

3. Become Located
in Gonad

aorta

embryonic
kidney

dorsal
mesentery

2. Migrate
in blood stream
and/or mesentery.

body
cavity

1. Primordial Sex Cells
become recognizable in
Yolk-sac Entoderm.

gut

FIGURE 33-1. Schema depicting the migration of totopotential germ cells from yolk sac toward the gonad. (Patton BM: Human Embryology, p 14. Philadelphia, Blakiston, 1947)

GENETICS

Recent karyotype studies of established ovarian and testicular cell lines have demonstrated the origin of the tumors before the first meiotic division and have shown that the genome on the short arm of chromosome 1 may be duplicated or lost (see also Chap. 2).[6,7] Malignant germ cell tumors have been associated with a wide variety of other abnormalities. For example, Hart and Burkons described six phenotypic females who had a 46XY karyotype and gonadal dysgenesis and gonadoblastomas or dysgerminomas mixed with endodermal sinus tumors or cystic teratomas.[8] Another family in which two phenotypically female 46XY siblings had gonadoblastomas and dysgerminoma has also been described. In another report, a normal 46XY male sibling developed a testicular tumor that proved to be choriocarcinoma with embryonal carcinoma and seminoma.[9] Ataxia-telangiectasia has also been associated with ovarian gonadoblastoma and contralateral dysgerminoma in one patient.[10] In addition, metastatic neuroblastoma arising in an immature ovarian teratoma[11] and hematologic malignancies associated with a mediastinal germ cell tumor have been reported.[12,13] Moreover, multiple instances of malignant germ cell tumors have been described in siblings, twins, and mothers and daughters, and even in three generations of one family.[14–16]

BIOLOGY

Markers

Since germ cell tumors are derived from totipotential cells, it might be anticipated that they would be associated with a variety of intracellular or extracellular products that could serve as tumor markers (see also Chap. 8).

Alpha-Fetoprotein (AFP)

AFP, an α_1-globulin, is the principal serum protein of the fetus. It is similar in size, structure, and function to serum albumen, which replaces it in later prenatal development and after birth.[17] It is first produced in the fetal yolk sac and later in the embryonic hepatocytes and gastrointestinal tract.[18] Maximal concentrations, measured at 3×10^6 ng/ml, are found at the 12th to 15th week of gestation. Full-term infants may have values of 5×10^4 ng/ml, with a rapid fall to 2×10^4 ng/ml within 24 hours.[19] Adult levels of less than 20 ng/ml are reached by 6 months of age.

Abelev and colleagues first demonstrated the association of AFP with malignant germ cell tumors.[20] It has since been reported that elevations of AFP occur with yolk sac tumors, since the fetal yolk sac is the source of physiologic AFP in early embryogenesis.[21] Elevations of AFP occur also with embryonal carcinoma.[22] Intracellular and intercellular hyaline droplets visible with light microscopy in these tumors have been shown to be AFP by immunofluorescent techniques.[23] However, AFP is not found in patients with pure dysgerminomas, pure choriocarcinomas, or mature teratomas.[24] In normal-weight newborns, children, and adults, the half-life of AFP is 5.5 days, whereas in low-birth-weight infants it is greater than 7.7 days; these values are important in determining whether a resected AFP-producing tumor has been totally removed.[19] Of note, AFP can also be elevated in other disease states, such as hepatic malignancy, hepatitis, certain gastrointestinal malignancies (see Chap. 35), and hereditary tyrosinemia, all of which can usually be distinguished easily from germ cell tumors.

Beta-Subunit Human Chorionic Gonadotropin (β-HCG)

Specialized placental cells can produce a glycoprotein, human chorionic gonadotropin, that is related to the continuing successful implantation of the fertilized egg and to a proper maternal-fetal relationship. This protein is composed of two polypeptide chains, alpha and beta, which resemble the structure of the pituitary gonadotropins. The alpha subunits of HCG are identical, but the beta subunits can be immunologically separated—this is the basis for a radioimmunoassay that detects small amounts of placental beta subunits separate from those of pituitary origin.[25]

Germ cell tumors with trophoblastic elements (choriocarcinomas), as well as gestational new growths of placental origin (pregnancy, as well as hydatiform moles) can be identified by the production of β-HCG. The choriocarcinoma invariably produces this hormone marker.[26] The half-life of the beta-subunit is only 45 minutes, and it therefore disappears rapidly if complete removal of the tumor is accomplished.

Other Markers

Lactate dehydrogenase isoenzyme-1 (LDH-1), a glycolytic enzyme that catalyzes the reaction between pyruvate and lactate, was elevated in seven of eight children with yolk sac tumors. Although not specific for these tumors, LDH-1 is rarely elevated in other malignancies in which other intermediate fractions of the isoenzyme are elevated. Elevation of LDH-1 is thought to result from its release into the blood from the tumor cells.[27] A monoclonal antibody for immunoassay of placental alkaline phosphatase has been predictive for the presence of seminomatous testicular disease and its recurrence.[28]

DNA and Chromosomes

Recently, new techniques have been described for predicting the biological behavior and prognosis of certain germ cell tumors. The majority of studies have been performed on adult testicular neoplasms (*i.e.,* teratomas and malignant germ cell tumors). Flow cytometry measurements of tumor cell DNA to determine the ploidy status of teratomas and germinomas were used by Quirke and coworkers,[29] who showed a DNA abnormality in testicular germ cell tumors and differences between subtypes of teratoma. It appears that certain DNA/RNA ratios and aneuploidy are associated with an unfavorable prognosis. Concomitant karyotyping and DNA flow cytometry have also been performed on malignant teratomas and their metastases after chemotherapy in an attempt to determine whether the metastases are of the same DNA index and have the same 1(12p) marker as the primary. Mature teratoma remaining after chemotherapy may appear deceivingly benign on histologic examination but may be genotypically malignant and potentially dangerous.[30] These studies appear promising for predicting response to therapy, planning further treatment, and determining prognosis.

Oncogenes

Unique segments of DNA preserved in the long course of evolution, as demonstrated by their presence in life forms from yeast to man, are involved in growth control (see Chap. 3). These oncogenes, when they are translocated or their copies amplified, or neighboring DNA segments are shifted, are thought to play a role in oncogenesis. Seeger and colleagues observed that genomic amplification of the N-*myc* oncogene correlates not only with the advanced stage of neuroblastoma at the time of diagnosis but also with rapid tumor progression.[31] Similarly, preliminary studies by Sikora and coworkers[32] have shown that flow cytometric assays for c-*myc* oncogene

products may be a helpful diagnostic and prognostic tool for evaluating germ cell tumors. This work was performed primarily on testicular and colonic tumors. The c-*myc* oncoprotein was probed with a mouse monoclonal antibody. The oncoprotein is apparently heat stable and unaffected by solvents because some of the determinations were performed on formalin-fixed paraffin-embedded tumors, making this a useful technique for evaluating archival tissue.

PATHOLOGY

It is thought that germ cell tumors arise from pluripotential or primordial germ cells that evolve into a variety of benign and malignant neoplasms.[33-35] Even though they are considered primarily germ cell in origin, this diverse group of tumors occurs in both gonadal and extragonadal sites.

The sex cord–stromal tumors (gonadal stromal tumors) originate from the sex cords and the stroma of the developing gonad. They are not derived from germ cells. Examples of this group include granulosa and theca cell tumors of the ovary, Sertoli and Leydig cell tumors of the testis, and stromal tumors of both gonads, occurring singly or in various combinations.[36,37] They are not discussed further in this chapter. The epithelial malignancies or carcinomas *per se* (*e.g.,* cystadenocarcinoma of the ovary), which are rare in children and appear to have a different biological behavior from germ cell tumors, are also not discussed in this chapter (see Chap. 35).

A workable classification for germ cell tumors of children appears in Table 33-1. The comparative characteristics of the different pathologic types of germ cell tumors are shown in Table 33-2.

Histopathology

Germinoma

This neoplasm was previously designated as seminoma when it occurred in the testis, dysgerminoma when it involved the ovary, and germinoma when it arose from extragonadal sites. Because the histology is the same regardless of the location of origin, the original names have been supplanted by the inclusive term "germinoma."

The ovary, anterior mediastinum, and pineal area are the most common sites for germinoma in the pediatric age group. Germinoma accounts for 10% of all ovarian tumors in children and approximately 15% of all germ cell tumors in all loca-

---

Table 33-1
Classification of Germ Cell Tumors in Children

I. Teratoma
   A. Mature
   B. Immature
   C. With malignant germ cell tumor component(s)*
II. Germinoma
III. Embryonal carcinoma
IV. Endodermal sinus (yolk sac) tumor
V. Choriocarcinoma
VI. Gonadoblastoma
VII. Polyembryoma

---

* Contains one or more of the malignant germ cell tumor components (II, III, IV, or V).

Table 33-2
Comparative Characteristics by Pathologic Types

| | | | | Markers | |
Tumor Type	Characteristic Histology	Relative Frequency	Most Common Locations	AFP	HCG
Germinoma	Large round cells, vesicular nuclei, clear eosinophilic cytoplasm; monotonous pattern	+	Ovary, anterior mediastinum, pineal, undescended testes	–	–
Embryonal carcinoma	Poorly differentiated, epithelial appearance; solid or glandular, anaplasia, necrosis	++	Testes, young adult	+	+
Endodermal sinus (yolk sac) tumor	Papillary, reticular or solid pattern; papillary projections with perivascular sheaths (Schiller–Duval bodies)	+++	Testes, infant; sacrococcygeal, ovary	+	–
Choriocarcinoma	Cytotrophoblasts (large round cells, clear cytoplasm, vesicular nuclei) and syncytiotrophoblasts (syncytia with abundant cytoplasm); hemorrhage, necrosis	+	Mediastinal, ovary, pineal	–	+
Teratoma	Immature to well-differentiated tissues foreign to anatomic site with lack of organization; benign or immature may contain other malignant components	++++	Sacrococcygeal midline structures	–	–
Polyembryoma	Embryoid bodies, resembling embryos with amniotic cavity, yolk sac, and embryonic disc	+	Ovary, anterior mediastinum	+	+
Gonadoblastoma	Large germ cells surrounded by smaller Sertoli cells containing hyaline bodies and calcium	+	Dysgenic gonads	–	–

tions.[33] These tumors are found more often in combination with other germ cell tumors than in the "pure" form. Germinoma is the chief malignancy found in dysgenetic gonads and undescended testes and is not infrequently seen in association with gonadoblastoma. It is not known why testicular germinomas are so much rarer in childhood than are ovarian germinomas.

Typically, germinoma has a rather uniform microscopic appearance consisting of sheets of large, round cells resembling primordial germ cells, with round vesicular nuclei and clear to finely granular eosinophilic staining cytoplasm. The cells are separated by slightly vascular fibrous septae containing lymphocytes and, occasionally, focal granuloma formations (Fig. 33-2). Markers for AFB and β-HCG are negative if no malignant germ cell elements other than germinoma are present. Carcinoembryonic antigen (CEA) is also negative. Antiferritin antibody is positive in most instances and therefore is useful in making the diagnosis.[38]

Embryonal Carcinoma

Embryonal carcinoma is defined as a poorly differentiated, malignant germ cell tumor consisting of embryonic-looking cells with an epithelial appearance displaying solid and glandular patterns (Fig. 33-3). Not infrequently, it does not exhibit a definite histologic picture but instead looks like a poorly differentiated or anaplastic carcinoma with extensive necrosis. Some studies have shown that embryonal carcinoma cells differentiate along somatic and extraembryonic lines. For example, the maturation of pulmonary embryonal carcinoma metas-

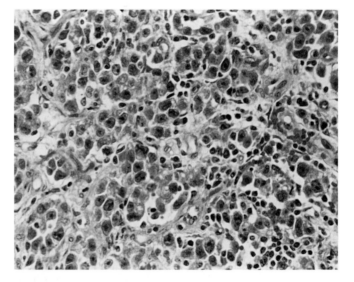

FIGURE 33-2. Germinoma of the ovary, 7-year-old girl. The tumor is composed of rather regular, round germ cells sprinkled with small darkly staining lymphocytes. (H & E; × 300)

tases to mature tissues that resemble a teratoma has been observed after bleomycin chemotherapy.

Dehner divides embryonal carcinoma into two histologic types, adult and infantile,[33,35] terming the latter "endodermal

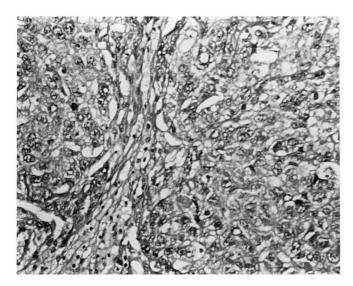

FIGURE 33-3. Embryonal carcinoma of the mediastinum. The patient was a 3½-year-old girl with an anterior mediastinal mass. Section shows nodules of irregular cells with variable vesicular nuclei and vacuolated cytoplasms. (H & E; × 200)

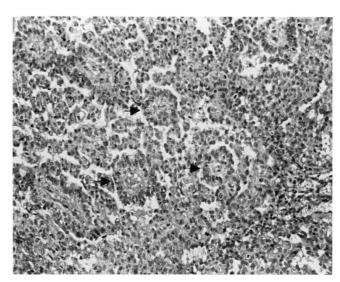

FIGURE 33-4. Endodermal sinus tumor of 2½-year-old girl with a rapidly growing sacrococcygeal mass. Arrows point to several perivascular cuffs of tumor cells (endodermal sinus structures) or Schiller–Duval bodies. The anti-α-fetoprotein immunoperoxidase stain was positive. (H & E; × 150)

sinus tumor." Perhaps the rationale for this concept is that it may be difficult if not impossible to distinguish between the two tumors histologically. If the tumor has endodermal sinus structures and stains positively for AFP by immunoperoxidase, then it is an endodermal sinus tumor. A similar problem exists when attempting to differentiate between embryonal carcinoma and cytotrophoblastic components of choriocarcinoma on hematoxylin and eosin section, particularly when only a small amount of material has been obtained by biopsy and syncytiotrophoblastic elements are not apparent. Perhaps this explains why some embryonal carcinomas show areas of positive staining for chorionic gonadotropin with monoclonal antibody or immunoperoxidase techniques.

Embryonal carcinoma is uncommon as a pure histologic pattern in infants and children but is not unusual in association with other germ cell tumors, such as teratoma and endodermal sinus tumor.

Endodermal Sinus Tumor

Endodermal sinus tumor (yolk sac carcinoma, yolk sac tumor), alone or in combination, is the most common malignant germ cell tumor found in the pediatric age group. The sacrococcygeal area is the major site of involvement in the newborn and infant; in older children and adolescents, the ovary is the chief location. Less common primary sites observed include the mediastinum, retroperitoneum, pineal area, and vagina. Testicular endodermal sinus tumors show two peaks of incidence, one in infancy and the other in adolescence.

Grossly endodermal sinus tumors have a pale tan-yellow, slimy appearance with grayish-red foci of necrosis and small cystic areas. The tumors tend to be very soft and mushy, falling apart on removal.

Several microscopic patterns have been described, ranging from solid nests of cells indistinguishable from embryonal carcinoma to distinct papillary and net-like reticular formations. Papillary projections are associated often with characteristic perivascular sheaths of cells, so-called endodermal sinus structures or Schiller–Duval bodies (Fig. 33-4). In addition, most well-differentiated tumors contain intracellular and extracellular hyaline droplets which are perodic acid-Schiff (PAS) and AFP positive, the latter demonstrated by immunoperoxidase (PAP) methods. One unusual form of endodermal sinus tumor (called the polyvesicular viteline tumor by Teilum[38]) displays hourglass-like vesicles with constrictions surrounded by a pale-staining stroma.

Choriocarcinoma

Choriocarcinoma is an uncommon, highly malignant germ cell neoplasm of extraembryonic differentiation with two distinct forms, *gestational* and *nongestational,* that differ in biological behavior and response to therapy. The gestational form arises from within the placenta and the nongestational form from the extraplacental tissues of a nongravid person. However, the histologic features of both forms are essentially the same. The neoplasm is found mainly in three situations in the pediatric age group, none of which is noted very often. The tumor is seen beyond infancy most frequently in the mediastinum and gonads. It may also be congenital, presenting in a young infant with disseminated metastases and elevated β-HCG levels resulting from a placental primary that has invaded villous vessels and entered the umbilical vein and fetal blood stream.[40] Finally, placental gestational choriocarcinoma may rarely be seen in an adolescent.

Microscopically, choriocarcinoma consists of two main components—cytotrophoblasts and syncytiotrophoblasts—with cells intermediate between the two. *Cytotrophoblasts* are composed of large, round cells with clear cytoplasms and variable vesicular nuclei, whereas *syncytiotrophoblasts* form syncytia or knots and contain much larger cells with abundant homogeneous-to-vaculated cytoplasms and dark irregular nuclei (Fig. 33-5). Cytoplasmic β-HCG is demonstrated by immunoperoxidase staining, but AFP is usually negative. Cytotrophoblasts and syncytiotrophoblasts are found next to one another, adjacent to dilated vascular sinusoids. Extensive hemorrhage and necrosis are characteristic.

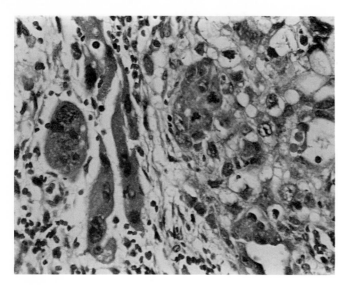

FIGURE 33-5. Choriocarcinoma of the ovary in a 10-year-old girl with an abdominal mass. Two populations of cells are present: the multinucleated giant cell syncytiotrophoblasts are situated on the left side of the field and the smaller vacuolated cytotrophoblasts on the right. (H & E; × 300)

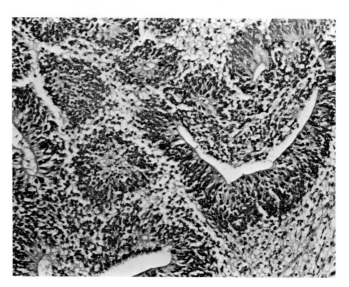

FIGURE 33-6. Immature teratoma of the stomach in a 6-month-old girl with an abdominal mass and feeding problems. The microscopic section shows embryonic appearing neuroglial elements forming neural tube-like structures. Mature elements such as skin and gut, also present in the tumor, are not shown. (H & E; × 150)

Polyembryoma

Polyembryoma is a very uncommon unusual germ cell tumor defined by Teilum as a "teratomatous tumor of the gonads containing myriads of embryoid bodies comparable to normal presomite embryos."[39] Microscopically, the embryoid bodies do look like tiny embryos composed of two vesicles resembling an amniotic cavity and a yolk sac, separated by a two- to three-cell layer embryonic disc. Furthermore, there are two germ cell tumors of the infant testis in the files of the Children's Hospital of Los Angeles (CHLA) consisting of both endodermal sinus tumor and polyembryoma elements. Immunoperoxidase techniques have shown that the polyembryoma stains positively for both AFP and β-HCG,[41] suggesting embryonic and extraembryonic differentiation. Little is known about the clinical behavior of this germ cell tumor because very few cases have been reported.

Gonadoblastoma

Gonadoblastoma was first described and named in 1953 by Scully,[42] who then reviewed and reported 74 cases in 1970.[43] It occurs almost exclusively in dysgenetic gonads, most often during the first two decades of life and in association with a Y chromosome karyotype.[39,44] The majority of affected individuals have either a 46XY or a mosaic 46XY/45XO karyotype.[35] Approximately one third of patients with gonadal dysgenesis develop gonadoblastoma, 40% of which are bilateral.[35,44] Gonadoblastoma could be considered an *in situ* malignancy because it does not spread. However, 25% to 30% of these tumors are associated with germinoma.[38] Grossly, the tumor is a tan, firm encapsulated mass, most of which contains small flecks of calcification that can be appreciated on radiographic studies. Gonadoblastoma displays a distinctive microscopic appearance, consisting of large germ cells surrounded by smaller, round, darkly staining Sertoli cells forming microfollicles and containing hyaline bodies and calcium deposits.[39] Talerman described a similar appearing, benign tumor in normal individuals, composed of germ cells and gonadal stromal cells.[45]

Teratoma

Teratoma is probably the most nebulous and controversial member of the germ cell tumor group. Classically, it is defined as a tumor composed of tissues derived from the three germinal layers of the embryo (endoderm, mesoderm, and ectoderm).[46,47] Gonzales-Crussi gives perhaps a somewhat broader definition: "neoplasms that originate in pluripotent cells and are composed of a wide variety of tissues foreign to the organ or anatomic site in which they arise."[34] Characteristically, the component tissues show a lack of organization and various stages of maturation. The lesion may be solid, multicystic, or formed about a single large cyst.[38,46] Sometimes it is difficult or impossible to distinguish between a mature teratoma and an abortive attempt at twinning (fetus *in fetu*). The majority of neonatal teratomas are found in the sacrococcygeal region and the cervical area (80% and 10%, respectively, in the CHLA study[48]). Other locations include the upper jaw (epignathus), nasopharynx, intracranial cavity, retroperitoneum, mediastinum, and gonads.

Teratomas have been classified histologically into three main types: mature, immature (embryonic components), and teratomas with malignant components.[48,49] The mature type consists of mature or well-differentiated tissues such as brain, skin, gastrointestinal tract, and bone. It is at the benign end of the spectrum. The immature teratoma is represented histologically by embryonic appearing neuroglial or neuroepithelial elements such as cells resembling medulloblastoma, ependymoma, or neural tubelike structures that are found in addition to mature components (Fig. 33-6).

The immature teratomas are associated with an increased incidence of malignancy, and their behavior is the least predictable of the three types. Further, they have been categorized microscopically into four grades, 0 through 3, depending on the amount of immature elements present and the degree of mitotic activity.[50] This grading system appears to be useful in evaluating immature teratomas occurring in older adolescents and adults, but in our experience is not as predictable in infants and children. Immature teratomas in the young tend to have a better prognosis than in older individuals. One example of this is the patient with an immature ovarian tumor and peritoneal neuroglial implants.[51,52] The majority of children with this condition probably have a favorable outcome. However, additional, more thorough clinicopathologic studies and careful follow-up data are required to determine how best to evaluate and treat children with this type of teratoma.

Teratomas with malignant germ cell elements contain one or more of the malignant germ cell tumors (germinoma, choriocarcinoma, endodermal sinus tumor or embryonal carcinoma), in addition to mature or immature tissues. Terms such as "teratocarcinoma" and "malignant teratoma," used frequently in the literature, are not only confusing but also inaccurate as to the specific type of malignancy present in the tumor, and should be avoided. It is important to note that in the newborn the majority of teratomas consist of mature or mature mixed with immature elements.[53] In this age group, the teratoma with malignant components is most likely to be found in the sacrococcygeal area, and the usual malignancies are endodermal sinus tumor and embryonal carcinoma.[54] The incidence of sacrococcygeal teratomas with malignant elements varies from one pediatric center to the next, ranging from 2.5%[3] to 10 times that figure.[55] In most instances, neonatal teratomas situated outside the sacrococcygeal (*e.g.*, in the nasopharynx, jaw, neck, mediastinum, or retroperitoneum) do not contain malignant germ cell tumor components.[3,48,54]

Several reports indicate that early diagnosis and complete resection of a sacrococcygeal teratoma including the coccyx provide the only means for cure.[49,54,55] Generally this appears to be the case, especially in young infants, but it is not true in all instances. The patient may return several months or even years later with a mass in the sacrococcygeal area which on biopsy proves to be a mature teratoma or a malignant germ cell neoplasm such as an endodermal sinus tumor. At present, it is impossible to determine whether this represents an old recurrence or a second primary. Other factors that enter into the picture are incomplete initial resection and sampling error by the pathologist. If only one or two microscopic sections are taken from a 1.5 kg teratoma, the likelihood of missing a malignant germ cell tumor component, if present, is quite high. Teratomas *per se* do not display positive staining for either AFP or HCG unless endodermal sinus tumor or trophoblastic components are present.[38]

CLINICAL CHARACTERISTICS AND PRESENTATION

The clinical presentations of germ cell tumors in children vary according to their locations and pathology. Their comparative presentations are summarized in Table 33-3.

Extragonadal Tumors

Sacrococcygeal

A summary from the literature reveals that 41% of germ cell tumors, both benign and malignant, occur in the sacrococcygeal region (Table 33-4).[35] Of these tumors, 70% are in females and just over half occur in neonates: 48% are benign, 29% are frankly malignant, and 23% have immature (also called embryonic) but not malignant components.[61] Altman and col-

Table 33-3
Comparative Clinical Presentations of Germ Cell Tumors

Tumor	Age	Relative Frequency	Symptoms	Findings	Pathology
Extragonadal					
Sacrococcygeal	Infants	41%	Constipation, neurologic abnormalities of bladder or lower extremities	Presacral mass with or without extension to buttocks or pelvis and abdomen	65% benign 5% immature 30% malignant
Mediastinal		6%	Cough, wheeze, dyspnea	Anterior mediastinal mass	Benign or malignant
Abdominal	<2 yr	5%	Secondary to pressure pain, GU obstruction, constipation	Often retroperitoneal; also stomach, omentum, liver	Benign or malignant
Intracranial	Children	6%	Headache, paralysis of upward gaze, incoordination	Pineal or supracellular tumors; AFP or HCG in CSF	Any type germ cell tumor
Head and neck	Infants	4%	Pressure-related; respiratory or swallowing difficulty	Large mass on physical examination	Usually benign
Vagina	<3 yr	1%	Blood-tinged vaginal discharge	Polyoid mass from vagina	Usually malignant
Gonadal					
Ovarian	10–14 yr	29%	Abdominal pain, nausea, vomiting, constipation, GU symptoms	Abdominal pelvic mass; calcifications in 50%; often + AFD or HCG	Any type germ cell tumor
Testicular	Infants, postpubertal	7%	Painless swelling of testis	Testicular mass; metastases to lung in infants	Any type germ cell tumor 82% malignant 18% benign Infants mostly yolk sac tumors

Table 33-4
Literature Summary: Sites of Germ Cell Tumors in Childhood, Benign and Malignant

Site	Year and Reference							Total	
	1969 Berry[3]	*1971* Partlow[56]	*1972* Carney[57]	*1975* Bale[58]	*1978* Mahour[59]	*1981* Marsden[60]	*1983* Tapper[55]	No.	%
Sacrococcyx	58	16	22	51	57	31	102	337	41
Ovary	10	18	5	16	51	45	94	239	29
Testis	7	4	3	7	6	25	8	60	7
Mediastinum, pericardium	5	2	17	5	4	5	11	49	6
Intracranial	5	4	7	5	4	13	9	47	6
Retroperitoneum	1	3	3	7	5	6	12	37	4
Neck	3	2		10	1	3	6	25	3
Head		3	1					4	<1
Stomach	2				1			3	<1
Uterus-vagina						3		3	<1
Spinal cord						3		3	<1
Bladder-prostate						2		2	<1
Liver									
Umbilical cord					1		2	3	<1
Total	91	52	58	107	133	137	254	832	100

(Modified from Dehner[35])

leagues[62] have classified the presentation of 398 patients with sacrococcygeal germ cell tumors in order of frequency as follows: Type I—predominantly external on the buttocks with a minimal presacral component; Type II—external with a significant intrapelvic component; Type III—external, with the predominant mass pelvic with extension into the abdomen; and Type IV—entirely presacral, without external presentation or significant pelvic extension (Fig. 33-7). Type I is the most common and the least likely to be malignant at diagnosis. Type III is the most likely to be malignant at diagnosis and Type IV the most likely to be overlooked. The diagnosis for the first three types can be made on physical examination, although the external mass may be subtle. In Type IV, urinary frequency or lower extremity weakness may occur, but it is usually a complaint of constipation that brings the infant to medical attention. The constipation is commonly handled with a formula change or a prescription for rectal suppositories. What is needed is a careful rectal examination with the examining finger directed posteriorly and sweeping the presacral fossa, searching for a firm discrete mass characteristic of a germ cell tumor. If a mass is found when the finger is directed anterior to the rectum toward the bladder, prostate, uterus, vagina, or perineum, the more likely diagnosis is rhabdomyosarcoma.

Skin-covered sacrococcygeal masses or presacral masses can present a problem in differential diagnosis (see also Chap. 5). Because germ cell tumors may have the potential to become malignant, accuracy and expediency are essential. The incidence of malignancy when the diagnosis was made before age 2 months was 10% in males and 7% in females. When the diagnosis was not made until after 2 months, 67% of males and 47% of females had malignant tumors.[62] Table 33-5 lists the differential diagnosis of skin covered lesions of the caudal spine and presacral masses.[63,64] The importance of the rectal examination to detect a presacral mass characteristic of germ cell tumors but also present in pelvic neuroblastoma and anterior meningocele cannot be overemphasized. The latter two growths, however, do not present externally. Lateral and anteriorposterior radiographs of the pelvis can reveal the calcifica-

tions found in over half of the teratomas. It is important to be aware also that lipomas can be associated with and adjacent to bone.[65] On lateral radiologic examination of the pelvis, anterior displacement of a gas-filled rectum characteristic of germ cell tumors can also be seen in anterior meningocele and neuroblastoma. Neuroblastomas commonly produce catecholamines. Lesions that are caudal to the sacrum radiographically are usually teratomas, although they may rarely occur in low meningoceles. Lipomeningoceles can be distinguished from lipomas by virtue of their association with neurologic deficits in the lower extremities, and from teratomas because on radiography they are posterior to the sacrum and do not displace the rectum. Meningoceles exhibit water density on radiographs or magnetic resonance images. Since meningoceles do not require immediate attention, whereas germ cell tumors may be or become malignant, this differentiation is critical. The mixed group of neural lesions that were skin-covered in the sacrococcygeal area in the Lemire series were myelocystoceles with cystic distention of the central canal (hydromyelia) or multiple cystic cavities related to neural elements.[63] This group of patients had neurologic deficits in the lower extremities and associated spina bifida, or sacral anomalies or agenesis.

STAGING FOR EXTRAGONADAL TUMORS. Although there is no generally accepted staging classification, the system shown in Table 33-6 is workable for achieving a description of extent of disease.

SURGICAL CONSIDERATIONS. Complete excision is necessary for sacrococcygeal tumors. For externally presenting tumors, a transsacral approach is the standard, whereas abdominal incision is necessary for large, fixed, primarily internal tumors; often, the two approaches are combined.[66] The coccyx must always be excised with the mass; failure to do so is associated with a high recurrence rate. The surgeon must be mindful of the possibility of intraspinal extension. Because the tumors are often cystic, the possibility of spill exists. For ex-

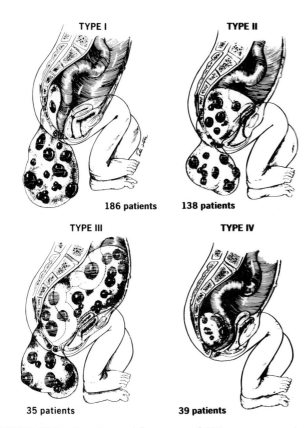

TYPE I

186 patients

TYPE II

138 patients

TYPE III

35 patients

TYPE IV

39 patients

FIGURE 33-7. Location and frequency of 398 sacrococcygeal teratomas in infants and children. Type I is predominantly external, minimal presacral (47%); type II is both external and intrapelvic (34%); type III is external, pelvic, and abdominal (9%); and type IV is only presacral (10%). (Altman RP, Randolph JG, Lilly JR: J Pediatr Surg 9:389–398, 1974)

Table 33-5
Presacral Masses and Skin-Covered Lesions of the Caudal Spine

Caudal Spine Lesions

Teratoma	Hemangioma
Pilonidal cyst	Duplication of the rectum
Lipomeningocele	Abscess
Lipoma	Bone tumor
Meningocele	Epidermal cyst
Mixed neural masses	Chondroma

Presacral Masses

Chordoma	Neuroblastoma
Lymphoma	Mucinoid carcinoma
Ependyoma	Glioma

(Modified from Lemire et al[63] and Werner and Taybi[64])

Table 33-6
Staging for Extragonadal Tumors

Stage I	Disease limited to one organ or structure completely resected at the time of the initial surgical procedure using a single incision
Stage II	Disease extending to structures adjacent to the primary tumor but completely resected at the time of the initial surgical procedure
	Tumors requiring more than one incision for removal but without tumor spillage during surgery
Stage III	A. Tumors with microscopic residual following surgery, due to spillage or extension of tumor to resection margins
	B. Tumors incompletely resected at surgery
Stage IV	Disseminated disease

tensive malignant tumors with sacral, rectal, and bowel involvement, excisional surgery should be postponed until a chemotherapeutic response has been achieved.

Mediastinal

Thoracic germ cell tumors are almost always located in the anterior superior mediastinum (see Chaps. 35 and 37).[67–70] Posterior mediastinal teratomas have been reported, and this rare possibility must be kept in mind.[71] The mediastinum is the second most frequent site of extragonadal germ cell tumors. The predominance of these locations is not surprising given that the urogenital ridge in the embryo extends from C6 to L4. Often, asymptomatic thoracic germ cell tumors may, however, produce symptoms of moderate to severe tracheobronchial compression. Coughing, wheezing, dyspnea, or chest pain all may occur when tumors are large.[71] Serious hemoptysis has been described in infants.[73] An insulin-producing mediastinal teratoma has been described in a 5-year-old boy.[74]

All tissue types have been reported but, curiously, endodermal sinus tumors occur mostly in males.[75,76] Lack and co-workers described 21 children with mediastinal germ cell tumors—13 boys and 8 girls with an average age of 7 years (range, 2 weeks to 16 years). Twelve tumors were pure teratoma, 5 contained embryonal carcinoma admixed with other germ cell components, and 4 were pure embryonal carcinoma.[77] Mediastinal teratomas appear as a dense well-rounded mass on chest radiographs, with calcifications present about 35% of the time (Figs. 33-8 and 33-9). The presence of a tooth

may be pathognomonic.[57] Computed tomography (CT) of the chest is the optimal imaging study. These tumors must be distinguished from other anterior mediastinal masses that occur in children: thymomas, thymic cysts, lymphomas, lymphangiomas, lipomas, bronchial and enteric cysts, and neurogenic tumors (see Chaps. 5 and 7).

SURGICAL CONSIDERATIONS. Most mediastinal germ cell tumors are in the anterior compartment and can be approached by unilateral thoractomy incision. A median sternotomy incision may be necessary for large, bilateral, invasive lesions. Again, it is necessary to remove contiguously involved tissues. The same principles hold for all germ cell tumors, no matter where they occur. Because they either are malignant or have the potential to become malignant, complete excision is necessary. Exceptions are the mature neuroglial implants of immature teratomas, which have been observed to outgrow their blood supply and eventually disappear. They may easily be mistaken for disseminated malignant disease.[44,51] Carter and associates reported that the immature teratomas of infants and young children behave as mass lesions and have good prognosis with excision, whereas those that occur in teenagers or young adults are highly malignant tumors (see Table 33-4).[78]

Abdominal

Abdominal germ cell tumors are usually located in the retroperitoneum, although tumors in the stomach,[79,80] omentum,[81]

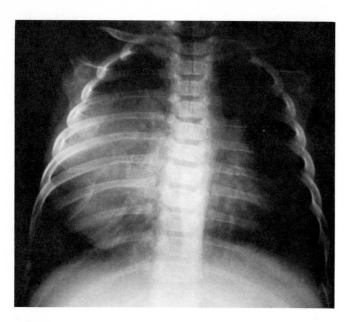

FIGURE 33-8. Four-month-old boy with mediastinal teratoma.

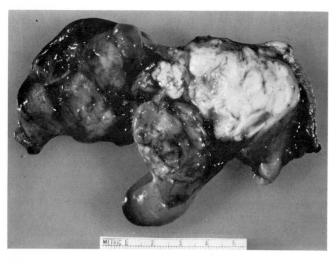

FIGURE 33-9. Surgical specimen from patient shown in Figure 33-8. An immature teratoma arises from the thymus.

and liver[82] have been described. Both hepatic and gastric teratomas typically occur in infancy. The retroperitoneum is the third most common extragonadal site. Retroperitoneal teratomas usually occur in children under 2 years.[83,84] Presenting symptoms are secondary to pressure and may include vague abdominal pain, constipation, or urinary difficulties.[85] The visualization of calcification of bone or teeth on radiologic study can be helpful in making the preoperative diagnosis.[86] Recurrent bleeding of the upper gastrointestinal tract in infants may be due to gastric outlet obstruction from a gastric teratoma. One must distinguish retroperitoneal germ cell tumor from Wilms' tumor, neuroblastoma, lymphoma and rhabdomyosarcoma.

Intracranial

Intracranial tumors comprise 6% of all germ cell tumors and approximately 0.5% to 2% of primary intracranial neoplasms.

Although most occur in the pineal area, about one fifth are located in the suprasellar or infrasellar regions (see also Chap. 24).[87] Tumors in this area may obstruct third ventricular outflow, causing hydrocephalus and subsequent headache. With anterior and caudal growth, the midbrain tegmentum is compressed, causing paralysis of upward gaze, better pupillary response to accommodation than to light, and convergence nystagmus (Parinaud's syndrome). With compression of the overlying thalamus, hemiparesis, incoordination, and movement and visual disorders may result. Tavcar and coworkers reported a patient with drop spinal metastases and cited three other reported patients with pineal endodermal sinus tumors.[88] Diabetes insipidtus may occur,[89] as may extracranial metastases to the lung[87] or to bone.[90] Intra-abdominal metastasis in an 8-year-old patient with an unfiltered ventriculoperitoneal shunt has also been observed.

In a series of 25 patients with pineal region tumors, all of whom underwent biopsy at the Children's Hospital in Philadelphia, 8 had germ cell tumors (5 embryonal carcinoma, 2 teratoma, and 1 germinoma). The other tumors were 8 pineal parenchymal tumors (pineoblastomas, pineocytomas), 8 glial tumors (astrocytomas, gangliogliomas) and one ganglio-neuroblastoma.[91] Germinomas occurred more frequently in the Children's Cancer Study Group study, in which 36 of 57 pineal tumor biopsies (63%) revealed a germinoma.[92] These studies point out the need to establish a specific diagnosis by biopsy because treatment for the various histologic types can be so different.

Intracranial germ cell neoplasms may produce markers in the plasma or CSF. Embryonal carcinoma produced AFP and β-HCG; choriocarcinoma produced β-HCG, and dysgerminoma produced no marker.[93] A plasma:CSF β-HCG ratio of less than 60 was found in 29 of 33 gestational choriocarcinoma patients with brain metastases, whereas in patients without CNS involvement the ratio was 286:1.[94] CSF markers may not reliably distinguish the various pineal area tumors but may be useful in following the progress of a specific tumor.[91]

Head and Neck

The oral cavity, pharynx, orbit, and neck account for approximately 6% of all germ cell tumors, and these tumors are almost always noted at birth. Orbital teratomas occur most commonly in females and are usually unilateral.[95,96] Germ cell tumors of the head and neck in children are almost always benign but may produce life-threatening symptoms due to obstruction.

Vaginal

Vaginal germ cell tumors are rare, almost always occur in children younger than 3 years, and are most commonly endodermal sinus tumors.[97-100] The patient presents with blood-tinged or bloody vaginal discharge. Vaginal examination, optimally done under anesthesia, reveals a polypoid, friable lesion arising from the vagina. This presentation is identical to that of a rhabdomyosarcoma of the vagina (sarcoma botyroides), so misdiagnosis is possible. Vaginal germ cell tumors may also be confused with clear cell carcinoma.[101]

Gonadal Tumors

Ovarian

Ovarian germ cell tumors account for 29% of all germ cell tumors and 1% to 1.6% of all childhood tumors (see Table

33-4).[102,103] When all ovarian tumors of childhood are included, 65% are benign teratomas, 5% are immature (embryonal) teratomas, and 30% are malignant tumors.[53] The predominance of germ cell neoplasms and the rarity of epithelial neoplasms in the ovarian tumors of children contrasts with the experience in adults, where epithelial cancers make up 87% to 90% of the tumors (see also Chap. 35).[104,105] Nonetheless, epithelial cancers can still occur in children, and in one family three teenage sisters died of undifferentiated ovarian carcinoma.[106,107] In several reviews of benign and malignant ovarian tumors in children, the frequency of germ cell tumors varied from 60% to 89%, with stromal–sex cord tumors (Sertoli–Leydig, granulosal–thecal, and undifferentiated) having a 10% to 13% incidence, and epithelial carcinomas, fibrosarcoma, and unclassified tumors comprising some 5% to 11%.[108–111] In these studies, all ages were represented but malignant tumors under age 10 were rare, whereas benign teratomas were described in all ages. Most benign tumors were in prepubertal patients, whereas the malignant tumors peaked just after 13 years. The peak incidence at the time of puberty supports the theory that increased ovarian activity from direct or indirect stimulation may release a latent factor resulting in new growth.

Abdominal pain, often chronic, is the most common presenting symptom, but if torsion of the tumor or fallopian tube occurs, then the pain can be acute and severe. Nausea and vomiting, sometimes accompanied by fever, may present with torsion. When an abdominal mass is not palpated or seen on imaging studies, a preoperative diagnosis of appendicitis is often considered. The possibility of an ovarian mass must always be entertained whenever the diagnosis of appendicitis is contemplated in girls or young women.[109] Slowly progressive abdominal enlargement, constipation, and genitourinary symptoms have all been described.[53] Tumors that secrete β-HCG may also cause breast enlargement and early pubic hair growth or menarche and cause a confusing presentation. For example, a 13-year-old patient with slowly progressive abdominal enlargement and a lower abdominal mass had a positive pregnancy test and was accused of being pregnant for several weeks before it was determined that her physical and laboratory findings were secondary to a β-HCG-producing mixed germ cell malignant ovarian tumor. Physicians should be aware of this rare possibility when a teenage pregnancy is suspected. Extraovarian spread occurs by direct extension to adjacent adnexa, but spread also occurs by tumor cells in ascitic fluid, or lymph nodes, or blood. When extraovarian spread occurs, the peritoneal surfaces of pelvic structures, the bladder, sigmoid colon, uterus, and fallopian tubes are most commonly involved, but spread to abdominal peritoneal surfaces including liver, diaphragm, mesentary, omentum, and small bowel also occurs.

Imaging studies reveal a calcified ovarian mass in about half of patients. These are the tumors most likely to be benign. In Ehren and coworkers' series, 71% of patients with benign teratomas had calcification on radiography.[53] A lower abdominal or pelvic mass without calcification occurs with both benign and malignant tumors. Evidence of urinary tract obstruction secondary to pressure from the tumor may also be seen. Abdominal ultrasound is an excellent and noninvasive imaging study that can give much information on the status of the ovaries and adnexa. Metastatic evaluation for patients suspected of malignant ovarian germ cell tumors should include CT scans of the chest and abdomen, radionuclide bone scans, and perhaps CT brain scans with contrast and pelvic MRI studies.

Elevated β-HCG levels occur with embryonal carcinoma and choriocarcinoma, and AFP is elevated with endodermal sinus tumors (see also Chap. 8).[112] These hormonal markers are of importance not only for diagnosis but also in following patients during treatment and evaluating possible recurrence.

STAGING OF OVARIAN TUMORS. Recognizing the relative rarity of malignant ovarian tumor in childhood, we have modified the ovarian cancer staging system adapted by the International Federation of Gynecology and Obstetrics (FIGO) as shown in Table 33-7. A difference in this staging system from that of FIGO is that children with ascitic fluid positive for tumor cells are placed in Stage III, reflecting the possibility that such patients are apt to have generalized disease in the abdomen as well as the pelvis, because in younger girls the ovaries are higher in the abdomen, not the pelvis.

SURGICAL CONSIDERATIONS. When an ovarian mass is found that might be malignant, the surgeon is obligated to determine the extent of disease because treatment and prognosis depend on staging. For small tumors, incisional biopsy with frozen specimen examination is recommended. For tumors larger than 5 cm, oophorectomy with frozen section is indicated. If germ cell malignancy is present, salpingo-oophorectomy is done. The other ovary is examined by a bivalve incision. If nodules are found, bilateral salpingo-oophorectomy is accomplished. The possibility of hysterectomy should then be considered. Ascitic fluid, if present, or peritoneal washings are sent for cytologic evaluation. The liver and subphrenic spaces are searched for evidence of tumor nodules. The omentum is biopsied; if it or the ascitic fluid is positive, omentectomy should be performed. If extensive tissue invasion has occurred so that removal of the tumor is not possible or would require an extensive and mutilating procedure, surgical treatment is delayed until the effects of chemotherapy can be determined.

Testicular

Testicular tumors in children comprise approximately 7% of all germ cell tumors and 1% of all childhood cancers.[113] Children under 15 years of age represent 0.5% to 5% of all patients with testicular tumors.[114–116] Therefore, only the busiest children's cancer center may see more than one such patient every year or two. The most common benign testicular neoplasm is a teratoma with mature elements. The most common malignancy is a germ cell tumor that has been variously described as infantile adenocarcinoma of the testis,[117] embryonal carcinoma,[118] orchioblastoma,[119] adenocarcinoma with clear cells,[120] and embryonal adenocarcinoma.[121] This confusion continues even today, where most pathologists would call these neoplasms either endodermal sinus tumor[122] or yolk sac tumor.[123]

Weissbach and colleagues[124] reported the incidence of the various types of testicular tumors in 1169 children and 1062

Table 33-7
Staging of Ovarian Tumors

Stage I	Diseases limited to one or both ovaries; capsule intact; peritoneal fluid negative for malignant cells
Stage II	Disease including or beyond the ovarian capsule with local pelvic extension; retroperitoneal nodes and peritoneal fluid negative for malignant cells
Stage III	Positive retroperitoneal nodes, malignant cells in the peritoneal fluid, or abdominal extension
Stage IV	Extra-abdominal dissemination

adults using both the German experience and a summary of the literature. In the children, 71% of the testicular tumors were of germ cell origin and 29% were nongerminal. In adults, the comparable figures were 92% and 8%. Of the germ cell tumors in children, 82% were malignant and 18% were pure teratomas and therefore benign. Yolk sac tumors were by far the most frequent of the germinal tumors in children, comprising 69% of the total, while other histologic types or mixtures represented 13%. In the latter group, seminomas were seen in 4% and embryonal carcinoma in 0.1% of the children; in adults, the figures were 43% and 37%, respectively. In 668 children with testicular tumors, local tumor extension, nodal stage and metastatic spread could be determined. More than 90% of children but only 39% of adults were free of metastases at diagnosis.

The tumor causes a slowly growing and painless testicular mass, which can be mistaken for an epididymitis or hydrocele. In examining the scrotal contents, the thumb and forefinger should be placed between the anterior testis and the posterior and superior epididymal and cord structures. The testis can then be made to slide between the examiner's fingers, and masses within the testis can then be felt and separated from abnormalities in the epididymis or cord. Making diagnosis more difficult, is the presence in approximately 25% of cases of an associated hydrocele,[125] which may transilluminate. Li and coworkers[126] noted that 21% of patients had an inguinal hernia. Other considerations in the differential diagnosis of intrascrotal masses are torsion, orchitis, epididymitis, and testicular infarct.[127]

The incidence of malignancy in the undescended testis has been reported to be 20 to 40 times higher than in the normally descended testis.[128] The increased incidence of cancer in the contralateral descended testicle in patients with unilateral cryptorchidism suggests that testicular cancer may result from an intrinsic testicular defect and that orchiopexy may not prevent its occurrence.[129]

Preoperative evaluation should include determinations of the serum markers AFP and β-HCG. Even if for some reason these important markers have not been obtained preoperatively, they should be determined when the patient is first seen so that their biological decay can be followed. CT of the chest and abdomen, looking for pulmonary metastasis or evidence of retroperitoneal adenopathy, and bone scan are the most sensitive ways to detect metastases. MRI produces the most detail in the pelvis and is the procedure of choice when optimal visualization of pelvic structures is necessary (see Chap. 7). Abdominal and pelvic ultrasound, which are excellent ways to follow patients with abdominal or pelvic disease, are easily performed, noninvasive, and less expensive. A prudent approach is to obtain both CT or MRI scans and ultrasound on the same day and then to follow the patient's progress with periodic ultrasound examinations.[130]

GROUPING OF TESTICULAR TUMORS.   A system for evaluating extent of disease specifically designed for testicular tumors in children, developed by the Committee on Tumors, Section of Urology, Academy of Pediatrics,[116] is presented in Table 33-8.

For pubertal boys, the staging system used for adults is most appropriate because histology and disease in this group are more like those in adults than in infants and very young children. A simple staging system used by Einhorn[131] for testicular cancer is as follows:

Stage I: Limited to testis alone.

Stage II: Testis and retroperitoneal nodes involved.

Stage III: Supradiaphragmatic involvement.

Table 33-8
*Grouping of Testicular Tumors in Children**

Group I	Tumor confined to the testis, AFP levels normal within 1 month after orchiectomy; chest radiograph and retroperitoneal imaging normal
Group IIA	Similar to Group I, but retroperitoneal lymph node dissection reveals unsuspected nodal metastases
Group IIB	Retroperitoneal metastasis demonstrated on imaging studies, AFP levels persistently elevated
Group III	Demonstrable metastases beyond the retroperitoneum

(From the Academy of Pediatrics[116])
* See text for staging system for pubertal boys.

SURGICAL CONSIDERATIONS.   Radical orchiectomy through an inguinal incision, with high ligation of the cord, is the initial treatment for all testicular tumors of infants and children. For patients without evidence of dissemination on imaging studies, controversy exists regarding the advisability of retroperitoneal lymphadenectomy. Because of the small numbers of patients available for study, prospective studies have not been done, and are unlikely to be done in a randomized fashion.[132] Sabio and colleagues[133] summarized the survival rates in children with testicular germ cell malignant tumors as follows: 25 of 52 with orchiectomy alone; 21 of 25 with orchiectomy and lymphadenectomy; and 25 of 30 with orchiectomy and radiotherapy.[121,134–137] These data are now more difficult to interpret because they were collected retrospectively from the literature of the 1960s and 1970s. In 1979, Bracken and colleagues, in a summary article, found that only 4 of 78 children who underwent retroperitoneal lymph node dissection had positive lymph nodes.[138]

Exelby,[125] limiting his recommendations to infants and children, advises orchiectomy without lymphadenectomy for children with embryonal adenocarcinoma of the infant testis (endodermal sinus tumor) when there is no evidence of hematogenous metastases. In his experience, none of 23 patients had retroperitoneal metastases, and 18 of 23 were long-term survivors. Duckett[139] makes similar recommendations for infants with endodermal sinus tumors (*i.e.,* radical orchiectomy) followed by monthly AFP assay and chest radiographs for 18 months. He does not recommend retroperitoneal lymphadenectomy, but states that a prospective randomized trial would be necessary to resolve the issue. Weissbach and colleagues[124] agreed and reported that with Stage I yolk sac tumors there was a correlation between age and prognosis. With orchiectomy as sole treatment, 73% of children younger than 2 years survived with no subsequent disease, whereas only 33% of those older than 2 years are disease-free. This suggests a more aggressive approach for children older than 2 years. All of 11 children who had lymph node dissection were found to have negative nodes in another study.[140] Kaplan and Firlit, on the other hand, reported that of 12 children with endodermal sinus tumors, all of whom had lymphadenectomy, 3 (all of whom were younger than 2 years) had positive nodes. An 8-month-old infant had a positive pulmonary hilar node. Those authors conclude that all children with yolk sac tumors should have extended unilateral lymphadenectomy for staging.[141]

The controversy regarding the adult population with Stage I testicular nonseminomatous germ cell tumors is equally intense and, because of the greater numbers involved, may help to focus the issues in pediatric tumors. Williams and Einhorn outline four treatment options: [1] retroperitoneal node dissection with or without chemotherapy, [2] radiotherapy with or without chemotherapy, [3] chemotherapy only, or [4] observation alone. They conclude that "standard" therapy for Clinical Stage I nonseminomatous germ cell tumor patients continues to be retroperitoneal lymph node dissection, which produces cure rates unparalleled in cancer treatment of adults, with negligible treatment mortality, and the avoidance of systemic therapy. Orchiectomy alone should be offered only in the context of a clinical trial.[142] Whitmore takes an almost identical position from the surgeon's point of view.[143] Another viewpoint is that of Glatstein, who suggests that with full modern staging, including lymphangiography and markers, and with the knowledge that excellent salvage therapy is available for patients with recurrence, patients with Clinical Stage I testicular cancer can be treated with orchiectomy, followed by careful monthly physical examinations and imaging studies.[144] Chemotherapy is the treatment of choice if there is recurrence. With this plan, the approximately 85% of patients in whom recurrence would not be expected would be spared lymphadenectomy or radiation as well as multiagent chemotherapy. The need for the patient to be compliant and reliable is stressed.[144] It is also recommended that a bipedal lymphangiogram be done; *this may be very difficult when this recommendation is extended to infants.* In a prospective study of 45 patients with Clinical Stage I nonseminomatous germ cell tumors treated with orchiectomy alone, 36 were continuously free of disease for a median duration of 19.5 months. Of the 9 patients who had relapsed, 7 were rendered disease-free with chemotherapy or surgery for a median duration of 7 months.[145]

Javadpour and colleagues recommend an alternative approach to adults with Clinical Stage I retroperitoneal disease, using a relatively brief procedure with fewer complications. The right caval nodes at the entrance of the right spermatic vein and the interaortocaval and left renal pedicle lymphatics are submitted for frozen section and, if negative, the ipsilateral spermatic vein is resected. Only if the samples nodes are positive is a limited formal lymphadenectomy performed.[146]

In summary, it may not be appropriate to carry over to children the data accumulated for adults, although the experience in that population is far greater than that with children. On the basis of the available data, a high inguinal orchiectomy alone is recommended for Stage I endodermal sinus testicular tumors in infants younger than 2 years and probably also in prepubertal children, provided markers fall to normal levels after surgery (remembering that normal adult values may not be reached until the age of 6 months) and initial imaging studies are all normal. These patients then need careful monthly monitoring with marker determinations and physical examinations. Ultrasound or CT scan of the retinoperitoneum and chest radiography or CT scan are recommended at 3-month intervals for at least 1 year after orchiectomy. Pubertal males should be treated in the same way as adults.

RADIATION THERAPY

The role of radiation therapy has not been established for pediatric germ cell tumors. Germinomas are known to be radiosensitive, and localized disease can be treated with radiation therapy.[147] However, germinomas rarely occur in childhood. Radiation is used chiefly as an attempt to salvage patients who either have not responded to chemotherapy or have relapsed after an initial response. Its effectiveness has yet to be established.

CHEMOTHERAPY

Benign Germ Cell Tumors

The treatment of benign germ cell tumors (mature teratomas) is surgical excision. They must be completely removed; otherwise, recurrence is the rule. This is especially important in sacrococcygeal teratomas, where removal of the coccyx is essential if recurrence is to be prevented. There is no role for chemotherapy or radiation. Periodic follow-up examinations and appropriate imaging studies are imperative. These tumors may recur if microscopic residual exists, or a malignant tumor may occur at a later time, perhaps because of undetected malignant elements in the original tumor.

Immature Germ Cell Tumors

The value of therapy beyond surgical excision for immature teratomas in children is not clear for all patients. Norris and colleagues[148] report that in 58 patients (median age = 18 years) with immature ovarian teratomas the histologic grade of the tumor was one of the major determinants of the likelihood of extraovarian spread. Once spread had occurred, the grade of the metastases was the major factor in determining prognosis. Their grading system is presented in Table 33-9.

The initial staging was also related to survival, and all 14 patients who were Stage I, Grade 1 survived with surgery alone. Stage I patients who had Grade 2 histology had a 70% survival but those with Grade 3 had only 33% survival. Until more data are available, children with immature ovarian teratoma Stage I, Grade 1, can be treated with surgery alone. Older children with higher stage disease and, perhaps, a higher-grade disease should receive chemotherapy. Gonzalez-Crussi and coworkers[149] have suggested that sacrococcygeal immature teratomas may exhibit similar behavior.

Malignant Germ Cell Tumors

Because of the rarity of malignant germ cell tumors in infants and children, much of what has been learned in the more common adult disease has been applied to the pediatric population. Before 1950, there was no effective therapy for malignant germ cell tumors and only a portion of those with complete surgical resection survived. In 1956, Li and colleagues[150] noted that in hypophysectomized mice with metastatic melanoma, HCG dropped to zero after treatment with aminopterin,

---

Table 33-9
Grading of Immature Ovarian Teratomas

Grade 0	All tissues mature; no mitotic activity
Grade 1	Some immaturity but with neuroepithelium absent or limited to one low-magnification field; not more than 1 focus in a slide
Grade 2	Immaturity present; neuroepithelium common but not more than 3 low-power microscopic fields in one slide
Grade 3	Immaturity and neuroectoderm prominent—more than 4 low-power fields per section

(Norris HJ, Zirkin HJ, Benson WL: Immature (malignant) teratoma of the ovary: A clinical and pathologic study of 58 cases. Cancer 37:2359–2372, 1976)

a folic acid antagonist. They reasoned that gestational choriocarcinoma, an HCG-producing tumor, might be similarly sensitive. Using a closely related folic acid antagonist, methotrexate, they produced a 47% complete response rate. Unfortunately, nongestational choriocarcinoma was not responsive to methotrexate. In 1960, Li and coworkers reported that disseminated testicular germ cell tumors had a 20% complete response to combination methotrexate, chlorambucil, and actinomycin D.[151] Until relatively recently, three fourths of females with Stage I endodermal sinus tumors of the ovary died within 2 years, despite resection of all visible disease.[152] Improved cure rates of both children and adults with ovarian germ cell tumors were first reported in 1969 and were usually achieved with combinations of vincristine, actinomycin D, and cyclophosphamide (VAC).[153–157]

Much of the subsequent work in the treatment of germ cell tumors has been done in young adults with testicular tumors because of the greater numbers of patients in this group than in children. In the 1970s, several single agents were found to produce significant response rates in disseminated testicular germ cell tumors. The Central Clinical Drug Evaluation Program evaluated mithramycin in 99 patients and found a 26% complete response plus partial response (CR + PR).[158] Actinomycin D as a single agent produced a 37% response rate with long-term survivals.[159] Samuels and Howe[160] reported a 52% CR + PR with vinblastine; Blum and colleagues showed a 32% CR + PR with bleomycin;[161] and Higby and coworkers[162] found a 28% CR with the use of cisplatin. Samuels and colleagues[163,164] combined vinblastine and bleomycin in a synergistic regimen for Stage III tumors. Vinblastine produces an arrest in the mitotic phase of the cell cycle, and bleomycin kills cells in M-phase.[165] When bleomycin was given by continuous infusion, a 52% CR was achieved. The justification for the continuous infusion was that the drug is cell-cycle specific and has a half-life of less than 2 hours.[166,167] In 1972 the Memorial Group in New York City started the first of many VAB (vinblastine, actinomycin D, and bleomycin) studies, which showed an overall response rate of 47% (22% CR + 25% PR) and a long-term disease-free rate of 13%. In VAB-II, high-dose platinum was added when it was found that prehydration and mannitol diuresis minimized renal toxicity and allowed the safe use of this highly effective agent in large doses.[168,169] Cyclophosphamide, Adriamycin, and chlorambucil were also added. The overall response rate was 96% and the CR was 62%, with a long-term disease-free rate of 45%. Einhorn and Donohue, aware of the effectiveness of single agents, combined cisplatin, vinblastine, and bleomycin (PVB) to produce a 70% CR, a 100% overall response rate, and 55% long-term disease-free survival. Patients at that time were treated for 2 years.[170] PVB combinations have come to be the standard to which other testicular treatment programs are compared. Subsequent prospective and randomized protocols by the Indiana group compared platinum with vinblastine at 0 to 4 mg/kg versus 0.3 mg/kg versus 0.2 mg/kg plus doxorubicin. The three treatment arms were comparable, with a 73% long-term CR.[171] A randomized study by the Southeastern Cancer Study Group failed to show any advantage to maintenance therapy for patients achieving a CR or NED (no evidence of disease) status after resection of benign teratoma with four courses of chemotherapy (Table 33-10).[172]

In ovarian germ cell tumors, comparison of PVB and VAC by retrospective analysis of published studies strongly suggests the superiority of PVB for ovarian germ cell tumors other than germinoma. The 1-year survival of Stage I patients is 73% with VAC and 100% with PVB, whereas with Stages II and III and recurrent patients, 1-year survival is 65% with VAC and 100% with PVB.[173] Taylor and coworkers[174] also summarized the liter

Table 33-10
PVB Regimen for Disseminated Testicular Cancer

Vinblastine	0.2 mg/kg IV d 1–2
Bleomycin	30 units IV weekly
Cisplatin	20 mg/m² IV d 1–5

Repeat every 3 weeks for 4 courses; no further maintenance if CR or NED with benign teratoma

(Einhorn LH, Williams SD, Troner M et al: The role of maintenance therapy in disseminated testicular cancer. N Engl J Med 305:727, 1981)

ature and added 14 of their patients. All 14 achieved a complete response, with only 1 having small macroscopic tumor at second-look surgery. One patient died of bleomycin toxicity; the remaining 13 were alive and disease-free from 20 months to more than 8 years. Those authors also conclude that for patients with Stages I and II disease there is no difference in survival for those with pure immature teratoma or mixed germ cell tumors treated with PVB versus VAC. There is an improved survival for patients with pure endodermal sinus tumors treated with PVB. In patients with Stage III or IV disease PVB confers an overall advantage, irrespective of cell type. PVB treatment for malignant ovarian germ cell tumors has become the new standard to which all other ovarian treatment programs in adults are compared.[175,176]

Therapeutic programs in children have confirmed many of the findings in adults. In 1976, Wolner and colleagues[177] reported almost 2-year median survival in 6 of 10 children with malignant ovarian tumors treated with surgery, radiation therapy, and chemotherapy with vincristine, actinomycin D, cyclophosphamide, and Adriamycin.[176] Cangir and coworkers showed that VAC was effective in Stages I and II ovarian tumors.[155] All 8 patients treated remained disease-free for 18 to 80+ months. Six of 37 Stage III but only 1 of 5 Stage IV patients had long-term survival. They concluded that adjuvant chemotherapy with VAC reduces the death rate significantly in children with ovarian germ cell malignancy and that radiation is not indicated in these tumors (except dysgerminoma) because they are not radiosensitive. Thomas reported 2 children with metastatic yolk sac tumors who failed VAC therapy but showed complete response to cisplatin, vinblastine, doxorubicin, and bleomycin. One child was tumor-free 2.5 years after stopping therapy; the other died with brain and bone metastases after 1 year of complete remission.[178] Green and associates reported encouraging results in 4 children with pelvic yolk sac tumors (1 testicular and 3 sacrococcygeal), all of whom responded to PVB induction, second-look surgery, and maintenance therapy for 13 months with VAC.[179] All were disease-free 7 to 22 months from diagnosis, even though one had multiple pulmonary metastases at diagnosis and one had gross residual disease after the first attempted resection. Investigators at Institut Gustave-Roussy in Villejuif, France, and Hopital General de Ninos, Buenos Aires, reported 35 children with nonseminomatous malignant germ cell tumors (12 ovarian, 6 testicular, 11 sacrococcygeal, 5 thoracic, and 1 abdominal). All children had either gross residual disease, gross lymph node involvement, or positive ascitic pleural fluid (Stage III, $N = 23$), or disseminated disease (Stage IV, $N = 12$). Treatment with vincristine, actinomycin D, cyclophosphamide, doxorubicin, cisplatin, and bleomycin led to a 63% disease-free survival with a median follow-up of 22 months (11 months to 5 years). This compares with a survival of only 21% in a similar group of patients treated from 1968 to 1977 with surgery, radiotherapy, and chemother

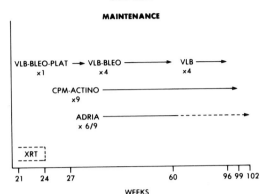

MALIGNANT GERM CELL TUMORS
CCG-861

FIGURE 33-10. Children's Cancer Group Study—861. Velban 6.5 mg/m² day 1; bleomycin 15 U/m² continuously days 1, 2, and 3; cisplatin (cis-platinum) 60 mg/m² day 3; actinomycin 0.015 mg/kg days 21–25; Cytoxan 600 mg/m² day 21; Adriamycin 40 mg/m² day 42. Repeat every 6 weeks for 2 years. Stop cisplatin after three courses and bleomycin after six courses.

Table 33-11
The CISCA$_{II}$/VB$_{IV}$ M. D. Anderson Program

CISCA
Cyclophosphamide 500 mg/m² IV d 1, 2
Doxorubicin 40–45 mg/m² IV d 1, 2
Cisplatin 100–120 mg/m² IV (2 hr) d 3

VB
Vinblastine 3 mg/m²/d IV (CI) d 1–5
Bleomycin 30 units IV (CI) d 1–5

Repeat for two courses beyond CR or a marker-negative stable mass

---

(Logothetis CJ, Samuels ML, Selig O et al: Improved survival with cyclic chemotherapy for non-seminomatous germ cell tumors of the testis. J Clin Oncol 3:326–335, 1985)

apy with methotrexate, actinomycin D, and cyclophosphamide at one of these institutions.[180] Infants with vaginal endodermal sinus tumors have been successfully treated with surgery and various combinations of VAC.[181,182]

The Children's Cancer Group recently reported 79 children with malignant germ cell tumors, excluding cranial and testicular locations and immature teratoma and germinoma histology—39% had widely disseminated metastases at diagnosis. This highly selected poor-risk group was treated with 9-week cycles of vinblastine, bleomycin, cisplatin, actinomycin D, cyclophosphamide, and doxorubicin (Fig. 33-10). A complete response was seen in 69% and a partial response in 29%; only 4% had no response or progressive disease. Four years from diagnosis, 45% remain free of disease. All 9 patients with Stages I and II ovarian tumors are disease-free.[183]

Prevention of relapse, treatment of the small percentage of initial failures, and salvage therapy for those who relapse, along with reduction of the considerable toxicity of chemotherapy regimens that so successfully treat most patients with germ cell tumors, are the goals of present clinical research. The epipodophyllotoxin VP-16-213 has single-agent activity in cisplatin-refractory patients. It is a spindle poison that induces a premitotic block and could, therefore, also be synergistic with bleomycin.[184] It has been used in salvage regimens with

cisplatin with or without bleomycin or doxorubicin.[171] The toxicities are significant, especially pulmonary toxicity from bleomycin. VP-16 and cisplatin offer potentially curative therapy for patients with resistant germinal tumors. In adults with refractory germ cell tumors who had been treated with intensive cisplatin-containing regimens, 80% responded to VP-16 plus cisplatin (43% CR, 27% PR), and 23% remained continuously disease-free for 20 to 39 months after completion of therapy in a Southeastern Cancer Study Group trial.[185]

High-dose platinum and ifosfamide regimens have been useful in salvage therapy and in front-line therapy for some high-risk adult groups.[186-189] Use of high-dose platinum is based on the steep dose–response relationship of cisplatin[169] and also on the fact that nephrotoxicity, but not antitumor effect, can be reduced in animals if cisplatin is administered in saline.[190] A program for advanced nonseminomatous germ cell tumors of the testis with cyclophosphamide, doxorubicin, cisplatin (CISCA) and a modified combination of vinblastine and bleomycin (VB) has produced a 92% CR with no relapses for a mean follow-up of 139 weeks (Table 33-11). No cardiotoxicity, clinical pulmonary toxicity, or renal failure occurred.[191] These studies may have applicability to pediatric germ cell malignancies, where long-term survival remains to be proven in reasonably large numbers of patients to be at the 80% to 90% range reported in adults with nonseminomatous testicular cancer.[180,183,192,193] A majority of children with germ cell tumors have extragonadal disease, so they may be like adults, in whom extragonadal disease carries a poorer prognosis.[194] Differences in age-related host factors and in type of pathology may account for differences in biology and response to therapy.

Increasingly aggressive approaches are being taken. High-dose melphalan, high-dose VP-16, high-dose cyclophosphamide, and rescue with autologous bone marrow transplantation have been attempted.[187,195,197] The last decade has seen malignant germ cell tumors, once almost always fatal, join the increasing rank of malignant diseases in childhood that can be cured in a majority of patients.

REFERENCES

1. Patten BM: Human Embryology, p 14. Philadelphia, Blakiston, 1947
2. Young JL, Miller RW: Incidence of malignant tumors in US children. J Pediatr 86:254–258, 1975

3. Berry CL, Keeling J, Hilton L: Teratoma in infancy and childhood: A review of 91 cases. J Pathol 98:241–252, 1969
4. Altman PR, Randolph JG, Lilly JR: American Academy of Pediatrics Surgical Section Survey—1973. J Pediatr Surg 9:389–398, 1974
5. Fraumani JF, Li FP, Dalager N: Teratomas in children: Epidemiologic features. J Natl Cancer Inst 51:1425–1430, 1973
6. Parrington JM, West LF, Povey S: The origin of ovarian teratomas. J Med Genet 21:4–12, 1984
7. Parrington JM, West LF, Povey S: Chromosome changes in germ cell tumors. In Jones WG, Ward AM, Anderson CK (eds): Germ Cell Tumors: II, pp 61–67 Oxford, Pergamon Press, 1986
8. Hart WR, Burkons DM: Germ cell neoplasms arising in gonadoblastomas. Cancer 43:669–678, 1979
9. Kingsbury AC, Frost F, Cookson CM: Dysgerminoma, gonadoblastoma and testicular germ cell neoplasia in phenotypically female and male siblings with 46XY genotype. Cancer 59:288–291, 1987
10. Goldsmith CI, Hart WR: Ataxia-telangiectasia with ovarian gonadoblasoma and contralateral dysgerminoma. Cancer 36:1838–1842, 1975
11. Block M, Gilbert E, Davis C: Metastatic neuroblastoma arising in an ovarian teratoma with long term survival: Case report and review of the literature. Cancer 54:590, 1984
12. Dement SH, Eggleston JC, Spivac JL: Associations between mediastinal germ cell tumors and hematologic malignancies: Report of two cases and review of the literature. Am J Surg Pathol 9:29–30, 1985
13. Larsen M, Evans WK, Shepherd FA: Acute lymphoblastic leukemia: Possible origin from a mediastinal germ cell tumor. Cancer 53:441–444, 1984
14. Trentini GP, Palmieri B: An unusual case of gonadic germinal tumor in a brother and sister. Cancer 33:250–255, 1974
15. Liber AF: Ovarian cancer in mother and 5 daughters. Arch Pathol 42:280–290, 1950
16. Jackson SM: Ovarian dysgerminoma in three generations. J Med Genet 4:112–113, 1967
17. Bergstrand CG, Czar B: Demonstration of a new protein fraction in serum from human fetus. Scand J Clin Lab Invest 8:174–178, 1956
18. Gitlin D, Pserricelli A: Synthesis of serum albumin, prealbumin, alpha-fetoprotein, alpha-1-antitrypsin and transferrin by the human yolk sac. Nature 228:995–997, 1970
19. Mizjewski GJ, Carter TP, Beblowski OW et al: Measurement of serum AFP in early infancy: Utilization of dried blood specimens. Pediatr Res 17:47–50, 1983
20. Abelev GI, Asseritova IV, Kraevsky N et al: Embryonal serum alpha-globulin in cancer patients: diagnostic value. Int J Cancer 2:551–558, 1967
21. Teilum G, Albrechtsen R, Norgaard-Pedersen B: The histogenetic-embryologic basis for reappearance of AFP in endodermal sinus tumors (yolk sac tumors) and teratomas. Acta Path Microbiol Scand 83:80–86, 1975
22. Talerman A, Haije WG, Baggerman L: Serum alpha-fetoprotein (AFP) in patients with germ cell tumors of the gonads and extragonadal sites: Correlation between endodermal sinus (yolk sac) tumor and raised serum AFP. Cancer 46:380–385, 1980
23. Teilum G, Albrechtsen R, Norgaard-Pedersen B: Immunofluorescent localization of alpha-fetoprotein synthesis in endodermal sinus tumor (yolk sac tumor). Acta Pathol Microbiol Scand 82:568–588, 1974
24. Norgaard-Pedersen B, Albrechtsen R, Teilum G: Serum alpha-foetoprotein as a marker for endodermal sinus tumour (yolk sac tumour) or a vitelline component of ''Teratocarcinoma.'' Acta Pathol Microbiol Scand 83:573–589, 1975
25. Vaitukatis JL, Braunstein GD, Ross GT: A radioimmunoassay which specifically measures human chorionic gonadotropin in the presence of human luteinizing hormone. Am J Obstet Gynecol 113:751–758, 1972
26. Perlin E, Engler JE, Edson M, et al: The value of serial measurements of both human chorionic gonadotropin and alpha-fetoprotein for monitoring germ cell tumors. Cancer 37:215–219, 1976
27. Kinumaki H, Takeuche H, Nakamura K: Serum lactate dehydrogenase isoenzyme-1 in children with yolk sac tumor. Cancer 56:178–181, 1985
28. Tucker DF, Oliver RTD, Ellard GA, et al: Testicular tumor marker applications of monoclonal antibodies to placental-like alkaline phosphatase. In Jones WG, Ward AM, Anderson CK (eds): Germ Cell Tumors II, pp 139–145. Oxford, Pergamon Press, 1986
29. Quirke P, Dyson JED, Sutton CK et al: Assessment of germ cell tumors of testis by flow cytometry and histopathology. In Jones WG, Ward AM, Anderson CK (eds): Germ Cell Tumors II, pp 45–54. Oxford, Pergamon Press, 1986
30. Ooosterhuis JE, de Jong B, Cornelisse CJ et al: Karyotyping and DNA flow cytometry of mature residual teratoma after intensive chemotherapy of disseminated nonseminomatous germ cell tumor of the testis: A report of two cases. Cancer Genet Cytogenet 22:149–157, 1986
31. Seeger RC, Brodeur BM, Sather H et al: Multiple copies of the N-myc oncogene in neuroblastomas are associated with rapid tumor progression. N Engl J Med 313:1111–1116, 1985
32. Sikora K, Evan G, Stewart J et al: Detection of the c-myc oncogene product in testicular cancer. Br J Cancer 52:171–176, 1985
33. Dehner LP: Gonadal and extragonadal germ cell neoplasia of childhood. Hum Pathol 14:493–511, 1983
34. Gonzalez-Crussi F: Extragonadal teratomas. Atlas of Tumor Pathology, 2nd Series, fascicle 18. Washington, DC, Armed Forces Institute of Pathology, 1982
35. Dehner LP: Gonadal and extragonadal germ cell neoplasms-teratomas in childhood. In Finegold M, Benington JL (eds): Pathology of Neoplasia in Children and Adolescents. Major Problems in Pathology, vol 18, pp 282–312. Philadelphia, WB Saunders, 1986
36. Scully RE: Tumors of the ovary and maldveloped gonads. Atlas of Tumor Pathology, 2nd Series, fascicle 16. Washington, DC, Armed Forces Institute of Pathology, 1979
37. Mostofi FK, Price EB Jr: Tumors of the male genital system. Atlas of Tumor Pathology, 2nd Series, fascicle 8. Washington, DC, Armed Forces Institute of Pathology, 1973
38. Taylor CR: Immunomicroscopy: A diagnostic tool for the surgical pathologist. In Bennington JL (ed): Major Problems in Pathology, vol 19, pp 208–215, Philadelphia, WB Saunders, 1986
39. Teilum G: Special Tumors of Ovary and Testis, 2nd ed. Copenhagen, Munksgaard, 1976
40. Witzleben CL, Bruninga G: Infantile choriocarcinoma: A characteristic syndrome. J Pediatr 73:374–378, 1968
41. Takeda A, Ishizuka T, Goto T, et al: Polyembryoma of ovary producing alpha-fetoprotein and HCG: Immunoperoxidase and electron microscopic study. Cancer 49:1878, 1982
42. Scully RE: Gonadoblastoma. A gonadal tumor related to the dysgerminoma (seminoma) and capable of sex hormone production. Cancer 6:455–463, 1953
43. Scully RE: Gonadoblastoma. A review of 74 cases. Cancer 25:1340–1356, 1970
44. Robboy SJ, Miller T, Donahue PK et al: Dysgenesis of testicular and streak gonads in the syndrome of mixed gonadal dysgenesis. Hum Pathol 13:700–716, 1982
45. Talerman A: The pathology of gonadal neoplasms composed of germ cells and sex cord stroma derivatives. Pathol Res Pract 170:24, 1980
46. Potter EL, Craig JM: Pathology of the Fetus and the Infant, 3rd ed. Chicago, Year Book Medical Publishers, 1975
47. Willis RA: The Borderland of Embryology and Pathology. Washington, DC, Butterworths, 1962
48. Isaacs H Jr: Perinatal (congenital and neonatal) neoplasms: A report of 110 cases. Pediatr Pathol 3:165–216, 1985
49. Mahour GH, Landing BH, Woolley MM: Teratomas in children: Clinicopathologic studies in 133 patients. Z Kinderchir 23:365–380, 1978
50. Robboy SJ, Scully RE: Ovarian teratoma with glial implants on the peritoneum. Hum Pathol 1:643–653, 1970
51. Favara BE, Franciosi RA: Ovarian teratoma and neuroglial implants on the peritoneum. Cancer 31:678–682, 1973
52. Nogales FF Jr, Favara BE, Major FJ et al: Immature teratoma of the ovary with a neural component (''solid'' teratoma): A clinicopathologic study of 20 cases. Hum Pathol 7:625, 1976
53. Ehren IM, Mahour GH, Isaacs H Jr: Benign and malignant ovarian tumors in children and adolescents: A review of 63 cases. Am J Surg 147:339–344, 1984
54. Dehner LP: Neoplasms of the fetus and neonate. In Naeye RL, Kissane JM, Kaufman N (eds): Perinatal Diseases. International Academy of Pathology Monograph no. 22, pp 286–345. Baltimore, Williams & Wilkins, 1981
55. Tapper D, Lack EE: Teratomas in infancy and childhood. A 54 year experience at the Children's Hospital Medical Center. Ann Surg 198:398, 1983
56. Partlow WF, Taybi H: Teratomas in infants and children. AJR 112:155–166, 1971
57. Carney JA, Thompson OP, Johnson CL et al: Teratomas in children: Clinical and pathological aspects. J Pediatr Surg 7:271, 1972
58. Bale PM, Painter DM, Cohen D: Teratomas in childhood. Pathology 7:208, 1975
59. Mahour GH, Landing BH, Woolley MM: Teratomas in children: Clinicopathological studies in 133 patients. Z Kinderchir 23:365, 1978

60. Marsden HB, Birth JH, Swindell R: Germ cell tumors of childhood: A review of 137 cases. J Clin Pathol 34:872, 1981

61. Whalen T, Mahour G, Landing B, Woolley MM: Sacrococcygeal teratomas in infants and children. Am J Surg 150:373, 1985

62. Altman RP, Randolph JG, Lilly JR: Sacrococcygeal teratoma: American Academy of Pediatrics Surgical Section Survey, 1973. J Pediatr Surg 9:389–398, 1974

63. Lemire RJ, Graham CB, Beckwith JB: Skin-covered sacrococcygeal masses in infants and children. J Pediatr 79:948–954, 1971

64. Werner JL, Taybi H: Presacral masses in children. Am J Roentgenol Radium Ther Nucl Med 109:403, 1970

65. Lassman JP, James CCM: Lumbosacral lipomas: Critical survey of 26 cases submitted to laminectomy. J Neurosurg Psychiatry 30:174, 1967

66. Ravitch MM: Sacrococcygeal teratoma. In Ravitch MM, Welch K, Benson CD et al (eds): Pediatric Surgery, vol 2, pp 1118–1127. Chicago, Year Book Medical Publishers, 1979

67. Luna MA, Valenzuela-Tamariz J: Germ-cell tumors of the mediastinum, postmortem findings. Am J Clin Pathol 65:450–454, 1976

68. Martini N, Golbey RB, Hajdu SE et al: Primary mediastinal germ cell tumors. Cancer 33:763–769, 1974

69. Sickles E, Belliveau RE, Wiernik PH: Primary mediastinal choriocarcinoma in the male. Cancer 33:1196–1203, 1974

70. Truong LD, Harris L, Mattioli C: Endodermal sinus tumor of the mediastinum: A report of seven cases and review of the literature. Cancer 58:730–739, 1986

71. Karl SR, Dunn J: Posterior mediastinal teratomas. J Pediatr Surg 20:508, 1985

72. Norohna PA, Noronha R, Rao DS: Primary anterior mediastinal endodermal sinus tumors in childhood. Am J Pediatr Hematol Oncol 7:312–316, 1985

73. Robertson J, Fee H, Mulder D: Mediastinal teratoma causing life-threatening hemoptysis. Am J Dis Child 135:148–150, 1981

74. Honicky R, dePapp EW: Mediastinal teratoma with endocrine function. Am J Dis Child 126:650, 1973

75. Gooneratne S, Keh P, Sreekanth S et al: Anterior mediastinal endodermal sinus tumor in a female infant. Cancer 56:1430, 1985

76. Kuzur ME, Cobleigh MA, Greco A et al: Endodermal sinus tumor of the mediastinum. Cancer 50:766–774, 1982

77. Lack EE, Weinstein HJ, Welch KJ: Mediastinal germ cell tumors in childhood. A clinical and pathologic study of 21 cases. J Thorac Cardiovasc Surg 89:826–835, 1985

78. Carter D, Bibro MC, Touloukian RJ: Benign clinical behavior of immature mediastinal teratoma in infancy and childhood: Report of two cases and review of literature. Cancer 49:398–402, 1982

79. Cairo MS, Grosfeld JL, Weethan RM: Gastric teratoma: Unusual cause for bleeding of the upper gastrointestinal tract in the newborn. Pediatrics 67:721–724, 1981

80. Purvis JM, Miller R, Blumenthal B: Gastric teratoma. J Pediatr Surg 14:86, 1979

81. Oronez NG, Manning JT Jr, Alyala AG: Teratoma of the omentum, abdominal wall and peritoneum. Cancer 51:955–958, 1983

82. Witte D, Kissane J, Askin F: Hepatic teratomas in children. Pediatr Pathol 1:81, 1983

83. Engel R, Eakins R, Fletcher B: Retroperitoneal teratoma: Review of the literature and presentation of an unusual case. Cancer 22:1068, 1968

84. Pantoja E, Lilobe T, Gonzales-Flores B: Retroperitoneal teratomas: Historical review. J Urol 115:520, 1976

85. Case Records of the Massachusetts General Hospital. N Engl J Med 303:1466, 1981

86. Lack EE, Travis WD, Welch KJ: Retroperitoneal germ cell tumors in childhood. Clinical and pathologic study of 11 cases. Cancer 56:602–608, 1985

87. Jennings CD, Powell DE, Walsh JW et al: Suprasellar germ cell tumor with extracranial metastasis. Neurosurgery 16:9–12, 1985

88. Tavcar D, Robboy SJ, Chapman P: Endodermal sinus tumor of the pineal region. Cancer 45:2646–2651, 1980

89. Dariano JA, Furlanetto TW, Costa SS et al: Suprasellar germinoma: Unusual clinical presentation. Surg Neurol 15:294–297, 1981

90. Gay JC, Janco RL, Lukens JN: Systemic metastases in primary intracranial germinoma. Cancer 55:2688, 1985

91. Packer RJ, Sutton LN, Rosenstock JG et al: Pineal region tumors of childhood. Pediatrics 74:97, 1984

92. Wara WM, Jenkin DT, Evans A et al: Tumors of the pineal and suprasellar region: Childrens Cancer Study Group Treatment Results 1960–1975. Cancer 43:698–701, 1979

93. Allen JC, Nissellbalum J, Epstein F: Alpha-fetoprotein and human chorionic gonadotropin determination in cerebrospinal fluid. J Neurosurg 51:368–374, 1979

94. Bagshawe KD, Harland S: Immunodiagnosis and monitoring of gonadotropin-producing metastases in the central nervous system. Cancer 38:112–118, 1976

95. Berlin AJ, Rich LS, Hahn JF: Congenital orbital teratoma. Childs Brain 10:208, 1983

96. Chang DF, Dallos RI, Walton OS: Congenital orbital teratoma: Report of a case with visual preservation. J Pediatr Ophthalmol Strabismus 17:88, 1980

97. Beller FK, Nienhaus H, Schmundt V et al: Endodermal germ cell carcinoma (endodermal sinus tumor) of the vagina in infant girls. J Cancer Res Clin Oncol 94:295–306, 1979

98. Young R, Scully RE: Endodermal sinus tumor of the vagina: A report of nine cases and review of the literature. Gynecol Oncol 18:380–392, 1984

99. Allyn OL, Silverberg SG, Salzberg AM: Endodermal sinus tumor of the vagina: Report of a case with a 7 year survival and literature review of so called "mesonephromas." Cancer 27:1231–1238, 1971

100. Andersen WA, Savio H, Durso N et al: Endodermal sinus tumor of the vagina. The role of primary chemotherapy. Cancer 56:1025–1027, 1985

101. Rezaizadeh M, Woodruff JD: Endodermal sinus tumor of the vagina. Gynecol Oncol 6:459–463, 1978

102. Bronsther B, Abrams MW: Ovarian tumors in childhood. Pediatr Annu 4:565, 1975

103. Lucraft HH: Ovarian tumors in children. A review of 40 cases. Clin Radiol 30:279–285, 1979

104. Barber RK: Ovarian cancer. Cancer 36:149, 1986

105. Richardson GS, Scully RE, Nikrui N et al: Common epithelial cancer of the ovary. N Engl J Med 312:415, 1985

106. McCrann DJ, Marchant DJ, Bardawil WA: Ovarian carcinoma in three teenage siblings. Obstet Gynecol 43:132–137, 1974

107. Hong SJ, Lurain JR, Tsukada Y et al: Cystadenocarcinoma of the ovary in a 4-year old. Cancer 45:2227–2230, 1980

108. Copeland LJ: Malignant gynecologic tumors. In Sutow WW, Fernbach DJ and Vietti TJ (eds): Clinical Pediatric Oncology, 3rd ed, p 745. St Louis, CV Mosby, 1984

109. Breen JL, Maxson WS: Ovarian tumors in children and adolescents. Clin Obstet Gynecol 20:607–623, 1977

110. Orr PS, Gibson A, Young OG: Ovarian tumors in children: A 27 year review. Br J Surg 132:5887–5889, 1986

111. Mahour GH, Woolley GH, Landing BH: Ovarian tumors in children: A 33 year experience. Am J Surg 63:367–370, 1976

112. Kurman RJ, Norris HJ: Embryonal carcinoma of the ovary: A clinicopathologic entity distinct from endodermal sinus tumor resembling embryonal carcinoma of the adult testis. Cancer 38:2420–2433, 1976

113. Altwein JE, Smith PJ, Basing R: Kindliche hoden tumoren: Inzidenz, entstehung, klinik and therapie. Akt Urol 12:139–145, 1981

114. Ericsson NO, Ivemaark B, Qvist O: Testicular and paratesticular tumors in infants and children. Z Kinderchir 6:308–314, 1969

115. Bergami F, Caione P, Rivosecchi M: Testicular tumors in infancy and childhood. Z Kinderchir 20:57–70, 1976

116. Tsuji I, Nakajima F, Nishida T et al: Testicular tumors in children. J Urol 110:127–129, 1973

117. Hodson JM, Perez-Mesa C: Infantile adenocarcinoma of the testis. J Urol 89:706–708, 1963

118. Sabio H, Burgart EO Jr, Farrow GM et al: Embryonal carcinoma of the testis of childhood. Cancer 34:2118–2121, 1974

119. Teoh TB, Steward JK, Willis RA: The distinctive adenocarcinoma of the infant's testis: An account of 15 cases. J Pathol Bacteriol 80:145–156, 1960

120. Manger D, Campbell JS, Wigglesworth FW: Testicular adenocarcinoma with clear cells occurring in infancy: A distinctive tumor. Can Med Assoc J 86:485–488, 1962

121. Young PG, Mount BM, Foote FE et al: Embryonal adenocarcinoma in the prepubertal testis: A clinicopathologic study of 18 cases. Cancer 26:1065–1075, 1970

122. Huntington RW Jr, Morgenstern NL, Sargent JA et al: Germinal tumors exhibiting the endodermal sinus pattern of Teilum in young children. Cancer 16:34–47, 1963

123. Teilum G: Endodermal sinus tumors of ovary and testis: Comparative morphogenesis of the so-called mesonephroma ovarii (Schiller) and extraembryonic (yolk sac-allantoic) structures of the rat's placenta. Cancer 23:1092, 1959

124. Weissbach L, Altwein JE, Stiens R: Germinal testicular tumors in childhood. Eur Urol 10:73–85, 1984

125. Exelby PR: Testicular cancer in children. Cancer 45:1803–1809, 1980

126. Li FP, Fraumeni JF Jr: Testicular cancers in children. J Natl Cancer Inst 44:1575–1582, 1972

127. Shapiro SR, Rabinowtiz J, Konrad P et al: Focal infarction of the testicle in a child simulating testicular tumor. J Urol 118:485–486, 1977

128. Whitaker RH: Management of the undescended testis. Br J Hosp Med 4:25–37, 1970

129. Martin DC: Malignancy in the cryptorchid testis. Urol Clin North Am 9:371–376, 1982

130. Burney BT, Klatte EC: Abdominal ultrasound and computed tomography in testicular cancer. In Einhorn LH (ed): Testicular Tumors: Management and Treatment, pp 83–115. New York, Masson Publishing, 1980

131. Einhorn LH, Williams SD: The management of disseminated testicular cancer. In Einhorn LH (ed): Testicular Tumors: Management and Treatment, p. 119. New York, Masson Publishing, 1980

132. Brosman SA: Testicular tumors in prepubertal children. Urology 13:581–588, 1979

133. Sabio H, Burgert EO Jr, Farrow GH et al: Embryonal carcinoma of the testis in childhood. Cancer 34:2118–2121, 1974

134. Matsumoto K, Nakauchi K, Fujita K: Radiation therapy for embryonal carcinoma of testis in childhood. J Urol 104:778–780, 1970

135. McCullough DL, Carlton CE, Seybold HM: Testicular tumors in infants and children—Report of 5 cases and evaluation of different modes of therapy. J Urol 105:140–148, 1971

136. Johnson DE, Kuhn CR, Guinn GA: Testicular tumors in children. J Urol 104:940–943, 1970

137. Tefft M, Vawter GF, Mitus A: Radiotherapeutic management of testicular neoplasms in children. Radiology 88:457–465, 1967

138. Bracken RB, Johnson DE, Cangir A et al: Regional lymph nodes in infants with embryonal carcinoma of testis. Urology 11:376–379, 1978

139. Duckett JW: Surgical aspects of testis tumors in children. In Hays DM (ed): Pediatric Surgical Oncology, pp 189–204. Orlando, Grune & Stratton, 1986

140. Hopkins GB, Jaffe N, Colodny A et al: The management of testicular tumors in children. J Urol 120:95, 1978

141. Kaplan WE, Firlit CF: Treatment of testicular yolk sac carcinoma in the young child. J Urol 126:663–664, 1981

142. Williams SD, Einhorn LH: Clinical Stage I testis tumors—The medical oncologist's view. Cancer Treat Rep 66:15–18, 1982

143. Whitmore WF Jr: Surgical treatment of clinical stage I nonseminomatous germ cell tumors of the testis. Cancer Treat Rep 66:5–10, 1982

144. Glatstein E: Optimal management of clinical stage I nonseminomatous testicular carcinoma: one oncologist's view. Cancer Treat Rep 66:11–14, 1982

145. Sogani PC, Whitmore WF, Herr HW et al: Orchiectomy alone in the treatment of clinical stage 1 nonseminomatous germ cell tumor of the testis. J Clin Oncol 2:267–270, 1974

146. Javadpour N, Moiley J: Alternative to retroperitoneal lymphadenectomy with preservation of ejaculation and fertility in stage I nonseminomatous testicular cancer: a prospective study. Cancer 55:1604–1605, 1985

147. Freel JH, Cassir JF, Pierce VIS et al: Dysgerminoma of the ovary. Cancer 43:798–205, 1975

148. Norris HJ, Zirkin HJ, Benson WL: Immature (malignant) teratoma of the ovary: A clinical and pathologic study of 58 cases. Cancer 37:2359–2372, 1976

149. Gonzalez-Crussi F, Winkler RF, Mirkin DL: Sacrococcygeal teratomas in infants and children: relationship of histology and prognosis in 40 cases. Arch Pathol Lab Med 102:420–425, 1978

150. Li MC, Hertz R, Spencer DB: Effect of methotrexate on choriocarcinoma and chorioadenoma. Proc Soc Exp Biol Med 96:361, 1956

151. Li MC, Whitmore WF, Golbey RB et al: Effects of combined drug therapy in treatment of testicular tumors. JAMA 174:245, 1960

152. Gallion H, Van Nagell JR, Powell DF: Therapy of endodermal sinus tumor of the ovary. Am J Obstet Gynecol 135:447–451, 1978

153. Wider FA, Marshall JR, Basridin CAE et al: Sustained remissions after chemotherapy for primary ovarian cancer containing choriocarcinoma. N Engl J Med 280:1439–1442, 1969

154. Smith JP, Rutledge F et al: Advances in chemotherapy of gynecologic cancer. Cancer 36:669–674, 1975

155. Cangir AI, Smith J, van Eys J: Improved prognosis in children with ovarian cancers following modified VAC (vincristine sulfate, dactinomycin and cyclophosphamide) chemotherapy. Cancer 42:1234–1238, 1978

156. Slayton RE, Hreshchyshyn MM, Silverberg SC et al: Treatment of malignant ovarian germ cell tumors: Response to vincristine, dactinomycin and cyclophosphamide. Cancer 42:390–398, 1978

157. Gershenson DM, Del Junco G, Herson J et al: Endodermal sinus tumor of the ovary: The M.D. Anderson experience. Obstet Gynecol 61:194–202, 1983

158. Hill GJ, Sedransk N, Rochlin D et al: Mithramycin (NSC 24559) therapy of testicular tumors. Cancer 30:900–908, 1972

159. Merrin CE, Murphy GP: Metastatic testicular carcinoma: single-agent chemotherapy (actinomycin D) in treatment. NY State J Med 654–657, 1974

160. Samuels ML, Howe CD: Vinblastine in the management of testicular cancer. Cancer 25:1009, 1970

161. Blum RH, Careter SS, Agre K: A clinical review of bleomycin—A new antineoplastic agent. Cancer 31:903, 1973

162. Higby DJ, Wallace HJ, Albert D et al: Diaminodichloro-platinum in chemotherapy of testicular tumors. J Urol 112:100, 1974

163. Samuels ML, Johnson DE, Holoye PY: The treatment of stage III metastatic germinal neoplasia of the testis with bleomycin combination therapy. Proc Am Assoc Cancer Res 14:89, 1973

164. Samuels ML, Holoye PY, Johnson DE: Bleomycin combination chemotherapy in the management of testicular neoplasia. Cancer 36:318, 1975

165. Barranacao SC, Humphrey RM: The effects of bleomycin on survival and cell progression in Chinese hamster cells in vitro. Cancer Res 31:1218–1223, 1971

166. Sikic BI, Collins JM, Mimnaugh EG et al: Improved therapeutic index of bleomycin when administered by continuous infusion in mice. Cancer Treat Rep 62:2011–2017, 1978

167. Samuels ML, Johnson DE, Holoye PY: Continuous intravenous bleomycin (NSC-125066) therapy with vinblastine (NSC 49842) in stage III testicular neoplasia. Chemother Rep 59:563–570, 1975

168. Cvitkovic E, Spaulding J, Bethune V et al: Improvement of cis-dichlorodiammineplatinum (NSC-119875): Therapeutic index in an animal model. Cancer 39:1357–1361, 1977

169. Hayes DM, Cvitkovic E, Golbey RB et al: High dose cis-platinum diammine dichloride: Amelioration of renal toxicity by mannitol diuresis. Cancer 39:1372–1381, 1977

170. Einhorn LH, Donohue JP: Cis-diaminodichloroplatinum, vinblastine and bleomycin combination chemotherapy in disseminated testicular cancer. Ann Intern Med 87:293, 1977

171. Einhorn LH, Williams SD: Chemotherapy of disseminated testicular cancer: a random prospective study. Cancer 46:1339–1344, 1980

172. Einhorn LH, Williams SD, Troner M et al: The role of maintenance therapy in disseminated testicular cancer. N Engl J Med 305:727, 1981

173. Carlson RW, Sikic BI, Turbow MM et al: Combination cisplatinum, vinblastine, and bleomycin chemotherapy (PVB) for malignant germ-cell tumors of the ovary. J Clin Oncol 10:645–651, 1983

174. Taylor MH, Depetrillo AO, Turner RA: Vinblastine, bleomycin and cisplatin in malignant germ cell tumors of the ovary. Cancer 56:1341–1349, 1985

175. Williams SD, Einhorn LH: Etoposide salvage therapy for refractory germ cell tumors: An update. Cancer Treat Rev 9:67–71, 1981

176. Lederman GS, Garnick MB, Canellos GP et al: Chemotherapy of refractory germ cell cancer with etoposide. J Clin Oncol 1:706–709, 1983

177. Wollner N, Exelby PR, Woodruff JM et al: Malignant ovarian tumors in childhood: Prognosis in relation to initial therapy. Cancer 37:1953–1964, 1976

178. Thomas WJ, Kelleher JF, Duval/Arnould B: Successful treatment of metastatic extragonadal endodermal sinus (yolk sac) tumor in childhood. Cancer 48:2371–2374, 1981

179. Green DM, Brecher ML, Grossi M et al: The use of different induction and maintenance chemotherapy programs for the treatment of advanced yolk sac tumors. J Clin Oncol 1:111–116, 1983

180. Flamant F, Schwartz L, Delons E et al: Nonseminomatous malignant germ cell tumors in children: Multidrug therapy in stages III and IV. Cancer 54:1687–1691, 1984

181. Copeland LJ, Sneige N, Ordonez G et al: Endodermal sinus tumor of the vagina and cervix. Cancer 55:2558–2565, 1985

182. Andersen WA, Sabio H, Durso N et al: Endodermal sinus tumor of the

vagina: The role of primary chemotherapy. Cancer 55:1025–1027, 1985

183. Ablin AR, Krailo M, Ramsay N et al: Malignant germ cell tumors in childhood: An outcome analysis. Proc Am Soc Clin Oncol 5:213, 1986

184. Rosencweig M, Von Holl DD, Henny JE et al: VM-26 and VP-16-213: A comparative analysis. Cancer 40:334–342, 1977

185. Hainsworth JD, Williams SD, Einhorn LH et al: Successful treatment of resistant germinal neoplasms with VP-16 and cisplatin: Results of a southeastern cancer study group trial. J Clin Oncol 3:666–671, 1985

186. Trump DL, Hortvet L: Etoposide and very high dose cisplatin: Salvage therapy for patients with advanced germ cell neoplasms. Cancer Treat Rep 69:259–261, 1985

187. Ozols RF, Deisseroth AB, Javadpour N et al: Treatment of poor prognosis nonseminomatous testicular cancer with a ''high-dose'' platinum combination chemotherapy regimen. Cancer 51:1803–1807, 1983

188. Loehrer PJ, Einhorn LH, Williams SD: VP-16 plus ifosfamide plus cisplatin as salvage therapy in refractory germ cell cancer. J Clin Oncol 4:528–536, 1986

189. Lederman GS, Garnick MB: Possible benefit of doxorubicin in patients with refractory germ cell cancer. Cancer 58:2393–2398, 1986

190. Litterst CL: Alterations in the toxicity of cis-dichlorodiammineplatinum and in tissue localization of platinum as a function of NaCl concentration in the vehicle of administration. Toxicol Appl Pharmacol 61:99–108, 1981

191. Logothetis CJ, Samuels ML, Selig O et al: Improved survival with cyclic chemotherapy for non seminomatous germ cell tumors of the testis. J Clin Oncol 3:326–335, 1985

192. Brodeur GM, Howrasth CB, Pratt CB: Malignant germ cell tumors in 57 children and adolescents. Cancer 48:1890–1898, 1981

193. Hawkins EP, Finegold MJ, Hawkins HK et al: Nongerminomatous malignant germ cell tumors in children: A review of 89 cases from the Pediatric Oncology Group, 1971–1984. Cancer 58:2579–2584, 1986

194. Israel A, Bosl GJ, Golbey RB et al: The results of chemotherapy for extragonadal germ-cell tumors in the cisplatin era: the Memorial Sloan-Kettering cancer center experience (1975–1982). J Clin Oncol 2:1073–1078, 1985

195. Blijham G, Spitzer G, Cirrincione C et al: The treatment of advanced testicular carcinoma with high dose chemotherapy and autologous marrow support. Eur J Cancer 17:441–444, 1981

196. Biron P, Phillip T, Maraninchi D et al: Massive chemotherapy and autologous bone marrow transplantation in progressive disease of nonseminomatous testicular cancer: A Phase II study on 15 patients. In Dicke KA, Spitzer G, Sander AR (eds): Proceedings, First International Symposium, Autologous Bone Marrow Transplantation, pp 203–210. University of Texas M. D. Anderson Hospital, 1985

197. Pico JL, Droz JP, Gouyette A et al: High dose chemotherapy followed by autologous bone marrow transplantation for poor prognosis non seminomatous germ cell tumors. Proc Am Soc Clin Oncol 4:107, 1985

thirty-four

Endocrine Tumors

George P. Chrousos

Endocrine tumors include neoplasms arising from endocrine organs, regardless of whether they secrete hormones, and tumors secreting hormones, regardless of the tissue of origin. The secretion of hormones by neoplasms of nonendocrine origin or by neoplasms arising from glands that normally secrete different hormones is called *ectopic* production (for overviews, see Refs. 1–11).

Endocrine tumors in children represent approximately 4% to 5% of all neoplasms observed in this age group.[5,12-17] Most of these tumors do not secrete hormones. Approximately 40% to 45% of childhood endocrine tumors arise from the gonads (germ cell tumors, testicular and ovarian tumors) (see Chap. 33), 30% from the thyroid gland, and 20% from the pituitary gland. The rest arise from all the other glands, including the parathyroids, the adrenal cortex and medulla, and the gastroenteropancreatic unit, as well as from nonendocrine tissues.

The majority of endocrine tumors in childhood are benign or low-grade malignant. A small percentage of gonadal and germ cell tumors, thyroid neoplasms, and adrenocortical tumors are characterized by high-grade malignancy. Malignant carcinomas of the parathyroids, the adrenal medulla, and the gastroenteropancreatic unit are rare.

A large percentage of endocrine tumors in childhood are of embryonic origin (germ cell tumors, craniopharyngiomas). Whereas the majority of neoplasms in this age group are sporadic, a small portion of certain endocrine tumors are familial, with some transmitted in a Mendelian fashion. Medullary carcinomas of the thyroid and pheochromocytomas can present in a familial fashion. Either or both may be associated with other endocrine tumors (pituitary gland, the parathyroids, the adrenal cortex, and the gastroenteropancreatic unit) or with tumors of the peripheral nervous system (mucosal neuromas). These associations constitute the syndromes of multiple endocrine neoplasia (MEN), which are genetically transmitted.[7-10] Pheochromocytomas can be associated with the phacomatoses (neurofibromatosis, tuberous sclerosis).

In this chapter, the endocrine tumors of the hypothalamic–pituitary unit, the thyroid gland, the parathyroid glands, the adrenal cortex and medulla (and adrenergic ganglia), and the gastroenteropancreatic unit (insulinomas, gastrinomas, glucagonomas, VIPomas, and somatostatinomas) are reviewed. Several features of these tumors are summarized in Table 34-1. Gonadal and germ cell tumors and the carcinoids are reviewed in Chapters 33 and 35. I also review briefly the ectopic hormone-secreting tumors and the MEN syndromes.

TUMORS OF THE HYPOTHALAMIC–PITUITARY UNIT

Definitions

Most pituitary tumors arise from the anterior pituitary (adenohypophysis) and are benign (adenomas). The majority do not secrete hormones. The most frequent

(*Text continues on p. 737*)

Table 34-1
*Endocrine Tumors in Children and Adolescents**

Tumor	Hormone Secreted	Incidence†	Genetics	Behavior, Spread	Syndrome	Diagnosis	Therapy	Ectopic Syndrome Equivalent
Hypothalamic–Pituitary Unit								
Hormone secreting adenomas								
Prolactinoma	PRL	Rare	MEN I	Benign, local	Galactorrhea, delayed puberty	↑PRL	Bromocriptine, surgery	PRL
Corticotropinoma	ACTH	Rare	MEN I	Benign, local	Cushing's syndrome	↑UFC, DST, CRH test, BIPSS	Surgical excision, radiotherapy, adrenalectomy, enzyme inhibitors, adrenolytics	CRH, ACTH
Somatotropinoma	GH	Rare	MEN I	Benign, local	Gigantism, acromegaly	↑GH, OGTT	Bromocriptine surgery, radiation	GRH, GH
Gonadotropinoma	LH, FSH	Rare		Benign, local	Precocious puberty	↑LH, FSH	Surgery	hCG
Thyrotropinoma	TSH	Rare		Benign, local	Hyperthyroidism	↑TSH, T₃, T₄	Surgery	
Nonhormone-secreting tumors								
Chromophobe adenomas	—	Rare		Benign, local	Pituitary hormone deficiencies	Pituitary CT, MRI	Surgery, radiation	
Craniopharyngiomas	—	1%		Benign, local	Pituitary hormone deficiencies	Pituitary CT, MRI	Surgery, radiation	
Thyroid								
Adenomas	±T₄, T₃	Common		Benign	± Hyperthyroidism	T₃, T₄, TSH, scintiscan	Surgery, T₄	AVP
Carcinomas	±T₄, T₃	1.5%		Malignant (differing spectrum) lymph nodes, lungs	Cervical lymphadenopathy, goiter	Thyroid scintiscan Chest x-ray, CT	↑Thyroglobulin	Thyroidectomy, ¹³¹I, T₄
Papillary		70–80% of thyroid cancers		Malignant (differing spectrum)	Cervical lymphadenopathy, goiter			

Follicular (mixed)		10–20% of thyroid cancers		Malignant (differing spectrum)	Cervical lymphadenopathy, goiter			
Anaplastic		Rare		Malignant (differing spectrum)	Cervical lymphadenopathy, goiter			
Medullary (C-cell)	Calcitonin	5–10% of thyroid cancers	Familial, MEN II$_a$ and II$_b$	Malignant (differing spectrum)	Cervical lymphadenopathy, goiter, diarrhea	↑Calcitonin (pentagastrin, calcium stimulation) ↑CEA	Thyroidectomy, regional node resection	Parathormone or ectopic PTH-like syndrome (OAF)

Parathyroids

Adenomas–hyperplasia	PTH	Rare	MEN I and II$_a$, familial hyperplasia–adenomatosis	Benign	Primary hyperparathyroidism (secondary and tertiary hyperparathyroidism)	↑Calcium, ↓phosphorus, nl or ↑PTH	Parathyroidectomy	
Carcinomas	PTH	Extremely rare (<1% of parathyroid tumors)	MEN I	Malignant–local lymph nodes, lungs and bone	Primary hyperparathyroidism	↑Calcium, ↓phosphorus, nl or ↑PTH	Parathyroidectomy	

Adrenal Cortex

Adenomas–hyperplasia	Cortisol, aldosterone, androgens, estrogens	Rare	MEN I	Benign	Cushing's syndrome, Cohn's syndrome, virilization, feminization	Hormone measurements, CT/MRI	Adrenalectomy	Adrenal rests (liver, testes, ovaries)
Micronodular disease	Cortisol	Rare		Benign	Cushing's syndrome	Hormone measurements, CT/MRI	Bilateral adrenalectomy	
Carcinomas	±Cortisol, aldosterone, androgens, estrogens	Rare		Malignant–local, liver, lungs, bone	Cushing's syndrome, Cohn's syndrome, virilization, feminization	Hormone measurements, CT/MRI	Adrenalectomy–tumor excision, o,p'DDD, aminogluethimide, ketokonazole, RU 486	

(continued)

Table 34-1 *(continued)*

Tumor	Hormone Secreted	Incidence†	Genetics	Behavior, Spread	Syndrome	Diagnosis	Therapy	Ectopic Syndrome Equivalent
Adrenal Medulla (and Adrenergic Ganglia)								
Adenomas–hyperplasia	Epinephrine, norepinephrine (dopamine)	Rare	Familial MEN II$_a$, II$_b$, phacomatoses	Benign	Hypertension	Epinephrine, norepinephrine, metanephrines, VMA, CT/MRI, angiography	Adrenalectomy Phenoxybenzamine ± propranolol Phentolamine, methyldopa	
Malignant pheochromocytoma	Epinephrine, norepinephrine (dopamine)	Rare (<2% of pheochromocytomas)		Malignant–local, liver, lungs, bone	Hypertension			
Gastroenteropancreatic Unit								
Insulinoma	Insulin	Rare	MEN I	Benign–malignant	Hypoglycemia	Fasting, CT/MRI Angiography	Surgery Diazoxide	
Gastrinoma	Gastrin	Rare	MEN I	Benign	Zollinger–Ellison syndrome	Plasma gastrin, secretin test	Surgery; H$_2$ blockers	
Glucagonoma	Glucagon	Rare	MEN I	Benign–malignant	Hyperglycemia, wasting, necrolytic rash	Plasma glucagon	Surgery	
VIPoma	VIP	Rare	MEN I	Benign	Watery diarrhea, hypokalemia	Plasma VIP	Surgery	Ectopic VIP (lungs–neural tumors)
Somatostatinoma	Somatostatin	Rare	—	Benign	Hyperglycemia	Plasma somatostatin	Surgery	

* ACTH = adrenocorticotropic hormone; AVP = vasopressin; BIPSS = bilateral inferior petrosal sinus sampling; CEA = carcinoembryonic antigen; CRH = corticotropin-releasing hormone; DST = dexamethasone suppression test; FSH = follicle-stimulating hormone; GH = growth hormone (somatotropin); GRH = growth hormone-releasing hormone; LH = luteinizing hormone; MEN = multiple endocrine neoplasia; nl = normal; OAF = osteoclast-activating factor; OGTT = oral glucose tolerance test; PRL = prolactin; PTH = parathormone; T$_3$ = triiodothyronine; T$_4$ = thyroxin; TSH = thyroid-stimulating hormone; UFC = urinary free cortisol; VIP = vasoactive intestinal polypeptide; VMA = vanilmandelic acid.
† Percentage of childhood cancers unless otherwise indicated.

tumor of pituitary origin is the nonhormone-secreting cranio-pharyngioma, which represents approximately 5% of all intra-cranial tumors in childhood (see also Chap. 24). The remain-ing tumors are rare (Table 34-1) (for overviews, see general Refs. 18–29).

Pituitary tumors are called *intrasellar* when they do not extend beyond the boundaries of the pituitary fossa and *supra-sellar* when they extend above the diaphragma sellae. Intrasel-lar tumors are called *microadenomas* when they are not de-tectable by radiologic techniques and *macroadenomas* when they are. Pituitary tumors that secrete hormones take the name of the hormone they secrete and the ending *-oma.* Thus, these tumors are divided into prolactinomas, corticotropinomas, so-matotropinomas, gonadotropinomas, and thyrotropinomas, se-creting respectively prolactin (PRL), corticotropin (ACTH), somatotropin (growth hormone, GH), gonadotropins (lutein-izing hormone, LH; follicle stimulating hormone, FSH), and thyrotropin (TSH). Each of these tumors produces a character-istic syndrome because of its secretion of excesses of the hor-mone(s) (see below). Nonhormone-secreting pituitary ade-nomas are not stained by either acid or basic stains and are called *chromophobe adenomas.*

Hypothalamic hormone-secreting tumors are extremely rare. Most reported cases have been described in adults.[30–32]

Clinical Presentation: General

All pituitary tumors may cause symptoms arising from pressure of the adjacent structures. Thus, headaches, visual distur-bances, and manifestations from one or more hypothalamic–pituitary hormone deficiencies can be the presenting symp-toms. The only exception is the development of hyperprolactinemia, a result of deficiency of the hypothalamic tubero-infudibular dopaminergic system, which is responsible for suppression of prolactin secretion.[24] Intracranial hyperten-sion and hydrocephalus may be found in these patients. The usual finding on ophthalmologic examination is bitemporal constriction of the visual fields (Fig. 34-1) because most su-prasellar pituitary tumors impinge on the crossing fibers of the optic chiasm. Other changes in the visual fields are possible, depending on the location of the tumor.

Deficiency of one or more pituitary or hypothalamic hor-mones may result from pressure by the pituitary tumor. De-pending on the hormone affected, different symptoms may arise. The tests required for the diagnosis of pituitary deficien-cies are summarized in Table 34-2 (for more details, see Refs. 33 and 34). The most frequently affected hormone is somato-tropin. Deficiency of this hormone leads to poor growth, hypo-glycemia, or both in younger children. The deficiency is diag-nosed by measuring the plasma GH concentration after stimulation with arginine–insulin, L-dopa, or glucagon. The attainment of symptomatic hypoglycemia (usually obtained by administration of 0.1 U/kg of regular insulin as an intravenous bolus) is a prerequisite for evaluating lack of response. Two abnormal tests (plasma GH elevations <6 ng/ml) are required for the diagnosis.

The next most frequently affected hormone is ACTH. De-ficiency of this hormone leads to secondary adrenal insuffi-ciency characterized by weakness, orthostatic hypotension, hyponatremia, and hypoglycemia in younger children. It is a life-threatening condition that should be diagnosed early. Diagnosis is made by measuring plasma cortisol 1 hour after adrenal stimulation with an intravenous bolus of 10 μg of ACTH 1–24 (Cortrosyn) per kilogram. A normal response (plasma cortisol ≥18 μg/dl) indicates the presence of non-atrophied adrenal glands. Pituitary ACTH deficiency would

have led to adrenal atrophy and a diminished cortisol re-sponse.

Gonadotropin and TSH deficiencies may occur in patients with pituitary tumors. The former is manifest as pubertal arrest or regression in children already in puberty or as delayed pu-berty in children affected prepubertally. Plasma LH and FSH are low for the age in these children, and bone age is delayed. Thyrotropin deficiency is manifest as poor growth, diminished performance at school, constipation, cold intolerance, dry skin, and other symptoms of hypothyroidism. Measurements of serum total T_4, free T_4, and TSH are required for the diagnosis.

Extension of a pituitary tumor into the hypothalamic para-ventricular nucleus may result in vasopressin (AVP) deficiency and diabetes insipidus (polyuria, polydipsia, dehydration, hy-pernatremia). The diagnosis of diabetes insipidus may require the water deprivation test.

Hormone-Secreting Tumors: Specific Endocrine Manifestations

Prolactinomas

Most of these tumors are microadenomas. Excess PRL secre-tion can cause galactorrhea and suppress the reproductive sys-tem in both males and females. The latter is manifest as de-layed or arrested puberty in both sexes. Primary or secondary amenorrhea may be caused by hyperprolactinemia. The diag-nosis is made by measuring plasma PRL concentrations (30 ng/ml is the upper limit of normal for most laboratories) (Table 34-3).[10,27,35–38] Prolactinomas may be seen in children with the McCune–Albright syndrome (precocious puberty, cu-taneous cafe-au-lait spots, and polyostotic fibrous dysplasia).

Corticotropinomas

Most of these tumors are microadenomas. Diffuse corticotro-phic cell hyperplasia has been described also. Excess pituitary ACTH secretion (Cushing's disease) produces hypercortiso-lism and the characteristic features of Cushing's syndrome, including growth arrest, pubertal arrest, weight gain, the char-acteristic phenotype (moon facies, buffalo hump, accumula-tion of supraclavicular fat), acne, purple skin striae, and weak-ness. Many patients complain of mood disturbances.[38,39]

The diagnosis of hypercortisolism is made by measuring 24-hour urinary free cortisol or 17-hydroxysteroid excretion. The latter should be corrected per gram of creatinine. The diagnosis of pituitary Cushing's disease is made by a series of endocrine tests (Table 34-3), which include the following:

1. The Liddle dexamethasone suppression test.[38,39] The patient has six sequential 24-hour urinary collections for measurement of 17-hydroxysteroids. The first two collections provide the baseline. During the following 2 days, the patient is given 2 mg of dexamethasone per day orally (30 μg/kg per day) divided every 6 hours. During the last 2 days, the patient is given 8 mg of dexamethasone per day orally (120 μg/kg per day) divided every 6 hours. Patients with Cushing's disease show characteristic suppression of their 17-hydroxysteroid excretion to less than 50% of baseline levels only on the high dose of dexamethasone. At this dose, neither patients with ectopic ACTH secretion nor patients with cortisol-secreting adrenal adenomas or carcinomas respond with suppression.
2. The corticotropin-releasing hormone (CRH) test.[38–41] Measurements of plasma ACTH and cortisol are obtained before and after intravenous administration of ovine CRH

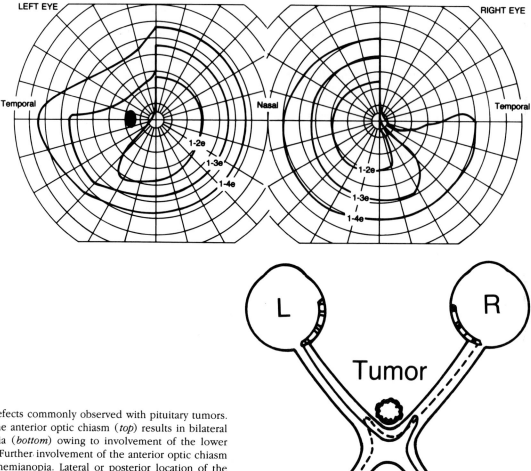

FIGURE 34-1. Visual field defects commonly observed with pituitary tumors. Impinging of the tumor on the anterior optic chiasm (*top*) results in bilateral superior temporal quadranopia (*bottom*) owing to involvement of the lower anterior crossing nasal fibers. Further involvement of the anterior optic chiasm results in bilateral temporal hemianopia. Lateral or posterior location of the tumor results in contralateral nasal or bilateral inferior temporal defects of the visual fields, respectively.

(1 μg/kg). Most patients with pituitary Cushing's syndrome respond with elevations of ACTH and cortisol, whereas most patients with the other categories of Cushing's syndrome do not respond.

3. Bilateral inferior petrosal sinus sampling.[41,42] The two inferior petrosal sinuses, which drain the pituitary gland, are catheterized, and blood is obtained simultaneously from both as well as from a peripheral vein. The presence of a concentration difference between either of the petrosal sinuses and the peripheral vein (ratio ≥1.6) confirms the pituitary source of ACTH. A difference in concentration in the two petrosal sinuses (ratio ≥1.6) suggests the location of the adenoma.

Somatotropinomas

Most of these tumors are macroadenomas. Excess GH secretion before epiphyseal fusion leads to gigantism and that after closure of the epiphyses to acromegaly. In addition to development of the characteristic phenotypes, hypersecretion of GH can be associated with carbohydrate intolerance or frank diabetes, arthropathy, and the carpal tunnel syndrome.[43–46] The diagnosis is made by measuring plasma levels of GH before and after ingestion of glucose (1.7 g/kg; glucose tolerance test). In the patients, the plasma GH concentration does not decrease after glucose administration as it does in normal persons (Table 34-3). Acromegaly has been observed in children with the McCune–Albright syndrome.

Table 34-2
Endocrine Tests for Evaluation of Pituitary Deficiencies

Hormone*	Tests	Response
GH	Arginine–insulin stimulation	GH >6 ng/ml
	L-Dopa stimulation	GH >6 ng/ml
	Glucagon stimulation	GH >6 ng/ml
ACTH	Cortrosyn stimulation	Cortisol ≥18 μg/dl
LH, FSH	LH–releasing hormone stimulation	LH and FSH nl for age
TSH	Plasma T$_4$, FT$_4$, T$_3$, TSH, TBG	—
	TRH stimulation	TSH nl for age
AVP	Water deprivation	Urinary osmolality ↓
		Serum osmolality ↑

* For abbreviations, see Table 34-1; also, FT$_4$ = free thyroxine; TBG = Thyroxine-binding globulin.

Gonadotropinomas

Hypersecretion of LH in a prepubertal boy leads to precocious puberty because of the excess stimulation of the Leydig cells and excessive production of testosterone. Gonadotropinomas secreting FSH are more frequent. Their presence is associated with visual disturbances and hypogonadism.[47,48]

Table 34-3
Endocrine Tests for Evaluation of Hormone Excess in Children and Adolescents

Hormone	Test*	Levels or Response
PRL	Serum PRL	High
ACTH	Urinary free-cortisol excretion	High
	Dexamethasone suppression test	Abnormal suppression
	CRH stimulation test	See text
	Bilateral inferior petrosal sinus sampling	See text
GH	Serum GH	High
	Oral glucose tolerance test	Abnormal suppression
Gonadotropins (LH, FSH)	Serum LH, FSH	High
	LH-releasing hormone stimulation	High
TSH	TSH, T_4, FT_4, T_3, TBG	High, TBG normal
	TRH stimulation test	See text
AVP	Plasma vasopressin	High
Thyroxine–triiodothyronine	Serum TSH, T_4, FT_4, T_3, TBG	TSH low, others high
Calcitonin	Calcitonin	High
	Calcium stimulation	Abnormal elevations
	Pentagastrin stimulation	Abnormal elevations
PTH	Parathormone	High
	Calcium, phosphorus	High Ca, low P
Cortisol	Urinary free cortisol, 17-hydroxysteroids	High
	Dexamethasone suppression test	Abnormal suppression
	CRH stimulation test	See text
Aldosterone	Urinary aldosterone	High
	Plasma aldosterone	High
Catecholamines	Urinary metanephrines, VMA	High
	Plasma epinephrine, norepinephrine	High
	Glucagon stimulation test	High catecholamine response
	Histamine stimulation test	High catecholamine response
	Clonidine suppression test	Abnormal suppression
Insulin	Plasma insulin and glucose	High insulin, low glucose
	Fasting (24–72 hours)	High insulin, low glucose
Gastrin	Plasma gastrin	High
	Secretin test	Abnormal elevations
Glucagon	Plasma glucagon	High
VIP	Plasma VIP	High
Somatostatin	Plasma somatostatin	High

* FT_4 = free thyroxine; TBG = thyroxine-binding globulin. Others as in Table 34.1.

Thyrotropinomas

Hypersecretion of TSH leads to hyperthyroidism. Plasma TSH, total T_4, and free T_4 are elevated (Table 34-3).[50-52] This acquired syndrome should be differentiated from the genetic syndrome of pituitary thyroid-hormone resistance with which it is biochemically identical.[53,54] Thyrotropinomas are macroadenomas and can be detected by radiologic procedures and magnetic resonance imaging (MRI). Unlike patients with thyroid-hormone resistance, patients with thyrotropinomas usually do not respond to TRH.[53,54]

Nonsecreting Tumors

Chromophobe Adenomas

These are rare tumors that are usually discovered because of their space-occupying manifestations, which may include elevations of plasma PRL concentrations as a result of pituitary stalk compression and insufficient dopaminergic suppression of the lactotrophs.[55] Occasionally, these tumors secrete glycoprotein-hormone (TSH, LH, FSH) α-subunit molecules, which are hormonally inactive.[56,57]

Craniopharyngiomas

These tumors arise from remnants of Rathke's pouch, the anlagen of the adenohypophysis. They are cystic tumors that expand locally. About two-thirds are calcified and can be seen on plain radiographs. They generally cause problems related to their location and pressure on or destruction of local structures. Headaches, visual disturbances, and panhypopituitarism are frequent manifestations. Occasionally, mild hyperprolactinemia is present because of pituitary stalk compression and inability of hypothalamic (tuberoinfudibular) dopamine to reach the lactotrophs and act as a PRL-inhibiting factor.[58-60]

Treatment and Prognosis

Surgery is always recommended for tumors that enlarge rapidly and threaten vision, regardless of the type of the tumor. Smaller tumors may be removed by transsphenoidal surgery. Larger tumors with suprasellar extensions may be removed by craniotomy or combined craniotomy and transsphenoidal surgery. Frequently, complete tumor excision is not feasible, and mere debulking is attempted.

Transspheroidal surgery is generally a low-risk procedure (Fig. 34-2).[61-64] Complications are rare and include total hypophysectomy and panhypopituitarism, caverous sinus hemorrhage, transient or permanent diabetes insipidus, cerebrospinal fluid leaks, and meningitis.

Transsphenoidal adenomectomy is the treatment of choice for corticotropinomas.[65] Lateralization of the plasma ACTH concentration difference during bilateral sampling of the inferior petrosal sinuses usually helps with localizing the adenoma to one side of the pituitary.[41,42] A proportion of corticotropinomas cannot be distinguished from normal pituitary tissue during surgery, in which case, hemipituitectomy of the side of the higher ACTH concentration is recommended. Cure is frequent, with no development of other pituitary hormone deficiencies.

Bromocryptine, a drug with potent dopamine agonist activity, is the treatment of choice for prolactinomas.[66,67] Doses ranging from 2.5 to 15 mg per day are frequently sufficient to correct the hyperprolactinemia and cause regression of the tumor. Years of treatment may be required for permanent cure. Bromocryptine, usually at higher doses (up to 25 mg/day), is occasionally helpful in the treatment of somatotropinomas and chromophobe adenomas.[68]

Generally, the pituitary adenomas and the craniopharyngiomas are radioresistant. However, radiotherapy in doses as high as 5000 cGy divided into 200-cGy fractions is given for the treatment of corticotropinomas and somatotropinomas if surgery has been unsuccessful.[38,39,69,70] Radiotherapy of craniopharyngiomas following subtotal excision may decrease the incidence of recurrences.

Corticotropinomas respond relatively well to radiation, with about 70% to 80% of children cured 1 to 2 years following therapy.[38,39,69] An alternative to radiation therapy is bilateral adrenalectomy. Patients are then committed to life-long glucocorticoid and mineralocorticoid replacement. The recommended doses are for hydrocortisone 12 to 15 mg/m² per day and for 9α-fluorocortisone 50 to 150 μg per day. In approximately 15% of patients so treated, Nelson's syndrome (pituitary ACTH-secreting macroadenoma, hyperpigmentation) develops within the 10 years after the adrenalectomy.[71] If the visual system is threatened, transsphenoidal surgery or radiation therapy is indicated.

Adrenolytic agents such as o,p′-DDD (mitotane or steroidogenesis enzyme inhibitors aminoglutethimide, metyra-

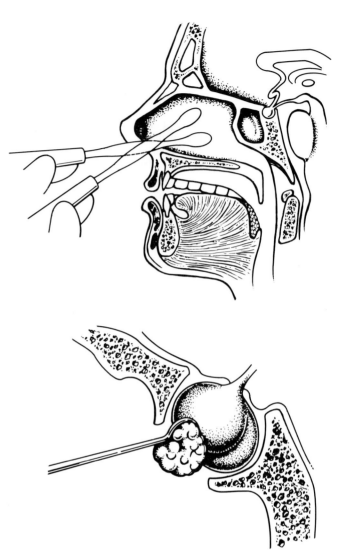

FIGURE 34-2. Transsphenoidal surgery. **Top.** The pituitary gland is approached through the sphenoid sinus. **Bottom.** Transsphenoidal exposure of the pituitary gland and adenomectomy. (Modified from Hardy J: Transsphenoidal surgery of hypersecreting pituitary tumors. In Kohler PO, Ross GT (eds): Diagnosis and Treatment of Pituitary Tumors, p 179. New York, American Elsevier, 1973)

pone trilostane, ketoconazole) may be employed also to control tne hypercortisolism.[38,39,72-75] Patients tolerate most of these drugs poorly, with ketoconazole being the best tolerated (10–15 mg/kg per day). This drug has some hepatotoxicity, however, and liver function should be monitored in patients receiving it.

When pituitary tumors are associated with pituitary hormone deficiencies, replacement treatments should be instituted. Such deficiencies may be absent before but develop after surgery. The replacement treatments include GH (0.2 U/kg subcutaneously three times weekly) for GH deficiency, hydrocortisone (oral 12–15 mg/m² per day basally or 30–100 mg/m² per day orally or parenterally during significant stress) for adrenal insufficiency, and thyroxine (2.2 μg/kg per day orally) for hypothyroidism. Testosterone enanthate (200 mg intramuscularly every 2 weeks) and one of various estradiol-progestin combinations may be employed for the treatment of male and female hypogonadism, respectively. DDAVP (0.1 ml intranasally as needed) is the treatment of choice for diabetes insipidus. Aqueous AVP (Pitressin) is available for subcutaneous administration (for more details on hormonal replacement therapies in children, see Refs. 1, 2, and 5).

The prognosis of patients with pituitary tumors is generally good. These tumors are benign, although some have a particular tendency to invade adjacent structures. Macroadenomas or craniopharyngiomas with suprasellar extensions are frequently difficult to remove completely. Treatment of these tumors by surgery or irradiation may add to the endocrine morbidity. Monitoring of visual function is crucial.

THYROID TUMORS

Definitions

Thyroid tumors are divided into adenomas and carcinomas (see Table 34-1).[76–79] Both adenomas and carcinomas can be hormone secreting, but the great majority of these tumors are hormonally inactive. Medullary carcinoma, a particular form of thyroid carcinoma that arises from the parafollicular cells (C cells) of the thyroid, produces calcitonin. Thyroid nodules can be spontaneous or associated with hyperstimulation of the thyroid by TSH or thyroid-stimulating immunoglobulins (TSI). The former are seen in situations such as iodopenic goiter or Hashimoto's thyroiditis, whereas the latter are seen in Graves' disease or mixed Graves'–Hashimoto's states. Only one nodule in 200 might harbor a thyroid cancer in adults, but the ratio in children may be much higher.

Thyroid carcinomas are malignant. Despite their histologic appearance, however, the clinical course is frequently benign.

Epidemiology and Genetics

Thyroid carcinomas represent approximately 1.5% of all tumors before the age of 15 and 7% of the tumors of the head and neck in childhood. Two-thirds of the cases occur in girls, with a peak incidence between 7 and 12 years.[80–91]

The role of neck irradiation in the development of thyroid cancer is not questioned.[85,92–100] Doses exceeding 150 cGy exert a carcinogenic effect with an average latency between irradiation and the appearance of thyroid carcinoma of 7 years. The incidence of thyroid cancer has decreased since the mid-1960s, when widespread application of radiotherapy to the neck was discontinued. The radiation was given in the neonatal period for enlarged thymus and later for tonsillitis, adenoid hypertrophy, pharyngitis, and skin diseases of the face and neck.

Medullary carcinomas of the thyroid can be familial. They also can be isolated or associated with MEN II[a] and II[b][7–10,101–104] (see below). At least 30% to 50% of medullary carcinomas are of the familial type, transmitted in an autosomal dominant mode. The rest occur sporadically.

Pathology

Most thyroid carcinomas in childhood are differentiated tumors.[80–91] Rarely, undifferentiated (anaplastic) carcinomas are found. Various differentiated types of thyroid carcinoma have been recognized, and different types may be found in combination. The relevant features of the various pathologic subtypes are noted in Table 34-4.

Papillary carcinoma is characterized by disseminated cancer foci in the gland.[77] The epithelial cells are arranged in the form of papillae containing fibrous tissue and vessels. Lymphocytic foci and psammoma bodies can also be found. This form occurs in younger children.

Follicular carcinoma is characterized by adenomatous, follicular formations of cells.[77] Nuclear abnormalities, capsular invasion, or vascular invasion differentiate this tumor from ordinary adenoma. This type of thyroid carcinoma occurs in older children.

Mixed forms of thyroid carcinoma are considered by some authors to be the most common. Most mixed types are included in the papillary cancer classification even if 90% of the specimen appears to be follicular.

Anaplastic (giant and spindle cell) carcinomas are extremely rare in children. They are characteristically undifferentiated and rapidly growing.[77]

Medullary carcinomas account for approximately 5% to 10% of all thyroid carcinomas. They are solid tumors composed of islets of regular undifferentiated-looking cells with abundant granular cytoplasm. The stroma contains abundant fibrotic tissue and various quantities of amyloid-like substance.[77,102]

Table 34-4
Types of Thyroid Carcinoma in Children and Adolescents

	Papillary (Mixed*)	Follicular	Anaplastic	Medullary
Incidence (% of total)	70	20	Rare	5–10
Age at onset (years)	<7	>7	Any	Any
Hormonal activity	—	— $(+T_3,T_4)$ $(+T_3,T_4)$	—	Calcitonin
Metastatic spread	Local, cervical and upper mediastinal lymph nodes, lungs	Local invasion, regional lymph nodes	Highly aggressive	Local invasion; regional lymph nodes; Lungs, bones, liver

* Most of these tumors are classified as papillary carcinomas.

Patterns of Spread

Local cervical and upper mediastinal lymph-node involvement by papillary cancer occurs in more than 50% of patients without necessarily implying a poorer prognosis.[80-91] The commonest site for distant metastases is the lung, and at least 20% of children with papillary thyroid cancer have pulmonary metastases at the time of diagnosis. Bone metastases from papillary cancers are uncommon, as are metastases to any site below the diaphragm.

Follicular carcinomas may be locally invasive but metastasize to regional lymph nodes far less commonly than do papillary cancers. However, they are more likely to spread to bone. Follicular carcinomas are more likely to be functional than are papillary cancers and may produce T_4, T_3, or both.

Anaplastic carcinomas of the thyroid are extremely malignant. They may evolve from a previously diagnosed papillary cancer. The growth of this type of carcinoma is explosive and may be accompanied by hypercalcemia.

Medullary carcinomas of the thyroid can invade locally or metastasize into the regional lymph nodes. Pulmonary, bone, and liver metastases can also be seen.

Clinical Presentation

The most common presenting complaint is anterior cervical adenopathy (see Chap. 5). The cervical mass may be discrete and may have been neglected for years before the physician decides to obtain a biopsy specimen. Frequently, the mass has been diagnosed as lymphadenitis or as a congenital branchial cyst. The second most common symptom is a firm, palpable thyroid nodule, either isolated or associated with a cervical lymph node. The combination of adenopathy and a thyroid nodule is found in approximately 50% of the cases. The patients are predominantly euthyroid, although rarely hyperthyroidism is seen.

Methods of Diagnosis

Tests of thyroid function usually confirm euthyroidism. Thyroid scintigrams performed with ^{125}I or ^{99}Tc usually show parenchyma with normal uptake and one or more "cold" nodules (Fig. 34-3). Rarely, "hot" nodules are seen. Discrepancies can be present between scintigrams taken with ^{125}I and ^{99}Tc. Very small nodules may not be imaged by one or both of the techniques. Chest radiographs or chest computed tomography (CT) should be obtained to look for metastases. Very high titers of antithyroglobulin or antimicrosomal antibodies make Hashimoto's thyroiditis likely, whereas low titers are not helpful diagnostically (Fig. 34-3).

A basal serum calcitonin assay can be helpful in pointing toward or away from medullary carcinoma. If the result is equivocal, or if suspicion of medullary carcinoma is high, a stimulation test using pentagastrin or calcium infusion should be performed. A stimulated calcitonin concentration three times higher than the upper limit of normal suggests the presence of medullary cancer or C-cell hyperplasia, a precancerous condition.[105]

It appears that, in general, the best single diagnostic test for the diagnosis of thyroid nodules is fine-needle aspiration.[106-108] The specimen obtained by this procedure may be unsatisfactory, however, in which case, a biopsy specimen obtained by excision of the enlarged cervical lymph node or of the isolated thyroid nodule may be required. For younger children, a biopsy rather than a fine-needle aspiration procedure is recommended.

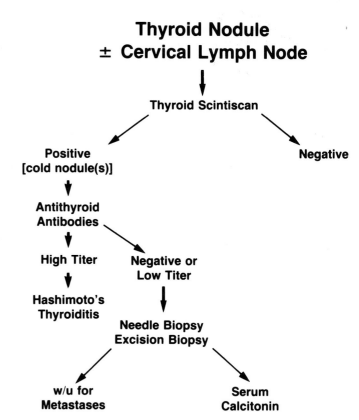

FIGURE 34-3. A proposed flow diagram for the diagnostic evaluation of thyroid nodules in children and adolescents.

Treatment

Surgery

Surgery is the treatment of choice for thyroid carcinoma.[76,77,79,109-114] Total thyroidectomy is not recommended except for obvious bilateral disease and for medullary cancer. The surgeon should decide whether to perform simple excision of an isolated nodule or of an entire lobe with resection of the isthmus. This practice diminishes the incidence of permanent morbidity (recurrent laryngeal nerve injury, hypoparathyroidism) associated with total thyroidectomy.

A similar conservative practice is recommended for lymph node dissection. The surgeon bases the decision on the appearance of the suspected lymph node chains and perhaps also on intraoperative examination of frozen sections. With this approach, the recurrent laryngeal nerve, jugular, carotid, and spinal chains are explored successively on the side of the nodule. The lymph node chains of the isthmus and the superior mediastinal nodes are usually removed.

Postoperatively, all patients are given replacement doses of thyroxine (2.2 μg/kg per day) to suppress TSH[115,116] and thus eliminate the growth-promoting effects of this hormone on the tumor.

Radioiodine

After surgical treatment of differentiated thyroid cancer, the decision whether to administer ^{131}I must be made. Most differentiated thyroid tumors take up ^{131}I, which provides high levels of radiation to the cancer cells. The presence of cancer outside the confines of the thyroid is a definite indication for such therapy. Because more than 20% of children will have lung metastases at the time of diagnosis that may or may not be apparent on chest radiographs, ^{131}I therapy is generally recommended in children.

Therapeutic doses of ^{131}I for metastases are administered only after ^{131}I dosimetry, thyroid ablation therapy, or both have been performed.[116-124] A formal dosimetry study is performed to determine whether thyroid ablation will be required before ^{131}I therapy and to select the therapeutic dose of the radioisotope. After oral administration of 1 mCi of ^{131}I, neck and whole-body scans are obtained on a rectilinear scanner at 24 and 48 hours, respectively. If metastatic disease is seen outside the bed of the thyroid, a full therapeutic dose rather than an ablative dose may be given. If no metastatic disease is seen outside the bed of the thyroid, ^{131}I-induced ablation of significant residual thyroid will be required to eliminate thyroid function and cause elevations in circulating TSH. The latter then stimulates tumor uptake of ^{131}I and enhances both the probability of its detection and its therapeutic effectiveness.

After proper preparation (avoidance of iodized substances, contrast preparations) and, usually, 4 weeks after surgery or 6 weeks after discontinuation of thyroxine replacement therapy, the patient is given a standard thyroid-ablation dose of 75 mCi of ^{131}I and is discharged on no thyroxine replacement. Six weeks later, standard scanning with 1 mCi of ^{131}I is repeated. If less than 0.3% of the dose is found in the thyroid at 48 hours, thyroid ablation has been successful. This occurs in approximately 80% of the cases. Plasma TSH is elevated in these patients without their being clinically hypothyroid. If no metastases are found, the patient is started on thyroid hormone replacement.

Iodine-131 therapy for metastatic disease is administered after successful thyroid ablation. Standard fixed therapeutic doses (150–200 mCi) may be given every 3 months after scanning. Alternatively, the dose may be calculated by previous dosimetry, with excellent results.

More than half of patients are cured by ^{131}I therapy. The majority of cures are obtained by one or two therapeutic doses, although some patients may require more.

The side effects of ^{131}I include transient bone-marrow suppression (decrease of circulating leukocytes and platelets with a nadir at about 6 weeks), nausea and vomiting, sialadenitis, pain in metastatic deposits, pulmonary fibrosis, and leukemia.[77,116] The sialadenitis may be permanent and leads to deterioration of the teeth. Azoospermia may occur, as well as decreased fertility.[125] Generally, with prior dosimetry, serious complications, such as radiation-induced pulmonary fibrosis and leukemia, occur much less frequently.

Other Treatment

In general, chemotherapy or external-beam radiation for metastatic differentiated and anaplastic thyroid cancer have been disappointing.[116,126] Adriamycin is the only proven active single agent, and the results are often temporary. Local control of anaplastic cancer of the thyroid has been rare until recently with a combination of low-dose (10 μg/m^2 per week) Adriamycin and external-beam radiation (200 cGy per fractions; total 5000 cGy).[116,127] This combination has also been successful in local control of bulky recurrences of differentiated cancer.[128]

Prognosis

The prognosis of patients with differentiated thyroid carcinoma is generally good. Patients should not be overtreated with extensive surgery and ^{131}I or external-beam radiation. Frequent monitoring of patients with differentiated thyroid cancer or medullary carcinoma of the thyroid is important. Physical examination, chest radiographs, and measurement of plasma concentrations of thyroglobulin and calcitonin or carcinoembryonic antigen (CEA) are important.[129-133] Patients may survive for many years with a good quality of life.[116-124,134] Repeat surgery, ^{131}I or both may be necessary between long asymptomatic intervals.

PARATHYROID TUMORS

Definitions

Parathyroid tumors include *adenomas,* usually found in one or, rarely, two glands; *hyperplasia,* usually affecting all four glands; and *carcinomas.*[8,9,135-149] Adenomas account for approximately 80% of parathyroid tumors, hyperplasia for 20%, and carcinoma for only a few cases. Parathyroid tumors secrete parathormone (PTH), which is responsible for the syndrome of primary hyperparathyroidism.

Parathyroid hyperplasia or adenomatous changes can also occur in conditions characterized by chronic hypocalcemia.[1-5,150,151] Such states include hypovitaminosis D, intestinal malabsorption of calcium, PTH resistance, and renal insufficiency. Parathyroid hyperplasia can also be found in familial hypocalciuric hypercalcemia, a benign autosomal dominant condition that requires no parathyroid surgery.[152,153]

Epidemiology and Genetics

Primary parathyroid tumors in childhood are rare. They can occur at any age from the neonate to the young adult. Most cases are not hereditary. However, familial parathyroid adenoma–hyperplasia states can be found.[1-5,139,145] These include [1] MEN I and MEN II$_a$ when associated with neoplasia of other glands (see below); [2] hereditary diffuse hyperplasia, a congenital hyperplasia of newborn infants almost always affecting the clear cells of the parathyroid glands and transmitted by either an autosomal recessive or a dominant mode; and [3] familial hyperplasia–adenomatosis, found in a few families containing an inordinate number of members with hyperparathyroidism without other endocrine manifestations.

Pathology

A number of pathologic variants have been described in the parathyroid glands of patients with primary hyperparathyroidism.[9,135,144,154] The predominant cell in parathyroid adenomas is the chief cell. Rarely, adenomas composed of oxyphil cells or a mixed population of chief and oxyphil cells are found. Whereas the normal parathyroid contains up to 50% fat, adenomatous or hyperplastic glands contain little or no fat. Classically, a capsule and a compressed rim of normal tissue are seen. The predominant cell in parathyroid hyperplasia is the chief cell. In a small percentage of cases, hyperplasia of the clear cell, a variant of the chief cell, is observed.

In parathyroid carcinomas, the tumor is larger than adenomatous or hyperplastic parathyroids.[137,140] Histologic examination reveals infiltration of the capsule and blood vessels as well as mitoses. Carcinomas of the parathyroids are slow growing and spread locally to the lymphatics. Distant hematogenous metastases are located in the lung, liver, and bone.

Clinical Presentation

Primary hyperparathyroidism can be associated with asymptomatic hypercalcemia, fortuitously diagnosed during an electrolyte check, or with the hypercalcemic syndrome.[1-5,147,149,155]

The latter may be manifest as polydipsia, polyuria, mental confusion, pruritus, headache, keratitis petrificans, band keratitis, and disseminated calcifications. Bone pain with demineralization and resorption cysts of the phalanges, subperiosteal zones, and lamina dura in the dental alveolae, as well as skeletal deformations and fractures may be present. Renal involvement with nephrolithiasis and nephrocalcinosis may develop, as may gastric ulcers and pancreatitis.

Diagnosis

The diagnosis is confirmed by demonstrating hypercalcemia, hypophosphatemia, elevation of serum alkaline phosphatase, and inappropriately high serum concentrations of PTH that cannot be suppressed by infusion of calcium.[1-5,147,149,155] Renal function may be impaired, manifest as alkalosis, AVP resistance, and sodium wasting. The electrocardiogram shows shortening of the QT interval. Bone radiographs reveal osteitis fibrocystica and findings compatible with rickets.

Adenomas of the parathyroid can be localized preoperatively by palpation, radiographs of the esophagus, arteriography, selective venous catheterization for determination of differences in plasma PTH concentrations, ultrasound imaging, and CT.[156-160]

Treatment and Prognosis

Treatment of adenomas consists of surgical removal after careful exploration of the cervical region.[9,161-169] The medical management of hypercalcemia is described in References 3, 4, 7, 155, and 170. If an abnormal parathyroid gland is removed, a second gland should be located and excised. If the second gland is normal in size and histology, a single adenoma is most likely, and further exploration is not necessary. If hyperplasia is suspected, or if the second gland is abnormal, all parathyroid glands should be located, and all but one should be excised totally. The remaining gland should be partially excised. If no glandular abnormalities are found in the cervical region, exploration of the mediastinum should be considered.[168] Some surgeons advocate transplantation of a portion of some of the parathyroid tissue into the muscle of the forearm to avoid hypoparathyroidism from delayed vascular failure in the portion of the gland left behind.[171,172]

Parathyroid carcinomas are resistant to radiation. Surgery is the treatment of choice.[137,140] Surgical morbidity of parathyroidectomy includes recurrent laryngeal-nerve injury and permanent hypoparathyroidism.

The postoperative course of patients treated with parathyroidectomy usually includes transient hypocalcemia in the first postoperative week.[173] If the bone disease has been severe, hypocalcemia may be profound and require treatment with calcium and vitamin D. Several months may be needed to decide whether permanent hypoparathyroidism has resulted from a compromised blood supply to the remaining parathyroid tissue.

ADRENAL TUMORS

Adrenal Cortical Tumors

Definitions

Adrenocortical tumors are divided into adenomas and carcinomas.[38,39,174-176] Both adenomas[177-188] and carcinomas[189-201] can secrete hormones or be hormonally inactive. The hormones secreted include cortisol, aldosterone, androgens, and estrogens as well as steroid biosynthesis intermediates (Fig. 34-4). Generally, adenomas are far more efficient than carcinomas in producing steroid hormones.

Regardless of hormone secretion, adenomas are generally

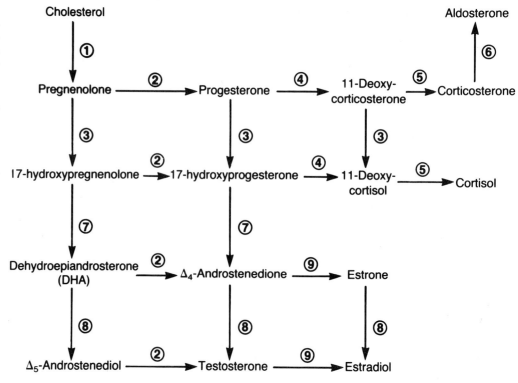

FIGURE 34-4. The adrenal steroidosynthesis pathway. Aldosterone, cortisol, androgens, and estrogens are manufactured from cholesterol after a series of enzymatic reactions. Numbers in circles represent enzymes: *1.* Cholesterol desmolase system; *2.* 3β-hydroxysteroid dehydrogenase-Δ5,Δ4-isomerase; *3.* 17α-hydroxylase; *4.* 21α-hydroxylase; *5.* 11β-hydroxylase; *6.* corticosterone methyloxidase types I and II; *7.* 17,20-desmolase; *8.* 17-ketosteroid reductase; *9.* aromatase. Enzymatic blocks are frequent in tumors, resulting in accumulation of one or more steroid precursors in plasma.

benign; carcinomas are malignant. Adrenal tumors can be found incidentally during adrenal CT or MRI scans or can be discovered in the course of evaluation for hypercortisolism, hyperaldosteronism, hyperandrogenism, or hyperestrogenism. One or more adrenal adenomas are frequently found during the course of ACTH-dependent Cushing's syndrome (Cushing's disease and, less frequently, in the ectopic ACTH-secretion syndrome). In this case, they are described as *macronodular adrenal hyperplasia* and should be distinguished from *micronodular adrenal disease,* a rare syndrome that afflicts primarily children and adolescents and is characterized by Cushing's syndrome and multiple "autonomous" cortisol-secreting small adenomas.[202-212] This syndrome is occasionally familial.[211] In one family, the disorder was associated with cardiac myxomas.[209]

Adrenal carcinomas frequently (50%–60%) secrete cortisol and, rarely, aldosterone, androgens, or estrogens.[189-201] About 40% of adrenocortical carcinomas secrete no active hormones, yet inactive steroid precursors, such as pregnenolone, 17-hydroxypregnenolone, and 11-deoxycortisol, or their metabolites can be found in the circulation and the urine, respectively. Occasionally, adrenocortical carcinomas secreting deoxycorticosterone or corticosterone cause hypokalemic alkalosis in the absence of hypercortisolism.[193,194] Generally, adrenocortical carcinomas are very inefficient in producing active hormones such as cortisol, and about 50% of them will have attained palpable size by the time they produce an endocrine syndrome.

Epidemiology

Adrenal adenomas and adrenocortical carcinomas causing Cushing's syndrome are rare tumors.[38,39] In older children and adolescents, they are responsible for 10% to 20% of cases of Cushing's syndrome, whereas in children younger than 5 years, they and ectopic ACTH-secreting tumors (see below) are together responsible for approximately 80% to 90% of cases of Cushing's syndrome.

Pathology

Adrenal adenomas are generally small, encapsulated, steroid-secreting tumors with characteristically increased smooth endoplasmic reticulum and lipid droplets inside the cells.[174-176] Frequently, few signs of malignancy can be found; however, numerous mitoses and pleomorphism can be seen without capsular invasion. Micronodular adrenal hyperplasia is characterized by the presence of small nodules dispersed in both adrenal glands.[202-212] The nodules contain a brown or black pigment. Macroscopically, they give the adrenal cortex a rugged appearance. The internodular parenchyma is hypotrophic.

In contrast, adrenocortical carcinomas are large by the time they are discovered.[174-176] They infiltrate neighboring tissues, such as the kidney capsule, and they spread locally. Cells are frequently characterized by numerous mitoses, scant cytoplasm, and pleomorphism. Areas of necrosis and hemorrhage within the tumor are common, and such hemorrhage can cause death.

Patterns of Spread

Local spread characterizes adrenocortical carcinomas. By the time they are discovered, 20% of the tumors are bilateral. Tumors spread into the kidneys, retroperitoneal and peritoneal space, the diaphragm, and the vena cava. Occasionally, the tumor will grow up into the right atrium. Intrahepatic spread is frequently observed. Lung and bone metastases are also common.

Endocrine Manifestations

The most common endocrine manifestation is Cushing's syndrome.[38,39] Distinguishing this from the other forms of Cushing's syndrome is relatively easy, as the tumor is identified radiologically by CT or MRI scans and no plasma ACTH is detectable because of pituitary ACTH suppression by the elevated plasma cortisol concentration. Adrenal adenomas or carcinomas fail to respond to low or high dexamethasone doses (see Table 34-3).

Other endocrine manifestations include hyperaldosteronism characterized by hypertension, hypokalemic alkalosis, and elevated plasma concentrations and 24-hour urinary excretion of aldosterone or other sodium-retaining corticoids. Hyperandrogenism, characterized by precocious puberty in the male or masculinization in the female, and hyperestrogenism, associated with feminization and hypogonadism in the male and precocious puberty in the female, may also be seen.

Diagnosis

Imaging procedures are the key to the diagnosis of adrenal tumors.[213-222] Adrenal ultrasound, CT, and MRI are excellent except for micronodular adrenal disease. Even in the latter condition, small rugged adrenal glands may be seen bilaterally. A radioactive iodocholesterol scan will allow imaging of cortisol-secreting adenomas but not of carcinomas or adrenal glands with micronodular disease.

Depending on the associated endocrine syndrome—hypercortisolism, hyperaldosteronism, hyperandrogenism, or hyperestrogenism—the diagnosis will be confirmed respectively by elevated 24-hour urinary free cortisol, urinary aldosterone, plasma androgens or urinary 17-ketosteroids, or plasma estrogens. In the rare case of "hyperaldosteronism" due to secretion of a steroid other than aldosterone with sodium-retaining properties, the plasma concentrations of steroid intermediates such as deoxycorticosterone and corticosterone should be measured (Fig. 34-4).

Treatment

The treatment of all primary adrenal tumors is surgical.[9,38,39,195,223-226] Adrenal adenomas should be removed with the whole ipsilateral adrenal gland, and the contralateral gland should be examined for tumor. Micronodular adrenal disease should be cured by bilateral adrenalectomy. Complete resection of the tumor is the treatment of choice for adrenal carcinoma. If complete resection cannot be achieved, as much as possible of the tumor should be removed. Solitary recurrences or metastases of adrenocortical carcinoma should be removed surgically if possible. Long-term disease-free status has been produced by complete resection of adrenocortical carcinoma, whereas long-term remissions have followed surgical resection of hepatic, pulmonary, or cerebral metastases.

Once it is known that the patient does not have surgically curable disease, therapy with o,p'-DDD is usually initiated. o,p'-DDD, an adrenocytolytic agent given at maximally tolerated oral doses (up to 16 g/day), ameliorates the endocrine syndrome in approximately two-thirds of the patients.[38,39,227-233] Tumor regression or arrest of growth has been observed on as many as one-third of the patients. However, mean survival does not appear to be altered, although there are patients with unresectable carcinomas who achieved long-term survival. The side effects include nausea, vomiting, diarrhea, skin reactions, and neurologic manifestations, primarily lethargy, somnolence, dizziness, and muscle weakness.

Occasionally, for the correction of hypercortisolism, steroid synthesis inhibitors (aminoglutethimide, metyrapone, ketoconazol) or glucocorticoid antagonists (RU 486) are required.[234-237] Patients taking mitotane (o,p'-DDD) may develop hypoaldosteronism or hypocortisolism, and fludrocortisone or hydrocortisone should be added as needed. Radiation therapy is occasionally helpful for palliation of metastases.[238]

After removal of an autonomous adrenal adenoma or carcinoma, a period of adrenal insufficiency ensues, during which glucocorticoids must be replaced.[38,39] This abnormality of the hypothalamic–pituitary–adrenal axis can last as long as 1 year. Perioperatively through the first 2 postoperative days, 100 mg per m^2 a day of hydrocortisone or its equivalent is given intravenously. Oral replacement doses of hydrocortisone, (12–15 mg/m^2 per day) are then initiated. Patients often complain of weakness at these doses. This regimen is maintained for 1 month and then tapered.

Tapering starts by doubling the daily dose and giving it on alternate days for 2 months. Then the patient is tested with a short ACTH-stimulation test (Cortrosyn 10 μg/kg intravenously with serum cortisol measured at 1 hour). If the response to this test is normal (plasma cortisol above 18 μg/dl), an attempt is made to discontinue hydrocortisone therapy. If the result is subnormal, the therapy is continued for another 2 months, and the test is repeated. During the period of adrenal insufficiency, patients should be given extra glucocorticoids in the form of replacement. During minor stress (febrile illness) they should double the daily dose. During major stress (trauma, surgery), they should be given ten times the replacement dose. All patients should wear medical alert badges indicating that they are receiving glucocorticoid replacement.

Prognosis

The prognosis of primary adrenal adenomas and micronodular adrenal disease is excellent. The prognosis of adrenal carcinoma is generally poor, with a mean survival of approximately 18 months. On occasion, highly aggressive tumors will progress rapidly over a period of a few months. Long survival (up to 10 years) has been described in some patients in whom vigilant monitoring and aggressive surgery for local recurrences or metastases was performed.

Adrenal Medulla and Adrenergic Ganglia

Definitions

Tumors of the adrenal medulla and adrenergic ganglia composed of chromaffin cells and secreting epinephrine, norepinephrine, or both and in some cases dopamine are called *pheochromocytomas*.[8,9,239-246] These tumors frequently give rise to endocrine manifestations such as hypertension, palpitations and hyperglycemia and should be contrasted with other tumors of the sympathetic system, such as neuroblastomas, which are composed of sympathetic cells and usually do not give rise to endocrine manifestations (see Chap. 28).

Epidemiology and Genetics

Pheochromocytomas of childhood are rare tumors.[247-251] They occur primarily between ages 6 and 14 years with possibly a slight predominance in boys. Less than 10% of these tumors are malignant. Most of pheochromocytomas occur sporadically;

however, they may also occur as a heritable disorder, either alone or, more commonly, associated with other endocrine tumors, particularly C-cell hyperplasia or medullary carcinoma of the thyroid (MEN II$_a$ and MEN II$_b$; see below). The transmission follows the pattern of an autosomal dominant gene with incomplete penetrance.

Pheochromocytomas can also be associated with the phacomatoses (neuro-fibromatosis, tuberous sclerosis), Lindau-von Hippel disease (retinal angiomatosis with cystic cerebellar hemangioblastomas) and Sturge–Weber disease (facial hemangioma with malformations of the brain and meninges).

Pathology and Patterns of Spread

Pheochromocytomas occur wherever chromaffin tissue is found.[239-251] Thus, in addition to the adrenal medulla, they are found in the organ of Zuckerkandl, which is particularly large in the fetus and gradually shrinks after delivery, and in association with sympathetic ganglia, nerve plexuses, and nerves. More than 95% of pheochromocytomas are found in the abdomen, and 85% of these are in the adrenal glands. Common extra-adrenal sites are sympathetic ganglia near the kidney and the organ of Zuckerkandl. The tumors may be multicentric; as many as one-third of affected children have multiple tumors.

Pheochromocytomas are usually small, most weighing less than 100 g.[239-251] They are vascular tumors and commonly contain cystic or hemorrhagic areas. The cells tend to be large and contain typical catecholamine-storage granules. Mitoses and multiple or pleomorphic nuclei can be found, as can extension of the tumor into the capsule or vessels. These findings do not indicate malignancy. Extensive local infiltration or metastases of the tumor and local recurrence or development of metastases after the initial operation can be used to define a malignancy.

The rare malignant pheochromocytomas can be associated with distant metastases. Bone, liver, lymph node, and lung metastases are the most common. Intracranial lesions have been reported also and are thought to be metastatic in origin.

Adrenal medullary hyperplasia has been described primarily in association with the MEN syndrome.

Endocrine Manifestations

Arterial hypertension is the cardinal sign, although it is found in only 70% to 80% of the cases. Most patients with functioning tumors have symptoms most of the time. These symptoms vary in intensity, however, and are perceived to be episodic or paroxysmal by half the patients. Thus, most patients with arterial hypertension have superimposed paroxysms.

Symptoms during paroxysms include headache, sweating, palpitations, anxiety, tremor, nausea and vomiting, abdominal or chest pain, and visual disturbances. Fatigue and exhaustion may follow a paroxysmal attack. Between paroxysms, increased sweating, cold hands and feet, weight loss, constipation, and low fever may be present. Polyuria and polydipsia may also be among the symptoms as a result of hyperglycemia. Clinical examination reveals hypertension and its consequences, namely increased heart size and retinopathy. Orthostatic hypotension may be observed also, a result of inadequately functioning neurovascular reflexes.

Diagnosis

Assays for catecholamines and their metabolites have simplified the diagnosis of pheochromocytoma (Fig. 34-5). In pa-

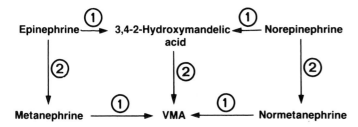

FIGURE 34-5. Catecholamine metabolism pathway. Numbers in circles represent metabolizing enzymes: *1.* Monoamine oxidase (MAO); *2.* catechol-o-methyltransferase (COMT).

tients with continuous hypertension or symptoms, plasma and 24-hour-urinary catecholamines and their metabolites are increased.[239–254] Plasma and urinary catecholamines, as well as urinary metanephrines and vanilmandelic acid, are usually sufficient to confirm the diagnosis. Malignant tumors may secrete large amounts of dopamine, leading to increased excretion of its metabolite, homovanillic acid, in the urine. Dopamine is also the principal active catecholamine produced by ganglioneuromas and neuroblastomas, leading to selectively elevated urinary homovanillic acid. It is important that during blood sampling and urine collections, drugs and foods that stimulate catecholamine secretion or interfere with the catecholamine assays be eliminated.

In patients with brief and infrequent paroxysms separated by symptom-free intervals, confirmation of the diagnosis may be difficult. Sampling of blood or timed urinary collections during a carefully observed episode may be necessary to confirm the diagnosis. In such cases, it may be useful to induce a paroxysm (see Table 34-3).[255,256] Such a procedure should be done under the supervision of an endocrinologist. Injection of 1 mg of glucagon intravenously will induce an attack in most patients with pheochromocytoma. In those cases in which glucagon fails to induce a paroxysm, histamine (25–50 μg) given intravenously may be tried. Histamine administration is frequently associated with flushing and severe headache. A diagnostic procedure of confirmatory value is the clonidine suppression test.[257] Clonidine, an α_2-adrenergic agonist, fails to decrease catecholamine secretion in patients with pheochromocytoma.

If the chemical tests are inconclusive, it may be useful to initiate a therapeutic trial with phenoxybenzamine hydrochloride, an α-adrenergic blocker (see below). A good sustained response suggests a need for reappraisal of the patient for pheochromocytoma.

Once the diagnosis of pheochromocytoma has been established, the tumor must be localized to facilitate its surgical removal. CT or MRI scanning is frequently sufficient.[217,218] A scintigraphic procedure in which ^{131}I-metaiodobenzyl-guanidine (MIBG) is injected, leads to detectable images of pheochromocytomas 24 to 72 hours later.[258,259] The procedure is specific and can detect pheochromocytomas not detected by CT. Not all pheochromocytomas will produce detectable images, however (see Chaps. 7 and 28).

Angiographic procedures (arteriography, venography) may be required for the localization of pheochromocytomas.[217] Patients should be adequately controlled with α-blockers, however, to avoid a paroxysmal attack during the procedure. Catecholamine measurements in blood samples obtained via percutaneous venous catheterization at various points along the inferior vena cava or renal, adrenal, and jugular veins can be of great value in locating small tumors.[217]

Treatment

As soon as the diagnosis has been confirmed, therapy with adrenergic antagonists should be initiated.[9,251,260–262] This treatment allows reduction of symptoms, lowering of blood pressure, amelioration of paroxysms, and expansion of the vascular bed and blood volume. A few days are required for preoperative preparation of patients. The agents used are primarily phentolamine (Regitine), a competitive α-antagonist; phenoxybenzamine (Dibenzyline), a noncompetitive α_1-adrenergic antagonist with a long effect (half-life 36 hours), and prazosin, a recently introduced α_1-antagonist with a shorter duration of action. Postural hypotension may be seen at the beginning of therapy with these agents. Occasionally, small doses of the β-blocker propranolol will be required to control tachycardia or arrhythmias. Such medical preparation of the patient decreases the risks of anesthesia and surgery.[9,263–267]

Abdominal tumors are approached transabdominally to allow exploration of both the adrenal glands and the abdominal sympathetic ganglia. When bilateral adrenal tumors are found, both adrenal glands are removed, and glucocorticoid and mineralocorticoid replacement is required (see above). The prognosis following successful surgery is excellent.

Patients with unresectable malignant tumors or metastases can be managed medically for long periods of time. Phenoxybenzamine or α-methyltyrosine, an inhibitor of tyrosine hydroxylase (the rate-limiting enzyme in catecholamine biosynthesis) can be employed. Long-term survival of such patients has been reported. Bone metastases respond well to radiation in terms of symptomatic relief. Chemotherapy or radiation therapy alone or in combination have been disappointing in patients with unresectable malignant pheochromocytomas.

TUMORS OF THE GASTROENTEROPANCREATIC UNIT

Definitions

The rare tumors that arise from endocrine cells of gastroenteropancreatic origin and that secrete peptide hormones have collectively been called *apudomas*. The term has prevailed because these tumors apparently arise from neuroectodermal cells that presumably have the ability to take up, decarboxylate, and store aromatic amine precursors (referred to as *a*mine *p*recursor *u*ptake and *d*ecarboxylation, or APUD).[8–10,268–273] Most apudomas are found in the pancreas, but a few occur in the wall of the gut or in the retroperitoneum. Most of these tumors probably arise from pluripotential stem cells (nesidioblasts) present in pancreatic ducts. Although many apudomas contain more than one type of endocrine cell and secrete more than one hormone, they are usually named after the hormone most responsible for the clinical manifestations.

The diagnosis of apudoma is made by measuring an elevated level of a gastroenteropancreatic hormone in the blood. Measurements are made on basal samples or after provocation (see Table 34-3) (see below).

Apudomas are generally difficult to find at laparotomy. Preoperative localization by CT, MRI, pancreatic arteriography, or percutaneous transhepatic venous sampling of portal vein tributaries for measurement of the suspected hormone(s) is frequently attempted.[8–10,270–274]

Approximately 50% of apudomas are malignant at the time of diagnosis. In general, apudomas are extremely rare in childhood. The most frequent type is the insulinoma. Gastrinoma, VIPoma, glucagonoma, and somatostatinoma occur less frequently. The overall incidence of concurrent endocrine tumors with apudomas is high; approximately 10% to 20% of patients with gastrinomas and 5% of patients with insulinoma are seen in the context of MEN I (see below).

Tumor Types

Insulinoma

Insulin-secreting tumors of the islets of Langerhans are called *insulinomas*.[275–281] Most of these tumors are single and benign. A small percentage are multiple, and a small percentage are malignant. Most insulinomas are located in the pancreas. Diffuse pancreatic β-cell hyperplasia or nesidioblastosis can also be associated with excess insulin secretion and hypoglycemia in children.[276,277,281–285]

The signs and symptoms are predominantly those of subacute glycopenia, primarily recurrent cerebral nervous system dysfunction at times of physical exertion or fasting. Acute hypoglycemia episodes with adrenergic discharge symptoms (sweating, hunger, tremor, seizures) can occur. Frequently, the patients are obese due to the lipogenetic and antilipolytic effects of insulin.[275–277,281]

Pancreatic β-cell tumors do not reduce their secretion of insulin in the presence of hypoglycemia.[275–277,281,285] Thus, a serum insulin level of 10 μU/ml or more with concurrent plasma glucose concentrations below 40 mg/dl suggests hyperinsulinism. Fasting of the patient with frequent sampling for plasma insulin and glucose concentrations is the best available test and provides the diagnosis in most patients. Alternatively, hypoglycemia caused by exogenous insulin (0.1 U/kg per hour intravenously) will fail to cause suppression of plasma C peptide (a marker of endogenous insulin secretion) to less than 50% the baseline value in patients with insulinomas.

The treatment of choice for insulin-secreting tumors is surgical resection. Preoperatively, and occasionally postoperatively, patients are treated with oral diazoxide (5–15 mg/kg per day, divided).[275–277,283] Side effects include sodium retention, which can be treated with concomitant thiazide administration; gastric irritation; and generalized hirsutism. If the surgeon cannot locate the tumor, a blind distal two-thirds pancreatectomy can be performed, although the success rate will be low.

Streprozotocin has proved beneficial in adult patients with islet-cell carcinomas.[286,287] Benign tumors respond poorly or not at all.

Gastrinoma

Gastrinomas are gastrin-secreting tumors that cause gastric acid hypersecretion and the Zollinger–Ellison syndrome.[8,9,288–290] Most gastrinomas occur in the pancreas; others are found in the duodenum and, rarely, in the antrum. Generally, gastrinomas are small and frequently are difficult to find even at laparotomy.

Gastrinomas are identified as malignant when metastases or blood vessel invasion is found. The histologic pattern is similar for malignant and benign tumors.

The symptoms of gastrinomas are manifestations of peptic ulcer disease and its complications. Some patients present with diarrhea due to passage of large amounts of acid into the duodenum.

Hypergastrinemia in the presence of acid hypersecretion is pathognomonic of gastrinoma.[8,9,273,274,289–294] Plasma gastrin levels usually exceed 500 pg/ml (normal <200 pg/ml). Patients with borderline hypergastrinemia (200–500 pg/ml)

should have the secretin stimulation test (2 U/kg intravenously bolus): a rise in plasma gastrin to more than 1500 pg/ml within 15 minutes is diagnostic. An upper gastrointestinal series usually shows ulceration of the duodenal bulb, prominent gastric rugal folds, and edema of the small-bowel mucosa. Selective angiography and CT scanning can sometimes demonstrate the pancreatic tumor.

Patients with gastrinomas should be started on H₂-blocking agents such as cimetidine or ranitidine.[8,9,295–300] This therapy is beneficial initially but becomes less effective with time. Tumor resection is ideal but is feasible in only a small percentage of patients. Laparotomy and removal of solitary tumors simultaneously with vagotomy may cure the patient or enhance the effectiveness of H₂-blocking agents.

Total gastrectomy remains the treatment of choice for patients with complications of ulcer disease and for those whose disease is not controlled satisfactorily by the H₂ blockers. These patients require life-long therapy with iron and vitamin B₁₂ replacement.

The prognosis of gastrinomas is generally good, and most patients lead a relatively normal life after gastrectomy. Most patients with malignant gastrinomas live for many years, whereas a few patients have aggressive, rapidly growing and metastasizing tumors. In this case, the patient may respond to streptozotocin.[301–304]

VIPoma

VIPomas are pancreatic tumors that secrete vasoactive intestinal peptide (VIP) and are associated with a syndrome of watery diarrhea, hypokalemia, and achlorhydria (pancreatic cholera).[8,9,305–314] In addition to VIP, serotonin, substance P, calcitonin, pancreatic polypeptide, and some of the prostaglandins may be present in high concentrations in the blood.

Complete removal of the tumor is curative. On occasion, the tumor cannot be found, and subtotal pancreatectomy is required. Malignant VIPomas may respond to streptozotocin.[315]

Glucagonoma

Glucagonomas are pancreatic tumors secreting glucagon.[8–10,316–323] The syndrome produced is characterized by migratory necrolytic dermatitis, weight loss, stomatitis, anemia, and hyperglycemia or frank diabetes mellitus. Glucagonomas can be benign and confined to the pancreas or malignant with metastases to the liver, regional lymph nodes, adrenal glands, or bones. Surgical removal is indicated if feasible.

Somatostatinoma

Somatostatinomas are pancreatic tumors secreting somatostatin.[8–10,324–327] The syndrome produced is characterized by hyperglycemia or frank diabetes mellitus, diarrhea, and malabsorption. Most somatostatinomas are malignant and give rise to hepatic metastases. Surgery is indicated if the disease is localized. Chemotherapy with streptozotocin may be helpful.

ECTOPIC HORMONE-SECRETING TUMORS

Definitions

Ectopically secreted hormones are peptides that cause endocrine syndromes similar to those caused by the entopically produced or exogenously administered "parent" hormones (see Table 34-1).[8–11,328,329] Frequently, however, ectopic hormones are biochemically different from the parent hormones. For example, tumors may manufacture large precursors that possess a fraction of the biologic activity of the parent hormone. Other times, the ectopic hormone cannot be confirmed as a moiety similar to the true hormone. When the chemical identity of the hormone cannot be confirmed, these hormones are given the name of the normal circulating hormone and the suffix -*like*.

Many of the ectopic hormone-secreting tumors have been described only in adults. It is theoretically possible, however, that they will also be found in children.

Ectopically Secreted Hormones and Endocrine Syndromes

Ectopic CRH-secreting tumors are rare and have been described only in adults (metastatic prostatic carcinoma, ganglioneuroma, lung carcinoma).[31,330-332] These tumors are associated with Cushing's syndrome. Ectopic ACTH-secreting tumors have been described in both adults and children on numerous occasions.[10,333-341] They are associated with severe Cushing's syndrome and are produced by carcinomas of the lung, thymus, pancreas, thyroid, adrenal medulla, and other tissues. Ectopic growth-hormone releasing hormone (GRH) secreting tumors have been described in adults and adolescents and are associated with gigantism and acromegaly.[30,342-350] A primary jejunal tumor with lymph node and liver metastases and a metastatic foregut carcinoid tumor have been reported to secrete GRH.

To date, no tumors ectopically secreting GH have been described in children. In adults, ectopic GH synthesis has been attributed to pancreatic, gastric, bronchial, and mammary carcinomas.[10,351-354] Ectopic chorionic gonadotropin (hCG), on the other hand, has been described in children, causing precocious puberty in boys by stimulating Leydig-cell function.[10] hCG is secreted by placental trophoblastic neoplasms, testicular and pineal tumors, hepatoblastomas, and carcinomas of the lung, stomach, pancreatic islet cells, and colon.[355-361] Some tumors secrete the inactive α-subunit, which then serves as a marker.[356,362] Such tumors include malignant insulinomas, gastrinomas, VIPomas, and intestinal or pulmonary carcinoids.

Ectopic AVP-secreting tumors producing the inappropriate antidiuretic-hormone syndrome cell have been reported in adults.[10,363] Several neoplasms, commonly small cell or oat cell carcinomas of the lung and carcinoma of the colon or, less commonly, prostatic or adrenocortical carcinomas, have been associated with ectopic AVP secretion.

Ectopic calcitonin secretion has been observed with bronchial carcinoids and with lung, breast, and other tumors.[363] This hormone does not produce an endocrine syndrome. Ectopic PTH or PTH-like substances have been described with many cancers.[364-367] Ectopic PTH is presumably a form of a PTH precursor that many antibodies raised against mature PTH fail to recognize. Osleoclast-activating factor (OAF) or some prostanoid substance stimulating bone resorption may be the PTH-like hormones.

No ectopic steroid or thyroid hormone syndrome exists, because it would entail the random synchronous activation of the multiple enzymes required for biosynthesis of steroid and thyroid hormones, respectively. However, adrenal rest tumors can be found in many ectopic areas, primarily the liver, pelvis, or testes that can secrete steroid hormones such as cortisol "ectopically."[335]

Many hormones of the gastroenteropancreatic unit are secreted ectopically by several tumors. A number of nonpancreatic tumors have been associated with hypoglycemia.[363] Such tumors are quite large at the time hypoglycemia is noted and

include retroperitoneal fibromas and fibro-sarcomas, some hepatomas, and some tumors of the adrenal cortex. The metabolic disturbances in these patients are profound, but no immunoreactive insulin has been found. Nonsuppressible insulin-like activity, presumably one or more growth factors, has been found in bioassays. The explanation that the hypoglycemia may also be due to excessive consumption of serum glucose by the tumor has been advanced.[368] Treatment includes surgical extirpation or irradiation of the tumor and frequent feedings, intravenous glucose infusions, or administration of glucocorticoids. Finally, ectopic secretion of gastrin, glucagon, somatostatin, and *VIP* has been described.[8,10,369-371]

MULTIPLE ENDOCRINE NEOPLASIA (MEN) SYNDROMES

Definitions

The MEN syndromes are familial disorders in which neoplastic changes arise simultaneously in more than one endocrine gland.[4-11,242,372-377] The neoplastic changes include hyperplasia, benign adenomas, and carcinomas. Three distinct patterns of glandular involvement, as well as overlapping or atypical combinations of gland involvement, have been described. The three combinations are referred to as MEN I,[375,378-387] MEN II$_a$,[388-394] and MEN II$_b$ (MEN III)[395-402] (Table 34-5).

Epidemiology and Genetics

The first two forms of MEN and approximately half of the cases of MEN II$_b$ are transmitted by an autosomal dominant mode with variable penetrance and variable expression. Thus, affected relatives with the same type of MEN syndrome may have different neoplasms that appear at different ages. It has been suggested that the different glands affected all have a common embryologic origin in APUD cells. However, not all MEN-affected organs originate from the neuroectoderm and thus do not all have a common embryologic origin. It is possible that affected individuals carry a mutant gene that is activated in susceptible tissues to produce neoplasia.[394]

Combinations of multiple endocrine tumors that do not fit any of the three distinct MEN syndromes may occur in a single individual.[403-407] An overlap syndrome characterized by pheochromocytoma and islet cell tumor has been described both in sporadic cases and in families. In the families, the pattern of inheritance is autosomal dominant.

Multiple Endocrine Neoplasia Type I (Wermer's Syndrome)

The parathyroids are the glands most frequently affected in MEN I.[375,378-387] Hyperparathyroidism, usually due to hyperplasia of all four glands, occurs in approximately 80% of patients. Islet cell tumors occur in approximately 70% to 80% of patients. About three-fourths of these tumors secrete gastrin and the remainder insulin. VIPomas, glucagonomas, and tumors secreting pancreatic polypeptide (PPomas) have also been reported. More than half of the gastrinomas, VIPomas, glucagonomas, and PPomas associated with MEN I are malignant, and 10% to 20% of the insulinomas are malignant.

Pituitary involvement in MEN I usually occurs as solitary adenoma. The most frequent adenomas are prolactinomas, and the second most frequent are somatotropinomas. Corticotropinomas are third most common but are rare. Chromophobe adenomas can occur also. Adrenocortical involvement includes silent adenomas, adrenocortical hyperplasia, cortisol-

Table 34-5
Comparison of Clusters of Involved Tumors in MEN Syndromes

Site of Origin	MEN I (Wermer's syndrome)	MEN II$_a$ (Sipple's syndrome)	MEN II$_b$*
Pituitary gland	Prolactinoma Somatotropinoma Corticotropinoma		
Thyroid gland		C-cell hyperplasia Medullary carcinoma	Medullary carcinoma
Parathyroid glands	Parathyroid hyperplasia–adenoma	Parathyroid hyperplasia–adenoma	
Adrenal cortex	Adrenal adenoma–hyperplasia		
Adrenal medulla		Pheochromocytoma	Pheochromocytoma
Gastroenteropancreatic unit	Gastrinoma Insulinoma VIPoma Glucagonoma PPoma		
Other	Lipomas Carcinoids		Mucosal neuromas, ganglioneuromas

* Characterized also by marfanoid habitus.

secreting adenomas, and, rarely, carcinomas. Both benign and malignant thymic and bronchial carcinoid tumors can be associated with MEN I. Single or multiple lipomas are observed in approximately half of MEN patients.

The clinical picture of the endocrine tumors that comprise the MEN I syndrome are generally the same as when these tumors are sporadic. Hyperparathyroidism, Zollinger–Ellison syndrome, hypoglycemia, pancreatic cholera, migratory necrolytic erythema, specific and nonspecific symptoms from pituitary adenomas, Cushing's syndrome (Cushing's disease), cortisol-secreting adrenal adenomas or ectopic-ACTH syndrome from gastrinomas (or carcinoids), carcinoid syndrome, and gigantism/acromegaly can occur.

Laboratory findings are those related to the specific hormone syndrome (see above). Similarly, therapy is directed toward each of the specific tumors and endocrine syndromes that are present (see above).

Multiple Endocrine Hyperplasia Type II$_a$ (Sipple's Syndrome)

The thyroid C cells are most frequently involved in these patients, with medullary carcinoma of the thyroid occurring in approximately 95% of the patients.[377,388-394] Pheochromocytoma occurs in approximately one-third of patients. These tumors are intra-adrenal and frequently bilateral and multifocal. Approximately one-fifth of patients develop frank hyperparathyroidism, mostly associated with parathyroid adenomas but also with hyperplasia.

The clinical and laboratory findings of MEN II$_a$ are those expected on the basis of the hormone(s) secreted by the tumors. Similarly, treatment is directed toward the individual tumors.

Multiple Endocrine Neoplasia Type II$_b$

All patients with MEN II$_b$ have some aspect of a distinctive marfanoid phenotype.[395-402] This is characterized by a slender body build, long and thin extremities, abnormal laxity of joints, and, in many cases, a high arched palate, pectus excavatum, or pes cavus. The facies is characterized by enlarged, thick lips, a result of imbedded mucosal neuromas. Mucosal neuromas are also observed on the surface of the lips and tongue and may be found on the eyelids and the cornea. Ganglioneuromas may be present diffusely at any level in the gastrointestinal tract, causing constipation or diarrhea due to abnormal control of intestinal motility.

Medullary thyroid carcinoma is particularly aggressive in MEN II$_b$ and occurs frequently within childhood (mean age 20 years), 10 to 15 years earlier than the mean age of presentation in MEN II$_a$. Pheochromocytomas behave similarly to those observed in MEN II$_a$.

Treatment of MEN II$_b$ includes standard therapy for medullary carcinoma of the thyroid and for pheochromocytoma. Superficial mucosal neuromas may be removed if they cause a cosmetic problem. Constipation or diarrhea should be treated symptomatically. As many as 30% of the patients require laparotomy and colon segment excision for megacolon.

Prognosis

The prognosis of patients with MEN I is generally good in the presence of a discrete parathyroid, pancreatic islet, or pituitary adenoma. Parathyroid hyperplasia occurs in approximately one-third of the patients. Pancreatic islet cell carcinoma and carcinoids are slowly progressive.

The prognosis of patients with MEN II$_a$ is also generally

good. The risk of postoperative recurrence of medullary thyroid carcinoma and pheochromocytoma is less if the tumor is excised early, before the disease becomes extensive. Hyperparathyroidism has a good prognosis.

The prognosis of patients with MEN II$_b$ is worse than that of those with MEN II$_a$. Medullary carcinomas in MEN II$_b$ are generally more aggressive and have a 50% 10-year survival rate.

Screening is of paramount importance in all three forms of MEN, as earlier therapy clearly improves the prognosis remarkably. Individuals at risk include patients with known MEN, a positive family history of MEN, ganglioneuromas and cutaneous neuromas, a marfanoid somatic phenotype, Zollinger–Ellison syndrome, parathyroid hyperplasia, multicentric medullary carcinoma of the thyroid, or multicentric or bilateral pheochromocytomas. Screening tests include measurements of serum calcium, gastrin, glucose, and prolactin in MEN I; basal and stimulated (calcium gluconate or pentagastrin) plasma calcitonin, 24-hour urinary free catecholamines, metanephrines and vanilmandelic acid, and serum calcium in MEN II$_a$; and basal and stimulated plasma calcitonin and 24-hour urinary free catecholamines, metanephrines, and vanilmandelic acid in MEN II$_b$ (see Table 34-3).

REFERENCES

1. Hung W, August GP, Glasgow AM: Pediatric Endocrinology. Garden City, Medical Examination Publishing Co, 1978
2. Frasier SD: Pediatric Endocrinology. New York, Grune & Stratton, 1980
3. Felig P, Baxter JD, Broadus AE, Frohman LA (eds): Endocrinology and Metabolism. New York, McGraw-Hill, 1981
4. Williams RH (ed): Textbook of Endocrinology. Philadelphia, WB Saunders, 1981
5. Job JC, Pierson M (ed): Pediatric Endocrinology. New York, John Wiley & Sons, 1981
6. Root AW, Diamond FD: The pituitary gland. In Kelley VC (ed): Practice of Pediatrics, pp 1–181. Philadelphia, Harper & Row, 1982
7. Rabin D, McKenna TJ: Clinical Endocrinology and Metabolism: Principles and Practice. New York, Grune & Stratton, 1982
8. Santen RJ, Manni A (eds): Diagnosis and Management of Endocrine-Related Tumors. Boston, Martinus Nijhoff, 1984
9. Edis AJ, Grant CS, Egdahl RH (eds): Manual of Endocrine Surgery. New York, Springer-Verlag, 1984
10. Root AW, Diamond FB, Duncan JA: Ectopic and Entopic Peptide Hormone Secreting Neoplasms of Childhood, pp 369–415. Chicago, Year Book Medical Publishers, 1985
11. Kohler PO (ed): Clinical Endocrinology. New York, John Wiley & Sons, 1986
12. Young JL Jr, Heise HW, Silverberg E et al: Cancer Incidence, Survival and Mortality for Children under 15 Years of Age. New York, American Cancer Society Professional Education Publication, 1978
13. Devesa SS, Silverman DT: Cancer incidence and mortality trends in the United States: 1935–1974. J Natl Cancer Inst 60:545, 1978
14. Henson MR, Mulvihill JJ: Epidemiology of cancer in the young. In Levine AS (ed): Cancer in the Young, pp 3–11. Paris, Masson, 1981
15. Gold EB: Epidemiology of pituitary adenomas. Epidemiol Rev 3:163, 1981
16. Pratt CB: Some aspects of childhood cancer epidemiology. Pediatr Clin North Am 32:541, 1985
17. Koos WT, Miller MH: Statistics of infancy and childhood tumors. In: Intracranial Tumors of Infants and Children, pp 9–27. St Louis, CV Mosby, 1971
18. Kohler PO, Ross GT (eds): Diagnosis and Treatment of Pituitary Tumors. New York, American Elsevier, 1973
19. Besser GM (ed): The hypothalamus and pituitary. Clin Endocrinol Metab 6:1–2, 1977
20. Tyrrell JB, Wilson CB: Pituitary syndromes. In Friesen SR (ed): Surgical Endocrinology: Clinical Syndromes, pp 304–328. Philadelphia, JB Lippincott, 1978
21. Martin JB, Reichlin S, Brown GM (eds): Clinical Neuroendocrinology. Philadelphia, FA Davis, 1978
22. Tolis G, Labrie F, Martin JB, Naftolin F (eds): Clinical Neuroendocrinology. New York, Raven Press, 1979
23. Post KD, Jackson I, Reichlin S (eds): The Pituitary Adenoma. New York, Plenum Medical Book Co, 1980
24. Krieger DT, Hughes JC (eds): Neuroendocrinology. Sunderland, MA, Sinauer Books, 1980
25. Frohman LA: Diseases of the anterior pituitary. In Felig P, Baxter J, Broadus A, Frohman L (eds): Endocrinology and Metabolism, pp 151–231. New York, McGraw-Hill, 1981
26. Daughaday WH: The adenohypophysis. In Williams RH (ed): Textbook of Endocrinology, 6th Ed, pp 73–116. Philadelphia, WB Saunders, 1981
27. Fraioli B, Ferrante L, Celli P: Pituitary adenomas with onset during puberty: Features and treatment. J Neurosurg 59:590, 1983
28. Tindall GT, Barrow DL: Disorders of the Pituitary. St Louis, CV Mosby, 1986
29. Page RB, Santen RJ: Approach to the pituitary tumor: Anatomic, diagnostic and surgical considerations. In Santen RJ, Manni A (eds): Diagnosis and Management of Endocrine-Related Tumors, pp 1–44. Boston, Martinus Nijhoff, 1984
30. Asa SL, Scheithauser BW, Bilboa JM et al: A case for hypothalamic acromegaly: A clinicopathological study of six patients with hypothalamic gangliocytomas producing growth hormone-releasing factor. J Clin Endocrinol Metab 58:796, 1984
31. Carey RM, Varma SK, Drake CK Jr et al: Ectopic secretion of corticotropin-releasing factor as a cause of Cushing's syndrome: A clinical, morphologic, and biochemical study. N Engl J Med 311:13, 1984
32. Price RA, Lee PA, Albright AL et al: Treatment of sexual precocity by removal of a luteinizing hormone–releasing hormone-secreting hematoma. JAMA 251:2247, 1984
33. Alsever RN, Gotlin RW: Handbook of Endocrine Tests in Adults and Children, pp 1–238. Chicago, Yearbook Medical Publishers, 1978
34. Eddy RL, Gilliland PF, Ibarra JD: Human growth hormone release: Comparison of provocative test procedures. Am J Med 56:179–185, 1974
35. Kleinberg DL, Noel GL, Frantz AG: Galactorrhea: A study of 235 cases, including 48 with pituitary tumors. N Engl J Med 296:589, 1977
36. Kirby RW, Kotchen TA, Rees ED: Hyperprolactinemia: A review of recent clinical advances. Arch Intern Med 139:1415, 1979
37. Koenig MP, Zuppinger K, Liechti B: Hyperprolactinemia as a cause of delayed puberty: Successful treatment with bromocriptine. J Clin Endocrinol 45:825, 1977
38. Loriaux DL, Cutler GB Jr: Diseases of the adrenal glands. In Kohler PO (ed): Clinical Endocrinology, pp 157–238. New York, John Wiley & Sons, 1986
39. Chrousos GP, Loriaux DL: Cushing's syndrome. In Rakel RE (ed): Conn's Current Therapy, pp 495–498. Philadelphia, WB Saunders, 1987
40. Chrousos GP, Schulte HM, Oldfield EH et al: The corticotropin-releasing factor stimulation test: An aid in the evaluation of patients with Cushing's syndrome. N Engl J Med 310:622, 1984
41. Chrousos GP, Schuermeyer T, Oldfield E et al: The clinical applications of corticotropin releasing factor. Ann Intern Med 102:344–358, 1985
42. Oldfield EH, Chrousos GP, Schulte HM et al: Preoperative lateralization of ACTH-secreting pituitary microadenomas by bilateral and simultaneous inferior petrosal sinus sampling. N Engl J Med 312:100, 1985
43. Haigler ED, Hershman JM, Meador CK: Pituitary gigantism: A case report and review. Arch Intern Med 132:588, 1973
44. Avruskin TW, San K, Tang S et al: Childhood acromegaly: Successful therapy with conventional radiation and effects of chlorpromazine on GH and prolactin secretion. J Clin Endocrinol 37:380, 1973
45. Daughaday WH, Cryer PE: Growth hormone hypersecretion and acromegaly. Hosp Pract 13(8):75, 1978
46. Whitehead EM, Shalet SM, Davies D et al: Pituitary gigantism: A disabling condition. Clin Endocrinol 17:271, 1982
47. Faggiano M, Criscuolo T, Perrone L et al: Sexual precocity in a boy due to hypersecretion of LH and prolactin by pituitary adenoma. Acta Endocrinol 102:167, 1983
48. Snyder PJ: Gonadotroph cell adenomas of the pituitary. Endocr Rev 6:552, 1985
49. Benoit R, Pearson–Murphy BE, Robert F et al: Hyperthyroidism due to a pituitary tumor with amenorrhea–galactorrhea. Clin Endocrinol 12:11, 1980
50. Yovos JG, Falco JM, D'Orisio TM et al: Thyrotoxicosis and a thyrotropin secreting pituitary tumor causing unilateral exophthalmus. J Clin Endocrinol Metab 53:338, 1981
51. Koide Y, Kugai N, Kimura S et al: A case of pituitary adenoma with possible simultaneous secretion of thyrotropin and follicle stimulating hormone. J Clin Endocrinol Metab 54:397, 1982

52. Smallridge RC, Smith CE: Hyperthyroidism due to thyrotropin-secreting pituitary tumors. Arch Intern Med 143:503, 1983

53. Kourides IA: Pituitary thyrotropin secretion in thyroid disorders. Thyroid Today 3:1, 1980

54. Weintraub BD (moderator): Inappropriate secretion of thyroid stimulating hormone. Ann Intern Med 95:334, 1981

55. Van Meter QL, Gareis FJ, Hayes JW et al: Galactorrhea in a 12 year old boy with a chromophobe adenoma. J Pediatr 90:756, 1977

56. Ridgway EC, Kilbansk A, Ladenson PW: Pure alpha-secreting pituitary adenomas. N Engl J Med 304:1254–1259, 1981

57. Klibanski A, Ridgway EC, Zerras NT: Pure alpha subunit secreting pituitary tumors. J Neurosurg 59:585, 1983

58. Matson DD, Crigler JF: Management of craniopharyngioma in childhood. J Neurosurg 30:377, 1969

59. Jenkins JS, Gilbert CJ, Ang V: Hypothalamic–pituitary function in patients with craniopharyngioma. J Clin Endocrinol 43:394, 1976

60. Thomasett MJ et al: Endocrine and neurologic outcome in childhood craniopharyngioma: Review of effect of treatment in 42 patients. J Pediatr 97:728, 1980

61. Hardy J: Transsphenoidal surgery of hypersecreting pituitary tumors. In Kohler PO, Ross GT (eds): Diagnosis and Treatment of Pituitary Tumors, p 179. New York, American Elsevier, 1973

62. Tyrrel JB, Brooks RM, Fitzgerald PA: Cushing's disease: Selective transsphenoidal resection of pituitary microadenomas. N Engl J Med 298:753–757, 1978

63. Arafah BM, Brodkey JS, Kaufman B et al: Transsphenoidal microsurgery in the treatment of acromegaly and gigantism. J Clin Endocrinol Metab 50:578, 1980

64. Zervas NT, Martin JB: Management of hormone-secreting pituitary adenomas. N Engl J Med 302:210, 1980

65. Styne DM, Grumbach M, Kaplan SL et al: Treatment of Cushing's disease in childhood and adolescence by transsphenoidal adenomectomy. N Engl J Med 310:889, 1984

66. Spark RF, Pallotta J, Maftolin F et al: Galactorrhea–amenorrhea syndromes: Etiology and treatment. Ann Intern Med 84:532, 1976

67. Parkes D: Bromocryptine. N Engl J Med 301:873, 1979

68. Wass JAH, Thorner MD, Moffis DV et al: Long-term treatment of acromegaly with bromocryptine. Br Med J 1:875, 1977

69. Jennings AS, Liddle GW, Orth DN: Results of treating childhood Cushing's disease with pituitary radiation. N Engl J Med 297:957, 1977

70. Roth J, Gorden P, Brace K: Efficacy of conventional pituitary irradiation in acromegaly. N Engl J Med 282:1385, 1970

71. Nelson DJ, Meakin JW, Thorn GW: ACTH-producing pituitary tumors following adrenalectomy for Cushing's syndrome. Ann Intern Med 52:560, 1960

72. Misbin RI, Canary J, Willard D: Aminoglutethimide in the treatment of Cushing's syndrome. J Clin Pharmacol 16:645, 1976

73. Orth DN: Metyrapone is useful only as adjunctive therapy in Cushing's disease. Ann Intern Med 89:128, 1978

74. Schteingart DE, Tsao HS, Taylor CI et al: Sustained remission of Cushing's disease with mitotane and pituitary irradiation. Ann Intern Med 92:613, 1980

75. Pont A, Williams PL, Loose DS et al: Ketoconazole blocks adrenal steroid synthesis. Ann Intern Med 97:370, 1982

76. Werner SC, Ingbar SH (eds): The Thyroid: A Fundamental and Clinical Text. New York, Harper & Row, 1978

77. De Groot LJ: Thyroid neoplasia. In De Groot LJ, Cahill GF, Odell WD (eds): Endocrinology, vol 4, pp 509–521. New York, Grune & Stratton, 1979

78. Hambruger J: The autonomously functioning thyroid adenoma. N Engl J Med 309:1512, 1983

79. Kaplan MM, Larsen PR (eds): Thyroid disease. Med Clin North Am 69:1985

80. Duffy BJ Jr, Fitzgerald PJ: Cancer of the thyroid in children: A report of 28 cases. J Clin Endocrinol 10:1296, 1950

81. Winship TH, Rosvoll RV: Childhood thyroid carcinoma. Cancer 14:734, 1961

82. Exelby PE, Frazell EL: Carcinoma of the thyroid in children. Surg Clin North Am 49:249, 1969

83. Winship TH, Rosvoll RV: Thyroid carcinoma in childhood: Final report on a 20 year study. Clin Proc Child Hosp Natl Med Cent 26:327, 1970

84. Block MA, Horn RC, Miller JM: Hazards in the diagnosis and management of certain thyroid nodules in children. Am J Surg 120:447, 1970

85. Harness JK, Thompson NW, Nishiyama RH: Childhood thyroid carcinoma. Arch Surg 102:278, 1971

86. Leichty C, Shirazi S: Carcinoma of thyroid in children. Surg Gynecol Obstet 134:595, 1972

87. Kirkland RT, Kirkland JL: Solitary thyroid nodules in 30 children and report of a child with a thyroid abscess. Pediatrics 51:85, 1973

88. Rallison ML, Dobyns BM, Keating FR et al: Thyroid nodularity in children. JAMA 233:1069, 1975

89. Buckwalter J, Colin G, Thomas C et al: Is childhood thyroid cancer a lethal disease? Ann Surg 181:632, 1975

90. Scott MD, Crawford JD: Solitary thyroid nodules in childhood: Is the incidence of thyroid carcinoma declining? Pediatrics 58:521, 1976

91. Anderson A, Bergdhal L, Boquist L: Thyroid carcinoma in children. Am J Surg 43:159, 1977

92. Hempelmann LH: Risk of thyroid neoplasms after irradiation in childhood: Studies of populations exposed to radiation in childhood show a dose response over a wide dose range. Science 160:159, 1960

93. Refetoff S, Harrison T, Karafinski ET et al: Continuing occurrence of thyroid carcinoma after radiation to the neck in infancy and childhood. N Engl J Med 292:171, 1975

94. McConahey WM, Hayles AB: Radiation to the head, neck, and upper thorax of the young and thyroid neoplasia. J Clin Endocrinol 42:1182, 1976

95. Favus MJ, Schneider AB, Stachura ME et al: Thyroid cancer occurring as a late consequence of head-and-neck irradiation. N Engl J Med 294:1019, 1976

96. Greenspan FS: Radiation exposure and thyroid cancer. JAMA 237:2089, 1977

97. Maxon HR, Thomas SR, Saenger EL et al: Ionizing radiation and the induction of clinically significant disease in the human thyroid gland. Am J Med 63:967, 1977

98. Schneider AB, Favus MJ, Stachura ME et al: Incidence, prevalence, and characteristics of radiation-induced thyroid tumors. Am J Med 64:243, 1978

99. Schneider AB, Pinsky S, Bekerman C et al: Characteristics of 108 thyroid cancers detected by screening in a population with a history of head and neck irradiation. Cancer 46:1218, 1980

100. Kaplan MM, Garnick MB, Gelber R et al: Risk factors for thyroid abnormalities after neck irradiation for childhood cancer. Am J Med 74:272, 1983

101. Hazard JB, Hawk WA, Crile G: Medullary (solid) carcinoma of the thyroid: A clinicopathologic entity. J Clin Endocrinol Metab 19:152, 1959

102. Williams ED, Brown CL, Doniach I: Pathological and clinical findings in a series of 67 cases of medullary carcinoma of the thyroid. J Clin Pathol 19:103, 1966

103. Melvin KEW, Tashjan AH: The syndrome of excessive thyrocalcitonin produced by medullary carcinoma of the thyroid. Proc Natl Acad Sci USA 59:1216, 1968

104. Hill CS, Ibanez ML, Samaan NA et al: Medullary (solid) carcinoma of the thyroid gland. Medicine 52:141, 1973

105. Wolfe HJ, Melvin KEW, Cervi–Skinner SJ et al: C-cell hyperplasia preceding medullary thyroid carcinoma. N Engl J Med 289:437, 1973

106. Walfish PG, Hazani E, Strawbridge HTG et al: A prospective study of combined ultrasonography and needle aspiration biopsy in the assessment of the hypofunctioning thyroid nodule. Surgery 82:474, 1977

107. Miller JM, Hamburger JI, Kim S: Diagnosis of thyroid nodules: Use of fine-needle aspiration and needle biopsy. JAMA 241:481, 1979

108. Miller JM: Evaluation of thyroid nodules: Accent on needle biopsy. Med Clin North Am 69:1603, 1985

109. Farrar WB, Cooperman M, James AG: Surgical management of papillary and follicular carcinoma of the thyroid. Ann Surg 192:701, 1980

110. Christensen SB, Ljungberg O, Tibblin S: Surgical treatment of thyroid carcinoma in a defined population: 1960–1977. Am J Surg 146:349, 1983

111. Ozaki O, Notsu T, Hirai K et al: Differentiated carcinoma of the thyroid gland. World J Surg 7:181, 1983

112. Block MA: Surgery of thyroid nodules and malignancy. Curr Probl Surg 20:113, 1983

113. Breaux EP, Guillamondegue OM: Treatment of locally invasive carcinoma of the thyroid: How radical? Am J Surg 140:514, 1980

114. Weber CA, Clark OH: Surgery for thyroid disease. Med Clin North Am 69:1097, 1985

115. Cady B, Cohn K, Rossi RL et al: The effect of thyroid hormone administration upon survival in patients with differentiated thyroid carcinoma. Surgery 94:978, 1983

116. Leeper RD: Thyroid cancer. Med Clin North Am 69:1079, 1985

117. Leeper RD: The effect of ^{131}I therapy on survival of patients with metastatic

papillary or follicular thyroid carcinoma. J Clin Endocrinol Metab 36:1143, 1973

118. Mazzaferri EL, Young RL, Oertel JE et al: Papillary thyroid carcinoma: The impact of therapy in 576 patients. Medicine 56:171, 1977

119. Beierwaltes WH: The treatment of thyroid carcinoma with radioactive iodine. Semin Nucl Med 8:79, 1978

120. Maxon H, Thomas SR, Hertzberg VS et al: Relation between effective radiation dose and outcome of radioiodine therapy for thyroid cancer. N Engl J Med 309:937, 1983

121. Samaan NA, Mahshwari YK, Nader S et al: Impact of therapy for differentiated carcinoma of the thyroid: An analysis of 706 cases. J Clin Endocrinol Metab 56:1131, 1983

122. Brown AP, Greening WP, McCready VR et al: Radioiodine treatment of metastatic thyroid carcinoma: The Royal Marsden Hospital experience. Br J Radiol 57:323, 1984

123. Samaan NA, Schultz PN, Haynie TP et al: Pulmonary metastasis of differentiated thyroid carcinoma: Treatment results in 101 patients. J Clin Endocrinol Metab 60:376–380, 1985

124. Benua RS, Cicale NR, Sonenberg M et al: The relation of radioiodine dosimetry to results and complications in the treatment of metastatic thyroid cancer. AJR 87:171, 1982

125. Sarker SD, Beierwaltes WH, Gill SP et al: Subsequent fertility and birth histories of children and adolescents treated with ^{131}I for thyroid cancer. J Nucl Med 17:460, 1976

126. Simpson WJ, Carruthers JS: The role of external radiation in the management of papillary and follicular thyroid cancer. Am J Surg 136:457, 1978

127. Kim JH, Leeper RD: Treatment of anaplastic giant and spindle cell carcinoma of the thyroid gland with combination Adriamycin and radiation therapy: A new approach. Cancer 52:954, 1983

128. Kim JH, Leeper RD: Combination Adriamycin and radiation therapy for locally advanced carcinoma of the thyroid gland. Int J Radiat Oncol Biol Phys 9:565, 1983

129. Schneider AB, Line BR, Goldman JM, Robbins J: Sequential serum thyroglobulin determinations, ^{131}I scans, and ^{131}I uptakes after triiodothyronine withdrawal in patients with thyroid cancer. J Clin Endocrinol Metab 53:1199, 1981

130. Echenique RL, Kasi L, Haynie TP et al: Critical evaluation of serum thyroglobulin levels and I-131 scans in post-therapy patients with differentiated thyroid carcinoma (concise communication). J Nucl Med 23:235, 1982

131. Pacini F, Pinchera A, Giani C et al: Serum thyroglobulin in thyroid carcinoma and other thyroid disorders. J Endocrinol Invest 3:283, 1980

132. Graze K, Spiler IJ, Tashjian AH et al: Natural history of familial medullary thyroid carcinoma. N Engl J Med 299:980, 1978

133. Saad MF, Fritsche HA Jr, Samaan NA: Diagnostic and prognostic values of carcinoembryonic antigen in medullary carcinoma of the thyroid. J Clin Endocrinol Metab 58:889, 1984

134. Beierwaltes WB, Nishiyama RH, Thompson NW et al: Survival time and "cure" in papillary and follicular thyroid carcinoma with distant metastases: Statistics following University of Michigan therapy. J Nucl Med 23:561, 1982

135. Roth SI: Pathology of the parathyroids in hyperparathyroidism: Discussion of recent advances in the anatomy and pathology of the parathyroid glands. Arch Pathol 73:495, 1962

136. Lloyd HM: Primary hyperparathyroidism: An analysis of the role of the parathyroid tumors. Medicine 47:53, 1968

137. Holmes EC, Morton DL, Ketcham AS: Parathyroid carcinoma: A collective review. Ann Surg 169:631, 1969

138. Bjernulf A, Hall K, Sjögren I, Werner I: Primary hyperparathyroidism in children. Acta Paediatr Scand 59:249, 1970

139. Goldbloom RB, Gillis DA, Prasad M: Hereditary parathyroid hyperplasia: A surgical emergency of early infancy. Pediatrics 49:514, 1971

140. Scantz A, Castleman B: Parathyroid carcinoma: A study of 70 cases. Cancer 31:600, 1973

141. Schneider AB, Sherwood LM: Calcium homeostasis, and the pathogenesis and management of hypercalcemic disorders. Metabolism 23:975, 1974

142. Mallette LE, Bilezikian JP, Heath DA, Aurbach GD: Primary hyperparathyroidism: Clinical and biochemical features. Medicine 53:127, 1974

143. Mannix H: Primary hyperparathyroidism in children. Am J Surg 129:528, 1975

144. Fialkow PJ, Jackson CE, Block MA, Greenwald KA: Multicellular origin of parathyroid adenomas. N Engl J Med 297:696, 1977

145. Marx SJ, Speigel AM, Brown EM, Aurbach GD: Family studies in patients with primary parathyroid hyperplasia. Am J Med 62:698, 1977

146. Heath H III, Hodgson SF, Kennedy MA: Primary hyperparathyroidism: Incidence, morbidity and potential economic impact in a community. N Engl J Med 302:189, 1980

147. Mundy GR, Cove DH, Fisken R: Primary hyperparathyroidism: Changes in the pattern of clinical presentation. Lancet 1:1317, 1981

148. Scholz DA, Purnell DC: Asymptomatic primary hyperparathyroidism: Ten year prospective study. Mayo Clin Proc 56:473, 1981

149. Clark OH, Arnaud CD: Hyperparathyroidism: incidence, diagnosis and problems. In Kaplan EL (ed): Surgery of the Thyroid and Parathyroids. Clinical Surgery International, vol 6, pp 144–157. Edinburgh, Churchill Livingstone, 1983

150. Slatopolsky E, Rutherford WE, Hoffsten FH et al: Nonsuppressible secondary hyperparathyroidism in chronic progressive renal disease. Kidney Int 1:38, 1972

151. David DS, Sakai S, Brenne BL et al: Hypercalcemia after renal transplantation: Long-term follow-up data. N Engl J Med 289:398, 1973

152. Marx SJ, Spiegel AM, Levine MA et al: Familial hypocalciuric hypercalcemia: The relation to primary parathyroid hyperplasia. N Engl J Med 307:416, 1982

153. Marx SJ, Attie MF, Speigel AM et al: An association between neonatal severe primary hyperparathyroidism and familial hypocalciuric hypercalcemia in three kindreds. N Engl J Med 306:257, 1982

154. Roth SI, Gallagher MJ: The rapid identification of "normal" parathyroid glands by the presence of intracellular fat. Am J Pathol 84:521, 1976

155. Lemann JL Jr, Donatelli AA: Calcium intoxication due to primary hyperparathyroidism: A medical and surgical emergency. Ann Intern Med 60:447, 1964

156. Eisenberg H, Pallotta J, Sherwood LM: Selective arteriography, venography and venous hormone assay in diagnosis and localization of parathyroid lesions. Am J Med 56:810, 1974

157. Doppman JL, Brennan MF, Koehler JQ, Marx SJ: Computed tomography for parathyroid localization. J Comput Assist Tomogr 1:30, 1977

158. Sommer B, Walter HF, Spelsberg F, Scherer U, Lissner J: Computed tomography for localizing enlarged parathyroid glands in primary hyperparathyroidism. J Comput Assist Tomogr 6:521, 1982

159. Reading CC, Charbneau JW, James EM et al: High resolution parathyroid sonography. AJR 139:539, 1982

160. Stark DD, Moss AA, Gooding GA, Clark H: Parathyroid scanning by computed tomography. Radiology 148:297, 1983

161. Edis AJ, Beahrs OH, van Heerden JA, Akwari OE: "Conservative" versus "liberal" approach to parathyroid neck exploration. Surgery 82:466, 1977

162. Sedgwick CE, Cady B: Surgical anatomy. In: Surgery of the Thyroid and Parathyroid Glands, pp 19–38. Philadelphia, WB Saunders, 1980

163. Anderberg B, Gillquist J, Larsson L, Lundstrom B: Complications to subtotal parathyroidectomy. Acta Chir Scand 147:109, 1982

164. Wang CA, Castleman B, Cope O: Surgical management of hyperparathyroidism due to primary hyperplasia. Ann Surg 195:384, 1982

165. Russell CF, Edis AJ: Surgery for primary hyperparathyroidism: Experience with 500 consecutive cases and evaluation of the role of surgery in the asymptomatic patient. Br J Surg 69:244, 1982

166. Tibblin S, Bondeson AG, Ljunberg O: Unilateral parathyroidectomy in hyperparathyroidism due to single adenoma. Ann Surg 195:245, 1982

167. Brennan MF, Doppman JL, Krudy AG et al: Assessment of techniques for reoperative parathyroid gland localization in patients undergoing reoperation for hyperparathyroidism. Surgery 91:6, 1982

168. Nathaniels EK, Nathaniels AM, Wang C-A: Mediastinal parathyroid tumors: A clinical and pathological study of 84 cases. Ann Surg 171:165, 1970

169. Flye MW, Brennan M: Surgical resection of metastatic parathyroid carcinoma. Ann Surg 193:425, 1981

170. Bilezikian JP: The medical management of primary hyperparathyroidism. Ann Intern Med 96:198, 1982

171. Wells SA Jr, Ellis GJ, Gunnels JC et al: Parathyroid autotransplantation in primary parathyroid hyperplasia. N Engl J Med 295:57, 1976

172. Edis AJ, Linos DA, Kao PC: Parathyroid autotransplantation at the time of reoperation for persistent hyperparathyroidism. Surgery 88:588, 1980

173. Kaplan EL, Sugimoto J, Yang H, Fredland A: Postoperative hypoparathyroidism: Diagnosis and management. In Kaplan EL (ed): Surgery of the Thyroid and Parathyroids. Clinical Surgery International, vol 6, pp 262–274. Edinburgh, Churchill Livingston, 1983

174. Karsner HT: Tumors of the adrenal. In: Atlas of Tumor Pathology, section VIII, fascicle 29. Washington, Armed Forces Institute of Pathology, 1950

175. O'Neal LW: Pathologic anatomy in Cushing's syndrome. Ann Surg 168:860, 1964

176. van Slooten H, Schaberg A, Smeenk D et al: Morphological characteristics of benign and malignant adrenocortical tumors. Cancer 55:766, 1985

177. Landau RL, Stimmel BF, Humphreys E et al: Gynecomastia and retarded sexual development resulting from a long-standing estrogen-secreting adrenal tumor. J Clin Endocrinol Metab 14:1097, 1954

178. Snaith AH: A case of feminizing adrenal tumor in a girl. J Clin Endocrinol Metab 18:318, 1958

179. Mortimer JG, Rudd BT, Butt WR: A virilizing adrenal tumor in a prepubertal boy. J Clin Endocrinol Metab 24:842, 1964

180. Scott WH Jr, Foster JH, Liddle G et al: Cushing's syndrome due to adrenocortical tumor: 11-year review of 15 patients. Ann Surg 162:505, 1965

181. Gabrilove JL, Sharma DC, Wotiz HH et al: Feminizing adrenocortical tumors in the male: A review of 52 cases including a case report. Medicine 44:37, 1965

182. Kenny FM, Yashida Y, Askari A et al: Virilizing tumors of the adrenal cortex. Am J Dis Child 115:445, 1968

183. Mathison DA, Waterhouse CA: Cushing's syndrome with hypertensive oritis and mixed cortical adenoma–pheochromocytoma. Am J Med 47:635, 1969

184. Halmi KA, Lascari AD: Conversion of virilization to feminization in a young girl with adrenal carcinoma. Cancer 27:931, 1971

185. Check JH, Rakoff AE, Roy BK: A testosterone-secreting adrenal adenoma. Obstet Gynecol 51:46s, 1978

186. Komiya I, Koizumi Y, Kobayashi R et al: Concurrent hypersecretion of aldosterone and cortisol from the adrenal cortical adenoma. Am J Med 67:516, 1979

187. Mimou N, Sakato S, Nakabayashi H et al: Cushing's syndrome associated with bilateral adrenal adenomas. Acta Endocrinol 108:245, 1985

188. Veldhuis JD, Sowers JR, Rogol AD et al: Pathophysiology of male hypogonadism associated with endogenous hyperestrogenisim. N Engl J Med 312:1371, 1985

189. Macfarlane DA: Cancer of the adrenal cortex: The natural history, prognosis and treatment in a study of fifty-five cases. Ann R Coll Surg Engl 23:155, 1958

190. Lipsett MB, Hert R, Ross GT: Clinical and pathophysiologic aspects of adrenocortical carcinoma. Am J Med 35:374, 1963

191. Hutter AM Jr, Kayhoe DE: Adrenal cortical carcinoma: Clinical features of 138 patients. Am J Med 41:572, 1966

192. Hayles AB, Hahn HB, Sprague RG et al: Hormone-secreting tumors of the adrenal cortex in children. Pediatrics 37:19, 1966

193. Fraser R, James VHT, Landon J et al: Clinical and biochemical studies of a patient with a corticosterone secreting adrenocortical tumour. Lancet 2:1116, 1968

194. Powell-Jackson JD, Calin A, Fraser R et al: Excess deoxycorticosterone secretion from adrenocortical carcinoma. Br Med J 2:32, 1974

195. Hajjar RA, Hickey RC, Samaan NA: Adrenal cortical carcinoma: A study of 32 patients. Cancer 35:549, 1975

196. Wohltmann H, Mathur RS, Williamson HO: Sexual precocity in a female infant due to a feminizing adrenal carcinoma. J Clin Endocrinol Metab 50:186, 1980

197. Didolkar MS, Bescher RA, Elias EG et al: Natural history of adrenal cortical carcinoma: A clinicopathologic study of 42 patients. Cancer 47:2153, 1981

198. Bertagna C, Orth DN: Clinical and laboratory findings and results of therapy in 58 patients with adrenocortical tumors admitted to a single medical center (1951 to 1978). Am J Med 71:855, 1981

199. Nader S, Hickey RC, Sellin RV et al: Adrenal cortical carcinoma: A study of 77 cases. Cancer 52:707, 1983

200. Henley DJ, Van Heerden JA, Grant CS et al: Adrenal cortical carcinoma: A continuing challenge. Surgery 94:926, 1983

201. Arteaga E, Biglieri EG, Kater CE et al: Aldosterone-producing adrenocortical carcinoma: Preoperative recognition and courses in three cases. Ann Intern Med 101:316, 1984

202. Klevit HD, Campbell RA, Blair HR et al: Cushing's syndrome with nodular hyperplasia in infancy. J Pediatr 68:912, 1966

203. Schletter FE, Clift GV, Meyer R et al: Cushing's syndrome in childhood: Report of two cases with bilateral adrenocortical hyperplasia, showing distinctive clinical features. J Clin Endocrinol Metab 27:22, 1967

204. Meador CK, Bowdoin B, Owen WC Jr et al: Primary adrenocortical nodular dysplasia: A rare cause of Cushing's syndrome. J Clin Endocrinol Metab 27:1255, 1967

205. Robinson MJ, Pardo V, Rywlin AM: Pigmented nodules (black adenomas) of the adrenal: An autopsy study of incidence, morphology and function. Hum Pathol 3:317, 1972

206. Robinson MJ: Pigmented nodules (black adenomas) of the adrenal gland. Arch Pathol 96:207, 1973

207. Ruder HJ, Loriaux DL, Lipsett MB: Severe osteopenia in young adults associated with Cushing's syndrome due to micronodular adrenal disease. J Clin Endocrinol Metab 39:1138, 1974

208. Josse RG, Bear R, Kovacs K et al: Cushing's syndrome due to unilateral nodular adrenal hyperplasia: A new pathophysiological entity? Acta Endocrinol 93:495, 1980

209. Schweizer–Cagianut M, Salomon F, Hedinger CE: Primary adreno-cortical nodular dysplasia with Cushing's syndrome and cardiac myxomas. Virchows Arch [Pathol Anat] 397:183, 1982

210. McArthur RB, Bahn RC, Hayles AB: Primary adrenocortical nodular dysplasia as a cause of Cushing's syndrome in infants and children. Mayo Clin Proc 57:58, 1982

211. Bohm N, Lippman–Grob B, von Pterykowski N: Familial Cushing's syndrome due to pigmented multinodular adrenocortical dysplasia. Acta Endocrinol 102:428, 1983

212. Shenoy BV, Carpenter BC, Carney JA: Bilateral primary pigmented nodular adenocortical disease: Rare cause of the Cushing syndrome. Am J Surg Pathol 8:335, 1984

213. Sample WF, Sarti DA: Computed tomography and gray scale ultrasonography of the adrenal gland: A comparative study. Radiology 128:377, 1978

214. Dunnick NR, Schoner EG, Doppman JL et al: Computed tomography in adrenal tumors. AJR 132:43, 1979

215. Gangury A, Pratt JH, Yune HY et al: Detection of adrenal tumors by computerized tomographic scan in endocrine hypertension. Arch Intern Med 139:590, 1979

216. White FE, White MC, Drury PL et al: Value of computed tomography of the abdomen and chest in investigation of Cushing's syndrome. Br Med J 284:771, 1982

217. Mitty HA, Yeh HC: Radiology of the Adrenals with Sonography and CT. Philadelphia, WB Saunders, 1982

218. Snell ME, Lawrence R, Litton D et al: Advances in the techniques of localisation of adrenal tumors and their influence on the surgical approach to the tumour. Br J Urol 55:617, 1983

219. Lieberman LM, Beierwaltes WH, Conn JW et al: Diagnosis of adrenal disease by visualization of human adrenal glands with ^{131}I-19-iodocholesterol. N Engl J Med 285:1387, 1971

220. Anderson BG, Beierwaltes WH: Adrenal imaging with radioiodocholesterol in the diagnosis of adrenal disorders. Adv Intern Med 49:327, 1974

221. Sarkar SD, Cohen EL, Beierwaltes WH et al: A new and superior adrenal imaging agent, ^{131}I-6β-iodomethyl-19-nor-cholesterol (NP-59): Evaluation in humans. J Clin Endocrinol Metab 45:353, 1977

222. Beierwaltes WH, Sisson JC, Shapiro B: Diagnosis of adrenal tumors with radionucleide imaging. Spec Top Endocrinol Metab 6:1, 1984

223. Roberts MS, Lattimer JK: The surgical treatment of Cushing's syndrome. JAMA 175:117, 1961

224. Egdahl RH: Surgery of the adrenal gland. N Engl J Med 278:939, 1968

225. Applequist P, Kostianinen S: Multiple thoracotomy combined with chemotherapy in metastatic adrenal cortical carcinoma: A case report and review of the literature. J Surg Oncol 24:1, 1983

226. Poter DA, Strott CA, Javadpour N et al: Prolonged survival following six pulmonary resections for metastatic adrenal cortical carcinoma: A case report. J Surg Oncol 25:273, 1984

227. Bergenstal DM, Hertz R, Lipsett MS, Moy RH: Chemotherapy of adrenocortical cancer with o,p'DDD. Ann Intern Med 53:672, 1960

228. Hutter AM, Kayhole DE: Adrenocortical carcinoma: Results of treatment with o,p'DDD in 138 patients. Am J Med 41:581, 1966

229. Hoffman DL, Mattox VR: Treatment of adrenocortical carcinoma with o,p'DDD. Med Clin North Am 56:999, 1972

230. Lubitz JA, Freeman L, Okun R: Mitotane use in inoperable adrenal cortical carcinoma. JAMA 223:1109, 1973

231. Downing V, Eule J, Juseby RA: Regression of an adrenal cortical carcinoma and its neovascular bed following mitotane therapy: A case report. Cancer 34:1882, 1974

232. Becker D, Schumacher OP: o,p'DDD therapy in invasive adrenocortical carcinoma. Ann Intern Med 82:677, 1975

233. Ostruni JA, Roginsky MS: Metastatic adrenal carcinoma: Documented cure with combined chemotherapy. Arch Intern Med 135:1257, 1975

234. Smilo RP, Earll JM, Forsham PH: Suppression of tumorous adrenal hyperfunction by aminoglutethimide. Metabolism 16:374, 1967

235. Child DE, Burke CW, Burley DM et al: Drug control of Cushing's syndrome:

Combined aminoglutethimide and metyrapone therapy. Acta Endocrinol 82:330, 1976

236. Contreras P, Altieri E, Liberman C et al: Adrenal rest tumor of the liver causing Cushing's syndrome: Treatment with ketoconazole preceding an apparent surgical cure. J Clin Endocrinol Metab 60:21, 1985
237. Nieman LK, Chrousos GP, Kellner C et al: Successful treatment of Cushing's syndrome with the glucocorticoid antagonist RU 486. J Clin Endocrinol Metab 61:536, 1985
238. Percarpio B, Knowlton AH: Radiation therapy of adrenal cortical carcinoma. Acta Radiat Ther Phys Biol 15:288, 1976
239. Malmehhac J: Activity of the adrenal medulla and its regulation. Physiol Rev 44:186, 1964
240. Hermann H, Mornex R: Human Tumors Secreting Catecholamines: Clinical and Physiopathological Study of the Pheochromocytomas, p 207. Oxford, Pergamon Press, 1964
241. Viser J, Axt R: Bilateral adrenal medullary hyperplasia: A clinico-pathological entity. J Clin Pathol 28:298, 1975
242. Greenspan FS, Forsham PH: Basic and Clinical Endocrinology, pp 311, 609. Los Altos, Lange, 1983
243. Manger WM, Gifford RW: Pheochromocytoma. New York, Springer, 1977
244. Modlin IM, Farndon JR, Shepherd A: Phaeochromocytomas in 72 patients: Clinical and diagnostic features, treatment and long term results. Br J Surg 66:456–465, 1979
245. Cryer PE: Physiology and pathophysiology of the human sympathoadrenal neuroendocrine system. N Engl J Med 303:436, 1980
246. St John Sutton MC, Sheps SG, Lie JT: Prevalence of clinically unsuspected pheochromocytoma. Mayo Clin Proc 56:354, 1981
247. Cone TE, Allen MS, Pearson HA: Pheochromocytoma in children. Pediatrics 19:44, 1957
248. Hume DM: Pheochromocytoma in the adult and in the child. Am J Surg 99:458, 1960
249. Robinson MJ, Kent M, Stocks J: Pheochromocytoma in childhood. Arch Dis Child 48:137, 1973
250. Frier DT, Tank ES, Harrison TS: Pediatric and adult pheochromocytomas. Arch Surg 107:252, 1973
251. Voorhess ML: Disorders of the adrenal medulla and multiple endocrine adenomatoses. Pediatr Clin North Am: 209–222, 1979
252. De Schaepdryver AF, Hooft C, Delbeke MJ et al: Urinary catecholamines and metabolites in children. J Pediatr 93:266, 1978
253. Bravo EL, Tarazi RL, Gifford RW, Stewart BH: Circulating and urinary catecholamines in pheochromocytoma: Diagnostic and pathophysiologic implications. N Engl J Med 301:682, 1979
254. Bravo EL: Pheochromocytoma: Current concepts in diagnosis, localization, and management. Primary Care 10:75, 1983
255. Sheps SG, Maher FT: Histamine and glucagon tests in diagnosis of pheochromocytoma. JAMA 205:895, 1968
256. Siqueira–Filho AG, Sheps SG, Maher FT et al: Glucagon-blood catecholamine test: Use in isolated and familial pheochromocytoma. Arch Intern Med 135:1227, 1975
257. Bravo EL, Tarazi RL, Fouad FM: Clonidine suppression test. N Engl J Med 305:623, 1981
258. Wieland DM, Brown LE, Tobes MX et al: Imaging the primate adrenal medullae with [^{123}I] and [^{131}I]meta-iodobenzylguanidine (concise communication). J Nucl Med 22:358, 1981
259. Sisson JL, Farger MS, Valk TW et al: Scintigraphic localization of pheochromocytoma. N Engl J Med 305:1217, 1981
260. Prichard BNC, Ross EJ: Use of propranolol in conjunction with alpha receptor blocking drugs in pheochromocytoma. Am J Cardiol 18:394, 1966
261. Nicholson JP Jr, Vaughn ED Jr, Pickering TG et al: Pheochromocytoma and prazosin. Ann Intern Med 99:477, 1983
262. Robinson RG, DeQuattro V, Grushkin CM et al: Childhood pheochromocytoma treatment with alpha methyl tyrosine for resistant hypertension. J Pediatr 91:143, 1977
263. Goldflien A: Pheochromocytoma: Diagnosis and anesthetic and surgical management. Anesthesiology 24:462, 1963
264. Ross EJ, Prichard BNC, Kaufman L et al: Preoperative and operative management of patients with pheochromocytoma. Br Med J 1:191, 1971
265. Harrison TS, Bartlett JD Jr, Seaton JF: Current evaluation and management of pheochromocytoma. Ann Surg 168:701, 1968
266. Samaan HA: Risk of operation in a patient with unsuspected pheochromocytoma. Br J Surg 57:462, 1970
267. Kaufman BH, Telander RL, Van Heerden JA et al: Pheochromocytoma in the pediatric age group: Current status. J Pediatr Surg 18:879, 1983

268. Pearse AGE, Takor–Takor T: Embryology of the diffuse neuroendocrine system and its relationship to the common peptides. Fed Proc 38:2288, 1979
269. Pearse AGE: The APUD concept and hormone production. Clin Endocrinol Metab 9:211, 1980
270. Bloom SR, Polak JM: Clinical aspects of gut hormones and neuropeptides. Br Med Bull 38:233, 1982
271. Friesen SR: Tumors of the endocrine pancreas. N Engl J Med 306:580, 1982
272. Bloom SR, Polak JM: Glucagonomas, vipomas and somatostatinomas. Clin Endocrinol Metab 9:285, 1980
273. Kolmannskog F, Schrumpf E, Valnes K: Computed tomography and angiography in pancreatic apudomas. Acta Radiol [Diagn] (Stockh) 23:365, 1982
274. Robins JM, Bookstein JJ, Oberman HA, Fajans SS: Selective arteriography in localizing islet cell tumors of the pancreas. Radiology 105:525, 1973
275. Service FJ, Dale AJ, Elveback LR et al: Insulinoma: Clinical and diagnostic features of 60 consecutive cases. Mayo Clin Proc 51:417, 1976
276. Cornblath M, Schwartz R: Disorders of Carbohydrate Metabolism in Infancy, 2nd Ed. Philadelphia, WB Saunders, 1976
277. Merimee TJ, Tyson JF: Hypoglycemia in man: Pathologic and physiologic variants. Diabetes 26:161, 1977
278. Tragl KH, Mayr WR: Familial islet-cell adenomatosis. Lancet 2:426, 1977
279. Turner RC, Lee ECG, Morris PJ et al: Localisation of insulinomas. Lancet 1:515, 1978
280. Wolfsdorf JI, Senior B: The diagnosis of insulinoma in a child in the absence of fasting hyperinsulinism. Pediatrics 64:496, 1979
281. Aynsley–Green A: Hypoglycemia in infants and children. Clin Endocrinol Metab 11:159, 1982
282. Yakovac WC, Baker L, Hummeler K: Beta cell nesidioblastosis in idiopathic hypoglycemia of infancy. J Pediatr 79:226, 1971
283. Balsam MJ, Baker L, Bishop HC et al: Beta cell adenoma in a child with hypoglycemia controlled with diazoxide. J Pediatr 80:788, 1972
284. Grampa G, Gargantini L, Girigolato PG et al: Hypoglycemia in infancy caused by beta cell nesidioblastosis. Am J Dis Child 128:226, 1974
285. Aynsley–Green A, Jenkins P, Tranier B et al: Plasma proinsulin and C-peptide concentrations in children with hyperinsulinaemic hypoglycaemia. Acta Paediatr Scand 73:359, 1984
286. Murray–Lyon IM, Cassar J, Coulson R et al: Further studies on streptozotocin therapy for a multiple-hormone producing islet cell carcinoma. Gut 12:717, 1971
287. Moertel CG, Hanley JA, Johnson LA: Streptotozotocin alone compared with streptozotocin plus fluorouracil in the treatment of advanced islet cell carcinoma. N Engl J Med 303:1189, 1980
288. Zollinger RM, Ellison EH: Primary peptic ulcerations of the jejunum associated with islet cell tumors. Ann Surg 142:709, 1955
289. Walsh JH, Grossman MI: Gastrin. N Engl J Med 292:1324 and 1377, 1975
290. McCarthy DM: Zollinger–Ellison syndrome. Annu Rev Med 33:197, 1982
291. Burcharth F, Stage JG, Stadil F et al: Localization of gastrinomas by transhepatic portal catheterization and gastrin assay. Gastroenterology 77:444, 1979
292. McGuigan JE, Wolfe MM: Secretin injection test in the diagnosis of gastrinoma. Gastroenterology 79:1324, 1980
293. Lamers CB: Clinical usefulness of the secretin provocation test. J Clin Gastroenterol 3:255, 1981
294. Romanus ME, Neal JA, Dilley WG et al: Comparison of four provocative tests for the diagnosis of gastrinoma. Ann Surg 197:608, 1983
295. Richardson CT, Feldman M, McClelland RN et al: Effect of vagotomy in Zollinger–Ellison syndrome. Gastroenterology 77:682, 1979
296. Drake DP, MacIver AG, Atwell JD: Zollinger–Ellison syndrome in a child: Medical treatment with cimetidine. Arch Dis Child 55:226, 1980
297. Bonfils S, Mignon M, Landor J: Management of Zollinger–Ellison syndrome. N Engl J Med 303:942, 1980
298. Peters MN, Richardson CT, Feldman M et al: Exploratory laparotomy, vagotomy, and cimetidine treatment of Zollinger–Ellison syndrome. Gastroenterology 82:1149, 1982
299. Wilson SD: The role of surgery in children with the Zollinger–Ellison syndrome. Surgery 92:682, 1982
300. Brennan MF, Jensen RT, Wesley RA et al: The role of surgery in patients with Zollinger–Ellison syndrome (ZES) managed medically. Ann Surg 196:239, 1982
301. Sadoff L, Franklin D: Streptozotocin in the Zollinger–Ellison syndrome. Lancet 2:504, 1975

302. Lamers CBH, Van Tongeren JH: Streptozotocin in the Zollinger–Ellison syndrome. Lancet 2:1150, 1975

303. Hayes JR, O'Connell N, O'Neill T et al: Successful treatment of malignant gastrinoma with streptozotocin. Gut 17:285, 1976

304. Stadil F, Stage G, Rehfeld JF et al: Treatment of Zollinger–Ellison syndrome with streptozotocin. N Engl J Med 294:1440, 1976

305. Bloom SR, Polak JM, Pearse AGE: Vasoactive intestinal polypeptide and watery diarrhoea syndrome. Lancet 2:14, 1973

306. Shield CF, Haff RD: The VIPoma: Further confirmation of VIP as the hormonal agent in the WDHA syndrome. Am J Surg 132:784, 1976

307. Ebeid AM, Murray PD, Fisher JE: Vasoactive intestinal peptide and the watery diarrhea syndrome. Ann Surg 187:411, 1978

308. Bloom SR, Mitchell SJ: Experimental evidence for VIP as the cause of the watery diarrhea syndrome. Gastroenterology 75:101, 1978

309. Modlin IM, Bloom SR: VIPomas and the watery diarrhea syndrome. S Afr Med J 54:53, 1978

310. Kaplan SJ, Holbrook CT, McDaniel HG et al: Vasoactive intestinal peptide secreting tumors of childhood. Am J Dis Child 134:21, 1980

311. Granot E, Deckelbaum RJ, Schiller M et al: Vasoactive intestinal peptide-secreting tumor appearing as growth failure. Am J Dis Child 137:1203, 1983

312. Long RG: Vasoactive intestinal polypeptide secreting tumors (vipomas) in childhood. J Pediatr Gastroenterol Nutr 2:122, 1983

313. Field M, Chang EB: Pancreatic cholera: Is the diarrhea due to VIP? N Engl J Med 309:1513, 1983

314. Bloom SR, Christofides ND, Delamarter J et al: Diarrhoea in vipoma patients associated with cosecretion of a second active peptide (peptide histidine isoleucine) explained by single coding gene. Lancet 2:1163, 1983

315. Kahn CR, Levy AG, Gardner JD et al: Pancreatic cholera: Beneficial effects of treatment with streptozotocin. N Engl J Med 282:941, 1975

316. Boden G, Owen OE, Rezvani I et al: An islet cell carcinoma containing glucagon and insulin: Chronic glucagon excess and glucose homeostasis. Diabetes 26:128, 1977

317. Binnick AN, Spencer SK, Dennison WL Jr et al: Glucagonoma syndrome. Arch Dermatol 113:749, 1977

318. Higgins GA, Recant L, Fischman AB: The glucagonoma syndrome: Surgically curable diabetes. Am J Surg 137:142, 1979

319. Khandekar JD, Oyer D, Miller HJ et al: Neurologic involvement in glucagonoma syndrome: Response to combination chemotherapy with 5-fluorouracil and streptozotocin. Cancer 44:2014, 1979

320. Leichter SB: Clinical and metabolic aspects of glucagonoma. Medicine 59:100, 1980

321. Stackpoole PW: The glucagonoma syndrome: Clinical features, diagnosis, and treatment. Endocr Rev 2:347, 1981

322. Stackpoole PW, Jaspan J, Kasselberry AG et al: A familial glucagonoma syndrome: Genetic, clinical and biochemical features. Am J Med 70:1017, 1981

323. Hendricks T, Jansen JBJM, Van Tongerer JHM: The glucagonoma syndrome: Stimulus induced plasma responses of circulating glucagon components IRG-9000 and IRG-3500. Acta Endocrinol 105:226, 1984

324. Larsson LI, Holst JJ, Kuhl C et al: Pancreatic somatostatinoma: Clinical features and physiological implications. Lancet 26:666, 1977

325. Ganda OP, Weir GC, Soeldner JS et al: "Somatostatinoma:" A somatostatin-containing tumor of the endocrine pancreas. N Engl J Med 296:963, 1977

326. Ganda OP, Soeldner JS: "Somatostatinoma:" Follow-up studies. N Engl J Med 297:1352, 1977

327. Krejs GJ, Orci L, Conlon JM et al: Somatostatinoma syndrome: Biochemical, morphologic and clinical features. N Engl J Med 30:285, 1979

328. Baylin SB, Mendelsohn G: Ectopic (inappropriate) hormone production by tumors: Mechanisms involved and the biological and clinical implications. Endocr Rev 1:45, 1980

329. Imura H: Ectopic hormone syndromes. Clin Endocrinol Metab 9:235, 1980

330. Asa SL, Kovacs K, Tindall GT et al: Cushing's disease associated with an intrasellar gangliocytoma producing corticotropin-releasing factor. Ann Intern Med 101:789, 1984

331. Belsky JL, Cuello B, Swanson LW et al: Cushing's syndrome due to ectopic production of corticotropin-releasing factor. J Clin Endocrinol Metab 60:496, 1985

332. Schteingart DE, Lloyd RV, Akil H et al: Cushing's syndrome secondary to ectopic corticotropin releasing-hormone–adrenocorticotropin secretion. J Clin Endocrinol Metab 63:770, 1986

333. Cohen RB, Toll GD, Castelman B: Bronchial adenomas in Cushing's syndrome: Their relation to thymomas and oat cell carcinomas associated with hyperadrenocorticism. Cancer 13:812, 1960

334. Prunty FTG, Brooks RV, Dure J et al: Adrenocortical hyperfunction and potassium metabolism in patients with "nonendocrine" tumors and Cushing's syndrome. J Clin Endocrinol Metab 23:737, 1963

335. O'Riordan JLH, Blanshard GP, Moxham A et al: Corticotrophin-secreting carcinomas. Q J Med 35:137, 1966

336. Strott CA, Nugent CA, Tyler FH: Cushing's syndrome caused by bronchial adenomas. Am J Med 44:97, 1968

337. Ratcliffe JG, Knight RA, Besser GM et al: Tumour and plasma ACTH concentrations in patients with and without the ectopic ACTH syndrome. Clin Endocrinol 1:27, 1972

338. Mason AMS, Ratcliffe JG, Buckle RM et al: ACTH secretion by bronchial carcinoid tumours. Clin Endocrinol 1:3, 1972

339. Forman BH, Marban E, Kayne RD et al: Ectopic ACTH syndrome due to pheochromocytoma: Case report and review of the literature. Yale J Biol Med 52:181, 1979

340. Styne DM, Isaac R, Miller WL et al: Endocrine, histological and biochemical studies of adrenocorticotropin-producing islet cell carcinoma of the pancreas in childhood with characterization of propiomelancortin. J Clin Endocrinol Metab 57:723, 1983

341. Lyons DF, Eisen BR, Clark MR et al: Concurrent Cushing's and Zollinger Ellison syndrome in a patient with islet cell carcinoma: Case report and review of the literature. Am J Med 76:729, 1984

342. Zafar MS, Mellinger RC, Fine G et al: Acromegaly associated with a bronchial carcinoid tumor: Evidence for ectopic production of growth hormone-releasing activity. J Clin Endocrinol Metab 44:66, 1979

343. Shalet SM, Beardwell CC, MacFarlane IA et al: Acromegaly due to production of a growth hormone-releasing factor by a bronchial carcinoid tumor. Clin Endocrinol 10:61, 1979

344. Frohman LA, Szabo M, Berelowitz M et al: Partial purification and characterization of a peptide with growth hormone-releasing activity from extra pituitary tumors in patients with acromegaly. J Clin Invest 65:43, 1980

345. Leveston SA, McKeel DW Jr, Buckley PJ et al: Acromegaly and Cushing's syndrome associated with a foregut carcinoid tumor. J Clin Endocrinol Metab 53:682, 1981

346. Thorner MO, Perryman RL, Cronin MJ et al: Somatotroph hyperplasia: Successful treatment of acromegaly by removal of a pancreatic islet tumor secreting a growth hormone-releasing factor. J Clin Invest 70:965, 1982

347. Guillemin R, Brazeau P, Bohlen P et al: Growth hormone releasing factor from a human pancreatic tumor that caused acromegaly. Science 218:585, 1982

348. Spiess J, Rivier T, Thorner M et al: Sequence analysis of a growth hormone releasing factor from a human pancreatic islet tumor. Biochemistry 21:6037, 1982

349. Scheithauer BW, Carpenter PC, Bloch B et al: Ectopic secretion of a growth hormone-releasing factor: Report of a case of acromegaly with bronchial carcinoid tumor. Am J Med 76:605, 1984

350. Von Werder K, Losa M, Muller OA et al: Treatment of metastasising GRF-producing tumor with a long-acting somatostatin analogue (letter). Lancet 2:282, 1984

351. Cameron DP, Burger HG, DeKretzer DM et al: On the presence of immunoreactive growth hormone in a bronchogenic carcinoma. Aust Ann Med 18:143, 1969

352. Greenberg PB, Beck C, Martin TJ et al: Synthesis and release of human growth hormone from lung carcinoma in cell culture. Lancet 1:350, 1972

353. Ghosh L, Ghosh BC, Das Gupta TK: Intracellular demonstration of growth hormone in human mammary carcinoma cells. Am J Surg 135:215, 1978

354. Kaganowicz A, Farkouh NH, Frantz AG et al: Ectopic human growth hormone in ovaries and breast cancer. J Clin Endocrinol Metab 48:5, 1979

355. Braunstein GD, Vaitukaitis JL, Carbone PP, Ross GT: Ectopic production of human chorionic gonadotropin by neoplasms. Ann Intern Med 78:39, 1973

356. Kahn CR, Rosen SW, Weintraub BD et al: Ectopic production of chorionic gonadotropin and its subunits by islet cell tumors: A specific marker for malignancy. N Engl J Med 297:565, 1977

357. Levine LS, Novogroder M, Saxena B et al: Primary intracranial hCG-producing germinoma in a boy with congenital adrenal hyperplasia. Acta Endocrinol 99:122, 1978

358. Vaitukaitis JL: Human chorionic gonadotropin: A hormone secreted for many reason. N Engl J Med 301:324, 1979

359. Oberg K, Wide L: hCG and hCG subunits as tumor markers in patients with endocrine pancreatic tumors and carcinoids. Acta Endocrinol 98:256, 1981

360. Sklar CA, Conte FA, Kaplan SL et al: Human chorionic gonadotropin-secreting pineal tumor: Relation to pathogenesis and sex limitation of sexual precocity. J Clin Endocrinol Metab 53:656, 1981

361. Arshad RR, Woo SY, Abbassi V et al: Virilizing hepatoblastoma: Precocious

sexual development and partial response of pulmonary metastases to cis-platinum. CA 32:293, 1982

362. Hietz PU, Kasper M, Kloppel G et al: Glycoprotein-hormone alpha-chain production by pancreatic endocrine tumors: A specific marker for malignancy. Immunocytochemical analysis of tumors of 155 patients. Cancer 51:277, 1983

363. Odell WD: Humoral manifestations of cancer. In Williams RH (ed): Textbook of Endocrinology, 6th Ed, pp 1228–1241. Philadelphia, WB Saunders, 1981

364. Raisz JG, Luben RA, Mundy GR et al: Effect of osteoclast activating factor from human leucocytes on bone metabolisms. J Clin Invest 56:408, 1975

365. Sherwood LM: The multiple causes of hypercalcemia in malignancy. N Engl J Med 303:1412, 1980

366. Stewart AF, Horst R, Deftos LJ et al: Biochemical evaluation of patients with cancer-associated hypercalcemia: Evidence for humoral and non-humoral groups. N Engl J Med 303:1377, 1980

367. Mundy GR, Ibbotson KJ, D'Souza SM et al: The hypercalcemia of cancer: Clinical implications and pathogenetic mechanisms. N Engl J Med 310:1718, 1984

368. Widmer V, Zapf J, Foresch ER: Is extrapancreatic tumor hypoglycemia associated with elevated levels of insulin-like growth factor II? J Clin Endocrinol Metab 55:833, 1982

369. Wolfe MM, Alexander RW, McGuigan JE: Extrapancreatic extraintestinal gastrinoma: Effective treatment by surgery. N Engl J Med 306:1533, 1982

370. Faurel JP, Bernard P, Saigot T et al: [A case of VIP and somatostatin-secreting phaeochromocytoma] (Fr). Nouv Presse Med 11:1483, 1982

371. El Shafie M, Samuel D, Klippel CH et al: Intractable diarrhea in children with VIP secreting ganglioneuroblastomas. J Pediatr Surg 18:34, 1984

372. Omenn GS: Ectopic hormone syndrome associated with tumors in childhood. Pediatrics 47:613, 1971

373. Harrison RS, Thompson NW: Multiple endocrine adenomatosis I and II. Curr Probl Surg 12(8):1, 1975

374. Schimke FN: Multiple endocrine adenomatosis syndromes. Adv Intern Med 21:249, 1976

375. Yamaguchi K, Kamaya T, Abe K: Multiple endocrine neoplasia type 1. Clin Endocrinol Metab 9:261, 1980

376. Sizemore GW, Heath H, Carney JA: Multiple endocrine neoplasia type 2. Clin Endocrinol Metab 9:299, 1980

377. Brunt LN, Wells SA Jr: The multiple endocrine neoplasia syndromes. Ann Chir Gynaecol 72:153, 1983

378. Underdahl LO, Woolner LB, Black BM: Multiple endocrine adenomas: Report of 8 cases in which parathyroids, pituitary and pancreatic islets were involved. J Clin Endocrinol Metab 13:20, 1953

379. Moldawer MP, Nardi GL, Raker JW: Concomitance of multiple adenomas of the parathyroids and pancreatic islets with tumor of the pituitary: A syndrome with familial incidence. Am J Med Sci 228:190, 1954

380. Wermer P: Genetic aspects of adenomatosis of endocrine glands. Am J Med 16:363, 1954

381. Wermer P: Endocrine adenomatosis and peptic ulcer in a large kindred: Inherited multiple tumors and mosaic pleiotropism in man. Am J Med 35:205, 1963

382. Haverback BJ, Dyce BJ: Gastrointestinal cancer syndromes: Gastrins, multiple endocrine adenomatosis, and the Zollinger–Ellison syndrome. Ann NY Acad Sci 230:297, 1976

383. Carlson HE, Levine GA, Goldberg NJ et al: Hyperprolactinemia in multiple endocrine adenomatosis, type I. Arch Intern Med 138:1807, 1978

384. Hutcheon DF, Bayless TM, Cameron JL, Beylin SB: Watery diarrhea mediated by different hormones in a multiple endocrine neoplasia type I kindred. Gastroenterology 74:1047, 1978

385. Veldhuis JD, Green JE, Kovacs E et al: Prolactin-secreting pituitary adenomas: Association with multiple endocrine neoplasia, type I. Am J Med 67:830, 1979

386. Reith KG, Brody SA: CT of the pituitary gland in multiple endocrine neoplasia type 1. Am J Neuroradiol 4:813, 1983

387. Hershon KS, Kelly WA, Shaw CM et al: Prolactinomas as part of the multiple endocrine neoplastic syndrome type I. Am J Med 74:713, 1983

388. Swinton NW Jr, Clerkin EP, Flint LD: Hypercalcemia and familial pheochromocytoma: Correction after adrenalectomy. Ann Intern Med 76:455, 1972

389. DePlaen JF, Boemer F, van Ypersele de Strihou C: Hypercalcemic phaeochromocytoma. Br Med J 2:734, 1976

390. Graze K, Spiler IJ, Tashjian AE et al: Natural history of familial medullary thyroid carcinoma: Effect of a program for early diagnosis. N Engl J Med 299:980, 1978

391. Ehrlichman RJ: Medullary thyroid carcinoma in Sipple syndrome. Johns Hopkins Med J 145:201, 1979

392. Brown JS, Steiner JS: Medullary thyroid carcinoma and the syndromes of multiple endocrine adenomas. D M 28:1, 1982

393. Lips KJM, van der Sluys Veer J, Struyvenberg A et al: Bilateral occurrence of pheochromocytoma in patients with the multiple endocrine neoplasia syndrome type 2A (Sipple's syndrome). Am J Med 70:1051, 1981

394. Babu VR, Van Dyke DL, Jackson CE: Chromosome 20 deletion in human multiple endocrine neoplasia types 2 A and 2 B: A double-blind study. Proc Natl Acad Sci USA 81:2525, 1984

395. Khairi MRA, Dexter RN, Burzynski NJ et al: Mucosal neuroma, pheochromocytoma and medullary thyroid carcinoma: Multiple endocrine neoplasia type 3. Medicine 54:89, 1975

396. Carney JA, Go VLW, Sizemore GW et al: Alimentary-tract ganglioneuromatosis: A major component of the syndrome of multiple endocrine neoplasia, type 2b. N Engl J Med 295:1287, 1976

397. Carney JA, Hayles AB: Alimentary tract manifestations of multiple endocrine neoplasia, type 2b. Mayo Clin Proc 52:543, 1977

398. Carney JA, Sizemore GW, Hayles AB et al: C-cell disease of the thyroid gland in multiple endocrine neoplasia, type 2b. Cancer 44:2173, 1979

399. Norton JA, Groome LC, Farrell RE et al: Multiple endocrine neoplasia type IIb: The most aggressive form of medullary thyroid carcinoma. Surg Clin North Am 59:109, 1979

400. Dyck PG, Carney JA, Sizemore GW et al: Multiple endocrine neoplasia type 2B: Phenotype recognition: Neurological features and their pathological basis. Ann Neurol 6:302, 1979

401. Kaufman FR, Roe TF, Isaacs H Jr et al: Metastatic medullary thyroid carcinoma in young children with mucosal neuroma syndrome. Pediatrics 70:263, 1982

402. Jones BA, Sisson JC: Early diagnosis and thyroidectomy in multiple endocrine neoplasia, type 2B. J Pediatr 102:219, 1983

403. Steiner AL, Godman AD, Powers SR: Multiple endocrine neoplasia type 2, and Cushing's disease. Medicine 47:371, 1968

404. Cameron D, Spiro HM, Landsberg L et al: Zollinger–Ellison syndrome with multiple endocrine adenomatosis type II. N Engl J Med 299:152, 1978

405. Carney JA, Go VLW, Gordon H et al: Familial pheochromocytoma and islet cell tumor of the pancreas. Am J Med 68:515, 1980

406. Nathan DM, Daniels GH, Ridgway EC: Gastrinoma and phaeochromocytoma: Is there a mixed multiple endocrine adenoma syndrome? Acta Endocrinol (Copenh) 93:91, 1980

407. Alberts WM, McMeekin JO, George JM: Mixed multiple endocrine neoplasia syndromes. JAMA 24:1236, 1980

thirty-five

Management of the Less Common Cancers of Childhood

Charles B. Pratt and Edwin C. Douglass

The preceding chapters have dealt with the principles of pediatric oncology in addition to the management of the more common tumors of childhood. This chapter deals with some of the less frequently encountered malignant tumors of childhood. Although much of the information presented may be more relevant to tumors of adults rather than to tumors of children, the basic principles of treatment remain the same. Pediatric hematologists–oncologists require some knowledge of the diagnosis, management, and treatment derived from the more extensive experience of medical, surgical, and radiation oncologists in dealing with these rare "adult tumors of childhood."

These tumors will be discussed in descending anatomic order from the nasopharynx through the trunk and to the skin. The references include pertinent information related to adult tumors as well as those involving children and adolescents.

NASOPHARYNGEAL CARCINOMA

Nasopharyngeal carcinoma, also known by the less satisfactory terms "lymphoepithelioma," "transitional cell carcinoma," and "epidermoid carcinoma," is a primary malignancy of nasopharyngeal epithelium first described as a separate entity by Regaud[1] and Schmincke[2] in 1921. Although it is a rare tumor, representing less than 1% of pediatric malignancies, it accounts for one-third of the nasopharyngeal neoplasms of childhood.[3] Approximately one-third of nasopharyngeal carcinomas of the undifferentiated type are diagnosed in adolescents or young adults.

Epidemiology

There are marked geographic differences in the distribution of nasopharyngeal carcinoma. Although the incidence is approximately 1:100,000 among the white population of Europe and North America, the incidence may be as high as 20:100,000 in southeast Asia, 25:100,000 in Hong Kong, and 8 to 10:100,000 in northern Africa.[4] In the United States, there may be an increased incidence of nasopharyngeal carcinoma among black teenagers.[5,6]

Biology

One of the most intriguing biologic characteristics of nasopharyngeal carcinoma is its association with Epstein–Barr virus (EBV) infection. EBV DNA can be demonstrated in the malignant cells in biopsy specimens of nasopharyngeal carcinoma (but not in the infiltrating lymphocytes), and these cells also express the EBV nuclear antigen (EBNA).[7,8] Patients with nasopharyngeal carcinoma may have markedly elevated antibody titers to various EBV antigens; of greatest specificity and clinical importance are the titers of IgA and IgG antibodies to the viral capsid antigen (VCA).[9,10] These titers usually correlate with the total tumor burden and decrease with successful therapy. Moreover, they tend to increase prior to the appearance of recurrent disease and thus are a useful indicator of disease activity.

Pathology

The World Health Organization (WHO) classification of nasopharyngeal carcinoma recognizes three subtypes: type 1—squamous cell carcinoma, type 2—nonkeratinizing carcinoma, and type 3—undifferentiated carcinoma (Table 35-1).[11] Most cases in childhood and adolescence are type 3, with a few type 2 cases. Type 1 cases are more typically found in the older adult population. Both types 2 and 3 are associated with elevated EBV titers, whereas type 1 is not.[12]

Both types 2 and 3 may be accompanied by an inflammatory infiltrate of lymphocytes, plasma cells, and eosinophils, which is often abundant, thus giving rise to the term "lymphoepithelioma." Two histologic patterns may occur: the Regaud type, with well-defined collections of epithelial cells surrounded by lymphocytes and connective tissue, and the Schmincke type, where the tumor cells are distributed diffusely and intermingle with the inflammatory cells. Both patterns may be present in the same tumor.[13]

Patterns of Spread

Nasopharyngeal carcinoma usually originates in the fossa of Rosenmuller and typically metastasizes initially to cervical lymph nodes. Cervical lymphadenopathy is, in fact, the initial complaint in many patients. Other types of spread include direct extension throughout the oropharynx, with epistaxis, trismus, Eustachian tube blockage, and hearing loss, and extension into the base of the skull, with cranial nerve palsies. Frequent sites of distant metastases are the lungs, mediastinum, bones, and visceral organs such as liver.

Clinical Presentations

Clinically significant cervical lymphadenopathy is present in most patients at diagnosis. Frequently, it is the only presenting symptom, and the diagnosis of nasopharyngeal carcinoma is often made by lymph node biopsy. Other presenting signs and symptoms are related to the local spread of the tumor as described above: trismus, epistaxis, chronic otitis media, hearing loss, and cranial nerve palsies. Metastatic spread may result in bone pain or symptoms related to organ dysfunction at sites of visceral metastases. A peculiar paraneoplastic syndrome of marked osteoarthropathy with joint swelling, clubbing, and bone and joint pain may occur with widespread disease or metastatic relapse (Fig. 35-1).

Differential Diagnosis

The differential diagnosis includes other malignancies that may present with primaries in the nasopharyngeal area (See also Chap. 5). The most common nasopharyngeal malignancy in childhood is rhabdomyosarcoma; non-Hodgkin's lymphoma, particularly Burkitt's lymphoma, may also present in this area. In children with a subtle or occult primary who present with lymphadenopathy, malignant lymphoma is often

Table 35-1
World Health Organization Classification of Nasopharyngeal Carcinoma[11]

Type	Pathologic Type	Occurrence in Childhood	EBV-Associated
1	Squamous cell	Rare	No
2	Nonkeratinizing	Uncommon	Yes
3	Undifferentiated	Usual	Yes

the first diagnosis and must be ruled out by careful examination of the pathologic material. Thyroid cancer may also present as cervical lymphadenopathy.

Evaluation

The evaluation of the child with nasopharyngeal carcinoma should delineate the extent of the primary tumor and any cervical metastases as well as rule out any distant metastatic spread. The size and location of cervical lymph nodes should be carefully noted, and indirect nasopharyngoscopy should be performed if the primary tumor is not obvious. Neurologic examination should pay special attention to the cranial nerves.

Computed tomography (CT) of the head and neck should include appropriate views of the brain with special attention to the base of the skull (see Chap. 7). CT of the chest and abdomen and radionuclide bone scanning should be done to search for metastatic disease. If there is invasion of the tumor through the base of the skull, a cerebrospinal fluid examination should be done in an attempt to identify tumor cells. Bone marrow examination is not necessary unless there is a strong suspicion of a myelophthistic process.

EBV titers should be assayed by a laboratory familiar with the full battery of EBV serology. The usual serologic examination obtained for acute EBV infection (monospot, EA, D titers) is not adequate. IgA and IgG anti-VCA are the most specific and useful, and direct consultation with the clinical laboratory is usually necessary to assure performance of this test or referral of the specimen to a laboratory where it is routinely performed.

Staging

The extent of the tumor at diagnosis is conveniently described by the tumor, node, metastasis (TNM) classification of the American Joint Committee on Cancer (Table 35-2).[14] Because of the very high incidence of lymph node metastasis at diagnosis, the vast majority of children and adolescents with nasopharyngeal carcinoma would be assigned by this system to the advanced Stages III and IV, which is of little value in assessing prognosis or planning therapy.

Ho has reviewed the problem of staging in nasopharyngeal carcinoma and proposed a modified classification scheme (Table 35-3).[15] His scheme takes into account the prognostic importance of tumorous nodes extending into the lower cervical and supraclavicular areas[16] and the uniformly poor prognosis of patients with metastatic disease at diagnosis.

Prognostic Considerations and Variables

Because it was designed to account for all oropharyngeal malignancies, including squamous cell carcinomas, in all age groups, the AJC stage grouping is of little help in assessing the

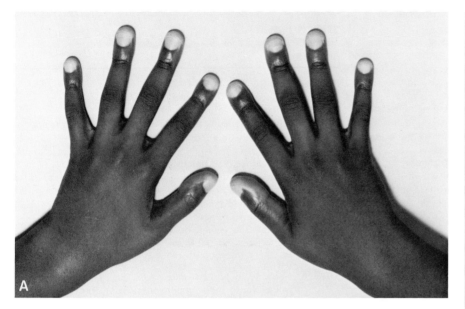

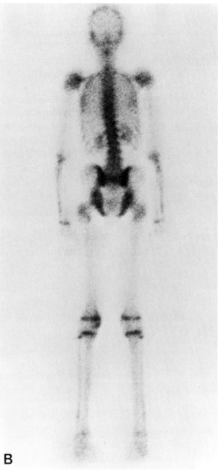

FIGURE 35-1. A. Digital clubbing. **B.** Periostitis with diffuse increased uptake on bone scan in a teenage boy with recurrent nasopharyngeal carcinoma associated with hypertophic osteoarthropathy (paraneoplastic syndrome).

prognosis of children and adolescents with nasopharyngeal carcinoma. It places more than 90% of patients in Stage III or IV and does not take into account the relatively good prognosis of many children with this disease, nor does it account for the lack of association between the T Stage and N Stage in this disease.

Survival on the basis of T Stage alone has been analyzed by several authors (Table 35-4). Jenkin and associates found a 75% overall survival rate in patients with T1–2 and 37% in those with T3–4.[23] Similarly, Lombardi and coworkers noted an 87% survival rate in T1–2 disease compared with 8% in T3–4,[25] and Ellouz and colleagues found survival rates of 54% in T1–2 and 25% in T3–4.[19] In our own series at St. Jude, we found a 78% disease-free survival rate (11 of 14 patients) in patients with T1–2 tumors.[30] Two of the three patients who died had metastatic disease at diagnosis. A 24% disease-free survival rate was found in patients presenting with T3–4 tumors. Analysis of our series according to Ho's classification and stage grouping shows 100% disease-free survival in Stages A and B (six of six patients), 41% in Stage C (9 of 13 patients), and zero in Stage D (three patients). No factors other than stage have correlated with prognosis.

Treatment

Surgery

The nasopharynx is a difficult area to approach surgically, and nasopharyngeal carcinoma has almost always spread beyond its confines at the time of diagnosis. Therefore, the principal role of surgery prior to other therapy is to obtain adequate diagnostic material from either an involved lymph node or the primary site. Myringotomy and tympanostomy tube insertion should be performed prior to radiation therapy if otitis media is present or expected. If there is evidence of surgically accessible residual disease following radiation therapy, this may be considered for resection.

Radiotherapy

Radiation remains the primary therapeutic modality for this disease. The primary volume should include the nasopharynx, posterior nasal cavity, posterior maxillary sinus, base of the skull including the sphenoid and cavernous sinuses, and the cervical lymphatics including the supraclavicular nodes (See also Chap. 11). Currently recommended dosages are 6000 to 7000 cGy.[31] If possible, radiation therapy with curative intent should be given for recurrent disease, either local or distant. This may provide long-term control or even apparent cure.

Chemotherapy

The role of chemotherapy in the treatment of nasopharyngeal carcinoma is much less clear than that of radiotherapy. Although some series of nasopharyngeal carcinoma in childhood have reported increased survival with chemotherapy using only historical controls,[28,29] there has been no adequate demonstration of increased disease-free survival in a randomized trial. Furthermore, adult patients with nasopharyngeal carci-

Table 35-2
Tumor, Node, Metastasis (TNM) Classification for Tumors of Nasopharynx

Primary Tumor
T0	No evidence of primary tumor
Tis	Carcinoma *in situ*
T1	Tumor confined to one site of nasopharynx or no tumor visible (positive biopsy only)
T2	Tumor involving two sites (both posterosuperior and lateral walls)
T3	Extension of tumor into nasal cavity or oropharynx
T4	Tumor invasion of skull, cranial nerve involvement, or both

Nodal Involvement
N0	No clinically positive node
N1	Single clinically positive homolateral node 3 cm or less in diameter
N2	Single clinically positive homolateral node more than 3 cm but not more than 6 cm in diameter, or multiple clinically positive homolateral nodes, none more than 6 cm in diameter
	N2a—Single clinically positive homolateral node more than 3 cm but not more than 6 cm in diameter
	N2b—Multiple clinically positive homolateral nodes, none more than 6 cm in diameter
N3	Massive homolateral nodes, bilateral nodes, or contralateral nodes
	N3a—Clinically positive homolateral nodes one more than 6 cm in diameter
	N3b—Bilateral clinically positive nodes
	N3c—Contralateral clinically positive nodes only

Distant Metastasis
M0	No evidence of metastasis
M1	Distant metastasis present

Stage Grouping, American Joint Committee
Stage I: T1, N0, M0
Stage II: T2, N0, M0
Stage III: T3, N0, M0 *or* T1 or T2 or T3, N1, M0
Stage IV: T4, N0 or N1, M0 *or* Any T, N2 or N3, M0 *or*
Any T, any N, MI

Table 35-3
Modified TNM Classification of Nasopharyngeal Carcinoma as Proposed by Ho[15]

Primary Tumor
T0	No evidence of primary tumor
Tis	Carcinoma *in situ*
T1	Tumor confined to nasopharyngeal mucosa or no tumor visible but biopsy positive
T2	Tumor extended to the nasal fossa, oropharynx, or adjacent muscles or nerves below base of the skull
T3	Tumor beyond T2 limits and subclassified as follows:
	T3a—Bone involvement below base of the skull
	T3b—Involvement of base of skull
	T3c—Involvement of cranial nerves
	T3d—Involvement or orbit, laryngopharynx, or infratemporal fossa

Nodal Involvement
N0	No clinically positive node
N1	Nodes wholly in the upper cervical level above lower third of the neck
N2	Nodes palpable in lower third of the neck or supraclavicular area

Distant Metastases
M	Distant metastasis present

This Classification Has an Accompanying Stage Grouping as Follows:
Stage A: T1 N0
Stage B: T1 N1; T2 N0 or N1
Stage C: T3 any N *or* N2 any T
Stage D: M

noma typically are entered into therapeutic trials with all cases of head and neck (upper aerodigestive tract) cancer, and the large proportion of squamous cell carcinomas in such trials may obscure the therapeutic benefits of chemotherapy in the small proportion of patients with nasopharyngeal carcinoma.

Nasopharyngeal carcinoma and other head and neck cancers are unquestionably responsive to several chemotherapeutic agents including cisplatin, 5-fluorouracil (5-FU), methotrexate, and bleomycin. Two basic regimens currently in use are the Price–Hill regimen[32] (vincristine, bleomycin, methotrexate, and 5-FU) and the cisplatin/5-FU infusion regimen as first used by Rooney and associates.[33] Despite the high response rate to these and other regimens, an overall improvement in survival in these adult trials remains to be shown.[34]

Children and adolescents with nasopharyngeal carcinoma may be appropriately treated by entry into adult therapeutic trials for head and neck cancer where data can be accumulated on the overall efficacy of chemotherapy. In addition, chemotherapy seems warranted in patients with recurrent disease. In these cases, an initial trial of chemotherapy to assess tumor responsiveness combined with subsequent radiotherapy to sites of disease may significantly prolong life or even cure rare cases. We have treated four adolescents who had recurrent

nasopharyngeal carcinoma with 5-FU, methotrexate, and radiation; all achieved a complete response, and two survive disease free 2 and 6 years from the initiation of chemotherapy.

Complications of Therapy

Xerostomia is the primary side effect of radiotherapy. This usually begins during treatment along with some mucositis and is almost always permanent. A self-limited sialadenitis may occur within a few months of completion of therapy. Later effects include fibrosis of the neck and trismus. Cranial nerve palsies are usually due to tumor but may be a late complication of fibrosis, and brachial plexus weakness may also occur. Marked muscular atrophy can be expected when children receive large doses of radiation, and we have observed one case of chronic shoulder drop and dislocation after treatment in early adolescence. Hypothyroidism is not uncommon after neck irradiation, and patients should have routine follow-up of thyroid functions. Long-term complications of chemotherapy are related to the particular drugs being used: cisplatin may cause chronic renal insufficiency; alkylating agents may cause sterility, particularly in males; and bleomycin may be responsible for pulmonary fibrosis. Chronic radiation changes will also be seen in the upper lobes after supraclavicular treatment.

Future Directions

The close relation between EBV and nasopharyngeal carcinoma has led to attempts at treatment with interferon[35,36] and acyclovir.[37] Increased knowledge of the biological role of EBV in this disease as well as in other cancers may lead to more

Table 35-4
Some Reported Series of Nasopharyngeal Carcinoma in Childhood and Adolescents (AJC TNM Clssification[14])

Year (Institution)	Number of Patients	Stage N1–3	T1–2	T3–4	M	Disease-free Survivors	Comments
				no. (%)			
1974 (MCV)[17]	9	9 (100)	5 (55)	4 (44)	0	4 (44)	
1976 (MD Anderson)[18]	10	10 (100)	2 (20)	8 (80)	0	6 (60)	
1978 (Tunis)[19]	82	68 (83)	15 (18)	67 (82)	3 (4)	26 (32)	12 cases paraneoplastic syndrome
1978 (Pittsburgh)[20]	7	7 (100)	ND	ND	0	1 (14)	
1980 (Toronto*)[21]	25	22 (88)	12 (48)	13 (52)	1 (4)	10 (40)	70% overall survival at 5 years
1980 (Sloan–Kettering)[22]	16	14 (88)	8 (50)	8 (50)	2 (12)	3 (19)	
1981 (CCSG†)	119	105 (88)	41 (34)	68 (66)	3 (2)	43 (32)	51% overall survival at 5 years
1982 (Michigan)[24]	10	8 (20)	2 (20)	8 (80)	0	5 (50)	
1982 (Milan)[25]	27	26 (96)	11 (41)	16 (59)	2 (7)	8 (40)	20 evaluable patients
1983 (Atlanta)[26]	27	24 (89)	11 (41)	16 (59)	2 (7)	16 (60)	64% overall survival at 5 years
1985 (New York)[27]	6	3 (50)	1 (16)	5 (84)	0	1 (16)	
1986 (Costa Rica)[28]	22	18 (82)	12 (55)	10 (45)	0	14 (63)	
1986 (Manchester)[29]	18	18 (100)	ND	ND	2 (9)	7 (38)	
1987 (St. Jude)[30]	31	29 (97)	14 (45)	17 (55)	3 (10)	15 (48)	58% overall survival at 5 years

* Series includes patients <30 years of age.
† Some patients in this series were previously reported.

specific and effective use of biological response modifiers either alone or in combination with conventional radiotherapy and chemotherapy.

ORAL AND OROPHARYNGEAL CANCER (SQUAMOUS CELL CARCINOMA) AND CANCER ASSOCIATED WITH SMOKELESS TOBACCO PRODUCTS

Oral squamous cell carcinoma in childhood and adolescence is an exceedingly rare event: a review of more than 1000 cases of oropharyngeal cancer at a single institution disclosed only one 10-year-old child and three teenagers.[38] The authors remarked on the rampant nature of squamous cell carcinoma in patients less than 40 years of age. All three teenagers died of disease. Squamous cell carcinoma of the tongue has been reported in a renal transplant recipient at age 26.[39] Squamous cell carcinoma is one of the malignancies which may appear at an early age in patients with Fanconi's anemia.[40]

Evidence is mounting of an increased use in the United States of smokeless tobacco products by preadolescent and adolescent boys (see Chap. 55).[41,42] Because of the known carcinogenic agents in smokeless tobacco[43] and the known association of oral carcinoma, primarily squamous cell carcinoma, with the use of smokeless tobacco products in older persons, oral cancer may become a potentially explosive problem for the present as well as the future if there is continued use of these products. Incidence figures for head and neck cancer under the age of 20 years are not available except for nasopharyngeal, parotid, and minor salivary gland carcinomas. It has been estimated that 8% to 36% of male high-school and college-age students regularly use smokeless tobacco products, the mean age of initiating the use of these products being 12 years.[44,45] The average use of chewing tobacco or snuff has been estimated at six times daily, with the average duration per dip or chew of 1 hour.

The association between cigarette smoking and multiple deleterious health conditions is well recognized, whereas the effects of smokeless tobacco are not so well recognized, even though these products contain potent carcinogens including aromatic hydrocarbons and nitrosamines.[43] Alterations in the texture, color, and contour of the mucosal lining as well as periodontal degeneration have been observed in more than half of teenagers surveyed for changes related to smokeless tobacco.[42] An additional survey indicated that characteristics of leukoplakia, a precancerous condition, occur in more than one-third of the users, and that other forms of ulcers, blisters, and gum, lip, and mouth lesions also occur.[45] It is not known whether the nicotine-related health hazards of smokeless tobacco are identical to those associated with smoking.

Pediatricians as well as health departments should mount concerted efforts in education and in the enactment of laws to prohibit advertisement of these products. Without such changes, we may expect an inordinate number of oral cancers in adolescent and young men within the next several decades.

AMELOBLASTOMA

Ameloblastoma, also known as adamantinoma, is a rare tumor that may arise in the mandible or maxilla and occasionally in the long bones.[46] The relationship of this tumor, which may be benign or malignant, to the development of the enamel of the teeth is recognized. Surgical excision is the treatment of choice. Local recurrence is more frequent for mandibular than for maxillary lesions. Sensitivity of recurrent tumors to irradiation is recognized; sensitivity to chemotherapy is unknown. Pulmonary metastases have been discovered many years after treatment of the primary tumor.

CARCINOMA OF THE LARYNX

Benign as well as malignant tumors of the larynx are rare. Benign tumors include polyps and papillomas, which may be associated with cough and hoarseness, dysphagia, and cervical lymphadenopathy. Probably the most common malignant tumor is rhabdomyosarcoma, the treatment of which is discussed in Chapter 30.

Squamous cell carcinoma of the larynx in children or adolescents should be managed along the guidelines established for this tumor in adults.[47,48] Surgery, irradiation, or both are the modalities of choice. In a recent review, the prognosis for 56 children with this rare disease was not clear; survival rates are not stage related. Rehabilitative efforts should begin with preoperative counseling, and an electronic speech device may be used immediately after operation. About 10% of laryngectomees develop satisfactory esophageal speech, which is accomplished by belching swallowed air to produce phonation. Prosthetic devices include the electrolarynx (a battery-powered tone generator) and pneumatic external reeds. The electrolarynx transmits sounds from the neck or mouth; speech from the neck type electrolarynx is more easily understood than that from the oral type. The American Cancer Society's involvement with rehabilitation of patients after laryngectomies includes information, support, and social outlets for these individuals patterned after those provided for adults. For survivors who were given radiation, long-term attention should also be directed to thyroid size and function.

LUNG CANCER

Primary pulmonary malignancies are extremely rare in childhood, but more than 100 cases have been reported.

Bronchogenic Carcinoma

The occurrence of bronchogenic carcinoma has been well documented in childhood. Most cases are of the undifferentiated or adenocarcinomatous type,[49] but squamous cell carcinomas have also been reported.[50,51] These cancers may occur in children of any age but more typically in adolescence.

The management of children with bronchogenic carcinoma should be according to reasonable adult guidelines with resection of operable tumors. Radiation therapy may be of some benefit in inoperable cases.

Bronchial "Adenomas"

The majority of cases reported as bronchial adenomas are in fact carcinoid tumors or slow-growing malignancies such as mucoepidermoid carcinomas or cylindromas.[52] All of these have been reported in childhood.[53-56] The primary treatment of these tumors is surgical resection.[55,56]

Pulmonary Blastoma

This rare pulmonary neoplasm tends to occur in a subpleural location.[57] It has been reported at all ages, but one-fourth of the more than 50 reported cases have been in children.[58] It was originally thought that this tumor was an embryonal malignancy of mesoblastic tissue,[59] but more recently, it has been proposed that pulmonary blastoma is a special form of pulmonary carcinosarcoma.[60] Pulmonary blastoma has been associated with cystic disease of the lung.[57] Large lesions (>5 cm) frequently recur or metastasize in spite of primary resection.[60] A response to a combination of vincristine, doxorubicin, and cyclophosphamide has been reported in one child.[61]

MESOTHELIOMA

The pleura, pericardium, and peritoneum are the primary sites of these tumors of the mesothelial surfaces.[62-68] Other tumors of children or adolescents have involved the testes[68] or auriculoventricular node.[69] Pleural mesotheliomas have also occurred as second malignant neoplasms.[69-71] These tumors have pleomorphic histologic appearances and may spread over the pleural and peritoneal surfaces but do not invade the underlying tissues deeply; however, these tumors may metastasize.

Many adults with mesotheliomas have a history of exposure to asbestos, which may be carcinogenic, either at industrial sites or within the environment. The amount of exposure required for risk is unknown, and information about the risk for children exposed to asbestos is not available. Annually, about 4000 cancer deaths in this country are related to exposure to asbestos.[64] Shipyard workers have had a greater incidence of pleural mesotheliomas in contrast to peritoneal tumors, which have occurred mainly in asbestos factory workers. The greatest incidence of cancer is that of insulation workers, who have developed lung cancer.

Benign and malignant mesotheliomas cannot be differentiated on histologic grounds. It should be understood that localized resection is curative and that a poor prognosis is associated with lesions that are diffuse or invasive and which recur. Treatment with doxorubicin and cisplatin has resulted in partial responses.[72] Radiation therapy may be used for palliation of pain.

THYMOMA

Primary malignant lesions involving the thymus include lymphomas, germ cell tumors, carcinoids, carcinomas, thymolipomas, and thymoma, most of which can be confused because of the similarity of the gross as well as microscopic appearance.[73,74]

To be identifiable as a thymoma, the epithelium of the thymus must undergo neoplastic change.[75] Both Hodgkin's and non-Hodgkin's lymphomas may involve the thymus gland and therefore must be differentiated from true thymomas. A neoplasm of the thymus is not considered to be a thymoma without the presence of the neoplastic epithelial components.[76]

Epidemiology

Thymomas are rare in adults as well as in children. Fewer than 10% of thymomas occur in patients less than 20 years of age.[73,77-83]

Various syndromes and diseases are associated with thymomas. Autoimmune or immune phenomena include myasthenia gravis, polymyositis, systemic lupus erythematosus, rheumatoid arthritis, hypogammaglobulinemia, cytopenias, and thyroiditis. Endocrine disorders associated with thymomas include hyperthyroidism, Addison's disease, and panhypopituitarism.[73,84,85]

The most frequent of the associated conditions are myasthenia gravis, red cell aplasia, and hypogammaglobulinemia.[85] Weakness and fatigability are the principal symptoms of myasthenia gravis; these symptoms may be relieved by acetylcholinesterase inhibitors. The association between myasthenia gravis and the thymus was recognized when histopathologic changes were found in the thymus of patients with this disease. The association between thymomas, the thymus, and myasthenia gravis remains troublesome for physicians who must treat these individuals, be they adults or children. Pure red cell aplasia is found in about 5% of patients with thymoma, whereas up to one half of patients with red cell aplasia have thymoma.[73] Hypogammaglobulinemia occurs in as many as 10% of patients with thymoma.[73]

Genetics

There are no genetically associated diseases that occur with significant frequency in patients with thymoma.

Pathology and Symptomatology

Thymomas are usually located in the anterior mediastinum and represent the most frequent neoplasms involving this compartment in adults.[73] Most tumors are discovered with the use of routine chest roentgenography or for reasons unrelated to tumor. These lesions generally are located anterior to the great vessels of the mediastinum, which may be displaced posteriorly by the tumor. The masses are usually round with smooth or lobulated margins and may protrude to one or both sides of the mediastinum. Calcifications may be seen.

Vague and nonspecific symptoms related to the chest may or may not be present.[77-83] These symptoms may include cough, dysphagia, tightness, pain, and dyspnea. A superior vena cava syndrome may accompany advanced lesions.

Pathogenesis and Natural History

Thymomas generally are slow-growing tumors. Although almost all are potentially invasive, metastasis to distant organs or regional lymph nodes is rare. Organs that have been involved have included bone, liver, kidney, brain, spleen, and colon. It is generally thought that thymomas in children have a more malignant course than those of adults.[80]

Diagnosis

Appropriate evaluation of patients suspected of having thymoma or other mediastinal tumors includes chest roentgenographs and CT. These studies will not differentiate thymomas from nonthymomatous masses but may differentiate cystic lesions from solid tumors. The differential diagnosis of other anterior mediastinal masses includes Hodgkin's disease and non-Hodgkin's lymphoma, thymolipoma, carcinoids, as well as germ cell tumors (primary seminoma, nonseminomatous and mixed germ-cell carcinomas), teratomas, and thymic carci-

nomas. In the Mississippi Valley, histoplasmosis should be included in the differential diagnosis of mediastinal tumors.

Staging

Staging of thymomas is based on the extent of invasiveness.[86,87] Burgh and colleagues[88] have proposed a staging scheme (Table 35-5).

Treatment

Thymomas are relatively radiosensitive.[93] Treatment with radiation is considered mandatory for patients with invasive thymomas, whether or not a complete resection is performed. Radiation may also be utilized as adjuvant therapy for patients with or without invasion. Dosage recommendations are based on the age of the child and the extent of invasiveness of the tumor. Dosages of 3500 to 4500 cGy delivered over 3 to 6 weeks are recommended for control of incompletely resected thymomas.[93]

Chemotherapy is generally reserved for patients with advanced-stage disease who have not responded to radiation or corticosteroid therapy. Doxorubicin and cisplatin are recognized as effective agents for the treatment of this tumor, although responses also have been reported with alkylating agents.[94-96] Other agents that have been used include vincristine, procarbazine, and bleomycin.

In studies of adults and children at large institutions, 5-year survival rates ranged from 65% to 83% for encapsulated tumors[73] and 30% to 54% for invasive tumors. The overall survival rate for patients with invasive thymoma and myasthenia gravis is about 10%.[97,98]

Complications of therapy may be related to the use of radiation. These complications may include pneumonitis, mediastinitis, pericarditis, and myocarditis.

TUMORS OF THE HEART

More than half of the primary tumors of the heart are benign; most are myxomas.[99-101] Neurofibromas may also involve the heart. More common, however, are metastatic tumors, such as rhabdomyosarcoma, melanoma, leukemia, and carcinomas.[101] These tumors may involve the pericardium, myocardium, or endocardium.[102] The symptoms may include arrhymias, cardiomegaly, pericardial effusions, and congestive failure. For malignant lesions, treatment may include pericardiocentesis, irradiation, and chemotherapy.

RENAL CELL CARCINOMA

Renal cell carcinoma (clear cell carcinoma, renal cell adenocarcinoma, hypernephroma) was first studied by Grawitz,[103] who believed that the tumor arose from ectopic adrenal tissue

---

Table 35-5
Proposed Staging Scheme for Thymomas Based on Extent of Invasion[88]

Stage I	Intact capsule or growth within the capsule
Stage II	Pericapsular growth into mediastinal fat
Stage III	Invasive growth into surrounding organs, intrathoracic metastases, or both

because of its microscopic similarity to adrenal. Because of this similarity, he named this tumor "hypernephroma," a misnomer that still is occasionally used today.

Renal cell carcinoma is the most common primary malignancy of the kidney in adults, accounting for 2% of adult cancer cases, but occurs only rarely in children. Data from the Third National Cancer Survey[3] show that the annual incidence rate of renal cell carcinoma in children is only 4 per 1 million compared with 117 per 1 million for Wilms' tumor (see Chap. 27). Referral patterns to the Armed Forces Institute of Pathology seem to indicate that in the second decade of life, the incidence of renal cell carcinoma may approach that of Wilms' tumor.[104] Although renal cell carcinoma in adults occurs with a male:female ratio of 2:1,[105] childhood series[106–109] show an approximately equally gender ratio.

Genetics

Renal cell carcinoma is seen in association with von Hippel–Lindau disease (hereditary angiomatosis of the retina and cerebellum).[110,111] The renal cysts that develop in this disease undergo malignant degeneration in as many as one-fourth of the cases. Renal cell carcinoma also has been reported in association with tuberous sclerosis,[108] a hereditary disease that is also characterized by the appearance of renal angiomyolipomas and cysts.

Familial renal cell carcinoma has been reported in association with a constitutional chromosomal translocation, t(3:8) (p14;q24).[112,113] Chromosome studies of nonfamilial tumors have shown a high incidence of abnormalities of chromosome 3.[114]

Pathology

Microscopically, the tumor tissue resembles renal tubules. Four major patterns of growth have been described: papillary, solid, cystic, and sarcomatoid. There is apparently little prognostic significance to these patterns, and several patterns are typically found within the same tumor.[14] In addition to these patterns of growth, three different types of cellular morphology may be identified: clear cells, granular cells, and sarcomatoid cells.[116]

Patterns of Spread

Renal cell carcinoma typically metastasizes by both hematogenous and lymphogenous spread. Lungs, bones, liver, lymph nodes, and the mediastinum are frequent metastatic sites.

Clinical Presentation

In contrast to Wilms' tumor, where an abdominal mass is often the presenting symptom, children with renal cell carcinoma typically present with abdominal or flank pain, gross hematuria, or both. The primary tumor is often not palpable nor is it visible on plain radiographs or even intravenous urography so that it must be demonstrated by ultrasound or CT (Fig. 35-2). A variety of paraneoplastic syndromes have been reported in adults, especially hepatic dysfunction that resolves after resection of the primary tumor.[117] Other syndromes appear due to ectopic production of various hormones including parathormone (hypercalcemia),[118] erythropoietin (polycythemia),[119] gonadotropin (gynecomastia),[120] and various other substances.

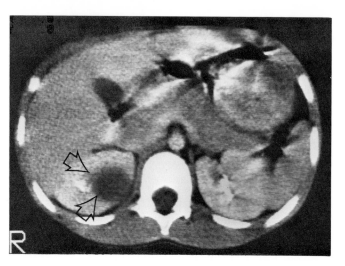

FIGURE 35-2.   Cystic renal lesion (*arrows*) in an 8-year-old boy who presented with hematuria. Pathologic study demonstrated a renal cell carcinoma.

These syndromes have not been a notable feature of renal cell carcinoma in childhood, however.

Children with renal cell carcinoma are typically older than the child with Wilms' tumor, with a median age at diagnosis of 11 years.[107,109] However, the diagnosis has been made in children as young as 14 months.

Differential Diagnosis

The obvious lesion to be considered in the differential diagnosis is Wilms' tumor, the most common renal neoplasm in childhood (see Chap. 27). Beckwith has pointed out the occasional difficulty in distinguishing Wilms' tumor from renal cell carcinoma.[121] Also to be considered are other space-occupying lesions of the pediatric kidney, including multilocular cysts, nephroblastomatosis, angiomyolipoma, congenital mesoblastic nephroma, benign stromal tumors, intrarenal neuroblastoma, renal teratoma, malignant rhabdoid tumor, clear-cell sarcoma, lymphoma (especially Burkitt's), and renal sarcomas (*e.g.,* rhabdomyosarcoma, liposarcoma) (also see Chap. 5).

Evaluation

Renal cell carcinoma should be considered particularly in the older child who presents with pain or hematuria and a renal lesion. Studies to be obtained include a complete blood count (anemia, erythrocytosis), biochemical profile (hypercalcemia), renal ultrasound with attention to the patency of the inferior vena cava, CT of the chest and abdomen with and without intravenous contrast infusion, and a bone survey and radionuclide bone scan.

Staging

Renal cell carcinoma in childhood has occasionally been staged according to the National Wilms' Tumor Study criteria. Although pediatric oncologists are most familiar with this staging system, it seems more appropriate to use one of the staging systems developed specifically for this tumor in adults (Tables

35-6 and 35-7). The TNM classification provides the most accurate description of disease extent.

Prognostic Considerations

The stage at diagnosis is the most important prognostic factor. Of the 37 children reported in two series,[107,109] the long-term survival rates were Stage I—11/11 (100%), Stage II—6/11 (66%), Stage III—3/7 (43%), and Stage IV—1/8 (12%). Although other variables such as tumor grade correlate with stage at diagnosis, they do not appear to be independent variables. Renal vein invasion, if the mass is resectable with the primary tumor, does not appear to affect prognosis adversely.[109] One large review reported an actuarial survival rate in 84 children of 60% at 2 years and 56% at 5 years.[106] Most recurrences and deaths occur within the first 2 years after diagnosis, but late recurrences are not infrequent.[108]

Treatment

Surgery

The primary therapy of localized renal cell carcinoma is unquestionably radical nephrectomy with resection of the kidney and tumor, the adrenal gland, surrounding perinephric fat, Gerota's fascia, and the regional lymph nodes.

Radiotherapy

The role of either preoperative or postoperative radiotherapy in the management of renal cell carcinoma is much less clear. Different series, both randomized and unrandomized, of adult patients have found both enhanced survival with the addition of radiotherapy and no difference in treated and untreated groups.[123] This situation is even less clear in children, where renal cell carcinoma is a much rarer disease. Empiric administration of postoperative radiotherapy (4000–4500 cGy in 150-cGy fractions) has been recommended for children with Stage III disease.[109] Radiotherapy can provide significant palliation to decrease pain, mass effects, or hematuria from unresectable primaries or metastatic disease.

Chemotherapy

No single chemotherapy agent or combination of agents has yet proved to be of significant benefit. However, renal cell carcinoma may prove amenable to therapy with biologic response modifiers. Responses have been seen after treatment with interferon,[124,125] and bolus or constant-infusion interleu-

kin-2 with lymphokine-activated killer cells has provided complete or partial responses in 15 of 42 patients.[126,127]

Current Therapy

Fortunately, at least 50% of pediatric patients with renal cell carcinoma are curable by surgery. Adjuvant radiotherapy remains controversial but should be considered when the disease has extended beyond the renal fossa. There is at present no satisfactory chemotherapy for renal cell carcinoma, but the further refinement and development of biologic response modifiers may provide a significant alternative for the treatment of this disease.

ADRENOCORTICAL CARCINOMA

Adrenocortical carcinoma is a rare tumor in children and accounts for less than 0.5% of childhood malignancies (see Chap. 1 and 34).[3] At St. Jude Children's Research Hospital, only five patients among more than 5000 patients with malignancies have had adrenocortical carcinoma. The appearance of this cancer in childhood may be associated with other developmental defects such as hemihypertrophy, genitourinary anomalies, or the Beckwith–Wiedemann syndrome; these same anomalies may also be associated with other cancers such as hepatoblastoma and Wilms' tumor (see Chap. 2).[129] Children who survive adrenocortical carcinoma may be at increased risk for second malignancies, including brain tumors, melanoma, and sarcomas.[130]

Most adrenocortical carcinomas are functional endocrine tumors, and symptoms are related to the particular hormones produced to excess: typically glucocorticoids (Cushing's syndrome), sex hormones (virilization or precocious puberty; rarely feminization) (Fig. 35-3), or mineralocorticoids (Conn's

Table 35-6

Staging Scheme for Renal Cell Carcinoma (Robson and Associates[122])

Stage A	Tumor confined to the kidney without involvement of perinephric fat
Stage B	Tumor with extension into perinephric fat but not beyond Gerota's fascia
Stage C	Metastases to regional lymph nodes or gross involvement of inferior vena cava
Stage D	Tumor involvement of adjacent organs other than adrenal gland or distant hematogenous and/or lymphatic metastases

Table 35-7

TNM Classification of Extent of Disease for Patients with Renal Cell Carcinoma[14]

Primary Tumor

T0	No evidence of primary tumor
T1	Small tumor; minimal renal and caliceal distortion or deformity; circumscribed neovasculature surrounded by parenchyma
T2	Large tumor with deformity or enlargement of kidney or collecting system
T3a	Large tumor involving perinephric tissues
T3b	Tumor involving renal vein
T3c	Tumor involving renal vein and infradiaphragmatic vena cava
T4	Tumor extending into neighboring organs or abdominal wall

Nodal Involvement

N0	No evidence of involvement of regional nodes
N1	Single, homolateral regional nodal involvement
N2	Involvement of multiple regional or of contralateral or bilateral nodes
N3	Fixed regional nodes (assessable only at surgical exploration)

Distant Metastases

M0	No known distant metastasis
M1	Distant metastasis present (specific sites)

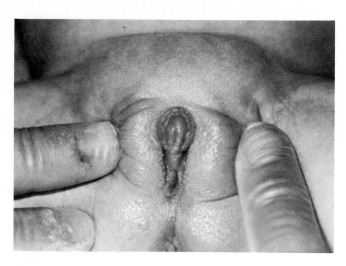

FIGURE 35-3. Clitoral hypertrophy in a 3-month-old female with adrenocortical carcinoma and virilism. This condition disappeared after resection of the abdominal tumor. The patient subsequently developed a medulloblastoma at age 8 years.

syndrome). Most adrenal tumors in children have been associated with either Cushing's syndrome, virilization, or both.[131] Almost all cases of Cushing's syndrome occurring in children are due to adrenocortical carcinoma.

Although various histologic criteria such as necrosis, calcifications, abnormal mitoses, vascular invasion, and capsular invasion have been used to differentiate malignant from benign adrenal tumors, it appears that the most significant factor in determining malignancy and prognosis is the size of the tumor at diagnosis. Tumors weighing less than 100 g have an excellent prognosis, whereas those weighing more than 500 g have a very poor prognosis.[131,132]

Metastasis of adrenocortical carcinoma occurs to regional lymph nodes, liver, or lung. The tumor also spreads locally to involve the kidney, adjacent blood vessels, and mesentery.

Clinical Presentation

The clinical presentation of an adrenocortical carcinoma is dependent upon its hormonal secretion pattern. Cushing's syndrome in a child less than 10 years of age should lead immediately to the diagnosis of adrenocortical carcinoma. The differential diagnosis of virilization includes other causes of isosexual precocity in boys and other virilizing tumors in girls.

Occasionally, adrenocortical carcinoma occurs without hormone secretion. These tumors typically present as an upper abdominal mass with pain and can be differentiated from neuroblastoma or Wilms' tumor only by histologic examination.

Treatment

Surgical excision is the treatment of choice for adrenocortical carcinoma. Patients with excess hormone production will have suppression of the contralateral adrenal gland and require perioperative corticosteroid coverage (see Chap. 34). Radiotherapy is not of value except for palliation of metastatic or unresectable disease. The single agent with any efficacy is o,p'-DDD (mitotane), a chemical derivative of DDT. Adult pa-

tients with adrenocortical carcinoma have shown objective tumor regression in as many as 61% of cases and decreased steroid production in 89%.[133] The median response duration is about 10 months. Effective therapy is associated with side effects that include anorexia, nausea, vomiting, diarrhea, lethargy, and somnolence.[133] Cures are unlikely. Aminoglutethimide, which inhibits the enzymatic conversion of cholesterol to 5-pregnenolone, has been used to alleviate the symptoms of corticosteroid excess.[134]

The prognosis of adrenocortical carcinoma in childhood is determined primarily by the initial size and thus the resectability of the tumor. Metastatic recurrence is likely for tumors weighing more than 500 g and possible for tumors in the 100- to 500-g range. Treatment of metastatic or unresectable disease with o,p'-DDD seems warranted, but there are no clear indications for adjuvant radiotherapy or chemotherapy in the absence of measurable disease or continued excess hormone production. Entry of patients with measurable disease into single-agent trials may yield information about responsiveness to other drugs.

CANCER OF THE STOMACH

Although cancer of the stomach is the sixth most common cause of cancer deaths in the United States,[135] with about 26,000 new cases being identified in 1987, this remains an exceptionally rare cancer of children and adolescents.[136-139]

Epidemiology

In 1936, gastric cancer was the leading cause of cancer-related deaths among American men.[140] At present, however, the death rate and frequency of this disease have declined worldwide.[141-144]

There is a marked variation of stomach cancer throughout the world, with the highest incidences being in Japan, Chile, and Iceland.[141] There is no apparent increased incidence of this cancer in children or adolescents in these countries. This cancer is more common in lower socioeconomic groups. About twice as many males as females are affected in this country and elsewhere.

Diet and gastric cancer have been studied in various countries (see Chap. 1, 2, and 55).[140] Gastric cancer is more common where there is a high-starch diet with low fruit and vegetable intake. The use of pickled, uncooked vegetables, salty sauces, and dried salted fish are associated with high risk; however, the use of unprocessed raw vegetables and raw fish does not seem to be associated with a higher incidence. Dietary nitrates, as are found in preserved and processed meats, have been implicated as a cause of gastric cancer.

Pernicious anemia, atropic achlorhydric gastritis, and other conditions that produce decreased gastric acidity are associated with a high risk of gastric cancer in adults.[140-143] Adenomatous polyps, gastric ulcers, and a history of gastric surgery may also be associated with an increased incidence of gastric cancer in adults. Fortunately, most of the above-mentioned associated conditions are rare in children and adolescents.[139]

Genetics

There are no recognized genetic syndromes associated with gastric cancer. Familial occurrence of this cancer is rare.[144]

Pathology

About 95% of the malignant neoplasms of the stomach are adenocarcinomas.[140] The term "gastric cancer" therefore is used to refer to adenocarcinoma of the stomach. Other, less frequent, tumors include lymphomas, adenoanthomas, squamous cell carcinomas, carcinoids, and leiomyosarcomas. The types of gastric adenocarcinomas include the papillary, tubular, mucinous, or signet-ring cell as well as adenosquamous carcinoma, squamous carcinoma, undifferentiated carcinoma, and unclassified carcinomas. Various of these tumors may be polypoid, fungating, or ulcerative lesions.

The gastric adenocarcinomas are classified according to the degree of histologic differentiation. About half of all stomach neoplasms are located in the distal stomach. Multicentric involvement has been reported.

Patterns of Spread

Gastric carcinomas spread via the lymphatics and blood vessels, by direct extension, and through seeding of peritoneal surfaces.[141,144] These lesions may infiltrate the submucosa, extend directly, and involve the duodenum or esophagus, omentum, liver, pancreas, or colon. Blood-borne metastases may involve the lungs, liver, or skin.

Clinical Presentation

Cancers of the stomach produce vague epigastric discomfort.[140,141,144] There may be associated weight loss or anorexia; iron deficiency anemia may be present with occult blood in the stool. Stomach cancer may also produce no symptoms until it has metastasized. For these reasons, individuals with weight loss, abdominal pain, nausea, vomiting, changes in bowel habits, anorexia, dysphasia, weakness, hematemesis, or other vague abdominal symptoms should be investigated.

Diagnosis

An upper gastrointestinal series is the most accurate method of identifying gastric carcinoma.[140,144] Fiberoptic endoscopy with biopsy and cytology study assure the correctness of the diagnosis. Areas of possible metastasis such as the supraclavicular lymph nodes may also suggest the diagnosis. By physical examination, hepatomegaly may be associated with gastric carcinoma, and a biopsy of the liver or other abdominal masses may be appropriate before diagnostic or therapeutic laparotomy.

In addition to an upper-gastrointestinal series, chest radiographs should be performed as well as CT. Various appropriate laboratory studies including blood chemistry determinations and complete blood counts should be performed.

Staging

The TNM classification is used for staging.[14] This information is obtained from surgical exploration as well as from clinical data when resection is not carried out. Partial or total gastric resection specimens permit pathologic staging, which considers the primary tumor, nodal involvement, and distant sites.[144] The tumor grades may also encompass well-differentiated, moderately well-differentiated, or poorly to very poorly differentiated tumors.

Prognostic Considerations and Variables

As expected, the prognosis for carcinoma of the stomach depends on the extent of disease as well as the treatment.[144] Both local and regional extension affect survival adversely. The best prognosis is for patients who have localized disease. For adults, survival relations have also been found with the size of the lesion, the age of the patient, operative mortality rates, age at operation, and pathologic stage. Little information exists relative to this tumor in patients under the age of 21 years.

Treatment

Surgical excision with appropriate margins is the procedure of choice for gastric carcinoma.[141,144] This operation should include a subtotal gastrectomy with resection of associated lymph nodes. It is recommended that total gastrectomy not be performed unless there is a potential for cure, as extended resections may be associated with an increased mortality rate without adding to the likelihood of cure.

The preferred methods for combining surgery and irradiation for gastric carcinoma differ. Preoperative, intraoperative, and postoperative radiation therapy all have been given; however, this tumor has long been regarded a radiounresponsive tumor, with the requirements for external-beam irradiation being greater than the tolerance of the surrounding tissues. Radiation therapy alone has had curative potential in only a small percentage of patients with resected residual or unresectable localized disease. The greatest benefits, have been with the use of the combination of radiation and chemotherapy following surgery. Preoperative irradiation may include multiple-field techniques, with the dosage limited by the tolerance of the organs and structures of the upper abdomen including the liver, kidneys, small intestine, and spinal cord.[143] Postoperative radiation dosages should aim for 4000 to 5000 cGy over 5 to 6 weeks delivered in 150- to 180-cGy fractions.[144] No data are available on radiation treatment results in children.

Effective chemotherapy regimens do not exist for gastric carcinoma.[141,144,145] Adjuvant chemotherapy continues to be investigated. Among the agents used are 5-FU or one of the nitrosoureas with and without doxorubicin or mitomycin C.[145-147] Combinations including 5-FU and a nitrosourea have produced responses for locally advanced or unresectable gastric carcinomas with metastases. Patients responding to these combinations apparently survive longer.[140] Again, no contemporary data are available on treatment results in children.

Complications of Therapy

Complications of therapy are related to the modalities used.[144] The association of radiation with surgery may lead to gastrointestinal complications, and the addition of chemotherapy may be associated with such complications as nausea, vomiting, weight loss, myelosuppression, mucositis, or diarrhea.

CANCER OF THE PANCREAS

Pancreatic cancers are rarely encountered in children and adolescents.[148] In adults, pancreatic cancer is the fourth most frequent cause of death from cancer, exceeded only by colon, lung, and breast cancers.[135] Pancreatic carcinomas are among the most aggressive of the visceral malignancies and account for about 25,000 deaths in the United States annually.[135] In frequency, pancreatic carcinoma is the seventh most common cancer in the United States.

The first reports of carcinoma of the pancreas in adults was issued by Bigsby in 1835.[148] Courvoiser was the first to notice a palpable gallbladder in the presence of painless jaundice as an indicator of pancreatic carcinoma.[148] The first resection of a pancreatic tumor was performed by Trendelenburg in 1882.[148] Whipple and his coworkers in 1935 described the surgical procedure for resection of tumors of the head of the pancreas and periampullary area; this procedure has since been modified but remains one of the accepted treatments of choice for tumors of this area.[149]

Epidemiology

The incidence of carcinoma of the pancreas has been rising slowly in this country since about 1920.[150]

Although cancers of the pancreas can occur at all ages, there is an increasing incidence in aging populations, with more than half of the deaths occurring past the age of 65 years.[148] There is a strong male predominance, although the gender ratio varies with age. There is a prevalence of earlier death among black individuals affected by this tumor; the age-adjusted incidence for pancreatic cancer is 10.9:100,000 for white males and 6.5:100,000 for white females, whereas the incidence for the black population is 14.0:100,000 for males and 7.9:100,000 for females. The worldwide incidence of this cancer is increasing, although this change may reflect to some extent improved diagnosis and elimination of confusion with other intra-abdominal malignancies. Low rates of this tumor are seen in Africa, South America, the Near East, and India and the highest rates in the United States and Australia.[150] Annual age-adjusted incidence ratio for all carcinomas in patients under the age of 20 years is 1.40 per 1 million; specific figures are not available for pancreatic carcinomas in this age group.

Genetics

There are no recognized genetic syndromes associated with pancreatic carcinoma in children or adolescents, although endocrine tumors of the pancreas may be associated with other hormone-producing tumors.

Biology

In recent years, there have been reports of the association of pancreatic carcinoma in adults with the intake of excessive amounts of coffee.[151] Various investigators have followed this lead, and some have been unable to substantiate a cause–effect relation.[152]

For adults, other possible associations of environmental factors with carcinoma of the pancreas have included lower socioeconomic groups, cigarette smoking, chronic pancreatitis, and prior diabetes mellitus. An increased incidence of pancreatic carcinoma in workers exposed to organic solvents and petroleum products has been reported.

Pathogenesis, Natural History, and Patterns of Spread

The causes of pancreatic carcinoma in children are unknown.[153-164] These tumors may arise in the head, body, or tail of the pancreas.[148] In most instances, the tumors are nonfunc-

tioning, and symptomatology differs according to the site of origin.[159,162]

Functioning tumors produce similar symptoms (see Chap. 34). Islet cell carcinomas[165-168] produce an overabundance of insulin, leading to hypoglycemia, which may be manifested by fatigue, restlessness, and malaise followed by clouding of the sensorium, staggering gate, hypothermia, and coma that may appear as intermittent attacks, most frequently in the early morning hours. Nonfunctioning islet cell tumors are usually associated with peptic ulcer disease and the elaboration of gastrin by the tumor.[148] Some patients develop watery diarrhea, hypokalemia, and achlorhydria.

The natural history of each of these tumors, as well as of the pancreatoblastoma,[169,170] is marked by clinical wasting and pain. Mechanical obstruction of the duodenum and gastric outlet by tumors of the head of the pancreas may be associated with obstructive jaundice and gastrointestinal hemorrhage. Venous obstruction may be associated with varices, hemorrhage, and ascites. Tumors of the body or tail of the pancreas may erode into the stomach and cause hemorrhage. Ascites is associated with involvement of the liver and peritoneum and may result in hepatic failure. These patients die because of progressive weight loss and anorexia.

Diagnosis

As with other tumors, the objective is to establish the diagnosis and the extent of disease, including the presence or absence of metastases.[156,157] Radiologic studies include contrast studies of the upper gastrointestinal tract,[148] abdominal ultrasonography,[157] and CT of the abdomen.[148] Accuracy of diagnosis with these latter two tests is greater than that of upper gastrointestinal barium studies. Primary tumors located in the head of the pancreas can cause deformity of the duodenal C-loop or the gastric antrum. This may be associated with mucosal abnormalities. CT of the abdomen is more reliable than ultrasonography in defining the suspected lesion, although ultrasonography may be more cost effective (see Chap. 7). The entire abdomen, including the pelvis, should be scanned, with concurrent use of iodinated contrast medium. The sensitivity of magnetic resonance imaging (MRI) for pancreatic carcinoma in children is yet to be determined. Retrograde endoscopic cholangiopancreatography may be useful[148]; this procedure involves direct cannulation of the duodenal papilla through the fiberoptic duodenoscope and an injection of contrast medium into both the common pancreatic duct and the common bile duct. Arteriography may be of value for patients being considered for surgical resection.

Various serum markers, including carcinoembryonic antigen (CEA), alpha-fetoprotein, (AFP), and pancreatic oncofetal antigen may be of value in the diagnosis and in follow-up (see also Chap. 8).[148,170,171] Other serum markers, including amylase, lipase, alkaline phosphatase, lactic dehydrogenase, transaminase, leucine aminopeptidase, and pancreatic ribonuclease, also may be valuable in diagnosing as well in following patients with this disease.

Pathology

The malignant tumors of the pancreas include those of duct cell origin (adenocarcinoma, squamous cell carcinoma), acinic cell origin (acinic cell carcinoma), connective tissue origin (e.g., liposarcoma), lymphatic origin (lymphoma), uncertain origin (malignant papillary cystic carcinoma, pancreatoblastoma), and islet cell origin (malignant insulinoma, glucagonoma, and gastrinoma).[148]

Staging

The surgical staging system for this cancer appears in Table 35-8.[14,172]

Prognostic Considerations and Variables

Only about 1% of adult patients with carcinoma of the pancreas survive. Slightly better results have been observed for children,[148] but most patients in the pediatric age group who develop this rare type of carcinoma expire, generally because the diagnosis is not made until after development of locoregional disease. Other factors influencing the prognosis include the lack of both radiosensitivity and chemosensitivity of most tumors of the pancreas.

The only potentially curable patients are those whose disease is diagnosed at an early stage, when tumor is confined to the body of the pancreas. For these patients, surgical resection provides the only chance for long-term disease-free survival.

Treatment

The principles of treatment of pediatric patients with pancreatic carcinoma have been derived from the adult experience, with various recommendations based on personal opinions.[148] The operations that have been developed since 1935 include pancreaticoduodenectomy,[149] total pancreatectomy, regional pancreatectomy, and distal pancreatectomy.[148] The standard operation for resection is the pancreaticoduodenectomy, also referred to as the Whipple procedure.[149] Patients selected for resection of the primary cancer must be free of evidence of disseminated malignancy, including involvement of the regional lymph nodes. These resections are complex technical procedures that necessitate significant postoperative monitoring and regulation of blood glucose levels, insulin administration, correction of metabolic abnormalities, and provision of nutritional support including intravenous hyperalimentation.[148] Following these operative procedures, there may be prolonged ileus and delayed return of gastrointestinal function. In addition to the management of the diabetic state, which may be particularly difficult, patients undergoing pancreatic resection must receive pancreatic enzymes with each meal.[148] Gastric hyperacidity may require treatment with cimetidine.

Results

Results are not available on the utility of radiation therapy for the treatment of pediatric patients with pancreatic carcinoma. For adults, treatment dosages have included 4500 cGy over a period of as much as 6 weeks.[148] These treatments may be associated with failure of tumor shrinkage or with local recurrence. Other complications include bowel obstruction, biliary obstruction, and biliary fistula. Various studies are being conducted in adults to determine the value of adjunctive conventional as well as intraoperative radiation therapy for localized pancreatic carcinomas.

Chemotherapy may also be tried for the treatment of localized or metastatic pancreatic carcinoma, although few agents

Table 35-8
Survival Staging System for Carcinoma of the Pancreas

Stage I	No direct extension, no nodal involvement; tumor localized within pancreatic capsule
Stage II	Direct extension into adjacent tissue with no lymph node involvement
Stage III	Regional lymph node involvement
Stage IV	Distant metastatic spread

have been successful in the treatment of measurable disease.[173] Single agents such as 5-FU, streptozotocin, mitomycin C, and doxorubicin have been associated with response rates of 7% to 36%.[174] Streptozotocin, a methylnitrosurea, is specifically toxic for pancreatic islet cells and has been associated with response rates of 35% or greater.[148] A combination of agents including 5-FU, doxorubicin, mitomycin C, and streptozotocin has yielded response rates as high as 48% in a small group of patients.[175] Unfortunately, other regimens such as 5-FU–doxorubicin–mitomycin C (FAM) have not been quite so successful.[176]

Combined-modality therapy has prolonged survival with palliation of symptoms for some patients with advanced disease. Chemotherapy appears to have some role in the management of unresectable pancreatic carcinoma, yet there is no knowledge as to whether chemotherapeutic agents and radiation therapy are synergistic.

CARCINOMA OF THE GALLBLADDER

This primary carcinoma rarely affects adults or children.[177] Signs, symptoms, and radiographic studies have been of little value in defining the diagnosis preoperatively. Most patients present with metastases to the liver and lymph nodes. Survival for adults with this cancer is 15% at 1 year, indicating the extremely poor prognosis.

For children and adolescents, a more common type of cancer involving the gallbladder would be rhabdomyosarcoma (see Chap. 30).

COLORECTAL CARCINOMA

Carcinoma of the large bowel is rare in individuals less than 20 years of age.

Epidemiology

Colonic cancer is more common in the western world than in rural Africa.[178] This difference is thought to be related to the relatively long transit time of fecal material in the bowels of persons consuming relatively low-fiber diets.[179,180]

Although there are about 145,000 new cases of colorectal carcinoma in adults annually,[135] the Surveillance, Epidemiology, and End Results (SEER) data suggest that only about 80 cases of colorectal carcinoma occur annually in the United States in individuals less than 20 years of age, since the incidence of this tumor is about 1 per 1 million in this group.[181] In children and adolescents, these tumors may occur at any site in the large bowel and are not usually associated with a family history of large-bowel cancer.[182] It is not known whether there is an increasing rate of colon cancer in young individuals or whether the median age of all individuals with colon cancer is decreasing. There is no known predisposition of colorectal carcinoma for gender. Most cases that occur under the age of 20 years occur at the median age of 15 years.[182] Geographically, in the United States, the largest number of cases has been reported from the Mississippi Valley.[182-185] Studies of some affected individuals have noted exposure of most of the young patients to pesticides and herbicides used in farming or dairy operations.[186] Young individuals with long-standing ulcerative colitis are at increased great risk; this risk increases with the duration and severity of colitis.[187] Black Americans have an increasing occurrence of the disease.[135] There is a shifting incidence of the sites of primary lesions from the left to the right side of the colon.[188]

Genetics

Several well-recognized conditions may be associated with the development of colorectal carcinoma in younger patients.[189-195] Familial polyposis, inherited as a dominant trait with 90% penetrance, is generally followed by the appearance of multiple cancers by the age of 37 years.[190] For affected individuals in these families, early diagnosis and colectomy can eliminate the risk. Other syndromes associated with colorectal cancer in young people include Turcot's syndrome,[196] Oldfield's syndrome,[197] and Gardner's syndrome[198] (Table 35-9) (see also Chap. 2). Recently, two younger patients with multiple colon carcinomas, polyposis coli, and neurofibromatosis have been reported.[199]

For children and adolescents, there is no evidence that a family history of bowel cancer confers a greater risk for their development of bowel cancer before the age of 20 years.[182] The same is true for persons under 20 belonging to families with hereditary colorectal cancer,[200] cancer family syndromes,[195] or familial juvenile polyposis.[193,194] Persons with the Peutz–Jegher syndrome may develop bowel cancer because of the risk associated with polyposis coli.[201,202]

Biology

The initial signs and symptoms associated with colorectal carcinoma in the young may be insidious.[182-185,203-206] A change in bowel habits such as constipation or diarrhea and change in the caliber of the stool may be observed prior to development of tarry stools or rectal bleeding. With changes in bowel habits, there may be a decrease in appetite and accordingly a decrease in weight.

Table 35-9
Syndromes Associated with Colorectal Carcinoma

Name	Description	Reference
Turcot's	Congenital abnormalities, brain tumors	196
Oldfield's	Multiple sebaceous cysts, polyposis	197
Gardner's	Multiple sebaceous cysts, exostoses, polyposis	198
Peutz–Jegher's	Mucocutaneous pigmentation of lips, perioral region, buccal mucosa, polyposis, ovarian granulosa cell tumors	201, 201

It must be remembered that the signs and symptoms of bowel cancer are related to the site in the large bowel where the primary tumor is located. Tumors involving the cecum and ascending colon, which may be associated with family colon cancer,[188] may develop into masses of tremendous size before symptoms appear. Tumors of the rectum or sigmoid are generally associated with changes in the caliber of the stool, hematochezia, and dyschezia. Because of the rarity of colorectal carcinoma under the age of 20 years, this diagnosis is seldom suspected and often delayed until individuals present with acute bowel symptoms that necessitate immediate abdominal exploration, at which time perforation of the large bowel may be observed along with multiple metastatic deposits. Intestinal obstructions due to tumor occurs more frequently in adolescents than in adults with this cancer.[205]

The natural history of colorectal carcinoma in the young differs slightly from that of adults in that the tumors of the young are frequently more advanced at diagnosis.[203] For this reason, the tumors may not be resected in an early stage and thus may spread throughout the peritoneal cavity to involve the omentum, peritoneum, mesenteric lymph nodes, liver, and ovaries and spread through the blood stream to the lungs and eventually to the brain, bones, or both. There is a propensity for peritoneal seeding in females to involve the ovaries, which may reach tremendous size due to tumor involvement.[185]

Hoener, in 1958, reviewed a collection of 262 patients with colorectal cancer before the age of 20 years. He reported that 50% of the neoplasms were mucoid adenocarcinoma, that delay in diagnosis was common, and that these circumstances adversely affected the prognosis.[203]

Ancillary Clinical Studies

The examination of the stool for occult blood often has positive results when no gross blood can be seen on the stool or to discolor the stools.[207] Studies of organ function generally are noncontributory, as are studies of the urine; anemia may be present due to blood loss or malnutrition. Biochemical assays of interest include CEA, which may or may not be elevated in relation to the production of this protein by the tumor. The frequency of positivity of this assay increases with increasing stage of disease. The CA 19-9 assay has been less valuable for following the extent of tumor involvement than the CEA assay, yet some tumors produce CA 19-9 in the absence of CEA production.[207] Liver function studies may be abnormal secondary to metastatic involvement of the liver, and abnormal pancreatic function studies may be related to metastases or obstructive jaundice.

Imaging Studies

Direct imaging of colorectal carcinomas located at any site is possible by way of direct or fiberoptic colonoscopy.[207] Evaluation of the large bowel should include the entire length because of the possibility of the colorectal carcinoma being found in association with polyps.

Conventional radiographic studies include barium enema with air contrast to define the tumor and the remainder of the colon (Fig. 35-4). This latter study coupled with CT of the abdomen and chest may define lesions that have spread to the liver, lungs, or enlarged lymph node areas as well as metastases that have involved the pelvis or are in the cul de sac. Radioisotope studies may include a bone scan or liver–spleen scan, both of which are used to determine spread of tumor to these parts. If the bone scan indicates abnormalities of various areas, bone marrow aspiration or biopsy may be appropriate to determine whether there has been spread to the marrow.

Pathology

The principal histologic categories of colorectal cancer are adenocarcinomas, mucinous or colloid adenocarcinomas, signet-ring adenocarcinoma, and scirrhous tumors.[207,208]

Colorectal carcinoma arises from the mucosal surface of the bowel, generally at the site of an adenomatous overgrowth or polyp.[207] The tumor may extend into the muscularis area, extend to the serosa, and perforate the serosa into omental fat, lymph nodes, liver, ovaries, and other loops of bowel. Some lesions grow to obstruct the bowel lumen. They may implant along an abdominal scar, at the anastomotic site, or throughout the peritoneum. Early reports of colorectal carcinomas in young patients indicate that obstruction was more frequent at presentation in children than in adults.[203,208]

Occasionally, more than one cancer is present simultaneously.[209] These lesions may have the same or different histology and be in the same or different stages. Carcinoma *in situ* may occur in one or more polyps.

The gross appearance of these lesions depends on the extent of involvement of the lumen of the bowel and the extent of the disease outside the bowel wall. These tumors are derived from endoderm, and therefore have all the cytologic characteristics of a carcinoma, but may be well-differentiated or poorly differentiated and contain pools of mucin (Fig. 35-5). The mucinous variety, which appears in approximately 15% of adult colorectal carcinomas,[208] is the predominant histologic variety in individuals under 20 years of age at the time of diagnosis.[181] Tumors may grow to huge sizes because of the pooling of mucin.

The differential diagnosis includes any tumor that can involve the large or small bowel, including leiomyosarcoma, malignant fibrous histiocytoma, malignant carcinoid, and metastatic tumor from other sites (see also Chap. 5 and 31).[207] Leiomyosarcoma or malignant fibrous histiocytoma are rare tumors, as are carcinoids. All may have similar presentations and metastases and may be identified only by histologic examination of the primary or metastatic sites. Acute appendicitis may be considered in the differential diagnosis where there is perforation of the bowel associated with intestinal obstruction.

Staging

Many staging systems have been proposed during the last 45 years.[207] The easiest to recall is Dukes' classification and as modified by Astler and Coller. For comparative purposes, the TNM classification of the American Joint Committee is used for reporting by tumor registries.[14] The TNM system is used before and after surgery. These staging systems are outlined in Table 35-10.

Treatment

General Surgical Principles

Biopsy is necessary for the diagnosis of colorectal carcinoma.[207] This may be obtained by colonoscopy or at laparotomy, at which time definitive surgery may or may not be feasible. The surgical staging procedures include biopsy of any known enlarged lymph nodes, biopsy of the ovaries in females, resection of the omentum, and biopsy of the liver. Complete surgical excision is the primary aim of the surgeon, with secondary aims being palliation by the resection of bulky tumors or metastases. Debulking provides little for the patient with extensive metastatic disease, however. Removal of single or multiple hepatic metastases may become a life-saving procedure for those rare individuals who have had excision of the large bowel and nodal dissections and who have metastases to the liver.

FIGURE 35-4. Left posterior oblique view of barium enema in an 11-year-old boy. The child had noted decreased stool caliber for 2 months with hematochezia. Gross constricting lesion ("apple-core") of sigmoid colon (*arrows*) was site of a mucinous adenocarcinoma. Note spasm proximal to tumor.

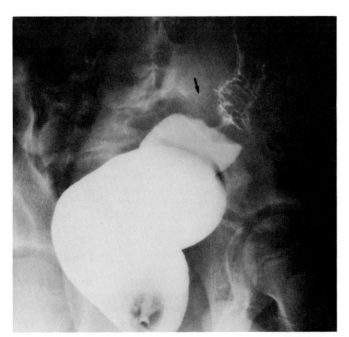

FIGURE 35-5. Histologic study of bowel lesion from patient whose tumor is shown in Figure 35-4. Tumor is mucinous adenocarcinoma, the most common histologic finding in patients with colorectal carcinoma before age 20 years.

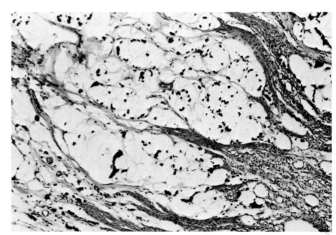

Table 35-10
Staging Schemes for Colorectal Carcinoma

Stage*				Description	Approximate 5-year Survival Rate (%)
Dukes	Astler-Coller	TNM	AJC		
A	A	T1 N0 M0	Ia	Lesion limited to submucosa, nodes negative	80
	B1	T2 N0 M0	Ib	Lesion into muscularis; nodes negative	70
B	B2	T2 N0 M0	IIa	Lesion transmural, nodes negative	60
	C1	T2 N1 M1	IIb	Lesion into muscularis; nodes positive	45
C	C2	T3 N1 M0	III	Nodes positive, lesion transmural	25
D	D	T3 N1 M1	IV	Metastases to liver, lung, bone; tumor unresectable	10

* TNM = tumor, node, metastasis; AJC = American Joint Committee.

Chemotherapy

When the primary tumor involves the rectosigmoid area and is considered nonresectable at the time of diagnosis, radiotherapy is often initiated in conjunction with chemotherapy prior to any surgical procedure.[207] The chemotherapy options are few, including the use of 5-FU with or without citrovorum factor[210] and one of the nitrosureas; for example, BCNU, CCNU, or streptozotocin.[207] Mitomycin C may also produce a favorable response in some of these tumors.[207] Such combined-modality therapy may provide a better environment for the surgeon to resect the primary tumor completely. Intraoperative radiation therapy has been advocated for disease known to have metastasized to the mesentery or mesenteric lymph nodes.[207] Intraoperative radiotherapy is delivered while the bowel is displaced from the peritoneal cavity.

A recent addition to the potentially effective treatments is interleukin-2 in combination with lymphokine-activated killer cells. In the study of Rosenberg and associates, one complete and two partial responses of pulmonary or hepatic metastases were observed among the 26 patients treated for metastatic colorectal carcinoma.[127]

The complications of therapy are sometimes difficult to separate from complications of the disease. Complications of disease may be nutritional or obstructive or be related to the effects of metastatic disease on other organs or systems. One of the less frequent complications of bowel cancer is the development of other cancers. The delivery of alkylating agents has increased the individual's risk of leukemia at some time following treatment.[211]

Future Considerations

Current therapy is unsatisfactory for several reasons. Colorectal carcinomas are detected after development of disease extension in adolescents.[182,204,205] Colon carcinoma is one of the most unlikely diagnoses for a teenager and is therefore unsuspected by the pediatrician, internist, or surgeon examining a patient with diffuse abdominal discomfort or mass. Another reason for concern is that surgery is the only modality known to be effective in providing cures. Adjuvant chemotherapy extends the life of individuals in the childhood years, yet few patients who present with extensive metastatic disease are cured, and adjuvant therapy has not proved to be of significant benefit.[207] Radiation has little to offer for this tumor except when the tumor involves the rectosigmoid or anal areas. However, irradiation of pulmonary or brain metastases of this tumor may provide therapeutic action as well as symptomatic relief for the sequelae of these metastases.[207]

Directions for treatment research include determination of the implications of the DNA labeling index for the response to chemotherapy, refinement of the tumor cloning assay for prediction of the response to treatment, determination of the import of specific histologies for the response to various chemotherapeutic agents, and greater integration of new therapeutic modalities in the management of these uncommon childhood tumors.

CARCINOID TUMORS

These epithelial tumors may be benign or malignant and may be located in the esophagus or bronchi or in the small or large bowel, pancreas, or ovary.[212-215] The most common site is the appendix, where most tumors are benign; benign carcinoids are the most common tumor of the appendix.[216,217]

Carcinoid tumors contain argentaffin cells derived from the Kulchitsky cells of the small intestine; these secretory cells are thought to have endocrine functions.[212] These tumors may produce symptoms referred to as the carcinoid syndrome,[218-221] characterized by elevated levels of serotonin in the blood and urine.[222] Affected patients have paroxysmal flushing, diarrhea, bronchoconstriction, peripheral vasomotor symptoms, and cyanosis. These symptoms are attributed to circulating 5-hydroxytyptamine (serotonin) and histamine. Urinary levels of 5-hydroxyindoleacetic acid are elevated.[222]

Treatment is primarily surgical resection when possible. If the tumor is malignant and has spread in a manner similar to colorectal carcinoma, chemotherapy may prove to be of benefit.[223] One of the 160 patients with carcinoma treated at St. Jude Children's Research Hospital had this diagnosis, with a primary site in the sigmoid colon. Intra-abdominal and pulmonary metastases were treated with doxorubicin, which effected a partial response.

NON-GERM-CELL OVARIAN CANCER

Most malignant ovarian tumors in adults are of epithelial origin. For children and adolescents, 60% of ovarian tumors are of germ-cell origin (see Chap. 33).[224]

The most common ovarian non-germ-cell tumors are granulosa–theca cell tumors and Sertoli–Leydig cell tumors (androblastoma, gynandroblastomas) derived from sex cord stroma. After the age of 15 years, about one-third of ovarian malignant neoplasms are epithelial. These malignant epithelial tumors include adenocarcinoma, cystadenocarcinoma, malignant endometrioid tumors, clear-cell (mesonephroid) tumors, and Brenner tumors as well as undifferentiated carcinomas.

The stage grouping for these and other malignant ovarian tumors is that recommended by the American Joint Committee on Cancer.[14] The prognosis is directly related to the stage of disease at the time of diagnosis.[225]

Treatment is stage related, with external-beam radiation therapy being used for resectable ovarian carcinoma beyond Stage IA.[223] In recent years, more attention has been focused on the use of chemotherapy, including intravenous as well as intraperitoneal use of such agents as cisplatin, doxorubicin, cyclophosphamide, 5-FU, hexamethylmelamine, and methotrexate given as two- to four-drug combinations. Complete responses have been achieved in 40% to 76% of patients with measureable advanced disease.[224]

CERVICAL, VAGINAL, AND VULVAR TUMORS

These tumors are extremely rare in children and adolescents. Rhabdomyosarcoma is the most common tumor of these sites; however, squamous cell tumors may also occur. Cervical squamous cell carcinoma has been observed more often with increasing age through adolescence.[226,227]

Clear-cell carcinomas of the vagina or cervix have been observed in the daughters of mothers who received diethyestilbesterol (DES) for the prevention of spontaneous abortion (see Chap. 1, 2, and 55).[228–231] Vaginal adenosis is also associated with these tumors. It is now recognized that about 70% of the young women with this condition had prenatal exposure to DES.[231] Treatment for clear-cell adenocarcinoma of these sites require vaginectomy, hysterectomy, and lymphadenectomy. The role of radiation is not clearly defined.[232,233]

Malignant tumors of the vulva have been reported as carcinoma, epidermoid carcinoma, adenocarcinoma, sarcoma, and rhabdomyosarcoma.[232,234] The principles for the treatment of these tumors depend on their site, stage, and pathologic features.

BREAST CANCERS

Breast tumors of children and adolescents are usually benign, yet carcinomas have been reported.[235–238] The most common tumor, which usually occurs after puberty, is fibroadenoma;

giant fibroadenomas are also called cytosarcoma phylloides.[236] Although the name of this tumor suggests malignancy and although these tumors may grow to such sizes as to suggest malignancy, most are benign. Other benign tumors include hypertrophy and intraductal papilloma. Most tumors, benign or malignant, present as a mass except for hypertrophy. They should be excised.[235]

Breast carcinomas, more common than breast sarcomas, have been reported in a few children. Both genders are affected equally. Most reviews of childhood breast carcinomas suggest that such cancers in children are less or no more malignant than those in young women and that at least half of these young patients survive with modified radical mastectomy alone. The histologic characteristics of cancer of the breast in children are commented on in the article by McDivitt and Stewart.[239] Recommendations regarding radiation therapy and chemotherapy for childhood and adolescent breast carcinoma are not available because no large series have been reported from contemporary times.

Whether a diagnosis of breast cancer under the age of 20 years in association with a family history of breast cancer is associated with an enhanced risk of development of a second primary breast cancer is unknown.[240,241]

CANCERS OF THE SKIN

Melanoma is the most common of the skin cancers in children. It is followed in frequency by basal cell and squamous cell carcinomas, which are usually referred to as nonmelanoma skin cancers.

Epidemiology

The most important stimulus for skin cancer is ultraviolet light, followed in frequency by chemical carcinogenesis, ionizing radiation, and immunodeficiency or immunosuppression.[242] Ultraviolet light was first mentioned in relation to skin cancer in 1894 and 1899 (see Chap. 2 and 55).[242] In 1906, Hyde[243] indicated that certain individuals were hypersensitive to the action of sunlight and had accelerated appearance of this hypersensitivity with such conditions as xeroderma pigmentosum.[244] Experimental skin cancer was produced in mice by exposure to ultraviolet light in 1928.[242] Epidemiologic data from various global latitudes has shown an increase in squamous cell and basal cell carcinomas in the white population closer to the equator.[235–248] Certain individual phenotypes are associated with greater susceptibility to skin cancer within any geographic area; these persons tend to have poor tanning ability with easy sunburning and often have blue eyes, light hair, and fair skin. There is no gender difference in the incidence of any types of skin cancer in the pediatric age groups.

There are two major effects of ultraviolet radiation on the skin that may be responsible for its carcinogenic effects. These are photochemical alteration of DNA and alterations in immunity.[242] As predicted, xeroderma pigmentosum cells in culture fail to repair ultraviolet damage to DNA secondary to lack of excision of thymine dimers.[249,250] Chemical carcinogens may also be associated with the development of basal cell and squamous cell carcinomas. This was first described by Pott, who noted the high incidence of carcinoma of the scrotal and penile skin in chimney sweeps in England.[242]

Ionizing radiation is also associated with carcinogenesis of the skin. Frieben first reported squamous cell carcinoma of the skin to be associated with radiation.[242] His report involved workers using early x-ray machines (Fig. 35-6). In children,

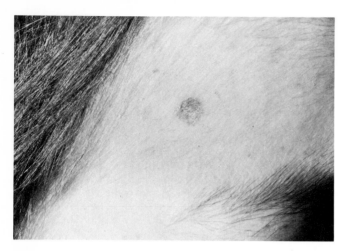

FIGURE 35-6. Basal cell carcinoma of the forehead in a 7-year-old boy who had received 2400-cGy prophylactic cranial irradiation as part of his treatment for acute lymphoblastic leukemia 5 years before he developed a second malignant neoplasm.

radiation-associated basal cell carcinomas generally have occurred in patients treated for acute lymphocytic leukemia with central nervous system prophylaxis or for Hodgkin's disease with mantle techniques.[251] The influence of cancer chemotherapeutic agents delivered with radiation therapy and the eventual diagnosis of nonmelanomatous skin cancers has not yet been assessed for survivors of childhood tumors.

The exact annual incidence of basal cell and squamous cell carcinomas in the United States is unknown because many of these affected individuals are treated in dermatologists' offices and because skin cancer other than melanoma is not generally a reportable disease. More than 450,000 cases of nonmelanoma skin cancer occur annually in the United States. The number of new cases of melanoma is about 26,000 annually.[135]

Basal cell carcinoma is the most common form of skin cancer in adults and accounts for 75% of the cases in the southern United States and more than 90% of the cases in the northern states.[242] Basal cell carcinomas also constitute a major element of the nevoid basal cell carcinoma syndrome, which also is characterized by jaw cysts, ovarian fibromas, palmar pits, and medulloblastoma.[244-248]

Squamous cell carcinomas have been observed in burn scars[257] and individuals with Fanconi's anemia.[258]

Melanoma is thought to represent 1% of cancers in the United States.[135] Although it represents only about 5% of cutaneous neoplasms, it accounts for approximately 65% of skin cancer deaths.[135] There is generally no gender predilection for melanoma, yet there are large numbers of melanomas on the lower extremities of women and a similar increase in truncal primaries in men. Melanoma is rare in people of black or Asian races, indicating the protective role of skin pigmentation.[256] Melanoma has also developed in burn scars (Fig. 35-7).[257]

Genetics

The first report of hereditary cutaneous melanoma was that of Norris in 1820.[242] Numerous pedigrees have since been published, and population-based surveys have indicated that first-degree blood relatives of melanoma patients are 1.7 times more likely to develop cutaneous melanoma than persons in the general population. It is estimated that 11% of melanomas

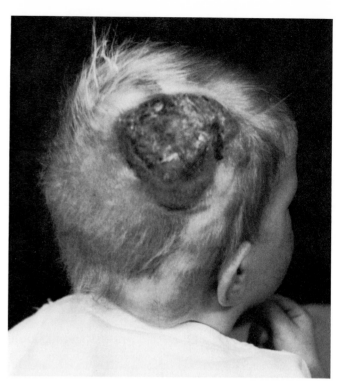

FIGURE 35-7. Melanoma of the scalp of a 4-year-old boy. Delay in diagnosis exceeded 1 year, and the patient died 6 months after diagnosis.

may be hereditary, with approximately 10 years' earlier occurrence of familial melanoma than of sporadic melanoma. Multiple primary melanomas have been reported.

The familial occurrence of melanoma in individuals with dysplastic nevus syndrome has been recognized in recent years (see Chap. 2).[259-262] Dysplastic nevi have irregular and indistinct borders, range in size from 5 to 12 mm, and have variegated tan to dark-brown pigmentation on a pink background. These nevi are usually located on the trunk but also may occur on the scalp or extremities. More than 25 such lesions are usually noted in adolescence and continue to appear even in older patients.

Patients with large congenital nevi are thought to have an increased risk of melanoma (Fig. 35-8).[263] About 10% of these lesions will develop into malignant melanoma. For this reason, these lesions should be removed, considering the consequences of surgery, the risk of melanoma, and the hazards to the affected individual.

Pathology

Cutaneous melanoma arises from melanocytes. Eleven types of extraocular melanoma have been described based on clinical and histologic groups.[242,264] The most common types are lentigo maligna melanoma, superficial spreading melanoma, nodular melanoma, and acral lentiginous melanoma. Most of the lesions are characterized by indolent peripheral enlargement of complex colored flat primary lesions. These lesions may undergo radial or vertical growth phases.

The signs and symptoms of malignant change include change in color (variegated), irregularity of borders, and irregularity of surface elevation.

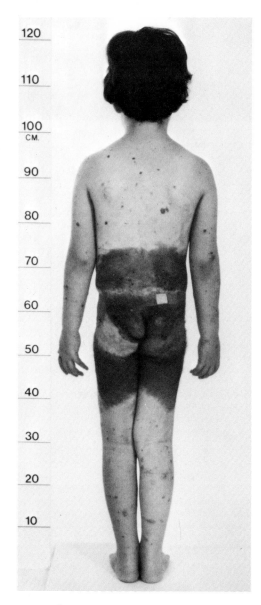

FIGURE 35-8. A 6-year-old boy with a "bathing trunk" nevus, present from birth. At age 5½ years, he was diagnosed as having a melanoma on a site on the left buttock. He developed inguinal lymph node metastasis 6 months after diagnosis and died 14 months after diagnosis.

The differential diagnosis includes congenital basal cell carcinoma, pigmented seborrheic keratosis, and the Spitz nevus (juvenile melanoma).[265]

The patterns of spread of melanoma in pediatric patients are in all ways similar to that of adults with the disease, with satellitosis and regional lymph nodes becoming involved prior to involvement of abdominal viscera, lungs, bone, or brain.[266]

Clinical Presentation

The more common types of melanomas are characterized by indolent, peripheral enlargement of relatively flat, complex colored primary lesions.[242] Such an indolent growth phase, which may take place over several years, is termed the radial growth phase, in which the tumor has little competence to

Table 35-11
Staging of Melanomas in Relation to Depth of Invasion[264]

Level I	All tumor cells are confined to epidermis with no invasion through basement membrane
Level II	Tumor cells penetrate through basement membrane into papillary dermis but do not extend to reticular dermis
Level III	Tumor cells fill papillary dermis and abut against reticular dermis without invasion of reticular dermis
Level IV	Extension of tumor cells between bundle of collagen characteristic of reticular dermis
Level V	Invasion into subcutaneous tissue

metastasize. The ability to metastasize is associated with penetration of the tumor into deeper cutaneous tissues (vertical growth phase).

There is no apparent difference in the site distribution of melanomas in children, adolescents, and adults.[266–272]

Basal cell carcinomas generally appear as nodular or nodular ulcerated lesions.[273] These tumors are generally found on the skin of the head or neck and rarely occur on the trunk or the extremities. They are generally asymptomatic except for crusting or bleeding with minor trauma. They are usually smooth, shiny, and translucent with prominent vessels seen beneath the surface. There is usually no tenderness or pain unless ulceration is noted. Rarely is melanin pigment present within these lesions. Individuals with a nevoid–basal cell carcinoma syndrome often have nodular lesions. Lesions that appear on the chest of trunk may be erythematous, beginning as a subtle erythematous plaque.

Squamous cell carcinomas usually are erythematous lesions with various degrees of scaling, crusting with similarity to eczema, psoriasis, infections, or trauma.[274] The lesions that appear on areas of the body exposed to sunlight develop with greater frequency on the nose, forehead, lower lips, backs of the hands, and helixes of the ear. Penile and anal carcinoma in the first decade of life are usually squamous cell carcinomas.[275,276]

Various studies have indicated a relation of tumor thickness to recurrence and to survival and the correlation of the depth of invasion of the primary tumor with survival (Table 35-11).[264] Other studies have indicated a relation of the primary site to survival as well as correlation of the lesion size with survival. In general, lesions of the extremities have a better outcome than lesions of the head and neck or trunk, and, as expected, the survival with localized disease is considerably better than with regional or metastatic disease. Survival decreases with greater depth of invasion and with the presence of lymph node metastases.[242,264]

Basal cell carcinomas are thought to arise from cells in the basal layer of the epidermis. These tumors are locally invasive but metastasize rarely, even to regional lymph nodes.[277] They may invade widely and deeply, extending through the subcutaneous tissues to involve neurovascular structures and occasionally invading bones. They may erode the skull and into the brain if untreated.

Squamous cell carcinomas tend to infiltrate more deeply than basal cell cancers and may infiltrate deeper structures.[242,278] Lymph node metastases are more common than with basal cell cancers, and metastases to lungs and liver by squamous cell carcinomas also are more common.[278]

Other more rare types of skin carcinomas are those which originate in hair follicles, sweat glands, and sebaceous cysts.[279] These tumors have a great propensity to metastasize early.

Treatment

Biopsy is necessary to determine the diagnosis of a skin cancer.[242] The decision about the definitive surgical procedure for a particular tumor depends on whether the tumor is a basal cell or squamous cell carcinoma or a melanoma and on the site and size of the primary tumor.[242] Excisional biopsy may be acceptable for the two former types of cancer, but wide excision, which may necessitate construction of skin flaps or grafts, is necessary for melanomas.[280]

Curettage or cryotherapy are reasonable treatments for primary basal cell carcinoma.[242] Microscopically controlled excision of skin carcinomas (basal cell and squamous cell) by the Mohs' technique (serial horizontal shave excisions followed by mapping of removed tissue for relation to wound, with frozen sections of the base of the infusion margins, followed by reexcisions as necessary) may be appropriate for lesions of the face.[281] Cryosurgery with liquid nitrogen continues to be investigated.

Basal cell and squamous cell carcinomas may be curable with surgery and radiation therapy.[242] Small lesions may respond to a single dose of 2200 cGy, whereas larger lesions may require fractionated dosages up to 6000 cGy.[242]

Treatment of melanomas is more challenging and requires greater consideration because of the greater potential of these tumors to metastasize.[280] The exact type of definitive surgery depends on the site, size, level of invasion, and extent of tumor (stage). Wide excision with skin grafting if necessary should be performed. When the regional lymph nodes are involved, chemotherapy with cyclophosphamide, dactinomycin, and vincristine has been of benefit to most adolescents so treated.[267] No good data relevant to adjuvant chemotherapy or immunotherapy exist for pediatric patients with melanoma. Palliative radiation may be of benefit to some patients.[280]

Future Considerations

Most probably, melanoma is a preventable cancer for children, adolescents, and adults. With a decrease in the enthusiasm for sun exposure by young people and with the judicious use of sunscreen products, a significant reduction in the frequency of both melanoma and nonmelanoma skin cancer may be expected.[281]

REFERENCES

1. Regaud C: Lympho-epitheliome de l'hypopharynx traite par la roentgentherapie. Bull Soc Franc Otorhinolaryng 34:209–214, 1921
2. Schmincke A: Uber lymphoepitheliale Geschwulste. Beitr Pathol Anat 68:161–170, 1921
3. Young JL, Miller RW: Incidence of malignant tumors in U.S. children. J Pediatr 86:254–258, 1975
4. Gastpar H, Wilmes E, Wolf H: Epidemiologic, etiologic and immunologic aspects of nasopharyngeal carcinoma. J Med 12:257–284, 1981
5. Green MH, Fraumeni JF, Hoover R: Nasopharyngeal cancer among young people in the United States: Racial variations by cell type. J Natl Cancer Inst 58:1267–70, 1977
6. Easton JM, Levine PH, Hyams VJ: Nasopharyngeal carcinoma in the United States: A pathologic study of 177 US and 30 foreign cases. Arch Otolaryngol 106:88–91, 1980
7. Klein G, Giovanella BC, Lindahl T et al: Direct evidence for the presence of Epstein–Barr virus DNA and nuclear antigen in malignant epithelial cells from patients with poorly differentiated carcinoma of the nasopharynx. Proc Natl Acad Sci USA 71:4747–4751, 1974
8. Huang DP, Ho JHC, Henle W et al: Presence of EBNA in nasopharyngeal carcinoma and control patients tissues related to EBV serology. Int J Cancer 22:266–274, 1978
9. Henle G, Henle W: Epstein–Bar virus-specific IgA serum antibodies as an outstanding feature of nasopharyngeal carcinoma. Int J Cancer 17:1–8, 1976
10. Naegele RF, Champion J, Murphy S, Henle G, Henle W: Nasopharyngeal carcinoma in American children: Epstein–Barr virus-specific antibody titer and prognosis. Int J Cancer 29:209–212, 1982
11. Shanmugaratnam K, Sobin L: Histological Typing of Upper Respiratory Tract Tumors, No. 19, pp 32–33. Geneva, World Health Organization, 1978
12. Neel HB, Pearson GR, Taylor WF: Antibodies to Epstein–Barr virus in patients with nasopharyngeal carcinoma and in comparison groups. Ann Otol Rhinol Laryngol 93:477–482, 1984
13. Rosai J: Oral cavity and pharynx. In Ackerman L (ed): Surgical Pathology, pp 165–166. St Louis, CV Mosby, 1981
14. Beahrs OH, Myers MH (eds): American Joint Committee on Cancer: Manual for Staging of Cancer, 2nd ed. Philadelphia, JB Lippincott, 1983
15. Ho JHC: Stage classification of nasopharyngeal carcinoma: A review. In de The G, Ito Y (eds): Nasopharyngeal Carcinoma: Etiology and Control, pp 99–113. Lyon, International Agency for Research in Cancer, 1977
16. Baker SR, Wolfe RA: Prognostic factors of nasopharyngeal malignancy. Cancer 49:163–169, 1982
17. Pick T, Maurer HM, McWilliams NB: Lymphoepithelioma in childhood. J Pediatr 84:96–100, 1974
18. Fernandez CH, Cangir A, Samaan NA, Rivera R: Nasopharyngeal carcinoma in children. Cancer 37:2787–2791, 1976
19. Ellouz R, Cammoun M, Ben Attia R, Bahi J: Nasopharyngeal carcinoma in children and adolescents in Tunisia: Clinical aspects and the paraneoplastic syndrome. In de The G, Ito Y (eds): Nasopharyngeal Carcinoma: Etiology and Control, pp 115–119. Lyon, International Agency for Research in Cancer, 1977
20. Deutsch M, Mercado R, Parsons JA: Cancer of the nasopharynx in children. Cancer 41:1128–1133, 1978
21. Berry MP, Smith CR, Brown TC et al: Nasopharyngeal carcinoma in the young. Int J Radiat Oncol Biol Phys 6:415–421, 1980
22. Jereb B, Huvos AG, Steinherz P, Unal A: Nasopharyngeal carcinoma in children: Review of 16 cases. Int J Radiat Oncol Biol Phys 6:497–491, 1980
23. Jenkin RDT, Anderson JR, Jereb B et al: Nasopharyngeal carcinoma: A retrospective review of patients less than thirty years of age. Cancer 47:360–366, 1981
24. Baker SR, McClatchey KD: Carcinoma of the nasopharynx in childhood. Otolaryngol Head Neck Surg 89:555–559, 1981
25. Lombardi F, Gasparini M, Gianni C et al: Nasopharyngeal carcinoma in childhood. Med Pediatr Oncol 10:243–250, 1982
26. Vita HC, Mendiondo OA, Shaw DL et al: Nasopharyngeal carcinoma in the second decade of life. Radiology 148:253–256, 1982
27. Bass IS, Haller JO, Berdon WE et al: Nasopharyngeal carcinoma: Clinical and radiographic findings in children. Radiology 156:651–654, 1985
28. Lobo–Sanahuja F, Garcia I, Carranza A, Camacho A: Treatment and outcome of undifferentiated carcinoma of the nasopharynx in childhood: A 13-year experience. Med Pediatr Oncol 14:6–11, 1986
29. Roper HP, Essex–Cater A, Marsden HB, Dixon PF, Campbell RHA: Nasopharyngeal carcinoma in children. Pediatr Hematol Oncol 3:143–152, 1986
30. Douglass EC: Unpublished observation
31. Huang AT, Crocker IR, Fisher SR, Walman MJ: Management of nasopharyngeal carcinoma. In Levine PH et al (eds): Epstein–Barr Virus and Associated Diseases, pp 644–659. Boston, Martinus Nijhoff, 1985
32. Price LA, Hill BT, Macrae KI: Increased survival in stage III and IV squamous cell carcinoma of the head and neck using an initial 24-hour combination chemotherapy protocol without cisplatin: 6 years follow-up. Prog Clin Biol Res 201:159–167, 1985
33. Rooney M, Kish J, Jacobs J, Kinzie J, Weaver A, Crissman J, Al-Sarraf M: Improved complete response rate and survival in advanced head and neck cancer after three-course induction therapy with 120-hour 5-FU infusion and cisplatin. Cancer 55:1123–1128, 1985
34. Taylor SG: Why has so much chemotherapy done so little in head and neck cancer? (editorial). J Clin Oncol 5:1–3, 1987
35. Connors JM, Andiman WA, Merigan TC: Treatment of nasopharyngeal carcinoma with interferon: Epstein–Barr virus serology and clinical results of a pilot study (abstract). Proc Am Soc Clin Oncol 23:198, 1982
36. Treuner J, Niethammer D, Dannecker G et al: Treatment of nasopharyngeal carcinoma in children with fibroblast interferon. In Grundman E et al (eds): Nasopharyngeal carcinoma: Cancer Campaign, pp 309–316. Stuttgart, Gustav Fischer Verlag, 1981

37. Sixbey JW, Thompson E, Douglass ED: Treatment of nasopharyngeal carcinoma with the antiviral drug 9-[(2-hydroxyethoxymethyl)]guanine: A case report. In Levine PH et al (eds): Epstein-Barr Virus and Associated Diseases, pp 660–665. Boston, Martinus Nijhoff, 1985

38. Son YH, Kapp DS: Oral cavity and oropharyngeal cancer in a younger population. Cancer 55:441–444, 1985

39. Lee YW, Gisser SD: Squamous cell carcinoma of the tongue in a nine year renal transplant survivor: A case report with a discussion of the risk of development of epithelial carcinoma in renal transplant survivors. Cancer 41:1–6, 1978

40. Reed K, Ravikuma TS, Gifford RRM, Grage TB: The association of Fanconi's anemia and squamous cell carcinoma. Cancer 52:926–928, 1983

41. Connolly GN, Winn DM, Hecht SS et al: The reemergence of smokeless tobacco. N Engl J Med 314:1020–1027, 1986

42. Jones RB: Smokeless tobacco: A challenge for the 80's. J Wisconsin Dental Assoc 10:717–721, 1985

43. Hoffmann D, Harley NH, Fisenne I, Adams JD, Brunnermann KD: Carcinogenic agents in snuff. JNCI 76:435–437, 1986

44. Marty PJ, McDermott RJ, Williams T: Patterns of smokeless tobacco use in a population of high school students. Am J Public Health 76:190–192, 1986

45. Poulson TC, Lindermuth JE, Greer RO Jr: A comparison of the use of smokeless tobacco in rural and urban teenagers. CA 34:248–261, 1984

46. Sedhew MK, Huvos AG, Strong EW et al: Proceedings: Ameloblastoma of maxilla and mandible. Cancer 33:324–333, 1974

47. Laurian N, Sadov R, Strauss M, Kessler. Laryngeal carcinoma in childhood: Report of a case and review of the literature. Laryngoscope 94:684–687, 1984

48. Deka BC, Deka AC: Carcinoma of the hypopharynx and larynx in a 12-year-old boy. Indian J Radiol 35:279–281, 1981

49. Anderson AE, Beuchner HA, Yager I, Ziskind MM: Bronchogenic carcinoma in young men. Am J Med 16:404, 1954

50. Niitu Y, Kubota H, Hasegawa S et al: Lung cancer (squamous cell carcinoma) in adolescence. Am J Dis Child 127:108, 1974

51. Las Salle AJ, Andrassy RJ, Stanford W: Bronchogenic squamous cell carcinoma in childhood: A case report. J Pediatr Surg 12:519–521, 1977

52. Askin FB: Lungs. In Kissane JM (ed): Pathology of Infancy and Childhood, pp 522–523. St Louis, CV Mosby, 1975

53. Verska JJ, Connolly JE: Bronchial adenomas in children. J Thorac Cardiovasc Surg 55:411–417, 1968

54. Weisel W, Lepley D: Tracheal and bronchial adenomas in childhood. Pediatrics 28:394–398, 1961

55. Okike N, Bernatz PE, Payne WS et al: Bronchoplastic procedures in the treatment of carcinoid tumors of the tracheobronchial tree. J Thorac Cardiovasc Surg 76:281–291, 1978

56. Leonardi HK, Jung–Legg Y, Legg MA, Neptune WB: Trancheobronchial mucoepidermoid carcinoma: Clinicopathological features and results of treatment. J Thorac Cardiovasc Surg 76:431–438, 1978

57. Weinblatt ME, Siegel SE, Isaacs H: Pulmonary blastoma associated with cystic lung disease. Cancer 49:669–671, 1982

58. Spencer H. Pulmonary blastoma. J Pathol Bacteriol 82:161–165, 1961

59. Stackhouse EM, Harrison EG, Ellis FH: Primary mixed malignancies of lung: Carcinosarcoma and blastoma. J Thorac Cardiovasc Surg 57:385–399, 1969

60. Fung CH, Lo JW, Yonan TN, Tilloy FJ, Hakami MM, Changer GW: Pulmonary blastoma: An ultrastructural study with a brief review of literature and a discussion of pathogenesis. Cancer 39:153–163, 1977

61. Kummet TD, Doll DC: Chemotherapy of pulmonary blastoma: A case report and review of the literature. Med Pediatr Oncol 10:27–33, 1982

62. Vogelzang NJ, Schultz SM, Iannucci AM, Kennedy BJ: Malignant mesothelioma: The University of Minnesota experience. Cancer 53:377–383, 1984

63. Lerner JH, Schoenfeld DA, Martin A et al: Malignant mesothelioma: The Eastern Cooperative Oncology Group (ECOG) experience. Cancer 52:1981–1985, 1983

64. Antman KH, Corson JM: Benign and malignant pleural mesothelioma. Clin Chest Med 6:127–140, 1985

65. Brenner J, Sordillo PP, Magill GB: Malignant mesothelioma in children. Med Pediatr Oncol 9:367–373, 1981

66. Kovalivker M, Motovic A: Malignant peritoneal mesothelioma in children: Description of two cases and review of the literature. J Pediatr Surg 20:274–275, 1985

67. Silberstein MJ, Lewis JE, Blair JD et al: Congenital peritoneal mesothelioma. J Pediatr Surg 18:243–245, 1983

68. Stein N, Henkes D: Mesothelioma of the testicle in a child. J Urol 135:794, 1986

69. Thorgeirsson G, Liebman J: Mesothelioma of the AV node. Pediatr Cardiol 4:219–223, 1983

70. Antman KH, Ruxer RL Jr, Aisner J, Vawter G: Mesothelioma following Wilms' tumor in childhood. Cancer 54:367–369, 1984

71. Anderson KA, Hurley WC, Hurley BT, Ohrt DW: Malignant pleural mesothelioma following radiotherapy in a 16-year-old boy. Cancer 56:273–276, 1985

72. Zidar B, Puch R, Schiffer L et al: Treatment of six cases of mesothelioma with doxorubicin and cisplatin (abstract). Proc Am Soc Clin Oncol 2:C-880, 1983

73. Rosenberg JC. Neoplasms of the mediastinum. In DeVita VT Jr, Hellman S, Rosenberg SA (eds): Cancer: Principles and Practice of Oncology, 2nd ed, pp 605–613. Philadelphia, JB Lippincott, 1985

74. Marino M, Muller–Haemelink HK: Thymoma and thymic carcinoma: Relation of thymoma epithelial cells to the cortical and medullary differentiation of the thymus. Virchows Arch 407:119–149, 1985

75. Swinborne–Sheldrake K, Gray GF Jr, Glick AD: Thymic epithelial neoplasms. South Med J 78:790–800, 1985

76. Levine GD, Rosai J: Thymic hyperplasia and neoplasia: A review of current concepts. Hum Pathol 9:495–515, 1978

77. Rose JS, McCarthy J, Mutchler RW, Velcek FT: Thymoma in childhood. NY State J Med 78:82–84, 1978

78. Bowie PR, Teteira OH, Carpenter B: Malignant thymoma in a 9-year-old boy presenting with pleuropericardial effusion. J Thorac Cardiovasc Surg 77:777–781, 1979

79. Furman WL, Buckley PJ, Green AA et al: Thymoma and myasthenia gravis in a 4-year-old child: Case report and review of the literature. Cancer 56:2703–2706, 1985

80. Dehner LP, Martin SA, Summer HW: Thymus related tumors and tumor-like lesions in childhood with rapid clinical progression and death. Hum Pathol 8:53–56, 1977

81. Ryniewicz B, Badurska B: Follow-up study of myasthenic children after thymectomy. J Neurol 217:133–138, 1977

82. Welch K Jr, Tapper D, Vawter GP: Surgical treatment of thymic cysts and neoplasms in children. J Pediatr Surg 14:691–698, 1979

83. Deshpanade GN, Fisher JE, Jewett TC Jr, Freeman AI: Malignant thymoma in an 8-month-old boy. J Surg Oncol 18:61–66, 1981

84. Drachman DB. Myasthenia gravis. N Engl J Med 298:136–142, 186–193, 1978

85. Souadjian JV, Enriquez P, Silverstein MN, Piepin JM: The spectrum of diseases associated with thymoma: Coincidence or syndrome? Arch Intern Med 134:374–379, 1974

86. Verley JM, Hollman KH: Thymoma: A comparative study of clinical stages, histologic features, and survival in 200 cases. Cancer 55:1074–1086, 1985

87. Masaoka A, Monden Y, Nakahara K, Tanioka T: Follow-up study of thymomas with special reference to their clinical stages. Cancer 48:2485–2492, 1981

88. Bergh NP, Gatzusky P, Larsson S et al: Tumors of the thymus and thymic region I: Clinicopathologic studies of thymomas. Ann Thorac Surg 25:91–98, 1978

89. Oosterhuis HJ: Thymectomy in myasthenia gravis: A review. Ital J Neurol Sci 4:399–407, 1983

90. Mulder DG, Hermann C Jr, Keesey J, Edwards H: Thymectomy for myasthenia gravis. Am J Surg 146:61–66, 1983

91. Hawkins JR, Mayer RF, Satterfield JR et al: Thymectomy for myasthenia gravis: 14 year experience. Ann Surg 201:618–625, 1985

92. Maggi G, Giacone G, Donadie M et al: Thymomas: A review of 169 cases with particular reference to results of surgical treatment. Cancer 58:765–766, 1986

93. Ariaratnam LS, Kalnicki S, Mincer F, Botstein C: The management of malignant thymoma with radiation therapy. Int J Radiat Oncol Biol Phys 5:77–80, 1979

94. Boston B: Chemotherapy of invasive thymoma. Cancer 38:49–52, 1976

95. Shetty MR, Arnora RK: Invasive thymoma treated with cisplatin (letter). Cancer Treat Rep 65:531, 1981

96. Daugaard G, Hansen HH, Rorth M: Combination chemotherapy for malignant thymoma. Ann Intern Med 99:189–190, 1983

97. Bernatz PE, Khonsari S, Harris EG Jr, Taylor WF: Thymoma: Factors influencing prognosis. Surg Clin North Am 53:885–892, 1973

98. Batata MA, Martini N, Huvos AG et al: Thymomas: Clinicopathologic features, therapy, and prognosis. Cancer 34:389–396, 1974

99. Chan HLS, Sonley MS, Moes CAF et al: Primary and secondary tumors of childhood involving the heart, pericardium and great vessels. Cancer 56:825–836, 1985

100. Smith C: Tumors of the heart. Arch Pathol Lab Med 110:371–374, 1986

101. Barnes WSF, Hunler AS, Stiller CA: Primary malignant cardiac tumors in children. Pediatr Hematol Oncol 3:347–356, 1986

102. Pratt CB, Dugger DL, Johnson WW, Ainger LE: Metastatic involvement of the heart in childhood rhabdomyosarcoma. Cancer 31:1492–1497, 1973

103. Grawitz PA: Die sogenannten Lipome der Niere. Virchows Arch [Pathol Anat] 93:39–63, 1883

104. Hartman DS, Davis CJ, Madewell JE, Friedman AC: Primary malignant renal tumors in the second decade of life: Wilms' tumor versus renal cell carcinoma. J Urol 127:888–891, 1982

105. Bennington JL, Beckwith JB: Tumors of the Kidney, Renal Pelvis and Ureter. Atlas of Tumor Pathology, fascicle 12. Washington, DC, Armed Forces Institute of Pathology, 1975

106. Castellanos RD, Aron BS, Evans AT: Renal adenocarcinoma in children: Incidence, therapy and prognosis. J Urol 111:534–537, 1974

107. Raney RB, Palmer N, Sutow W, Baum E, Ayala A: Renal cell carcinoma in children. Med Pediatr Oncol 11:90–98, 1983

108. Chan HS, Daneman A, Gribbin M, Martin DJ: Renal cell carcinoma in the first two decades of life. Pediatr Radiol 13:324–328, 1983

109. Lack EE, Cassady JR, Sallan SE: Renal cell carcinoma in childhood and adolescence: A clinical and pathological study of 14 cases. J Urol 133:822–828, 1985

110. Horton WA, Wong V, Eldridge R: Von Hippel–Lindau disease: Clinical and pathologic manifestation in 9 families with 50 affected members. Arch Intern Med 1136:769–777, 1976

111. Kaplan C, Sayre GP, Greene LF: Bilateral nephrogenic carcinomas in Lindau–Von Hippel disease. J Urol 86:36–42, 1961

112. Cohen AJ, Li FP, Berg S et al: Hereditary renal cell carcinoma associated with a chromosomal translocation. N Engl J Med 301:592–595, 1979

113. Wang N, Perkins KL: Involvement of band 3p14 in t(3:8) hereditary renal carcinoma. Cancer Genet Cytogenet 11:479–481, 1984

114. Yoshida MA, Ohyashik K, Ochi H et al: Cytogenetic studies of tumor tissue from patients with nonfamilial renal cell carcinoma. Cancer Res 46:2139–2147, 1986

115. Sibley RK, Rosai J: Urinary tract/kidney, renal pelvis, and ureter. In Ackerman L (ed): Surgical Pathology, pp 801–802. St Louis, CV Mosby, 1981

116. Paulson DF, Perez CA, Anderson T: Cancer of the kidney and ureter. In DeVita VT Jr, Hellman S, Rosenberg SA (eds): Cancer: Principles and Practice of Oncology, 2nd ed, p 896. Philadelphia, JB Lippincott, 1985

117. Ramos CV, Taylor HB: Hepatic dysfunction associated with renal carcinoma. Cancer 29:1287–1292, 1972

118. Goldberg MF, Tashjian AH, Order SE: Renal adenocarcinoma containing a parathormone-like substance and associated with marked hypercalcemia. Am J Med 367:805–814, 1964

119. Hewlett JS, Hoffman GC, Senhauser DA, Battle JD: Carcinoma of the kidney producing multiple hormones. J Urol 106:820–822, 1971

120. Golde DW, Schambelan M, Weintraub BD, Rosen SW: Gonadotropin-secreting renal carcinoma. Cancer 33:1048–1053, 1974

121. Beckwith JB: Wilms' tumor and other renal tumors of childhood. In Finegold ML (ed): Pathology of Neoplasia in Children and Adolescents, pp 313–318. Philadelphia, WB Saunders, 1986

122. Robson CJ, Churchill BM, Anderson W: The results of radical nephrectomy for renal cell carcinoma. J Urol 101:297–301, 1969

123. Paulson DF, Perez CA, Anderson T: Cancer of the kidney and ureter. In DeVita VT Jr, Hellman S, Rosenberg SA (eds): Cancer: Principles and Practice of Oncology, 2nd ed, p 903. Philadelphia, JB Lippincott, 1985

124. Vugrin D, Hood W, Taylor W, Laszlo J: Two trials of lymphoblastoid alpha-interferon (IFN) in patients with advanced renal carcinoma (abstract). Proc Am Soc Clin Oncol 3:153, 1984

125. Strayer DR, Weisband J, Carter WA, Brodsky I: Renal cell carcinoma and leukocyte interferon: Correlation between sensitivity in a clonogenic assay and clinical response (abstract). Proc Am Soc Clin Oncol 3:158, 1984

126. Rosenberg SA, Lotze MT, Muul LM: Observations on the systemic administration of autologous lymphokine-activated killer cells and recombinant interleukin-2 to patients with metastatic cancer. N Engl J Med 313:1485–1492, 1985

127. Rosenberg SA, Lotze MT, Muul LM et al: Progress report on the treatment of 157 patients with advanced cancer using lymphokine-activated killer cells and interleukin-2 or high-dose interleukin-2 alone. N Engl J Med 316:889–897, 1987

128. West WH, Tauer KW, Yanelli JR et al: Constant-infusion recombinant interleukin-2 in adoptive immunotherapy of advanced cancer. N Engl J Med 316:898–905, 1987

129. Sotelo–Avila C, Gooch WM: Neoplasms associated with the Beckwith–Wiedemann syndrome. In Rosenberg HS, Bolande RP (eds): Perspectives in Pediatric Pathology, vol 3. Chicago, Year Book Medical Publishers, 1976

130. Levine GW: Adrenocortical carcinoma in two children with subsequent primary tumors. Am J Dis Child 132:238–240, 1978

131. Humphrey GB, Pysher T, Holcombe J et al: Overview on the management of adrenocortical carcinoma (ACC). Cancer Treat Rev 17:349–358, 1983

132. Cagle PT, Hough AJ, Pysher TJ et al: Comparison of adrenal cortical tumors in children and adults. Cancer 57:2235–2237, 1986

133. Lubitz JA, Freeman L, Okun R: Mitotane in inoperable adrenal cortical carcinoma. JAMA 223:1109–1111, 1973

134. Schteingart DE, Cash R, Coon JW: Aminoglutethimide and metastatic adrenal cancer. JAMA 198:1007–1010, 1966

135. American Cancer Society: Cancer Facts and Figures—1987. New York, American Cancer Society, 1987

136. Ludwig R, Stromeyer H, Willich E: Tumors of the stomach in children (meeting abstract). Nineteenth Congress of the European Society of Pediatric Radiology, April 22–24, 1982, Prague, Czechoslovakia. European Society of Pediatric Radiology, 1982

137. Schwartz MG, Sgaglione NA: Gastric carcinoma in the young: Overview of the literature. Mt Sinai J Med (NY) 51:720–723, 1984

138. Goto S, Ikeda K, Ishii E, Miyazaki S, Shimizu S, Iwashita A: Carcinoma of the stomach in a 7-year-old boy: A case report and a review of the literature on children under 10 years of age. Z Kinderchir 39:137–140, 1984

139. Black RE: Linitis plastica in a child. J Pediatr Surg 20:86–87, 1985

140. Mayer RJ, Rosoff CB, Feldman MI: Cancer of the stomach. In Cancer Manual, 6th ed, pp 176–183. Boston, American Cancer Society, Massachusetts Division, 1982

141. Moertel CG: The stomach. In Holland JF, Frei E (eds): Cancer Medicine, pp 1527–1540. Philadelphia, Lea & Febiger, 1973

142. Haenszel W, Correa P: Developments in the epidemiology of stomach cancer over the past decade. Cancer Res 35:3452–3459, 1975

143. Nobrega FT, Sedlack JD, Sedlack RE, et al: A decline in carcinoma of the stomach: A diagnostic artifact? Mayo Clin Proc 58:255–260, 1983

144. McDonald JS, Cohn I Jr, Gunderson LL: Cancer of the stomach. In DeVita VT Jr, Hellman S, Rosenberg SA (eds): Cancer: Principles and Practice of Oncology, 2nd ed, pp 659–690. Philadelphia, JB Lippincott, 1985

145. Macdonald JS, Schein PS, Wooley PV et al: 5-Fluorouracil, doxorubicin and mitomycin (FAM) combination chemotherapy for advanced gastric cancer. Ann Intern Med 93:533–536, 1980

146. Comis RL, Carter SK: A review of chemotherapy in gastric cancer. Cancer 34:1576–1586, 1974

147. Levi JA, Dalley DN, Aroney RS: Improved combination chemotherapy in advanced gastric cancer. Br Med J 2:1471–1473, 1979

148. Sindelar WF, Kinsella TJ, Mayer RJ: Cancer of the pancreas. In DeVita VT Jr, Hellman S, Rosenberg SA (eds): Cancer: Principles and Practice of Oncology, 2nd ed, pp 691–739. Philadelphia, JB Lippincott, 1985

149. Whipple AO, Parsons LB, Mullins CR: Treatment of carcinoma of the ampulla of Vater. Ann Surg 102:763–779, 1935

150. Fontham ETH: Epidemiology of cancer of the pancreas. In Correa P, Haenszel W (eds): Epidemiology of Cancer of the Digestive Tract, pp 243–259. The Hague, Martinus Nijhoff, 1982

151. MacMahon B, Yen S, Trichopoulos D et al: Coffee and cancer of the pancreas. N Engl J Med 304:630–633, 1981

152. Wynder EL, Hall NEL, Polansky M: Epidemiology of coffee and pancreatic cancer. Cancer Res 43:3900–3906, 1983

153. Hayman W, Neerlaub RC, Johnson TS: Pancreatic carcinoma in childhood: Report and review. J Pediatr 65:1711–1720, 1964

154. Masterson JB, Bowie JD, Port RB et al: Carcinoma of the pancreas occurring in a child: A case report with description of gray scale ultrasound findings. J Clin Ultrasonogr 6:189–190, 1978

155. Kissane JM: Carcinoma of the pancreas in childhood. Newsletter Natl Pancreas Cancer Project 6:30, 1981

156. Humphrey GB, Bukowski, RM, Dehner LP et al: Diagnosis, pathology, prognosis and treatment of childhood pancreatic malignancies (abstract). Proc Am Soc Clin Oncol 1:177, 1982

157. Hecht ST, Brasch RC, Styne DM: CT localization of occult secretory tumors in children. Pediatr Radiol 12:67–71, 1982

158. Lack EE, Cassady JR, Levey R, Vawter GF: Tumors of the exocrine pancreas in children and adolescents: A clinical and pathologic study of eight patients. Am J Surg Pathol 7:319–327, 1983

159. Robey G, Daneman A, Martin DJ: Pancreatic carcinoma in a neonate. Pediatr Radiol 13:284–286, 1983

160. Tersigni R, Arena L, Alessandroni L et al: Pancreatic carcinoma in childhood: Case report of long survival and review of the literature. Surgery 96:560–566, 1984

161. Smith JH, Baugh C, Rippun T: Obstructive jaundice secondary to pancreatic adenocarcinoma in a 7-year-old male. J Pediatr Surg 20:184–185, 1985

162. Lewis MA, Lilleyman JS, Variend S: Benign metastatic islet cell tumor of the pancreas. Med Pediatr Oncol 13:97–100, 1985

163. Reed DN Jr, Turcotte JG: Papillary epithelial neoplasm of the pancreas in the pediatric population. J Surg Oncol 32:182–183, 1986

164. Bowlby LS: Pancreatic adenocarcinoma in an adolescent male with Peutz–Jeghers syndrome. Hum Pathol 17:97–99, 1986

165. Schimke RN: The multiple endocrine neoplasms syndromes. Cancer Treat Rev 17:249–264, 1983

166. Viniki AI, Strodel WE, O'Doridro TM: Endocrine tumors of the gastroentero-pancreatic axis. Cancer Treat Rev 20:305–345, 1984

167. Carney JA, Go VL, Gordon H et al: Familial pheochomocytoma and islet cell tumor of the pancreas. Am J Med 68:515–521, 1980

168. Tareishi R, Wada A, Ishigiro S et al: Coexistence of bilateral pheochromo-cytoma and pancreatic islet cell tumor: Report of a case and review of the literature. Cancer 42:2928–2934, 1978

169. Horie A, Yaro Y, Kofoo Y, Mirva I: Morphogenesis of pancreatoblastoma: Infantile carcinoma of the pancreas. Cancer 39:247–254, 1977

170. Iseki M, Suzuki T, Koizumi Y et al: Alpha-fetoprotein-producing pancreato-blastoma: A case report. Cancer 57:1833–1835, 1986

171. Sharma MP, Gregg JA, Loewenstein MS et al: Carcinoembryonic antigen (CEA) activity in pancreatic juice of patients with pancreatic carcinoma and pancreatitis. Cancer 38:2457–2461, 1976

172. Cancer of the Pancreas Task Force: Staging of cancer of the pancreas. Cancer 47:1631–1637, 1981

173. Carmprodon R, Quentanilla E: Successful long-term results with resection of pancreatic carcinoma in children: Favorable prognosis for an uncommon neoplasm. Surgery 95:420–426, 1984

174. Horton J, Gelber RD, Engstrom P et al: Trials of single-agent and combination chemotherapy for advanced cancer of the pancreas. Cancer Treat Rep 65:65–68, 1981

175. Bukowski RM, Schacter LP, Grappe CW et al: Phase II trial of 5-fluorouracil, Adriamycin, mitomycin C, and streptozotocin (FAM-5) in pancreatic carci-noma. Cancer 50:197–200, 1982

176. Smith FP, Hoth DF, Levin B et al: 5-Fluorouracil, Adriamycin and mitomycin-C (FAM) chemotherapy for advanced carcinoma of the pancreas. Cancer 46:2014–2018, 1980

177. Kelly TR, Chamberlain TR: Carcinoma of the gallbladder. Am J Surg 143:737–741, 1982

178. Correa P, Haenszel W: The epidemiology of large-bowel cancer. Adv Cancer Res 26:1–141, 1978

179. Howell MA: Diet as an etiological factor in the development of cancers of the colon and rectum. J Chronic Dis 28:67–80, 1975

180. Wynder EL, Shigematsu T: Environmental factors of cancer of the colon and rectum. Cancer 20:1520–1561, 1967

181. Young YL, Percy CL, Asire AJ (eds): Surveillance, Epidemiology and End Results: Incidence and Mortality Data, 1973–1977. National Cancer Insti-tute Monograph 57. Washington, DC, US Government Printing Office, 1981

182. Pratt CB, George SL: Epidemic colon cancer in children and adolescents? In Correa P, Haensze W (eds): Epidemiology of Cancer of the Digestive Tract, pp 127–146. The Hague, Martinus Nijhoff, 1982

183. Pratt, CB, Rivera G, Shanks E et al: Colorectal carcinoma in adolescents: Implications regarding etiology. Cancer 40(suppl):2464–2472, 1977

184. Odone V, Chang L, Caces J et al: The natural history of colorectal carci-noma in adolescents. Cancer 49:1716–1720, 1982

185. Rao BN, Pratt CB, Fleming ID et al: Colon carcinoma in children and adoles-cents: A review of thirty cases. Cancer 55:1322–1326, 1985

186. Caldwell GC, Cannon SB, Pratt CB, Arthur RD: Serum pesticide levels in childhood colorectal carcinoma patients. Cancer 48:774–778, 1981

187. Hinton JM: Risk of malignant change in ulcerative colitis. Gut 7:427–432, 1966

188. Abrams JS, Reines HD: Increasing incidence of right-sided lesions in colorec-tal carcinoma. Am J Surg 137:522–526, 1979

189. Sherlock P, Lipkin M, Winauer SJ: Predisposing factors in carcinoma of the colon. Adv Intern Med 20:121–150, 1975

190. Reed TE, Neel JV: A genetic study of multiple polyposis of the colon (with an appendix deriving a method of estimating relative fitness). Am J Hum Genet 7:236–259, 1955

191. McKusick VA: Genetics and large-bowel cancer. Am J Dig Dis 19:954, 1964

192. Bussey HJR: Gastrointestinal polyposis. Gut 11:970–978, 1970

193. Stemper TJ, Kent TH, Summers RW: Juvenile polyposis and gastrointestinal carcinoma: A study of a kindred. Ann Intern Med 83:639–646, 1975

194. Haggitt RC, Pitcock JA: Familial juvenile polyposis of the colon. Cancer 26:1232–1238, 1970

195. Lynch HT, Giurgis H, Schwartz M et al: Genetics and colon cancer. Arch Surg 106:669–675, 1973

196. Turcot J, Despies JP, St Pierre F: Malignant tumors of the central nervous system associated with familial polyposis of the colon: Report of two cases. Dis Colon Rectum 2:465–468, 1959

197. Oldfield MC: The association of familial polyposis of the colon with multiple sebaceous cysts. Br J Surg 41:534–541, 1954

198. Gardner EJ: Follow-up study of a family group exhibiting dominant inheri-tance for a syndrome including intestinal polyps, osteomas, fibromas, and epidermal cysts. Am J Hum Genet 14:376–390, 1962

199. Pratt CB, Parham D, Rao BN, Fleming ID: Adolescent colorectal carcinoma, polyposis coli and neurofibromatosis (abstract). Proc Am Soc Cancer Res 28:254, 1987

200. Lynch HT, Lynch PM: Heredity and gastrointestinal tract cancer. In Lipkin M, Good RA (eds): Gastrointestinal Tract Cancer. New York, Plenum, 1978

201. Jeghers H, McKusick VA, Katz JH: Generalized intestinal polyposis and melanin spots of the oral mucosa, lips and digits. N Engl J Med 241:993–1005, 1949

202. Chabalko JJ, Fraumeni JF Jr: Colorectal cancer in children: Epidemiologic aspects. Dis Colon Rectum 18:1–3, 1975

203. Hoerner MT: Carcinoma of the colon and rectum in persons under twenty years of age. Am J Surg 96:47–53, 1958

204. Middlekamp JN, Haffner H: Carcinoma of the colon in children. Pediatrics 32:558–571, 1963

205. Sessions RT, Reddell DH, Kaplan HJ, Foster JH: Carcinoma of the colon in the first two decades of life. Ann Surg 162:279–284, 1965

206. Pillay SP, Augorn IB, Baker LW. Colorectal carcinoma in young black pa-tients: A report of eight cases. J Surg Oncol 10:125–132, 1978

207. Sugarbaker PH, Gunderson LL, Wittes RE: Colorectal cancer. In DeVita VT Jr, Hellman S, Rosenberg SA (eds): Cancer: Principles and Practice of Oncology, 2nd ed, pp 795–884. Philadelphia, JB Lippincott, 1985

208. Symonds DA, Vickery AL Jr: Mucinous carcinoma of the colon and rectum. Cancer 37:1891–1900, 1976

209. Moertel CG: Multiple primary neoplasms: Their incidence and significance. Recent Results Cancer Res 7:1–107, 1966

210. Madajewicz S, Petelli N, Rustum YM et al: A phase I–II trial of high-dose calcium leucovorin and 5-fluorouracil in advanced colorectal carcinoma. Cancer Res 44:4667–4669, 1984

211. Boice JD Jr, Green MH, Killen JY Jr et al: Leukemia and preleukemia after adjuvant treatment of gastrointestinal cancer with semustine (methyl-CCNU). N Engl J Med 309:1079–1084, 1983

212. Macks C: Carcinoid Tumors, pp 1–124. Boston, GK Hall, 1979

213. Buchino JJ, Groff DB: Epithelial tumors of the large intestine in children. In Spratt JS (ed): Neoplasms of the Colon, Rectum and Anus: Mucosal and Epithelial, pp 331–340. Philadelphia, WB Saunders, 1984

214. Spratt JS: Carcinoids. In Spratt JS (ed): Neoplasms of the Colon, Rectum and Anus: Mucosal and Epithelial, pp 261–267. Philadelphia, WB Saunders, 1984

215. McDougall JC, Unni K, Gorenstein A, O'Connell EJ: Carcinoid and muco-epidermoid carcinoma of bronchus in children. Ann Otol Rhinol Laryngol 89:425–427, 1980

216. Patterson K, Chandra RS, Kapur S: Appendical carcinoid tumors in child-hood: A report of 2 cases. Clin Proc Child Hosp Natl Med Cent 37:13–17, 1981

217. Anderson A, Bergdahl L: Carcinoid tumors of the appendix in children: A report of 25 cases. Acta Chir Scand 143:173–175, 1977

218. King MD, Young DG, Hann IM, Patrick WJ: Carcinoid syndrome: An unusual cause of diarrhea. Arch Dis Child 60:269–271, 1985

219. LaFeila G, Baxter RA, Tavadia HB, Harper DR: Multiple colonic carcinoid tumors in a child. Br J Surg 71:843, 1984

220. Sabback MS, O'Brien PH: Clinical study of 81 gastrointestinal carcinoid tumors. South Med J 72:386–390, 1979

221. Chow CW, Sane S, Campbell PE, Center RF: Malignant carcinoid tumors in children. Cancer 49:802–811, 1982

222. Yang K, Ulich T, Cheng L, Lewin KJ: The neuroendocrine products of intes-

tinal carcinoids: An immunoperoxidase study of 35 carcinoid tumors stained for serotonin and eight polypeptide hormones. Cancer 51:1918–1926, 1983

223. Moertel CG, Hanley JA: Combination chemotherapy trials in metastatic carcinoid tumor and the malignant carcinoid syndrome. Cancer Clin Trials 2:327–334, 1979

224. Young RC, Knapp RC, Fuks Z, DiSaia PJ: Cancer of the ovary. In DeVita VT Jr, Hellman S, Rosenberg SA (eds): Cancer: Principles and Practice of Oncology, 2nd ed, pp 1083–1117. Philadelphia, JB Lippincott, 1985

225. Tobias JS, Griffiths CT: Management of ovarian carcinoma: Current concepts and future prospects. N Engl J Med 294:818–823 and 882–887, 1976

226. Dillon MB, Rosenshein NB, Parmley TH et al: The diagnosis and management of cervical intraepithelial neoplasia in the patient under the age of twenty-one. Int J Gynaecol Obstet 19:97–102, 1981

227. Dakel A, Van Iddekinge B, Leiman G: Invasive squamous cell carcinoma of the cervix in a 15-year-old girl: A case report and review of the literature. S Afr Med J 61:628–629, 1982

228. Herbst AL, Robboy SJ, Scully RE, Poskanzer DC: Clear-cell adenocarcinoma of the vagina and cervix in girls: Analysis of 170 registry cases. Am J Obstet Gynecol 119:713–724, 1974

229. Fletcher GH, Delcos L, Wharton JT, Rutledge FN. Tumors of the vagina and female urethra. In Fletcher GH (ed): Textbook of Radiotherapy, p 959. Philadelphia, Lea & Febiger, 1980

230. Ostergard DR: DES-related vaginal lesions. Clin Obstet Gynecol 24:379–384, 1981

231. Melnick S, Cole P, Anderson D, Herbst A: Rates and risks of diethylstilbesterol-related clear-cell carcinoma of the vagina and cervix: An update. N Engl J Med 316:514–516, 1987

232. Huffman JW, Dewhurst CJ, Casparo VJ: Tumors of the vulva and vagina during childhood. In: The Gynecology of Childhood and Adolescence. 2nd ed, pp 225–258. Philadelphia, WB Saunders, 1981

233. Norris HJ, Bagley GP, Taylor HB: Carcinoma of the infant vagina: A destructive tumor. Arch Pathol 90:473–379, 1970

234. Cario GM, House MJ, Paradinas FJ: Squamous cell carcinoma of the vulva in association with mixed vulvar dystrophy in an 18-year-old girl: Case report. Br J Obstet Gynaecol 91:87–90, 1984

235. Herrmann JH: Tumors and other enlargements of the breast. In Ariel IM, Pack GT (eds): Cancer and Allied Diseases of Infancy and Childhood, chap 7. Boston, Little, Brown, 1960

236. Bower R, Bell MJ, Ternberg JL: Management of breast lesions in children and adolescents. J Pediatr Surg 11:337–346, 1976

237. Festenstein H: Adenocarcinoma of the breast in a South African Bantu boy aged 14. S Afr Med J 34:517–518, 1960

238. Lippitt WH, Medart WS Jr, Ramsey SN: Breast cancer in a 10-year-old girl. Surgery 68:395–396, 1970

239. McDivitt RW, Stewart FW: Breast carcinoma in children. JAMA 195:388–390, 1966

240. Lynch HT, Guirgis H, Brodkey F et al: Early age of onset in familial breast cancer. Arch Surg 111:126–131, 1976

241. Anderson DE, Badzioch MD: Bilaterality in familial breast cancer patients. Cancer 56:2092–2098, 1985

242. Haynes HA, Mead KW, Goldwyn RM: Cancers of the skin. In DeVita VT Jr, Hellman S, Rosenberg SA (eds): Cancer: Principles of Practice of Oncology, 2nd ed, pp 1343–1369. Philadelphia, JB Lippincott, 1985

243. Hyde JN: On the influence of light in the production of cancer of the skin. Am J Med Sci 131:1–22, 1906

244. Robbins JH, Kraeman KH, Lutzner MA et al: Xeroderma pigmentosum: An inherited disease with light sensitivity, multiple cutaneous neoplasms and abnormal repair. Ann Intern Med 80:221–248, 1974

245. Holman CD, Armstrong BK: Cutaneous malignant melanoma and indicators of total accumulated exposure to the sun: An analysis separating histogenetic types. JNCI 73:75–82, 1984

246. Green A, Siskind V, Bain C, Alexander J: Sunburn and malignant melanoma. Br J Cancer 51:393–397, 1985

247. Hicks N, Zack M, Caldwell GG, McKinley TW: Life-style factors among patients with melanoma. South Med J 78:903–908, 1985

248. Holman CD, Armstrong BK, Heenan P: Relationship of cutaneous melanoma to individual sunlight-exposure habits. JNCI 76:403–414, 1986

249. Cleaver JE: Defective repair replication of DNA in xeroderma pigmentosum. Nature 218:652–656, 1968

250. Kobayashi M, Satoh Y, Irimajiri T et al: Skin tumors in xeroderma pigmentosum (I). J Dermatol (Tokyo) 9:319–322, 1982

251. Pratt CB: Unpublished observations

252. Heimler A, Friedman E, Rosenthal AD: Naevoid basal cell carcinoma syndrome and Charcot–Marie–Tooth disease: Two autosomal dominant disorders segregating in a family. J Med Genet 15:288–291, 1978

253. Southwick GJ, Schwartz RA: The basal cell nevus syndrome: Disasters occurring among a series of 36 patients. Cancer 44:2294–2305, 1979

254. Gundlach KK, Keihn M: Multiple basal cell carcinomas and keratocysts: The Gorlin and Goltz syndrome. J Maxillofac Surg 7:299–307, 1979

255. Cramer H, Niederdallmann H: Cerebral giantism associated with jaw cyst basal cell naevoid syndrome in two families. Arch Psychiatr Nervenkr 233:111–124, 1983

256. Morar G, Burris R: Cancer of the skin in blacks: A review of 128 patients with basal-cell carcinoma. Cancer 47:1436–1438, 1981

257. Novick M, Gard DA, Hardy SB, Spira M: Burn scar carcinoma: A review and analysis of 46 cases. J Trauma 17:809–817, 1977

258. Kennedy AW, Hart WR: Multiple squamous-cell carcinomas in Fanconi's anemia. Cancer 50:811–814, 1982

259. Kopf AW, Hellman LJ, Rogers GS et al: Familial malignant melanoma. JAMA 256:1915–1919, 1986

260. Greene MH, Clark WH Jr, Tucker MA et al: Acquired precursors of cutaneous malignant malanoma: The familial dysplastic nevus syndrome. N Engl J Med 10:91–97, 1985

261. Greene MH, Clark WH Jr, Tucker MA et al: High risk of malignant melanoma in melanoma-prone families with dysplastic nevi. Ann Intern Med 102:458–465, 1985

262. Nordlund JJ, Kirkwood J, Horget BM et al: Demographic study of clinically atypical (dysplastic) nevi in patients with melanoma and comparison subjects. Cancer Res 45:1855–1861, 1985

263. Quaba AA, Wallace AF: The incidence of malignant melanoma (0 to 15 years of age) arising in "large" congenital nevocellular nevi. Plast Reconstr Surg 78:174–181, 1986

264. Clark WH Jr, Ainsworth AM, Bernandino EA et al: The developmental biology of primary human malignant melanomas. Semin Oncol 2:83–103, 1975

265. Briggs JC: Melanoma precursor lesions and borderline melanomas. Histopathology 9:1251–1262, 1985

266. Pratt CB, Palmer MK, Thatcher N, Crowther D: Malignant melanoma in children and adolescents. Cancer 47:392–397, 1981

267. Hayes FA, Green AA: Malignant melanoma in childhood: Clinical course and response to chemotherapy. J Clin Oncol 2:1229–1234, 1984

268. Flemming AF, Ruggins N: Malignant melanoma in childhood. Br J Plast Surg 38:432–434, 1985

269. Bader JL, Li FP, Olmstead PM et al: Childhood malignant melanoma: Incidence and etiology. Am J Pediatr Hematol Oncol 7:341–345, 1985

270. Moss DM, Grant–Kels JM: Significant melanocytic lesions in infancy, childhood and adolescence. Dermatol Clin 4:29–44, 1986

271. Naraysingh V, Busby GO: Congenital malignant melanoma. J Pediatr Surg 21:81–82, 1986

272. Melvik MK, Urdanetak LF, Al-Jurf AS et al: Malignant melanoma in childhood and adolescence. Am Surg 52:142–147, 1986

273. Rahbari H, Mehregan AH: Basal cell epithelioma (carcinoma) in children and teenagers. Cancer 49:350–353, 1982

274. Harvey RA, Chaglassian T, Knapper W, Goulian D: Squamous cell carcinoma of the skin in adolescence: Report of a case. JAMA 238:513, 1977

275. Narasinharao KL, Chatterjee H, Veliath AJ: Penile carcinoma in the first decade of life. Br J Urol 57:358, 1984

276. Daugherty BG, Evans HL: Carcinoma of the anal canal: A study of 79 cases. Am J Clin Pathol 83:159–164, 1985

277. Blewitt RW: Why does basal cell carcinoma metastasize so rarely? Int J Dermatol 19:144–146, 1980

278. Amer FC, Hickey RC: Metastases from squamous cell skin cancer of the extremities. South Med J 75:920–923, 1982

279. Civatte J, Tsoitis G: Adnexal skin carcinomas. In Andrade R, Gumport SL, Popkin GL et al (eds): Cancer of the Skin, pp 1045–1068. Philadelphia, WB Saunders, 1976

280. Mastrangelo MJ, Baker AR, Katz HR: Cutaneous melanoma. In DeVita VT Jr, Hellman S, Rosenberg SA (eds): Cancer: Principles of Practice of Oncology, 2nd ed, pp 1371–1422. Philadelphia, JB Lippincott, 1985

281. Mohs FE, Jones DJ, Koranda FC: Microscopically controlled surgery for carcinomas in patients with nevoid basal cell carcinoma syndrome. Arch Dermatol 116:777–779, 1980

282. Stern RS, Weinstein MC, Baker SG: Risk reduction for non-melanoma skin cancer with childhood sunscreen use. Arch Dermatol 122:537–545, 1986

thirty-six

The Acquired Immune Deficiency Syndrome (AIDS)

Philip A. Pizzo,
Janie Eddy, and
Judith Falloon

Knowledge of and experience with the acquired immune deficiency syndrome (AIDS) are becoming increasingly important for the pediatric hematologist–oncologist for a variety of reasons. First, the incidence of AIDS in children is increasing. Although just over 1000 cases of pediatric AIDS had been reported to the Centers for Disease Control (CDC) as of June 1988, it is projected that this number will exceed 3000 by 1991, with some estimates projecting upward of 10,000 HIV-infected children.[1] Second, some of these children (e.g., cancer patients with transfusion-related infection or children with hemophilia) are already in the care of pediatric hematologists–oncologists or may be referred to them for evaluation of clinical findings suggestive of a hematologic or oncologic disorder. Third, the finding that AIDS is associated with a retrovirus, now referred to as the human immunodeficiency virus (HIV), is likely to have important implications for oncology.[1-11] Indeed, many of the basic biological insights gained from this retroviral disorder may have therapeutic implications for cancer, and many of the treatment concepts used in cancer are applicable or relevant to the design of therapeutic strategies for pediatric AIDS. Indeed, AIDS stands at the interface between immunology, infectious disease, and oncology.

DEFINITION OF AIDS IN CHILDREN

Case definition criteria for AIDS in children were established by the CDC and were subsequently modified when it became clear that AIDS in children is different from the syndrome as seen in adults.[12,13] The initial CDC case definition of pediatric AIDS (Table 36-1) was restrictive, requiring a documented opportunistic infection or histologically confirmed lymphoid interstitial pneumonitis, thus resulting in an underreporting of AIDS in children.[13] For example, it has been estimated that as many as 70% of children with clearly HIV-related disease do not meet the initial CDC criteria for AIDS.[14] Moreover, HIV-positive children may have died from bacterial infection or unbiopsied interstitial pneumonitis without having fulfilled the CDC definition of AIDS. The initial CDC definition also excluded children who were receiving immunosuppressive therapy, even though such patients could clearly have been infected from blood products.[15]

In order to improve the epidemiologic tracking of AIDS-related morbidity and mortality, to simplify reporting, and to increase the sensitivity and specificity of the definition of AIDS in a manner consistent with current clinical practice, the CDC revised its surveillance case definition effective September 1, 1987.[16] In the revised system, AIDS is defined according to whether laboratory evidence supports HIV infection (e.g., HIV antibody in children older than 15 months; HIV antibody plus increased serum immunoglobulin and either reduced absolute lymphocyte count, depressed CD4 lymphocyte count, decreased CD4:CD8 ratio in children less than 15 months of age; the presence of HIV serum antigen, positive culture for HIV, or another highly specific test for HIV). Conversely,

---

Table 36-1
CDC Case Definition for AIDS in Children

Child Must Have Had
1. Reliably diagnosed disease at least moderately indicative of underlying cellular immunodeficiency, and
2. No known cause of underlying cellular immunodeficiency or other reduced resistance reported to be associated with that disease.

Specific Conditions That Must be Excluded Are
1. Primary immunodeficiency diseases including severe combined immunodeficiency, DiGeorge syndrome, Wiskott–Aldrich syndrome, ataxia-telangiectasia, graft-versus-host disease, neutropenia, neutrophil function abnormality, agammaglobulinemia, and hypogammaglobulinemia with raised IgM
2. Secondary immunodeficiency associated with immunosuppressive therapy, lymphoreticular malignancy, or starvation, and
3. Congenital infections such as toxoplasmosis or herpes simplex virus infection in the first month after birth or cytomegalovirus infection in the first 6 months after birth.

Diseases Accepted as Sufficiently Indicative of Underlying Cellular Immunodeficiency (Same as Those Used in Defining AIDS in Adults) Are
Pneumocystis carinii pneumonia; chronic cryptosporidiosis; disseminated toxoplasmosis; extraintestinal strongyloidiasis; chronic isosporiasis; candidiasis (esophageal, bronchial, or pulmonary); extrapulmonary cryptococcosis; disseminated histoplasmosis; noncutaneous, extrapulmonary, or disseminated atypical mycobacterial infection; cytomegalovirus infection; chronic mucocutaneous or disseminated herpes simplex virus infection; extrapulmonary or disseminated coccidioidomycosis; nocardiosis; progressive multifocal leukoencephalopathy; Kaposi's sarcoma; B-cell non-Hodgkin's lymphoma; or primary lymphoma of the brain.

A histologically confirmed diagnosis of chronic lymphoid interstitial pneumonitis is indicative of AIDS unless tests for HIV are negative.

---

laboratory evidence can be negative or inconclusive. Within each laboratory category, patients can be scored as having AIDS if certain indicator diseases (*e.g.,* opportunistic infections, recurrent bacterial infections, Kaposi's sarcoma, lymphoid interstitial pneumonia, progressive multifocal leukoencephalopathy, HIV encephalopathy, lymphoma of the brain and certain other non-Hodgkin's lymphomas, HIV wasting syndrome) are present. Unlike previous CDC case definitions, a presumptive diagnosis of indicator diseases may be acceptable.

In the revised surveillance system, the definition of AIDS in children differs from that in adults in the following ways. First, multiple or recurrent bacterial infections or lymphoid interstitial pneumonitis are indicative of AIDS with HIV-seropositive children older than 15 months of age. Second, for children younger than 15 months of age whose mothers are seropositive, the laboratory criteria for AIDS must also include elevated immunoglobulin and either a low lymphocyte count, a low CD4 count, or a decreased CD4:CD8 ratio.

The spectrum of HIV infection ranges from asymptomatic seropositivity to critical illness. A variety of signs and symptoms have been used to describe children who have not had opportunistic infections or documented lymphoid interstitial pneumonitis under the heading of AIDS-related complex (ARC) (Table 36-2).[17] The terminology may be abandoned as newer case definitions are employed. The CDC also recently developed a classification schema for HIV infection in children (Table 36-3).[18]

EPIDEMIOLOGY

Evidence that HIV is the etiologic agent of AIDS and ARC includes data linking the presence of antibody or the recovery of HIV from blood with an AIDS-related illness.[3,5–7,19,20] Be-

cause HIV infection in infants and children is a recent occurrence in the United States, detailed epidemiologic data are lacking, and a detailed understanding of the natural history of HIV-related disease is still evolving.[21]

In adults, the principal routes for HIV infection are close sexual contact, particularly homosexual contact; the sharing of contaminated needles by intravenous drug abusers; and the receipt of infected blood or blood products.[22–25] HIV infection in children also has been associated with blood transfusion, this route of transmission accounting for approximately 13% of AIDS in the pediatric population.[26–34] Another 5% of childhood AIDS patients have acquired HIV from treatment for severe hemophilia A with Factor VIII concentrate.[23] A few pediatric cases have been associated with sexual abuse.[14,35]

Transplacental and Perinatal Transmission

Approximately 80% of children with AIDS have a parent with established ARC or AIDS or one who is at increased risk of acquiring HIV infection.[36] In infants and children with putative transplacental transmission of HIV, mothers generally have had a history of intravenous drug abuse or prostitution or multiple sex partners; have had sex with a partner who had homosexual encounters or who was HIV positive (*e.g.,* hemophiliac); have originated from a geographic region where heterosexual transmission is thought to play a significant role in transmission (*e.g.,* Haiti, central Africa); or have themselves become infected by blood transfusion.[11,16,17,36–47] Although women who have transmitted HIV transplacentally are usually seropositive or culture positive, they can be asymptomatic.[42]

The incidence of *in utero* transmission from seropositive or culture-positive mothers has not yet been defined but appears to be in the range of 50% to 65%.[14,40,42,48–50] HIV has been

Table 36-2
Clinical and Laboratory Findings in ARC

Clinical
Oral candidiasis
Failure to thrive
Hepatosplenomegaly
Lymphadenopathy
Diarrhea
Bacterial infections
Encephalopathy
Microcephaly, neurologic abnormalities
Cardiomyopathy
Eczematoid rash
Salivary gland enlargement

Laboratory
Increased immunoglobulins
Decreased CD4:CD8 ratio, increased CD4 and CD8 lymphocytes
Decreased lymphocyte response to mitogens or antigens
Impaired antibody synthesis after immunization
Anemia, leukopenia, thrombocytopenia
Increased circulating immune complexes
Increased transaminases
Cutaneous anergy
Decreased thymulin
Antibody to HIV

Table 36-3
Classification System for HIV Infection in Children Younger Than 13 Years of Age

P-0[2] *   **Indeterminate infection** in perinatally exposed children younger than 15 months of age who have antibody to HIV

P-1   **Asymptomatic infection**
    A[†] Normal immune function
    B   Abnormal immune function
    C   Immune function not tested

P-2   **Symptomatic infection**
    A Nonspecific findings
    B Progressive neurologic disease
    C Lymphoid interstitial pneumonitis
    D Secondary infectious diseases
        D-1[‡] Those listed in CDC definition of AIDS
        D-2   Recurrent serious bacterial infections
        D-3   Others (oral candidiasis, recurrent herpes stomatitis, multidermatomal or disseminated herpes zoster)
    E Secondary cancers
        E-1 Those listed in CDC definition of AIDS
        E-2 Others
    F Other diseases possibly due to HIV infection (hepatitis, cardiomyopathy, nephropathy, anemia, thrombocytopenia, dermatologic disease)

* Class.
† Subclass.
‡ Category.

---

isolated from the tissues of 14- to 20-week fetuses as well as from cord blood.[48,51,52] Of interest, monozygotic twins in whom only one twin was infected have been described.[14,17,48,53] It currently appears that the incubation period may be shorter in infants who have acquired infection transplacentally than in children who have transfusion-related AIDS, but this may change over time.[22,54]

Perinatal infection of the newborn via breast milk from an HIV-infected mother, although rare to date, can occur. HIV has been cultured from cell-free breast milk, and infection has been reported in a breastfed child who had been born by cesarean section to a woman given contaminated blood postpartum.[55,56]

The question of whether perinatal infection can occur at birth and whether it is more likely with vaginal than with cesarean delivery has been raised. There are well-documented cases of infected children born by cesarean section, and there are no data to support the contention that vaginal delivery increases the risk of transmission to an infant.[36,55-57,57a]

Infants may be more susceptible to HIV infection than adults, at least when the exposure is from contaminated blood products. In a study of transfusion-related AIDS, infants accounted for 10% of such AIDS cases even though they had received less than 2% of the blood transfusions.[24] In addition, the interval between transfusion and the diagnosis of AIDS appears to be shorter in children (mean 21 and median 14 months) than in adults (mean 32 and median 30 months). The interval until symptoms become evident also is shorter for the infants (a mean of 15 and a median of 8 months compared with a mean of 27 and a median of 26 months in adults).

Blood Product Transmission

The first cases of AIDS in hemophiliacs receiving HIV-contaminated factor replacement were reported in 1981. Since then, surveillance studies from a number of medical centers indicate that 34% to 74% of hemophiliacs are HIV seropositive.[58-66] The incidence of seropositivity is related to the number of units of factor VIII received. Patients receiving less than 400 U/kg per year have a 34% frequency of seroconversion compared with 93% of those receiving more than 1000 U/kg per year.[67] The introduction of heat-inactivated donor-screened factor concentrates has now eliminated this route of transmission for hemophiliacs. Nonetheless, a large number of hemophiliacs are now HIV seropositive, and it is unclear how many of these individuals will progress to symptomatic AIDS. Many of these individuals have lymphadenopathy, increased immunoglobulin, decreased CD4 cells, and low CD4:CD8 ratios. Although some of these findings may be a consequence of factor replacement *per se* (since they have also been observed in HIV-negative hemophiliacs who have received heat-inactivated factor VIII), they may be a harbinger of eventual illness.[59] To date, the incidence of symptomatic HIV infection in seropositive hemophiliacs has remained lower than expected (*i.e.,* approximately 1%); however, anecdotal reports suggest that this pattern may be changing, and that a higher rate of illness in seropositive individuals might be anticipated in the immediate future.

Transfusion-related AIDS has also been associated with red-blood cell, platelet, and leukocyte transfusions. Although routine testing has made the blood supply safe in the United States since the spring of 1985, children given transfusions before that time are still at risk. Pediatric cancer patients often fall within this risk category, and a number of such cases have been identified. Detailed prevalence data are unavailable, however, and the length of the incubation period remains uncertain.[68-70,70a]

GENETICS

The expression of HIV infection may be influenced by genetic traits and other cofactors. Although preliminary, recent studies suggest that HIV induces cytotoxic lymphocytes that recognize and kill HIV-infected cells and that may be restricted by class I HLA (transplantation) antigens.[71,72] These observations may help to clarify why certain individuals infected with HIV have AIDS whereas others appear to remain stable. Environmental factors and infections with other agents such as cytomegalovirus (CMV) or Epstein–Barr virus (EBV) may serve as epigenetic (see Chap. 2) cofactors.[72a]

Transplacental transmission represents an acquired congenital infection. Because congenital infections with a variety of microorganisms (*e.g.,* rubella, cytomegalovirus, *Treponema pallidum, Toxoplasma gondii*) have been associated with congenital malformations, it is notable that a dysmorphic syndrome has been reported among 20 children with AIDS or ARC who were born to intravenous drug-abusing mothers.[73,74] Growth failure was observed in 75%, microcephaly in 70%, ocular hypertelorism in 50%, prominent boxlike forehead in 75%, flat nasal bridge in 70%, mild obliquity of the eyes in 65%, long palpebral fissures with blue sclerae in 60%, short nose with flattened columella in 75%, well-formed triangular philtrum in 75%, and prominent upper vermilion border in 60%. Although these data are provocative, it must be noted that not all investigators have observed this dysmorphism.[74a,74b] It is important that control groups consisting of siblings of affected patients, children with postnatal infection, and children with the same racial and socioeconomic background be examined.

BIOLOGY

Virology

The etiologic agent of AIDS is the retrovirus now referred to as HIV, previously denoted human T-cell lymphotrophic virus type III (HTLV-III), lymphadenopathy-associated virus (LAV), or the AIDS-related virus (ARV).[3–7,75] Like other retroviruses, HIV has RNA as its genetic material and utilizes the enzyme reverse transcriptase to assemble DNA from its RNA template. HIV is related to the lentiviruses, a group of nontransforming cytopathic retroviruses that includes visna virus, caprine arthritis encephalitis virus, and the equine infectious anemia virus.[76–78] HIV appears to be closely related to the simian T-cell lymphotropic virus (STLV-III), which causes a disease similar to AIDS in subhuman primates. Recently, another lymphotropic retrovirus, HIV-2 (also called LAV-2 or HTLV-4), has been isolated in West Africa from patients with an immunodeficiency syndrome similar to AIDS.[79–84]

Like other retroviruses, HIV includes the *gag, pol,* and *env* genes, which encode for the core protein, reverse transcriptase, and envelope, respectively. In addition, the HIV genome includes the *tat* and *trs/art* genes, both of which appear to serve as post-transcriptional or translational regulators of HIV synthesis.[85,86] Two other genes, *3orf* and *sor,* also distinguish HIV from other retroviruses. The function of these genes and their products is not yet known.

HIV infects both the CD4$^+$ (CD4 helper–inducer) lymphocyte and the monocyte. Infection begins with the attachment and binding of the HIV envelope glycoprotein to the CD4 molecule (the probable receptor for HIV) on the CD4$^+$ lymphocyte. After fusion with the cell membrane, the virus penetrates into the cell and is uncoated in the cytoplasm (Fig. 36-1). The viral RNA is then transcribed into DNA by the viral-

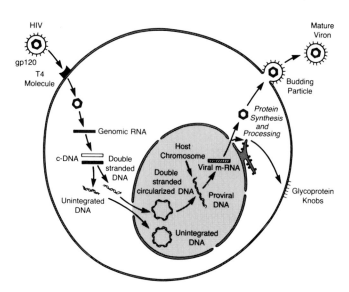

FIGURE 36-1. Entry, uncoating, integration into a proviral form, activation and budding of HIV from a CD4 lymphocyte. (Ho D, Pomerantz RJ, Kaplan JC: Pathogenesis of infection with human immunodeficiency virus. N Engl J Med 317:278–286, 1987)

encoded reverse transcriptase. Next, some of the DNA is circularized and transported to the nucleus, where it is integrated with the host's DNA during a cell division. The majority of the DNA remains unintegrated in the cytoplasm. When the infected cell is activated, the proviral HIV DNA is transcribed to messenger RNA and then translated to viral proteins. Some of these proteins are cleaved and glycosylated, and genomic RNA and viral proteins are synthesized. The proteins are transported through the endoplasmic reticulum and Golgi apparatus, with subsequent viral assembly and then release by budding through the plasma membrane.

HIV replication is cytopathic to the CD4$^+$ cell, and the depletion of these helper–inducer cells is central to the pathophysiology of AIDS, presumably because of the integral role these cells play in cellular immunity. Cofactors such as the cytomegalovirus may contribute to enhanced destruction of the CD4$^+$ cells.

In addition to CD4$^+$ cells, HIV can also infect monocytes and macrophages that express the CD4 antigen. These cells are less susceptible to HIV cytotoxicity and may thus serve as a reservoir of persistent infection. Infections of the monocyte/macrophage can be associated with the disease process by altering the pulmonary macrophages (potentially contributing to infections with *Pneumocystis carinii* or the syndrome of lymphocytic interstitial pneumonitis) or by serving as a transport vehicle for carrying HIV to the central nervous system, an important target organ in children with HIV infections.

Immunology

As noted, depletion of the CD4$^+$ helper–induced cell is a central component of AIDS, particularly in adults. Although this is also true in children, abnormalities of the immune response can be demonstrated that differ from those described in adults.[17,87] For example, infants are less frequently lymphopenic and can have normal lymphocyte mitogenic and antigenic responses and normal distribution of T-cell subsets even when suffering fatal bacterial and opportunistic infections.[17,28,38,48,88–92]

Abnormal humoral immunity, on the other hand, is present in most HIV-infected children and appears to antedate T-cell abnormalities.[14,92,93] Elevated serum immunoglobulin, especially IgG but also IgD, IgA, or IgM, is the most notable laboratory manifestation of abnormal B-cell function, but hypogammaglobulinemia or deficiencies of IgG subclasses (IgG, IgG3, IgG4) have also been described in HIV-infected children, particularly late in the course of illness.[17,26-28,37,38,87,94-98] B-cell numbers can be elevated, and increased numbers of cells that spontaneously secrete immunoglobulin have been noted along with decreased immunoglobulin secretion following stimulation.[26,38,92] Circulating immune complexes have been described.[28,31,37,56,95,96] Other abnormalities include reduced *in vitro* lymphocyte proliferative responses to pokeweed mitogen and *Staphylococcus* Cowan A strain; a poor primary antibody response to new antigens or diminished secondary responses after immunization with diphtheria or tetanus toxoid or pneumococcal polysaccharide vaccine; and deficiencies in isoagglutinins.[11,14,56,87-89,92,94-99]

Cell-mediated immunity, on the other hand, appears less compromised in the early stages of childhood HIV infection.[14] A reversal of the ratio of CD4$^+$ (helper–inducer) to CD8$^+$ (suppressor–cytotoxic) cells is common, reflecting a decrease in the numbers and percentages of CD4$^+$ cells and an increase in CD8$^+$ cells.[17,26,37,38,88,94,98,100] However, some pediatric patients have normal or increased helper:suppressor ratios.[87] Other abnormalities of cell-mediated immunity include diminished lymphocyte mitogenic response to phytohemagglutinin and concanavalin A and to specific antigens, but these can be normal in infected infants.[37,38,48,95,99] Cutaneous anergy has also been observed, as well as defective suppressor T-cell function, an increase in circulating thymosin α1, low circulating thymulin activity, decreased alpha and gamma interferon production, and deficient natural killer-cell activity.[17,19,37,56,87,98-101]

PATHOLOGY

Although data are limited, characteristic abnormalities have been described in children dying from HIV infection.[102-105] The thymus can be small, with lymphocyte depletion and decreased numbers of Hassall's corpuscles, a mononuclear or plasma cell infiltrate obscuring the corticomedullary junction, and calcification or microcystic changes of Hassall's corpuscles.[98,105] Abnormalities in thymic epithelium have been described, including abnormal architecture with necrosis, areas of thymulin-negative cells, a decrease in some differentiation antigens, and the presence of immunoglobulin and complement.[106]

Lymph node biopsy can reveal follicular hyperplasia, with or without lymphocyte depletion of the paracortical zone, atrophy of follicles with absence of germinal centers, and lymphocyte depletion of the paracortical zone.[48,102] Giant cells have also been described in lymph nodes from HIV-infected children.[102] Prominent lymphoid infiltrates have been seen in other organs, including the spleen, kidneys, intestine, liver, adrenals, and skeletal muscle.[104,107-109] These lymphocytes can be polyclonal B cells, and, in some cases, lymphocytes have been seen invading blood vessels in a lympoproliferative pattern.[104]

Persistent salivary gland enlargement is seen in about 20% of the pediatric cases, often in association with pulmonary interstitial infiltrates.[48,89,107] Affected children can have serologic evidence of Epstein–Barr virus (EBV) infection, and the EBV genome has been found in salivary gland tissue.[109] Lymphocytic infiltrates have been seen on biopsy of affected glands.[48]

CLINICAL MANIFESTATIONS

To date, most cases of pediatric AIDS have been geographically restricted, occurring primarily in New York, New Jersey, Florida, and California, predominantly in blacks or Hispanics and often with a drug-abusing parent.[11,21,39,110-112] Because these very populations are generally prone to high-risk pregnancies, the features seen in these children may not apply to all HIV-infected infants.

The incubation period in children has been variable, ranging from approximately 4 to 6 months in congenitally infected infants to longer than 5 years in some transfusion-infected children.[26,32,39,48,88,113] There is, however, likely to be variation from this mean as experience and natural history data continue to accrue.[113a,113b] Most cases of pediatric HIV infection occur in young children, with 50% of pediatric AIDS diagnosed during the first year of life and 82% by 3 years of age.[11,21] Opportunistic infections have been reported in infants less than 1 month of age.[48]

In infants and young children, the characteristic feature of HIV infection include low birth weight or failure to thrive, generalized lymphadenopathy, hepatomegaly, splenomegaly, chronic or recurrent diarrhea, mucocutaneous candidiasis, fevers, interstitial pneumonitis, parotitis, digital clubbing, chronic eczematoid dermatitis, recurrent bacterial and viral infections, opportunistic infections, and neurologic abnormalities.[14,17,26,28,37,38,89,90,114,115] Lymphocytic interstitial pneumonitis, parotitis, and bacterial infections are more typical of HIV infection in children than in adults.

Infectious Complications

The pattern of infection reflects the B- and T-cell alterations observed in HIV-infected children. Moreover, children are less likely than adults to develop infection with latent organisms, such as toxoplasma. *Pneumocystis carinii,* on the other hand, is a common opportunistic pathogen in children and has been described in 52% of the cases reported to the CDC.[8] HIV-infected children also have a high incidence of chronic EBV infection characterized by persistent high-titer antibodies to viral capsid antigen and the early antigen and an abnormal antibody response to nuclear antigen.[37,116,117] Chronic ulcerative infections with the varicella–zoster virus have also been noted.

Recurrent bacterial infections are more common in children with AIDS or ARC than in HIV-infected adults and include sepsis, meningitis, pneumonia, cellulitis and skin abscesses, urinary tract infections, and chronic otitis media.[13,17,28,48,91,94] The most common infecting organisms are *Streptococcus pneumoniae, Haemophilus influenzae,* and *Salmonella.* Children with AIDS who have been hospitalized are also subject to a broad range of nosocomial pathogens, including group D streptococci, *Escherichia coli, Enterobacter, Citrobacter,* and *Pseudomonas.* It is also important to recognize that there are no differences in the patterns of infection that occur in children with AIDS versus those with ARC. This underscores the fact that terms such as AIDS and ARC may be semantic when applied to pediatric patients.

Noninfectious Complications

Encephalopathy

A characteristic encephalopathy that can progress to dementia has been seen in many, possibly the majority of, children with HIV-related disease.[17,48,89,118-122,122a,122b] Involvement of the central nervous system is probably a consequence of the entry of HIV-infected monocytes. Disease manifestations may reflect damage to neural cells by monokines or proteolytic enzymes. Alternatively, encephalopathic and neurologic abnormalities can be the result of blockade of neuroleukin receptors by the gp120 envelope glycoprotein of HIV or of damage to infected astrocytes or microglial cells.[85]

Affected patients may present with either developmental delay or a loss of motor milestones or intellectual abilities; infants may have acquired microcephaly.[118,119,122,123,123a] Most children with encephalopathy have concomitant focal abnormalities, including pyramidal tract signs, paresis, ataxia, pseudobulbar palsy, or rigidity.[118–121] Seizures may occur but are not a prominent feature.[118,123] Of interest, severe encephalopathy has been noted in a seronegative infant in whom HIV cultures were subsequently positive, thus compounding the diagnostic difficulties that may be faced in children.[124] Computed tomographic scans of symptomatic children show cerebral atrophy and ventricular enlargement, often with calcification of the basal ganglia or areas of calcification or attenuation of white matter.[118–123] Cerebrospinal fluid is usually normal but may show a mild pleocytosis or protein elevation.[118–120]

Pathologic examination of brain tissues from children with encephalopathy has shown cerebral atrophy with inflammatory-cell infiltration, multinucleated cells, microglial nodules, calcification of vessels (most prominent in basal ganglia), and white matter changes.[118–125,125a] Cortical gray matter is largely spared, and neuronal loss is rare. HIV viral particles, DNA sequences and RNA, and HIV antigen have been demonstrated in brain tissue and cerebrospinal fluid.[118,122,126–128] These data underscore the fact that the brain is an important target organ during HIV infection and is both the site of active disease and a potential sanctuary for latent virus.

Pulmonary Disease

A chronic interstitial pulmonic process has been described in children with HIV infection that is generally referred to as lymphoid interstitial pneumonitis or pulmonary lymphoid hyperplasia.[14,48,102–104] This entity is distinctly uncommon in adults with AIDS. The pneumonitis has a chronic progressive course that can result in dyspnea and hypoxia.[107] The pulmonary picture must be differentiated from infection, although the only way to establish the diagnosis definitively is by histologic examination. Certain clinical features (*e.g.,* generalized lymphadenopathy, salivary gland enlargement, and digital clubbing) are more closely associated with interstitial pneumonitis than with interstitial pneumonia caused by *Pneumocystis carinii,* and children with pneumonitis are less likely to be febrile or to have abnormal auscultory findings and more likely to have hypergammaglobulinemia and lower lactate dehydrogenase (LDH) levels than children with *Pneumocystis* pneumonia.[107]

Histologic examination of the lungs of patients with lymphoid interstitial pneumonitis reveals peribronchiolar or parenchymal mononuclear cells forming nodules that may have germinal centers (*i.e.,* pulmonary lymphoid hyperplasia) or a diffuse interstitial and peribronchial infiltration with lymphocytes and plasma cells.[102–107] Immunoperoxidase staining for kappa and lambda light chains shows the lymphocytic infiltrates to be polyclonal.[103,109] Some children have persistently elevated antibodies to EBV, an abnormal response to EBV nuclear antigen, or the presence of EBV DNA in lung tissues, suggesting to some investigators that this virus may be etiologically linked to this pulmonary process.[48,107,109,116,129] Alternatively, HIV RNA has been identified in lung tissue from children with lymphoid interstitial pneumonitis, raising the possibility that the lung may be another target of HIV infection.[130,130a]

Cardiac Abnormalities

Congestive heart failure has been described in children perinatally infected with HIV and has included both left-sided and right-sided abnormalities.[131] Echocardiographic abnormalities have been described, including left ventricular dysfunction in 45% to 74% of the affected patients and pericardial effusion in 18% to 22%. Periodic screening with echocardiograms has been recommended, although the value of such surveillance is unknown. Whether these cardiac abnormalities are related to direct HIV damage is uncertain.

Immunohematologic Abnormalities

Children with HIV infection can present with an immune thrombocytopenia and bleeding.[17,28,48,88,132] Coombs'-positive anemias and immune leukopenias have also been described and may be related to abnormal humoral immunity.[17,20,54,133]

Less Common Abnormalities

Other laboratory abnormalities include anemia, abnormal liver function tests, and an elevation in LDH.[28,38,134,135] In four children with AIDS or ARC who had hepatomegaly and abnormal serum transaminase levels, histologic examination of the liver revealed both lobular and portal changes with evidence of hepatocellular and bile duct damage, sinusoidal cell hyperplasia, and T_8 lymphocyte infiltration as well as changes consistent with chronic active hepatitis.[135] Nodular lymphoid aggregates in portal triads have been described.[102,104] In adults, a nephropathy with proteinuria and azotemia is associated with AIDS; this has been observed in advanced HIV infections in children.[136,136a]

Malignancies Associated with HIV Infection in Children

Although Kaposi's sarcoma is a common manifestation of AIDS in homosexual men, it accounts for only 1% of the pediatric AIDS cases reported to the CDC.[8] In children, the lymphadenopathic form of Kaposi's sarcoma has been described.[137] Lymphomas considered to be associated with HIV infection have been described in children but are not common.[28,48,116,117]

METHODS OF DIAGNOSIS

The primary method of serodiagnosis is the enzyme-linked immunosorbent assay (ELISA). In adults, the sensitivity of the ELISA is between 93.4% and 99.6%, with a specificity of 99.2% to 99.8%.[138,139] Because false-positive results occur, a positive ELISA test should be repeated and confirmed by Western blot (see Chap. 3) or immunofluorescence assay, especially in low-prevalence populations. Although virus culture is generally less sensitive than serologic testing, HIV has been cultured from seronegative individuals, including asymptomatic children.[17,124,140] This test is particularly important during the period that follows infection but precedes the production of antibody. The time to seroconversion after infection is not precisely known but is estimated to be 1 to 3 months in adults.[141–145] Children may also be HIV seronegative if they have a congenital or acquired defect in antibody production. In addition, HIV-infected children with hypogammaglobulinemia and children who have become seronegative when terminally ill have been described.[14,17,48,95]

A significant diagnostic problem arises in the neonatal or young infant because of the passive transfer of maternal antibody. IgM antibody cannot be used to differentiate maternal from infant infection.[14,17,18,87,146,146a,146b,146c-148] Antibody to HIV has been found in the cord blood of babies born to HIV-seropositive mothers, and antibody that is presumed to be of maternal origin can persist for more than 6 months.[14] Thus, seropositivity in infants cannot be used to prove HIV infection, although it certainly can identify an infant at risk. Gammaglobulin administration can also be a source of passively acquired antibody to HIV and false-positive serology.[148]

At present, the prognostic significance of seropositivity and the numbers of seropositive children who will develop clinical disease are not known. However, there is no indication that a seropositive immune and noninfectious state exists. Antibody does not appear to be protective but rather serves as a marker for the presence of infectious virus; the duration of infection is not known, but infection appears persistent.[149] The utility of examining children for neutralizing antibody to HIV also is unknown.[150,151]

Ultimately, the diagnosis of HIV-related disease in children rests on several factors: a presentation with a suggestive clinical picture, especially interstitial lung disease, recurrent bacterial infections, thrush, or failure to thrive; a characteristic immunologic picture manifested as a polyclonal hypergammaglobulinemia and T-cell immunodeficiency; the demonstration of epidemiologic risk, especially with an HIV-seropositive, P24 antigen-positive or culture-positive mother or one who has T-cell immune abnormalities; the absence of an established primary or secondary immunodeficiency; and either the presence of antibody to HIV or HIV isolation.[18,88,93,152] The diagnosis of HIV infection in children younger than 15 months, and especially younger than 6 months, of age can be difficult, however, because antibody status may not be meaningful at this age, and characteristic immune abnormalities may not yet have developed. In addition, primary congenital immunodeficiency diseases (*e.g.,* adenosine deaminase deficiency, purine nucleotide phosphorylase deficiency) always must be ruled out.

PROGNOSTIC CONSIDERATIONS AND VARIABLES

Because prevalence studies have not yet been performed in children, the number of asymptomatic seropositive or culture-positive children is unknown. Moreover, the number of infected asymptomatic children who will progress to symptomatic disease and the number of ARC patients who will develop opportunistic infections or malignancies are unknown. It appears that opportunistic infections occur later in the course of HIV-infected children than of HIV-infected adults, but the mortality rate in children with AIDS or ARC is high.[93]

Prognosis has been correlated in one study with the presence or absence of normal antigen-induced lymphocyte proliferation. Patients with abnormal proliferative responses also had anergy to several antigens as well as poorer antibody responses and the absence or disappearance of antibodies to HIV core proteins. Although the numbers of patients were small, patients with normal proliferative responses were all alive and stable, whereas patients with abnormal proliferative responses were more likely to have had opportunistic infections and failure to thrive, and all were either dead or seriously ill. There were also more cases of lymphoid interstitial pneumonitis (diagnosed clinically and by bronchoalveolar lavage) in the group with the better prognosis.

In a life table analysis of 64 children with AIDS reported to the New York City Department of Health,[153] 59 of whom were presumed vertically infected, two distinct courses were distinguished: [1] children with a history of *Pneumocystis* pneumonia, in whom the onset of symptoms occurred at a mean age of 5.5 months (range, birth to 29 months) and in whom pneumonia was diagnosed at a mean of 11 months (range 2–53 months); and [2] children with other opportunistic infections whose mean age at the onset of symptoms was 14.3 months (range 1–60 months) with opportunistic infection presenting at a median of 31.4 months (range 3–77 months). The children with *Pneumocystis* pneumonia had a median survival time of 9 to 12 months after birth, whereas children without this infection had a median survival time of 31.5 months. The survival after opportunistic infection was similar for both: median of less than 3 months with 75% dead within 1 year.

Children with an opportunistic infection in the first year of life rarely survive beyond the second year, and the number of congenitally infected children who are asymptomatic for longer than 3 years is small.[14,48,153] Children with lymphoid interstitial pneumonitis may have a better prognosis, with survival to school age reported.[14,48,107] On the other hand, children with progressive encephalopathy appear to have a poor prognosis.[118] Although follow-up has not been long enough to obtain a true estimate of the mortality rate, more than 61% of reported children with AIDS are known to have died.[8]

TREATMENT AND MANAGEMENT CONSIDERATIONS

General Supportive Care

Hospital Care

Children with HIV infection encounter many of the same problems as children with cancer, including repeated infections, nutritional deficiencies, fatigue, and the need for repeated hospitalizations. During hospitalization, children with AIDS, like those with cancer, require comprehensive medical and psychosocial support and a respect for confidentiality. There are, however, unique aspects to the care of children with HIV infection. For example, medical personnel bring their own feelings, values, fears, and beliefs into the patient relationship and may experience internal conflicts when faced with differing sexual and social behavior in the child's family. Concerns about the transmission of HIV to other patients or to the medical staff may also be present. In any event, caring for a child with a fatal illness for which current interventions are limited produces stress and feelings of helplessness, frustration, anger, sadness, and loss for medical care personnel.

Because a serious concern of medical staff and patients centers on the transmission of HIV, continuing multidisciplinary education is critical. Among the information that should be included in educational programs are blood and body fluid precautions, cleaning procedures for blood and body fluid spills, and current information about the risk of transmission. The risk to health care workers of contracting HIV infection in the workplace appears small.[154,155,155a] In a prospective surveillance of 938 health care workers who had a documented parenteral or mucous membrane exposure to blood and body fluids of AIDS or ARC patients, two possibly occupationally acquired seropositives and no established illness were noted after a mean follow-up of 15 months.[154] Nearly half of these exposures might have been prevented if recommendations for the protection of medical personnel had been strictly observed.[156-159] Nonetheless, because occupationally acquired cases have been reported after accidental needlestick or, very rarely, after mucocutaneous blood contamination, continued vigilance and surveillance are mandatory.[155,160,161] In particular, all hospital personnel should be informed about and urged to utilize the CDCs recommendations for "universal precautions" that include blood and body fluid precautions in the handling of needles and other sharp instruments from all patients, including those in whom HIV status is known, as well as patients who have not been tested (Table 36-4).

Care at Home

In the home environment, many of the same concerns about infection, nutrition, rehabilitation, and transmissibility arise. A thorough assessment of the home and the parents' ability to care for the affected child, especially if the parent(s) are also infected, is necessary. Current studies of families and household contacts of infected patients have not demonstrated horizontal transmission of HIV.[34,114-116] Nonetheless, failure to observe caution might result in infection. For example, a seronegative mother who cared for her transfusion-infected infant became seropositive after heavy exposure to blood, secretions, and excreta without the use of gloves and adequate handwashing.[162] Although the risk for infection by inoculation through skin or mucosal surfaces is extremely small, the possibility does exist and underscores the need for continued education and scrupulous care. Although HIV is present in very small quantities in tears and saliva, transmission by means of these body fluids has not been observed.[163,164]

Families need counseling for dealing with the stress that AIDS produces, particularly that due to social stigmatization

---

Table 36-4
Recommendations for Preventing Transmission of HIV in the Workplace

1. Sharp items (*e.g.,* needles, scalpel blades) should be considered potentially infective and handled with extreme care to prevent accidental injuries.
2. Disposable syringes and needles, scalpel blades, and other sharp items should be placed into puncture-resistant containers located as close as practical to the area in which they were used. To prevent needlestick injuries, needles should not be recapped, purposefully bent, broken, removed from disposable syringes, or otherwise manipulated by hand.
3. When the possibility of exposure to blood or other body fluids exists, routinely recommended precautions should be followed. The anticipated exposure may require gloves alone, as in handling items soiled with blood or equipment contaminated with blood or other body fluids, or may also require gowns, masks, and eye coverings when performing procedures involving more extensive contact with blood or potentially infective body fluids, as in some dental or endoscopic procedures or postmortem examinations. Hands should be washed thoroughly and immediately if they accidentally become contaminated with blood.
4. To minimize the need for emergency mouth-to-mouth resuscitation, mouth pieces, resuscitation bags, or other ventilation devices should be strategically located and available for use in areas where the need for resuscitation is predictable.
5. Pregnant health care workers are not known to be at greater risk of contracting HIV infections than those who are not pregnant; however, if a health care worker develops HIV infection during pregnancy, the infant is at increased risk of infection resulting from perinatal transmission. Because of this risk, pregnant health care workers should be especially familiar with precautions for preventing HIV transmission.

---

and financial needs. Families may also need assistance with such ancillary issues as day care, foster care, or school arrangements. The impact on other family members of living with and caring for an HIV-infected child may need to be dealt with.

Care in the Community

Concerns of the community generally revolve around the availability and utilization of resources for health care and financial support, transmissibility (especially in day care centers and schools), and education. Health guidelines on school attendance suggest that decisions be made on a case-by-case basis with a view to both the potential risk that the infected child poses and the risk to the child of contracting infections at school. Among the issues to be considered are the child's socialization skills, including the ability to control body secretions and biting behavior, and the presence of oozing skin lesions or transmissable diseases (*e.g.,* varicella–zoster). Clearly, all child care personnel and educators, regardless of the setting, should follow accepted guidelines for the handling of blood and body fluids, including the wearing of disposable gloves and the use of disposable towels and tissues and a dilute bleach solution for disinfection. Although the data are limited, they suggest that live vaccines should be avoided in children with symptomatic HIV infection.

Care in School

Current data suggest that, with rare exceptions, children with HIV infection should be allowed to attend school in an unrestricted manner. As with cancer patients receiving chemotherapy, exposure to infections such as varicella–zoster should be avoided, and parents or health providers should be notified of any such exposure (see also Chap. 39). Schools should adopt routine procedures for handling blood and body fluids as noted above. However, a student's records should be confidential and privacy maintained. School attendance for children with HIV disease is supported by Public Law 94-142 (see Chap. 51) because AIDS has been recognized as a handicap.

In addition to providing education to children with HIV infection, schools have a role in educating all students and school personnel about HIV infection and the known routes of transmission. Indeed, the school should serve as a reliable source of information about AIDS to children and teenagers, including education about drug abuse and safe sex practices.[168]

Antiretroviral Therapy

Targets for antiviral therapy are based on the life cycle of HIV (see also Fig. 36-1). Indeed, each stage of viral replication, processing, and assembly serves as a potential target for antiretroviral therapy (Table 36-5). The desirable properties of antiretroviral agents include efficacy, penetration into sanctuary sites (particularly the central nervous system), ease of administration (especially since long courses of therapy are likely to be necessary), and tolerable toxicity. In many ways, these properties are similar to those of effective anticancer agents.

Evaluation of potential antiretroviral agents should be comprehensive and include clinical, immunologic, and virologic assessment. Among the clinical features that should be evaluated are changes in the incidence of bacterial and opportunistic infections and improvements in central nervous system symptomatology, lymphadenopathy, fever, wasting, or hematologic abnormalities. Immunologic measures that can be monitored include the absolute number of $CD4^+$ lymphocytes, delayed cutaneous hypersensitivity reactions, quantitative immunoglobulin levels, and antigen stimulation assays, among others. Although crucial, virologic assessment is difficult at present because of technical limitations in the quantitative viral assays.

Limited antiretroviral intervention has been explored in children to date, but several agents have been tested in adults (Table 36-6). The first drug reported to have activity *in vitro* against HIV was suramin, an antiparasitic agent known since the 1920s and used for African trypanosomiasis and onchocerciasis.[166–170] Suramin had been shown in 1979 to inhibit reverse transcriptase and thus became a candidate for the therapy of AIDS. Unfortunately, clinical trials showed no benefit, and the toxicity associated with this agent has dismissed it from further study.

The most promising agent to date is 3'-azido-3' deoxythymidine (AZT) recently approved by the U.S. Food and Drug Administration and released by Burroughs-Wellcome as Retrovir for adults with AIDS who have had an opportunistic infection with *Pneumocystis carinii* or who have symptomatic ARC with low CD4+ counts. AZT is a thymidine analogue that is phosphorylated to its active triphosphate form by cellular ki-

nases and is a strong inhibitor of reverse transcriptase. When AZT triphosphate is incorporated into viral DNA by reverse transcriptase, its 3' substitution prevents further 5' to 3' phosphodiester linkages, terminating the chain. After *in vitro* studies showed that AZT inhibits HIV reverse transcriptase and prevents its cytopathic effects, a Phase I study of AZT was conducted in 23 adults with ARC or AIDS. Both intravenous and oral administration were studied, showing that the bioavailability of AZT given orally is about 60%, that there is excellent penetration into the cerebrospinal fluid, and that the half-life is approximately 1 hour, necessitating frequent dosing. The principal side effects of AZT are hematologic, primarily depression of the white blood cell count and a macrocytic anemia.[166–170] Headaches occur in half of the adults treated with AZT.

A randomized, double-blind, placebo-controlled study of AZT has been conducted in 282 HIV-infected adults with a history of *Pneumocystis* pneumonia. A number of benefits were observed in this study, primarily a significant decrease in the mortality rate in treated patients, as well as fewer opportunistic infections; improvements in performance status, weight, symptoms, and number of T helper cells; and development of positive skin tests. The differences in the mortality rates between treated and placebo groups prompted withdrawal of the placebo, and follow-up studies a year later confirm that AZT-treated patients have better survival rates than those who were treated with placebo.[171,172] As in the Phase I trials, AZT therapy was not without toxicity; side effects included nausea, insomnia, myalgias, severe headaches, and, most importantly, bone marrow toxicity with anemia or neutropenia that necessitated an alteration in dose, withdrawal of the drug, or transfusion.[173] In addition to the benefits documented in this study, AZT appears promising as treatment for the neurologic syndromes associated with AIDS in adults, with improvements seen in patients with chronic dementia or peripheral neuropathy.[174] Studies of AZT in other adult populations are in progress, as are studies of AZT in combination with other drugs.

Because of the promise shown by AZT in HIV-infected adults, Phase I trials of AZT in children with AIDS or ARC have been initiated. In studies at the National Cancer Institute, modes of administration include continuous intravenous infusion by means of a portable infusion pump and Hickman or Broviac catheter or orally in older children able to take oral medications reliably.[175] In the study evaluating continuous intravenous delivery of AZT, 21 children with symptomatic (CDC

Table 36-5
Stages in Life Cycle of HIV That Might be Targets for Antiretroviral Therapy

Stage	Potential Intervention
Binding to target cell	Antibodies to the virus or cell receptor
Early entry into target cell	Drugs that block fusion or interfere with retroviral uncoating
Transcription of RNA to DNA	Reverse transcriptase inhibitors
Integration of DNA into host genome	Drugs that inhibit gene-mediated "integrase" function
Expression of viral genes	Use of "antisense" constructs; inhibitors of *tat* or *trs/art* gene expression
Viral component production and assembly	Myristylation, glycosylation, and protease inhibition or modification
Budding of virus	Interferons

Table 36-6
Antiretroviral Agents Studied in HIV Infection

Drug	Route	Mode of Action	CSF Penetration	Side Effects
Suramin	IV	RT inhibitor	No	Fever, skin reactions, neutropenia, renal and adrenal toxicity
HPA23	IV	RT inhibitor	No	Thrombocytopenia, hepatotoxicity
Phosphonoformate	IV	RT inhibitor	Yes	Possible acute renal failure
Ribavirin	IV, PO	Guanosine analogue	Yes	Anemia
Azidothymidine (AZT)	IV, PO	Chain terminator; RT inhibitor	Yes	Megaloblastic anemia, neutropenia, headache
Dideoxycytidine (DDC)	IV	Chain terminator; RT inhibitor	Yes	Rash, peripheral neuropathy, neutropenia, thrombocytopenia
AL721	PO	Extracts cholesterol from cell membranes	Unknown	None observed
Interferon	IM	Inhibits assembly and release of virus	Poor	Fever, bone marrow suppression, flu-like symptoms

class P2) ranging in age from 14 months to 12 years, were enrolled. A notable aspect of this study was that 13 of 21 (62%) of the children entering this trial had evidence of neurodevelopmental abnormalities before beginning AZT. Dramatic improvement occurred in all 13 children. Moreover, serial IQ measurement before therapy and after 3 and 6 months of AZT showed a significant improvement ($p < .005$) in the overall IQ score, and included improvement in both verbal IQ ($p < 0.05$) and performance IQ ($p < 0.02$). Of note, 6 children without detectable evidence of encephalopathy prior to AZT also showed improvements ($p < 0.01$) in IQ scores from baseline compared to 6-month follow-up, suggesting that cognitive impairment may be among the earliest manifestations of AIDS encephalopathy in children, underscoring the need for modalities that will treat the central nervous system, even in patients who do not have neurodevelopmental deficits. Phase II pediatric studies of AZT and other antiretroviral agents are under way.

Other nucleoside analogues that act as chain terminators are also being examined *in vitro* and *in vivo*. Of these, 2'3'-dideoxycytidine (DDC) is among the most potent. *In vitro* studies of DDC showed that at low concentrations, helper–inducer T cells are completely protected from the cytopathic effect of HIV. Clinical Phase I studies in adults are being completed. The National Cancer Institute is conducting Phase I studies of DDC in children.

A number of other modalities are also being explored. HPA23 (ammonium 21-tungsto-98-antimoniate) is a competitive inhibitor of reverse transcriptase. Little clinical experience exists. Ribavirin, a guanosine analogue that may act on posttranscriptional processing, has been given to a small number of affected children both orally and parenterally.[176] The infants developed mild anemia, with no clinical improvements noted. Further trials of ribavirin in children are in progress. Phosphonoformate (Forcarnet, PFA), another inhibitor of reverse transcriptase, has been well tolerated in adults having cytomegalovirus infection. Clinical trials in adults have been initiated, but no experience in children with AIDS or ARC is available. AL721, a lipid compound composed of neutral glycerides, phosphatidylcholine, and phosphatidylethanolamine in a 7:2:1 ratio, shows *in vitro* activity against HIV. Clinical experience is sparse.

Immunologic Reconstitution

Another therapeutic approach that has been explored in AIDS is immunoreconstitution with agents such as interferons, interleukin-2 (IL-2), thymic factors, lymphocyte transfusions, isoprenosine, and bone-marrow transplantation.[177,178]

Interferon and Interleukin

Interferon has an inhibitory effect on HIV replication and has induced transient increases in immunologic function. Of interest, in patients with Kaposi's sarcoma, remissions have been seen when lesions are limited to the skin. On the other hand, even though IL-2 production is deficient in patients with AIDS and defects in CD4 function can be partially reversed *in vitro* by the addition of IL-2, clinical studies have not demonstrated beneficial effects of IL-2 in adults with AIDS.

Immunoglobulins

On the basis of the propensity of children with AIDS or ARC to develop recurrent bacterial infections with encapsulated organisms and their recognized deficits in humoral immunity, the use of prophylactic intravenous immunoglobulin has been advocated.[88,100,178,179,179a] Controlled clinical trials have not been reported, but a multi-institutional randomized study in symptomatic HIV-infected children is currently underway.

In one study, 14 AIDS or ARC patients with recurrent bacterial infections who were nonrandomly given immunoglobulin were compared with 27 untreated controls.[178] Over an average follow-up of 20 months, there were fewer febrile episodes and fewer episodes of sepsis in the treated group: 1 versus 18 cases of sepsis. Improvement was observed in all of the treated patients, whereas all but three untreated patients either deteriorated or died. Moreover, increases in CD4 lymphocytes and in lymphocyte proliferative responses and decreases in circulating immune complexes and LDH were noted in the children receiving immunoglobulin. No effect was seen on the number of lymphocytes. In a small series, four of five children treated with immunoglobulin had normalization of pokeweed mitogen-driven immunoglobin secretion.[100] A decrease in the frequency and severity of bacterial and viral infections has also been reported in children receiving intravenous immunoglobulin.

Other Measures

Corticosteroids have been used with some success for the treatment of children with progressive lymphoid interstitial pneumonitis, although controlled data are unavailable.[56,179] Importantly, increased *Pneumocystis* infections have not been observed with the use of steroids, but experience has been very limited.

Syngeneic and allogeneic bone-marrow transplantation has been attempted but with limited benefit, most likely because of the failure to control the retroviral infection. Studies evaluating pretreatment with AZT followed by syngeneic bone-marrow transplantations in identical twins are currently in progress.

FUTURE CONSIDERATIONS

Future issues involve three basic areas: earlier diagnosis, better therapy, and prevention by vaccination. Early diagnosis will allow treatment to begin before significant immunologic impairment has occurred. In children with transplacentally transmitted infection, this would mean treatment at, or even before, birth. Better therapy can be achieved by development of improved and specific antiretroviral agents that will most likely be used in combination, perhaps with adjunct immunomodulators. The development of a safe and effective anti-HIV vaccine is among the highest priorities. The heterogeneity of the envelope region of HIV is just one of the problems that must be overcome with vaccine development. Many approaches are being intensively pursued.[180,181]

Whereas the goal of stopping transmission of HIV may be met in the future by an effective vaccine, the present challenge is to limit the spread of HIV infection. This requires an intensive educational program about the epidemiology and transmission of HIV and safe sex practices. For the pediatric community, education of children and teenagers, as well as of women of childbearing age and pregnant women, is essential if the current spread of HIV is to be curtailed.[182–184]

REFERENCES

1. Barnes DM: Grim projections for AIDS epidemic. Science 232:1589–1590, 1986
2. Coffin J, Haase A, Levy JA et al: Human immunodeficiency viruses. Science 232:697, 1986

3. Gallo RC, Salahuddin SZ, Popovic M et al: Frequent detection and isolation of cytopathic retroviruses (HTLV-III) from patients with AIDS and at risk for AIDS. Science 224:500–503, 1984

4. Barre-Sinoussi F, Chermann JC, Rey F et al: Isolation of a T-lymphotropic retrovirus from a patient at risk for acquired immune deficiency syndrome (AIDS). Science 220:868–871, 1983

5. Laurence J, Brun-Vezinet F, Schutzer SE et al: Lymphadenopathy-associated viral antibody in AIDS: Immune correlations and definition of a carrier state. N Engl J Med 311:1269–1273, 1984

6. Levy JA, Hoffman AD, Kramer SM et al: Isolation of lymphocytopathic retroviruses from San Francisco patients with AIDS. Science 225:840–842, 1984

7. Broder S, Gallo RC: A pathogenic retrovirus (HTLV-III) linked to AIDS. N Engl J Med 311:1292–1297, 1984

8. Update: Acquired immunodeficiency syndrome—United States. MMWR 35:757–766, 1986

9. Provisional Public Health Service inter-agency recommendations for screening donated blood and plasma for antibody to the virus causing acquired immunodeficiency syndrome. MMWR 34:1–5, 1985

10. Survey of non-U.S. hemophilia treatment centers for HIV seroconversions following therapy with heat-treated factor concentrates. MMWR 36:121–124, 1987

11. Immunization of children infected with human T-lymphotropic virus type III/lymphadenopathy-associated virus. MMWR 35:595–606, 1986

12. Update: Acquired immunodeficiency syndrome (AIDS)—United States. MMWR 32:688–691, 1984

13. Revision of the case definition of acquired immunodeficiency syndrome for national reporting—United States. MMWR 34:373–375, 1985

14. Rubinstein A, Bernstein L: The epidemiology of pediatric acquired immunodeficiency syndrome. Clin Immunol Immunopathol 40:115–121, 1986

15. Anderson KC, Gorgone BC, Marlink RG et al: Transfusion-acquired human immunodeficiency virus infection among immunocompromised persons. Ann Intern Med 105:519–527, 1986

16. Centers for Disease Control: Revision of the CDC surveillance case definition for acquired immunodeficiency syndrome. MMWR 36(Suppl 15):1S–15S, 1987

17. Pahwa S, Kaplan M, Fikrig S et al: Spectrum of human T-cell lymphotropic virus type III infection in children: Recognition of symptomatic, asymptomatic, and seronegative patients. JAMA 255:2299–2305, 1986

18. Classification system for human immunodeficiency virus (HIV) infection in children under 13 years of age. MMWR 36:225–236, 1987

19. Sarngadharan MG, Popovic M, Bruch L, Schüpbach J, Gallo RC: Antibodies reactive with human T-lymphotropic retroviruses (HTLV-III) in the serum of patients with AIDS. Science 224:506–508, 1984

20. Safai B, Sarngadharan MG, Groopman JE et al: Seroepidemiological studies of human T-lymphotropic retrovirus type III in acquired immunodeficiency syndrome. Lancet 1:1438–1440, 1984

21. Rogers MF, Thomas PA, Starcher ET et al: Acquired immunodeficiency syndrome in children: Report to the Centers for Disease Control National Surveillance, 1982–85. Pediatrics 79:1008–1014, 1987

22. Curran JW, Morgan WM, Hardy AM et al: The epidemiology of AIDS: Current status and future prospects. Science 229:1352–1357, 1985

23. Blattner WA, Biggar RJ, Weiss SH, Melbye M, Goedert JJ: Epidemiology of human T-lymphotropic virus type III and the risk of the acquired immunodeficiency syndrome. Ann Intern Med 103:665–670, 1985

24. Peterman TA, Jaffe HW, Feorino PM et al: Transfusion-associated acquired immunodeficiency syndrome in the United States. JAMA 254:2913–2917, 1985

25. Redfield RR, Markham PD, Salahuddin SZ et al: Heterosexually acquired HTLV-III/LAV disease (AIDS-related complex and AIDS): Epidemiologic evidence for female-to-male transmission. JAMA 254:2094–2096, 1985

26. Thomas PA, Jaffe HW, Spira TJ et al: Unexplained immunodeficiency in children: A surveillance report. JAMA 252:639–644, 1984

27. Ammann AJ, Cowan MJ, Wara DW et al: Acquired immunodeficiency in an infant: Possible transmission by means of blood products. Lancet 1:956–958, 1983

28. Scott GB, Buck BE, Leterman JG, Bloom FL, Parks WP: Acquired immunodeficiency syndrome in infants. N Engl J Med 310:76–81, 1984

29. Church JA, Isaacs H: Transfusion-associated acquired immune deficiency syndrome in infants. J Pediatr 105:731–737, 1984

30. Wykoff RF, Pearl ER, Saulsbury FT: Immunologic dysfunction in infants infected through transfusion with HTLV-III. N Engl J Med 312:294–296, 1985

31. O'Duffy JF, Isles AF: Transfusion-induced AIDS in four premature babies. Lancet 2:1346, 1984

32. Lange JMA, van den Berg H, Dooren LJ et al: HTLV-III/LAV infection in nine children infected by a single plasma donor: Clinical outcome and recognition patterns of viral proteins. J Infect Dis 154:171–174, 1986

33. Shannon K, Ball E, Wasserman RL et al: Transfusion-associated cytomegalovirus infection and acquired immune deficiency syndrome in an infant. J Pediatr 103:859–863, 1983

34. Lifson AR, Rogers MF, White C et al: Unrecognized modes of transmission of HIV: Acquired immunodeficiency syndrome in children reported without risk factors. Pediatr Infect Dis 6:292–293, 1987

35. Leiderman IZ, Grimm KT: A child with HIV infection. JAMA 256:3094, 1986

36. Cowan MJ, Hellmann D, Chudwin D et al: Maternal transmission of acquired immune deficiency syndrome. Pediatrics 73:382–386, 1984

37. Rubinstein A, Sicklick M, Gupta A et al: Acquired immunodeficiency with reversed T4/T8 ratios in infants born to promiscuous and drug-addicted mothers. JAMA 249:2350–2356, 1983

38. Oleske J, Minnefor A, Cooper R et al: Immune deficiency syndrome in children. JAMA 249:2345–2349, 1983

39. Rogers MF: AIDS in children: A review of the clinical, epidemiologic and public health aspects. Pediatr Infect Dis 4:230–236, 1985

39a. Pahwa S, Kaplan M, Fikrig S et al: Spectrum of human T-cell lymphotropic virus type III infection in children. Recognition of symptomatic, asymptomatic, and seronegative patients. JAMA 255:2299–2305, 1986

40. Recommendations for assisting in the prevention of perinatal transmission of human T-lymphotropic virus type III/lymphadenopathy-associated virus and acquired immunodeficiency syndrome. MMWR 34:721–732, 1985

41. Martin K, Katz BZ, Miller G: AIDS and antibodies to human immunodeficiency virus (HIV) in children and their families. J Infect Dis 155:54–63, 1987

42. Scott GB, Fischl MA, Klimas N et al: Mothers of infants with the acquired immunodeficiency syndrome: Evidence for both symptomatic and asymptomatic carriers. JAMA 253:363–366, 1985

43. Ragni MV, Urbach AH, Kiernan S et al: Acquired immunodeficiency syndrome in the child of a haemophiliac. Lancet 1:133–135, 1985

44. Joncas JH, Delage G, Chad Z, Lapointe N: Acquired (or congenital) immunodeficiency syndrome in infants born of Haitian mothers. N Engl J Med 308:842, 1983

45. Vilmer E, Fischer A, Griscelli C et al: Possible transmission of a human lymphotropic retrovirus (LAV) from mother to infant with AIDS. Lancet 2:229–230, 1984

46. Ragni MV, Spero JA, Bontempo FA, Lewis JH: Recurrent infections and lymphadenopathy in the child of a hemophiliac: A survey of children of hemophiliacs positive for human immunodeficiency virus antibody. Ann Intern Med 105:886–887, 1986

47. Antibody to human immunodeficiency virus in female prostitutes. MMWR 36:157–161, 1987

48. Rubinstein A: Pediatric AIDS. Curr Probl Pediatr 16:361–409, 1986

49. Luzi G, Ensoli B, Turbessi G, Scarpati B, Aiuti F: Transmission of HTLV-III infection by heterosexual contact. Lancet 2:1018, 1985

50. Chiodo F, Ricchi E, Costigliola P et al: Vertical transmission of HTLV-III. Lancet 1:739, 1986

51. Jovaisas E, Koch MA, Schäfer A, Stauber M, Löwenthal D: LAV/HTLV-III in a 20-week fetus. Lancet 2:1129, 1985

52. Sprecher S, Soumenkoff G, Puissant F, Degueldre M: Vertical transmission of HIV in 15-week fetus. Lancet 2:288–289, 1986

53. Menez-Bautista R, Fikrig SM, Pahwa S, Sarangadharan MG, Stoneburner RL: Monozygotic twins discordant for the acquired immunodeficiency syndrome. Am J Dis Child 140:678–679, 1986

54. Bernstein LJ, Rubinstein A: Acquired immunodeficiency syndrome in infants and children. Prog Allergy 37:194–206, 1986

55. Thiry L, Sprecher-Goldberger S, Jonckheer T et al: Isolation of AIDS virus from cell-free breast milk of three healthy virus carriers. Lancet 2:891–892, 1985

56. Ziegler JB, Cooper DA, Johnson RO, Gold J: Postnatal transmission of AIDS-associated retrovirus from mother to infant. Lancet 1:896–898, 1985

57. Lapointe N, Michaud J, Pekovic D, Chausseau JP, Dupuy J-M: Transplacental transmission of HTLV-III virus. N Engl J Med 312:1325–1326, 1985

57a. Lepage P, Van de Perre P, Carad M et al: Postnatal transmission of HIV from mother to child. Lancet 2:400, 1987

58. Sullivan JL, Brewster FE, Brettler DB et al: Hemophiliac immunodeficiency: Influence of exposure to factor VIII concentrate, LAV/HTLV-III and herpes viruses. J Pediatr 108:504–510, 1956

59. Gill JC, Menitove JE, Anderson PR et al: HTLV-III serology and hemophilia: Relationship with immunologic abnormalities. J Pediatr 108:511–516, 1986

60. Levine PH: The acquired immunodeficiency syndrome in persons with hemophilia. Ann Intern Med 103:723–726, 1985

61. Jason JM, Evatt BL, Chorba TL, Ramsey RB: Acquired immunodeficiency syndrome in hemophiliacs. Scand J Haematol 33:349–356, 1984

62. Carr R, Veitch SE, Edmond E et al: Abnormalities of circulating lymphocyte subsets in haemophiliacs in an AIDS-free population. Lancet 1:1431–1434, 1984

63. Wolff LJ, Borzy M, Kamoun M, Lourien EW: Alteration of T-lymphocyte subpopulations in children, youth and adults with hemophilia A. Scand J Haematol 33:375–377, 1984

64. Goldsmith JC, Dewhurst S, Hedenskog M, Casareale D, Volsky DJ: High prevalence and high titers of LAV/HTLV-III antibodies in healthy hemophiliacs in the midwestern United States. Am J Med 81:579–583, 1986

65. Umid T, Cohen IJ, Pecht M et al: Impaired immune regulation in children and adolescents with hemophilia and thalassemia in Israel. Am J Pediatr Hematol Oncol 6:371–378, 1984

66. Shannon BT, Roach J, Cheek–Lulten M, Ruymann FB: HTLV-III status and abnormalities in T-lymphocyte distribution in children with hemophilia A. Diagn Immunol 4:37–42, 1986

67. Jones P, Hamilton PJ, Bird G et al: AIDS and haemophilia: Morbidity and mortality in a well-defined population. Br Med J 291:695–699, 1985

68. Paul R, Dobkin D, Mauerer H, Noah Z, Yogev R: Acquired immunodeficiency syndrome in a thalassemic child. Pediatr Infect Dis 5:274–276, 1986

69. Anderson KC, Gorgone BV, Marlink RG et al: Transfusion-acquired human immunodeficiency virus infection among immunocompromised persons. Ann Intern Med 105:519–527, 1986

70. Peterson TA, Joffe HW, Feorino PM et al: Transfusion-associated acquired immunodeficiency syndrome in the United States. JAMA 254:2913–2917, 1985

70a.Hilgartner MVˇ: AIDS in the transfused patient. Am J Dis Child 141:194–198, 1987

71. Walker BD, Chakaabarti S, Moss B et al: HIV-specific cytotoxic T-lymphocytes in seropositive individuals. Nature 328:345–348, 1987

72. Plata F, Autran B, Martins LP et al: AIDS virus-specific cytotoxic T-lymphocytes in lung disorders. Nature 328:348–351, 1987

72a.Haverkos HW: Factors associated with the pathogenesis of AIDS. J Infect Dis 156:251–257, 1987

73. Marion RW, Wiznia AA, Hutcheon RG, Rubinstein A: Human T-cell lymphotropic virus type III (HTLV-III) embryopathy: A new dysmorphic syndrome associated with intrauterine HTLV-III infection. Am J Dis Child 140:638–640, 1986

74. Marion RW, Wiznia AA, Hutcheon RG, Rubinstein A: Fetal AIDS syndrome score: Correlation between severity of dysmorphism and age at diagnosis of immunodeficiency. Am J Dis Child 141:429–431, 1987

74a.Iosub S, Bamji M, Stone RK, Gromisch DS, Wasserman E: More on the immunodeficiency virus embryopathy. Pediatrics 80:512–516, 1987

74b.Qazi QH, Sheikh TM, Fikrig S, Menikoff H: Lack of evidence for craniofacial dysmorphism in perinatal human immunodeficiency virus infection. J Pediatr 112:7–11, 1988

75. Popovic M, Sarngadharan MG, Read E, Gallo RC: Detection, isolation and continuous production of cytopathic retroviruses (HTLV-III) from patients with AIDS and pre-AIDS. Science 224:497–500, 1984

76. Sonigo P, Alizon M, Staskus K et al: Nucleotide sequence of the visna lentivirus: Relationship to the AIDS virus. Cell 42:369–382, 1985

77. Stephens RM, Casey JW, Rive NI: Equine infectious anemia virus, gag and pol genes: Relatedness to visna and AIDS virus. Science 231:589–594, 1986

78. Gonda MA, Wong-Staal F, Gallo RC et al: Sequence homology and morphologic similarity of HTLV-III and visna virus, a pathogenic lentivirus. Science 227:173–177, 1985

79. Clavel F, Guétard F, Brun–Vezinet et al: Isolation of a new human retrovirus from West African patients with AIDS. Science 233:343–346, 1986

80. Clavel F, Mansinho K, Charmaret S et al: Human immunodeficiency virus type 2 infection with AIDS in West Africa. N Engl J Med 316:1180–1185, 1987

81. Brun–Vezinet F, Rey A, Katlama C et al: Lymphadenopathy-associated virus type 2 in AIDS and AIDS-related complex: Clinical and virologic features in four patients. Lancet 1:128–132, 1987

82. Clavel F, Guyader M, Guétard D et al: Molecular cloning and polymorphism of the human immune deficiency virus type 2. Nature 324:691–695, 1986

83. Guyader M, Emerman M, Sonigo P et al: Genome organization and trans-activation of the human immunodeficiency virus type 2. Nature 326:662–669, 1987

84. Kanki PJ, Barin F, M'Boup S et al: New human T-lymphotropic retrovirus related to simian T-lymphotropic virus type III (STLV-III$_{AGM}$). Science 232:238–243, 1986

85. Ho D, Pomerantz RJ, Kaplan JC: Pathogenesis of infection with human immunodeficiency virus. N Engl J Med 317:278–286, 1987

86. Gallo RC: The AIDS virus. Sci Am 256:46–56, 1987

87. Ammann AJ, Levy J: Laboratory investigation of pediatric acquired immunodeficiency syndrome. Clin Immunol Immunopathol 40:122–127, 1986

88. Shannon KM, Ammann AJ: Acquired immune deficiency syndrome in childhood. J Pediatr 106:332–342, 1985

89. Blanche S, Le Deist F, Fischer A et al: Longitudinal study of 18 children with perinatal LAV/HTLV III infection: Attempt at prognostic evaluation. J Pediatr 109:965–970, 1986

90. Rosner F, Forgel M, Telsey A et al: Acquired immunodeficiency syndrome (AIDS) in infants and children: Report of nine cases. Biomed Pharmacother 39:350–355, 1985

91. Harnish DG, Hammerberg O, Walker IR, Rosenthal KL: Early detection of HIV infection in a newborn. N Engl J Med 316:272–273, 1987

92. Pahwa S, Fikrig S, Menez R, Pahwa R: Pediatric acquired immunodeficiency syndrome: Demonstration of B lymphocyte defects in vitro. Diagn Immunol 4:24–30, 1986

93. Ammann AJ: The acquired immunodeficiency syndrome in infants and children. Ann Intern Med 734–737, 1985

94. Bernstein LJ, Krieger BZ, Novick B, Sicklick MJ, Rubinstein A: Bacterial infection in the acquired immunodeficiency syndrome of children. Pediatr Infect Dis 4:472–475, 1985

95. Bernstein LJ, Ochs HD, Wedgwood RJ, Rubinstein A: Defective humoral immunity in pediatric acquired immunodeficiency syndrome. J Pediatr 107:352–357, 1985

96. Maloney MJ, Guill MF, Wray BB, Lobel SA, Ebbeling W: Pediatric acquired immune deficiency syndrome with panhypogammaglobulinemia. J Pediatr 110:266–267, 1987

97. Church JA, Lewis J, Spotkov JM: IgG subclass deficiencies in children with suspected AIDS. Lancet 1:279, 1984

98. Rubinstein A, Novick BE, Sicklick MJ et al: Circulating thymulin and thymosin-α_1 activity in pediatric acquired immune deficiency syndrome: In vivo and in vitro studies. J Pediatr 109:422–427, 1986

98a.Pawha R, Good RA, Pawha S: Prematurity, hypogammaglobulinemia, and neuropathology with human immunodeficiency virus (HIV) infection. Proc Natl Acad Sci USA 84:3826–3830, 1987

98b.Honda WS, Sun NCJ, Heiner DC: Isolated IgG4 subclass deficiency and malignant lymphoma in a child with acquired immunodeficiency syndrome. Am J Dis Child 141:398–399, 1987

99. Borkowsky W, Steele CJ, Grubman S et al: Antibody responses to bacterial toxoids in children infected with human immunodeficiency virus. J Pediatr 110:563–566, 1987

100. Gupta A, Novick BE, Rubinstein A: Restoration of suppressor T-cell functions in children with AIDS following intravenous gamma globulin treatment. Am J Dis Child 140:143–146, 1986

101. Sarin PS, Sun DK, Thornton AH, Naylor PH, Goldstein AL: Neutralization of HTLV-III/LAV replication by antiserum to thymosin α_1. Science 232:1135–1137, 1986

102. Joshi VV, Oleske JM, Minnefor AB et al: Pathology of suspected acquired immune deficiency syndrome in children: A study of eight cases. Pediatr Pathol 2:71–87, 1984

103. Joshi VV, Oleske JM, Minnefor AB et al: Pathologic pulmonary findings in children with the acquired immunodeficiency syndrome: A study of ten cases. Hum Pathol 16:241–246, 1985

104. Joshi VV, Oleske JM: Pulmonary lesions in children with acquired immunodeficiency syndrome: A reappraisal based on data in additional cases and follow-up study of previously reported cases. Hum Pathol 17:641–642, 1986

105. Joshi VV, Oleske JM: Pathologic appraisal of the thymus gland in acquired immunodeficiency syndrome in children: A study of four cases and a review of the literature. Arch Pathol Lab Med 109:142–146, 1985

106. Savino W, Dardenne M, Marche C et al: Thymic epithelium in AIDS: An immunohistologic study. Am J Pathol 122:302–307, 1986

107. Rubinstein A, Morecki R, Silverman B et al: Pulmonary disease in children with acquired immune deficiency syndrome and AIDS-related complex. J Pediatr 108:498–503, 1986

108. Goldman HS, Ziprkowski MN, Charytan M, Rubinstein A, Morecki R: Lym-

phocytic interstitial pneumonitis in children with AIDS: A perfect radiographic–pathologic correlation. AJR 145:868, 1985

109. Case records of the Massachusetts General Hospital: Weekly clinicopathological exercises. N Engl J Med 314:629–640, 1986

110. Education and foster care of children infected with human T-lymphotropic virus type III/lymphadenopathy-associated virus. MMWR 34:517–521, 1985

111. Acquired immunodeficiency syndrome (AIDS) among blacks and Hispanics —United States. MMWR 35:655–666, 1986

112. Thomas PA, Lubin K, Milberg J et al: Cohort comparison study of children whose mothers have acquired immunodeficiency syndrome and children of well inner city mothers. Pediatr Infect Dis 6:247–251, 1987

113. Maloney MJ, Cox F, Wray BB et al: AIDS in a child 5½ years after a transfusion. N Engl J Med 312:1256, 1985

113a. Kelly DA, Hallett RJ, Saeed A, Morgan G, Levinsky RJ, Strobel S: Prolonged survival and late presentation of vertically transmitted HIV infection in childhood. Lancet 1:806–807, 1987

113b. Medley GF, Anderson RM, Cox DR, Billard L: Incubation period of AIDS in patients infected via blood transfusion. Nature 328:719–721, 1987

114. Berkowitz CD: AIDS and parasitic infections, including *Pneumocystis carinii* and cryptosporidiosis. Pediatr Clin North Am 32:933–952, 1985

115. Barbour SD: Acquired immunodeficiency syndrome of childhood. Pediatr Clin North Am 34:247–268, 1987

116. Andiman WA, Eastman R, Martin K et al: Opportunistic lymphoproliferations associated with Epstein–Barr viral DNA in infants and children with AIDS. Lancet 2:1390–1393, 1985

117. Katz BZ, Andiman WA, Eastman R, Martin K, Miller G: Infection with two genotypes of Epstein–Barr virus in an infant with AIDS and lymphoma of the central nervous system. J Infect Dis 153:601–604, 1986

118. Epstein LG, Sharer LR, Oleske JM et al: Neurologic manifestations of human immunodeficiency virus infection in children. Pediatrics 78:678–687, 1986

119. Belman AL, Ultmann MH, Horoupian D et al: Neurological complications in infants and children with acquired immune deficiency syndrome. Ann Neurol 18:560–566, 1985

120. Epstein LG, Sharer LR, Joshi VV et al: Progressive encephalopathy in children with acquired immune deficiency syndrome. Ann Neurol 17:488–496, 1985

121. Price RW, Navia BA, Cho E-S: AIDS encephalopathy. Neurol Clin 4:285–301, 1986

122. Ultmann MH, Belman AL, Ruff HA et al: Developmental abnormalities in infants and children with acquired immune deficiency syndrome (AIDS) and AIDS-related complex. Dev Med Child Neurol 27:563–571, 1985

122a. Price RW, Brew B, Sidtis J, Rosenblum M, Scheck A, Cleary P: The brain in AIDS: Central nervous system HIV–I infection and AIDS dementia complex. Science 239:586–592, 1988

122b. Belman A, Diamond G, Dickson O et al: Pediatric acquired immunodeficiency syndrome: Neurologic syndromes. Am J Dis Child 142:29–35, 1988

123. Belman AL, Lantos G, Horoupian D et al: AIDS: Calcification of the basal ganglia in infants and children. Neurology 36:1192–1199, 1986

123a. Gabuzda DH, Hirsch MS: Neurologic manifestations of infection with human immunodeficiency virus. Clinical features and pathogenesis. Ann Intern Med 107:383–391, 1987

124. Ragni V, Urbach AH, Taylor S: Isolation of human immunodeficiency virus and detection of HIV DNA sequences in the brain of an ELISA antibody-negative child with acquired immune deficiency syndrome and progressive encephalopathy. J Pediatr 110:892–894, 1987

125. Sharer LR, Epstein LG, Cho E-S et al: Pathologic features of AIDS encephalopathy in children: Evidence for LAV/HTLV-III infection of brain. Hum Pathol 17:271–284, 1986

125a. Epstein LG, Berman CZ, Sharer LR, Khademi M, Desposito F: Unilateral calcification and contrast enhancement of the basal ganglia in a child with AIDS encephalopathy. AJNR 8:163–165, 1987

126. Salahuddin SZ, Markham PD, Popovic M et al: Isolation of infectious human T-cell leukemia/lymphotropic virus type III (HTLV-III) from patients with acquired immunodeficiency syndrome (AIDS) or AIDS-related complex (ARC) and from healthy carriers: A study of risk groups and tissue sources. Proc Natl Acad Sci USA 82:5530–5534, 1985

127. Epstein LG, Sharer LR, Cho E-S et al: HTLV-III/LAV-like retrovirus particles in the brains of patients with AIDS encephalopathy. AIDS Res 1:447–454, 1984

128. Shaw GM, Harper ME, Hahn BH et al: HTLV-III infection in brains of children and adults with AIDS encephalopathy. Science 227:177–181, 1985

129. Fackler JC, Nagel JE, Adler WH, Mildvan PT, Ambinder RF: Epstein–Barr virus infection in a child with acquired immunodeficiency syndrome. Am J Dis Child 139:1000–1004, 1985

130. Chayt KJ, Harper ME, Marselle LM et al: Detection of HTLV-III RNA in lungs of patients with AIDS and pulmonary involvement. JAMA 256:2356–2359, 1986

130a. Resnick L, Pitchenik AE, Fisher E, Croney R: Detection of HTLV-III/LAF-specific IgG and antigen in broncheoalveolar lavage fluid from two patients with lymphocytic interstitial pneumonitis associated with AIDS-related complex. Am J Med 82:553–556, 1987

131. Steinherz LJ, Brochstein JA, Robins J: Cardiac involvement in congenital acquired immunodeficiency syndrome. Am J Dis Child 140:1241–1244, 1986

132. Saulsbury FT, Boyle RJ, Wykoff RF, Howard TH: Thrombocytopenia as the presenting manifestation of human T-lymphotropic virus type III infection in infants. J Pediatr 109:30–34, 1986

133. McCance–Katz EF, Hoecker JL, Vitale NB: Severe neutropenia associated with anti-neutrophil antibody in a patient with acquired immunodeficiency syndrome-related complex. Pediatr Infect Dis 6:417–418, 1987

134. Silverman BA, Rubinstein A: Serum lactate dehydrogenase levels in adults and children with acquired immune deficiency syndrome (AIDS) and AIDS-related complex: Possible indicator of B-cell lymphoproliferation and disease activity. Am J Med 78:728–736, 1985

135. Duffy LF, Daum F, Kahn E et al: Hepatitis in children with acquired immune deficiency syndrome: Histopathologic and immunocytologic features. Gastroenterology 90:173–181, 1986

136. Rao TKS, Friedman EA, Nicastri AD: The types of renal disease in the acquired immunodeficiency syndrome. N Engl J Med 316:1062–1068, 1987

136a. Pardo V, Meneses R, Ossa L et al: AIDS-related glomerulopathy: Occurrence in specific risk groups. Kidney Int 31:1167–1173, 1987

137. Buck BE, Scott GB, Valdes–Dapena M, Parks WP: Kaposi sarcoma in two infants with acquired immune deficiency syndrome. J Pediatr 103:911–913, 1983

138. Petricciani JC: Licensed tests for antibody to human T-lymphotropic virus type III: Sensitivity and specificity. Ann Intern Med 103:726–729, 1985

139. Status report on the acquired immunodeficiency syndrome: Human T-cell lymphotropic virus type III testing. JAMA 254:1342–1345, 1985

140. Salahuddin SZ, Groopman JE, Markham PD et al: HTLV-III in symptom-free seronegative persons. Lancet 2:1418–1420, 1984

141. Marlink RG, Allan JS, McLane MF et al: Low sensitivity of ELISA testing in early HIV infection. N Engl J Med 315:1549, 1986

142. Cooper DA, Gold J, Maclean P et al: Acute AIDS retrovirus infection: Definition of a clinical illness associated with seroconversion. Lancet 1:537–540, 1985

143. Needlestick transmission of HTLV-III from a patient infected in Africa. Lancet 2:1376–1377, 1984

144. Esteban JI, Shih JW-K, Tai C-C et al: Importance of Western blot analysis in predicting infection of anti-HTLV-III/LAV positive blood. Lancet 2:1083–1086, 1985

145. Ho DD, Sarngadharan MG, Resnick L et al: Primary human T-lymphotropic virus type III infection. Ann Intern Med 103:880–883, 1985

146. Johnson JP, Nair P, Alexander S: Early diagnosis of HIV infection in the neonate. N Engl J Med 316:273–274, 1987

146a. Harnish DG, Hammerberg O, Walker IR, Rosenthal KL: Early detection of HIV infection in a newborn. N Engl J Med 316:272–273, 1987

146b. Krilov LR, Kamani N, Hendry RM, Wittek AE, Quinnan GV: Longitudinal serologic evaluation of an infant with acquired immunodeficiency syndrome. Pediatr Infect Dis J 6:1066–1067, 1987

146c. Borkowsky W, Krasinski K, Paul D, Moore T, Bebenroth D, Clondwan S: Human-immunodeficiency-virus infection in infants negative for anti-HIV by enzyme-linked immunoassay. Lancet 1:1168–1171, 1987

147. Di Maria H, Courpotin C, Rouzioux C et al: Transplacental transmission of human immunodeficiency virus. Lancet 2:215–216, 1986

148. Wood CC, Williams AE, McNamara JG et al: Antibody against the human immunodeficiency virus in commercial intravenous gammaglobulin preparations. Ann Intern Med 105:536–538, 1986

149. Feorino PM, Jaffe HW, Palmer E et al: Transfusion-associated acquired immunodeficiency syndrome: Evidence for persistent infection in blood donors. N Engl J Med 312:1293–1296, 1985

150. Robert–Guroff M, Brown M, Gallo RC: HTLV-III-neutralizing antibodies in patients with AIDS and AIDS-related complex. Nature 316:72–74, 1985

151. Weiss RA, Clapham PR, Cheingsong–Popov R et al: Neutralization of human T-lymphotropic virus type III by sera of AIDS and AIDS-risk patients. Nature 316:69–72, 1985

152. Wykoff RF: Classification of HTLV-III/LAV-related diseases in children. J Infect Dis 153:1181–1182, 1986

153. Lampert R, Milberg J, O'Donnell R, Kristal A, Thomas P: Life table analysis of children with acquired immunodeficiency syndrome. Pediatr Infect Dis 5:374–375, 1986

154. McCray E, Cooperative Needlestick Surveillance Group: Occupational risk of the acquired immunodeficiency syndrome among health care workers. N Engl J Med 314:1127–1132, 1986

155. Update: Evaluation of human T-lymphotropic virus type III/lymphadenopathy-associated virus infection in health-care personnel—United States. MMWR 34:575–578, 1985

155a.Friedland GH, Klein RJ: Transmission of the human immunodeficiency virus. N Engl J Med 317:1125–1135, 1987

156. Acquired immune deficiency syndrome (AIDS): Precautions for clinical and laboratory staffs. MMWR 31:577–580, 1982

157. Acquired immunodeficiency syndrome (AIDS): Precautions for health-care workers and allied professionals. MMWR 32:450–451, 1983

158. Summary: Recommendations for preventing transmission of infection with human T-lymphotropic virus type III/lymphadenopathy-associated virus in the workplace. MMWR 34:681–695, 1985

159. Recommendations for preventing transmission of infection with human T-lymphotropic virus type III/lymphadenopathy-associated virus during invasive procedures. MMWR 35:221–223, 1986

160. Stricof RL, Morse DL: HTLV-III/LAV seroconversion following a deep intramuscular needlestick injury. N Engl J Med 314:1115, 1986

161. Oksenhendler E, Harzic M, Le Roux J-M, Rabian C, Clauvel JP: HIV infection with seroconversion after a superficial needlestick injury to the finger. N Engl J Med 315:582, 1986

162. Apparent transmission of human T-lymphotropic virus type III/lymphadenopathy-associated virus from child to mother providing health care. MMWR 35:75–79, 1986

163. Groopman JE, Salahuddin SZ, Sarngadharan MG et al: HTLV-III in saliva of people with AIDS-related complex and healthy homosexual men at risk for AIDS. Science 226:447–449, 1984

164. Fujikawa LS, Salahuddin SZ, Palestine AG et al: Isolation of human T-lymphotropic virus type III from the tears of a patient with the acquired immunodeficiency syndrome (AIDS). Lancet 2:529–530, 1985

165. Goedert JJ: What is safe sex? Suggested standard linked to testing for human immunodeficiency virus. N Engl J Med 316:1339–1342, 1987

166. Yarchoan R, Broder S: Progress in the development of antiviral therapy in HTLV-III associated diseases. In DeVita VT Jr, Hellman S, Rosenberg SA (eds): Important Advances in Oncology 1987, pp 293–311. Philadelphia, JB Lippincott, 1987

167. Yarchoan R, Broder S: Development of antiretroviral therapy for the acquired immunodeficiency syndrome and related disorders: A progress report. N Engl J Med 316:557–564, 1987

168. Mitsuya H, Broder S: Strategies for antiviral therapy in AIDS. Nature 325:773–778, 1987

169. DeVita VT, Broder S, Fauci AS, Kovacs JA, Chabner BA: Developmental therapeutics and the acquired immunodeficiency syndrome. Ann Intern Med 106:568–581, 1987

170. Hirsch M, Kaplan JC: Treatment of human immunodeficiency virus infections. Antimicrob Agents Chemother 31:839–843, 1987

171. Barnes DM: Promising results halt trial of anti-AIDS drug. Science 234:15–16, 1986

172. Fischl MA, Richman DD, Grieco MH et al: The efficacy of azidothymidine (AZT) in the treatment of patients with AIDS and AIDS-related complex: A double-blind, placebo-controlled trial. N Engl J Med 371:185–191, 1987

173. Richman DD, Fischl MA, Grieco MH et al: The toxicity of azidothymidine (AZT) in the treatment of patients with AIDS and AIDS-related complex: A double-blind, placebo-controlled trial. N Engl J Med 317:192–197, 1987

174. Yarchoan R, Berg G, Brouwers P et al: Response of human immunodeficiency-virus-associated neurological disease to 3'-azido-3'-deoxythymidine. Lancet 1:132–135, 1987

175. Pizzo PA, Eddy J, Falloon J et al: Continuous infusion of azidothymidine in children with AIDS: A Phase I Study. Presented at the Interscience Conference on Antimicrobial Agents and Chemotherapy, New York, 1987

176. Blanche S, Fischer A, Le Deist F et al: Ribavirin in HTLV-III/LAV infection of infants. Lancet 1:863, 1986

177. Lane HC, Fauci AS: Immunologic reconstitution in the acquired immunodeficiency syndrome. Ann Intern Med 103:714–718, 1985

178. Calvelli TA, Rubinstein A: Intravenous gamma-globulin in infant acquired immunodeficiency syndrome. Pediatr Infect Dis 5:S207–S210, 1986

179. Charytan M, Krieger BZ, Wiznik A et al: Treatment of AIDS associated lymphoid interstitial pneumonitis with intravenous gammaglobulin and prednisone (abstract). Pediatr Res 19:401A, 1985

179a.Ochs HD: Intravenous immunoglobulin in the treatment and prevention of acute infections in pediatric acquired immunodeficiency syndrome patients. Pediatr Infect Dis J 6:509–511, 1987

180. Francis DP, Petricciani JC: The prospects for and pathways toward a vaccine for AIDS. N Engl J Med 313:1586–1590, 1985

181. Vogt M, Hirsch MS: Prospects for the prevention and therapy of infections with the human immunodeficiency virus. Rev Infect Dis 8:991–1000, 1986

182. MacDonald KL, Danila RN, Osterholm MT: Infection with human T-lymphotropic virus type III/lymphadenopathy-associated virus: Considerations for transmission in the child day care setting. Rev Infect Dis 8:606–612, 1986

183. American Academy of Pediatrics, Committee on School Health, Committee on Infectious Diseases: School attendance of children and adolescents with human T-lymphotropic virus III/lymphadenopathy-associated virus infection. Pediatrics 77:430–432, 1986

184. Additional recommendations to reduce sexual and drug abuse-related transmission of human T-lymphotropic virus type III/lymphadenopathy-associated virus. MMWR 35:152–155, 1986

Management of Problems Arising at Diagnosis and During Treatment

part

five

thirty-seven

Oncologic Emergencies

Beverly Lange,
Giulio D'Angio,
Arthur J. Ross III,
James A. O'Neill, Jr., and
Roger J. Packer

Emergencies in oncology arise in three ways: [1] a space-occupying lesion causes pressure or obstruction (a mechanical emergency); [2] leukemia or a tumor creates life-threatening metabolic or hormonal problems; or [3] cytopenias arise from the effects of the disease or treatment on the bone marrow. This chapter deals first with mechanical emergencies by region and second with metabolic emergencies. The reader is referred to other chapters for discussions of emergencies related to infection (see Chap. 39), anemia, hemorrhage, thrombosis (see Chap. 38), and pain (see Chap. 44).

THORACIC EMERGENCIES

Superior Vena Cava Syndrome and Superior Mediastinal Syndrome

Definition

The term *superior vena cava (SVC) syndrome* (SVCS) refers to the signs and symptoms of compression or obstruction of that major vessel. The term *superior mediastinal syndrome* (SMS) is used when tracheal compression also occurs. The signs of SVC obstruction dominate the clinical presentation in adults; in children, tracheal compression and respiratory embarrassment also occur with SVC obstruction. Hence, in pediatric practice, the terms SVCS and SMS have become almost synonymous. Without prompt treatment or with injudicious positioning or use of anesthesia, death may occur suddenly from cardiac or respiratory arrest.

Etiology

Janin and coworkers[1] reviewed the world literature and Issa and associates[2] analyzed 150 recent pediatric cases to determine the frequency and the causes of SVCS in childhood and adolescence (Table 37-1). Historically, SVCS or SMS has been uncommon. Between 1757 and 1904, 252 cases of SVCS were reported, three of which were in children.[1] Between 1904 and 1949, another 250 cases of SVCS were added to the literature; one was in a child.[3] More recently, D'Angio and colleagues reported nine cases among 607 children and adolescents with malignant solid tumors.[4] These studies emphasize the rarity of SVCS in pediatrics. However, if one calculates the frequency of SVCS or SMS in pediatric patients with malignant anterior mediastinal tumors, it would appear to be about 12% at presentation.[4-6]

In the past, infections, especially syphilis or tuberculosis, aortic aneurysm, and malignant tumor were the most common causes of SVCS. Now the most common cause in pediatric practice is vascular thrombosis complicating cardiovascular surgery for congenital heart disease, shunting for hydrocephalus, or catheterization for venous access.[1] Malignant tumors are the most common primary cause of SVCS, and most of these are non-Hodgkin's lymphomas (see

Table 37-1
Causes of Superior Vena Cava Obstruction in Childhood: Review of 150 Cases

	Number of Cases
Mediastinal tumors ($N = 24$)	
Non-Hodgkin's lymphoma	16
Neuroblastoma	2
Ewing's sarcoma of rib	2
Hodgkin's disease	1
Malignant degeneration of bronchogenic cyst	1
Unspecified malignant tumors	2
Ventriculoatrial shunt for hydrocephalus	8
Congenital heart disease and cardiovascular surgery ($N = 106$)	
Mustard repair of transposition of great arteries	8
Superior vena cava-to-right pulmonary artery anastomosis	97
Repair of supradiaphragmatic total anomalous pulmonary venous connection	1
Mediastinal fibrosis ($N = 8$)	
Histoplasmosis	7
Granuloma	1
Miscellaneous	4
Thrombosis of superior vena cava	3
Hydrocephalus	1
Total	150

(Issa PY et al: Superior vena cava syndrome in childhood. Pediatrics 71:337–341, 1983. Reproduced by permission of Pediatrics)

Chapters 20 and 21). Mediastinal granulomas, usually from histoplasmosis, are the second most frequent primary cause.[7] The distribution of cases in the review of Issa and colleagues, most of which are reported after 1971, is shown in Table 37-1.

Pathophysiology

The anatomy of the mediastinum is illustrated in Figure 37-1. The SVC is a thin-walled vessel with low intraluminal pressure. Thus, it cannot resist mechanical compression from without, and, once conditions favoring clot formation have been introduced, it is prone to thrombosis. The SVC is surrounded by lymph nodes that drain the right side and lower left side of the chest and by the thymus in the anterior superior mediastinum. Part of the SVC is within the pericardial reflection. When the thymus or nodes become involved with tumor or infection, they compress the vena cava. The adjacent pericardium and coronary vessels and collateral vessels may be involved with tumor and clot. The trachea and right main-stem bronchus are relatively rigid compared to the vena cava, but in children, these structures, too, may be compressed by tumor. Also, the relatively small intraluminal diameter of the infant's trachea and bronchi can accommodate little edema before obstructive symptoms occur. The end-result of compression, clotting, and edema is that air flow as well as blood flow is reduced. Blood return from the head, neck, upper thorax, and arms is diminished or stopped altogether; collateral vessels enlarge to compensate but often fail to do so adequately.

Evaluation and Differential Diagnosis

Common symptoms of SMS are cough, hoarseness, dyspnea, orthopnea, and chest pain. Less frequent but more sinister are

anxiety, confusion, lethargy, headache, distorted vision, a sense of fullness in the ears, and, especially, syncope. Symptoms may be aggravated when the patient lies supine or flexes as for a lumbar puncture.

Signs of SMS include swelling, plethora, and cyanosis of the face, neck, and upper extremities; suffusion and edema of the conjunctiva; diaphoresis; wheezing; and stridor. The veins on the chest wall may be engorged. If the right arm is raised above the patient's head, the brachial veins remain full. Signs of pleural effusion and of pericardial effusion may coexist with those of SVC obstruction. In adults with SVCS, spinal cord compression is an associated, albeit unusual, finding; it has not been reported in children.[8] In adults, onset of SVCS caused by malignant tumor is often insidious; in children and adolescents, by contrast, symptoms often progress rapidly over days.

Chest radiographs show a mass in the anterior superior mediastinum. Pleural and pericardial effusions may be apparent. More than half the children with Hodgkin's disease have tracheal compression on chest radiography.[9]

History, physical examination, and chest radiographs should be sufficient to generate a differential diagnosis and a plan for management. Secondary benign cardiovascular lesions can be excluded by history, and histoplasmosis can almost be ruled out in nonendemic areas. In endemic areas, histoplasma complement-fixing antibody titers exceeding 1:32 are suggestive of infection.[10] When vascular and infectious causes are eliminated, lymphoma becomes the most likely diagnosis.

When a lymphoma or another malignant disease is the probable cause of SMS, one would like to obtain a tissue diagnosis, but doing so may cause problems.[11] Children with SVCS or SMS tolerate the necessary procedures poorly. They may suffer irreversible cardiac arrest when placed in a position that further embarrasses venous return or air flow; for example, when the child is placed supine for preoperative sedation and general anesthesia. General anesthesia in particular causes cardiovascular and respiratory changes that aggravate SVCS and SMS. First, it may be impossible to intubate the child. Second, with anesthesia, abdominal muscle tone increases, respiratory muscle tone decreases, the caudal movement of the diaphragm disappears, bronchial smooth muscle relaxes, and lung volume is greatly reduced.[12] These changes increase the effects of extrinsic compression of the SVC. Venous return, reduced by the peripheral vasodilatation caused by sedatives, may never be restored.[13] Uncontrollable hemorrhage at the biopsy site has been often cited as a major complication, but in practice it is a relatively rare problem.[14] Finally, even when sedation, anesthesia, and biopsy proceed uneventfully, extubation may be exceedingly difficult or impossible. Patients may require mechanical ventilation until the tumor bulk has been reduced.

Because of the risks of anesthesia, diagnosis should be obtained by the least-invasive means possible. A peripheral blood count may show leukemia/lymphoma syndrome, as may a marrow aspiration performed with the patient sitting. Pleurocentesis or pericardiocentesis may offer immediate relief as well as diagnostic material. Peripheral node biopsy may be possible in the older child or adolescent, but sedation may be hazardous, and consideration must be given to whether the distressed, anxious patient can tolerate the emotional and physical stress needed to obtain tissue. Lymph node aspiration is faster and less invasive than open biopsy. There are, however, few data on the safety and efficacy of this technique in children with SMS.[15] A number of recent reports suggest a stepwise approach to diagnosis.[12,16] An algorithm appropriate for pediatric patients is shown in Figure 37-2.

Computed tomography (CT) of the chest to delineate tracheal size, upright and supine echocardiography, and a flow volume loop may help evaluate anesthetic risk. Obviously, patients who cannot tolerate these procedures are not candidates

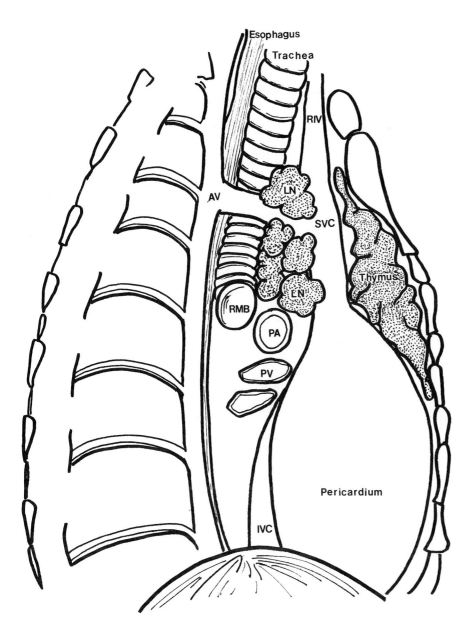

FIGURE 37-1. Anatomic relationships in the mediastinum that predispose to superior vena cavae and tracheal compression. AV = azygous vein; LN = lymph node; SVC = superior vena cava; IVC = inferior vena cava; RIV = right innomerate vein; RMB = right main bronchus; PA = pulmonary artery; PV = pulmonary vein.

for general anesthesia. However, if the tumor is not chemosensitive or radiosensitive, surgery may be inevitable. In this case, surgery should be performed with the patient in the semi-Fowler's position with preparations for change of position to lateral or prone and with cardiopulmonary bypass facilities and a rigid bronchoscope on standby.[12]

Therapy

Establishing a tissue diagnosis before therapy is sometimes impossible. In this case, it may be in the patient's best interest to receive empiric prebiopsy therapy. Traditionally, this therapy has been irradiation, but chemotherapy may offer certain advantages. Lymphoblastic lymphoma is exquisitely radioresponsive: doses as low as 200 cGy can cause such rapid dissolution of the tumor that only ghost cells are found at biopsy. An additional problem is postradiation respiratory deterioration, presumably from tracheal swelling. The phenomenon of postirradiation deterioration seems limited to children and adolescents, perhaps because of the greater compressibility of the respiratory structures in younger patients, the inability of relatively narrower lumens to accommodate edema, and the

greater edema at onset because of the more rapidly progressive tumors in the younger age group.

Two radiation field arrangements may circumvent the problems of swelling and tumor dissolution. Both are designed to minimize radiation scatter to the periphery of the mass and to the supraclavicular lymph nodes. The first is a small field centered on the trachea and not including the lateral edges of the tumor mass. The second is bilateral opposing fields using a small field to include the trachea, SVC, and proximal right auricle. Which of the two is preferable depends largely by the size of the mass. The objective is to make biopsy proof of the diagnosis possible when the anesthesia risk has lessened. The daily dose is governed by the presumed radiosensitivity of the tumor: 100 cGy the morning or the evening of diagnosis and a similar dose or double that amount in the afternoon or the following morning—that is, approaching twice-a-day radiation. The total dose is governed by the response. Many patients improve within 12 hours after the first dose. There is no need for high doses for this purpose.

Among 19 patients reported by Loeffler and associates who had emergency prebiopsy radiation for mediastinal masses, the histologic specimen was rendered uninterpretable

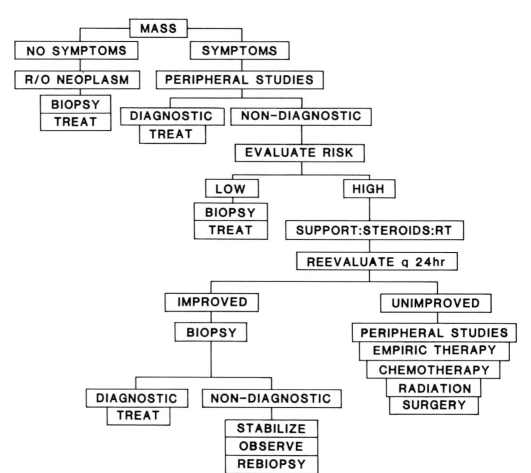

FIGURE 37-2. Algorithm for approach to diagnosis in pediatric patients with superior vena cava (SVC) or superior mediastinal syndrome (SMS).

in eight.[15] Seven of eight were treated empirically for Hodgkin's disease or non-Hodgkin's lymphoma. Four have not relapsed; three relapsed with the disease they were assumed to have; and the one untreated patient developed recurrent seminoma. The authors point out that patient management was not altered by prebiopsy therapy or by continued empiric therapy.

Although radiation has traditionally been used for empiric therapy of SVCS or SMS, chemotherapeutic agents including steroids, cyclophosphamide, or both in combination within an anthracycline and vincristine are reasonable alternatives. Chemotherapy, like radiation, may confound diagnosis.[15] The histologic picture may be rendered uninterpretable within 48 hours of chemotherapy or radiation. Failure to persist with treatment for the presumed lymphoma, even if a histologic diagnosis is not made, may allow the disease to progress to a more advanced stage.[14,16] Chemotherapy is readily available and does not have the same long-term morbidity as radiation. The advantages of empiric chemotherapy may become more apparent as radiation is used less and less in young patients with non-Hodgkin's lymphoma or Hodgkin's disease (see Chaps. 20 and 21). However, chemotherapy should be started with a commitment to continuation of therapy for the presumed diagnosis.[16] Although most chemotherapy- and radiotherapy-sensitive anterior mediastinal tumors in children are lymphomas, dysgerminomas and seminomas may also respond. Alpha-fetoprotein or, less commonly, human chorionic gonadotropin (hCG) assays may help to differentiate these from lymphomas.

When small fields and low doses of radiation are used and when the biopsy site is well removed from the region of maxi-

mum irradiation, open biopsy proceeds safely and with success. In the rare cases in which the patient's symptoms become life-threatening because of apparent edema during empiric irradiation, a course of prednisone at 40 mg/m² daily divided into four doses may be unavoidable. One other situation in which chemotherapy rather than irradiation is indicated is acute T-cell lymphoblastic leukemia with a very high white blood cell count and a mediastinal mass causing SMS or SVCS (see Chap. 16). The intrathoracic complications of T-cell acute lymphocytic leukemia may be difficult to distinguish from those of lymphoblastic lymphoma.[17] Chemotherapy treats both life-threatening problems: SVCS and hyperleukocytosis (see section on hyperleukocytosis). However, if renal failure is impending, irradiation is the treatment of choice for the SVCS or SMS until renal function is adequate (see section on tumor lysis syndrome).

If the tumor fails to respond, it may be one of the benign lesions listed in Table 37-1. If symptoms progress, they may rarely be caused by an unresponsive tumor such as teratoma or by extensive clotting or increasing chylous effusion from damage to the lymphatics by tumor. In the latter case, withdrawal of fluid and complete elimination of fat from the diet are necessary.[18]

Pleural and Pericardial Effusions

Definition

Effusions are classified as exudates or transudates. Exudates may be caused by local invasion or metastatic spread of tumor or by infection and transudates, by a sympathetic response to tumor in the chest or abdomen or by fluid overload, heart failure, or hypoproteinemia. Chylous effusion can occur from obstructed lymphatics. Exudates have protein concentrations exceeding 2.5 g/dl, a specific gravity greater than 1.015, and a high cell count. Transudates have low protein, low specific gravity, and low cell counts.

Evaluation

Small, clinically silent pleural and pericardial effusions are often detected on radiographs as part of the evaluation of the extent of disease in patients with leukemia, lymphoma, sarcoma, and Wilms' tumor (see Chaps. 16, 20, 21, 27, and 30). Thoracentesis is indicated when fluid is needed to exclude infection, to establish the stage or possibly the diagnosis, to relieve respiratory or cardiac distress, or to eliminate a potential reservoir for drugs such as methotrexate. Fluid should be sent for measures of protein content, specific gravity, and lactic dehydrogenase and for cell count, cytology study, culture, and assays of appropriate immunologic and biologic markers.

Therapy

In an untreated child in respiratory distress, it may be sufficient to remove fluid once, because the fluid may not reaccumulate after specific therapy is started. In children with resistant disease, recurrent effusion may compromise the duration and quality of life. A number of sclerosing agents, including nitrogen mustard, quinacrine, dactinomycin, talc, bleomycin, and tetracycline, have been injected into pleural and pericardial cavities to cause irritation and adhesions and thus prevent reaccumulation of fluid.[19,20] Tetracycline seems to be the most effective and to have the fewest side effects. The effusion is drained, and 500 to 1000 mg of tetracycline in 20 ml of 0.9% saline is instilled into the cavity. It may be necessary to repeat the procedure daily for several days to achieve control. Tetracycline prevented reaccumulation of pericardial fluid in 15 of 22 patients[21] and in 30 of 33 patients.[22] Intrapleural tetracycline achieved control in 10 of 12 effusions, was associated with less pain and fever than quinacrine,[23] and proved far superior to a control solution of pH 2.8.[24] If tetracycline fails, surgical pleurectomy or pericardiectomy may be necessary, but surgery entails greater morbidity and mortality rates in the patient with resistant metastatic disease.[19,20]

Cardiac Tamponade

Definition

Cardiac tamponade is inability of the left ventricle to maintain output, usually because of extrinsic pressure or, rarely, because of an intrinsic mass.

Etiology and Pathogenesis

Tamponade is caused by compression by pericardial fluid, by constrictive fibrosis from previous irradiation, and by primary tumors of the cardiac muscle or pericardium. Tamponade of the right cardiac chambers can occur when intracardiac masses such as a Wilms' tumor thrombus fill the chambers or extend from the renal vein through the tricuspid valve.

Pericardial effusion with tamponade is a rare presentation of malignancy. In their review of 26 cases of tamponade at presentation, Fraser and associates cite three that are relevant

to pediatrics: a 15-year-old with leukemia, a 17-year-old with lymphoma, and a 25-year-old with rhabdomyosarcoma.[25]

Evaluation and Differential Diagnosis

The history of symptoms is important: gradual accumulation of fluid allows the pericardium to stretch to accommodate a large volume, whereas rapid accumulation of several hundred milliliters can cause tamponade. Symptoms of impending tamponade resemble those of heart failure: cough, chest pain, dyspnea, orthopnea, and hiccoughs. Plethora and cyanosis may be present. A pulsus paradoxus greater than 10 mm is abnormal and one greater than 20 mm indicates serious compromise. Radiographs may show a typical "water-bag" cardiac shadow. Pericardial effusion can be confirmed by echocardiography of the posterior wall, where there will be two echoes, one from the cardiac muscle and one from the pericardium.[19]

Tamponade must be differentiated from congestive heart failure, infections, myocarditis, and therapy-induced cardiomyopathy. Patients with constrictive pericarditis may have friction rubs, diastolic murmurs, and atrial arrythmia.[19] Chest radiography will show a small heart. The ECG may have flattened or inverted T waves and electrical atrial and ventricular alternans.

Therapy

Supportive care for malignant pericardial effusion consists of hydration, oxygen, and positioning the patient to maximize cardiac output. Diuretics are usually contraindicated. The specific treatment of cardiac tamponade is immediate removal of fluid under echocardiographic guidance. A sclerosing agent should not be instilled if the patient has had no treatment for the tumor. Supportive care for constrictive pericarditis is the same as for tamponade from effusion. The definitive treatment for constrictive pericarditis is surgical: pericardiectomy or pericardial window. The indications are tamponade from constrictive pericarditis or persistent symptomatic effusion unresponsive to steroids or other medical management.

In most patients with a Wilms' tumor thrombus extending into the right side of the heart, the mass does not occlude the chambers, and therapy with dactinomycin and vincristine may reduce the size of thrombus within a week (also see Chap. 27). If hypotension or cardiac arrest occurs, open heart surgery is indicated. Indeed, the review by Nakayama and associates suggests that primary surgery should be used whenever possible and, in centers with adequate facilities for cardiopulmonary bypass, may be preferable to preoperative chemotherapy.[26]

ABDOMINAL EMERGENCIES

Definition of the Problem

The important issue in the assessment of an acute abdomen in a child with cancer is whether the child requires an operation. Until the last decade, the medical literature was replete with document of disastrous results in children with leukemia who developed abdominal complications.[27,28] The outcome of surgical intervention was particularly disappointing because the prevailing approach entailed managing an abdominal complication with intensive medical therapy in any and every way possible to avoid surgical intervention.

The current approach is more optimistic and aggressive. Appropriate surgical intervention is often life-saving. Since most abdominal emergencies present as an acute abdomen, early collaborative evaluation and continuing consultation are mandatory (see also Chap. 10).

Etiology and Pathophysiology

Although a child with cancer can develop an acute abdomen for the same reasons as any other child of the same age, such as volvulus in an infant or appendicitis in an older child,[29] an acute abdomen unrelated to the underlying malignancy is exceptional. There are many causes of abdominal emergencies that are almost unique to the immunocompromised host: esophagitis, gastric hemorrhage, typhlitis, perirectal abscess, hemorrhagic pancreatitis, and massive acute hepatic enlargement from tumor.

Abdominal emergencies in the child with cancer, as in any child, arise because of inflammation, mechanical obstruction, hemorrhage, and perforation.[30-33] Processes that are localized in healthy children, however, may be generalized in the neutropenic or immunosuppressed child. Moreover, the inflammatory response may be blunted by a lack of cells to mediate inflammation. Obstruction may result from a mass effect or chemotherapy-induced ileus. Hemorrhage may result from thrombocytopenia, coagulopathy, mucosal ulceration, or abnormal tumor vessels. Perforation may result from localized ulceration and segmental necrosis. Wound healing may be slow because of the effects of malnutrition and chemotherapy, most notably corticosteroids, on fibroblast proliferation and collagen production.[34,35]

Evaluation and Differential Diagnosis

Pain is the principal symptom of an acute abdominal process, no matter how compromised the patient. It is important to understand the location, quality, and timing of pain in relation to the primary diagnosis, recent medications, or previous surgery. Changes in vital signs including fever, hypertension or hypotension, and tachycardia; the presence of blood in vomitus or stool; abdominal distention; or cessation of passage of flatus are less specific indications of an acute abdomen.

Before abdominal examination, one must spend sufficient time to gain the patient's trust to allow an adequate assessment. It is best to perform as much of the examination as possible without causing discomfort. Observation is painless. Does the child lie motionless on the bed, or is he willing to move about? Does the child wince with cough, movement, or motion of the bed? Does the child's abdomen appear scaphoid or distended? Are there scars or areas of fullness to give a clue to the cause of the discomfort?

Auscultation can help differentiate ileus from obstruction. Complete absence of bowel sounds or waves, rushes, and paroxysms are more likely indications of obstruction, whereas an occasional tinkle or drip-drop plunking sound are often heard in ileus.[35] Chemotherapeutic agents such as vincristine cause constipation, ileus, and distention but rarely cause obstruction.

Gentle palpation during auscultation is an excellent and diverting diagnostic tool. Spasm, guarding, and tenderness can be assessed with gentle examination. Encouraging the child to participate may make the examination easier. However, a child's cooperation may be deceptive: the sickest child may cooperate because he is too weak to do otherwise.

Rectal examination is mandatory. It can detect pelvic, perianal, and anorectal disease and is an essential means of evaluat-

ing the peritoneal cavity. Thrombocytopenia, neutropenia, and pain are not contraindications to a gentle rectal examination—using the fifth finger in infants, for example. Pain detected on rectal examination may be the result of generalized serositis or mucositis.

Diagnostic Studies

Selective use of diagnostic studies and laboratory aids may distinguish the child who requires immediate surgical intervention from one who will benefit more from conservative medical management.

Serial blood counts can help to differentiate hemorrhage, local inflammation, and sepsis in situations where pus and abscess formation may not develop because of neutropenia. Blood cultures may indicate the presence of an abscess, especially when they are persistently positive despite treatment with appropriate antibiotics. Electrolyte changes may show metabolic deficits from fluid shifts before these are apparent clinically. Abdominal paracentesis and diagnostic lavage may give information about extraluminal bleeding, intestinal perforation, or infection. Table 37-2 presents the differential diagnosis of acute intra-abdominal processes based on peritoneal fluid findings in normal hosts. In neutropenic patients, the presence of any neutrophils is suggestive of infection or perforation, whereas their absence does not rule out these conditions.

Diagnostic radiologic studies begin with supine, erect, and left lateral decubitus abdominal films (also see Chap. 7).[36] Obstruction, especially high small-bowel obstruction, pneumatosis intestinalis, and free air, can be seen in these studies. A chest film may help distinguish an ileus associated with pneumonitis from an intra-abdominal process. A barium swallow study may help diagnose esophagitis. On the other hand, barium enemas are rarely indicated in the evaluation of a compromised child with an acute abdomen; direct examination with endoscopy or colonoscopy has tended to replace contrast studies in the evaluation of gastrointestinal bleeding in compromised as well as in healthy children.[36] Abdominal sonography (US), CT, magnetic resonance imaging (MRI), and angiography may all be helpful in locating and characterizing mass lesions. However, each study must be interpreted in light of the clinical findings.

Specific causes of abdominal emergencies in children with cancer are discussed below by region.

Table 37-2

Laboratory Criteria for Positive Peritoneal Lavage (Intestinal Perforation or Hemorrhage)

	Positive	*Indeterminate*	*Negative*
RBC/mm³	≥100,000	50,000–100,000	<50,000
WBC/mm³	≥500	100–500	0–100*
Amylase (mg/dl)	175	75–175	<75
Bile	+	−	−
Intestinal contents	+	−	−
Bacteria, yeast, *etc.* (Gram stain/ culture)	+	−	−

* Absence of WBC in neutropenic patient may not rule out perforation.

Esophagus

Esophagitis

The most common esophageal problem seen in children with cancer is esophagitis. This condition is discussed in Chapter 39.

Esophageal Varices

Varices can develop as an effect of hepatotoxic therapy. They may occur weeks or months after daunomycin and 6-thioguanine for acute nonlymphocytic leukemia or after transplantation or years later as a result of methotrexate-induced hepatic fibrosis. Variceal bleeding is brisk; it is appropriately treated with a systemic infusion of vasopressin at a rate of 0.2 and 0.4 units per minute.[32] Patients with bleeding varices also may require the use of a Sengstaken–Blakemore tube. Sclerotherapy is occasionally useful, and a splenorenal shunt may be a last resort.

Stomach

Children with cancer are prone to multiple punctate shallow gastric and duodenal ulcers: "stress ulcers" or "Cushing's ulcers." Children taking high-dose corticosteroids and those with increased intracranial pressure are at especially high risk. These ulcers may present with exsanguinating hemor-

rhage.[37–39] Children receiving steroids for posterior fossa tumors should be treated empirically with antacids and cimetidine.[40] Medical management of bleeding consists of antacids, lavage, and correction of thrombocytopenia and coagulation abnormalities. Operation for bleeding uncontrolled by medical management must be individualized but most often entails vagotomy, pyloroplasty, and oversewing of the ulcer.

Small Intestine

Dewar and coworkers have characterized four distinct types of bowel lesions in leukemic patients: [1] mucosal hemorrhagic necrosis; [2] leukemic infiltration, which may cause necrosis, intussusception, and obstruction; [3] agranulocytic necrosis, typically seen with typhlitis (see section on large intestine), which may be a form of pseudomembranous enterocolitis; and [4] fungal lesions.[41] Thrombocytopenia or coagulopathy may contribute to a bleeding tendency in these children. Children may have acute massive hemorrhage from fungal ulcers in the small bowel. Candidial jejunal ulcers may cause bleeding in bone-marrow transplant recipients.[28] Antifungal therapy should be started empirically, but primary resection and anastomosis may be required. Treatment decisions must be based on the patient's anatomy, prior therapy, nutrition, and coagulation status.[42]

Small-bowel obstruction from primary or metastatic cancer is rare in children. The differential diagnosis of small-bowel obstruction in the child who has had adjuvant therapy or

FIGURE 37-3. Flat (**A**) and erect (**B**) abdominal radiographs in a 3-year-old white girl 6 days after removal of a Wilms' tumor. Radiographic evidence of a complete small bowel obstruction is present. Jejunal–ileal intussusception was found at laparotomy and manually reduced. The child recovered promptly.

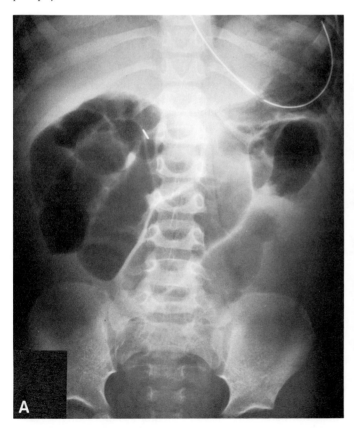

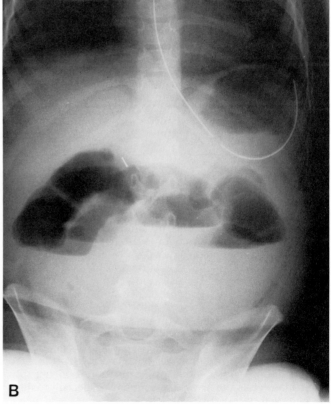

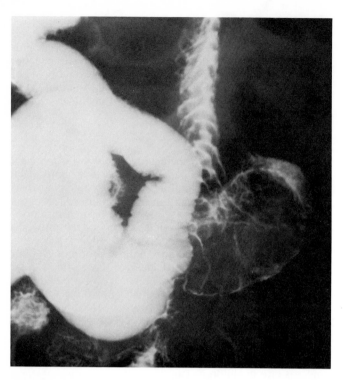

FIGURE 37-4.   Contrast study of the patient depicted in Figure 37-3 demonstrating a filling defect that represents a small bowel intussusception.

previous abdominal surgery includes vinca alkaloid-induced obstipation, adhesions or stricture, and intussusception. Small-bowel intussusception frequently occurs days to weeks postoperatively (Figs. 37-3 and 37-4).

Small-bowel obstruction is managed initially with a nasogastric tube for decompression. History, physical examination, and radiographs that document obstipation can help differentiate vincristine-related ileus from a surgical abdomen. A Miller–Abbott or other long intestinal tube alone may be sufficient in the child who is recently postoperative; however, its use is unwarranted in the child who has had an abdominal procedure in the distant past except for early decompression pending definitive surgery.

Typhlitis

Right lower-quadrant pain in the child with cancer may be from appendicitis; however, in the neutropenic child, typhlitis is the major concern. Typhlitis, from the Greek *typhlon* meaning cecum, is a necrotizing colitis localized to the cecum. Bacterial invasion of the mucosa may progress from inflammation to full-thickness infarction and perforation. *Clostridium septicum* is the single bacterial species most commonly implicated, and gram-negative bacteria (particularly *Pseudomonas aeruginosa*) can also cause this syndrome.[43,44] Typhlitis occurs only in the setting of severe neutropenia. Wagner and associates found that 10% of patients with leukemia have typhlitis at autopsy.[45] Shamberger and coworkers found that one-third of patients with acute myelogenous leukemia had documented typhlitis during induction therapy.[46] This figure is higher than that in most series and may reflect a regimen especially toxic to the intestinal tract. Typhlitis also occurs in transplant recipients. Radiographic studies may demonstrate pneumatosis in-

testinalis or nonspecific bowel-wall thickening (Figs. 37-5 and 37-6). Diffuse thickening of the cecal wall on CT scan in a neutropenic patient with fever and right lower quadrant pain is highly suggestive of typhlitis.[47]

Treatment of typhlitis is controversial.[45,46,48,49] The mortality rate ranges from 50% to nearly 100% with either operative or supportive treatment. Recently, Shamberger and associates proposed four criteria for surgical intervention in typhlitis: [1] persistent gastrointestinal bleeding despite resolution of neutropenia and thrombocytopenia and correction of clotting abnormalities; [2] evidence of free intraperitoneal perforation; [3] clinical deterioration requiring support with vasopressors or large volumes of fluid, suggesting uncontrolled sepsis from intestinal infarction; and [4] development of symptoms of an intra-abdominal process, which, in the absence of neutropenia, would normally require operation.[46] Pneumatosis and localized peritoneal signs are not sufficient to warrant exploration in the absence of one or more of the four guidelines. Using these criteria, 80% of patients can be managed medically with broad-spectrum antibiotics to cover gram-negative pathogens and clindamycin to treat gastrointestinal anaerobes (see Chap. 39). In children who require operation, diversion is the best treatment.

Patients who do not fit the description of typhlitis but yet have signs and symptoms of enterocolitis may have antibiotic-related pseudomembranous or clostridial enterocolitis.[49] The evaluation, management, and operative guidelines outlined above for typhlitis hold up well when dealing with these syndromes. However, these conditions are often generalized processes that are difficult to manage in any fashion (see Chap. 39).

Perirectal Abscess

Anorectal pain, tenderness, and discomfort with bowel movements may indicate a perirectal abscess or fistula. Perirectal abscesses occur in patients with chronic neutropenia, especially those with myeloid leukemia. Superficial lesions are obvious; deeper lesions require careful rectal examination (also see Chap. 39). In a neutropenic patient, the abscess may not be palpable; the only physical finding may be brawny woody edema with a dense cellulitic reaction. Most of these infections are caused by a mixture of aerobes and anaerobes. Initial therapy should include antibiotics to cover gram-negative bacilli, enterococcus and anaerobes (see Chap. 39). Sitz baths may help relieve pain. If the abscess or induration is well circumscribed or progresses on antibiotic therapy, incision and drainage can be attempted. However, not all patients require surgical intervention, and early aggressive medical management may eliminate the need for incision and drainage, particularly while the patient is neutropenic. Careful follow-up evaluation of the patient is important, but repeated rectal examinations should be avoided.

Acute rectal obstruction is rare. However, presacral teratomas and pelvic sarcomas may occlude the rectum. Use of a stool softener and passage of a small well-lubricated rectal tube may help until specific treatment of the tumor reduces the mass effect.

Cholecystitis and Biliary Obstruction

Inflammation of the liver and biliary tract can present as localized right upper-quadrant pain or jaundice.[50] Acute cholecystitis and, particularly, acute acalculous cholecystitis occur in children who are septic, stressed, and volume depleted. Ultra-

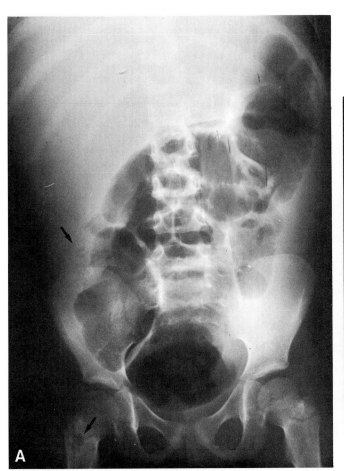
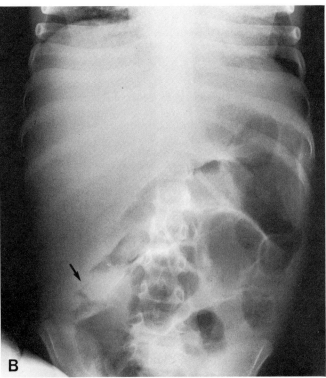

FIGURE 37-5.   Flat (**A**) and upright (**B**) abdominal radiographs of a 5-year-old girl with marrow aplasia who developed abdominal pain and right lower quadrant tenderness. Fullness and heme positive diarrhea were noted. Radiographs demonstrate a right lower quadrant mass and extraluminal gas (*arrow*). Also visible is an osteomyelitis of the right femur. The child was operated on for suspected typhlitis, which was confirmed by exploratory laparotomy. She underwent a right colectomy with end ileostomy. Her operative procedure was tolerated well.

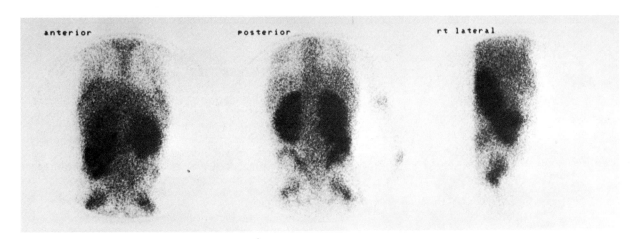

FIGURE 37-6.   A gallium scan of the patient in Figure 37-5 shows increased radionuclide uptake in the right lower quadrant.

sonography or CT scan can differentiate calculous from acalculous cholecystitis. Hydration, broad-spectrum antibiotics, and nasogastric decompression will usually treat the acute process of cholecystitis. Antibiotics should cover gram-negative bacilli and, in the neutropenic patient, fungi. Sludge in the biliary tree, often seen in the acute setting and sometimes associated with pancreatitis, may disappear once the patient is fully resuscitated. Biliary obstruction as a result of primary tumor is rare, although lymphoma and neuroblastoma occasionally block biliary flow and rhabdomyosarcoma of the common duct has been described.

Acute Massive Hepatomegaly in Neuroblastoma

Massive hepatomegaly may complicate Stage IV-S neuroblastoma in the neonate (see Chaps. 10 and 28). Unless there is life-threatening respiratory embarrassment, supportive care and observation are sufficient until the disease resolves spontaneously. If hepatomegaly compromises respiratory function, the therapeutic options include chemotherapy and irradiation and, rarely, surgical enlargement of the abdominal wall with a Silastic patch.[51] The irradiation technique involves lateral portals with the child supine and fields encompassing most of the liver but sparing the ovaries and kidneys and extending from the dome to the posterior portion of the right hepatic lobe. The midplane dose is 150 cGy given on three successive days.

Hemorrhagic Pancreatitis

Children with acute lymphoblastic leukemia treated with L-asparaginase can develop hemorrhagic pancreatitis.[52] Sterile pancreatitis may be followed by superinfection with either bacteria or fungi. Nasogastric drainage, maintenance of hydration, and antibiotics are essential support.

The indications for and the timing of surgical drainage of a pancreatic abscess depend on the child's condition and the appearance of the process on sequential US and CT examinations.[53,54] Whereas an area of phlegmon can be treated conservatively, localized abscess and pancreatic dissolution require emergency open drainage. A CT scan with contrast medium may show phlegmon as a diffuse homogeneous area, whereas abscess may appear as a loculation or loculations of various densities within the pancreatic substance. When pancreatitis develops into a pseudocyst, supportive care permitting maturation of the cyst beyond 6 weeks will often facilitate effective internal drainage. Percutaneous CT-guided drainage may also be effective.

GENITOURINARY EMERGENCIES

Hemorrhagic Cystitis

Definition

Hemorrhagic cystitis consists of painful urination with leukocytes, erythrocytes, or clots in the urine because of bleeding and inflammation of the bladder.

Etiology and Pathophysiology

Cyclophosphamide and ifosfamide are the most common causes.[55-58] Cystitis may occur hours or years after cyclophosphamide administration. The early phases of cystitis are mucosal edema, ulceration, subendothelial telangectasia, and sub-

mucosal fibrosis.[56,57] Late developments are bladder fibrosis with reflux and hydronephrosis. Damage is caused by an acrolein dye that is a byproduct of cyclophosphamide metabolism. With stasis of acrolein-containing urine, damage can occur to the collecting system and ureters as well.[56]

Evaluation and Differential Diagnosis

The diagnosis is made by history and urinalysis. Ultrasonography may demonstrate a boggy, edematous, hemorrhagic bladder or possibly a fibrotic bladder with hemorrhage. Direct examination may be necessary to locate large areas of bleeding. Immediate treatment consists of hydration, transfusion, correction of thrombocytopenia and coagulation abnormalities, and removal of clots via a catheter or cystoscopically. Spasm may be controlled with belladonna and opium suppositories. Concurrent bladder irradiation and chemotherapy with radiomimetic agents should be stopped.[58]

Patients who continue to bleed should have endoscopy with electrocoagulation of the bleeding areas, but occasionally this is unsuccessful. An alternative treatment involves instilling a 0.25% solution of formalin into the bladder via a Foley catheter while the patient is under anesthesia.[59] The absence of ureterovesical reflux must be demonstrated prior to this treatment, because formalin can damage the ureters and kidneys. In those patients with reflux, alum instillation is preferred. Formalin therapy carries risks of severe complications including obstruction, extravasation, and bladder contraction; however, in the desperate situations of uncontrollable bladder hemorrhage, this treatment should be tried before proceeding to emergency cystectomy.[58]

Hemorrhagic cystitis can be prevented by acidification of the urine with ascorbic acid before infusing cyclophosphamide, vigorous hydration during and after treatment, and, most successfully, by the use of intravenous or, when tolerated, oral sodium-2-mercaptoethanesulfonate (MESNA).[60]

Urinary Flow Obstruction

Lesions of the spinal cord and bulky pelvic tumors, including retroperitoneal sarcomas and lymphomas, ovarian tumors, and bladder-wall rhabdomyosarcomas, and benign masses such as bowel duplication may cause acute urinary retention. All have characteristic radiographic and sonographic appearances. Vinca alkaloids, narcotic analgesics, and phenothiazines may also cause urinary retention. The initial management of the obstruction consists of catheterization or nephrostomy.

NEUROLOGIC EMERGENCIES

These emergencies may result from a direct effect of the malignancy, as a secondary effect of dysfunction of another organ system, or as a sequela of treatment. Neurologic emergencies in children with cancer can be classified as [1] acute alterations in consciousness, [2] cerebrovascular accidents (CVAs), [3] seizures, and [4] spinal cord compression. A detailed history with special attention to the treatment and an understanding of the metastatic pattern of the particular malignancy are crucial in making a prompt, correct diagnosis.

A frequent mistake in evaluating a child with cancer and an acute neurologic deficit is the omission of a careful, detailed neurologic examination. The child is often considered too weak, too uncooperative, or in too much pain to be put through a formal neurologic evaluation. Often, the reason for the child's malaise and discomfort lies in the central nervous system (CNS) impairment itself, and specific treatment will result in resolution of those symptoms. Furthermore, without neurologic localization of the deficit, unnecessary, potentially harmful investigations may be carried out, further delaying diagnosis and increasing discomfort.

Acute Alterations in Consciousness

Acute alterations in consciousness consist of lethargy, stupor, and coma.

Etiology

Acute alterations in consciousness often occur in the child with cancer who is medically unstable either because of systemic illness or primary CNS dysfunction. Table 37-3 lists the causes of acute alterations in consciousness in children with cancer over a 5-year period at the Children's Hospital of Philadelphia.

Pathogenesis

A state of full awareness depends on the integrity of the cerebral hemispheres and the ascending reticular activating system (ARAS), a polysynaptic neuronal network lying in the central core of the brainstem, thalamus, and hypothalamus.[61] The ARAS receives input from and projects to all portions of the CNS. Coma or other forms of alteration in consciousness result either from diffuse derangement of cerebral function or damage to the ARAS. The latter is most commonly caused by increased intracranial pressure or by a localized cortical mass, both of which may cause herniation or compression of the brainstem with disruption of the ARAS.[61]

Evaluation and Differential Diagnosis

The emergency evaluation of coma begins with assessment of vital signs followed by examination for evidence of cerebral herniation and signs of increased intracranial pressure and focal neurologic deficits. To determine whether there is herniation, special attention is given to breathing pattern, pupillary size and reactivity, extraocular movements, spontaneous motor function, and the response of the patient to verbal or physical stimuli. Clinical findings can localize the level of the brain involved (Tables 37-4 and 37-5).[61] A diffuse increase in intracranial pressure may cause a symmetric downward displacement of the brain through the tentorial opening, called rostrocaudal or central herniation, with gradual orderly failure of diencephalic and brain-stem functions. In contrast, uncal herniation results from lateralized mass lesions that shift the brain and compress the third nerve and lateral midbrain. Uncal herniation tends to be less predictable and more rapid. Brainstem dysfunction may ultimately occur, but in a less stereotyped fashion, with sparing of certain brain-stem functions such as pupillary responses despite compromise of lower brain-stem functions such as breathing. In the later stages of herniation, symptoms of the two forms often overlap. Metabolic disturbance can also cause signs of increased pressure and of central herniation but more frequently changes mentation.

A complete blood count, serum glucose and electrolytes, hepatic and renal function tests, and a coagulation profile should be obtained. After correction of vital signs and treatment of increased intracranial pressure, patients with presumed mass lesions or those with unexplained coma should undergo emergency CT scanning without and with intravenous

Table 37-3

Etiology of Acute Alterations in Consciousness in 61 Children with Systemic Cancer at Children's Hospital of Philadelphia, 1981–1986*

Intracranial hemorrhage excluding infarction	3
Cerebrovascular accident	3
Metastatic disease	15
Primary CNS fungal or bacterial infection	8
Viral encephalitis	6
Sepsis/disseminated intravascular coagulation	9
Metabolic abnormality	7
Leukoencephalopathy	3
Other†	4
Unknown	3

* Excluding postictal patients.
† Oversedation (2), somnolence postradiotherapy (1), and hemorrhage (1).

Table 37-4

Syndrome of Uncal Herniation

Pattern	Breathing Pattern	Pupillary Size/Reactivity	Oculocephalic/Oculovestibular Response	Motor Response to Noxious Stimuli
Early third nerve	Normal	Unilateral moderately dilated pupil (usually to side of lesion); dilated pupil reacts sluggishly	Full or dysconjugate	Appropriate (fends off) or unilateral hemiparesis
Late third nerve	Central hyperventilation or Cheyne–Stokes	Unilateral widely dilated pupil (usually to side of lesion); unreactive	Dysconjugate (absent, late); eye with dilated pupil does not move	Decorticate or decerebrate (may be asymmetric)
Midbrain, upper pons	Central hyperventilation	Bilateral midposition pupils, unreactive	Impaired or absent	Bilateral, decerebrate

(Plum F, Posner JB: Diagnosis of Stupor and Coma, Philadelphia, FA Davis, 1980; reprinted from Packer RJ, Berman PH: Coma. in Fleisher G, Ludwig S [eds]: Textbook of Pediatric Emergency Medicine, pp 87–101. Baltimore, Williams & Wilkins, 1983)

Table 37-5
Central Syndrome of Rostrocaudal Deterioration

Pattern	Breathing Pattern	Pupillary Size/Reactivity	Oculocephalic/Oculovestibular Response	Motor Response to Noxious Stimuli
Early diencephallic	Cheyne–Stokes	Small pupils; reactive	Full doll's eye; full ipsilateral (toward side of ice water irrigation) tonic deviation	Appropriate (fends off stimuli) or rigidity
Late diencephallic	Cheyne–Stokes	Small pupils; reactive	Full doll's eye (easy to obtain); full ipsilateral tonic deviation (easy to obtain)	Decorticate posture
Midbrain, upper pons	Central hyperventilation	Midposition, ± irregular pupils; unreactive	Impaired, dysconjugate	Decerebrate posture
Lower pons, upper medulla	Shallow or ataxia	Pinpoint; unreactive	Absent	No response

(Plum F, Posmer JB: Diagnosis of Stupor Coma, Philadelphia, FA Davis, 1980; reprinted from Packer RJ, Berman PH: Coma. In Fleisher G, Ludwig S [eds]: Textbook of Pediatric Emergency Medicine, pp 87–101. Baltimore, Williams & Wilkins, 1983)

contrast medium (the latter provided there is no hyperviscosity or hyperosmolarity; see Chap. 7). Lumbar puncture is more safely performed after a mass lesion has been ruled out.

Focal intracranial mass lesions that cause coma in children with cancer include infarctions, hemorrhages, metastases, and abscesses. Acute thrombotic or, rarely, embolic CVAs can cause neurologic deterioration (see section on cerebrovascular accidents).[63] Subdural hematomas and intracranial hemorrhages may complicate platelet-resistant thrombocytopenia.[63] Metastatic spread of tumor to the CNS occurs late in the disease in children with sarcomas, lymphomas, and primary renal tumors. Children with cancer who are myelosuppressed or immunosuppressed are prone to fungal or bacterial brain abscess (see Chap. 39). Diagnosis may be difficult because fever and meningismus may be absent.

If focal lesions are not found, diffuse lesions must be considered. Infections can affect the brain diffusely. Viral encephalitis, most commonly from varicella or herpes simplex, may result in acute coma. Metabolic derangements that alter consciousness include anoxia, ischemia, hepatic and renal failure, and electrolyte abnormalities. Intracranial disseminated intravascular coagulation (DIC) may occur without evidence of systemic hematologic abnormalities; the diagnosis may be difficult early in the process.[63] Leukemic meningitis and hyperleukocytosis are relatively infrequent causes of acute alterations in consciousness. A postictal state is also a possible cause of coma. Deterioration and obtundation are commonly seen in a child previously treated with a neurotoxic agent such as radiation or methotrexate. The CNS of such patients is essentially primed for neurologic compromise, and relatively mild metabolic derangements or sedative drugs can cause a degree of suppression of consciousness that seems out of proportion to the acute insult. Such a multifactorial cause of coma is especially common in children with leukemia who have received extensive CNS therapy and in patients who have undergone bone-marrow transplant.[64] However, before a complex etiology for coma is accepted, focal mass lesions and other treatable processes must be ruled out.

Therapy and Recommendations

If the vital signs of the child are not normal, life-threatening respiratory and circulatory disturbances must be corrected. Symptoms or signs of increased intracranial pressure should be managed with measures to decrease that pressure, including

hyperventilation, intravenous dexamethasone (1–2 mg/kg), and possibly infusion of mannitol in a 20% solution at 1.25 to 2 g/kg. The effects of intravenous dexamethasone may be delayed. Hyperventilation sufficient to decrease the partial pressure of blood carbon dioxide to 20 to 25 mm Hg reduces cerebral blood flow. Excessive hyperventilation may result in too drastic a decrease in blood flow and relative ischemia of the brain.

If a mass lesion or acute hydrocephalus is demonstrated on CT and medical management fails to reduce the pressure, surgical intervention may be indicated. If bacterial meningitis is suspected, antibiotics should be given before CT. If the patient has thrombocytopenia or a coagulopathy, it should be corrected before lumbar puncture or surgery.

Cerebrovascular Accidents

Etiology

Three percent of children with non-CNS primary malignancies develop cerebrovascular compromise. Children with leukemia are at greatest risk.[49] Cerebrovascular accident may be secondary to direct or metastatic spread of tumor, to antineoplastic agents, to hematologic abnormalities, or to primary CNS infections (Table 37-6). In children with cancer, CVA is most frequently due to cerebral arterial or venous thrombosis or to intracerebral hemorrhage; embolic causes are unlikely.

When a CVA occurs at the onset of illness, it is most commonly associated with disease-related coagulation abnormalities. During treatment, most strokes can be related to a specific chemotherapeutic agent. At the end stages of disease, sepsis, DIC, CNS infection, and progressive tumor are common causes. Strokes occurring months to years after children have apparently become free of disease are most likely secondary to radiation-induced vascular damage.

Pathogenesis

L-asparaginase has been associated with venous thrombosis or lateral and sagittal sinus thrombosis near the end of induction therapy (see Chap. 16).[65] Smaller arterial thrombosis may also occur, and there may be a combination of hemorrhage and thrombosis. L-asparaginase-associated events are believed to be caused by a rebound hypercoagulable state following drug-

Table 37-6
Etiology of Cerebrovascular Accidents in Children with Cancer

Malignancy-related
    Leptomeningeal disease
    Metastatic disease
    DIC
Chemotherapy-related
    L-asparaginase
    Methotrexate (?)
Radiation-related
    Large-vessel occlusion
    Mineralizing microangiopathy
Infections
    Bacterial meningitis
    Fungal meningitis

(Packer RJ, Rorke LB, Lange BL et al: Cerebrovascular accidents in children with cancer. Pediatrics 76:194–201, 1985. Reproduced by permission of Pediatrics)

induced imbalance in production of coagulation and anticoagulation factors (see Chap. 38).[65] Patients with L-asparaginase-associated strokes have received subsequent courses of the drug without sequelae, strongly suggesting that L-asparaginase toxicity does not have an allergic basis.[65]

Children with acute nonlymphocytic leukemia, especially those with acute promyelocytic leukemia, acute monoblastic leukemia, or high white cell counts, are at especially high risk for strokes (see section on hyperleukocytosis and Chap. 38).[65-70] Leukemic promyelocytes and monoblasts contain poorly characterized procoagulants,[65-67] and as these cells lyse, the procoagulant is released, causing DIC and CVA. The CVA usually occurs early in the illness and may even be the presenting symptom. Myelodysplasia or leukemia with peripheral hypereosinophilia and acute megakaryoblastic leukemia are also associated with an increased risk of stroke.

Intracranial DIC is probably the least-recognized cause of CVA.[61,63] DIC-associated strokes occur primarily in children with lymphoreticular malignancies. Intracranial DIC may present as a diffuse encephalopathy with or without seizures. Because it most frequently occurs in an ill, septic child, the child's neurologic deterioration is often misdiagnosed as a metabolic encephalopathy or a CNS relapse. If the DIC process remains localized, laboratory evidence of intravascular coagulation may be delayed for as long as 48 hours after the onset of symptoms or may not be manifest at all.[63,71] Nonbacterial thrombotic endocarditis is the leading cause of strokes in adults with cancer; however, it is yet to be linked to strokes in pediatric patients.[71,72]

Radiation therapy may cause delayed large- and small-vessel occlusions.[73,74] Total doses of radiotherapy in excess of 5500 cGy or dose fractions of 250 to 350 cGy have been related to large-vessel occlusions. The peak incidence of large-vessel occlusions is at 6 months to 3 years after treatment, but occlusions may take place many years later. Rare patients develop a CVA after lower doses or conventional fractions of radiation (180–200 cGy). In these cases, CVA has been considered an idiosyncratic event. More commonly, radiotherapy causes small focal vascular occlusions. Mineralizing microangiopathy with dystrophic calcification is seen histopathologically in many children who have died of cancer but is rarely reported in children who have received less than 2000 cGy. The addition of intrathecal methotrexate and cytosine arabinoside (cytarabine) may increase the risk of damage.

Hemorrhagic CVAs usually occur preterminally, especially in children with neuroblastoma metastatic to the dura and in those with platelet-resistant thrombocytopenia. Neuroblastoma may also cause lateral and transverse sinus thrombosis by compression from metastases to the calvarium adjacent to the venous channels.

High-dose methotrexate can cause acute focal neurologic deficits. Initially, this was postulated to be on a vascular basis. However, recent evidence suggests that this syndrome is more likely due to acute intracellular metabolic derangements.[75,76]

Evaluation and Differential Diagnosis

Cerebrovascular accidents usually present as acute impairments in motor function or speech, often with associated seizures. A major CVA, such as a sagittal sinus thrombosis or a brain-stem stroke, can also cause significant obtundation. It may be impossible to distinguish between a CVA and a postictal state if focal seizures occur, but if symptoms do not clear within 24 hours after the ictus, the patient should be considered to have structural CNS damage until proved otherwise. Children with multiple small infarctions from intracranial DIC commonly have a stuttering, subacute onset of symptoms.

In evaluating a child with cancer and a presumed CVA, one must consider the type of tumor, the extent and status of the disease, the antineoplastic treatment, and any associated medical complications. In a critically ill child with extensive uncontrollable cancer, no specific evaluation may be indicated. However, laboratory studies may still help in managing the child, in helping the family understand the disease process, and thus in long-term decision-making.

After the child has been medically stabilized, CT should be performed without and with contrast medium. In patients with small subcortical or small vessel infarcts, the initial scan may be normal or show nonspecific changes. In these cases, the study may need to be repeated 7 to 10 days later to document infarction and demonstrate the full extent of damage.[78] Care should be taken to evaluate the torcular region of the calvarium and dura, especially in children with neuroblastoma, to rule out the possibility of sinus thrombosis.

If the CT scan does not show a focal mass lesion, lumbar puncture can be performed for analysis of opening pressure, protein, and glucose and for cell count, cytology, and culture. Children who have received cranial irradiation or neurotoxic drugs should have the myelin basic protein level in the cerebrospinal fluid measured because elevated values may be helpful in the diagnosis of leukoencephalopathy.[79,80] The same precautions discussed previously should be taken at the time of lumbar puncture.

Arteriography can help in confirming a specific diagnosis but is rarely needed at the onset of symptoms. It is most useful in documenting the presence of partial sagittal sinus thrombosis or radiation vasculitis. Similarly, digital subtraction angiography is helpful in the diagnosis of sagittal sinus thrombosis, but the diagnosis usually can be made on the basis of other tests.

Therapy and Recommendations

Management of a CVA is supportive in most cases. The management of patients with nonmetastatic sagittal sinus thrombosis includes corticosteroids and hyperosmolar agents to decrease the intracranial pressure. The use of anticoagulants is potentially detrimental because they may cause extension of the venous infarct. Some authors recommend twice-daily fresh frozen plasma or infusions of antithrombin III concentrate for patients with L-asparaginase CVA or with profound coagulation abnormalities while they are receiving this drug.[81,82] However, it is apparent that almost all patients receiving this drug have coagulation abnormalities, and it is difficult to determine which ones will suffer a CVA.[83] Treatment of DIC associated with acute promyelocytic leukemia or monoblastic leukemia consists of platelet and plasma transfusions and possibly low-dose heparinization when there is laboratory evidence of DIC (see Chap. 38).[68-70] In children with neuroblastoma metastatic to the torcula region, emergency radiation to the sinus area (*e.g.,* 300 cGy per day for 3 days) can resolve the symptoms rapidly. In the child with an intracerebral hemorrhage, surgical intervention may be lifesaving, but since many of these patients are severely thrombocytopenic and at the end stage of their disease, operative relief is seldom warranted.

Management of radiation-induced vascular change is primarily supportive. When large areas of focal necrosis are present, surgical debulking may be rewarding.[84] Although both hyperbaric oxygenation and anticoagulation have been recommended for the treatment of radiation-induced vasculitis, their efficacy is unproved.[85]

Seizures

Seizures are transient involuntary alterations of consciousness, behavior, motor function, sensation, or autonomic function.

Etiology and Pathogenesis

A seizure is caused by an excessive rate in hypersynchrony of discharges from a group of cerebral neurons. Table 37-7 lists

Table 37-7
Causes of Seizures in 46 Children with Systemic Cancer at Children's Hospital of Philadelphia, 1981–1986

Metastatic disease	14
Cerebrovascular disease	4
Primary CNS infection	5
Treatment sequelae	9
Metabolic abnormality	3
Other	7
Unknown	4

the etiologies of seizures in children with cancer. Metastatic spread of tumor usually occurs late in the course of disease. Cerebrovascular accidents and primary CNS infections result from therapy- or disease-induced complications including those attributable to vincristine, intrathecal methotrexate, cisplatin, or cytosine arabinoside. Antineoplastic therapy can cause convulsions, especially in children who have received cranial irradiation. Radiation-induced small-vessel disease, cerebral necrosis, and leukoencephalopathy are associated with seizures. Metabolic abnormalities from disease or treatment predispose to seizures, either focal or generalized, especially in patients who have received previous CNS therapy and have underlying structural brain injury.

Evaluation of Differential Diagnosis

A seizure must always be viewed as a symptom of an underlying pathologic process. The investigation of the seizure is similar to that previously discussed for encephalopathy and CVA and should take place as soon as the seizure is controlled. CT without and with contrast is indicated. MRI is extremely sensitive for the detection of treatment-related CNS damage and may show abnormalities not seen by CT.[86] Cerebrospinal fluid analysis after CT is an integral part of the evaluation. Electroencephalography localizes the origin of the seizure and may demonstrate electrical seizure activity that may not be obvious clinically.

Therapy and Recommendations

Most seizures are self-limited, although occasionally a prolonged seizure requires emergency management.[87-89] Initially, the adequacy of ventilation and circulation must be assured; anticonvulsants are then given (Table 37-8). Of special note are drugs that cause respiratory depression or hypotension. These problems are managable, but they may require a level of cardiac and respiratory support that is undesirable in patients with end-stage disease.

Most children with cancer and seizures require antiepileptic medication for at least a few days after the seizure. Phenytoin or phenobarbital, when used to stop the seizure, may be continued through the first few days. In cases of CNS infection and metabolic seizures, these medications can be withdrawn relatively soon (1 week to 1 month) after correction of the

Table 37-8
Anticonvulsants for Status Epilepticus in Children with Cancer

Anticonvulsant	Dose (mg/kg)	Onset of Action	Advantages	Disadvantages
Diazepam	0.2–0.3 IV (max 10 mg total) at 1 mg/min; may repeat in 20 min (max 3 doses)	Seconds–minutes	Rapid onset of action	Short duration of action (15–20 minutes); respiratory depression; hypotension
Lorazepam	0.05 IV over 2 min	Seconds–minutes	Rapid onset of action; longer duration than diazepam	Respiratory depression; hypotension
Phenytoin	10 IV at 30–50 mg/min	Seconds–minutes	Minimal sedation; rapid onset of action	Cardiac depression
Phenobarbitol	10 IV or IM (max 150 mg)	20–30 minutes	Good intramuscular absorption	Respiratory depression; delayed effect; long half-life (53–118 hours)
Paraldehyde	0.3 with 0.3 ml/kg mineral oil rectally	Minutes	For seizures resistant to other medications; little respiratory depression	Rectal route of administration

underlying abnormality if the follow-up electroencephalogram shows no epileptiform activity and there is no residual focal CNS deficit.

Spinal Cord Compression

Etiology

Four per cent of children with cancer develop spinal cord dysfunction, which is nearly always due to tumor-related compression.[90,91] Another 5% to 10% of patients develop back pain that must be distinguished from spinal cord compression. Sarcomas account for 43% to 65% of metastatic spinal cord disease in childhood, and neuroblastoma, lymphomas, and leukemias account for the most of the rest.[90,91] Spinal cord disease develops in 10% to 12% of patients with sarcomas and 3% to 4% percent of patients with lymphoma. Treatment-related myelitis may also cause neurologic compromise and cannot readily be distinguished from spinal cord compression by clinical criteria alone (see Chaps. 11 and 50).[91] Although it is not life-threatening in most patients, cord compression causes severe neurologic morbidity.[90-94]

Pathogenesis

The spinal cord and cauda equina may be compressed by tumor in the epidural or subarachnoid space or by metastatic spread to the cord parenchyma. Epidural compression is by far the most common. Metastatic involvement of the vertebral bodies and secondary compression of the spinal cord, the most frequent mode in adults with cancer, is uncommon in childhood.[93] Tumor is more likely to cause spinal cord compression by infiltrating through the intravertebral foramina.[91]

Evaluation and Differential Diagnosis

Although more likely to occur in the terminal phases of widely metastatic malignancy, spinal cord compression may be the presenting sign of cancers such as neuroblastoma, lymphomas, or, rarely, sarcoma. Back pain occurs in 80% of children with compression and may be either local or radicular.[91] Any child with cancer and back pain should be considered to have spinal cord compression until proved otherwise. Detailed neurologic examination with attention to extremity strength, reflexes, anal tone, and determination of a sensory level is mandatory. Localized tenderness to percussion is found in 80% to 90% of pa-

tients,[91] and the level of maximal spinal tenderness is a reliable localizing sign. At the time of diagnosis, most patients with spinal cord compression have significant objective loss of motor strength in the extremities. Sensory loss or a sensory level may be difficult to document. Based on clinical findings, the level of spinal cord involvement can usually be determined (Table 37-9); however, the absence of weakness or sensory abnormalities cannot be relied on to exclude spinal cord compression.

After the neurologic examination, spine radiographs should be obtained (see Chap. 7). More than 85% of adult cancer patients with spinal cord involvement have abnormal plain spine radiographs,[92,93] but less than one-half of children show abnormalities. A normal bone scan does not exclude epidural disease, and this study is not appropriate in the patient with progressing neurologic dysfunction.[91] A positive bone scan is helpful in localization but cannot distinguish between back pain due to local bone involvement and that due to spinal cord compression. Cerebrospinal fluid laboratory studies, although important in the evaluation of subarachnoid disease, are nonspecific and nonlocalizing in children with epidural disease. The protein concentration is elevated in patients with complete spinal cord block, but protein may be normal in patients with partial obstruction. Lumbar myelography has been the standard for diagnosis. Metrizamide CT is an alternative but requires imaging levels to demonstrate the presence or lack of disease. With either myelography[92] or metrizamide CT, every attempt should be made to do a complete study to determine the rostral and caudal extent of tumor involvement, since the lesion may include multiple vertebral levels either continuously or discontinuously. Thus, if a complete block is demonstrated by lumbar myelography, contrast medium must be introduced at C1-C2 to define the upper extent.

Magnetic resonance imaging with a surface coil has recently been proved useful in evaluating spinal cord disease in children (see Chap. 7).[94] Epidural disease is well seen on MRI, which can also demonstrate associated intraparenchymal spread of tumor. However, it is as yet unclear whether MRI can detect small lesions compressing nerve roots in the cauda equina region. Any child who is nonambulatory at the time of clinical presentation, independent of the duration of dysfunction prior to evaluation, should undergo emergency myelography or MRI. Close observation is indicated in the child with local back pain and no evidence of myelopathy on examination. Plain radiographs of the spine or bone scans, or both may be useful in these children to help identify a local cause for the

---

Table 37-9
Clinical Localization of Epidural Cord Compression

	Location		
Sign	*Spinal Cord*	*Conus Medullaris*	*Cauda Equina*
Weakness	Symmetric; profound	Symmetric; variable	Asymmetric; may be mild
Tendon reflexes	Increased or absent	Increased knee; decreased ankle	Decreased; asymmetric
Babinski	Extensor	Extensor	Plantar
Sensory	Symmetric; sensory level	Symmetric; saddle	Asymmetric; radicular
Sphincter abnormality	Spared until late	Early involvement	May be spared
Progression	Rapid	Variable; may be rapid	Variable; may be rapid

pain. However, many of these patients will need myelography or MRI at some point during the investigation.

Therapy and Recommendations

An algorithm for the evaluation of patients with cancer and back pain is shown in Figure 37-7. If the history and physical examination suggest progressive or severe spinal cord dysfunction, dexamethasone (1–2 mg/kg intravenously) is given followed by immediate myelography.[95–97] MRI with a surface coil may be substituted for myelography for many patients unless small nerve root lesions are thought likely.[94] If the signs of spinal cord involvement are equivocal or if there is no evidence of progression of neurologic dysfunction, a lower dose of dexamethasone (0.25–0.5 mg/kg orally) every 6 hours is recommended. Myelography is performed within the next 24 hours.

If an epidural mass is demonstrated, then the spinal cord must be decompressed immediately. Although corticosteroids reduce edema rapidly and result in neurologic improvement, they are not an alternative to spinal decompression. Both local radiotherapy and surgical decompression can be used; in studies to date, there is little evidence to recommend one form of therapy over the other.[93,96]

A clear indication for surgery is the unknown primary. In the child with epidural disease without known dissemination, surgery offers the dual benefit of decompression plus identification of the tumor type. In adults with cancer in whom spinal cord compression most often results from vertebral body involvement and secondary epidural spread, vertebral body resection may be needed to decompress the cord.[92] However, since pediatric tumors more frequently enter the spinal canal by way of the intervertebral foramina, laminectomy and posterior decompression usually suffice.

Radiation therapy is chosen when the diagnosis is known, especially when the tumor type is radioresponsive. The portal should include the full volume implicated on myelogram plus one vertebral body above and below the visualized tumor. Supervoltage techniques are used, and three daily doses of 400 cGy each are given with concomitant dexamethasone. An additional four to nine 200-cGy fractions are given for totals of 2000 to 3000 cGy. The choice of total dose depends on tumor histology. Radioresponsive lesions such as non-Hodgkin's lymphoma receive the lower dose, whereas most other solid tumors are given the higher dose.

Recently, a third alternative, chemotherapy, has been suggested for patients with spinal cord compression.[98] This treatment has been effective in patients with asymptomatic epidural disease. The usefulness of this approach in patients with acutely symptomatic disease is unclear.

The prognosis for recovery in patients with spinal cord compression depends on the neurologic findings when treatment is begun. Patients who are ambulatory at the time treatment is started usually remain ambulatory.[96,98] In adults, patients who are nonambulatory at the time of treatment rarely regain function.[96] However, in a recent series, one-half of the children who were nonambulatory at the beginning of treatment regained the ability to walk after emergency treatment, reflecting the greater resilience of childhood tissues.[91] Every attempt should be made to diagnose and treat spinal cord compression as early as possible.

HYPERLEUKOCYTOSIS

Hyperleukocytosis is defined as a peripheral white blood cell count exceeding 100,000/μl.

Etiology

Hyperleukocytosis occurs in 9% to 13% of children with acute lymphocytic leukemia, 5% to 22% of children with acute nonlymphocytic leukemia, and virtually all children with chronic myelogenous leukemia in the chronic phase (see Chaps. 16 and 17).[99–101] Hyperleukocytosis can cause death by CNS hemorrhage or thrombosis (see section on cerebrovascular accidents), pulmonary leukostasis, and the metabolic derangements that accompany tumor lysis (see section on tumor lysis syndrome). Table 37-10 shows that intracerebral hemorrhage and pulmonary leukostasis are more likely to complicate acute nonlymphocytic than acute lymphocytic leukemia, whereas

FIGURE 37-7. Algorithm for evaluation of back pain in the child with proven or probable malignancy.

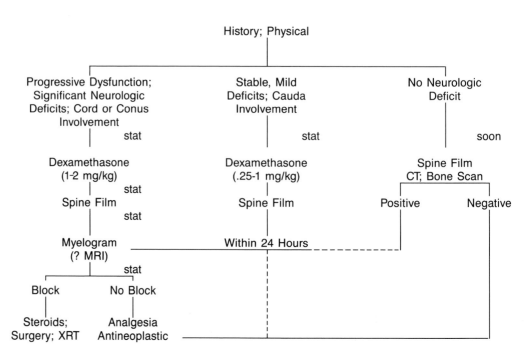

Table 37-10
Early Complications in Patients with Hyperleukocytosis

	ALL (N = 161)	ANLL (N = 73)	p Value*
Metabolic†	22	4	0.08
Hyperkalemia	16	2	
Decreased calcium/increased phosphorus	15	3	
Acute renal failure	5	4	
Respiratory	0	6	<0.001
Hemorrhagic	4	14	<0.001
CNS	2	9	
Gastrointestinal	0	2	
Pulmonary	2	3	
Pericardial	0	1	
Death	8	17	<0.001

(Bunin NJ, Piu CH: Differing complications of hyperleukocytosis in children with acute lymphoblastic or acute nonlymphoblastic leukemia. J Clin Oncol 3:1590–1595, 1985. Copyright © 1985 Grune & Stratton, Inc)
* For comparison of frequencies of the indicated complication in patients with acute lymphocytic leukemia versus those with acute nonlymphocytic leukemia.

the reverse is true of tumor lysis. Among 234 children with hyperleukocytosis, 23% of 73 patients with acute nonlymphocytic leukemia died during the early induction phase, whereas 5% of 161 patients with acute lymphocytic leukemia died during this time.[99] The risk of death increases greatly when the leukocyte count exceeds 300,000/μl.

Pathogenesis

Hyperleukocytosis increases blood viscosity by leading to blast cell aggregates and thrombi in the microcirculation (see Chap. 38).[101] The viscosity depends on the packed erythrocyte and the packed leukocyte volumes. Myeloblasts are relatively large (350–450 μm^3); lymphoblasts are smaller (250–350 μm^3). Blasts are not easily deformable and tend to trap plasma between them. The poor perfusion and anaerobic metabolism of the blasts within the microcirculation can contribute to lactic acidosis.[102] A packed cell volume of leukocytes exceeding 20% to 25% increases the bulk viscosity of blood.[101] The effects of trapped plasma and high white cell counts are likely to become apparent in the microcirculation at lower volumes of packed cells.

Fritz and associates first described the pathology of the effects of hyperleukocytosis on the cerebral vasculature.[70] In patients with counts greater than 300,000/μl, those investigators found local proliferation of cells within the cerebral vasculature and within the brain itself, resulting in damage to vessels and secondary hemorrhage. Tryka and coworkers characterized the pathology of pulmonary leukostasis as "leukemic cell lysis pneumonopathy": degenerating aggregates of blasts in the vessels and interstitium releasing their intracellular contents, which damage alveoli diffusely.[103]

Evaluation and Differential Diagnosis

Many children will have no particular signs or symptoms other than those of leukemia, but some will show signs of hypoxia and acidosis with dyspnea, blurred vision, agitation, confusion, delirium, and stupor. Physical examination may reveal plethora and cyanosis, papilledema, retinal artery or retinal vein disten-

tion, and ataxia.[101,104] Priapism occurs rarely,[105] and clitoral engorgement has been described once.[106] A number of investigators have found that hypoxia may be symptomatic in as many as 50% of children with chronic myelogenous leukemia.[101,107]

Therapy and Recommendations

Management of hyperleukocytosis has not been investigated in controlled studies. Hydration, alkalinization, and allopurinol should start immediately. Specific antileukemic therapy should begin as soon as life-threatening complications have been corrected (see tumor lysis section). If the platelet count is less than 20,000/μl, platelet transfusions can be given because cerebral hemorrhage is a definite risk and platelets will not add substantially to blood viscosity. Packed red cells, by contrast, must be given only with caution because they will increase viscosity.[108] The hemoglobin level should not be raised above 10 g/dl.

The use of exchange transfusion and leukopheresis is controversial. If a patient has congestive heart failure from the effects of hyperleukocytosis and anemia, partial exchange transfusion will correct the anemia and may correct hyperviscosity.[109,110] Frozen erythrocytes or those less than 5 days old should be used to assure adequate levels of 2,3-diphosphoglycerate.

Leukopheresis has been advocated by some investigators both to correct metabolic abnormalities and to reduce viscosity.[110–112] Its purpose is to reduce tumor bulk and the metabolic load on the kidneys. In two large uncontrolled series, leukopheresis did seem to prevent severe tumor lysis syndrome in patients with acute lymphocytic leukemia.[99,113] The procedure is usually well tolerated, but nonetheless, leukopheresis may fail to reduce the leukocyte count substantially. For example, Cuttner and associates found that 5 of their 22 patients with acute nonlymphocytic leukemia had less than a 30% reduction in white cell count following leukopheresis; none of the five achieved remission.[112] Other problems associated with leukopheresis are the need for anticoagulation, difficulty with access in small children, and limited availability in many institutions.[114] Whether leukopheresis reduces the risk of CNS hemorrhage in acute nonlymphocytic leukemia is unknown.

Several investigators have suggested that immediate cranial irradiation to 400 cGy be given to prevent CNS hemorrhage.[115,116] This recommendation is based on anecdotal experience. Gilchrist and associates reported that five of six children with hyperleukocytosis died of CNS hemorrhage with 6 days of diagnosis, whereas none of 11 who were irradiated died.[115] However, the risk of CNS hemorrhage in acute lymphocytic leukemia is small: none occurred in 136 patients with counts between 100,000 and 400,000/μl.[99] At this point, most pediatric oncologists do not recommend irradiation in either type of leukemia but instead favor prompt specific cytoreductive measures and aggressive correction of metabolic abnormalities.

METABOLIC EMERGENCIES

Tumor Lysis Syndrome

The *tumor lysis syndrome* consists of the metabolic triad of hyperuricemia, hyperkalemia, and hyperphosphatemia. Secondary renal failure and symptomatic hypocalcemia are common complications.

Etiology

Tumor lysis occurs before therapy or 1 to 5 days after the start of specific cytotoxic therapy in tumors that have a high growth fraction and that are exquisitely sensitive to chemotherapy. It is seen most commonly in Burkitt's lymphoma, which has a doubling time of 38 to 116 hours,[117] and in T-cell leukemia/lymphoma, which has a labeling index about three times that of pre-B-cell acute lymphocytic leukemia (see Chap. 20).[118] The syndrome generally does not occur in acute nonlymphocytic leukemia or in nonlymphomatous solid tumors; it may complicate chronic myeloid leukemia.

In their review of 37 patients with Burkitt's lymphoma, Cohen and associates defined those factors that predispose to severe metabolic derangements: bulky abdominal tumors, elevated pretreatment serum uric acid and lactic dehydrogenase concentrations, and poor urine output.[119] Azotemia occurred in 14 of the 37 patients and hyperphosphatemia in 24 patients. Andreoli and coworkers found that relatively older age (10.4 ± 5.4 years) correlated with development of renal failure in children with acute lymphoblastic leukemia.[120] This may in part be due to the progressive decline in the fractional excretion and clearance of uric acid that accompanies advancing age throughout childhood.[121] Although tumor lysis syndrome usually occurs in the setting of a large tumor burden, Andreoli and coworkers did not find high white cell count to be a predictor of renal failure,[120] and Yolken and Miller describe hyperuricemia and renal failure as the presenting manifestations of occult hematologic malignant processes.[122]

Pathophysiology

The tumor lysis syndrome is a direct result of the degradation of malignant cells and of inadequate renal function. All three metabolites involved—uric acid, phosphorus, and potassium—are excreted by the kidney. A certain amount of spontaneous degradation of malignant cells takes place before treatment starts; successful treatment accelerates the process. Elevated uric acid comes from breakdown of nucleic acids. Uric acid, which has a pKa of 5.4, exists in a soluble, monovalent form at physiologic pH but can precipitate in the collecting ducts in the acid environment of the kidney.[125] Lactic acidosis secondary to poor tissue oxygenation in patients with high white cell counts may contribute to uric acid deposition. Uric acid also precipitates in the ureters, but frank urate lithiasis is unlikely in the setting of acute hyperuricemia in childhood cancer.

Phosphates are released when tumor cells lyse. Lymphoblasts are especially rich in phosphate, having four times the content of normal lymphocytes.[124] When the calcium–phosphorus product exceeds 60, calcium phosphate precipitates in the microvasculature. These precipitates can lead to renal failure. The second major consequence of hyperphosphatemia is hypocalcemia and seizures.[125]

Finally, potassium, the principal intracellular cation, is released with tumor cells lysis. Hyperkalemia also can result from secondary renal failure.

Evaluation and Differential Diagnosis

In a patient at risk for tumor lysis syndrome, pertinent historical information includes the time of onset of symptoms referable to the malignancy, abdominal pain or fullness, back pain, changes in the amount of urine, and symptoms of hypocalcemia, including anorexia, vomiting, cramps, spasms, tetany, seizure, and alterations in consciousness. Special attention during the physical examination should be given to blood pressure, cardiac rate and rhythm, abdominal masses, presence of pleural effusions or ascites, and signs of cerebral anoxia. The following laboratory studies should be ordered immediately: complete blood count; serum sodium, potassium, chloride, bicarbonate, calcium, phosphorus, uric acid, urea nitrogen and creatinine; and urinalysis. If there are mass lesions in the abdomen or if there is renal failure, ultrasonography of the abdomen and retroperitoneum should be done immediately. If the serum potassium is 7.0 mEq/liter or more, there is danger of life-threatening ventricular arrhythmia. An ECG therefore should be done. It may show QRS widening and peaked T waves. However, when the white cell count is high, the serum potassium can be artifactually elevated by spontaneous lysis of leukocytes, platelets, and red cells ("pseudohyperkalemia"). In pseudohyperkalemia, there are no cardiac or ECG changes, and the actual potassium concentration can be determined from plasma rather than serum.

In patients with disseminated intra-abdominal Burkitt's lymphoma, tumor lysis and renal failure may be present at diagnosis because of renal parenchymal involvement with tumor, large pelvic masses causing obstructive uropathy, poor venous return because of compression, and rapid turnover of tumor cells.

Therapy and Recommendations

Metabolic stability must be achieved before treatment proceeds, but if treatment is delayed the tumor burden increases. Prevention of renal failure entails hydration, alkalinization, and allopurinol (Table 37-11). Patients should receive two to four times the maintenance fluid volume as 5% glucose in 0.25 N saline with 50 to 100 mEq of sodium bicarbonate per liter to produce a urine pH of 7.0 to 7.5 with a specific gravity of no more than 1.010. Hydration and alkalinization promote uric acid and phosphate excretion. Allopurinol inhibits xanthine oxidase, the enzyme that forms uric acid from the purine degration products hypoxanthine and xanthine. In the presence of allopurinol, uric acid formation is reduced and hypoxanthine and xanthine excretion are increased. Generally, potassium should not be added to the intravenous solution. Sodium bicarbonate should be withdrawn when cancer treatment

Table 37-11
Metabolic Management of Disseminated Burkitt's Lymphoma

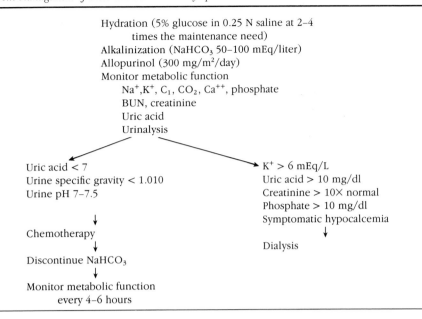

Hydration (5% glucose in 0.25 N saline at 2–4
times the maintenance need)
Alkalinization ($NaHCO_3$ 50–100 mEq/liter)
Allopurinol (300 mg/m²/day)
Monitor metabolic function
    Na^+, K^+, C_1, CO_2, Ca^{++}, phosphate
    BUN, creatinine
    Uric acid
    Urinalysis

Uric acid < 7
Urine specific gravity < 1.010
Urine pH 7–7.5

Chemotherapy

Discontinue $NaHCO_3$

Monitor metabolic function
every 4–6 hours

K^+ > 6 mEq/L
Uric acid > 10 mg/dl
Creatinine > 10× normal
Phosphate > 10 mg/dl
Symptomatic hypocalcemia

Dialysis

starts: at pH above 7.5 hypoxanthine stones may occur; at pH 8 or above, calcium phosphate may crystallize within the kidney.

For most patients, this regimen of hydration, alkalinization, and allopurinol suffices to prevent clinically significant tumor lysis and renal failure, but there are exceptions. Andreoli and associates have explained some cases of renal failure on the basis of the effects of allopurinol in altering purine excretion.[120] The solubility of all three metabolites is enhanced at alkaline pH. At pH 5.0, the solubility of uric acid is 150 mg/liter, that of xanthine 50 mg/liter, and that of hypoxanthine 115 mg/liter. At pH 7.0, uric acid solubility is increased to 2000 mg/liter, that of xanthine to 130 mg/liter, and that of hypoxanthine to 1500 mg/liter. In the presence of allopurinol, Andreoli and associates found a 174% increase in uric acid excretion, a 1630% increase in hypoxanthine excretion, and a 1460% increase in xanthine excretion, which exceeded its solubility limit. Despite these enormous increases in urinary filtration of purine metabolites, the solubility limit of xanthine was exceeded in 16 of 19 children with acute lymphocytic leukemia, and 4 developed renal failure. These children had significantly higher pretherapy serum uric acid and post-treatment xanthine concentrations. Thus, in some patients, the shift from uric acid to xanthine excretion may predispose to xanthine precipitation. Those authors believe that other factors, such as rapid release of organic phosphates such as ATP, may affect intrarenal hemodynamics.[120] Hydration is probably the most critical factor in preventing renal failure.

Frank or impending renal failure requires additional therapeutic measures. Hyperkalemia usually presents the most immediate threat to life. All potassium intake should be stopped, and Kayexalate (1 g/kg orally with 50% sorbitol), a potassium-binding resin, should be started.[128] Calcium gluconate (100–200 mg/kg per dose) can induce shift of potassium intracellularly and stabilize myocardial conduction. Insulin (0.1 U/kg of regular insulin) with 2 m/kg of 25% glucose in water as an intravenous bolus also induces intracellular influx of potassium.[128] If hyperkalemia and renal failure cannot be controlled, dialysis should be started. Hemodialysis is preferable

to peritoneal dialysis because uric acid is better removed by the former. The indications for dialysis are in Table 37-11. Fildes and coworkers have recently reviewed the management of renal failure in children.[129]

Because tumor lysis occurs often in the setting of a high white cell count, some authors have advocated leukopheresis, exchange transfusion, or low-dose steroids to reduce the metabolic consequences of massive tumor lysis. These methods have not been subjected to any controlled analysis (see section on hyperleukocytosis).

Hypercalcemia

Hypercalcemia refers to a serum calcium greater than 10.5 mg/dl. Normally, serum calcium must be maintained between 9.0 and 10.5 mg/dl. Levels above 12.0 mg/dl disturb virtually every organ system, and levels above 20 mg/dl can be fatal.

Etiology

Hypercalcemia commonly complicates metastatic breast, lung, and kidney carcinoma; T-cell leukemia; and multiple myeloma in adults. It is, however, an infrequent complication of pediatric cancer. The childhood tumors associated with hypercalcemia are acute lymphoblastic leukemia, non-Hodgkin's lymphoma, neuroblastoma, Ewing's sarcoma.[130-134] Le Blanc and coworkers have defined three other distinct groups apparently at high risk of hypercalcemia: patients with undifferentiated lymphoblastic lymphoma widely metastatic to bone, adolescents with rhabdomyosarcoma metastatic to breast and marrow, and infants with renal tumors with rhabdoid histology.[131] Dickersin and associates describe hypercalcemia in five adolescent girls with small-cell carcinoma of the ovary.[132]

Pathogenesis

The effects of hypercalcemia on the various systems interact with one another to create a vicious cycle: as anorexia, nausea, and vomiting develop, polyuria begins; the combination leads to dehydration; dehydration, in turn, impairs gastrointestinal and renal function; and impaired renal function aggravates hypercalcemia. In a detailed study of seven children with hypercalcemia, Harguindey and associates found all to have elevated blood urea nitrogen and uric acid levels, normal or increased phosphorus concentration, and metabolic alkalosis.[130]

Most malignant hypercalcemia results from excessive bone resorption. Normal calcium homeostasis is maintained by a balance between bone deposition and bone resorption. The latter is stimulated by parathyroid hormone, prostaglandin E_2, polypeptide growth factors, osteoclast-activating factor, and osteoclasts, which are derived from mononuclear phagocytes.[135] The hypercalcemia of cancer patients is mediated by these same factors, and the tumor itself can be the source.[136] The diversity of metabolic interactions of these and other factors with one another and with metastatic bone lesions is not yet fully understood.

Ectopic parathormone production is a rare cause of hypercalcemia.[136–139] Ramsay and associates demonstrated parathormone production *in vitro* by marrow and cerebrospinal fluid blasts of a 15-year-old with acute lymphoblastic leukemia and hypercalcemia.[137] Zidar and coworkers found that blasts from a 25-year-old with acute myeloblastic leukemia synthesized parathormone *in vitro;* a freeze–thawed preparation of these blasts contained high levels of parathormone.[138] However, others have failed to detect parathormone in many types of malignant cells.[130,140] Strewler and colleagues showed that some patients' tumors secrete substances that bind to the parathormone receptor and function as parathormone.[141] These receptor-binding substances are immunologically distinct from normal parathormone.

Ectopic production of prostaglandin E_2 has been implicated in hypercalcemia of breast cancer and a variety of carcinomas but not that of pediatric tumors.[142] Osteoclast-activating factor is produced by mitogen- or antigen-stimulated lymphocytes; it acts locally to induce resorbtion of bone and requires close contact with bone.[137] Osteoclast-activating factor has been associated with hypercalcemia in patients with multiple myeloma or Burkitt's lymphoma.[143,144]

Some leukemias secrete hematopoietic colony-stimulating factors that have bone-resorbing properties and may cause hypercalcemia in patients with hematopoietic malignancies.[136] Members of the family of transforming growth factors such as epidermal growth factor and transforming growth factor-B cause malignant hypercalcemia in rodents and are implicated in hypercalcemia of some human cancers.[136]

Recently, Breslau and associates described three patients with non-Hodgkin's lymphoma, hypercalcemia, and renal failure without metastatic bone disease. The patients' tumors produced 1,25-dihydroxyvitamin D (calcitrol).[145] The calcitrol stimulated bone resorption and increased calcium absorption from the intestine.

Evaluation and Differential Diagnosis

Gastrointestinal, renal, neuromuscular, and cardiovascular symptoms dominate the clinical picture of malignant hypercalcemia (Table 37-12). The diagnosis is made on the basis of the serum calcium level and the presence of cancer. Other factors that may coexist in cancer patients to cause hypercalcemia or exacerbate tumor-mediated hypercalcemia include use of thiazide diuretics, oral contraceptives, tamoxiphen, antacids with calcium carbonate, or lithium; hypervitaminosis A or D; renal disease; granulomatous disease; adrenal insufficiency; fractures; and immobilization.

Table 37-12
Signs and Symptoms of Hypercalcemia of Malignancy

Gastrointestinal
Anorexia
Nausea
Vomiting
Constipation
Ileus
Neuromuscular
Lethargy
Apathy
Depression
Fatigue
Hypotonia
Obtundation
Stupor
Coma
Cardiovascular
Bradycardia
Arrhythmia
Digitalis toxicity
Renal
Polyuria
Nocturia

Therapy and Recommendations

Acute hypercalcemia or calcium levels of greater than 14 mg/dl require immediate correction. First, intravascular volume must be restored with normal saline. For a serum calcium less than 14 mg/dl, saline repletion with standard furosemide diuresis may suffice. With higher serum calcium levels, a more vigorous forced diuresis has been recommended for adults using volumes of normal saline up to three times maintenance with furosemide (2–3 mg/kg) every 2 hours.[146] Sodium and calcium are excreted by the kidney, and both cations are reabsorbed in the proximal collecting tubule and loop of Henle, where furosemide has its greatest blocking action. This forced diuresis requires precise monitoring of intravascular volume and of serum and urine electrolytes; profound fluid shifts and potassium and magnesium losses may accompany sodium, calcium, and fluid excretion. By the forced diuresis method, serum calcium can be reduced a mean of 3 mg/dl in 48 hours. However, other therapy is necessary if the calcium concentration is rising rather than falling in the first 6 to 12 hours.

Glucocorticoids in doses equal to 1.5 to 2.0 mg/kg of prednisone per day can reduce serum calcium in those diseases where hypercalcemia is mediated by osteoclast-activating factor, prostaglandin E_2, and calcitrol or in the lymphoid neoplasms where steroids treat the tumor directly. Steroids require 2 to 3 days to take effect. Salmon calcitonin, on the other hand, acts within hours to reduce serum calcium by inhibiting bone resorption. Unfortunately, resistance to exogenous calcitonin develops within days, but the combined use of steroid and calcitonin may provide control for longer periods. Mithramycin, an antineoplastic antibiotic, lowers calcium within days but is too cytotoxic for long use.[147]

Oral phosphorus is effective in controlling chronic but not acute elevation of serum calcium. Intravenous phosphorus is contraindicated because of metastatic calcification. Diphosphonates were originally developed to reduce calcium deposits in pipes used in plumbing.[148] Recently, a number of diphosphonates have been found to inhibit bone formation.

Those effective in the treatment of acute and chronic hypercalcemia include dichloromethylene diphosphonate and aminohydroxypropylidine diphosphonate.[149,150] These agents take effect within 2 to 7 days, and the effects last for several weeks. Prolonged use of dichloromethylene diphosphonate inhibits bone remineralization and may be associated with secondary leukemia,[151] but these may not be problems with short-term use. Gallium nitrate is the most recent antihypercalcemic agent: it inhibits accelerated bone turnover and reduces serum calcium and urinary calcium and hydroxyproline excretion.[152] Bone can remineralize in the presence of gallium nitrate.

Hemodialysis or peritoneal dialysis can also reduce serum calcium. In general, dialysis is reserved for those patients with renal failure.

Syndrome of Inappropriate Secretion of Antidiuretic Hormone (SIADH)

The SIADH is characterized by continuous release of antidiuretic hormone (ADH) without any relation to plasma osmolality.

Etiology

SIADH can occur with CNS injury or disease; with stress, pain, surgery, or positive pressure ventilation; with lung infection, inflammation, and tumor, especially small-cell carcinoma in adults; and with other tumors such as lymphoma or gastrointestinal carcinoma.[154] Aside from the CNS and postoperative cases, the most common cause of SIADH in pediatric oncology is either vincristine or cyclophosphamide. In the case of vincristine, SIADH usually coincides with severe neurotoxicity, which suggests a direct effect of vincristine on the supraoptic nuclei, where ADH is synthesized.[155] Cyclophosphamide reduces free-water clearance, and this effect may be especially troublesome in the face of the aggressive hydration used to prevent cystitis.[156,157]

Pathophysiology

ADH causes the kidneys to conserve water and to concentrate urine. The clinical consequences of inappropriate ADH secretion are those of hyponatremia and water intoxication.

Evaluation and Differential Diagnosis

The symptoms of SIADH are fatigue, weight gain, lethargy, confusion, seizures, and coma. A sudden drop in serum sodium to less than 120 mmol/liter in less than 24 hours may be fatal. With more gradual decrements or after 1 or 2 days of hyponatremia, the brain adapts by extruding water and electrolytes; chronic SIADH thus may be well tolerated.[153]

To make the diagnosis of SIADH, it is necessary to document a urine osmolality inappropriately high for the serum osmolality and to exclude renal, adrenal, or thyroid disease and simple hypotonic dehydration.

Therapy and Recommendations

Fluid restriction is the mainstay of therapy of chronic SIADH or of acute SIADH if the sodium is above 120 mmol and the patient is asymptomatic.[158,159] If fluid restriction is not possible when the patient is having seizures, furosemide (1 mg/kg) and 3% saline to replace sodium losses can correct the situation in 6 hours.[160] Weizman and associates found that only the addition of deoxycortisone acetate (4 mg/m² per day) to furosemide and hypertonic saline could raise serum sodium in a 6-year-old girl with SIADH following surgery for craniopharyngioma.[161] Recently, there has been some concern that too rapid a correction of sodium can cause further neurologic deterioration and death: a rate of correction 2 mmol per hour is recommended.[159]

REFERENCES

1. Janin Y, Becker J, Wise L, Schneider K et al: Superior vena cava syndrome in childhood and adolescence: A review of the literature and report of three cases. J Pediatr Surg 17:290–295, 1982
2. Issa PY, Brinhi ER, Janin Y, Slim MS: Superior vena cava syndrome in childhood. Pediatrics 71:337–341, 1983
3. McIntire FT, Sykes EM Jr: Obstruction of the superior vena cava: A review of the literature and report of two personal cases. Ann Intern Med 30:925–960, 1949
4. D'Angio GJ, Mitus A, Evans AE: The superior mediastinal syndrome in children with cancer. Am J Roentgenol Radium Ther Nucl Med 93:537–544, 1965
5. Porkony WJ, Sherman J, Idriss FS: Mediastinal masses in infants and children. J Thorac Cardiovasc Surg 68:869–875, 1974
6. King RM, Telander RL, Smithson WA: Primary mediastinal tumors in children. J Pediatr Surg 17:512–517, 1982
7. Pate JW, Hammon J: Superior vena cava syndrome due to histoplasmosis in children. Ann Surg 161:778–785, 1985
8. Carabell SC, Goodman RL: Superior vena cava syndrome. In DeVita VT Jr, Hellman S, Rosenberg SA (eds): Principles and Practice of Oncology, 2nd Ed, pp 1855–1860. Philadelphia, JB Lippincott, 1985
9. Mandell GA, Lantieri R, Goodman LR: Tracheobronchial compression in Hodgkin's lymphoma in children. AJR 139:1167–1170, 1983
10. Gaebler JW, Kleiman MB, Cohen M et al: Differentiation of lymphoma from histoplasmosis in children with mediastinal masses. J Pediatr 104:706–710, 1984
11. Lockich JJ, Goodman RL: Superior vena cava syndrome. JAMA 213:58–61, 1975
12. Neuman GC, Weingarten AE, Abramowitz RM et al: The anesthetic management of the patient with an anterior mediastinal mass. Anesthesiology 60:144–147, 1984
13. Keon TC: Death on induction of anesthesia for cervical node biopsy. Anesthesiology 55:471–472, 1981
14. Abmann F: A reassessment of the clinical implications of the superior vena cava syndrome. J Clin Oncol 2:961–969, 1984
15. Klein TS, Neil HS: Lymphadenopathy and aspiration biopsy cytology. Cancer 53:1076–1081, 1984
16. Halpern S, Chatten J, Meadows AT et al: Anterior mediastinal masses: Anesthesia hazards and other problems. J Pediatr 102:407–410, 1983
17. Mitchell CD, Gordon I, Chessels JM: Clinical, hematologic, and radiological feature in T-cell malignancy in childhood. Clin Radiol 257–261, 1986
18. Halpern S, Gewitz, Lange B: Nutritional management of malignant chylous effusion. Am J Dis Child 135:170–171, 1981
19. Mauch PM, Ultmann JE: Treatment of malignant pericardial effusions. In DeVita VT Jr, Rosenberg S, Hellman S (eds): Principles and Practice of Oncology, 2nd Ed, pp 2141–2149. Philadelphia, JB Lippincott, 1985
20. Leff A, Hopewell PC, Costello J: Pleural effusion from malignancy. Ann Intern Med 88:532–537, 1978
21. Shepard FA, Ginsberg JS, Evans WK et al: Tetracycline sclerosis in the management of malignant pericardial effusion. J Clin Oncol 13:1678–1682, 1985
22. Davis S, Rambotti P, Grignani F: Intrapericardial tetracycline sclerosis in the treatment of malignant pericardial effusion: An analysis of thirty-three cases. J Clin Oncol 2:631–636, 1984
23. Bayly TC, Kisner DL, Sybert A et al: Tetracycline and quinacrine in the control of malignant pleural effusions. Cancer 41:1188–1192, 1978
24. Zaloznik AJ, Oswald SG, Langin M: Intrapleural tetracycline in malignant pleural effusions. Cancer 51:752–755, 1983
25. Fraser RS, Viloria JB, Want N-S: Cardiac tamponade as a presentation of extracardiac malignancy. Cancer 45:1697–1704, 1980
26. Nakayama DK, Delorimer AA, O'Neill JA et al: Intracardiac extension of Wilms' tumor: Report of National Wilms' Tumor Study Group. Ann Surg 24:693–697, 1986

27. Exelby PR, Ghandchi A, Lansigan N et al: Management of the acute abdomen in children with leukemia. Cancer 35:826–829, 1975

28. Sherman NJ, Williams K, Willy MM: Surgical complications in the patient with leukemia. J Pediatr Surg 8:235–244, 1973

29. Hatch EI: The acute abdomen in children. Pediatr Clin North Am 32:1151–1164, 1985

30. Schaller RT, Schaller JF: The acute abdomen in the immunologically compromised child. J Pediatr Surg 18:937–944, 1983

31. Kuffer R, Fortner J, Murphy M: Surgical complications in children undergoing cancer therapy. Ann Surg 167:215, 1968

32. Rasmussen BL, Freeman JS: Major surgery in leukemia. Am J Surg 130:647–651, 1975

33. Prolla JC, Kirsner JB: The gastrointestinal lesions and complications of the leukemias. Ann Intern Med 61:1084–1103, 1964

34. Ferguson M: The effect of antineoplastic agents in wound healing. Surg Gynecol Obstet 154:421–429, 1982

35. Cope Z: The Early Diagnosis of the Acute Abdomen, 14th Ed. London, Oxford University Press, 1972

36. Kirchner SG, Horev G: Diagnostic imaging in children with acute chest and abdominal disorders. Pediatr Clin North Am 32:1363–1382, 1985

37. Welch CE, Malt RA: Surgery of the stomach, duodenum, gallbladder and bile ducts. N Engl J Med 316:999–1007, 1987

38. Athanasoulis CA, Baum S, Waldman AC et al: Control of acute gastric mucosal hemorrhage: Intraarterial infusion of posterior pituitary extracts. N Engl J Med 290:597–603, 1974

39. Baum S, Athanasoulis CA, Waltman AC et al: Angiographic diagnosis and control of gastrointestinal bleeding. Adv Surg 7:149–198, 1973

40. Ross AJ III, Siegel KR, Bell W et al: Massive gastrointestinal hemorrhage in children with posterior fossa tumors. J Pediatr Surg 22:633–636, 1987

41. Dewar GJ, Lim CN, Michal Y, Shyn B et al: Gastrointestinal complications in patients with acute and chronic leukemia. Can J Surg 24:67–71, 1981

42. Localio SA, Stone A, Friedman M: Surgical aspects of radiation enteritis. Surg Gynecol Obstet 129:302–307, 1969

43. Rifkin GD: Neutropenic enterocolitis and Clostridium septicum infection in patients with agranulocytosis. Arch Intern Med 1:834–835, 1980

44. Hopkins DG, Kushner JP: Clostridial species in the pathogenesis of necrotizing enterocolitis in patients with neutropenia. Am J Hematol 14:289–295, 1983

45. Wagner M, Rosenberg H, Fernbach D et al: Typhlitis: A complication of leukemia in childhood. Am J Roentgenol 109:341–350, 1970

46. Shamberger RC, Weinstein HJ, Delorey M et al: The medical and surgical management of typhlitis in children with acute nonlymphocytic (myelogenous) leukemia. Cancer 57:603–609, 1986

47. Frick MP, Maile CW, Crass JR et al: Computed tomography of neutropenic colitis. AJR 143:763–765, 1984

48. Moir CR, Scudamore CH, Benny WB: Typlitis: Selective surgical management. Am J Surg 151:563–566, 1986

49. Bartlett JG, Chang TW, Gurwith M et al: Antibiotic associated pseudomembranous colitis due to toxin-producing clostridia. N Engl J Med 298:531–534, 1978

50. Touloukian RJ: Hepatic infections and abscesses. In Welch KJ, Randolph JG, Ravitch MM, O'Neill JA, Rowe MI (eds): Pediatric Surgery, 4th Ed, pp 1071–1073. Chicago, Year Book Medical Publishers, 1986

51. Schnaufer L, Koop CE: Silastic abdominal patch for temporary hepatomegaly in stage IV-S neuroblastoma. J Pediatr Surg 10:73–75, 1975

52. Caniano DA, Browne AF, Boles ET: Pancreatic pseudocyst complicating treatment of acute lymphoblastic leukemia. J Pediatr Surg 20:452–455, 1985

53. Gonzolez AC, Bradley EL, Clements JL: Pseudocyst formation in acute pancreatitis: Ultrasonographic evaluation of 99 cases. Am J Roentgenol 127:315–317, 1976

54. Coleman BG, Arger PT, Rosenberg HK et al: Gray scale sonographic assessment of pancreatitis in children. Radiology 146:145–150, 1983

55. Mahboubi S, Duckett JN, Spackman TJ: Ureteritis cystica after treatment of cyclophosphamide-induced hemorrhagic cystitis. Urology 7:521–523, 1976

56. Chaviano AH, Gill WB, Ruggiero KJ et al: Experimental Cytoxan cystitis and prevention by acetylcysteine. J Urol 134:598–600, 1985

57. Johnson WW, Meadows DC: Urinary bladder fibrosis and telangectasia associated with long-term cyclophosphamide therapy. N Engl J Med 284:290–294, 1971

58. Erschler WB, Gilchrist KW, Citrin DL: Adriamycin enhancement of cyclophosphamide induced bladder injury. J Urol 123:121–122, 1980

59. Shrom SH, Donaldson MH, Duckett JW, Wein AJ: Formalin treatment for intractable hemorrhagic cystitis: A review of the literature with 16 additional cases. Cancer 38:1785–1789, 1976

60. Droller MJ, Saral R, Santos G: Prevention of cyclophosphamide-induced hemorrhagic cystitis. Urology 20:256–258, 1982

61. Plum F, Posner JB: The Diagnosis of Stupor and Coma, 3rd Ed. Philadelphia, FA Davis, 1980

62. Packer RJ, Berman PH: Coma. In Fleisher G, Ludwig S (eds): Textbook of Pediatric Emergency Medicine, pp 87–101. Baltimore, Williams & Wilkins, 1983

63. Packer RJ, Rorke LB, Lange BL et al: Cerebrovascular accidents in children with cancer. Pediatrics 76:194–201, 1985

64. Wiznitzer M, Packer RJ, August CM et al: Neurologic complications of bone marrow transplant in childhood. Ann Neurol 16:569–576, 1984

65. Sandler RM, Liebman HA, Patch MJ et al: Antithrombin III and activated factor X activity in patients with acute promyelocytic leukemia and disseminated intravascular coagulation treated with heparin. Cancer 51:681–685, 1983

66. Wada H, Nagano T, Tomeoku M et al: Coagulant and fibrinolytic activities in leukemic cell lysates. Thromb Res 30:315–322, 1983

67. Gralnick HR, Abrell E: Studies of the procoagulant and fibrinolytic activity of promyelocytes in acute promyelocytic leukemia. Br J Haematol 24:89–98, 1973

68. Kantarjian HM, Keating MJ, Walters RS et al: Acute promyelocytic leukemia: MD Anderson Hospital experience. Am J Med 80:789–797, 1986

69. McKee IC, Collins RDD: Intravascular leukocyte thrombi as a cause of morbidity and mortality in leukemia. Medicine 53:463–478, 1974

70. Fritz RD, Forkner CE, Freireich EJ et al: The association of fatal hemorrhage and blastic crisis in patients with acute leukemia. N Engl J Med 261:59–64, 1959

71. Collins RC, Al-Mondhindry H, Chernick NL et al: Neurologic manifestations of intravascular coagulation in patients with cancer. Neurology 25:795–806, 1975

72. Schwartzman RJ, Hill JB: Neurologic complications of disseminated intravascular coagulation. Neurology 32:791–797, 1982

73. Painter MJ, Chutorian AM, Hilal SK: Cerebrovasculopathy following irradiation in childhood. Neurology 25:189–194, 1975

74. Rosenberg DA, Chernick NL, Deck MDF: Cerebral necrosis following radiotherapy of extracranial neoplasms. Ann Neurol 1:339–357, 1977

75. Allen JC, Rosen GR: Transient cerebral dysfunction following chemotherapy for osteogenic sarcoma. Ann Neurol 3:441–444, 1978

76. Walker RJ, Allen JC, Rosen G, Caparros B: Transient cerebral dysfunction secondary to high dose methotrexate. J Clin Oncol 4:1845–1850, 1986

77. Jaffe N, Takaue Y, Anzae T, Robertson R: Transient neurologic disturbances induced by high-dose methotrexate treatment. Cancer 56:1356–1360, 1985

78. Zimmerman RA, Bilaniuk LT: Computed tomography of primary and secondary craniocerebral neuroblastoma. AJNR 1:431–434, 1980

79. Ganji D, Reamon GH, Cohen SR et al: Leukoencephalopathy and elevated levels of myelin basic protein in the cerebrospinal fluid of patients with acute lymphoblastic leukemia. N Engl J Med 303:19–21, 1980

80. Broder LE, Carter SK: Meningeal Leukemia. New York, Plenum Press, 1972

81. Priest JP, Ramsey NKC, Latchaw RE et al: Thrombotic and hemorrhagic strokes complicating early therapy for childhood acute lymphoblastic leukemia. Cancer 46:1548–1554, 1980

82. Zaunschirm A, Muntean W: Correction of hemostatic imbalances induced by L-asparaginase therapy in children with acute lymphoblastic leukemia. Pediatr Haematol Oncol 3:19–25, 1986

83. Bezeaud A, Drouet L, Leverger G et al: Effect of L-asparaginase therapy for acute lymphoblastic leukemia on plasma vitamin K-dependent coagulation factors and inhibitors. J Pediatr 108:698–701, 1986

84. Edwards MS, Wilson CB: Treatment of radiation necrosis. In Gilbert HA, Kagan AR (eds): Radiation Damage to the Nervous System: A Delayed Therapeutic Hazard, pp 129–145. New York, Raven Press, 1980

85. Rizzoli HG, Pagnanelle DM: Treatment of necrosis of the brain: A clinical observation. J Neurosurg 60:589–594, 1984

86. Packer RJ, Zimmerman RA, Bilaniuk LT: Magnetic resonance imagining (MRI) in the evaluation of treatment related central nervous system (CNS) damage. Cancer 58:33–38, 1986

87. Dodson WE, Prensky AL, DeVivo DC: Management of seizure disorders: Selected aspects, part 1. J Pediatr 89:527–534, 1976

88. Porter RJ: Epilepsy: One Hundred Elementary Principles. London, WB Saunders, 1984

89. Walker JE, Homan RW, Vasko MR et al: Lorazepam in status epilepticus. Ann Neurol 6:207–213, 1979

90. Lewis DW, Packer RJ, Raney B et al: Incidence, presentation and outcome of spinal cord diseases in child with systemic cancer. Pediatrics 78:438–443, 1986

91. Baten M, Vannucci RC: Intraspinal metastatic disease in childhood cancer. J Pediatr 90:207–212, 1977

92. Posner JB: Secondary neoplastic disease. In Diseases of the Nervous System: Clinical Neurology, pp 1155–1168. Philadelphia, WB Saunders, 1986

93. Ch'ien LT, Kalwinsky DK, Peterson G et al: Metastatic epidural tumors in children. Med Pediatr Oncol 10:455–462, 1982

94. Packer RJ, Zimmerman RA, Sutton LN et al: Magnetic resonance imaging (MRI) of spinal cord disease of childhood. Pediatrics 78:251–256, 1986

95. Gilbert RW, Kim J, Posner JB: Epidural spinal cord compression from metastatic tumor: Diagnosis and treatment. Ann Neurol 3:40–51, 1978

96. Rodriguez M, Dinapoli RP: Spinal cord compression: With special reference to metastatic epidural tumors. Mayo Clin Proc 55:442–448, 1980

97. Portenoy RK, Lipton RB, Foley KM: Back pain in the cancer patient: An algorithm for evaluation and management. Neurology 37:134–138, 1987

98. Hayes FA, Thompson FI, Hvizdala E et al: Chemotherapy as an alternative to laminectomy and radiation in the management of epidural tumor. J Pediatr 104:221–224, 1981

99. Bunin NJ, Piu CH: Differing complications of hyperleukocytosis in children with acute lymphoblastic or acute nonlymphoblastic leukemia. J Clin Oncol 3:1590–1595, 1985

100. Coccia PF, Bleyer WA, Siegel SE et al: Development and preliminary findings of Children's Cancer Study Group Protocols (161, 162 and 163) for low-, average- and high-risk acute lymphoblastic leukemia in children. In Murphy SB, Gilbert JR (eds): Leukemia Research: Advances in Cell Biology and Treatment, pp 241–250. New York, Elsevier Science Publishing, 1983

101. Lichtman MA, Rowe JM: Hyperleukocytic leukemias: Rheological, clinical, and therapeutic considerations. Blood 60:279–283, 1982

102. Field M, Block JB, Levin R et al: Significance of blood lactate elevations among patients with acute leukemia and other neoplastic proliferative disorders. Am J Med 40:528–545, 1966

103. Tryka AF, Godleski JJ, Fanta CH: Leukemic cell lysis pneumonopathy: A complication of treated myeloblastic leukemia. Cancer 50:2763–2770, 1982

104. Hess CE, Nicholas AB, Hynt WB, Suratt PM: Pseudohypoxemia secondary to leukemia and thrombocytosis. N Engl J Med 301:361, 1979

105. Steinhardt GF, Steinhardt E: Priapism in children with leukemia. Urology 18:604, 1981

106. Williams DL, Bell BA, Ragab AH: Clitorism at presentation of acute non-lymphocytic leukemia. J Pediatr 107:754–756, 1985

107. Rowe JM, Lichtman MA: Hyperleukocytosis and leukostasis: Common features of childhood chronic myelogenous leukemia. Blood 63:1230–1234, 1984

108. Harris AL: Leukostasis associated with blood transfusion in acute myeloid laeukemia. Br Med J 2:1169–1171, 1978

109. Kamen BA, Summers CP, Pearson HA: Exchange transfusion as a treatment for hyperleukocytosis, anemia, and metabolic abnormalities in a patient with leukemia. J Pediatr 96:1045–1046, 1980

110. Del Vasto F, Caldore M, Russo F, Bertuccioli A, Pellegrini F: Exchange transfusion in leukemia with hyperleukocytosis. J Pediatr 100:1000, 1982

111. Carpentieri U, Patten EV, Chamberlin PA, Young AD, Hitter ME: Leukopheresis in a 3-year-old child with lymphoma in leukemic transformation. J Pediatr 94:919–921, 1979

112. Cuttner J, Holland JF, Norton L, Ambinder E, Button G, Meyer RJ: Therapeutic leukopheresis for hyperleukocytosis in acute myelocytic leukemia. Med Pediatr Oncol 11:76–78, 1983

113. Maurer HS, Steinherz PG, Gaynon PS et al: Management of hyperleukocytosis (HL) in childhood with acute lymphoblastic leukemia (abstract). Proc Am Soc Clin Oncol 4:172, 1985

114. Ablin AR: Managing the problem of hyperleukocytosis in acute leukemia. Am J Pediatr Hematol Oncol 6:287–291, 1984

115. Gilchrist GS, Fountain KS, Dearth JC, Smithson20WA, Burgert EO: Cranial irradiation in the management of extreme leukemic leukocytosis complicating childhood acute lymphocytic leukemia. J Pediatr 98:257–259, 1981

116. Wiernick PH, Serpick AA: Factors affecting remission and, survival in adult acute nonlymphocytic leukemia (ANLL). Medicine 49:505–513, 1970

117. Iverson OH, Iverson U, Ziegler JL, Bluming AZ: Cell cycle kinetics in Burkitt's lymphoma. Eur J Cancer 10:155–163, 1974

118. Dow LF, Chang LJA, Tsiatis AA: Relation of pretreatment lymphoblast proliferative activity and prognosis in 87 children with acute lymphoblastic leukemia. Blood 59:1197–1202, 1982

119. Cohen LF, Balow JE, Magrath IT, Poplack DG, Ziegler JL: Acute tumor lysis syndrome. Am J Med 68:486–491, 1980

120. Andreoli SP, Clark JH, McGuire WA, Bergstein JM: Purine excretion during tumor lysis in children with acute lymphocytic leukemia receiving allopurinol: Relationship to acute renal failure. J Pediatr 109:292–298, 1986

121. Stapleton FB, Linshaw MA, Hassanein K, Gruskin AB: Uric acid excretion in normal children. J Pediatr 92:911–914, 1978

122. Yolken RH, Miller DR: Hyperuricemia and renal failure: Presenting manifestations of occult hematologic malignancies. J Pediatr 89:775–777, 1976

123. Klinenberg JR, Kippen I, Bluestone R: Hyperuricemic nephropathy: Pathologic features and factors influencing urate deposition. Nephron 14:88–98, 1975

124. Rigas DA, Duerst ML, Jump ME et al: The nucleic acids and other phosphorus compounds of human leukemic leukocytes: Relation to cell maturity. J Lab Clin Med 48:356–378, 1956

125. Zusman J, Brown DM, Nesbit ME: Hyperphosphatemia, hyperphosphaturia and hypocalcemia in acute lymphoblastic leukemia. N Engl J Med 289:1335–1340, 1973

126. Holland MR, Jacobs AG, Kitis G: Pseudohyperkalemia in acute lymphocytic laeukemia. Lancet 2:1139, 1976

127. Holland P, Holland NH: Prevention and management of acute hyperuricemia in childhood leukemia. J Pediatr 72:358–366, 1968

128. Allegretta GJ, Weisman SJ, Altman AJ: Metabolic and space-occupying consequences of cancer and cancer treatment. Pediatr Clin North Am 32:601–611, 1985

129. Fildes RD, Springate JE, Feld LG: Acute renal failure: II. Management of suspected and established disease. J Pediatr 109:567–571, 1986

130. Harguindey S, DeCastro L, Barcos M, Getaz EP, Henderson ES, Freeman A: Hypercalcemia complicating childhood malignancies. Cancer 44:2280–2290, 1979

131. Leblanc A, Caillaud JM, Harmann O et al: Hypercalcemia preferentially occurs in unusual childhood tumors. Cancer 54:2132–2136, 1984

132. Dickersin RG, Kline IW, Scully RE: Small cell carcinoma of the ovary with hypercalcemia: A report of eleven cases. Cancer 49:188–197, 1982

133. Al-Rashid RA, Cress C: Hypercalcemia associated with neuroblastoma. Am J Dis Child 133:838–841, 1979

134. Spiegel A, Greene M, Magrath I et al: Hypercalcemia with suppressed parathyroid hormone in Burkitt's lymphoma. Am J Med 64:691–695, 1978

135. Raisz LG, Kream BE: Regulation of bone formation. N Engl J Med 309:29–35, 1983

136. Mundy GR, Ibbotson KJ, D'Souza SM, Simpson EL, Jacobs JW, Martin TJ: The hypercalcemia of cancer. N Engl J Med 310:1718–1727, 1984

137. Ramsay NKC, Brown DM, Nesbit ME, Coccia PF, Krivit W, Krutzik S: Autonomous production of parathyroid hormone by lymphoblastic leukemia cells in culture. J Pediatr 94:623–625, 1979

138. Zidar BL, Shadduck RK, Winkelstein A, Zeigler Z, Hawker CD: Acute myeloblastic leukemia and hypercalcemia. N Engl J Med 13:692–694, 1976

139. Jayaraman J, David R: Hypercalcemia as a presenting manifestation of leukemia: Evidence of excess PTH secretion. J Pediatr 90:609–610, 1977

140. Simpson EL, Mundy GR, D'Souza SM, Ibbotson KJ, Bockman R, Jacobs JW: Absence of parathyroid hormone messenger RNA in nonparathyroid tumors associated with hypercalcemia. N Engl J Med 309:325–330, 1983

141. Strewler GJ, William RD, Nissenson RA: Human renal carcinoma cells produce hypercalcemia in the nude mouse and a novel protein recognized by parathyroid hormones receptors. J Clin Invest 71:769–774, 1983

142. Demers LM, Allegra JC, Harvey HA et al: Plasma prostaglandins in hypercalcemic patients with neoplastic disease. Cancer 39:1559–1562, 1977

143. Mundy GR, Luben RA, Raisz LG et al: Bone-reabsorbing activity in supernatants from lymphoid cell lines. N Engl J Med 290:867–871, 1974

144. Mundy GR, Raisz LG, Cooper RA, Schechter GP, Salmon SE: Evidence for the secretion of an osteoclast-stimulating factor in myeloma. N Engl J Med 291:1041–1046, 1974

145. Breslau NA, McGuire JL, Zerwekh JE, Frenkel EP, Pak CYC: Hypercalcemia associated with increased serum calcitriol levels in three patients with lymphoma. Ann Intern Med 100:1–6, 1984

146. Suki WN, Yium JJ, Minden MV et al: Acute treatment of hypercalcemia with furosemide. N Engl J Med 283:836–840, 1970

147. Stapleton FB, Lukert BP, Linshaw MA: Treatment of hypercalcemia associated with osseous metastases. J Pediatr 89:1029–1030, 1976

148. Raisz LG: New diphosphonates to block bone resorption. N Engl J Med 302:347–348, 1980

149. Siris ES, Sherman WH, Baquiran DC et al: Effects of dichloromethylene diphosphonate on skeletal mobilization of calcium in multiple myeloma. N Engl J Med 302:310–315, 1980

150. Body JJ, Borkowski A, Cleeran A, Bijvoet OLM: Treatment of malignancy-associated hypercalcemia with intravenous aminohydroxypropylidine diphosphonate. J Clin Oncol 4:1177–1183, 1986

151. Elomaa I, Blomquist C, Grohn P: Long-term controlled trial with diphosphonate in patients with osteolytic bone metastases. Lancet 1:146–149, 1983

152. Warrell RP, Alcock NW, Bockman RS: Gallium nitrate inhibits accelerated bone turnover in patients with bone metastases. J Clin Oncol 5:292–298, 1987

153. Rymer MM, Fishman RA: Protective adaptation of brain to water intoxication. Arch Neurol 28:49–54, 1973

154. Moses AM: Diabetes insipidus and ADH regulation. Hosp Pract 37–44, 1977

155. Nicholson RG, Feldman W: Hyponatremia in association with vincristine therapy. Can Med Assoc J 106:356–357, 1972

156. Harlow PJ, DeClerck YA, Shore NA et al: A fatal case of inappropriate ADH secretion induced by cyclophosphamide therapy. Cancer 44:896–898, 1979

157. DeFronzo RA, Braine H, Colvin OM, Davis PJ: Water intoxication in man after cyclophosphamide therapy: Time course and relation to drug activation. Ann Intern Med 78:861–869, 1973

158. Miyagawa CI: The pharmacologic management of the syndrome of inappropriate secretion of antidiuretic hormone. Drug Intell Clin Pharm 20:527–531, 1986

159. Narins RG: Therapy of hyponatremia: Does haste make waste? N Engl J Med 314:1573–1574, 1986

160. Hantman D, Rossier B, Zohlman R, Schrier R: Rapid correction of hyponatremia in the syndrome of inappropriate secretion of antidiuretic hormone: An alternative treatment to hypertonic saline. Ann Intern Med 78:870–875, 1973

161. Weizman Z, Goitein K, Amit Y, Wald U, Landau H: Combined treatment of severe hyponatremia due to inappropriate antidiuretic hormone secretion. Pediatrics 69:610–612, 1982

thirty-eight

Hematologic Supportive Care

George R. Buchanan

The close association of oncology and hematology is nowhere more apparent than in the supportive care provided to children with hematologic malignancies (leukemia and lymphoma) and solid tumors. Many aspects of supportive care of the child with cancer are strictly hematologic in nature, for they must deal with the multiple hematologic complications of the primary disease and its treatment.[1,2] The most important of these, bone marrow failure, will be the primary focus of this chapter.

The specific purpose of this review is to discuss the hematologic complications of childhood cancer and their treatment from the standpoint of pathophysiology, differential diagnosis, and practical aspects of management. The primary emphasis will be on transfusion support with erythrocytes and platelet concentrates. However, other applicable supportive measures will be addressed briefly.

MANAGEMENT OF ANEMIA IN THE PEDIATRIC CANCER PATIENT

Pathophysiology

Anemia is the most common and readily managed of the hematologic complications of childhood cancer. The ease of its treatment is due primarily to the relatively long survival of red blood cells (120 days), with the hemoglobin declines usually being gradual and productive of only minimal symptoms. In addition, the longer storage time (35 days) and ease of administration of erythrocytes makes red cell transfusion support an uncomplicated process.

The primary cause of anemia in the pediatric cancer patient is diminished red blood cell production. This may be due to [1] replacement of the bone marrow by malignant cells (either leukemic blasts or, less commonly, aggregates of solid tumor cells); [2] aplasia secondary to chemotherapeutic drugs; [3] the poorly understood pathophysiologic events that constitute the anemia of chronic disease; and [4] specific inhibitors of erythropoiesis.

Whether anemia is secondary to replacement of the bone marrow or to chemotherapy-induced hypoplasia, the usual rate of decline in the child's hemoglobin concentration is 0.8 to 1.0 g/dl per week (*i.e.,* 1/120th of the total red cell mass per day). Reductions more rapid than this indicate bleeding or hemolysis (see below). The diagnosis of anemia in such a setting is usually made without difficulty, and bone marrow examination to define its presence is not required unless a marrow aspirate is necessary for diagnosis or monitoring of the underlying malignancy. The reticulocyte count is inappropriately low, and leukopenia, thrombocytopenia, or both often coexist. Patients with cancer also generally have a component of the anemia of chronic disease, characterized by defective iron reutilization and diminished serum concentrations of erythropoietin.[3,4] Hence, patients with newly diagnosed solid malignant tumors, even without marrow infiltration, often have mild hypoproliferative anemia.

Table 38-1
Hemolytic Anemia in Children with Cancer

Pathophysiology	Laboratory Findings	Clinical Example(s)
Extrinsic erythrocyte disorder		
Microangiopathic (mechanical) process	Schistocytes and helmet cells on peripheral blood smear	Disseminated intravascular coagulation (*e.g.*, septicemia, acute promyelocytic leukemia)
		Thrombotic thrombocytopenic purpura-like syndrome due to mithramycin[9]
Immune-mediated process	Microspherocytes Positive antiglobulin (Coombs') test	Hodgkin's disease Drugs (*e.g.*, teniposide)[10] Transfused isohemagglutinins
Intrinsic erythrocyte deficit (unrelated to cancer)	Variable	Sickle cell anemia, hereditary spherocytosis, *etc.*

The production of specific cellular or humoral inhibitors by tumor cells as a cause of anemia is controversial.[3] Inhibitory substances may play a role in the severe and temporarily reversible pancytopenia seen as a preleukemic condition in children who ultimately develop acute lymphoblastic leukemia.[5,6] The transient pure red-cell aplasia seen in some leukemic children[7,8] may also be a result of inhibited erythropoiesis due to immunologic or other mechanisms.

A second mechanism of anemia is external blood loss in association with thrombocytopenia, usually epistaxis or from the gastrointestinal tract. Such bleeding is usually obvious clinically, but continued occult gastrointestinal bleeding may be responsible for striking hemoglobin declines in the thrombocytopenic subject, with the consequent need for intensive transfusion support. Blood loss may also result from diagnostic surgical procedures (*i.e.*, resection of Wilms' tumor or neuroblastoma) or from repetitive blood sampling for diagnostic tests or monitoring.

Hemolysis as a significant cause of anemia (Table 38-1), resulting either from mechanical factors or from antibody binding to the erythrocyte membrane, occurs relatively infrequently in the pediatric cancer patient. Mild immune-mediated hemolysis sometimes results from isohemagglutinins in plasma in which transfused platelets are suspended.[11] For instance, if blood group O platelets are administered to a type A recipient, anti-A in the transfused plasma may coat the recipient's erythrocytes, resulting in a positive antiglobulin test and in low-grade hemolysis. There may be subsequent difficulties in crossmatching for red blood cell transfusions because of the alloantibody remaining in the patient's plasma. This problem can be avoided completely by providing ABO and Rh type-specific platelets (see below).

Indications for Red Blood Cell Transfusion Support

The decision to transfuse or not to transfuse a red blood cell-containing product into a child with cancer must be made with a firm understanding of the normal and expected range of blood values in the pediatric population. Children have lower hemoglobin and red blood cell size measurements than adults, with values rising slowly from infancy to early adolescence and little variation between the genders[12] (Table 38-2). Red blood cell measurements also differ among races, with normal values being slightly lower in blacks than in whites. In adolescents,

Table 38-2
Age-Related Definition of Anemia in Pediatric Patients

Age	Lower Limit of Normal Hemoglobin Value (g/dl) Below Which Child Would Be Considered Anemic	
Newborn infant		13.5
3 months		9.5
1–3 years		11.0
4–8 years		11.5
8–12 years		11.5
12–16 years		12.0*
Adult	Males	13.5
	Females	12.5

* During and after puberty, hemoglobin values in boys rise progressively to reach adult levels.

the hemoglobin measurement depends more on the Tanner stage of sexual maturity than on chronologic age. Standard pediatric hematology references should be consulted for determining the specific range of hematologic values in an individual patient. Table 38-2 provides lower limits of normal hemoglobin values in children of various ages.

No one would argue with the need to administer packed red blood cells to a child with cancer who has symptomatic anemia. With hemoglobin values below 6 to 7 g/dl, tissue oxygen delivery is suboptimal, and most children exhibit malaise, lassitude, decreased activity, irritability, or some combination thereof. More controversial is whether transfusions should be administered to children with hemoglobin values in the 7 to 10 g/dl range, a level at which similar symptoms may occur but often without convincing evidence that anemia is their cause. Children with small degrees of anemia (hemoglobin values greater than 10 g/dl) would not require transfusion support.

A number of factors need be considered when one is assessing whether a transfusion is to be given. Unless the child with moderate to severe anemia has attendant symptoms, transfusion should not be routine if either recovery from chemotherapy-induced myelosuppression or leukemic remission is imminent. Such children have polychromasia and nucleated red blood cells on the peripheral smear and an elevated and progressively rising reticulocyte count. Moreover, the child with anemia need not be given a transfusion if the subsequent chemotherapy cycle or regimen is not likely to be intensive and cause further myelosuppression. Children on nonintensive chemotherapy programs should not routinely receive transfusion support for mild anemia.

On the other hand, there are certain clinical situations in which red blood cell replacement therapy should be given even if the anemia is not markedly symptomatic. For example, optimal oxygen-carrying capacity is desirable during intensive radiation therapy, since radiotherapy is most effective in an oxygen-rich environment in which free-radical formation is enhanced. Thus, even mild to moderate anemia should be corrected by red blood cell transfusions during radiation treatment. Another situation in which more aggressive red cell transfusion support might be advised is the child with only a modest degree of anemia (hemoglobin 8–10 g/dl) who is receiving or has just received an intensive cycle of chemotherapy that predictably will cause temporary marrow aplasia. Entering the expected 1- to 2-week-long phase of myelosuppression with a normal or near-normal hemoglobin value reduces the likelihood that severe anemia will occur shortly thereafter, particularly when thrombocytopenia is also anticipated. Maintaining a higher hemoglobin level provides "reserve" in case the patient suddenly has severe epistaxis or gastrointestinal bleeding.

RED BLOOD CELL TRANSFUSION REPLACEMENT THERAPY

Whole Blood

Although whole blood was the principal red blood cell-containing product used before the 1960s, component therapy is preferred at this time. Therefore, whole blood is almost never used except in cases of brisk external hemorrhage or for exchange transfusion for hyperleukocytosis.[13] Even in the former situation, the combination of packed red blood cells and either crystalloid, fresh frozen plasma, or plasma protein fraction is frequently delivered as an alternative.

Packed Red Blood Cells

The treatment of choice for children with cancer who are anemic and require transfusion is packed red blood cells, which comprise the sedimented or centrifuged erythrocytes from one unit of single-donor whole blood.[2] Currently, the blood is drawn in one of several anticoagulants, usually citrate–phosphate–dextrose (CPD)–adenine, and stored for up to 35 days. The product has a hematocrit of approximately 80% (hemoglobin 25 g/dl).

Red blood cell transfusions for children should always be ordered in milliliters per kilogram of body weight rather than in whole units. The "standard" transfusion volume, irrespective of the age of the child, is 10 ml/kg of body weight. This amount raises the child's hemoglobin by 2.5 to 3 g/dl. The maximum volume of red blood cells that can be safely administered in one transfusion is 15 ml/kg, but this should be ordered only if the patient is hemodynamically stable. Children with severe anemia (hemoglobin value less than 5 g/dl), particularly when either congestive heart failure or hypertension is present, should receive smaller repeated transfusions, perhaps accompanied by a diuretic. Multiple transfusions of 3 to 5

ml/kg, each administered over 3 hours and separated by a period of several hours to allow cardiovascular stabilization, restore oxygen-carrying capacity within 24 hours. Rapid provision of a large volume of erythrocytes in such circumstances may result in pulmonary edema.

A partial exchange transfusion is sometimes preferable to single or repetitive packed red blood cell transfusions.[2,14] This procedure requires adequate venous access (ideally, two indwelling catheters) and is conducted by withdrawing the patient's blood and administering packed red cells alternately in increments of 10 to 50 ml, depending on the weight of the patient. Several investigators have proposed formulas or nomograms that permit calculation of the optimal amount of blood to be exchanged in order to reach the desired post-transfusion hemoglobin value.[14,15] Packed red blood cells are preferable to whole blood when exchange transfusion is being conducted as treatment for severe anemia.

The advantage of partial exchange transfusion is that the anemia may be corrected rapidly and isovolemically.[14] This approach is particularly advisable in the severely anemic child with congestive heart failure, especially when the need for vigorous hydration is apparent, for example, the child with newly diagnosed leukemia with hyperleukocytosis (white blood cell count exceeding 100,000/mm^3) who has hyperuricemia and other metabolic features of the tumor lysis syndrome (see Chap. 37). Correction of the anemia and removal of toxic metabolites may occur following the exchange, and intensive intravenous hydration might then be given safely without the risk of pulmonary edema. The disadvantage of such an exchange procedure relates to difficulties with venous access.

Washed Leukocyte-Poor or Frozen Packed Red Blood Cells

Packed erythrocytes that have been washed with saline and thus rendered relatively free of leukocytes, platelets, and plasma components are rarely if ever indicated in pediatric cancer patients. Their use certainly minimizes exposure to leukocyte, platelet, and plasma alloantigens, thus reducing subsequent allergic and febrile transfusion reactions in patients on long-term hypertransfusion programs (e.g., with thalassemia major).[16] However, nearly all children with cancer who need intensive red blood cell support also receive transfused platelets, which contain multiple HLA and platelet-specific antigens and are suspended in plasma with additional soluble alloantigens. Most pediatric centers have not utilized thawed and washed previously frozen red blood cells[17] for the same reasons.

Irradiated Blood Products

This subject is addressed below in the discussion of graft-versus-host disease as a complication of blood transfusion therapy.

Other Treatment for the Anemic Patient

The child with a malignant disorder who is anemic often benefits from therapy other than transfusion replacement. Iron deficiency or other nutritional deficits may coexist, particularly in the young infant with an abnormal diet containing excessive quantities of milk or the older child who has continuing external blood loss. Other specific treatment for anemia includes chemotherapy for remission of the primary malignancy and, of course, withdrawal of offending drugs in the setting of drug-induced immunohemolytic anemia.

Supplemental oxygen is often overlooked as a simple means of providing additional oxygen-carrying capacity to the anemic patient. Although hyperbaric oxygen is not practical, use of a mask or nasal prongs to deliver humidified 40% oxygen is often comforting to the patient and may deliver symptomatic relief in instances of life-threatening anemia prior to or during the necessary blood transfusions.

Many children with anemia require no treatment at all. The numerous physiologic mechanisms that compensate for anemia (tachycardia, increased stroke volume, hyperventilation, vasodilatation, and rightward shift in the oxyhemoglobin-dissociation curve) appear to function effectively even in the hypermetabolic setting of advanced malignant disease.

PATHOPHYSIOLOGY OF HEMORRHAGE IN THE CHILD WITH MALIGNANT DISEASE

Hemorrhage occurs whenever the normal hemostatic mechanism is impaired as a result of a defect in one or more of its three major components: blood vessels, circulating platelets, and soluble coagulation proteins. Thrombocytopenia is by far the most common bleeding complication encountered by the pediatric oncologist. The principal form of hematologic support for this problem is platelet transfusion, so most of this discussion will focus on that modality.

PLATELET TRANSFUSION

Pathophysiology of Thrombocytopenia

Thrombocytopenia, defined as a platelet count less than 175,000/mm³, results from one or more of four basic mechanisms: decreased production, increased destruction, hypersplenism (splenic sequestration), or loss following extensive transfusion replacement or apheresis. Diminished production of platelets is nearly always due to reduced megakaryocytes accompanying replacement of the bone marrow by leukemia or neuroblastoma or aplasia secondary to chemotherapy or radiation. Other lineages (red blood cells and granulocytes) usually are affected also. Thrombocytopenia due to increased peripheral destruction with inadequate marrow compensation may occur either on an immune basis or because of mechanical

factors. Immune-mediated thrombocytopenia, with features identical to idiopathic thrombocytopenic purpura, has been described in children with leukemia and other forms of cancer but is probably coincidental.[18,19] Immune complexes may be deposited on the platelet membrane during bacterial or viral infection and frequently result in platelet injury or ingestion by fixed mononuclear phagocytes in the spleen. Also, the severe thrombocytopenia accompanying dactinomycin (actinomycin D) therapy has recently been shown to be due in part to immunologic factors and to be responsive to prednisone.[20] Thrombocytopenia resulting from mechanical platelet injury is seen primarily in disseminated intravascular coagulation (DIC) complicating acute nonlymphocytic leukemia (ANLL) or large solid tumors such as neuroblastoma. Hypersplenism as a cause of thrombocytopenic hemorrhage is uncommon except in instances of massive splenomegaly, as in Langerhans' cell histiocytosis, erythrophagocytic syndromes, and juvenile chronic myelogenous leukemia.

Historical Perspective

Prior to a quarter of a century ago, the only form of transfusion support for the thrombocytopenic cancer patient was freshly drawn whole blood. This treatment was often ineffective because of the small number of platelets within the transfused product.[21] Thus, severe external or intracranial hemorrhage was a common cause of death in children with leukemia. By the mid-1960s, it had been proved that the risk of hemorrhage in the thrombocytopenic patient was directly related to the platelet count (Table 38-3) and that provision of blood products containing platelets was an effective means of stopping hemorrhage.[22] Within several years, the practice of separating platelet concentrates from freshly drawn units of donor blood became standard practice, and platelet transfusion support to the thrombocytopenic cancer patient demonstrably reduced hemorrhagic morbidity and mortality rates.

During the 1970s, two major controversies evolved regarding the use of platelet transfusions: [1] the optimal methods to store platelet concentrates in the blood bank prior to their administration to a recipient, and [2] whether platelet concentrates should be given "prophylactically" to thrombocytopenic patients who are not bleeding. Although research during the past 10 to 15 years has resulted in successful resolution of the first issue—superiority of room-temperature-stored platelets[23]—the latter subject—prophylactic versus therapeutic platelets—remains much argued.

Table 38-3
Relation Between Platelet Count and Extent of Hemorrhage in Children with Cancer

Platelet Count (per mm³)	Usual Type and Severity of Hemorrhage*			
	Bruising	Petechiae	Mucosal Bleeding†	Intracranial Bleeding
>100,000	0	0	0	0
50,000–100,000	+	+	0	0
20,000–50,000	++	++	+	0
5,000–20,000	+++	+++	++	Rare
<5,000	++++	++++	+++	Most episodes

* Relative scale of frequency and severity: 0 = extremely rare or not at all, + = infrequent and/or mild, ++ = common and usually mild, +++ = extremely common and/or moderately severe, ++++ = invariable and potentially severe.
† Epistaxis, gingival bleeding, hematuria, metrorrhagia.

Platelet Procurement and Storage

Platelets administered to children with cancer are derived from single units of whole blood from which platelet-rich plasma is removed in a closed system. The platelets are then separated from most of the plasma following centrifugation at 3000 rpm for 10 minutes. Freshly drawn platelets are usually not used immediately (unless they are derived from a single apheresis donor), so some method of storage is necessary. In current practice, platelets may be stored for up to 5 days at 24°C as long as they are suspended in a relatively large volume (50–60 ml) of plasma containing CPD–adenine as the anticoagulant and are gently agitated throughout the storage period. The platelets are stored in specially designed plastic bags that permit entry of oxygen, thus enhancing aerobic metabolism of the metabolically active platelets and preventing accumulation of lactic acid, with its deleterious effects on viability.[23]

Although platelets stored in such a matter are hemostatically effective, they acquire a mild "storage lesion" characterized by diminished ability to aggregate immediately after transfusion, sometimes resulting in a period of several hours before normal hemostasis is achieved. At one time, it was suggested that storage of platelets at 4°C was preferable since prompt cessation of bleeding and correction of the bleeding time test occurred following transfusion. However, these 4°C-stored platelets survive in the recipient just a few hours. Therefore, nearly all blood banks now utilize 20° to 24°C rather than 4°C storage.[23]

Although the defect in platelet prostaglandin synthesis induced by aspirin is clinically significant in certain settings,[24] "aspirinated" platelets from donors who have taken the drug within several days of donation will aggregate normally if the recipient also receives one or more units from donors who have not used aspirin.

Frozen platelets have been used in adults with acute non-lymphocytic leukemia in remission, from whom autologous platelets were harvested, separated, suspended in a cryopreservative, and frozen.[25] They were then later thawed, washed, and reinfused during periods of severe thrombocytopenia accompanying intensive consolidation chemotherapy or following relapse. Satisfactory platelet recovery and survival ensued. However, concerns about toxicity of the cryoprotective agents and the great expense associated with the procedure has made this approach impractical, particularly for pediatric patients.

As described further below, platelets may be obtained by apheresis techniques from a single donor (often a family member) in order to improve platelet recovery and survival in cases of suspected or proven alloimmunization.

Method of Administration

Platelets should be infused rapidly (usually over 20–40 minutes) through a standard platelet transfusion filter (170 μm diameter) designed to remove large aggregates. Each unit generally contains approximately 10^{11} platelets in a volume of 30 to 70 ml. In very young children or when volume overload is present, some of the accompanying plasma can be removed in the blood bank by gentle centrifugation immediately before the transfusion. This is not desirable as a routine, however, because some platelets are lost or damaged in the process.

Typing and crossmatching procedures for platelets are unfortunately neither clinically applicable nor widely available.[26] Although much has been learned during the past two decades about the structure and function of platelet-specific and HLA antigens on the platelet surface, serologic tests to define their presence and to measure reproducibly antibodies directed against them are performed only in a few research laboratories.

It is usually desirable to request platelets from a donor of the same ABO and Rh red cell type as the recipient. Although A and B antigens are expressed to only a slight extent if at all on platelets, infusion of ABO-incompatible platelets can result in a positive antiglobulin test and low-grade hemolysis due to isohemagglutinins in the plasma or erythrocytes contaminating the platelet concentrate. Moreover, ABO-incompatible platelets have a slightly shorter survival than matched cells.[27] Nevertheless, when ABO-matched platelets are not available, mismatched platelets should be administered. Although Rh antigens are not expressed on platelets, Rh-positive platelets should not be given to Rh-negative female recipients who are likely to survive into adulthood.

The "dose" of platelets (number of units ordered) depends on the weight of the child and the post-transfusion platelet count desired. Theoretically, the 1-hour post-transfusion increment should be 10,000 to 12,000 platelets/mm³ per m² of body surface area. Therefore, a 30-kg (1.0-m²) child who receives 4 units of platelets would be expected to exhibit a rise in platelet count of 40,000 to 48,000/mm³ above the baseline value. This calculation does not always prove useful clinically since there are multiple variables that affect platelet recovery that are not easily quantified, such as infection, prior alloimmunization, or injury to the platelets during procurement, storage, or transfusion. The aim should be to stop or prevent hemorrhage, not necessarily to achieve and maintain a normal platelet count. A dose of 1 unit per 6 to 8 kg of body weight usually suffices to stop hemorrhage and raise the platelet count to greater than 30,000/mm³ for 24 hours or more. For practical purposes, a minimum of 2 units should always be ordered for infants, 3 units for toddlers, 4 units for young children, and 6 to 8 units for preadolescents and adolescents.

The response to a platelet transfusion may be assessed by measuring the increment in platelet count 1 and 24 hours after the infusion.[1] However, 1-hour post-transfusion platelet counts are not usually indicated because of the extra fingerstick that is required. Achievement of a normal survival of the transfused platelets (7–10 days) is rarely a realistic goal because of the many confounding variables. The best indication that the platelet transfusion has been effective is cessation of hemorrhage and absence of new bleeding signs or symptoms during the ensuing days. The bleeding time has been used to document the hemostatic effectiveness of transfused platelets in experimental trials but is rarely if ever practical in thrombocytopenic children.

Indications for Platelet Transfusions

One of the most controversial subjects in pediatric oncology is platelet transfusion support, particularly prophylactic use in the nonbleeding thrombocytopenic patient. There is no doubt about the need for intensive platelet support in a child with leukemia or receiving cytotoxic chemotherapy who has severe (platelet count less than 20,000/mm³) thrombocytopenia and extensive cutaneous, mucosal, or internal bleeding. Transfusions should be provided on a regular basis (usually every 24–72 hours) until the bleeding ceases and the patient's bone marrow recovers. Platelet transfusion support is most effective when the child does not manifest fever or other evidence of infection and when alloimmunization is absent.

Some children with cancer and more modest degrees of thrombocytopenia (platelet count 20,000–100,000/mm³) may be at risk of local hemorrhage at the site of an invasive procedure, such as a surgical incision, lumbar puncture, or bone marrow aspiration. Unfortunately, little information is available regarding what level of platelet count is "safe" for performance of a lumbar puncture without a prior platelet transfusion. A minimal platelet level of 50,000/mm³ has been recommended by some workers. Although in the vast majority of circumstances, bone marrow and lumbar puncture can be performed with safety even when the platelet count is less than 20,000/mm³, platelet transfusion is still recommended for a patient whose platelet count is <20,000/mm³. Concern about the extremely rare complication of spinal epidural hemorrhage and paraplegia following lumbar puncture does not justify routine platelet transfusion support in every thrombocytopenic patient prior to this commonly performed and important diagnostic procedure.

A useful measurement of primary hemostasis in the patient with mild to moderate thrombocytopenia is the bleeding time[28] measured using one of the new disposable spring-loaded devices. The results may assist with the decision regarding whether platelet transfusions should be given prior to a major surgical procedure. Severe hemorrhage would not be expected if the bleeding time is less than 15 minutes, the typical value when the platelets are normal in function and greater than 40,000 to 50,000/mm³ in number.

Prophylactic Platelet Transfusions

In thrombocytopenic patients with cancer and other hematologic conditions, the risk and severity of hemorrhage is related primarily to the platelet count (see Table 38-3). Severe hemorrhage is uncommon until the platelet count falls below 20,000/mm³, and even at or below this level, most children exhibit only crops of petechiae and a bruising tendency. Most instances of intracranial hemorrhage are associated with platelet counts less than 5,000/mm³. Nevertheless, many oncology centers routinely provide platelet concentrates to children with leukemia, lymphoma, or solid tumors whose platelet counts are below an arbitrarily defined critical level, usually 20,000/mm³.[1,2] Such "prophylactic" platelet transfusions, given solely on the basis of the platelet count rather than because of coexisting hemorrhage, account for a large percentage of the total units of blood transfused in many oncology units.

The controversy surrounding use of prophylactic platelets has recently been summarized by an excellent review by Feusner.[29] Some of the pros and cons of prophylactic platelet transfusions for counts below 20,000/mm³ are provided in Table 38-4. Advocates of prophylactic platelet transfusions justify their position by preferring to prevent mucosal or internal hemorrhage rather than having to deal with its consequences. Moreover, since one cannot predict with certainty when intracranial hemorrhage will occur in the child with marked thrombocytopenia, such disastrous events can likely be prevented by maintaining the count greater than 20,000/mm³. Also, it has been proposed that microvascular integrity may be better maintained when small numbers of platelets are constantly present to "nurture" the vascular endothelium.[30]

Opponents of prophylactic platelets invoke their great expense, associated strains on blood bank resources, and—most especially—the numerous side effects (alloimmunization, transfusion reactions, and hepatitis) resulting from this more intensive form of transfusion replacement (Table 38-4).[26,31,32] Also, it has been observed that intracranial or severe mucosal bleeding rarely is a sudden event in a patient with a stable platelet count of 5,000 to 20,000/mm³ in the absence of warning signs such as a sudden increase in cutaneous bleeding, blood blisters in the mouth, or retinal hemorrhages. If platelet transfusions are not given prophylactically to all subjects with severe thrombocytopenia but rather are reserved for patients with these warning signs or counts below 5,000/mm³, it might be possible to prevent fatal hemorrhagic events with far fewer transfusions.

A controversial issue such as this is ideally addressed by randomized controlled studies that generate statistically sound data. However, prophylactic platelet transfusions has been difficult to evaluate in a controlled fashion, since the undesired end point, intracranial hemorrhage, is, fortunately, a rare event

Table 38-4
*Pros and Cons of Prophylactic Platelet Transfusions**

Reasons for	*Reasons Against*
Hemorrhage from all sites reduced by maintaining platelet count >20,000/mm³	Unnecessary since life-threatening bleeding rarely occurs without warning in a stable afebrile thrombocytopenic host
Risk of fatal intracranial hemorrhage practically eliminated	Fatal intracranial hemorrhage is extremely rare unless platelet count is <5,000/mm³
Psychological benefits of preventing minor hemorrhage rather than treating it once it occurs	Platelets administered therapeutically for mucosal or internal bleeding just as effective as platelets given prophylactically
Alloimmunization, hepatitis, and other side effects not increased appreciably since most affected patients are heavily transfused anyway	Lack of controlled studies proving efficacy
	Expense
	Greater likelihood of alloimmunization and allergic reactions
	Increased incidence of infectious complications, especially non-A, non-B hepatitis

* Defined as a transfusion administered to a patient with marrow failure due to cancer or its treatment who is not exhibiting clinical hemorrhage (except for bruises and petechiae) but who has a platelet count <20,000/mm³.

and because potential study patients are heterogeneous with regard to underlying disease, chemotherapy and antibiotic regimens, age, and other variables. Nevertheless, several randomized trials or retrospective reviews have been conducted.[33–35] Those studies that support the use of prophylactic platelets have suggested that the risk of hemorrhage is less in patients who do than in those who do not receive prophylactic platelets.[33–35] However, other investigators are able to identify no benefit from prophylactically administered platelets and recommend instead selective transfusion support for specific hemorrhagic complications.[31,32,36–38] Unfortunately, all of the studies conducted thus far are small, faulty in design, or both, and the results sometimes have been reported only as abstracts.

Although many pediatric oncologists continue to order platelet concentrates for all patients with platelet counts under 20,000/mm³, this author reserves them for the specific clinical situations summarized in Table 38-5. A recent National Institutes of Health Consensus Development Conference has addressed this subject and also has suggested that 20,000/mm³ is too high a level for prophylactic platelet transfusions to be given to the nonbleeding (except for petechiae and bruising) patient without fever, infection, or need for invasive procedures.[26] Further study of this important issue is clearly indicated.

Single-Donor Platelets

Platelets for transfusion are usually obtained from multiple random donors. An attractive, if less practical and more expensive, alternative is the procurement of a large number of platelets (equivalent to 8 to 10 units) from a single donor by using apheresis technology.[39] The rationale for the use of a single donor is several-fold. Side effects, such as alloimmunization, should be reduced in view of the limited number of donor exposures.[40–41] Although selective use of single donors also allows for administration of matched or type-specific platelets, crossmatching tests using lymphocytotoxicity, immunofluorescence, or other assays provide inconsistent results and are not widely available. Partial or fully HLA-matched platelets from a

relative (often a parent) or an unrelated individual derived from a large donor pool (available in a few regional blood centers) are sometimes the only effective therapy in the alloimmunized thrombocytopenic recipient. However, this approach is costly and has a number of logistical shortcomings, including problems identifying appropriate donors because of nonuniform compatibility tests and the rarity of completely HLA-matched individuals in the general population.[39,42]

Platelet Dysfunction

Abnormal platelet function as a cause of hemorrhage in children with cancer is infrequent. Aspirin and aspirin-containing drugs are nearly always avoided by such patients, and remarkably few other prescription or over-the-counter drugs have been conclusively shown to affect platelet function in a clinically significant manner.[43] Certain penicillin derivatives (i.e., carbenicillin and ticarcillin) and cephalosporins (i.e., moxalactam) used by pediatric oncologists have been reported to impair platelet aggregation and prolong the bleeding time.[44–46] However, although bleeding signs have been observed in adults, the semisynthetic penicillins used widely in thrombocytopenic children with cancer have not been reported to cause a bleeding tendency. Some chemotherapeutic agents, including L-asparaginase and vincristine, may impair platelet aggregation,[47] but these effects, too, are unlikely to be important clinically. If platelet dysfunction is thought to contribute to a child's bleeding tendency, then platelet transfusions represent the treatment of choice.

Other Supportive Care Measures for the Patient with Severe Thrombocytopenia

In addition to platelet transfusion support, certain nonspecific local measures may be of value: [1] avoidance of intramuscular injections and deep (i.e., femoral and jugular) venipunctures, [2] use of firm local pressure in the case of epistaxis or bleeding from puncture wounds, [3] application of Gelfoam, desiccated collagen preparations, or topical thrombin for lesions of the

---

Table 38-5
Recommended Indications for Platelet Transfusion Support in Children with Cancer

In the Presence of Significant* Hemorrhage	*In the Absence of Significant* Hemorrhage (i.e., prophylactically)*
Thrombocytopenia of any severity (usually significant hemorrhage does not occur if the platelet count is >20,000/mm³ unless other factors are present, i.e., infection, local anatomic lesion)	Before major surgical procedure if platelet count is <50,000/mm³
	Before lumbar puncture or minor surgical procedure if platelet count is <20,000/mm³
Suspected platelet dysfunction (e.g., aspirin) irrespective of platelet count	In febrile patient with platelet count <20,000/mm³, especially in a child with acute nonlymphocytic leukemia
	Platelet count <5,000/mm³ with little likelihood of imminent (within 1–2 days) rise

* Significant hemorrhage is defined as follows: recurrent or severe epistaxis, gingival bleeding, extensive buccal "blood blisters," gross gastrointestinal hemorrhage (not just occult blood in stool), retinal bleeding, extensive *new* cutaneous bleeding, suspected or proven internal hemorrhage. Bruises and scattered petechiae are not considered clinically significant hemorrhage.

oral mucous membranes. Although popular in the past, anterior nasal packs are now generally avoided because of the local discomfort and the risk of infection. Epsilon-aminocaproic acid (Amicar), a fibrinolytic inhibitor, would not be expected to enhance primary hemostasis greatly, but some clinicians attest to its utility in thrombocytopenic patients with mucosal hemorrhage.[48] Desmopressin (DDAVP) enhances the adhesion of platelets to vascular subendothelium and has been a valuable adjunct or even substitute for blood transfusions in some hemorrhagic disorders.[49] The drug shortens the bleeding time in mildly thrombocytopenic patients, but it is of no demonstrable value in patients with platelet counts below 50,000/mm³.[49] Prednisone in low doses (5–10 mg) is often used to reduce hemorrhage in thrombocytopenic patients as a consequence of its nonspecific effects on capillary stability.[30] Estrogens are of value for severe menometrorrhagia.

PLASMA PRODUCTS

Pathophysiology of Blood Coagulation

The body's chief defense against excessive hemorrhage from large blood vessels is rapid deposition of an insoluble fibrin clot produced by a complicated sequence of reactions involving more than a dozen soluble plasma proteins. These reactions have been divided conveniently, but somewhat artificially, into intrinsic and extrinsic coagulation systems, which are respectively measured by two screening tests, the partial thromboplastin time (PTT) and the prothrombin time (PT). Further discussion of the biochemistry, pathophysiology, and laboratory measurement of these factors cannot be provided here because of space limitations; standard hematology textbooks should be consulted for details.

Disseminated Intravascular Coagulation

Disseminated intravascular coagulation is characterized by inappropriate and excessive activation of blood coagulation, with consumption and utilization of clotting factors and platelets, resulting in hemorrhage (usually from multiple sites), hemolytic anemia, and, occasionally, a thrombotic tendency.[50] In children with cancer, DIC is seen primarily in patients with gram-negative septicemia, newly diagnosed or relapsing ANLL,[51] and, less frequently, in disseminated neuroblastoma[52] and other metastatic solid tumors.[53] A syndrome resembling DIC has also been reported in children with familial erythrophagocytic lymphohistiocytosis.[54] Some of the initial descriptions of DIC included patients with acute promyelocytic leukemia, the M3 variant of ANLL according to the French–American–British classification.[55] Yet DIC is also observed in other forms of ANLL (particularly M5 or monomyelocytic disease) and in children with acute lymphoblastic leukemia with hyperleukocytosis.[51,56] In one recent series of pediatric patients with ANLL, DIC had prognostic significance in that its presence was independently associated with failure to achieve remission.[51]

As shown in Table 38-6, the laboratory diagnosis of DIC is made by demonstrating prolongation of both PT and PTT and a reduced platelet count. Necessary confirmatory test results include decreased fibrinogen and elevated levels of fibrin degradation products. Specific factor assays, fibrinopeptide A measurements, or other, more elaborate, studies are usually not required.

The primary therapy for DIC is management of the underlying neoplastic or complicating infectious disease.[50] When DIC accompanies bacterial septicemia, the mortality rate is high, usually not from bleeding but from endotoxic shock. Platelet and fresh frozen plasma transfusions should be given to patients with DIC who have mucosal or internal hemorrhage. Although these transfusions may be of transient benefit, the bleeding may resume within 24 hours unless the triggering mechanism is brought under control; thus, transfusion support may be required for many days.

Heparin was once widely used as therapy for DIC but is infrequently recommended now except in patients with acute promyelocytic leukemia. Several small series of patients with this form of leukemia have received low-dose continuous heparin infusions (approximately 150–200 units/kg per day) during the initial induction phase of treatment, and the results have been favorable.[57,58] However, neither standard nor low-dose heparin has ever been evaluated in carefully controlled studies, and a recent trial from Boston reported high induction rates and few hemorrhagic or thrombotic complications in adults with M3 ANLL who were managed *without* heparin.[59] Therefore, the issue is not yet resolved. Fortunately, acute promyelocytic leukemia is an infrequent form of ANLL in children.

Liver Disease

Patients with impaired hepatocellular function from any cause commonly have a bleeding tendency, resulting primarily from decreased synthesis of multiple blood coagulation factors in the liver.[60] Children with cancer occasionally develop severe hepatitis, cirrhosis, or both as a consequence of transfusion-related infection, biliary obstruction, or hepatotoxicity of chemotherapeutic agents. Thrombocytopenia resulting from portal hypertension-induced hypersplenism is a common accompaniment. Although recommended management consists of fresh frozen plasma in the event of hemorrhage or prior to invasive procedures,[61] few efficacy data are available.

Vitamin K Deficiency

Vitamin K promotes the gamma-carboxylation of glutamic acid residues on Factors II (prothrombin), VII, IX, and X. This postsynthetic modification allows these molecules to bind calcium, a prerequisite for phospholipid-mediated reactions in the coagulation cascade. Vitamin K deficiency may result from diminished intake, decreased intestinal absorption, suppression of the bowel microflora by broad-spectrum antibiotics (resulting in diminished synthesis of endogenous vitamin K), and the presence of vitamin K antagonists, which interfere with its action at the cellular level.[61] In children with cancer, vitamin K deficiency occurs infrequently. Although patients with severe protein–calorie malnutrition are usually provided with enteral or parenteral vitamin K supplements, stores can sometimes be depleted in patients with neoplastic disease.[62] Vitamin K deficiency also occurs in some patients receiving certain of the new beta-lactam antibiotics as therapy for febrile episodes during periods of severe neutropenia.[62] Several of these agents, especially moxalactam and cefamandole, interfere directly in the carboxylation reaction mediated by vitamin K.[46]

Vitamin K deficiency is easily diagnosed in the appropriate clinical setting[50] (see Table 38-6). The PT and PTT are both prolonged, with the PT elevation being proportionately greater because of the short half-life of Factor VII. The fibrinogen concentration and platelet count are normal. Therapy consists

Table 38-6
Diagnosis and Management of Clinically Significant Coagulation Disturbances in the Child with Cancer

	Most Frequent Clinical Settings	Abnormal Screening Tests	Other Diagnostic Studies*	Management Approaches	
				Standard and Accepted	Infrequently Used and/or Investigational
DIC	Septicemia ANLL (M3 variant) Any leukemia with WBC count > 100,000/mm³ Disseminated neuroblastoma	Increased PT, PTT Decreased platelet count Short survival of transfused platelets	Reduced fibrinogen Elevated fibrin degradation products	Treatment of underlying problem (*i.e.,* chemotherapy for tumor, antibiotics for infection) Platelet and fresh frozen plasma transfusions	Heparin Cryoprecipitate
Vitamin K deficiency	Severe malnutrition in advanced cancer Use of certain cephalosporins	Increased PT, PTT Normal platelet count and fibrinogen	None usually required	Vitamin K (1–5 mg orally or IV)	Fresh frozen plasma
L-asparaginase-induced coagulopathy	Cerebrovascular accident Large-vessel thrombosis or (rarely) unexplained hemorrhage	Increased PT, PTT Reduced fibrinogen	Reduced antithrombin III Reduced protein C and protein S	Supportive care Temporarily discontinue L-asparaginase	Fresh frozen plasma Antithrombin III concentrate
Liver dysfunction	Gastrointestinal or other hemorrhage Jaundice and hepatomegaly	Increased PT, PTT Platelet count and fibrinogen variable Other liver function tests abnormal	None usually required	Fresh frozen plasma	—

* Multiple coagulation factors are decreased in most cases, but their measurement is rarely necessary in clinical practice.

of oral or parenteral vitamin K, 1 to 5 mg, depending on the child's age. Drugs that interfere with vitamin K action should probably be avoided in children with cancer, since effective alternative antimicrobial agents are available.

L-Asparaginase

Ever since L-asparaginase was first used clinically, laboratory evidence of coagulopathy has been noted as a side effect. Because the drug inhibits the synthesis of several proteins containing asparagine (see Chap. 9), it exerts effects on the hepatic synthesis of numerous asparagine-rich blood coagulation factors and inhibitors. Fibrinogen, Factor V, and many of the vitamin K-dependent factors are reduced in a dose-dependent fashion, resulting in strikingly abnormal laboratory coagulation screening tests.[63,64] Plasminogen deficiency[65] and altered patterns of Factor VIII–von Willebrand factor multimers[66] also exist following L-asparaginase therapy. The drug also inhibits the synthesis of the physiologic inhibitors of the activated blood coagulation proteins, antithrombin III, protein C, and protein S.[64,67,68] This balanced reduction of procoagulants and inhibitors results in L-asparaginase having few clinically apparent effects on hemostasis.

The most frequently reported complication of L-asparaginase treatment on blood coagulation has been cerebrovascular accidents, occurring in 1% to 3% of children with acute lymphoblastic leukemia who receive multiple doses of the drug.[63] This stroke syndrome is characterized by focal neurologic findings, seizures, abnormalities on computed tomography scan consistent with hemorrhagic infarction, and striking alterations in coagulation screening tests and levels of inhibitors.[63] Whether the primary event is intracranial hemorrhage or infarction due to large-vessel thrombosis is sometimes unclear. The laboratory findings in children with strokes are not significantly different from those in patients receiving L-asparaginase who do not develop neurologic signs or symptoms.[67] For instance, both antithrombin III and protein C are decreased in patients receiving L-asparaginase whether or not they develop strokes. A recent study of a large series of children receiving L-asparaginase has shown that an altered pattern of von Willebrand factor multimers is the only laboratory abnormality that correlates with thrombosis.[66]

The management of the patient with hemorrhagic/thrombotic strokes due to L-asparaginase is strictly supportive. There are no studies endorsing the use of fresh frozen plasma or antithrombin III concentrates. An important feature of this complication is the relatively good prognosis of these children, many of whom subsequently receive additional L-asparaginase without untoward effects.[69]

Miscellaneous Coagulation Disturbances in Children with Cancer

Laboratory evidence of a coagulopathy has recently been noted in children receiving high doses of human lymphoblastoid interferon.[70] Although levels of vitamin K-dependent factors were somewhat reduced in these patients, convincing evidence of vitamin K deficiency was not demonstrated. With the increasing use of interferon preparations in children with cancer, further study of this subject is warranted.

Another unusual coagulation protein abnormality is the acquired von Willebrand's defect noted in some children with Wilms' tumor.[71] This does not appear to be associated with abnormal bleeding.

General Principles of Management of Coagulation Disturbances

Children with cancer who have altered laboratory tests of hemostasis but little or no hemorrhage do not require any treatment whatsoever.[50] Although fresh frozen plasma has been used to treat coagulation disorders in children and adults, it has also been ordered inappropriately as a volume expander and as "prophylaxis" for patients with minimal coagulation abnormalities.[72] Its major indication in pediatric cancer patients is for DIC; rarely, it is indicated for bleeding due to liver failure. The usual dose of fresh frozen plasma is 10 to 15 mg/kg administered over 1 to 2 hours and repeated every 12 to 24 hours as necessary to stop hemorrhage.

Specifically purified (to inactivate viruses) plasma concentrates containing Factor VIII or the prothrombin complex (Factors II, VII, IX, and X) should not be used in children with cancer unless they also happen to have hemophilia. Several cases of high-grade diffuse malignant lymphoma have recently been described in hemophiliacs as a result of acquired immune deficiency syndrome (AIDS) due to the human immunodeficiency virus (HIV). Cryoprecipitate, which contains mainly Factor VIII and fibrinogen, has been recommended for bleeding patients with DIC, but fresh frozen plasma is preferable since it contains a wider spectrum of the depleted factors.[50] Cryoprecipitate may be useful, however, to correct the severe hypofibrinogenemia complicating some of the erythrophagocytic disorders.

As with hemorrhage complicating thrombocytopenia, application of local pressure and other nonspecific supportive measures should, when indicated, complement the use of blood products.

GRANULOCYTE TRANSFUSIONS

A form of hematologic support used extensively during the 1970s was granulocyte transfusions. However, during the past few years, the transfusion of granulocytes, obtained by apheresis techniques from normal donors, has been used infrequently because of improvements in other aspects of supportive care (especially liberal use of more effective antibiotics) and in view of several controlled trials showing no efficacy. Because granulocyte transfusions are an aspect of the management of life-threatening infection, they are discussed further in Chapter 39. The side effects of granulocyte transfusions are similar to those observed following other blood products and are discussed below.

APHERESIS PROCEDURES

Current technology permits safe, rapid, and nearly isovolemic removal of large quantities of plasma or cellular elements from the circulation by means of continuous-flow centrifugation. In pediatric oncology, apheresis procedures are used as therapy for patients with excessive numbers of abnormal cells or to remove cells from normal blood donors for replacement therapy for a thrombocytopenic or granulocytopenic recipient.

Erythrocytopheresis, plasmapheresis, and plateletpheresis are not used therapeutically in pediatric patients due to the extreme rarity of polycythemia vera, macroglobulinemia, and essential thrombocythemia. However, leukopheresis is sometimes carried out for children with acute leukemia who have presenting white blood cell counts in excess of 100,000/mm^3, although the height of the white count at which this intervention is undertaken differs among institutions. Patients with ANLL, in particular, are at risk of intracerebral or pulmonary leukostasis, DIC, or the severe metabolic derangements of the tumor lysis syndrome when hyperleukocytosis exists[2,51] (see Chap. 37). Continuous- or intermittent-flow centrifugation techniques have removed large quantities of leukocytes from such children. The procedure is most feasible for patients over 5 years of age in whom venous access is more easily achieved and usually results in a marked (but often transient) reduction of the leukocyte count. An effective alternative measure—particularly for younger patients—is simple exchange transfusion with fresh whole blood using manual techniques.[13] The controversy regarding whether these cell removal procedures need to be performed in the child with newly diagnosed leukemia and hyperleukocytosis is addressed in Chapter 37.

The use of apheresis techniques to remove platelets from normal adult donors is discussed elsewhere in this chapter.

COMPLICATIONS OF BLOOD TRANSFUSION SUPPORT

It is beyond the scope of this chapter to provide a detailed discussion of the myriad complications of blood transfusions. Standard infectious disease or transfusion medicine reference sources should be consulted. However, the following brief survey will address the two most common side effects in the child with cancer: abnormal immunologic responses and transmission of infectious agents.

Immunologic Complications of Blood Transfusions

Transfusion Reactions

Every blood transfusion carries a risk of an untoward immunologic reaction. Transfusion reactions can be classified as either hemolytic or nonhemolytic. Hemolytic transfusion reactions usually result from infusion of blood that is incompatible at the ABO or Rh locus.[73] The most common cause of life-threatening hemolytic reactions is clerical or nursing error (*i.e.,* incorrect matching, mislabeling, or administering the blood to the wrong patient). Minor hemolytic events are seen frequently in children receiving intensive platelet support with ABO-incompatible platelets (described above). Hemolytic transfusion reactions manifest as high fever, chills, back or abdominal pain, dark urine, pallor, and jaundice. Abnormal laboratory results include hemoglobinuria, hemoglobinemia, hyperbilirubinemia, increase in anemia, spherocytes on the peripheral blood smear, and a positive antiglobulin test. Specimens of the recipient's and donor's blood should be submitted promptly to the blood bank for analysis. Management consists of vigorous hydration and mannitol diuresis to maintain urine flow until the hemoglobinuria resolves.

Nonhemolytic transfusions reactions are much more common; they are frequently a nuisance but not particularly serious. They most commonly result from alloantibodies in the recipient's plasma that react against HLA or other antigens on platelets and leukocytes in the transfused products. Therefore, these reactions are observed more commonly in multitransfused patients. Clinical features include fever, chills, and urticaria or a diffuse macular rash. The symptoms usually begin shortly after the initiation of the offending transfusion. Laboratory tests are unnecessary, although in some cases, steps need be taken to exclude a hemolytic reaction. Treatment consists of discontinuing the transfusion temporarily and ordering diphenhydramine or another antihistamine and acetaminophen. Clinical evidence of the reaction usually resolves within a few minutes. Often, the platelet transfusion can be resumed without further untoward effects. However, if the patient reacts a second time, then the remainder of the unit should be discarded. Heavily transfused patients who frequently have minor reactions may benefit from premedication with diphenhydramine and acetaminophen.

Refractory State Secondary to Alloantibodies

Some children who receive multiple blood transfusions develop antibodies against HLA antigens that immediately destroy all platelets containing these antigens that are subsequently transfused. The result is little or no post-transfusion platelet recovery, and the child may therefore be at risk of uncontrollable hemorrhage. The time course of alloimmunization leading to the refractory state is variable.[74] In some cases, it may result from only several transfusions. On the other hand, 30% to 50% of multitransfused patients never develop alloantibodies.[75] The diagnosis is made by confirming the absence of the expected increment in platelet count 1 hour after the transfusion.[26] Patients who exhibit other mechanisms of platelet destruction (i.e., mechanical factors or autoantibodies) usually have a satisfactory 1-hour post-transfusion platelet count, even though subsequent platelet survival may be markedly reduced. Alloimmunization should be suspected if the transfusion has no effect on the bleeding tendency.

Laboratory tests for the purpose of identifying the offending anti-HLA antibodies are not widely available. Little can be done to avoid the refractory state except for ordering platelets and other blood components judiciously. Use of single-donor platelets, obtained by apheresis techniques from a family member or another individual who shares common HLA antigens with the patient, may delay the onset of alloimmunization[40,41] and clearly represents the best therapeutic approach for the refractory patient.[26] Completely HLA-matched platelets are ideal, but they are usually unavailable for pediatric patients except in unusual circumstances when they can be obtained from a regional blood center that has a large registry of HLA-matched donors. Even completely HLA-matched platelets are sometimes ineffective in the refractory patient, implicating other antibodies (e.g., against platelet-specific antigens). Providing a specially processed leukocyte-poor platelet product or performing plasma exchange to remove alloantibody[76] are current investigational approaches to this problem.

Pharmacologic agents that block the reticuloendothelial system have been useful in other forms of immune-mediated thrombocytopenia, so they have been tried in alloimmunized patients as a means of obtaining better platelet recovery and survival. Although corticosteroids are unfortunately of no value in this setting, recent attention has focused on the use of intravenous gamma globulin (IV GG), which is frequently effective in raising the platelet count in children with idiopathic thrombocytopenic purpura.[77] The results of IV GG thus far in alloimmunized subjects are contradictory. Several groups of investigators have reported that IV GG (at a dose of 1.0 mg/kg intravenously over 4 hours) immediately before transfusion of random-donor platelets to a refractory patient results in improved platelet recovery and control of hemorrhage.[78,79] However, only small numbers of patients were included in these trials, and Schiffer and his colleagues in a larger study of adult patients have shown no benefits with IV GG.[80] At present, this expensive form of therapy remains investigational.

Fortunately, alloimmunization to HLA or platelet-specific antigens is not as common a problem in pediatric cancer patients as in subjects with severe aplastic anemia who are persistently and chronically thrombocytopenic. Patients with cancer develop the refractory state less often because the immunosuppressive effects of the chemotherapeutic agents blunt the production of alloantibodies.[81]

Graft-Versus-Host Disease

The graft-versus-host (GVH) reaction is characterized by the toxic effects of immunocompetent donor lymphocytes on certain target organs in an immunosuppressed recipient (also see Chap. 48). Cutaneous reactions, liver dysfunction, diarrhea, and severe infection are the most frequent clinical features.

Controversy exists regarding the frequency of GVH disease as a consequence of intensive chemotherapy in multitransfused patients who do not receive a bone marrow transplant. Many chemotherapy regimens used in children with leukemia and solid tumors cause profound immunosuppression, similar in magnitude to that seen following marrow transplantation. Thus, GVH disease might be expected in such children following blood transfusion. A number of case reports have described GVH disease in children receiving chemotherapy for neuroblastoma, other solid tumors, and lymphoma.[82,83] No information is available, however, about the actual incidence of this complication or the associated risk factors. Current evidence points to GVH being a rare occurrence.

Studies of children with congenital immunodeficiency have shown that irradiation of blood products prior to their administration renders the lymphocytes within the unit nonviable, thus preventing GVH. A dose of 1500 to 5000 rad (15–50 Gy) is an effective lymphocytotoxic dose and does not affect the function of granulocytes or platelets.[2,82,84]

The need to provide irradiated blood products to chemotherapy recipients who have not been given transplants is unclear. Some investigators believe that all children with cancer who receive intensive chemotherapy should receive only irradiated blood products. In other centers, blood products given to all children with cancer are irradiated as a routine, yet in many other institutions, blood products are never irradiated, even when they are used for patients with diseases for which highly immunosuppressive treatment is used.

Available data do not currently support the recommendation that blood products be irradiated routinely except for transfusion after marrow transplantation, since clinically significant GVH disease seems to be rare. Many blood banks do not have an irradiation source readily available; thus delays may occur if the product has to be transported elsewhere to receive irradiation before its administration to the patient. On the other hand, if an irradiation source is readily available in the blood bank, it seems prudent to use it routinely, since no harm is done to cells other than lymphocytes.

Infectious Complications of Transfusion Support

The infectious complications of blood transfusions in children with cancer are similar in type and severity to those in patients without malignant disease who are exposed to a similar number of donors (also see Chap. 39). As a rule, the risk of transfusion-related infection is proportional to the number of units of blood products received. Thus, more heavily treated patients, such as children receiving multiple transfusions of random-donor platelets, have a higher rate of infection. The following section reviews transfusion-associated infection only briefly. Current reference sources should be consulted for further information.

Bacterial Infection

Bacterial contamination of blood products is fortunately rare. However, it still occurs, primarily in platelet concentrates that may become contaminated during long room-temperature storage.[85] This complication should be suspected in the recipient who develops high fever, extreme toxicity, and cardiovascular collapse immediately following a transfusion. The mortality rate is extremely high.

Post-Transfusion Hepatitis

Hepatitis is, unfortunately, a frequent result of blood transfusions in children with cancer. The pathophysiology and the natural history of hepatitis are probably similar to those in other transfusion recipients, but in view of concomitant immunosuppression due to chemotherapy and the hepatotoxicity of some antineoplastic agents, the potential for serious liver disease exists.[86]

Hepatitis B was formerly the most common type of transfusion-related hepatitis, but it is now less frequent in this country because of the near-exclusive use of volunteer blood donors who are screened for hepatitis B by sensitive laboratory tests. Hepatitis B is now estimated to account for less than 10% of cases of post-transfusion hepatitis. A high incidence of acute and chronic hepatitis B has been reported in children with leukemia,[86] and the risk of chronic hepatitis and cirrhosis (and possibly of hepatocellular carcinoma) has provoked concern.[87] However, most reports of hepatitis B are from Italy (where the infection is extremely common) or describe patient populations from the 1970s, when donor testing was insensitive or not routine.[86–89]

Non-A, non-B (NANB) hepatitis is the most common form of post-transfusion hepatitis today in the United States.[90–92] Its incidence following exposure to volunteer donor blood has been as high as 1% to 3% per transfused unit. An anicteric subclinical course occurs in most patients. Approximately 40% to 70% of patients with acute NANB hepatitis develop chronic persistent or chronic active disease; up to 20% of these latter subjects may develop cirrhosis.[91,92] Thus, NANB represents a potentially serious problem.

NANB hepatitis is a diagnosis of exclusion, since there are no specific serologic tests. Widely accepted diagnostic criteria include ALT (alanine–leucine aminotransferase) values at least 2.5 times the upper limit of normal on two or more occasions 1 to 6 months after a blood transfusion. Because many chemotherapeutic agents (including methotrexate, 6-mercaptopurine, cytarabine, and L-asparaginase) are hepatotoxic, it is diffi-

cult to define the actual incidence of NANB hepatitis in children with cancer who receive intensive transfusion support. Several studies in leukemic children suggest that chemical or histologic evidence of hepatitis is a frequent occurrence.[93,94] A recent study in children with acute lymphoblastic leukemia in remission has shown that ALT elevations, previously ascribed to methotrexate or other chemotherapeutic agents, correlate with transfusion history (number of donor exposures) more than with other variables.[95] The number of children with cancer who develop end-stage liver disease as a complication of its treatment is fortunately small at this time, but further follow-up of at-risk patients is necessary. Also, there is currently little information about whether post-transfusion hepatitis has an influence on the child's response to chemotherapy or on the natural history of the neoplasm.[86]

Cytomegalovirus Infection

Cytomegalovirus (CMV) is a ubiquitous member of the herpesvirus group. It is transmitted by blood and blood products as well as by other routes. Its protean clinical manifestations include hepatitis, an infectious mononucleosis-like illness, and, in bone-marrow transplant recipients, a usually fatal form of interstitial pneumonia. Patients with cancer frequently acquire this infection via contaminated blood products derived from seropositive donors whose transfused leukocytes contain the virus. Prevention of CMV infection in seronegative bone-marrow transplant recipients has been attempted in some centers by using only CMV antibody-negative donors. This approach creates logistical difficulties for the blood bank, since only 20% to 30% of adults are seronegative. Other preventive measures used in transplant recipients include IV GG or hyperimmune CMV globulin preparations. Both modalities are investigational at this time.

Human Immunodeficiency Virus Infection

During the past several years, it has been conclusively shown that HIV (formerly called LAV and HTLV-III) is the cause of AIDS. As described in detail in Chapter 36, this viral agent attacks helper T-lymphocytes, resulting in profound immunoincompetence. The HIV-infected host is susceptible to a wide array of opportunistic infections (most commonly *Pneumocystis carinii* pneumonia), as in congenitally immunodeficient patients. In the early and mid-1980s, transfusion-related HIV infection resulting in AIDS became a serious problem.[96] Among infected individuals were some patients with cancer who received blood products contaminated with the virus.[97] In 1985, it became uniform practice in blood banks to screen donors for HIV infection using questionnaires and extremely sensitive laboratory tests. Therefore, at present, seroconversion in blood recipients should be extremely rare.

Other Complications of Blood Transfusion Support

Transfusion-related hemochromatosis or iron overload causes difficulties only rarely in pediatric cancer patients due to the years of exposure to red blood cells necessary to cause toxic injury to the heart, liver, and pancreas. The problem of venous access, a form of transfusion-related complication, is discussed elsewhere in this volume.

CONCLUSION

Despite the risks, inconveniences, and expense of blood transfusion support, provision of donor erythrocytes and platelets to children with cancer has allowed delivery of the intensive cytotoxic treatments that have proved to be curative in an ever-increasing percentage of cases. Hematologic supportive care will continue to remain a key modality in the armamentarium of the pediatric oncologist.

REFERENCES

1. Skelton J, Pizzo PA: Problems of intensive therapy in childhood cancer. Cancer 58:488–503, 1986
2. Allegretta GJ, Weisman SJ, Altman AJ: Hematologic and infectious complications of cancer and cancer treatment. Pediatr Clin North Am 32:613–629, 1985
3. Doll D, Weiss RB: Neoplasia and the erythron. J Clin Oncol 3:429–446, 1985
4. Lee GR: The anemia of chronic disease. Semin Hematol 20:61–80, 1983
5. Homans AC, Cohen JL, Mazur EM: Aplastic presentation of childhood lymphoblastic leukemia: Evidence for cellular inhibition of normal hematopoietic progenitor cells (abstract). Blood 68(suppl 1):200a, 1986
6. Sills RH, Stockman JA III: Preleukemic states in children with acute lymphoblastic leukemia. Cancer 48:110–112, 1981
7. Sallan SE, Buchanan GR: Selective erythroid aplasia during therapy for acute lymphoblastic leukemia. Pediatrics 59:895–898, 1977
8. de Alarcon PA, Miller ML, Stuart MJ: Erythroid hypoplasia: An unusual presentation of childhood acute lymphocytic leukemia. Am J Dis Child 132:763–764, 1978
9. Doll D, Ringenberg QS, Yarbro JW: Vascular toxicity associated with antineoplastic agents. J Clin Oncol 4:1405–1417, 1986
10. Habibi B, Lopez M, Serdaru M et al: Immune hemolytic anemia and renal failure due to teniposide. N Engl J Med 306:1091–1093, 1982
11. Pierce RN, Reich LM, Mayer K: Hemolysis following platelet transfusions from ABO-incompatible donors. Transfusion 25:60–62, 1985
12. Dallman P, Siimes MA: Percentile curves for hemoglobin and red cell volume in infancy and childhood. J Pediatr 94:26–31, 1979
13. Strauss RA, Gloster ES, McCallister JA et al: Acute cytoreduction techniques in the early treatment of hyperleukocytosis associated with childhood hematologic malignancies. Med Pediatr Oncol 13:346–351, 1985
14. Nieburg PI, Stockman JA III: Rapid correction of anemia with partial exchange transfusion. Am J Dis Child 131:60–61, 1977
15. Berman B, Krieger A, Naiman L: A new method for calculating volumes of blood required for partial exchange transfusion. J Pediatr 94:86–89, 1979
16. Hughes ASB, Brozovic B: Leucocyte depleted blood: An appraisal of available techniques. Br J Haematol 50:381–386, 1982
17. Chaplin H Jr: The proper use of previously frozen red blood cells for transfusion. Blood 59:1118–1120, 1982
18. Amylon MD, Link MP, Glader BE: Immune thrombocytopenia associated with acute nonlymphocytic leukemia. J Pediatr 105:776–778, 1984
19. Rao S, Pang EJM: Idiopathic thrombocytopenic purpura in acute lymphoblastic leukemia. J Pediatr 94:408–409, 1979
20. Hodder FS, Kempert P, McCormack S et al: Immune thrombocytopenia following actinomycin-D therapy. J Pediatr 107:611–614, 1985
21. Gardner FH: Preservation and clinical use of platelets. In Williams WJ, Beutler E, Erslev AJ, Lichtman MA (eds): Hematology, 3rd Ed, pp 1556–1563. New York, McGraw-Hill, 1983
22. Gaydos AL, Freireich EJ, Mantel N: The quantitative relation between platelet count and hemorrhage in patients with acute leukemia. N Engl J Med 266:905–909, 1962
23. Murphy S: Platelet storage for transfusion. Semin Hematol 22:165–177, 1985
24. Kaneshiro MM, Mielke CH Jr, Kasper CK et al: Bleeding time after aspirin in disorders of intrinsic clotting. N Engl J Med 281:1039–1042, 1969
25. Schiffer CA, Aisner J, Wiernik PH: Frozen autologous platelet transfusion for patients with leukemia. N Engl J Med 299:7–12, 1978
26. Consensus Conference: Platelet transfusion therapy. JAMA 257:1777–1780, 1987
27. Duquesnoy RJ, Anderson AJ, Tomasulo PA et al: ABO compatibility and platelet transfusions of alloimmunized thrombocytopenic patients. Blood 54:595–599, 1979
28. Harker LA, Slichter SJ: The bleeding time as a screening test for evaluation of platelet function. N Engl J Med 287:155–159, 1972
29. Feusner J: The use of platelet transfusions. Am J Pediatr Hematol Oncol 6:255–260, 1984
30. Kitchens CS, Pendergast JF: Human thrombocytopenia is associated with structural abnormalities of the endothelium that are ameliorated by glucocorticosteroid administration. Blood 67:203–206, 1986
31. Ilett S, Lilleyman JS: Platelet transfusion requirements of children with newly diagnosed lymphoblastic leukaemia. Acta Haematol 62:86–89, 1979
32. Solomon J, Bofenkamp T, Fahey J: Platelet prophylaxis in acute non-lymphoblastic leukaemia. Lancet 2:267, 1978
33. Murphy S, Litwin S, Herring L: Indications for platelet transfusion in children with acute leukemia. Am J Hematol 12:347–356, 1982
34. Higby DJ, Cohen E, Holland JF: The prophylactic treatment of thrombocytopenic leukemic patients with platelets: A double blind study. Transfusion 14:440–446, 1974
35. Roy AJ, Jaffe N, Djerassi I: Prophylactic platelet transfusions in children with acute leukemia: A dose response study. Transfusion 13:283–290, 1973
36. Van Eys J, Thomas D, Olivos B: Platelet use in pediatric oncology: A review of 393 transfusions. Transfusion 18:169–173, 1978
37. Aderka D, Praff G, Santo M et al: Bleeding due to thrombocytopenia in acute leukemias and reevaluation of the prophylactic platelet transfusion policy. Am J Med Sci 291:147–151, 1986
38. Balopole W, Beutler E: The incidence of hemorrhage in thrombocytopenic patients (abstract). Clin Res 35:186A, 1987
39. Eisenstaedt R: Blood component therapy in the treatment of platelet disorders. Semin Hematol 23:1–7, 1986
40. Sintnicolaas K, Sizoo W, Haije WG: Delayed alloimmunisation by random single donor platelet transfusions: A randomised study to compare single donor and multiple donor platelet transfusions in cancer patients with severe thrombocytopenia. Lancet 1:750–753, 1981
41. Gmür J, von Felten A, Osterwalder B et al: Delayed alloimmunization using random single donor platelet transfusions: A prospective study in thrombocytopenic patients with acute leukemia. Blood 62:473–479, 1983
42. Schiffer CA, Slighter SJ: Platelet transfusion from single donors. N Engl J Med 307:245–247, 1982
43. Buchanan GR, Martin V, Levine PH et al: The effects of "anti-platelet" drugs on bleeding time and platelet aggregation in normal human subjects. Am J Clin Pathol 68:355–359, 1977
44. Brown CH III, Natelson EA, Bradshaw MW et al: The hemostatic defect produced by carbenicillin. N Engl J Med 291:265–270, 1974
45. Ballard JO, Barnes SG, Sattler FR: Comparison of the effects of mezlocillin, carbenicillin, and placebo on normal hemostasis. Antimicrob Agents Chemother 25:153–156, 1984
46. Sattler FR, Weitekamp MR, Ballard JO: Potential for bleeding with the new beta-lactam antibiotics. Ann Intern Med 105:924–931, 1986
47. Pui CH, Jackson CW, Chesney C et al: Sequential changes in platelet function and coagulation in leukemic children treated with L-asparaginase, prednisone, and vincristine. J Clin Oncol 1:380–385, 1983
48. Gardner FH, Helmer R III: Aminocaproic acid: Use in control of hemorrhage in patients with amegakaryocytic thrombocytopenia. JAMA 243:35–37, 1980
49. Mannucci PM: Desmopressin (DDAVP) for treatment of disorders of hemostasis. Prog Hemost Thromb 8:19–45, 1986
50. Buchanan GR: The bleeding child. In Dickerman J, Lucey J (eds): The Critically Ill Child: Diagnosis and Medical Management, pp 212–228. Philadelphia, WB Saunders, 1985
51. Ribeiro R, Pui CH: The clinical and biological correlates of coagulopathy in children with acute leukemia. J Clin Oncol 4:1212–1218, 1986
52. Scott JP, Morgan E: Coagulopathy of disseminated neuroblastoma. J Pediatr 103:219–222, 1983
53. Sills RH, Stockman JA III, Miller ML et al: Consumptive coagulopathy: A complication of therapy of solid tumors in childhood. Am J Dis Child 132:870–872, 1978
54. McClure P, Strachan P, Saunders E: Hypofibrinogenemia and thrombocytopenia in familial hemophagocytic reticulosis. J Pediatr 85:67–70, 1974
55. Gralnick HR, Bagley J, Abrell E: Heparin treatment for the hemorrhagic diathesis of acute promyelocytic leukemia. Am J Med 52:167–174, 1972
56. Champion LAA, Luddy RE, Schwartz AD: Disseminated intravascular coagulation in childhood acute lymphocytic leukemia with poor prognostic features. Cancer 41:1642–1646, 1978
57. Daly PA, Schiffer CA, Wiernik PH: Acute promyelocytic leukemia—Clinical management of 15 patients. Am J Hematol 3:347–359, 1980
58. Drapkin RL, Gee TS, Dowling MD et al: Prophylactic heparin therapy in acute promyelocytic leukemia. Cancer 41:2484–2490, 1978
59. Goldberg MA, Ginsburg D, Mayer RJ et al: Is heparin administration necessary during induction chemotherapy for patients with acute promyelocytic leukemia? Blood 69:187–191, 1987
60. Kelly DA, Tuddenham EGD: Haemostatic problems in liver disease. Gut 27:339–349, 1986

61. Phillips LL: Transfusion support in acquired coagulation disorders. Clin Haematol 13:137–150, 1984

62. Jones PG, Strother V, Rolston KVI et al: Hypoprothrombinemia in patients with cancer receiving cefoperazone and mezlocillin. Arch Intern Med 146:1397–1399, 1986

63. Priest JR, Ramsay NKC, Steinherz PG et al: A syndrome of thrombosis and hemorrhage complicating L-asparaginase therapy for childhood acute lymphoblastic leukemia. J Pediatr 100:984–989, 1982

64. Bezeaud A, Drouet L, Leverger G et al: Effect of L-asparaginase therapy for acute lymphoblastic leukemia on plasma vitamin K-dependent coagulation factors and inhibitors. J Pediatr 108:698–701, 1986

65. Kucuk O, Kwaan HC, Gunnar W et al: Thromboembolic complications associated with L-asparaginase therapy. Cancer 55:702–706, 1985

66. Pui CH, Chesney CM, Weed J et al: Altered von Willebrand factor molecule in children with thrombosis following asparaginase–prednisone–vincristine therapy for leukemia. J Clin Oncol 3:1266–1272, 1985

67. Pui CH, Chesney CM, Bergum PW et al: Lack of pathogenetic role of proteins C and S in thrombosis associated with asparaginase–prednisone–vincristine therapy for leukaemia. Br J Haematol 64:283–290, 1986

68. Buchanan GR, Holtkamp CA: Reduced antithrombin III levels during L-asparaginase therapy. Med Pediatr Oncol 8:7–14, 1980

69. Clavell LA, Gelber RD, Cohen HJ et al: Four-agent induction and intensive asparaginase therapy for treatment of childhood acute lymphoblastic leukemia. N Engl J Med 315:657–663, 1986

70. Mirro J Jr, Kalwinsky D, Whisnant J et al: Coagulopathy induced by continuous infusion of high doses of human lymphoblastoid interferon. Cancer Treat Rep 69:315–317, 1985

71. Scott JP, Montgomery RR, Tubergen DG et al: Acquired von Willebrand's disease in association with Wilms' tumor: Regression following treatment. Blood 58:665–669, 1981

72. Blumberg N, Laczin J, McMican A et al: A critical survey of fresh-frozen plasma use. Transfusion 26:511–513, 1986

73. Lichtiger B, Perry–Thornton E: Hemolytic transfusion reactions in oncology patients: Experience in a large cancer center. J Clin Oncol 2:438–442, 1984

74. Dutcher JP, Schiffer CA, Aisner J et al: Alloimmunization following platelet transfusion: The absence of a dose–response relationship. Blood 57:395–398, 1981

75. Howard JE, Perkins HA: The natural history of alloimmunization to platelets. Transfusion 18:496–503, 1978

76. Bensinger WI, Buckner CD, Clift RA et al: Plasma exchange for platelet alloimmunization. Transplantation 41:602–605, 1986

77. Bussel JB: Intravenous immunoglobulin therapy for the treatment of idiopathic thrombocytopenic purpura. Prog Hemost Thromb 8:103–125, 1986

78. Becton DL, Kinney TR, Chaffee S et al: High-dose intravenous immunoglobulin for severe platelet alloimmunization. Pediatrics 74:1120–1123, 1984

79. Atrah HI, Sheehan T, Gribben J et al: Improvement of post platelet transfusion increments following intravenous immunoglobulin therapy for leukaemic HLA-immunized patients. Scand J Haematol 36:160–164, 1986

80. Schiffer CA, Hogge DE, Aisner J et al: High-dose intravenous gammaglobulin in alloimmunized platelet transfusion recipients. Blood 64:937–940, 1984

81. Holohan T, Terasaki PI, Deisseroth AB: Suppression of transfusion-related alloimmunization in intensively treated cancer patients. Blood 58:122–128, 1981

82. Pflieger H: Graft-versus-host disease following blood transfusions. Blut 46:61–66, 1983

83. Woods W, Lubin B: Fatal graft versus host disease following a blood transfusion in a child with neuroblastoma. Pediatrics 67:217–221, 1981

84. Moroff G, George VM, Siegl AM et al: The influence of irradiation on stored platelets. Transfusion 26:453–456, 1986

85. Anderson KC, Lew MA, Gorgone BC, Martel J et al: Transfusion-related sepsis after prolonged platelet storage. Am J Med 81:405–410, 1986

86. Ratner L, Peylan–Ramu N, Wesley R: Adverse prognostic influence of hepatitis B virus infection in acute lymphoblastic leukemia. Cancer 58:1096–1100, 1986

87. Locasciulli A, Vergani G, Uderzo C: Chronic liver disease in children with leukemia in long-term remission. Cancer 52:1080–1087, 1983

88. Locasciulli A, Alberti A, Rossetti F: Acute and chronic hepatitis in childhood leukemia: A multicentric study from the Italian Pediatric Cooperative Group for Therapy of Acute Leukemia (AIL-AIEOP). Med Pediatr Oncol 13:203–206, 1985

89. Vergani D, Masera G, Moroni G: Histological evidence of hepatitis-B-virus infection in children with negative serology in children with acute leukaemia who develop chronic liver disease. Lancet 2:361–364, 1983

90. Wick M, Moore S, Taswell H: Non-A, non-B hepatitis associated with blood transfusion. Transfusion 25:93–101, 1985

91. Koretz RL, Stone O, Mousa M: Non-A, non-B posttransfusion hepatitis—A decade later. Gastroenterology 88:1251–1254, 1985

92. Shih JW, Esteban Mur JI, Alter HJ: Non-A, non-B hepatitis: Advances and unfulfilled expectations of the first decade. Prog Liver Dis 8:433–452, 1986

93. Locasciulli A, Alberti A, Barbieri R: Evidence of non-A, non-B hepatitis in children with acute leukemia and chronic liver disease. Am J Dis Child 137:354–356, 1983

94. Malone W, Novak R: Outcome of hepatitis in children with acute leukemia. Am J Dis Child 134:584–587, 1980

95. Hetherington ML, Buchanan GR, Sartain P: Transaminase elevation during therapy for acute lymphoblastic leukemia (ALL) correlates with prior transfusion of blood products (abstract). Blood 68(suppl 1):298a, 1986

96. Peterman T, Jaffe H, Feorino P: Transfusion-associated acquired immunodeficiency syndrome in the United States. JAMA 254:2913–2917, 1885

97. Groopman JE, Hammer SM, Sallan SE et al: Human T-lymphotropic virus type III infection in previously immunocompromised hosts. J Clin Oncol 4:540–543, 1986

thirty-nine

Infectious Complications in the Pediatric Cancer Patient

James W. Hathorn and
Philip A. Pizzo

The relation between malignancy, the immunocompromised host, and infectious morbidity and death is well established.[1-4] With the use of more intensive, and potentially curative, treatment regimens, a larger number of children are being rendered immunocompromised. The infectious complications that can occur are life-threatening and may limit the benefits of antineoplastic therapy. It is imperative, therefore, for the pediatric oncologist to be familiar with the factors contributing to infection and to be knowledgeable about the infectious syndromes that are likely to occur and the procedures and drugs available to treat or prevent them.

NATURE OF THE IMMUNOCOMPROMISED HOST

The child with cancer may be immunocompromised because of the underlying malignancy as well as by the antineoplastic therapy administered to treat it. Moreover, specific malignancies may be associated with immune deficits that predispose to infection with particular pathogens. For example, patients with Hodgkin's disease or non-Hodgkin's lymphomas often have abnormalities of the cellular immune system that heighten their risk for viral infections (*e.g.*, Herpes simplex, varicella–zoster) and fungal infections (*e.g.*, *Cryptococcus*). On the other hand, therapeutic modalities such as corticosteroids, cytotoxic chemotherapy, and localized or wide-field irradiation result in further deficiencies of host defense. The net consequence of these interrelated abnormalities of immune function is the immunocompromised cancer patient.

Interactions Among Altered Microbial Attachment, Colonization, and Enhanced Susceptibility to Infection

One of the most important factors increasing the risk of infection among hospitalized cancer patients is the altered nature of their colonizing organisms. The attachment of a microbial pathogen to an epithelial surface is the first step in the initiation of an infectious process.[5,6] There is now ample evidence that such attachment is mediated by a specific lock-and-key mechanism, whereby ligand molecules (adhesions) on the surface of the microbe interact with complementary molecules (receptors) on the epithelial cell surface. The biochemical structures of adhesions are variable and include proteins (*E. coli, Neisseria gonorrhoeae*), the lipid portion of a glycolipid (*Streptococcus pyogenes*), and carbohydrates (many cariogenic streptococci).

In healthy individuals, integumentary and mucosal attachment sites are populated with relatively innocuous "normal" flora consisting predominantly of aerobic gram-positive and a variety of anaerobic organisms.[5-7] Within 24 hours of hospitalization, seriously ill patients undergo a change in their indigenous microflora toward one of aerobic gram-negative organisms.[8,9] The specific reason for this altered pattern of colonization is unclear; it is partly mediated by a change in the nature of the epithelial receptors. Antibiotics also promote changes in bacterial adherence and colonization.[8-14]

The organisms colonizing the patient are integrally related to the pattern of infections that ultimately occur in the cancer patient. Indeed, greater than 80% of the microbiologically documented infections that occur in patients with acute nonlymphocytic leukemia are caused by organisms that are part of the endogenous microflora, usually at sites at or near the source of infection.[10] Furthermore, approximately half of the responsible pathogens are acquired by the patient only after the initial admission to the hospital. Thus, efforts to reduce the enhanced risk of infectious morbidity and death in cancer patients might appropriately be directed to the factors that modulate the attachment of microorganisms to mucosal receptors.[7]

An intact integument represents the first line of defense against exogenous microbial pathogens, not merely as a mechanical barrier but as a complex arrangement of specialized cells of the skin and the respiratory, gastrointestinal, and genitourinary mucosa. For example, ciliated and mucus-producing cells of the respiratory tract, acid- and enzyme-producing cells of the gastrointestinal tract, and bactericidal fatty acids and secretory immunoglobulins displayed by epidermal cells are specific adaptations that enhance defense against exogenous organisms. The mucosal and epidermal cells also contain both specific and nonspecific receptors for the attachment of microorganisms.[5-7]

Any factor that bypasses or disrupts this integumentary barrier will enhance susceptibility to infection. The integrity of this barrier may be disrupted by local tumor invasion or as a result of surgery, radiation, or cytotoxic chemotherapy. Additionally, a large number of procedures (including finger sticks, venipunctures, bone-marrow aspirations, and insertion of venous access devices) can disrupt the integument and provide a nidus for colonization and the eventual dissemination of pathogens.

Cellular Immune Dysfunction

Quantitative or qualitative abnormalities of the cellular aspects of the immune response predispose to infections with a broad array of pathogens (Table 39-1). The effector cells of the immune response include polymorphonuclear leukocytes (PMNs), lymphocytes (T, B, and natural killer [NK] cells), peripheral blood monocytes, and fixed tissue macrophages (including the cells of the spleen and reticuloendothelial system). The cells that are more severely affected by disease or therapy-mediated immune dysfunction are the PMNs, monocytes, and lymphocytes. The cells of the reticuloendothelial system are relatively less sensitive to the toxic effects of antineoplastic therapy and provide at least a rudimentary framework for the maintenance of cellular immunity even in the face of profound cellular immunosuppression.

Polymorphonuclear Leukocytes

The single most important determinant of susceptibility to bacterial and fungal pathogens is the number of circulating neutrophils. The more profound and protracted the granulocytopenia, the greater the likelihood of a serious infection.[11] Granulocytopenia may be secondary to the disease itself (*e.g.,* acute leukemia or aplastic anemia) but is more commonly a consequence of cytotoxic chemotherapy or radiotherapy. Not only is the absolute level of granulocytopenia a crucial deter-

Table 39-1
Predominant Pathogens in Pediatric Cancer Patients

Bacteria—Gram-Positive
  Staphylococci (coagulase-negative; coagulase-positive)
  Streptococci (alpha-hemolytic; group D)
  Corynebacterium
  Listeria

Bacteria—Gram-Negative
  Enterobacteriacea
    Pseudomonads (multiply resistant species)
    Anaerobes

Fungi
  Candida spp.
  Aspergillus spp.
  Phycomycetes
  Cryptococcus

Viruses
  Herpes simplex
  Varicella–Zoster
  Cytomegalovirus
  Epstein–Barr virus
  Respiratory syncytial virus
  Adenoviruses
  Influenza
  Rotavirus

Other
  Pneumocystis carinii
  Toxoplasma gondii
  Strongyloides stercoralis
  Cryptosporidia

minant of susceptibility to infection, but the rate of decline is an important variable as well. Thus, a patient with aplastic anemia may be at a lesser risk of a serious infection than is the patient with a similar degree of granulocytopenia induced by chemotherapy. It is important to remember, however, that in the pediatric cancer patient, granulocytopenia rarely occurs as an isolated perturbation of the immune system. Additional disease-related or therapeutically mediated abnormalities of the immune response, alterations of microbial colonization secondary to broad-spectrum antimicrobial therapy, and mucosal or iatrogenic anatomic defects caused by cytotoxic therapies usually occur in concert, markedly increasing the patient's susceptibility to infection (Fig. 39-1).

In addition, qualitative abnormalities of neutrophil function may occur as a consequence of the underlying malignancy (especially acute leukemias) or secondary to antineoplastic therapy. For example, the neutrophils from patients with leukemias and lymphomas have suboptimal chemoattractant responsiveness, bactericidal activity, and superoxide production.[12,13] Antineoplastic chemotherapy and radiotherapy also cause qualitative abnormalities of neutrophil function.[14-16] Finally, deficiencies of neutrophil function iatrogenically induced by the administration of various medications (*e.g.,* opiates, corticosteroids, or antibiotics) may have a detrimental effect.[17,18]

Patients with either quantitative or qualitative defects of their PMNs are subject primarily to infections with bacteria and fungi. Gram-positive and gram-negative bacteria and invasive fungi (especially *Candida* and *Aspergillus*) are the most common pathogens.

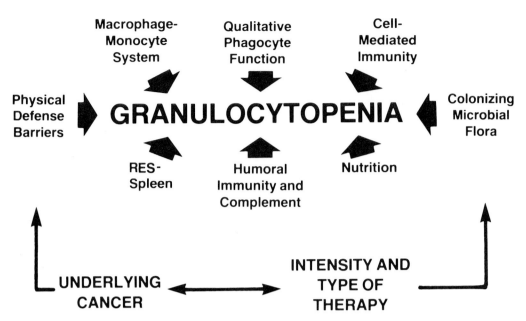

FIGURE 39-1. Interactions of the defense matrix that delineates the compromised host.

Lymphocytes

Disease- or treatment-induced abnormalities of lymphocytes can affect both the humoral and the cellular arm of the immune response. Certain malignancies, such as chronic lymphocytic leukemia or multiple myeloma, result in a significant alteration of the humoral limb of the immune response.[19,20] Patients with Hodgkin's disease and non-Hodgkin's lymphomas have an impaired cellular immune response.[21] Children with the acquired immune deficiency syndrome (AIDS) suffer from a profound abnormality of lymphocyte function affecting both T and B cells (see Chap. 36).

Deficiencies in lymphocyte function may be induced by corticosteroids, cytotoxic chemotherapy, and radiotherapy.[18,19,22] Additionally, some pathogens such as cytomegalovirus (CMV) that infect patients with altered cellular immunity further suppress the host's defenses and so contribute to bacterial or fungal superinfections.[23,24]

Patients with defects in humoral immunity are particularly susceptible to infections by encapsulated bacteria, especially *Streptococcus pneumoniae, Haemophilus influenzae,* and *Neisseria meningitidis.*[24a] Patients with deficiencies of cellular immunity are prone to fungal, viral, and intracellularly replicating bacterial pathogens (*e.g., Listeria monocytogenes, Salmonella* species).

Spleen and Reticuloendothelial System

The spleen and fixed tissue cells of the reticuloendothelial system act both as a mechanical filter and as an immune effector organ. The spleen is the principal organ involved in the production of antibody to polysaccharide antigens and also acts as a filter to remove damaged cells and opsonin-coated organisms from the circulation.[25] Splenectomized patients are deficient in antibody production when challenged with particulate antigens, have decreased levels of IgM and properdin (a component of the alternate complement pathway), and are deficient in the phagocytosis-promoting peptide tuftsin.[26] Splenectomized patients are at increased risk for fulminant and rapidly fatal septicemia due to encapsulated bacterial pathogens such as *S. pneumoniae, H. influenzae,* and *N. meningitidis.*[27,28]

Other Factors Contributing to the Immunocompromised State

A number of additional factors in the child with cancer can exacerbate the immunocompromised state. For example, alterations in central nervous system function or decreased levels of awareness, obstruction of a hollow viscus, and the depressed nutritive states common with malignancy all can enhance susceptibility to infectious complications.

Obstruction of the biliary tree, gastrointestinal or genitourinary tracts, or respiratory passages by either a primary or a metastatic tumor mass can promote an infection by the organisms colonizing the site of obstruction. Similarly, diminution or obliteration of the gag reflex secondary to local neural infiltration or a decreased level of cognition markedly increases the risk of aspiration pneumonia. Aspirated pharyngeal organisms (most commonly gram-negative aerobes) can colonize, invade, and disseminate from a pulmonary source. The risk of an aspiration pneumonia and subsequent disseminated infection is heightened by decreased mucosal clearance mechanisms and damage mediated by antineoplastic therapy.

The compromising effect of a malnourished state on immune function is well documented.[29,30] Although the precise effects of specific or generalized nutritional deficiencies in cancer patients have been difficult to elucidate, it is clear that nutritional deficiencies impact on B and T lymphocytes, PMNs, mononuclear phagocytes, and complement system function.

MANAGEMENT OF THE FEBRILE CANCER PATIENT

Fever (most commonly defined as a temperature greater than 38° C) is common among children with cancer.[31] The molecule responsible for the production of fever, known as interleukin-1 (IL-1), has recently been cloned and sequenced.[32] The monocyte–macrophage is believed to be the most important source of physiologically relevant IL-1. However, other phagocytic cells (including PMNs and fixed tissue cells of the reticuloendothelial system) as well as keratinocytes, gingival and corneal epithelial cells, renal mesangial cells, and astrocytes, are also capable of producing interleukin-1-like molecules.[33] Interleukin-1 mediates an array of metabolic, endocrinologic, neurologic, and immunologic functions common to the acute-phase inflammatory response, the sum effect of which is a unified host response against an infectious insult. These effects include, either directly or indirectly, the production of fever, polymorphonuclear leukocytosis, hepatic synthesis of acute-phase reactants, activation of T and B lymphocytes, and the metabolic changes (mobilization of amino acids, decreased serum iron and zinc, and increased serum copper) that inhibit bacterial replication.[32,33]

Although fever in the cancer patient is frequently due to an infection, noninfectious causes must also be considered. Pyrogenic medications (particularly cytotoxic agents such as bleomycin and cytosine arabinoside), blood products, allergic reactions, and the malignant process itself are potential sources of a febrile response. Nonetheless, in a granulocytopenic patient, fever may be the first and only sign of infection;[31,34] other clinical signs and symptoms frequently indicative of an infectious process (*i.e.,* pain, erythema, and swelling) may be blunted or even absent. Although the definition of granulocytopenia is somewhat arbitrary, most oncologists consider patients with an absolute granulocyte count (consisting of PMNs plus band forms) of 500/mm^3 or less to be neutropenic. Also, from a practical standpoint, patients whose absolute count is between 500/mm^3 and 1000/mm^3 but falling due to antineoplastic therapy should be considered neutropenic.

Evaluation of the Febrile but Non-Neutropenic Patient

The evaluation of a febrile non-neutropenic cancer patient should include a careful history and physical examination, but empirical therapy is rarely indicated. However, the association of infectious syndromes with specific defects of cell-mediated or humoral immunity should be recognized. For example, children receiving maintenance chemotherapy are at increased risk for *Pneumocystis carinii* pneumonia, and patients with defects in cell-mediated immune function may develop cryptococcal meningitis. Thus, although the presence of granulocytes precludes the necessity for routine empirical antibiotics, it does not exclude infectious agents as the cause for fever.

In general, bacterial cultures of the blood (two specimens obtained through separate venipuncture sites) and urine should be obtained. Patients with localizing symptoms or signs should undergo the appropriate diagnostic procedures: aspiration for culture and gram stain of accessible sites of cellulitis, stool cultures in patients with diarrhea, and lumbar puncture for patients with meningeal irritation. If a site of infection is not defineable, antibiotics are not necessary, but the patient should be followed for clinical or microbiologic evidence of infection. If an infectious etiology for fever has been effectively eliminated and the elevated temperature is felt to be a "tumor fever" (rare in children), a trial of naproxen or ibuprofen is indicated.

Patients with an indwelling venous access (Hickman–Broviac) catheter who become febrile, even if they are non-neutropenic, present a special problem. The incidence of infectious complications in patients with intravascular devices can be high. Blood cultures should be obtained from each port of a multilumen catheter as well as from at least one peripheral venipuncture site.[35] The patient should then be started on an antibiotic regimen designed to cover the most commonly encountered line-related pathogens (*i.e., Staphylococcus aureus, S. epidermidis, Bacillus* spp., gram-negative aerobes). Vancomycin in combination with either an aminoglycoside or an appropriate third-generation cephalosporin (*e.g.,* ceftazidime, cefoperazone) offers appropriate coverage. These antibiotics should be continued for a 48- to 72-hour trial. If the preantibiotic blood and line cultures turn out to be negative, the

antibiotics may be withdrawn; if the cultures are positive, a full therapeutic course is necessary (Fig. 39-2).

Evaluation of the Febrile Neutropenic Patient

The initial evaluation of the febrile neutropenic patient necessitates an expeditious and meticulous physical examination, with particular attention to those sites that are commonly the source of infection in granulocytopenic patients. This includes scrupulous examination of skin (particularly sites of intravenous access), lungs, and both the perioral and perirectal areas.

Several important points regarding the evaluation of febrile neutropenic patients must be emphasized. First, the initial evaluation will yield a clinically or microbiologically defined site of infection in less than half of neutropenic children who become febrile.[31,36] This statistic probably reflects the short period of time that elapses between the onset of fever, evaluation, and initiation of empirical therapy. Second, even subtle indications of inflammation must be considered as presumptive signs of infection in the presence of granulocytopenia.[34] For example, mild perirectal erythema and tenderness may be the harbinger of a perirectal cellulitis. Also, slight erythema and serous discharge at the exit site of a Hickman catheter may herald a tunnel or exit infection. Accordingly, any clinically suspicious and accessible site of infection should be aspirated for culture and gram staining. It must be stressed that it is generally not possible to differentiate granulocytopenic patients who turn out to have a bacteremia from those with unexplained fever.[31] Indeed, as many as 50% of patients ultimately found to be bacteremic lack any specific physical findings to suggest such a diagnosis.

After the initial history and physical examination, all febrile neutropenic patients should have two sets of peripheral blood cultures from separate venipuncture sites, as well as cultures from all lumens of indwelling venous catheters. A routine urinalysis and culture should be performed. Patients with diarrhea should have a stool culture. Although the yield of routine chest radiographs in asymptomatic neutropenic patients is small, the study should be performed, since it provides an important baseline for comparison with later films, which may present only subtle indications of a pneumonic process. Following this evaluation, all febrile neutropenic patients should be promptly placed on broad-spectrum antibiotics.

Empirical Antibiotic Therapy

The prompt initiation of empirical antibiotics when the neutropenic cancer patient becomes febrile has been the single most important advance in the management of the immunocompromised host. Prior to this policy, the mortality rate of gram-negative infections (especially with *Pseudomonas aeruginosa, E. coli,* and *Klebsiella pneumoniae*) approached 80%.[37-39] Since the widespread utilization of effective empirical antibiotics, the overall mortality rate has dropped to 10% to 40%.[36,40-44]

What are the criteria upon which an empirical antibiotic regimen should be based? Between 85% and 90% of pathogens associated with new fevers in immunosuppressed patients are bacteria.[31,44] However, because both gram-positive and gram-negative bacteria (as well as mixed infections) can be responsible, the empirical regimen must be broad in spectrum, provide bactericidal drug levels, and be as nontoxic and as simple to administer as possible. These requirements have usually necessitated the combination of two or more antibiotics. The

(*Text continues on p. 845*)

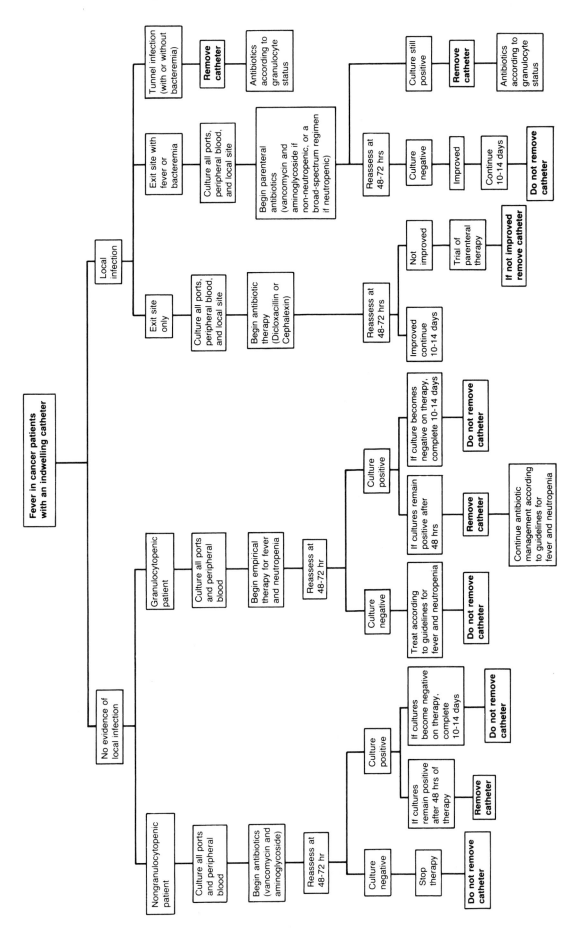

FIGURE 39-2. Algorithm for the management of fever in the cancer patient with an indwelling catheter.

Table 39-2
Commonly Used Antimicrobial Agents for Pediatric Cancer Patients

Antibiotic	Trade Name	Major Indications	Usual Daily Dosage (IV) (mg/kg)	Daily Dosage Schedule	Usual Maximum Dose per Day (g)
Penicillins					
Penicillin G	Benzathin Permapen Bicillin	*S. pneumoniae, S. pyrogenes, S. viridens, S. bovis Neisseria,* most anaerobes (except *B. fragilis*)	25–500,000 U/kg	q4h	20
Isoxozyl penicillins	Staphcillin, Celbenin	*S. aureus,* streptococcus	1–300	q4h	12
Methicillin			1–300	q4h	12
Nafcillin	Unipen		1–300	q4h	12
Oxacillin	Prostaphin, Bactocill				
Aminopenicillin					
Ampicillin	Omipen Principen Polycillin Penbritin	*S. faecalis, L. monocytogenes, Hemophilus, E. coli. Salmonella, Proteus*	2–400	q4h	12
Carboxypenicillins					
Carbenicillin	Pyopen, Geopen	*P. aeruginosa, Enterobacter, Proteus, Serratia, Acinetobacter, Providentia* Anaerobes (including some *Bacteroides* sp. some *Clostridium* sp., *Peptostreptococcus, Fusobacter*)	500	q4h	36
Ticarcillin	Ticar		300	q4h	21
Extended-spectrum penicillins					
Mezlocillin	Mezlin	Same as carboxypenicillin plus *Klebsiella* sp.	300	q4h	21
Piperacillin	Pipercil	Same as mezlocillin plus increased activity against *P. aeruginosa*	300	q4h	21
Azlocillin	Azlin	Same as piperacillin	300	q4h	21
Cephalosporins					
First generation					
Cephalothin	Keflin	*E. coli, Klebsiella, Proteus, Hemophilus, S. aureus, S. epidermidis, Streptococcus*	170	q4h	12
Cefazolin	Kefzol, Ancef	Similar to cephalothin, more active against *Klebsiella, E. coli*	50	q6h	2–6
Second generation					
Cefamandole	Mandol	More active against *Hemophilus, Klebsiella, E. coli, Enterobacter* sp., *Proteus;* less active against gram-positive cocci	100–200	q4h	6–12
Cefoxitin	Mefoxitin	Same as cephalothin plus *Proteus* sp. and anaerobes (including *B. fragilis*)	200	q4h	6–12
Cefuroxime	Zinacef	Similar to cefamandole, penetrates into CSF	25	q6h	4–5

(continued)

Table 39-2 (continued)

Antibiotic	Trade Name	Major Indications	Usual Daily Dosage (IV) (mg/kg)	Daily Dosage Schedule	Usual Maximum Dose per Day (g)
Cephalosporins (continued)					
Third generation					
Cefotaxime	Claforan	Same as cephalothin plus *Enterobacter* sp., indole-positive *Proteus*, *H. influenza*, *Citrobacter* sp., *Serratia* sp., and some *P. aeruginosa* and *Bacteroides* sp.	200	q4h	12
Moxalactam	Moxam	Same as cefotaxime but better anaerobe coverage (including *B. fragilis*)	200	q8h	12
Cefoperazone	Cefobid	Same as moxalactum but with better *P. aeruginosa* activity	200	q8h	12
Ceftizoxime	Cefizox	Same as moxalactam	200	q8h	12
Ceftazidime	Fortaz Tazidime Tazicef	Same as cefoperazone but with less anaerobic activity; most active agent against *P. aeruginosa*	100	q8h	6
Carbapenems					
Imipenem/ cilastatin	Primaxin	In addition to the *Enterbacteriaceae* and *P. aeruginosa*, primaxin has efficacy against *S. aureus,* Group D streptococci, many coagulase-negative staphylococci, listeria, and anaerobes. Only *P. maltophilia* and *P. cepacia* are not covered.	50–60	q6h	3–4
Monobactems					
Aztreonam	Azactam	Broad gram-negative but no gram-positive coverage. Is not cross-reactive with other *β*-lactams so can be used in penicillin or cephalosporin allergic patients	100–150	q6h	4–6
Aminoglycosides					
Gentamicin	Garamycin	*P. aeruginosa, Enterobacteriaceae, Enterococcus* (with ampicillin)	3–6	q6–q8h	
Tobramycin	Nebicin	Similar to gentamicin (except not as active against *Enterococcus* with ampicillin). Most active for *P. aeruginosa*	3–6	q6–q8h	
Amikacin	Amikin	*Serratia, Proteus, Pseudomonas, Enterobacteriaceae, Providentia*	15	q8–12h	

(continued)

Table 39-2 (*continued*)

Antibiotic	Trade Name	Major Indications	Usual Daily Dosage (IV) (mg/kg)	Daily Dosage Schedule	Usual Maximum Dose per Day (g)
Aminoglycosides (*continued*)					
Miscellaneous					
Chloramphenicol	Chloromycetin	*Hemophilus, B. fragilis, S. pneumoniae, Neisseria, Salmonella, Klebsiella,* most anaerobes, *Rickettsia*	50–100	q6h	3–6
Erythromycin	Ilotycin Gluceptate	*Legionella, mycoplasma*	30–50	q6h	6
Clindamycin	Cleocin	*B. fragilis, Clostridium, S. pneumoniae, S. viridans, S. pyrogenes, S. aureus*	30	q6h	2,400
Vancomycin	Vancocin	*C. difficile, S. aureus, S. epidermidis, S. fecalis,* multiply resistant *Corynebacterium, S. bovis*	25–40	q8–12h	3
Trimethoprim-sulfamethoxazole (1:5 ratio)	Bactrim Septra	*P. carinii, S. aureus, S. pneumoniae, S. pyrogenes, Salmonella, Serratia, Hemophilus, Neisseria*	10–20 as trimethoprim	q8–12h	960 as trimethoprim
Antiparasitic Agents					
Pentamidine	Lomidine	*P. carinii*	4 (IM)	Once/day	3
Thiabendazole	Mintezol	*Strongyloides,* visceral larva migrans	50	q12h	
Antifungal Agents					
Amphotericin	Fungizone	*Candida, Aspergillus, Zygomycetes, Torulopsis, Cryptococcus, Histoplasma*	0.5–1.0	Once/day	
5-Fluorocytosine	Flucytosine, Ancobon	*Cryptococcus, Candida, Torulopsis, Chromomycosis*	50–150	q6h	
Clotrimazole	Lotrimin	*Candida* sp., dermatophytes	50 mg (trouces)		
Miconazole	Monistat	*Candida* sp., *Aspergillus* sp., *Zygomycetes, Torulopsis, Cryptococcus, Pseudallescheria, Blastomyces, Coccidioides, Histoplasma, Paracoccidiodes, Sporothrix*	7–13	q8h	
Ketoconazole	Nizoral	Similar to miconazole	5–10 mg/kg/day (PO)	qid	
Antiviral Agents					
Adenosine arabinoside (ara-a)	Vidarabine	H. simplex, varicella zoster	10–15 mg/kg/day	12-h infusion	
Acycloguanosine	Acyclovir	H. simplex, varicella zoster	750 mg/m²/day (*H. simplex*) 1,500 mg/m²/day (VZV)	q8h	
Interferons (IF$_\alpha$, IF$_\beta$, IF$_\gamma$)		H. simplex	1×10^4 5×10^5 U/kg/day	qid	

availability of third-generation cephalosporins and carbapenems may offer an alternative to combination regimens, however, since a number of these agents provide, as single agents, an exceedingly broad range of activity, including both gram-positive and gram-negative bacteria, as well as bactericidal levels (Table 39-2).[45-47] Moreover, unlike the aminoglycosides, these newer beta-lactam antibiotics have minimal toxicity and do not require monitoring of serum levels.

At present, combination therapy is still considered the standard of care. A number of regimens, generally consisting of a cephalosporin, an aminoglycoside, and/or an extended-spectrum penicillin, have been employed.[47a] No particular combination regimen has proved clearly superior, and the regimen that is chosen at a given institution should reflect specific epidemiologic considerations (*e.g.,* local resistance patterns) as well as cost.

The potential of a single antibiotic (monotherapy) for the empirical management of the febrile neutropenic patient is attractive because of its ease of administration, lower cost, and lesser toxicity. To assess the efficacy of a monotherapeutic regimen, a prospective randomized trial was initiated at the National Cancer Institute (NCI) that compared monotherapy (ceftazidime) with combination therapy with cephalothin, carbenicillin, and gentamicin for the initial empirical management of 550 episodes of fever and neutropenia.[36] The antibiotic regimens were evaluated at both early (72 hours) and late (*i.e.,* at the resolution of granulocytopenia) points. The early evaluation was performed specifically to assess the efficacy of the antibiotics during the time when they were truly being utilized in an empirical manner; that is, prior to the availability of definitive microbiologic data. The responses were categorized as successful (with or without modifications of the initial regimen) if the patient survived the episode of neutropenia, and as failures if the patient died while neutropenic. There was no significant difference in terms of success (with or without modifications) for patients randomized to ceftazidime or the combination regimen among patients classified as having either an unexplained fever or a clinically or microbiologically documented infection. However, a significantly greater number of modifications was required among the patients randomized to ceftazidime (58 of 282 [21%] versus 29 of 268 [11%], P_2 = 0.002 by χ^2). This increased need for antibiotic modifications at the early evaluation reflected the need for anaerobic coverage among the patients randomized to ceftazidime who developed necrotizing gingivitis or perirectal cellulitis as well as the greater need for vancomycin for patients with documented gram-positive infections especially those due to *S. epidermidis.*

The results at the overall evaluation demonstrated equivalent success rates for the two regimens for patients classified as having either an unexplained fever or a documented infection. The percentage of patients treated successfully without the need for modification of the initial antimicrobial therapy was predictably less than that at the early evaluation. Patients with documented infections required changes in antimicrobial therapy more often than patients with unexplained fever, but the need was the same (59%) for patients randomized to either monotherapy or combination therapy. Therefore, in terms of the overall outcome and the frequency with which modifications of the initial empirical regimen were necessary, monotherapy with ceftazidime was as effective as combination therapy with cephalothin, carbenicillin, and gentamicin.

Despite these results and the encouraging findings of other investigators,[48-50] several concerns must be raised. First, the relative lack of activity of third-generation cephalosporins against gram-positive organisms, particularly the coagulase-negative staphylococci, has prompted a number of investigators to advocate inclusion of vancomycin in the primary regimen.[51,52] Second, several investigators have argued for the inclusion of an aminoglycoside in the initial regimen, not only to maximize the activity against gram-negative pathogens but also to decrease the emergence of resistant organisms. However, analysis of the NCI data fails to substantiate these concerns. Without doubt, in recent years gram-positive bacteria have become increasingly problematic and were isolated in 75 of the 550 episodes (14%) in the recent NCI study. Fifty-three of these isolates were from the preantibiotic evaluation (*i.e.,* primary infections). The remaining 22 isolates were responsible for secondary (or "breakthrough") infections. Vancomycin was ultimately required in 26 of the 53 (49%) primary infections but was added after the identification of a resistant isolate in 14 of 17 cases. There were no deaths or significant morbidity associated with the addition of vancomycin after the identification of an organism resistant to the initial regimen. Thus, the routine inclusion of vancomycin in the initial empirical therapy would have overtreated most patients, needlessly exposed them to a potentially toxic compound, and increased the cost without improving the overall clinical response. Thus, it seems more appropriate to withhold vancomycin until it is clearly necessary.[53] On the other hand, if there is a high incidence of methicillin-resistant coagulase-positive staphylococci (*i.e.,* Staph. aureus) at a given hospital, inclusion of vancomycin in the initial antibiotic regimen would be appropriate.

In the NCI study, 36 of 282 patients (13%) randomized to ceftazidime required an aminoglycoside at some time during the episode of neutropenia.[36,54] Two-thirds of these patients (24 of 36) received the aminoglycoside because of prospectively designed protocol modifications for clinical deteriorations or breakthrough bacteremias. Patients with documented infections received aminoglycosides somewhat more frequently than did patients with unexplained fevers (16 of 92 [17%] compared with 20 of 190 [11%], respectively). Clearly, however, most patients (87%) never required an aminoglycoside, and the inclusion of one as part of the initial empirical therapy would have unnecessarily exposed the patients to potential ototoxicity and nephrotoxicity.

Ultimately, the decision regarding the appropriate empirical regimen must be individualized at each institution. Oncology centers have different patterns of microbial isolates and antibiotic resistance, and this must be taken into account. Nevertheless, there is mounting evidence that the initial empirical management of a febrile, neutropenic cancer patient may be accomplished with a single antibiotic—especially selected third-generation cephalosporins. Regardless of the regimen chosen, however, the clinician must recognize the indications for, and appropriately employ, the modifications essential to ensure a successful outcome (Table 39-3).

Adjuncts to Antibiotic Therapy

The prophylactic or therapeutic replacement of granulocytes has been explored as an adjunct to antibiotic therapy for neutropenic patients. Five prospectively randomized, controlled clinical trials have investigated the efficacy of daily prophylactic granulocyte transfusions for patients undergoing induction chemotherapy for acute leukemia or bone marrow transplantation.[55-59] The two trials conducted at UCLA did not demonstrate a decrease in the frequency of infections or an enhancement of either remission or survival rates.[55,58] However, these trials utilized a relatively low daily dose of transfused granulocytes (median of 0.5×10^{10} per day) that had been harvested by

Table 39-3
Modification of Initial Antimicrobial Regimen for Febrile Neutropenic Cancer Patients

Clinical Event	Possible Modifications
Breakthrough bacteremia	If gram-positive isolate (*e.g., Staph. epidermidis*), add vancomycin
	If gram-negative isolate (*i.e.,* presumably resistant), switch to new regimen
Catheter-associated infection	Add vancomycin (as well as gram-negative coverage if not already being given)
Severe oral mucositis or necrotizing gingivitis	Add specific antianaerobic agent (*e.g.,* clindamycin or metronidazole)
Esophagitis	Trial of oral clotrimazole, ketoconazole, or IV amphotericin B
Pneumonitis	
Diffuse or interstitial	Trial of trimethoprim–sulfamethoxazole and erythromycin (plus broad-spectrum antibiotics if the patient is granulocytopenic)
New infiltrate in a granulocytopenic patient also receiving antibiotics	If granulocyte count is rising, watch and wait
	If granulocyte count is not recovering, biopsy to establish diagnosis; if biopsy cannot be done, add amphotericin B empirically
Perianal tenderness	If patient is already receiving broad-spectrum antibiotics, add a specific antianaerobic agent
	If patient is not on antibiotics, begin broad-spectrum therapy with anaerobic coverage
Persistent fever and neutropenia	Continue antibiotics and after 1 week of persistent fever and neutropenia, add systemic antifungal therapy empirically

a discontinuous-flow centrifugation leukapheresis without steroid premedication of the donors. Whether the low dose accounts for the lack of clinical efficacy is speculative, although a dose–response relation between the number of transfused leukocytes and the clinical response has been demonstrated in both animal models and early human trials using leukocytes collected from donors with chronic myelogenous leukemia.[60-62]

Despite conflicting data, it is probable that the daily administration of a sufficient number of properly collected leukocytes (*i.e.,* greater than $10^{10}/m^2$ per day) would reduce the incidence of infectious complications among neutropenic patients. However, such an approach is neither economically nor medically feasible with our current technology. Additionally, the nature and severity of the potential adverse effects to the patient (*e.g.,* transmission of cytomegalovirus, alloimmunization, pulmonary toxicity) and donor argue against transfusion use.[63-67]

Several well-designed, prospectively randomized clinical trials have investigated the therapeutic utility of transfused granulocytes.[68-73] Unfortunately, the interpretation of the results is complicated by the disparate techniques used for leukocyte collection (including filtration leukapheresis and continuous and discontinuous centrifugation leukapheresis), the absence of histocompatibility information, the different numbers of transfusions and doses, and inconsistent criteria for the institution of therapy and evaluation of results. Nonetheless, the weight of evidence suggests a beneficial role for granulocytes in neutropenic patients with documented bacteremia

(particularly that due to gram-negative aerobes) who are not expected to recover marrow function within a several-day period. In recent years, however, the relevance of this database has been questioned because of advances in induction regimens for patients with acute leukemia, and, most importantly, because of the availability of more efficacious antimicrobial regimens. There has been no recent documentation that therapeutic granulocyte transfusions would further improve the short- or long-term survival of infected neutropenic patients. Furthermore, the cost considerations and potential for adverse reactions are similar to those cited for prophylactic granulocyte transfusions. Thus, current data do not support the use of granulocyte transfusions for neutropenic patients.[74,75]

It is possible that improvement in biotechnology may make the collection of leukocytes or monocytes more successful. An alternative approach is to use recombinant granulocyte–macrophage colony-stimulating factor(s) (GM-CSF) to accelerate neutrophil recovery following cytotoxic therapy. Preclinical data show considerable promise, and a number of clinical trials are currently under way.[33,76,77,77a]

MANAGEMENT OF THE NEUTROPENIC PATIENT WITH UNEXPLAINED FEVER

A large proportion of neutropenic cancer patients who become febrile will not have a clinically or microbiologically identifiable cause for their initial fever.[31,36] Although some of these patients may have become febrile in response to a medication or blood product or because of their underlying malignant process, it is probable that the majority have an occult infection, the site of which remains undefined because they are rapidly evaluated and given effective empirical therapy. Despite the frustration inherent in not defining the site of the infection and the possibility that early empirical antibiotics are masking infection, the reduced morbidity and mortality rates associated with this approach make it justifiable.

Having started antibiotics empirically, the question of how long to continue them when a site of infection has not been defined is often problematic. Stopping antibiotic therapy too early can lead to clinical deterioration in patients who remain granulocytopenic, particularly when they are persistently febrile.

Patients with fever of unexplained origin can be divided into low- and high-risk groups. Low-risk patients resolve their granulocytopenia within 1 week of starting antibiotics. These patients do well when antibiotics are continued until the granulocyte count recovers to about 500/mm³.[31] The dilemma pertains to the high-risk patients who remain neutropenic for more than 1 week. The management of these patients has been addressed in a series of prospective clinical studies which stratified them according to whether they had defervesced after the initiation of broad-spectrum antibiotics or remained persistently febrile (Fig. 39-3).[78,79] Within 3 days of stopping antibiotics on day 7 in patients who had defervesced on therapy, 41% again became febrile; the new isolate(s) were sensitive to the antibiotics that had been withdrawn. In contrast, no subsequent infections were observed in the patients who continued antibiotics. However, these data did not define whether antibiotics should be continued until the final resolution of neutropenia or whether a specific limited course of antibiotic therapy, as if the patient had an occult site of infection, might suffice. Therefore, in an ongoing study, we have tried to evaluate the appropriate duration of antibiotic therapy by continuing antibiotics for afebrile but persistently granulocytopenic patients for a full 14-day course as if they had an occult infectious etiology for their fever and then randomizing them to either stop antibiotics or to continue treatment until the resolution of the granulocytopenia. We have observed that after day 14, approximately one-third of the patients either stopping or continuing antibiotic therapy become febrile again; because patients randomized to discontinue antibiotics responded to the

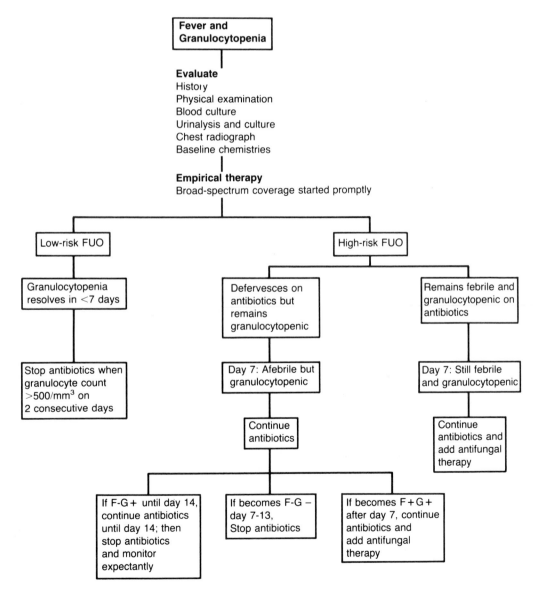

FIGURE 39-3. Algorithm for the initial management of the child who has unexplained fever and neutropenia.

reinstitution of therapy when a new fever developed, it seems reasonable to continue patients with unexplained fever on a standard 14-day treatment course if they remain granulocytopenic and then to stop the antibiotic therapy, recognizing that approximately 30% will require further intervention.

Empirical Antifungal Therapy

The situation is more complicated for patients who remain persistently granulocytopenic and febrile despite antibiotic therapy. In a randomized clinical trial, we observed that 56% of patients with unexplained fever who remained febrile after receiving empirical antibiotics developed complications within 3 days of stopping therapy. Of these, 38% became hypotensive. However, simply continuing antibiotics in the face of persistent fever and granulocytopenia was also not satisfactory, since 31% of these patients eventually developed invasive fungal infections. It is not possible to determine whether these fungal infections were the cause of the patient's persistent fever or a consequence of their continued antibiotic therapy and long-term granulocytopenia. However, patients with persistent fever and granulocytopenia did best when their antibiotic therapy was continued and amphotericin B was added empirically.

Thus, the rationale for the empirical use of an antifungal compound is based on several lines of reasoning. First, the antemortem diagnosis of even disseminated fungal disease is difficult in an immunocompromised host. Second, withholding antifungal therapy pending a definitive diagnosis frequently allows dissemination to occur prior to the institution of therapy,[80] whereas the outcome of a fungal infection in an immunocompromised patient is improved by early institution of therapy. Last, it is possible to identify patients who are at greatest risk for invasive mycoses. Thus, neutropenic patients who remain febrile despite a 4- to 7-day trial of broad-spectrum antimicrobial therapy are particularly prone to fungal disease.[81,82] The use of empirical antifungal therapy would be expected to provide a dual benefit: the suppression of the fungal overgrowth that inevitably accompanies broad-spectrum antimicrobial therapy and the early treatment of subclinical, localized mycotic disease.

Further support for the empirical institution of antifungal therapy comes from several retrospective studies. Burke and coworkers used amphotericin B in patients with acute leukemia with recurrent or persistent fever despite antibiotic coverage with gentamicin and carbenicillin.[81] Stein and colleagues used amphotericin B (at 0.4 mg/kg per day) for patients with persistent or recrudescent fever after a week of antimicrobial therapy during induction therapy for acute myelogenous leukemia.[82] Both of these studies found a decrease in deaths due to invasive mycoses relative to historical control groups.

Despite the theoretical and clinical evidence substantiating the efficacy of empirical antifungal therapy, the widespread acceptance and clinical use of this information have been hindered by the significant toxicity of amphotericin B. Fever, nephrotoxicity, hepatotoxicity, chilling reactions, and electrolyte imbalances (particularly hypokalemia) are frequently associated with the administration of this drug. Less toxic alternatives are desirable. The imidazoles are a class of antifungal agents that are broad in spectrum, low in toxicity, and easily administered. Of the currently available imidazoles, ketoconazole is the most appropriate candidate. An NCI study randomized 72 patients who remained febrile and neutropenic after 7 days of antimicrobial therapy to receive either amphotericin B (at 0.5 mg/kg per day) or ketoconazole (800 mg/day).[83] The results were similar in terms of the duration of fever following the antifungal randomization, the number of documented fungal infections, the number of patients requiring crossover due to intolerance, and the overall outcome scored as success (*i.e.,* survival) or failure (*i.e.,* death from invasive fungal infection). However, once the diagnosis of an invasive fungal infection was documented, disease progression was likely unless the patient received amphotericin B.

Fainstein and associates corroborated these findings in a study of 172 neutropenic patients who remained febrile for 72 to 96 hours after the institution of empirical antibiotic therapy and who were randomized to receive either amphotericin B (0.6–1.0 mg/kg daily) or ketoconazole (200 mg orally every 6 hours).[84] In this study, there was no difference between the two regimens in the response of patients with documented, "probable," or "possible" fungal infections. However, patients with documented infections due to *C. tropicalis* responded more often to amphotericin B (five of eight patients) than to ketoconazole (none of eight patients). Unfortunately, the unusual design and response criteria in this study hinder its correlation with previously established data. Recently, Winegard and co-workers evaluated parenteral miconazole as an empirical antifungal agent and demonstrated that its use, compared to a placebo, reduced significantly the incidence of invasive fungal infections.[84a]

Questions remain regarding the optimal point at which to initiate antifungal therapy. The arbitrary designation of day 7 avoids the overuse of antifungal agents in patients who are slow to defervesce with empirical antibiotics or those who recover their granulocyte counts before day 7. The potential value of alternative antifungal compounds (*e.g.,* liposome-encapsulated amphotericin B, itraconazole, fluconazole) remains to be established by prospectively randomized clinical trials.[84b–84e]

In summary, empirical antifungal therapy is indicated for patients who remain neutropenic and febrile (or who recrudesce) despite 1 week of broad-spectrum antibiotics. It appears that ketoconazole is a useful alternative to amphotericin B as an empirical agent, but a confirmed invasive fungal infection mandates the use of amphotericin B. The optimal duration of empirical antifungal therapy is based on clinical experience. For patients who remain neutropenic, antifungal therapy should be continued until the resolution of granulocytopenia. Persistence or recrudescence of fever should prompt a meticulous investigation for nonfungal infectious causes (*e.g.,* bacterial or viral superinfections). Patients who develop a documented fungal infection should be treated according to established clinical guidelines for the offending pathogen (generally 2 g of amphotericin B).

EVALUATION AND MANAGEMENT OF THE NEUTROPENIC PATIENT WITH A DOCUMENTED INFECTION

Bacteremia

Approximately 20% of febrile neutropenic cancer patients have a bacteremia at the time of presentation.[36,40] The site of origin for these bacteremic episodes differs significantly from that observed in a general hospital setting, where the genitourinary tract is the most common site. Among immunocompromised patients, the respiratory tract is the most commonly identified site of origin (25%), followed by perianal and perioral cellulitis, the gastrointestinal tract, and the genitourinary tract (each approximately 10%). Unfortunately, there is no clinically reliable method by which to identify prospectively those febrile neutropenic patients who are bacteremic.[31]

Until the late 1970s, gram-negative aerobic organisms (especially *Pseud. aeruginosa, E. coli,* and *K. pneumoniae*) were the most frequently isolated pathogens. During the past several years, the pattern of infections has shifted, and gram-positive bacteria are now isolated as often as gram-negatives at most cancer centers. Among the gram-positive pathogens, *Staph. aureus, Staph. epidermidis,* and *Streptococcus* spp. (including the group D) are the most commonly isolated. Species of *Corynebacterium* (*e.g.,* CDC group JK, *Coryn. diphtheriae,* and *Coryn. equi*) and *Bacillus* are less frequently isolated and tend to occur in patients with long episodes of granulocytopenia or indwelling vascular access devices, respectively.[85] *E. coli, K. pneumoniae,* and *Pseud. aeruginosa* remain the most frequently isolated gram-negative bacilli, although more resistant species (*e.g.,* non-aeruginosa pseudomonads, *Serratia marcescens,* Enterobacteriaceae) are occasionally encountered. For reasons that are unclear, the incidence of infections (including bacteremias) due to *Pseud. aeruginosa* has been decreasing in recent years. Of note, the morbidity and mortality rates of infections with gram-positive bacteria (especially the coagulase-negative staphylococci) are less than those due to gram-negative pathogens.

The most important therapeutic intervention for patients ultimately shown to be bacteremic is the prompt initiation of empirical antibiotics. Necessary modifications of this regimen should be based on the antimicrobial sensitivity pattern of the bloodstream isolate (see Table 39-3). The minimal duration of therapy for bacteremic patients is 10 to 14 days, although patients with persistent neutropenia or infection are likely to require longer treatment courses.

Pathogen-Directed or Broad-Spectrum Therapy?

The optimal management of the neutropenic patient with a defined infection poses a difficult dilemma. That is, should the patient continue to receive a broad-spectrum antibiotic regimen, or can the antibiotic(s) be narrowed to a pathogen-directed therapy? Continuing broad-spectrum therapy maintains antimicrobial activity against a wide range of gram-positive and gram-negative pathogens and may eradicate, or at least suppress, second bacterial infections. However, this approach may allow the proliferation of resistant bacteria and fungi and result in breakthrough (secondary) bacteremias or disseminated mycoses. Alternatively, the advantage of pathogen-directed therapy is a lessened impact on the patient's microbial flora, potentially decreasing the risk of infection with multiply resistant bacteria or fungi.

A retrospective study conducted at the NCI reviewed 78 neutropenic patients with gram-positive (primarily *S. aureus*) bacteremia who received either specific therapy with nafcillin or oxacillin or continued broad-spectrum therapy.[86] Patients who remained granulocytopenic for less than 1 week did well regardless of the drug chosen. However, among patients with granulocytopenia of greater than 7 days, 47% of those who received specific therapy developed a second infection with a gram-negative aerobe. A prospectively randomized trial has revealed no significant difference between patients treated with narrow or broad-spectrum coverage with respect to the occurrence of second infections, new fevers, or death. However, a greater number of patients treated with a narrowed antibiotic regimen required a subsequent modification of therapy.[87]

Therefore, current recommendations for the management of immunosuppressed (and particularly neutropenic) patients with a documented bacterial infection can be summarized as follows. For those patients whose duration of neutropenia is expected to be less than 7 days, a narrowed antimicrobial regimen may be safely employed. On the other hand, for patients with more prolonged episodes of neutropenia, there seems to be no advantage (and potential disadvantages) to narrowing the initial empirical regimen. If the empirical regimen is narrowed (*e.g.,* for simplification of fluid administration or due to cost constraints), the patient's course must be carefully monitored for evidence of recrudescent fever, progression of an infectious process, or clinical deterioration. Any such change should immediately prompt the reexpansion of antimicrobial coverage.

Catheter-Associated Bacteremia

With the increased use of indwelling venous access devices, catheter-associated bacteremic episodes have become more frequent.[35] The diagnosis of a catheter-related bacteremia is made by documentating positive blood cultures from the catheter lumen(s) and a peripheral venous site. The colony count from the sample obtained from the lumen is ordinarily greater than that from the peripheral site.

Most (approximately 80%) of catheter-associated infections caused by coagulase-positive staphylococci can be controlled without removal of the catheter. It is imperative, however, to obtain follow-up blood cultures from both the catheter and peripheral sites to document the eradication of the infection. If blood cultures remain positive despite 24 to 48 hours of appropriate antimicrobial therapy, the catheter should be removed. Patients should receive a 10- to 14-day course of therapy unless there is evidence of an intravascular infection. If the patient has a multilumen catheter, the antibiotic infusions should be rotated to include all ports and lumens.

Ears, Nose, and Sinus Infections

A meticulous examination is critical in the initial evaluation of a febrile neutropenic patient, and repetitive examinations are especially important in the neutropenic patient who has persistent fever.

Ears

Children with cancer may, of course, develop the same infectious problems as nonimmunocompromised patients. For example, as in the immunocompetent child, otitis media may follow a viral upper respiratory illness.

Clinical findings suggestive of an ear infection range from the classic complaints (ear pain, drainage, fever, irritability) to minimal symptomatology (slight tympanic erythema) in profoundly neutropenic children. Diagnostic tympanocentesis is generally not feasible because of the thrombocytopenia usually present in children who are neutropenic. Although the most likely pathogens are identical to those isolated from an immunocompetent host (*i.e., S. pneumoniae* and *H. influenzae*)*,* neutropenic patients are also susceptible to gram-positive or gram-negative bacteria that may have colonized the oropharynx and nasopharynx.[88] Therefore, antibiotic coverage in the neutropenic patient must be broad spectrum unless a specific pathogen has been identified. Patients should receive 10 to 14 days of therapy. Children with anatomical alterations (*e.g.,* local tumor growth) or treatment-induced abnormalities (*e.g.,* radiation damage) of the external or middle ear or eustachian tubes are particularly susceptible to recurrent infectious episodes.

Although mastoiditis has become uncommon, the immunosuppressed child with an abnormality of the middle ear (*e.g.*, due to rhabdomyosarcoma) is at risk for the development of mastoiditis. Such patients should undergo appropriate evaluation (including x-ray films and computed tomography [CT] scans of the involved area), particularly if they have symptoms or signs (*e.g.*, localized erythema, swelling, and tenderness) referrable to the mastoid.

Sinusitis

Patients with obstruction of the sinuses by tumor (*e.g.*, nasopharyngeal carcinomas, Burkitt's lymphoma, or rhabdomyosarcomas) are especially at risk for acute or chronic sinusitis. Younger children and infants are less susceptible because of the lack of development of all but rudimentary sinusoidal air spaces. In the immunocompetent or non-neutropenic child, *S. pneumoniae, H. influenzae,* and *Branhamella catarrhalis* are the most common pathogens.[89] In an immunocompromised (and particularly neutropenic) patient, gram-negative aerobes (including *Pseud. aeruginosa*) and anaerobic bacterial species are more frequently found.[90–92] Fungal pathogens (*e.g., Aspergillus* spp., *C. albicans,* and *Mucor*) are particularly worrisome causes of sinusitis in the immunocompromised host.[93–95] Patients with acute leukemia and other disorders with long periods of neutropenia (*e.g.*, aplastic anemia) are especially prone to fungal sinusitis.

The diagnosis of acute sinusitis is usually suggested by complaints of facial pain, local tenderness, and (assuming a patent outlet and an adequate granulocyte count) purulent nasal drainage. With involvement of the ethmoid sinus, edema of the eyelids and excessive tearing may also be noted. In young children, a nonproductive cough and fetid breath may indicate a sinus infection.[89] However, in an immunosuppressed patient, many of the classic symptoms and signs may be absent, and a high index of suspicion must be maintained, particularly in a persistently febrile, granulocytopenic patient receiving broad-spectrum antibiotics. Any sinus tenderness in a neutropenic child should be pursued with sinus x-ray films and a detailed nasopharyngeal examination, since even subtle findings on physical examination (*e.g.*, minimal crusting on nasal turbinates) may be indicative of an invasive fungal lesion.

In children over 1 year of age, radiologic examination of the sinuses remains the most sensitive diagnostic test.[96] The findings of sinus opacity, an air–fluid interface, or mucosal thickening are strongly correlated with an acute infection. In patients with chronic sinusitis, radiographic findings are less helpful because of the persistence of abnormalities related to the chronic infection. Serial CT scans may prove helpful in the immunosuppressed patient with chronic sinusoidal disease and may facilitate detection of bony erosion common to the indolent fungal pathogens.

Therapy must be tailored to the clinical situation. Acute sinusitis in a non-neutropenic individual is best managed with amoxicillin plus clavulanic acid (Augmentin) or trimethoprim–sulfamethoxazole.[97] For neutropenic patients, broad-spectrum antimicrobial therapy is necessary. If a neutropenic patient with sinusitis does not improve with 72 hours of treatment, aspiration or biopsy of the sinus should be performed. For patients with chronic or recurrent sinusitis, particularly those with a local tumor mass or damage secondary to radiotherapy, an antral window may be necessary to allow adequate drainage.

The diagnosis and treatment of a fungal sinusitis in neutropenic patients remains difficult, and the definitive diagnosis is dependent on histopathologic documentation of tissue invasion. Fungal sinusitis due to *Aspergillus* or *Mucor* can progress to the rhinocerebral syndrome, with invasion through the cribiform plate and into the central nervous system. Early institution of amphotericin B is imperative. Surgical debridement of involved tissue is often required in an effort to remove necrotic and inflammatory material. Even with these aggressive therapeutic maneuvers, a successful outcome is most dependent on the recovery of an adequate granulocyte count.

Management of Documented Infections of the Respiratory Tract

Infections of the respiratory tract are among the most common complications in the immunosuppressed cancer patient. A number of factors account for the frequency and severity of these infections. First, the shift in the pattern of colonization of the upper airway provides a ready source of pathogenic species in direct proximity to the lower respiratory tract. Second, the altered mucosal and humoral immune mechanisms (*e.g.*, subnormal ciliary function, decreased secretory immunoglobulins) provide for less effective clearance of aspirated organisms. Third, the absence or suboptimal functioning of the phagocytic effector cells (PMNs, pulmonary macrophages) permits the establishment of a local infection and, frequently, hematogenous dissemination of the organisms.

One of the principal problems in the management of pulmonary infiltrates in an immunocompromised host is the fact that the potential etiologies are so numerous. Both infectious and noninfectious etiologies must be considered, including progression of the underlying malignancy, drug reactions, emboli, and hemorrhage secondary to vascular erosion or severe thrombocytopenia (Table 39-4). The most practical approach for the evaluation of an immunocompromised patient with a pulmonary infiltrate is to categorize patients according to the anatomic distribution of the infiltrative lesion (localized versus diffuse) and the granulocyte count (neutropenic or not). This classification permits expeditious evaluation, identification of likely pathogens, and prompt institution of appropriate therapy to optimize the chances for a successful outcome (Fig. 39-4).

Diagnostic Approach to the Immunocompromised Patient with Pneumonia

The initial evaluation of the child with a suspected pneumonia should include a chest radiograph, blood cultures, hematologic indices, arterial blood gases, and collection and examination of available culture material. Unfortunately, sputum is usually not available in granulocytopenic patients.[34] In patients with a compatible history and physical examination, consideration should be given to skin testing for tuberculosis. It is generally wise to store an acute-phase serum specimen for serologic testing or viral titers.

A definitive diagnosis is established by noninvasive means in a relative minority of patients who present with pulmonary infiltrates. The question of when an invasive diagnostic procedure is necessary and which procedure should be performed is a common yet difficult problem. Diagnostic techniques have ranged from transtracheal aspiration to transthoracic or transbroncheal aspirations and biopsies to the gold standard, open lung biopsy. In recent years, bronchoalveolar lavage has come into vogue since it has a low morbidity and can be safely per-

Table 39-4
Differential Diagnosis of Pneumonia in Cancer Patients

Localized Infiltrate	Diffuse Infiltrate
Non-neutropenic Patients	
Bacteria: *Strep. pneumoniae, Haemophilus,* mycobacteria	Parasites: *P. carinii, T. gondii, Strongyloides*
Mycoplasma	Bacteria: mycobacteria, *Nocardia, Legionella, Chlamydia* (including TWAR).
Fungi: *Cryptococcus, Histoplasma, Coccidioides*	Mycoplasma
Viruses: respiratory syncytial virus, adenovirus	Viruses: H. simplex, varicella–zoster, cytomegalovirus, measles, influenza, adenovirus
Underlying tumor	Fungi: *Aspergillus, Candida, Zygomycetes, Cryptococcus*
Drugs: busulfan, bleomycin, cyclophosphamide, methotrexate, cytosine arabinoside	Radiation pneumonitis
Radiation	Drugs
Neutropenic Patients	
Bacteria: Any gram-positive or gram-negative, mycobacteria, *Nocardia*	Bacteria: Any gram-positive or gram-negative, mycobacteria, *Nocardia, Legionella, Chlamydia*
Fungi: *Aspergillus, Zygomycetes, Candida, Cryptococcus, Histoplasma*	*Mycoplasma*
Viruses: H. simplex, varicella–zoster	Fungi: *Candida, Aspergillus, Zygomycetes, Cryptococcus, Histoplasma*
Drugs (see above)	Parasites: *P. carinii, T. gondii, Strongyloides*
Radiation	Viruses: H. simplex, varicella–zoster, cytomegalovirus, measles, influenza, adenovirus, RSV
	Radiation pneumonitis
	Drugs

formed, in experienced hands, in patients with platelet counts as low as 30,000/mm³.[98,98a,98b] However, transbronchial biopsy should not be performed in patients whose platelet count is less than 50,000/mm³. If the diagnosis cannot be established with a lavage, the next procedure to consider is the open lung biopsy.

Localized Pulmonary Infiltrate in a Non-neutropenic Patient

The causes of a localized pulmonary infiltrate in a non-neutropenic cancer patient are similar to those in an immunocompetent child. Common bacterial, viral, and mycoplasmal organisms are most frequently isolated (see Table 39-4), and therapeutic considerations are similar to those for an immunocompetent child.[99]

Non-neutropenic patients who are receiving immunosuppressive therapy (including corticosteroids) and patients with AIDS are at risk for tuberculosis and atypical mycobacterial disease. Specific mycobacterial identification is especially important in AIDS patients because of the frequency of atypical isolates (particularly *M. avium intracellulare*) (see Chap. 36). Children with documented *M. tuberculosis* should receive 9 to 12 months of therapy with at least two effective antituberculous agents (isoniazid and rifampin). The management of atypical mycobacterial disease is more complex, and decisions regarding the relative roles of effective antimycobacterial therapy (*e.g.,* ansamycin, clofazamine), surgery, and palliative therapy must be individualized.

Less commonly encountered etiologies for a localized pulmonary infiltrate in a non-neutropenic patient include progression of the underlying malignancy, an atelectatic segment of lung (generally due to compromise of the airway by adjacent tumor), and a localized reaction to a chemotherapeutic agent (particularly methotrexate, cyclophosphamide, or bleomycin). However, such drug reactions are more commonly manifest as diffuse interstitial pulmonary processes.

Localized Pulmonary Infiltrate in a Neutropenic Patient

In addition to the pathogens causing a localized infiltrate in the non-neutropenic patient, an array of opportunistic pathogens must be considered in the differential diagnosis if a neutropenic patient has a localized infiltrate. In essence, any gram-positive or gram-negative organism, as well as a variety of fungal, parasitic, and even viral pathogens, can be responsible (see Table 39-4). In patients with relatively short (less than 14-day) durations of neutropenia, bacterial pathogens predominate. Patients with longer periods of neutropenia, or those of a particular clinical setting (*e.g.,* following allogeneic bone-marrow transplantation), are more prone to develop a fungal (*Candida* or *Aspergillus*) or viral (CMV) process. Unless the clinical presentation suggests otherwise, it is appropriate to initiate a 48- to 72-hour trial of broad-spectrum antibiotics before proceeding to an invasive diagnostic procedure. If the patient has stabilized or improved by 72 hours, a 10- to 14-day course of treatment is necessary. If the patient has not stabilized or improved, a bronchoalveolar lavage or open lung biopsy should be performed (see Fig. 39-4).

A less common but nevertheless important pathogen to consider as the cause of localized pneumonia in an immunosuppressed host is *Legionella*.[100–103] *Legionella* species are ubiquitous and usually found in water, including air conditioning cooling towers and hospital shower heads.[104,105] Aero-

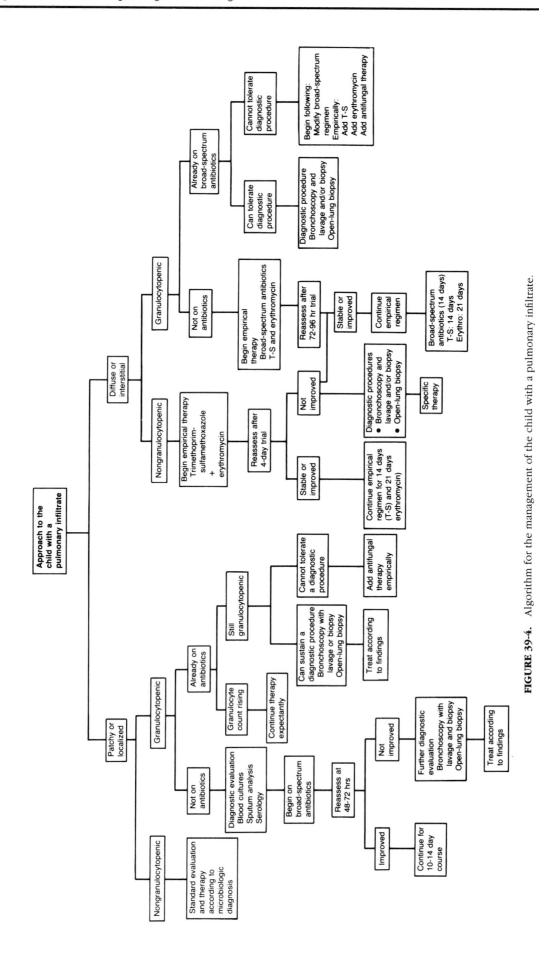

FIGURE 39-4. Algorithm for the management of the child with a pulmonary infiltrate.

solization of contaminated water is probably the most common mechanism of transmission, and nosocomial infections have been described.

Although legionellosis is a multisystem disease (including the gastrointestinal, central nervous, and cardiovascular systems), the lung is the primary target organ. The incubation period ranges from 2 to 10 days (median 4 days), although immunosuppressed patients tend to have shorter incubation periods and a more abrupt onset of symptoms. The initial symptoms are generally nonspecific and include malaise, anorexia, lethargy, and headache. A nonproductive cough develops in 90% of patients, usually after a lag of 2 to 3 days. Diarrhea, which occurs in approximately 50% of patients, may either precede or follow the respiratory symptoms.

Fever is usually the initial sign of *Legionella* infection and is generally unremitting in the absence of effective therapy. Two-thirds of patients will manifest a pulse deficit (relative bradycardia), and one-third will have some degree of neurologic dysfunction ranging from disorientation, depression, hallucinations, and seizures to lethargy, stupor, and coma.[106-108] Physical examination may reveal either hyperreactive or hyporeactive deep tendon reflexes, nystagmus, peripheral sensory or motor neuropathies, and, rarely, signs of meningeal irritation.

The initial radiographic abnormality generally is a patchy, alveolar infiltrate involving a single lobe. If translobar consolidation occurs, it usually involves contiguous rather than non-adjacent segments.[109] Cavitary lesions or abscess formation is unusual except in infections with *L. midadei.*

The most rapid and accurate means of diagnosis is a direct fluorescent antibody test performed on respiratory tract secretions, pulmonary tissue from biopsy specimens, pleural fluid, or even pus. However, not all serotypes are detectable, and a negative test does not eliminate *Legionella* as a diagnostic consideration. Culturing of the organism on a charcoal–yeast-extract-enhanced medium requires 2 to 7 days.

Erythromycin (40–50 mg/kg per day [maximum of 4 g] in four divided doses for 3 weeks) is the treatment of choice. The drug should be administered intravenously for the first several days in seriously ill patients; the oral route may be used as the patient responds. Patients unable to tolerate erythromycin should receive doxycycline (5 mg/kg per day in two doses). Rifampin (20 mg/kg per day in two doses) may be given in addition to erythromycin or doxycycline for seriously ill patients. Response is usually prompt, with a resolution of fever and subjective improvement within 24 to 48 hours.

Nocardia asteroides and *Nocardia brasiliensis* may also present as a localized pulmonary infiltrate, although miliary and microcavitary patterns have been described in cancer patients.[110-112] Importantly, approximately 30% of patients with a pulmonary infection due to *Nocardia asteroides* will have cutaneous and central nervous system (usually brain abscesses) infections as well. Diagnosis is dependent on positive cultures or histopathologic demonstration of tissue invasion by the organisms. Sulfadiazine (100 mg/kg per day for 6 months) is the therapy of choice. The mortality rate of disseminated disease remains approximately 30%.

The most frequently encountered cause of a localized pulmonary infiltrate in the patient with protracted neutropenia is a fungal pneumonia, particularly when the patient already is receiving broad-spectrum antibiotics.[113] *Candida* species (especially *C. albicans* and *C. tropicalis*), *Aspergillus* spp., and the phycomycetes (*i.e., Mucor, Rhizopus*) are the pathogens most often responsible.[114-117] Other fungi, including *Histoplasma capsulatum, Coccidioides immitis,* and *Cryptococcus neoformans,* may also cause pneumonia in immunocompromised patients, although infections with these organisms are more

commonly manifest as a diffuse or nodular pulmonary pattern.[118-120] The clinical, laboratory, and radiographic features of fungal pathogens are indistinguishable from those of other pulmonary processes, and definitive diagnosis is dependent on microbiologic or histopathologic confirmation in specimens obtained from transbronchial or open lung biopsy.

Candida pneumonia generally manifests as a progressive pulmonary infiltrate in a patient with persistent fever and neutropenia. Hematogenous seeding of the lungs, usually from the gastrointestinal tract, is the most common route of infection, resulting in involvement of multiple (often bilateral) pulmonary segments. Aspiration of oropharyngeal contents, especially in heavily colonized patients, may also cause a *Candida* bronchopneumonia. There is no particular radiographic pattern diagnostic of *Candida* pneumonia, and findings range from normal-appearing to localized, often perihilar, infiltrates to a miliary-type pattern.[116] The diagnosis of pulmonary candidiasis, like that of disseminated candidiasis in general, remains problematic.[122] Positive blood cultures are rare even with disseminated disease, and negative cultures cannot be used as a diagnostically useful exclusion.[121] Current antigen, antibody, and cell-wall component assays are not helpful. The presence of a sputum culture positive for *C. albicans* is not diagnostically useful, but the isolation of *C. tropicalis* from multiple sites (*e.g.,* sputum, urine, and stool) has been correlated with invasive disease.[123] In most instances, however, definitive diagnosis requires histopathologic confirmation.

The incidence of pulmonary infections due to *Aspergillus* spp. has increased in recent years and has been noted in clusters in certain hospitals.[124-128] The most common scenario is that of a profoundly and persistently neutropenic patient who develops a localized, progressive pulmonary infiltrate while receiving broad-spectrum antibiotics.[115] Infections due to *A. fumigatus* and *A. flavus* are the most common, presumably initiated via inhalation of airborne spores. Cultures of the anterior nares may be helpful in identifying those patients at increased risk for invasive pulmonary disease due to *A. flavus.*[127] Because of the tendency for *Aspergillus* spp. to invade blood vessels, a necrotizing bronchopneumonia is characteristic, and there is the possibility of life-threatening hemoptysis. Disseminated aspergillosis occurs in approximately 30% of the cases, with involvement of the central nervous system, liver, kidneys, skin, and spleen. Despite this propensity for widespread disease, blood cultures are virtually never positive.

Diagnosis of aspergillosis by noninvasive measures remains suboptimal, although recent reports suggest that positive cultures of sputum or bronchoalveolar lavage specimens in a patient with long-term fever and neutropenia and a progressive infiltrate is highly associated with *Aspergillus* pneumonia.[128] Despite numerous initially optimistic reports, antigen and antibody methods of detection have not proved as sensitive as had been hoped and are too often falsely negative. Thus, a definitive diagnosis still requires histologic confirmation or a positive bronchoalveolar lavage culture obtained in a clinically relevant setting.

Control of an *Aspergillus* pneumonia requires an early diagnosis and prompt intervention.[119] Optimal therapy is with amphotericin B. Recent studies suggest that doses of 1 to 1.5 mg/kg per day be given to ensure response, although this schedule has not been tested in a randomized clinical trial.[127a] Although also not proved, the addition of 5-fluorocystosine (100–150 mg/kg per day in three doses) may be helpful. When 5-fluorocytosine is given, blood levels of the drug should be measured. Even with appropriate pharmacologic intervention, the most important prognosticator of a successful outcome is the return of adequate numbers of granulocytes.

The phycomycetes, especially *Mucor* and *Rhizopus* species, can cause a pulmonary infiltrate that is similar to that associated with *Aspergillus.* These organisms may also cause sinus infections and rhinocerebral syndrome. Systemic dissemination to the liver, pancreas, central nervous system, myocardium, kidney, and gastrointestinal tract occurs in approximately 50% of patients. Diagnosis requires documentation of tissue invasion. Therapy consists of amphotericin B (1.0 mg/kg per day) and aggressive surgical debridement, although treatment results remain poor unless granulocyte recovery ensues.

Diffuse Pulmonary Infiltrates in a Non-neutropenic Cancer Patient

Diffuse pulmonary infiltrates can be caused by bacterial, viral, fungal, and protozoal pathogens; the probability of various pathogens is influenced by whether the patient is neutropenic (see Table 39-4). A non-neutropenic patient with a diffuse pulmonary infiltrate is unlikely to have a bacterial or fungal process. Perhaps the most commonly encountered infection in this setting is *P. carinii* pneumonia.[128] This infection is believed to result from a reactivation of latent cysts, since essentially 100% of normal children possess detectable antibody to the organism.[129] However, patient-to-patient transmission has been suggested by reports of nosocomial clusterings of cases.[130] It is also possible that certain chemotherapeutic regimens predispose patients to interstitial infiltrates caused by *P. carinii.*[131] Confirmation of patient-to-patient transmission will have dramatic epidemiologic ramifications, particularly with regard to the isolation precautions used for AIDS patients.

Patients with *Pneumocystis* pneumonia most commonly present with fever, a nonproductive cough, tachypnea, and hypoxemia. The time course of the symptoms ranges from a chronic, indolent course (characteristic of AIDS patients) to an acute, fulminant presentation.[132] Rales are not usually detectable on auscultation. Radiographic examination usually reveals bilateral fluffy alveolar infiltrates, often originating at the hilum and extending peripherally. Rarely, the chest radiograph is atypical, ranging from normal to a lobar or nodular infiltrate. Pleural effusions are rare.

Diagnosis of *Pneumocystis* pneumonia requires demonstration of cysts or trophozoites in pulmonary material from patients with a clinically compatible course, as cysts have been found in asymptomatic, previously healthy individuals autopsied following traumatic deaths. In patients with AIDS (including children), positive specimens may be obtained from sputum samples, since the cyst burden is high, whereas in cancer patients, cysts are best demonstrated by broncheoalveolar lavage or open lung biopsy. Serologic confirmation remains of questionable value.

In clinical situations in which the likelihood of *Pneumocystis* pneumonia is great, the choice is either to proceed with a diagnostic procedure or to administer an empirical course of trimethoprim–sulfamethoxazole. In centers where bronchoalveolar lavage is readily available, it is the procedure of choice for establishing the diagnosis. However, if this procedure is not available or if the patient's clinical or hematologic status does not permit its use, an empirical trial of trimethoprim–sulfamethoxazole plus erythromycin (for *Legionella*) is recommended rather than proceeding directly to open lung biopsy. This recommendation is based on the results of a randomized NCI trial demonstrating that in non-neutropenic patients with diffuse infiltrates, empirical therapy is as safe and effective as an open lung biopsy.[133,134] However, it must be remembered that a response to trimethoprim–sulfamethoxazole may not be apparent for 4 to 5 days, although stabilization or slight improvement in alveolar air exchange generally occurs within 72

to 96 hours. Patients who do not respond should be given pentamidine. Recently, the antifolate trimetrexate has shown promising efficacy in the treatment of *P. carinii* pneumonia in adult AIDS patients who have not responded to trimethoprim–sulfamethoxazole or pentamidine.[134]

A number of viruses can cause a diffuse interstitial infiltrate in non-neutropenic patients. Cytomegalovirus pneumonitis is the most common and is most frequently observed following allogeneic bone-marrow transplantation. Reactivation of latent virus, or acquisition of CMV from blood product transfusions in seronegative patients, are the most important risk factors.[135,136] Other herpes viruses (*e.g.,* varicella–zoster, Herpes simplex) may also cause a diffuse pneumonitis, but this usually occurs as a consequence of visceral dissemination from dermatomal or cutaneous disease. Rarely, the measles virus and other common respiratory viruses (*e.g.,* respiratory syncytial virus, adenovirus, rhinovirus, and enterovirus) have caused diffuse pulmonary infiltrates in immunosuppressed patients. With the exception of the association between CMV and diffuse pneumonitis among allogeneic transplant recipients, there are no distinguishing clinical or pathologic features to identify the exact etiology of a diffuse viral pneumonitis. Unfortunately, therapy for CMV pneumonitis (including trials of acyclovir, DHPG, and interferons), alone or in combination, has been ineffective.[137] Although initially promising, the use of specific or pooled immunoglobulins to prevent CMV pneumonia in patients undergoing bone-marrow transplantation has also proved ineffective.[138]

Diffuse Pulmonary Infiltrates in a Neutropenic Patient

In addition to *P. carinii* and CMV, both gram-positive and gram-negative bacteria and several fungi can cause interstitial infiltrates in neutropenic patients. Thus, broad-spectrum antibiotics and trimethoprim-sulfamethoxazole are necessary if empiric therapy is administered. Again, failure of the patient to improve necessitates lung biopsy and consideration of antifungal therapy.

Management of Documented Infections of the Gastrointestinal Tract

The gastrointestinal tract is a frequent source of infection in the neutropenic patient for several reasons. First, the gastrointestinal mucosa is in direct contact with the external environment. Normally, it acts as a mechanical barrier against penetration by invading pathogens, but this barrier can be disrupted by tumor invasion or damage from chemotherapy or radiotherapy. Second, the mucosal ulceration induced by these treatments offers a potential site for bacterial, fungal, and viral colonization, invasion, and, ultimately, infection. Furthermore, the normal microbial balance of the gastrointestinal tract is altered by serious illness, mechanical factors (*e.g.,* surgery, altered motility), and, especially, antimicrobial therapy, further contributing to colonization and infection.

Oral Cavity

The most common mucosal infection encountered in the immunosuppressed cancer patient is thrush, a superficial oral infection due to *C. albicans.*[139] Such lesions usually appear as whitish plaques with slightly raised, indurated borders. This infection is easily controlled in most cases by topical antifungal agents such as clotrimazole troches. If there is no response to topical therapy, low-dose amphotericin B (0.1–0.5 mg/kg per day) should be given for 5 to 7 days.[139a] Despite their relatively benign appearance and ease of control, such superficial fungal infections may serve as a nidus for systemic dissemination and contribute to poor nutrition.

Herpes simplex is the most common viral pathogen isolated from mucosal lesions.[140,141] Clinically, such lesions usually appear as clear vesicular eruptions, frequently in clusters or "crops," on an erythematous base. However, lesions may be nondescript and can be confused with the stomatotoxicity usually attributed to chemotherapy. Diagnosis may be confirmed by culture (requiring 24–72 hours) or may be made presumptively by the identification of multinucleated giant cells (positive Tzanck preparation) or by a positive fluorescent-antibody reaction. Unlike the self-limited and relatively innocuous presentation in an immunocompetent host, herpetic stomatitis may be a serious complication in an immunosuppressed patient. The severity of the local tissue involvement, inflammation, and eschar formation has deleterious consequences, not only because the areas may serve as a nidus for bacterial superinfections, but also because of the compromise of nutritional status mediated by the disruption of oral intake and deglutition. Acyclovir (750 mg/m² per day given every 8 hours) is the preferred treatment because of its infrequent toxicity, ease of administration, and documented efficacy in reducing the duration of viral shedding and shortening the time to healing.[142] Seropositive patients undergoing bone marrow transplantation or induction regimens for acute leukemia should receive prophylactic acyclovir, either orally or parenterally.[141]

Without specific local or systemic indications of infection, management of areas of mucosal ulceration should be directed toward palliation (e.g., bicarbonate mouthwash, regular dental care). Unfortunately, there is no evidence that maintenance of oral hygiene reduces the incidence or severity of oral mucositis, although it is probably beneficial.

Periodontal disease (including both gingivitis and periodontitis) is especially problematic among adults, as the incidence of periodontal disease in the general population increases with age. However, periodontal disease and gingivitis may be found among pediatric cancer patients and is related to the adverse effects of the antineoplastic therapy on the host defense mechanisms normally operative in the oral mucosa. Gingivitis is an inflammation of the superficial structures of the mucosal epithelium, whereas periodontitis describes an involvement of the supportive structures of the tooth. Peterson and colleagues prospectively evaluated 38 febrile patients receiving therapy for acute nonlymphocytic leukemia and documented a 32% incidence of oral infections.[143,143a] The periodontium was the most common site, and cultures of infected sites revealed mixed aerobic and anaerobic flora. The presence of marginal or necrotizing gingivitis, characterized by an erythematous periapical gingiva, is caused by anaerobes and should be treated with specific antianaerobic agents such as clindamycin or metronidazole.

Esophagitis

Clinically significant esophagitis may be the result of both infectious and noninfectious etiologies. For example, a syndrome clinically identical to infectious esophagitis occurs in patients who have received extensive chest wall or mediastinal irradiation. An infectious esophagitis most commonly occurs among patients who have been granulocytopenic and receiving antibiotics for several days. Patients most often present with a subacute onset of retrosternal burning chest pain and odynophagia. Fungal, viral, and bacterial organisms can all

cause an infectious esophagitis in the immunocompromised host.[144,145]

The occurrence of infectious esophagitis in a non-neutropenic individual is rare. In fact, in non-neutropenic patients, esophagitis is most commonly due to chemical irritation of the distal esophagus by refluxed gastric contents (e.g., in association with chemotherapy-induced emesis). These patients are best managed with judicious use of antacids, histamine antagonists (cimetidine, ranitidine), or both. If the non-neutropenic patient has persistent esophageal discomfort, esophagoscopy with brushings for culture and biopsy should be done. In non-neutropenic patients with AIDS, herpetic or candidal esophagitis is the most common infection.

For the neutropenic patient who presents with complaints referrable to the esophagus, it is best to begin broad-spectrum antimicrobial therapy and oral clotrimazole (10-mg troches five times daily). If patients have persistence or worsening of the esophageal complaints after 48 hours of therapy, they should be given a trial of low-dose amphotericin B (0.1–0.5 mg/kg per day for 5 days). Only 50% of patients with candidal esophagitis will have oropharyngeal evidence of fungal disease, and therefore the absence of oral lesions cannot be used as an argument against the presence of candidal esophagitis. If the patient has persistent symptoms after 48 hours of intravenous amphotericin B, it is unlikely that *Candida* is the etiologic agent. Although some advocate esophagoscopy to clarify the course of therapy, the procedure is not without risk (bacteremia and bleeding), and a reasonable alterative is an empirical course of acyclovir (750 mg/m² per day, given at 8-hour intervals), since the second-most-likely pathogen (or copathogen) is Herpes simplex. If the patient responds, acyclovir should be given for 5 to 7 days. The barium swallow lacks sensitivity and specificity and so does not generally add to the clinical evaluation of the patients.

Intra-abdominal Infections

The clinical presentation of even common intra-abdominal processes such as appendicitis or infectious diarrheal syndromes can be altered by granulocytopenia and compounded by complications of cancer or its treatment. For example, obstructive lesions may be due to primary or metastatic cancer (lymphoma), cholangitis or a conjugated hyperbilirubinemia may be due to extrahepatic biliary obstruction by tumor (e.g., rhabdomyosarcoma), and chronic abdominal pain or diarrheal syndromes may be secondary to bowel-wall infiltration by malignant disease or infection.

Intra-abdominal complaints must be expeditiously evaluated with a thorough abdominal and pulmonary examination, including a judiciously performed rectal examination. It must be underscored, however, that repetitive rectal examination must not be performed in the neutropenic patient, as bacteremia and local infection may result. Appropriate studies include routine hematologic and serum chemistry values as well as amylase, total and direct bilirubin, and flat and upright abdominal radiographs. Additional diagnostic procedures such as abdominal or pelvic ultrasound or CT scans should be pursued in the appropriate settings. As a rule, invasive diagnostic or radiographic procedures such as barium enema and endoscopy should be avoided in the neutropenic patient.

Several intra-abdominal infections are virtually restricted to the cancer patient. Foremost among these is typhlitis or necrotizing enterocolitis, an inflammatory cellulitis involving the cecum.[146,147] Typhlitis most commonly occurs in association with chronic granulocytopenia and broad-spectrum antimicrobial therapy in patients with acute leukemia, although any granulocytopenic patient is at risk. Patients most often present with subacute or acute onset of right lower-quadrant abdominal pain, which frequently becomes generalized over a several-hour period, along with fever, diarrhea, and prostration. The etiologic agents responsible for typhlitis include gram-negative bacillary organisms, especially clostridia or *P. aeruginosa*. Optimal management includes supportive care, adjustment of antimicrobial therapy to cover resistant gram-negative and anaerobic species, and aggressive surgical intervention to resect necrotic bowel. Despite such aggressive measures, the mortality rates remain 30% to 50%.[148]

An infrequently encountered clinical syndrome is peritonitis and bacteremia due to *Clostridia* spp. Patients with clostridial peritonitis classically have a fulminant clinical course with fever, tachycardia, abdominal wall ecchymoses and crepitance, and significant hemolysis.[149] *C. perfringens* and *C. septicum* are the two most frequently isolated organisms. Recently, however, a less fulminant bacteremic syndrome due to *C. tertium* has been described.[150] Most of these patients have been granulocytopenic children with acute leukemia maintained on broad-spectrum antimicrobial therapy for long periods (*e.g.,* 17 days). The gastrointestinal tract is most often implicated as the source of infection. Importantly, however, the majority of these isolates have been relatively resistant to the pencillins, cephalosporins, and clindamycin and necessitate the use of vancomycin.

Antibiotic-associated colitis has long been associated with the administration of clindamycin, ampicillin, and broad-spectrum beta-lactam antibiotics. The organism *C. difficile* has been isolated as the causative agent in the majority of cases.[151] The symptomatic disease is related to toxin production by the organism.[152] In cancer patients, both antineoplastic agents and antibiotics increase the risk.[153] Patients classically present with acute generalized abdominal pain, fever, leukocytosis, and watery or mucoid, foul-smelling diarrhea. A high index of suspicion is necessary because of the occurrence of similar abdominal symptomatology in cancer patients receiving chemotherapy or periabdominal radiation. Cancer patients with diarrhea with or without fever and abdominal pain should be evaluated with both stool cultures for *C. difficile* and toxin assays. Toxin production, and not just a culture positive for *C. difficile,* is necessary for diagnosis, since as many as 42% of hospitalized patients receiving antibiotics will be culture positive but not toxin positive.[153]

Treatment of documented *C. difficile*-associated colitis requires either oral vancomycin (125 mg four times daily for 10–14 days) or metronidazole (250 mg four times daily for 10 days). There is a 10% to 20% rate of relapse, although the majority of patients will respond to a second course with either the same or alternate therapy. It is important to remember that *C. difficile* may be nosocomially transmitted, and patients who are culture and toxin positive should be placed on enteric precautions.

An infrequently encountered clinical problem is a hyperinfection syndrome caused by the intestinal nematode *Strongyloides stercoralis.*[154] The clinical syndrome of fever, nausea, vomiting, diarrhea, and abdominal pain is caused by the invasion and ulceration of the gastrointestinal mucosa by the filariform larvae. Chemotherapy is thought to promote the maturation of these larvae from a quiescent rhabditiform stage. Polymicrobial sepsis may accompany the intestinal invasion, presumably as a result of the ulcerated mucosa. Overwhelming pulmonary and meningeal involvement has been described in immunocompromised patients. Diagnosis requires demonstration of the larvae in feces or duodenal fluid and should be sought in patients who have resided in subtropical climates or

endemic regions. Treatment of asymptomatic infestation is accomplished with thiabendazole (25 mg/kg twice daily for 2 days). Immunocompromised patients with the hyperinfection syndrome should be treated for 2 to 3 weeks, although the mortality rate remains high despite such long-term treatment.

Hepatic Infections

Hepatitis may be caused by a variety of infectious agents, including those that infect the liver primarily (*e.g.,* hepatitis A, B, non-A, non-B, and the delta agent) and secondarily (Herpes simplex, CMV, Epstein–Barr virus, Coxsackie B virus, adenovirus, toxoplasmosis, and *C. albicans*).

Non-A, non-B hepatitis is now the most commonly encountered blood-transmissable hepatitis among cancer patients. Since the widespread utilization of efficacious screening methods to detect hepatitis B, non-A, non-B hepatitis accounts for 85% to 90% of all cases of post-transfusion hepatitis.[155] Clinically, non-A, non-B hepatitis closely resembles hepatitis B, with an insidious onset and a long relapsing course. It is currently unclear whether non-A, non-B hepatitis is produced by a single or several transmissable agents. There is substantial evidence of a chronic carrier state, and chronic sequelae may occur in as many as 50% of infected individuals.[156] Alpha-interferon has recently been shown to be effective in patients with non-A, non-B hepatitis.[157]

Hepatitis B may result in both acute and chronic infections, including chronic active, chronic persistent, and asymptomatic carrier states. The incidence of hepatitis B was previously as high as 10% to 20% among cancer patients, but with the introduction of effective prophylactic measures as well as efficient screening methods to detect infected donors, the number of patients affected has fallen dramatically. It is important to remember that immunosuppressive therapy may increase the likelihood of development of a chronic carrier state among individuals infected with hepatitis B, making it important to know the patient's hepatitis status prior to initiating antineoplastic therapy.[158]

The delta agent, an incomplete RNA virus, requires prior or coinfection with the hepatitis B virus to be manifest clinically. Therefore, hepatitis due to the delta agent occurs only in three circumstances: [1] as a superimposed infection in a patient with active hepatitis B; [2] as an acute hepatitis in a chronic hepatitis B carrier; and [3] as a chronic infection in a chronic hepatitis B carrier.[159] Although hepatitis caused by the delta agent has been noted among multiply transfused patients, its incidence will presumably also decrease as the prevalence of hepatitis B diminishes.

A number of viruses may involve the liver secondarily as part of a more widespread systemic infection. The Epstein–Barr virus, CMV, herpes simplex, rubella, rubeola, mumps, adenovirus, and Coxsackie B virus have been associated with hepatic enzyme elevations. The hepatic dysfunction attending these secondary infections is generally self-limited and less severe than that associated with primary viral hepatitis. However, fulminant hepatic necrosis, coma, and death have been described with several of these agents (especially of the herpesvirus group) in the immunocompromised host.

All cancer patients with clinical or biochemical evidence of hepatitis should undergo a serologic evaluation to attempt to characterize the etiologic agent. Serum tests for anti-HAV (IgM), HBsAg, and anti-HBc (IgM) will identify those patients with hepatitis A or B. Patients with a negative antibody screen will have either non-A, non-B or delta or a hepatitis due to another infectious or noninfectious cause. In addition to viral infection, hepatic enzyme elevation or hyperbilirubinemia can occur with bacterial sepsis, fungal infection of the liver (especially *Candida* or *Aspergillus*) or toxoplasmosis.

In addition to the morbidity (including fever, nausea, emesis, arthritis, arthralgia) and deaths directly attributable to hepatitis, significant alteration in hepatic function can affect the pharmacokinetics of antineoplastic agents, especially those metabolized or excreted by the liver (methotrexate, Adriamycin). Therapy of hepatitis is primarily supportive, with bed rest and avoidance of further hepatic insult the mainstay of therapy. Patients with hepatitis due to Herpes simplex should receive acyclovir. As noted above, chronic non-A, non-B hepatitis can be treated with alpha-interferon.

Hepatic Candidiasis

During the past several years, a syndrome referred to as hepatic candidiasis has become increasingly recognized.[160–162] It is characterized by the presence of bull's eye lesions in the liver on ultrasound or CT scan (Fig. 39-5). These lesions are not apparent in patients who are neutropenic but rather become recognizable at the time of neutrophil recovery. Patients have persistent fever at the time of recovery from an episode of neutropenia, frequently with right upper-quadrant discomfort, nausea, and an elevated serum alkaline phosphatase. The lesions are granulomas consisting of an inner core of necrosis (where the yeast and pseudophyphae can be found) surrounded by a ring of inflammatory cells and an outer ring of fibrosis. These imaged lesions change over time and with treatment and on resolution become calcified, an important end point of therapy. The diagnosis is based on a high index of suspicion and must be confirmed with liver biopsy.

Hepatic candidiasis poses a therapeutic challenge. Long courses of treatment are necessary, with the average amount of amphotericin B administered close to 5 g. Experimental data suggest that the combination of amphotericin B with 5-fluorocytosine is preferable.[102] Serial biopsy may be necessary to confirm resolution of infection. It is also worth noting that the lesions may be below the limit of resolution of current imaging techniques; thus, in high-risk patients with a negative abdominal ultrasound or CT scan, a biopsy may still be necessary to confirm or rule out hepatic candidiasis. Although experience is preliminary, magnetic resonance imaging of the liver may be more sensitive than CT or ultrasound. In the future, liposome-amphotericin B might speed recovery from hepatic candidiasis.[84b]

Perirectal Cellulitis

The overall incidence of perirectal cellulitis has decreased in recent years, presumably because of the early use of empirical antibiotics when granulocytopenic patients become febrile. Nonetheless, the risk for perianal cellulitis remains, especially for patients with chronic (greater than 7 days) and profound (<100/mm^3) granulocytopenia. Predisposing factors include perirectal mucositis due to chemotherapy or localized radiotherapy, hemorrhoids, anal fissures, and any type of rectal manipulation (barium enema, anoscopy, sigmoidoscopy). Accordingly, constipation should be avoided, since passage of hard stool promotes the formation of anal fissures and increases the risk of perianal infections.

The most common pathogens in perirectal cellulitis are aerobic gram-negative bacilli (*P. aeruginosa, K. pneumoniae, E. coli*), the group D streptococci, and bowel anaerobes. Because of the involvement of anaerobic organisms, antibiotic coverage must include a specific antianaerobic agent such as clindamycin or metronidazole in addition to the broad-spectrum aerobic coverage. Therapy should start at the first complaints of tenderness and ideally before florid symptoms of cellulitis develop. Additional supportive measures include sitz baths three or four times daily, stool softeners, a low-bulk diet, and avoidance of unnecessary rectal manipulation, especially repetitive digital examinations. Surgical intervention should be restricted to those cases that demonstrate persistence of erythema or induration or progressive involvement of the ischiorectal fossa despite optimal antimicrobial therapy.[163,164]

Infections of the Central Nervous System

Infections of the central nervous system are surprisingly infrequent in children with cancer. Nevertheless, patients who present with symptoms or signs suggestive of central nervous system dysfunction must be expeditiously evaluated with the appropriate physical, laboratory, and radiographic examinations. Evaluation of cerebrospinal fluid from cancer patients should include aerobic culture and gram stain, cryptococcal antigen determination, fungal culture, and cytology in addition to the routine studies (cell count and differential, protein, glucose). The spectrum of potential infections includes shunt (*e.g.,* Ommaya reservoir) infections, meningitis or meningoencephalitis, encephalitis, and brain abscesses.

Shunt Infections

Intraventricular shunts (ventriculoatrial and ventriculoperitoneal) and Ommaya reservoirs are associated with an increased incidence of central nervous system infection. The responsible pathogens are most commonly those colonizing the adjacent skin: coagulase-positive and -negative staphylococci, *Corynebacterium* spp., and enterococci; rarely, they are gram-negative bacilli.[165,166] Patients may be totally asymptomatic, in which case the diagnosis may be made by noting cerebrospinal fluid cultures repetitively positive for the same organism, or patients may have fever, headache, increased intracranial pressure, and meningismus. The majority of patients with Ommaya reservoir infections can be treated successfully without the need to remove the device.[166]

Meningitis and Meningoencephalitis

Meningitis or meningoencephalitis is most frequently encountered in patients with impaired cell-mediated immunity and is typically caused by fungal (*Cryptococcus neoformans*) or bacterial (*Listeria monocytogenes*) pathogens. *Cryptococcus neoformans* causes a meningoencephalitis that is typically indolent in onset. The most common presenting complaints are headaches, altered mental state, low-grade intermittent fever, and, rarely, meningismus.[167] Examination of the cerebrospinal fluid demonstrates a mild mononuclear pleocytosis (40–400/mm^3) and minimally decreased glucose. Only 50% of patients will have organism detectable by an india ink preparation, and the most reliable means of diagnosis is documentation of cryptococcal antigen in serum or cerebrospinal fluid.[168] Therapy of cryptococcal meningitis or meningoencephalitis includes the combination of amphotericin B (0.3–0.5 mg/kg per day) and oral 5-fluorocytosine (150 mg/kg per day given every 6 hours) for 4 to 6 weeks.[169,170]

Listeria monocytogenes is a motile, gram-positive rod that causes several distinct clinical syndromes in humans, including meningitis. Patients with impaired cell-mediated immunity, and especially those with defects of T-cell-mediated immune function, are especially susceptible.[171] Although the

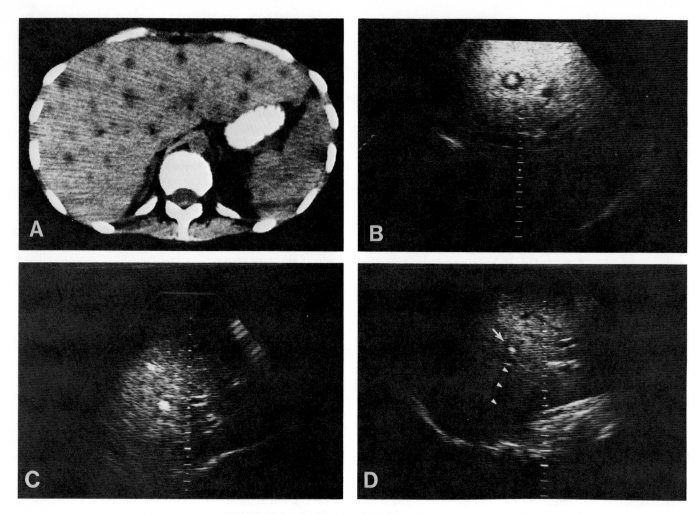

FIGURE 39-5. **A.** CT scan of the liver shows numerous rounded areas of decreased attenuation, compatible with the diagnosis of hepatic candidiasis. This is a nonspecific finding. **B.** Ultrasound examination in the same patient shows the typical "bull's-eye" lesion of candidiasis characterized by a central echogenic nidus surrounded by a radiolucent halo. This is seen early in the natural history of the disease. **C.** The radiolucent halo is now less obvious than in *B.* This illustrates the variable appearances of candida abscesses on ultrasound studies at different times in the same patient. **D.** Late in the course of the disease, the microabscesses become denser (*arrow*). Note the acoustical shadow posterior to the lesion, caused by attenuation of the sound beam (*arrowheads*). (Thaler M, Bader J, O'Leary T, Pizzo PA: Hepatic candidiasis in immunocompromised patients. Ann Intern Med 108:88–100, 1988)

organism can be isolated from soil, dust, water, sewage, and contaminated foods (especially cheese and dairy products), the exact mode of transmission in most immunocompromised patients is unclear. Community outbreaks have occurred, and hospital-associated case clustering has been described in immunosuppressed patients.[172] The most common presentation is a subacute course of low-grade fever and personality changes. Focal neurologic signs are occasionally present. Laboratory findings include a mild to moderate cerebrospinal fluid pleocytosis (6,000–12,000 cells/mm³) and may include a predominance of either PMNs or mononuclear cells. Protein levels are generally elevated (100–300 mg/dl), and glucose levels are usually, but not invariably, decreased. Diagnosis must be based on a high index of suspicion. Ampicillin or penicillin provide the optimal treatment and should be continued for 3 to 6 weeks, as relapses have been reported after

shorter courses.[173] It is important to remember that third-generation cephalosporins are inactive against *Listeria.*

Encephalitis

A variety of viral, bacterial, parasitic, fungal, and rickettsial agents can be associated with encephalitis or encephalomyelitis. However, the relative prevalence of the various etiologic agents is altered in immunodeficient patients. For example, patients with humoral immune abnormalities, especially hypogammaglobulinemia, may have a chronic encephalitis due to poliovirus or echovirus,[174,175] whereas patients with abnormalities of cell-mediated immunity are more commonly afflicted by encephalitis due to measles or adenovirus.[176] Cancer patients as a group are susceptible to encephalitis due to the herpesvirus group (Epstein–Barr, CMV, varicella–zoster, Herpes simplex).

Patients with encephalitis or encephalomyelitis commonly present with signs of meningeal irritation (fever, headache, nuchal rigidity) and evidence of altered mentation. Confusion may progress to stupor and finally to coma. Focal neurologic signs and seizures are relatively common. Cerebrospinal fluid examination may demonstrate a pleocytosis (10–2000 cells/mm³), with a predominance of mononuclear cells. An increased number of red cells has been reported with Herpes simplex encephalitis. Protein levels are usually elevated, and the glucose characteristically remains within the normal range except for a decreased level in mumps infection.

For the cancer patient with either focal neurologic deficits or altered mentation, it is important to differentiate between an infectious, metabolic, toxic, and neoplastic etiology. Unfortunately, specific diagnosis of encephalitis in an immunocompromised patient is difficult. Acute and convalescent serum antibody titers should be measured, and specific cerebrospinal fluid antibody may be detected in cases of mumps, Herpes simplex, and varicella–zoster. Because definitive diagnosis of Herpes simplex encephalitis requires a brain biopsy, and because the clinician's therapeutic armamentarium against most causes of encephalitis is limited, empirical administration of acyclovir (1500 mg/m² per day given every 8 hours) to the cancer patient with signs and symptoms suggestive of encephalitis seems warranted.[177]

A treatable central nervous system infection that can present as an encephalitis in an immunosuppressed child or as a mass lesion in the AIDS patient is caused by the obligate intracellular parasite *Toxoplasma gondii.*[178] Toxoplasmosis may represent either newly acquired or reactivated infection and is rarely limited to the central nervous system, usually occurring in concert with fever, lymphadenopathy, hepatitis, pneumonitis, myocarditis, and pericarditis. The cerebrospinal fluid typically manifests a mononuclear pleocytosis, elevated protein, and a normal glucose concentration. A battery of serologic tests are available for the diagnosis of toxoplasmosis in the immunocompetent host, but most of these are limited in their applicability to the immunosuppressed patient due to suboptimal antibody responses. The definitive diagnosis requires demonstration of the parasite within tissue sections.

Treatment of active toxoplasmosis should include the combination of pyrimethamine and sulfadiazine or triple sulfa therapy (trisulfapyrimidines–sulfamerazine, sulfamethazine, and sulfadiazine). In immunodeficient patients, therapy should be continued for 4 to 6 weeks after the resolution of all clinical symptoms and signs. Trimetrexate is being studied for the treatment of toxoplasmosis.[134]

Brain Abscesses

The important differential diagnosis in a cancer patient with evidence of a focal (mass) lesion within the central nervous system is between metastatic or primary malignancy and a brain abscess. Predisposing factors for brain abscesses include contiguous infected sites such as otitis, sinusitis, or dental abscesses; a history of penetrating cranial trauma; congenital cardiac disease; bacterial endocarditis; and pulmonary infections. In addition to the usual aerobic and anaerobic bacteria responsible for abscesses in immunocompetent individuals, fungal and nocardial species are particularly prone to cause disease in an immunosuppressed patient. These infections are usually associated with pulmonary infiltrates.

Early evaluation and specific diagnosis are crucial in the management of brain abscesses, as effective antimicrobial or neurosurgical therapy is available. Diagnosis is commonly made by radiographic demonstration of a localized mass followed by an open or closed procedure to aspirate or resect the localized lesion.

Infections of the Genitourinary Tract

The genitourinary tract is infrequently the source of infection in the immunocompromised child. However, local obstruction due to tumor, neurologic dysfunction mediated by spinal cord compression or medications (vincristine, narcotics), and local therapeutic maneuvers (radiotherapy, surgery, or bladder catheterization) can predispose cancer patients to genitourinary infection. Most commonly, gram-negative aerobic bacilli (including *E. coli, Klebsiella* spp., *Proteus.* spp., *P. aeruginosa*) and enterococci will be the causative agents.

An important distinction must be made between a pathogen and a colonizing organism when interpreting the results of urine cultures obtained from an immunocompromised (and particularly a neutropenic) patient. In a non-neutropenic individual, a colony count of greater than 10⁵/ml of a single organism is considered diagnostic of a urinary tract infection in a symptomatic individual. In neutropenic patients, a colony count greater than 10³/ml of a single organism may be considered diagnostic of a urinary tract infection if the patient is symptomatic (dysuria, urgency, frequency, fever). In a neutropenic patient, colony count greater than 10⁵/ml of a single organism should prompt antibiotic intervention whether or not the patient is symptomatic. Obviously, the presence or absence of white cells in the urine must not be relied on as a diagnostic criterion in the neutropenic patient.

The distinction between colonization and tissue invasion is particularly difficult for fungal pathogens. Fungal colonization is especially prevalent among patients with indwelling urinary catheters or those receiving broad-spectrum antimicrobial therapy. Unlike the typical situation with bacterial pathogens, where clinical signs and symptoms are present, if not florid, fungal invasion of the genitourinary tract may be insidious. The repetitive isolation of a particular fungal species (usually *C. albicans, C. tropicalis,* or *C. glabrata*) in association with fever, deteriorating renal function, and, rarely, flank pain should prompt the institution of systemic amphotericin B. Heavily colonized bladders or superficial bladder infections manifested by persistence of positive urine cultures despite removal of predisposing factors may be effectively treated by instillation of amphotericin B (50 mg in 1 liter of 5% dextrose in water daily) into the bladder.

Infections of the Cardiovascular System

Cardiovascular infections are relatively uncommon among cancer patients, probably because of the early institution of broad-spectrum antimicrobial therapy.[179] However, cancer patients who have predisposing factors for a cardiovascular infection such as dental abscesses, a history of intravenous drug abuse, or congenital cardiac anomalies are at risk. Additionally, endovascular infections are more likely with the increased utilization of indwelling venous access catheters. Although gram-positive bacterial species (enterococcus, viridans or beta-hemolytic streptococci, and *S. aureus*) are most commonly causative of endovascular infections, aerobic gram-negative bacilli and fungi may also cause disease.[180] These latter pathogens are particularly difficult to eradicate, and morbidity and mortality remain discouragingly high.

The clinical manifestations of endocarditis in the immuno-suppressed patient are generally similar to those in an immunocompetent patient. Nonspecific complaints of fever, chills, malaise, fatigue, night sweats, and weight loss are common. Unfortunately, these complaints are nondescript, and the degree of diagnostic specificity that may be ascribed to them is slight. In most instances, therefore, the diagnosis must be made on the basis of the physical and laboratory evaluation. The numerous physical stigmata of endocarditis should be sought (heart murmurs, splinter hemorrhages, Roth's spots, splenomegaly), but the diagnosis is confirmed by the isolation of an organism from multiple blood cultures.

The complications of endovascular infections are similar to those described for patients without cancer. Valvular insufficiency resulting in congestive heart failure, emboli, and renal failure are the most serious. Fungal endocarditis is particularly likely to cause large-vessel embolization. Patients with *Candida* or *Aspergillus* endocarditis are candidates for valve replacement.

Therapy must be directed at the specific pathogen. The isolation of *S. aureus* or *S. epidermidis* from multiple blood samples, even if the patient has an indwelling catheter, is not a sufficient criterion for prolonged antibiotic therapy unless a valvular infection can be confirmed. A standard 10- to 14-day therapy will suffice for these patients.

Infections of the Skin

The skin can be infected primarily or in association with bacteremia (*e.g., P. aeruginosa, Aeromonas hydrophilia, Serratia marcesens*); fungemia (*Aspergillus*,[180a] *Candida, Mucor, Cryptococcus, Histoplasma*); or viremia (Herpes simplex, varicella–zoster, CMV). Skin lesions may permit the early diagnosis of an established infection, and new lesions should be aspirated or biopsied and the material stained (Gram, wet mount, methylene blue) and cultured. If the lesions are vesicular, the base should be scraped, smeared on a glass slide, and stained with Wright or Giemsa and examined for multinucleated giant cells that imply a herpes infection (Tzanck test).

Primary varicella is a significant concern for the child with cancer, since the mortality rate in untreated patients ranges from 7% to 20%, usually because of visceral dissemination to the liver, lung, and central nervous system.[181] Severe abdominal pain, back pain, or evidence of inappropriate antidiuretic hormone secretion may herald multisystem involvement, indicating the need for prompt use of acyclovir.[182]

An important objective in the care of children with cancer is the prevention of primary varicella. Careful education of the parents, child, and school to avoid exposure to known cases of chickenpox is essential. In order to anticipate and plan for prompt intervention, it is important to know the child's history of varicella (or antibody status) before initiating chemotherapy. If a seronegative child is exposed to varicella, defined by the Centers for Disease Control as either a continuous household contact, a playmate contact (generally >1 hour of play indoors), or a hospital contact, varicella–zoster immune globulin should be administered promptly, no later than 96 hours after exposure. Children who have received ablative therapy associated with bone marrow transplantation should receive immune globulin regardless of their immune status. Although a preliminary study has suggested that passive immunization with pooled intravenous immunoglobulins may be an alternative, definitive data are lacking.

Of current interest for the child with cancer is the role of the live attenuated varicella vaccine. A controlled trial has shown this vaccine to be 100% protective and safe in normal children, and although it is undergoing evaluation in children with leukemia as part of a multi-institutional study, it remains to be determined how safe this vaccine will be in more intensively immunosuppressed children and whether antibody titers will remain protective during long and repeated courses of cytotoxic chemotherapy.[183]

PREVENTION OF INFECTION IN CHILDREN WITH CANCER

In a multitude of clinical trials investigating the efficacy of various measures to prevent or reduce infection, the most important anti-infective measure identified has been the simplest: careful handwashing practices.[184] A number of approaches have been taken to decrease the acquisition of new organisms or to suppress those already colonizing the cancer patient (Table 39-5). Unfortunately, no method has stood out as singularly effective, each having promise and problems (Table 39-6). Unfortunately, as new preventive strategies are evaluated, they appear promising initially, but as additional studies are conducted, their beneficial results become less clear.[185]

Preventing the Acquisition of New Organisms

Because it has been well documented that nearly 85% of the organisms responsible for infections in patients with cancer are derived from the endogenous flora and that nearly half of this flora are acquired from the hospital environment, much attention has been directed toward preventing the acquisition of potential pathogens. Inanimate objects within the hospital

---

Table 39-5
Methods for Preventing Infection in Cancer Patients

Prevent Acquisition and/or Suppress or Eliminate Microbial Flora	Improve or Modify Host Defenses
Isolation	**Immunization**
Simple or reverse isolation	Active
Isolation with HEPA air	*Pseudomonas*
filtration	*S. pneumoniae*
Prophylactic antibiotics	Passive
Nonabsorbable antibiotics	J-5 core glycolipid
Trimethoprim-	Pooled immunoglobulins
sulfamethoxazole	Specific
Selective decontamination	**Cell-component replacement**
Quinolones	Leukocyte transfusions
Prophylactic antivirals	**Accelerate granulocyte**
Acycloguanosine	**recovery**
Amantadine	Lithium
Prophylactic antifungals	GM-CSF
Nystatin	
Imidazoles	
Prophylactic antiparasitics	
Thiabendazole	
Trimethoprim-	
sulfamethoxazole	
Combination–comprehensive	
Total protected isolation	

Table 39-6

Effectiveness and Acceptability of Various Measures for Reducing Acquisition of New Organisms

	TPE	Nonabsorbable Antibiotics	TMP–SMX	Selective Decontamination	Quinolones
Protect Against					
Exogenous sources	Yes	No	No	No	No
Endogenous sources					
Nares	Yes	No	No	No	Yes
Oropharynx	Yes	±	No	Yes	Yes
Lower respiratory tract	±	No	±	±	Yes
GI tract	Yes	Yes	Yes	Yes	Yes
Perianal	Yes	±	±	±	±
Skin	Yes	No	No	No	No
Central venous catheter	No	No	No	No	No
Peripheral catheters	No	No	No	No	No
Systemic Effect	±	No	Yes	Yes	Yes
Efficacy					
Reduced infection	Yes	No	±	±	Yes
Decreased fever	Yes	No	No	No	No
Reduced need for antibiotics	No	No	No	±	Yes
Improve survival	No	No	No	No	No
Compliance					
Well tolerated?	No	No	±	?	Yes
Impact on efficacy	Yes	Yes	Yes	?	No
Liabilities					
Emergence of resistance	Yes	Yes	Yes	Yes	Yes
Side effects					
Interfere with other drugs	Yes	Yes	Yes	No	No
Bone marrow suppression	No	No	Yes	Yes	No
Specific organ toxicity	No	No	Yes	Yes	Yes
Cost					
For drugs/regimen	High	High	Low	High	High
For surveillance	High	High	High	High	High
Reduced need for hospitalization/other drugs	No	No	No	±	?

* Trimethoprim–sulfamethoxazole.

environment (faucet aerators, shower heads, respirators, plants, floors) are reservoirs of pathogenic organisms. However, most epidemiologic studies (albeit most commonly investigating nonimmunocompromised patients) suggest that transmission from such inanimate sources usually requires a human vector. Therefore, the simplest yet most efficacious intervention that can be performed is adherence to strict handwashing precautions. In reality, the easiest way to enforce such a policy is to educate the child and parents to disallow contact with anyone who has neglected to wash his or her hands.

A second maneuver to decrease the acquisition of new organisms is to maintain a cooked diet during periods of granulocytopenia, with avoidance of fresh fruits and vegetables and nonprocessed dairy products, since these foods are naturally contaminated with gram-negative bacteria especially *K. pneumoniae, E. coli,* and *Pseud. aeruginosa.*[186,187]

Environmental sources can contribute to fungal (especially *Aspergillus* spp.) and bacterial (*Legionella*) colonization and infection. In medial centers where *Aspergillus* is a significant problem, special air filtration systems such as high-efficiency particulate air filters (HEPA) or water-purification systems may prove helpful.

Although the technique of reverse isolation has often been used, it does not significantly reduce the acquisition of new organisms in an environment where handwashing techniques are strictly followed.[188] Therefore, there is no compelling reason to enforce this policy, particularly since the extra expense, time consumption, and inconvenience are not balanced by a beneficial effect.

The total protective environment (TPE) is a comprehensive regimen designed to reduce the patient's endogenous microbial burden while preventing the acquisition of new organisms (see Table 39-6). A sterile environment is created in a clean-air room with constant positive-pressure air flow. It is maintained by an aggressive program of surface decontamination and sterilization of all objects that enter the room and by an intensive regimen to disinfect the patient including oral nonabsorbable antibiotics, skin antiseptics, antibiotic sprays and ointments, and a low-microbial diet. The TPE can indeed reduce the number of infections in profoundly granulocytopenic individuals.[189] However, it is expensive, and because of the improvement in treating established infections, it does not offer a survival advantage to patients. Thus, total protected isolation is not necessary for the routine care of cancer patients. However, it may be of value to patients undergoing bone marrow transplantation or those patients who are likely to experience periods of 30 or more days of profound neutropenia.

Prophylactic Antibiotics

Antibacterial Prophylaxis

A large number of clinical trials have been conducted to investigate the utility of prophylactic antibiotic regimens in immunocompromised patients. A number of strategies have been explored, including systemic prophylaxis, gastrointestinal decontamination, and selective gastrointestinal decontamination (maintenance of "colonization resistance"). Unfortunately, the interpretation of many of these trials is difficult because of poor study design (many were uncontrolled), nonuniform patient groupings, and failure to report or document the extent of compliance with the prophylactic regimens.[185,190]

Because the gastrointestinal tract is the source of many of the pathogens causing microbiologically defined infections, investigators have evaluated the efficacy of reducing the endogenous gastrointestinal flora with oral nonabsorbable antibiotics. This technique has not been especially valuable and is fraught with problems. The antimicrobial agents utilized (e.g., vancomycin, gentamicin, polymyxin B, nystatin, framycetin, and colistin) are unpalatable and poorly tolerated, making compliance a significant liability, especially among patients receiving emetogenic chemotherapy (see Table 39-6). Equally disturbing has been the emergence of resistant bacterial strains among patients receiving aminoglycoside-containing regimens. Therefore, prophylactic regimens aimed solely at reducing the endogenous gastrointestinal flora cannot be recommended.

A modified technique is the selective decontamination of the gastrointestinal tract with antibiotics that preserve the anaerobic flora while reducing the aerobic bacteria. This tactic is based on experimental data showing that the preservation of the anaerobic flora of the gastrointestinal tract provides colonization resistance against aerobic and fungal organisms.[191,192] Although initial clinical trials provided evidence of a reduction of infections in patients undergoing induction therapy for acute leukemia, efficacy has not been definitely established.[193,194] The most commonly investigated agent has been trimethoprim–sulfamethoxasole. Early trials of the utility of this preparation in children and adults demonstrated a reduction in all infections and in bacteremic episodes. However, a large number of follow-up clinical trials have yielded conflicting results.[190,195–200] The reasons for the contradictory results are unclear, although factors such as variability in study design, nonuniform patient populations, and failure to monitor compliance properly have played a part. The potential for reduction in infectious morbidity and mortality must be balanced against the prolongation of granulocytopenia and emergence of resistant organisms noted with the prophylactic utilization of trimethoprim–sulfamethoxazole.[200,201] Successful use of this approach requires close microbiologic monitoring in order to adjust the antimicrobial regimen properly for resistant or newly emerging species. Such surveillance is costly in both time and money.

More recently, prophylactic trials of a derivative of nalidixic acid, the quinolone antibiotic norfloxacin, have shown promising results in bone marrow transplant recipients.[202] Additional clinical trials will be needed to assess the generalized applicability of these results to other immunocompromised patients. Similar studies with fluorinated quinolones such as ciprofloxacin have also shown promising results, but confirmatory studies in larger numbers of patients are necessary.[203] At present, the quinolones cannot be used in children less than 18 years old because of putative joint toxicity.

Antifungal Prophylaxis

Because of the increasing incidence of invasive mycoses in immunocompromised hosts, antifungal prophylaxis has also been studied. The most frequently evaluated agents are nystatin, amphotericin B, miconazole, clotrimazole, and ketoconazole. It is important to realize that the majority of prophylactic regimens have been aimed at a reduction of invasive infections due to *Candida* species and by virtue of the antifungal activity of the agents employed would not be expected to have a significant impact against *Aspergillus* or *Mucor* mycoses.

As in the studies of antibiotic prophylaxis of bacterial infections, interpretation of existing data is difficult, since studies suffer from variable patient inclusion criteria, disparate dosage regimens, nonuniform response criteria, and lack of appropriate controls. An added problem is the inherent difficulty in the definitive diagnosis of a fungal infection in an immunocompromised patient. Within these limitations, however, several conclusions regarding antifungal prophylaxis can be proffered. First, when an adequate dose of an antifungal agent has been administered, there has been a consistent decrease in fungal colonization (especially that due to *Candida* spp.).[204] However, decreased colonization has not reduced the incidence of invasive mycotic disease, although a decrease in superficial infection has been noted in some studies. Second, several studies employing prophylactic empirical antifungal regimens have noted a shift in the colonization pattern of fungal organisms, generally toward more resistant fungi. Thus, the prophylactic regimens may eradicate the susceptible fungi (particularly *C. albicans*) while permitting overgrowth and ultimate invasion by more resistant species, especially *Aspergillus*. This trend will need to be monitored closely in future studies.

Overall, the potential benefits of prophylactic antifungal therapy must be balanced against the toxicities, epidemiologic considerations, and relative efficacy of the regimen employed. Until clear benefit can be proved, widespread chemoprophylaxis against fungi should not be attempted.

Antiviral Prophylaxis

Two antiviral agents can be used for selective prophylaxis. First, amantidine has proven prophylactic activity against influenza A (although not influenza B) and may be successful in the immunocompromised host. Second, parenteral or oral acyclovir is effective against Herpes simplex infections.[141] This prophylaxis has proved especially valuable among patients undergoing bone marrow transplantation or induction therapy for acute leukemia. Acyclovir-resistant strains have been noted, however, and the significance of such isolates will need assessment in future trials. Unfortunately, no effective prophylaxis or treatment is available for the most serious of the viral pathogens, CMV.

Other Prophylaxes

In centers where *P. carinii* occurs with some frequency, the administration of trimethoprim–sulfamethoxazole has reduced the incidence of infection. However, not all children undergoing cancer treatment require such prophylaxis. Rather, this should be influenced by the patient's underlying disease (leukemia versus solid tumors), the intensity or immunosuppressive potency of the therapy being delivered, and the medical center where treatment is being administered. Although the initial recommendations were for daily prophylactic therapy, recent studies have suggested that twice- or thrice-weekly dosage is effective and less toxic.[205]

Active and Passive Immunization

As a general rule, live attenuated viral vaccines should not be administered to immunosuppressed children. Although an initial antibody response may be elicited, the concurrent administration of cytotoxic chemotherapy is associated with a rapid decline of titers. Recently, a live varicella–zoster vaccine has been successful when administered to children with acute leukemia receiving maintenance chemotherapy.[206]

Trials have evaluated the efficacy of active immunization against commonly encountered pathogens such as the influenza virus and *S. pneumoniae*. Such trials have been only partially successful because of the inability to maintain an adequate degree of protection in the face of repetitive immunosuppressive insults.

Passive immunization with varicella–zoster immune globulin reduces the incidence of pneumonitis and encephalitis and decreases the mortality rate (from 5%–7% to 0.5%) in immunocompromised patients with primary varicella infection. Immunosuppressed children who are seronegative or possess low-titer anti-varicella antibody should receive 1 vial of globulin per 15 kg of body weight within 72 hours after exposure to a potentially infectious source.

A number of investigators have evaluated the efficacy of passive immunization with either high-titer antibody directed against the core glycolipid of Enterobacteriaceae (J-5 antiserum) or pooled intravenous gamma globulin preparations.[207] The rationale for this approach is drawn from several observations. First, patients with defective antibody production, such as those with chronic lymphocytic leukemia or multiple myeloma, have an enhanced susceptibility to bacterial infection. Second, antibody levels fall in patients receiving cytotoxic chemotherapy, and patients who develop gram-negative bacteremia have lower levels of antibody than patients who do not develop infections.[208] The results of early clinical trials with the J-5 antiserum have been encouraging. A double-blind, randomized, placebo-controlled trial involving patients with documented gram-negative bacteremia demonstrated enhanced survival among patients receiving the antiserum.[209] A second placebo-controlled study using prophylactic J-5 antiserum in surgical patients at high risk for gram-negative bacteremia demonstrated a reduction in infectious complications but no survival advantage among the recipients.[210] Unfortunately, preparation of such an antiserum is time- and labor-intensive and costly, and passive immunization with the J-5 antiserum will remain an investigational approach until a clear advantage can be defined.

Pooled immunoglobulin preparations proved valuable in decreasing the incidence of *H. influenzae* infections in high-risk children, but the efficacy of prophylactic intravenous gamma globulin in other bacterial infections has not been established. A trial is currently in progress at the NCI investigating the prophylactic role of intravenous gamma globulin in neutropenic cancer patients. Other investigators are evaluating hyperimmune antisera or monoclonal antibodies both to prevent and to treat bacterial infection.

Perhaps the most exciting development is the recent cloning and purification of molecules that can activate neutrophils or monocytes (interferons, tumor necrosis factor) or accelerate recovery from neutropenia (GM-CSF). The use of these agents offers the prospect of abbreviating or attenuating the risk of serious infection in patients receiving cytotoxic chemotherapy. Moreover, if these agents are successful in reducing serious infectious complications, they may permit the delivery of chemotherapy in schedules that maximize tumoricidal activity while minimizing toxicity.

REFERENCES

1. Bodey G: Infection in cancer patients: A continuing association. Am J Med 81(suppl 1A):11–26, 1986
2. Sculier JP, Weerts D, Klastersky J: Causes of death in febrile granulocytopenic cancer patients receiving empiric antibiotic therapy. Eur J Cancer Clin Oncol 20:55–60, 1984
3. Chang HY, Rodriguez V, Narbone G et al: Causes of death in adults with acute leukemia. Medicine (Baltimore) 55:259–268, 1976
4. Pizzo PA: Granulocytopenia and cancer therapy: Past problems, current solutions, future challenges. Cancer 54:2649–2661, 1984
5. Beachey EH: Bacterial adherence: Adhesion–receptor interactions mediating the attachment of bacteria to mucosal surfaces. J Infect Dis 143:225–245, 1981
6. Shibl AM: Effect of antibiotics on adherence of microorganisms to epithelial cell surfaces. Rev Infect Dis 7:51–65, 1985
7. Schoolnik GK, Lark D, O'Hanley P: Bacterial adherence and anticolonization vaccines. In Remington JS, Schwarz MN (eds): Current Clinical Topics in Infectious Diseases, vol 6, pp 85–102. New York, McGraw-Hill, 1985
8. Johanson WG, Pierce AK, Sanford JP: Changing pharyngeal bacterial flora of hospitalized patients: Emergence of gram-negative bacilli. N Engl J Med 281:1137–1140, 1969
9. Johanson WG, Woods DE, Chaudhuri T: Association of respiratory tract colonization with adherence of gram-negative bacilli to epithelial cells. J Infect Dis 139:667–673, 1979
10. Schimpff SC, Young V, Greene W et al: Origin of infection in acute non-lymphocytic leukemia: Significance of hospital acquisition of potential pathogens. Ann Intern Med 77:707–714, 1972
11. Bodey GP, Buckley M, Sathe YS, Freireich EJ: Quantitative relationships between circulating leukocytes and infection in patients with acute leukemia. Ann Intern Med 64:328–340, 1966
12. Pickering LK, Anderson DC, Choi S et al: Leukocyte function in children with malignancy. Cancer 35:1365–1371, 1975
13. McCormak RT, Nelson RD, Bloomfield CD et al: Neutrophilic function in lymphoreticular malignancy. Cancer 44:920–926, 1979
14. Pickering LK, Ericsson CD, Kohl S: Effect of chemotherapeutic agents on metabolic and bactericidal activity of polymorphonuclear leukocytes. Cancer 42:1741–1746, 1978
15. Curnutte JT, Boxer LA: Clinically significant phagocytic cell defects. In Remington JS, Swartz MN (eds): Current Clinical Topics in Infectious Diseases, vol 6, pp 103–156. New York, McGraw-Hill, 1985
16. Baehner RL, Neiberger RG, Johnson DG et al: Transient bactericidal defect of peripheral blood phagocytes from children with acute lymphoblastic leukemia receiving craniospinal irradiation. N Engl J Med 289:1209–1213, 1973
17. Tubaro E, Borelli G, Croce C et al: Effect of morphine on resistance to infection. J Infect Dis 148:656–666, 1983
18. Dale DC, Petersdorf RG: Corticosteroids and infectious disease. Med Clin North Am 57:1277–1287, 1973
19. Hersh E, Gutterman J, Mavligit GM: Effect of haematologic malignancies and their treatment on host defense factors. Clin Haematol 5:425–448, 1976
20. Fahey JL, Scoggins R, Utz JP et al: Infection, antibody response, and gamma globulin commponents in multiple myeloma and macroglobulinemia. Am J Med 35:698–707, 1973
21. Fisher RI, DeVita VT, Bostick F: Persistent immunologic abnormalities in long term survivors of advanced Hodgkin's disease. Ann Intern Med 92:595–599, 1980
22. Donaldson SS, Glatstein E, Vost KL: Bacterial infections in pediatric Hodgkin's disease: Relationship to radiation, chemotherapy, and splenectomy. Cancer 41:1949–1958, 1978

23. Mackowiak PA: Microbial synergism in human infections. N Engl J Med 298:21–26 and 83–87, 1979
24. Rouse BT, Horohov DW: Immunosuppression in viral infections. Rev Infect Dis 8:850–873, 1986
24a. Cooper M: B lymphocytes: Normal development and function. N Engl J Med 317:1452–1456, 1987
25. Rosse WF: The spleen as a filter. N Engl J Med 317:705–706, 1987
26. Spirer Z, Zakuth V, Diamant S et al: Decreased tuftsin concentration in patients who have undergone splenectomy. Br Med J 2:1574–1576, 1977
27. Eraklis AJ, Kevy SV, Diamond LK et al: Hazard of overwhelming infection after splenectomy in childhood. N Engl J Med 276:1225–1229, 1967
28. Chilcote RR, Baehner RL, Hammond D et al: Septicemia and meningitis in children splenectomized for Hodgkin's disease. N Engl J Med 295:798–800, 1976
29. Keusch GT: Nutrition and infection. In Remington JS, Swartz MN (eds): Current Clinical Topics in Infectious Disease, vol 5, pp 106–123. New York, McGraw-Hill, 1984
30. Good RA, Weat A, Fernandes G: Effects of nutritional factors on immunity. In Verhoef J, Peterson PK, Quie P (eds): Infections in the Immunocompromised Host—Pathogenesis, Prevention, and Therapy. Developments in Immunology, vol 11, pp 95–128. Amsterdam, Elsevier/North-Holland Biomedical Press, 1980
31. Pizzo PA, Robichaud KJ, Wesley R, Commers JA: Fever in the pediatric and young adult patient with cancer: A prospective study of 1001 episodes. Medicine (Baltimore) 61:153–165, 1982
32. Dinarello CA, Cannon JG, Mier JW et al: Multiple biologic activities of human recombinant interleukin 1. J Clin Invest 77:1734–1739, 1986
33. Dinarello CA, Mier JW: Lymphokines. N Engl J Med 317:940–945, 1987
34. Sickles EA, Greene WH, Wiernike PH: Clinical presentation in granulocytopenic patients. Arch Intern Med 135:715–719, 1975
35. Hiemenz J, Skelton J, Pizzo PA: Perspective on the management of catheter related infections in cancer patients. Pediatr Infect Dis J 5:6–11, 1986
36. Pizzo PA, Hathorn JW, Hiemenz JW et al: A randomized trial comparing ceftazidime alone with combination antibiotic therapy in cancer patients with fever and neutropenia. N Engl J Med 315:552–558, 1986
37. McCabe WR, Jackson GG: Gram-negative bacteremia. Arch Intern Med 110:847–855, 1982
38. Freid MA, Vosti KL: The importance of underlying disease in patients with gram negative bacteremia. Arch Intern Med 121:418–423, 1968
39. Bryant RE, Hood AF, Hood CE et al: Factors affecting mortality of gram-negative bacteremia. Arch Intern Med 127:120–128, 1971
40. EORTC International Antimicrobial Therapy Project Group: Three antibiotic regimens in the treatment of infection in febrile granulocytopenic patients with gram-negative bacteremia. Am J Med 68:643–648, 1980
41. Love LJ, Schimpff SC, Schiffer CA, Wiernik PH: Improved prognosis for granulocytopenic patients with gram-negative bacteremia. Am J Med 68:643–648, 1980
42. Young LS: Combination or single-drug therapy for gram-negative sepsis. In Remington JS, Swartz MN (eds): Current Clinical Topics in Infectious Diseases, vol 3, pp 177–205. New York, McGraw-Hill, 1982
43. Klastersky J, Zinner SH: Synergistic combination of antibiotics in gram-negative bacillary infections. Rev Infect Dis 4:294–301, 1982
44. Schimpff SC: Overview of empiric antibiotic therapy for the febrile neutropenic patient. Rev Infect Dis 7(suppl 4):5734–5740, 1985
45. Pizzo PA, Thaler M, Hathorn J et al: New β-lactamase antibiotics in the granulocytopenic patient: New options and new questions. Am J Med 79:75–82, 1985
46. Birnbaum J, Kaham FM, Kropp H, Macdonald JS: Carbapenems: A new class of beta-lactam antibiotics. Discovery and development of imipenem/cilastatin. Am J Med 78(suppl 6A):3–21, 1985
47. Neu HC: β-Lactam antibiotics: Structural relationships affecting in vitro activity and pharmacologic properties. Rev Infect Dis 8(suppl 3):S237–S259, 1986
47a. The EORTC International Antimicrobial Therapy Cooperative Group: Ceftazidime combined with a short or long course of amikacin for empirical therapy of gram-negative bacteremia in cancer patients with granulocytopenia. N Engl J Med 317:1692–1698, 1987
48. Bolivar R, Fainstein V, Etting L et al: Cefoperazone for the treatment of infection in patients with cancer. Rev Infect Dis 5(suppl 1):S181–S187, 1983
49. de Pauw BE, Kauw F, Muytjens H et al: Randomized study of ceftazidime versus gentamicin plus cefotaxime for infections in severely granulocytopenic patients. J Antimicrob Chemother 12(suppl A):593–599, 1983
50. Young L: Empirical antimicrobial therapy in the neutropenic host (editorial). N Engl J Med 315:580–581, 1986
51. Karp JE, Dick JD, Angelopoulos C et al: Empiric use of vancomycin during prolonged treatment-induced granulocytopenia: Randomized, double-blind, placebo-controlled clinical trial in patients with acute leukemia. Am J Med 81:237–242, 1986
52. Kramer BJ, Ramphal R, Rand K: Randomized comparison between two ceftazidime containing regimens and cephalothin–gentamicin–carbenicillin in febrile granulocytopenic cancer patients. Antimicrob Agents Chemother 30:64–68, 1986
53. Rubin M, Hathorn JW, Marshall D, Gress J, Pizzo PA: Gram-positive infections and the use of vancomycin in 550 episods of fever and neutropenia. Ann Intern Med 108:30–35, 1988
54. Hathorn JW, Rubin M, Pizzo PA: Empirical antibiotic therapy in the febrile neutropenic cancer patient: Clinical efficacy and impact of monotherapy. Antimicrob Agents Chemother 31:971–977, 1987
55. Winston DJ, Ho WG, Gale PR: Prophylactic granulocyte transfusion during chemotherapy of acute nonlymphocyte leukemia. Ann Intern Med 94:616–622, 1981
56. Strauss RG, Connett JE, Gale RP et al: A controlled trial of prophylactic granulocyte transfusions during initial induction chemotherapy for acute myelogenous leukemia. N Engl J Med 305:597–603, 1981
57. Ford JM, Cullen MH, Roberts MM et al: Prophylactic granulocyte transfusions: Results of a randomized controlled trial in patients with acute myelogenous leukemia. Transfusion 22:311–316, 1982
58. Winston DJ, Ho WG, Young LS, Gale PR: Prophylactic granulocyte transfusions during human bone marrow transplantation. Am J Med 68:893–897, 1980
59. Clift RA, Sanders JE, Thomas ED, Williams B, Buchner CD: Granulocyte transfusions for the prevention of infection in patients receiving bone marrow transplants. N Engl J Med 298:1052–1057, 1982
60. Applebaum FR, Bowles CA, Makuch RW, Deisseroth AB: Granulocyte transfusion therapy of experimental Pseudomonas septicemia: Study of cell dose and collection techniques. Blood 52:323–331, 1978
61. Epstein RB, Chow HS: An analysis of quantitative relationships of granulocyte transfusion therapy in canines. Transfusion 21:360–362, 1981
62. Morse EE, Freireich EJ, Carbone PP, Bronson W, Frei E: The transfusion of leukocytes from donors with chronic myelogenous leukemia to patients with leukopenia. Transfusion 6:183–192, 1966
63. Winston DJ, Ho WG, Howell CL et al: Cytomegalovirus infections associated with leukocyte transfusions. Ann Intern Med 93:671–675, 1980
64. Schiffer CA, Aisner J, Daly PA, Schimpff SC, Wiernik PH: Alloimmunization following prophylactic granulocyte transfusion. Blood 54:766–774, 1978
65. Wright DG, Robichaud KJ, Pizzo PA, Deisseroth AB: Lethal pulmonary reactions associated with the combined use of amphotericin B and leukocyte transfusions. N Engl J Med 304:1185–1189, 1981
66. Karp DD, Ervin TJ, Tuttle S, Gorgone BC, Lavin P, Yunis EJ: Pulmonary complications during granulocyte transfusions: Incidence and clinical features. Vox Sang 42:57–61, 1982
67. Maguire LC, Strauss RG, Koepke JA, et al: The elimination of hydroxyethyl starch from the blood of donors experiencing single or multiple intermittent-flow centrifugation leukopheresis. Transfusion 21:347–353, 1981
68. Herzig RH, Herzig GP, Graw RG, et al: Granulocyte transfusion therapy for gram-negative septicemia. N Engl J Med 296:701–705, 1977
69. Higby DJ, Yates JW, Henderson ES, Holland JF: Filtration leukophoresis for granulocyte transfusion therapy: Clinical and laboratory studies. N Engl J Med 292:761–766, 1975
70. Alavi JB, Root RK, Djerassi I et al: A randomized clinical trial of granulocyte transfusions for infection in acute leukemia. N Engl J Med 296:706–711, 1977
71. Volger WR, Winton EF: The efficacy of granulocyte transfusions in neutropenic patients. Am J Med 63:548–555, 1977
72. Winston DJ, Ho WG, Gale RP: Therapeutic granulocyte transfusions for documented infections. Ann Intern Med 97:509–512, 1982
73. Schiffer CA: Granulocyte transfusion therapy. Cancer Treat Rep 67:113–119, 1983
74. Schiffer CA: Current status of granulocyte transfusion therapy. In Remington JS, Swartz MN (eds): Current Clinical Topics in Infectious Diseases, vol 5, pp 189–209. New York, McGraw-Hill, 1984
75. DiNubile MJ: Therapeutic role of granulocyte transfusions. Rev Infect Dis 7:232–243, 1985
76. Mayer P, Lam LC, Obenaus H, Liehl LE, Besemer J: Recombinant human GM-CSF induces leukocytosis and activates peripheral blood polymorphonuclear neutrophils in nonhuman primates. Blood 70:206–213, 1987

77. Nienhuis AW, Donohue RE, Karlsson S et al: Recombinant human granulo-cyte–macrophage colony stimulating factor (GM-CSF) shortens the period of neutropenia after autologous bone marrow transplantation in a primate model. J Clin Invest 80:573–577, 1987

77a.Weisbart RH, Kwan L, Golde DN, Gasson JC: Human GM-CSF primes neutrophils for enhanced oxidative metabolism in response to the major physiological chemoattractants. Blood 69:18–21, 1987

78. Pizzo PA, Robichaud KJ, Gill FA et al: Duration of empiric antibiotic therapy in granulocytopenic cancer patients. Am J Med 67:194–200, 1979

79. Pizzo PA, Robichaud RJ, Gill FA et al: Empiric antibiotic and antifungal therapy for cancer patients with prolonged fever and granulocytopenia. Am J Med 72:101–111, 1982

80. Pennington JE: Successful treatment of *Aspergillus* pneumonia in hematologic neoplasia. N Engl J Med 295:426–427, 1976

81. Burke PJ, Braine HG, Rathbun HK et al: The clinical significance and manage-ment of fever in acute myelocytic leukemia. Johns Hopkins Med J 139:1–12, 1976

82. Stein RS, Kayser J, Flexner J: Clinical value of empirical amphotericin B in patients with acute myelogenous leukemia. Cancer 50:2247–2251, 1982

83. Hathorn JW, Gress J, Thaler M et al: Empirical antifungal therapy among febrile neutropenic cancer patients: Amphotericin B versus ketoconazole (submitted)

84. Fainstein V, Bodey GP, Elting L et al: Amphotericin B or ketoconazole therapy of fungal infections in neutropenic cancer patients. Antimicrob Agents Chemother 31:11–15, 1987

84a.Winegard JA, Vaughan WP, Braine HG, Merz WG, Saral R: Prevention of fungal sepsis in patients with prolonged neutropenia: A randomized, dou-ble-blind, placebo-controlled trial of intravenous miconazole. Am J Med 83:1103–1110, 1987

84b.Lopez-Berestein G, Budey G, Frenkel LS, Mehta K: Treatment of hepatosple-nic candidiasis with liposomal-amphotericin B. J Clin Oncol 5:310–317, 1987

84c.Goner A, Arathoon E, Stevens DA: Initial experience in therapy for progres-sive mycoses with itraconazole, the first clinically studied triazole. Rev Infect Dis 9:S77–S86, 1987

84d.Arndt C, Walsh IJ, McCally CL, Balis FM, Pizzo PA, Poplack DG: Cerebro-spinal fluid penetration of fluconazole. J Infect Dis 157:178–180, 1988

84e.Saag MS, Dismukes WE: Azole antifungal agents: Emphasis on new tria-zoles. Antimicrob Agents Chemother 32:1–8, 1988

85. Cotton DJ, Gu V, Hiemenz J, MacLowry J, Longo D, Pizzo P: *Bacillus* bacteremias in an immunocompromised patient population: Clinical features, therapeutic interventions, and relationship to chronic intravascular catheters in sixteen cases. J Clin Microbiol 25:672–674, 1987

86. Pizzo PA, Ladisch, Robichaud K: Treatment of gram positive septicemia in cancer patients. Cancer 45:206–207, 1980

87. Cotton D, Marshall D, Gress J et al: Pathogen-specific vs broad-spectrum antibiotics for granulocytopenic patients with proven infection. Proc 24th Intersci Conf Antimicrob Agents Chemother, 1984, p 158

88. Bluestone CK, Klein JO: Otitis media with effusion, atelectasis, eustachian tube dysfunction. In Bluestone CD, Stool SE (eds): Pediatric Otolaryngology, p 356. Philadelphia, WB Saunders, 1983

89. Wald ER, Milmoe GJ, Bowen AD et al: Acute maxillary sinusitis in children. N Engl J Med 304:749–754, 1981

90. Frederick J, Braude AI: Anaerobic infection of the paranasal sinuses. N Engl J Med 290:135–137, 1974

91. Caplan ES, Hoyt NJ: Nosocomial sinusitis. JAMA 247:639–641, 1982

92. McGill TJ, Simpson G, Healvy GB: Fulminant aspergillosis of the nose and paranasal sinuses: A new clinical entity. Laryngoscope 90:748–754, 1980

93. Meyer RD, Rosen P, Armstrong D: Phycomycosis complicating leukemia and lymphoma. Ann Intern Med 77:871–879, 1972

94. Berkow RL, Weisman SJ, Provisor AJ et al: Invasive aspergillosis of parana-sal tissues in children with malignancies. J Pediatr 103:49–53, 1983

95. Stevens MH: Primary fungal infections of the paranasal sinuses. Am J Oto-laryngol 2:348–357, 1981

96. Kovatch AL, Wald ER, Ledesma–Medina J et al: Maxillary sinus radiographs in children with non-respiratory complaints. Pediatrics 73:306–308, 1984

97. Wald E: Sinusitis. In Nelson JD (ed): Current Therapy in Pediatric Infectious Disease, p 6. Toronto, BC Decker, 1986

98. Stover DE, Zamm MB, Hajdu SI, Lange N, Gold J, Armstrong D: Bronchoal-veolar lavage in the diagnosis of diffuse pulmonary infiltrates in the immuno-compromised host. Ann Intern Med 101:1–6, 1984

98a.Tharpe JE, Baughman RP, Frome PT, Wesseler TA, Stoneck JL: Bronchoal-veolar lavage for diagnosing acute bacterial pneumonia. J Infect Dis 155:855–861, 1987

98b.Kahn FW, Jones JM: Diagnosing bacterial respiratory infection by bron-choalveolar lavage. J Infect Dis 155:862–869, 1987

99. Iacuone JJ, Wong KY, Bove KE et al: Acute respiratory illness in children with acute lymphoblastic leukemia. J Pediatr 90:915–919, 1977

100. Meyer RD, Edelstein PH: Legionella pneumonias. In Pennington JE (ed): Respiratory Infections: Diagnosis and Management, pp 283–297. New York, Raven Press, 1983

101. Myerowitz RL, Pasculle AW, Dowling JN et al: Opportunistic lung infection due to "Pittsburgh pneumonia agent." N Engl J Med 301:953–958, 1979

102. Muldoon RL, Jaecker DL, Kiefer HK: Legionnaires' disease in children. Pediat-rics 67:329–332, 1981

103. Anderson RD, Lauer BA, Frazer DW et al: Infections with Legionella pneu-mophilia in children. J Infect Dis 143:386–390, 1981

104. Tobin J, Beare J, Dunnill MS et al: Legionnaires' disease in a transplant unit: Isolation of the causative agent from shower baths. Lancet 2:118–121, 1980

105. Kirby BD, Snyder KM, Meyer RD, Feingold SM: Legionnaires' disease: Report of sixty-five nosocomially acquired cases and review of the literature. Medicine (Baltimore) 59:188–205, 1980

106. Maskill MR, Jordan EC: Pronounced cerebellar features in Legionnaires' disease. Br Med J 283:276, 1981

107. Shetty KR, Cilyo CL, Starr BD, Harter DH: Legionnaires' disease with pro-found cerebellar involvement. Arch Neurol 37:379–380, 1980

108. Harris LF: Legionnaires' disease associated with acute encephalomyelitis. Arch Neurol 38:462–463, 1981

109. Kirby BD, Peck H, Meyer RD: Radiograph features of Legionnaires' disease. Chest 76:562–565, 1979

110. Young LS, Armstrong D, Blevins A et al: *Nocardia asteroides* infection complicating neoplastic disease. Am J Med 50:356–367, 1971

111. Palmer DL, Harvey RL, Wheeler JK: Diagnostic and therapeutic consider-ations in *Nocardia asteroides* infection. Medicine (Baltimore) 53:391–401, 1974

112. Smego RA, Gallis HA: The clinical spectrum of *Nocardia brasiliensis* infec-tion in the United States. Rev Infect Dis 6:164–180, 1984

113. Commers JC, Robichaud K, Pizzo PA: New pulmonary infiltrates in granulo-cytopenic patients being treated with antibiotics. Pediatr Infect Dis J 3:423–428, 1984

114. Edwards JE, Lehrer RI, Stiehm ER et al: Severe candidal infections: Clinical perspective, immune defense mechanisms, and current concepts of therapy. Ann Intern Med 89:91–106, 1978

115. Young RC, Bennett JE, Vogel CL et al: Aspergillosis: The spectrum of the disease in 98 patients. Medicine (Baltimore) 49:147–173, 1970

116. Krick JA, Remington JS: Opportunistic invasive fungal infections in patients with leukemia and lymphoma. Clin Haematol 5:249–310, 1976

117. Meyer RD, Rosen P, Armstrong D: Phycomycosis complicating leukemia and lymphoma. Ann Intern Med 77:871–879, 1972

118. Kauffman CA, Israel KS, Smith JW et al: Histoplasmosis in immunosup-pressed patients. Am J Med 64:923–931, 1978

119. Deresinski SC, Stevens DA: Coccidioidomycosis in compromised hosts: Ex-perience at Stanford University Hospital. Medicine (Baltimore) 54:377–395, 1974

120. Kaplan MS, Rosen PP, Armstrong D: Cryptococcosis in a cancer hospital: Clinical and pathological correlates in forty-six patients. Cancer 39:2265–2274, 1977

121. Young RC, Bennett JE, Gealhoed GW et al: Fungemia with compromised host resistance: A study of 70 cases. Ann Intern Med 80:605–617, 1974

122. Gold JW: Opportunistic fungal infections in patients with neoplastic disease. In Brown AE, Armstrong D: Infectious Complications of Neoplastic Disease: Controversies in Management, pp 111–121. New York, Yorke Medical Books, 1985

123. Wingard JR, Merz WG, Saral R: Candida tropicalis: A major pathogen in immunocompromised patients. Ann Intern Med 91:539–543, 1979

124. Meyer RD, Young LS, Armstrong D, Yu B: Aspergillosis complicating neo-plastic disease. Am J Med 54:6–15, 1973

125. Rinaldi MG: Invasive aspergillosis. Rev Infect Dis 5:1061–1077, 1983

126. Aisner J, Schimpff SC, Bennet JE et al: *Aspergillus* infection in cancer pa-tients: Association with fireproofing materials in new hospitals. JAMA 235:411–412, 1976

127. Aisner J, Schimpff SC, Wiernik PH: Treatment of invasive aspergillosis: Rela-tion of early diagnosis and treatment to response. Ann Intern Med 86:539–543, 1977

127a.Burch PA, Karp JE, Merz WG et al: Favorable outcome of invasive asper-gillosis in patients with acute leukemia. J Clin Oncol 5:1985–1993, 1987

128. Hughes WT: *Pneumocystis carinii* pneumonia. N Engl J Med 297:1381–1383, 1977

129. Meuwissen JH, Tauber I, Leeuwenberg AD et al: Parasitologic and serologic observations of infection with Pneumocystis in humans. J Infect Dis 136:4349, 1977

130. Ruebush TK, Weinstein RA, Baehner RL et al: An outbreak of *Pneumocystis* pneumonia in children with acute lymphocyte leukemia. Am J Dis Child 132:143–148, 1978

131. Browne M, Hubbard S, Longo DL et al: Excess prevalence of *Pneumocystis carinii* pneumonia in lymphoma patients with chemotherapy. Ann Intern Med 104:338–344, 1986

132. Kovacs JA, Hiemenz JW, Macher AM et al: *Pneumocystis carinii* pneumo-nia: A comparison of clinical features in patients with the acquired immune deficiency syndrome and patients with other immune diseases. Ann Intern Med 100:663–671, 1984

133. Browne MJ, Potter D, Gren J et al: A randomized trial of open lung biopsy versus empiric antimicrobial therapy in cancer patients with diffuse pulmonary infiltrates (submitted)

134. Allegra CJ, Chabner BA, Tuazon CU et al: Trimetrexate for the treatment of *Pneumocystis carinii* pneumonia in patients with the acquired immunodefi-ciency syndrome. N Engl J Med 317:978–985, 1987

135. Adler SP: Transfusion-associated cytomegalovirus infections. Rev Infect Dis 5:977–993, 1983

136. Hersman J, Meyers JD, Thomas ED et al: The effect of granulocyte transfu-sions on the incidence of cytomegalovirus infection after allogeneic marrow transplantation. Ann Intern Med 96:149–152, 1982

137. Meyers JD, McGuffin RW, Bryson YG et al: Treatment of cytomegalovirus pneumonia after marrow transplant with combined vidarabine and human leukocyte interferon. J Infect Dis 146:80–84, 1982

138. Bowden RA, Sayers M, Flournoy N et al: Cytomegalovirus immune globulin and seronegative blood products to prevent primary cytomegalovirus infec-tion after marrow transplantation. N Engl J Med 314:1006–1010, 1986

139. Kostiala I, Kostiala AAI, Kahanpaa A, Elonen E: Acute fungal stomatitis in patients with hematologic malignancies: Quantity and species of fungi. J Infect Dis 146:101, 1982

139a.Medoff G: Controversial areas in antifungal chemotherapy: Short course and combination therapy with amphotericin B. Rev Infect Dis 9:403–407, 1987

140. Lam MT, Pazin GJ, Armstrong JA, Ho M: Herpes simplex infection in acute myelogenous leukemia and other hematologic malignancies: A prospective study. Cancer 48:2169–2171, 1981

141. Saral R: Acyclovir prophylaxis of herpes simplex virus infections: A random-ized double-blind controlled trial in bone marrow transplant patients. N Engl J Med 305:63–67, 1981

142. Meyers JD, Wade JC, Mitchell CD et al: Multicenter collaborative trial of intravenous acyclovir for treatment of mucocutaneous herpes simplex infec-tion in the immunocompromised host. Am J Med 73:229–235, 1982

143. Peterson DE, Overholser CD: Increased morbidity associated with oral in-fection in patients with acute nonlymphocytic leukemia. Oral Surg 51:390–393, 1982

143a.Peterson D, Minah GE, Overholser CD: Microbiology of acute periodontal infection in myelosuppressed cancer patients. J Clin Oncol 5:1461–1468, 1987

144. Walsh TJ, Belitsos N, Hamilton SR: Bacterial esophagitis in immunocompro-mised patients. Arch Intern Med 146:1345–1348, 1986

145. Buss DH, Scharyj M: Herpes virus infection of the esophagus and other visceral organs in adults: Incidence and clinical significance. Am J Med 66:457–462, 1979

146. Varki AP, Armitage JO, Feagler JR: Typhlitis in acute leukemia: Successful treatment by early surgical intervention. Cancer 43:695–697, 1979

147. Skibber JM, Matler GJ, Lotze MT, Pizzo PA: Right lower quadrant compli-cations in young patients with leukemia: A surgical perspective. Ann Surg 206:711–716, 1987

148. Shaked A, Shinar E, Freund H: Neutropenic typhlitis: A plea for conserva-tion. Dis Colon Rectum 26:351–352, 1983

149. Wynne JW, Armstrong D: Clostridial septicemia. Cancer 29:215–221, 1972

150. Thaler M, Gill V, Pizzo PA: Emergence of *Clostridium tertium* as a pathogen in neutropenic patients. Am J Med 81:596–600, 1986

151. Larson HE, Price AB, Honour P et al: *Clostridium difficile* and the aetiology of pseudomembranous colitis. Lancet 1:1063–1066, 1978

152. Bartlett JG, Chang TW, Gurwith M et al: Antibiotic-associated pseudo-membranous colitis due to toxin producing clostridia. N Engl J Med 298:531–534, 1978

153. Elstner CL, Lindsay AN, Book LS, Matson JM: Lack of relationship of *Clostrid-ium difficile* to antibiotic-associated diarrhea in children. Pediatr Infect Dis 2:364–366, 1983

154. Scowden EB, Schaffner W, Stone WJ: Overwhelming strongyloidiasis: An unappreciated opportunistic infection. Medicine (Baltimore) 57:527–544, 1978

155. Dienstag JL: Non-A, non-B hepatitis I: Recognition, epidemiology, and clini-cal features. Gastroenterology 85:439–462, 1983

156. Tabor E, Gerety RJ, Drucker JA et al: Transmission of non-A, non-B hepatitis from man to chimpanzee. Lancet 1:463–465, 1978

157. Hoofnagle JH, Mullen KD, Jones B et al: Treatment of chronic non-A, non-B hepatitis with recombinant human alpha interferon: A preliminary report. N Engl J Med 315:1575–1578, 1986

158. Hoofnagle JH, Dusheiko GM, Schafer DF et al: Reactivation of chronic hepatitis B virus infection by cancer chemotherapy. Ann Intern Med 96:447–449, 1982

159. Rizzetto M, Purcell RH, Gerin JL: Epidemiology of HBV-associated delta agent: Geographical distribution of anti-delta and prevalence in polytrans-fused HBsAg carriers. Lancet 1:1215–1218, 1980

160. Haron E, Feld R, Tuffnell P, Patterson B, Hasselbach R, Matlow A: Hepatic candidiasis: An increasing problem in immunocompromised patients. Am J Med 83:17–26, 1987

161. Thaler M, Bader J, O'Leary T, Pizzo PA: Hepatic candidiasis in cancer patients: The evolving picture of the syndrome. Ann Intern Med 108:88–100, 1988

161a.Haron E, Feld R, Tuffnell P, Patterson B, Hasselback R, Matlow A: Hepatic candidiasis: An increasing problem in immunocompromised patients. Am J Med 83:17–26, 1987

162. Thaler M, Bader J, O'Leary T, Pizzo PA: An experimental model of candi-diasis in rabbits with prolonged neutropenia. J Infect Dis (in press)

163. Barnes SG, Sattler FR, Ballard JO: Improved survival after drainage of perirectal infections in patients with acute leukemia. Ann Intern Med 100:515–518, 1984

164. Glenn J, Cotton D, Wesley R, Pizzo PA: Anorectal infections in patients with malignant diseases. Rev Infect Dis 10:42–52, 1988

165. Schoenbaum SC, Gardner P, Shillito J: Infections of cerebrospinal fluid shunts: Epidemiology, clinical manifestations and therapy. J Infect Dis 131:543–552, 1979

166. Browne M, Dinndorf P, Perek D et al: Infections complications of intraventric-ular reservoirs in cancer patients. Pediatr Infect Dis J 6:182–189, 1987

167. Kaplan MS, Rosen PP, Armstrong D: Cryptococcosis in a cancer hospital: Clinical and pathological correlates in forty-six patients. Cancer 39:2265–2274, 1977

168. Diamond RD, Bennet JE: Prognostic factors in cryptococcal meningitis: A study of 111 cases. Ann Intern Med 80:176–181, 1974

169. Bennett JE, Dismukes WE, Duma RJ et al: Amphotericin B and flucytosine in cryptococcal meningitis. N Engl J Med 201:126–131, 1979

170. Dismukes WE, Cloud G, Gallis HA et al: Treatment of cryptococcal meningi-tis with combination amphotericin B and flucytosine for four as compared with six weeks. N Engl J Med 317:334–341, 1987

171. Lavetter A, Leedom JM, Mathies AE et al: Meningitis due to *Listeria mono-cytogenes*. N Engl J Med 285:598–603, 1971

172. Gantz NM, Myerwitz RL, Medieros AA et al: Listeriosis in immunosup-pressed patients: A cluster of eight cases. Am J Med 58:637–643, 1975

173. Gordon RC, Barrett FF, Yow MD: Ampicillin treatment of listeriosis. J Pediatr 77:1067–1070, 1970

174. Davis LE, Bodian D, Price D et al: Chronic progressive poliomyelitis second-ary to vaccination of an immunosuppressed child. N Engl J Med 297:241–245, 1977

175. Wilfert CM, Buckley RM, Mokanakumar T et al: Persistent and fatal central nervous system echovirus infections in patients with agammaglobulinemia. N Engl J Med 296:1485–1489, 1977

176. Roos RP, Graves MC, Wollmann RL et al: Immunologic and virologic studies of measles inclusion body encephalitis in an immunosuppressed host: The relationship to subacute sclerosing panencephalitis. Neurology 31:1263–1270, 1981

177. Whitley RJ, Soong S-J, Dolin R et al: Adenosine arabinoside therapy of biopsy-proved herpes simplex encephalitis. N Engl J Med 297:289–294, 1977

178. Ruskin J, Remington JS: Toxoplasmosis in the compromised host. Ann Intern Med 84:193–199, 1976

179. Ladisch SL, Pizzo PA: S. aureus sepsis in children with cancer. Pediatrics 61:231–234, 1978

180. Howat AJ, Todd CEC, Scott CA: Two cases of endocarditis due to Candida albicans discovered at autopsy. J Infect Dis 147:1122–1123, 1983

180a.Primary cutaneous aspergillosis associated with Hickman intravenous catheters. N Engl J Med 317:1105–1108, 1987

181. Feldman S, Lott L: Varicella in children with cancer: Impact of antiviral therapy and prophylaxis. Pediatrics 80:465–472, 1987

182. Shepp DH, Dandliker PS, Myers JD: Treatment of varicella–zoster virus infection in severely immunocompromised patients: A randomized comparison of acyclovir and vidarabine. N Engl J Med 314:208–212, 1986

183. Gelb LD, Dohner DE, Geighon AA et al: Molecular epidemiology of live, attenuated varicella virus vaccine in children with leukemia and in normal adults. J Infect Dis 155:633–640, 1987

184. Albert RK, Condie F: Handwashing patterns in medical intensive care units. N Engl J Med 304:1465–1466, 1981

185. Pizzo PA: Considerations for preventing infectious complications in cancer patients. Rev Infect Dis (in press)

186. Remington JS, Schimpff SC: Please don't eat the salads. N Engl J Med 304:433–435, 1981

187. Pizzo PA, Purvis D, Waters CW: Microbiological evaluation of food items for patients undergoing gastrointestinal decontamination and protected isolation. J Am Diet Assoc 81:272–279, 1982

188. Nauseef WM, Maki DG: A study of the value of simple protective isolation in patients with granulocytopenia. N Engl J Med 304:448–453, 1981

189. Pizzo PA: Do results justify the expense of protected environments? In Wiernik P (ed): Controversies in Oncology, pp 267–277. New York, John Wiley & Sons, 1982

190. Pizzo PA: Antibiotic prophylaxis in the immunosuppressed patient with cancer. In Remington JS, Swartz MN (eds): Current Clinical Topics in Infectious Diseases, 4th Ed, pp 153–167. New York, McGraw–Hill, 1983

191. Waaij D van der, Berghuis–de Vries JN, Lekkerkerk–van der Wees JEC et al: Colonization resistance of the digestive tract in conventional and antibiotic-treated mice. J Hyg (Lond) 69:405–411, 1971

192. Waaij D van der, Berghuis–de Bries JN: Selective elimination of Enterobacteriaciae species from the digestive tract in mice and monkeys. J Hyg (Camb) 72:205–211, 1974

193. Guiot HFL, Brock PJ van den, Meer JWM van der, Furth R van: Selective antimicrobial modulation of the intestinal flora of patients with acute nonlymphocytic leukemia: A double blind placebo controlled study. J Infect Dis 147:615–623, 1983

194. Sleijfer DT, Mulder NK, de Vries–Hospers HG et al: Infection prevention in granulocytopenic patients by selective decontamination of the digestive tract. Eur J Cancer 16:859–869, 1980

195. Gurwith MJ, Brunton JL, Lank BA: A prospective controlled investigation of prophylactic trimethoprim/sulfamethoxazole in hospitalized granulocytopenic patients. Am J Med 66:248–256, 1979

196. Weiser B, Lange M, Fialkow MA et al: Prophylactic trimethoprim–sulfamethoxozole during consolidated chemotherapy for acute leukemia: A controlled trial. Ann Intern Med 95:436–438, 1981

197. Dekker A, Rozenberg–Arsha M, Sixma JJ et al: Prevention of infection by trimethoprim–sulfamethoxazole plus amphotericin B in patients with acute nonlymphocytic leukemia. Ann Intern Med 95:555–559, 1981

198. Kauffman CA, Leipman MJ, Bergman AG et al: Trimethoprim–sulfamethoxazole prophylaxis in neutropenic patients: Reduction of infections and effect on bacterial and fungal flora. Am J Med 74:599–607, 1983

199. Gaultieri RJ, Donowitz GR, Kaiser CE et al: Double-blind randomized study of prophylactic trimethoprim–sulfamethoxazole in granulocytopenic patients with hematologic malignancies. Am J Med 74:934–940, 1983

200. Wade JC, DeJongh CA, Newman KA et al: Selective antimicrobial modulation as prophylaxis against infection during granulocytopenia: Trimethoprim–sulfamethoxazole versus nalidixic acid. J Infect Dis 147:624–634, 1983

201. Wilson JM, Guinery DG: Failure of oral trimethoprim–sulfamethoxazole prophylaxis in acute leukemia: Isolation of resistant plasmids from strains of Enterobacteriaceae causing bacteremia. N Engl J Med 306:16–20, 1982

202. Karp JE, Merz WG, Hendricksen C et al: Oral norfloxacin for prevention of gram-negative bacterial infections in patients with acute leukemia and granulocytopenia. Ann Intern Med 106:1–7, 1987

203. Dekker AW, Rozenberg–Arska M, Verhoes J: Infection prophylaxis in acute leukemia: A comparison of cifrofloxacin with trimethoprim–sulfamethoxozole and colistin. Ann Intern Med 106:7–12, 1987

204. Meunier F: Prevention of mycoses in immunocompromised patients. Rev Infect Dis 9:408–416, 1987

205. Hughes WT, Rivera GK, Schell MJ, Thornton D, Lott L: Successful intermittent chemoprophylaxis for Pneumocystis carinii pneumonitis. N Engl J Med 316:1627–1632, 1987

206. Gershon A: Live attenuated varicella vaccine. J Pediatr 110:154–157, 1987

207. Peter G, Pizzo PA, Robichaud KK et al: Possible protective effect of circulating antibodies to the shared glycolipid of enterobacteriaceae in children with malignancy. Pediatr Res 13:466, 1979

208. Ziegler EJ, McCutchon JA, Fierer JA et al: Treatment of gram-negative bacteremia and shock with human antiserum to mutant Escherichia coli. N Engl J Med 307:1254–1230, 1982

209. Baumgartner JD, Glauser MP, McCutcheon JA et al: Prevention of gram-negative shock and death in surgical patients by antibody to endotoxin core glycolipid. Lancet 2:59–63, 1985

210. Metcalf D: The molecular biology and functions of the granulocyte–macrophage colony stimulating factors. Blood 67:257–267, 1986

forty

Nutritional Supportive Care

Jeffrey A. Norton and Jane Peter

CANCER CACHEXIA IN THE PEDIATRIC PATIENT

Definition, Incidence, and Treatment Implications

Cancer cachexia is a syndrome that includes the final deterioration of late cancer and the distant systemic effects of any phase of cancer.[1] It is a common manifestation of a malignant tumor[2] and has grave implications for the quality of life, length of survival, and permissible aggressiveness of treatment.

The term "cachexia" is derived from two Greek words, *kakos* and *hexis,* meaning simply "poor condition." The clinical features include host tissue wasting, anorexia (decline in food intake), asthenia (weakness), anemia, hypoalbuminemia, hypoglycemia, lactic acidosis, hyperlipidemia, impaired liver function, glucose intolerance, elevated gluconeogenesis, skeletal muscle atrophy, visceral organ atrophy or hypertrophy, and anergy.[2-4] The particular combination of features varies with tumor type and patient, but the central characteristic is progressive depletion of vital host tissue, resulting in emaciation. Because of the variability in occurrence and clinical presentation, some tumors are thought not to cause cachexia, whereas others, such as Ewing's sarcoma, cause significant cachexia.[5,6]

The incidence of cachexia differs with the progression and extent of malignancy. In children with cancer, the frequency of malnutrition at the time of diagnosis is no greater than that seen in children with benign diseases.[7,8] However, in children with progressive and metastatic malignant disease, the incidence of cachexia is as high as 40%.[8] Among more than 3000 adults with cancer, 54% had lost weight and 32% had lost greater than 5% of their preillness weight.[9] Once weight loss occurs in adults[9] and children,[7] the prognosis is poorer and the survival shorter.

Etiology

Relative Hypophagia

A controversy in cachexia is whether tissue depletion arises predominantly from depressed food intake or from elevated energy expenditure.[10,11] The only way tissue depletion can occur is by nutrient intake falling short of energy demand. In normal animals, a change in metabolic cost is usually followed by a corresponding change in food intake. This happens with an increase in energy expenditure due to exercise,[12] temperature,[13] caloric density of food,[14] and pregnancy or lactation;[15] however, it fails to happen with cancer. In the pediatric patient, this problem is amplified because host growth raises the metabolic demand.

The question of tumor-induced change in host energy expenditure remains unanswered because it is impossible to separate the tumor from the host. It is also probable that one answer does not apply to all tumors and all hosts, since individual tumor types and individual host metabolism differ greatly. One group of investigators recently concluded that increased energy expenditure had little impact on cachexia.[16] However, another group, that studied a homogeneous population of young sarcoma patients, did find elevated resting energy expenditure compared to controls.[17] Fortunately, an absolute answer is not critical; the important observation is that food intake fails to support the energy expenditure, and host tissue thus becomes depleted.

Anorexia can be a direct consequence of cancer treatment. The nausea, vomiting, and anorexia induced by chemotherapeutic agents can be severe. Indeed, in the pediatric patient population, cancer treatment results in a greater degree of anorexia than does the cancer itself.[18,19] Both chemotherapy[18] and radiotherapy[19] induce these nutritional complications.

There may also be an alteration in taste perception in children with cancer. The most significant change appears to be a lower threshold for bitter-tasting foods, which may explain the observed aversion to meat and other protein foods.[20,21] Alterations in taste perception have also been reported as a consequence of cancer chemotherapy.[22]

Abnormal Metabolism

PROTEIN. The central abnormality of nitrogen metabolism is the ability of the tumor to incorporate nitrogen at the expense of the host.[4] Moreover, because the host usually has an inappropriate reduction in nitrogen intake, the source of nitrogen for tumor growth is host skeletal muscle.[23] Both accelerated host protein degradation and reduced synthesis contribute to the skeletal muscle depletion.[24-26] It is possible that the internal redistribution of nitrogen starts before any decline in nitrogen (food) intake. This implies that host nitrogen depletion is not caused totally by reduced food intake but may also entail a tumor-specific metabolic abnormality.

CARBOHYDRATES. Starting with the demonstration of lactic acid production by tumors,[27,28] reduced blood glucose,[27] elevated blood lactate,[29] abnormal glucose tolerance,[30] and changes in glucose turnover, pool size, and half-life,[29-32] there is ample evidence of disordered carbohydrate metabolism in cachexia. Hypoglycemia and lactic acidosis may appear only in a minority of cancer patients.[33] However, lactic acidosis can be the cause of unexplained metabolic acidosis in pediatric cancer patients who are receiving parenteral or enteral glucose.[34] Elevated glucose turnover and Cori cycle activity (gluconeogenesis from lactate) may be linked to progressive weight loss and an elevated metabolic rate.[33] Clear changes in carbohydrate metabolism have been detected in animals with minimal tumor burdens prior to cachexia.[29] Some of this change is probably a reflection of tumor metabolism, but some represents action of the tumor on host metabolism. Attempts to separate tumor and host effects have not yielded clear results. The two most common abnormalities of carbohydrate metabolism in treated pediatric cancer patients are glucose intolerance, which is thought to be secondary to insulin resistance,[30] and lactic acidosis, which occurs during glucose infusion.[34] Both of these abnormalities can become clinical problems and so must be considered when managing these patients.

LIPID. Hyperlipidemia and depletion of lipid stores are the main gross abnormalities of fat metabolism in patients with cancer.[35] Evidence for change in plasma free fatty acids is equivocal. Hyperlipidemia may be present in some patients with cancer and absent in others. The coexistence of hyperlipidemia and depletion of lipid stores has led to the hypothesis that the basic abnormality of lipid metabolism in cachexia is increased mobilization and decreased deposition of fat. There have been several demonstrations of a circulating lipolytic fac-

tor in cachexia,[36] and extracts of tumors have shown lipolytic effects.[37] Both the clearing of the hyperlipidemia and the stimulation of adipose gain by exogenous insulin in the tumor-bearing organism suggest that lipogenic mechanisms are not impaired by the presence of tumor but rather that abnormalities in insulin activity may be involved.[38] Recent work[39] showed that tumor-bearing animals are intolerant of administered lipid, which raises serum triglyceride levels, and that the addition of glucose fails to prevent the triglyceride increase. Increased lipolytic activity was also demonstrated in sera of tumor-bearing animals and was not due to hypoglycemia or hypoinsulinemia.[39]

Plasma lipoprotein line width as measured by proton magnetic resonance is significantly reduced in patients with cancer compared with patients with diseases not involving tumors and patients with benign tumors.[40] The biological mechanism for this change is not clear, but a host response to the malignant tumor is suggested because the change is not tumor specific. The host mediator is not known; possibilities include a newly described proteolipid[41] and cachectin, which, among its properties, changes certain aspects of host lipoprotein metabolism.[42]

Table 40-1 lists the nutritional and metabolic abnormalities associated with cancer cachexia and contrasts them with changes seen during simple starvation and sepsis. During simple starvation, the body adapts to food deprivation and minimizes nitrogen loss.[43] During sepsis, host dissolution may be mediated by factors such as cachectin[44] that cause marked tissue wasting and increased nitrogen loss.[45] With cancer, the nitrogen loss and host dissolution are intermediate between those of sepsis and starvation.[46]

Substrate Utilization and Tumor Growth

Indirect evidence that total parenteral nutrition (TPN) stimulates tumor growth comes from a prospective randomized study of conventional oral nutrition and TPN in pediatric pa-

Table 40-1
*Nutritional and Metabolic Comparison of Starvation, Sepsis, and Cancer**

	Starvation	Sepsis	Cancer
Anorexia	Present	Present	Present
Weight loss	Present	Present	Present
Resting energy expenditure	↓↑	↑↑	↑ or ↓
Blood glucose	↓	↑↑	↑ or ↓
Blood lactate	Normal	↑	↑
Serum insulin	↓	↓	↑ or ↓
Insulin resistance	Absent	↑↑	↑
Glucose tolerance	↓	↓↓	↓
Gluconeogenesis	↓	↑↑	↑
Glucose recycling (Cori cycle)	↓	↑↑	↑
Urinary nitrogen	↓	↑↑	Normal
Protein turnover	↓	↑↑	↑
Protein synthesis	↓	↑↑	↑
Protein catabolism	↓	↑↑	↑
Lipolysis	↑	↑↑	↑
Lipogenesis	↓	↓	↓
Cachectin	Absent	Present	Unknown

* Modified from Reference 46 and compiled primarily from References 43 through 46.
↑↑ = increased; ↑↑ = greatly increased; ↓ = decreased; ↓↓ = greatly decreased.

tients undergoing aggressive chemotherapy.[47] Fourteen patients were randomized to conventional nutrition and 18 to TPN. As expected, the TPN group received significantly more calories and nitrogen during the study than did the control group. The proportion of responders to chemotherapy in the two groups was not statistically different, but the duration of remission was significantly shorter for the TPN group than for the control group.[47] This indirect evidence of increased tumor growth suggests that TPN may be detrimental to some cancer patients, but this study had small numbers of patients with different tumor types. In the rat with sarcoma, TPN at increasing dosages correspondingly increases growth as more substrate is provided.[48] Similarly, by tumor biopsies and cell kinetics, TPN appears to increase the growth of head and neck squamous cell cancers.[49] These studies provide some evidence that nutritional substrate may increase tumor growth, but a consensus conference on results in humans concluded that there is no clear evidence of TPN-stimulated tumor growth.[50]

^{18}F-2-deoxyglucose and positron emission tomography (PET) scanning were used recently to quantitate glucose consumption by large extremity sarcomas in children.[51] Glucose consumption rates from 6 to 15 mg/100 g per minute were found. These high rates are similar to those of brain tumors, where the glucose consumption rate appears to correlate with the histologic grade of tumor: the higher the glucose consumption of a tumor, the poorer the prognosis and possibly the greater the cachectic effect. Glucose uptake by human sarcomas correlates directly with excised tumor size.[52] Amino acids are also released at a lesser rate from the extremity bearing a sarcoma, implying tumor uptake.[52] Glucose and amino acid consumption by tumors can place a large metabolic demand on the host to produce substrate and metabolize toxic end-products.

Hypothesis for Cachexia

A recent hypothesis suggests that cancer cachexia is a direct consequence of the common feature of all malignant tumors: growth. The uncontrolled continued growth of tumors places a demand on the host for essential nutrients that causes muscle wastage and anorexia.[53] The cause of cachexia in young cancer patients is multifactorial (Fig. 40-1), but there appear to be five major contributors. First, abnormal host metabolism of glucose, nitrogen, and lipid leads to inefficient use of nutrients. Second, the tumor consumes vital nutrients for its own growth. Third, the host tissue requires extra nutrients to support normal growth. Fourth, anticancer therapy itself has significant nutritional morbidity. Fifth, the host fails to consume enough nutrients to meet expenditures. The net result of these five forces is cancer cachexia, which results in host weight loss and asthenia. Cachexia is one of the major sources of morbidity for young cancer patients and as such mandates aggressive treatment. In addition, cachexia worsens the response to anticancer therapy.[9]

OUTCOME OF NUTRITIONAL SUPPORT

Total parenteral nutrition or enteral nutrition (EN) using complete or elemental formulations can maintain adequate nutrition and promote growth of a starving patient without cancer or sepsis. If a patient has a functional impairment of the gastrointestinal tract, TPN or possibly EN can completely maintain him. He retains the benefits of adequate nutrition and maintains normal activity and energy expenditure, including the ability to groom himself and engage in activities of interest such as play,

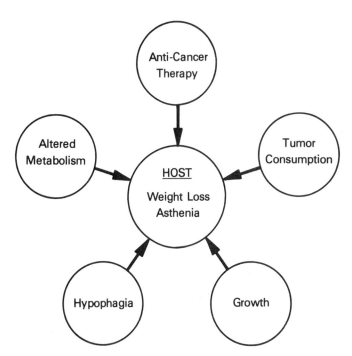

FIGURE 40-1.   Schematic representation of the origin of cachexia in a young patient with cancer.

reading, writing, and arts. Adequate nutrition reverses previous malnutrition and promotes growth, which is important in young patients, who have additional demands for "catch-up" growth following a period of inadequate nutritional intake.

It is clear that enteral or parenteral nutrition can totally maintain an otherwise healthy patient. The question here is whether it can maintain a young growing patient with cancer who is undergoing chemotherapy, surgery, or radiation therapy. Cancer places inordinate demands on young patients, in whom it may be impossible to maintain adequate oral nutrition. Any malignancy in which fevers commonly occur, such as leukemia or lymphoma, greatly increases whole-body protein turnover.[54] In addition, chemotherapy itself, which is essential to the treatment of some malignant diseases, greatly increases whole-body protein turnover and places additional energy and metabolic demands on the host.[55]

The results of studies designed to discover whether malnourished cancer patients can be re-fed using TPN or EN are contradictory. Generally, the studies indicate that it is possible to feed these patients, but it may not be possible to preserve or restore vital host protein mass. Esophageal cancer patients with marked (20%) weight loss who have not had additional treatment can be re-fed successfully by either the oral or the parenteral route.[56] However, another study, which examined the effects of 4 weeks of TPN in patients with small-cell lung cancer undergoing aggressive chemotherapy, found that TPN increases body fat and potassium but not body nitrogen, indicating that TPN cannot reverse host nitrogen loss.[57] The difference in outcome of these studies may be caused by chemotherapy's detrimental action on nitrogen metabolism[55] and the inability of TPN to retard it.

The inability of TPN to restore lean body mass in the face of aggressive chemotherapy and cancer may provide insight into the results of trials with TPN and cancer treatment. In cancer patients, there have been no therapeutic advantages of nutritional support[46,58]: TPN has not increased the amount of chemotherapy administered, it has not improved disease-free interval or survival, and it has not improved tolerance for radiation therapy.[46,58] In the patients with childhood malignancies undergoing chemotherapy with or without radiation therapy, TPN did not improve survival,[59–61] nor did it decrease measurable therapeutic toxicity.[59–62]

Some authors emphasize the problems associated with TPN in the oncology patient;[58] others[63] point out we should not let these problems blind us to the benefits. Present nutritional support regimens may not be adequate for patients receiving aggressive chemotherapy with associated changes in nitrogen metabolism.[55] It is clear that death ensues between 60 and 70 days of total starvation and that current TPN will prevent this complication in oncologic patients with long-term inadequate nutritional intake. New generations of parenteral formulas may be more efficacious in the oncology patient. Until then, however, we must not use TPN in patients undergoing short-term therapy with minimal nutritional morbidity. In patients with existing cachexia and weight loss who are undergoing complex therapy with nutritional morbidity, such as total-body radiation with autologous bone-marrow transplantation, TPN is indicated to conserve protein and prevent death from starvation. If a growing patient loses greater than 5% of body weight and has inadequate food intake, TPN is indicated until adequate oral intake can be resumed. Death from starvation can occur when a patient drops below 20% to 30% of his or her usual weight, and TPN should be used to prevent this as long as reasonable cancer-treatment options are available (Fig. 40-2).

EVALUATION OF NUTRITIONAL STATUS AND GUIDELINES FOR SUPPORT

Indices of Nutritional Status

Standard Measurements

The initial measurements needed for assessing the nutritional status are age, height, weight, and, in children younger than 3 years old, head circumference. Any recent weight loss of 5% or greater, including dehydration, requires further investigation.[64] It is important to record the usual weight and any recent change in weight. Values of height for age, weight for age, weight for height, and head circumference for age (if applicable) are plotted against the National Center for Health Statistics growth curves, which depict standards derived from U.S. populations of healthy children. Any measurement below the tenth percentile should be investigated as a sign of growth impairment due to inadequate nutrition. A weight-for-height value below the fifth percentile may reflect acute malnutrition, whereas a height-for-age value below than the fifth percentile may reflect chronic malnutrition. Any percentile value that has changed significantly from previous measurements should be investigated. In the pediatric cancer patient, current or previous chemotherapy may depress growth.[65] Hereditary influences should also be considered. These simple measurements are the best indicators for a decision regarding nutritional support. If a patient has lost 5% of body weight, nutritional support is indicated.

FIGURE 40-2. Algorithm that guides the nutritional support of the pediatric cancer patient.

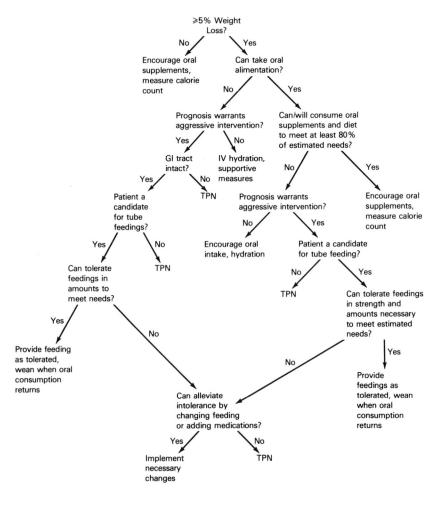

Investigational Measurements

Serum proteins are common laboratory measures of nutritional status: total protein, albumin, transferrin, prealbumin, and retinol-binding protein. The total lymphocyte count is also used (Table 40-2). Whereas each measure offers a certain advantage, albumin is probably the most common.[67] A concentration of albumin less than 3.0 g/dl may reflect protein–calorie malnutrition; however, infection, impaired liver function, certain chemotherapy, and overhydration can all depress serum albumin.[68] Also, with a turnover of approximately 14 days, serum albumin responds slowly to changes in nutritional status.[69]

Serum transferrin (mg/dl) can be measured directly or determined indirectly from a measurement of total iron-binding capacity (TIBC; μg/dl):

$$\text{Transferrin} = \frac{\text{TIBC}}{1.45}$$

While the half-life of transferrin is only 8 to 10 days, values will be artificially elevated by iron deficiency anemia or chronic blood loss. Retinol-binding protein has a half-life of only 12 hours, and prealbumin has a half-life of 2 to 3 days. Both measurements are good indicators of nutritional repletion in children[67,69] and may be utilized more often in the future. The total lymphocyte count is an unreliable indicator of nutritional status in most cancer patients because of the effects of chemotherapy on blood counts.[70,71]

The creatinine:height index is an indicator of muscle mass. Because creatinine is a product of muscle metabolism, the urinary excretion of creatinine is proportional to lean body mass. The index is obtained by multiplying the 24-hour urinary creatinine output by 100 and dividing by the ideal urinary creatinine excretion for an individual of the same height and gender. Values for ideal urinary creatinine excretion can be obtained from tables published by Viteri and Alvarado.[72] A range of 90% to 100% of the standard is generally accepted as normal.[73] The difficulties in obtaining accurate results from this test include problems in obtaining complete 24-hour urine

collections, and the requirement for normal renal function. Infection increases urinary creatinine excretion and may result in an artificially elevated measurement.

Methods are available for assessing body composition. Anthropometrics and total body potassium have been measured to examine the body composition of cancer patients. The results indicate that in young patients with solid tumors, changes in major body compartments can precede changes in body weight.[17] Anthropometric tests assess protein and fat compartments by measurement of mid-arm circumference and skinfold thickness at the triceps, biceps, subscapular, and suprailiac sites. Two of these measurements, triceps skinfold (TSF) and midarm circumference, can be used to determine arm muscle area from the following formula:[70]

$$\text{Arm muscle area (mm}^2) = \frac{\pi}{4} \frac{(\text{arm circumference} - \text{TSF})^2}{\pi}$$

The TSF measurements are taken on the nondominant arm halfway between the olecranon and the acromion process. A skinfold caliper is used to measure in millimeters the thickness of the skinfold pinched at the back of the arm, taking care to include only skin and subcutaneous fat. Measurements are then compared with tables of established normal values for age and gender.[70] A percentile value of less than 10% for arm muscle area is indicative of muscle depletion, whereas a triceps skinfold of greater than 90% may reveal excess fat stores. Anthropometrics can help ascertain the nature of weight gain or loss. For example, the child who has had repeated cycles of weight gain and loss may be at a preillness weight yet may have lost significant muscle mass and gained adipose tissue. For accurate anthropometric measurements, it is important to use meticulous technique. When serial measurements are needed, the same investigator should perform all measurements. A caliper is needed to measure skinfolds, and a nonstretchable tape is used to measure arm circumference (Table 40-2).

Total body potassium is an index of body cell mass. Potassium-40 is a naturally occurring radioisotope present as a small proportion of the total body potassium. Sensitive whole-body

---

Table 40-2
Normal Values for Serum, Anthropometric, and Body Composition Measurements

| | Serum | | | | Anthropometrics[66] * | | | | | | Composition† | |
| | Total Protein (g/dl) | Albumin (g/dl) | Transferrin (mg/dl) | | Triceps Skin Fold (mm) | | Arm Circumference (mm) | | Arm Muscle Area (mm²) | | Body Cell Mass (% TBW) | |
					M	F	M	F	M	F	M	F
Premature	4.3–7.6				–	–‡	–	–	–	–	–	–
Infant	4.6–7.4				10	10	160–165	155–165	1200–1400	1200–1400	–	–
Child	6.8–8.0	3.5–5.0	210–450	(4–8 yr)	8–9	10–11	170–175	170–185	1500–1800	1500–1700		
				(9–12 yr)	10–11	12–13	190–220	190–220	2200–2600	2100–2600	–	–
				(13–16 yr)	8–11	14–18	230–260	230–255	3400–4400	3000–3300		
Adult	6.0–7.8	3.4–5.0	200–400		9–12	19–25	280–330	260–330	5200–6400	3300–4000	36	33

* Figures represent approximately 50th percentile for each group.
† From Moore FD et al: The Body Cell Mass and Its Supporting Environment. Philadelphia, WB Saunders, 1963.
‡ Data not available.
§ Total-body potassium (mEq) $\times$ 8.33 = body cell mass.

Table 40-3
Deficiency Characteristics of Selected Vitamins and Minerals[67-71]

Vitamin or Mineral	Daily Requirement	Deficiency Symptoms	Factors Associated with Deficiency	Associated Characteristics	Normal Values for Determination of Status
Thiamine	0.5 mg/1000 kcal	Confusion, anorexia, weakness, peripheral paralysis, tachycardia, enlarged heart	Long-term TPN, chronic febrile infections	Deficiency symptoms may mimic symptoms of chemotherapeutic toxicity; urinary excretion is used to measure status	μg excreted/g creatinine: 4–16 yr ≥121 7–12 yr ≥181 13–15 yr ≥151 Adults ≥60
Biotin	100–300 mg	Anorexia, nausea, vomiting, dermatitis, glossitis	Long-term use of antibiotics without adequate dietary replacement; often not adequately supplemented by TPN solutions	Intestinal microflora contributes to stores of biotin; urinary excretion is used to measure status	30–60 μg excreted/24 hours
Riboflavin	0.6 mg/1000 kcal or 1.2 mg	Cheilosis, dermatitis, angular stomatitis, photophobia	Inadequate intake	Light sensitive. Possibly synthesized by intestinal microflora; urinary excretion is used to measure status	μg excreted/g creatinine 1–3 yr ≥500 4–6 yr ≥300 7–9 yr ≥270 10–15 yr ≥200 Adults ≥80
Niacin	11.3–13.3 mg of niacin equivalents	Pellagra	Diets low in niacin and in tryptophan; 60 mg tryptophan is equivalent to 1 mg niacin	Large amounts of nicotinic acid may cause flushing, decreased utilization of muscle glycogen, decreased mobilization of fatty acids; urinary excretion of N-methylnicotinamide determines status	μg N-methylnicotimamide excreted/g creatinine adults ≥1.6
Pyridoxine	Infants: 3–6 mg Children and adults: 2 mg	Infants: Convulsions, weight loss vomiting, irritability Adults: Dermatitis, confusion, EEG abnormalities, glossities, cheilosis	Inadequate intake	Use of oral contraceptives may increase need; urinary excretion of xanthurenic acid after a tryptophan load determines status	Net increase in xanthurenic acid excretion <25 mg/day
Folate	Infants: 5 mg/kg Children: 8–10 mg/kg Adults: 400 mg	Macrocytic, megaloblastic anemia	Inadequate intake; use of methotrexate, phenytoin, oral contraceptives	Synthesized by intestinal bacteria. Deficiency systoms may result from a B-12 deficiency; serum folate is measured to determine status	≥6.0 ng folate/ml serum
Iron	Children: 10–15 mg Adolescents and adults: 18 mg	Hypochromic, microcytic anemia	Inadequate intake, long-term TPN without adequate supplementation, frequent blood drawing	Low serum iron will demonstrate deficiency prior to onset of anemia	<2 yr ≥30 μg iron/100 ml 2–5 yr ≥40 μg/100 ml 6–12 yr ≥50 μg/100 ml 13–adult ≥60 μg/100 ml ≥40 μg/100 ml

(continued)

Table 40-3 *(continued)*

Vitamin or Mineral	Daily Requirement	Deficiency Symptoms	Factors Associated with Deficiency	Associated Characteristics	Normal Values for Determination of Status
Magnesium	Infants: 50–70 mg Adults: 300 mg	Neuromuscular dysfunction, tremors, convulsions	Persistent vomiting or diarrhea, prolonged TPN, gastrointestinal diseases and malabsorption, poor intake	Requirements are altered by the presence of renal disease, diuretic use, or inflammatory bowel disease; depressed serum levels indicate deficiency	1.8–3 mg/100 ml
Zinc	Children: 6 mg Adults: 15 mg	Dermatitis, taste changes, poor wound healing, poor appetite	Prolonged TPN without adequate supplementation; inadequate intake	Deficiency may occur with fat malabsorption; serum zinc levels are used to measure status.	101–139 µg/100 ml

counters can measure ^{40}K, which can then be used to estimate total-body potassium and body cell mass, which is the metabolically active tissue component that must be preserved to maintain life[74] (Table 40-2). Other isotope methods can be used to assess body composition (total body water, neutron activation analysis for lean body mass[57]). However, such methods are available only in research environments, and they do not usually help in day-to-day management questions. Repeated anthropometric measurements, on the other hand, can be very useful in clinical settings.

Manifestations of Vitamin and Mineral Deficiency States

Whereas it is unusual for a patient to present with an isolated nutrient deficiency, marginal deficiencies of several vitamins and minerals can occur in groups who are at risk. Patients on intravenous nutritional support without use of gastrointestinal function for an extended period, patients who have sustained radiation or surgical damage to an area of the intestine, and patients with chronic infections who are on antibiotics are especially susceptible to nutrient deficiencies due to malabsorption or lack of adequate supplementation. Protein–calorie malnutrition can be readily diagnosed by examining weight change, serum proteins, dietary history, and anthropometrics. Specific nutrient deficiencies can be masked by the effects of therapy, however, and are more difficult to identify. Suspicion should be maintained in young cancer patients receiving chemotherapy; certain deficiencies are more commonly found in these patients (Table 40-3).[75–79]

In addition, several nutrients warrant special consideration, as deficiencies in children and infants receiving TPN have been documented. Thiamine deficiency has been found in children on long-term parenteral nutrition; the peripheral neuropathy that can accompany this deficiency mimics chemotherapeutic toxicity. Infantile rickets has been observed in low-birth-weight infants; inadequate vitamin D, calcium, and phosphate have all been implicated.[80] Carnitine deficiency has been identified as a possible cause of impaired fat utilization in young children who do not have the reserves or synthetic ca-

pacity of adults.[81,82] Carnitine is an essential nutrient for children but is frequently omitted from TPN solutions.

Guidelines for Protein and Calorie Needs

Whereas the Harrison–Benedict formula and other equations have been used to estimate caloric needs in adults, no standard formulas are available for children under 18 years of age. The Recommended Dietary Allowance of the National Academy of Science categorized by age, gender, and body weight can serve as an initial estimation of caloric need.[79] Although the Recommended Dietary Allowance includes factors for activity that may not apply to the hospitalized child, this increase may be appropriate because of the extra calories a cancer-bearing child may need due to fever, active tumor metabolism, or host metabolism (Table 40-4). These guidelines serve as an initial estimate of protein and calorie requirements. Nitrogen balance and actual energy balance can be measured to ensure that the desired results have been achieved. Alternatively, monitoring changes in weight or serum proteins can give an indication of the adequacy of the prescribed regimen.

Who Needs Nutritional Support?

An assessment of nutritional status requires a physical (weight, height) and laboratory (protein, albumin) examination and an accurate dietary history (Table 40-5). If the child has been receiving cyclic chemotherapy, his or her eating pattern may be altered to avoid periods of nausea. Also, it is not uncommon for sleeping and waking hours to be reversed: the child may sleep through chemotherapy infusions during the day, which will limit hospital meal intake. Diarrhea may be a chronic problem due to irritation of the intestinal mucosa from radiation or chemotherapy.[83] Alternatively, constipation may be a problem because of low dietary fiber intake, lack of activity, or use of narcotic pain medication.

Aggressive nutritional support should be considered in patients who cannot maintain food intake to meet energy de-

Table 40-4
Recommended Intakes of Calories and Protein for Infants and Children (derived from RDA[71])

Age (Years)		kcal/kg Body Weight*	Protein (g/kg Body Wt)
0–0.5		110–120	2.2
0.5–1		100–110	2.0
1–3		90–100	1.8
4–6		80–90	1.5
7–10		75–85	1.2
11–14	M	60–70	1.0
	F	50–60	
15–18	M	45–55	0.8
	F	35–45	

* Factors that increase caloric requirement: fever (12% for each degree over 37°C), surgery (20%–30%), sepsis (40%–50%), growth failure (50%–100%).

Table 40-5
Important Factors in Assessing Dietary History

Appetite or recollection of actual food intake
Recent weight change
Specific food aversion or intolerance
Limited or monotonous diet
Altered taste sensation
Chronic constipation or diarrhea
Use of nutritional supplements
Sleeping periods that interfere with meal hours
Treatment schedule that interferes with meal hours
Medications that affect appetite or gastrointestinal tract

mands. It has been reported that 25% of children undergoing abdominal or pelvic radiation with chemotherapy can be expected to become malnourished.[84] If the child has sustained an injury to the gastrointestinal lining resulting in malabsorption, a trial of a low-residue, low-fat, lactose-free diet may be helpful in alleviating symptoms.[83,85] Elemental diets such as Vital HN or Vivonex may be easily absorbed but are unpalatable. In cases of oral or esophageal mucositis, topical anesthetics along with clear, cool (not hot or cold), nonacidic beverages are often tolerated as the first step in feeding. Clear-liquid protein- and vitamin-fortified supplements such as Citrotein can provide protein. If the diet cannot be advanced to include calorically denser liquids, tube feeding infused below the point of irritation or parenteral nutrition should be considered. Any child who has sustained a weight loss of 5% over a 1-month period or less, has an albumin of 3.0 g/dl or lower, and is receiving treatment expected to prevent adequate nutrient consumption is a candidate for aggressive complete enteral or parenteral nutritional support (see Fig. 40-2).

ENTERAL NUTRITIONAL SUPPORT

Indications for Use

When the voluntary intake of food is inadequate to meet caloric needs, calorically dense oral feedings in the form of special milkshakes or supplements should be the first step. There

are a wide variety of oral supplements available that offer easy administration and minimal preparation. If the child has a functional gastrointestinal tract, enteral supplementation offers many advantages over intravenous feeding, including avoidance of deep-vein catheters and maintenance of gut mucosal integrity. Intestinal mucosa can become significantly atrophied if the patient takes nothing enterally for an extended period of time.[86]

Oral Supplements

Pharmaceutical companies are continually developing new products in accord with the latest nutritional research findings. Solutions differ in caloric density, osmolality, and formulation. These products should be used to augment the patient's usual diet to provide sufficient nutrients to meet individually estimated needs. Table 40-6 lists some of the more common preparations and their indications for use. Modular components are also available, allowing the clinician to tailor make solutions to an individual patient's needs by separately prescribing the amount of protein, fat, and carbohydrate. Regular foods can also be supplemented with individual nutrient components.

The greatest limitation to the use of oral supplements in the pediatric cancer population is patient acceptance. Milkshakes made with familiar products, possibly supplemented with Polycose, a carbohydrate supplement composed of glucose polymers or other nondetectable modular components, are usually most easily tolerated. The soy-based formulas can be useful for the child who is lactose-intolerant and come flavored to improve palatability. The presence of mouth or esophageal sores will limit tolerance for oral supplements of any kind, and diarrhea may be aggravated by hyperosmolar or lactose-containing products. Encouragement from the staff and family can help improve patient compliance with taking oral supplements.

Tube Feedings

A small soft tube is passed through the nasopharynx and stomach into the small intestine (this task can be facilitated by the use of fluoroscopy), and elemental feedings are provided as a constant infusion. Initially, the solution is infused at half-strength, and the volume given is increased slowly until maintainance volumes are being provided. Finally, the concentration of the solution is increased until the required caloric needs are met. If diarrhea is encountered during the increase in volume or concentration, the physician should decrease the volume or concentration, respectively. If adequate calorie needs cannot be provided by tube feeding because of diarrhea or large gastric residuals, TPN should be considered (see Fig. 40-2).

The solution should be low in osmolality, nutritionally complete, and, preferably, lactose free. Commercial preparations made from blenderized foods, such as Compleat–Modified, contain soluble fiber, which is helpful in managing both constipation and diarrhea, and are given as boluses into the stomach. Other commonly used formulas are the soy-based, 1 to 2 Cal/ml solutions. If the feeding tube has been placed in the small bowel, an elemental or peptide formula is recommended. Although these feedings require minimal digestion, they are generally much higher in osmolality.

The most common complications of tube feedings are diarrhea and delayed gastric emptying. Constipation can occur with long-term use of a product low in residue, but it is rarely a problem. When managing diarrhea, it is important to establish

Table 40-6
Selected Tube Feeding and Oral Supplement Products

Name	kcal/ ml	mOsm/ kg H₂O	Protein/Fat/ Carbohydrate (g/liter)	Na/K⁺ (mEq/liter)	Sources Protein	Fat	Carbohydrate	Special Properties and Indications for Use
Vital-HN	1	460	42/11/185	20/34	Whey, soy, meat protein hydrolysates; free amino acids	Safflower oil, MCT oil	Hydrolyzed corn starch; sucrose	Useful for malabsorption maldigestion; contains free amino acids and peptides; 1500 ml provides RDA for vitamins; flavored; especially useful as a jejunostomy feeding
Vivonex Ten	1	630	38/3/206	20/20	ʟ-Amino acids, high branched-chain	Safflower oil	Maltodextrin; modified starch	Branched-chain-enriched, elemental formula; 2000 ml provides RDA for vitamins; flavored; especially useful as a tube feeding, for malabsorption/ maldigestion
Amin-Aid	2	1095	19/46/366	<15/<16	Crystalline essential amino acids	Soy oil, lecithin, monoglyceride, and diglycerides	Maltodextrin; sucrose	Low-electrolyte, essential amino acid formula for renal disease; flavored; for oral or tube feeding
Hepatic-Aid	1.1	560	44/36/169	<15/<6	Crystalline amino acids; high branched-chain	Soy oil, lecithin, monoglycerides and diglycerides	Maltodextrin; sucrose	Low-electrolyte, high branched-chain amino acid formula for liver disease; flavored; for oral or tube feeding
Ensure	1	450	37/37/145	37/40	Na and Ca caseinate; soy protein isolate	Corn oil	Hydrolyzed corn starch; sucrose	Nutritionally complete; 1890 ml provides RDA for vitamins; flavored; lactose-free; for oral or tube feeding
Ensure Plus	1.5	600	55/53/200	50/60	Na and Ca caseinate; soy protein isolate	Corn oil	Hydrolyzed corn starch; sucrose	Nutritionally complete; 1600 ml provides RDA for vitamins; lactose-free; flavored; for oral or tube feeding
Compleat– Modified	1	300	43/37/141	29/36	Beef; Ca caseinate; vegetables	Corn oil	Hydrolyzed cereal solids; fruit and vegetable puree	Nutritionally complete; 1500 ml provides RDA for vitamins; lactose-free; isotonic; blenderized tube feeding
Osmolite	1	300	37/39/145	24/26	Ca and Na caseinate; soy protein isolate	MCT oil; corn oil; soy oil	Hydrolyzed corn starch	Nutritionally complete; 1890 ml provides RDA for vitamins; lactose-free; isotonic; unflavored; for oral or tube feeding

whether the problem preceded initiation of the feeding, as it may be the result of an underlying infection or medications.

The rate and strength at which to initiate tube feeding will depend on the osmolality of the product and the individual tolerance of the patient. In general, beginning a tube feeding at half strength with a rate of 50 ml per hour is reasonable; the volume and strength are then advanced as rapidly as tolerated to meet the calculated requirement. If tube feeding is being started after the patient has had nothing by mouth for an extended period, the absorptive areas along the intestinal wall may be atrophied. It may then take several days of slow nutrient infusion for regeneration to occur, during which time mild diarrhea will be observed. The initial step in controlling diarrhea is decreasing the concentration of the feeding. The feeding should be given at room temperature and hung for no longer than the time recommended by the manufacturer to prevent bacterial contamination.[85] If diarrhea persists beyond 2 to 3 days with a diluted product, a trial of a more elemental feeding or of one containing soluble fiber may be helpful, starting at a concentration that is iso-osmotic or less. Antidiarrheal agents can also be used.

Hyperosmolar nonketotic coma can occur with hyperosmolar tube feedings, and this complication must be avoided by monitoring serum electrolytes and glucose. Delayed gastric emptying is usually managed by decreasing the rate of infusion or switching to a low-fat solution.

Clinical conditions that contraindicate the use of tube feeding include a nonfunctional gastrointestinal tract or obstruction, gastrointestinal bleeding, severe ulcerations that may be irritated by the tube, persistent nausea and vomiting, or severe uncontrollable diarrhea. Individual preference plays a part; some clinicians use tube feeding when others prefer parenteral feeding. If possible, tube feeding is the initial approach (see Fig. 40-2).

PARENTERAL NUTRITIONAL SUPPORT

Indications for Use

Unfortunately, the pediatric cancer patient sometimes cannot ingest, digest, or absorb food via the gastrointestinal tract. In general, use of the gastrointestinal tract for alimentation, including a small feeding tube placed into the small intestine, is desirable; but for some patients, it is not acceptable (see Fig. 40-2). Even with a functional gastrointestinal tract, some physicians prefer to begin with parenteral nutrition, which can be given safely to these high-risk patients with low white blood cell and platelet counts. Total parenteral nutrition serves as a reliable source of nutrients. Since TPN does not appear to improve survival or response to therapy, the only indication for it is to maintain normal body composition in a growing patient and to prevent starvation. In a patient with normal reserves, death from total starvation occurs in 60 to 70 days if adequate fluids are provided. Therefore, TPN is not indicated in patients with reasonable baseline status who have only mild anorexia and vomiting associated with cycles of chemotherapy or other treatments. The percentile value of weight for height and age should provide a standard reference, and if a patient is more than 5% below usual weight, nutritional support is indicated. Aggressive treatment regimens with nutritional morbidity are also a factor in deciding whether to use nutritional support (see Fig. 40-2). If a patient will have chronic nausea and vomiting (30 days or greater) while undergoing antitumor treatment, parenteral nutritional support is indicated. Nutritional support is not effective in decreasing therapy complications or in im-

proving survival or response to therapy. It is indicated to attempt to maintain or improve the composition of a cachectic patient who must undergo a treatment that may further reduce the body cell mass. In its current form, TPN can maintain vital body mass in some patients receiving anticancer treatment. A cancer patient should not die from starvation with current methods of parenteral support.

Solution Composition

Numerous intravenous solutions for parenteral nutrition are now available. A synthetic amino acid source (5% amino acids) is required, and an energy source, usually glucose (20%–25%), is also administered (Table 40-7). In pediatric patients, it is recommended to give 30% of the nonprotein calories as fat administered daily as a 10% or 20% lipid solution. Peripheral amino acid solutions are not indicated because they cannot maintain positive nitrogen balance. Special amino acid solutions are available for patients in hepatic or renal failure but are rarely indicated. Hepatic solutions are useful to reverse hepatic coma in patients with severe hepatic encephalopathy. Renal failure solutions are used to limit dialysis in patients with acute renal failure (blood urea nitrogen exceeding 100 mg/dl). Branched chain-enriched solutions have been used in stressed oncology patients and may improve nitrogen balance.[87] Although the value of adding albumin to the TPN solution is unproved, it can be safely added to diminish insulin binding to the container.

Trace metals are administered daily to prevent deficiency. Recommended dosages are listed in Table 40-8. Vitamin deficiencies are common in young patients receiving vitamin-free TPN. One vial of MVI-12 (USV Laboratories) generally provides adequate vitamin maintainance levels without toxicity,[88] and in these patients with frequent blood drawing or other loss, 12.5 mg daily of parenteral iron (Inferon; Merrill National Laboratories, Cincinnati, Ohio) also is necessary (Table 40-8).[89] Insulin can also be added to maintain glucose homeostasis. Many recommend adding insulin only for glucose intolerance (greater than 200 mg/dl), but experimental data in animals[90] and humans[91] indicate that added insulin may improve nutrient utilization and so preserve host tissues. There-

---

Table 40-7
General Formulations for TPN: Amounts per Day

Age (yr)	Fluid (ml/kg)	Calories (kcal/kg)*	Electrolytes (mEq/kg)†
0–1	130	90–120	
1–8	80–120	75–90	
9–15	50–75	60–75	
>15	50	30–55	
All			
Na			2.0–4.0
K			1.5–2.0
Ca phosphate			0.15–0.20
Mg			0.15–0.25

* Calorie composition: 20% to 30% fat (as a 10% or 20% lipid supplement infused once daily), 50% to 60% carbohydrate (usually 20%–25% dextrose [glucose] by weight), and 10% to 20% protein (amino acids; usually 5% by weight).
† Not age dependent; formulas apply to all ages.

Table 40-8
Recommended Vitamin and Trace Element Dosage for TPN

Vitamin or Trace Element	Daily Dose*
A	3,300 IU
D	200 IU
E	12–15 IU
C	100 mg
Folate	400 µg
Niacin	40 mg
Riboflavin	3.6 mg
Thiamin	3 mg
B6	4 mg
B12	5 mg
Pantothenic acid	15 mg
Biotin	60 µg
Zinc	5 mg
Copper	1.4 mg
Manganese	0.5 mg
Iodine	56 mg
Chromium	16 µg
Selenomethionine	200 µg
Iron	12.5 mg

* Dosage recommended for adults but used safely in children.

fore, it is better to maintain blood sugar below 125 mg/dl and add insulin as necessary to do it.

Technical Considerations

Venous access remains a problem in all pediatric oncology patients as a result of patient size plus repetitive venous puncture for administration of chemotherapy and monitoring of hematologic toxicity. TPN requires a central site of infusion because of the high osmolality of the solution, and the subclavian route is the preferred site. It is better to create the access in the operating room with either general or local-standby anesthesia and fluoroscopic control. We use multilumen catheters and allow administration of drugs and sampling of blood through the other ports.

Permanent venous access catheters such as a Hickman or indwelling catheters such as the Port-a-cath are inserted more easily through the internal jugular than the subclavian vein (see Chap. 10). The difference is that permanent catheters require venous dilatation and introducers for percutaneous placement. Fewer life-threatening and technical complications are possible with the internal jugular approach. Several studies indicate that internal permanent catheters have fewer infectious complications than exiting catheters. However, internal catheters take longer to insert and also require a second operation to remove. Any of these catheters can be used for TPN.

Subclavian vein thrombosis is a more common complication than initially expected in patients with TPN or long-term venous access. It should be considered a possibility if one has difficulty puncturing a subclavian vein or detects swelling of an upper extremity. The diagnostic procedure of choice is an upper-extremity venogram. If thrombosis is found, it is recommended to remove the catheter and treat the patient with systemic heparin until the swelling resolves or for at least 7 to 10 days. Pulmonary emboli have been documented from subcla-

vian vein thrombosis. An incidence of subclavian vein thrombosis as high as 10% has been described in patients with cancer undergoing chemotherapy and nutritional support.[92]

Fever is a common accompaniment of chemotherapy, especially in patients with a white blood cell count less than 500/mm[3] (see Chap. 39). Most of the time, the fever is not caused by the catheter, and when the white count recovers, the fever disappears.[93] However, if there is any evidence that the catheter is the source of sepsis and the infection cannot be eradicated with antibiotic therapy, we do not hesitate to remove the catheter. Septic thrombophlebitis of the subclavian vein is a life-threatening complication that must be avoided. It requires excision of the subclavian vein as well as a long course of antibiotics.

Metabolic complications such as hyperchloremic acidosis, hyperosmolar nonketotic coma, and lactic acidosis can occur during TPN in cancer patients. These complications are less frequent when clinicians remain vigilant. Early detection of metabolic complications makes potential life-threatening complications easily correctable.

Guidelines for Administration in Children and Infants

The percentages of calories from each of the major nutrients should approach the percentages recommended for an oral diet: 30 for fat, 50 to 60 for carbohydrate, and 10 to 20 for protein (see Table 40-7). Total calorie and protein requirements are estimated in Table 40-4. Thirty per cent of calories are provided as fat emulsion (Intralipid, Liposyn). No more than 4 g/kg of body weight per day of fat emulsion is given to children, and no more than 3 g/kg of body weight per day is given to adults. Excessive administration of carbohydrate is avoided to reduce the risk of glucose intolerance and fatty liver.[94,95] Serum triglycerides are checked weekly to verify normal lipid clearance, which may be impaired in cachexia.[39]

Fluid Volumes for Age and Body Size

Guidelines for providing adequate fluid intake must take into account many factors. Generally, children tolerate larger fluid volumes than adults; 1.5 ml/kcal per day for infants, and 1 ml/kcal per day for adults is considered reasonable under ordinary circumstances.[79] In terms of body weight, this calculates as approximately 130 ml/kg per day for ages 0 to 12 months, 80 to 120 ml/kg per day for 1 to 8 years, 50 to 75 ml/kg per day for 8 to 15 years, and about 50 ml/kg per day for over 15 years (see Table 40-7). Factors that will increase needs include fever, diarrhea, hyperventilation, vomiting, or polyuria. Patients who are comatose or are taking diuretics need especially careful monitoring, as do patients with cardiovascular or renal disease. Children receiving TPN may need excess fluids in order to provide adequate calories.[96]

Special Complications Related to Total Parenteral Nutrition

Metabolic abnormalities can develop as a consequence of TPN. Most abnormalities are alleviated by manipulation of the solution composition and by careful monitoring of laboratory values.

The most common abnormal finding in patients on intravenous feeding is abnormal liver function test results (Table 40-9), which occur frequently in patients who have received TPN for 1 week or longer.[94] These mild abnormalities will return to normal when the feeding is discontinued. In the cancer patient, elevated liver enzymes may be a reflection of the disease, and the concurrent administration of parenteral nutrition can make mild abnormalities worse.

The etiology of the liver function abnormalities observed during TPN is not precisely known; however, several theories exist. Excess carbohydrate administration is associated with fatty infiltration and excess liver glycogen deposition. One treatment is reducing the amount of carbohydrate and replacing those calories with lipid emulsion.[95] An imbalance of amino acids or omission of certain amino acids from standard protein solutions has also been proposed as a reason for elevated liver enzymes.[97] Taurine deficiency has been identified as a possible cause of cholestasis in infants, potentially leading to liver dysfunction.[98] Fat emulsion may also transiently raise liver enzyme concentrations, a change that may be related to a lack of carnitine or other factors.[81,82] The abnormalities of liver function with TPN are mild (Table 40-9); greater abnormalities usually indicate another cause of liver toxicity.

Cholestasis after an extended period of parenteral feeding has been reported and is reversed by cholecystokinin or oral fat in small amounts.[80,98,99] Premature infants are at high risk for this complication. It has been suggested that providing a small amount of oral fat to stimulate the gallbladder helps prevent cholestasis; it has been theorized that this problem, too, is related to carnitine deficiency. The most effective treatment is to decrease the parenteral feeding as soon as possible and resume enteral feeding.

Glucose intolerance and lactic acidosis[34] can occur with administration of large volumes of carbohydrate. Many cancer patients exhibit a diabetic-type glucose tolerance curve,[100] which can exacerbate hyperglycemia. The standard treatment is exogenous insulin, usually directly in the parenteral nutrition solution. Enough insulin must be added to compensate for the portion that will adhere to the glass or plastic container. Alternatively, albumin can be added.

The influence of parenteral feeding on pulmonary status has been studied. Two major concerns have been identified: the effect of parenteral nutrition on respiratory quotient and the possibility of lipid accumulation in the alveoli.[101] High carbohydrate loads will measurably increase oxygen demand, which may lead to difficulty in weaning ventilator-dependent patients. Replacing a portion of the administered carbohydrate calories with fat emulsion is a standard treatment.

OUTPATIENT NUTRITIONAL MANAGEMENT

Basic Nutritional Care

Nutritional intervention is probably most effective when the child is receiving treatment as an outpatient or is between cycles of therapy. Access to the child's favorite foods is easier then, and the interruptions for tests and scheduled treatment are removed. Moreover, children frequently associate the hospital environment with the side effects they have experienced on chemotherapy and may develop anticipatory nausea and vomiting. During the outpatient period, emphasis should be placed on maximizing calorie and protein intake for the child who is nutritionally depleted and on weight maintenance for the child who is adequately nourished or overweight. Exercise or activity should be encouraged to maintain lean body mass.

There is some evidence that patients can help protect themselves from infections by avoiding all raw vegetables and salads during periods of neutropenia. This proposal comes from a study reporting isolation of *Enterobacter, Klebsiella, Pseudomonas,* and other bacteria from salads. The presence of bacteria was attributed to both contamination by food service workers and the natural flora of the vegetables.[102] The significance that this restriction would have for preventing infection is unclear, particularly in the absence of other precautionary measures.

A well-balanced diet is always prudent for any child, especially one who is undergoing cancer treatment. If a child becomes significantly malnourished, however, intake of adequate calories and protein becomes a high priority. If this goal can be accomplished only with the high-fat, high-carbohydrate "junk food" preferred by many children, this should be permitted, supplemented with high protein foods and a general multivitamin preparation. When the acute weight loss has been corrected, a varied diet composed of adequate amounts of fruits, vegetables, starches, lean meats, and dairy products should be substituted.

Sometimes, even provision of favorite foods may not coax the child to eat, even in the absence of obvious physical causes. Anorexia may stem from other factors such as poor pain control, taste changes, and depression. With adolescents, suspicion should be maintained that anorexia nervosa may underlie the disease process. Although it is often difficult to distinguish anorexia of emotional from that of organic cause, the possibil-

Table 40-9
Impact of TPN on Liver Function[94]

Duration of TPN (wk)	Total Bilirubin (mg/dl)	Direct Bilirubin (mg/dl)	SGOT (IU/liter)	SGPT (IU/liter)	LDH (IU/liter)	Alkaline Phosphatase (IU/liter)
0 (normal range)	<1.4	<0.3	<30	<42	<250	<120
1*	1.5	1.3	50	75	400	160
2	1.5	1.5	42	73	300	180
3	2.5	1.5	45	77	300	200
4	1.4	2.0	42	60	400	220
5	1.3	1.1	40	60	300	200
6	1.8	1.0	43	60	300	200
7	2.0	1.5	50	60	500	220

* Elevation greater than that indicated here probably marks another cause of reduced liver function such as occult sepsis.

ity of a psychological component should be addressed with the patient if physical examination fails to produce an organic basis for restricted food intake. In patients with anorexia nervosa as a component, the first emphasis must be on returning the patient to a stable condition and continuing antineoplastic therapy. Once the patient is stabilized, psychiatric intervention by an individual familiar with eating disorders may be necessary. Control of the tumor and control of the anorexia nervosa must be dealt with as separate issues.

There are chemotherapeutic regimens that promote excessive weight gain, particularly those that involve steroids. Retrospective studies of children in long-term remission from acute lymphocytic leukemia indicate that excess weight gain can start during treatment and persist long into remission.[103] The most effective approach to avoid excessive weight gain is prompt counseling after intensive treatment as the child progresses to maintenance chemotherapy. This approach provides the child with a single goal during each treatment period. Food restriction during stressful periods such as intensive treatment may make treatment more difficult. When dietary restrictions are implemented, the goal is weight maintenance, which prevents any stunting of overall growth because of inadequate nutrition.

Home Tube Feeding

The use of home tube feeding is recommended for the outpatient with malnutrition due to poor appetite. The criteria for selecting who should be placed on home tube feeding are similar to the criteria for deciding which inpatients may benefit from a tube feeding coupled with an assessment of the ability of the family to manage the feeding outside the hospital. Severe oral or esophageal ulcerations or radiation injury to the gastrointestinal tract contraindicate use; however, there remain a significant number of malnourished patients who can benefit from outpatient tube feedings. Some patients will object to the discomfort of frequent nasogastric tube placements and to the appearance of the tube if it is left in position between feedings.[104] These disadvantages are outweighed by the risks and expense of home TPN.[46] Tube feeding offers the additional advantage of maintaining the intestinal absorptive villi.

Home tube feeding can usually be managed by the family with adequate training. A responsible adult is designated to place the tube and administer the solution. Feeding pumps are helpful but not necessary. Proper sanitary measures are emphasized, including care of the bag and the tubing and the length of time the solution may be left at room temperature. Commercial solutions (see Table 40-6) are easy to use, although mixtures also can be prepared using blended or baby foods.[86,105] As with inpatients on tube feeding, the patient should be weighed regularly and laboratory values monitored for any symptoms of nutritional inadequacy.

Home Total Parenteral Nutrition

For the malnourished patient who is not responsive to oral repletion and not a candidate for home tube feeding, home parenteral nutrition can reverse malnutrition while allowing the patient time out of the hospital.[106] Teaching should begin prior to discharge from the hospital. The designated home health care agency works with the hospital health care team to establish solution composition and provide effective patient education. Complete solutions are supplied by the health care agency or delivered to the patient as components for mixing at home. Laboratory values are monitored regularly, and the results are used to determine any adjustments in solution composition. The patient should be weighed daily to confirm the appropriateness of fluid volume and nutrient content.[107]

Home TPN can be delivered in either a cyclic or a continuous fashion; administration over 8 to 12 hours during the evening allows more freedom of movement, if the larger fluid volumes can be tolerated.

The decision to administer home parenteral nutrition is based on medical feasibility and prognosis. Although it can be argued that home parenteral feeding should not be used to delay the inevitable death from underlying disease, the decision becomes more difficult when effective palliation can be achieved, and nutritional support may significantly improve the patient's last months of life. As a guideline, the patient should have an estimated survival of 12 weeks to be considered for home parenteral nutrition.

Vitamin, Macrobiotic, and Other Unconventional Diet Therapies

The search for an effective treatment for cancer has led researchers to look at the effect of vitamins on the growth of malignancies. Vitamin A in high doses has been used in patients with acute myelogenous leukemia as part of the consolidation regimen and may have a role in cancer treatment when used pharmacologically with other chemotherapeutic drugs.[108] As a vitamin supplement, however, high doses of vitamin A are hepatotoxic. Vitamin C has also been studied as a treatment for cancer and can be consumed in amounts 8 to 10 times the Recommended Dietary Allowance without serious consequence. However, its utility in the treatment of malignancy has not been supported in controlled trials.[109] Epidemiologic studies have suggested that selenium and zinc have a protective effect against certain types of tumors.[110]

Generally, excess amounts of any vitamin or mineral should be discouraged due to the potential for toxicity, especially in patients receiving hepatotoxic drugs. A general multivitamin, formulated for the patient's particular age group, given between cycles of therapy seems at present to be the most prudent advice.

Repeatedly, various diets are promoted as a treatment for cancer, either in combination with or in lieu of conventional therapy.[111] One diet that continues to surface is the "macrobiotic" diet, which proposes that all cancers are the result of a chemical "imbalance" in the body and are treatable by restoring the proper "balance" with dietary manipulations. No controlled studies as yet support the use of macrobiotics to treat or control cancer, although studies and reports have been done on the nutritional consequences. The majority of difficulties with these diets arise when the diet is deficient in certain nutrients; cases of scurvy, folate, and protein deficiency have been reported.[112] Vegetarian diets are also frequently promoted as being beneficial to cancer patients; however, such a diet eliminates the principal sources of absorbable iron in the American diet. A diet high in fruits and vegetables is generally high in bulk and low in protein and calories, and it is especially difficult for the pediatric patient to meet his or her nutritional needs on such a diet. Eliminating dairy products removes the chief source of dietary calcium, an especially important nutrient for the growing child.

Any diet used by patients with cancer should provide adequate nutrients to allow tolerance to therapy with proven antineoplastic activity. Both radiation and chemotherapy can cause significant nutritional depletion; a dietary regimen that compounds the problem by providing inadequate nutrients or toxic excesses of nutrients should be avoided. A professional trained in nutrition should be consulted to examine any unusual dietary regimen for nutritional adequacy.

REFERENCES

1. Norton JA, Peacock JL, Morrison SD: Cancer cachexia. CRC Crit Rev Oncol Hematol 7:289, 1987
2. Costa G: Cachexia: The metabolic component of neoplastic disease. Prog Exp Tumor Res 3:321, 1963
3. Strain AJ: Cancer cachexia in man: A review. Invest Cell Pathol 2:181, 1979
4. Midler GB: Neoplastic diseases: Some metabolic aspects. Annu Rev Med 4:187, 1953
5. Carter P, Carr D, van Eys J et al: Energy and nutrient intake of children with cancer. J Am Diet Assoc 82:610, 1983
6. Carter P, Carr D, van Eys J, Coody D: Nutritional parameters in children with cancer. J Am Diet Assoc 82:616, 1983
7. Donaldson SS, Wesley MN, DeWys WD et al: A study of the nutritional status of pediatric cancer patients. Am J Dis Child 135:1107, 1981
8. Van Eys J: Nutrition and cancer: Physiological interrelationships. Annu Rev Nutr 5:435, 1985
9. DeWys WD, Begg D, Lavin PT et al: Prognostic effect of weight loss prior to chemotherapy in cancer patients. Am J Med 69:491, 1980
10. Mider GB: Some aspects of nitrogen and energy metabolism in cancerous subjects: A review. Cancer Res 11:821, 1951
11. Waterhouse C, Fenninger LD, Keutmann EM: Nitrogen exchange and caloric expenditures in patients with malignant neoplasm. Cancer 4:500, 1951
12. Mayer J, Marshall NB, Vitale JJ et al: Exercise, food intake and body weight in normal rats and genetically obese adult mice. Am J Physiol 177:544, 1954
13. Brobeck JR: Food and temperature. Recent Prog Hormone Res 16:439, 1960
14. Morrison SE: Feeding response to change in absorbable food fraction during growth of Walker 256 carcinosarcoma. Cancer Res 32:968, 1972
15. Morrison SE: The total energy and water metabolism during pregnancy in the rat. J Physiol (Lond) 134:650, 1956
16. Hansell DT, Davies JWL, Burns HJG: The relationship between resting energy expenditure and weight loss in benign and malignant disease. Ann Surg 203:240, 1986
17. Peacock JL, Inculet RI, Corsey R, Norton JA: Resting energy expenditure and body cell mass alterations in sarcoma patients. Surg Forum 37:11, 1986
18. Ohnuma T, Holland JF: Nutritional consequences of cancer chemotherapy and immunotherapy. Cancer Res 37:2395, 1977
19. Donaldson SS: Nutritional consequences of radiotherapy. Cancer Res 37:2407, 1977
20. DeWys WD: Taste and feeding behavior in patients with cancer. Curr Concepts Nutr 6:131, 1977
21. DeWys WD: Anorexia as a general effect of cancer. Cancer 43(suppl):2013, 1979
22. Carson JS, Gormican A: Taste acuity and food attitudes of selected patients with cancer. J Am Diet Assoc 70:361, 1977
23. Norton JA, Lowry SF, Brennan MF: Effect of work-induced hypertrophy on skeletal muscle of tumor- and nontumor-bearing rats. J Appl Physiol 46:6540, 1979
24. Goodlad GAJ, Clark CM: Leucine metabolism in skeletal muscle of the tumor-bearing rat. Eur J Cancer 16:1153, 1980
25. Heber D, Chleboroski TR, Ishibachi DE, Herrold JN, Block JB: Abnormalities in glucose and protein metabolism in non-cachectic lung cancer patients. Cancer Res 42:4815, 1982
26. Norton JA, Shamberger R, Stein TP, Milne GWA, Brennan MF: The influence of tumor-bearing on protein metabolism in the rat. J Surg Res 30:456, 1981
27. Cori CF, Cori FT: The carbohydrate metabolism of tumors. J Biol Chem 65:397, 1925
28. Gullino RM, Granthan FM, Courtney AM: Glucose consumption by transplanted tumors in vivo. Cancer Res 27:1031, 1967
29. Burt ME, Lowry SF, Gorschboth C, Brennan MF: Metabolic alterations in a noncachectic animal tumor system. Cancer 47:2138, 1981
30. Norton JA, Maher M, Wesley R, Whjite D, Brennan MF: Glucose intolerance in sarcoma patients. Cancer 54:3022, 1984
31. Arbeit JM, Burt ME, Rubinstein IV, Gorschboth CM, Brennan MF: Glucose metabolism and the percentage of glucose derived from alanine: Response to exogenous infusion in tumor-bearing and non-tumor-bearing rats. Cancer Res 42:4936, 1982
32. Waterhouse C, Jeanpretre N, Keilson J: Gluconeogenesis from alanine in patients with progressive malignant disease. Cancer Res 39:1968, 1979
33. Holroyd CP, Reichard GA: Carbohydrate metabolism in cancer cachexia. Cancer Treat Rep 65(5):55, 1981
34. Goodgame JT, Pizzo P, Brennan MF: Iatrogenic lactic acidosis: Association with hypertonic glucose administration in a patient with cancer. Cancer 42:800, 1979
35. Begg RW: Tumor–host relations. Adv Cancer Res 5:1, 1958
36. Kitada S, Hays EF, Mead JF: A lipid mobilizing factor in the serum of tumor-bearing mice. Lipids 15:168, 1980
37. Masumo H, Yamasaki N, Okuda H: Purification and characterization of a lipolytic factor (toxohormone-L) from cell free fluid of ascites sarcoma 180. Cancer Res 41:284, 1981
38. Schein PS, Kisner DD, Hatter D, Blecher M, Hamosh M: Cachexia of malignancy: Potential role of insulin in nutritional management. Cancer 43:2070, 1979
39. Devereaux DF, Redgrave TG, Tilton M, Hollander D, Deckers PJ: Intolerance to administered lipids in tumor-bearing animals. Surgery 96:414, 1984
40. Fossel ET, Carr JM, McDonagh J: Detection of malignant tumors: Water-suppressed proton nuclear magnetic resonance spectroscopy of plasma. N Engl J Med 315:1369, 1986
41. Wieczorek AJ, Rhyner C, Block LH: Isolation and characterization of an RNA–proteolipid complex associated with the malignant state in humans. Proc Natl Acad Sci USA 82:3455, 1985
42. Beutler B, Cerami A: Cachectin and tumor necrosis factor as two sides of the same biological coin. Nature 320:584, 1986
43. Cahill GF Jr: Starvation in man. N Engl J Med 282:668, 1970
44. Tracey KJ, Beutler B, Lowry SF et al: Shock and tissue injury induced by recombinant human cachectin. Science 234:470, 1986
45. Meguid MM, Brennan MF, Aoki TT et al: Hormone substrate interrelationships following trauma. Arch Surg 109:776, 1974
46. Brennan MF: Total parenteral nutrition in the cancer patient. N Engl J Med 305:375, 1981
47. Shamberger RC, Brennan MF, Goodgame JT et al: A prospective, randomized study of adjuvant parenteral nutrition in the treatment of sarcomas: Results of metabolic and survival studies. Surgery 96:1, 1984
48. Popp MB, Wagner SC, Brito OJ: Host and tumor responses to increasing levels of intravenous nutritional support. Surgery 94:300, 1983
49. Baron PL, Larence W, Chan WMY, White FKN, Banks WL: Effects of parenteral nutrition on cell cycle kinetics of head and neck cancer. Arch Surg 121:1282, 1986
50. Brennan MF, Copeland EM: Panel report on nutritional support of patients with cancer. Am J Clin Nutr 34:1199, 1981
51. Kern KA, Brunetti A, Norton JA et al: Metabolic imaging of human extremity musculoskeletal tumors by PET. J Nucl Med 29:181, 1988
52. Norton JA, Burt ME, Brennan MF: In vivo utilization of substrate by human sarcoma-bearing limbs. Cancer 45:2934, 1980
53. Lazo PA: Tumor–host metabolic interaction and cachexia. FEBS Lett 187:189, 1985
54. Klein CL, Camitta BM: Increased whole-body protein turnover in sick children with newly diagnosed leukemia or lymphoma. Cancer Res 43:5586, 1983
55. Herrmann VM, Garnick MB, Moore FD, Wilmore DW: Effect of cytotoxic agents on protein kinetics in patients with metastatic cancer. Surgery 90:381, 1981
56. Burt ME, Borschboth CM, Brennan MF: A controlled, prospective, randomized trial evaluating the metabolic effects of enteral and parenteral nutrition in the cancer patient. Cancer 49:1092, 1982
57. Shike M, Russell D, Detsky A et al: Changes in body composition with small-cell lung cancer: The effect of total parenteral nutrition as an adjunct to chemotherapy. Ann Intern Med 101:303, 1984
58. Koretz RL: Parenteral nutrition: Is it oncologically logical? J Clin Oncol 2:534, 1984
59. van Eys J, Copeland EM, Cangir A et al: A clinical trial of hyperalimentation in children with metastatic malignancies. Med Pediatr Oncol 8:63, 1980
60. Donaldson SS, Wesley MN, Gharrini F et al: A prospective randomized clinical trial of total parenteral nutrition in children with cancer. Med Pediatr Oncol 10:129, 1982
61. Gharrini F, Shils ME, Scott BF et al: Comparison of morbidity in children requiring abdominal radiation and chemotherapy, with and without total parenteral nutrition. J Pediatr 101:530, 1982
62. Shamberger RC, Pizzo PA, Goodgame JT et al: The effect of total paren-

teral nutrition on chemotherapy-induced myelosuppression. Am J Med 74:40, 1983

63. Apelgren KN, Wilmore DW: Parenteral nutrition: Is it oncologically logical? —A response. J Clin Oncol 2:539, 1984

64. Mize CE, Cunningham C, Teitell BC et al: Undernutrition in pediatric inpatients: Repeated nutritional status evaluation. Nutr Suppl Serv 4:4, 1984

65. Pendergrass TW, Foulkes MA, Robison LL, Nesbit ME: Stature and Ewing's sarcoma in childhood. Am J Pediatr Hematol Oncol 6:33, 1984

66. Frisancho AR: Triceps skinfold and upper arm muscle size norms for assessment of nutritional status. Am J Clin Nutr 27:1052, 1974

67. Grant A: Nutritional Assessment Guidelines. Seattle, Cutter Medical, 1979

68. Merritt RJ, Kalsh M, Roux LD, et al: Significance of hypoalbuminemia in pediatric oncology patients: Malnutrition or infection? JPEN 9:303, 1985

69. Tilkian SM, Conover MB, Tilkian AG: Clinical Implications of Laboratory Tests. St Louis, CV Mosby, 1983

70. van Eys J, Hilliard J: Nutritional status and immune function in childhood cancer. Nutr Cancer 2:61, 1980

71. Ramirez I, van Eys J, Carr D et al: Immunologic evaluation in the nutritional assessment of children with cancer. Am J Clin Nutr 41:1314, 1985

72. Viteri FE, Alvarado J: The creatinine:height index: Its use in the estimation of the degree of protein depletion and repletion in protein malnourished children. Pediatrics 46:696, 1976

73. Meredith HV: Childhood studies on thickness of skin and subcutaneous adipose tissue at arm back: A review. Hum Biol 57:525, 1985

74. Moore FD: Energy and maintenance of body cell mass. JPEN 4:228, 1980

75. Norton JA, Peters ML, Wesley R et al: Iron supplementation of total parenteral nutrition: A prospective study. JPEN 7:457, 1983

76. Mock DM, Baswell DL, Baker H et al: Biotin deficiency complicating parenteral alimentation: Diagnosis, metabolic repercussions, and treatment. J Pediatr 106:762, 1985

77. Gillis J, Murphy FR, Boxall LBH, Pencharz PB: Biotin deficiency in a child on long-term total parenteral nutrition. JPEN 6:308, 1982

78. Ovesen L: Vitamin therapy in the absence of obvious deficiency: What is the evidence? Drugs 27:148, 1984

79. National Research Council: Recommended Dietary Allowances, 9th ed. Washington, DC, National Academy of Sciences, 1980

80. Toomey F, Hoag R, Batton D, Vain N: Rickets associated with cholestasis and parenteral nutrition in premature infants. Radiology 142:85, 1982

81. Rubecz I, Sandor A, Hamar A, Mestyan J: Blood levels of total carnitine and lipid utilization with and without carnitine supplementation in newborn infants. Acta Paediatr Hung 25:165, 1984

82. Worthley LIG, Fishlock RC, Snoswell AM: Carnitine balance and effects of intravenous L-carnitine in two patients receiving long-term total parenteral nutrition. JPEN 6:717, 1984

83. Donaldson SS, Jundt S, Ricour C et al: Radiation enteritis in children. Cancer 35:1167, 1975

84. Donaldson SS, Wesley MN, Ghavimi F et al: A prospective randomized clinical trial of TPN in children with cancer. Med Pediatr Oncol 10:129, 1982

85. Hyams JS, Batrus CL, Grand RJ, Sallan SE: Cancer chemotherapy-induced lactose malabsorption in children. Cancer 49:646, 1982

86. Torosian MH, Rombeau JL: Feeding by tube enterostomy. Surg Gynecol Obstet 150:918, 1980

87. Bonau RA, Ang SD, Jeevanandam M, Daly JM: High branched-chain amino acid solutions improve nitrogen balance in stressed patients. Surg Forum 36:49, 1985

88. Inculet RI, Norton JA, Nichoalds GE et al: Water-soluble vitamins in cancer patients on parenteral nutrition: A prospective study. JPEN 11:243, 1987

89. Norton JA, Peters ML, Wesley R et al: Iron supplementation of total parenteral nutrition: A prospective study. JPEN 7:457, 1983

90. Moley JF, Peacock JE, Morrison SD, Norton JA: Insulin reversal of cancer-induced protein loss. Surg Forum 36:416, 1985

91. Burt NE, Aoki TT, Gorschboth CM, Brennan MF: Peripheral tissue metabolism in cancer-bearing man. Ann Surg 198:685, 1983

92. Valdivieso M, Bodney GP, Benjamin RS et al: Role of intravenous hyperalimentation as an adjunct to intensive therapy for small cell bronchogenic carcinoma: Preliminary observations. Cancer Treat Rep 65(suppl 5):145, 1981

93. Maher MM, Henderson DK, Brennan MF: Central venous catheter exchange in cancer patients undergoing TPN. J Natl Intravenous Ther Assoc 5:54, 1982

94. Wagman LD, Burt ME, Brennan MF: The impact of total parenteral nutrition on liver function tests in patients with cancer. Cancer 49:1249, 1982

95. Wagner WH, Lowry AC, Silberman H et al: Similar liver function abnormalities occult in patients receiving glucose-based or lipid-based parenteral nutrition. Am J Gastroenterol 78:199, 1983

96. Kerner JA: Manual of Pediatric Parenteral Nutrition. New York, John Wiley & Sons, 1983

97. Bower RH: Hepatic complications of parenteral nutrition. Semin Liver Dis 3:218, 1983

98. Cooper A, Betts J, Pereira G, Zeigler M: Taurine deficiency in the severe hepatic dysfunction complicating total parenteral nutrition. J Pediatr Surg 19:462, 1984

99. Wilmington PF: Cholestasis associated with total parenteral nutrition in infants. Hepatology 5:693, 1985

100. Heber D, Byerley LO: Known metabolic abnormalities in the cancer patient. Nutr Suppl Serv 5:11, 1985

101. Wesson DE, Rich RH, Zlotkin SH, Pencharz PB: Fat overload syndrome causing respiratory insufficiency. J Pediatr Surg 19:777, 1988

102. Remington SJ, Schimpff SC: Please don't eat the salads. N Engl J Med 304:433, 1981

103. Sainsbury CPQ, Newcombe RG, Hughes IA: Weight gain and height velocity during prolonged remission from acute lymphocytic leukemia. Arch Dis Childh 60:832, 1985

104. Padilla GV, Grant M, Wong H et al: Subjective distresses of nasogastric tube feeding. JPEN 3:53, 1979

105. Greene HL, Helinek GL, Folk CC et al: Nasogastric tube feeding at home: A method for adjunctive nutritional support of malnourished patients. Am J Clin Nutr 34:1131, 1981

106. Lenssen P, Moe GL, Cheney CL et al: Parenteral nutrition in marrow transplant recipients after discharge from the hospital. Exp Hematol 11:974, 1983

107. Bayer LM, Bauers CM: Preparing patients for home parenteral nutrition. Pat Counsel Health Ed 4:174, 1980

108. Lie SO, Slordahl SH: Vitamin A and/or high-dose Ara-C in the maintenance of remission in acute myelogenous leukaemia in children? Scand J Haematol 33:256, 1984

109. Olson RE: Ascorbic acid does not cure cancer. Nutr Rev 43:146, 1985

110. Schrauzer GN: Selenium and cancer: A review. Bioinorgan Chem 5:275, 1976

111. Greenwald P: Manipulation of nutrients to prevent cancer. Hosp Pract 19:119, 1984

112. Bowman BB, Kushner RF, Dawson SC, Levin B: Macrobiotic diets for cancer treatment and prevention. J Clin Oncol 2:702, 1984

forty-one

Psychiatric and Psychological Support of the Child and Adolescent with Cancer

Shirley B. Lansky,
Marcy A. List, and
Chris Ritter–Sterr

In the past decade, technologic advances have effected dramatic improvements in the survival rates of children with cancer. In light of this medical success, the focus of pediatric oncology now includes a heightened awareness of the multiple psychiatric and psychological implications of cancer in childhood. The child's adaptation during disease and treatment and the quality of life as a long-term survivor are of paramount concern. For the child with cancer, successful outcome in all psychosocial arenas hinges on early assessment, prevention, and intervention.

This chapter surveys the phases of illness from diagnosis and treatment through reentry into the community to long-term survival. Predictable points of stress and potential disruptions are presented. For each phase, developmental implications and appropriate psychological and psychiatric support measures are discussed.

INITIAL DIAGNOSTIC PERIOD: A TIME OF CRISIS

Most children with a suspected malignancy are referred to a tertiary care facility for definitive diagnosis and initiation of treatment. This is a period of intense activity and extreme stress. Families are faced with the diagnosis of cancer and the fears that it arouses. They are frightened by the life-threatening illness and by the unfamiliar environment of a large medical center. Guilt is pervasive as parents search for causes, often looking for past errors of omission or commission.

In the midst of this distress, parents must begin to learn about the many aspects of their child's illness. They will be faced with the prognostic implications and the many necessary diagnostic and treatment procedures. The parents' education includes familiarization with the names of various tests, chemotherapeutic agents, and side-effects, as well as understanding possible surgical interventions. In addition, parents and child must learn about general hospital and clinic routines (see Chap. 46).

Certain techniques are useful in helping families absorb this large volume of new information. Frequent repetition of material allays anxiety and facilitates learning.[1] To avoid misunderstandings, it is also important that, whenever possible, both parents receive information simultaneously. This approach promotes open discussion and sharing and helps to avoid one parent bearing the total responsibility for mastering the new language of disease and treatment.

The initial presentation of the diagnosis to the child is also critical. It is this encounter that sets the stage for the future relationships among the child, parents, and treatment team. All children should be told about the diagnosis by their parents or by the physician with parents present. Later, older children will benefit from private discussions about their disease and treatment with the medical staff as they develop trust in and comfort with their caretakers.[2] Children should be given honest and accurate information about their illness and explanations of specific treatments and medications. Educational materials written for young patients[3,4] are helpful supplements to verbal discussions. Although presenting too much information may be overwhelming, presenting too little allows the imagination to take over, bringing on additional anxiety.[5]

There is an array of written materials for children and their parents. Some have limited audience appeal, but a few have stood the test of time. No complete list can be presented here because this is such a rapidly changing body of information. However, the best sources continue to be the American Cancer Society, the Leukemia Society of America, the National Cancer Institute, and the Candlelighters Foundation. One publication that has been used widely for the past 10 years is *You and Leukemia: A Day at a Time,* by Lynn Baker (Philadelphia, W. B. Saunders). Materials acceptable to adolescents are in short supply. A pamphlet distributed by the Leukemia Society —*What It Is That I Have, Don't Want, Didn't Ask For, Can't Give Back, and How I Feel About It*—is one of the few publications addressing the questions of development and sexuality that are of such great concern to the teenager. Other materials, such as films and videotapes, are also available from the sources listed above (see also Chap. 46).

The child's and family's ability to effectively assimilate and use illness-related information is also influenced by individual and family characteristics. Early assessment of the whole family is thus important to comprehensive care. Evaluation begins with a careful history of the child that includes questions about developmental tasks, school performance, and school functioning.[6] A description of family demographics outlines family members' ages, sex, and any special problems.

A detailed discussion of family issues, including assessment and management, appears in Chapter 42. In understanding the child's reaction to illness, it is helpful to consider the current context of both family and child. In addition to the new stresses and anxieties imposed by the diagnosis of cancer, both the child and family may be coping with a variety of ongoing pressures.[7] These factors must be identified. A sample list of possible stress factors is presented in Table 41-1.

The magnitude of these stressors, individually or in combination, has a significant impact on the family's ability to deal with the new illness (see also Chap. 42). It is impossible, however, to identify specific factors that place a particular family or child at risk. Each child and family reacts very differently; for some, the stress of a move may be incapacitating, whereas for others it may be exciting and handled relatively smoothly. The family's previous manner of coping with major events may best predict their way of coping with cancer. Thus, an exploration of the child's and family's past management style and effectiveness, particularly with experiences of serious illness or death, is most helpful in anticipating and providing support for current adaptation.[8]

Table 41-1
Stress Factors Impacting on Child and Family

Illness Related	Nonillness Related
Cost	Job or school change
Separations	Move or relocation
Disruption of usual routines (school, job)	Marital problems or divorce
	School problems
General burdens (traveling, sleep interruption)	Family illness, injury, or death
	Financial problems
Unfamiliar caretakers	Family problems
Isolation from peers	
Threat of death	

The Child's Reaction to Diagnosis and Initiation of Treatment: Developmental Considerations

A diagnosis of cancer is traumatic for all children, but the child's age and developmental level significantly influence his or her experience of illness-related events. Children will be particularly upset when circumstances interfere with their unique developmental needs.

Young Children

The young child's immediate concerns revolve around hospitalization, separation from parents, and fear of medical procedures. Toddlers and preschoolers are particularly sensitive to separations and changes in familiar routines. These young patients may view hospitalization and disruption of usual daily life as punishment. This perception is further reinforced by the experience of painful and invasive medical procedures. The fact that trusted parents allow this treatment is quite confusing for the child.

Hospitalized young children need constant reassurance from their parents that they will not be abandoned and that hospitalization and medical interventions are not a form of punishment. The young child's concerns about body boundaries, along with fears of mutilation, require special attention in relation to all medical procedures, from temperature-taking to lumbar punctures. Before any medical procedure, children should receive a brief, honest description of what the procedure is, how it will be done, and the intensity and duration of any pain involved (see also Chap. 46).[9]

Behavioral interventions are also effective in reducing the child's anxiety and distress surrounding medical procedures.[9-11] A system of positive incentive in combination with strategies of attentional distraction can help the child control fear before and during tests or treatments. The presentation of a valued reward may elicit the extra motivation to cooperate (*e.g.,* to try and remain still). It is important that expectations for the child's behavior be realistic and allow the child to experience success.

Children often want to be "brave" and not fight medical procedures. They will welcome the physician's help in controlling their fears. Such help may take the form of attentional distraction, emotive imagery, or hypnosis. During painful procedures, children can be engaged and distracted through storytelling, fantasy play, intellectual challenges, and video games. A more structured desensitization or emotive imagery procedure is most useful when the child's fears are not directly linked to aversive procedures. This technique is first introduced away from the treatment area. The aim is to teach the child mastery of the feared situation through repeated fantasy, for example, imagining how a favorite storybook hero would cope. The fantasy is designed to elicit motivation to master the pain rather than avoid it. Finally, hypnosis can be employed to train the child to refocus attention on images or thoughts that are unrelated to the source of distress. All these techniques succeed by diverting the child's attention away from the feared procedure and toward more positive activity.

When surgery is planned, the child needs special preparation. Visits to the operating and recovery rooms and familiarization with the surgical personnel and surgical garb (*i.e.,* masks and gowns) help ease the child's fear and lessen the shock of the strange environment. The child also needs to be prepared for the consequences of surgery. Discussions about amputation or other resulting disabilities or deformities must begin very early. This kind of trauma is best handled when children have several days to assimilate the information, voice their fears, and adjust expectations in light of further explanations. Other amputees are of considerable assistance in allaying some of the child's anxiety. Finally, as with all intensive and painful procedures, physical comforting is reassuring.

The stress of illness and hospitalization can cause regression in all patients. For the young child, regression might take the form of loss of newly acquired skills (*e.g.,* toilet training, speech, self-feeding). Previously discarded behaviors, such as thumb-sucking or clinging, may reemerge. Parents should be helped to understand this regression as part of the child's efforts to cope. It is most helpful to avoid either scolding or being overly tolerant of these behaviors. Adaptive regressive behaviors generally subside after the acute phase of illness. At times, however, regressive patterns will become more entrenched and can become serious problems. For example, while increased dependency between parent and child is inevitable, this can lead to more extreme symbiotic regression, a maladaptive behavior pattern that is difficult to change. This and other behaviors of concern will be discussed in detail later.

School-Age Children

In the school-age child, diagnosis and initiation of therapy arouse many of the same feelings and fears seen in the preschooler. Separation, strange people, an unfamiliar environment, fears of abandonment and punishment, and threats to body integrity are all major concerns of the school-age child.

School-age children cope with the stress of illness in a variety of ways. They may have a very delayed initial reaction or may respond immediately with acute anxiety or panic. Other reactions include psychosomatic complaints, nightmares, labile emotions, regression, or "adult acceptance."

School-age children are likely to be quite verbal about their illness, requesting information about all aspects of the disease and treatment. They often pose difficult questions about the reasons for and causes of their illness. Children at this age also experience pride of mastery from the learning associated with their illness. They enjoy learning the proper labels for their disease, treatments, and medications and can use this information effectively on returning to school.

This is a developmental period of vigorous inquiry, and the diagnosis of a severe illness, with all the associated anxiety, prompts a barrage of questions. From the outset, these questions should be answered in a simple straightforward approach. (A sample exchange might be: Q: "Why are we going to the university hospital?" A: "Because Dr. Jones thinks you may have a serious illness." Q: "What kind of serious illness?" A: "It may be a blood disease called leukemia." Q: "Does that mean I am going to die?" A: "We are going to the university because they have special treatments for leukemia that have cured many children.")

Parents often need to engage in specific scripting because they are not used to conveying stressful information to their children. It is important to start this process at the first encounter. If the family's usual practice is to avoid issues, the child will learn that asking questions produces discomfort in his or her parents, which increases the child's personal distress.

Once the physician has formed a working relationship with the child, a special education session between physician and child, without the parent, provides an opportunity to correct any misconceptions or offer more detailed information to the child. Obviously, the amount of detail presented depends on the age, comfort level, and sophistication of the child. This approach may lead to a warm bond between doctor and child that can enhance compliance with both procedures and treatment. Although some parents may feel threatened by this ex-

clusion, most will be grateful that the physician is sharing the educational task.

Compared to preschoolers, school-age children have heightened concerns about privacy. Their extreme modesty can interfere with medical exams and procedures. Within reason, every attempt should be made to respect their need for privacy.

The major activity of these children is school. School begins the processes of working toward independence from parents, establishing peer relationships, and acquiring academic skills. The physical and emotional concomitants of life-threatening illness result in a significant disruption in school attendance and performance (see section on Return to School, as well as Chap. 51).

Adolescence

For the adolescent, in a state of transition between childhood and adulthood, illness presents unique issues. Focal concerns about independence, appearance, acceptance, sexuality, and future plans are immediately confronted. The adolescent's strivings toward autonomy and self-determination are inevitably threatened by the forced dependence, compliance, and loss of control accompanying the illness and treatment. Most adolescents are self-conscious about their appearance and emerging sexuality. These issues assume an even greater significance in the face of such physical changes as hair loss, weight alterations, and mutilating surgery.[12] Concerns about infertility may be misconstrued, may result in fears of impotence or frigidity, and may increase the chances that the adolescent will develop a distorted image of his or her own sexuality. The sense of physical weakness and vulnerability similarly interferes with the adolescent's maintenance of peer interactions.

School life is also disrupted. Both social and academic pursuits are interrupted, delayed, or critically altered by frequent and prolonged school absences. Feelings of isolation or embarrassing physical changes may make it difficult for the adolescent to return to school or maintain adequate attendance (see Return to School). Finally, long-established plans or expectations about career or family may require reconsideration in light of physical limitations, academic difficulties, and questions related to fertility and parenthood.

Each adolescent responds to these stresses differently, and the same child may react differently at different times. Emotions ranging from depression and withdrawal to agitation are common. For some adolescents, verbal expression is important. For others, behavioral outlets for feelings are more commonly used. Initially, some adolescents may respond with questions that are general rather than personal.[13,14] Concerns may center on causation and prevention, new research and treatments, statistics about recurrence and survival, and payment of medical bills. For others, more personal issues, such as their specific treatment plan, the effect of treatment on appearance, and disruption in family, peer, and school activities, emerge as immediate concerns (see Chaps. 42 and 52).

Although these specific issues need to be individually evaluated and addressed periodically throughout treatment and follow-up, several initial strategies help facilitate the adolescent's mastery.[15] Whenever possible, the adolescent should be treated within a pediatric rather than adult cancer facility. Pediatric units typically place a greater emphasis on psychosocial and developmental needs of the patient and have extended assistance and resources (*e.g.,* child life workers, psychologists, and nutritionists). At diagnosis, adolescents indicate a desire for simple, understandable explanations from the physician, with reassurance about possible treatments.[12] From this point on, it is critical that the adolescent be allowed and encouraged to participate in medical decisions. Within the limits of the particular treatment center, the adolescent can be given control over the scheduling of treatments and procedures, permitted to see radiographs or test results, and involved actively in discussions of alternate treatments. Particularly for the older adolescent,[14] these experiences can be helpful. Both group support and individual contacts should be available to be used when the adolescent is ready (see section on Play). Finally, parent education should focus on helping parents encourage their children to maintain active participation in daily activities, including school and extracurricular programs. Parents must learn to give themselves and their adolescents permission to argue, voice opinions, and engage in normal, developmentally appropriate intrafamily combat.

Costs

Very few families undergo the rigors of years of cancer treatment and follow-up without considerable economic stress. Financial burdens begin at diagnosis and extend well beyond the time of illness (see Chap. 43).

The cost of treatment can be divided into direct medical charges and nonmedical out-of-pocket expenses. Nonmedical costs, including extra food and clothing, transportation, family care, lodging, and miscellaneous items, have a greater immediate impact on the family's budget. Two independent surveys of these expenditures, one in Kansas and the other in England, have reported virtually identical results.[16,17] Approximately half the families indicated that out-of-pocket expenses plus loss of pay amounted to at least 26% of their weekly family budgets. Four factors influenced nonmedical expenses. For obvious reasons, hospitalization (as opposed to outpatient treatment or no contact) and distance from the treatment center were associated with higher expenses. As the child's ability to engage in normal activities deteriorated, expenses increased. Costs also increased with family size; the more children in the family, the greater the expense of caring for them in the parents' absence. Single-parent families also had considerable expense, presumably related to child care for siblings when the patient was being treated at the medical center. These out-of-pocket expenses are not covered by third-party carriers, and most are not even deductible for income tax purposes. Studies with adult cancer patients have yielded similar results.

Direct medical costs for cancer treatment are prohibitive. Outpatient medical costs vary with diagnosis, with a large spread between those cancers requiring intensive treatment and those that involve only routine follow-up. In families whose children eventually died of their illness, mean annual medical costs amounted to almost twice the mean annual income. The diagnostic and terminal stages of illness accounted for more than 50% of these charges. The major source of payment of these bills was insurance. However, outstanding debts to the cancer center as long as 3½ years after the child's death were frequent.[18,19]

Half of the families experience costs related to their child's illness that amount to at least one third of their monthly income—this is more than the level described as "catastrophic."[20] This total financial burden is made up of medical charges not covered by third-party carriers, nonmedical out-of-pocket costs, and loss of pay. This economic impact adds significantly to the family's overall distress. Even when the financial hardship is less extreme, it has long-lasting deleterious effects on all family members because of the depletion of resources over an extended period. Parents and siblings are de-

prived of basic needs because such a large proportion of the family budget goes toward the care of the sick child. There are no simple solutions for the financial plight of these families. Early assessment of socioeconomic vulnerability might include evaluation of third-party coverage, the availability of community resources, and job-related issues.[21] At best, such an assessment will uncover possible supports. At the least, it will serve to forewarn families about the magnitude of future expenses.[22]

THE ADAPTATION PERIOD: REENTRY

After the initial acute phase of illness, attention turns toward reentry or "getting back to normal." The focus is on making the child's life as normal as possible while continuing with medical treatment protocols. When children have been hospitalized for initiation of treatment, leaving the safety of the hospital environment evokes anxiety in them and in their parents (see Chap. 42).

Discharge Planning

Thorough discharge planning is essential. Parents should be given a phone number where they can reach medical personnel at any time. Medication schedules need to be reviewed and the first outpatient clinic appointment set up. The oncology team should review with parents possible symptoms that necessitate immediate action.

Anticipatory guidance is also a vital part of discharge planning. Forewarning about possible reactions of friends, family, and school personnel may help children and parents deal with situations that arise. Families should anticipate a wide variety of responses, ranging from complete rejection to excessive sympathy. They can also be reminded about the myths that some people still hold, such as the belief cancer is contagious. Families should be encouraged to deal honestly with others. They may benefit from rehearsing short "scripts" describing the illness, treatment, and side-effects.

Also important at discharge is a complete assessment of the child's intellectual, cognitive, and neuropsychological functioning. A baseline evaluation that describes strengths and weaknesses in specific rather than global terms is critical to accurately determine the influence of disease progression and treatment effects. As soon as possible after diagnosis, and continuing at regular intervals as part of long-term follow-up, each child requires a complete neuropsychological assessment, including IQ testing and achievement testing.[8,23,24]

Testing can be done by a psychometrist, psychologist, or neuropsychologist. If these services are not available at the medical center, school psychologists and counselors may facilitate referrals to outside agencies. Any changes in functioning relative to baseline should be carefully evaluated. Children with suspected learning disabilities may be further assessed to differentiate among retardation, specific learning disorders, emotional disturbances, and immaturity.[6] Appropriate interventions or placements can then be established.

Results of testing need to be shared with the medical care team, parents, teachers, and the children themselves. Children are often aware of changes, perhaps noticing that tasks which once were simple now require considerable effort. They are often relieved to have such perceptions confirmed, particularly when explanations include a description of strengths and reassurances that the child is not lazy or stupid. It is important that all involved understand the implications of test results for the child's daily life and future academic achievement. Appropriate goals and expectations can be set accordingly.

Other concerns associated with reentry depend on the child's age and developmental level. The first priority is to reestablish patterns and routines of daily life that have been disrupted by initial treatment or hospitalization. For young children, familiar routines revolving around bedtime, toileting, feeding, naps, and playing provide a sense of control and security. For older children and adolescents, attention should be paid to reestablishing the child's role in the family. Chores that were previously the child's responsibility should be retained if possible. Special limitations caused by the illness or treatment may require some redefinition of roles among the family members. Of utmost importance, however, is the child's sense of belonging to the family unit. Fears of replacement or displacement are common in ill children.

Discipline is another area that may be disrupted. Parents often become quite lax in their expectations of ill children. At the same time, they may become overprotective or overindulgent. If this cycle continues, significant behavioral problems will result. Even ill children need firm and consistent limits, with predictable disciplinary measures carried out if they do not comply with the set limits. Lack of limits leads to a sense of lack of control and insecurity in all children, particularly those threatened by a serious illness.

Return to School

A child's life is organized around school, and successful reentry demands a rapid return to this environment. School provides for the development of academic abilities as well as peer contacts and social activities. A child who misses as little as 4 weeks of school in 1 year may encounter problems in building the skills necessary for academic progress. Similarly, a month away from one's peers interferes with the shared experiences that make up friendships. For the child with cancer, school plays the additional and vital role as the most immediate and important part in normalizing his or her life and counteracting the anxiety, depression, and isolation that may accompany illness and treatment.[25-28] Thus, successful rehabilitation must start with the reestablishment of these usual routines (see Chap. 51).

Children with cancer often have difficulty returning to school and maintaining attendance.[29,30] They show high rates of absenteeism and school refusal, missing an average of 21 to 45 days per year.[31,32] Long-term survivors have reported school absenteeism to be one of the most significant and disruptive consequences of having cancer.

Reasons for the child's missing school extend beyond the unavoidable absences associated with clinic visits, hospitalizations, and treatment side-effects. Children must also cope with fears of death, the reactions of others, fatigue, and activity restriction, as well as changes in physical appearance caused by weight gain or loss, alopecia, or amputation. Resulting anxieties and embarrassment significantly contribute to the child's reluctance to attend school.[27] The frequent development of a dependent-protective relationship between the parent and child may also reinforce school absences.[33]

Interventions facilitating the child's school experiences are imperative.[34] The first step is one of prevention, by establishing a system for early and ongoing communication among the family, school, and medical personnel. Early detection and treatment of problems are the goals. To be most effective, such a program can begin at diagnosis, with documentation of prediagnosis levels of achievement and attendance, and baseline assessment of current functioning (achievement and neuropsy-

chological testing). It is important to arrange for continuity of classwork directly through the child's school or, when necessary, through hospital schools or homebound teachers. At the same time, to minimize feelings of isolation, patients and their families can be encouraged to maintain contact with the child's school friends and teachers. The patient, classmates, and school personnel all need to be prepared for the child's return to the classroom.

For the patient, concerns about appearance and the reactions, questions, or misunderstandings of classmates will be foremost. Opportunities to rehearse explanations or possible answers often decrease anxiety. It is usually best to tell the child to respond to questions or comments briefly, directly, and honestly. Questions the child may be asked include: "Where have you been?" "What's wrong with you?" "Why do you wear a wig?" "Why are you bald?" "What happened to your leg?" "Can I catch it?" "Can you still go to school [ride your bike]?" The child might benefit from practicing possible explanations, such as: "I have been out of school because I have cancer. I have cancer in my leg [blood]. I had an operation on my leg to take out the cancer. I am getting chemotherapy, special medicine to get rid of the cancer. I have no hair [wear a wig] because the chemotherapy [medicine] makes my hair fall out. After I stop taking the medicine, my hair will grow back. Cancer is not contagious. No one can catch it from being around me or playing with me. I can do most of the stuff I always did. Sometimes I might be a little tired because of the medicine I take." The child's specific response will depend on his or her comfort and developmental level.

In addition, it can be helpful for teachers to obtain permission from the family to prepare the class in advance for the child's return by describing events openly and answering questions honestly. Alternatively, some children are interested in talking to their class as a group. Presentations or projects, such as a show-and-tell for young children or science or health projects for older children, may be used to inform the class about the disease and its treatment.[35-37]

School personnel need information about childhood cancer and its specific implications for school. The importance of successful school experiences can be emphasized and appropriate behavioral and academic expectations discussed.[38] Teachers require a description of the child's medical status, treatment side-effects, prognosis, and daily functioning. Specific information about any physical changes or restrictions, potential absenteeism, and treatment schedules will further alleviate the teacher's own anxieties and uncertainties.[27] Conferences, workshops, and phone contacts all have been found useful in conveying this material. Teachers have responded with reassurance and appreciation for such opportunities to ask questions and clarify misconceptions.[39-42]

Play

Play occupies a central role in the mental and physical growth of all children. Serious illness and its accompanying stress and physical restriction interrupt natural play and socialization.[43,44] Specific developmental tasks, such as the toddler's exploratory behaviors or the adolescent's identification with peers, may be diverted. Parents may be fearful of injury or anxious about their child being with other children. An important task for the oncology team is to encourage the child to resume previous play as much as possible and to participate in available supervised experiences.

In many pediatric oncology centers, the child with cancer has access to a number of established supportive activities. These opportunities range from hospital or clinic playrooms to structured groups to special summer camps. The child's participation in such play and recreational programs is important, beginning at diagnosis and continuing through treatment and remission to long-term survival. Over the course of illness, these activities may assume varying functions, helping to prepare the child for medical procedures, forestalling major developmental disruptions, and facilitating the child's reentry into his or her community of peers.

Hospital and clinic playrooms provide the patient with a child-centered environment. They offer a safe place, a setting free from medical procedures in which the patient can restore, in part, normal aspects of living. Play activities provide a much needed source of pleasure and a medium for self-exploration and expression. They offer the patient an opportunity for mastery and control as opposed to the passivity and dependence enforced by illness. Play may reduce anxiety by helping the child overcome fears and cope with frustrations. Finally, playroom activities encourage the social interaction that is particularly important in counteracting the isolation facing the child with cancer.[45,46]

Playrooms and play groups can vary in degree of structure and the extent to which the primary purpose is recreational, educational, or preparatory. Activities must be selected to appeal to children at different developmental levels. For instance, whereas dolls and arts and crafts may interest young or school-age children, adolescents might be more attracted by cooking, music, or organizing special parties. In addition to any other materials, playrooms should be equipped with regular hospital equipment, including syringes, needles, surgical gloves, masks, and IV tubing. This equipment is helpful not only in free play but in teaching or preparing a child for upcoming medical procedures. For example, the child may try on a surgical mask or listen to a nurse's heart with a stethoscope. Because all pediatric oncology patients receive multiple needle punctures, some manner of supervised needle play is a part of most playrooms. Here, children are given the opportunity to copy their nurse or doctor and perform spinal taps, do bone marrow aspirations, and start intravenous lines on dolls. Even very young children become extremely adept at explaining procedures to their "patient," telling the "patient" what it will feel like and then carrying out the procedures. Nurses, child life specialists, or other playroom staff are available for supervision, encouragement, and demonstration.[44-46]

A child's play activities can also be employed as an index of performance status or physical disability, an important outcome consideration in treatment and rehabilitation planning. A recently constructed performance scale for children uses play and activity as the measure of performance. The scale is rated by the parent, and scores indicate the degree to which the child engages in his or her usual play activities. Its purpose is to monitor change in functional status in response to disease and treatment effects, relapse, or remission.[47]

More specifically, the play performance scale describes ten levels of performance in terms of active play, degree of physical limitation, and degree of independent functioning. These distinctions are combined to form a hierarchy ranging from fully active, normal (score 100) to moderately restricted (score 50–60), to completely disabled (score 10 or less). To obtain a measure of overall functioning, ratings are made on the basis of the child's activity over the period of a week. Parents are asked to think about their child's play and activity over the week and indicate which description is the "best fit." The scale is appropriate for use with inpatients and outpatients ages 1 to 16 years.

To date, the psychometrics of the scale have been tested on a sample of 98 pediatric oncology patients and two groups of healthy, well children. There was a high degree of agreement between the mother's and father's ratings and ratings on the scale were meaningful, that is, they appeared to accurately reflect functional status. The play performance scale distinguished patients from healthy children as well as detecting more modest differences in functioning, for example, between inpatients and outpatients.[48]

Future research endeavors include longitudinal studies, with repeated administration of the scale from diagnosis through various phases of illness and treatment. In this way it can be determined whether, as expected, disease-related changes such as hospitalization or cessation of treatment are reflected in changes in play-performance ratings. It might be interesting to use multiple ratings to generate individual profiles that would describe a child's response. Many additional questions about the functional impact of particular treatment protocols, the child's adaptability, and individual differences in response to treatment are open for study.

In addition to play groups, various events and outings aid in reducing the stresses of cancer and promote a sense of normality. Field trips may be initiated, taking into account the interest and developmental needs of children at various ages (e.g., for young children, trips to the zoo or circus; for older children, attending musical or sporting events). Other special activities provide opportunities for new skill acquisition. For example, the older school-age child or adolescent who has had an amputation and then learns to snow ski or begins to lift weights will feel proud, more competent, and more comfortable with the body changes he or she has to endure.[45]

Finally, special summer camp programs provide a sense of accomplishment and belonging.[49,50] They offer the child a variety of normal camping experiences (horseback riding, archery, swimming, hiking) while providing necessary medical supervision and maintaining ongoing treatment regimens. The child who, for example, is embarrassed by baldness or afraid to play ball again may find him- or herself swimming across the lake or putting up a tent after a day-long canoe trip. Camp may be the first time the child has been away from home since diagnosis. It is an important moment for both child and parent. Both may begin to see the patient as less vulnerable, more capable, and more independent. And while the child is enjoying the camp, the family gets a break from the day-to-day stresses and worries with which they have been living. The camping experience also provides a unique opportunity for the child to be with a group of children who have shared similar medical experiences and represent a spectrum of disease states. There are usually long-term survivors as well as children in the late stages of disease. The child can see that he or she is not alone in coping with this disease and can share experiences with others who understand.

Compliance

Ongoing compliance with medical regimens is an important part of living with and adapting to cancer. This includes following prescribed drug protocols, enduring multiple medical procedures, and adhering to appointment schedules. Recent reports suggest that noncompliance is a significant problem in pediatric oncology, with rates of medical noncompliance ranging from 33% to 59%.[51-55] Noncompliance is serious; it can hinder or negate attempts to provide optimal treatment and compromise the young patient's chances of survival.

In addition to influencing therapeutic outcome, noncompliance affects other aspects of cancer therapy: medications may be misjudged as ineffective, unnecessary diagnostic tests ordered, and alternative treatments initiated. Undetected noncompliance also precludes reliable assessment of new or experimental treatment regimens, resulting in erroneous conclusions. Finally, the extent to which noncompliance contributes to poorer outcomes in certain groups of patients (*e.g.,* adolescents with leukemia) remains an unanswered question.

To date there have been relatively few comprehensive studies of compliance issues in pediatric oncology populations. However, there are several circumstances surrounding the treatment of childhood cancer that probably contribute to poor compliance. These include the aversiveness of procedures, the complexity and prolonged nature of drug protocols, and the patients' age.[56–59]

The aversiveness of medical procedures and treatment side-effects, even if accepted initially, may interfere with long-term compliance as symptoms improve and disease remission is obtained.[60] Children with cancer do not habituate to painful medical procedures, and anxiety may only intensify with repeated clinic visits or hospitalizations.[62,63] Treatment failures may also result in noncompliance as discouragement and hopelessness set in (see section on Refusal of Therapy).

One recent investigation more specifically addressed compliance questions.[54] That study examined the level of medication compliance and the reasons for noncompliance among adolescent and pediatric cancer patients on chemotherapy. Forty-six patients, ages 2½ to 23 years (mean = 6.8 years) and 40 parents were extensively interviewed at four points during therapy (up to 50 weeks from diagnosis). Separate parent-child interviews were conducted for patients older than 10 years (N = 22; mean age = 17 years). Serum bioassays were used to corroborate self-reported compliance.

Results suggested that occasional or serious noncompliance occurs in approximately one third of children and adolescents with cancer. Noncompliance increased slightly over the duration of treatment and was greatest at 20 weeks; adolescents were less compliant overall than younger children. Compliance was not related to sex of the patient, stage of disease, satisfaction with physician-related information, or the number of medications and doses. Rather, it was the patient's understanding of medication and dose schedules that distinguished compliers from noncompliers. Noncompliance was also more frequent when patients and parents disagreed as to who was responsible for administering the medication. Finally, when asked about their noncompliant behavior, patients most often attributed missed doses to forgetfulness, whereas parents most often suggested that busy schedules interfered. These findings are consistent with earlier reports that increased family size, with accompanying increased activity, is negatively related to compliance.[61]

Other studies also target the adolescent as being at greatest risk for noncompliance. Compared to younger children, adolescents were found to be less compliant with oral medication[55] and, in general, less cooperative with their medical care.[64] Several reasons for this have been suggested. Compliance is enhanced when the parent assumes responsibility for medication administration, which is more likely with younger children. And, although the adolescent is beginning to assume some adult responsibilities, these are probably carried out somewhat inconsistently. Confusion about who is responsible for certain functions increases the chances of missing appointments or medication doses. Noncompliance may also be one attempt to maintain and exert control in the face of the forced dependence and restrictiveness of illness. Alternatively, noncompliance may represent the adolescent's denial of illness and its life-threatening consequences.[65]

The following suggestions are offered as strategies for enhancing the adolescent's cooperation and compliance with treatment procedures. First, as discussed previously, it is extremely important that the adolescent be included as an active participant in treatment-related decision making. To the extent that he or she is capable, the adolescent should be given as much choice as is possible (*e.g.,* scheduling treatments when they will least interfere with other activities). Increasing the adolescent's sense of control will increase compliance. Second, the oncology team can help the family to set clear expectations and clarify roles. Decisions about who will be responsible for administering medications or remembering appointments should be made early, before problems arise. In this regard, it can be helpful to both physicians and adolescents to set up a contract, a system of expected behavior and consequent reward.[52,58,59] Third, medical personnel should provide written directions and make sure that patients understand medication schedules. It may also help to set up "cueing" procedures to remind adolescents when it is time to take their medication. For example, the patient can learn to identify a daily routine that can be linked to pill taking. Finally, if necessary, other family members or friends can be recruited to assume supportive or supervisory roles.

The Child at Risk: Specific Problems

Many children cope reasonably well with "reentry" and successfully adapt to the demands of living with cancer. There are some children, however, who have trouble adjusting and who continue to experience disturbance and distress. Surveillance and monitoring of problems will help alert the medical team to needs for intervention. The most frequent early problems requiring systematic attention and psychiatric referral include severe depression, symbiotic regression, and school refusal.

Any child diagnosed with cancer may at times appear depressed. The child may have trouble sleeping or eating, be excessively anxious or sad, or be silent and withdrawn. These behaviors often reflect the shock, fear, distress, and exhaustion accompanying the diagnosis of cancer. However, if symptoms are persistent, continuing after remission is achieved, and include uncharacteristic feelings of hopelessness and worthlessness, further evaluation is warranted. Once a full medical evaluation has determined that there is no physical cause for the child's symptoms, a psychiatric consultation may be helpful. In many cases, the child's depression will respond to psychotherapeutic interventions; in other instances, more intensive treatment, including antidepressant medications, will be necessary.[66]

A particularly difficult behavior pattern to change, once it has been established, is a symbiotic relationship between the sick child and a parent, usually the mother.[34] The pair becomes an inseparable dyad, with the child continuing to regress and becoming progressively dependent on the parent. Extreme separation anxiety occurs in both child and parent. The pair may isolate themselves in the child's hospital room or, after discharge, remain in seclusion at home. They may withdraw from all social contacts, including other family members. At times, the child's medical care may be obstructed, as the parent and child resist even the involvement of physicians and nurses. This seriously maladaptive behavior can be prevented by early attention to and active initiation of mother-child separations. Playrooms, play groups, and special activities offer ideal opportunities to effect separations. At the same time, parents can be encouraged to participate in parent groups. This experience provides a forum for voicing concerns, as well as a reason for separating from the child.

The child who is reluctant and ultimately refuses to go to school is at risk for future academic and social difficulties. For these children, the support of family, classmates, and educators is not enough. When a child's school absences continue and are unrelated to disease and treatment, more vigorous intervention is necessary. At this point, psychiatric consultation is warranted to assist the child and family in increasing and maintaining school attendance.

RELAPSE OR RECURRENCE: A SECOND CRISIS

Although an increasing number of children with cancer are able to achieve and maintain freedom from disease, some will inevitably experience a relapse or recurrence of their disease. In some ways, this second crisis can be more devasting than the initial stress of diagnosis.[67,68] Denial of the illness and fantasies of cure are now much more difficult to maintain. Families faced with reinitiation of treatment must start over again, but with a smaller chance for successful outcome. Encouraging the family to once again adopt a positive attitude toward treatment is a challenge to the oncology team. Yet families generally gain a sense of hope from the knowledge that there is some action to be taken against the disease. The period of relapse or recurrence is another in which communication among the child, family, and oncology team is essential. Yet, because all involved are dealing with their feelings of failure, communication may be hampered. Support must be given to staff members who, in turn, provide the most support for the child and family. At this point, perhaps more than ever before, parents require the availability of team members.

Alternative Treatments and Refusal of Therapy

The recurrence of disease may be an impetus for parents to seek alternative treatments (see Chaps. 15, 42, and 53). Newspapers, magazines, fund-raising events, and television talk shows disseminate information about cancer research "breakthroughs" and unconventional treatment in such a dramatic way that it is difficult for the general public to evaluate the reports. The result is that relatives and friends may encourage the family to transfer the child to a more prestigious cancer center or to seek experimental treatments.

In most instances, parents continue treatment with their current medical team and refuse to subject their child to unproven methods. Nonetheless, they may experience guilt and anxiety about rejecting a possible "miracle cure." The treatment team can help to minimize this stress by discussing with the family the facts of any treatment information they have received.

Some parents do pursue unproven methods of treatment or faith healing. The approach to this situation depends on the child's prognosis.[69] For the child with a good prognosis, it is important to explain carefully to the family all the information about achieving that good prognosis with conventional therapy. Should parents remain adamant in their refusal, the help of the juvenile court can be enlisted. Use of the child abuse and neglect statutes may be the only way to ensure that a child with a treatable disease receives appropriate therapy. Such measures should be taken only after all efforts have been exhausted to secure the parents' willing participation in the treatment regimen. When the prognosis is poor, regardless of conventional treatment, and the parents seek unconventional treatment or faith healing, review of the illness with the family is again indicated. Even if the parents pursue alternative treatments, they should be reassured that the medical care team remains interested in them and the child's welfare and is willing to provide any care needed.

When the child (usually the adolescent) refuses treatment, the underlying motivations include hopelessness about

the outcome, feelings of helplessness, distress with the side-effects of treatment, or a combination thereof. By refusing treatment, some adolescents will be asserting their independence once again and demonstrating that they are in charge of their own destiny (see Chap. 15). This is another situation in which preventive measures are far more effective than trying to intervene in a crisis. Preventive measures involve including the adolescent in the discussion and decision-making process from the beginning. Participation in a group for teenagers is also effective because the members confront one another when poor decisions are being made, just as they provide support for one another in coping. When an adolescent actively refuses treatment, the treatment staff need to calmly sort out which factors are operating and proceed in an orderly manner to discuss them. If the patient feels that the parent is making all the decisions and the refusal is an attempt to assert him- or herself, this can usually be handled in a straightforward manner by getting the parents to withdraw a bit and permit the adolescent to have the primary role in communicating with the staff. For those who feel that treatment is hopeless, the risk/benefit ratio must be presented clearly, particularly when the treatment is palliative. The distress and discomfort of side-effects are the most common reasons for refusal of treatment and most difficult for the adults (family and treatment team) to deal with because these feelings are viewed as being narcissistic and shortsighted. The adolescent is dealing in the here and now, not in the future. A mental health professional not directly involved in the child's care can be of assistance in such instances. In addition, careful evaluation and creative approaches to management of symptoms (*e.g.,* changing the venue of the chemotherapy for patients with severe anticipatory nausea and vomiting) can be implemented. For a few patients, the life-threatening nature of the illness may not have been clearly presented or fully understood. In this case, a factual account of what can be expected without treatment, including progression of the disease and death, may bring the patient to a point where he or she has to look at the future. Obviously, this is the least desirable method.

TERMINAL ILLNESS

Despite medical advances, there are still children who will inevitably succumb to their cancer. The realization that treatments have failed and that the child will die is difficult. The task of the oncology team is to continue to provide appropriate care for the child while attending to the needs of the family. Comprehensive care for the dying child involves maximizing both physical and emotional comfort (see Chaps. 42, 43, 46, and 49). Open communication, pain control, and the maintenance of familiar routines all convey a sense of security that is important in reassuring the dying child. The family also needs ongoing emotional support as well as specific information and assistance with difficult decisions and preparations. Painful decisions must be made regarding home versus hospital care for the dying child, autopsy, and funeral arrangements. The decision-making process can be facilitated through open discussion ahead of time. How the family handles such events and concerns clearly affects the child. These interactions, family interventions, and follow-up contact with the family after the child dies are discussed in detail in Chapter 42. This section focuses on the child and how the caregiver most effectively and compassionately cares for the dying child.

To the extent possible, the child should be encouraged to participate in normal daily routines. Continued attendance at school (even if part-time) and involvement in family functions counteract boredom and boosts morale. The child's day can be organized so that even when confined to bed, he or she remains an important contributor to his or her world. Preserving familiar behaviors and schedules also minimizes the child's experience of him- or herself as a burden.

Talking to the Dying Child

In the past, it was frequently assumed that children did not understand death and that creating an atmosphere of cheerful normality would protect the child from the seriousness of the illness. In striking contrast, more recent reports clearly indicate that even when they are not told, young as well as older children are aware of both the seriousness of their disease and the possibility that they will die.[70] The child may not spontaneously voice suspicions or ask questions, sensing the discomfort of parents and caretakers. Such silence only exacerbates the child's fearful fantasies and can establish a pattern of growing isolation. The oncology team can play a central role in helping dying children to express their questions and concerns.

What does one say to the dying child? How do you help? Children generally have two major questions. The first is, "Am I going to die?" When the answer is understood to be yes, the second question is, "When?" It is often helpful to point out to the child that there are some things that can be done and others that cannot be done regarding the illness. Telling the child that cure is no longer a possibility is the most difficult but also the most important message to convey. It is easy for caregivers to camouflage difficult messages in professional jargon. One must give the child this particular message in an open, straightforward manner without going to the extreme of appearing overly blunt or uncaring. Especially now, the child needs the sense of security and trust maintained through honest communication.

In telling the child that cure is no longer possible, one must also leave room for hope. In this circumstance, the hope is redirected from cure to comfort. Comfort includes having around them the people they love, being free from further diagnostic or treatment procedures, and having their pain controlled. Although the adolescent may need some time alone, one of the young patient's greatest fears is being abandoned by or separated from family and friends. If the child is in the hospital, a nonrestrictive visiting policy for family should be provided, and interaction with friends and other patients encouraged. Even children being cared for at home will need repeated reassurances that they will not be left alone. Providing comfort also involves acknowledgment and acceptance of the range of feelings that will come and go. The child should be told that it is all right to feel confused, sad, or angry—and to talk about these feelings or, at times, to remain silent.

Pain Control

Of utmost concern to all children and parents is how much pain they will have to endure (see Chap. 44). One of the child's most frequent questions is "Will it hurt?" This will be asked about medical interventions and will be introduced again in discussions about dying. It is the responsibility of the health care team to guarantee the child the most effective pain management available. This means freedom from intense pain without unnecessary sedation. Proper pain control enables the child to enjoy the environment actively. At one stage, it may enable the child to attend school; at a late stage, relative freedom from pain makes it possible for the child to interact with others at home or in the hospital.[71] The following is a summary of the principles of effective pain management for the child.[11,66,72–76]

1. The child may have difficulty describing pain in ways that are immediately meaningful to the physician; determining the source and severity of the pain may thus be complicated.
2. Analgesics should be administered on a regular basis before the effects of the previous dose have worn off.
3. When nonnarcotic agents are no longer effective, narcotic analgesics should be employed; addiction or dependence in terminally ill patients is rare.
4. Pain may be intensified by sleep disturbance, anxiety, or depression. The judicious use of adjuvant psychotropic medication (*e.g.,* hypnotics, benzodiazepines, tricyclic antidepressants) often results in improved pain control.
5. When psychoactive drugs are used with children, baseline blood workups (hepatic, renal function) and careful monitoring of side-effects (*e.g.,* electrocardiograms when cardiotoxic agents are employed) are crucial.
6. The child may respond with discomfort or fear to common drug side-effects (*e.g.,* the grogginess or disorientation associated with some sedatives); attention to the child's unique experience is important.

Once the more immediate problem of pain control has been resolved, the child and family turn to other aspects of the experience of terminal illness. This is the time when the child begins the process of saying goodbye. Reviewing relationships and talking over shared experiences may become part of the child's interactions with friends, parents and siblings. Many children will have thought about their death and funeral and, with a little encouragement, will convey this information and their special requests and wishes. For example, some children ask that their special belongings be distributed to the people they feel will find them equally important, usually siblings. The gesture of distributing some of the child's belongings serves to inform the siblings that their brother or sister is dying. It also provides clear evidence to the dying child that he or she will not be forgotten.

Most of the concepts and activities discussed here involve parents and other family members as well as the health care team. The family's specific needs and level of comfort and communication dictate the nature and extent of the caregivers' initiative and ongoing involvement (see Chap. 42). In general, however, the task of the care team is to promote open dialogue between the parents and the child. The first step is to tell the parents they can and should talk with their child. The second is to help the parents with what they might say and what the child's responses might be. Finally, the medical team's participation and investment in caring for the dying child is extremely important to, and greatly appreciated by, *all* families, even those who appear to be coping well on their own.

COMPLETION OF THERAPY

The completion of therapy is another point of extreme stress. Discontinuation of treatment encourages an increased sense of hope for extended survival. Yet this hope is clouded by anxiety from several sources. First, the child and family can no longer cling to the routine of taking medication to maintain security and optimism. Parents often feel that they are not actively fighting the disease and that relapse is therefore more likely. Families also fear a loss of contact with the treatment team.

Families require extra support and education at this junction. Physicians must outline reasons for discontinuation of therapy, the possibility of relapse with or without treatment, and the risks of continuing therapy any longer than necessary.[77] Treatment options in the event of a relapse should be explained to the parents. Families can also be reassured by the knowledge that the child is still very much a patient and that he or she will be monitored as closely as before.[78]

LONG-TERM SURVIVORS

The anxiety felt when therapy is completed dissipates slowly as months pass and the child remains free of disease.[79] As concern about recurrent disease diminishes, other worries take its place. These include fears about long-term sequelae of the illness and treatment (see Chap. 50). Long-term survivors of childhood cancer face serious future physical and psychosocial risks, many of which are as yet unknown.

The survivor must first cope with medical sequelae, ranging from changes in appearance (*e.g.*, obesity, physical disabilities left by surgery), to defects in major organ systems (*e.g.*, cardiac, liver, renal), to worries about fertility, progeny, and the risk of second malignant neoplasms.[80-96] Routine follow-up of the long-term survivor should include screening for these potential late effects as well as age-appropriate education regarding special lifetime health risks and necessary health maintenance practices.

Potential disruptive effects of childhood cancer and its treatment extend into other areas of the survivor's life. Developmental disruptions experienced during treatment have undeniable implications for future psychosocial adjustment. The degree to which these disruptions affect the child's later adjustment varies. Increasing time since disease onset and younger age at diagnosis seem to be related to fewer subsequent adjustment problems.[97] Older children and adolescents may be particularly sensitive to interruptions in their developing peer and intimate relationships, school and extracurricular activities, and plans for future lifestyle and occupation.[98] Reports of psychosocial adjustment are conflicting; descriptions of relatively high rates of psychiatric symptomatology[97,99,100] contrast with hypotheses that overall adjustment is not affected by the experience of childhood cancer.[85,94,101]

Specific educational and occupational achievements and choices may be affected by cancer survival. The academic ability of the long-term survivor may potentially be affected by intellectual deficits[80,104-107] and learning problems. Cancer therapy, specifically cranial irradiation, has been associated with problems in attention and concentration, performance under pressure, visual and auditory memory, and mathematical skills. Language skills appear to be relatively unaffected.[102,108-112] These potential learning problems, coupled with disruptions in school attendance, may limit the child's educational achievement and occupational attainment.

Recommendations for intervention include baseline assessment and periodic monitoring of neuropsychological functioning. Continuous evaluation of academic performance as a part of regular aftercare permits prompt identification of learning disabilities that may not appear for several years. Once identified, learning problems can be dealt with through an educational program tailored to the individual child's specific areas of strength and weakness.

Even when they are successful in overcoming learning and educational barriers, long-term survivors may encounter difficulties in the workplace as a result of their cancer history. Hiring discrimination, ineligibility for health and life insurance, and employers' attitudes about cancer may all complicate the cancer survivor's entry into the work force.[111,112]

CONCLUSION

Clinicians have become increasingly alert to the multiple and varied implications of childhood cancer. The child with cancer is now recognized as a child at risk for future difficulties—medical, psychiatric, and psychosocial. It is evident that coping with and adjusting to a life-threatening disease significantly alters a child's life. The child and family are challenged by the immediate crises and developmental disruptions as well as the spectrum of long-term sequelae.

This chapter highlights the need for a comprehensive and preventive approach that begins with early assessment and continues with ongoing evaluation of stresses throughout all phases of illness. Each phase raises unique concerns, ranging from acute anxiety and fear at diagnosis to difficulty in resuming previous activities during treatment and remission to the uncertainties of long-term survival. The medical care team's attention to these changing needs and use of appropriate psychological and psychiatric support measures will minimize immediate distress and facilitate the child's future adjustment.

REFERENCES

1. Johnson FL, Rudolph L, Hartmann J: Helping the family cope with childhood cancer. Psychosomatics 21:244–251, 1979
2. Cotter JM, Schwartz AD: Psychological and social support of the patient and family. In Altman AR (ed): Malignant Disease of Infancy, Childhood, and Adolescence. Philadelphia, WB Saunders, 1978
3. Baker LS, Roland CG, Gilchrist GS: You and Leukemia: A Day at a Time. Philadelphia, WB Saunders, 1978
4. Kjosness MA, Rudolph LA (eds): What Happened to You Happened to Me. A Booklet for Young People with Cancer. Seattle, The Children's Orthopedic Hospital and Medical Center, 1980
5. Ross JW: The role of the social worker with long-term survivors of childhood cancer and their families. Soc Work Health Care 7:1–13, 1982
6. Ruccione K, Fergusson J: Late effects of childhood cancer and its treatment. Oncol Nurs Forum 11:54–64, 1984
7. Moore IM, Kramer RF, Perin G: Care of the family with a child with cancer. Diagnosis and early stages of treatment. Cancer Nurs Perspect 13:60–66, 1986
8. Nir Y: Psychologic support of children with soft tissue and bone sarcomas. Natl Cancer Inst Monogr 56:145–148, 1981
9. Sun Han Y, McLone DG: Pain in children with spinal cord tumors. Childs Brain 11:36–46, 1984
10. Barbour LA, McGuire DB, Kirchhoff KT: Nonanalgesic methods of pain control used by cancer outpatients. Oncol Nurs Forum 13:56–60, 1986
11. Foley KM: The treatment of pain in the patient with cancer. Cancer 36:195–215, 1986
12. Orr DP, Hoffmans MA, Bennetts G: Adolescents with cancer report their psychosocial needs. J Psychosoc Oncol 2(2):47–59, 1984
13. Pfefferbaum BJ, Levenson PM: Adolescent cancer patient and physician responses to a questionnaire on patient concerns. Am J Psychiatry 139:348–351, 1982
14. Levenson PM, Pfefferbaum BJ, Copeland DR, Silberberg Y: Informational preferences of cancer patients, ages 11–20 years. J Adolesc Health Care 3:9–13, 1982
15. Spinetta JJ, Deasy-Spinetta P, McLaren HH, Kung FH, Schwartz DB, Hartman GA: The adolescent's psychosocial response to cancer. In Tebbi CK (ed): Major Topics in Pediatric and Adolescent Oncology. Boston, GK Hall Medical Publishers, 1983
16. Lansky SB, Cairns NU, Clark GM et al: Childhood cancer: Nonmedical costs of the illness. Cancer 43:403–408, 1979
17. Bodkin DM, Pigott TJ, Mann JR: Financial burden of childhood cancer. Br Med J 284:1542–1544, 1982
18. Lansky SB, Black JL, Cairns NU: Childhood cancer: Medical costs. Cancer 52:762–766, 1983
19. Cairns NU, Clark GM, Black J, Lansky SB: Childhood cancer: Nonmedical costs of the illness. In Spinetta J, Deasy-Spinetta P (eds): Living with Childhood Cancer. St Louis, CV Mosby, 1981

20. Tucker MA: Effect of heavy medical expenditures on low income families. Public Health Rep 85:419–425, 1970

21. Adams–Greenly M: Psychological staging of pediatric cancer patients and their families. Cancer 58:449–453, 1986

22. Evans AE: Practical care for the family of a child with cancer. Cancer 35:871–875, 1975

23. Pfefferbaum–Levine B, Copeland DR, Fletcher JM, Reid HL, Jaffe N, McKinnon WR: Neurologic assessment of long-term survivors of childhood leukemia. Am J Pediatr Hematol Oncol 6:123–128, 1984

24. LeBaron S: Neuropsychological assessment of children with medulloblastoma. Biomedicine 36:405–407, 1982

25. Zwartjes WJ: Education of the child with cancer. In Proceedings of the National Conference on the Care of the Child with Cancer, pp 150–156. Boston, American Cancer Society, 1978

26. Henning J, Fritz GK: School re-entry in childhood cancer. Psychosomatics 24:261–269, 1983

27. Moore IM, Triplett JL: Students with cancer: A school nursing perspective. Cancer Nurs 3:265–270, 1980

28. Sposto R, Hammond GD: Survival in childhood cancer. Clin Oncol 4:195–204, 1985

29. Lansky SB, Lowman JT, Vats T et al: School phobia in children with malignant neoplasms. Am J Dis Child 129:42–46, 1975

30. Stehbens JA, Kisker CT, Wilson BK: School behavior and attendance during the first year of treatment for childhood cancer. Psychol Sch 20:223–228, 1983

31. Lansky SB, Cairns NU, Zwartjes W. School attendance among children with cancer: A report from two centers. J Psychosoc Oncol 1:75–82, 1983

32. Cairns NU, Klopovich P, Hearne E, Lansky SB: School attendance of children with cancer. J Sch Health 152–155, 1982

33. Lansky SB, Gendel M: Symbiotic regressive behavior patterns in childhood malignancy. Clin Pediatr 17:133–138, 1978

34. Katz ER, Kellerman J, Rigler D et al: School intervention with pediatric cancer patients. J Pediatr Psychol 2:72–76, 1977

35. Greene P: The child with leukemia in the classroom. Am J Nurs 75:86–87, 1975

36. Komp D, Crocket J: Educational needs of the child with cancer. Presented at the American Cancer Society Second National Conference on Human Values and Cancer, Chicago, 1977

37. Klopovich P, Rosen D, Cairns N et al: Cancer in the Classroom: How Do You Cope? (A Teacher's Guide to Cancer in Children). Kansas City, KS, Mid-American Cancer Center, University of Kansas Medical Center, 1980

38. Deasy–Spinetta P: The school and the child with cancer. In Spinetta JJ, Deasy–Spinetta P (eds): Living with Childhood Cancer. St Louis, CV Mosby, 1981

39. Deasy–Spinetta P, Spinetta JJ: The child with cancer in school: Teacher's appraisal. Am J Pediatr Hematol Oncol 2:89–94, 1980

40. Wear ET, Blessing P: Child with cancer—Facilitating the return to school. In Peluson B, Kellogg C (eds): Current Practice in Oncologic Nursing, pp 222–230. St Louis, CV Mosby, 1976

41. Ross JW, Scarvalone SA: Facilitating the pediatric cancer patient's return to school. Soc Work 27:256–261, 1982

42. Ross JW: Resolving nonmedical obstacles to successful school re-entry for children with cancer. J Sch Health 54:84–86, 1984

43. Adams MA: A hospital play program. Helping children with serious illness. Am J Orthopsychiatry 46:416–424, 1976

44. Gibbons MB, Boren H: Stress reduction: A spectrum of strategies in pediatric oncology nursing. Nurs Clin North Am 20:83–103, 1985

45. Taylor MM, Williams HA: Use of therapeutic play in the ambulatory pediatric hematology clinic. Cancer Nurs 3:433–437, 1980

46. McEvoy M, Duchon D, Schaefer DS: Therapeutic play group for patients and siblings in a pediatric oncology ambulatory care unit. Top Clin Nurs Apr:10–18, 1985

47. Lansky LL, List MA, Lansky SB, Cohen ME, Sinks LF: Toward the development of a play-performance scale for children (PPSC). Cancer 56:1837–1840, 1985

48. Lansky SB, List MA, Lansky LL, Ritter–Sterr C, Miller DR: Measurement of performance in childhood cancer patients. Cancer (in press)

49. Friedman FB: Kids with cancer go to camp. Cancer News, Spring/Summer, 1982

50. Dasson ME: A chance to be normal again. Cancer Nurs Dec:453–459, 1982

51. Lansky SB, Smith SD, Cairns NU, Cairns GF: Psychological correlates of compliance. Am J Pediatr Hematol Oncol 5:87–92, 1983

52. Dolgin MJ, Katz ER, Doctors SR, Siegel SE: Caregivers' perceptions of medical compliance in adolescents with cancer. J Adolesc Health Care 7:22–27, 1986

53. Smith SD, Cairns NU, Sturgeon JK, Lansky SB: Poor drug compliance in an adolescent with leukemia. Am J Pediatr Hematol Oncol 3:297–300, 1981

54. Tebbi CK, Cummings KM, Zevon MA, Smith L, Richards M, Mallon J: Compliance of pediatric and adolescent cancer patients. Cancer 58:1179–1184, 1986

55. Smith SD, Rosen D, Trueworthy RC: A reliable method for evaluating drug compliance in children with cancer. Cancer 43:169–173, 1979

56. Shope JT: Medication compliance. Pediatr Clin North Am 28:5–21, 1981

57. Haynes RB: Determinants of compliance. The disease and the mechanics of Rx. In Haynes RB, Taylor DW, Sackett DL (eds): Compliance in Health Care, pp 49–62. Baltimore, Johns Hopkins University Press, 1979

58. Jay S, Litt IF, Durant RH: Compliance with therapeutic regimens. J Adolesc Health Care 5:124–136, 1984

59. Litt IF, Cuskey WR: Compliance with medical regimens during adolescence. Pediatr Clin North Am 27:3–15, 1980

60. Becker MH, Maiman LA, Kirscht JP et al: Patient perceptions and compliance. In Haynes RB, Taylor DW, Sackett DL (eds): Compliance in Health Care, pp 78–109. Baltimore, Johns Hopkins University Press, 1979

61. Gordis L, Markowitz M, Lilienfeld A: Studies in the epidemiology and preventability of rheumatic fever: IV. A quantitative determination of compliance in children on oral penicillin prophylaxis. Pediatrics 43:173–182, 1969

62. Katz ER, Kellerman J, Siegel SE: Behavioral distress in children with cancer undergoing medical procedures: Developmental considerations. J Consult Clin Psychol 48:356–365, 1980

63. Spinetta JJ, Maloney LJ: Death anxiety in the outpatient leukemic child. Pediatrics 65:1034–1037, 1975

64. Jamison RN, Lewis S, Burish T: Cooperation with treatment in adolescent cancer patients. J Adolesc Health Care 7:162–167, 1986

65. Zeltzer LK: The adolescent with cancer. In Kellerman J (ed): Psychological Aspects of Childhood Cancer, pp 70–79. Springfield, IL, Charles C Thomas, 1980

66. Pfefferbaum–Levine B, DeTrinis RB, Young MA, VanEys J: The use of psychoactive medications in children with cancer. J Psychosoc Oncol 2:65–71, 1984

67. Jones PG: Malignant disease in childhood: The problems in general practice. Aust Fam Physician 6:234–241, 1977

68. Kupst MJ, Tylke L, Thomas L, Mudd ME, Richardson C, Schulman JL: Strategies of intervention with families of pediatric leukemia patients: A longitudinal perspective. Soc Work Health Care 8:3–47, 1982

69. Lansky SB, Vats T, Cairns NU: Refusal of treatment. Am J Pediatr Hematol Oncol 1:277–282, 1979

70. Spinetta JJ: The dying child's awareness of death: A review. Psychol Bull 81:256–260, 1974

71. Chapman JA, Goodall J: Dying children need help too. Br Med J 1:593–594, 1979

72. American College of Physicians, Health and Public Policy Committee: Drug therapy for severe, chronic pain in terminal illness. Ann Intern Med 99:870–873, 1983

73. McGivney WT, Crooks GM: The care of patients with severe chronic pain in terminal illness. JAMA 251:1182–1188, 1984

74. Newburger PE, Sallan SE: Chronic pain: Principles of management. J Pediatr 98:180–189, 1981

75. Halperin EC, Cos EB: Radiation therapy in the management of neuroblastoma: The Duke University Medical Center experience 1967–1984. Int J Radiat Oncol Biol Phys 12:1829–1837, 1986

76. Brunnquell D, Hall M: Issues in the psychological care of pediatric oncology patients. Am J Orthopsychiatry 52:32–44, 1982

77. Pfefferbaum B, Lucas RH: Management of acute psychological problems in pediatric oncology. Gen Hosp Psychiatry 1:215–218, 1979

78. Ross JW: Social work intervention with families of children with cancer: The changing critical phases. Soc Work Health Care 3:257–272, 1978

79. Peck B: Effects of childhood cancer on long-term survivors and their families. Br Med J 1:1327–1329, 1979

80. Meadows AT, Krejmas NL, Belasco JB: The medical cost of cure: Sequelae in survivors of childhood cancer. In vanEys J, Sullivan M (eds): Status of the Curability of Childhood Cancers. New York, Raven Press, 1980

81. Li FP: Follow-up survivors of childhood cancer. Cancer 39:1776–1778, 1977

82. Li FP: Second malignant tumors after cancer in childhood. Cancer 40:1899–1902, 1977

83. Li FP, Cassady JR, Jaffe N: Risk of second tumors in survivors of childhood cancer. Cancer 35:1230–1235, 1975

84. Li FP, Myers MH, Heise HW, Jaffe N: The course of 5-year survivors of cancer in childhood. J Pediatr 93:185–187, 1978

85. Li FP, Stone R: Survivors of cancer in childhood. Ann Intern Med 84:551–553, 1976

86. D'Angio GJ: The child cured of cancer: A problem for the internist. Semin Oncol 9:143–149, 1982

87. D'Angio GJ: Early and delayed complications of therapy. Cancer 51:2515–2518, 1983

88. Jaffe N: Non-oncologic sequelae of cancer chemotherapy. Radiology 114:167–173, 1975

89. Biancaniello T, Meyer RA, Wong KY, Sagar C, Kaplan S: Doxorubicin cardiotoxicity in children. J Pediatr 97:45–50, 1980

90. Dawson WB: Growth impairment following radiotherapy in childhood. Clin Radiol 19:241–256, 1968

91. Jaffe N, Toth BB, Hoar RE, Ried HL, Sullivan MP, McNeese MD: Dental and maxillofacial abnormalities in long-term survivors of childhood cancer: Effects of treatment with chemotherapy and radiation to the head and neck. Pediatrics 73:816–823, 1984

92. Brown IH, Lee TJ, Eden OB, Bullimore JA, Savage DCL: Growth and endocrine function after treatment for medulloblastoma. Arch Dis Child 58:722–727, 1983

93. Zee P, Chen CH: Prevalence of obesity in children after therapy for acute lymphoblastic leukemia. Am J Pediatr Hematol Oncol 814:294–299, 1986

94. Holmes HA, Holmes FF: After ten years, what are the handicaps and life styles of children treated for cancer? Clin Pediatr 14:819–823, 1979

95. Li FP, Fine W, Jaffe N, Holmes GE, Holmes FF: Offspring of patients treated for cancer in childhood. J Natl Cancer Inst 62:1193–1197, 1979

96. Green PE, Ferguson JH: Nursing care in childhood cancer. Am J Nurs 82:443–446, 1982

97. Koocher GP, O'Malley JE, Gogan JL, Foster D: Psychological adjustment among pediatric cancer survivors. J Child Psychol Psychiatry 21:163–173, 1980

98. Kellerman J, Zeltzer L, Ellenberg L, Dash J, Rigler D: Psychological effects of illness in adolescence. 1. Anxiety, self-esteem and perception of control. J Pediatr 97:126–131, 1980

99. Koocher GP, O'Malley JE: The Damocles Syndrome, pp 74–84. New York, McGraw-Hill, 1981

100. Lansky SB, List MA, Ritter–Sterr C: Psychosocial consequences of cure. Cancer 58:529–533, 1986

101. Teta MJ, Del Po MC, Kasl SV, Meigs JW, Myers MH, Mulvihill JJ: Psychosocial consequences of childhood and adolescent cancer survival. J Chronic Dis 39:751–759, 1986

102. Rowland JH, Glidewell RF, Sibley RF et al: Effects of different forms of central nervous system prophylaxis on neuropsychologic function in childhood leukemia. J Clin Oncol 2:1327–1335, 1984

103. Browers P, Riccardi R, Poplack D, Fedio P: Attentional deficits in long-term survivors of childhood acute lymphoblastic leukemia (ALL). J Clin Neuropsychol 6:325–336, 1984

104. Duffner PK, Cohen ME, Thomas P: Late effects of treatment on intelligence of children with posterior fossa tumors. Cancer 51:233–237, 1983

105. Eiser C: Intellectual abilities among survivors of childhood leukemia as a function of CNS irradiation. Arch Dis Child 53:391–395, 1978

106. Lansky SB, Cairns NU, Cairns GF, Stephenson L, Lansky LL, Garvin G: Central nervous system prophylaxis: Studies showing impairment in verbal skills and academic achievement. Am J Pediatr Hematol Oncol 6:183–190, 1984

107. Robison LL, Nesbit ME, Sather HN, Meadows AT, Ortega JA, Hammond GD: Factors associated with IQ scores in long-term survivors of childhood acute lymphoblastic leukemia. Am J Pediatr Hematol Oncol 6:115–120, 1984

108. Copeland DR, Fletcher JM, Pfefferbaum-Levine B, Jaffe N, Ried HL, Maor M: Neuropsychological sequelae of childhood cancer in long-term survivors. Pediatrics 75:745–753, 1985

109. Pfefferbaum-Levine B, Copeland DR, Fletcher JM, Ried HL, Jaffe N, McKinnon WR: Neuropsychologic assessment of long-term survivors of childhood leukemia. Am J Pediatr Hematol Oncol 6:123–127, 1984

110. Meadows AT, Massari DJ, Ferguson J, Gordon J, Littman P, Moss K: Declines in IQ scores and cognitive dysfunctions in children with acute lymphocytic leukemia treated with cranial irradiation. Lancet 2:1015–1018, 1981

111. Fobair P, Hoppe RT, Bloom J, Cox R, Varghese A, Spiegel D: Psychosocial problems among survivors of Hodgkins disease. J Clin Oncol 4:805–814, 1986

112. Feldman F: Work and Cancer Health Histories. American Cancer Society, California Division, 1980

forty-two

Psychosocial Support for the Family of the Child with Cancer

Stephen P. Hersh and
Lori S. Wiener

The diagnosis of cancer has an immediate and lasting impact on the family. It presents a major developmental challenge to the family, as well as the child. Families must endure the transition from feeling in control of their lives to constant feelings of uncertainty. The need to relinquish control and depend on the medical system for answers and cure requires enormous adjustment. No family member is left unaffected.

Because of advances in pediatric oncology over the past 15 years, most children with cancer survive for extended periods of time. Many are cured. Even with cure, the impact on the family often persists. Marriage, careers, and relationships with others will be significantly affected. Some families will become more cohesive, developing increased strengths and a positive redefinition of values.[1,2] Others, often those with preexisting vulnerabilities, suffer various degrees of chronic disequilibrium.

Understanding the challenge that cancer and its treatment present to the family system requires an awareness of our social system, its mythologies, its pluralism and its problems. There is a stigmatizing folklore associated with cancer, which includes loss of control, fears of death and disfigurement, images of punishment for unnamed transgressions, and guilt.[3] When one combines this folklore with the extraordinary family-destabilizing social changes over the past 30 years, little imagination is needed to understand how much cancer tests the strength of a family system. These social changes include [1] the continuing movement away from the influence of traditions over daily life; [2] the powerful, intrusive influence of the media (magazines, movies, newspapers, radio, television) on the expectations and ideas of individuals; [3] the dramatic increase in the number of families in which both parents work outside the home; [4] the increases in divorce and remarriage rates;[4] [5] the dramatic increase in single-parent families;[5] [6] the increased reliance on various forms of day care; [7] the increased delegation by parents to the school system of responsibilities for training children in behaviors and values; [8] the progressive increase in the number of years spent in school rather than in work;[6] [9] the gradual reduction in family size and in time spent together;[6] and [10] the increasing rates of substance abuse, suicide, and arrests for juvenile delinquency. These changes coexist with another, harsher reality: there is no universal law protecting families who have a child or adolescent with cancer from sequentially or simultaneously having other problems.

This chapter addresses the impact of childhood cancer on the family. The disease process and treatments are examined in relation to the predictable points of stress identified in Chapter 41. Special attention is directed toward families with preexisting vulnerabilities and to the known effects on siblings. Interventions and strategies aimed at building on family strengths, providing support, handling stresses, and enhancing adaptive coping skills are reviewed.

PRINCIPLES AND ESSENTIAL KNOWLEDGE FOR HEALTH PROFESSIONALS

The developmental stages and tasks of human beings influence perceptions, understandings, and behaviors during life crises. The capacities of individuals to function, cope with stress, and to survive evolve over time. That evolution rests on a foundation of metabolic, motor, affective, language, cognitive, and social capacities in the context of accumulated experience. Norms of behavior exist within each culture. Medical personnel must always be aware that behaviors vary when there is loss of integrity of the central nervous system (CNS), poor nutrition, abnormal physiology, or significantly distorting life experiences such as abandonment, abuse, chronic unemployment, alcoholism, or other substance abuse.

People of all ages share the same complex range of responses to stress. At the neurophysiologic level, neocortical perceptions (such as being given the information that one's child has cancer) influence subcortical activity and other CNS functions, including the pituitary–adrenal axis, blood flow, vascular permeability, smooth muscle activity, respiration, and temperature. Simultaneously, general physiologic, peripheral nerve, and organ states affect the CNS at its various levels. Psychological concomitants of these responses coexist with thoughts and are identified as fear, guilt, tension, anxiety, "foggy-headedness," anger or rage, hopelessness, or depression. Behavioral responses follow. No matter how disguised, these responses in some way fall into the categories of alerting, fight, and flight.

The individual reactions described above interact to affect the functioning and behaviors of the entire family system; those behaviors in turn affect the perceptions and behaviors of the individual. A family's belief systems, history, and material resources influence its level of trust and experience of control over the realities it has faced. These in turn influence the family's image of itself (as intact, well-functioning, and strong, or as fragmented, troubled, and insecure). Experiences determine a family's capacity to adapt and tolerate many forms of stress. Past experiences that have shaken the family's confidence in having some control over events make the family more vulnerable to dysfunction in the face of new stresses. The family is a crucible within which not only are children molded, but all members are continuously "reworked". Behaviors, fears, and values are learned within the family. The behavior and beliefs of family members powerfully influence the ways in which children and adults respond to new situations and to experiences such as discomfort, separation, loss of function, fear, guilt, and pain. Children affect parents by their reactions, just as anxiety, fears, feelings of guilt, and loss of control in parents and grandparents are all transmitted to children.

Families are best understood in terms of overlapping "systems" of behaviors, needs, perceptions, values, and resources (cognitive-experiential, as well as material). When one observes the interactions within a family, one must see them not only in terms of the interactions between parents and children but among the various other possible combinations (*e.g.,* parental; an only child; both parents with each individual child; child and siblings; children and grandparents; grandparents and parents). Power balances and shifts occur during times of crisis. Expectations shift. The family reevaluates its organizing principles and beliefs. Universally, families have certain experiences which trigger or stimulate their attention (alerting response) and signal a potential loss of control. Such signals range from the obvious—a change in health status, such as a diagnosis of cancer, physical changes (*e.g.,* Cushingoid), or disfigurement (*e.g.,* amputation)—to more subtle changes, such as reduced activity level, pain, or changes in appetite or eating habits.

In recent years, health-care professionals have recognized the complexity of delivering care to the child and family facing cancer. No one health professional can completely meet a family's needs. Through collaborative, multidisciplinary efforts, a health care team can provide comprehensive care that supports the entire family through the disease course. The team can anticipate the psychological adjustment of families and plan appropriate interventions. An essential component of this approach includes an assessment of the family's strengths and vulnerabilities (Table 42-1). This information can be gathered and synthesized over a series of one to three intake meetings, each lasting 45 to 90 minutes. The sessions should be conducted by a member of the treatment team, preferably a skilled mental health professional. The setting should be as relaxed and nonthreatening as possible. Intake is the optimal time for identification of families who are at high risk for the development of significant psychosocial problems over the course of the child's illness. We define significant problems as the following: the development of clinical psychiatric symptoms (*e.g.,* anxiety, depression, patterns of impulsive behaviors and poor judgment, sleep cycle disruptions); obvious impairment in school or work performance; family system dysfunction (*e.g.,* scapegoating, lack of communication, alienation, social isolation); and noncompliance or overt sabotage of medical care. Families at high risk for these problems tend to share certain characteristics (Table 42-2).

INITIAL DIAGNOSTIC PERIOD: A TIME OF CRISIS

Diagnosis

How the diagnosis of cancer is presented to parents and their child significantly influences not only initial responses but the attitudes that will affect collaboration, compliance, and trust over the course of the illness.[3,7,8] Sophisticated oncologists develop an empathetic but direct style of disclosing a cancer diagnosis, tailoring that style to the characteristics and needs of each family, patient, and situation. The need to repeat information cannot be overemphasized (see Chap. 41 for details on informing parents and child of the diagnosis).

> "It just doesn't feel real. I can't believe this is happening."
>
> "I feel numb. I'm doing what I need to do but it doesn't feel like enough."
>
> "I just don't understand how this happened. A kid doesn't just 'get' cancer. There had to be a way that this could have been prevented."
>
> "I'm scared. There are so many things to think about. She could die. . . . She really could die. And yet, here I am thinking about what this could do to my marriage."

These comments were made at a support group for parents whose children had recently been diagnosed with malignancy. Parents perceive themselves as providers for their children, whom they are supposed to protect from fear, hurt, and pain.[9] The diagnosis of cancer represents an assault on a parent's identity and sense of adequacy as guardian.[1] Shock, disbelief, guilt, anger, and fear are the usual emotional reactions experienced by parents following their child's diagnosis. In response to these emotions, most parents struggle toward understanding

Table 42-1
Suggested Areas of Inquiry for Outlining the Family's Strengths and Vulnerabilities

Illness and History

How the illness presented itself

Was the illness identified and diagnosed rapidly?

Did parents feel a sense of competence in their handling of the situation?

Stage of child's disease at diagnosis and prognosis

Previous child and family experiences with physical health problems and trauma, behavioral and psychological problems

Family's ways of coping with any previous health or mental health problems, especially family's cohesiveness and communication style

The Child Patient as a Person

Preillness relationships with parents, siblings, peers, significant others

As seen by parents, the child's basic trust, sense of self, ability to deal with separation, level of self care, ability to use fantasy and play, orientation toward and ability to effectively deal with others, curiosity

Preillness functioning in school, plus any existing standardized test information (*e.g.,* WRAT, CATs, WISC)

Energy level, moods, sleeping and eating habits pre- and postillness

Adherence to family beliefs and values

Parent in whom child confides when he or she has a problem

How child responds to diagnosis

The Parents

Family constellation/extended nuclear family

Length of marriage

Relationship with one another before the diagnosis: level of collaboration in parenting, any prior actual or contemplated separations, sexual adjustment, differences in coping styles and communication patterns, trust, mutual respect

Physical health, previous losses, mental health, alcohol or drug abuse, self-esteem

Comfort with parent role, nurturant interests and capacities, abilities to set limits and allow independence, knowledge of child's nonverbal cues, awareness of importance of role-modeling, knowledge of growth and development, ability to be protective yet separate

Ability to express range of feelings (sadness, anxiety, guilt, fear)

Feelings toward the patient

Opinions about sharing medical information with the child

Emotional and physical symptoms since child's diagnosis

Attitudes toward and knowledge and understandings of cancer

Religious beliefs

Expectations about the future

Siblings

Ages and sex

Health

Social (family, community, school) adjustment

Perceptions of parents' attitudes toward them

Quality of current and past relationship to ill child

Role and responsibilities in family

Ability to express feelings

Understanding of illness

How informed about illness and by whom?

Degree of involvement in the diagnosis, treatment, and care

Capacity to ask questions

Parent in whom child confides when he or she has a problem

Environment

Housing

Sleeping arrangements within home

Number of moves over child's lifetime

Quality of neighborhood and community support

Financial status

Amount of television viewing

Involvement within the community prior to illness

Distance in miles and travel time to treatment center

Grandparents

Number

Ages

Physical and mental health

Residence

Social adjustment

Understanding of cancer

Sources of information about cancer

Expectations and sense of the future

Relationship to own children and to grandchildren; trust in and respect for children's autonomy and functioning as parents

Availability and ability to be supportive

---

the diagnosis and recommended treatments. Driven by a wish to reverse the implications of the diagnosis, families may seek second or third opinions, as well as spending long hours in libraries. They may selectively talk only to those acquaintances or relatives who promote unrealistic hope or who encourage disbelief in what the doctors have told them. Initial disbelief allows the reality to be approached and integrated at a pace that does not overwhelm defenses.[10] Thus, disbelief at first is protective. It reduces what might otherwise be intolerable anxiety, guilt, and anger.

As the diagnosis is accepted, guilt and anger become significant emotions. They may be directed in many ways. Anger in particular may be directed at doctors, other staff members, or the hospital at large. Those who were involved in the initial presentation of the diagnosis, a presentation that radically alters the family's life, may, for a short time, be the focus of significant negative feelings. Guilt is expressed in ruminations as parents seek reasons for cancer occurring in their child.

Many parents pass through a period of self-blame, reflecting on transgressions they may have committed (their ruminations) and for which they feel they are now being punished. They may begin searching for evidence that they failed to pay sufficient attention to early signs of less than optimal health in their child. Some parents may berate themselves for not taking complaints seriously enough, for example, for having children when "cancer runs in the family," for smoking during pregnancy, or for living in a "Love Canal" type area where industrial pollutants exist. Careful listening and support by the staff is of great importance to these families. They need reassurance (even if they verbalize no direct expressions of guilt) that they are not responsible for causing the disease.[11,12] Such interventions release parental energies for use in providing the extensive emotional support needed by their sick child or adolescent and his or her siblings. Recognizing their children's needs and having their thoughts structured by the treatment plan, parents often show a transition into a period of intense activity.

Table 42-2
Factors That Place Families at High Risk

- Single parents or two-parent families functioning as a single-parent family (*e.g.,* spouse travels frequently, is a "workaholic," or works more than one job or shift)
- Preexisting chronic health or mental health problems
- Parent incapacitated by health or mental health problem or substance abuse
- Economic problems: rural or urban poor; overextended (debts) middle-class family; job loss and minimal or no health insurance
- Separation; divorce
- Step-family system
- Chronic (unresolved) conflicts: parent–parent; parent–patient; parent–other children; sibling–sibling; grandparents–parents; grandparent–child
- Language differences: immigrant; foreign national; significantly different subculture
- Families away from their cultural support network because of the child's need for medical treatment

They rapidly absorb information about the disease and its treatment while they mobilize their own support systems.

A very important task for parents is deciding when, how, and what to tell their child about his or her diagnosis. Children, as well as parents, later recall vividly what took place when the diagnosis was revealed. Ideally, the parents should be the ones to share this information with their child. Parents need much guidance in this task. They often use euphemisms and attempt to protect their child from the harsh realities of the diagnosis and the illness itself. They need help in understanding how to communicate information about the nature of the illness and the changes in appearance and energy, and why it must be presented both honestly and calmly. Often, parents find it hard to believe that such communication promotes understanding and trust. They need repeated explanation that this approach, tailored to the age and developmental level of the child, avoids the distortions of secrets held, promises not kept, and misinformation given.[13] Family stress can be considerably alleviated once the child understands and accepts the diagnosis; this paves the way for more open communication within the family.[14-16]

Initiation of Treatment

A new adaptive equilibrium in the family occurs as treatment is initiated. This equilibrium incorporates the illness, as the family reaches for a new sense of normalcy. Treatment fosters parental confidence, with a sense of hope for the future.[17] As one mother stated, "After I found out what needed to be done, I felt like I had something to hold on to . . . a chance for a cure. Almost immediately, I felt as if I had some control back . . . now we had something to fight with."

Along with the feelings of relief, optimism, and improved mood, the initiation of treatment stimulates anxiety, particularly concerning side-effects. Eliciting from families their understanding and expectations of the illness and diagnostic and treatment procedures and correcting these as needed with further education and explanations become essential activities. Misunderstandings commonly occur at this time because of the "selective" hearing of the parents as well as their assumptions about how busy physicians are. Some parents tend to retain in conscious memory information that reinforces their hopeful-

ness while failing to recall information with negative implications. Perceiving the physician as "too busy" gives the parent a comfortable reason to avoid confirmation of valid fears about the child's condition. Coping with the treatment process is often affected by the length of the prediagnostic period: a rapid diagnosis, without uncertainty, demands much less of the family resources than a prolonged prediagnostic period of professional uncertainty. Equally important, the physician needs to reclarify for the family the nature of his or her involvement throughout the treatment process: how much care he or she will administer directly; what will be done by others; and his or her supervisory role. Such precise communication often makes the difference between a compliant family that becomes engaged in the treatment process and a highly noncompliant one. Noncompliant families are expensive in terms of their demands on the physician's time, anxiety-provoking to the patient, and distressing to other families and to medical staff.

Informed Consent

Informing parents and their child about treatments falls in the same arena as informing them about the diagnosis of cancer (see also Chaps. 15, 41, and 53). The approach used, the setting, the need for repetition, and the awareness of each family's unique strengths and limitations, all remain important. Parents fear the complications of procedures and treatments. Especially if the child feels and looks well, parents tend to want to postpone interventions that seem "risky" to them but are considered necessary by physicians. This desire, especially when combined with the unsettled feeling caused by not fully understanding the information presented through consent forms, can further threaten physician–family relationships. Careful explanations of the disease and its treatment that are tailored to the understanding of each family will significantly improve compliance. It is a positive sign of coping and adaptation when the family asks questions, openly expresses concern, and actively seeks to increase sophistication about the child's disease and treatment.[18] Parents should be encouraged to take notes; we suggest offering them pads and pencils. Note-taking will assist them in recall and in formulating questions. For parents who are not literate or who speak another language, it is important to have in attendance a team member assigned as a patient advocate or a translator. Only the physician(s) involved in the child's treatment should be responsible for informed consent. Nine steps can assist families through this process:[18,19]

1. A full explanation of the treatments and associated procedures must be presented. The language should avoid professional images and jargon, explaining in lay images and words those professional terms that are unavoidable.
2. The purposes and expected benefits of the treatments need to be listed.
3. Common morbidities from procedures as well as common morbidities and side-effects of treatments should be outlined. Overinforming verbally (*e.g.,* presenting extensive lists of all possible side-effects) generates confusion and anxiety. It should be avoided.
4. Alternative treatments need to be acknowledged and discussed.
5. At this point, the physician should stop and review both questions and psychological reactions with the parents. This recognition of the parents' feelings and thoughts invariably enhances their reaction to the physician. It also helps to quiet anxiety. This is the time to inquire about the known or expected reactions from grandparents, other relatives and friends; these caring individuals may

pressure the parents with their own disbelief about the diagnosis, their anxieties, and advice. Learning about such pressures helps the physician to more clearly understand the parents' questions and emotional responses.[18]

6. The voluntary nature of treatment must be made clear.
7. Parental awareness of the right to withdraw from treatment should be explained carefully, including the meaning of withdrawal "against medical advice." Describe, if necessary, those situations in which the physician will vigorously pursue treatment over parental objections, even to the point of obtaining a court order supporting treatment.
8. The above steps are summarized in the patient's medical chart; at the least, the date, time, and those present when informed consent was obtained are noted.
9. Written consent forms are signed where appropriate or required.

Consent forms almost always cause the families considerable stress. Studies reveal that the majority of consent forms "obfuscate, intimidate, and alienate."[3] The readability of these forms is often at a college or higher educational level.[3] In clinical research settings, the realities of informed consent are compounded by requests to participate in randomized treatment trials; such trials tend to restimulate guilt in parents and to provoke feelings of helplessness, anxiety, and anger.[8,14,20] Parents fear the complications of procedures and treatments. Their desire to postpone these interventions—especially in a child who *seems* well—coupled with being unsettled by not fully understanding information presented through consent forms, threatens physician–family relationships.

Nausea, vomiting, and hair loss usually accompany the use of chemotherapy agents. Infections and toxicity may also occur. Highly visible side-effects (hair loss, muscle weakness, ataxia) or severe toxicity (neutropenia with infection) generate guilt in parents about their having given their consent for treatment. As one parent described it, "I can't stand watching the chemo being administered. I feel as if I'm permitting my son to be poisoned." Many parents struggle with the changes in their child's appearance: "I know she's the same person and I love her every bit as much as I always have. But she looks so different. Only a few weeks ago she was standing on the stage of her school play singing. Her hair looked so beautiful and her eyes sparkled so. I can't let her see how much her appearance bothers me. Truly, my biggest consolation is how well she's handling all of this."

Unfortunately, for some patients, amputation may be the best or only treatment for the disease. Although numerous effects on the patient undergoing an amputation have been noted in the literature, many health care professionals tend to overlook the effect that an amputation may have on parents.[18] The loss of a child's limb is experienced as a loss for the parents as well. Parents mourn this loss, and they need time to accommodate to the resultant disfigurement and to integrate the modified body image of their child (see also Chaps. 41 and 46). As one mother stated, "I'll do anything to save his life— including an amputation. But I feel as if I'm losing something that is mine too. I love his leg like I love all of him. People don't seem to understand that."

Parents welcome the opportunity to discuss their feelings about their child, the changes in their child's condition and appearance, and the changes taking place in their own lives with someone who knows the child's situation and who they feel can be sensitive to their own personal struggles.[21] Thus, true informed consent is a process that extends beyond a few formal meetings and printed consent forms.

In summary, complexities of the diagnostic period call on all the family's resources and all the clinical skills of the medi-

cal staff. Families often need assistance preparing for the long siege of illness. They need to learn the value of dealing openly with serious illness and the importance of maintaining a balance between the needs of the sick child and those of other family members.[13] Parents who are under emotional stress and facing financial burden are apt to neglect or postpone necessary care for their own or the siblings' health. Efforts need to be made to obtain information regarding current health problems of all family members in an attempt to prevent future crises and to conserve the family's energies and emotional resources.[22]

Despite severe stress, most family members tend to manifest considerable resiliency throughout the disease course. They learn to accept the child's diagnosis realistically. Many are able to hold a neutral, if not optimistic, view of their lives while acknowledging the life-threatening nature of the illness.[15] A number of factors influence how a particular family copes. These include the personality make-up of individual family members, the family's background, how previous crises have been managed, and the current economic and social situation.[10,14,16,23] Coping does not mean absence of problems, severe emotional upsets, or the occasional use of defensive measures or behaviors. Acute stress reactions are normal. Families benefit from being informed that their own responses are understandable and appropriate. Throughout the disease course, each family will demonstrate a range of responses along a spectrum of adaptability. Ideally, problems in adaptation are immediately identified at each stage of the process (diagnosis, informed consent, initiation of treatment). Table 42-3 presents the spectrum of warning signs and problems in adaptation. It is imperative that all maladaptive responses be identified early and that psychosocial intervention be obtained. Such interventions may include crisis intervention, insight-oriented psychotherapy, the use of psychotropic medication or other treatments such as behavioral techniques (which address specific problems) and supportive therapy for the family.

The initial coping style manifested by the family can be used as a significant indicator of its long-term adaptability.[24] Therefore, it is best to have a thorough understanding of how the family functions prior to the diagnosis as well as at the time of crisis. This allows the health professional to assess the impact of the diagnosis on the family, identify behaviors that may indicate future problems, and plan how to offer help most effectively.[17] It is often helpful to engage the family in predicting how they will cope with future crises. Families then feel forewarned and prepared and are able to adapt more effectively to stresses that occur throughout the treatment process. Evaluation of family functioning is best formulated at the time of diagnosis or on entry into a new medical environment. However, such "intakes" need to be ongoing in order to assess family functioning at the different stress points throughout the child's disease course.

ADAPTATION PERIOD

Given the improved survival rate in childhood cancer, health care professionals emphasize normalcy throughout the treatment and adaptation period. This creates a "burden of normalcy"[8] as the family is faced with the task of reorganizing itself, changing previous priorities and expectations, and reassigning roles. Optimally, both parents are physically and emotionally available to share the responsibility of the child's care. Unfortunately this is often not the case, and the increased burden of care falls more on one parent.[25] Families who live in communities without a major cancer treatment center face additional problems: the need to travel long distances for treatment; separation from home and most supports during a

Table 42-3
Spectrum of Adaptation During Diagnostic Period

Adaptive Responses	*Early Signs of Problems in Coping*	*Maladaptive Responses*
Parents and other family members understand diagnosis and prognosis[22]	Forgetting or intermittently denying diagnosis or its implications and prognosis (*i.e.,* can't remember disease or treatments)	Unquestioning acceptance and unreserved compliance, or massive denial/refusal to accept diagnosis and explanations
Ability to seek information from medical staff, ask questions, take notes, seek second and third opinions	Inability to ask questions, or frantic activity, repeatedly asking the same questions	"Shopping" (seeking more than a third opinion) for a better, more acceptable diagnosis while avoiding potentially curative treatments
Ability to engage in necessary and appropriate explanations to patient and siblings; ability to make changes in lifestyle and life rhythms to accommodate the demands of diagnostic processes and treatments	Passive, slowly reactive	Parents unable to perform ordinary tasks on behalf of patient, siblings, themselves, or family system
Ability to express feelings within family and with appropriate health care professionals (physician, primary nurse, social worker, hospital clergy)	Too busy to talk or "think about" feelings; partial withdrawal from one another within family (veil of silence); no expression to health care professionals	Only rudimentary communication among family members; increasing self-blame, guilt, and depression; use of "splitting" defenses as in excessive criticism of some staff while aggrandizing others;[23] assaultive anger directed at physicians, nurses, the "system"

stressful and frightening time; and the strain on finances due to transportation, child care and accommodations, all combined with rising medical costs.

Cost

The economic impact of cancer therapy has a direct and significant effect on the entire family's ability to cope (see also Chaps. 41 and 43). Expenses begin to mount prior to diagnosis and extend throughout the course of the child's treatment. Even for those families who have medical insurance, out-of-pocket cash expenses are substantial. These include items such as parking, transportation, long-distance telephone calls to doctors and family members, meals, temporary housing near the hospital, laundry, wigs, childcare for siblings, and new clothing if the treatment center is located in a different climatic zone or if the child loses or gains a significant amount of weight.

Early assessment of the family's financial situation is essential in order to lessen future economic stress on the family. This is best done by the social worker. The assessment should include the specifics of third party insurance coverage (in-cluding military or CHAMPUS) and the name of the insurance representative; and whether or not the family is in need of or eligible for social security benefits, specific state benefits, Medicaid, or resources available within the hospital or community. Many families find it helpful to keep a record of all incurred expenses. Chapter 43 provides a more complete discussion of financial issues and resources.

Parental Adjustment

A study by Cook[26] found that both parents (or the single parent) tend to remain at the hospital during the initial diagnosis and first therapeutic interventions. Once the first crisis passes, the mother is likely to assume the burden of day-to-day care of the child. Mothers are likely to stay overnight during subsequent hospitalizations, while the fathers are often responsible for the care of the child's siblings and other home-related matters. Mothers continue to remain responsible for the outpatient visits.

Decisions regarding a shift of roles in the support, management, and care of the home and family appear to be influenced by several factors. These include where treatment is provided, the financial and task burdens it causes, whether both parents are employed, the age of the affected child and siblings, and, most importantly, the ability of the parents to communicate openly and to share tasks.[25] Open communication allows spouses to negotiate the reallocation of roles more effectively, resulting in a more cohesive, less conflictual family environment.[20]

A mutually supportive marital relationship is a significant variable in the family's ability to cope with the stress imposed by childhood cancer.[27] Nevertheless, parents are often reluctant to take time to meet their own individual needs or those of their spouse.[28] Many parents tend to be overprotective and to include the sick child in most of their activities. Fife[29] identified several reasons for this additional strain on the marriage, including [1] the parents' need to "make the child as happy as possible"; [2] a sense of guilt regarding the child's disease; [3] fear of leaving the child alone or in someone else's care (compounded by the fear of permanent separation and loss of one's child); and [4] parents becoming so caught up in their day-to-day stress that they tend to disregard the importance of their own needs or those of other family members.

The separation of a family (the mother and patient at the hospital and the siblings and father at home) can cause significant stress and may also strain marital ties.[22] Some parents may be apart from their spouses for the first time and be faced with the difficult task of making decisions independently. When both partners are forced to give up roles that were exclusively theirs and assume new ones, problems arise when they remain emotionally invested in their relinquished roles.[30] "Dissynchrony of coping styles may occur.[31] This often leads to family members becoming isolated from one another while experiencing a feeling of abandonment and lack of empathy.[32] For example, mothers often perceive their husbands as being disengaged or disinterested. When differences of coping styles are identified and addressed, tension within the marriage and family is often considerably alleviated. It is also important to know whether both parents understand the diagnosis in the same way, whether the plan for treatment was mutually decided upon, whether the parents have compatible ways of dealing with stress and adapting, whether they are able to understand and support one another, and whether one parent feels he or she is doing all the work while the other feels left out.[16] Parents must be treated by the staff as individuals with their own lifetime of experience and needs while also recognizing their particular role within the family structure. Attempts at understanding the past personal and family history of each parent are essential in order to avoid severing of family ties. This will also enhance the family's ability and willingness to place their trust in the hospital staff.

Because usually it is the patient's mother who is most often at the treatment facility, her strengths and vulnerabilities can be identified more readily than those of the child's father. Unfortunately, fathers tend to receive less support, have limited opportunity to share their concerns with others, and tend to feel guilty as well as excluded from the daily aspects of the child's life and care. When given the opportunity to do so, fathers often describe the difficulty of having to perform at work and at home, of constantly having to alter work schedules due to family obligations, of missing life "as it was", and of feeling helpless.

It is essential to involve both parents in the program of care. This can be done by: [1] including the father in as many of the early discussions as possible; [2] enabling him to express his particular concerns; and [3] helping him to become more familiar with the day-to-day responsibilities that his wife will have while looking after their child.[14] Concomitantly, attempts must continually be made to keep communication open between the parents. It is important for both parents to feel they have firsthand knowledge of their child's medical progress and that their involvement is essential to the well-being of their child. Parents often benefit from support groups where families can learn from each other how to meet their own needs as well as those of their sick child. They also benefit from individual or family therapy where the issues of communication, intimacy, or differences in coping styles can be addressed and hopefully resolved.[17,32] The Candlelighters Foundation as well as the American Cancer Society and its local chapters may also be a source of support for families interested in self-help groups within their home community and for those who wish to obtain a bibliography of reading materials and films pertaining to their child's disease (see also Chap. 46 for resource information).

Early Remission and Ongoing Treatment

Following the induction of therapy, there is often a period of remission or tumor regression. The child is able to go home for extended periods of time, returning to the hospital on a scheduled basis to receive chemotherapy or radiation treatments. This process may continue for a number of years.

Particularly when the initial hospital admission has been lengthy, families anxiously await the day their child is well enough to return home. Some parents, however, find this a particularly stressful time. The hospital is often perceived as a safe environment, a place where the child's medical needs are continuously met. For the first time, parents may feel powerless and question their ability to care for their child's physical well-being.

The health care staff can help ease the transition from hospital to home. A schedule of follow-up visits should be given to the family along with a copy of the protocol and necessary blood work. Parents should be told what to do if the child has a fever or appears ill, and necessary time for questions needs to be alloted. Also, families find it exceptionally helpful to visit the outpatient clinic or treatment facility and to meet the new staff before the child's discharge (see sections on discharge planning in Chaps. 41 and 46).

Once home, parents attempt to sustain as normal a life as possible within the confines of the diagnosis.[33] A new day-to-day routine must be established encompassing the needs of the marital relationship and the well siblings, in addition to the sick child. When the affected child is confined at home due to fatigue, pain, low blood cell counts, or low morale, stress within the family increases considerably. Parents may not be able to return to their work or to meet other commitments. At the same time, the child, probably bald and possibly cushingoid or disfigured in other ways, must confront the reactions of siblings, relatives, neighbors, and peers. These challenges are most dramatic for adolescent patients.[34] Parents, concerned about the responses of others, may not receive the comfort expected from relatives and friends. This may be attributed to fears surrounding separation and death, anxiety about "not knowing what to say," or misconceptions about cancer in general. As a result, parents may feel they can no longer relate to some of the people they had previously relied on for emotional support. A sense of angry disappointment and feelings of isolation may evolve into withdrawal, further threatening the family's equilibrium. This can be avoided by specific interventions. Parents benefit from having staff members and other families prepare them for the possible reactions, ranging from support to avoidance, that they may encounter from others. They also profit from having the opportunity to "rehearse" how they will describe the illness, treatments, and prognosis to family, friends, and school personnel prior to their child's discharge.

When it is time for the child to return for further treatment, some parents feel resentful at again having to yield some of their parental responsibilities to the medical system. Others look forward to being assured that their child is doing well or will be receiving treatments that can cure the disease. These responses are appropriate. Soon, most families will become actively involved in the treatment process. This entails settling into the routine of the hospital or clinic visits while obtaining a comprehensive grasp of the medical treatments and procedures. It is important to remember that all individuals have their own way of handling stress and coping with crises. Some parents may be perceived as a "tower of strength" throughout the diagnosis and early treatment period, only to "fall apart" temporarily following successful induction therapy.[17] This should not be mistaken as maladaptive behavior. Rather it occurs because some individuals, after the initial impact of the disease has been absorbed, find themselves only then becoming aware of the chronic, life-threatening nature of the disease. At this point, parents may begin to mourn the loss of their child's health and their previous life. Families find the support of relatives, friends, and faith as well as the honesty of the physicians and nurses helpful. They often benefit from talking to a nonmedical person about the disease, a person who can help them anticipate and cope with the hospital system and treatment. They also profit from talking to other parents who have been through a similar experience, from learning to take "one day at a time," and from talking with other children who have done well.

The continuum of coping responses seen during the reentry period is described in Table 42-4. A number of variables correlate with family coping during the period of remission.[35] These include open communication about the illness within the family, an attitude of living in the present, lack of other concurrent stresses (marital, financial, illness of other family members), the quality of relationships among family members; previous adaptive coping with the illness, coping of other family members, and adequacy of the support system. During remission and treatment, maladaptive coping often occurs in families who had significant difficulties coping at the time of diagnosis. Maladaptive coping may be expressed through many symptoms, including an excessive concern about relapse and death, inability to allow the child to return to everyday activities, interpersonal strife, continuous crying and generalized anxiety/worrying, behavioral symptoms in the well siblings, poor compliance with clinic visits or treatments, refusal to interact with other patients or families, and an ongoing pessimism about the unfairness of life in general. In more extreme situations, magical thinking, regressive forms of behavior, or withdrawal from reality will be evident (see Table 42-4). Interventions during remission need to be tailored to the specific needs of the individual family members. Families who have adapted well can benefit from individual or family supportive counseling to find ways in which the family can further unite and develop even stronger ties. In contrast, poor adaptation necessitates ongoing intensive intervention by an experienced mental health professional which provides the individual family member or the family as a whole with support, limits, and structure (see Table 42-5).

With the passage of time, most families develop a new kind of stability in their lives. They become more hopeful that the remission will last and may again begin to make plans for the future. An infection or unexpected treatment side-effect necessitating hospitalization interferes with family adjustment.[36] Family members briefly find themselves experiencing once again many of the feelings they had at the time of diagnosis. When the physical health of the child is restabilized and time between visits is lengthened, families may then begin to worry that the details of their child's "case" have been forgot-

Table 42-4
Spectrum of Adaptation During Remission

Adaptive Responses	Early Signs of Problems in Coping	Maladaptive Responses
Parents and other family members able to communicate openly about the illness and how it is affecting their lives	Family members feel estranged from one another and unable to establish a comfortable "new normalcy" within the family	Inter- and intrapersonal disequilibrium evidenced by behavioral problems in well siblings, difficulties in problem solving, and marital discord
Return to work and school, family and community life; make plans for future	Feelings of estrangement; having to force selves to return to work, school, family, and community life; refusal to think about future	Inability to return to work, school, family, and community life; estrangement, isolation; no plans for future
Able to assist patient with transitions, social acceptance, self-image, health-enhancing behaviors while engaging in normal limit-setting	General pessimism; difficulty in following through on the various parental responsibilities; fear of setting limits; feeling of "walking on eggs"	Withdrawal from parental responsibilities, especially vis-á-vis patient, or overindulging patient in every way
Able to call on medical team, other family, or community resources for any needed support	Little to no spontaneous interactions with support networks, combined with feelings of loneliness and isolation	Avoidance of medical staff, family and community supports

Table 42-5
Issues Addressed in Interventions for Parents and Siblings During Diagnostic and Adaptation Period

Education
    The disease and its management
    Care: activities of daily living, finances, nutrition, physical activity,
        touching and holding
    Stress management training

Mobilization of Resources and Environmental Change
    Transportation/travel
    Day care
    Employment problems

Self-Help Groups
    Education resource information
    Isolation/legitimization
    Channeling of feelings and advocacy

Psychiatric Interventions
    Family therapy
        Feelings
        Communication
        Dealing with separation
        Dealing with regression
        Goal setting
        Preexisting conflicts
    Marriage counseling
        Feelings
        Role changes
        Case management
    Individual psychotherapy
        Anxiety
        Depression
        Working through feelings of helplessness and hopelessness
        Enhance strengths, promote growth
    Group therapy
        Feelings of isolation/support
        Helplessness
        Separation
        Goal setting
    Behavior therapy
        Anxiety
        Phobias
        Sleep disorders
    Medication
        Anxiety
        Panic reactions
        Depression

ten. Such feelings may be more exaggerated in teaching hospitals where physicians frequently rotate assignments. These feelings are surmountable. Most families are eager to have the support and understanding of their physician, and like to be thought of as special.[37] Therefore, it is important that attention also be given to the emotional needs of families whose child is in remission. Systematic referrals to community-based advocacy and support services (*e.g.,* Candlelighters, ACS) aid in adjustment during this less stressful but difficult phase.

PARENTAL EXPECTATIONS AND DISCIPLINE

As treatment continues, fears related to the disease are less prominent, and other concurrent stresses are perceived as more troublesome.[38] Mothers and fathers often find themselves in a quandary as to how to "parent" their own child. Treating the child as "normal" requires parents to return to pre-illness expectations—achievement, independence, and responsibility for specific chores—all of which should result in the child becoming a well-functioning and responsible adult.[39] However, feelings of uneasiness, guilt, and anxiety about the disease and possible relapse may interfere with the parents' ability to act in the child's best interest. Their expectations for their child may range from high to low.

> "I thought because his treatments were going well, he should be able to continue football practice and be as content and easygoing as before. It wasn't until I found him alone sobbing one day that I realized that my expectations were unrealistic. . . . I just wanted him to be normal . . . like before".

> "I remember when I turned 15 and my mother took me to the Social Security office. We didn't need the money but she told me that it was better to apply for disability now so I could be assured of an income later on. I assumed this meant that I could never be well enough to work and that I would be permanently sick. She was wrong—there are plenty of things I can do. . . . That wasn't fair".

Many parents find themselves feeling frustrated when faced with excessive dependency on the part of their children.[40] At the same time, parents tend to encourage dependency, to overindulge or overprotect their child, and they find it difficult to administer any discipline. This exacerbates the child's perception of him- or herself as different and "singled-out," placing the child in an uncomfortable position with peers and siblings, who resent the "extra attention." Such attention also may be perceived by the child as meaning that the prognosis is worse than he or she had been told. Children who encounter overprotectiveness in one parent and overindulgence in another, or both reactions alternately in the same parent, are forced to understand and cope with this inconsistency.[41] Children with a chronic or life-threatening disease are especially sensitive to changes in their parents' behavior and attitudes, as these create the "atmosphere" within which children understand and cope with their disease. The child has already lost his or her health and is fearful of losing parental love as well. When a parent becomes uncharacteristically lenient or upset, one may hear the child playfully request that the "real" parent return. Children often feel relieved when the discipline resumes, for it brings with it a sense of normalcy and parental control missing from their current life situation.

Parents appreciate the suggestions of physicians, social workers, nurses, and other parents concerning their child's behavior. They need to be informed of what the child can and cannot realistically do in comparison to abilities before the cancer diagnosis. This includes decisions on returning to school and outside activities. Parents need to be encouraged to allow the child to live as full and normal a life as possible within the restrictions imposed by the disease. They need to find a balance between overindulging the child and setting too many limits.[42] Parents feel less guilty saying "no" to their child when such behavior has been sanctioned by the physician or other significant persons on the health care team.

Completion of Therapy

Following successful completion of therapy, the family may be full of joy, pride, and a sense of accomplishment. However, they may also experience a concomitant sense of anxiety, sadness, and fear, recalling other patients who have relapsed or died. Separation from the treatment team on whom they have depended generates uneasiness.

Families require additional education and support at this point. They often describe feeling insecure and helpless when therapy is not being administered. Parents benefit from a review of the treatment protocol and the reasons why therapy is being discontinued. They want to be told about treatment options that will be available if the disease recurs. They need to be reassured that they will in no way be responsible nor will they have "failed" if the cancer returns. At this point, the physician and other staff members can be especially helpful by explaining to the family the meaning of the word "cure," by discussing the follow-up care that will be provided, and by reviewing symptoms that should be reported without delay. Changes and growth that have taken place in each family member should also be discussed at this time, allowing for a sense of achievement while preparing the family for the challenges of long-term survival (see Chaps. 50–52).

RELAPSES AND RECURRENCES: A SECOND CRISIS

Parents often describe the first relapse or recurrence as the most difficult time to bear, especially when treatment appeared to be going well and no obvious symptoms were present, or when the remission was of long duration. Following confirmation of a relapse, feelings of shock, anxiety, disbelief, fear, guilt, anger, and sadness are common. The crisis and stress of the diagnosis are reactivated, the threat to life relived, and new adjustments are required.[42,43] The following statements represent only a few of the many reactions that parents have following their child's first relapse.

> "I was not prepared for the disease to come back. Not yet . . . Not so soon. We were just starting to get our feet back on the ground."

> "I really thought it was a mistake. She felt and looked so well. But the doctor showed me her old chest x-ray and put it next to the new one. Then I knew. It was happening all over again."

> "As I told my daughter, we got through it before and we would get through it again. We have a lot of faith in God and in the doctors. . . . But I'd be lying if I said we weren't scared."

> "That poor kid—after everything he's gone through. I don't know if I could watch him go through that again. I feel like I lied to him—by telling him the treatments would make him well. They made him sick and the lumps came back anyway. This is the beginning of the end. I just know it."

Krulik calls the time between the first relapse (recurrence) and second remission or failure as the midstage of illness.[44] Unfortunately, some children do not survive past this point. Hopes for another treatment response are rekindled when the family is encouraged to begin reinduction or another treatment regimen promptly.[45] Attempts to re-create stability and equilibrium within the family are difficult. Intensive treatments once again limit the family's time for other activities. Work habits, social activities, friendship patterns, relationships within the family, and expression of feelings are again altered.[1] Within the hospital environment itself, the family may experience a change of identity. Krulik points out, "[The family] can no longer belong to the 'successful' remission group receiving similar treatment protocols. It is as if the relapse has singled

them out. From this point, their child's treatment is more individualized and their ability to draw some comfort and control from the benchmarks of other children's experiences is gone."[44] The family may also sense a change in the attitudes of health care team members, who may be struggling with feelings of disappointment, frustration, sadness, and possibly defeat. As one father expressed it, "After Pammy relapsed, the doctor told us what needed to be done. He was very nice and all . . . but it was different this time. His enthusiasm was gone. And so was the closeness we felt with him in the past."

Following the recurrence of disease, some families may question whether they should seek other treatments, new second opinions, or whether they should try some unorthodox method of therapy. At the same time, the physician may decide that it is in the child's best interest to be referred to another treatment center for participation in a particular randomized clinical trial. The request to consider such a referral may challenge the trust between family and physician, particularly if the family interprets the referral as being sent away because their child's case is now "hopeless."[46] This can be worked through and confidence reestablished when a pattern of open, honest communication is encouraged and maintained. The physician needs to reassure the child and family that the relationship that he or she has with the family will not be severed.[46] A commitment to care for the emotional needs of the patient and family, to provide pain control if necessary, and not to abandon the family if the disease progresses, is essential. Each family will be searching for ways to cope with the renewed threat to life and to emotional equilibrium. At relapse, increased psychosocial support and exploration of family's strengths help many to discover new hope and courage.[42]

Most families manage to cope adequately through the different treatment processes. Once again, they need to develop a new sense of "normalcy" and stability in their lives. The degree of stability is dependent on treatment side-effects, the length of time the child needs to remain hospitalized, and on such concurrent stresses as financial pressures, career obligations, and family problems. The altered prognosis will elicit feelings of sadness and fears of separation and loss; yet, an investment in "going on" persists. Maladaptive coping is manifested by an overly pessimistic attitude about the future that may immobilize parents in their day-to-day functioning. Emotional or physical withdrawal from the child, inability to normalize the child's life, or refusal to follow through with medical care are other signs indicating the need for immediate intervention (see Table 42-6). Crisis intervention with individual or family sessions can help the family alter the maladaptive coping behavior.

If another remission is achieved, the termination of active treatment will often activate a crisis situation that requires additional education and support from the staff. Parents fear another relapse and the lack of future treatment options. As one mother stated, "I'm petrified. I've been through this before and the disease came back. At least with chemo, we have a hold on the disease. I can't help but think that ending the treatment will eventually result in ending my son's life." It is essential for the treatment team to remain in close contact with the family. Not only is frequent medical follow-up required, but the quality of the family's life needs continual assessment as the family copes with fear and tremendous uncertainty.[41]

Successive relapses and the introduction of Phase I and Phase II trials will considerably tax the family's coping abilities (see also Chaps. 9 and 15). Most families maintain some hope with each new treatment, although this is often interspersed with feelings of powerlessness and uncertainty. The family may vacillate between wanting "to do everything possible" and the desire to provide only comfort and peace. As side-ef-

Table 42-6
Spectrum of Adaptation During Relapse

Adaptive Responses	Early Signs of Problems in Coping	Maladaptive Responses
Accepting as normal the reactions of shock, anxiety, disbelief, fear, guilt, anger, and sadness; being able to express and share these feelings within the family	Continuous crying; ruminating about all the fearful possibilities that could occur; sleep disorders; withdrawal from one another	Withdrawal emotionally and physically from sick child or other family members; blaming others for the relapse or other angry scapegoating
Mobilization of selves and the family system to understand the new medical situation and support the patient in treatments directed at obtaining a new remission	Slow response to news of relapse and pessimistic attitude; absence of information seeking or questioning behaviors	Withdrawal from all supports with refusal to try for new remission despite medical advice; immobilization with or without clinical symptoms of anxiety, depression, severe sleep disorder; inability to deal with daily responsibilities

fects become more frequent and as more difficult treatment decisions need to be made, tension within the family escalates. The home may no longer provide the family with a reprieve from hospital life. Little time may be available for family members to communicate their expressions of fear, anxiety, and anger. Parents, often eager to acquire the necessary skills to care for their sick child at home, may begin to question their physical and emotional ability to do so.

Important interventions during this time include providing extended family and community supports; creating an atmosphere in the hospital and at home where family members can talk through their concerns and where decisions can be made, and ensuring the availability of the entire oncology treatment team for support, information, guidance, and encouragement.

TERMINAL ILLNESS

When Treatment Is No Longer Effective

Currently, the course of cancer for many children and adolescents remains a series of treatment responses and relapses leading to a time when established treatments are no longer effective. A small number of patients remain refractory to all treatments. Whatever the clinical course, during the terminal phase of illness there comes a time when aggressive treatment only increases or prolongs suffering.[18] When that time comes is based on several factors: the specific form of cancer, the child's physiology; the child's and family's threshold of tolerance for physical pain and loss of control; their levels of hope and hunger for life; fatigue; and religious and other beliefs.[47] When the experienced physician feels the time to offer palliative care has arrived, a meeting with the family is indicated. The clinician needs to elicit from parents their understanding of the situation, selectively sharing impressions with them. The child may or may not attend this meeting, depending on his or her developmental stage and other circumstances. If the child is not present, the physician or parents should later broach this

issue directly with him or her. The patient and family need to be told what may happen, physically and emotionally, if they choose to stop all treatments (*e.g.,* when and how the child may die). It is essential that the staff who have been a support to the child and family during the course of the disease be present at these meetings. The use of hospice care may be raised for the first time. When the family is in agreement, treatment should then be allowed to become palliative.[48]

The principles of palliative treatment and terminal care are guided by concern for the physical and psychological comfort of the patient, the patient's family system, and its members. Chapter 49 discusses treatment of the terminally ill child; our focus remains on the family.

Once it is clear that treatment is no longer effective, hope ebbs and parents begin the process of accepting that their child will die. They may experience preparatory (anticipatory) grief. Many of their thoughts will focus on preparing for death (this may include rehearsing the funeral in their imaginations) while continuing to hope for cure or recovery.[49] This is a time when parents are again very vulnerable to nontraditional or even fraudulent healers and healing rituals. Feeling moments of hopefulness while simultaneously thinking of the child's funeral generates guilt. Guilt can be diminished by simply informing the parents of the normalcy of these responses.

Struggling with their own anticipations and fears of separation and death, the family may need assistance in refocusing on their child's thoughts and concerns. Many parents find themselves unable to discuss the imminence of death with their child.[10] They often believe that the child is unaware of his or her fatal prognosis and impending death. Share, in reviewing the literature, has found two opposing modes of communication at this time.[50] She describes these as "the protective approach in which the ill child is shielded from knowledge of the disease diagnosis and prognosis; and, the open approach, which encourages provision of an environment in which the child feels free to express concerns and ask questions about his or her condition."[50] Research has shown that children who exhibited a higher level of adaptation to the illness were members of families in which open discussion was allowed and maintained.[51] Waechter, who conducted a study of hospitalized and fatally ill children, states that giving a child the opportunity to discuss issues related to death does not heighten death anxiety.[52] In fact, her findings support the prediction that "understanding, acceptance, and conveyance of permission to discuss any aspect of the illness, decreases feelings of isolation and alienation from parents and other meaningful adults and gives the child the sense that his or her illness is not too terrible to discuss."[52]

In published accounts, parents themselves have documented with great feeling the self-awareness of their dying children. Well-known examples include books by John Gunther, Doris Lund, Mickie Sherman, and Nancy Roach.[53-56]

When given the opportunity, children most frequently ask what death will be like: what will happen to them after they die, if the "bad things" they have done or thought will cause them to be punished, whether their parents will be all right, when they will again be with those closest to them, and whether they will experience much pain. Parents benefit from being informed of these thoughts. Depending on the child's religious upbringing, other spiritual concerns and questions may arise. For example, a child experiencing considerable guilt and conflict or feelings of isolation may become frightened and preoccupied about whether "the devil is in my heart" or whether "God will stop watching over me." Consultation with a chaplain specializing in work with terminally ill children can allay the child's fears and bring to the child and family a renewed sense of comfort and peace. Parents often need help understanding their child's questions and providing answers that are at a level consistent with the child's developmental stage and knowledge of his or her disease. Some children do keep most of their thoughts about death to themselves. Sometimes this is due to fear of emotional abandonment by family members and significant others who the child perceives will find the added emotional burdens of his or her awareness and fears unbearable.[57] Mental health professionals, through play, art, drama, and therapeutic conversation, can ascertain the child's private perceptions and concerns. Through such techniques, the professional can correct distortions, dispel fantasies, and promote self-esteem through mastery of fears.[58] Parents should be encouraged to participate in such processes.

As death approaches, it is important to help families feel that they have done all they could for their child. Parents, trying to hold on to any control they might have, may seem less cooperative or easily frustrated and annoyed. These are appropriate responses, given the sequence of experiences leading to the terminal phase of illness. Families struggle with the additional stress of living with dying.[59] One needs to respect each family's readiness, delicately balancing life issues with those related to death and loss. Sensitive assistance should be given to the family with difficult decisions and preparations. Parents need repeated reassurance about the importance of their vigil with the child, and how this vigil reduces their child's feelings of isolation and abandonment through the moment of death.

The terminal phase of illness is an especially crucial time to involve all significant family members. As separation anxiety is heightened, feelings of helplessness and despair may prevail. Family members often find it helpful to participate in the child's physical and emotional care. This care can take place either in the hospital or at home. It can involve everything from having a sibling help the child eat to a parent administering medications and oxygen. It is important to remember that family members vividly recollect these terminal events. They can either be plagued by them or find solace in their remembrance.[50] Parents, siblings, and others close to the child benefit greatly from having someone available with whom to share their thoughts, fears, and concerns, whether rational or irratio-

nal. As Kubler-Ross has stated; "If we tolerate their anger, whether it is directed at us, at the deceased or at God, we are helping them take a great step toward acceptance without guilt."[10]

There is no way to prepare a parent completely for his or her child's death. Even on the day of death, some parents continue to have moments of hope. No matter how much a family feels "ready," the death may be experienced as a shock. After the child's death, it is important for the family to have time alone with the child's body. This gives them a chance to express some parting words in private, to observe the child lying peacefully without discomfort, and to obtain a much needed sense of finality.[42] The emptiness of returning home with the child's belongings but without the child hurts deeply.[42] However, amidst the sadness, many parents experience a feeling of relief that their child's long ordeal is over, and that death has brought an end to suffering and a sense of tranquility and peace.[48]

On Passive and Active Euthanasia

"Helping a child on his way" and "ending the child's suffering" are whispered or unspoken issues during the terminal stage of illness. More open and frank appraisal of these issues by health professionals is long overdue. One of this country's most respected pediatric psychiatrists has said, "I consider active euthanasia unthinkable. It implies an unwarranted assumption of infallibility on the part of the physician (spontaneous remissions have occurred in the sickest patients)."[18] Yet, in referring to heroic measure to save a comatose terminally ill child he states, "Passive euthanasia (negative euthanasia) is a different matter."[18]

Although such practices are neither publicly acknowledged nor professionally sanctioned, some physicians of terminally ill adult cancer patients offer them the option of shortening their suffering. For example, this may be accomplished through instructions not to treat new infections, not to employ resuscitation, to withdraw steroids in CNS tumor patients, or to decrease or remove supplementary oxygen; or even through self-administered medications to induce prolonged sleep. Similar approaches are cautiously used at times by those treating pediatric oncology patients. These realities are rarely openly discussed in pediatric oncology (see Chap. 15).

Although many agree that children should not be allowed to die in agony, children sometimes do die that way.[61] The physician should at least be open to parents who wish to inquire about helping their child to die in comfort. The physician can serve as a very special listener, selectively interpreting and responding to the parent's concerns. Often, the "treatment" in such situations is allowing the parents to think out loud with a nonjudgmental professional, expressing their fears, worries, and wishes for a reasonably pain-free, swift death. When the physician becomes aware that a parent has made a decision to ease the pain of dying through more aggressive use of pain medications or removal of treatments that slow the pace of the dying process but in no way influence its outcome, that physician must test the parent's wishes against his or her professional evaluation of the child's status. If the physician finds his or her perceptions concordant with those of the parent, we believe it appropriate to stand by that parent. Parents obviously have the most control in these situations when their terminally ill child is either at home or in a hospice.

After the child's death, the involved professional needs to be available to the parents. It will take time for them to place even a "passive euthanasia" decision in the perspective of their lives and values. This working through of the decision may, like the mourning process, extend over several years. For example, 3 years after her son's death, a mother shared the following thoughts:

"I still don't know how to say I did my best and that was enough . . . I still feel a sadness about this whole situation . . . assisting him to die . . . you had to do it but you hated to have to do it . . . he was on the verge of hemorrhaging or choking to death like he almost did that afternoon . . . when it came time to take the (oxygen) mask off, I had to do it; I didn't want to ask anyone else to . . . you're not causing him to die, but you are. . . ."

Such actions of "passive euthanasia" are taken out of love and perhaps a feeling in some that they do not have the "infinite strength" to stand vigil over the terminal suffering of their child. Be aware that the echoes and emotional doubts over these actions linger. As health professionals we should be there to listen, quietly and acceptingly.

Bereavement in the Family

The death of a child is one of life's great tragedies and it disrupts a family system in multiple ways. In our society, the bereavement process may have even greater consequences than in earlier times because of the absence of general familiarity with death and its rituals. Death in children accounts for less than 5% of mortality in this country.[62] Cancer deaths account for 18% of that pediatric mortality.[62] This means that families who lose a child to cancer are a rather isolated minority, with relatively few social supports for their grief.

The child's death marks the major milestone in a bereavement process initiated when the cancer diagnosis was first heard (see Chap. 49). Varying degrees of family disruption consequent to such a death have been identified.[59,60,63,64] Included are rates of marital separation and divorce ranging from 23% to 60%.[65,66] One study comparing bereavement in parents to bereavement over the death of a parent or spouse found "more intense grief reactions of somatic types, greater depression . . . anger and guilt with accompanying feelings of despair."[67] Lewis identifies "sudden" (guilt and mourning), "acute" (anger, overidealizing, fantasy), and "chronic" (remorse, relief, and guilt) reactions.[68] The bereavement process continues in undulating waves, perhaps for as long as 3 to 5 years after a child's death.[69-71]

The parents suffer from both the loss of the child and the loss of what the child represented to them. In our culture, children represent continuity of their parents' lives (generativity).[72] Children also are vessels into which parents tend to pour hopes and dreams not only for the child but for themselves through the child's growth. Mothers and fathers will differ from one another in their responses, as will individual parents, based on their own personalities, life experiences, and beliefs. The impact of the loss often varies with the age of the child: a "different kind of pain" is associated with the death of younger and older children.[72] The older the child, the more experience the family has had with him or her, the more formed his or her personality, the greater the effects on the family system and the individuals within it, and the more extensive the memories.

A child's death may precipitate guilt in parents in reaction to feelings they perceive as negative toward the child. These usually involve wishes that "it would all finally end."[68] When this kind of guilt is left unresolved, unexposed, and unexamined, it is a significant psychological risk factor for the parent. Other special vulnerabilities involve the deceased child's role in the family. For example, the more emotionally dependent the family was on the child and the more the child was viewed by one or both parents as an emotional extension of self (in a need-fulfillment or symbiotic sense), the more disruptive his or her death will be to the family system.[59,73] The same is true for a child who served as the essential bond between parents, or one who was the "communicator" for spouses in conflict.

In a study measuring effective coping following the death of a child from cancer, Spinetta and colleagues found that certain family coping efforts during the course of the illness can make a difference in their adaptation after the death. Better adjustment was seen in [1] parents who had a viable and ongoing "significant other" to turn to for help during the course of the illness; [2] those who had an open and responsive communication with the child during the illness and who gave their child the information and emotional support he or she needed; and [3] those who had a consistent philosophy of life that helped the family to accept the diagnosis and cope with its consequences. Participation in the care of the child during his or her life is associated with healthier bereavement responses. Similarly, attendance on the child during the dying process through home care or hospice care makes a significant difference, attenuating guilt feelings and anger.

Siblings should be informed by the parents of the dying child's status and of the child's death (if they are not present). This should be done in a way that is tailored to siblings' developmental stages. They too will have immediate and long-term reactions. These reactions will vary based on factors that include the quality of their relationship with the deceased and the sex of the deceased and of the bereaved. "Same sex as the deceased" siblings are always at higher risk for failure in working through the loss. In the absence of guidance, and depending on family dynamics, they may feel it necessary to take on the identity of the deceased.

Families generally do not seek professional help for dealing with the upheaval and sadness of bereavement. They do, however, tend to benefit from the opportunity to reflect on and review the illness–dying–death experience until acceptance occurs.[16] When the atmosphere is accepting, families may return over a period of many years for spontaneous visits to the oncology service where their child was treated. Ongoing availability and interest in the health of these families should not stop at the point of the child's death.[1,16,43,74]

SPECIAL FAMILY CONSIDERATIONS AND VULNERABILITIES

Many of the challenges and issues presented previously are those faced by all "cancer families" and are clearly beyond the demands of daily living. All families have preexisting conflicts and problems, but certain family situations and vulnerabilities can be anticipated by the health care team in order to avert potential problems in coping. This section addresses those considerations.

Siblings

The effects of childhood cancer on well siblings deserve special attention. Several studies that have attempted to illuminate this issue tend to report predominantly adverse effects. Withdrawal, sleep disturbances, enuresis, crying, envy, guilt, preoccupation with their own health, somatic complaints, antisocial behavior, depression, fearfulness, separation anxieties, and poor school performance have been noted.[63,75-78] However, unless a crisis has occurred, problems with siblings are rarely brought to the attention of the oncology staff. Perhaps our evaluations do not emphasize enough the importance of siblings in the overall emotional management of the child. Also, their problems may appear temporary and less burdensome compared with the difficulties facing their ill brothers or sisters.[79]

Envy and rivalry between children exist in every family. In fact, hostile feelings between siblings are far more frequent in childhood than the literature would indicate.[80] Following the diagnosis of cancer and throughout the treatment process, healthy siblings often feel additional resentment because of the special care and parental attention given to the sick child. As a result, the healthy sibling may be fraught with jealousy and subsequently experience guilt for escaping the affliction. This guilt may be further reinforced by the belief that the illness would not have occurred if he or she had treated the sibling more kindly. The following statements represent some of the reactions children have had to a sibling's diagnosis of cancer.

"I pushed my brother down and he hurt his leg and now he has a big tumor in it."

"I get so mad at my sister sometimes. She gets away with everything. I can't help feeling guilty for all the times I told her I wished she'd get sick and die."

As the child proceeds throughout treatment, the healthy sibling often feels a sense of isolation and deprivation. Frequent hospitalizations can result in the temporary loss of the child's sibling, in addition to one or both parents, to an environment that is highly charged with emotion.[81] Often, healthy siblings share less of the parents' time and interest, and may begin to question if they still are loved. Most siblings attempt in one way or another to earn a status similar to the ill child. Latency-age children may ask whether they can also "have some chemotherapy." Most siblings complain of and become concerned about any aches and pains they develop. Some healthy children may wish they were the ones with the disease, while others fear the day that they too will develop cancer. Lengthy hospitalizations or limited financial resources may cause siblings to be deprived of basic needs, including parental supervision. Emotional withdrawal or self-destructive acts serve as dramatic indications that the sibling is assuming more responsibility than is appropriate for his or her developmental level.[20] This may be more quietly evidenced by repeated excuses to be away from the home. An extreme example of self-destructive behavior and maladaptive coping is the well sibling who takes the sick child's medicines, or runs in front of a moving vehicle in order to also be treated in the hospital. Siblings who engage in dangerous behavior or activities are demonstrating serious difficulty coping with the current home and medical situation. In such situations, intervention by an experienced mental health professional is essential. This should be introduced and encouraged by the physician or members of the health care team who have the family's trust and confidence.

Feelings of isolation are exacerbated for siblings if the family moves to be closer to the treatment facility. The healthy sibling will experience a loss of community and of friends and playmates, and will need to adapt to the changes and stress of starting in a new school. This sense of loss may be somewhat lessened in larger families when the burden of care can be distributed among several children. Although siblings often feel neglected when parental attention is focused on the ill child (and upset by having their life circumstances altered),

most fear confronting their parents with negative feelings.[82] This results in an increased sense of isolation from their family, and at times a sense of personal failure. Oncology staff and other health care professionals can assist families considerably by directing their attention to the needs of their well children and by encouraging open communication among all family members.

Several other measures can be helpful in easing the emotional stress on siblings. The parents or treatment team need to discuss the affected child's diagnosis, treatment, and prognosis with siblings at a level they can easily understand.[83] Siblings need to be prepared for the physical changes that their brother or sister will undergo and for the possible role realignments in the family. It is essential that siblings feel that their thoughts, concerns, and questions are important and acceptable. This includes feelings of anger toward their parents and jealousy or hostility toward the sick child. Siblings need to be reassured that they will be kept up-to-date on their brother's or sister's treatment progress and, whenever possible, included in the patient's care and management. When treatment requires parental absence from home, a regularly scheduled time should be arranged for the parents and siblings to talk by telephone. This helps lessen separation anxiety and provides the sibling with a sense of belonging, consistency, and inclusion in the sick child's care.

There have been few investigations concerning children's reactions to the death of a sibling from cancer. Spinetta and coworkers[2] found that siblings' symptoms or unresolved feelings persisted in the majority of families, including crying spells, health fears, feelings of remorse and guilt, and refusal to discuss the deceased child even 2 or 3 years following the death. In a study based on parental report, Lewis[7] reported that more than half of the siblings required some sort of medical consultation following the death of the affected child. In a study based on psychiatric patients, Cain and colleagues[84] found the surviving children had a heightened awareness and fear of death, feeling that it could strike someone close to them, at any time or themselves, when they reached the same age as the dead sibling. All authors agreed that the experience of a child's death has a profound effect on his or her siblings. The factors that determine a child's immediate and long-term reactions to the death of a sibling are multiple. These factors, identified in the studies reported, include the level of communication with the sibling during his or her life; the parents' explanation of the diagnosis, treatment, and prognosis to the surviving child; the child's ability to express both positive and negative feelings about the sibling and his or her disease and hospitalizations; the age, sex, and developmental level of the surviving sibling; the child's preexisting relationship with the sibling and parents; the parents' reactions to the death and their subsequent attitude toward their remaining children.

It is only in recent years that the siblings of children with cancer have been recognized as having special needs of their own. We need to identify these needs, intervene when appropriate, involve and inform them whenever possible, and not view them solely under the shadow of the sick child's affliction.[79] Support for the healthy siblings should occur at the time of diagnosis, throughout the course of the illness, and as part of the bereavement program, if the child should die. The strengths and vulnerabilities of each well sibling should be included in the initial family assessment (see Table 42-1). If at all possible, the well siblings should also attend the early family conferences. The siblings' early involvement minimizes feelings of family isolation and establishes an atmosphere of honesty and openness that sets the stage for further communications among family members.[85]

Marital Disharmony

The crisis evoked by childhood cancer taxes every marriage. Parents who have supported each other through previous crises, who can share with one another expressions of sadness, anger, frustration, and hope, and who are able to make their child's illness a priority often eventually find their relationship strengthened. For others, the stress of a child's cancer exacerbates previous marital problems, especially those of long duration. The child's parents may appear to be emotionally distant, coping with the situation in isolation from each other or using it to fight their unresolved battles. Such marital disharmony negatively affects the entire family's emotional adjustment to the disease and requires mental health intervention.[86]

Divorce

If the child's parents are separated or divorced, special efforts need to be made to keep both parents informed about the child's diagnosis, treatments, and progress. Parents who have maintained a friendship following separation or divorce tend to have a less intense experience of loss.[87] They also tend to find the stresses associated with the disease and treatment less severe than do those parents who continue to have difficulty communicating or being in the same place together. The latter situation often presents a dilemma for staff. In an attempt to gain a sense of control and feel included in the child's care, some parents tend to vie for alignments with certain staff members. It is essential that the staff not get enmeshed in the family system by splitting their alliances between parents. In such cases, it is often the child who gets caught in the middle and is left feeling guilty, alone and without family or staff support. The health care team also needs to be aware of custody decisions, parental visitation arrangements, and possible remarriage and step-family relationships.

Single Parents

A major problem for most single-parent families is task overload.[87] Single parents often find themselves in a situation of financial hardship. Struggling to work, provide childcare, maintain a home, have a personal life, and possibly deal with visitation arrangements can be most difficult. When a child develops a life-threatening or chronic illness, single parents may feel especially isolated, alone, and without an adequate support system to meet the crisis (see Chap. 53). They are often without another person with whom they can share the responsibility of the sick child's care or the daily decisions that need to be made. Following diagnosis and throughout the treatment process, single parents often describe themselves as feeling overwhelmed, incompetent, indecisive, guilty, and sad. They may also experience considerable anger toward former mates, who may provide little if any emotional or financial assistance, or even toward other families who seem to have "less problems" than they do.

The health care team can assist single-parent families by identifying their economic, psychological, social, and support resources early in the child's treatment. Each family member's strengths and weaknesses must be assessed. Parents need to be encouraged to turn to staff, extended families, or other non-family supports for help in decision making, reassignment of home responsibilities, and financial assistance (especially travel and childcare costs) when needed. Individual and family counseling often helps single parents find the strength needed to cope with the daily demands and often overwhelming stress with which they are confronted. With caring and sensitive intervention, these families may discover new resources within themselves, within their families, and with their extended or nonfamily supports that can be used again through the course of the child's illness.[88]

Preexisting Psychopathology

Preexisting psychopathology in any family member adds to the challenge of dealing with a chronic, life-threatening condition. Determining whether or not a preexisting condition is a significant drain on the family system and presents a potential disruption of the prescribed treatments for the cancer patient is based on four factors: the family member involved, the form of psychopathology, the seriousness of the psychopathology and its responsiveness to treatment, and the willingness of the individual involved to accept treatment. Consider the gamut of disorders: anxiety disorders and phobias, depression, developmental disorders, presenile psychoses and dementias, antisocial and other severe personality disorders, the schizophrenias, and the various forms of substance abuse. Any one in and of itself can deplete a family's time, exhaust its emotional resources, and drain it financially. The consequences are very different if one of the parents is ill than if a sibling or grandparent is affected. Obtaining a history of problems before the onset of the child cancer patient's illness is essential orienting information for the health care team because even dramatic psychiatric symptoms can be reactive, at least in part, to the stresses and disruptions of the cancer diagnosis and treatment course. When the behaviors of family members present patterns that raise questions about psychopathology, it is wise to seek a consultation with a social worker, psychologist, or a psychiatrist.

Cultural Differences and Considerations

When considering family vulnerability and crisis, the effects of cultural attitudes are of increasing importance in countries with a significant immigrant population.[89] Cultural attitudes are outgrowths of value orientations, which vary considerably from one culture to another.[90] Such differences will affect how each family perceives and responds to illness, treatment, and death. For example, different cultures have different expectations of the medical system, different beliefs and attitudes about patient care and disease causation, and about death and rituals of death. The effects of cultural barriers on communication also have a major impact on the family's response to their child's illness and their ability to place trust in the health care team (see also Chap. 54).[91]

The failure of the medical team to consider sociocultural factors in the child's care often results in misunderstanding, confusion, and alienation. Learning about the beliefs, attitudes, and behaviors of the family's ethnic group enhances the therapeutic alliance. This can be accomplished by carefully exploring with the family their understanding of the illness, their expectations of the staff and of the treatment being offered, and the role of religion in their daily lives. Further, medical staff should determine whether [1] conflict exists between religious beliefs and treatment decisions; [2] the parents can meet their child's need for information; [3] problems exist because of language differences or difficulty using the supports available within the medical environment or community; [4] parents are able to accept assistance from others whose lifestyles differ from their own; and [5] parents respond better to informal or formal interactions with staff. Families are often eager to share with staff information about the family structure, culture, roles within the family, and belief systems when an interest is expressed. Once this information has been elicited, it may be possible to mobilize available sources of support that could further reduce the stress of being in a foreign environment and assist in the family's adjustment. If the family does not speak English, regularly scheduled meetings with the family are essential. These meetings should include the child's physician(s), nurse, and social worker, as well as a staff member or reliable volunteer who speaks the language, understands the culture, and is trusted by the family. Such meetings will avoid communication breakdown and enhance the quality of patient–family–staff relations.

CONCLUSION

Despite the life-disrupting and life-threatening nature of childhood cancer, most families display remarkable resilience in adaptation.[92] Mobilizing the strengths of families adds enormously to the effectiveness of the oncology treatment team. Even vulnerable families have strengths that can be tapped by the team. However, ignoring signs of significant vulnerabilities or frank dysfunction can wreak havoc with the most brilliant treatment protocols. Oncologic diseases are chronic processes, so comprehensive psychosocial care begins with early assessment of family strengths and vulnerabilities and continues throughout and beyond the course of the disease.

The need for an ongoing multidisciplinary approach to the psychosocial care of families is basic to responsible modern treatment. Interventions and strategies aimed at identifying the continuum of coping responses, building on family strengths, assisting families with special needs, and enhancing adaptive coping skills are essential to facilitating family growth through the crises generated by childhood cancer.

REFERENCES

1. Futterman EH, Hoffman I: Crisis and adaptation in the families of fatally ill children. In Anthony EJ, Koupernik E (eds): The Child in His Family, pp 127–143. New York, John Wiley & Sons, 1973
2. Spinetta JJ, Swarner JA, Sheposh JP: Effective parental coping following the death of a child from cancer. J Pediatr Psychol 6:251–263, 1981
3. Hersh SP: Psychological aspects of patients with cancer. In DeVita VT Jr, Hellman S, Rosenberg SA (eds): Principles and Practice of Oncology, 2nd ed, pp 2051–2066. Philadelphia, JB Lippincott, 1985
4. Bronfenbrenner U: Who cares for America's children. In Vaughan VD, Brazelton TB (eds): The Family—Can It Be Saved? pp 3–32. Chicago, Year Book Medical Publishers, 1976
5. Hersh SP: Crucible of strength and "nest of vipers." In Brazelton TB, Vaughan VD (eds): The Family: Setting Priorities, pp 303–315. New York, Science & Medicine Publishing, 1979
6. Eisenberg L: Youth in a changing society. In Vaughan VD, Brazelton TB (eds): The Family—Can It Be Saved? pp 59–66. Chicago, Year Book Medical Publishers, 1976
7. Grossman HJ, Simmons JE, Dyer AR, Work HH: The Physician and The Mental Health of the Child: I. Assessing Development and Treating Disorders Within a Family context, p 52. Monroe, WI, American Medical Association, 1979
8. Pfefferbaum BJ: Mental health aspects of neoplasm in children. In Grossman HJ, Stubblefield RL (eds): The Physician and the Mental Health of the Child: II. The Psychosocial Concomitants of Illness, pp 113–118. Monroe, WI, American Medical Association, 1980
9. Wolfenstein M: Fun mortality: An analysis of recent child training literature. In Mead M, Wolfenstein M (eds): Childhood in Contemporary Culture, pp 168–178. Chicago, The University of Chicago Press, 1955
10. Kubler-Ross E: On Death and Dying, pp 39–180. New York, Macmillan, 1969

11. Evans AE, Edins G: If a child must die . . . . N Engl J Med 278:138–142, 1968
12. Stephens JA, Lascari AD: Psychological follow-up of families with childhood leukemia. J Clin Psychol 30:394–397, 1974
13. Kaplan DM: Interventions for acute stress experiences. In Spinnetta JJ, D Deasy-Spinetta P (eds): Living with Childhood Cancer, pp 41–49. St Louis, CV Mosby, 1981
14. Johnson FL, Rudolph LA, Hatmann JR: Helping the family cope with childhood cancer. Psychosomatics 20:241–251, 1979
15. Susman EJ, Hersh SP, Nannis ED, Strope BE, Woodruff PJ, Pizzo PA, Levine AS: Conceptions of cancer: The perspectives of child and adolescent patients and their families. J Pediatr Psychol 7:253–261, 1982
16. Koch CB, Herman J, Donaldson MH: Supportive care of the child with cancer. Semin Oncol 1:81–86, 1974
17. Ross JW: Social work intervention with families of children with cancer: The changing critical phases. Soc Work Health Care 3:257–272, 1978
18. Prugh DG: The Psychosocial Aspects of Pediatrics, pp 92–112, 483–498. Philadelphia, Lea & Febiger, 1983
19. Carparulo F, Kempton W: Sexual health needs of the mentally retarded adolescent female. Issues Health Care Women 3:35–46, 1981
20. Vess JD, Moreland JR, Schwebel AI: An empirical assessment of the effects of cancer on family role functioning. J Psychosoc Oncology 3(1):1–16, 1985
21. Howarth RV: The psychiatry of terminal illness in children. Proc R Soc Med 65:1039–1040, 1972
22. Taylor G: Helping families cope when a child has cancer. Med Times 109(9):24s–27s, 1981
23. Christ G, Adams MA: Therapeutic strategies at psychosocial crisis points in the treatment of childhood cancer. In Christ AE, Flomenhaft K (eds): Childhood Cancer: Impact on the Family, pp 109–128. New York, Plenum, 1984
24. Kaplan DM, Smith A, Grobstein R, Fishman SE: Family mediation of stress. Soc Work 18(1-C):60–69, 1973
25. Burr CK: Impact on the family of a chronically ill child. In Hobbs N, Perrin JM (eds): Issues in the Care of Children with Chronic Illness, pp 24–40. San Francisco, Jossey-Bass, 1985
26. Cook JA: Influence of gender on the problems of parents of fatally ill children. J Psychosoc Oncol 2(1):71–91, 1984
27. Hamovitch MB: The Parent and the Fatally Ill Child, p 112. Los Angeles, Delmar, 1964
28. Fife BL: Childhood cancer is a family crisis: A review. J Psychosoc Nurs Ment Health Serv 18(10):29–34, 1980
29. Fife BL: Reducing parental overprotection of the leukemic child. Soc Sci Med 12:117–122, 1978
30. Freund BL, Siegel K: Problems in transition following bone marrow transplantation: Psychosocial aspects. Am J Orthopsychiatry 56:244–252, 1986
31. Christ G: "Dis-synchrony" of coping among children with cancer, their families and the treating staff. In Christ A, Flomenhaft K (eds): Psychosocial Family Interventions in Chronic Pediatric Illness, pp 85–96. New York, Plenum, 1982
32. Adams-Greenly M: Psychological staging of pediatric cancer patients and their families. Cancer 58:449–453, 1986
33. McQuown L: The Parents of children with cancer. A view from those who suffer most. In Spinetta JJ, Deasy-Spinetta P (eds): Living with Childhood Cancer, pp 198–208. St Louis, CV Mosby, 1981
34. Zeltzer L, LeBaron S, Zeltzer P: The adolescent with cancer. In Blum RW (ed): Chronic Illness and Disabilities in Childhood and Adolescence, pp 375–394. Orlando, Grune & Stratton, 1984
35. Kupst MJ, Schulman JL, Maurer H, Honig G, Morgan E, Fochtman D: Coping with pediatric leukemia: A two year follow-up. J Pediatr Psychol 9(2):149–163, 1984
36. Ross JW: The role of the social worker with long term survivors of childhood cancer and their families. Soc Work Health Care 7(4):1–13, 1982
37. Kirkpatrick J, Hoffman I, Futterman EH: Dilemma of trust: Relationship between medical care givers and parents of fatally ill children. Pediatrics 54:169–175, 1974
38. Kalnins IV, Churchill MP and Terry GE: Concurrent stresses in families with a leukemic child. J Pediatr Psychol 5(1):81–92, 1980
39. Bluebond-Langner M: The Private Worlds of Dying Children, p 223. Princeton, NJ, Princeton University Press, 1978
40. Heffron WA, Bommelaere K, Masters R: Group discussions with the parents of leukemic children. Pediatrics 52:831–840, 1973
41. Levine AS, Hersh SP: The psychosocial concomitants of cancer in young patients. In Levine AS (eds): Cancer in the Young, pp 367–387. New York, Masson Publishing, 1982

42. Adams DW, Deveau EJ: Coping With Childhood Cancer. Where Do We Go From Here? pp 66–71. Alexandria, VA, Prentice-Hall, 1984
43. Holland J: Psychological aspects of oncology. Medi Clin North Am 61:737–748, 1977
44. Krulik T: Helping parents of children with cancer during the midstage of illness. Cancer Nurs 5:441–445, 1982
45. Kupst MJ, Tylke L, Thomas L, Mudd ME, et al: Strategies of intervention with families of pediatric leukemia patients: A longitudinal perspective. Soc Work Health Care 8(2):31–47, 1982
46. Levine RJ: Referral of patients with cancer for participation in randomized clinical trials: Ethical considerations. CA 36(2):95–99, 1986
47. Hersh SP: Views on the psychosocial dimensions of cancer and cancer treatment. In Ahmed PI, Coelho GV (eds): Toward a New Definition of Health, pp 175–190. New York, Plenum Press, 1979
48. Chapman JA, Goodall J: Helping a child to live whilst dying. Lancet 1:753–756, 1980
49. Frantz TT: When your child has a life-threatening illness. Washington, DC, Association for the Care of Children's Health and the Candlelighters Foundation, 1983
50. Share L: Family communication in the crisis of a child's fatal illness: A literature review and analysis. Omega 3(3):187–201, 1972
51. Spinetta JJ, Maloney LJ: The child with cancer: Patterns of communication and denial. J Consult Clinical Psychol 46:1540–1541, 1978
52. Waechter EH: Children's awareness of fatal illness. Am J Nurs 71:1168–1172, 1971
53. Gunther J: Death Be Not Proud. New York, Harper & Row, 1949
54. Lund D: Eric. New York, JB Lippincott, 1974
55. Sherman M: The Leukemic Child. DHEW Pub No (NIH) 76-863. Washington, DC, US Government Printing Office, 1976
56. Roach N: The Last Day of April. New York, American Cancer Society, 1977
57. Greenham DE, Lohmann RA: Children facing death: Recurring patterns of adaptation. Health Soc Work 7(2):89–94, 1982
58. Adams–Greenly M: Helping children communicate about serious illness and death. J Psychosoc Oncol 2(2):61–72, 1984
59. Herz F: The impact of death and serious illness on the family life cycle. In Carter EA, McGoldrick M (eds): The Family Life Cycle: A Framework for Family Therapy, pp 223–240. New York, Gardner Press, 1980
60. Tietz W, McSherry L, Britt B: Family sequelae after a child's death due to cancer. Am J Psychother 32:417–425, 1978
61. Howell DA: A child dies. J Pediatr Surg 1:2, 1966
62. Owen G, Fulton R, Marknsen E: Death at a distance: A study of family survivors. Omega 13:191–225, 1982–1983
63. Binger CM, Ablin AR, Feuerstein RC et al: Childhood leukemia: Emotional impact on patient and fam J Med 280:414–418, 1969
64. Morrow GR, Hoagland A, Carnrike CLM: Social support and parental adjustment to pediatric cancer. J Consult Clin Psychol 49:763–765, 1981
65. Kaplan DM, Grobstein R, Smith A: Predicting the impact of severe illness in families. Health Work 1(3):71–81, 1976
66. Lansky SB, Cairns NU, Hassanein R, Wehr J, Lowman JT: Childhood cancer: Parental discord and divorce. Pediatrics 62(2):184–188, 1978
67. Sanders C: A comparison of adult bereavement in the death of a spouse, child and parent. Omega 10:303–322, 1979–1980
68. Lewis M, Lewis DO: Death and dying in children anilies. In Grossman HJ, Stubblefield RL (eds): The Physician and the Mental Health of the Child: II. The Psychosocial Concomitants of Illness, pp 121–129. Monroe, WI, American Medical Association, 1980
69. Rando T: An investigation of grief and adaptation in parents whose children have died from cancer. J Pediatr Psychol 8:3–20, 1983
70. Levar I: Mortality and psychopathology following the death of an adult child: An epidemiologic review. Isr J Psychiatric Relat Sci 19:23–38, 1982
71. Rees WD, Lutkins SG: Mortality of bereavement. Br Med J 1:13–16, 1967
72. Hersh SP: Reactions to particular types of bereavement. In Osterweis M, Solomon F, Green M (eds): Bereavement Reactions, Consequences, and Care, pp 71–96. Washington, DC, National Academy Press, 1984
73. Bowen M: Family reaction to death. In Guerin PJ (ed): Family Therapy: Theory and Practice, pp 335–348. New York, Gardner Press, 1976
74. Lewis IC: Leukemia in childhood: Its effects on the family. Aust Pediatr J 3:244–247, 1967
75. Binger CM: Childhood leukemia—Emotional impact on siblings. In Anthony EJ, Koupernick E (eds): The Child and His Family, pp 195–209. New York, John Wiley & Sons, 1973
76. Lavigne JV, Ryan M: Psychologic adjustment of siblings of children with chronic illness. Pediatrics 63:616–627, 1979
77. Taylor SC: The effect of chronic childhood illnesses upon well siblings. Matern Child Nurs J 9(2):109–116, 1980
78. Bergmann T, Wolfe S: Observations of the reactions of healthy children to their chronically ill siblings. Bull Phila Assoc Psychoanal 21:145–161, 1971
79. Kennedy H: Growing up with a handicapped sibling. Psychoanal Study Child 40:255–274, 1985
80. Colonna AB, Newman LM: The psychoanalytic literature on siblings. Psychoanal Study Child 38:285–308, 1983
81. Adams MA: Helping the parents of children with malignancy. J Pediatr 93:734–738, 1978
82. Cairns NU, Clark GM, Smith SD, Lansky SB: Adaptation of siblings to childhood malignancy. J Pediatrics 95:484–487, 1979
83. Blotcky AD: Helping adolescents with cancer cope with their disease. Semin Oncol Nurs 2(2):117–122, 1986
84. Cain AC, Fast I, Erickson ME: Children's disturbed reactions to the death of a sibling. Am J Orthopsychiatry 34:741–751, 1964
85. Perin GM, Kramer RF: The child and family facing death. In Waechter EH, Phillips J, Holaday B (eds): Nursing Care, pp 1333–1355, Philadelphia, JB Lippincott, 1985
86. Murstein BI: The effects of long term illness of children on the emotional adjustment of parents. Child Development 31:157–171, 1960
87. Beal EW: Separation, divorce, and single-parent families. In Carter EA, McGoldrick M (eds): The Family Life Cycle: A Framework for Family Therapy, pp 241–264. New York, Gardner Press, 1980
88. Burns CE: The hospitalization experience and single-parent families: A time of special vulnerability. Nurs Clin North Am 19(2):285–293, 1984
89. Tiller JWG, Ekert H, Richards WS: Family reactions in childhood acute lymphoblastic leukemia in remission. Aust Pediatr J 13:176–181, 1977
90. Spiegel JP: Cultural variations in attitudes toward death and disease. In Grosser GH, Wechsler H, Greenblatt M (eds): The Threat of Impending Disaster, pp 283–299. Cambridge, MA, MIT Press, 1964
91. Thoma MA: The effects of a cultural awareness program on the delivery of health care. Health Soc Work 2(3):124–136, 1977
92. Hamburg DA: Coping behavior in life-threatening circumstances. Psychother Psychosom 23:13–25, 1974

forty-three

Financial Issues in Pediatric Cancer

Shirley Bonnem and Judith Ross

Within the past two decades, pediatric oncologists have become involved increasingly with the financial aspects of their patients' care. Starting in the mid-1960s with Medicaid and its myriad required forms, concern for costs has become an integral part of medical practice. With the numerous health maintenance organizations (HMOs) and other forms of payment, clinics have become inundated with financial record-keeping related to patient care. For families, the financial burden of the child with cancer has emerged as a major source of stress, second only to the disease itself.[1]

A 1981 study of 569 children with malignancies in the Philadelphia, southern New Jersey, and Delaware area determined that about 95% of all medical costs were paid from private, public, or charitable resources. Medical expenses that were the responsibility of the families amounted to about $1000 each year. Moreover, all nonmedical disease-related expenses were borne by the family.[2]

Modern treatment of pediatric cancer is conducted according to a protocol, and variables such as stage, age, and selected risk factors are used to determine the therapeutic regimen. Treatment of some patients involves periodic or prolonged inpatient admissions, whereas other children can be managed exclusively as outpatients. All therapies produce side-effects; neutropenia and the resulting opportunistic infections and other iatrogenic life-threatening conditions may necessitate hospitalization (see Chap. 39).

The complexities of treatment and its sequelae are matched by the variety of public and private insurance programs. Some plans completely cover the cost of inpatient stays but barely support outpatient care, whereas others emphasize outpatient treatment. Many insurance companies are altering their approach to the chronically ill child. Pediatric experts are employed, providers are contacted early, and the least expensive care for clients is promoted. New flexibility has resulted in innovative care plans, and increasing numbers of patients are being managed at home with chemotherapy, hyperalimentation, and antibiotics.

Hospital billing systems also present problems, particularly when there are several billing departments within one institution. If a child is seen in an oncology clinic and receives blood work, a physical examination, radiographs, and chemotherapy, the parents may receive bills from five or more billing offices. Further, surgeons, orthopedists, ophthalmologists, and other specialists who routinely see oncology patients each bill separately. These practices can be very confusing to the parents, who may need help understanding how to submit bills to insurers and how to sort out benefit checks when payments are sent to them.

Resources are available in the community to help families confronting serious pediatric illness, but services are limited and do not meet all needs. Without guidance regarding available programs and application procedures, and an advocate to present the case to appropriate agencies, many families would not receive the benefits to which they are entitled.

The involvement of the social worker at the time of diagnosis is a key to optimum results (see also Chaps. 41 and 42). The hospital administration, through its public relations and development staffs, can be of further benefit to the oncology service and its pediatric patients.

PAYMENT IN HEALTH CARE

In the past, hospitals charged reimbursement agencies whatever costs they incurred. Little thought was given to the number of tests that might be ordered for a given patient, the length of time that patient spent in the hospital or, indeed, whether hospitalization was necessary at all.

All of this changed a few years ago with two developments that reversed the way hospitals were paid for their services (see Table 43-1). Instead of receiving money for care that had been rendered, hospitals were to be paid flat rates beforehand. The United States Congress made this change through passage of the Social Security Amendments of 1983, in which the pricing system became a method of payment to hospitals that predetermines, by diagnosis-related groups (DRGs), the rate hospitals receive for inpatient treatment. If their cost is lower than the DRG reimbursement, hospitals keep the difference; if it is above the fixed price, they must absorb the loss. Many insurance companies and Blue Cross organizations have now adopted such "prospective pricing systems" of paying for health care.

The development of DRGs by two Yale University professors, who divided illnesses into 472 (current) categories based on body systems, resulted in a near revolution in health care provision to the poor. The impact in pediatric health care has been felt only in those states that used DRG reimbursement methodology for children; federal law had exempted pediatric institutions from the prospective payment system. As an example of the application of this principle, if a child is admitted to a medical center with a primary diagnosis of leukemia, subsequent admissions, no matter what the cause and no matter how expensive the necessary treatment, are labeled as "leukemia" for payment purposes.

The discrepancies in DRG payments and costs of treating sick children prompted the National Association of Children's Hospitals and Related Institutions, Inc. (NACHRI) to undertake a study to delineate these differences.[4] Funded in part by NACHRI itself, the Health Care Financing Administration

---

Table 43-1
Financial Glossary

Case mix index—The relative costliness of treating an average case in a specific hospital in comparison to the statewide or nationwide cost of treating a case.

Children's diagnostic-related groups (CDRGs)—Clinical or pediatric classification system based on a study by NACHRI. The study has demonstrated that DRGs as originally designated do not reflect true costs incurred in pediatric hospitals or pediatric units in university hospitals. Implementation of the results of the study will depend on providers and payers and will occur at varying times throughout the country.

Coherence—Patient groups that are expected to have certain clinical responses resulting in similar patterns of resource use.

Co-morbidity—A preexisting condition that, because of its presence with the specific principal diagnosis, is thought to increase the length of stay.

Diagnostic-related groups (DRGs)—A patient classification system used as the basis for setting prices in the prospective pricing system. The DRG method groups hospital cases into 472 clinically coherent classifications. The system was developed under the leadership of Yale University Professors John D. Thompson and Robert B. Fetter.

Exempt providers—Hospitals that are exempt from the prospective payment system. Nationally this term applies to children's, psychiatric, rehabilitation, and long-term care hospitals. It also includes distinct-part rehabilitation or psychiatric units of general hospitals.

Grouper—A calculation determining the DRG based on principal diagnosis and procedures performed.

Group rate—A payment rate per case based on the average of all hospitals in a group. Hospitals are divided into five groups based on teaching status, size, and other factors.

Hospital specific—A payment rate per case derived from the actual cost to the institution.

International Classification of Diseases, 9th Revision, Clinical Modification (ICD-9-CM)—A coding system used to classify patients according to their diagnosis and treatment.

Major diagnostic category (MDC)—Division of ICD-9-CM codes into a system of categories related to the body's organ systems.

There are 23 MDCs. Patient grouping according to principal diagnosis forms the basis of the DRG grouping.

Outliers—Those patients having either [1] longer lengths of stay (day outliers) or [2] higher costs (cost outliers) in relation to the average patient discharge within the same DRG.

Patient discharge under PPS—[1] formally released from the hospital; [2] transferred to another hospital or a unit within the same hospital that is excluded from the PPS; [3] died in the hospital.

Peer review organizations (PROs)—The 1982 TEFRA legislation contained the Peer Review Improvement Act, which created a new federal authority to fund utilization review and quality control organizations. These PROs replace the old Professional Standard Review Organizations and under the new payment system are responsible for determining the medical necessity, appropriateness of delivery setting, and conformance to accepted standards of quality of all hospital patient care services.

Primary diagnosis—The diagnosis that requires the most intensive use of hospital resources. This may or may not be the admitting (principal) diagnosis. For example, if a patient is admitted for minor surgery and subsequently suffers a myocardial infarction, the MI would be the primary diagnosis, while the surgery would be the principal diagnosis.

Principal diagnosis—The diagnosis which, after study, has been found to necessitate a patient's admission to the hospital.

Prospective Payments Assessment Commission (ProPAC)—an independent commission that advises the Department of Health and Human Services.

Prospective pricing system (PPS)—Prospective pricing began with Congressional passage of the Social Security Amendments of 1983. The pricing system is a payment method that predetermines by DRGs the rate hospitals receive for inpatient treatment. If their cost is lower than the predetermined rate, hospitals keep the difference. If their costs are above the fixed price, hospitals absorb the loss.

Waiver—States may be exempt from the national PPS if they have an alternative payment system that meets the government's requirements.

(HCFA), and the Pew Memorial Trust, NACHRI recently completed an analysis of this study demonstrating that children's hospitals and university hospitals treat a broader and more specialized range of children's conditions and, therefore, are more costly than community hospitals. For example, children's hospitals and specialized pediatric programs care for most of the pediatric heart and cancer cases. Accordingly, NACHRI has recommended to HCFA a set of DRGs for children (CDRGs). Implementation has not yet taken place.

Prepayment

Prepayments may be required by certain medical institutions, particularly in the case of foreign nationals who are not eligible for public aid. In rare instances, hospitals demand prepayments or deposits from the parents of a child who is not covered by medical insurance. Such practices have been protested. Many hospitals were built with Hill-Burton Act funds and are required under this act to provide free or reduced cost health care to medically indigent patients.[4] Some institutions will facilitate applications for medical assistance and Supplementary Security Income (SSI) rather than turn a child away. Social workers can assist further with applications to other programs.

Commercial Insurance

Commercial insurance, offered by *for-profit* companies (*e.g.,* Prudential, Travelers, John Hancock, and Aetna), usually pays between 80% and 100% of pediatric cancer care after deductibles are met. A deductible is the minimum required amount, usually $100 or $200, that the family must pay before the insurance benefit is computed. For example, if the total medical bill is $5000 and the insurance company pays 80% after a $100 deductible is satisfied, then the company would reimburse 80% of $4900, or $3920. The parents are then responsible for the remaining $1080 (including the $100 deductible). Some insurance policies cover completely the cost of inpatient care and outpatient drugs, as well as physicians' charges for administering them. The administration of blood products (but not the actual products themselves) is covered, as are bone marrow aspirations and lumbar punctures. Hospitals may accept installment payments for the remaining charges, and in some instances will accept the insurance benefit as payment in full.

Health Maintenance Organizations

HMOs are a type of prepaid group health practice that provides basic and supplemental health maintenance and treatment services to subscribers. Fees are preset, regardless of the services provided. The emphasis is on prevention of illness. Federal financial support for the establishment of HMOs was provided under Title XIII of the United States Public Health Service Act of 1973, with amendments in 1976 and 1978 that reduced restrictions. There are now more than 300 HMOs in the United States, with more than 15 million members.[5]

Civilian Health and Medical Program of the Uniformed Services (CHAMPUS)

CHAMPUS covers military personnel and their families and usually requires a written statement from providers to the effect that services are not available in a local military hospital. CHAMPUS coverage is usually comprehensive.

Blue Cross and Blue Shield

Blue Cross and Blue Shield are a collection of nonprofit corporate entities that operate regionally to pay for health care for subscribers on a contractual basis. Blue Cross covers hospital costs and Blue Shield, physician fees. One or more states or only a portion of a state may be included in a region. Contracts may be arranged with hospitals and with physicians. Typically, all hospitals in a region have established contracts with Blue Cross. In Pennsylvania, New York, and Washington, D.C., for example, there are no nonparticipating hospitals. However, not all physicians have contracts with Blue Shield. If contractual arrangements exist, the hospital or the physician bills Blue Cross or Blue Shield directly and is paid directly, accepting the payment that has been agreed on for the particular category of service. If no contractual agreement exists with the physician, the patient is responsible for paying the doctor and, by submitting bills and insurance forms, can receive direct reimbursement from the insurance company for covered services.

As a rule, "the Blues" pay benefits to their subscribers in terms of service. Service benefits are not defined in terms of dollars. Therefore, if a subscriber is entitled to 40 days of inpatient hospitalization, reimbursement is provided regardless of the actual hospital charges. Charges may vary from hospital to hospital or even within a hospital (as with the cost of a standard bed versus an intensive care bed). The contract agrees to pay for whatever the hospital does, as long as the person is eligible for benefits. Subscribers' policies or entitled benefits can be limited or quite generous, depending on the type of coverage the family has, with variations in deductibles and other copayments and in maximum numbers of paid hospital days. Most subscribers participate through employer-subsidized groups, but some arrange Blue Cross and Blue Shield coverage privately. Many plans have attached major medical policies that operate like commercial insurance.

Blue Cross pays for hospital costs for inpatient care and for clinic visits (but not physician's office visits) for chemotherapy. If billing is through a physician's private office rather than through a hospital system, Blue Shield would pay for chemotherapy visits but not for physical examinations. Some Blue Shield plans pay for chemotherapy and its administration, whereas others only cover the physician charges. If there is a major medical policy, visits not paid by Blue Shield are covered, usually after a yearly deductible and up to 80% or, sometimes, 100%.

Blue Cross is conducting an experimental program of paying for inpatient care on a case basis—similar to the DRG payment system. This arrangement involves payment of a specific dollar amount as contracted per admission, regardless of the actual number of days in hospital, and is being used in selected regions.

Payment for Experimental Therapy

For children enrolled on studies supported by the National Cancer Institute (NCI), drugs that are not available commercially are supplied. These are agents under investigation and would not be paid for by insurance companies. However, drugs that are available commercially, although they may be prescribed as part of a research protocol, are not provided by the government and are usually covered by insurance. Blue Cross on occasion has questioned hospital admissions for experimental care, taking the position that research dollars should be available from NCI, but the NCI does not provide funds for patient care.

On the whole, commercial insurance companies and Blue Cross and Blue Shield have been willing to pay for therapy when it can be shown that, although the suggested treatment is part of a research protocol, it is the only reasonable treatment for the child. Because relationships exist between regional insurance programs and providers, a letter or a phone call can often facilitate approval for benefits. When negotiations are unsuccessful, the medical justification for specific treatments may need to be determined by a review committee.

LIMITATIONS TO HEALTH CARE PAYMENT

A major drawback in health care reimbursement for children with chronic or disabling conditions is that insurance companies generally define care in terms of the needs of children who are acutely ill, and it is more difficult to define benefits for children in other categories. Another problem occurs with respect to coverage for institutional care, such as nursing homes, rehabilitation centers, and the like, which are not extensively provided for.

Often insurance plans refuse coverage for conditions that existed before the purchase of the policy. Thus, if the child's condition was diagnosed before the insurance became effective, the company would not pay for medical bills related to the condition, including sequelae of the disease or its treatment. Usually the company will cover cancer conditions after a waiting period of 1 year or less. Some group plans do not have restrictions for prior conditions, but insurance policies purchased directly from Blue Cross and Blue Shield almost always contain such restrictions. For this reason, parents may want to consider purchasing a separate policy for a youngster who would be dropped from their own insurance within a year because of age (most policies cover dependent children until they are 19 or complete college)—especially if they know that the child will not be eligible for other benefits such as Medicaid or SSI. At the time the youngster is no longer covered by the parents' insurance, his or her own policy would be in effect.

Problems have occurred also with HMOs when the preferred center for pediatric cancer treatment has not contracted with the HMO. HMOs have at times insisted that a child be treated at an institution that has no pediatric program because of contractual agreements with that hospital. HMOs may not be willing to pay for treatment that they regard as experimental. Conversely, some HMOs are willing not only to fund experimental therapy but also to pay for transportation when such treatment is not available locally.

Bone Marrow Transplantation

Bone marrow transplantation (BMT) is now regarded as a standard therapy for many leukemic conditions and is covered by insurance companies and Medicaid. However, when BMT is used as a treatment for neuroblastoma and other diseases, insurance companies and Medicaid programs in some states refuse payment. It may be necessary to pursue the matter in court to force payment on the grounds that in particular cases transplantation is the only reasonable treatment. This has been successful in several cases.

ECONOMIC CONSIDERATIONS AND IMPEDIMENTS

Nonmedical financial pressures can affect a family's ability to care for the child while maintaining a family life. For some families, the effort to provide basic necessities can be a constant struggle, and the illness and its risks pale by comparison to the perils of hunger and dispossession. In such families, decisions regarding treatment, both initial and palliative, may be based on criteria that change in relation to the "crisis of the day." Thus, compliance with medical care can be inconsistent.

For some families, extreme poverty is compounded by other social and health problems such as disorganization, lack of education, sibling maladjustment, family violence, alcoholism, and drug abuse. With the onset of illness, the need for basic goods and services intensifies. Housing can be a major problem; for the urban poor in particular, housing is often substandard and in short supply. The need for clean, safe, and uncrowded living quarters becomes critical when a child is seriously ill and immunosuppressed. Often regarded as a basic necessity, even the telephone is beyond the means of some families. When there is no way to call for help, the child's life is placed in jeopardy.

For families who do have phone service, enormous telephone bills resulting from calls to the hospital can present a financial strain. Parents want to make contact with family members or friends to receive emotional support and to provide an update on the child's condition.[1] The extended family may also be poor and unable to provide material help. Because social welfare programs do not extend coverage to meet most of these additional needs and expenses, the financially distressed family undergoes considerable hardship and worry.

Finally, a mistrust of institutions, which is not uncommon among poor people, can inhibit the development of relationships with caretakers and of positive attitudes toward treatment. Poor people are afraid of being guinea pigs and may wonder whether their child would fare differently if they were wealthy.

Families in the lower middle class and middle class are also economically vulnerable. If the father becomes unemployed permanently through disability, or loses a position and cannot find another that pays as well, the family's standard of living plummets at the same time that its need for extra funds increases. These are "the new poor, displaced from dying industries and struggling to get by on low paying jobs or welfare."[6] Elderly grandparents, or other chronically or terminally ill family members, can further strain available resources. For those without a financial cushion, one disaster can cause significant financial distress.

In a study of medical costs and out-of-pocket expenses for families of children with cancer, conducted by The Children's Hospital of Philadelphia, more than one third of the families' gross annual income was spent on disease-related costs. Families spent similar amounts in out-of-pocket costs for medical, continuing, and one-time expenses. For those in the lowest quartile, out-of-pocket costs were 47.9% of mean family income. For all families, only 10.8% of out-of-pocket costs were medical (*i.e.,* physician charges and insurance copayments).[2]

Nonmedical costs can wreak havoc on a budget. These can include the purchase of extra clothing (because of weight fluctuations), buying wigs, and eating in restaurants because the family is pressed for time or is away from home. Additional expenses include the cost of travel to and from either the community in which the hospital is located or, if local, the hospital itself. Parking poses another expenditure. Lodging for parents and possibly for siblings during a child's hospitalization can result in a large outlay of money.

The financial distress imposed by nonmedical expenses was aided in 1974 with the opening of the first Ronald McDonald House in Philadelphia. There are now 86 Ronald McDonald Houses in the United States, 10 in Canada, 2 in Australia and 2 in Europe. The houses provide, at a nominal cost, an informal setting with homelike amenities for families. They are maintained by local owner-operators of McDonald's restaurants and committees of volunteers.

When such facilities are not available or siblings must remain in their own home for other reasons, the cost of additional child care can be a serious problem.[1] This is especially true when parents cannot take time off from work or there are no other family members who will or can help when a sick child needs his or her parents during hospitalization or while attending an ambulatory clinic.

ASSISTING THE FAMILY

The Role of the Social Worker

The social worker is the member of the multidisplinary team who is usually designated to make a psychosocial assessment and to address the family's material requirements (see also Chaps. 42 and 43). Determinations regarding the necessity for specific services such as transportation, assistance with medical expenses, housing, child care, and often financial support (for food, utilities, or other items) are not made in a vacuum. It is necessary to gain a thorough understanding of the family and how it operates, including relationships, pertinent history, and the available resources, both emotional and economic. Thus, unmet needs must be identified, problems or vulnerable areas revealed, and potential resources explored. Contact with a social worker should occur early in the course of the first hospitalization so that a positive connection can be formed and problems dealt with on a timely basis.[7]

Merely referring a family for assistance or providing services may not be an effective means of solving problems because so many factors contribute to the family's receptivity and ability to make use of help that is offered. Social work intervention involves providing not only information about eligibility, entitlements, and available programs of assistance, but also counseling to facilitate self-awareness of behavior and motives and to promote realistic planning. Counseling addresses feelings that interfere with successful management of financial aspects or willingness to follow through with referrals. When family members accept the social worker as a trustworthy and helpful professional, efforts to assist them can be productive.

Families overburdened by chronic financial distress or with ingrained patterns of disorganization who have been unsuccessful in negotiating bureaucratic and institutional systems are often mistrustful and resistant to attempts to help them. However, because of the cancer and its threat to their child, even hostile or suspicious parents may be open to establishing a relationship and will respond favorably to social work intervention. Direct work with deprived families or advocacy on their behalf with landlords, law enforcement authorities, schools, and child welfare and other agencies demands an enormous expenditure of the social worker's time, yet this may be the only way to ensure that the child receives medical care and lives in a wholesome environment. It is not unusual for parents to become more responsive to the medical staff and receptive to treatment once they have benefited from, or felt reassured by, the social worker's efforts to ease their living situation. As a member of the health care team who focuses on the needs of the whole family, the social worker functions as a "goodwill ambassador," representing and reinforcing the team's concern for the family's well-being.

As an advocate for the child and for the family, the social worker should interpret to other team members the social and physical environment of the home for discharge from the hospital, follow-up treatment, and home care. Compliance with continued therapy is not automatic and can be thwarted if the staff's expectations are not congruent with actual conditions in the home. Parents are often reluctant to voice opposition to doctors' directives, even though they may be unable or unwilling to follow them.

The oncology social worker fills an important role as intermediary with agencies to assist families in obtaining all of the services to which they are entitled. Thus, the social worker must be knowledgeable about existing programs and willing to be aggressive and persistent in pursuing them for the family. Social work coverage is important not just at the time of the diagnosis but on a continuing basis, as economic circumstances can fluctuate drastically during and beyond the course of treatment. Parents are likely to bring their problems, on a timely basis, to a social worker whom they already know and who may have proved helpful in the past.

Community Resources and the Public Welfare System

While publicly funded programs of financial support do exist, resources are extremely limited and qualification guidelines are restrictive, usually based on outdated standards of income needed for subsistence. As a result, many who genuinely need help are excluded. The average monthly benefit per family (three persons) in the nation as a whole is $313, ranging from $91 in Mississippi to $542 in Alaska.[8] Application procedures are confusing and often degrading. Interpretation of vague guidelines varies considerably, so that acceptance or rejection may depend on who reviews the application. In the past few years, spending cutbacks have produced altered and even more stringent eligibility requirements and reductions in coverage, and have created the need for repeated reexamination of entitlement. Frequently, the personnel who staff large public agencies find it difficult to keep track of the complex and ever-changing regulations.

Families may already be receiving some type of financial aid when a malignancy is diagnosed (Table 43-2). Unfortunately, these services, especially cash grants, do not expand to meet the increased needs. At The Children's Hospital of Philadelphia, for instance, 14% to 18% of newly diagnosed cancer patients are receiving medical assistance, as opposed to 35% for hospital inpatients as a whole. These figures vary, of course, from region to region.

Medical Assistance, or *Medicaid,* is a medical insurance program that was established as part of the Social Security Act of 1966 to provide medical care for the blind, aged, disabled, and members of families with dependent children. The program is administered and funded by each state with matching federal funds. In 1983, 54% was funded federally and the remainder by individual states.[8]

Medicaid is a blanket label for different programs and is not consistent from state to state. Federal law requires that states participate and that certain services are provided. Among these are inpatient and outpatient hospital care, laboratory and radiology services, skilled nursing care, home health care for persons 21 and older, and early and periodic screening programs for persons younger than 21.[9] Some states provide only what is federally mandated, whereas others offer more comprehensive programs of health care.

Eligibility for Medicaid is based primarily on income. Families receiving *Aid to Families with Dependent Children* (*AFDC*) automatically receive Medicaid, and some low-income working families can be accepted into the program. Outstanding medical bills are considered a part of eligibility determinations.

Medicaid reimbursement to providers varies considerably among states. In some areas, only a percentage of actual costs are reimbursed; in others, Medicaid pays dollar for dollar. Some programs will not pay physicians fees, as for the administration of chemotherapy, but others do. Under Medicaid, certain procedures or equipment may require prior approval and some drugs used for cancer patients (*e.g.,* oral morphine) are not automatically covered.

State and local welfare agencies typically offer important services, although programs differ substantially. In some states,

Table 43-2
Specific Resources and Programs

Financial aid—Public assistance, in the form of limited cash grants and food stamps, is available to needy, dependent children and their families through state and county public agencies under AFDC. Eligibility requirements are stringent. Applications are taken at local offices of the Department of Human Services.

Medicaid—A locally administered program funded by each state and the federal government. It provides health benefits to recipients of public assistance and to other persons (who may be employed) meeting financial eligibility requirements. Entitlements vary and may be restrictive in some eligibility categories. Not all equipment, drugs, or services are covered, and rates of reimbursement to medical providers usually are lower than rates paid by private insurance companies. Some states are experimenting with health maintenance plans, a trend that no doubt will become widespread. In most areas Medicaid pays for medical transportation, usually through reimbursement of travel expenses. Applications are taken at local Departments of Human Services.

Supplementary Security Income (SSI)—A federally funded program that entitles eligible recipients (the patient, not the family) to a modest cash grant and to Medicaid. For children under the age of 18, eligibility is based on parents' income. Medical conditions, in specific categories which include malignancies, that would prevent employment if the child were an adult and that are likely to continue for at least 12 months or to be terminal may meet eligibility guidelines. Claims that are rejected may be appealed and will be granted a hearing with a Social Security administrative law judge. Families can request free legal assistance with the appeal through Legal Aid. SSI will cover patients hospitalized after a full calendar month, regardless of the parents' income, although it will likely be discontinued after discharge if other requirements are not met. Applications for SSI are taken at the Social Security Administration and, under certain circumstances, at the hospital where the child is admitted (if the hospital has arranged for a Social Security representative to be on site during specified hours, or if prolonged hospitalization prevents parents from going to the Social Security office to file a claim). When approved, benefits are retroactive to the date of initial request. In some states, Medicaid covers for 90 days prior. Even if the child is covered through the parents' private insurance plan, if income eligibility can be met, it is advantageous to apply for SSI. It will provide a cash grant and supplement existing coverage so no out-of-pocket medical expenses are billed to the family.

National societies—The American Cancer Society (ACS), the Leukemia Society of America, and others combine research and public and professional education with services to patients. Local chapters are widespread but services vary considerably. The *Leukemia Society* helps patients with a diagnosis of leukemia, lymphoma or Hodgkin's disease, while the *ACS* covers all cancer patients. Assistance with selected expenses related to treatment, such as chemotherapy or home care, and provision of services, such as equipment or transportation, educational materials, or support groups may be available. The ACS National Advisory Committee on Childhood Cancer promotes the cause of pediatric cancer patients through recommendations for national and local activities. ACS has also provided funds for special camps, educational programs and even seed money to establish The Association of Pediatric Oncology Social Workers, a professional organization. Both organizations promote and arrange educational programs for professionals and the lay

public. Local chapters of the Leukemia Society may be located by writing to 211 East 43rd Street, New York, NY 10017. National Headquarters for ACS is located at Tower Place, 3340 Peachtree Road, Atlanta, GA 30026. Telephone (404) 320-3333.

Crippled Children's Program—This and other programs administered under state departments of health offer a wide range of health-related services to children with crippling and chronic illness. Eligibility usually is based on the medical condition and family income.

State and local hospitalization—Programs may be offered in some states that do not have crippled children's programs and may pay for hospital costs for children who are not eligible for Medicaid or SSI.

Private foundations and charities—Some national and local charities provide limited emergency help to families, usually in the form of cash grants. These groups usually do not pay for medical care but will offer support for nonmedical bills. Some will pay for transportation, rent, baby sitting, or utilities. Certain foundations offer aid specifically to pediatric cancer patients and their families; others have a more diverse client population. Amounts of cash grants vary but usually are under $1000.

Make a Wish organizations—These national and local groups offer one-time trips, gifts, or other items to seriously or terminally ill children.

Candlelighters' Childhood Cancer Foundation—A nationally based group that lobbies and provides information and referral services to parents. The national organization offers advice and sometimes assists families experiencing difficulties with insurance companies, hospitals, or the military. Two newsletters are published regularly (one for parents and one for teens). Local chapters conduct support groups and carry on a variety of activities. The national headquarters is located at 2025 I Street, NW, Suite 1011, Washington, DC 20006.

Home-based services—Hospice care, visiting nurse services, and home care are available in each community. Programs vary and not all have specially trained pediatric workers.

Vocational Rehabilitation Bureaus—Under a federally mandated program cofunded with states, vocational counselling, testing, and training are provided and higher education is funded for eligible clients. BVR also funds prostheses and other physical aids. Young adult and recovered pediatric cancer patients can benefit from these services.

Corporate Angel Network (CAN)—At no cost, transports ambulatory, medically authorized patients to specialized treatment centers or to their homes, in available seats on corporate aircraft. Arrangements can be made through Mrs. Priscilla Blum, Westchester County Airport, Hangar F, White Plains, NY 10604; (914) 328-1313

Developmental disabilities or protection and advocacy networks—State programs established through Public Laws 9103 and 95602, and with matching federal funds, provide an independent and private network for safeguarding education and employment rights for developmentally disabled citizens. In some areas Education Law Centers have been established by this program. Young cancer patients who need educational advocates to ensure appropriate school placements can benefit from this program. Developmental Disabilities Offices can be located through state government offices.

Compassionate Friends—This self-help organization offers mutual support for parents of children (of any age) who have died. Many local chapters exist and can be located in the white pages of the telephone book.

for example, crippled children's programs provide, or pay for, extensive services, such as physical therapy, nutritional support, and home care, but coverage is not extended to most children with cancer (amputees being an exception) because the criteria employed to define "handicapped" are so restrictive. In some of the states where pediatric cancer patients are included in crippled childrens programs, there is a 12-month waiting period; in others, so few services are offered that benefits are negligible. Elsewhere, such programs do not exist. Even when programs have been established, they may not be advertised or widely known, or they may be funded so minimally that only a few children can be covered.

SSI, which is based on family income, entitles recipients to a cash grant that is federally administered and to medical assistance that is administered by the state. Eligibility for this and other programs can be restrictive, albeit less so than programs funded by states or municipalities. Here again, applications are subject to interpretation. One of the guidelines for SSI specifies that children may be considered eligible if their medical condition would render them unable to work if they were employed adults and if their disability is expected to last 1 year or to be fatal. Also, the child's condition must be considered under one of the specified categories. Eligibility for a pediatric cancer patient would depend on the judgment of the person receiving the application, as well as the way information is presented by the medical institution. If the medical problem does not fall clearly within a definite category, it is still possible to prove eligibility, but the burden of proof lies with the doctor and the hospital.

Establishing eligibility may take considerable tenacity. For example, a child with a chiasmatic glioma could be rejected for benefits because the tumor is not malignant (although many consider it malignant because of its site). Nonmalignant brain tumors can be eligible if the resulting neurologic or visual dificits meet requirements under those categories. Without detailed documentation of these deficits, or if the child has not been so affected, the application would be denied even though treatment would be similar to that of malignant tumors, with identical financial and social costs for the family. As a rule, SSI workers request copies of the inpatient hospital record to determine eligibility, but such records may not contain the desired information, or it may be presented in a form that is unsuitable for documentation. In the case of the child with the chiasmatic glioma, a resulting Marcus Gunn pupil could qualify him for SSI, but the inpatient record of his diagnostic admission might not clearly indicate the accommodative reflex deficit.

Funeral Expenses

The struggle to pay for health care and other related expenses may not end with the child's death, and parents still face the unhappy problem of paying for the funeral, which can be a major expenditure. If the family has life insurance for the child, this can help defray the costs. Health insurance policies do not, however, pay funeral expenses. SSI and public welfare programs sometimes provide a modest amount (usually $300 to $500) that is not adequate to cover the costs in today's economy. In the case of public assistance, the grant may not be usable because of the restrictions imposed by some states that prevent the family from accepting other monies. In other words, if the family arranges a funeral for $1000 and they receive a $700 grant from a charity, they are not entitled to the $300 welfare benefit. If the welfare grant is used, the funeral director must agree to accept it as payment in full. Charities and foundations often help pay for funerals and cemetery costs, and funeral directors may reduce fees for needy families. How-

ever, the need for help is greater than the resources of these groups.

PUBLIC RELATIONS AND DEVELOPMENT ACTIVITIES

In addition to the efforts of a multidisciplinary team of physicians, nurses, social workers, and ancillary personnel, the hospital's administration may be able to assist families in obtaining financial support through its public relations and development staffs. Often, they are overlooked or not called on in time to secure maximum assistance. It is important for the entire management group in the hospital to understand parental feelings of guilt and responsibility when their child has cancer. Unusual behavior can sometimes result. These feelings may manifest themselves in complaints to the administration regarding high costs associated with hospitalization. The need for financial assistance can be the real message behind the complaints.

Effective public relations is necessary to lay the groundwork for fund-raising activities or for grass-roots lobbying efforts. Public relations should *not* be confused with publicity. Publicity is a public relations tool, sometimes the most visible aspect of the public relations program. Hence, the confusion and mistaken interchange of terms.[10] No other disease entity evokes as much public response to pleas for funds as childhood cancer because of its widespread association with death. A word of caution: the necessity of being nonexploitive in publicity efforts is paramount when trying to raise money.

A close working relationship with the oncology staff serves as a constant reminder of the special circumstances surrounding families coping with the problem of childhood cancer. Also, working together reinforces the role of oncology staff within the institution. New philanthropic opportunities that arise through the development office can be shuttled more easily to the cancer service when the fundraising arm of the hospital is knowledgeable about cancer and its impact on families.

Not infrequently, parents of children who do not survive cancer are the ones who set up special funds for others whose children are suffering. Who better than they would understand the monetary problems faced by these families.

The authors wish to thank Mr. Steven Sieverts, Vice-President, Health Care Finance, Blue Cross–Blue Shield, National Capitol Area for providing helpful information about Blue Cross and Blue Shield.

REFERENCES

1. Lansky SB, Cairns NU, Clark GM, Black J: Children's cancer, nonmedical costs of the illness. Cancer 43:403–408, 1979
2. Bloom BS, Knorr RS, Evans AE: The epidemiology of disease expenses the cost of caring for children with cancer. JAMA 253:2393–2397, 1985
3. The Children's Hospitals Case Mix Classification System Project, Project Summary and Recommendations. National Association of Children's Hospitals and Related Institutions, October 1986
4. Hill Burton Act, Title 42, Section 291 et seq., August 13, 1946. Amended 1974
5. Mayer TR, Mayer GG: HMO's: Origins and developments. N Engl J Med 312:590–594, 1985
6. Ansberry C: Desperate straits. The Wall Street Journal, January 5, 1987
7. Ross J: Social work intervention with families of children with cancer: The changing critical phases. Soc Work Health Care 3:257–271, 1978
8. Statistical Abstracts of the United States, p 381. Washington, DC, US Census Bureau, Bureau of the Census, 1986
9. Encyclopedia of Social Work. New York, National Association of Social Workers, 1987
10. Bonnem S: Introduction. In Riggs L (ed): The Health Care Facility's Public Relations Handbook, p 3. Rockville, MD, Aspen Systems, 1982

forty-four

Management of Childhood Cancer Pain

Angela W. Miser and
James S. Miser

The International Association for the Study of Pain has defined pain as "an unpleasant sensory and emotional experience associated with actual or potential tissue damage or described in terms of such damage. Pain is always subjective. Each individual learns the application of the word through experiences related to injury in early life. It is unquestionably a sensation in a part or parts of the body, but it is also always unpleasant and therefore an emotional experience."[1] In addition to tissue damage, other factors, such as anger, fear, depression, loss of self-esteem, cultural aspects,[2,3] and internalization of parental fears and feelings, play an important role in the child's overall pain experience. Although the child with cancer may experience pain arising from causes other than the malignancy itself (*e.g.,* therapy-related pain) the major emphasis of this chapter is on cancer-derived pain.

PATHOPHYSIOLOGY OF PAIN

Pain impulses are initiated by noxious stimuli that cause the release of ions or specific organic substances including histamine, prostaglandins, or other peptides. These sensitize or activate nociceptors, which appear to be specific, undifferentiated nerve endings in the skin or deeper tissues. Pain impulses are carried centrally by large myelinated A-delta or unmyelinated fibers; cell bodies of these fibers are located in the dorsal root ganglia of the spinal cord. After entry through the dorsal root of the spinal cord, these afferent sensory nerves may ascend or descend in Lissauer's tract for a few segments before synapsing in specific laminae of the dorsal horn. Within the dorsal horn, there appears to be extensive interaction and cross-modulation mediated by short interneurons, many of which are inhibitory.

Ascending central pathways carry the pain impulses rostrally. The neospinothalamic tract, which projects to the ventral, lateral, and posterior thalamus and then synapses with neurons projecting to the somatosensory cortex, is primarily responsible for the perception of pain intensity and localization. The phylogenetically older paleospinothalamic tract projects diffusely to the reticular formation and medial thalamus, with final projection to the frontal cortex, and is primarily responsible for the perception of dull, poorly localized pain impulses and for motivational and emotional components of the pain experience.

More recent work has demonstrated the importance of an extensive descending inhibitory system, including a pathway originating in the periaqueductal gray nuclei in the midbrain and descending by the raphe magnus and dorsolateral funiculus to the dorsal horn of the spinal cord, and a pathway from the locus ceruleus to the dorsal horn. The role of neurotransmitters in the transmission (substance P)[4] and modulation (serotonin, dopamine, norepinephrine, and the endogenous opioid peptides β-endorphin, enkephalins, and dynorphin) of pain stimuli is being intensively studied. Opioid receptors,[5,6] which are stereospecific binding sites capable of binding endogenous and exogenous opioids, have been found extensively in the periaqueductal gray region of the midbrain and the dorsal horn of the spinal cord. These receptors mediate the pharmacologic properties of opioid analgesics, and many subtypes have been identified, including the high-affinity and low-affinity mu, delta, kappa, sigma, and epsilon receptors.

PREVALENCE AND ETIOLOGY OF PAIN ASSOCIATED WITH CANCER

Pain experienced by the child with cancer can be of one or more of four basic etiologies (Table 44-1): cancer-related, treatment-related, procedure-related, and incidental.[7]

Several studies have documented a high incidence of pain in adults with malignancy;[8,9] however, these data cannot necessarily be extrapolated to children, whose spectrum of malignancies is entirely different. Pediatric data are sparse, but a large retrospective Italian survey indicated that moderate to severe pain is a common symptom during the course of cancer diagnosis and treatment in children.[10] A prospective study of the selected, generally high-risk cohort of children and young adults treated at the Pediatric Branch of the National Cancer Institute (NCI),[7] in which procedure-related pain was excluded, confirmed a high prevalence of pain, with roughly 50% of inpatients and 25% of outpatients experiencing pain at any given time. In this population, however, therapy-related pain predominated, in contrast to the overwhelming preponderance of tumor-related pain found in adult series. This was true even in pediatric patients with active malignancy.

The different spectra of pain experienced by children with cancer compared to adults may be in part due to the generally more aggressive multimodality regimens used in most pediatric malignancies, which lead to significant treatment-related morbidity. Further, the high initial response rate of childhood malignancies to intensive treatment results in the rapid disappearance of tumor-related pain in most children. This was reflected in a second prospective NCI study[11] of children and young adults with cancer: although 78% were experiencing cancer-related pain at initial presentation and pain had been present for a median of 74 days, the pain persisted for a median of only 10 days after cancer therapy was begun. Finally, children with unresponsive or refractory malignancies generally experience a rapid demise. Thus, true chronic pain, as defined by persistence for longer than 6 months, appears to be less common in pediatric than adult oncology.

EVALUATION OF THE CHILD WITH PAIN

Because the optimal evaluation and treatment of childhood pain frequently requires input from a variety of medical subspecialities, the establishment of multidisciplinary "pain teams" for children (to include pediatric oncologists, radiation therapists, surgeons, anesthesiologists, nurses, pharmacists, teachers, psychiatrists, social workers, dietitians, pastoral workers, physical therapists, and play therapists) can be a major advance in both care of the individual child and in fostering pediatric pain research.

In evaluations of pain in the child with cancer, two important principles deserve emphasis. First, although some investigators have proposed that, because of the immaturity of the central nervous system, neonates are unable to fully experience pain,[12] more recent observations in newborns[13] support the working hypothesis that children of any age feel pain when an appropriate stimulus is applied. Therefore, appropriate analgesic intervention is required for all age groups. Second, there is no evidence from the literature or from medical practice to indicate that fabricated complaints of pain in a child with cancer are more than an extreme rarity. Therefore, complaints of pain in a child with malignancy should be appropriately investigated and, because diagnostic studies of malignant lesions may occasionally be initially negative,[14] continuing vigilance is required even if initial studies are unrevealing.

A thorough evaluation of pain requires investigation of its etiology, location, intensity, duration, and prior treatment.

Etiology and Location: Pain Syndromes

It is critical to diagnose accurately not only the etiology of the pain (see Table 44-1) but also the precise location of the causative lesion, particularly distinguishing referred from local pain.

Tumor-related pain[15] most commonly arises from malignant deposits in bone that usually, but not invariably,[14] are accompanied by changes on plain radiographs or radionuclide scans. Extreme pain on movement, especially in conjunction with localized swelling, may indicate pathologic fracture. Bone invasion at sites closely approximating a nerve pathway (e.g., pelvic foramina, vertebral column, skull) may be accompanied by nerve compression or destruction. Although many malignant soft tissue masses are painless, pain often accompanies impingement on adjacent bone or nervous tissue, capsular distention, or hollow viscus obstruction.

Involvement of the nervous system is also associated with specific pain syndromes, including headache and vomiting with early morning exacerbation from intracranial tumor deposits, and localized spine or radiating pain, with or without concomitant neurologic changes, from cord compression or invasion. Meningeal leukemia or carcinomatosis frequently manifests with headache and signs of raised intracranial pressure in conjunction with diffuse back pain that may radiate to the extremities and be exacerbated by back or neck flexion. Recognized syndromes affecting the peripheral nervous system include plexopathies (brachial, lumbar, and sacral), in which there may be referred limb pain and accompanying autonomic changes, and peripheral neuropathy, wherein paresthesias, hyperesthesias, and dysesthesias may accompany motor weakness in the distribution of the peripheral nerves involved. Deafferentation pain arising from injury to nerve or spinal cord frequently has a characteristic superficial burning

Table 44-1
Major Causes of Pain in Children with Cancer

Category	Major Examples
Cancer-related	Bone invasion; soft tissue invasion with or without viscus obstruction; invasion of central or peripheral nervous systems
Treatment-related	Mucositis; postoperative infection; radiation dermatitis; abdominal pain from protracted vomiting; prolonged post-lumbar-puncture headache; neuropathic, including phantom limb pain and drug-induced peripheral neuropathy
Procedure-related	Lumbar puncture; bone marrow biopsy or aspiration
Incidental	Trauma

(dysesthetic) or shooting quality. Alterations in autonomic nervous system activity can also cause painful syndromes, such as that found in reflex sympathetic dystrophy.[16]

Intensity: Pain Assessment and Measurement

Pain measurement involves assessment of both quality and intensity. Description of the quality of the pain is limited by the child's maturity and vocabulary[17]; tests such as the McGill Pain Questionnaire, in which descriptive terms such as "sharp," "lancinating," and "burning" are used both qualitatively and quantitatively, may be used in older children.[18]

Measurement of pain intensity in children is controversial, and no well-established guidelines are available. Three general methods have been espoused: assessment of changes in physiologic parameters, assessment based on health care professionals' observations and parental report, and self-report by the child.

Changes in physiologic parameters such as heart rate, respiratory rate, and sweating, while reported in adults to be a feature of acute rather than chronic pain,[19] may be less reliable in the child with cancer, in whom confounding features such as anxiety, infection, and chemotherapy administration play an important role.

Observational assessment by health care professionals involves evaluation of verbal complaints of the child, the presence of specific pain behaviors (*e.g.,* failure to move a painful extremity, rubbing or pulling at the painful site, crying during a particular movement, general fretfulness),[20,21] and functional changes (*e.g.,* sleep, play, sports, school attendance), as well as physical examination of the painful site, laboratory and radiographic evaluation where appropriate, and report from child care providers. Although various formal scales rating pain intensity according to the manifestation of specific pain behaviors[22-24] have been advocated for use in procedure-related pain, these are primarily research tools, and no comparable behavioral scales for chronic pain have been developed. Further, although this observational method is the one most commonly used in clinical practice, its accuracy depends on factors such as the clinical experience of the health care provider, his or her rapport with the patient, and the time spent in the evaluation process. Indeed, the literature indicates that health care providers often underestimate the pain experienced by their patients.[24-27]

Pain measurement based on patient self-report is limited to the child who is old enough and sufficiently mature to understand the testing procedure and to express himself or herself in a standardized and reproducible fashion. Two-year-olds are the youngest children reported capable of this form of pain measurement.[28] Major concerns with the use of this method, particularly in young children, are the child's paucity of prior experience with painful stimuli on which to base comparative statements such as "little" or "much," the willingness to cooperate with repeated testing, and the effect of confounding variables such as anxiety and cultural factors. Nonetheless, several such methods have been advocated (Table 44-2). It should be stressed that although these methods have been used in clinical studies, not all have undergone rigorous scientific evaluation. Further testing in several centers to assess the validity and reproducibility of, and degree of patient cooperation with, these tests is in progress and hopefully will result in the formulation of well-established guidelines for their use.

As an overall guideline, although pain measurement in the preverbal child must of necessity be based entirely on parental report and physician or nurse observation and examination, older children can be given the opportunity to express their pain in both qualitative and quantitative terms so that the

health care provider can have the broadest possible data base on which to formulate a treatment plan.

Duration of Pain and Prior Treatment

Particularly helpful features of the prior pain history include allergy or intolerance to specific drugs, recently used effective or ineffective regimens, drug dosages used, and patient or parental biases against a particular drug (*e.g.,* morphine may be rejected because of connotations with addiction, whereas hydromorphone may be acceptable). Further, because narcotic withdrawal symptoms have been reported following abrupt discontinuation of therapeutic narcotics given for periods as short as 1 week,[33] the duration and intensity of prior opioid use should be noted.

Finally, it should be stressed that in the rare instance when there is reason to doubt the genuineness of the child's complaint of pain, a "placebo trial" is both meaningless and unjustifiable, because roughly 30% of a general population experiencing pain will report relief from a placebo injection.[34]

DEVELOPMENT OF A TREATMENT PLAN: THERAPEUTIC STRATEGIES

As part of the development of an analgesic treatment regimen, the role of anticancer treatment should be evaluated. Surgical intervention (*e.g.,* for relief of cord compression), local irradiation, or systemic chemotherapy can provide rapid pain relief from tumor shrinkage. In cases where such treatment is not indicated or ineffective, or while anticancer therapy is being initiated, other analgesic interventions may be used. The basic pain-relieving strategies available are [1] analgesic drugs; [2] anesthetic blocks and inhalational agents; [3] noninvasive techniques such as hypnosis, relaxation, and transcutaneous electrical nerve stimulation; and [4] neurosurgical techniques.

In addition, the child experiencing cancer pain and his or her family require intensive ongoing supportive counseling to cover such topics as the cause and significance of the pain, the child's change in body image, his or her dependence on analgesic medications or other forms of pain relief, school absenteeism, or other related issues.

The interventions chosen for an individual patient will depend on the strategies available at the treatment center and on the clinical situation. In particular, the choice of treatment depends on the etiology and location of the pain; the intensity of the pain; the anticipated duration of the pain (*e.g.,* pain of 1 to 2 weeks' duration or less that will rapidly decrease in intensity, as from chemotherapy-responsive or radiosensitive tumor or postoperative pain, may be managed with a short-acting analgesic drug given on an "as needed" (PRN) basis, whereas pain of longer duration is generally managed optimally using a regularly scheduled analgesic drug, perhaps with a longer analgesic action); and the life expectancy of the child, which is of particular importance when considering neuroablative surgery.

Administration of Analgesic Drugs

As in adult oncology, the administration of analgesic drugs forms the mainstay of pain control in childhood malignancy. Drugs may be given as the sole form of pain management, as adjuncts to other analgesic strategies, or as an initial intervention during diagnostic evaluation or the initiation of other treatment regimens. Analgesic drugs (Table 44-3) may be considered in three groups: nonsteroidal anti-inflammatory drugs

Table 44-2
*Pediatric Pain Measurement Tools Using Patient Self-Report**

Type	Description/Examples	Methodology/Limitations
Visual analogue scale[29]	Pain thermometer[30]	Marking a point on a 100-mm line from "no pain" to "severe pain, as bad as it can be"; age $\geq$ 8 yr for comprehension of test
Picture scales	Smile faces;[22,28] pictures of painful stimuli[26]	Selection of appropriate picture
Number rating scales	Numbers representing no pain (1) to excruciating pain (5)[22]	Selection of appropriate number
Verbal descriptor scales	Descriptive words (*e.g.,* mild, moderate, severe, excruciating) according to child's understanding	Selection of appropriate word
Color-coded scales	Eland color tool;[31] identification of colors associated with no, mild, moderate, severe pain	Selection of appropriate color crayon(s) to color location and intensity of pain on body diagram
Manual quantitative methods	Hester's poker chip technique[32]	Selection of number of poker chips representing intensity of pain (4 = excruciating); age $\geq$ 4 yr for comprehension
Cross-modality matching methods[29]	Pressure gauge concealed in puppet	Hand-grip force represents pain intensity
Qualitative measures	McGill Pain Questionnaire[18]	Selection of words describing pain; adult vocabulary required

* Some of these measures are validated; others are not.

(NSAIDs) or aspirin-like drugs, opioids (weak narcotic and mixed agonist/antagonist drugs, or potent narcotics), and adjuvant drugs.

Several general principles are helpful in planning optimal drug use. First, the route of drug administration should be carefully selected. Under most circumstances, the oral route is preferable when feasible. Many analgesics can be prepared in pleasant-tasting liquid vehicles to increase patient compliance. Where oral medication is not tolerated, the parenteral route is the most often used alternative. Too few agents have been adequately studied following sublingual administration to permit reliable usage guidelines. Rectal administration yields equivalent analgesia to oral dosing and is occasionally indicated. However, this route should be avoided in the neutropenic child, in whom minor rectal trauma can lead to perirectal cellulitis.

Second, drugs appropriate for the type and severity of the pain should be selected. The concept of the analgesic ladder (Fig. 44-1), as recommended by the World Health Organization,[35] illustrates the principle of administering an analgesic drug of appropriate strength to treat the pain. Mild pain may be controlled with an NSAID, whereas moderate to severe pain usually require the use of a weak or strong narcotic. Adjuvant drugs appropriate to the clinical situation may be used at each step of the ladder. Should a patient fail to achieve pain relief with an adequate trial of a drug at one level of the ladder, a change should be made to a drug on a higher level rather than to another drug on the same level. In each group of drugs, detailed knowledge of the pharmacokinetics and clinical features of one or two drugs will be adequate under most circumstances.

Third, for management of all but acute, rapidly changing pain, drugs should be administered on a regular schedule ("by the clock") based on the plasma half-life of the drug and on individual patient response. This permits an even level of pain control and avoids the suffering and anxiety experienced with PRN administration, which requires that the patient experience breakthrough pain in order to receive another dose of drug. Drugs with a short plasma half-life, such as codeine and morphine, generally require administration every 4 hours, whereas

Table 44-3
Nonsteroidal Anti-inflammatory Drugs and Narcotics Commonly Used in Pediatrics

Drug (trade name)	Administration	Comments
NSAIDs		
Acetaminophen (Tylenol)	65 mg/kg/day PO, divided doses every 4 h	These preparations lack gastric ulcerogenic effect and do not inhibit platelet function; both have antipyretic effect and may mask infection-associated fever
Choline magnesium trisalicylate (Trilisate)	25 mg/kg every 12 h PO (adult dose, 1125 mg every 12 h)	
Weak Narcotics		
Codeine	0.5–1 mg/kg PO every 4 h	No increased analgesia with dosage escalation
	0.7–1.3 mg/kg IM every 4 h	
Strong Narcotics		
Short half-life (1.5–5 hr)		
Morphine	0.3 mg/kg PO every 4 h	Dosage may be escalated to increase analgesic effect
	0.1–0.15 mg/kg IV or IM every 4 h	
Long half-life (12–25 h)		
Methadone (Dolophine)	0.6 mg/kg/day PO, divided doses every 4–6 h	Dosage may be escalated to increase analgesic effect; accumulation may occur, resulting in delayed respiratory depression
	0.3–0.45 mg/kg/day IV or IM, divided doses every 4–6 h	
Sustained-release morphine (MS Contin; Roxanol SR)	0.9 mg/kg every 12 h PO	Dosage titration performed initially with regular oral morphine, followed by change to sustained release preparation at 70%–100% total daily dose
	0.6 mg/kg every 8 h PO	

drugs with longer half-lives, such as methadone and levorphanol, can be successfully administered every 6 to 8 hours.

Fourth, the drug dosage and schedule should be titrated to individual patient needs. Although NSAIDs and weak narcotics have a ceiling effect of analgesia (*i.e.,* further escalation in drug dose above recommended levels leads to increasing toxicity without improved analgesia), the strong narcotics have no defined interpatient maximum dose, thus permitting progressive dosage escalation as required, provided that no dose-limiting toxicity, particularly respiratory depression, is encountered.

Fifth, drug side effects (outlined below and in Table 44-4) should be anticipated and appropriately managed.

Sixth, should dosage reduction be clinically indicated, this should be done slowly because abrupt discontinuation of narcotics after treatment periods as short as a week may precipitate a classical withdrawal syndrome,[33] and sudden cessation of benzodiazepines or barbiturates given as adjuvant drugs may also precipitate characteristic withdrawal symptoms, including seizures.[36]

Finally, the choice of analgesic drugs should be discussed with parents or child. Many misconceptions surround the need for strong narcotics and the possibility of inducing "addiction," particularly when widely known drugs such as morphine are prescribed. Tolerance to an opioid drug has developed when, after repeated administration, decreased drug effect is noted, or increasingly larger doses must be administered to maintain drug efficacy. This generally occurs only after prolonged administration, usually by the parenteral route, and rarely poses a clinical problem. Physical dependence refers to an altered physiologic state produced by the repeated administration of a drug that necessitates the continued administration of the drug to prevent the appearance of a stereotypical withdrawal or abstinence syndrome characteristic of the drug. Although this is usually apparent only after regular drug use of several weeks' duration, it may occur following short, intensive courses of narcotics and can be avoided by tapering drug doses over several days. Psychological dependence or "addiction" involves a behavioral pattern of drug use characterized by overwhelming involvement with the use of a drug (compulsive use) and the securing of its supply, and a high tendency to relapse after withdrawal.[36] Psychological dependence is rarely if ever produced by pharmacologic management of cancer pain,[7,37] and families should receive appropriate reassurance.

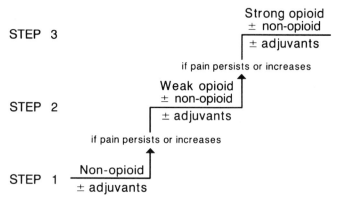

FIGURE 44-1. The analgesic ladder for cancer pain management. (Adapted from Cancer Pain Relief, World Health Organization, 1986)

Thus, there is no medical rationale or justification for withholding appropriate narcotics to "save them for something worse," and these definitions should be transmitted, where appropriate, to the family.

Classes of Analgesic Drugs

NSAIDs and Aspirin-like Drugs

All aspirin-like drugs are analgesic, antipyretic, and anti-inflammatory, and their therapeutic effect is derived, at least in part, from the inhibition of prostaglandin synthesis. None has been shown definitely superior to any other; all are effective in the management of mild to moderate pain. Because of their antipyretic properties, they must be used circumspectly in the neutropenic child, in whom suppression of fever may mask a potentially life-threatening infection. Most NSAIDs, including aspirin, cause gastric irritation and an increased bleeding tendency, primarily on the basis of drug-induced platelet dysfunction; thus the use of most drugs in this class should be extremely limited in cancer patients. Acetaminophen produces neither of these effects and is generally considered the agent of choice in this drug category (see Table 44-3). Choline salicylate, which is available alone or in combination with magnesium salicylate (Trilisate), also reportedly produces minimal gastric irritation and no increase in bleeding tendency, and has the advantage of twice daily administration.

Narcotics

A narcotic is indicated for a child experiencing pain unresponsive to an NSAID or for whom an NSAID is contraindicated. Narcotics may be considered in two classes: weak narcotics, including codeine and the mixed agonist–antagonist drugs; and strong narcotics (see Table 44-3). All have a similar spectrum of side effects, as outlined below and in Table 44-4. Several good reviews of narcotic use in adults are available[38,39]; data in children are limited.

Weak Narcotics and Mixed Agonist–Antagonist Drugs. These narcotics are effective in the treatment of mild to moderate pain, but their efficacy shows a ceiling effect, so that escalation above the recommended dose tends to yield increasing toxicity without added analgesia. They may be used alone or in combination with an NSAID.

The opioid agonist codeine is the most commonly used agent in this group. Propoxyphene is structurally related to methadone and may accumulate on repeated dosing; large

Table 44-4
Narcotic Side-Effects

Side-Effect	*Management*
Respiratory depression	Reduction in narcotic dose
Respiratory arrest	Naloxone 0.01–0.1 mg/kg IV or IM. Small frequent doses of diluted naloxone or naloxone drip preferable for patients on chronic narcotic therapy to avoid severe, painful withdrawal syndrome. Repeated doses often required until narcotic effect subsides. Intubation may be required because naloxone frequently induces vomiting
Drowsiness/sedation	Frequently subsides after a few days without dosage reduction; amphetamine useful in adults (inadequate pediatric data)
Constipation	Prophylactic laxatives indicated
Nausea/vomiting	Change to a different narcotic may alleviate symptoms; hydroxyzine or a phenothiazine drug often beneficial but may cause increased sedation
Euphoria, confusion, nightmares, hallucinations	Reassurance only, if symptoms mild; change to a different narcotic may avoid symptoms
Allergic Phenomena Urticaria	Change to opioid of different structure (*e.g.,* morphine to methadone) required
Itching	Antihistamine (*e.g.,* hydroxyzine) often beneficial
Multifocal myoclonus; seizures	Generally occur only during extremely high-dose therapy; reduction in opioid dose indicated if possible
*Related Manifestations** Tolerance	Escalate drug dosage as required. If clinically problematic, change to a different drug or route of administration may be indicated
Physical dependence	Taper drug doses slowly to avoid withdrawal symptoms[33]
Psychological dependence ("addiction")	Rarely induced by therapeutic use of narcotics in cancer patients[7,37]

* See text.

doses have been associated with convulsions. Use in children is not recommended because of inadequate dosage and toxicity data.

Mixed agonist–antagonist drugs such as pentazocine, nalbuphine, and butorphanol may produce undesirable psychotomimetic effects, and may precipitate narcotic withdrawal in patients being managed on pure opioid agonists. Although it was initially hoped that use of these drugs would not lead to physical or psychological dependence, both may occur. Data on the use of most of these agents in children are extremely sparse. However, buprenorphine, widely available for parenteral use and of limited availability in sublingual form, has been studied in children[40] and appears to be promising for outpatient management of mild to moderate cancer-related pain. The potential for producing psychotomimetic effects appears to be very low with this agent.

Strong Narcotics.   A strong narcotic, with or without an NSAID, is indicated for the treatment of moderate to severe pain. Unlike weak narcotics, strong narcotics have no definable fixed dosage range. Rather, the dose can be escalated as required to achieve adequate pain relief, provided that dose-limiting toxicity, particularly respiratory depression, is not encountered. As with other analgesic drugs, oral administration is generally preferred whenever possible. For simplicity, these drugs may be divided into two pharmacokinetic groups: the short-acting agents such as morphine and hydromorphone (half-lives of 1.5–5 hours) and the long-acting agents such as methadone and levorphanol (half-lives of 12–25 hours). The sustained-release preparations of oral morphine may also be considered long-acting agents.

Short-Acting Strong Narcotics.   Oral morphine has been considered the gold standard of pain control in cancer patients for many years[41,42]; the drug is also available for rectal[43,44] and parenteral administration.[45–47] After an oral dose, morphine is readily absorbed from the gastrointestinal tract but undergoes significant first-pass metabolism in the liver, so that during chronic administration a subcutaneous dose is 2 to 3 times as potent as the same dose given orally.[45] In adults, reported analgesic doses range from 2.5 mg to more than 100 mg every 4 hours.[41,42] In children, a starting dose of 0.3 mg/kg orally every 4 hours, with titration as required, has been used effectively. Sustained release oral morphine preparations may be given at 8- to 12-hour intervals rather than every 4 hours to permit uninterrupted sleep. These preparations are in tablet form, so they are unsuitable for the very young child. Clinical experience, primarily in adults, indicates that initial dosage titration using regular oral morphine every 4 hours followed by conversion to the sustained release preparation, given every 8 to 12 hours in a total 24-hour milligram dose 70% to 100% of the total 24-hour regular oral morphine dose, is optimal.[48]

Hydromorphone (Dilaudid) is available for oral, rectal, and parenteral administration. In adult studies, an intramuscular dose of 1.5 to 2 mg of hydromorphone is roughly comparable in analgesic effect to 10 mg of intramuscular morphine. The drug has a parenteral to oral relative analgesic potency of roughly 2:1.[49] Reports of use in children are anecdotal.

Meperidine (Demerol) is rarely indicated in cancer patients because it carries no major advantage over other short-acting potent narcotics, and chronic use has been associated with seizure activity caused by accumulation of the toxic metabolite normeperidine.[50] Where prescribed, meperidine should be limited to brief courses.

Long-Acting Strong Narcotics.   Methadone (Dolophine) is a synthetic drug whose pseudopiperidine ring configuration confers opioid activity.[51] For management of cancer pain in adults, doses of 2.5 to 10 mg every 4 hours are recommended by the manufacturer. For initial management in children, 0.6 mg/kg per 24 hours divided into oral doses every 4 to 6 hours

and followed by titration as required is a safe and effective regimen.[52] Although most texts suggest an oral-to-parenteral dosage conversion of 2:1,[53] recent work has indicated a much higher oral bioavailability in most patients,[54] so that a parenteral dose of 75% of the oral dose is probably more appropriate in most cases. The major potential hazard of methadone relates to its long half-life; the drug may accumulate over the first 2 to 4 days of therapy, leading to overdosage.[55] Therefore, close contact should be maintained with the patient during the initial phase of methadone therapy or following dose escalation. Great caution should be exercised when a narcotic with a long half-life is used in a patient with a rapidly changing clinical condition or with metabolic complications; in such circumstances, a drug with a shorter half-life is usually preferable.

Levorphanol (Levo-Dromoran) has properties and clinical indications very similar to those of methadone when used in adults. Inadequate data are available in children to recommend treatment guidelines.

ALTERNATIVE MODES OF ADMINISTRATION OF STRONG NARCOTICS.   Continuous Intravenous and Subcutaneous Narcotic Infusions.   Continuous intravenous and subcutaneous infusions of morphine[56–58] have been found to provide adequate analgesia in children failing to achieve pain relief with other strategies. Indications for the use of parenteral narcotics include inability to tolerate oral medication and severe or rapidly worsening pain, where titration with oral drugs is too slow to provide adequate pain relief. Indications for a continuous narcotic infusion rather than intermittent boluses include "peaks and valleys" of both side-effects and pain control following intermittent narcotic injections, commonly encountered where narcotic pulses are required more often than every 6 hours; severe pain that is not controlled by frequent narcotic boluses; and absence of an intravenous line, in which case a continuous subcutaneous narcotic infusion[57] provides an alternative to frequent needle punctures. Both continuous subcutaneous infusion, using a small portable syringe pump and long, low-volume tubing, and continuous intravenous infusion, delivered by an infusion pump into a long-term intravenous line, are suitable for home care. The starting dose for a continuous infusion can be calculated from the total preceding 24-hour dose requirement divided evenly over the succeeding 24-hour period, or an arbitrary dose of 0.05 mg/kg per hour can be initiated, followed by titration as required. Although a child may start with a continuous subcutaneous infusion, the most common approach is to initiate a continuous intravenous infusion, adjust the dose to individual patient requirements, and then switch to the subcutaneous route on an equal milligram basis. Particular caution should be exercised when high hourly doses of morphine are required; under these circumstances, preservative-free morphine should be used to avoid somnolence from accumulation of the preservative chlorobutanol.[59] Further, there is a suggestion that acutely ill patients, for instance, those having recently undergone bone marrow transplantation and those receiving other drugs known to cause central nervous system depression (e.g., ifosamide), exhibit increased narcotic side-effects, particularly respiratory depression. A narcotic infusion should be avoided in these patients if possible, or used with extreme caution if pain control is not being achieved by other means.[57] Although other narcotics can be administered as a continuous infusion,[60] particularly when morphine is contraindicated, these require individual tailoring because no pediatric guidelines are available.

Patient-Controlled Analgesia (PCA).   A PCA pump[61] connected to an indwelling intravenous line permits the patient to trigger delivery of a preset narcotic bolus as required for pain relief. A minimal interval of bolus administration is programmed into the pump to prevent excessive usage. Although most of the data on this device have been obtained in postoperative adults, some centers have found the PCA method useful in cancer patients.[62] Data on PCA in children are anecdotal, but in older children with malignancy this technique, used either alone or combination with a continuous narcotic infusion, may occasionally be useful.

Transdermal Narcotic Infusion. The delivery of a continuous opioid infusion by a transdermal therapeutic system placed on the skin surface is currently undergoing investigation. This promises to be a major advance for the child who requires a continuous narcotic infusion because the system avoids the use of needle, syringe, and pump.

Intrathecal, Intraventricular, and Epidural Narcotic Administration. These approaches[63-66] have been found useful in adult cancer patients experiencing pain, particularly in the pelvis or lower limbs, that is difficult to control with systemic narcotics. Indications for the use of these routes of narcotic administration are not well defined, but anecdotal data in children indicate that, despite its invasive nature, this method of drug administration can be valuable in pediatric patients.

NARCOTIC SIDE-EFFECTS. All opioid drugs exhibit the same spectrum of side-effects, which should be anticipated whenever a narcotic is prescribed (see Table 44-4). In an individual patient, however, a particular toxicity may be apparent with one narcotic but not another, so that a change of drug may avoid a toxic manifestation. For example, a patient may experience vomiting or nightmares with the use of morphine but not hydromorphone.

Adjuvant Drugs

Unlike the NSAID and narcotic drug groups, the use of adjuvant drugs for pain control has generally been derived from

Table 44-5
Adjuvant Analgesic Drugs

Drug Class	Drug, Dosage	Indications	Comments
Corticosteroids	Various drugs and doses advocated, (*e.g.,* dexamethasone 6–12 mg/m²/ day)	Raised intracranial pressure, spinal cord or nerve compression; prolonged post-LP headache; widespread metastases	Effect may be short-lived
Antidepressants and anticonvulsants[67-69]	Amitriptyline 0.5–1 mg/kg HS Carbamazepine, phenytoin	Neuropathic pain (*e.g.,* postherpetic, vincristine-induced, radiation plexopathy, tumor invasion of nerve)	Action may be from inhibition of neuronal uptake and increase in synaptic serotonin[69]; pain relief and improved sleep within 3–5 days; doses subtherapeutic for depression
Neuroleptics	Chlorpromazine, prochlorperazine, methotrimeprazine	Nausea; confused, combative child	Consider concurrent use of antiparkinsonian drug (*e.g.,* diphenhydramine) to avoid oculogyric crisis if high doses or prolonged course used
		Enhancement of narcotic analgesia	Only methotrimeprazine (only parenteral drug available) has documented analgesic properties; other drugs may limit narcotic use by enhancing sedation
Anxiolytic sedatives	Benzodiazepines (*e.g.,* diazepam, oxazepam, lorazepam)	Acute anxiety, muscle spasm	No analgesic properties; sedative effect may limit narcotic use; lorazepam (short-acting) often considered drug of choice; most except lorazepam and oxazepam are converted to active metabolites, causing very prolonged action; withdrawal syndrome precipitated by abrupt discontinuation after prolonged use
	Antihistamines (*e.g.,* hydroxyzine)	Anxiety, nausea, narcotic-induced pruritus	May potentiate analgesia
Psychostimulants	Amphetamines	Opioid-induced somnolence, potentiation of narcotic analgesia[70]	No studies available in children

anecdotal experience or uncontrolled trials. Therefore, evidence for their efficacy and treatment guidelines are more tenuous. Suggested clinical use of these agents is outlined in Table 44-5.

Anesthetic Nerve Blocks and Inhalational Agents

Although temporary or permanent nerve blocks have a well-established place in the relief of pain in adult cancer patients, they are rarely indicated in children because of the terror induced by invasive procedures and because the most common fatal childhood malignancies are either widespread (leukemia, lymphoma, metastatic neuroblastoma) or confined to the central nervous system. Modalities include peripheral nerve blocks, primarily for the chest and abdominal wall, where interruption of both motor and sensory components will not pose a functional problem; autonomic blocks, such as lumbar sympathetic blocks for lumbosacral plexus pain; and epidural and intrathecal blocks for pain in the sacrum, lumbosacral plexus, abdomen, and perineum. The reader is referred to standard texts for details of indications and procedures.[71]

In trigger point injections, saline or local anesthetic is injected into specific, localized, painful, soft tissue areas occasionally found in children with musculoskeletal pain secondary to tumor in deeper structures.[72,73] The noninvasive local application of a cold stimulus has been advocated as an alternative management approach.[74,75]

Nitrous oxide is useful during the performance of brief, painful procedures, and has also been used in adults with terminal cancer pain as an adjunct to systemic analgesic drugs.[76] A patient-controlled machine[77,78] that delivers a fixed 50% nitrous oxide–50% oxygen combination and is fitted with a scavenger device to vent exhaled gases into a regular wall suction unit has provided good analgesic efficacy in children undergoing painful procedures. However, concern regarding excessive exposure of medical personnel to nitrous oxide may limit the use of this modality.

Noninvasive Techniques

Hypnosis. Hypnosis in children with cancer has been studied primarily during painful procedures, and is effective in the relief of pain and anxiety in many children willing to use this technique.[25,79,80] Once trained in the procedure, children can use hypnosis for relief of pain of any etiology.[79]

Other Approaches. Relaxation,[80] biofeedback,[81] and transcutaneous electrical nerve stimulation (TENS)[82] have been found useful under some circumstances for pain relief, but the inadequate data available in children do not permit formal treatment recommendations.

Neurosurgical Techniques

Neurosurgical techniques can be categorized as either destructive, (a nerve pathway is ablated by chemical, neurosurgical, or other techniques) or neurostimulatory (electrodes are stereotactically placed to activate pain inhibitory pathways). Such interventions may occasionally be useful in the preterminal child with localized tumor-associated pain that is refractory to other analgesic modalities. Because destructive procedures may produce late neuropathic pain, these should be avoided in the child whose malignancy is potentially cured. Because of the invasiveness of the procedures, the disseminated nature of most pediatric malignancies by the time they give rise to pain of extended duration, and the fulminant nature of most childhood malignancies once they become refractory to anticancer

therapy, pain-relieving neurosurgical intervention is rarely performed in pediatrics. The reader is referred to neurosurgical texts or descriptions of analgesia in the adult cancer patient for a detailed discussion of this modality.[83,84]

REFERENCES

1. IASP Subcommittee on Taxonomy: Pain terms: A list with definitions and notes on usage. Pain 8:249–252, 1980
2. Merskey H, Spear FG: The concept of pain. J Psychosom Res 11:59–67, 1967
3. Wolff BB: Cultural factors and the response to pain. Am Anthropol 70:494–501, 1968
4. Nicholl RA: Substance P as a transmitter candidate. Annu Rev Neurosci 3:227–268, 1980
5. Goodman RR, Pasternak GW: Multiple opiate receptors. In Kuhar MJ, Pasternak GW (eds): Analgesics: Neurochemical, Behavioral and Clinical Perspectives. New York, Raven Press, 1984
6. Iwamoto ET, Martin WR: Multiple opioid receptors. Med Res Rev 1:411–440, 1981
7. Miser AW, Dothage JA, Wesley RA et al: The prevalence of pain in a pediatric and young adult cancer population. Pain (in press)
8. Daut RL, Cleeland CS: The prevalence and severity of pain in cancer. Cancer 50:1913–1918, 1982
9. Oster MW, Vizel M, Turgeon LR: Pain of terminal cancer patients. Arch Intern Med 138:1801–1802, 1978
10. Cornaglia C, Massimo L, Haupt R et al: Incidence of pain in children with neoplastic diseases. Pain 2:S28, 1984
11. Miser AW, McCalla J, Dothage JA et al: Pain as a presenting symptom in children and young adults with newly-diagnosed malignancy. Pain 29:85–90, 1987
12. Merskey H: On the development of pain. Headache 10:116–123, 1970
13. Owens ME, Todt EH: Pain in infancy: Neonatal reaction to a heel lance. Pain 20:77–86, 1984
14. Thrupkaew A, Henken R, Quinl JL: False negative bone scans in disseminated metastatic diseases. Radiology 113:383–386, 1975
15. Foley KM: Pain syndromes in patients with cancer. Adv Pain Res Ther 2:59–75, 1979
16. Bernstein BH, Singsen BH, Kent JT et al: Reflex neurovascular dystrophy in childhood. J Pediatr 93:211–215, 1978
17. Savedra M, Gibbons P, Tesler M et al: How do children describe pain? A tentative assessment. Pain 14:95–104, 1982
18. Melzack R: The McGill pain questionnaire: Major properties and scoring methods. Pain 1:277–299, 1975
19. Foley KM: The treatment of cancer pain. N Engl J Med 313:84–95, 1985
20. Katz ER, Varni JW, Jay SM: Behavioral assessment and management of pediatric pain. Prog Behav Modif 18:163–193, 1984
21. Dothage JA, Arndt C, Miser AW: Use of a continuous intravenous morphine infusion for pain control in an infant with terminal malignancy. J Assoc Pediatr Oncol Nurs 3:22–24, 1986
22. LeBaron S, Zeltzer L: Assessment of acute pain and anxiety in children and adolescents by self-reports, observer reports, and a behavioral checklist. J Consult Clin Psychol 52:729–738, 1984
23. McGrath PJ, Johnson GR, Goodman JT et al: The development and validation of a behavioral pain scale for children: The Children's Hospital of Eastern Ontario Pain Scale (CHEOPS). Pain (Suppl 2):S24, 1984
24. Teske K, Daut RL, Cleeland CS: Relationships between nurses' observations and patients' self-reports of pain. Pain 16:289–296, 1983
25. Hilgard J, LeBaron S: Relief of anxiety and pain in children and adolescents with cancer: Quantitative measures and clinical observations. Int J Clin Exp Hypn 30:417–442, 1982
26. Lollar DJ, Smits SJ, Patterson DL: Assessment of pediatric pain; An empirical perspective. J Pediatr Psychol 7:267–277, 1982
27. Marks RM, Sachar EJ: Undertreatment of medical inpatients with narcotic analgesics. Ann Intern Med 78:173–181, 1973
28. Pothmann J, Goepel R: Comparison of the visual analog scale (VAS) and the Smiley analog scale (SAS) for the evaluation of pain in children. Pain (Suppl 2):S25, 1984
29. Gracely RH: Psychophysical assessment of human pain. In Adv Pain Res Therapy 3:805–824, 1979
30. Szyfelbein SK, Osgood PF, Carr DB: The assessment of pain and plasma beta-endorphin immunoreactivity in burned children. Pain 22:173–182, 1985
31. Eland JM: The child who is hurting. Semin Oncol Nurs 1:116–122, 1985

32. Hester NK: The preoperational child's perspective to immunization. Nurs Res 28:250–255, 1979

33. Miser AW, Chayt KJ, Sandlund JT et al: Narcotic withdrawal syndrome in young adults after the therapeutic use of opiates. Am J Dis Child 140:603–604, 1986

34. Levine JD, Gordon NC: Influence of the method of drug administration on analgesic response. Nature 312:755–766, 1984

35. World Health Organization: Cancer Pain Relief. Geneva, World Health Organization, 1986

36. Jaffe JH: Drug addiction and drug abuse. In Gilman AG, Goodman LS, Gilman A (eds): The Pharmacological Basis of Therapeutics, 6th ed, pp 535–584. New York, Macmillan, 1980

37. Kanner RM, Foley KM: Patterns of narcotic drug use in a cancer pain clinic. Ann NY Acad Sci 362:161–172, 1981

38. Foley KM: The practical use of narcotic analgesics. Med Clin North Am, pp 1091–1104, 1982

39. Levy MH: Pain management in advanced cancer. Semin Oncol 12:394–410, 1985

40. Massimo L, Haupt R, Zamorani ME: Control of pain with sublingual buprenorphine in children with cancer. Eur Paediatr Haematol Oncol 2:224, 1985

41. Walsh TD: Oral morphine in chronic cancer pain. Pain 18:1–11, 1984

42. Neumann PB, Henriksen H, Grosman N et al: Plasma morphine concentrations during chronic oral administration in patients with cancer pain. Pain 13:247–252, 1982

43. Ellison NM, Lewis GO: A pharmacokinetic comparison of rectal morphine sulfate (RMS) suppositories and oral morphine sulfate (OMS) solution. Proc Am Soc Clin Oncol 3:89, 1984

44. Brook–Williams P, Hoover LH: Morphine suppositories for intractable pain. Can Med Assoc J 126:14, 1982

45. Sawe J, Dahlström B, Paalzow L et al: Morphine kinetics in cancer patients. Clin Pharmacol Ther 30:629–635, 1981

46. Dahlstrom B, Bolme P, Feychting H et al. Morphine kinetics in children. Clin Pharmacol Ther 26:354–365, 1979

47. Nahata MC, Miser AW, Miser JS et al: Variations in morphine pharmacokinetics in children with cancer. Dev Pharmacol Ther 8:182–188, 1985

48. Homesley HD, Welander CE, Muss HB et al: Dosage range study of morphine sulfate controlled-release. Am J Clin Oncol 9:449–453, 1986

49. Vallner JJ, Stewart JT, Kotzan JA et al: Pharmacokinetics and bioavailability of hydromorphone following intravenous and oral administration to human subjects. J Clin Pharmacol 21:152–156, 1981

50. Kaiko RF, Foley KM, Grabinski P et al: Central nervous system excitatory effects of meperidine in cancer patients. Ann Neurol 13:180–185, 1983

51. Verebely K, Volavka J, Mule S et al: Methadone in man: Pharmacokinetic and excretion studies in acute and chronic treatment. Clin Pharmacol Ther 18:180–190, 1975

52. Miser AW, Miser JS: The use of oral methadone to control moderate and severe pain in children and young adults with malignancy. Clin J Pain 1:243–248, 1985

53. Beaver WT, Wallenstein SL, Houde RW et al: A clinical comparison of the analgesic effects of methadone and morphine administered intramuscularly, and of orally and parenterally administered methadone. Clin Pharmacol Ther 8:415–426, 1967

54. Nilsson MI, Meresaar U, Änggård E: Clinical pharmacokinetics of methadone. Acta Anaesth Scand Suppl 74:66–69, 1982

55. Ettinger DS, Vitale PJ, Trump DL: Important clinical pharmacologic considerations in the use of methadone in cancer patients. Cancer Treat Rep 63:457–459, 1979

56. Miser AW, Miser JS, Clark BS: Continuous intravenous infusion of morphine sulfate for control of severe pain in children with terminal malignancy. J Pediatr 96:930–932, 1980

57. Miser AW, Davis DM, Hughes CS et al: Continuous subcutaneous infusion of morphine in children with cancer. Am J Dis Child 137:383–385, 1983

58. Miser AW, Moore L, Greene R et al: Prospective study of continuous intravenous and subcutaneous morphine infusions for therapy-related or cancer-related pain in children and young adults with cancer. Clin J Pain 2:101–106, 1986

59. DeChristoforo R, Corden BJ, Hood JC et al: High-dose morphine infusion complicated by chlorbutanol-induced somnolence. Ann Intern Med 98:335–336, 1983

60. Portenoy RK, Moulin DE, Rogers A et al: IV infusion of opioids for cancer pain: Clinical review and guidelines for use. Cancer Treat Rep 70:575–581, 1986

61. Bennett RL, Batenhorst RL, Bivins BA et al: Patient-controlled analgesia: a new concept of postoperative pain relief. Ann Surg 195:700–705, 1982

62. Baumann TJ, Batenhorst RL, Graves DA et al: Patient-controlled analgesia in the terminally ill cancer patient. Drug Intell Clin Pharm 20:297–301, 1986

63. Krames ES, Gershow J, Glassberg A et al: Continuous infusion of spinally administered narcotics for the relief of pain due to malignant disorders. Cancer 56:696–702, 1985

64. Onofrio BM, Yaksh TL, Arnold PG: Continuous low-dose intrathecal morphine administration in the treatment of chronic pain of malignant origin. Mayo Clin Proc 56:516–520, 1981

65. Leavens ME, Hill CS, Cech DA et al: Intrathecal and intraventricular morphine for pain in cancer patients: Initial study. J Neurosurg 56:241–245, 1982

66. Wang JK: Intrathecal morphine for intractable pain secondary to cancer of pelvic organs. Pain 21:99–102, 1985

67. Taub A, Collins WF: Observations on the treatment of denervation dysesthesia with psychotropic drugs: Postherpetic neuralgia, anesthesia dolorosa, peripheral neuropathy. Adv Neurol 4:309–315, 1974

68. Rosenblatt RM, Reich J, Dehring D: Tricyclic antidepressants in treatment of depression and chronic pain: Analysis of the supporting evidence. Anesth Analg 63:1025–1032, 1984

69. Feinmann C: Pain relief by antidepressants: Possible modes of action. Pain 23:1–8, 1985

70. Forrest WH, Brown BW, Brown CR et al: Dextroamphetamine with morphine for the treatment of postoperative pain. N Engl J Med 296:712–715, 1977

71. Cousin MJ, Bridenbaugh PO (eds): Neural Blockade in Clinical Anesthesia and the Management of Pain. Philadelphia, JB Lippincott, 1980

72. Sola AE: Myofascial trigger point therapy. Resident Staff Physician August: 38–45, 1981

73. Travell J: Myofascial trigger points: Clinical review. Adv Pain Res Ther 1:919–926, 1976

74. Mennell JM: The therapeutic use of cold. J Am Osteopath Assoc 74:1146–1158, 1975

75. Bates T, Grunwaldt E: Myofascial pain in childhood. J Pediatr 53:198–209, 1958

76. Fosburg MT, Crone RK: Nitrous oxide for refractory pain in the terminally ill. JAMA 250:511–513, 1983

77. Flomenbaum N, Gallagher EJ, Eagen K: Self-administered nitrous oxide: An adjunct analgesic. JACEP 8:95–97, 1979

78. Stewart RD, Paris PM, Stoy WA et al: Patient-controlled inhalational analgesia in prehospital care: A study of side effects and feasibility. Crit Care Med 11:851–855, 1983

79. Olness K: Imagery (self-hypnosis) as adjunct therapy in childhood cancer. Clinical experience with 25 patients. Am J Pediatr Hematol Oncol 3:313–321, 1981

80. Zeltzer L, LeBaron S: Hypnosis and nonhypnotic techniques for reduction of pain and anxiety during painful procedures in children and adolescents with cancer. J Pediatr 101:1032–1035, 1982

81. Turk DC, Meichenbaum DH, Berman WH: Application of biofeedback for the regulation of pain: A critical review. Psychol Bull 86:1322–1341, 1979

82. Ventafridda V, Sganzerla EP, Fochi C et al: Transcutaneous nerve stimulation in cancer pain. In: Bonica JJ (ed): Advances in Cancer Pain, pp 509–515. New York, Raven Press, 1979

83. Foley KM, Sundaresan N: Management of cancer pain. In DeVita VT Jr, Hellman S, Rosenberg SA (eds): Cancer: Principles and Practice of Oncology, 2nd ed, pp 1940–1961. Philadelphia, JB Lippincott, 1985

84. Friedberg S: Neurosurgical treatment of pain caused by cancer. Med Clin North Am 59:481–485, 1975

forty-five

Management of Nausea and Vomiting

Carol M. Cronin and Stephen E. Sallan

The intensification of both chemotherapy and radiation therapy programs has resulted in increased toxicity to cancer patients. This problem has grown over the years with the introduction of combined treatment modalities and more specific antitumor agents. One of the most common manifestations, nausea and vomiting, is considered to be the most troublesome and debilitating side-effect patients experience. In cancer patients, nausea (the feeling of the imminent need to vomit) and vomiting (the forceful expulsion of gastric contents) are not the mild, self-limiting symptoms commonly associated with other disease states. Rather, they are severe and often prolonged symptoms associated with numerous unpleasant sequelae ranging from wound dehiscence to dehydration requiring hospitalization. Far too often, these symptoms become debilitating and patients are physically incapable of receiving further chemotherapy or are so psychologically distressed that they or their parents may refuse subsequent treatments.

Over the past decade, advances in the understanding of the physiology and pharmacology of nausea and vomiting have led to a better ability to control these symptoms. In addition, increased recognition of these side-effects as potentially life-threatening and increased education regarding antiemesis have resulted in a marked decrease in the intensity of these symptoms. Although complete control may not yet be available for all patients, proper use of the available agents will provide improved relief for most.

PHYSIOLOGY OF VOMITING

All vomiting occurs through the vomiting center located in the medullary lateral reticular formation.[1] This center receives afferent input from five main sources: [1] the chemoreceptor trigger zone (CTZ); [2] vagal and other sympathetic afferents from the viscera; [3] midbrain receptors of intracranial pressure; [4] the labyrinthine apparatus; and [5] higher central nervous system (CNS) structures (*e.g.,* the limbic system). It is crucial that the origin of vomiting be identified before any therapy is established. In addition to chemotherapy, other causes of vomiting common to pediatric cancer patients include stretching of the capsule of an organ, vestibular reflexes (motion sickness), inflammation of the gastrointestinal tract (gastritis, gastroenteritis), and increased intracranial pressure.

Chemotherapy-Induced Vomiting

The majority of the vomiting experienced by cancer patients is induced by chemotherapeutic agents that either directly stimulate the vomiting center or, most commonly, stimulate the CTZ, a distinct medullary center located in the floor of the fourth ventricle. The nature of the interaction of these toxic substances with the CTZ is unknown; once stimulated, the CTZ activates the vomiting center to produce nausea and vomiting. The CTZ has no autonomous capability to produce vomiting.

Animal studies of CTZ ablation suggest that chemotherapeutic agents induce nausea and vomiting by CTZ stimulation.[2] Participation of the forebrain and peripheral mechanisms has also been demonstrated.[3] However, there are major species differences. Thus, one can only infer the site of action in humans by extrapolation from animal studies and by clinical observations.[2] Radiation-induced nausea and vomiting appears to be mediated through both CTZ and peripheral mechanisms.[4] The neurochemistry of vomiting remains obscure. The CTZ contains H_1 and H_2 histamine receptors, and its anatomic surroundings are rich in histamine. H_1 antagonists such as dimenhydrinate have antiemetic activity limited to motion sickness and vestibular disorders.[2] H_2 antagonists are not effective antiemetics. Other neurotransmitters possibly involved in the control of vomiting are dopamine and acetylcholine. Apomorphine, the classic CTZ stimulant, has dopaminomimetic properties, and its action is blocked by phenothiazines, which are potent dopamine blockers.[5] The phenothiazines also have anticholinergic and antihistaminic effects, but their antiemetic efficacy correlates best with dopamine-blocking activity.[6] Nitrogen mustard, a potent emetic, has cholinergic activity, and centrally acting anticholinergic drugs such as scopolamine are effective antiemetics.[7,8] A role for endogenous opiates is suggested by the mixed emetic–antiemetic effects of narcotic analgesics, which are blocked by naloxone, by the emetic properties of naloxone itself, and by the concentration of opiate receptors in the CTZ.[9,10]

The vomiting center, in turn, has a series of efferent pathways, which include phrenic nerves to the diaphragm, spinal nerves to abdominal musculature, and visceral nerves to the stomach and esophagus (Fig. 45-1). These efferent pathways respond to the centrally mediated stimulation in the vomiting center and act to induce actual vomiting.

FIGURE 45-1. Connections between the chemoreceptor trigger zone (CTZ), vomiting center (VC), and efferents of vomiting. (Newburger PE, Sallan SE: Symptom control in childhood malignancy. Pain and vomiting. *In* Care of the Child with Cancer. American Cancer Society, 1979)

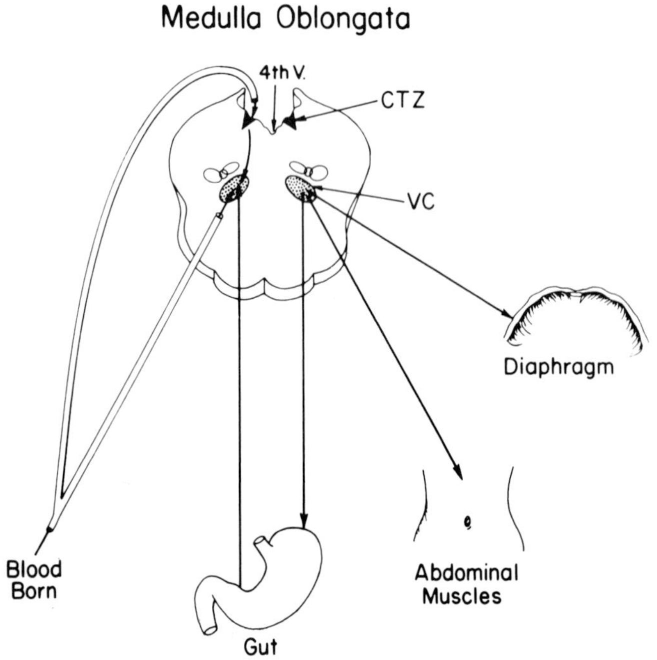

Medulla Oblongata

Radiation-Induced Emesis

The mechanism for radiation-induced vomiting is more obscure. Although the emetogenic potential of radiation therapy is principally site-dependent, the mechanism of inducing toxicity is centrally mediated, because these symptoms respond to centrally active agents. Whether or not the central stimuli are restricted to the CTZ is unclear because there are anecdotal reports that patients respond to dimenhydrinate, an agent that works directly on the labyrinthine apparatus. It has been postulated that there may also be a direct effect on the CTZ from leftover circulating protein fractions; however, this has not been demonstrated.

Disease-Induced Emesis

Nausea and vomiting results from various sequelae of the disease. Metastatic disease may produce tumor exudate or sloughing of tissue which, in turn, produces toxic central effects. Increased intracranial pressure or obstruction may also initiate nausea and vomiting. The exact mechanism is not clearly defined. However, these states respond to both surgical and pharmacologic intervention.

CLINICAL PRESENTATION

There is great variability both in the symptoms that present and in their intensity. This variability is a result of the different treatment modalities employed, as well as the variability between patients in response to identical regimens. Therefore, it is important to evaluate the emetogenic potential of the modality being used before initiating antiemetic therapy. The symptoms range from nausea to retching and vomiting and tend to occur in a cyclic fashion if not properly treated early in therapy. Retching is identical to vomiting in that the same physiologic mechanisms are occurring, but there is no expulsion of gastric contents. Clinically, retching is often perceived by the patient to be more debilitating than vomiting because the abdominal musculature can be significantly strained and no relief is achieved.

The cyclic nature of these symptoms becomes particularly critical when anticipatory or psychogenic patterns of nausea and vomiting develop. Anticipatory (psychogenic) vomiting—the onset of nausea and vomiting before the administration of chemotherapy—may begin at any time before treatment. This pattern, which may occur in as many as 25% of patients receiving chemotherapy, is often difficult to treat because it is a conditioned response. Therefore, prevention of vomiting during early courses of therapy is important. Specific approaches to treating anticipatory nausea and vomiting are discussed later.

PRINCIPLES OF THERAPY

To provide effective treatment of nausea and vomiting it is necessary to identify the underlying cause of the symptoms and to maintain a receptor site blockade of the CTZ or vomiting center during CNS stimulation. To successfully block these receptor sites, therapy must be prophylactic, continuous, and individualized.

Prophylactic antiemetic therapy, initiated before treatment with chemotherapeutic drugs or radiation, is designed to block the receptor site prior to stimulation by the emetic agent.

If the emetic stimuli are noniatrogenic, as with infection or metabolic derangement, it is not possible to initiate therapy before symptoms become established. However, nausea and vomiting in patients with malignancy is most commonly treatment-related, so a planned approach to prophylactic antiemetic therapy is indicated.

All of the antiemetic agents are more effective when administered prophylactically. The actual time frame for initiating prophylactic therapy is variable and depends on the patient's previous patterns of nausea and vomiting, the chemotherapeutic agent being administered, and, most importantly, the route of administration used for the antiemetic. Clinical experience suggests that when antiemetics are administered parenterally (intramuscularly, intravenously, or subcutaneously), one complete dose should be given before therapy, whereas enteral administration (oral or rectal) necessitates at least two complete doses before therapy to achieve clinically effective blood levels. Although the rectal route of drug administration is not generally preferred in this patient population because of their susceptibility to infection, it can be used in non-neutropenic patients receiving antiemetic therapy at home. However, routine precautions for rectal administration in neutropenic patients should be observed.

Once clinically effective blood levels are achieved, it is essential to maintain them by treating patients on a continuous rather than as-needed (PRN) basis. This maintains the receptor site blockade, thereby preventing breakthrough vomiting. When parenteral antiemetic therapy is indicated, a loading dose followed by a continuous infusion offers a reliable method of maintaining a scheduled regimen. With enteral therapy, scheduled doses must be administered in a timely fashion, regardless of whether symptoms appear. The duration of this follow-up therapy is determined by both the patient's previous patterns of nausea and vomiting and the expected duration of emetic activity of the stimulus.

An additional requirement for a successful antiemetic regimen is individualization of therapy. The psychological status of the patient plays a major role in developing effective therapy. The efficacy of placebo and the negative effects of a vomiting roommate demonstrate the importance of suggestion.[11] Recently, greater attention has been afforded to this area in the form of attempts to predict which patients may be more prone to these symptoms and to better utilize nonpharmacologic interventions to treat these symptoms. It has been shown that susceptibility to motion sickness is a predictor of the side-effects of cancer therapy that may prove useful as a clinical marker of the need for more intensive side-effect management.[12] It also has been demonstrated that after the initial treatment course, it is possible to predict the development of anticipatory symptoms using post-treatment nausea and vomiting, tastes of drugs during injections, and anxiety before injections as markers.[13] Hypnosis or systematic desensitization may serve as important adjuncts to a good antiemetic regimen.[14] In a study of 51 children aged 6 to 17 years, intervention with both hypnosis and supportive counseling was associated with significant reduction in nausea and vomiting and in the extent to which these symptoms bothered patients.[15] Conditioned responses, such as vomiting on arrival in the clinic, are difficult to control, but a setting that is free of the sight or smell of food removes at least one stimulus. Because anxiety contributes to nausea, reassurance, quiet, and privacy are also important adjuncts to therapy.

Even the best antiemetic regimen will fail if it is not tailored to meet the individual patient's needs. Discussion with the patient of various options, such as oral versus parenteral therapy, inpatient versus outpatient therapy, and soporific versus nonsoporific therapy, helps to improve patient compliance. All of these factors should be considered in selecting an antiemetic regimen.

Knowledge of the emetogenic potential and patterns of vomiting associated with the various chemotherapeutic agents helps to predict the severity and duration of the anticipated symptoms. Table 45-1 lists some of the antineoplastic agents most commonly used in children, in decreasing order of relative ability to induce emesis. The variability in emetogenic potential of these agents is great. The agents at the lower end of the scale may induce moderate nausea accompanied by no vomiting or mild vomiting, whereas those at the upper end may produce debilitating nausea accompanied by severe vomiting. The severity of vomiting also differs between patients. Some patients may experience 20 retching or vomiting episodes a day for 5 days, while others may have 50 episodes over a span of a few hours. The time of onset is also variable between drugs and in different patients. Symptoms may appear immediately (as with nitrogen mustard) or may be delayed by 6 to 12 hours (cyclophosphamide or dactinomycin). When these agents are used in combination, the potential for more pronounced and prolonged emesis increases, and antiemetic therapy should be adjusted accordingly.

Nausea and vomiting associated with radiation therapy is not as clearly defined. Whenever radiation is applied to the abdominal area, as in Hodgkin's disease, nausea and vomiting ensues.

Pharmacologic Approaches

Antiemetic agents can be classified into many different groups. No one agent is clearly superior in children. In addition, specific dosing parameters are unavailable for children because these agents have not received clinical evaluation in the pediatric population. Table 45-2 outlines various antiemetic agents in the order in which they are discussed. The dosage recommendations presented are the result of our clinical experience and should serve only as a guideline for establishing proper antiemetic regimens. Each child should be individually evaluated on the basis of body surface area and ability to handle central nervous system drugs.

Phenothiazines

Phenothiazine-type drugs remain the mainstay of therapy among the commercially available agents. At the usual therapeutic doses, many phenothiazines appear to depress CTZ activity and also may directly depress the vomiting center.[2] These

Table 45-1
Chemotherapeutic Agents Listed by Decreasing Relative Emetogenic Potential

Cisplatin
Imidazole carboxamide
Nitrogen mustard
Actinomycin D (dactinomycin)
High-dose cytosine arabinoside (cytarabine)
Cyclophosphamide
Nitrosoureas
Anthracyclines
Etoposide
Bleomycin
Vinblastine
High-dose methotrexate

Table 45-2
*Antiemetic Agents**

Agent	Antiemetic Activity	Routes of Administration	Frequency	Side-Effects†
Chlorpromazine (Thorazine)	Minimal	PO, PR, IV, IM	4–6 h	Orthostatic hypotension, sedation, EPS
Prochlorperazine (Compazine)	Moderate	PO, PR, IV, IM	4 h	EPS, agitation
Thiethylperazine (Torecan)	Marked	PO, PR, IV, IM	6–8 h	EPS, agitation
Perphenazine (Trilafon)	Marked	PO, IV, IM	4 h	EPS, agitation
Promethazine (Phenergan)	Minimal	PO, PR, IV, IM	4–6 h	Sedation
Metoclopramide (Reglan)	Marked	IV	2–3 h	EPS, sedation
Droperidol (Inapsine)	Marked	IV, IM	Infusion	Somnolence, agitation
Dexamethasone (Decadron)	Moderate	PO, IV	8 h	
Trimethobenzamide (Tigan)	Minimal	PO, PR, IM	6–8 h	
Tetrahydrocannabinol (Marinol)	Moderate	PO	4 h	Drowsiness, dysphoria, high

* See text for dosage recommendations.
† EPS = extrapyramidal symptoms.

drugs act on both the central and autonomic nervous systems. They are widely distributed throughout the body and are 90% bound to plasma proteins. Metabolism is primarily by way of the liver, with metabolites excreted in the urine, bile, and feces.

Two distinct chemical classes of phenothiazines exist, each with its own therapeutic and toxic characteristics. The aliphatic class, of which chlorpromazine (Thorazine) is the prototype, has limited antiemetic activity and is associated with a high incidence of orthostatic hypotension, sedation, prolongation of the sedative effects of narcotics and barbiturates, and blood dyscrasias. The piperazine class, which includes prochlorperazine (Compazine), thiethylperazine (Torecan), and perphenazine (Trilafon), has pronounced antiemetic activity but is associated with an increased incidence of extrapyramidal effects. Although most clinicians prescribe prochlorperazine or chlorpromazine, thiethylperazine and perphenazine are much more effective antiemetics, at least in experimental animals. Evidence in dogs indicates that the efficacy of perphenazine, at nontoxic doses, is 24 times greater than that of chlorpromazine and 8 times greater than prochlorperazine in preventing apomorphine-induced emesis.[16] Further, the relative antiemetic activity of perphenazine increases as the emetic stimulus increases in intensity. It has been suggested that the increased antiemetic activity of perphenazine may be due to its greater affinity for, and tighter binding with, receptors in the CTZ. Thiethylperazine acts to decrease both the incidence of nausea and vomiting and the severity of the symptoms, resulting in enhanced antiemetic activity.

The major disadvantage of these agents is the development of extrapyramidal reactions or agitation, most commonly associated with intravenous administration. The incidence of these reactions can be decreased, however, by administering the IV solution slowly, over 45 to 60 minutes, and by concomitantly administering an antihistamine such as diphenhydramine (Benadryl). These side-effects can appear up to 48 hours after discontinuation of therapy. Although one dose of diphenhydramine is usually sufficient to allay these symptoms, the patient may require repeat doses for up to 48 hours. A second dose of diphenhydramine should always be administered 4 hours after the first to ensure continued efficacy. Occasionally, patients fail to respond to diphenhydramine and require treatment with benztropine (Cogentin).

The doses and routes of administration vary among the different phenothiazines. Thiethylperazine, available for intravenous, intramuscular, oral, and rectal administration, should

be given in 10 mg doses every 6 to 8 hours for children 12 years or older and 5 mg for younger children. It is not recommended for children younger than 2 years. The recommended loading dose of perphenazine is 2 to 5 mg IV over 60 minutes, depending on the age of the child. The loading dose can be followed by either a continuous infusion of 0.25 to 0.5 mg/hr or an oral dose of 2 to 4 mg every 4 hours. Prochlorperazine is considered to be the safest phenothiazine in children younger than 5 years. It has only minimal antiemetic efficacy, and is used primarily for its sedative effect, in a dose of 5 mg/m². Promethazine (Phenergan), used most commonly for vestibular symptoms or gastritis-like symptoms in young children, may be effective for very young children experiencing chemotherapy-induced vomiting. The dose of promethazine used is 0.25 to 0.5 mg/pound IV over 60 minutes every 4 to 6 hours.

Metoclopramide

Metoclopramide (Reglan), a procainamide derivative, has both central and peripheral antiemetic actions: it inhibits apomorphine-induced vomiting and accelerates gastric emptying. It has undergone extensive evaluation in patients receiving cisplatin chemotherapy. Because of its short half-life, it must be administered frequently.[17-19] The standard regimen in adults has been 2 mg/kg 30 minutes before chemotherapy and again at 1.5, 3.5, 5.5, and (sometimes) 8.5 hours after chemotherapy. Although published trials suggest the necessity of the 2 mg/kg dose, a large accumulation of anecdotal evidence suggests that efficacy can be obtained at 0.75 mg/kg to 1.0 mg/kg. Our experience has shown that a dose of 1 mg/kg IV over 60 minutes every 3 to 4 hours for a total of five doses is effective. Clinical evaluations of the antiemetic effect of orally administered metoclopramide are currently under way. Extrapyramidal symptoms are also seen with metoclopramide and are usually well-controlled with diphenhydramine.

Droperidol

Droperidol (Inapsine), a butyrophenone, is a potent inhibitor of the CTZ. One of the main advantages of droperidol is its minimal effects on the cardiovascular and respiratory systems when used in high doses. Numerous studies have been conducted to evaluate the efficacy and toxicity of this agent, using doses ranging from 0.5 mg to 2.5 mg as single or multiple doses, or by continuous infusion.[20] Overall, these studies have found droperidol to be somewhat effective, with reported toxicities ranging from hypotension and occasional instances of tachycardia to somnolence and agitation. Extrapyramidal effects do occur but are not reported as often as with the phenothiazines. In more recent studies, higher doses of droperidol (10 mg) have produced better antiemetic control with fewer reported toxicities.[21] This finding may be ascribed to the anecdotal speculation that droperidol has two therapeutic windows, thereby allowing the higher dose to be more effective.

Experience with droperidol in young children is very limited. In older children, a loading dose of 10 mg IV over 60 minutes followed by a continuous infusion of 2 mg/hour is recommended. Droperidol is not available in an oral dosage form. Again, concomitant use of diphenhydramine is recommended. The other butyrophenone commonly used as an antiemetic is haloperidol (Haldol). It is not suggested for use in children.

Steroids

Although the mechanism of their action is not understood, steroids have been used, with some success, as antiemetic agents. Dexamethasone is the most extensively evaluated steroid, with doses ranging from 5 to 48 mg in single and multiple doses.[22-24] It appears to be most effective when used in combination with other agents. One study of patients considered resistant to metoclopramide showed a significant decrease in both the number of vomiting episodes and mean duration of vomiting when dexamethasone was added to the metoclopramide regimen.[25] Overall, dexamethasone appears to be a safe, effective adjunct to antiemetic regimens and should be evaluated further. Depending on the age of the child, a loading dose of 10 to 20 mg IV administered over 20 minutes followed by 6 to 10 mg IV or PO every 6 hours is recommended.

Miscellaneous Agents

Many antihistamines have antiemetic properties, but there is no correlation between antihistaminic potency and antiemetic activity.[26] Both dimenhydrinate (Dramamine) and diphenhydramine are effective antiemetics for motion sickness and may be used in combination with other antiemetic therapy to potentiate effectiveness or to decrease toxicity.[27,28] The exact mechanism of action of these agents is unknown; however,

they appear to act by blocking labyrinthine impulses and they do not antagonize apomorphine-induced emesis.[29,30] Clinical experience suggests that the antihistamines, particularly dimenhydrinate, may be effective in controlling the chronic nausea that often accompanies progressive disease, but we have not yet rigorously tested this hypothesis.

Trimethobenzamide (Tigan) is an ethanolamine antihistamine that exerts its primary action on the CTZ. Although it has been reported to be an effective antiemetic, some investigators have found it to be less effective than placebo.[31,32] Because its efficacy appears to be inversely proportional to the intensity of the emetic stimulus, it is not recommended for cancer chemotherapy-induced vomiting.[33]

The cannabinoids, the active ingredients of marijuana, have proven antiemetic properties. Delta-9-tetrahydrocannabinol (THC) has been shown to be more effective than both placebo and prochlorperazine in preventing vomiting in patients receiving antineoplastic drugs.[34-37] Although the exact mechanism of action is unknown, THC is thought to exert its antiemetic effect through CNS depression. Interest in the cannabinoids has led to the development of synthetic analogues of THC, one of which is now commercially available as dronabinol (Marinol). Although cannabinoids are not considered first-line therapy, they have been proved effective in children, in doses ranging from 2.5 to 7.5 mg/m². [37] Side-effects range from drowsiness to dysphoria, the most common side-effect being the development of a "high."[35]

Although they have no direct antiemetic activity, barbiturates are often used for their sedative effects when patients experience breakthrough vomiting midcourse. Because aspiration may occur, this approach is recommended only in a controlled setting when all other therapeutic avenues have been exhausted.

As more effective antiemetic agents have been identified, clinicians have tended to group different agents in an attempt to increase efficacy. This approach is effective when diphenhydramine or dexamethasone is added to a regimen. However, combinations of direct-acting agents (metoclopramide, droperidol, and phenothiazines) are not recommended because of the increased risk of toxicity.

One agent that has proved particularly useful in combination is lorazepam (Ativan).[38,39] It is important to note that lorazepam has little or no direct antiemetic activity. Rather, it pro-

Table 45-3
*Stepwise Approach to Antiemetic Therapy**

| | Patient Age | | | |
Step	0–2 Years	2–4 Years	4–8 Years	8–16 Years
First choice	Promethazine	Prochlorperazine	Thiethylperazine	Thiethylperazine or perphenazine
If unsuccessful, try or add:				
First	Diphenhydramine	Dexamethasone	Metoclopramide	Metoclopramide
Second		Diphenhydramine	Perphenazine and dexamethasone	Droperidol
Third			Metoclopramide and dexamethasone	Any one of the above agents with dexamethasone
Fourth				THC

* Concomitant use of diphenhydramine is recommended with a phenothiazine, metoclopramide or droperidol. Metoclopramide, phenothiazines, and droperidol should not be used in combination. Lorazepam may be added to control anticipatory vomiting, as described in text.

duces anterograde amnesia and is therefore very useful in allaying anticipatory nausea and vomiting by causing patients to forget their previous experiences with chemotherapy.[40] Lorazepam should always be used in combination with an antiemetic. The dose of lorazepam is 0.025 to 0.05 mg/kg IV or PO, administered as a one-time dose 30 minutes before chemotherapy.[39,40]

Approach to Therapy

Table 45-3 outlines a general stepwise approach to antiemetic therapy based on patient age. If the first choice agent fails, it is important to switch to second-line therapy early in the treatment course to prevent the development of anticipatory/psychogenic tendencies. If switching to an alternative agent is not successful, increasing the dose of the agent may increase efficacy; however, the risk of inducing toxicity also increases. More commonly, addition of a second agent such as diphenhydramine or dexamethasone to potentiate the primary antiemetic proves more beneficial. Success or failure of a particular regimen is ultimately determined by the patient's acceptance of future courses of chemotherapy. Although complete elimination of symptoms may not be possible in all patients, a substantial reduction in both the degree and duration of symptoms can usually be achieved, making the treatment more tolerable.

There is no one antiemetic agent currently available that will totally prevent chemotherapy-induced nausea and vomiting in all patients. However, careful evaluation of the individual patient's needs and of previous patterns of nausea and vomiting, followed by implementation of prophylactic and continuous therapy and a willingness to try alternative agents, is certain to increase the effectiveness of any antiemetic program.

REFERENCES

1. Wang SC, Borison HL: A new concept of organization of the central emetic mechanism: Recent studies on the sites of action of apomorphine, copper sulfate, and cardiac glycosides. Gastroenterology 22:1–12, 1952
2. Wang SC: Emetic and antiemetic drugs. In Root WS, Hofmann FE (eds): Physiological Pharmacology, vol 2, pp 255–328. New York, Academic Press, 1965
3. Borison, HL, Brand D, Orkand RK: Emetic action of nitrogen mustard in dogs and cats. Am J Physiol 192:410–416, 1958
4. Wang, SC, Renzi AA, Chinn SI: Mechanism of emesis following X-irradiation. Am J Physiol 193:335–339, 1958
5. Jaffe JH, Martin WR: Narcotic analgesics and antagonists. In Goodman LS, Gilman A (eds): The Pharmacologic Basis of Therapeutics, 5th ed, pp 245–283. New York, Macmillan, 1975
6. Byck R: Drugs and the treatment of psychiatric disorders. In Goodman LS, Gilman A (eds): The Pharmacologic Basis of Therapeutics, 5th ed, pp 152–200. New York, Macmillan, 1975
7. Hunt CC, Philips FS: The acute pharmacology of methyl-bis (2-chloroethyl)amine. J Pharmacol Exp Ther 95:131–143, 1949
8. Sawicka J, Sallan SE: Transdermal therapeutic system scopolamine: Prevention of vomiting associated with cancer chemotherapy (abstr). Proc Am Soc Clin Oncol 18:302, 1977
9. Costello DJ, Borison HL: Naxolone blocks narcotic self-blockage of emesis in cats. J Pharmacol Exp Ther 203:222–230, 1977
10. Snyder SH: Opiate receptors in the brain. N Engl J Med 296:266–271, 1977
11. Parson JA, Webster JH, Dowd J: Evaluation of the placebo effect in the treatment of radiation sickness. Acta Radiol 56:129–140, 1961
12. Morrow GR: The effect of a susceptibility to motion sickness on the side effects of cancer chemotherapy. Cancer 55:2766–2770, 1985
13. Nerenz DR, Lefventhal H, Easterlilng DV, Love RR: Anxiety and drug taste as predictors of anticipatory nausea in cancer chemotherapy. J Clin Oncol 4:224–233, 1986
14. Morrow GR, Morrell C: Behavioral treatment for the anticipatory nausea and vomiting induced by cancer chemotherapy. N Engl J Med 307:1476–1480, 1982
15. Zelter L, LeBaron S, Zelter PM: The effectiveness of behavioral intervention for reduction of nausea and vomiting in children and adolescents receiving chemotherapy. J Clin Oncol 2:683–690, 1984
16. Wang SC: Perphenazine, a potent and effective antiemetic. J Pharmacol Exp Ther 123:306–310, 1958
17. Strum SB, McDermed JE, Opfell RW et al: Intravenous metoclopramide. An effective antiemetic in cancer chemotherapy. JAMA 247:2683–2686, 1982
18. Swann IL, Thompson EN, Querishi K: Domperidone or metoclopramide in preventing chemotherapeutically induced nausea and vomiting. Br Med J 2:1188–1189, 1979
19. Gralla RJ, Itri LM, Piswko SE et al: Antiemetic efficacy of high-dose metoclopramide: Randomized trials with placebo and prochlorperazine in patients with chemotherapy induced nausea and vomiting. N Engl J Med 305:905–909, 1981
20. Lamb HC, Cox FM: Clinical use of droperidol in patients with chemotherapy induced nausea and vomiting. Oncol Nurs Forum 9(3):23–25, 1982
21. Wilson JP: Results of high-dose droperidol from Walter Reed Army Medical Center, Washington, D.C. Presented at The Clinical Management of Emesis in the Cancer Patient, New Brunswick, NJ, 1982
22. Khan AB, Bucklew CA, Leventhal BG: Effectiveness of Decadron and Thorazine in prevention of nausea and vomiting induced by chemotherapy in pediatric patients. Proc Am Soc Clin Oncol 199(2):78, 1983
23. Bruera ED, Roca E, Cedaro L et al: Improved control of chemotherapy-induced emesis by addition of dexamethasone to metoclopramide in patients resistant to metoclopramide. Cancer Treat Rep 67:381–383, 1983
24. Drapkin RL, Sokol GH, Paladine WJ et al: The antiemetic effect and dose response of dexamethasone in patients receiving cisplatinum. Proc Am Soc Clin Oncol 199:61, 1982
25. Cassileth PA, Lusk EJ, Torri S et al: Antiemetic efficacy of dexamethasone therapy in patients receiving cancer chemotherapy. Arch Intern Med 143:1347–1349, 1983
26. Chinn HI, Smith PK: Motion sickness. Pharmacol Rev 7:33–82, 1955
27. Gay LN, Carliner PE: The prevention and treatment of motion sickness. Bull Johns Hopkins Hosp 84:470–487, 1949
28. Nickerson M: Dramamine. Science 111:312–313, 1950
29. Jaju BP, Wang SC: Effects of diphenhydramine and dimenhydrinate on vestibular neuronal activity of cat: A search for the locus of their antimotion sickness action. J Pharmacol Exp Ther 176:718–723, 1971
30. Wyant GM: A comparative study of eleven antiemetic drugs in dogs. Can Anaesth Soc J 9:399–407, 1962
31. Bardfield P: A controlled double-blind study of trimethobenzamide, prochlorperazine and placebo. JAMA 196:796–798, 1966
32. Dobkin A, Evers W, Israel J: Double-blind evaluation of metoclopramide, trimethobenzamide and a placebo as postanesthetic antiemetics following methoxyflurane anaesthesia. Can Anaesth Soc J 15:80–91, 1968
33. Wolfson B, Torres-Kay M, Foldes F: Investigation of the usefulness of trimethobenzamide for the prevention of postoperative nausea and vomiting. Anesth Analg 41:172–177, 1962
34. Sallan SE, Zinberg NE, Frei E III: Antiemetic effect of delta-9-tetrahydrocannabinol in patients receiving cancer chemotherapy. N Engl J Med 293:795–797, 1975
35. Sallan SE, Cronin CM, Zelen M et al: Antiemetics in patients receiving chemotherapy for cancer. N Engl J Med 302:134–138, 1980
36. Chang AE, Shiling DJ, Stillman RC et al: A prospective evaluation of delta-9-tetrahydrocannabinol as an antiemetic in patients receiving adriamycin and cytoxan chemotherapy. Cancer 47:1746–1751, 1981
37. Ekeret H, Waters KD, Jurk IH et al: Amelioration of cancer chemotherapy-induced nausea and vomiting by delta-9-tetrahydrocannabinol. Med J Aust 2:657–659, 1979
38. Kris MG, Gralla RJ, Clark RA et al: Consecutive dose-finding trials adding lorazepam to the combination of metoclopramide plus dexamethasone. Improved subjective effectiveness over the combination of diphenhydramine plus metoclopramide plus dexamethasone. Cancer Treat Rep 69:1257–1262, 1985
39. Bishop JF, Oliver IN, Wolf MM: Lorazepam: A randomized, double-blind, crossover study of a new antiemetic in patients receiving cytotoxic chemotherapy and prochlorperazine. J Clin Oncol 2:691–695, 1984
40. Laszlo J, Clark RA, Hanson DC: Lorazepam in cancer patients treated with cisplatin: A drug having antiemetic, amnesic and anxiolytic effects. J Clin Oncol 3:864–869, 1985

forty-six

Nursing Support of the Child with Cancer

June L. McCalla and Sheila Judge Santacroce

The management of cancer in children has become increasingly complex and sophisticated. Treatment that results in considerable instability in the child's physical condition may require prolonged or repeated hospitalizations. Nursing care demands range from expertise in intensive care management to family counseling skills. Care is given in a variety of settings: hospitals, outpatient clinics, schools, home, or hospice. There are, therefore, broad opportunities for pediatric oncology nurses to positively influence the quality of life for children and their families.

PRINCIPLES OF CARE

Family-Centered Approach

The family is the unit of care in pediatric oncology nursing practice (see also Chaps. 41 and 42). The child is the identified patient, the reason why the family enters the health care delivery system, and the reason why family-oriented nursing is needed. The rationale for family-centered nursing is based on the premise that the healthy family will nurture the child in an optimal way no matter what the child's special problems are.[1] Certain principles are fundamental to family-centered nursing care. First, the family is viewed as a system which recognizes that disruption or change in one part of the family causes change in other areas as well. Second, nursing care focuses on all members of the family, even when immediate nursing care is being directed only to a particular person. Third, consideration is given to the physical, emotional, cognitive, and social needs of each person within the family unit. Finally, the needs of the family as a whole, as well as those of individual members, are considered.[2]

The overall impact of chronic illness on a child and family is a result of interactions among three systems: community, family, and child. Periodic reassessment includes analyses of both the family subsystems (parent, child, siblings) and suprasystems (social contacts, relatives, community). Nurses need to plan specific long-term interventions that provide for continuity of care and participation of the child and family.[3] The psychosocial effects of illness and hospitalization are considered in a developmental framework.[4,5] Comprehensive models for responsible pediatric nursing practice have been developed and implemented.

Although nursing care differs during each phase of the illness, the roles that nurses assume can be summarized as follows: [1] support system for the child and family throughout the course of the illness; [2] educator of family members regarding knowledge of the disease, its treatment, and the psychological reactions of others; and [3] coordinator, liaison, and advocate of the family, along with other members of the health care team.[6] This is best accomplished by a multidisciplinary approach to care.

(*Text continues on p. 942*)

Table 46-1
Educational Resources for the Professional

Title or Organization	General Description	Source
General Psychosocial Issues		
Poster E, Fore C (eds): Meeting Psychosocial Needs of Children and Families in Health Care, 1985 (100 pp)	Discusses needs of family members, hospitalized child, and children with chronic conditions.	Association for Care of Children's Health (ACCH) 3615 Wisconsin Avenue, NW Washington, DC 20016
Petrillo M, Sanger S: Emotional Care of Hospitalized Children: An Environmental Approach, 2nd ed., 1986 (450 pp)	Describes emotional needs of hospitalized children and outlines developmental approaches for preparing children for specific health care experiences.	Medical Books J. B. Lippincott Company East Washington Square Philadelphia, PA 19105
American Academy of Pediatrics: Hospital Care of Children and Youth, 1986 (288 pp)	Describes recent developments in hospital management, medical technology, financing, cost containment, architecture, and emotional needs of hospitalized children.	ACCH 3615 Wisconsin Avenue, NW Washington, DC 20016
Committee for Development of Guidelines, Metropolitan Affiliate of Association for Care of Children's Health: Psychosocial Policy Guidelines For Administration of Pediatric Health Care Facilities, 1980 (23 pp)	Prepared for use by administrators in children's health care facilities. Outlines specific recommendations for application of pediatric health care principles relating to family involvement, preparation for health care experiences, participation by child and family in decision-making, environment, and daily structure.	ACCH 3615 Wisconsin Avenue, NW Washington, DC 20016
Thompson, R: Psychosocial Research on Pediatric Hospitalization and Health Case: A Review of the Literature, 1985 (324 pp)	Review of more than 300 research studies published since 1965. Topics include responses to hospitalization and health care, separation, impact of hospital environment, and value of play and preparation.	ACCH 3615 Wisconsin Avenue, NW Washington, DC 20016
Association for Care of Children's Health: Educational Resources for Pediatric Health Care, 1986 (14 pp)	This interdisciplinary, international association promotes quality psychosocial health care for children and their families.	ACCH 3615 Wisconsin Avenue, NW Washington, DC 20016
Cancer Diagnosis: A Time of Crisis		
Association of Pediatric Oncology Nurses. Fochtman D, Foley G (eds): Nursing Care of the Child with Cancer. 1982 (371 pp)	Discusses nursing implications of common issues in pediatric cancer, including diagnostic and staging procedures, treatment, physical and psychological care, and multidisciplinary team.	Medical Books Little, Brown & Company Boston, MA
Droske SC, Francis SA: Pediatric Diagnostic Procedures with Guidelines for Preparing Children for Diagnostic Tests, 1981 (293 pp)	Contains developmental guidelines and outlines appropriate methods of preparation for 53 common diagnostic procedures.	ACCH 3615 Wisconsin Ave., NW Washington, DC 20016
Association for Care of Children's Health: Annotated Media Bibliography 1985 (138 pp)	Lists and describes films, videotapes, film strips, and cassettes related to psychosocial health care, with emphasis on preparation and disease management.	ACCH 3615 Wisconsin Avenue, NW Washington, DC 20016
Office of Cancer Communications, National Cancer Institute: Coping With Cancer: A Resource for the Health Professional, 1980 (145 pp)	Discusses impact of cancer on adults and young persons, including adolescent's special concerns. Additional sections discuss family coping, coping by health professionals, and financial aspects.	Office of Cancer Communications NCI National Institutes of Health Bethesda, MD 20892
Association of Pediatric Oncology Nurses: APON: Cancer Chemotherapy Handbook. 1985 (56 pp)	Handbook designed as both reference guide and educational tool; includes "Special Nursing Care for Children Receiving Chemotherapy."	Association of Pediatric Oncology Nurses 1311A Dolley Madison Boulevard McLean, VA 22101

(continued)

Table 46-1 (*continued*)

Title or Organization	General Description	Source
Cancer Diagnosis: A Time of Crisis (*continued*)		
Oncology Nursing Society: Cancer Chemotherapy Guidelines and Recommendations for Nursing Education and Practice, 1984	Discusses professional nurse preparation, guidelines for chemotherapy administration, care of the patient receiving chemotherapy, and recommendations for safeguarding the caregivers.	Oncology Nursing Society 3111 Banksville Road Pittsburgh, PA 15216
Office of Cancer Communications, NCI: Publication List for Professionals, 1987	List of all NCI publications useful for health care professionals.	Office of Cancer Communications NCI National Institutes of Health Bethesda, MD 20892
American Cancer Society: Publications and Media Listing For Professionals, 1987	List and brief description of publications and media resources useful for health care professional education programs.	American Cancer Society 90 Park Avenue New York, NY 10016
Leukemia Society of America, Inc: Professional education programs and publications	Voluntary organization newsletter with medical and chapter news. Society funds research into causes and cures and provides public and professional education.	Leukemia Society of America, Inc. 800 Second Avenue New York, NY 10017
Albright L, McCalla J, and members of Multidisciplinary Team: Preparation of Patients for Amputation, 1986	Specific guidelines for preparation of child or adolescent for amputation; specifies responsibilities of each member of the multidisciplinary team.	Pediatric Oncology Cancer Nursing Service Clinical Center National Institutes of Health Bethesda, MD 20892
Reentry to Home and Community		
Nathanson M: Organizing and Maintaining Support Group for Parents of Children with Chronic Illness and Handicapping Conditions, 1986 (102 pp)	Handbook for parents and professionals forming and working in support groups. Sections address getting started, organizing, structuring, maintaining.	ACCH 3615 Wisconsin Avenue, NW Washington, DC 20016
Kleinberg S: Educating The Chronically Ill Child, 1982 (335 pp)	Details needs of children with chronic illness and suggests educational strategies to meet these needs.	ACCH 3615 Wisconsin Ave., NW Washington, DC 20016
McCollum A: The Chronically Ill Child: A Guide for Parents and Professionals, 1981 (273 pp)	Discusses developmental and family impact of chronic illness. Designed to help parents and professionals to anticipate needs and plan solutions.	ACCH 3615 Wisconsin Ave., NW Washington, DC 20016
National Cancer Institute, et al: Students with Cancer: A Resource for the Educator, 1980 (24 pp)	Explanations of disease, treatment; suggested approaches for dealing with student, classmates, parents; guidelines for school reentry.	Office of Cancer Communications NCI Building 31, Room 10A18 Bethesda, MD 20892
Association for Care of Children's Health and Division of Maternal and Child Health, PHS, USDHHS: Homecare for Children with Serious Handicapping Conditions: Report on a Conference, 1984 (117 pp)	Articles on pediatric home care, including financing, continuing education, and approaches for assessing and building family skills.	ACCH 3615 Wisconsin Avenue, NW Washington, DC 20016
Association for Care of Children's Health: Homecare for Children: A Selected Bibliography, 1984	Annotated references on topics related to children with serious handicaps and health conditions.	ACCH 3615 Wisconsin Ave., NW Washington, DC 20016
Terminal Care		
Kubler-Ross E: On Death and Dying: What the Dying Have To Teach Doctors, Nurses, Clergy and Their Own Families, 1970 (289 pp)	Describes attitudes toward death and dying; five stages through which dying person progresses; and impact on patient's family.	Medical Books Macmillan Company 866 Third Avenue New York, NY 10022

(continued)

Table 46-1 *(continued)*

Title or Organization	General Description	Source
Terminal Care (continued)		
Kubler-Ross E: Death: The Final Stage of Growth, 1975 (175 pp)	Collection of views on death and dying from a variety of professionals; personal accounts of dying individuals and their families. Describes how through an acceptance of our finiteness, we can grow, for death provides a key to the human experience.	Human Development Books: A Series in Applied Behavioral Science Prentice-Hall, Inc. Englewood Cliffs, NJ
Ahmed P (ed): Living and Dying With Cancer, 1981 (314 pp)	Leading cancer researchers provide a conceptual model for caring for the cancer patient and for defining and assessing adaptive tasks and coping skills. Examines major strategies for coping with severe emotional stress related to disease process, threat of recurrence, and probability of death.	Coping With Medical Issues Series Elsevier North Holland, Inc. 52 Vanderbilt Avenue New York, NY 10017
Children's Hospice International	Promotes hospice support through pediatric care facilities; has information clearinghouse; sponsors seminars and lectures for professionals; issues publications, newsletter, and cassette tapes.	Children's Hospice International 501 Slater's Lane #207 Alexandria, VA 22314
National Hospice Organization: NHO Bibliography of Children's Literature on Death and Dying; also Standards for Quality Care	NHO sponsors conferences, monitors legislation, works to gain insurance coverage for hospice care; publishes and distributes books, pamphlets, and bibliographies; sets standards for quality care.	National Hospice Organization 1901 North Fort Myer Drive, Suite 402 Arlington, VA 22209

Multidisciplinary Team

The goal of treatment is to achieve a truly cured child, one who not only has no evidence of disease but who is mentally healthy and can function at an age-appropriate level in society.[7]

Members of the multidisciplinary care team have equal responsibility for the welfare of the child but different tasks to perform. Team members include physicians, nurses, social workers, child life workers, school teachers, recreation therapists, psychologists, psychiatrists, rehabilitation therapists, and chaplains (see also Chaps. 41, 42, and 44).[8] Parent consultants —parents of former pediatric oncology patients—are also team members at some institutions. These people, who have coped with the many aspects of a potentially fatal illness, now serve as staff members. Their primary responsibilities are to act as liaison and advocates for the families and children with cancer.[9] The nurse acts as team coordinator and facilitates communication among team members. The nurse also assists team members to provide services by appropriate scheduling of the patient's activities, and records the patient's progress.

As pediatric oncology has become an established area of clinical specialization, the patient's psychosocial needs have been recognized as being of equal importance to physical needs. Health care policies must be developed in which the psychosocial needs of pediatric patients and their families are seriously acknowledged, sympathetically considered, and appropriately satisfied.[10] The demands of care require honest, open communication among the child, the family, and the staff. A variety of resources are available to assist in policy development and implementation (see Table 46-1).

All members of the health care team participate in providing services aimed at improving patient family functioning and promoting health. One method of facilitating care is through participation in multidisciplinary rounds. Rounds must be scheduled on a regular basis. Responsibility for conducting the rounds may be assumed by one discipline or rotated among several. The focus of individual rounds may vary from case presentations to policy revision or presentation of a unit or service problem. During rounds, the topic is explored and recommendations made. Evaluation of problem resolution or policy revision at future rounds is essential. Multidisciplinary rounds may also be used for staff support.

SCOPE OF PEDIATRIC ONCOLOGY NURSING PRACTICE

The dynamic, evolutionary nature of nursing practice has been well described.[11] The responsibilities and accountability of professional nurses are specified in licensing and credentialing requirements.[12] Nurses are autonomous in their practice, within boundaries outlined through Nurse Practice Acts at the state level. They are legally accountable for their actions. Current trends within the profession include emphasis on professionalism, expanded or advanced nursing practice, and primary nursing.[13]

The practice of nursing is defined in standards established by the profession. The establishment, maintenance, and improvement of standards ensures that service of a high quality will be provided. Pediatric oncology nursing practice is defined as direct service to children and their families. It is an integral part of a multidisciplinary, coordinated approach to the child and his family.[14] In addition, professional nurses are guided by the profession's code of ethics and have accepted accountability for the protection of human rights of consumers within the health care system.[15,16]

The Pediatric Oncology Nurse as Clinician

Primary Nursing

Primary nursing is a system of delivery of nursing care that ensures continuity of care. The identifying elements of the system of primary nursing are as follows:[17]

The primary nurse voluntarily enters into a relationship with a consenting child and family and works with the entire family in establishing mutual care goals.

The primary nurse is accountable for planning 24-hour delivery of nursing care and for evaluating the effectiveness of the plan and of the care delivered.

The primary nurse–family relationship is one that endures over the course of a child's illness. Continuity is ensured through communication among all caregivers and ongoing discussions with the family.

The primary nurse works toward promoting normal growth and development in the child and toward achieving the highest possible state of health.

The primary nurse assists the entire family in developing effective coping mechanisms.

Primary nursing is well suited for implementation in pediatric oncology. The diagnosis of a chronic, potentially fatal illness in a child has a significant impact on all family members. The entire family can be assisted through the establishment of a consistent and ongoing relationship with a primary nurse who is a member of the medical care team. The primary nurse in pediatric oncology is experienced in assessing and intervening in common complications of cancer and its treatment, in administering chemotherapy, and in providing sophisticated supportive care.[18] The relationship between the primary nurse and the family is a means of providing continuity of care from diagnosis and initial treatment, over the course of repeated hospitalizations for further therapy and treatment of complications, to reentry into school and the local community; in a few cases this may extend until the time of death.

Communication is essential among all "primary nurses" involved in the care of a child and family—the inpatient nurse, the ambulatory care nurse, the nurse in the home hospital or pediatrician's office, and the school nurse. As the child transfers from one area to another, each nurse keeps the other informed of the child's problems and progress. These nurses share an understanding of each other's work and concerns. This is achieved through phone contact, written care plans, documentation of nursing actions and, when feasible, site visits. The extra efforts exerted on behalf of the child and family go a long way toward fostering professional collegiality as well as promoting the family's comfort and well-being.

Advanced Roles in Pediatric Oncology

Advanced roles in pediatric oncology nursing have grown out of the need to support and enhance the development of the primary nurse, to provide avenues for professional advancement, to support biomedical research, and to create options for

delivery of patient care in a variety of settings. The *chemotherapy nurse* is a pediatric oncology nurse who has demonstrated expertise in phlebotomy and has experience in the use of alternate venous access devices, and who has formally or independently acquired the knowledge necessary to practice according to an institution's standards regarding safe administration of chemotherapy. The chemotherapy nurse may be a primary nurse on an inpatient unit or in an ambulatory care setting, or a member of a cadre of nurses administering therapy in an oncologist's office or clinic. The *clinical nurse specialist* is an experienced pediatric oncology nurse who has completed a master's level educational program in pediatric or oncology nursing. The clinical specialist uses advanced knowledge and clinical skills to provide expert care to a defined patient population and serves as a pediatric oncology nurse consultant to families, to the health care team, and to the community. The clinical specialist participates in nursing staff development, particularly in practice areas. The *pediatric nurse practitioner* has completed a university-based master's level program or an institutional certificate program. These programs emphasize physical assessment skills, knowledge of growth and development, and preparation for safely assuming physician-delegated tasks such as bone marrow aspirations and lumbar punctures. The pediatric nurse practitioner independently cares for well children who have completed therapy and those on therapy who have acute, minor complaints. The practitioner cares for children in chronic and terminal phases of their cancer under the guidance of a pediatric oncologist using standing orders, medical and nursing protocols, and nursing care plans. The nurse practitioner counsels and advises patients and their families, identifies support resources in the community, and collaborates with outside agencies providing funding, services, and supplies.[19] He or she may also be the coordinator of a multidisciplinary team brought together to address patient care concerns, such as the evaluation of the late effects of cancer and cancer therapy.[20] The pediatric nurse practitioner is an ideal coordinator of a pediatric home care or hospice care team.

Nursing Responsibilities

Preparation for Possible Cancer Diagnosis

Members of the health care team can help the child and family cope with the diagnosis and treatment of cancer (see Chaps. 41 and 42). For professional nurses, this assistance begins with the first patient or family contact. An initial nursing history is collected and an assessment is made of the child's current health status and the emotional state of both child and family. This initial contact may be brief, but it enables the nurse to develop a tentative plan for nursing interventions. It is essential for the nurse to be present when the possibility of a cancer diagnosis is first presented to the family by the physician. Nursing responsibilities include clarifying and reinforcing information given by the physician, as indicated by patient and family responses. In addition, the nurse promotes open discussion and encourages family members to voice their questions and concerns. The nurse also initiates referrals to other members of the multidisciplinary team (*e.g.,* the social worker). Finally, the nurse documents the information given, the patient's and family's response, and the plans that were made.

It is customary for the physician to describe necessary diagnostic and staging procedures during the first interview. It

(*Text continues on p. 946*)

Table 46-2
Educational Resources for Children, Adolescents, and Families

Title or Organization	General Description	Source
General Medical and Psychosocial Issues		
Association for Care of Children's Health: A Child Goes To The Hospital, 1981 (16 pp)	Suggestions for parents preparing their child for hospitalization; includes guidelines for evaluating pediatric facilities and an annotated bibliography.	ACCH 3615 Wisconsin Avenue, NW Washington, DC 20016
Association for Care of Children's Health: Preparing Your Child for the Hospital: A Checklist, 1981 (4 pp)	A six-point checklist to help parents prepare their children for hospitalization.	ACCH 3615 Wisconsin Avenue, NW Washington, DC 20016
Association for Care of Children's Health: For Teen-agers: Your Stay In The Hospital, 1981 (4 pp)	Designed to help acquaint adolescents with hospital routines, policies, staff members, and common medical terms; annotated bibliography.	ACCH 3615 Wisconsin Avenue, NW Washington, DC 20016
Braznic D: Becky's Story, 1981 (32 pp)	Encourages siblings of hospitalized children to explore and understand their own reactions, needs and emotions.	ACCH 3615 Wisconsin Avenue, NW Washington, DC 20016
Association for Care of Children's Health: Selected Books for Children and Teen-agers about Hospitalization, Illness and Handicapping Conditions, 1984 (16 pp)	Annotated bibliography.	ACCH 3615 Wisconsin Avenue, NW Washington, DC 20016
Cancer Diagnosis: A Time of Crisis		
Bracken JM: Children With Cancer: A Comprehensive Guide for Parents, 1986 (407 pp)	Written by reference librarian and parent of child who survived cancer. Describes childhood cancers, available treatments, how to cope with changes in family, and where to go for help. Appendix explains common medical terms and lists sources of help in U. S. and other countries.	Oxford University Press 200 Madison Avenue New York, NY 10016
Candlelighters Childhood Cancer Foundation, Inc.	An international organization of parents whose children have had cancer. Provides guidance, emotional support, information, and referral to local and regional resources.	Candlelighters Childhood Cancer Foundation, Inc. 2025 I Street, NW, Suite 1011 Washington, DC 20006
National Cancer Institute: Publication List for the Public, 1987	Listing of all NCI publications useful for nonprofessionals.	Office of Cancer Communications NCI Building 31, Room 10A18 Bethesda, MD 20892
American Cancer Society	Volunteer organization offering programs of education, patient service, information, rehabilitation, and referral to local and regional resources.	American Cancer Society 90 Park Avenue New York, NY 10016 (National Office)
Leukemia Society of America, Inc.	Volunteer organization offering financial assistance, education, information, referrals to other sources of help.	Leukemia Society of America, Inc. 800 Second Avenue New York, NY 10017
National Cancer Institute, Cancer Information Service	A network of regional information offices that provide accurate personalized answers to cancer-related questions from patients, families, the general public, and health professionals; provides information and referral to local and regional resources.	Cancer Information Service NCI Building 31 National Institutes of Health Bethesda, MD 20892
Frantz TF: When Your Child Has A Life-Threatening Illness, 1983 (23 pp)	Topics include initial reactions, hope, communication, other children, impact on marriage and single-parent families.	ACCH 3615 Wisconsin Avenue, NW Washington, DC 20016
National Cancer Institute: Talking to Your Child About Cancer, 1986 (15 pp)	Discusses who should tell, when to tell, and what to tell, depending on developmental stage.	Office of Cancer Communications NCI Building 31, Room 10A18 Bethesda, MD 20892

(continued)

Table 46-2 (continued)

Title or Organization	General Description	Source
Cancer Diagnosis: A Time of Crisis (continued)		
National Cancer Institute: When Someone In Your Family Has Cancer, 1986 (15 pp)	Describes changes in the family when a family member has cancer. Includes general discussion of cancer treatment.	Office of Cancer Communications NCI Building 31, Room 10A18 Bethesda, MD 20892
National Cancer Institute: Hospital Days—Treatment Ways. Hematology-Oncology Coloring Book, 1983 (28 pp)	Designed to familiarize child with procedures and experiences in hospital environment.	Office of Cancer Communications NCI Building 31, Room 10A18 Bethesda, MD 20892
National Cancer Institute: Young People with Cancer: A Handbook for Parents, 1983 (93 pp)	Describes diseases, treatment, health issues, common medical procedures, coping methods; lists sources of information, support, and assistance.	Office of Cancer Communications NCI Building 31, Room 10A18 Bethesda, MD 20892
National Cancer Institute: Help Yourself—Tips for Teenagers with Cancer (booklet, audiotapes, user's guide), 1983	Describes impact of diagnosis, treatment, coping. Lists additional resources.	Office of Cancer Communications NCI Building 31, Room 10A18 Bethesda, MD 20892
National Cancer Institute: Chemotherapy and You: A Guide To Self-Help During Treatment, 1985 (65 pp)	Describes chemotherapy treatment, managing side-effects, nutrition, and follow-up care.	Office of Cancer Communications NCI Building 31, Room 10A18 Bethesda, MD 20892
National Cancer Institute: Radiation Therapy and You: A Guide to Self Help During Treatment, 1985 (36 pp)	Discusses radiation treatment, what to expect, managing side-effects, nutrition and follow-up care.	Office of Cancer Communication NCI Building 31, Room 10A18 Bethesda, MD 20892
Bowen J: When You Visit The ICU (coloring book), 1981	A coloring book to use in preparing children for a stay in the ICU.	ACCH 3615 Wisconsin Avenue, NW Washington, DC 20016
Jeter KF: These Special Children: The Ostomy Book for Parents of Children with Colostomies, Ileostomies and Urostomies, 1982 (192 pp)	A resource book for parents of children with ostomies; designed to "inform, counsel and comfort." Explains ostomies, impact on child depending on developmental stage; lists additional resources for information and equipment.	Bull Publishing Company Box 208 Palo Alto, CA 94302
Reentry to Home and Community		
Association for Care of Children's Health: Preparing Your Child For Repeated or Extended Hospitalizations, 1981 (16 pp)	Guidelines for self-education, using support services, cooperating with hospital staff, and understanding the emotional and developmental needs of the chronically ill child.	ACCH 3615 Wisconsin Avenue, NW Washington, DC 20016
Association for Care of Children's Health: The Chronically Ill Child and Family In The Community, 1981 (6 pp)	Focuses on family life, managing medical care, school, and finances; annotated bibliography designed to help parents.	ACCH 3615 Wisconsin Avenue, NW Washington, DC 20016
Jones ML: Home Care For The Chronically Ill or Disabled Child: A Manual and Sourcebook for Parents and Professionals, 1985 (416 pp)	Describes a parent's perspective on home care issues, including organizing the home, financial planning, and techniques for general and specific conditions.	ACCH 3615 Wisconsin Avenue, NW Washington, DC 20016
Terminal Illness		
National Institute of Mental Health: Talking To Children About Death, 1979 (16 pp)	Guidelines for communicating with children about death, with discussions of age-related understanding of death and mourning.	Superintendent of Documents U. S. Government Printing Office Washington, DC 20402
Forrari MS: A Look At Death, 1978	Designed for children ages 4–10. Text and photographs present concept of death, the importance of grief, and customs of mourning.	Lerner Awareness Series Lerner Publications Company Minneapolis, MN

(continued)

Table 46-2 (continued)

Title or Organization	General Description	Source
Terminal Illness (continued)		
Schoff HS: The Bereaved Parent, 1982 (146 pp)	Offers guidelines and suggestions to help parents cope with every stage of grief.	Penguin Books 625 Madison Avenue New York, NY 10022
Kubler-Ross E: On Death and Dying, 1970 (289 pp)	Describes attitudes towards death and dying; five stages through which dying person progresses; impact on patient's family.	Medical Books Macmillan Company 866 Third Avenue New York, NY 10022
Children's Hospice International	Volunteer organization that promotes hospice support through pediatric care facilities; has information clearinghouse; issues publications, newsletters, and cassette tapes.	Children's Hospice International 501 Slater's Lane #207 Alexandria, VA 22314
National Hospice Organization: NHO Bibliography of Children's Literature on Death and Dying	NHO sponsors conferences, monitors legislation, works to gain insurance coverage for hospice care; publishes books, pamphlets, and bibliographies; sets standards for quality care.	National Hospice Organization 1901 North Fort Myer Drive, Suite 402 Arlington, VA 22209

is the nurse's responsibility to prepare the child and family for these procedures in a manner that provides adequate information and permits the child to maintain some degree of autonomy, self-esteem, competence, and trust in self and others.[21] Health care providers must take into consideration the child's age and cognitive development in preparing children for any procedure (see Table 46-2).[22–24] *Young children* (preschool) are best prepared with brief, simple, concrete information based on the senses (*e.g.,* "Is it going to hurt?" "Will I need to hold still?"). A simple demonstration using a doll to show what will be done is helpful. *School-age children* are able to understand cause and effect relationships. These children are interested in the purpose of the procedure and will also benefit from a description of behavior required during the procedure (*e.g.,* "You will need to lie very still on the table with your head inside the machine."). Nurses can help by giving verbal descriptions using drawings, dolls, and patient education booklets and films. *Adolescents* have adult thought processes. They are best able to cope with procedures when they understand the reasons why they are necessary.

During the teaching sessions, the patient and family are informed of necessary preparations for each procedure and a written personal procedure schedule is developed. At this time, parents are informed of procedures during which their attendance is limited, such as computed tomography (CT) scans. All teaching is conducted in an honest, open atmosphere that promotes the expression of questions and concerns. The nurse must be alert to any clues of unexpressed concerns. For example, a mother may be fearful of accompanying her child during a procedure. She needs to be assured that while her presence is welcome, it is not mandatory, and that the staff will be available to support the child. It is helpful for the nurse to conclude the teaching sessions with written information that includes the nurse's name and telephone number.

A major responsibility for the nurse during this period is to serve as a child advocate. The nurse acts as a liaison with staff in other hospital departments who are unfamiliar with children's needs and concerns. For example, the nurse may ask the tech-

nicians who operate magnetic resonance imaging scanner to turn on the machine so that the child can hear the noise before the test begins. It may be necessary for the nurse to remind hospital personnel that procedures performed on a child should be preceded by warning and explanation. Staff may also need reminders to respect "safe times," such as nap times, and "safe areas," such as playrooms, lounges, or other public areas.

The nurse who spends long periods of time with the child and family is cognizant of stress limitations and has a responsibility to promote the use of appropriate preparation or local anesthesia for procedures. Appropriate preparation for procedures or radiation therapy may require drug administration or relaxation techniques. Some children benefit from the administration of medication such as meperidine, chlorpromazine, promethazine with dextromethorphan, or chloral hydrate prior to bone marrow aspirations or lumbar punctures (see Chap. 44). Noninvasive methods, such as imagery, deep breathing, distraction, or hypnosis (by a trained therapist) have been found to be effective in the older child and are probably underused. The benefits of these methods are minimal risk and return of control to the child.[25]

The nurse also supports the child and family during procedures by inviting family members to be present whenever possible. If this is not possible, as during radiologic procedures, family members are invited to wait nearby.

Facilitation of Adjustment to the Diagnosis

Each family's response to stress is a function of cultural and family influences (see also Chap. 42).[26] During the diagnostic and staging evaluations, the nurse continues to collect data about the child's physical, developmental, and emotional status, as well as the coping skills of, and support available for, family members. With this information, the nurse is prepared to participate in the family conference when the physician explains the diagnosis and outlines plans for treatment. Other members of the health care team may also be present.

Even if they suspect what the diagnosis will be, few parents are prepared to have their worst fears confirmed. The physician customarily explains the diagnosis, intended treatment, and prognosis. This discussion with the family is oftentimes candid and tempered with realistic hope. Treatment alternatives and their advantages and disadvantages may be reviewed at this time. Parents are not usually able to retain this information, and they need to be told that these explanations will be repeated many times.

From the time of diagnosis, the parents face many decisions, including what to tell the child. There is general agreement that children should be told as much about their illness as their age allows them to understand. The child may learn the diagnosis from the physician or from the parents. At the earliest opportunity, the nurse needs to explore the child's understanding of the diagnosis; the child should know the name of the disease and have at least a beginning concept of the treatment planned. The nurse also reinforces or clarifies information given to the parents and assesses the need for crisis intervention. Previous methods of coping will influence the family's initial reaction to the diagnosis. Nursing staff and social workers collaborate to assist family members in mobilizing resources and suggesting ways to reduce stress.

A nurse assists the child and family to gain control over the physical setting of an unfamiliar hospital environment by providing tours of the unit, including bathroom and rooming-in facilities and family visiting areas, and explaining the patient communication system. At this time, the nurse also reviews the orientation booklet (or unit guidelines) and introduces the new child and family to other members of the health care team. Another way to reduce stress is to schedule periodic family interviews to answer questions and clarify information. During all interactions with parents and child, the nurse attempts to establish a basis of honest and open communication that encourages questions and respects psychological defenses.

The family may require assistance with treatment decisions. The nurse is able to facilitate this process by providing appropriate resources, serving as liaison to other members of the health care team, acting as a nonjudgmental listener, and facilitating communication to all concerned. At times, it is necessary for the child to be treated at another facility. The nurse then helps to prepare the patient for transfer and prepares necessary documentation for nursing staff at the new facility.

Preparation for Treatment

Treatment may need to begin soon after parents and child are informed of the diagnosis. Regardless of the type of cancer and therapy, treatment is a lengthy process. The nurse must develop and implement a patient and family educational program. Most treatment of childhood cancer is initiated in the hospital. This is a time of stress. Young children need to have a basic understanding of necessary procedures and treatment processes to facilitate their acceptance and participation. Adolescents and parents require a more sophisticated understanding (see Chap. 41). The assimilation of information regarding the disease and therapy takes time. Some essential information needs to be given early, in simple language, with plans for reinforcement at a later time. Experience suggests that the child and family require approximately 9 months to adapt to the change in lifestyle that may result from the diagnosis of cancer.[27] In the meantime, medical and nursing staff educate the patient and family about the illness and its treatment, and the patient and family educate the medical and nursing staff about the patient and how the therapy and its effects can best be managed so as to have a minimal effect on the family's lifestyle.[28] A teaching plan is developed with both short-term

and long-term goals, specific nursing actions to meet those goals, and periodic evaluations of progress toward goal achievement.

CHEMOTHERAPY. The patient and family need to be informed of the treatment schedule, the names of the drugs, any necessary preparation, and the route and time of delivery (see also Chap. 9). They should be prepared for the side-effects of therapy and the time frame within which these effects may be experienced. Patient education booklets, information sheets, and film strips have been developed to assist the nurse with patient and family education (see Table 46-2). All, however, are designed to be used in conjunction with personal reinforcement by the nurse over an extended period. The questions and concerns of the newly diagnosed patient are different from those of the patient during remission maintenance therapy.

RADIATION THERAPY. Preparation for radiation therapy also requires patient and family education (see also Chap. 11). It is helpful for the nurse to arrange a visit to the department, with a review of the equipment to be used, and liaison with a nursing staff member there. Very young children will require sedation or anesthesia during radiation therapy, and this needs to be arranged in advance. Patient and family members need to be informed of necessary preparations for radiation therapy, such as "simulation" (use of special radiographic equipment to locate the exact place on the body where therapy will be given). During simulation, the technologist marks the skin with colored, indelible ink to define the treatment area. Radiation therapy staff members provide the majority of patient and family teaching; the child's nurse reinforces this education and needs to be informed of the treatment schedule, expected side-effects, and plans for follow-up care. The nurse has an obligation to provide liaison with the radiation therapy department and the patient and family members. Booklets have been developed to help with patient and family education (see Table 46-2).

SURGERY. The need for preparation for surgery is well documented (see also Chap. 10). Many community and children's hospitals have developed prehospitalization tours, guidelines, and preparation programs to ensure that children and families will be prepared prior to surgery. Books and audiovisual materials are also available to assist the nurse with preoperative preparation (see Table 46-1). All patient teaching must be based on the child's developmental age. It is helpful for the nurse to be present when the surgeon explains the surgical procedure to child and family. This permits the nurse to use the surgeon's words and explanations in preoperative teaching to clarify and reinforce information the surgeon has provided. The nurse should also be present during the anesthesiologist's visit to the child. It is most helpful if the nurse reviews the child's status with the anesthesiologist before the visit. Generally, the anesthesiologist will not have a longstanding relationship with the child and family and will benefit from the knowledge and approach of those who know the family best.[29] A number of booklets, information sheets, dolls, kits, and films have been developed to assist the nurse in preparing a child for surgery (see Table 46-2). All are designed to be used in conjunction with the nurse's individualized teaching plan. Children should be shown the recovery room where their parents will visit them after surgery. If the child will be taken to an intensive care unit (ICU), the nurse should arrange for the child to visit this area and meet the staff members there.

The child's nurse has a responsibility to ensure that all

preparations have been completed before surgery. Both child and family members should have knowledge of the personnel and equipment involved in postoperative care and of the sensations that will be experienced after surgery. For example, the nurse may explain, "You will have a tube in your mouth and won't be able to talk, but a nurse will always be there." Parents are usually allowed to accompany a child to the door of the operating room. They must be shown the designated waiting area and be assured that the surgeon will meet them there. Visiting policies in both the recovery room and surgical ICU must be explained. Both child and parents need to be informed of the expected time period before the child will be returned to his or her hospital room and of the normal surgical recovery period. The family also requires assurance that members of the health care team will be available to assist them throughout the surgical experience.

Prevention of Complications

Infection

Infection in the child with cancer is a common occurrence and a major cause of death (see Chap. 39). Perhaps the most important role of the pediatric oncology nurse is the prevention of infection through meticulous patient care, frequent inspection of the child and environment, heightened awareness of infection potential, and family education concerning measures to prevent infection and the need to report the occurrence of fever.

The hospital environment itself puts children at risk for infection. Handwashing before and after patient contact plays an important role in reduction of microbial transmission. Hospital equipment and the patient room should be cleansed carefully. Visitors should not be limited but are asked not to visit if they have an ongoing or recent infection.

The child's skin and mucous membranes should be inspected daily for signs of infections. The neutropenic child may not show the usual signs of infection; therefore, the index of suspicion for any change in a wound, catheter exit site, or lesion must be high. Manipulations of oral, perineal, and rectal mucosa are restricted: rectal temperatures, enemas, and suppositories are avoided in neutropenic or potentially neutropenic children. Mouth care and perineal hygiene must be meticulous. The child's temperature is monitored carefully in the hospital and at home: changes can occur quickly.

The same good hygiene principles are followed at home. Families are taught when to expect neutropenia following therapy, how and when to monitor the child's temperature, to avoid persons with known infection, and to be alert for physical or behavioral changes in the child. Immunosuppressed children should not receive any live virus vaccines, such as poliomyelitis and measles vaccines, or be exposed to others who have been vaccinated and are shedding virus.

Varicella presents a danger to the child with cancer. The dissemination of virus throughout internal organs can cause encephalitis, hepatitis, pancreatitis or pneumonia, and may be fatal. Parents of children with cancer must inform their child's teacher, school nurse, and the parents of playmates about this danger and ask to be notified when classmates or playmates develop chickenpox (see also Chap. 51). The incubation period of varicella is 10 to 21 days. Patients are considered contagious 1 to 2 days before and until all lesions have become crusted (usually 6 days after the onset of rash in the nonimmunosuppressed child). Continuous household contact, playmate contact (one or more hours of play indoors), and hospital contact (shared room or prolonged face-to-face contact with a contagious person) are considered significant exposures for which varicella-zoster immune globulin (VZIG) is indicated. If exposure occurs, the physician or nurse must be notified and VZIG given, preferably within 48 hours and not more than 96 hours after exposure. If a second exposure to varicella should occur more than 3 weeks after the child has received VZIG, another dose is given.[30]

Children with cancer who develop primary varicella infection are hospitalized and treated with acyclovir. At-risk contacts of these children are notified and treated with VZIG if necessary. Immunocompromised children are considered contagious until new lesions stop appearing and all old lesions are crusting and dry. Strict isolation is indicated for the duration of the illness. The child in isolation presents a challenge to the entire multidisciplinary team.

The nurse inspects the child's skin daily for evidence of new lesions and infection from scratching. Measures are taken to relieve itching (topical and systemic medications, loose-fitting clothing) and eliminate scratching (mitting, trimming of nails). Adequate hydration is maintained, particularly during febrile periods and throughout the course of treatment with acyclovir. Fever is controlled with the use of acetaminophen or sponging. The child is carefully observed for any evidence of dissemination of varicella. Two months after recovery from chickenpox, immune status against varicella should be determined and documented. The presence of antibody is useful information should further exposures to virus occur.[31]

Varicella-zoster persists in a latent form after primary infection. Reactivation results in the development of vesicular lesions along the distribution of a sensory dermatome. The eruption of lesions may be preceded by localized pain. Lesions in an immunocompromised host may not have a typical vesicular appearance, and a high index of suspicion is essential to early diagnosis. These patients are placed in strict isolation, and their care is similar to that of children with primary varicella-zoster.

Fever is the most common sign of infection in a child with cancer. Parents are taught to notify the nurse or physician immediately when the child has a fever (any one temperature of 38.5°C orally or three temperatures of 38.0°C at least 4 hours apart within 24 hours). Children who are potentially neutropenic or who have an indwelling catheter are seen for further evaluation (see Chap. 39). A nursing history and assessment are performed to elicit even subtle signs of infection. Specimens for culture are collected from the throat, nares, urine, and stool, and at least two blood samples are obtained for culture. If there is an indwelling catheter or subcutaneous port in place, blood is obtained from each lumen, as well as peripherally, and labeled appropriately for culture. Any wound, lesion, or catheter exit site should be cultured. A radiograph of the chest is obtained and the child is placed on broad-spectrum antibiotics without delay.

The nursing care of the child hospitalized for fever and neutropenia is focused on continued observation for early signs of sepsis. Vital signs are monitored at least every 4 hours for changes in pulse (becoming weak and fast), shallow and rapid respirations, falling blood pressure, drop in temperature, change in level of consciousness, and fall in urine output. Antibiotic doses should be checked by the nurse and delivered on schedule. If a catheter culture is positive, antibiotics should be delivered through each of the lumens on a rotating schedule. The child should be observed for any potential reaction to the drugs, such as rash. The child should be kept comfortable. Acetaminophen is given for a temperature greater than 38.5°C after the physician is notified and cultures obtained. A tepid sponge or tub bath may bring down the temperature. Any interventions that cause chilling and further temperature elevation are avoided. The patient should be discouraged from bundling in heavy blankets and clothing. The physician should be notified of any rapid rise in temperature. The child should be observed for any evidence of irritability, hallucinations, or tremors. Fluids are encouraged as tolerated. The skin is inspected, lungs auscultated, and all dressings changed daily. Finally, the child and family need support during this medical emergency, and opportunities for discussion and continued information sharing should be offered.

Bleeding

A child with cancer may be at risk for bleeding because of thrombocytopenia or coagulopathy (see also Chap. 38). The potential for bleeding may be lessened through family and staff education. For example, aspirin and aspirin-containing products must be avoided. Razors should not be used. A soft toothbrush is preferable because it helps to prevent gum injury. Contact sports are discouraged when platelet counts are low. Pressure is applied to injury or needle puncture sites. The platelet count and coagulation profile should be checked before any invasive procedures, including intramuscular injection, bone marrow aspiration, or spinal tap, and before administering medications. Parents are also taught to manage minor anterior nasal bleeding by pinching nostrils together and are instructed to come to the hospital if this does not control the bleeding. When a child with a low platelet count is hospitalized, measures are taken to prevent injury (*e.g.,* keeping side rails up to prevent a fall from bed), and secretions are inspected and tested for evidence of blood. Blood pressure and pulse rate are monitored for evidence of internal bleeding. When packed cell or platelet transfusions are necessary, nursing department procedures for administration of blood products should be followed. The rate of infusion is guided by the child's weight and physical condition.

Alteration in Fluid Balance

Children with cancer are at risk for fluid and electrolyte imbalances caused by the disease process, the cancer therapy, and their complications (see Chap. 37). These imbalances can become severe and life-threatening. The nurse should be aware of the critical imbalances that may take place (overhydration, decreased vascular volume, hypercalcemia, hypocalcemia, hyperphosphatemia, hyperuricemia, and hyperkalemia), their causes, signs, symptoms, and potential medical management.[32] He or she needs to continually monitor fluid intake and output, weight, and tissue turgor, and must be aware of recent blood and urine laboratory values that can be indicative of impending difficulties. The nurse must realize the potential dangers of these imbalances and intervene immediately, according to medical orders.

Nausea and vomiting are side-effects of cancer therapy that also affect fluid balance (see Chap. 45). Potentially noxious stimuli should be removed from the environment. Chemotherapy is preceded by an antiemetic regime or relaxation imagery, and the child is positioned to prevent aspiration should vomiting occur. Careful monitoring of fluid intake and output is essential for the child receiving chemotherapy.

Diarrhea resulting from chemotherapy and radiation therapy affects fluid and electrolyte balance. Stools are measured and tested for the presence of frank or occult blood. The weight of the child is followed daily. A bland diet is initiated and antispasmodic drug therapy ordered. Intravenous fluid and electrolyte therapy are administered to correct imbalances (see also Chap. 40).

Alterations in Nutrition

Maintenance of good nutritional status is necessary for the child with cancer in coping with the physical stress of illness, lessening the risk of sepsis, and facilitating the healing of wounds postoperatively.[33] Cancer and side-effects of therapy (nausea, vomiting, anorexia, stomatitis) interfere with a child's ability to take in adequate calories. Prevention of stomatitis is attempted by arriving at an oral care regimen that is acceptable to the child and will be done regularly. The mouth should be inspected frequently for signs of viral or fungal infection so that medical interventions may be initiated. Parents are encouraged to prepare and offer foods that the child is familiar with and enjoys.

When these interventions fail and debilitating weight loss occurs, intravenous hyperalimentation should be initiated by the physician (see Chap. 40). Central venous access is obtained and line placement checked before initiation of an infusion. Line connections are Luer-locked or taped and entered only after careful cleansing with povidone-iodine (Betadine). The line insertion site should be cleansed with Betadine and dressed at regular intervals. The rate of the hyperalimentation infusion needs to be carefully regulated. Urine is tested for sugar and acetone, and a careful record of intake and output, as well as weight, is kept. A hyperalimentation infusion is never ended abruptly; to prevent hypoglycemia, the rate is titrated downward. Long-term home parenteral nutrition is now an option for those children who are otherwise medically stable but who need continued intravenous nutritional support.[34]

Management of Pain

The single greatest problem regarding pain in children is making professionals aware of its potential. Children experience the same types of cancer-related pain that adults do (see also Chap. 44). Nurses often witness the pain experienced by young patients but may have difficulty in objectively communicating their observations. Tools have been developed to assist professionals in assessing pain in those children who are developmentally unable to express their discomfort or are reluctant to do so. Nurses working with children need to be familiar with these tools, with children's perceptions of pain and its causes, and with behavioral changes seen in children with pain.

No one pain intervention will help all children, and the challenge is to find the combinations that are most effective for each child. Nurses are responsible for assessing the effectiveness of pain management plans, administering analgesics, and monitoring their success. Flow sheets can be used to summarize all data about pain and other useful information, such as the relationship between timing of analgesic administration and degree of pain relief. Nurses may have unrealistic fears about drug addiction in children or about the safety of using "large" doses of narcotics. Professional education about these issues is critical to changing attitudes toward pain and pain relief in children.

Terminal Care

There may come a time in the course of a child's struggle with cancer when treatment options have been exhausted and nursing interventions must focus on supporting the family in their decision to forego further therapy. The goal should be to maximize the child's comfort, at home or in the hospital, and to be sensitive to the family's need for guidance in making decisions that they can live with long after the child's death. Community and hospital-based hospice programs are available to assist families with the management of pain and symptoms and provide the support of professionals skilled in the coordination of home care services (see Chap. 49). Plans for discharge care are made with the family by the primary nurse, social worker, and physician. All families need the assurance that they will not be abandoned and may return to the hospital at any time for respite or long-term care (see Tables 46-1 and 46-2).

Facilitating Reentry into the Home Community

In most cases, the initial treatment results in a period of disease remission. As the child begins to look and feel well, all family members struggle to cope with the emotional impact of a cancer diagnosis. Guidelines for nursing intervention have been developed that incorporate assessments of the family's current emotional state into a care plan designed to facilitate adjustment to a life-threatening chronic illness.[35] Nurses need to plan specific interventions that foster the child's development and normal family functioning. This includes encouraging the child to engage in his or her own daily care activities to the fullest extent possible. In addition, health care settings should provide the opportunity for the child to participate in developmentally appropriate educational, recreational, and social activities.[36] The stress and pressure of coping with a child's life-threatening illness can be overwhelming (see Chaps. 41 and 42). The hope is that the remission will go on for years and the child will be cured, but the fear is that the cancer will return and the child will die.[27] Support groups for parents and family members can be most helpful. Such groups may be sponsored by an institution (*e.g.,* hospital nursing and social work departments) or by organizations such as the Candlelighters Foundation. Publications are also available to assist parents but should always be used in conjunction with patient education programs (see Table 46-2).

Preparation for Discharge

When treatment regimens have stabilized the child's status, preparations for hospital discharge begin. Resources in the family and community are identified. The child's local pediatrician and nurse should be contacted and a liaison is established with hospital personnel. Treatment will be continued for an extended period of time. The more complete the treatment program, the more interference there will be with a family's rehabilitation and reintegration. Many children and families will benefit from referral to public health nurses in the home community. The referring nurse first contacts the community health nurse by phone to inform her of the child's illness, treatment plan, specific reason for referral, future goals, and a plan of care. This is followed by more specific written documentation and reference material. Names and telephone numbers of resource individuals and the child's specific follow-up schedule are included. It is essential for the referring nurse to periodically inform the community health nurse of any changes in the child's disease and status and to maintain open and ongoing communication.[37]

Preparation for discharge includes assessing and reinforcing the family's progress toward understanding the diagnosis, the treatment program for the next few weeks, and the side-effects of therapy that may occur during the next few weeks, as well as identifying support individuals in the home community. The nurse also reviews plans for home care and discusses possible emergency care with the parents before the child's discharge. Simple rehearsal of these plans helps to reduce anxiety. The nurse constantly stresses to the parents that they are competent and able to care for their child at home. Instructions are given verbally, but all teaching is reinforced with written patient information sheets and discharge care plans that family members and community caretakers will use as reference materials. The discharge care plan must clearly identify hospital resource people and provide telephone numbers. Thorough instruction by oncology team members enables the majority of families to leave the hospital with the basic skills to care for their child.[26]

Return to School

The reentry process for the pediatric cancer patient involves returning to family, friends, and community while still undergoing rigorous medical treatment.[38] Reentry is stressful for both parent and child. The goals are for the child to resume normal activities and for family members to resume family roles and responsibilities. These goals, however, must be accomplished in collaboration with the medical treatment plan, which requires periodic visits to the physician's office or hospital clinic. It takes time to adjust to a changed lifestyle. Preparation for discharge includes not only discussion of physical care but also the gradual resumption of normal activities. For the child, this means return to school at a time when he or she may perceive a change in body image and worry about the reactions of friends. At first, most children are reluctant to return to school. Parents may also be hesitant because of fear that the child may become ill or be injured and may request a homebound teacher. The child's nurse is the appropriate person to assess the concerns of child and family about school reentry. Nurses planning school reentry need to develop a plan to help normalize the school experience. Return to the classroom signals resumption of the child's usual life routine. The treatment team needs to encourage the return to school and outline its benefits. The nurse must listen to the child describe his or her fears. Socialization with peers is what most children like best about school, and fear of peer rejection is usually their greatest concern. The nurse must listen to what the child feels would be helpful and find out from the child how much information about the disease may be shared with classmates.[39] This nurse can then initiate a school reentry program, with the permission of the child and family.

A formal school reentry program consists of preparing the child and school personnel for the return to school, a classroom presentation, and program follow-up (see also Chap. 51).[40] The nurse should begin by contacting the school nurse, describing the child's health care needs, and requesting the school nurse's assistance in coordinating plans for the student's return to class and meeting health care needs in the educational setting. It is appropriate for the school nurse to contact the child's teachers and discuss the program. Each program is individualized to address the special needs and concerns of a particular child but includes information about the child's disease, its treatment, and obvious side-effects.

With the cooperation of school personnel, a classroom presentation is conducted, usually by the child's primary nurse, although additional staff members such as a child life and recreational therapist may participate. Presentations vary according to the developmental level of the classmates and may include the use of puppets, booklets, or films. In addition to the formal presentation, questions and conversations with the child's classmates are encouraged. The child patient may choose to be present or may request that the program be conducted while he or she is absent. Teachers are especially concerned about the treatment schedule, potential side-effects, and effects of disease or therapy on appearance, behavior, and limitations on activities. Classmates' concerns vary with age and developmental status. The nurse is careful to include topics suggested by the child or family. Teachers are asked to be aware of questions and concerns subsequent to the presentation.

Follow-up occurs with the child and family on an informal basis when the child returns for subsequent clinic visits. Teachers are contacted by the primary nurse to determine how the child is progressing. Evaluations of reentry programs have generally been positive. Observers have noted that the child with cancer receives support from classmates and social acceptance is enhanced.

Continued school attendance for the child receiving treatment may be complicated by frequent absences for medical reasons, overprotection and overindulgence by parents, limitations on physical activity, and social isolation.[41] These obstacles can be overcome with strong family reinforcement and positive support from educators and caretakers. The goal of Public Law 94-112 is to allow each child to participate in regular classroom activities as much as possible while providing the extra support services and facilities needed because of the child's handicap or disability. A number of approaches may be used in the education of children with special needs, and the participation of the school nurse is essential.[42,43] School nurses need and want information about students who return to school. These nurses have a commitment to continuity of care. Their primary responsibilities are to help the students cope and to serve as resources for school staff.

Preparation for Completion of Therapy

The nursing goals for a child with a chronic illness are to prevent secondary effects, help parents in their role as advocates for their children, teach self-care and parenting skills, and facilitate communication with and support for the family.[44] As the child's treatment progresses, the nurse periodically assesses the progress of child and family toward these goals. Without professional intervention, dependency, change in self-concept, passivity, and anxiety are inevitable side-effects of a chronic illness.[45] With periodic reassessment, however, appropriate interventions to foster growth and development of the child and functional family coping may be instituted.

Completion of the prescribed course of therapy begins another period of crisis for both child and family. There is relief that treatment is finished, but also fear that, without treatment, the disease will recur.[26] Ideally, several months in advance, the nurse should begin preparing the child and family for discontinuing therapy. During routine clinic visits, the nurse discusses the treatment schedule and assures family members of the oncology team's belief in the treatment's success. The nurse also encourages family members to voice their questions and concerns. Parents are relieved to learn that their worry about disease recurrence is common and appropriate. Children also have fears about discontinuing treatment and are concerned about the residual effects of the disease and of therapy. Parental response is the key factor affecting the way a child responds to changes in appearance.[46] If the parent has a positive attitude, the child will have a positive attitude.

For a long time, the child has been forced to adapt to illness and to accept treatment as a way of life. Now the child must be taught that therapy is being discontinued because he or she is doing well. The return to normal living needs to be gradual, however, or the child may be overwhelmed by the expectations of others (see Chaps. 41 and 52). Children learn to become comfortable in the sick role, and this new period needs to be approached with support and consideration. With psychological support from nurses and other team members, children and families can survive the cancer experience without serious adjustment problems.[46]

It is a nursing responsibility to ensure that the child who has completed therapy receives careful periodic evaluations. Although the possibility of disease relapse is well known to pediatric oncology nurses, the potential problems that may arise from late effects of disease or therapy are less familiar. Nurses must first become educated about these physiologic and psychological posttherapeutic disabilities. Nursing assessments will then include screening for the most common late effects during follow-up visits and ensuring proper referral when new problems are identified. It is also a nursing responsibility to provide patient and family education about the need for careful, complete follow-up care.[47]

The Pediatric Oncology Nurse in Education

Preparing the New Employee

When preparing a nurse for practice in a pediatric oncology setting, it is essential to assess his or her professional knowledge and background as well as personal experience with children, families, chronic and acute illness, cancer, cancer therapy, and death. Nurses who care for children with cancer are specialists in the practice of both pediatric and oncology nursing. Content related to both specialties should be provided during an orientation period that includes both clinical and didactic components.

The learning needs of the professional new to pediatric oncology nursing are at two levels: first, information needed to correctly and safely perform the day-to-day technical routines and nursing procedures, and second, that needed to carry out the nursing process, to set priorities, and to acquire a theoretic knowledge base. A nurse preceptor serves the new employee as a professional role model and offers opportunities for the practice and acquisition of skills, providing close supervision and continuous feedback to the preceptee and the supervisor. A preceptor is a full-time employee who has demonstrated theoretic knowledge as well as clinical and interpersonal skills and is interested in teaching new employees. The preceptor coordinates a workshop providing instruction in needs assessment, teaching strategies, feedback, and evaluation techniques. An outline of a formal orientation program is used as a guide during the orientation period. The *clinical nurse educator* is available to the preceptor as a resource in the orientation of newly employed nursing staff and also develops, coordinates, and implements continuing education programs for all nursing staffs.

Preparing Nurses for Expanded Roles

Professional nurses who are primary nurses to children with cancer in inpatient and outpatient settings can enhance their skills and expand their practice by acquiring the knowledge and ability to administer intravenous push chemotherapy. In most states, the employing institution determines standards of nursing practice as guidelines in the administration of these drugs. The Oncology Nursing Society has developed a framework of information relevant to the administration of chemotherapeutic agents, outlining both educational content and nursing practice issues that should be addressed in any education program designed to prepare registered nurses to administer these agents and to care for patients who have received them. The emphasis in such programs is on the development of clinical proficiency in assessment and management of individual patient situations.[29] Table 46-3 outlines the areas in which knowledge and skills are acquired by the nurse qualified to administer chemotherapy.

After the nurse has successfully completed the educational program, there are repeated opportunities to develop skill in management of the patient receiving chemotherapy, to review emergency procedures, and to demonstrate clinical competency in the administration of chemotherapy under the supervision of a preceptor who has current institutional approval and who demonstrates skill in chemotherapy administration.

Professional Certification

As nursing grows more complex and as nurses become more sophisticated in their practice, nurses in both journeymen and advanced roles have the option of validating their qualifications through professional certification. Certification assures the public that the individual has mastered a body of knowledge and acquired skills in a specialty area. Table 46-4 lists organizations offering certification in areas related to the practice of pediatric oncology nursing.

The Pediatric Oncology Nurse in Administration

Staffing Patterns

Health care today is in a new era. Nursing and hospital administrators face the challenge of providing cost-effective, high-quality care to increasingly ill hospitalized patients who have complex care needs. Pediatric oncology patients require care by a highly skilled nursing staff. Treatment is aggressive, physical care is complex, and technology is a part of the everyday hospital environment. Psychosocial issues require constant assessment and intervention throughout the course of a child's illness. Studies have shown that registered nurses using a primary nursing model can deliver cost-effective care by significantly reducing the number of inpatient hospital days. Staff spend a greater portion of time in direct patient care, communication, and workable discharge planning.[49]

Models have been developed to estimate nursing care requirements related to medical diagnoses and to nursing pro-

---

Table 46-3

Skills Acquired from Educational Programs Preparing Nurses to Administer Chemotherapy

Before administering chemotherapy, the nurse should be able to do the following:

Demonstrate familiarity with cancer chemotherapeutic agents (pharmacokinetics, dosage, interactions, stability, administration, side effects, toxicities and latent effects)

Interpret laboratory values that determine need for delay in treatment administration or dose adjustment

Educate patients about their treatment

Plan for the management of treatment side effects

Plan for potential extravasation or anaphalaxis

Understand and initiate the institution's procedure for nursing interventions in emergency situations

Verify the appropriateness of the drug dosage ordered by the physician by verifying the dose with the protocol and checking it with a second person

When applying knowledge in a clinical setting, the nurse should be able to do the following:

Prepare drugs safely and dispose of unused drugs as a hazardous waste

Select an appropriate vein through which to administer chemotherapy, perform the venipuncture, and anchor the needle safely

Administer drugs according to the facility's procedure

Document drug administration and the patient's reaction to treatment

---

Table 46-4

Professional Certification Programs Related to Pediatric Oncology Nursing

Organization	Program (designation)	Recertification
American Nurses Association, Inc. Center for Credentialing Services 2420 Pershing Road Kansas City, MO 64108 (816) 474-5720	Child and Adolescent Nurse Pediatric Nurse Practitioner Nursing Administration (R.N., C)	5-year period, renewal by continuing education or reexamination
The National Board of Pediatric Nurse Associates and Practitioners 414 Hungerford Drive, Suite 310 Rockville, MD 20850 (301) 340-8213	Pediatric Nurse Practitioner (C.P.N.P.)	6-year period, renewal by Board-approved continuing education programs, reexamination, or annual self-assessment exercises
The Oncology Nursing Certification Corporation 1016 Greentree Road Pittsburgh, PA 15220-3125 (412) 921-7373	Oncology Nursing, Generalist (O.N.C.)	4-year period, renewal by reexamination only

cess standards (*i.e.,* measures a prudent nurse would take in a given situation).[50] These models, together with average unit census and average patient acuity, provide a means of predicting the workload of a nursing unit. The predicted workload is used to determine the daily staffing pattern (nursing staff required for 24 hours for the average daily workload of the specific unit). This then is the basis for the personnel budget (full-time equivalents, positions, and employment costs). The staffing pattern distributes the staff by shift, considering the type, amount, and desired quality of work to be done at various points throughout the day. Communication and coordination with other departments are important when developing staffing patterns and projecting workloads. The purpose of the unit and the institution, as well as the services and the types of care families expect, are also considered when developing a staffing pattern.

Effective staffing programs incorporate evaluation of nursing services provided and the impact of staffing on the quality of care into routine assessments of the program. Approaches to measuring quality of care fall into three categories:

Structural—Do the prerequisites for care (staff, space) exist?
Process—Are the necessary nursing tasks performed?
Outcome—Is patient welfare ensured?

Whichever quality assurance method is used, minimally acceptable levels are determined and a monitoring system established. Whether acceptable quality levels are achieved is considered in determining whether existing staffing patterns (for the unit and for each shift) should be continued. Adjustments are made to reflect additional staff and nursing time needed to provide quality care and meet unit goals.[51]

Staff Support

Nursing administrators are challenged with providing a caring environment for the practice of pediatric oncology nursing as well as for ensuring the quality of care for children and their families. The practice of pediatric oncology nursing is stressful and can be emotionally burdensome. Serious illness or death in a child seems an event out of the natural order. Family and friends of staff often find the subject of childhood cancer distressing and are unwilling to listen to or discuss feelings about workplace issues. There is competition among nursing staff, between disciplines, and with patients' parents, and constant internal and external demands to keep pace with technologic and therapeutic advances in order to maintain professional credibility and provide state-of-the-art care.

Quality of nursing care is directly related to the physical and emotional health of the nursing staff. A unit-based nursing staff support group with the stated goal of enhancing function in the workplace is one strategy for promoting the emotional health of a staff. The support group is a forum for validating feelings and perceptions, for promoting peer support, and for exploring stressful aspects of the professional environment and experiences of working with children with cancer and their families.[52] Another strategy for promoting emotional health in staff is varying the work routine to provide respite from stressful work situations. A rotation to another unit (*e.g.,* an ICU or an outpatient clinic), where new but highly transferable skills may be learned, can be productive. Other approaches include class attendance, library time, and time to work on a group or individual project. Staff can be involved in recruitment at conferences or on the unit as part of the inter-

viewing process. Some staff members find professional speaking opportunities satisfying and an affirmation of their expertise. Staff may choose to become involved in pediatric oncology community issues by writing, participating in professional organizations, working to influence legislation, and serving in patient advocacy roles. Some staff members find spending time with healthy children essential to maintaining their perspective on the incidence of childhood cancer. Regardless of the strategies used and the administrative supports available, each nurse must gain insight into personal coping behaviors. Maintaining competency, demonstrating commitment to practice, and communicating knowledge, concern, and respect for each person promote team function and foster quality patient care.

The Pediatric Oncology Nurse in Research

Participation in Medical Research

One of the roles of the nurse caring for children in a medical research environment is to support the family and to facilitate communication among all team members participating in the decision to offer and accept therapy. Nurses can promote open communication between families and investigators, answering questions, addressing concerns and ensuring that informed consent is an ongoing process.[53,54]

Nurses play an important role in medical research by delivering therapy in a manner prescribed by the physician and consistent with the research protocol. Nurses are in a position to accrue data related to the patient's response to treatment, to observe the patient throughout the day, to communicate concerns about patient responses to treatment, to note trends, and to document their observations in the nursing record.

The *research nurse/data manager* plays a critical role in managing clinical data collected in support of a cancer treatment protocol. The nurse ensures that both institutional permission to conduct the study and consent from the patient or legal guardian have been obtained. Nurses monitor the recruitment of appropriate patients and enter them on study after required baseline data are complete. The nurse ensures that randomization, therapy, and data collection are done according to protocol specifications in all institutions participating in the study and is active in evaluating response to therapy and in the reporting of results. The nurse has an ongoing responsibility for patient, family, and professional staff education concerning participation in medical research studies.[37]

Participation in Nursing Research

The growth of pediatric oncology as a nursing specialty depends on the ability of nurses to develop a body of scientific knowledge on which practice can be based. There is a need for nursing research in areas that will generate new knowledge concerning the diagnosis and treatment of human responses to actual or potential health problems related to childhood cancer and its treatment.[56] Nursing research has been conducted in the areas of utilization of home care resources,[57] the late effects of central nervous system therapy,[58] and the management of pain in children.[59] Other areas for concern include the effects of the occurrence of cancer in a child on siblings and other family members; sexuality and fertility in survivors of childhood cancer; the feasibility of alternate and innovative means of nursing care delivery to children with cancer; and the development of patient acuity tools for pediatric oncology care settings.

CONCLUSION

The trends and issues in cancer care will continue to influence pediatric oncology nursing practice, education, administration, and research. There are many opportunities for pediatric oncology nurses to positively influence the quality of life for children and their families.

Pediatric oncology nurses can best meet the challenges of the future by first defining what it is that nurses and nurses alone do to meet the needs of children with cancer and their families. They must stay current with medical and technologic advances and be ready to provide safe, cost-effective care in the home, hospital, or outpatient setting. They must look for opportunities in new areas related to cancer (*e.g.*, acquired immunodeficiency syndrome) to which oncology nursing skills may be applied and which will afford opportunities for research and expanded practice. Nurses must continue to seek professional acknowledgment for expertise in a practice area by seeking the appropriate credentials. They must also play an active role in setting health policy, influencing health legislation, and disseminating information in the community to ensure the public's continued access to health care services provided by nurses and other health care professionals.

REFERENCES

1. Burns C: Perspectives on family centered child nursing. In Fore C, Poster E (eds): Meeting Psychosocial Needs of Children and Families in Health Care, pp 12–19. Washington, DC, Association for Care of Children's Health, 1985
2. Sciarillo WG: Using Hymovich's framework in the family-oriented approach to nursing care. Am J Maternal Child Nurs 5:242–248, 1980
3. Leonard BJ: Psychosocial dimensions of chronic illness. In Mott S, Fazekas N, James S: Nursing Care of Children and Families: A Holistic Approach, pp 978–999. Menlo Park, CA, Addison-Wesley, 1985
4. King J, Ziegler S: The effects of hospitalization on children's behavior: A review of the literature. Child Health Care 10(1):20–28, 1981
5. Association for Care of Children's Health: Education Resources for Pediatric Health Care. Washington, DC, Association for Care of Children's Health, 1985
6. Whaley LF, Wong DL: The child with a potentially terminal illness. In Whaley LF, Wong DL (eds): Nursing Care of Infants and Children, pp 943–1031. St Louis, CV Mosby, 1983
7. Van Eys J: The Truly Cured Child: The New Challenge In Pediatric Cancer Care. Baltimore, University Park Press, 1977
8. Van Eys J, Copeland D: The staffing conference on pediatric oncology. In Christ AE, Flomerhalft K (eds): Childhood Cancer: Impact on Family, pp 87–104. New York, Plenum Press, 1984
9. Pitel AU et al: Parent consultants in pediatric oncology. Children's Health Care 14(1):46–51, 1985
10. Committee for Development of Guidelines, Metropolitan Washington Affiliate of Association for Care of Children's Health: Psychosocial Policy Guidelines for Administration of Pediatric Health Care Facilities. Washington, DC, Association for Care of Children's Health, 1980
11. American Nurses Association: Nursing—A Social Policy Statement. Kansas City, MO, American Nurses Association, 1980
12. Fickeissen JL: Getting certified. Am J Nurs 85:265–269, 1985
13. Pidgeon U, Sander C: Nurses' perceptions of pediatric nursing functions. Child Health Care 10(4):125–130, 1982
14. American Nurses Association, Division on Maternal and Child Health Nursing Practice and Association of Pediatric Oncology Nurses: Standards of Pediatric Oncology Nursing Practice. Kansas City, MO, American Nurses Association, 1978
15. American Nurses Association: Code for Nurses with Interpretive Statements. Kansas City, MO, American Nurses Association, 1985
16. American Nurses Association, Commission on Nursing Research: Human Rights Guidelines for Nurses in Clinical and Other Research. Kansas City, MO, American Nurses Association, 1985
17. Spitzer A: Primary nursing in childhood cancer as applied in Israel. Cancer Nurs 8(2):89–95, 1985
18. Foley GV: The team caring for the child with cancer. In Fochtman D, Foley GU (eds): Nursing Care of the Child with Cancer. Boston, Little, Brown, 1982
19. Raulin AM, Shannon KA: PNP's: Case managers for technology dependent children. Pediatr Nurs 12:338–339, 1986
20. McCalla JL: A multidisciplinary approach to identification and remedial intervention for adverse late effects of cancer therapy. In Gibbon MD (ed): Symposium on Pediatric Oncology. Nurs Clin North Am 20:83–103, 1985
21. Wear ET, Covey J, Brush M: Facilitating children's adaptations to intrusive procedures. In Fochtman D, Foley GU (eds): Nursing Care of the Child with Cancer, pp 61–80. Boston, Little, Brown, 1982
22. Hellier A, Ptak H, Cerreto M: CATS inside my brain: Children's understanding of the cerebral computed tomography scan procedure. Child Health Care 14(4):211–217, 1986
23. Droske SC, Francis JA: Pediatric Diagnostic Procedure with Guidelines for Preparing Children for Clinical Tests. New York, John Wiley & Sons, 1981
24. Petrillo M, Sanger S: Preparing children and parents for diagnostic and surgical procedures and teaching about illness. In Emotional Care of Hospitalized Children, An Environmental Approach, 2nd ed, pp 207–301. Philadelphia, JB Lippincott, 1980
25. Hockenberry MJ: Preparation for intrusive procedures in children. J Assoc Pediatr Oncol Nurses 3(4):28, 1985
26. Hockenberry MJ: Crisis points in cancer. In Hockenberry MJ, Coody DK (eds): Pediatric Oncology and Hematology, pp 432–449. St Louis, CV Mosby, 1986
27. Hall M, Havelin K, Conatser C: The Challenges of Psychological Care. In Fochtman D, Foley G (eds): Nursing Care of the Child With Cancer, pp 312–354. Boston, Little, Brown, 1982
28. Wilbur JR: A picture essay—Treating cancer in children. In 1978 Medical and Health Annual, pp 278–279. Chicago, Encyclopaedia Britannica, 1978
29. Hall SC: The pediatric cancer patient and general anesthesia. J Assoc Pediatr Oncol Nurses 1(2):8–14, 1984
30. Committee on Infectious Diseases: Red Book 1986. Elkridge, IL, American Academy of Pediatrics, 1986
31. Couillard-Getreur DL: Herpes-zoster in the immunocompromised patient. Cancer Nurs 5:361–370, 1982
32. Cunningham SG: Fluid and electrolyte disturbances associated with cancer and its treatment. Nursing Clin North Am 17:579–593, 1982
33. Hinson LR: Nutritional assessment and management of the hospitalized patient. Crit Care Nurse 5(2):53–60, 1985
34. Konstantinides NN: Home parenteral nutrition: A viable alternative for patients with cancer. Oncol Nurs Forum 12(1):23–29, 1985
35. Peter MA: Quality Assurance Programs in Nursing. Philadelphia, JB Lippincott, 1980
36. Committee for Development of Guidelines, Metropolitan Washington Affiliate of Association for Care of Children's Health: Psychosocial Policy Guidelines for Administration of Pediatric Health Care Facilities. Washington, DC, Association for Care of Children's Health, 1980
37. Klopovich P, Suenram D, Cairns N: A common sense approach to caring for children with cancer: The community health nurse. Cancer Nurs 40:201–208, 1980
38. Kagen-Goodheart L: Re-entry: Living with childhood cancer. Am J Orthopsychiatry 47:651–658, 1977
39. Chekiyn J, Deegan M, Reid J: Normalizing the return to school of the child with cancer. J Assoc Pediatr Oncol Nurses 3(2):20–24,34, 1986
40. McCormick D: School re-entry program for oncology patients. J Assoc Pediatr Oncol Nurses 3(3):13–17, 25, 1986
41. National Cancer Institute in Cooperation with Washington, DC, Metropolitan Candlelighters and Department of Pediatric Hematology-Oncology at University of Kansas Medical Center: Students with Cancer: A Resource for the Educator. NIH Publ no 80-2086. Bethesda, MD, National Cancer Institute, 1980
42. Kleinberg S: Facilitating the child's entry to school and coordinating school activities during hospitalization. In Home Care for Children with Serious Handicapping Conditions: A Report on a Conference Held May 21, 1984, Houston, TX. Washington, DC, Association for Care of Children's Health, 1984
43. Moore IM, Triplet JL: Students with cancer: A school nursing perspective. Cancer Nurs 3(4):265–270, 1980
44. Whaley LF, Wong DL: Children, their families, and the nurse. In Whaley LF,

Wong DL (eds): Nursing Care of Infants and Children, 2nd ed, pp 3–77. St Louis, CV Mosby, 1983

45. Ack M: Psychosocial effects of illness, hospitalization and surgery. Child Health Care 11(4):132–136, 1983

46. Arneson SW, Triplett JL: How children cope with disfiguring changes in their appearance. Am J Maternal Child Nurs 3:366–370, 1978

47. Waskerwitz MJ, Fergusson J: The late effects of cancer treatment in children. In Hockenberry MJ, Coody DK (eds): Pediatric Hematology and Oncology: Perspectives in Care, pp 469–492. St Louis, CV Mosby, 1986

48. Oncology Nursing Society Guidelines and Recommendations for Nursing Education and Practice. Oakmont, PA, Oncology Nursing Society, 1984

49. Minyard K, Wall J, Turner R: RN's may cost less than you think. J Nursing Admin 16(5):28–34, 1986

50. Grohar ME, Meyers J, McSweeney M: A comparison of patient acuity and nursing resource use. J Nursing Admin 16(6):19–23, 1986

51. Gallagher J: Developing a powerful and acceptable nurse staffing system. Nurs Management 18(3):45–49, 1987

52. Gibbons MG, Boren H: Stress reduction. A spectrum of strategies in pediatric oncology nursing. Nurs Clin North Am 20:83–103, 1985

53. Cogliano–Shutta NA: Pediatric Phase I clinical trials: Ethical issues and nursing considerations. Oncol Nurs Forum 13(2):29–32, 1986

54. Verzemmeks IL, Nash D: Ethical issues related to pediatric care. Nurs Clin North Am 19:319–328, 1984

55. Antonelli DM: Data management and the cancer treatment protocol. Cancer Nursing 4:477–478, 1982

56. Grant MM, Padilla GV: An overview of cancer nursing research. Oncol Nurs Forum 20(1):58–69, 1983

57. Lauer ME, Mulhern RK, Hoffman RG, Camitta BM: Utilization of hospice/homecare in pediatric oncology: A national survey. Cancer Nurs 9:102–107, 1986

58. Moore IM, Kramer J, Albin A: Late effects of central nervous system prophylactic leukemia therapy on cognitive function. Oncol Nurs Forum 4(13):45–53, 1986

59. Broome ME: The child in pain: A model for assessment and intervention. Crit Care Q 8(1):47–55, 1985

forty-seven

Rehabilitation of the Child with Cancer

Lynn H. Gerber and Helga Binder

Rehabilitation is a process designed to restore, maintain, or prevent the decline of function that may result from a disability. Function is defined broadly and includes physical, social, psychological, vocational, and educational activity.

It is estimated that a significant number of patients with cancer have functional disabilities that are amenable to rehabilitation interventions.[1] There are barriers to comprehensive rehabilitation that are often the result of the primary physician's failure to identify functional problems, which stems from a lack of knowledge of rehabilitation and its usefulness for cancer patients. The goal of this chapter is to help the pediatrician (or other pediatric specialist who treats children with cancer) gain a clear understanding of what rehabilitation is and what it can offer the child with cancer. The physician should be able to identify functional problems and make appropriate referrals to rehabilitation specialists.

Rehabilitation evaluations and treatments are of necessity comprehensive and address issues of mobility, activities of daily living, stamina, speech and language, and behavior. These assessments are done by a team of professionals from multiple disciplines. Most medical facilities provide rehabilitation services. The most common team structure includes a physician (oncologist or physiatrist), social worker, physical therapist, occupational therapist, nurse, and psychologist.[2] Others who may be included are speech pathologists, vocational or educational counselors, dietitians, and chaplains. Each medical facility may vary the particulars of the team model, but most use conferences to present each individual professional's findings and develop a comprehensive therapeutic plan designed to maximize the child's functional abilities. Table 47-1 provides a list of a typical rehabilitation team members and their responsibilities.

All rehabilitation team members must be familiar with the impact of the tumor and of its biological properties on function at specific stages (*e.g.*, acute, chronic, or terminal). They should be aware of the effects that cancer treatments (surgery, radiation, and chemotherapy) have on function and on the child's quality of life and development. Although much of the effort rehabilitation medicine invests in patient care is directed toward maximizing physical performance, all caregivers share responsibility for the psychosocial needs of the child and for alerting family and school to the role they play in reaching a good functional outcome for the child.

The child with cancer presents a unique challenge to the rehabilitation specialist because his needs and skills change constantly; the progression of needs may create previously unidentified problems. It is critical that rehabilitation team members continue to monitor the child's functional change so that the interventions can be synchronized with the child's developmental needs.

Table 47-1
The Cancer Rehabilitation Team

Member	Roles
Physiatrist	Diagnose neuromusculoskeletal impairment and developmental delay
	Assess impact or impairments on function
	Develop multidisciplinary treatment plan to maximize function
	Prescribe prosthetics, orthotics
Physical therapist	Evaluate strength, range of motion, posture, mobility
	Develop treatment plans designed to improve deficits or prevent decline using heat, cold, hydrotherapy, electricity, gait aids
	Ambulation training for amputees and children needing orthoses
Occupational therapist	Evaluate hand function, independence in activities of daily living, and educational status
	Develop treatment plans designed to improve upper extremity strength and function
	Provide adaptive equipment to promote independence
	Train in use of upper extremity prosthesis and orthoses
Speech pathologist	Evaluate language production and comprehension
	Evaluate oral motor status and swallowing
	Develop strategies to augment cognitive function, speech, and swallowing
Rehabilitation nurse	Evaluate patient's (family's) comprehension of the treatment plan and ability to take medication and maintain proper hygiene
	Educate family and patient for hospital and home treatment
Social worker	Evaluate family and community support to meet parents' needs
	Counsel in family dynamics, coping strategies, financial and community resources
Psychologist	Evaluate psychological adjustment to illness and body changes
	Counsel with respect to stress management and coping strategies
	Provide biofeedback and relaxation training for stress management in age-appropriate children
Vocational counselor	Evaluate impact of tumor on education and employment
	Review school or work site for accessibility
	Identify school and career interests
	Counsel with respect to proper educational and job placement
	Recommend retraining or reeducation when appropriate
	Inform patients of appropriate legislation pertaining to handicapping conditions

REHABILITATION EVALUATION

The physiatric evaluation of a child with cancer combines many aspects of a pediatric, neurologic, and orthopedic examination, with emphasis on delineation of functional limitations and their impact on the child's development.[3] The result should be a realistic plan for remedial approaches to assist the child in developing as normally as possible and in the least restrictive environment.

Like every medical examination, the rehabilitation examination begins with a thorough history. In contrast to the usual pediatric examination, previous illnesses are of less interest than premorbid lags or strengths in the acquisition of language, fine and gross motor skills, and personal-social style, and the ways in which the malignancy has led to functional limitations and—especially in infants and young children—in developmental regression. An accurate assessment of a child's premorbid functional status is the basis for a realistic rehabilitation plan. For instance, a child who has never had athletic interests will be less functionally and emotionally impaired by a permanent limp than a child whose whole life revolved around competitive sports.

In the case of a very young or very fearful child, the initial assessment is a good time for observing the child unobtrusively; appropriate toys requiring gross and fine motor skills, language, and interaction with caretakers must be provided toward this end. Attention, motivation, endurance, and specific limitations will be readily apparent, as will behavioral aberrations.

Spontaneous play often leads naturally into the formal functional and developmental assessment, which is the unique element of the physiatric evaluation. Prehension and visual-motor and visual-preceptual skills can be observed, and an assessment of cognitive and language development can easily be gained during table-top activities using paper and pencil, blocks, puzzles, and form boards.[4] The physiatrist should also observe the child undressing, which provides an opportunity to evaluate balance and coordination.

The assessment of gross motor skills begins with a gait assessment, which, for example, may reveal hemiparetic or ataxic gait patterns associated with central nervous system (CNS) tumors; this evaluation can be enhanced by asking the child to perform more demanding motor tasks, such as running, hopping, and skipping. More intricate age-appropriate motor tasks will also bring out gross incoordination of the type commonly seen after whole-brain irradiation. Chemotherapy-related neuropathy may result in a steppage gait due to drop foot, whereas children with pain due to soft tissue or bone tumors may limp or refuse to walk at all.

The orthopedic aspect of the physiatric examination is the musculoskeletal examination, which begins with observation of the child's posture and spinal alignment in sitting and standing positions, with special concern for head tilts, scoliosis, or kyphosis. Because posture and joint alignment in the lower extremities change with age, it is necessary that the examiner be familiar with normal postures at certain ages, such as hyperlordosis in the 3-year-old and valgus knees in the 4-year-old.[5]

In the case of scoliosis, it is important to establish whether it is functional (due to pelvic obliquity and perhaps an underlying leg length discrepancy) or structural, and whether there is associated pain and paraspinal muscle spasm. Mobility of the spine is assessed, again paying attention to associated pain. Extremity length and girth measurements reveal asymmetries. The examination concludes with inspection and palpation of muscles and subcutaneous tissues and active and passive range of motion measurements of the major joints, again attending to associated pain and muscle spasm. (Assessment of muscle strength is discussed later.)

The neurologic examination[6] should include evaluation of cranial nerves III, IV, VI, VII, VIII, IX, and X in all children who can be expected to have deficits, primarily those patients with posterior fossa tumors. The neurologic examination must be age-specific; children under age 3 cannot follow specific instructions, whereas school-age children can be tested as adults. However, even in infants, the presence and absence of vision can usually be established; malalignment of the eyes at rest and with visual pursuit of a toy is easily visible, as are nystagmus and limitations in extraocular movements. A visual field defect or diplopia is often suspected by the parents if a child tends to ignore stimuli from one side or tilts the head when focusing. Even small children will close one eye when this eliminates diplopia. Facial paralysis is obvious. Accurate testing of hearing for children under 5 years of age should be done by an audiologist. Gross hearing loss in the infant can be established by using rattles or bells. Total or partial paralysis of the 9th and 10th nerves can be suspected if the child has profound trouble handling secretions and shows return of food from the nose and aspiration. The gag may be absent or depressed; vocalizations may have a nasal quality.

Neuromuscular testing consists of testing of muscle strength, tone, and reflexes. In children younger than 4 or 5 years, formal manual muscle testing is usually not possible. Observation of spontaneous antigravity movements and functional testing is used instead.[7] In very young infants, primary reflexes such as the Moro or grasp provide valuable information about strength of the muscles involved in the response. Pulling the child up from supine will give good information about neck and shoulder flexors and adductors, the biceps, wrist, and finger flexors, as well as abdominal muscle strength. Holding a child in axillary suspension gives information about the strength of the shoulder depressors. Letting a child jack-knife forward while holding him or her around the hips permits assessment of neck and back extensor strength as the child struggles to raise himself or herself. Observation of how a child assumes the kneeling and standing position and of the gait allows assessment of hip girdle and lower extremity strength. In short, there is almost endless variety in functional assessment of strength. However, children are also very clever at substitutions, and a casual observer may be fooled. Quantitative testing in preschool children requires a very experienced examiner because of the wide range of normal variations in strength. However, comparison with the normal side will usually permit quite reliable quantitation.[3] Tone, unless extremely high or low, may have to be assessed several times, but the movement patterns observed during functional assessment are usually helpful.

Deep tendon reflexes are more easily elicited in the lower extremities because children tend to tense their arms or withdraw them forcefully. Hypo- or hyperreflexia is easily estab-lished, but subtle reflex asymmetries may be difficult to discern if the child cannot or will not cooperate. Abdominal, cremasteric, and anal reflexes are easily elicited and information in children with spinal lesions.

Testing of sensation is limited to pinprick in the preschool child. An intelligent young school-age child can be expected to give accurate information about vibration and position sense. In the young child, inability to stand still and a wide-based ataxic gait may indicate sensory or proprioceptive loss. Cortical sensation testing and formal cerebellar function testing can be accomplished by 6 to 8 years of age.[8,9]

Electrodiagnostic evaluation can substantiate and delineate the clinical findings if lower motor neuron problems have been established.[10] In a child with a spinal cord tumor, for instance, all signs of active denervation as well as decreased recruitment of motor unit action potentials compatible with the degree of weakness will be found in the weak extremity, as well as the paraspinal muscles. Children with vincristine-induced neuropathy will show varying degrees of demyelination or axonal loss and slowing of nerve conduction velocities. In patients with facial nerve paralysis secondary to posterior fossa or brain-stem tumors, it is important to establish evidence of nerve continuity, degree of denervation, and evidence of reinnervation in order to predict the chance for recovery.

With all the gathered information in hand, the physiatrist must then decide on the most appropriate therapies, appliances (e.g., orthoses, prostheses), and changes in the home and school environment that will permit the patient to function as normally and comfortably as possible. This decision is usually made with the help of the rehabilitation team and is then presented to patients (if they are old enough) or to their parents. It is very important to explain what rehabilitation problems have to be anticipated and how, from experience, they are best solved. It is imperative to be honest, but one should focus on positive and hopeful aspects of outcome rather than just possible complications. It is especially helpful if children and families can meet a patient with a similar malignancy who has undergone surgery and treatment and is actively involved in a rehabilitation program.

IMPACT OF TUMOR ON FUNCTION

Age-Specific Concerns

It can be generally stated that the younger the child at the time of cancer diagnosis, the more complex the rehabilitation problems. Pediatric oncology patients are growing, developing human beings and are therefore physically, cognitively, and emotionally vulnerable to all insults interfering with normal growth and development. Development is threatened not only by a deadly disease but also by therapies that result in a high degree of morbidity.

An exception are two tumor types that affect the extremely young child and have very favorable outcomes when treated in the first year of life—neuroblastoma[11] and Wilms' tumor.[12] A very young child will not remember the discomfort associated with the treatment. Growth and development, although temporarily arrested, may progress in a normal fashion with minimal or no sequelae once the child has successfully completed treatment, particularly if radiation was not used. The recognition of late sequelae has resulted in modification of radiotherapeutic techniques, producing a lower incidence of these sequelae.

The impact of a malignancy on the physical, cognitive, and emotional development of a child differs according to age groups because specific problems must be anticipated at the various stages of development.

Infancy and Preschool Years

Partial or complete limb ablation, excision and radiation of bone and soft tissue tumors, laminectomies, and radiation of the spine produce major musculoskeletal problems at this age because of the tremendous growth potential left. Very young children are also extremely sensitive to chemotherapy, especially with vincristine, which may cause profound neuropathy and hypotonia leading to temporary loss of acquired motor skills and even inability to feed orally, with very slow recovery over weeks to months.[13] Cognitive development will be permanently impaired in a considerable number of children under the age of 8 years who require radiation or radiation plus intrathecal methotrexate for treatment or prophylaxis of CNS leukemia or for treatment of brain tumors. The deficits range from mild loss of cognitive ability to profound retardation in a previously normal child.[14–22]

Personal-social development in infants and young children will be temporarily halted or may even regress during treatment for a malignancy. These changes may persist in those children who have suffered a permanent cognitive deficit. However, children who survive cognitively intact but physically impaired tend to make a remarkable functional recovery because of their inherent ability to adapt and to compensate for skills that had not yet been firmly established at the time of tumor impact.

Preadolescence

Musculoskeletal problems in the preadolescent child are still considerable because of the remaining growth potential of spine and limbs. Adaptation to a functional deficit is more difficult because dominance is firmly established and balance and coordination skills have been perfected. True retraining must take place; this is easier than in the adult, but not as natural as in the infant.

Because brain growth and myelination are largely completed, the cerebrospinal axis is less sensitive to radiation, and cognitive development appears to proceed normally in the majority of cases, unless tumor location and removal lead to impairment.

Personal-social development is severely affected at this age because the child's normal ability to function quite independently in the areas of mobility and self-care are, at least temporarily, markedly impaired. The child will become much more dependent on his caretakers, who may become overly protective. Children in this age group are not very accepting of mobility or adaptive aids and are frequently unwilling participants in rehabilitation, particularly if exercises are to be performed with the help of the parents.

Adolescence

Musculoskeletal problems become less difficult to handle in older children because extremity and spinal growth are largely completed. However, adolescents seem to have more severe sensory-motor neuropathies associated with vincristine therapy which, although reversible, may persist for months and considerably impair ambulation and fine motor activity.[13] Cognitive deficits resulting from therapy are rare, except in cases of brain tumors.

Personal-social functioning in the adolescent tends to be less related to actual loss of physical ability than to emotional state. The adolescent is a human being with established physical strengths and weaknesses, who may have to completely change his lifestyle and career goals, as in the case of an athlete or musician who has lost a limb. Emotional problems in the pediatric cancer patient are discussed in detail in Chapter 41. However, since the ability to successfully participate in a rehabilitation program depends to a large part on the patient's emotional state, these problems are mentioned briefly here.

Except in the very young infant, emotional problems must be expected and are related to diagnosis, as far as the child is able to comprehend it; pain and stress associated with treatment procedures; temporary and lasting bodily changes; long and repeated hospitalizations; and reentry into society, often with permanent physical or neurologic deficits.[23,24]

Emotional and behavioral problems can severely affect the child's rehabilitation, especially in preadolescence and adolescence, when self-image and fitting into the peer group are extremely important.[25] School phobia[26] is frequent, especially when the child has visible physical or noticeable functional changes, such as scars, a prosthesis, or the need for other mobility aids such as canes or a wheelchair.

Impact of the Natural History of Tumors on Function

Rehabilitation interventions may differ as the child progresses through the phases of cancer. Initially, child and family may need support and education about the future process rather than actual physical therapeutic interventions. As time progresses, the long-term effects of treatment and persistent or recurrent tumor may warrant different interventions. The phase-specific events can be divided into early or initial phase, chronic or intermittent phase, and terminal phase.

Early Phase

Many pediatric tumors are curable, but some cures are achieved at great cost to the growing child. Table 47-2 summarizes the childhood tumors that most commonly prompt referral for rehabilitation intervention, and the functional problem the tumor is likely to present during the initial stage. At the time of presentation, children may not be febrile, weak, or clinically ill. When this is the case, the rehabilitation process is best begun immediately because patient cooperation and participation in his treatment are likely to be good at this time. Instruction in ambulation with crutches or in exercise is more easily given if the patient is pain-free and mobile, so preoperative or preradiation intervention is highly desirable.

Once definitive treatment is begun, the nature of the problems changes. Those undergoing ablative surgery need to recover from surgery and adapt to a major change in body image and function. Soft tissue resections and radiation, *en bloc* resections, and implants produce less radical body image changes, but often have a more protracted hospital course; thus, ongoing rehabilitation is necessary to reduce extremity edema and mobility problems.[27]

If definitive treatment is radiation therapy to the extremity, the brain, or a vital organ, the rehabilitation staff can see the patient during the initial treatment phase. The purposes of such visits are to support and comfort the child and family and to begin preventive stretching and strengthening to body parts being irradiated. Radiation causes skin and underlying soft tissue to react with some degree of fibrosis and a stretching program often helps to maintain a functional range of motion (ROM), minimizing the risk of contracture.

The majority of children with cancer are likely to be re-

Table 47-2
Presenting Symptoms Frequently Seen in Some Childhood Cancers

Tumor	Presenting Symptoms	Deficits	Treatments
Bone tumor Soft tissue tumor	Extremity pain Stiffness Limp Limited daily activity	Bone lesions Extremity mass	ROM, strengthening exercise Mobility aids Orthoses/prostheses Education Pain management

Brain tumor
  Posterior fossa
 	
  Hemispheric lesion
	Vomiting
	Headache
	Mental or behavioral change
	Visual problems
	Balance and coordination problems
	Seizures
	Weakness
		Cranial nerve deficit
		Ataxia
		Mild hemiparesis
		
		Stroke-like picture
			ROM, strengthening and
			  functional exercise for
			  upper and lower
			  extremities
			Orthoses, mobility devices
			Adaptive equipment
			Speech and oral–motor
			  therapy
			Special education

Spinal cord tumor	Weakness Stiffness or spasticity Limited daily activity Incontinence or constipation Numbness, tingling Scoliosis or torticollis	Paraparasis Hemiparesis Sensory loss Muscle atrophy Neurogenic bowel/bladder Scoliosis	ROM, strengthening and functional exercise Gait training Orthoses Bladder/bowel training Intermittent catheterization

ceiving chemotherapy, occasionally in conjunction with radiation and surgery. Many of these regimens last 1 to 2 years or longer and create a chronic, often intermittent, relationship with the oncology program. Some of these children have illnesses that may require multiple operations, parenteral nutrition, and management of other medical problems (*e.g.,* hormonal, cardiorespiratory); ongoing rehabilitation support is often necessary to maintain strength, mobility, stamina, and independent function. Some data suggest that ongoing exercise is necessary to aid the incorporation of amino acids delivered parenterally into protein.[28]

Chronic Phase

Chronic continuous or intermittent illness usually requires an ongoing rehabilitation program that addresses management of fatigue, weakness, and pain. The growing child will need frequent evaluation of braces, crutches, and prostheses to ensure proper fit.

Musculoskeletal changes are among the relatively common delayed effects of radiation. Patients who have received radiation to the vertebrae before age 10 are likely to develop kyphosis and scoliosis.[29,30] The scoliosis is clearly structural; if it exceeds 25°, it should be evaluated by an orthopedist for possible correction.

Radiation of long bones for solid tumors of the extremity is often associated with limb shortening and fibrosis of soft tissue when the total dose exceeds 5000 cGy.[31–33] Treatment should include an ROM program that continues to prevent joint contracture and corrects the leg length discrepancy. A limb length difference in excess of 1.5 cm accompanied by functional scoliosis and limp should be corrected with an external lift to balance the pelvis and reduce compensatory scoliosis.

Whole-brain irradiation, particularly in younger children, may cause brain atrophy and neuropsychological dysfunc-

tion.[34] Radiation myelitis, with spasticity at levels below the radiation or frank quadriplegia or paraplegia, also requires referral for training to maximize independence.[35] Some antineoplastic drugs are associated with impairment of the neuromusculoskeletal system, and children so affected can often be helped by rehabilitation.

Peripheral neuropathy can result from vincristine, vinblastine, or cisplatin therapy. This sensorimotor neuropathy is often partial and may be reversible.[13] Mild strengthening exercises, use of adaptive equipment (foot drop splint), and education of the child to use visual rather than sensory cues for daily activity are the therapeutic interventions used.

Several chemotherapeutic agents—particularly actinomycin D, Adriamycin, and streptozocin—can cause severe tissue necrosis if they extravasate. In addition to the immediate local care needed, if the necrosis occurs around a joint, it is most important to ensure that the joint is in a functional position if the extremity needs to be immobilized. During the healing phase, motion should be initiated as soon as possible to gain function. Range of motion is an essential intervention if a functional recovery is to occur because the lesion, much like a burn, will heal with scarring. Tendons and joint capsules contract as a result of healing or of immobility, and joint contracture occurs.

Children receiving intrathecal medication, particularly those who have received cranial irradiation, are at risk of developing CNS deficits, including cerebellar, cranial nerve, and cortical damage.[36] These children may also become delayed in physical growth and development.[37] We are just beginning to learn more of the delayed effects on cognitive development.[22,25]

Finally, bone marrow transplantation can result in a graft versus host syndrome that is associated with skin changes not unlike scleroderma. Joint contractures and muscle atrophy can result from this and should be treated. Children with this syndrome do very well with hydrotherapy or therapeutic pool activity that permits ROM to all extremities. A warm pool also permits relaxation and buoyancy of limbs, thereby reducing the effort of motion.

Terminal Phase

Children who have unresectable, incurable, or untreatable cancers are in need of rehabilitation intervention to control pain, preserve independence and support age-appropriate behavior. Heat, cold, and transcutaneous electrical nerve stimulation (TENS) units are often helpful in controlling bone and soft tissue pain. Bed positioning, isometric exercise, active ROM, and the use of proper supportive cushioning materials to maintain skin integrity in the bed-bound patient are helpful. Protective ambulation using crutches and canes is essential for patients with metastatic lesions that have destroyed cortex of weight bearing bones. A summary of chronic and terminal phase rehabilitation needs is presented in Table 47-3.

TUMOR OR TREATMENT-RELATED CNS DEFICITS

CNS Tumors

The rehabilitation approach to children with brain and spinal cord tumors varies according to tumor type and severity of symptoms at the time of diagnosis. Although children with inoperable or widely disseminated CNS tumors and no hope of cure are not candidates for restorative rehabilitation, they should receive physiatric attention for generalized conditioning, prevention of contractures and deformities and, if appropriate, pain-relieving physical therapy modalities.

Almost all CNS tumors are initially treated by surgical excision, complete or incomplete, which may be followed by radiation, chemotherapy, or both, depending on the tumor type. In the immediate postoperative period, nurses under the supervision of a physiatrist customarily provide skin care, postural drainage, and contracture-preventing positioning and passive ROM exercises of paralyzed limbs. They can also apply prefabricated or custom-made splints for the distal extremities and, in the case of flaccid paralegia or quadriplegia, elastic stockings to prevent venostasis.

Once the patient is medically stable, wounds are healed, and the oncologic protocol has been decided, the patient should be thoroughly assessed by the physiatrist and short-, intermediate-, and, if possible, long-term rehabilitation goals should be established and discussed with the patient, family, and rehabilitation team. These will differ considerably, of course, depending on the patient's neurologic deficit and age, which in turn determine growth and potential for development.

The patient treated for supratentorial or hemispheric tumor will usually present with a stroke-like picture consisting of spastic hemiparesis or quadriparesis, hemisensory deficit, possible hemianopsia, aphasia, dysarthria, and parietal lobe deficits, in any combination. Children with tumors in the vicinity of the optic chiasm may be partially or completely blind. Tumors involving the basal ganglia frequently cause involuntary movements. Children treated for infratentorial tumors tend to show mild flaccid hemiparesis, ataxia, and cranial nerve palsies, and often have ventriculoperitoneal shunts. Cerebral edema associated with the surgery may initially aggravate the functional deficit and may also cause mental depression.

These neurologic deficits should be addressed by physical therapy, which may begin with facilitated movement of a partially paralyzed limb and advance to strengthening exercises, progressive bed mobility, sitting balance, and finally ambulation. At that time, mobility aids such as braces, walkers, or canes are introduced.

During this period, the occupational therapist tries to improve the strength and function of the upper extremity and introduces adaptive aids such as special eating utensils. He or she can also apply the expertise needed to feed a child with impaired oral-motor function. The occupational therapist's knowledge of sensory-motor integration techniques is very valuable in evaluating a child and treating deficits in cortical sensation, visual-motor, and visual-perceptual skills, in preparation for school reentry. Language deficits are usually much less severe than those observed in adults, but attention span, motivation, and memory often interfere with rehabilitation.

Once the rehabilitation program is well established and the family is familiar with all aspects of the child's care, the child is usually discharged home and ongoing therapy is arranged through community agencies. If the child is not well enough to attend school, a home tutor will be requested; very specific instructions for remedial teaching techniques must be provided to school or homebound teachers. Physiatric follow-up has to remain very close in order to detect neurologic and functional changes and to adapt the rehabilitation program accordingly.

Once patients complete the cancer treatment program and their neurologic and functional status stabilize, the emphasis is on preventing musculoskeletal problems during the growing years, especially contractures and deformities of paralyzed or spastic limbs and spinal curvatures, by ongoing physical and occupational therapy and optimal bracing. Nonambulatory pa-

---

Table 47-3
Rehabilitation Needs of Children with Tumors in Chronic or Terminal Phases

Condition	Deficit	Treatment
Laminar flow status	Decreased sensory stimulation Limited mobility	Sensory stimulation ROM and isometric exercise Support functional independence
Bed bound	Deconditioning Contractures Skin breakdown Regression	Isometric and ROM exercises (active or active assisted) Frequent turning Proper mattress Sensory stimulation Socialization
Chemotherapy	Cardiomyopathy Neuropathy (sensory and motor)	Maintain physiologic condition Orthoses Adaptive equipment
Radiation	CNS—Mental retardation or learning disability Spine—Myelitis, scoliosis or torticollis Limb—Fibrosis, contractures, pain, stiffness	Special education Continued active ROM exercises

tients need appropriate wheelchair prescriptions. All children will be reintegrated as much as possible into their home and school environment and will receive the needed therapies as part of their school day. Long-term follow-up reports of patients treated for brain tumors indicate that the physical handicaps may be fairly subtle, particularly following posterior fossa tumors. More debilitating are distractibility, poor memory, and learning disabilities.[38-43] Behavioral problems are common. Thus, the role of the physiatrist in long-term follow-up of brain tumor patients often focuses less on monitoring motor deficits and more on securing the most appropriate school and home environment, with support and counseling for the patient as well as the family.

Spinal Cord Tumors

Most children with these tumors require an extensive laminectomy and postoperative spinal radiation. The child's functional deficit may be substantial in the immediate postoperative period because of the surgery and associated spinal cord swelling. The shorter the history and the less the neurological deficit, the better the outlook for functional recovery.[38,45]

The outlook for 5-year survival increases with lower levels of spinal involvement.[46] The rehabilitation approach varies greatly depending on the patient's functional deficits, which may range from partial paralysis of one limb to paraplegia or quadriplegia. Neurogenic bladder and bowel problems are almost always present.

In the case of flaccid or spastic monoparesis, the emphasis is on strengthening and bracing, and the eventual functional outcome can be expected to be favorable. Partial or complete quadriplegia or paraplegia, must be treated like a spinal cord injury. Physical therapy begins with strengthening exercises for trunk and extremities and progress to bed mobility and ambulation if feasible. If spasiticity sets in and cannot be controlled with splints, inhibitive casts for upper and lower extremities can be applied, and tone-reducing medication may be used (dantrolene sodium, 0.5 mg/kg b.i.d.; this increased slowly to 3.0 mg/kg q.i.d., not to exceed 100 mg q.i.d.). Liver function tests must be performed regularly, and the lowest effective dose should be used. Dantrolene may be used for intractable spasticity in children with brain tumors. Baclofen is increasingly accepted for use in older children with spasticity due to spinal cord lesions.

Occupational therapy attends to improve upper extremity function, provides the most appropriate assistive and seating devices, and helps the family to adapt the home environment to the child's needs, particularly if the patient is wheelchair-bound.

Initial bowel and bladder management may fall to the physiatrist or the urologist. If the child is incontinent, frequent checks of residual urine following voiding are mandatory. If incontinence persists for more than a few days, or the child is unable to void, clean intermittent catheterization will be instituted. Cystometrograms should be performed at intervals to follow the status of the neurogenic bladder.

Before the patient is discharged, the family or caretakers are instructed in all aspects of the child's care. Rehabilitation in most cases continues in the community with supervision by the physiatrist.

If the child has a persistent paraplegia or quadriplegia, follow-up usually takes place in a spina bifida clinic, because the services of so many disciplines (neurosurgery, physiatry, urology, and usually orthopedics) are needed.

The physiatrist is concerned with the development of a scoliosis, especially if the laminectomy was extensive, the child is young, and trunk muscle strength is asymmetric. Initially the curvature may be contained in a spinal orthosis, but spinal fusion may be required once the child reaches adolescence.

Flaccid and spastic paralyses of the limbs are equally difficult to handle in the growing child and usually require bracing, occasionally preceded by chemical neurolysis of the spastic adductors of the hips or by orthopedic surgery for soft tissue releases, obturator neurectomies, or hip stabilization procedures.

In flaccid monoparesis, a considerable leg length discrepancy may develop. Children who cannot ambulate have to be carefully fitted with standing aids (parapodium, Motostand) or mobility devices such as manual or powered wheelchairs. As the child gets older, the danger of decubiti increases markedly, particularly in the nonambulatory patient, and the child must take most of the responsibility for weight relief while sitting as well as for contracture prevention.

Like children who have been treated for a brain tumor, these patients should return to school as soon as possible and should receive the needed therapy there. However, unlike many patients after brain surgery, they should be academically mainstreamed because they usually do not develop cognitive impairment or learning disabilities.

Both groups of patients should be encouraged to participate in recreational and other social activities as much as possible—particularly while still undergoing cancer therapy. Especially valuable are camp experiences with other cancer victims, which permit children to freely discuss their feelings with similarly afflicted peers and often help the parents to be less overprotective.[47]

Unfortunately, there are no long-term follow-up studies of cancer patients describing physical development in any detail, and the very high rates of good functional outcome in survivors of cerebrospinal cancers, for instance, are most likely due to the fact that subtle physical handicaps were not noted as deficits.[38,40,45] Even less likely to be noted are learning disabilities and abnormal behaviors.

TUMOR- OR TREATMENT-RELATED MUSCULOSKELETAL DEFICITS

Nearly all tumors that affect children can involve the musculoskeletal system, either primarily or secondarily. The most frequent sites of involvement are the lower extremities, followed by the upper extremities and head, neck, and trunk. The most frequent presenting sign is pain, followed by functional loss caused by the tumor or its treatment.

Preventive Measures

The child who is confined to bed is at risk for developing decubiti, muscle wasting, and joint contractures from disuse. In addition, deconditioning of the cardiovascular system and loss of ability to resume an upright position can occur within a week. Children kept on bed rest because of surgery or significant illness often regress and do not maintain self-care and other daily activity skills.

The physiatrist can review bed positioning, instruct staff in proper posture to avoid knee flexion contractures and heel cord tightening, and stress the need for bed mobility to minimize the possibility of developing decubiti. Chest physical therapy can be initiated if needed.

Restorative Measures: Prostheses

Lower Extremity

Children with amputations of the lower extremity including below knee, above knee, and hip disarticulations or hemipelvectomy can become functional ambulators with the use of prostheses (Fig. 47-1). Even children with metastatic disease and poor prognosis can benefit from prosthetic use.

The influential work of Burgess radically changed the management of amputees in this country.[48] The application of a plaster cast to the stump at the time of amputation has decreased the amount of time required to shape a stump to a sufficiently mature condition to permit the fitting of a final prosthesis.[49] This has benefited children with cancer immeasureably by enabling them to be upright and ambulatory quickly and has enhanced their quality of life. There is evidence suggesting that rigid dressings also decrease postoperative pain and phantom limb symptoms (Fig. 47-2).[50]

CHOICE OF PROSTHESIS. The prescription of a prosthesis requires some knowledge of the child's needs, including daily routines and desires and the environment in which he or she lives. Options for below knee amputees include exoskeletal units with strap or wedge suspensions and feet that compress at the heel or have an axis of rotation. The above knee prosthesis can be exoskeletal or endoskeletal. The latter is a metal tube with a soft foam cover. Very active children should receive an exoskeletal unit, because the soft cover of the endoskeletal prosthesis tears easily and will not withstand playground activity. An articulated ankle is necessary for walking on uneven terrain or for sports activities that require medial/lateral motion. The knee component most frequently prescribed for

young children is a single axis knee. It is safe, reliable, and durable. One shortcoming is that the knee does not permit the leg to speed up or slow down as gait cadence changes. For older children who want to run or participate in stop–start activity, a hydraulic unit is prescribed. It is heavier than the single axis and not quite as reliable, and is often prescribed for experienced or trained amputees. A hydraulic unit is rarely prescribed for hip disarticulation or hemipelvectomy patients (Fig. 47-3).

PROSTHETIC TRAINING. The lower extremity amputee should have early and ongoing rehabilitation. Early intervention is important to promote confidence, a positive attitude toward physical activity, and development of good standing and sitting posture, and to prevent deconditioning. An exercise program is begun that stretches hip and knee flexors to prevent flexion contractures and knee contractures. Strengthening of leg and thigh muscles is begun, and patients are taught how to wrap the stump in order to maintain its shape so it can fit into the prosthetic socket.

Ambulation training is begun in order to toughen the stump and train the child to tolerate prosthetic use, and to learn normal stride patterns, how to fall and get up from ground, to climb stairs, and to care for the stump and the prosthesis. Children are able to assume some responsibility for their own rehabilitation. Frequent return visits are mandatory to ensure that the prosthesis fits properly and the limb is the proper length; significant leg length discrepancies resulting from poor prosthetic fit will lead to a compensatory scoliosis.

Children are encouraged to engage in as much athletic activity as they desire, with the exception of contact sports. Children should swim and boat without the prosthesis. Snow

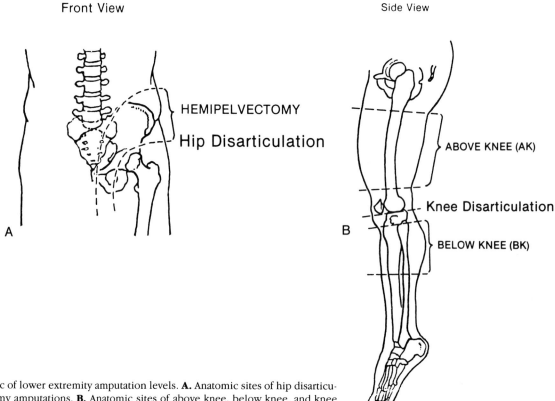

Front View   Side View

HEMIPELVECTOMY

Hip Disarticulation

ABOVE KNEE (AK)

Knee Disarticulation

BELOW KNEE (BK)

A   B

FIGURE 47-1. Schematic of lower extremity amputation levels. **A.** Anatomic sites of hip disarticulation and hemipelvectomy amputations. **B.** Anatomic sites of above knee, below knee, and knee disarticulation amputations.

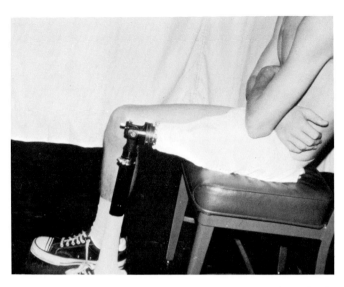

FIGURE 47-2. Rigid plaster above knee socket with polyvinyl chloride pylon attached.

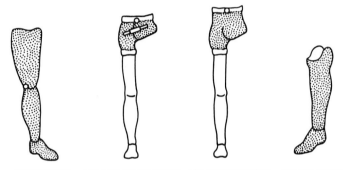

ABOVE KNEE　　HIP DISARTICULATION　　HEMIPELVECTOMY　　BELOW KNEE

FIGURE 47-3. Schematic of lower extremity prostheses. Depicted are the Above-knee suction socket, the Canadian-style hip disarticulation and hemipelvectomy, and the below-knee patellar tendon-bearing supracondylar prostheses.

skiing for children with above knee or higher level amputations should be done in a one-legged fashion. Several athletic associations have been developed for handicapped children and are a resource for training, equipment, and group activity.[51]

A review of the physical environment at home and school that considers access as well as safety is very helpful. Occupational therapists play an important role in recommending adaptive equipment for safety in the bathroom and improved function in the classroom.

Upper Extremity

Upper extremity prosthetic components offer some options as well. Patients with amputations of the upper extremity below the elbow usually have good prosthetic options and functional outcome. This is not the case for above elbow level amputations, including shoulder disarticulation and forequarter amputation, although many children adapt to one-handed activities (Fig. 47-4). The below elbow prosthesis can be equipped with an artificial hand or a hook. Either can be powered mechanically, by shrugging the shoulder, or myoelectrically.

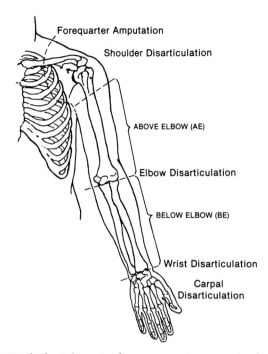

FIGURE 47-4. Schematic of upper extremity amputation levels.

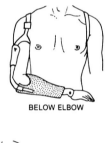

BELOW ELBOW

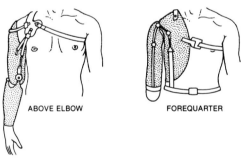

ABOVE ELBOW　　　　　FOREQUARTER

FIGURE 47-5. Schematic of upper extremity prostheses: below elbow, above elbow, and forequarter prostheses.

Children with higher level amputations can be offered a prosthetic option that combines mechanical and electrical power input, but training to use these devices in a functional way is often not rewarding (Figs. 47-5, 47-6).

Children with upper extremity amputation are good rehabilitation candidates. Cosmetically, a hand as a terminal device is often the most desirable component. Unfortunately, the hand is not a very functional unit. Despite its appearance, the hook is preferable, and we often recommend it to children who will accept it (Fig. 47-7). Another option is the myoelectric unit. This unit is powered by energy from a contracting

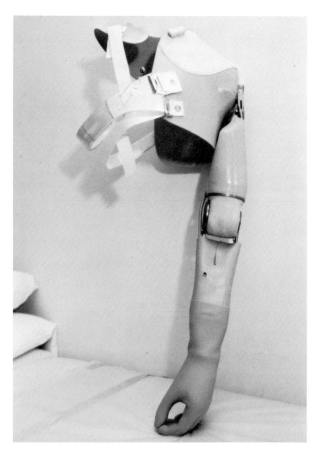

FIGURE 47-6.   Forequarter prosthesis with mechanical elbow and myoelectric terminal device.

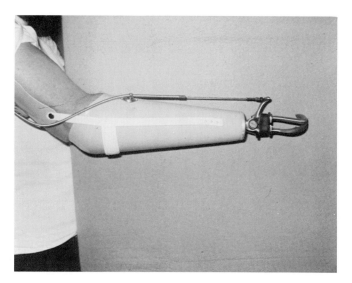

FIGURE 47-7.   Below-elbow prosthesis with hook as terminal device.

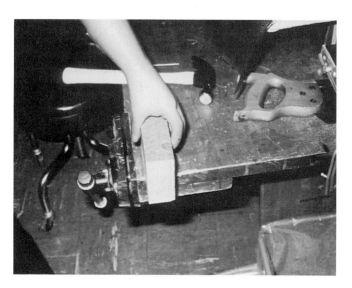

FIGURE 47-8.   Below-elbow prosthesis with myoelectric hand as terminal device.

muscle—often the brachialis—which causes an opening and closing of the hand. Myoelectric units can be used to power elbows as well as terminal devices, but the terminal device is more difficult to use and less functional than the hook (Fig. 47-8). There is as yet no consensus on whether the myoelectric unit is more functional than the mechanical unit. If the surgical level is above elbow or forequarter, we do not prescribe a prosthesis; one-handed activities are often the rehabilitative therapy of choice. We strongly urge a surgical procedure to preserve hand function, when possible. The Tikhoff–Linberg procedure resects proximal tumor, including bone and soft tissue, but leaves the distal unit intact.[52]

Training in activities of daily living for the one-armed child focuses on role-related needs; adapted equipment, such as plates with suction cups, knives with rocker blades, and Velcro fasteners or button hooks, can be provided.[53,54]

Orthoses

Limb support and joint stability are often problems for the cancer patient. Whether paresis results from tumor invasion of nerve, surgical excision of neuromuscular structures, or chemotherapy, the paretic limb should be supported in a position of comfort and greatest function. Splints and braces can control motion in order to minimize deformity and pain. A variety of hand and wrist splints are used. The functional wrist splint supports the wrist in a neutral position, permitting free

use of fingers. This is often used in radial nerve palsies. A "C" splint can help support thumb and index fingers in a position that permits pinch and grasp. A tenodesis splint utilizes the principle that wrist position can help control finger function and provides wrist extension in order to produce finger flexion and wrist flexion to produce finger extension.

Lower extremity orthoses can be used to unweight a painful area or provide stability. A patellar tendon-bearing brace can unweight a painful or paretic foot. An ischial weight-bearing long leg brace can provide limb support for the entire lower extremity and can unweight the entire limb by distributing weight across the upper rim of the brace, which sits under the ischium and upon which the patient sits. Patients with anterior tibialis weakness who walk with a foot drop can benefit from the use of an ankle-foot orthosis designed to keep the foot in neutral position. Often this brace is made of plastic and fits into the shoe, but if the instability is both in eversion–inversion and dorsi–plantar flexion, a double upright, Klenzak-type brace or one with flares over the malleoli is needed. Braces to control knee instability most often need to include the knee, ankle, and foot. A knee cage or elastic wrap with side stays is not sufficient to control knee motion.

If sensation is impaired or if position sense is diminished as a result of chemotherapy, a cane or crutch is recommended to enhance feedback. The upper extremity or the eyes are able to substitute for the sensory loss.

Often a child will prefer to use crutches rather than be slowed down by a prosthesis or orthosis. The comfortable walking speed is higher using gait aids than a prosthesis at the above knee or hip disarticulation/hemipelvectomy level. However, the use of a prosthesis is helpful in balancing the pelvis and minimizing scoliosis. It offers proprioceptive feedback for upper and lower extremity amputees and should be encouraged, when feasible.

Pain Management

Children with musculoskeletal problems that are due primarily to pain rather than loss of a limb or neuromuscular excision should be referred to rehabilitation specialists for evaluation of pain management. Musculoskeletal pain often responds to application of heat and cold, or postural interventions. These are particularly useful in the presence of muscle spasm. A splint or orthosis may reduce joint pain by limiting motion. The use of transcutaneous nerve stimulation has also been shown effective in treating cancer pain. Radicular, pleuritic, and incisional pain are often responsive to this modality (see Chap. 44).

Edema Management

Children who have had interruption of lymphatic drainage for surgical exploration or radiation therapy are likely to develop lymphedema of the treated extremity. Direct invasion of tumor (lymphoma or solid tumors) occasionally causes lymphedema. Edema management should be initiated as early as possible, with education about maintaining the extremity in a position in which gravity can help drain the limb and about frequent use of muscle relaxation–contraction to pump fluid out. If circumferential measures indicate a significant fluid retention, an elastic stockinette can be prescribed. We usually do this at an increase of 2 cm over the unaffected side. If the increase is greater, the use of compression pumps followed by a customized compression garment is recommended. This regimen has been reported to be useful in controlling edema.[57]

Exercise

Muscle atrophy and weakness resulting from disuse are often easily reversed with a strengthening exercise program, usually beginning with isometric contractions. As strength improves, a dynamic program can be initiated with some form of resistive exercise using weights or a weight system (*e.g.,* Nautilus) or a dynamometer (*e.g.,* Cybex). Joint contractures are best prevented by proper positioning and an active stretching program, but active assistive or passive stretching may be needed. The use of serial plaster casting or a brace with a dial lock or a continuous passive ROM machine can be used to relieve contractures. A stretching program is often accompanied by local heat to increase tendon elasticity or can be done in a therapeutic pool or with ultrasound delivered in water. Evidence exists to support the efficacy of superficial heat or deep heat in treating contractures.

When nutritional status is poor or chemotherapy directly affects cardiac performance, endurance and stamina are decreased; this may further thwart efforts to strengthen weak muscles. The outcome is a generalized deconditioning. An aerobic cardiovascular exercise program is added to the rehabilitation goals and often uses bicycle ergometry, arm ergometry, or progressive ambulation. The benefits of conditioning include increased stamina and strength, and evidence suggests that there is an antidepressant effect in adults that may also be true for children.[58]

An exercise program for children with cancer should be supervised by trained staff, familiar with the effects of chemotherapy, radiation, and tumor on the musculoskeletal and cardiopulmonary status of children. Often, a conditioning program is performed concomitly with isometric or range of motion exercise. The initial program begins at a level of exercise that can be done comfortably by the patient. This may be as low as 1 or 2 mets (a met is a measure of work equal to 3.5 ml oxygen/kg body weight/min). A level of 2 to 3 mets is needed for routine daily activity, whereas 7 to 8 mets are needed for running. The patient should be monitored by heart rate and rhythm, if necessary, and blood pressure.

Metastases to long bones, especially those of the lower extremity, are often evaluated from the perspective of their potential for fracture. When there is 50% or more cortical destruction, the bone is thought to be at significant risk for fracture and the limb should be unloaded with a crutch and the patient taught a three-point gait (the gait pattern that most unweights the limb). A brace designed to unweight the limb can be used also, such as a patellar tendon-bearing brace to unload the foot.

The musculoskeletal problems of the child with metastatic disease can be formidable. The psychological effects of recurrence are often profound and, coupled with associated physical problems, may overwhelm patient and family. Regardless of stage, the rehabilitation goals are to make the patient as comfortable and functional for as long a time as possible.

Educational and Occupational Counseling

Children with handicapping conditions are protected from discrimination under Section 504 of the Rehabilitation Act. The law states that schools must make a reasonable effort to accommodate handicapped children and must offer them access to regular public education.[59] Often, children with physical disability are shunted into special educational programs designed for those with intellectual impairments (see Chap. 51). In addition, children with cancer diagnoses may be considered uninsurable for health costs either as part of their family insurance plan or as adults applying for their own policy. The military assumes that persons with cancer histories are not fit for active duty.

Rehabilitation professionals are well versed in the laws pertaining to the rights of the handicapped and can advise patients and families about them. These professionals are uniquely qualified to counsel patients about educational and work environments, educate school administrators and employers about prognosis and performance capabilities of the cancer patient, and support patients in the pursuit of their legal rights under federal and state laws.[60]

Given the high likelihood of cure of childhood tumors, children should be supported and encouraged to lead as full and normal a life as possible, physically, educationally, vocationally, and socially. The rehabilitation team is uniquely qualified to help achieve these goals.

NEW DIRECTIONS IN REHABILITATION

Considerable effort is being directed toward developing lightweight thermoplastic materials to be used in orthoses and prostheses for children. These new materials will increase the likelihood of patient acceptance because of improved cosmetic appearance and ease of use. Motor-driven prostheses, using a small battery or myoelectrically powered systems, have been developed for upper extremity use. Computers are being used in the design and manufacture of these units.

Functional electrical stimulation is a technique whereby denervated muscle is stimulated to contract using an external source of electricity. This has been used primarily for persons with spinal cord injury to help them achieve some upright activity and weight bearing. Application to upper extremity function is also being evaluated. Some preliminary work is being done to assess the potential of implantable systems for restoring motion.

Development of new methods of enhancing the independence of handicapped children and making classrooms wheelchair-accessible are important areas requiring additional innovation. Small, easily maneuvered motorized wheelchairs are available for mobility independence. New materials have made these units lightweight and portable. Updates in key issues in the field of physical medicine and rehabilitation, with emphasis on research developments, are available.[61]

REFERENCES

1. Lehmann JF, De Lisa JA, Warren CG et al: Cancer rehabilitation: Assessment of need, development and evaluation of a model of care. Arch Phys Med Rehabil 59:410–419, 1978
2. Harvey RF, Jellinck HM, Habeck RV: Cancer rehabilitation: An analysis of 36 program approaches. JAMA 247:2127–2131, 1982
3. Molnar GE, Kellerman WC: History and examination. In Molnar GE (ed): Pediatric Rehabilitation. Baltimore, Williams & Wilkins, 1985
4. Knobloch H, Pasamanick B: Gesell and Amatruda's Developmental Diagnosis, 3rd ed. Hagerstown, MD, Harper & Row, 1974
5. Lowrey GH: Growth and Development of Children, 7th ed. Chicago, Year Book Medical Publishers, 1978
6. Baird HW, Gordon EC: Neurological Evaluation of Infants and Children. Clinics in Developmental Medicine Nos. 84/85: Spastics International Medical Publications. Philadelphia, JB Lippincott, 1983
7. Johnson EW: Examination for muscle weakness in infants and small children. JAMA 10:1306–1313, 1958
8. Denckla MB: Development of speed in repetition and successive finger movements in normal children. Dev Med Child Neurol 15:635–645, 1973
9. Denckla MB: Development of coordination in normal children. Dev Med Child Neurol 16:729–741, 1974
10. Kimura J: Electrodiagnosis in Diseases of Nerve and Muscle: Principles and Practice. Philadelphia, FA Davis, 1983
11. Lopez-Ibor B, Schwartz AD: Neuroblastoma. Pediatr Clin North Am 32:755–778, 1985
12. Green DM: The diagnosis and management of Wilm's tumor. Pediatr Clin North Am 32:735–751, 1985
13. Allen JC: The effects of cancer therapy on the nervous system. J Pediatr 93:903–909, 1978
14. Bamford FN, Morris Jones P, Pearson D et al: Residual disabilities in children treated for intracranial space-occupying lesions. Cancer 37:1149–1151, 1976
15. Hirsch JF, Renier D, Czernichow P et al: Medulloblastoma in childhood. Survival and functional results. Acta Neurochir 48:1–15, 1979
16. Moss HA, Nannis ED, Poplack DG: The effects of prophylactic treatment of the central nervous system on the intellectual functioning of children with acute lymphocytic leukemia. Am J Med 71:47–52, 1981

17. Chin HW, Maruyama Y: Age at treatment and longterm performance results in medulloblastoma. Cancer 53:1952–1958, 1984
18. Li FP, Winston KR, Gimbrere K: Follow-up of children with brain tumors. Cancer 54:135–138, 1984
19. Silverman CL, Palkes H, Talent B et al: Late effects of radiotherapy on patients with cerebellar medulloblastoma. Cancer 54:825–829, 1984
20. Eiser C, Landsdown R: Retrospective study of intellectual development in children treated for acute lymphoblastic leukemia. Arch Dis Child 52:525–529, 1977
21. Eiser C: Intellectual abilities among survivors of childhood leukaemia as a function of CNS radiation. Arch Dis Child 53:391–395, 1978
22. Pfefferbaum-Levine B, Copeland DR, Fletcher JM et al: Neuropsychologic assessment of longterm survivors of childhood leukemia. Am J Pediatr Hematol Oncol 6:123–128, 1984
23. Katz ER, Kellerman J, Siegel SE: Behavioral distress in children with cancer undergoing medical procedures: Developmental considerations. J Consult Clin Psychol 48:356–365, 1980
24. Clapp MJ: Psychosocial reactions of children with cancer. Nurs Clin North Am 11:73–93, 1976
25. Van Dongen-Melman JEWM, Sanders-Woustra JAR: Psychosocial aspects of childhood cancer: A review of the literature. J Child Psychol Psychiatry 27:145–180, 1986
26. Lansky SB, Lowman JT, Vats T et al: School phobia in children with malignant neoplasms. Am J Dis Child 129:42–46, 1975
27. Lampert MH, Gerber LH, Glatstein E et al: Soft tissue sarcoma: Functional outcome after wide local excision and radiation therapy. Arch Phys Med Rehabil 65:477–480, 1984
28. Altman AJ, Schwartz AD: Nutritional Consequences of Cancer in Malignant Diseases of Infancy, Childhood and Adolescence, 2nd ed. Philadelphia, WB Saunders, 1983
29. Parker RG, Berry HG: Late effects of therapeutic irradiation on the skeleton and bone marrow. Cancer 37:1162–1171, 1976
30. Risenborough EJ, Grabias SL, Burton RF et al: Skeletal alterations following irradiation for Wilm's tumor with particular reference to scoliosis and kyphosis. J Bone Joint Surg [Am] 58:2232, 1979
31. Jentzsch K, Binder H, Cramer H et al: Leg function after radiotherapy for Ewing's sarcoma. Cancer 47:1267–1278, 1981
32. Lewis RJ, Marcove RC, Rosen G: Ewing's sarcoma: Functional effects of radiation therapy. J Bone Joint Surg 59:325–331, 1977
33. DeSmet A, Kulins L, Fayos J et al: Effects of radiation on growing long bones. AJR 127:935–939, 1976
34. Inati A, Sallan SE, Cassady JR et al: Efficacy and morbidity of central nervous system "prophylaxis" in childhood acute lymphoblastic leukemia: Eight year's experience with cranial irradiation and intrathecal methotrexate. Blood 61:297–303, 1983
35. Wara WM, Phillips TL, Sheline GE et al: Radiation tolerance of the spinal cord. Cancer 35:1558, 1975
36. Meadows AT, Evans AE: Effects of chemotherapy on the central nervous system: A study of parenteral methotrexate in long-term survivors of leukemia and lymphoma in childhood. Cancer 37:1079–1085, 1976
37. Weiss HD, Walker MD, Wiernik PH: Neurotoxicity of commonly used antineoplastic agents. N Engl J Med 291:127–133, 1974
38. Milhorat TH: Pediatric Neurosurgery. Philadelphia, FA Davis Co, 1979
39. Gjerris F: Clinical aspects and longterm prognosis of infratentorial intracranial tumours in infancy and childhood. Acta Neurol Scand 57:31–52, 1978
40. Gol A: Cerebellar astrocytomas in children. Am J Dis Child 106:55–58, 1963
41. Danoff BF, Cowchock S, Marquette C et al: Assessment of the longterm effects of primary radiation therapy for brain tumors in children. Cancer 49:1580–1586, 1982
42. Duffner PK, Cohen ME, Thomas P: Late effects of treatment on the intelligence of children with posterior fossa tumors. Cancer 51:233–237, 1983
43. Giuffre R, Caroli F, Deffini R et al: Longterm follow up of 40 children operated on for primary intracranial tumors. Neurochirurgica 25:119–123, 1982
44. Madon E, Besencon L, Brach del Prever A et al: Results of a multi center retrospective study on pediatric brain tumors in Italy. Tumori 72:285–292, 1986
45. DeSousa AL, Kalsbeck JE, Mealey J Jr et al: Intraspinal tumors in children. J Neurosurg 51:437–445, 1979
46. Farwell JR, Dohrmann GJ: Intraspinal neoplasms in children. Paraplegia 15:262–273, 1978
47. Hvizdala EV, Miale TD, Barnard PJ: A summer camp for children with cancer. Med Pediatr Oncol 4:71–75, 1978

48. Burgess E, Romano R: The management of amputees using immediate post surgical prosthesis. Clin Orthop 57:132, 1968

49. Thorpe W, Gerber LH, Lampert M et al: A prospective study of the rehabilitation of the above knee amputee with rigid dressings. Clin Orthop 143:133–137, 1979

50. Kegel B, Carpenter M, Burgess E: A survey of lower limb amputees: prosthesis, phantom sensations, psychosocial aspects. Bull Prosthet Res 10:43, 1977

51. Kegel B: Physical fitness. J Rehabil R D Clin Suppl 1:1–125, 1985

52. Malawer MM, Sugarbaker PH, Lampert MH et al: The Tikhoff Linberg procedure: Report of 10 patients. Surgery 97:518–528, 1985

53. Hale G (ed): Source Book for the Disabled. Philadelphia, WB Saunders, 1979

54. Kreisler N, Kreisler T: Catalog of Aids for the Disabled. New York, McGraw-Hill, 1982

55. Bates JAV, Nathan PW: Transcutaneous electrical nerve stimulation for chronic pain. Anesthesia 35:817–822, 1980

56. Magora F, Aladjemoff L, Tannenbaum J et al: Treatment of pain by transcutaneous electrical stimulation. Acta Anaesthesiol Scand 22:587–592, 1978

57. Pierson S, Pierson D, Swallow R et al: Efficacy of graded elastic compression in the lower leg. JAMA 249:242–243, 1983

58. Mellion MB: Exercise therapy for anxiety and depression. Postgrad Med 77(3):59–62, 91–93, 1985

59. Summary of Existing Legislation Relating to the Handicapped. US Department of Education Publ. no. E-80-22014. Washington, DC, US Government Printing Office, 1980

60. Kaplan D: Employment Rights: History Trends and Status in Law. Reform in Disability Rights, vol 2. Berkeley, CA, Disability Rights Education and Defense Fund, 1987

61. Rehabilitation R&D Progress Reports. Office of Technology Transfer (153D), VA Administration Medical Center, 50 Irving St, Washington, DC 20422

forty-eight

Bone Marrow Transplantation in Pediatric Oncology

Norma K. C. Ramsay

Bone marrow transplantation has evolved over the past decade to become an established treatment modality for a number of pediatric diseases, including immunologic, hematologic, and oncologic disorders. The first successful bone marrow transplants were performed in 1968 in infants with severe combined immunodeficiency (SCID).[1,2] Subsequently, bone marrow transplantation (BMT) was used successfully in patients with severe aplastic anemia.[3-7] It is now considered the treatment of choice for newly diagnosed patients with severe aplastic anemia who have a sibling matched at the major histocompatibility locus, and survival in these patients is greater than 70%.[8-10] The early success of BMT in SCID and severe aplastic anemia prompted its use in hematologic malignancies. In the early 1970s, BMT was performed in patients with end-stage leukemia.[11-13] Although there was a high rate of mortality from infections, transplant-related complications, and recurrent leukemia, approximately 10% of the patients were long-term survivors. This small group of surviving end-stage patients warranted the use of BMT earlier in the course of the disease. The scope of diseases for which marrow transplantation is currently used includes acute and chronic leukemias, lymphomas, and certain solid tumors, as well as inherited metabolic storage disorders, neutrophil function defects, osteopetrosis, and selected hemoglobinopathies such as thalassemia major.

This chapter reviews the current status of bone marrow transplantation in pediatric oncology with specific discussion of its use in acute lymphoblastic leukemia (ALL), acute nonlymphoblastic leukemia (ANLL), chronic myelogenous leukemia, (CML), lymphoma, and neuroblastoma, and other solid tumors (Table 48-1). In addition to discussing specific disorders, the BMT process, donor selection, and complications are described.

BONE MARROW TRANSPLANT PROCESS

Donor Typing

In oncologic disorders, BMT is used to restore normal hematopoiesis following high-dose chemoradiotherapy directed at eradicating the malignancy. The very high doses of chemotherapy and radiation therapy used are ablative to the patient's normal bone marrow. These patients require marrow infusion for hematopoietic reconstitution. The second purpose of the pretransplant preparative therapy is to suppress patients' immune systems so that they will accept the bone marrow graft.

The source of marrow may be the patient (autologous transplant), an identical twin (syngeneic transplant), or a histocompatible donor, most frequently a sibling (allogeneic transplant). The majority of transplants performed have been allogeneic, using marrow from a sibling matched at the major histocompatibility locus. Significant progress has occurred over the past two decades in defining the

Table 48-1
Indications for Bone Marrow Transplantation in Children with Malignancies, by Disease Status

Disease	Allogeneic BMT	Autologous BMT
Leukemia		
ANLL	First remission or first relapse	Second remission
ALL	Second or third remission	Second or third remission
CML	Chronic or accelerated phase	Chronic or accelerated phase
Non-Hodgkin's lymphoma	Recurrent or refractory	Recurrent or refractory
Hodgkin's disease	—	Failure of two treatment modalities
Neuroblastoma*	At time of initial complete or partial response	At time of initial complete or partial response

* Stage III or Stage IV patients.

genetic makeup of the major histocompatibility complex (MHC) in man. This complex, also referred to as the human leukocyte antigen (HLA) system, contains a set of genes that are usually inherited as one group or haplotype. The HLA region is located on the short arm of chromosome 6 (Fig. 48-1).[14] People inherit a maternal and paternal copy of chromosome 6. Each sibling has a 25% chance of inheriting the same genetic material from the parents as did the patient; with current family size, the overall likelihood of an individual having an HLA-identical sibling is approximately 35%.

The HLA system consists of genes encoding Class I molecules, including HLA-A, HLA-B, and HLA-C, and Class II molecules within the HLA-D region, which currently consists of at least seven genes (see also Chap. 4).[15,16] The HLA phenotype of a patient is determined by a series of serologic and cellular techniques that identify the different major loci. The Class I antigens as well as some of the Class II antigens are defined serologically by their reactivity to a panel of typing sera.[17,18] Monoclonal antibodies are being used increasingly to replace heterologous sera in tissue-typing panels. D-region identity is determined by the mixed lymphocyte culture (MLC), which is a test of lymphocytic proliferation.[19] Because the genes of the MHC are inherited as a haplotype, the finding of identical HLA-A and B typing in full siblings conveys a greater than 95% probability that they are identical for all MHC antigens and will be found to be nonreactive in the MLC test.

Donor Selection

The source of bone marrow in most cases of BMT is an HLA-identical, MLC-nonreactive sibling donor (allogeneic). In rare cases an identical twin donor (syngeneic) is the source of donor marrow or a patient may act as his or her own donor (autologous).

Bone marrow is usually obtained from the donor under general anesthesia in the operating room. Multiple bone marrow aspirations are performed. The usual site for bone marrow harvest is the posterior iliac crests bilaterally. No fatalities have occurred in donors, and the risk of potentially life-threatening complications has been less than 1%.[20] Young children are used as donors; at our institution, marrow has been successfully obtained from a 5-month-old donor. There may be the potential risks of blood transfusion because sufficient marrow is often obtained to warrant transfusion of the donor. In many cases, the marrow donor donates a unit of blood before the procedure to decrease the risk of transfusion-related disease. The number of cells obtained at donor harvest is based on the recipient's weight. Usually, a dose of 2 to 4 × 10^8 nucleated cells/kg recipient weight is obtained for transplant. In the case of autologous BMT, a lower cell dose may be adequate. In most cases, the bone marrow is infused directly into the recipient

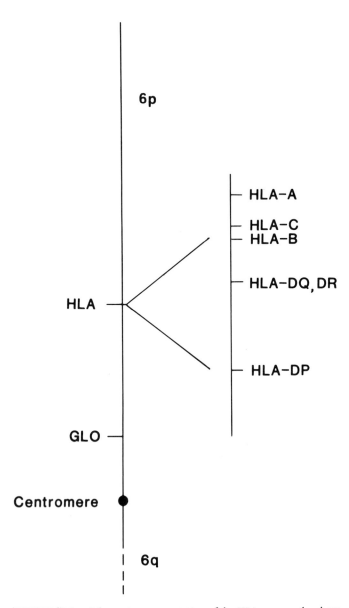

FIGURE 48-1. Schematic representation of the HLA gene on the short arm of chromosome 6.

through an indwelling catheter. If the marrow is obtained from the patient (autologous), it is usually cryopreserved until the patient is prepared for transplant. Cryopreservation techniques for bone marrow are well established and allow marrow to be reinfused into the patient at a later time.[21] A major ABO incompatibility between donor and recipient is not a contraindication for transplant and may be overcome by a variety of methods.[22-24] If antibodies are directed against donor erythrocytes, (*e.g.,* donor A, recipient O), the risks include hemolysis of erythrocytes in the marrow or possible failure of engraftment because of ABO antibodies directed against stem cell antigens. The latter complication does not present a problem, and transplantation is done successfully across major ABO incompatibility combinations.[22-26] Hemolysis of erythrocytes can be a problem when major ABO incompatibility exists between donor and recipient, so that erythrocytes are removed from the marrow prior to transplant by a variety of methods.[27] The alternative approach to this problem is to remove the antibody from the patient by plasma exchange using blood cell separators.[24-26] If antibody is still detectable, ABO-incompatible erythrocytes may be given before transplantation of the marrow.[28] If a minor ABO incompatibility is present, the donor plasma contains antibodies against the recipient erythrocytes and may cause hemolysis of recipient erythrocytes if the volume of plasma is large. This problem can be avoided by removing the plasma from the donor bone marrow by centrifugation.[29] This concentrated bone marrow has no adverse effect on the success of engraftment.[28]

In most cases, the bone marrow is administered to the patient directly or cryopreserved for future use. In the last several years, special *ex vivo* treatment of bone marrow has been used. The two major indications for *ex vivo* treatment are [1] removal of T-lymphocytes in an effort to decrease graft-versus-host disease (GVHD), and [2] removal of malignant cells in autologous marrow. The agents used for *ex vivo* marrow treatment include monoclonal antibodies combined with complement, monoclonal antibodies linked to toxins, and drugs such as 4-hydroperoxycyclophosphamide. Further discussion of these techniques is in the sections on leukemia and GVHD.

PRETRANSPLANT CONDITIONING

Patients undergoing BMT for malignancy are conditioned or prepared for transplant using high-dose chemoradiotherapy. This therapy is designed to eliminate residual malignant cells. In addition, it is immunosuppressive and allows acceptance of

the marrow graft by the patient. The doses of radiation therapy and chemotherapy used are intentionally marrow ablative. Following conditioning, which lasts approximately a week, donor bone marrow is infused. At this time pancytopenia occurs and lasts from 2 to 6 weeks until the donor marrow engrafts and produces sufficient hematopoietic cells. These patients are extremely immunosuppressed and myelosuppressed and are kept in isolation rooms or, in some institutions, in laminar air flow rooms during this time. Supportive care is essential and includes the use of frequent erythrocyte and platelet transfusions, antibiotic therapy, and numerous other measures. All blood products, including plasma, must be irradiated to prevent GVHD. Patients are at risk for mortality associated with infections, especially opportunistic infections (discussed in the section on Complications). The BMT procedure is schematically depicted in Figure 48-2.

GRAFT-VERSUS-HOST DISEASE AND ITS PREVENTION

Patients who receive allogeneic marrow are at risk for the development of GVHD once the marrow engrafts. This potential for GVHD is mediated by immunocompetent cells in the marrow graft, presumably T-lymphocytes that are capable of injury to the host (foreign) tissues.[29,30] GVHD may occur in an acute form or progress to a chronic condition (see section on Complications). Because of its potentially devastating effects, major efforts have been directed at the prevention of GVHD. GVHD prophylaxis has been either *in vivo,* by administration of agents early after transplant; or *ex vivo,* involving removal of T-cells from donor marrow (Table 48-2). The agents most frequently given to patients following transplant for GVHD prophylaxis have been methotrexate, steroids, antithymocyte globulin (ATG), and cyclosporin A. Methotrexate alone posttransplant was the initial form of GVHD prophylaxis used, but combinations of agents are currently being evaluated in an effort to decrease the incidence of GVHD. Immunologic agents, such as ATG, in combination with methotrexate did not result in decreased GVHD in two series,[31,32] but the combination of methotrexate, ATG, and prednisone was associated with decreased GVHD when compared with methotrexate alone.[33]

More recently, the immunosuppressive agent cyclosporine has been evaluated alone or in combination with methotrexate for the prevention of GVHD.[34-36] Combination therapy has been associated with less GVHD and improved survival.

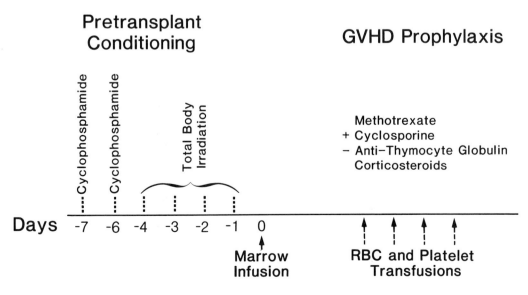

Pretransplant Conditioning

GVHD Prophylaxis

Methotrexate
+ Cyclosporine
− Anti-Thymocyte Globulin
Corticosteroids

Cyclophosphamide
Cyclophosphamide
Total Body Irradiation

Days   -7   -6   -4   -3   -2   -1   0

Marrow
Infusion

RBC and Platelet
Transfusions

FIGURE 48-2. Schematic representation of marrow transplantation. Pretransplant preparation consists of combined chemoradiotherapy. Total body irradiation is given in fractionated doses as shown or as a single dose. GVHD prophylaxis is administered posttransplantation unless T cells have been removed *ex vivo* from the donor marrow. Transfusions are given post-transplantation as needed.

Table 48-2
Approaches to Preventing Graft-Versus-Host Disease

In Vivo Therapy*
  Methotrexate
  Anti-thymocyte globulin
  Corticosteroids
  Cyclophosphamide
  Cyclosporine

Ex Vivo Therapy
  Monoclonal antibodies ± complement
  Monoclonal antibody–ricin conjugates
  E-rosette depletion
  Soybean lectin agglutination
  Elutriation

---

* These have been used as single agents or in combination.

Ex vivo depletion of T-cells has been performed using monoclonal antibodies directed against T-lymphocytes, either in the presence of complement or linked to toxins such as ricin. Differential binding to lectins has been also used for T-cell removal. The initial findings in animal studies that *ex vivo* removal of immunocompetent cells can prevent GVHD[30,37,38] has prompted the evaluation of this approach in humans. Several methodologies of T-cell removal are being evaluated for the prevention of GVHD. In matched patients, this approach has been associated with less GVHD.[39,40] However, these regimens have been associated with the problems of rejection or nonengraftment in some series, especially in the mismatched setting.[39–45] The problem of rejection may be overcome using more intensive conditioning regimens. The possibility of an increased relapse rate following this approach to GVHD prevention has also been raised.[46,47] Further studies are needed to evaluate the role of T-cell depletion and its impact on GVHD, rejection, and posttransplant relapse.

The occurrence of GVHD in patients with malignancy may have a beneficial graft-versus-tumor effect. In some reports, patients who develop GVHD post-transplant have a lower relapse rate than those who do not.[48,49] Further support for a graft versus tumor effect comes from studies of syngeneic transplantation, where the relapse rate is higher than in the allogeneic setting.[50] (GVHD prophylaxis is discussed in more detail in the Complications section).

ONCOLOGIC DISEASES TREATED BY MARROW TRANSPLANTATION

Leukemia

Acute Nonlymphoblastic Leukemia

ALLOGENEIC. Although induction remission rates for patients with ANLL have improved over the past several years, long-term disease-free survival rates have been disappointing for patients treated with chemotherapy. One approach using intensive reinduction cycles of chemotherapy has been more encouraging (see also Chap. 17).[51,52] For patients younger than 18 years, the actuarial probability of continuous complete remission at 3 years is 56%; however, older patients have a poorer outcome. For patients ages 18 to 50 years, the probability of continuous complete remission at 5 years decreases to 27%.[52] Marrow ablative chemoradiotherapy followed by donor marrow infusion was first used by

investigators at the Fred Hutchinson Cancer Center for patients with end-stage disease.[11] Of 54 end-stage patients treated with BMT, 6 were long-term survivors (6–10 years) on no maintenance therapy.[53] This initial study prompted the evaluation of BMT earlier in the course of the disease.

Subsequently, in Seattle, patients in first remission were transplanted with a similar preparative regimen; 10 of 19 patients were survivors at 10 years posttransplantation.[54,55] These patients were conditioned for transplant with cyclophosphamide, 60 mg/kg for 2 days, and 10 Gy total body irradiation. With more aggressive pretransplant conditioning, morbidity and mortality increased and survival was not improved.[56]

In children, survival obtained following bone marrow transplantation for ANLL in first remission has been excellent because there is less morbidity and mortality related to GVHD in young patients. In 38 children under the age of 17 transplanted in first remission, a disease-free survival rate of 64% was reported and the relapse rate was less than 20%.[57]

Several centers have reported their results of BMT for ANLL in first remission. Conditioning with cytosine arabinoside, cyclophosphamide, and total body irradiation resulted in disease-free survival of 60% in 33 children and young adults. In patients younger than 20 years, the only cause of death was leukemic relapse.[58]

Transplantation in first remission is superior to transplantation in second remission in most centers.[59] However, in one series, the disease-free survival for patients transplanted in second remission did not differ from that seen in patients transplanted in first remission.[60] Patients transplanted in third remission or in relapse with the same conditioning regimen, however, had significantly poorer survival.

Factors prognostic for survival can be evaluated now that larger numbers of patients have been transplanted. In one series of 39 children and young adults transplanted in first remission, a high initial leukocyte count ($\geq20,000/\mu l$) and monocytic morphology (French–American–British M4, M5a) were associated with a higher relapse rate.[61] Disease-free survival in these patients was 55% at 3 years, with the latest relapses occurring at 2 years post-transplant. The International Bone Marrow Transplant Registry evaluated factors associated with early mortality in 85 patients transplanted in first remission from a variety of centers.[62] Mortality at 6 months post-transplant was associated with the occurrence of moderate or severe GVHD and the use of high dose rates of total body irradiation (>2.5 cGy/min).

A preparative regimen for transplant that does not utilize total body radiation has been used successfully by investigators at the Johns Hopkins Oncology Center.[63] Chemotherapy alone (busulfan and cyclophosphamide) resulted in a 44% 2-year survival rate in 18 patients transplanted in first remission. No relapses occurred in this group of first-remission patients.

Now that BMT has been clearly shown to result in disease-free survival rates of 45% to 65% for ANLL patients transplanted in first remission (Table 48-3), comparison of conventional chemotherapy with BMT is important. In a study reported from Seattle, first-remission patients who lacked a donor ($N = 46$) received maintenance chemotherapy and were compared to 33 patients who were transplanted.[64] As expected, initial mortality was higher in the transplanted group; however, the long-term disease free survival was superior in the transplanted patients. The Kaplan-Meier estimate of 5-year disease-free survival was 49% for the transplanted patients versus 20% for the chemotherapy-treated patients. There are other such comparisons,[65,66] but many difficulties are encountered in each of these studies.[67] In a prospective study in adults, 23 transplanted patients

Table 48-3
Allogeneic BMT for ANLL Patients

Center*	Preparative Regimen†	Number of Patients	Age (yr) Range	Age (yr) Median	Remission Status	2-Year Disease-Free Survival (%)
Seattle[57]	CTX + TBI	38	0.8–17	—	First	64
Seattle[59]	CTX + TBI	24	2–30	22	Second	24
City of Hope[58]	CTX + ara-C + TBI	33	7–41	28	First	60
MSKCC[60]	CTX + TBI	30	1–38	20	First	64
		11	6–40	16	Second	55
		3	11–24	20	Third	35
		26	2–43	24	(Relapse)	10
Minnesota[61]	CTX + TBI	39	1–40	14	First	55
Hopkins[63]	Busulfan + CTX	18	13–41	23	First	44
		17	6–37	22	First or second	29
CCSG[69] ‡	CTX + TBI	92	N.A.		First	49
UCLA[68]	CTX + TBI	23	15–41	25	First	40§

* MSKCC = Memorial Sloan-Kettering Cancer Center; CCSG = Children's Cancer Study Group; UCLA = University of Caifornia, Los Angeles.

† CTX = cyclophosphamide; TBI = total body irradiation.

‡ This multi-institutional study includes some patients reported in other series.

§ This figure represents survival, not disease-free survival.

had a significantly lower relapse rate than 44 patients treated with chemotherapy. However, the actuarial survival at 4 years was not significantly different.[68] One trial in children compared BMT to two different maintenance regimens.[69] In this study of 347 children, all patients received identical induction therapy. Patients with matched sibling donors were transplanted, whereas those without donors were randomized to one of two chemotherapy maintenance regimens. The disease-free survival rate at 3 years is significantly better in the transplanted patients (49%) than the chemotherapy-treated patients (36%).[69]

This randomized study comparing BMT with maintenance chemotherapy for first-remission ANLL patients, combined with single-arm BMT studies from a number of institutions, clearly indicates that BMT is the treatment of choice for pediatric patients with ANLL in first remission. Since only one third of patients have a matched donor, the use of autologous BMT for first-remission ANLL patients needs to be evaluated.

AUTOLOGOUS. With the excellent long-term disease-free survival obtained using allogeneic BMT in first-remission ANLL patients has come interest in the use of autologous marrow for patients without an HLA-matched sibling donor. Usually, the marrow is harvested and stored during remission and then reinfused following marrow ablative therapy. Marrow has been "cleaned up" or purged using monoclonal antibodies or[70] *ex vivo* chemotherapy;[71,72] in some cases, unpurged marrow has been used (Table 48-4).[73,74]

Unpurged Marrow. The use of autologous remission bone marrow without any form of purging has yielded different results in different centers. In 12 first-remission patients given unpurged marrow after preparation with cyclophosphamide and total body irradiation, the predicted 3-year disease-free survival is 58%.[75] Survival at 2 years is 22% in another series of 13 ANLL patients transplanted in first remission and given similar preparative therapy.[73] One possible explanation for the discrepant results is that better survival was seen in patients transplanted later in first remission, indicating that these selected patients were at lower risk for recurrent leukemia.

Purging with Chemotherapy. The efficacy of cyclophosphamide metabolites as purging agents was first demonstrated by Sharkis in a rat model, wherein marrow contaminated with leukemic cells was successfully purged using 4-hydroperoxy-cyclophosphamide.[76] This agent does not require liver activation and thus is an excellent candidate for *ex vivo* purging. Excellent results using this approach have been obtained in 25 second- and third-remission ANLL patients following preparation of the patients with busulfan and cyclophosphamide or cyclophosphamide and total body irradiation. Although the actuarial relapse rate was 46%, the actuarial disease-free survival rate was 43%.[72] These results were very similar to those seen in patients undergoing allogeneic BMT using the same conditioning regimen.[73]

Purging with Monoclonal Antibodies. The use of monoclonal antibodies for purging marrow of ANLL patients has been more limited because of the difficulty in developing monoclonal antibodies that are selective for ANLL cells but spare hematopoietic precursors, particularly those of myeloid lineage. A recent report described the results of 10 patients whose marrow was harvested in first to third remission and who were transplanted in second or third remission using marrow purged with two monoclonal antibodies (PM-81 and AML-2-23) plus complement. Full marrow reconstitution occurred in 8 patients; 2 patients had failure of marrow recovery. Although follow-up is short, 7 patients remain disease-free.[70]

The role of autologous BMT for ANLL patients is currently limited. Comparison with postinduction chemotherapy in a prospective study is needed. The advantages of autologous transplant include fewer deaths from infection and absence of GVHD. These advantages must be weighed against a potentially higher relapse rate, as is seen in patients receiving bone marrow from an identical twin.[50] The lack of GVHD in autologous and syngeneic transplants may be responsible for the

Table 48-4
*Autologous BMT for Patients with ANLL in Remission**

Center	Patient Age Range (yr)	Purging Agent	Preparative Regimen	Remission Status	Disease-Free Survival		
					Number of Patients	Actuarial (%)	Follow-up Range or Median (mo)
Unpurged Marrow							
Glasgow[75]	18–53	—	CTX + TBI	First	7/12	58	6.5–35
Seattle[73]	14–37	—	CTX + TBI	First	3/13	22	26–50
Purged with Chemotherapeutic Agents							
Johns Hopkins[72]	4–53	4-Hydroperoxycyclo-phosphamide (4HC)	Busulfan + CTX	Second Third	8/20 3/5	43	14
Paris[71]	13–50	Mafosfamide	CTX + TBI ± ara-C ± VP-16-213	First and second	6/15	NA	9–56
Purged with MoAbs							
Dartmouth[70]	16–44	MoAbs PM-81 and AML-2-23 and C'	CTX + TBI	Second ($N = 6$), third ($N = 2$); second early relapse ($N = 2$)	7/10	NA	2–21 10

* NA = data not available; C' = complement; MoAbs = monoclonal antibodies.

higher relapse rate, as a beneficial graft versus tumor effect has been observed in allogeneic transplants.[48,49] A prospective study comparing these modalities is clearly warranted.

Acute Lymphoblastic Leukemia

ALLOGENEIC. Children with ALL are in most cases successfully treated with chemotherapy (see Chap. 16). Over 60% of children with ALL are now cured with intensive induction regimens followed by 2 to 3 years of maintenance therapy.[77–79] Therefore, intensive therapy using BMT is not warranted for the majority of children with ALL. However, certain factors at diagnosis portend a very poor prognosis, such as the presence of the Philadelphia chromosome[80] or the presence of a t(4;11) chromosomal abnormality.[81] For such patients, BMT in first remission may be warranted. For most children, however, BMT is initially considered following an on-therapy relapse. Although second remissions may be prolonged, ultimate survival is usually poor when patients are treated with chemotherapy.[82] Two recent reports, however, have shown improved survival for patients treated with chemotherapy following a bone marrow relapse, especially for those with long initial remissions (see Chap. 16).[83,84]

Bone marrow transplantation has been successfully used in combination with chemoradiotherapy in a number of centers for patients with ALL who have relapsed (Table 48-5).[85–91] In most cases, donors have been matched siblings and transplant has been performed in second or third marrow remission. The majority of series report combined results for transplanted children and adults, although three series have reported results for children alone.[86,88,89] Boys who develop an isolated testicular relapse while receiving chemotherapy also have a poor long-term survival, with the majority of patients ultimately relapsing in the bone marrow and dying of their disease.[92,93] For these patients, BMT should be considered once a second remission is achieved.

An isolated relapse in the central nervous system (CNS) is associated with subsequent relapse in other sites in over 50% of patients.[94] Long-term survival is poor because of systemic relapse as well as recurrent CNS disease, and for this reason BMT is frequently performed.

The appropriateness of transplanting patients who experience a bone marrow relapse after the completion of maintenance chemotherapy remains controversial. The timing of an off-therapy relapse may be important in deciding appropriate therapy, in that patients who relapse within 6 months of cessation of therapy have a relatively poor long-term prognosis compared to patients who relapse at a later point after discontinuation of maintenance therapy.[95]

The majority of reports have evaluated the use of allogeneic transplantation in ALL patients in second or later remissions. In comparing these reports, it is important to consider patient selection and timing of transplantation. Patients undergoing transplant more recently have usually failed more intensive initial chemotherapy than was received by patients reported in earlier series. Although the influence of this variable is difficult to measure, it is reasonable to assume that current patients may have more resistant disease. Certain factors have been reported to have prognostic importance in allogeneic bone BMT for ALL. Patients with a high leukocyte count at diagnosis ($>50,000/\mu l$) and those with prior extramedullary disease had poorer disease-free survival post-transplant.[88] In another series, patients transplanted in third or later remissions had poorer survival than those transplanted in second remission.[68] For the former patients, several factors predicted for a poorer prognosis, including a high leukocyte count at diagnosis, short initial remission (<1 year), and age greater than 10 years at transplant.[87] A short initial remission ("fast disease") has been demonstrated in another series to be associated with poorer post-transplant survival than that observed in patients transplanted after a longer initial remission ("slow disease").[96]

All of the reported allogeneic studies are single-arm transplant studies. However, two reports have compared in a

Table 48-5
Allogeneic BMT for Patients with ALL

Center	Patient Age (yr)		Preparative Regimen*	Remission Status	2-Year Disease-Free Survival		
	Range	Median			Number of Patients	Actuarial (%)	Follow-up Range or Median (yr)
Seattle[86,90]	5–16	8	CTX + 10 Gy TBI	Second	4/14	38	7–10
				≥Third	4/10		
Seattle[89]	2–17	N.A.	CTX + 9–10 Gy TBI or fTBI 12–15 Gy	First–fifth	15/51	33	2–9
				Relapse	5/63	10	3–10
MSKCC[87]	1–36	N.A.	11 × 1.2 Gy TBI + CTX	Second	14/22	62.5	2
				Third or fourth	5/15	26.7	1⅓
				Relapse	4/15	26.7	NA
Minnesota[88,96]	3–26	14	CTX + 7.5 Gy TBI	Second or third	5/15	33	5–7
Minnesota[49]	3–47	14	CTX + 8 × 1.65 Gy TBI	First–third	13/40	30	2.5
Cleveland[98]	3–15	6.5	ara-C + 6 × 2 Gy TBI	Second	11/18	59†	4
City of Hope[91]	6–36	18	11 × 1.2 Gy TBI + VP-16-213	>Second	3/5	NA	<1
				Relapse	4/8		<1

* fTBI = fractionated total body irradiation.
† This figure represents survival, not disease-free survival.

nonrandomized study the results of transplant at their institutions with the results for a group of similar children with ALL treated with continued chemotherapy.[86,88] In both reports, children with ALL undergoing transplant in second to fourth remission had superior disease-free survival compared to patients treated with chemotherapy. Further follow-up of these series has shown that disease-free survival continues to be superior in the transplanted patients, with follow-up longer than 4 years.[90,97] In one study, 5 of 15 transplanted patients are alive in continuous complete remission, whereas only 1 of 23 patients treated with conventional chemotherapy remains alive in continuous complete remission.[97]

The occurrence of GVHD, although a cause of significant post-transplant morbidity and even mortality, has been associated with higher relapse-free survival.[48] In a series of 114 children with ALL who were transplanted in remission (N = 51) or relapse (N = 63), both the presence of remission status at transplant and the presence of chronic GVHD predicted improved survival. Acute or chronic GVHD and transplant during remission were both associated with significantly fewer relapses post-transplant.[89] Initial leukocyte counts and prior extramedullary disease were not of prognostic importance in this series. In another series of 40 children and adults with ALL, transplanted in remission, the presence of acute GVHD was associated with a reduction in post-BMT relapses.[49] This study evaluated the effect of posttransplant maintenance chemotherapy with oral 6-mercaptopurine and methotrexate in a randomized trial and found that post-transplant maintenance therapy did not improve survival or decrease the relapse rate, in contrast to earlier preliminary data.[88]

Although posttransplant complications, including infection and GVHD, impact on long-term survival following allogeneic transplantation, the major reason for failure in patients with ALL who are transplanted is post-BMT leukemic relapse, which occurs in 25% to 50% of the patients. Lower relapse rates occur following BMT in ANLL and CML. Although prolonged relapse-free survival occurs in some patients, more effective antileukemic preparative therapy is clearly needed for the majority of ALL patients. Novel approaches of using the graft versus leukemia effect may also improve relapse-free survival.

In most series, the preparative regimen has included cyclophosphamide and total body irradiation, given as a single fraction or fractionated in various schedules. The disease-free survival in various studies ranges from 30% to 40%. Two preparative regimens given to second-remission ALL patients show promise with respect to a decreased relapse rate.[87,98] The Memorial Sloan-Kettering Cancer Center has shown improved disease-free survival in second-remission patients given hyperfractionated total body irradiation followed by cyclophosphamide.[87] Disease-free survival of patients in third or later remission treated in this manner yields results similar to other series. Another small series of second-remission children with ALL transplanted after preparation with high-dose ara-C and fractionated total body irradiation has demonstrated a low relapse rate and excellent disease-free survival.[98] Patients with ALL who fail initial chemotherapy should be transplanted if a donor is available.

AUTOLOGOUS. The majority of transplants for children with ALL have been performed using an HLA-identical, MLC-compatible sibling donor. Because only about 30% of patients have a matched sibling donor, alternative donors are being investigated. Some patients are being transplanted using matched unrelated donors or less than fully matched family donors; some method of T-cell depletion is typically used.[99,100] Two centers have been evaluating the use of autologous bone marrow combined with purging of residual leukemic cells with monoclonal antibodies,[101,102] and others have used the pharmacologic agents ASTA-Z 7557[103] and 4-hydroperoxycyclophosphamide (Table 48-6).[104]

The majority of autologous transplants for children with ALL have involved the use of bone marrow purged with mono-

Table 48-6
Autologous BMT for Patients with ALL

				Disease-Free Survival		
Center	Purging	Remission Status	Preparative Regimen	Number of Patients	Actuarial (%)	Follow-up Range or Median
Dana-Farber[105]	J5* + C′	Second or third	CTX + VM-26 + ara-C + TBI	9/30	27 (2 yr)	45 mo
Minnesota[102,111]	BA-1, 2, 3† + C′	Second or third	CTX + TBI 8 × 1.65 Gy	6/28	21 (2 yr)	3–5 yr
	BA-1, 2, 3 + C′	First–third	TBI 8.5 Gy + ara-C	6/13	25 (1 yr)	<1 yr
Johns Hopkins[104]	4HC dose escalation	Second–fourth	CTX + TBI 3 Gy × 4	2/21	NA	>2 yr

* J5 is anti-CD10.

† BA-1 is anti-CD24; BA-2 is anti-CD9; BA-3 is anti-CD10.

clonal antibodies and complement. Monoclonal antibodies have been produced against antigens present on the surface of leukemic cells, and a number of trials worldwide are testing the efficacy of this approach.

At the Dana-Farber Cancer Institute, remission bone marrow is treated *ex vivo* with the anti-CALLA monoclonal antibody J5 and complement. Patients are conditioned for transplant with VM-26, ara-C, cyclophosphamide, and 8.5 cGy total body irradiation. The initial report demonstrated that hematologic reconstitution occurred.[101] The series has been expanded to 30 patients who have an event-free survival at 5 years of 30% ± 8%; median follow-up of disease-free survivors is 52 months. In this series, an initial remission of longer than 24 months was associated with significantly improved survival.[105]

At the University of Minnesota, *ex vivo* elimination of leukemic cells has involved three antibodies—BA-1 (anti-CD24),[106] BA-2 (anti-CD9),[107] and BA-3 (anti-CD10/CALLA)[108]—and complement. These three antibodies were chosen because they do not react with hematopoietic cells and they bind the majority of non-T-ALL cells.[109,110] Two clinical trials using bone marrow purged in this method have been carried out in the past several years.[102,111] Two sequential preparative regimens were used to condition patients in second or later remission for BMT before reinfusion of purged autologous bone marrow.

There are several conclusions that can be made from these two studies: [1] engraftment occurs readily after reinfusion of monoclonal antibody-purged bone marrow, [2] post-transplant mortality due to complications is very low, [3] the relapse rate is high (70%–75%), and [4] a percentage (20%–25%) of patients appear to be cured with this methodology. Longer follow-up of the initial study[102] reveals that 6 of 28 patients transplanted in second or third remission remain disease-free 3 to 5 years after transplant.

The high incidence of recurrent leukemia following autologous BMT may be related to multiple factors. Persistent leukemia in the patient accounts for some relapses, because identical preparative regimens in allogeneic patients are also associated with a high relapse rate. Another reason for an increased relapse rate in patients undergoing autologous transplantation is the presence of undetectable residual contaminating leukemic cells in the purged bone marrow. The ability to perform fresh leukemic cell progenitor assays may be helpful in answering this question in the future.[112,113] An additional factor that may be responsible for the higher relapse rates in autologous transplants compared to allogeneic transplants for ALL is the absence of a graft versus leukemia effect in the autologous as compared to the allogeneic setting.[48,49]

A patient who relapses following BMT for ALL will not be cured. Reinduction therapy, however, has been successful in a large percentage of patients, with some patients maintaining remissions for longer than a year. In one study, the complete remission rate was 56% in 53 patients who were retreated with chemotherapy following a posttransplant relapse.[114] The area of autologous BMT for ALL remains investigational, and prospective studies comparing retreatment with chemotherapy should be compared with autologous BMT.

Chronic Myelogenous Leukemia

ALLOGENEIC. Although CML, a myeloproliferative stem cell disorder, accounts for less than 5% of the cases of leukemia in children, it should be addressed when discussing BMT in children.

There are two types of CML seen in children that differ markedly in their characteristics and natural history (see Chap. 18). Juvenile CML occurs in very young children, frequently presents more like an acute leukemia, and has been ineffectively treated with chemotherapy.[115] Bone marrow transplantation has provided successful therapy.[116] Adult CML is the more common type of CML in children and is identical to the disease in adults. Most information on CML is derived from series of adults that usually include a few children. A characteristic finding in these patients is the presence of the Philadelphia chromosome, which is helpful is following disappearance of the leukemic clone.[117]

Since conventional chemotherapy does not alter the course of CML, transplantation following high-dose chemoradiotherapy has been evaluated, and success was initially reported using identical twin donors.[118] This early series was extended to 12 patients who experienced a complete clinical and cytogenetic remission, with disappearance of the Philadelphia chromosome, following BMT.[119] The first allogeneic transplants in CML were performed in patients in blast crisis. These reports were encouraging in that the Philadelphia chromosome could be eradicated in some patients; however, disease-free survival was poor in these patients with advanced disease.[120,121]

Bone marrow transplantation was subsequently performed at an earlier stage of disease in patients in accelerated phase, when the leukemic clone could be eradicated; leukemic relapse remained a problem.[122]

A number of centers have been evaluating BMT for patients in the chronic phase of the disease who have matched donors.[123-129] Complete remission, with eradication of the malignant clone, is achieved, and disease-free survival in these patients is very promising.

In a recent report, compiling results from a number of centers, the International Bone Marrow Transplant Registry evaluated prognostic factors in patients transplanted for CML.[126] The stage of disease at the time of transplant was the most important variable. The 3-year survival for patients transplanted in chronic phase was 63% compared to 36% for patients transplanted in accelerated phase and 12% for those transplanted in blast crisis. Similar results were reported from a single center.[127] The causes of death after transplant differ with the stage of disease at the time of transplant. For patients in chronic phase, interstitial pneumonia was the major cause of death, and for patients transplanted in accelerated phase or blast crisis, relapse was the major cause of death.[128] Younger age (<30 years) and absence of severe GVHD were also associated with better survival. Patients transplanted less than 1 year after diagnosis also had superior survival when compared to patients transplanted at a later time in chronic phase.[128] In a smaller series, the stage of disease at transplant was also important for improved disease-free survival, but patient age was not of prognostic significance.[129]

Although the presence of myelofibrosis and osteosclerosis in CML patients has been reversed in transplanted CML patients,[130,131] severe marrow fibrosis has been associated with significantly slower marrow recovery and prolonged dependence on platelet and erythrocyte transfusions.[132]

The role of splenectomy before BMT in patients with CML has recently been analyzed. Although there was no difference in the post-transplant survival of patients who had and had not undergone splenectomy, differences occurred in engraftment parameters and transfusion requirements.[133] Recovery of granulocytes was more rapid in the splenectomized patients. Also, platelet transfusions were given for a mean of 10 days in the splenectomized group as compared to 20 days for nonsplenectomized patients.

The studies of allogeneic BMT for CML clearly indicate its efficacy for patients transplanted in the chronic phase (Table 48-7). In this stage of the disease, the major reasons for nonsurvival are GVHD and infection. The current survival rates are 50% to 70%, with persistent eradication of the Philadelphia-positive leukemic clone, suggesting cure of these patients. With improved methods of GVHD prevention, survival rates should improve further. Transplantation of CML patients in the accelerated phase is clearly inferior to transplantation earlier in the disease course; however, it does offer improved survival over current conventional therapy. Although the initial CML transplants were performed in blast crisis patients, survival is very poor and this practice should not continue.

AUTOLOGOUS. Although allogeneic BMT provides curative therapy for CML patients, it is restricted to the 30% to 40% of patients with a sibling donor matched at the major histocompatibility locus. For CML patients without a donor, autologous BMT has been attempted with reinfusion of untreated bone marrow. Cells were harvested in chronic phase and reinfused following high-dose chemoradiotherapy administered when the patient was in blast crisis.[134,135] In a study of 11 patients (10 in blast crisis) treated with autologous marrow harvested during chronic phase, the outcome was poor, with only 1 patient surviving disease-free. It is possible that autologous transplantation before the development of advanced disease, combined with marrow treatment, may improve the results of autologous grafting in CML.

Non-Hodgkin's Lymphoma

Current therapeutic programs provide excellent disease-free survival for non-Hodgkin's lymphoma (NHL) in most children (see Chap. 20).[136,137] Patients who relapse or have refractory lymphoma, however, may benefit from high-dose chemoradiotherapy coupled with infusion of allogeneic, syngeneic, or autologous marrow. Initial reports of syngeneic and allogeneic transplant in NHL are limited but encouraging.

Table 48-7
Allogeneic BMT for Patients with CML

Center*	Preparative Regimen	Stage of Disease†	2-Year Survival		
			Number of Patients	Actuarial (%)	Median Follow-up (mo)
Minnesota[123]	CTX + fTBI 1.3 cGy	CP	20/29	64	25
		AC	9/28	30	25
Seattle[128]	CTX + TBI (single dose or fTBI)	CP	38/67	49	NA
		Second CP	7/12	58	
		AP	11/46	15	
		BC	7/42	14	
Hammersmith[129]	CTX + fTBI	CP	38/52	72	25
		AP + second CP	4/18	18	
IBMTR[126]	Various	CP	25/39	63	NA
		AP	21/56	36	
		BC	2/22	12	

* IBMTR = International Bone Marrow Transplant Registry.

CP = chronic phase; AP = accelerated phase; BC = blast crisis.

Syngeneic transplantation for NHL has been reported by the Seattle transplantation team.[138] Four of eight transplanted patients remained in remission from 2 to 11 years after transplant.[139,140]

Allogeneic transplantation was evaluated as therapy for 20 patients with advanced or refractory NHL. Only 4 patients survived, and the risk of recurrent disease following cyclophosphamide, total body irradiation, and allogeneic transplantation was 75%.[141] Allogeneic BMT was used as therapy for 10 children and young adults (ages 4–29 years) with disseminated Burkitt's lymphoma or T-cell lymphoblastic lymphoma.[141] Five of the 10 patients remain alive in long-term remission without maintenance therapy.

The use of autologous transplantation in NHL has been more extensively evaluated. Since many patients with NHL do not have marrow involvement, this approach is particularly attractive. Preparative regimens have used chemotherapy combined with total body irradiation or high-dose chemotherapy alone. Studies of autologous BMT in NHL are combined series of children and adults, with the majority of patients being adults.

The initial reported studies of autologous BMT in NHL used a preparative regimen (BACT) consisting of BCNU, ara-C, 6-thioguanine, and high-dose cyclophosphamide, with infusion of autologous marrow in some patients.[142,143] Four patients were cured of their disease, remaining disease-free 5½ to 7½ years after autologous transplantation having initially failed conventional chemotherapy.[140]

In a series of 17 children and adults with NHL who received autologous BMT after preparation with BACT and, in some patients, additional total body irradiation, 7 patients remain in continuous complete remission with a median follow-up of 16 months after transplantation.[144] An analysis of 50 poor-prognosis NHL patients transplanted at several centers using different preparative regimens demonstrated that long-term disease-free survival could be achieved in some patients who were chemotherapy-responsive after relapse.[145] Patients who were resistant to chemotherapy, however achieved complete responses of only short duration, with poor disease-free survival.

Phillips reported a series of 27 NHL patients prepared with high-dose cyclophosphamide and total body irradiation.[146] Engraftment occurred, but progressive lymphoma was a major cause of failure. Five of the patients remained free of disease for 1½ to 6 years.

A series of 16 children with relapsed NHL has been reported by Hartmann and colleagues.[147] These children with Burkitt's lymphoma or lymphoblastic lymphoma failed initial chemotherapy and subsequently were treated with high-dose chemotherapy and autologous BMT. Five children remained in continuous complete remission with a median follow-up of 2½ years.

Although other successful autologous bone marrow transplants in NHL have been reported, the numbers of patients are too small for any meaningful conclusions.[148–150] A recent survey indicated that over 1000 patients with NHL or Hodgkin's disease have received autologous BMT.[151]

The role of bone marrow purging for autologous BMT in NHL is currently being evaluated. Monoclonal antibodies plus complement or chemotherapeutic agents such as 4-hydroperoxycyclophosphamide have been evaluated as purging reagents in NHL.[152–154] Although preliminary trials have demonstrated adequate engraftment, follow-up is too short to evaluate outcome data.[152–156] The role of BMT for NHL remains to be clarified. There are no clearly superior preparative regimens, and the optimal timing of BMT is not defined in this heterogeneous group of diseases. Thus, the role of autologous transplant also needs further delineation.

Hodgkin's Disease

Current therapeutic approaches are very successful in children with Hodgkin's disease (see Chap. 21).[157] Patients who fail two treatment modalities, however, are usually not cured.[158] For these patients, intensive therapy followed by autologous marrow infusion has been attempted. Bone marrow transplant for relapsed or refractory Hodgkin's disease has been performed following chemotherapy alone or combined with total body irradiation.[159–162] Only occasional pediatric patients are included in some reports. Few patients with refractory Hodgkin's disease have received allogeneic transplants, and conclusions from these initial studies performed in advanced patients are limited. Remission—prolonged in a few cases—have been achieved in some patients with refractory Hodgkin's disease, although failures are frequent in these intensively pretreated patients. The role of BMT in patients with Hodgkin's disease has yet to be determined and is currently very limited.

Solid Tumors

Neuroblastoma

The survival for children with disseminated neuroblastoma at diagnosis has not improved over the past 20 years despite treatment with chemotherapy, surgery, and irradiation (see Chap. 28). Although initial responses occur, the disease relapses in most cases and the long-term survival is less than 20%.[163] The success of BMT in childhood leukemia[57] led investigators to evaluate high-dose chemotherapy and radiation therapy followed by infusion of autologous or donor bone marrow as treatment for patients with neuroblastoma.

Initial studies evaluated the use of high-dose melphalan or other chemotherapeutic agents followed by autologous BMT.[164,165] These studies provided encouragement for this approach because long-term survival was achieved in some patients.

The role of BMT in the treatment of neuroblastoma is currently being evaluated in several centers. In one study, ten patients with recurrent Stage IV neuroblastoma received local radiation therapy, supralethal chemotherapy, and total body irradiation followed by allogeneic or autologous BMT.[166] Two of four patients who received allogeneic grafts are in complete remission at 3 and 4½ years, and two of six patients who received autologous grafts are in complete remission at 22 and 35 months. This study suggests that some patients with relapsed neuroblastoma may be cured with this approach.

The development of techniques to purge bone marrow of tumor cells is important for the use of autologous BMT in neuroblastoma because the majority of patients with Stage IV neuroblastoma have marrow involvement. The technique developed by Kemshead uses monoclonal antibodies bound to polystyrene microspheres containing magnetite and is being used to remove tumor cells from bone marrow of patients with neuroblastoma.[167] This technique was used in a series of Stage IV neuroblastoma patients other than 1 year, in combination with consolidation using intensive chemoradiotherapy and BMT performed within 12 months of diagnosis.[168] Of 56 patients entered on study, 37 patients were transplanted, 35 of whom received autografts. The marrow of 32 patients was purged using immunomagnetic techniques. The relapse rate in the entire group of patients was 32% and the acute toxic death rate was 19%. Progression-free survival at 32 months for patients transplanted in complete remission or very good partial remission was 44% compared to 13% for patients transplanted in partial remission. Very good partial remission was defined as removal of more than 90% of the tumor at surgery, normal catecholamines, and normal marrow with an improved bone scan.

Another approach to bone marrow transplantation in neuroblastoma has been the use of two intensive chemotherapy regimens and autologous BMT without total body irradiation.[169]

The timing of BMT in neuroblastoma patients is important. In one report, transplantation of patients before the development of progressive disease yielded significantly better survival than transplantation after progressive disease developed.[170]

The conditioning regimens used in BMT for neuroblastoma have been intensive, leading to a high death rate from toxicity.[168,171] Still, recurrent neuroblastoma occurs in a number of patients. Future approaches will need to address these problems in order to define the role of BMT for neuroblastoma in children. Currently, it is recommended that newly diagnosed children with Stage IV neuroblastoma undergo BMT in the first few months after diagnosis, preferably at a time of maximum response and before disease progression.

Ewing's Sarcoma and Brain Tumors

Bone marrow transplantation combined with intensive chemoradiotherapy is being investigated for patients with recurrent Ewing's sarcoma (see also Chap. 31). In most cases, autologous marrow has been used because marrow involvement is unusual in these malignancies. High-dose melphalan followed by autologous marrow infusion produced partial responses of short duration in some Ewing's sarcoma patients.[165,172,173]

Bone marrow transplantation following high-dose chemotherapy, usually with nitrosoureas, is being evaluated in recurrent brain tumors, particularly malignant gliomas. In one series of 36 children and adults, prolonged disease-free survival was noted in an occasional patient.[174] Although responses were obtained in 44% of 29 patients transplanted after progressive disease, only 2 patients had prolonged disease-free survival. Three of nine patients treated with BMT as adjuvant therapy had prolonged disease-free survival. The role of BMT in brain tumors needs further evaluation.

COMPLICATIONS

Graft-Versus-Host Disease

Graft-versus-host disease is a pathologic process wherein donor T-lymphocytes are activated *in vivo* and produce damage to recipient target organs by either direct or indirect effects.[19,175] In humans, the clinical syndrome of acute GVHD consists of weight loss, diarrhea, skin rash, and liver dysfunction. GVHD occurs in 30% to 70% of patients receiving MHC-identical sibling transplants[176-177] and consists of an acute and chronic form (Table 48-8).

Acute GVHD is a clinical syndrome of rash, cholestatic liver dysfunction, and diarrhea that occurs at the time of engraftment or shortly thereafter. Increasing recipient age has been associated with an increased risk of GVHD, so that the

Table 48-8
Clinical Features of Graft-Versus-Host Disease in BMT Patients

System	Acute	Chronic
Skin	Maculopapular rash Erythroderma Desquamation and bullae	Pigmentary changes Thickening of the skin Scleroderma Nail changes
Liver	Jaundice	± Jaundice
Gastrointestinal tract	Diarrhea Abdominal pain Nausea, vomiting	Dysphagia Weight loss Oral dryness and ulcers
Eye	—	Photophobia Eye pain Dry eyes
Lung	—	Symptoms of obstructive lung disease
Other	—	Myasthenia gravis Vaginal strictures/ stenosis

risk is less in children than in adults.[33,178,179] There is also an increased risk of acute GVHD with an increased degree of HLA nonidentity between host and donor marrow.[180] Female donors and opposite-sex donors have been associated with increased GVHD.[178-180] In patients with aplastic anemia, those with HLA-B18 had increased acute GVHD, and patients who received buffy coat infusions had a higher incidence of chronic GVHD.[181,182]

The clinical picture of acute GVHD needs to be distinguished from other complications, particularly infections. The rash of acute GVHD is a maculopapular eruption that frequently evolves to a confluent, erythematous rash involving most of the skin.[183] Histologic findings include basal cell vascular degeneration with necrosis of epidermal cells (single cell necrosis) and, in severe cases, separation of the dermal–epidermal junction.[184,185]

Liver dysfunction consists primarily of cholestatic changes. Hyperbilirubinemia frequently occurs with less dramatic changes in hepatocellular enzymes, and the histologic findings include bile duct damage with relative sparing of parenchymal tissue. Portal or central vein endothelialitis has been described.[186-188]

Gastrointestinal GVHD is manifested by diarrhea that may be severe and is often associated with crampy abdominal pain. Although rectal biopsy is helpful in making the diagnosis, the effects of chemotherapy and irradiation may be difficult to differentiate in the first 3 weeks post-transplant.[189] The characteristic findings of GVHD of the rectum include necrosis of individual cells in the crypts, which may progress to dropout of entire crypts and loss of the epithelium.[190] Upper gastrointestinal involvement with GVHD may be manifested by anorexia, nausea, and vomiting and is associated with involvement of the esophagus, stomach, and duodenum.[191]

Graft-versus-host disease is a clinicopathologic syndrome that must be distinguished from other post-transplant complications, especially those due to chemoradiotherapy and infections. Histologic examination of material from affected organs is helpful in making this diagnosis. The severity of acute GVHD is usually graded I to IV according to the criteria developed by the Seattle transplant team (Table 48-9). The overall grade of acute GVHD has been correlated with outcome.[176]

Chronic GVHD occurs later in the transplant course, typically after day 100.[177] It may represent persistence of acute GVHD or occur *de novo* in a patient who did not have acute GVHD.[192,193] The clinical manifestations are summarized in Table 48-8. Skin involvement in chronic GVHD may be localized or generalized. In the generalized form, an erythematous rash progresses to poikiloderma, with hyperpigmentation and sclerodermatous changes. Joint contractures may occur.[193,194] The liver is commonly involved in chronic GVHD, with predominantly cholestatic changes; pathologic evaluation reveals loss of bile ducts and periportal fibrosis.[195,196]

Xerostomia and oral mucosal ulceration are frequent manifestations of chronic GVHD.[197–199] Xerophthalmia, photophobia, and eye pain may be seen in chronic GVHD, associated with a variety of ocular pathologic states.[200,201] Esophageal involvement is seen in patients with extensive chronic GVHD and may be manifested by dysphagia or pain on swallowing; radiographic findings include webs and strictures.[202]

Gynecologic manifestations of GVHD include vaginal inflammation, sicca, and stenosis.[203] Other rare manifestations of chronic GVHD include myasthenia gravis and polymyositis.[204,205] A small number of patients with chronic GVHD develop obstructive lung disease that is very resistant to therapy. Histologically, a pattern of obliterative bronchiolitis is seen.[206,207]

Because of the morbidity and mortality associated with GVHD, tremendous effort has been directed at its prevention (see Table 48-2). Preventive techniques have involved either *in vivo* immunosuppressive therapy aimed at eliminating T-lymphocytes or *ex vivo* removal of T-lymphocytes from donor marrow using a variety of purging techniques. *In vivo* therapy has involved post-transplant immunosuppression with methotrexate, ATG, steroids, and cyclosporine, used alone or in combination. Methotrexate alone post-transplant was initially evaluated based on studies in dogs and is frequently compared to other regimens.[208] Although one group reported no difference in GVHD in patients who received methotrexate compared to those who received no methotrexate,[209] a recent study reported hyperacute GVHD in patients receiving no post-transplant immunosuppression.[210] The addition of ATG and prednisone to methotrexate significantly decreased the incidence of acute GVHD in one series[33] but not in others.[31,32]

Cyclosporine, a potent immunosuppressive agent, has been associated with less GVHD.[211–213] Although cyclosporine is not myelotoxic, allowing faster engraftment, it does produce renal toxicity, neurotoxicity, and hypertension.[214–216] When cyclosporine was evaluated as a single agent, there was less acute GVHD in patients with ANLL but not CML, and survival did not differ.[34,35]

Currently, combination therapy with methotrexate and cyclosporine is being evaluated and in leukemic patients has resulted in less acute GVHD and improved survival when compared to cyclosporine alone.[36]

Because of the continuing occurrence of GVHD despite the use of these post-transplant immunosuppressive agents, coupled with their associated toxicity, recent studies have been evaluating the removal of donor T-lymphocytes *ex vivo* before marrow infusion. Animal studies have demonstrated that *ex vivo* removal of immunocompetent cells can prevent GVHD and allow transplantation across major and minor histocompatibility barriers.[30,37,38]

The removal of mature T-lymphocytes using the soybean agglutinin was described by Reisner and colleagues.[217] This technique has been effective when transplanting patients with SCID using haploidentical donors. However, engraftment problems were seen in a series of leukemic patients who received haploidentical grafts.[41,42]

T-cell removal has been accomplished by using monoclonal antibodies alone[43,44] or with complement,[39,40] or monoclonal antibodies linked to a toxin such as ricin.[45] When monoclonal antibodies were used alone, the incidence of GVHD was not decreased. Combining monoclonal antibodies with complement has resulted in decreased GVHD in matched patients. When partially matched donors were used, however, GVHD and nonengraftment occurred.

In a series of 17 matched patients transplanted with donor marrow depleted of T-cells using a "cocktail" of monoclonal antibodies linked to ricin, 4 patients experienced graft rejection. No severe GVHD was observed.[45]

Table 48-9
Clinical Staging and Grading of Acute Graft-Versus-Host Disease

	Clinical Feature or Severity			Functional Impairment
	Skin	Liver	Gut	
Stage				
+	Maculopapular rash <25% body surface	Bilirubin 2–3 mg/dl	Diarrhea 500–1,000 ml/day	—
++	Maculopapular rash 25%–50% body surface	Bilirubin 3–6 mg/dl	Diarrhea 1,000–1,500 ml/day	—
+++	Generalized erythroderma	Bilirubin 6–15 mg/dl	Diarrhea > 1,500 ml/day	—
++++	Desquamation and bullae	Bilirubin > 15 mg/dl	Pain or ileus	—
Grade*				
I	+ to ++	0	0	0
II	+ to +++	+	+	+
III	++ to +++	++ to +++	++ to +++	++
IV	++ to ++++	++ to ++++	++ to ++++	+++

(Sullivan KM: Acute and chronic graft-versus-host disease in man. Int J Cell Cloning 4[suppl 1]:42–93, 1986. Reprinted with permission of AlphaMed Press.)
* Grade I = mild; II = moderate; III = severe; IV = life-threatening.

The problem of rejection has varied in different series but is increased in leukemic patients when various forms of T-cell depletion are used. This is true whether donors are matched or mismatched, but rejection is especially prevalent in recipients of mismatched marrow. The intensity of the conditioning regimen appears to play a role in the engraftment problem, with more intense regimens associated with a higher rate of engraftment.

Increased relapses have also been observed in two small series of T-cell-depleted transplants for leukemia.[46,47] The impact of T-cell depletion on relapse rates needs further evaluation.

Donor T-cells can now be removed from marrow with a variety of techniques. These techniques have decreased the incidence of GVHD in matched patients, but further studies are needed to evaluate the impact of potentially increased relapse rates and nonengraftment with these regimens. Increased intensity of conditioning regimens combined with T-cell depletion techniques should allow successful transplantation across histocompatibility barriers that previously made transplantation impossible.

Until recently, allogeneic BMT has been restricted to patients with a donor matched at the major histocompatibility locus. Several different approaches are currently being explored for the majority of patients who do not have donors. Mismatched family donors have been used with only cyclosporine for GVHD prophylaxis, with a not unexpected high incidence of GVHD.[218] The Seattle team evaluated 105 patients with hematologic malignancies who were transplanted with haploidentical donors using standard methotrexate for GVHD prophylaxis.[219] Acute GVHD occurred earlier and more often in this group of patients than in matched transplant recipients. However, in the group of patients who were phenotypically but not genotypically identical for HLA-A, HLA-B, and HLA-D the risk of GVHD was not different from that of the control group of 728 similar patients concurrently receiving grafts from HLA genotypically identical siblings. Survival of the leukemic patients transplanted in remission was also comparable in the two groups.

The newer methods of *ex vivo* T-cell depletion are being evaluated in mismatched transplants.[42,220–222] The post-transplant complications of nonengraftment and severe GVHD are increased, but more intensive conditioning has facilitated engraftment. A disturbing complication is post-transplant immunoblastic lymphoproliferative disorders in T-cell-depleted mismatched transplants.[223] The overall incidence of this complication is not yet clear.

The use of phenotypically identical unrelated donors is currently being evaluated in several centers. Mechanisms of searching a large population of potential donors are now available.[224] Registries of HLA-typed donors willing to donate bone marrow have frequently been developed from a file of blood or apheresis donors. In one program, 70% of previously HLA-typed donors agreed to participate in a bone marrow donor program. Until recently, requests for an unrelated donor search were directed to a few programs with donor files. However, a national program is now available that will expedite national searches. This larger pool will also provide potential donors for larger numbers of patients. Successful unrelated but matched allogeneic marrow transplants have been reported in a limited number of patients with acute and chronic leukemia. GVHD occurred in 6 of 8 patients in one series.[100,225] The role of matched, unrelated donors in BMT requires evaluation in more patients, which should be possible with the development of the national registry.

Infections

Infections caused by multiple etiologic agents are a major source of morbidity and mortality in BMT recipients (see also Chap. 39). The cytoreductive regimen results in profound myelosuppression of relatively short duration (weeks) and immunosuppression that persists for months. If GVHD occurs, immunologic dysfunction persists even longer.

Three post-transplant periods have been described that are characterized by a high incidence of specific infections (Fig. 48-3).[226] In the first 2 to 4 weeks, profound granulocyto-

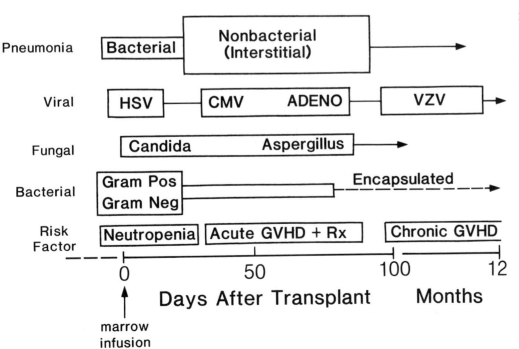

FIGURE 48-3. Occurrence of infections at specific times after transplantation. (Reprinted with permission from Myers JD: Infections in marrow recipients. In Principles and Practice of Infectious Diseases, 2nd ed, p 1674. New York, John Wiley & Sons, 1985)

penia exists, with susceptibility to bacterial and fungal infections.[227-229] Infections may be due to common pathogens, such as gram-positive bacteria, or to less common pathogens, such as aspergillus. These problems are seen despite the aggressive use of antibiotics and amphotericin in these febrile, neutropenic patients. The role of laminar air flow rooms in transplantation is not clear; their use has been shown to decrease the incidence of GVHD in patients undergoing BMT for severe aplastic anemia but not for leukemia.[230]

After the first month, when neutropenia is less common, the risk of viral infections, particularly cytomegalovirus (CMV), is high. CMV is the most common infectious cause of death in allogeneic transplantation, often resulting in CMV pneumonia.[231] It occurs more frequently in patients who are seropositive before BMT. In seronegative patients, significant risk factors include positive serology of the marrow donor and the use of granulocyte transfusions from seropositive donors. In all patients, the occurrence of acute GVHD increased the risk of CMV infection.[232]

Several approaches have been taken to prevent CMV infection, which presumably occurs from reactivation of endogenous virus or, in seronegative patients, from infection acquired through transfusion of blood products.[233] The administration of hyperimmune globulin prophylactically[234-237] and the use of antiviral agents have yielded variable results.[234] The use of blood products from CMV-negative donors may be an effective prophylactic approach for CMV-negative recipients.[238]

Other localized or disseminated viral infections that occur at this time include adenovirus, herpes virus, and polyoma viruses.[239-242]

Infections occurring after the first 3 months are often seen in patients with chronic GVHD that is associated with prolonged immunosuppression. Herpes zoster infections and late infections due to pneumococcus frequently occur in such patients.[242,243]

Interstitial Pneumonitis

Interstitial pneumonitis is one of the most important transplant complications because of its frequency and high fatality rate. In a recent analysis of 932 patients with leukemia by the International Bone Marrow Transplant Registry, the incidence of interstitial pneumonitis was 35%, with a fatality rate of 24%.[244] In this large multi-institutional study, six factors were associated with an increased risk of interstitial pneumonitis: use of methotrexate rather than cyclosporine post-transplant, older age, severe GVHD, long interval from diagnosis to transplantation, lower performance ratings before transplantation, and high dose rates of irradiation in patients given methotrexate.

Although the clinical picture of rapid onset of tachypnea associated with bilateral interstitial infiltrates is a common presentation, multiple etiologic agents have been implicated in the pathogenesis of this complication. Cytomegalovirus is the most common pathogen: other etiologic agents include *Pneumocystis carinii* and herpes simplex virus.[245] In a large number of cases, no pathogen is identified ("idiopathic interstitial pneumonitis"). Radiation to the lungs likely plays a role in the development of interstitial pneumonitis.[246]

Late Effects, Second Malignancies, and Post-transplant Lymphomas

The increasing population of long-term survivors of BMT in childhood necessitates delineation of the late effects of this procedure. The potential sequelae of the disease, treatment,

and complications are important. The main areas that have been evaluated in children include growth and endocrinologic (*e.g.,* gonadal and thyroid) function.[247-249]

Children transplanted for malignancies usually receive high-dose total body irradiation. As a group, these children experience decreased height velocity following BMT.[247-249] Thyroid dysfunction is seen in 40% to 50% of patients.[247-249] Gonadal dysfunction or failure is common, and patients who were prepubertal before BMT have delayed development of secondary sex characteristics.[249] It is important that children who are survivors of transplant have close follow-up for these effects, with appropriate hormonal replacement as required.

The development of cataracts following transplantation with total body irradiation has been reported in the majority of patients.[250] Fractionated total body irradiation may be associated with a lower incidence of cataracts than single-dose total body irradiation.

As the number of long-term survivors of BMT increases, the occurrence of second malignancies in a proportion of patients is to be expected. Patients receive high-dose chemotherapy, often in combination with total body irradiation and usually with additional post-BMT immunosuppressive drugs. All of these modalities have been associated with the development of malignancies in other situations.

A review outlining the details of 20 second malignancies reported before 1984 described three different groups.[251] In the first group were six patients who had recurrence of leukemia identical to that of their original disease, but occurring in donor cells. The second group consisted of seven patients who developed lymphoproliferative malignancies that differed from their original disease. In the patients who were evaluated, EBV-genome or EBV-associated antigens were present. These EBV-related lymphomas have been well described in organ transplant recipients and in immunodeficient patients. The disorder appears to vary from a polyclonal to monoclonal disorder and in some cases may be responsive to antiviral therapy.[252] The third group of six patients developed solid tumors, two of which occurred in the brain of children previously irradiated for ALL. Long-term survivors of ALL treated with radiation and chemotherapy without BMT have also had an increased incidence of brain tumors.[253]

These late effects of therapy are devastating, and as long-term survival improves, conditioning regimens will need to be evaluated for their long-term impact.

FUTURE DIRECTIONS

Since its initial use as curative therapy for infants with inherited immunodeficiency disorders, bone marrow transplantation has become the primary treatment modality for patients with various types of malignancies as well as quantitative and qualitative defects of bone-marrow-derived cell populations. The ability to deliver high-dose chemotherapy, with or without radiotherapy followed by marrow rescue, has made BMT the treatment of choice for patients with ANLL in first remission and for CML patients in chronic phase when a matched donor is available. For patients with ALL who relapse and for selected first-remission ALL patients, BMT represents an important treatment option that currently compares favorably to chemotherapeutic regimens. More recently, initial promising results for poor-risk Stage III and Stage IV neuroblastoma have been attained. Retrieval therapy for non-Hodgkin's and Hodgkin's lymphomas have yielded results worthy of further investigation. The role of allogeneic and autologous BMT in many of these disease processes will be more clearly defined in the next decade. Until that time, transplantation will remain the mainstay of therapy for certain patients with malignant disorders, and its role in advanced stages of malignancies will be increasingly explored.

Progress is being made in overcoming the major limitations of BMT. The previous absolute prerequisite for a histocompatible sibling donor may soon be successfully and routinely avoided by the use of better prophylactic regimens and improved therapeutic strategies for GVHD. T-cell depletion of donor grafts as a means of GVHD prophylaxis has already been shown efficacious in preventing GVHD in the histocompatible sibling donor setting. Expanded efforts to modify the current techniques for T-cell depletion may produce a more successful outcome in recipients of donor marrow from histoincompatible donors. Graft rejection, which has been the major complication of these techniques in the mismatched setting, is being intensively studied in preclinical and clinical systems. The use of improved cytoreductive regimens or more specific or limited T-cell depletion may allow bone marrow transplantation across the HLA barrier without GVHD and with full donor cell engraftment. The use of recombinant growth and differentiating factors that are now entering clinical trials may further enhance hematopoietic recovery. For those patients who develop GVHD, more effective therapeutic regimens would lessen the morbidity and mortality associated with this complication. Anti-T-cell antibodies linked to toxins are being studied in trials in BMT patients. Preliminary results are encouraging. In the meantime, autologous BMT will be more extensively explored as an option for those patients who lack a histocompatible sibling donor. Marrow purging techniques for autologous BMT are being evaluated for tumor cell elimination prior to marrow reinfusion. Combinations of monoclonal antibody purging and chemotherapy are being tested. Novel cytoreductive regimens for ablation of malignant cells are being piloted. These efforts are particularly important because recurrence of malignancy is the single most problematic complication after BMT for patients with ALL and for those with more advanced stages of malignancy. Antibodies directed against leukemia-associated antigens and conjugated to drugs, radionucleotides, or toxins may provide the added antileukemia effect necessary to significantly decrease the rate of malignancy relapse after BMT. Advances in gene insertion techniques, currently being explored for the therapy of inherited metabolic disorders and immunodeficiency diseases, may provide a method of preventing recurrences after transplantation. The insertion of drug-resistant genes in the donor marrow could potentially permit the administration of chemotherapy after BMT, without compromise to the newly engrafted marrow. Conceivably, genes that turn off the growth of malignant cells could be inserted into the autologous marrow graft before bone marrow transplantation. However, these strategies will not be applicable for a considerable period of time.

In conclusion, the current success of bone marrow transplantation and the likely extension of this procedure as the primary treatment modality for patients with malignancies are justification for the continued use of bone marrow transplantation as a curative procedure for patients with malignancies.

REFERENCES

1. Gatti RA, Meuwissen HJ, Allen HD et al: Immunological reconstitution of sex-linked lymphopenic immunological deficiency. Lancet 2:1366–1369, 1968
2. Bach FH, Albertini RJ, Anderson JL et al: Bone marrow transplantation in patients with the Wiskott-Aldrich syndrome. Lancet 2:1364–1366, 1968
3. Camitta BM, Thomas ED, Nathan DG et al: Severe aplastic anemia: A prospective study of the effect of early marrow transplantation on acute mortality. Blood 48:63–70, 1976
4. Camitta BM, Thomas ED, Nathan DG et al: A prospective study of androgens and bone marrow transplantation for treatment of severe aplastic anemia. Blood 53:504–514, 1979
5. Storb R, Thomas ED, Buckner CD et al: Allogeneic marrow grafting for treatment of aplastic anemia. Blood 43:157–180, 1974
6. UCLA Bone Marrow Transplant Team: Bone marrow transplantation in severe aplastic anemia. Lancet 2:921–923, 1976
7. Ramsay NKC, Kim T, Nesbit ME et al: Total lymphoid irradiation and cyclophosphamide as preparation for bone marrow transplantation in severe aplastic anemia. Blood 55:344–346, 1980
8. Storb R, Prentice RL, Thomas ED et al: Factors associated with graft rejection after HLA-identical marrow transplantation for aplastic anemia. Br J Haematol 55:573–585, 1983
9. Ramsay NKC, Kim TH, McGlave P et al: Total lymphoid irradiation and cyclophosphamide conditioning prior to bone marrow transplantation for patients with severe aplastic anemia. Blood 62:622–626, 1983
10. Champlin RE, Feig SA, Sparkes RS et al: Bone marrow transplantation for identical twins in the treatment of aplastic anemia: Implications for the pathogenesis of the disease. Br J Haematol 56:455–463, 1984
11. Thomas ED, Buckner CD, Banaji M et al: One hundred patients with acute leukemia treated by chemotherapy, total body irradiation, and allogeneic marrow transplantation. Blood 49:511–533, 1977
12. Graw RG, Yankee RA, Rogentine GN et al: Bone marrow transplantation from HLA-matched donors to patients with acute leukemia. Transplantation 14:79–90, 1972
13. UCLA Bone Marrow Transplant Team: Bone marrow transplantation in acute leukemia. Lancet 2:1197–1200, 1977
14. Francke U, Pellegrino MA: Assignment of the major histocompatibility complex to a region of the short arm of chromosome 6. Proc Natl Acad Sci USA 74:1147–1151, 1977
15. Bodmer J, Bodmer W: Histocompatibility 1984. Immunol Today 5:251–254, 1984
16. Trowsdale J, Young JAT, Kelly AP et al: Structure, sequence and polymorphism in the HLA-D region. Immunol Rev 85:5–43, 1985
17. van Rood JJ, van Leeurven A, Keuning JJ et al: The serological recognition of the human MLC determinants using a modified cytotoxicity technique. Tissue Antigens 5:73–79, 1975
18. Dupont B, Hansen JA, Good RA, O'Reilly RJ: Histocompatibility testing for clinical bone marrow transplantation. In Ferrara GB (ed): HLA System—New Aspects, p 153. New York, Elsevier-North Holland Biomedical, 1977
19. Bach FH, van Rood JJ: The major histocompatibility complex. N Engl J Med 295:806–813, 1976
20. Bortin M, Buckner C: Major complications of marrow harvesting for transplantation. Exp Hematol 11:916–921, 1983
21. Wells J, Sullivan A, Cline M: A technique for separation and cryopreservation of myeloid stem cells from human marrow. Cryobiology 16:201–210, 1979
22. Bensinger WI, Buckner CD, Thomas ED, Clift RA: ABO-incompatible marrow transplants. Transplantation 33:427–429, 1981
23. Blacklock HA, Gilmore MJML, Prentice HG et al: ABO incompatible bone marrow transplantation: removal of red blood cells for donor marrow avoiding recipient antibody depletion. Lancet 1:1061–1064, 1982
24. Lasky LC, Warkentin PI, Kersey JH et al: Hemotherapy in patients undergoing blood group incompatible bone marrow transplantation. Transfusion 23:277–285, 1983
25. Gale RP, Feig S, Ho W et al: ABO blood group system and bone marrow transplantation. Blood 50:185–194, 1977
26. Buckner CD, Clift RA, Sanders JE et al: ABO-incompatible marrow transplants. Transplantation 26:233–238, 1978
27. Braine HG, Sensenbrenner LL, Wright SK et al: Bone marrow transplantation with major ABO blood group incompatibility using erythrocyte depletion of marrow prior to infusion. Blood 60:420–425, 1982
28. Berkman EM, Caplan SN, Kim CS: ABO-incompatible bone marrow transplantation: preparation by plasma exchange and in vivo antibody absorption. Transfusion 18:504–508, 1978
29. Billingham RE: The biology of graft-versus-host reactions. In The Harvey Lecture Series 62, 1966–1967, pp 21–78. New York, Academic Press, 1968
30. Vallera D, Soderling C, Carlson G, Kersey J: Bone marrow transplantation across major histocompatibility barriers in mice. Effects of elimination of T cells from donor grafts by pre-treatment with monoclonal Thy 1.2 plus complement or antibody alone. Transplantation 31:218–222, 1981
31. Weiden PL, Doney K, Storb R, Thomas ED: Antihuman thymocyte globulin for prophylaxis of graft-versus-host disease. A randomized trial in patients with

leukemia treated with HLA-identical sibling marrow grafts. Transplantation 27:227–230, 1979

32. Doney KC, Weiden PL, Storb R, Thomas ED: Failure of early administration of antithymocyte globulin to lessen graft-versus-host disease in human allogeneic marrow transplant recipients. Transplantation 31:141–143, 1981

33. Ramsay NKC, Kersey J, Robison L et al: A randomized study of prevention of acute graft-versus-host disease. N Engl J Med 306:392–397, 1982

34. Deeg HJ, Storb R, Thomas ED et al: Cyclosporine as prophylaxis for graft-versus-host disease: A randomized study in patients undergoing marrow transplantation for acute nonlymphoblastic leukemia. Blood 65:1325–1334, 1985

35. Storb R, Deeg HJ, Thomas ED et al: Marrow transplantation for chronic myelocytic leukemia: A controlled trial of cyclosporine versus methotrexate for prophylaxis of graft-versus-host disease. Blood 66:698–702, 1985

36. Storb R, Deeg HJ, Whitehead J et al: Marrow transplantation for leukemia: A controlled trial of a combination of methotrexate and cyclosporine versus cyclosporine alone for prophylaxis of acute graft-versus-host disease. N Engl J Med 314:729–735, 1986

37. Rodt H, Theirfelder S, Eulitz M: Anti-lymphocytic antibodies and marrow transplantation III. Effect of heterologous anti-brain antibodies on acute secondary disease in mice. Eur J Immunol 4:15–19, 1974

38. Korngold LR, Sprent J: Lethal graft-versus-host disease after bone marrow transplantation across minor histocompatibility barriers in mice. Prevention by removing mature T cells from marrow. J Exp Med 148:1687–1698, 1978

39. Prentice HG, Blacklock HA, Janossy G et al: Depleton of T-lymphocytes in donor marrow prevents significant graft-versus-host disease in matched allogeneic leukaemic marrow transplant recipients. Lancet 1:472–476, 1984

40. Trigg ME, Billing R, Sondel PM et al: Clinical trial depleting T lymphocytes from donor marrow for matched and mismatched allogeneic bone marrow transplants. Cancer Treat Rep 69:377–386, 1985

41. Reisner Y, Kapoor N, Kirkpatrick D et al: Transplantation for severe combined immunodeficiency with HLA-A, B, D, DR incompatible parenteral marrow cells fractionated by soybean agglutinin and sheep red blood cells. Blood 61:341–348, 1983

42. O'Reilly RJ, Collins NH, Kernan N et al: Transplantation of marrow-depleted T cells by soybean lectin agglutination and E-rosette depletion: Major histocompatibility complex-related graft resistance in leukemic transplant recipients. Transplant Proc 17:455–459, 1985

43. Filipovich AH, Ramsay NKC, Warkentin P et al: Pretreatment of donor bone marrow with monoclonal antibody OKT3 for prevention of acute graft-versus-host disease in allogeneic histocompatible bone marrow transplantation. Lancet 1:1266–1269, 1982

44. Prentice H, Janossy G, Skeggs D et al: Use of anti-T-cell monoclonal antibody OKT3 to prevent graft-versus-host disease in allogeneic bone marrow transplantation for acute leukaemia. Lancet 1:700–703, 1982

45. Filipovich AH, Vallera DA, Youle RJ et al: Graft-versus-host disease prevention in allogeneic bone marrow transplantation from histocompatible siblings: A pilot study using immunotoxins for T-cell depletion of donor bone marrow. Transplantation 44:62–69, 1987

46. Apperly JF, Jones L, Arthur C et al: Incidence of relapse after T-cell depleted marrow transplant for chronic granulocytic leukemia in first chronic phase. Blood 68(Suppl 1):270a, 1986

47. Mitsuyasu RT, Champlin RE, Ho WG et al: Prospective randomized trial of ex vivo treatment of donor bone marrow with monoclonal anti-T-cell antibody and complement for prevention of graft-versus-host disease: A preliminary report. Transplant Proc 17:482–485, 1985

48. Weiden PL, Flournoy N, Thomas ED et al: Anti-leukemic effect of graft versus host disease in human recipients of allogeneic marrow grafts. N Engl J Med 300:1068–1073, 1979

49. Weisdorf DJ, Nesbit ME, Ramsay NKC et al: Allogeneic bone marrow transplantation for acute lymphoblastic leukemia in remission: Prolonged survival associated with acute graft versus host disease. J Clin Oncol 9:1348–1355, 1987

50. Gale RP, Champlin RE: How does bone marrow transplantation cure leukaemia? Lancet 2:28–30, 1984

51. Weinstein HJ, Mayer RJ, Rosenthal DS et al: Treatment of acute myelogenous leukemia in children and adults. N Engl J Med 303:473–478, 1980

52. Weinstein HJ, Mayer RJ, Rosenthal DS et al: Chemotherapy for acute myelogenous leukemia in children and adults: VAPA update. Blood 62:315–319, 1983

53. Thomas ED, Clift RA, Buckner CD et al: Marrow transplantation for patients with acute nonlymphoblastic leukemia who achieve a first remission. Cancer Treat Rep 66:1463–1466, 1982

54. Thomas ED, Buckner CD, Clift RA et al: Marrow transplantation for acute nonlymphoblastic leukemia in first remission. N Engl J Med 301:597–599, 1979

55. Thomas ED: Marrow transplant for acute nonlymphoblastic leukemia in first remission: A followup. N Engl J Med 308:1539, 1983

56. UCLA Bone Marrow Transplantation Group: Bone marrow transplantation with intensive combination chemotherapy/radiation therapy (SCARI) in acute leukemia. Ann Intern Med 86:155–161, 1977

57. Sanders JE, Thomas ED, Buckner CD et al: Marrow transplantation for children in first remission of acute non-lymphoblastic leukemia: An update. Blood 66:460–462, 1985

58. Forman SJ, Spruce WE, Farbstein MJ et al: Bone marrow ablation followed by allogeneic marrow grafting during first complete remission of acute non-lymphocytic leukemia. Blood 61:439–442, 1983

59. Buckner CD, Clift RA, Thomas ED et al: Allogeneic marrow transplantation for patients with acute nonlymphoblastic leukemia in second remission. Leuk Res 6:395–399, 1982

60. Dinsmore R, Kirkpatrick D, Flomenberg N et al: Allogeneic bone marrow transplantation for patients with acute nonlymphocytic leukemia. Blood 63:649–656, 1984

61. Bostrom B, Brunning R, McGlave P et al: Factors predicting relapse following bone marrow transplantation (BMT) for acute nonlymphocytic leukemia (ANLL). Blood 65:1191–1196, 1985

62. Bortin MM, Gale RP, Kay HEM, Rimm AA, for the Advisory Committee of the International Bone Marrow Transplant Registry: Bone marrow transplantation for acute myelogenous leukemia: Factors associated with early mortality. JAMA 249:1166–1175, 1983

63. Santos GW, Tutschka PJ, Brookmeyer R et al: Marrow transplantation for acute nonlymphocytic leukemia after treatment with busulfan and cyclophosphamide. N Engl J Med 309:1347–1353, 1983

64. Applebaum FR, Dahlberg S, Thomas ED et al: Bone marrow transplantation or chemotherapy after remission induction for adults with acute nonlymphoblastic leukemia. Ann Intern Med 101:581–588, 1984

65. Powles RL, Morgenstern G, Clink HM et al: The place of bone marrow transplantation in acute myelogenous leukemia. Lancet 2:1047–1050, 1980

66. Begg CB, McGlave PB, Bennett JM et al: A critical comparison of allogeneic bone marrow transplantation and conventional chemotherapy as treatment for acute nonlymphocytic leukemia. J Clin Oncol 2:369–378, 1984

67. Gale RP: Progress in acute myelogenous leukemia. Ann Intern Med 101:702–705, 1984

68. Champlin RE, Ho WG, Gale RP et al: Treatment of acute myelogenous leukemia: A prospective controlled trial of bone marrow transplantation versus consolidation chemotherapy. Ann Intern Med 102:285–291, 1985

69. Nesbit M, Buckley J, Lampkin B et al: Comparison of allogeneic bone marrow transplantation with maintenance chemotherapy in previously untreated childhood acute non-lymphocytic leukemia. Proc Am Soc Clin Oncol 6:163, 1987

70. Ball ED, Mills LE, Coughlin CT et al: Autologous bone marrow transplantation in acute myelogenous leukemia: In vitro treatment with myeloid cell-specific monoclonal antibodies. Blood 68:1311–1315, 1986

71. Gorin NC, Douay L, Laporte JP et al: Autologous bone marrow transplantation using marrow incubated with ASTA Z 7557 in adult acute leukemia. Blood 67:1367–1376, 1986

72. Yeager AM, Kaizer H, Santos GW et al: Autologous bone marrow transplantation in patients with acute non-lymphocytic leukemia, using ex vivo marrow treatment with 4-hydroperoxycyclophosphamide. N Engl J Med 315:141–147, 1986

73. Stewart P, Buckner CD, Bensinger W et al: Autologous marrow transplantation in patients with acute nonlymphocytic leukemia in first remission. Exp Hematol 13:267–272, 1985

74. Gorin NC: Autologous bone marrow transplantation in acute leukemia. J Natl Cancer Inst 76:1281–1287, 1986

75. Burnett AK, Tansey P, Watkins R et al: Transplantation of unpurged autologous bone marrow in adult myeloid leukemia in first remission. Lancet 2:1068–1070, 1984

76. Sharkis SE, Santos GW, Colvin M et al: Elimination of acute myelogenous cells from marrow and tumor suspensions in the rat with 4-hydroperoxycyclophosphamide. Blood 55:521–523, 1980

77. Niemeyer CM, Hitchcock-Bryan S, Sallan SE: Comparative analysis of treatment programs for childhood acute lymphoblastic leukemia. Semin Oncol 12:122–130, 1985

78. Nesbit ME, Sather HN, Robison LL et al: Randomized study of three years

versus five years of chemotherapy in childhood acute lymphoblastic leukemia. J Clin Oncol 1:308–316, 1983

79. Riehm H, Gadner H, Henze G et al: Acute lymphoblastic leukemia: Treatment results in three BFM studies (1970–1981). In Murphy SB, Gilbert JR (eds): Leukemia Research: Advances in Cell Biology and Treatment, pp 251–260. New York, Elsevier, 1983

80. Priest JR, Robison LL, McKenna RW et al: Philadelphia chromosome positive childhood acute lymphoblastic leukemia. Blood 56:15–22, 1980

81. Arthur DC, Bloomfield CD, Lindquist LL et al: Translocation 4;11 in acute lymphoblastic leukemia: Clinical characteristics and prognostic significance. Blood 52:96–99, 1982

82. Baum E, Nachman J, Ramsay N et al: Prolonged second remissions in childhood acute lymphocytic leukemia: A report from the Children's Cancer Study Group. Med Pediatr Oncol 11:1–7, 1983

83. Chessels JM, Rogers DW, Leiper AD et al: Bone marrow transplantation has a limited role in prolonging second marrow remission in childhood lymphoblastic leukemia. Lancet 1:1239–1241, 1986

84. Rivera GK, Buchanan G, Bovett JM et al: Intensive retreatment of childhood acute lymphoblastic leukemia in first bone marrow relapse: A pediatric oncology group study. N Engl J Med 315:273–278, 1986

85. Blume K, Beutler E, Bross K et al: Bone marrow ablation and allogeneic marrow transplantation in acute leukemia. N Engl J Med 302:1041–1046, 1980

86. Johnson FL, Thomas ED, Clark BS et al: A comparison of marrow transplantation with chemotherapy for children with acute lymphoblastic leukemia in second or subsequent remission. N Engl J Med 305:846–851, 1981

87. Dinsmore R, Kirkpatrick D, Flomenberg N et al: Allogeneic bone marrow transplantation for patients with acute lymphoblastic leukemia. Blood 62:381–388, 1983

88. Woods WG, Nesbit ME, Ramsay NKC et al: Intensive therapy followed by bone marrow transplantation for patients with acute lymphocytic leukemia in second or subsequent remission: Determination of prognostic factors. Blood 61:1182–1189, 1983

89. Sanders JE, Flournoy N, Thomas ED et al: Marrow transplant experience in children with acute lymphoblastic leukemia: An analysis of factors associated with survival, relapse and graft-versus-host disease. Med Pediatr Oncol 13:165–172, 1985

90. Johnson FL, Sanders J, Thomas ED: Long-term follow-up after bone marrow transplantation in acute lymphoblastic leukemia. Lancet 1:380–381, 1987

91. Blume KG, Forman SJ, O'Donnell MR et al: Total body irradiation and high-dose etoposide: A new preparatory regimen for bone marrow transplantation in patients with advanced hematologic malignancies. Blood 69:1015–1020, 1987

92. Nesbit ME, Robison LL, Ortega JA et al: Testicular relapse in childhood acute lymphoblastic leukemia: Association with pretreatment patient characteristics and treatment. A report from Childrens Cancer Study Group. Cancer 45:2009–2016, 1980

93. Sullivan MP, Perez CA, Herson J et al: Radiotherapy (2500 rad) for testicular leukemia: Local control and subsequent clinical events: A Southwest Oncology Group Study. Cancer 46:508–515, 1980

94. Nesbit ME, D'Angio JG, Sather HN et al: Effect of isolated central nervous system leukemia on bone marrow remission and survival in acute lymphoblastic leukemia. Lancet 1:1386–1389, 1981

95. Sallan SE, Hitchcock-Bryan S: Relapse in childhood acute lymphoblastic leukemia after elective cessation of initial treatment: Failure of subsequent treatment with cyclophosphamide, cytosine arabinoside, vincristine, and prednisone (COAP). Med Pediatr Oncol 9:455–462, 1981

96. Poynton CH, Joshi R, Giangrande PLF, Barrett AJ: Acute lymphoblastic leukemia (ALL): Prevention of relapse after allogeneic transplantation (abstr). Proc Am Soc Clin Oncol 4:158, 1985

97. Woods WG, Ramsay NKC, Kersey JH: Long-term followup of individuals undergoing allogeneic bone marrow transplantation for acute lymphoblastic leukemia. J Clin Oncol 4:1015–1016, 1986

98. Coccia PF, Strandjord SE, Warrentin PI et al: High-dose cytosine arabinoside and fractionated total–body irradiation: An improved preparative regimen for bone marrow transplantation of children with acute lymphoblastic leukemia in remission. Blood 71:888–893, 1988

99. Hansen JA, Clift RA, Beatty PG et al: Marrow transplantation from donors other than HLA genotypically identical siblings. In Gale RP (ed): Recent Advances in Bone Marrow Transplantation, pp 739–756. New York, Alan R Liss, 1983

100. Gingrich RD, Howe CWS, Goeken NE et al: The use of partially matched, unrelated donors in clinical bone marrow transplantation. Transplantation 39:526–532, 1985

101. Ritz J, Sallan SE, Bast RC et al: Autologous bone marrow transplantation in CALLA-positive acute lymphoblastic leukemia after in vitro treatment with J5 monoclonal antibody and complement. Lancet 2:60–63, 1982

102. Ramsay NKC, LeBien T, Nesbit M et al: Autologous bone marrow transplantation for patients with acute lymphoblastic leukemia in second or subsequent remission: Results of bone marrow treated with monoclonal antibodies BA-1, BA-2, BA-3 plus complement. Blood 66:508–513, 1985

103. Herve P, Tamayo E, Lamy B et al: In vitro treatment of autologous marrow cells collected in leukemic patients using cyclophosphamide derivative (abstr). Exp Hematol 11:10, 1983

104. Kaizer H, Stuart RH, Brookmeyer R et al: Autologous bone marrow transplantation in acute leukemia: A phase I study of in vitro treatment of marrow with 4-hydroperoxycyclophosphamide to purge tumor cells. Blood 65:1504–1510, 1985

105. Sallan S: Personal communication

106. Abramson CS, Kersey JH, LeBien TW: A monoclonal antibody (BA-1) reactive with cells of human B lymphocyte lineage. J Immunol 126:83–88, 1981

107. Kersey JH, LeBien TW, Abramson CS et al: A human leukemia-associated and lymphohemopoietic progenitor cell surface structure identified with monoclonal antibody. J Exp Med 153:726–731, 1981

108. LeBien TW, Boue DR, Bradley JG et al: Antibody affinity may influence antigenic modulation of the common acute lymphoblastic leukemia antigen in vitro. J Immunol 129:2287–2292, 1982

109. Kersey J, Goldman A, Abramson C et al: Clinical usefulness of monoclonal antibody phenotyping of childhood acute lymphoblastic leukemia. Lancet 2:1419–1423, 1982

110. LeBien TW, Ash RC, Zanjani ED et al: In vitro cytodestruction of leukemic cells in human bone marrow using a cocktail of monoclonal antibodies. In Neth R, Gallo RC, Greaves MF, et al (eds): Modern Trends in Human Leukemia, pp 112–116. New York, Springer-Verlag, 1983

111. Ramsay N, Nesbit M, McGlave P et al: Autologous bone marrow transplantation for patients with acute lymphoblastic leukemia in second or subsequent remission: Results of bone marrow treated with monoclonal antibodies BA-1, BA-2, BA-3 and complement using two sequential preparative regimens. In Gale RP, Champlin R (eds): Recent Advances in Bone Marrow Transplantation, vol 53. New York, Alan R Liss, 1987

112. Uckun FM, Gajl-Peczalska KJ, Kersey JH et al: Use of a novel colony assay to evaluate the cytotoxicity of an immunotoxin containing pokeweed antiviral protein against blast progenitor cells freshly obtained from patients with common B-lineage acute lymphoblastic leukemia. J Exp Med 163:347–368, 1986

113. Uckun FM, Gajl-Peczalska K, Meyers DE et al: Marrow purging in autologous lymphoblastic leukemia: Efficacy of ex vivo treatment with immunotoxins and 4-hydroperoxycyclophosphamide against fresh leukemic marrow progenitor cells. Blood 69:361–366, 1987

114. Bostrom B, Woods WG, Nesbit ME: Successful reinduction of patients with acute lymphoblastic leukemia who relapse following bone marrow transplantation. J Clin Oncol 5:376–381, 1987

115. Mays JA, Neerhout RC, Bogby GC, Koler RD: Juvenile chronic granulocytic leukemia. Am J Dis Child 134:654–658, 1980

116. Sanders JE, Buckner CD, Thomas ED et al: Allogeneic marrow transplantation for children with juvenile chronic myelogenous leukemia. Blood 71:1144–1146, 1988

117. Lawler SD: The cytogenetics of chronic granulocytic leukemia. Clin Haematol 6:55–75, 1977

118. Fefer A, Cheever MA, Thomas ED et al: Disappearance of Ph[1]-positive cells in four patients with chronic granulocytic leukemia after chemotherapy, irradiation, and marrow transplantation from an identical twin. N Engl J Med 300:333–337, 1979

119. Fefer A, Cheever MA, Greenberg PD et al: Treatment of chronic granulocytic leukemia with chemoradiotherapy and transplantation of marrow from identical twins. N Engl J Med 306:63–68, 1982

120. Doney KC, Buckner CD, Thomas ED et al: Allogeneic bone marrow transplantation for chronic granulocytic leukemia. Exp Hematol 9:966–971, 1981

121. McGlave PB, Miller WG, Hurd DD et al, for the University of Minnesota Bone Marrow Transplant Team: Cytogenetic conversion following allogeneic bone marrow transplantation for advanced chronic myelogenous leukemia. Blood 58:1050–1052, 1981

122. McGlave PB, Arthur DC, Weisdorf D et al: Allogeneic bone marrow trans-

plantation as treatment for accelerating chronic myelogenous leukemia. Blood 63:219–222, 1984

123. McGlave P, Arthur D, Haake R et al: Therapy of chronic myelogenous leukemia with allogeneic bone marrow transplantation. J Clin Oncol 7:1033–1040, 1987

124. Clift RA, Buckner CD, Thomas ED et al: Treatment of chronic granulocytic leukemia in chronic phase by allogeneic marrow transplantation. Lancet 2:621–622, 1982

125. Speck B, Gratwohl A, Nissen C et al: Allogeneic bone marrow transplantation for chronic granulocytic leukemia. Blut 45:237–242, 1982

126. Speck B, Bortin M, Champlin R et al: Allogeneic bone marrow transplantation for chronic myelogenous leukemia. Lancet 1:665–668, 1984

127. Fefer A, Clift RA, Thomas ED: Allogeneic marrow transplantation for chronic granulocytic leukemia. J Natl Cancer Inst 76:1295–1299, 1986

128. Thomas ED, Clift RA, Fefer A et al: Marrow transplantation for the treatment of chronic myelogenous leukemia. Ann Intern Med 104:155–163, 1986

129. Goldman JM, Apperley JF, Jones L et al: Bone marrow transplantation for patients with chronic myelogenous leukemia. N Engl J Med 314:202–207, 1986

130. McGlave PB, Brunning RD, Hurd DD, Kim TH: Reversal of severe myelofibrosis and osteosclerosis following allogeneic bone marrow transplantation for chronic myelogenous leukemia. Br J Haematol 52:189–194, 1982

131. Oblon DJ, Elfenbein GJ, Braylin RC et al: Reversal of myelofibrosis associated with chronic myelogenous leukemia after allogeneic bone marrow transplantation. Exp Hematol 11:681–685, 1983

132. Rajantie J, Sale GE, Deeg HJ et al: Adverse effect of severe marrow fibrosis on hematologic recovery after chemoradiotherapy and allogeneic bone marrow transplantation. Blood 67:1693–1697, 1986

133. Banaji M, Bearman SI, Buckner CD et al: The effects of splenectomy on engraftment and platelet transfusion requirements in patients with chronic myelogenous leukemia undergoing marrow transplantation. Am J Hematol 2:275–283, 1986

134. Goldman JM, Johnson SA, Islam A et al: Hematological reconstitution after autografting for chronic granulocytic leukemia in transformation. The influence of previous splenectomy. Br J Hematol 45:223–231, 1980

135. Vellekoop L, Zander AR, Kantarjian HM et al: Piperazinedione, total body irradiation, and autologous bone marrow transplantation in chronic myelogenous leukemia. J Clin Oncol 4:906–911, 1986

136. Anderson JR, Wilson JF, Jenkin DT et al: Childhood non-Hodgkin's lymphoma. The results of a randomized therapeutic trial comparing a 4-drug regimen (COMP) with a 10-drug regimen (LSA$_2$-L$_2$). N Engl J Med 308:559–565, 1983

137. Murphy SB, Bowman WP, Abromowitch M et al: Results of treatment of advanced stage Burkitt's lymphoma and B-cell (SIg+) acute lymphoblastic leukemia with high-dose fractionated cyclophosphamide and coordinated high dose methotrexate and cytarabine. J Clin Oncol 4:1732–1739, 1986

138. Appelbaum FR, Fefer A, Cheever MA et al: Treatment of non-Hodgkin's lymphoma with marrow transplantation in identical twins. Blood 58:509–513, 1981

139. Appelbaum FR, Thomas ED, Buckner CD et al: Treatment of non-Hodgkin's lymphoma with chemoradiotherapy and allogeneic marrow transplantation. Haematol Oncol 1:149–157, 1983

140. Appelbaum FR, Thomas ED: Review of the use of marrow transplantation in the treatment of non-Hodgkin's lymphoma. J Clin Oncol 1:440–447, 1983

141. O'Leary M, Ramsay NKC, Nesbit ME et al: Bone marrow transplantation for non-Hodgkin's lymphoma in children and young adults. Am J Med 74:497–501, 1983

142. Appelbaum FR, Deisseroth AB, Graw RG et al: Prolonged complete remission following high dose chemotherapy of Burkitt's lymphoma in relapse. Cancer 41:1059–1063, 1978

143. Appelbaum FR, Herzig GP, Ziegler JL et al: Successful engraftment of cryopreserved autologous bone marrow in patients with malignant lymphoma. Blood 52:85–95, 1978

144. Philip T, Biron P, Herve P et al: Massive BACT chemotherapy with autologous bone marrow transplantation in 17 cases of non-Hodgkin's malignant lymphoma with a very bad prognosis. Eur J Cancer Clin Oncol 19:1371–1379, 1983

145. Philip T, Biron P, Maraninchi D et al: Massive chemotherapy with autologous bone marrow transplantation in 50 cases of bad prognosis non-Hodgkins lymphoma. Br J Haematol 60:599–609, 1985

146. Phillips GL, Herzig RH, Lazarus HM et al: Treatment of resistant malignant lymphoma with cyclophosphamide, total body irradiation, and transplanta-

tion of cryopreserved autologous marrow. N Engl J Med 310:1557–1562, 1984

147. Hartmann O, Pein F, Beaujean F et al: High dose polychemotherapy with autologous bone marrow transplantation in children with relapsed lymphomas. J Clin Oncol 2:979–985, 1984

148. Kaizer H, Wharam MD, Munoz RJ et al: Autologous bone marrow transplantation in the treatment of selected human malignancies: The Johns Hopkins Oncology Center Program. Exp Hematol 7:309–320, 1979

149. Gorin NC, David R, Stachowiak J et al: High dose chemotherapy and autologous bone marrow transplantation in acute leukemias, malignant lymphomas and solid tumors. Eur J Cancer 17:557–568, 1981

150. Spitzer G, Vellekoop L, Zander A et al: Autologous bone marrow transplantation in leukemia and lymphoma. J Exp Clin Cancer Res 3:317–332, 1983

151. Armitage JO, Gale RP: Bone marrow autotransplantation in man: Report of an international cooperative study. Lancet 2:960–962, 1986

152. Hurd D, LeBien T, Petersen B et al: Intensive therapy and autologous bone marrow support for the treatment of refractory non-Hodgkin's lymphoma (abstr). Proc Am Soc Clin Oncol 5:193, 1986

153. Favrot M, Philip I, Philip T: Monoclonal antibodies and complement as purging procedure in Burkitt's lymphoma. In Dicke KA, Spitzer G, Zander AR (eds): Autologous Bone Marrow Transplantation, pp 389–401. Houston, University of Texas MD Anderson Hospital and Tumor Institute, 1985

154. De Fabritis P, Bregni M, Lipton J et al: Elimination of clonogenic Burkitt's lymphoma cells from human bone marrow using 4-hydroperoxycyclophosphamide in combination with monoclonal antibodies and complement. Blood 65:1064–1070, 1985

155. Anderson KC, Nadler LM: Bone marrow transplantation in the therapy of non-Hodgkin's lymphomas. In DeVita VT Jr, Hellman S, Rosenberg SA (eds): Important Advances in Oncology 1986, pp 287–310. Philadelphia, JB Lippincott, 1986

156. Gulati S, Fedorciw B, Gopal A et al: Autologous stem cell transplant for poor prognosis diffuse histiocytic lymphoma. In Dicke KA, Spitzer G, Zander AR (eds): Autologous Bone Marrow Transplantation, Proceedings of the First International Symposium, pp 75–81. Houston, University of Texas MD Anderson Hospital and Tumor Institute, 1985

157. Jenkin RDT, Berry MP: Hodgkin's disease in children. Semin Oncol 7:202–211, 1980

158. Harker WG, Kushlan P, Rosenberg SA: Combination chemotherapy for advanced Hodgkin's disease after failure of MOPP:ABVD and B-CAve. Ann Intern Med 101:440–446, 1984

159. Jagannath S, Dicke KA, Armitage JO et al: High dose cyclophosphamide, carmustine, and etoposide and autologous bone marrow transplantation for relapsed Hodgkin's disease. Ann Intern Med 104:163–168, 1986

160. Wolff SN, Phillips GL, Fay JW et al: Treatment of advanced Hodgkin's disease with intensive chemoradiotherapy and autologous bone marrow transplantation (abstr). Blood 66(suppl):246a, 1985

161. Philip T, Dumont J, Teillet F et al: High dose chemotherapy and autologous bone marrow transplantation in refractory Hodgkin's disease. Br J Cancer 53:737–742, 1986

162. Appelbaum FR, Sullivan KM, Thomas ED et al: Allogeneic marrow transplantation in the treatment of MOPP-resistant Hodgkin's disease. J Clin Oncol 3:1490–1494, 1985

163. Rosen EM, Cassady JR, Frantz CN et al: Neuroblastoma: The Joint Center for Radiation Therapy/Dana-Farber Cancer Institute/Children's Hospital Experience. J Clin Oncol 2:719–731, 1984

164. Pritchard J, McElwain TJ, Graham-Pole J: High dose melphalan with autologous bone marrow rescue for treatment of advanced neuroblastoma. Br J Cancer 45:86–94, 1982

165. Graham-Pole J, Lazarus HM, Herzig RH et al: High dose melphalan therapy for the treatment of children with refractory neuroblastoma and Ewing's sarcoma. Am J Pediatr Hematol Oncol 6:17–26, 1984

166. August CS, Serota FT, Koch PA et al: Treatment of advanced neuroblastoma with supralethal chemotherapy, radiation and allogeneic or autologous marrow reconstitution. J Clin Oncol 2:609–616, 1984

167. Treleaven JG, Gibson FM, Ugelstad J et al: Removal of neuroblastoma cells from bone marrow with monoclonal antibodies conjugated to magnetic microspheres. Lancet 1:70–73, 1984

168. Philip T, Bernard JL, Zucker JM et al: High-dose chemoradiotherapy with bone marrow transplantation as consolidation treatment in neuroblastoma: An unselected group of stage IV patients over one year of age. J Clin Oncol 5:266–271, 1987

169. Hartmann O, Kalifa C, Beaujean F et al: Treatment of advanced neuroblas-

toma with two consecutive high-dose chemotherapy regimens and ABMT. In Evans A, D'Angio GT, Seeger RC (eds): Advances in Neuroblastoma Research, pp 565–568. New York, Alan R Liss, 1985

170. Seeger R, Lenarsky C, Moss T et al: Bone marrow transplantation for poor prognosis neuroblastoma (abstr). Proc Am Soc Clin Oncol 6:221, 1987

171. D'Angio GJ, August C, Elkins W et al: Metastatic neuroblastoma managed by supralethal therapy and bone marrow reconstitution. Results of a four-institution Children's Cancer Study Group pilot study. In Evans A, D'Angio GJ, Seeger RC (eds): Advances in Neuroblastoma Research, pp 557–563. New York, Alan R Liss, 1985

172. Cornbleet MA, Carringham RET, Prentice HG et al: Treatment of Ewing's sarcoma with high dose melphalan and autologous bone marrow transplantation. Cancer Treat Rep 65:241–244, 1981

173. Kanfer EJ, Petersen FB, Buckner CD et al: Phase I study of high-dose dimethylbusulfan followed by autologous bone marrow transplantation in patients with advanced malignancy. Cancer Treat Rep 71:101–102, 1987

174. Phillips GL, Wolff SN, Fay JW et al: Intensive 1,3-Bis(2-chloroethyl)-1-nitrosourea (BCNU) monochemotherapy and autologous marrow transplantation for malignant glioma. J Clin Oncol 4:639–645, 1986

175. Santos GW, Cole JL: Effects of donor and host lymphoid and myeloid tissue injections in lethally x-irradiated mice treated with rat bone marrow. J Natl Cancer Inst 21:279–293, 1958

176. Glucksberg H, Storb R, Fefer A et al: Clinical manifestations of graft-versus-host disease in human recipients of marrow from HLA-matched sibling donors. Transplantation 18:295–304, 1974

177. Sullivan K: Graft-versus-host disease. In Blume KG, Petz LD (eds): Clinical Bone Marrow Transplantation, pp 91–129. New York, Churchill–Livingstone, 1983

178. Storb R, Prentice RL, Thomas ED: Treatment of aplastic anemia by marrow transplantation from HLA identical siblings. Prognostic factors associated with graft versus host disease and survival. J Clin Invest 59:625–632, 1977

179. Bross DS, Tutschka PJ, Farmer ER et al: Predictive factors for acute graft-versus-host disease in patients transplanted with HLA-identical bone marrow. Blood 63:1265–1270, 1984

180. Bortin MM: Risk factors for acute graft-versus-host disease. Exp Hematol 13:406, 1985

181. Storb R, Doney KC, Thomas ED et al: Marrow transplantation with or without donor buffy coat cells for 65 transfused aplastic anemia patients. Blood 59:236–246, 1982

182. Storb R, Prentice RL, Hansen JA, Thomas ED: Association between HLA-B antigens and acute graft-versus-host disease. Lancet 2:816–819, 1983

183. Hood AF, Soter NA, Rappeport J, Gigli I: Graft-versus-host reactions. Cutaneous manifestations following bone marrow transplantation. Arch Dermatol 113:1087–1091, 1977

184. Lerner KG, Kao GF, Storb R, Buckner CD et al: Histopathology of graft-vs-host reaction (GvHR) in human recipients of marrow from HLA-matched sibling donors. Transplant Proc 6:367–371, 1974

185. Sale GE, Lerner KG, Barker EA et al: The skin biopsy in the diagnosis of acute graft-versus-host disease in man. Am J Pathol 89:621–635, 1977

186. Shulman HM, McDonald GB: Liver disease after marrow transplantation. In Sale GE, Shulman HM (eds): *The Pathology of Bone Marrow Transplantation*, pp 104–135. New York, Masson, 1984

187. Snover DC, Weisdorf SA, Ramsay NK et al: Hepatic graft versus host disease: a study of the predictive value of liver biopsy in diagnosis. Hepatology 4:123–130, 1984

188. McDonald GB, Shulman HM, Sullivan KM, Spencer GD: Intestinal and hepatic complications of human bone marrow transplantation: Part I. Gastroenterology 90:460–477, 1986

189. Epstein RJ, McDonald GB, Sale GE et al: The diagnostic accuracy of the rectal biopsy in acute graft-versus-host disease: A prospective study of thirteen patients. Gastroenterology 78:764–771, 1980

190. Sale GE, Shulman HM, McDonald GV, Thomas ED: Gastrointestinal graft-versus-host disease in man. A clinicopathologic study of the rectal biopsy. Am J Surg Pathol 3:291–299, 1979

191. Snover DC, Weisdorf SA, Vercellotti GM et al: A histopathologic study of gastric and small intestinal graft-versus-host disease following allogeneic bone marrow transplantation. Hum Pathol 16:387–392, 1985

192. Simes MA, Hohansson E, Rapola J: Scleroderma-like graft-versus-host disease as late consequence of bone marrow transplantation. Lancet 2:831–832, 1977

193. Shulman HM, Sullivan KM, Weiden PL et al: Chronic graft-versus-host syndrome in man: A clinicopathological study of 20 long-term Seattle patients. Am J Med 69:204–217, 1980

194. Sullivan KM, Shulman HM, Storb R et al: Chronic graft-versus-host disease in 52 patients: Adverse natural course and successful treatment with combination immunosuppression. Blood 57:267–276, 1981

195. Yau JC, Zander AR, Srigley JR et al: Chronic graft-versus-host disease complicated by micronodular cirrhosis and esophageal varices. Transplantation 41:129–130, 1986

196. Berman M, Rabin M, O'Donnell et al: The liver in long-term survivors of marrow transplant-chronic graft-versus-host disease. J Clin Gastroenterol 2:53–63, 1980

197. Rodu B, Gockerman JP: Oral manifestations of the chronic graft-v-host reaction. JAMA 249:504–507, 1983

198. Barrett AP, Bilous AM: Oral patterns of acute and chronic graft-vs-host disease. Arch Dermatol 120:1461–1465, 1984

199. Schubert MM, Sullivan KM, Morton TH et al: Oral manifestations of chronic graft-v-host disease. Arch Intern Med 144:1591–1595, 1984

200. Jack MK, Jack GM, Sale GE et al: Ocular manifestations of graft-v-host disease. Arch Ophthalmol 101:1080–1084, 1983

201. Franklin RM, Kenyon KR, Tutschka PJ et al: Ocular manifestations of graft-vs-host disease. Ophthalmology 90:4–13, 1983

202. McDonald GB, Sullivan KM, Plumley TF: Radiographic features of esophageal involvement in chronic graft-vs-host disease. AJR 142:501–506, 1984

203. Corson SL, Sullivan K, Batzer F et al: Gynecologic manifestations of chronic graft-versus-host disease. Obstet Gynecol 60:488–492, 1982

204. Smith CIE, Aarli JA, Biberfeld P et al: Myasthenia gravis after bone marrow transplantation. Evidence for a donor origin. N Engl J Med 309:1565–1568, 1983

205. Anderson BA, Young PV, Kean WF et al: Polymyositis in chronic graft vs host disease. A case report. Arch Neurol 39:188–190, 1982

206. Kurzrock R, Zander A, Kanojia M et al: Obstructive lung disease after allogeneic bone marrow transplantation. Transplantation 37:156–162, 1984

207. Serota FT, August CS, Koch PA et al: Pulmonary function in patients undergoing bone marrow transplantation. Med Pediatr Oncol 12:137–143, 1984

208. Storb R, Epstein RB, Graham TC, Thomas ED: Methotrexate regimens for control of graft-versus-host disease in dogs with allogeneic marrow grafts. Transplantation 9:240–246, 1970

209. Lazarus HM, Coccia PF, Herzig RH et al: Incidence of acute graft-versus-host disease with and without methotrexate prophylaxis in allogeneic bone marrow transplant patients. Blood 64:215–220, 1984

210. Sullivan KM, Deeg HJ, Sanders J et al: Hyperacute graft-vs-host disease in patients not given immunosuppression after allogeneic marrow transplantation. Blood 67:1172–1175, 1986

211. Borel JF, Feurer C, Gubler MU, Stahelin H: Biological effects of cyclosporin A: A new anti-lymphocytic agent. Agents Actions 6:468–475, 1976

212. Powles RL, Clink HM, Spence D et al: Cyclosporin A to prevent graft-versus-host disease in man after allogeneic bone marrow transplantation. Lancet 1:327–329, 1980

213. Tutschka PJ, Beschorner WE, Hess AD, Santos GW: Cyclosporin-A to prevent graft-versus-host disease: A pilot study in 22 patients receiving allogeneic marrow transplants. Blood 61:318–325, 1983

214. Hows JM, Chipping PM, Fairhead S et al: Nephrotoxicity in bone marrow transplant recipients treated with cyclosporin A. Br J Haematol 54:69–78, 1983

215. Thompson CB, June CH, Sullivan KM, Thomas ED: Cyclosporine neurotoxicity is associated with hypomagnaesemia. Lancet 2:1116–1120, 1984

216. Loughran TP, Deeg HJ, Dahlberg S et al: Incidence of hypertension after marrow transplantation among 112 patients randomized to either cyclosporine or methotrexate as graft-versus-host disease prophylaxis. Br J Haematol 59:547–553, 1985

217. Reisner Y, O'Reilly R, Kapoor N, Good RA: Allogeneic bone marrow transplantation using stem cells fractionated by lectins: VI. In vitro analysis of human and monkey bone marrow cells fractionated by sheep red blood cells and soybean agglutinin. Lancet 2:1320–1324, 1980

218. Powles RL, Morgenstern GR, Kay HEM et al: Mismatched family donors for bone marrow transplantation as treatment for acute leukemia. Lancet 1:612–615, 1983

219. Beatty PG, Clift RA, Mickelson EM et al: Marrow transplantation from related donors other than HLA-identical siblings. N Engl J Med 313:765–771, 1985

220. Sondel PM, Hank JA, Molenda J et al: Relapse of host leukemic lymphoblasts following engraftment by an HLA-mismatched marrow transplant:

Mechanisms of escape from the "graft versus leukemia" effect. Exp Hematol 13:782–790, 1985

221. Trigg ME, Sondel PM, Billing R et al: Mismatched bone marrow transplantation in children with hematologic malignancy using T lymphocyte depleted bone marrow. J Biol Response Mod 4:602–612, 1985

222. Trigg ME, Billing R, Sondel et al: Clinical trial depleting T lymphocytes from donor marrow for matched and mismatched allogeneic bone marrow transplants. Cancer Treat Rep 69:377–386, 1985

223. Bozdech MJ, Finlay JL, Trigg ME et al: Monoclonal B-cell lymphoproliferative disorders following monoclonal antibody (CT2) T cell depleted allogeneic bone marrow transplantation (abstr). Blood 62:218c, 1983

224. McCullough J, Rogers G, Dahl R et al: Development and operation of a program to obtain volunteer bone marrow donors unrelated to the patient. Transfusion 26:315–323, 1986

225. Hansen JA, Clift RA, Thomas ED et al: Transplantation of marrow from an unrelated donor to a patient with acute leukemia. N Engl J Med 303:565–567, 1980

226. Meyers JD, Atkinson K: Infection in bone marrow transplantation. Clin Haematol 12:791–811, 1983

227. Winston DJ, Gale RP, Meyer DV, Young LS and the UCLA Transplantation Group: Infectious complications of human bone marrow transplantation. Medicine 58:1–31, 1979

228. Peterson PK, McGlave P, Ramsay NKC et al: A prospective study of infectious diseases following bone marrow transplantation: Emergence of Aspergillus and cytomegalovirus as the major causes of mortality. Infect Control 4:81–89, 1983

229. Peterson PK, McGlave P, Ramsay NKC et al: Empirical antibacterial therapy in febrile, granulocytopenic bone marrow transplant patients. Antimicrob Agents Chemother 26:136–138, 1984

230. Storb R, Prentice RL, Buckner CD et al: Graft-versus-host disease and survival in patients with aplastic anemia treated by marrow grafts from HLA-identical siblings. Beneficial effect of a protective environment. N Engl J Med 308:302–307, 1983

231. Meyers JD, Flournoy N, Wade JC et al: Biology of interstitial pneumonia after marrow transplantation. In Gale RP (ed): Recent Advances in Bone Marrow Transplantation, pp 405–423. New York, Alan R Liss, 1983

232. Meyers JD, Flournoy N, Thomas ED: Risk factors for cytomegalovirus infection after human marrow transplantation. J Infect Dis 153:478–488, 1986

233. Hersman J, Meyers JD, Thomas ED et al: The effect of granulocyte transfusions on the incidence of cytomegalovirus infection after allogeneic marrow transplantation. Ann Intern Med 96:149–152, 1982

234. Winston DJ, Pollard RB, Ho WG et al: Cytomegalovirus immune plasma in bone marrow transplant recipients. Ann Intern Med 97:11–18, 1982

235. O'Reilly RJ, Reich L, Gold J et al: A randomized trial of intravenous hyperimmune globulin for the prevention of cytomegalovirus (CMV) infections following marrow transplantation: Preliminary results. Transplant Proc 15:1405–1411, 1983

236. Meyers JD, Leszczynski J, Zaia JA et al: Prevention of cytomegalovirus infection by cytomegalovirus immune globulin after marrow transplantation. Ann Intern Med 98:442–446, 1983

237. Meyers JD, Wade JC, McGuffin RW et al: The use of acyclovir for cytomegalovirus infections in the immunocompromised host. J Antimicrob Chemother 12(suppl B):181–193, 1983

238. Harris R, Neudorf S, McGill M: CMV-negative blood products for prevention of cytomegaloviral pneumonia in seronegative transplant recipients: A study of 50 patients. In Gale RP, Champlin R (eds): Recent Advance in Bone Marrow Transplantation. UCLA Symposium on Molecular and Cellular Biology, pp 577–581. New York, Alan R Liss, 1987

239. Filipovich AH, Blazar BR, Ramsay NKC et al: Allogeneic bone marrow transplantation for X-linked lymphoproliferative syndrome. Transplantation 42:222–224, 1986

240. Neiman PE, Reeves W, Ray G et al: A prospective analysis of interstitial pneumonia and opportunistic viral infection among recipients of allogeneic bone marrow grafts. J Infect Dis 136:754–767, 1977

241. Arthur RR, Shah KV, Baust SJ et al: Association of BK viruria with hemorrhagic cystitis in recipients of bone marrow transplants. N Engl J Med 315:230–234, 1986

242. Atkinson K, Meyers JD, Storb R et al: Varicella-zoster virus infection after marrow transplantation for aplastic anemia and leukemia. Transplantation 29:47–50, 1980

243. Winston DJ, Schiffman G, Wang DC et al: Pneumococcal infections after human bone marrow transplantation. Ann Intern Med 91:835–841, 1979

244. Weiner RS, Bortin MM, Gale RP et al: Interstitial pneumonitis after bone marrow transplantation: Assessment of risk factors. Ann Intern Med 104:168–175, 1986

245. Meyers JD, Flournoy N, Wade JC et al: Biology of interstitial pneumonia after marrow transplantation. In Gale RP (ed): Recent Advances in Bone Marrow Transplantation, pp 405–423. New York, Alan R Liss, 1983

246. Keane TJ, VanDyk J, Rider WD: Idiopathic interstitial pneumonia following bone marrow transplantation: the relationship with total body irradiation. Int J Radiat Oncol Biol Phys 7:1365–1370, 1981

247. Sklar CA, Ramsay NKC: Endocrine dysfunction after successful bone marrow transplantation. Clin Oncol 4:345–352, 1985

248. Shapiro RS, Robison LL, Kim TH et al: Thyroid dysfunction following bone marrow transplant: Long-term followup of 53 pediatric patients. J Cell Biochem 10(suppl):250, 1986

249. Sanders JE, Pritchard S, Mahoney P et al: Growth and development following marrow transplantation for leukemia. Blood 68:1129–1135, 1986

250. Deeg HJ, Flournoy N, Sullivan KM et al: Cataracts after total body irradiation and marrow transplantation: A sparing effect of dose fractionation. Int J Radiat Oncol Biol Phys 10:957–964, 1984

251. Deeg HJ, Sanders J, Martin P et al: Secondary malignancies after marrow transplantation. Exp Hematol 12:660–666, 1984

252. Shapiro RS, Pietryga D, Blazar BR et al: B-cell lymphoproliferative disorders following bone marrow transplantation. In Gale RP, Champlin R (eds): Recent Advances in Bone Marrow Transplantation, UCLA Symposia on Molecular and Cellular Biology. New York, Alan R Liss (in press)

253. Albo V, Miller D, Leiken S et al: Nine brain tumors as a late effect in children cured of acute lymphoblastic leukemia from a single protocol study. Proc Am Soc Clin Oncol 4:172, 1985

forty-nine

Management of the Terminally Ill Child

Doris A. Howell and Ida M. Martinson

The death of a child is never acceptable to parents, family, or caregiving professionals. The loss of a life that has not yet been truly lived seems unbearable. The physician's concentration on cure is favored by all, but never more intensely than when a disease is identified as life-threatening and the family hopes desperately to avoid a fatal outcome. The professionals involved frequently perceive a child's death of cancer as failure. Yet the dying child both needs and deserves the optimal attention that a multidisciplinary care team can provide.

In this chapter, "terminal illness" is defined as the period when a child's death is imminent (*i.e.,* likely to occur within 2 to 6 weeks). The focus is on salient issues in the preterminal, terminal, and post-terminal phases. It is assumed that supportive and palliative care should be given, regardless of whether the child remains on treatment. Specific segments identify and discuss management issues related to children of various ages as well as to parents, siblings, grandparents and other affected persons, and to health professionals. Selection of the most appropriate location—hospital, home, or hospice—for the child's final days or weeks of life is also explored, and suggestions to aid the decision-making process are offered.

PRETERMINAL MANAGEMENT

As the disease advances from life-threatening to fatal, a point is reached where hope for recovery or significant reprieve is no longer realistic. The ability of the family and staff to cope throughout this phase reflects the extent of the mutual trust that has developed between them over the course of the illness. During this preterminal phase, three critical questions need to be addressed: Should therapeutic treatment be continued? When will death occur? Where should the child spend the final days of life?

Resolution of these questions will help facilitate the best possible death for the child. The question of whether therapeutic treatment should be continued requires serious consideration by the primary physician. When chemotherapy or other treatment is no longer effective, the decision to discontinue cure-oriented treatment must be faced. Although it is not possible to predict precisely when death will occur, the family needs to be included in the acknowledgement of impending death, and the advantages and disadvantages of various locations for the child's final days should be discussed.

The parents and child need to explore alternatives and express their preferences. The involved professionals carry the responsibility for ongoing attentiveness to the principles of good medical care, whether in the form of curative or supportive care in the hospital, hospice, or home setting. Consensus and an accompanying plan of action will permit the terminal phase to be calmer and less frightening for the child and family.[1-3]

In addition to determining answers to these questions, each involved party

991

—child, parents, siblings, grandparents, and health professionals—needs to deal with specific issues to prepare effectively for the approaching terminal phase.

Child

In the United States, most children and many parents have never been exposed to death. Increased sophistication in technology and intensive therapeutic regimens has resulted in hospitalization of most terminally ill patients. This practice prevents children from understanding death as a natural event and from experiencing the closure of the normal life cycle.

In a society that seeks to protect children from exposure to death, most children encounter death only through the drama of television. Their parents' limited familiarity with death further deepens the mystery. Even the euphemisms parents may use in describing death, such as "passing away" or "going to Heaven," evade the reality of death.

Realization of Impending Death

Many observers have noted that children who are dying have a level of maturity "far beyond their years." Children seem to know intuitively the seriousness of their illness, even when this has not been discussed with them. This awareness is not necessarily related to age or to intellectual ability. However, a child's awareness of approaching death varies with developmental age.

Toddlers cannot conceptualize death, but fear separation from parents and other loved ones and need reassurance and comfort.

Preschoolers understand that they are very sick and are not getting better. Their comprehension of the meaning of death may be limited, yet Bluebond-Langer found that children as young as age 3 not only know that they will eventually die, but also know when their illness is preterminal.[4] Both preschoolers and toddlers are likely to express themselves only in symbolic ways, demonstrating awareness and emotions through play activities.[5]

School-age children are usually able to understand that death is approaching. They are astute observers and pick up clues from adults' conversation, behavior, and body language. They also talk openly with other children in the hospital or clinic and observe and draw conclusions from the fate of these peers.

Adolescents are acutely aware of the implications of their diagnosis, their condition, and the failure of various treatments. The adolescent is fully and painfully aware of the finality of death.

Need for Open Communication

Although dying children are very likely aware of what is happening, they may not ask direct questions or seem to want to talk about the matter much. This is often a response to adults who, hoping to protect the child, evade the whole topic of death and carry out a game of pretense. Such behavior deceives the dying child not at all; the child is, as Wass puts it, "thrown into an ironic role reversal and goes along with the game pretending that all is well to protect his parents."[6]

Most experts now suggest that parents work to adopt an open, honest approach to communication. This may be very difficult, especially if this style of interaction has not been a family pattern in the past. However, when parents and children do not talk openly, the results can be unfortunate. Children may feel isolated from their parents and experience great loneliness. Lacking straight answers to their questions (or to the questions they leave unasked to protect their parents), preschoolers and school-age children may develop fears and fantasies about their illnesses. Young children may also interpret painful procedures and separation from parent during hospitalization as a punishment for some bad behavior. Thus dying children can feel frightened, isolated, and guilty unless there is a parent or other beloved adult who is willing to listen and respond to their fears and concerns. Such pain adds unnecessarily to the agony of the dying process.

Most dying teenagers continue to proceed through the adolescent maturational process, with its attendant rebellion. Open communication with teenagers that provides them the opportunity to share the many feelings they may have about adolescence, illness, and dying can be very helpful. Some teenagers may be able to talk more openly with a trusted adult other than their parent.

Need for Trust and Support

Honesty and a supportive approach are necessary to establish a basis of trust between the child and the adults important to him or her. Consistent, honest answers to questions will identify the respondent as a trusted and caring person. Such trust and support improve the child's ability to cope with emotional crises and physiologic changes, and provide the security of being inside the confidence of family and caregivers, not isolated or abandoned.

Parents

When their child is diagnosed with a potentially fatal disease, the parents' primary reaction is disbelief, quickly followed by anguish and despair. These emotions ebb and flow throughout the entire illness, not in any prescribed sequence but rather in response to the child's changing condition. Even the strongest of parents will become exhausted, both emotionally and physically, by the stresses and strains of making decisions about their child's care, answering the questions of the ill child and of any well siblings, keeping the household running, and finding money to pay for medical and related expenses. Thus, parents need support and understanding from professionals as well as from friends and other family members.

Need for Emotional and Practical Support

It is easy for parents to become overwhelmed by stress, but, as marital partners, they need to be able to support each other both emotionally and practically. Efforts to keep communicating and to allow room for varying feelings at different times are very important, yet the need for one parent to be at the hospital while the other is at home often prevents parents from spending time together and makes it difficult for them to share feelings and help each other. If parents are unable to help each other, the ensuing resentment and discontent may build, with resultant long-term problems in or dissolution of the marriage.

Role in Caring for the Child

The sense of devastation imposed by the life-threatening situation is usually diminished only by increased efforts to fight against the disease, which are often inappropriate in the preterminal phase, or by the opportunity to provide care for the child. Parents should be given chances to help take care of their child during both the preterminal and terminal phases, whether the child is in a hospital, hospice, or home setting.

The family's ability to provide care will expand when they are reminded that they know the child's needs and desires better than anyone else does. A booklet for parents entitled "Home Care: A Manual for Parents" is available from Children's Hospice International (see also Chap. 46).[7]

Need for Information

Throughout the course of a child's life-threatening illness, health professionals must assess the parents' understanding of the disease and prognosis, and their ability to cope with all aspects of the illness, including death. Staff must be prepared to assist the parents in communicating each stage of the illness, including death, to the child. Explaining the developmental stages to parents can help them to evaluate their own child's level of comprehension and to provide the child with an appropriate level of information.

Parents will ask about the process of dying repeatedly during the preterminal phase. Their questions need to be answered appropriately, based on the child's current status. Changes that may occur as death approaches and the needs of the child at that time should be explained. All questions about death from the parents—and from the child—should be answered openly and honestly by professional caregivers.

As the disease progresses, the parents accrue both professional consultants and friends among other parents of ill children. As they gain more knowledge, their questions will become less global and more immediate. This is particularly true during the preterminal stage, as parents realize that death is approaching. If professionals and family members have had open exchanges and ongoing collaboration throughout the child's illness, there should be no surprises but rather a continuing consensus as to the course of events and the child's condition.

Approach of Terminal Phase

When the terminal phase of the child's life is imminent, the staff and parents need to acknowledge the situation together and to share this knowledge with the child if he or she has not preceded them in this awareness. Ultimately, the deteriorating physical status and the failing response to treatment reveal to the nurses and physicians that there is no further realistic expectation of a remission or recovery. Professionals should inform the parents gently but clearly; they should not assume that the parents are interpreting signs and symptoms in the same way that professionals are.

Parents usually press to know how long the child can be expected to live. With the proviso that no one can predict exactly when a person will die, a careful "guesstimate" can provide the family with a time frame within which to make plans. This assists parents in maintaining some control over events; they can make plans for optimal use of their time with the dying child while also making appropriate arrangements regarding their jobs, child care for siblings, and intermittent respite for themselves.

Siblings

The weight of grief borne by the parents of a child with a terminal illness is so heavy that the pain, fear, and confusion felt by the siblings can be easily ignored or given superficial attention (see also Chap. 42). It is understandable that the needs of well siblings receive a lower priority, but parents need to be aware that these children may not only be grieving for the dying child but also fearing that they too will become ill and die. Like the sick child, the well siblings will "read" the parents' behavior and become more upset and frightened if they realize they are not being told the truth or are being dealt with evasively.

Children have difficulty absolving themselves of guilt when illness strikes a sibling with whom they have shared a normal love/hate relationship. In addition to these unspoken, and often unspeakable, fears, the sibling may also experience jealousy of the sick child, who consumes the majority of the parents' time and energy. Siblings (except those who are very young) will gain security if they are incorporated in the family tragedy and called on to perform tasks to help their sick brother or sister. The siblings need ample opportunity to talk, to know that they are being heard, and to be allowed to play a meaningful role during this difficult experience.

Grandparents

Parents and children may assume that grandparents, by virtue of their age, are more experienced, stronger, and inured to death. However, they, too may have had limited experience with this particular kind of loss. Grandparents may have a special problem if they have felt bereft as a result of the distancing from their own adult child and grandchildren.

There are many tasks the grandparents can perform on behalf of the parents, patient, or siblings that will make them feel needed and helpful without being a burden. To exclude them from involvement is to deny them an opportunity to exorcise their grief over the death and impending loss.

Professionals

The Physician's Multiple Roles

The pediatrician and pediatric oncologist, trained in curative medicine, face the impending death of the child patient with little preparation for filling the variety of expected roles listed below.

Coordinator. Although the physician's primary role must be to deliver the most appropriate medical treatment, he or she must also function as an effective coordinator for the multiple consultants utilized, and must communicate their input to the family.

Sounding board. The physician and nurse must serve as a sounding board for the patient's anxieties and fears, the parents' concerns, and the agendas of other health personnel involved in the child's care. The interpersonal skills of the physician and nurse must be honed in order to orchestrate the emotions and reactions of patient, parents, relatives, and health caretakers so that the resultant atmosphere of collaboration and cohesion will sustain morale.

Developmental consultant. The physician or nurse trained in behavioral pediatrics can recognize the developmental stage of the patient even though the child is ill, and can evaluate the expected degree of comprehension and the changing coping mechanisms the child will use in progressing along the developmental pathway. Sharing this information with the parents permits the family, the physician, and the nurse to work in unison to provide appropriate responses and support to the child.

Risk of Distancing

Through the active treatment stage of the disease, physicians may feel competent and secure in their actions. With increasing failure of the disease to respond to treatment, the physician often suffers anxiety and may cope with this by distancing himself or herself from the deteriorating patient. The physician is then unable to fulfill the role of counselor and comforter. Some physicians become overtly angry and ineffective, but this may not be evident until the terminal phase, when the patient and family need them the most.

Unfortunately, medicine has labeled the terminal phase of illness as that period of time when the patient's downhill course appears to be irreversible and curative treatment is replaced with caring and supportive services. The risk to the patient of this definition is that the physician may conclude that his or her major responsibility is completed and thus may abrogate continuing responsibility to the nursing staff, who seem more competent in providing such care. A more positive relationship for physicians is possible. In partnership with the nurse, the physician serves as consultant, interpreting nursing observations, altering medications in response to these observations of changing need, and fostering family sharing and bonding.[8]

The parents often become even more desperate in the face of what feels like abandonment by the physician. In this situation, the nurses are caught between the two behaviors at a time when, despite their own grief, they must continue to provide all necessary services and treatments and to sustain the child and family. The resulting stress can adversely affect the dying child by increasing fear and apprehension.

The nursing staff wants, and the dying child requires, the continuing concern and involvement of the physician throughout the preterminal and terminal phases. Although the disease may be incurable, the physical and emotional needs of the child not only persist but may well increase as death approaches. Thus, health professionals must retain stewardship of the child's death.[9]

Impact on Nursing Staff

In many ways, the nursing staff carries the heaviest emotional burden in the preterminal and terminal phases (see also Chap. 46). They identify with the patient and commit long hours to meeting the child's physical needs and providing the ongoing emotional support necessary to help the child and parents to ultimately accept death.

Physicians, nurses, and other health professionals must work together as a team so that they can support each other and together provide outlets to release and deal with their feelings. By accepting denial, anger, guilt, frustration, and depression as normal reactions, health professionals can gain personal strength that can be transmitted to the child and family through effective action as well as empathy.

Coping and Support Mechanisms

A supportive work setting is essential for the health care team members to optimize their coping skills and obtain needed support.[10] Table 49-1 describes several mechanisms which can facilitate this process. The periodic revision of goals and the organized procedures of analysis and evaluation leading to constructive decisions provide comfort and sustenance to the staff in their difficult roles during the preterminal and terminal phases.

PLANNING FOR TERMINAL CARE

When there is consensus that the terminal phase is near, the patient and family should be encouraged to decide where the child's final days will be spent. Whether it be the security of the

Table 49-1
Facilitating Mechanisms for Health Care Team Members

Mechanism	Purpose
Case conferences	Develop a basic, individualized, flexible care plan to accommodate changing needs
Staff meetings	Provide consultants or professional associates, from outside the immediate situation, to promote fresh insight
Work environment	Encourage verbal and nonverbal reinforcements for work well done
Evaluation sessions	Establish time to analyze generic problem, discuss and incorporate new modalities of care, and develop plan to incorporate new suggestions for improvement
Time tables	Schedule sessions regularly to measure care experiences against stated goals
Staff support	Incorporate professional psychiatric and advanced nursing consultants as support for staff

hospital and its staff or the intimacy and comfort of the home with supportive help, health professionals must support the family's decision and be accepting of a possible change of mind should circumstances change.

Regardless of where the terminal phase of life is spent, the same high quality of management, with adherence to established standards, should be practiced.[11] The home or hospice care of the dying child should follow the same management plan as for the hospitalized child. The patient's primary physician should maintain responsibility for medical care and remain readily available to the patient and parents.

The choice of location for the child's terminal days or weeks is the parents', but it is heavily influenced by professional opinion and the available options. A staff aware of community resources and willing to assist the family through all circumstances will be rewarded by increased responsibility and strength on the part of the parents as they regain a level of control in the decision-making process.

Hospital Care

Parents who wish hospital care for their child—whether because of a difficult home situation or because of fears that they cannot cope away from the security of the hospital staff—should have that wish respected. Also, an essential element of home and hospice care is the need to reassure the family that the child may be readmitted to the hospital at any time they so request. Such admissions should be expedited, with complete exchange of pertinent information relative to the patient and his or her comfort. The family needs to perceive home, hospice, and hospital as part of the continuum of care.

Movement Toward Out-of-Hospital Care

Pediatricians are now beginning to plan for a smooth transition from the heavily medicine-controlled, hospital-based style of care that has been in place for over 5 decades to thoughtful discharge to home and to the community. Until efforts were made to accommodate families and dying children, taking a child home to die was discouraged by professionals and only rarely attempted by courageous parents.[12] The beneficial effect of home death has now been supported by a series of excellent studies demonstrating parents' coping capacities and the impact of the site of death on the remaining family members.[13–15]

These critical studies and others[1,6,16] have substantiated to a large degree that not only do children prefer to live out their lives at home, but they and their families gain significantly from the experience and the survivors experience a much shorter and smoother period of bereavement, with less significant pathology.

The goal of both home care for the terminally ill and the majority of hospice programs is to maintain patients in their own homes, permitting them or their families to have the lead role in determining the care they are to receive. The family needs to be fully informed as to all of the available supportive services in the community so that they can select the assistance that best meets their needs.

Unfortunately, although the 1985 survey by McCann inquiring about hospice care for children quoted 59% of the 515 respondent programs as stating they provided hospice services for children, direct questioning of a representative percentage of such programs has shown that, although there was no exclusion of child patients in the admission policy, none had ever been enrolled.[17] However, increasing numbers of pediatric cancer centers are expanding their scope of practice to include home hospice services in the continuum of care and to encourage parents to take their child home during the terminal phase.

Home Care

For those able and willing to choose home care, multiple services and support from the community or agencies and the collaborative services of the child's primary physician and nurse will be a necessity. The staff should facilitate this choice and accommodate parents' preparations for assuming the responsibility for terminal care. In transferring the child from hospital to home, it is essential that support staff accept the parents as the primary care givers and view their own roles as those of teacher, counselor, and supplemental caregiver.

It is not easy for the professional to function in a secondary role, but this is of prime importance to the parents. The psychological and emotional milieu around dying children is so heavily charged that the supportive role is essential to achieve optimal care. The parents themselves must be the primary care-givers or they will not feel they have fulfilled their parental duty or have the solace of knowing they did all they could to care for their child.

Before World War II, the care of the dying was the responsibility of the family. With the national dispersion of the extended family, the nuclear family is often isolated and neighbors and friends replace family members in providing assistance.

The comfort of the child in his final days depends on the availability and competency of services that can be tapped to assist the family. The type of out-of-hospital care available to each child will depend on community resources.

Most families will need, in addition to 24-hour-per-day nursing availability, the assistance of social work, clergy, and homemaker services. Wherever they have been established, hospice programs provide this wide scope of services through the combined efforts of professional and volunteer caregivers. Because only about 3000 currently are in existence in the United States, the Visiting Nurse Association, Public Health Nursing, and private home health care agencies provide some of these needed services. Historically, they have concentrated on restoring patients to function, not on the care of the dying

person. Very few have been able to provide 24-hour nursing services, and because they have been rarely called upon to care for children, these agencies do not tend to hire pediatric-trained nurses.

The field of home care is changing rapidly, with extended nursing hours and supplementation by professionals from other disciplines. The gap between the more ideal services provided in hospice care and community home care programs is rapidly diminishing. Regardless of the source of home care, the quality of the care that is given should meet the highest standards.

National and international resources for home and hospice care are as follows:

Children's Hospice International
 1101 King Street, Suite 131
 Alexandria, Virginia 22314
 (203) 684-0330
National Association for Home Care
 519 C Street, N.E.
 Stanton Park
 Washington, D.C. 20002
 (202) 547-7420
National Hospice Organization
 1901 North Fort Myer Drive, Suite 402
 Arlington, Virginia 22209
 (703) 243-5900

Hospice Care

History

Hospice care—traceable to before the birth of Christ—began with a religious connotation and has fluctuated in popularity in accord with the occurrence of wars, pestilence, and other scourges. The modern hospice philosophy and provision of care is credited to England and, in particular, to Saunders for her pioneer efforts to alleviate pain and reduce the suffering of dying persons.[18,19] "Hospice" does not refer primarily to a specific place but to a concept of care that places the needs and desires of the patient foremost and encompasses his or her family or significant others. The breadth of service differs from that of traditional home health services that provide nursing care to the patient. Focusing on the patient and the family as the unit of care, hospice programs strive to fulfill the physical, emotional, and spiritual needs of the patient and extend beyond the patients' life to provide bereavement support to the survivors. Key elements of the hospice philosophy and essentials of care are listed in Table 49–2.

The British hospice programs were developed initially within or in association with existing hospitals. St. Christopher's Hospice, funded in part by grants from the National Health Service and public contributions, opened as a free-standing facility in London in 1967. In the United States, the hospice concept did not find a comfortable home within the modern tertiary care hospital. The American concentration on technology placed the emphasis on cure, with little attention given to palliation. The hospice "movement" increased in popularity in the United States, when the public, demanding to have more of a voice in decisions concerning their bodies, began to turn from hospitalization and sought home care when facing irreversible disease. Parents with terminally ill children found far greater difficulty separating from the security of the hospital, but slowly they too began to heed the pleas of their dying child to be at home.

Table 49-2
Essential Elements of Hospice Care

The multidisciplinary team concentration on the entire family as the unit of care

The availability of all services 24 hours a day, 7 days a week

The critical role of the patient's primary care physician in the treatment plan and continuous medical support when needed

The central role of the professional nurse in the coordination, assessment, and provision of services for patient and family

The provision of resources for meeting spiritual and psychosocial needs

The relief of physical pain and other stressful bodily symptoms

The recognition and alleviation of physical, mental, and emotional suffering of patient and family

The supportive services of staff trained in anticipatory grief and their continued help to the survivors throughout the bereavement

Standards

Because of its grass-roots beginning in the United States hospice care has evolved into as many forms as there are programs. Fortunately, the development of standards of care is bringing order to the variability and quality of services. A growing number of states have now established specific hospice legislation.

The Joint Commission on Accreditation of Hospitals published the first standards for the rapidly growing hospice movement in 1984.[20] The second edition of the Hospice Standards Manual (1986) reflects the continuing evolution of hospice care and increasing experience of hospice staff in implementing the standards.[11] The new standards place increasing importance on quality assurance as a management tool.

Legislation

Hospice care for adult patients in the United States grew slowly in the 1970s but has increased dramatically in the past 3 years since the Tax Equity and Fiscal Responsibility Act of 1982 (TEFRA) enacted the Medicare hospice benefit, making hospice services reimbursable for Medicare-eligible patients with terminal disease (see also Chap. 43). Although by 1983 only 13 insurance companies had extended their policies to reimburse for hospice services, the impetus given by the Health Care Financing Administration's support of the hospice legislation has stimulated an increase in the number of hospice programs to over 1500.[17] These are predominantly home care programs.

Although far from ideal and rife with limitations and penalties, the new legislation offers enough reimbursement to enable home care agencies and health care professionals to provide home or hospice care as an alternative to hospital care for dying patients.[21] Almost simultaneously, the implementation of rates of reimbursement for hospital charges on the basis of predetermined diagnosis-related groups has led to earlier hospital discharge for many patients, thereby favoring the use of home nursing and hospice care for the irreversibly or terminally ill.

In pediatrics, however, the legislative changes affecting reimbursement are limited to Medicare patients. Reimbursement for home or hospice care through the Crippled Children's Services, now funded through their respective State Maternal and Child Health block grants, may in some cases be reduced because such care must compete for the limited resources.

The hospice philosophy of care has also emphasized reducing the financial worry to the family: lack of funds should never deprive a patient of hospice care. However, the changes in hospice financing from community charity to increasing third-party reimbursement has spawned growing numbers of for-profit hospices which defies this basic principle.

The lack of eligibility of most children for Medicare reimbursement has made the financing of hospice services for children too expensive for many programs. However, in April 1986, federal legislation expanded Medicaid benefits so that states willing to amend their existing Medicaid programs and provide matching funds may provide assistance to dying children. A danger exists that in states unable to provide matching funds, hospice service will remain unreimbursed, especially for the poor.

Pediatric Programs

Although hospice care has become increasingly widespread for adults, hospice care specifically for children has been very limited and highly inconsistent in services.[22] The work of Martinson and colleagues, which demonstrated the feasibility of providing adequate supportive home care to children with terminal cancer and permitting them to live out their lives in familiar surroundings, stimulated the impetus for home care, and exemplified the principles of the hospice philosophy.[23]

The hospice concept promotes the patient and family as the unit of care and therefore the determinants of the care in fatal disease. The confidence of Martinson and Lauer and colleagues in the ability of parents to bear the burden of providing such care, given professional support, has spurred a rise in home care for a wide variety of disabled children, including those who are ventilator-dependent.[13,15]

There are few pioneer programs providing care exclusively to children. One such model program is St. Mary's Hospital for Children in Bayside, New York, where a 10-bed unit for terminally ill children with a life expectancy of less than 1 year occupies a floor of this hospital for chronic diseases.[24] Some children's hospitals, referral centers for childhood cancer, are developing models of care through their hospital home care departments, community agency contracts, or local hospice programs.

The reasons given for the slow growth of hospice care for children have been the lack of trained personnel who are comfortable with sick children; the severe emotional strain of a child's death; and the reluctance of parents to accept assistance, preferring to be all things to their dying child. Lauer and colleagues report that parents who have rejected home care in favor of a return to the hospital give as a major reason the home care nurses' lack of knowledge and experience in caring for a child.[14]

Because cancer is the major cause of death from disease in children, some hospice programs limit their care to cancer patients. As in adults, cancer in children lends itself to a more precise estimation of life expectancy, so that hospice services can be designated for those for whom death is anticipated in less than 6 months. Parents may remain tenaciously optimistic, rejecting death as an outcome until quite late in the illness, so that most home or hospice care for children is delayed until the last 3 or 4 weeks of life.

Criteria for admitting children to hospice care are basically the same as those for adults, with the exception of the parents serving as spokespersons for the younger child. Unlike adult patients, curative therapy is rarely discontinued except in the immediate preterminal stage. For the sake of the grieving parents, palliation is added to the therapeutic regimen unless the treatment is the cause of pain or stress.

The acquired immune deficiency syndrome (AIDS) (see Chap. 36) has led to a specific need for increased hospice services to serve the mounting number of infected infants as well as young adults. The multiple problems and needs of such patients utilize all facets of hospice care and, in high density areas, are threatening to overwhelm the capacity and resources of the local hospice programs. At least three large cities have responded to this rising volume by establishing hospice programs exclusively for AIDS patients.

TERMINAL PHASE

During the terminal stage the physical, mental, social, and spiritual well-being of the child and family becomes the focus of care.[16] In this section the needs and roles of the child, family, and caregivers in the child's last days and weeks of life are presented.

Child

Assessment

Each child in the terminal phase needs an individualized care plan developed by the health care team that addresses all pertinent physical and emotional health needs. When thorough, competent, and loving care is provided, the family will have less worry and can concentrate on enriching and sharing the last moments of their child's life.

The anticipated life expectancy should be used as a guideline in writing the care plan. Guidelines should reflect the degree of life support measures that the family wishes to use. The plan must include sufficient time for the family to gain nursing skills and to acknowledge their child's impending death.

Table 49-3 lists health care team activities facilitated by information derived from the assessment process. Physical maintenance should include [1] adequate hydration, nutrition, elimination, skin integrity, and metabolism; and [2] amelioration of discomfort caused by pain, nausea, vomiting, ascites, or iatrogenic effects of therapy.

Concern for the child's mental health involves providing him or her with the opportunity to ventilate anxiety, depression, anger, and fear. Social and spiritual support are also important, although the degree varies markedly from patient to patient, dependent upon available resources.

When the child's death is imminent, the care plan is modified to focus exclusively on providing comfort. A balanced diet and adherence to rules are no longer pertinent. For the child who is expected to live longer, the plan will include health maintenance and prevention of avoidable health deterioration. The plan should be designed around the parents' usual pattern of care which is familiar and comforting to the child and strengthens the parents' confidence in their continuing role as primary caregivers.

Physical Problems

Children dying of malignancy suffer from numerous physical symptoms, such as pain, anxiety, constipation, nausea and vomiting, temperature imbalance, and skin irritation. Tables 49-4 and 49-5 summarize management techniques for handling these problems (see also Chaps. 37–40, 44, and 45).

Emotional Support

Children of all ages fear abandonment in the course of serious illness. This becomes particularly critical during the final stages of the illness. Unfortunately, many children have already experienced loss by the distancing of friends or relatives who

Table 49-3
Patient Care Team Responsibilities

Identify and evaluate acute health problems in the child and family

Develop an appropriate care plan for the dying child

Plan for the family's role in comfort care

Design and offer strategies to assist the parents and other family members through the pain and loss

have found the illness and its prognosis too difficult to bear. It is essential to reassure children frequently that the family and the key staff, whom they trust and depend on for relief of symptoms, will not desert them and will be there to address every need.

The staff must not break this trust, no matter how emotionally painful the circumstances may be. With dying patients, behaviors such as touching and holding speak better than words, and parents and even siblings should be encouraged to lie on the bed and comfort the child through their closeness. Private rooms undoubtedly promote this intimacy but pose the danger of isolating the patient away from the attention and ministrations of the staff, which in itself conveys a message of desertion.

As death approaches, the patient gives an ambiguous message of wanting the staff visible and supportive but not wanting the stressful or painful treatments, tests, or procedures. This is not an easy role for staff, who are action oriented. It requires concentrated effort to alter care plans in order to accommodate the patient with the least discomfort and disruption.

Need for Control

One of the most serious stresses experienced by children with cancer and by their parents is the loss of control over even small matters. This loss permeates all aspects of the family's life, so that every decision seems to hinge on the wish of the physician. Opportunities need to be made for the child and the family to participate in decision making and to feel that they have control over the situation.

Methods of risk assessment can help staff reach decisions based on the pros and cons for the patient rather than on adherence to a protocol. Contract making with the patient often develops into a collaborative *quid pro quo* relationship that is satisfying to the patient at a time of few pleasures. Staff carry the responsibility of being sensitive to risk factors, particularly those which might affect the family members after the patient's death.[25]

Family

Parents

During the final stage, the parents vacillate between hope for a miracle and recognition of the obvious, and they begin preparing for the transition to loss. During this period, most parents express a variety of fears that can be overwhelming if not talked through with a supportive staff. As much as they want to have the child live, they want him to live as a normal, healthy child. Therefore, they fear prolonging the inevitable death as well as extending the pain and agony. With the fear of losing control and not being able to cope, they resist help from others who could take over some of their responsibilities. They are frequently afraid to leave the child for fear he or she will die while they are away.

Table 49-4
Symptom Management

Symptom	Cause	Relief
Pain	Bone metastases Nerve compression Hollow viscus or retroperitoneal tumor spread Chemotherapy, surgery, radiation therapy	Pain management—see Chap. 44 See Chap. 37 Aggressive pain management Lower analgesic requirement by altering therapy

Bleeding*	Thrombocytopenia
	Coagulopathy
		Medical care
		    Coagulation factors
		    Transfusion of blood products
		(See Chapter 38)
		Nursing care
		    Local pressure
		    Gel foam
		    Packing
		    Topical thrombin
		    Ice pack

Dyspnea	Advanced disease with space occupation or encroachment	Oxygen Opiates Positioning Suctioning Moist, controlled environment

Seizures	Primary or metastatic CNS tumor	Anticonvulsants
		    Phenytoin
		    Phenobarbital
		    Chloral hydrate
		See Chap. 37

Anorexia/dehydration	Swallowing difficulty Apathy	Ice chips Fluid sips Small amounts of palatable food IV fluids (See Chap. 40)

Mouth sores	Secondary to chemotherapy or poor hygiene	Good oral hygiene
		    Petroleum jelly to cracks
		    Mouth wash
		    2% viscous lidocaine
		    2% Cetacaine spray
		Drugs
		    Diphenhydramine
		    Mild narcotics

Constipation	Inactivity
	Poor nutrition
	Chemotherapy
	Narcotics
		Stool softeners
		    Colace,
		    Dulcolax
		Glycerine suppositories
		Metamucil
		Digital removal
		Enemas

Skin breakdown	Combination of decreased activity poor nutrition, neurologic problems	Preventive care
		    Frequent turning
		    Repositioning
		    Massage
		    Special mattress and bed
		    Heel protectors

Insomnia and restlessness	Bladder or bowel distention	Long-acting morphine at night, with or without chlorpromazine
Cough	Lung infections Poor circulation	Steady, well-humidified air Mild narcotics to allay exhaustion Antibiotics as needed
Itching	Limited fluid intake Increased cachexia	Antihistamines Topical steroids
Terminal muscle twitching	Unknown	Diazepam, with or without morphine, and/or chlorpromazine
"Death rattle"	Accumulation of secretions in posterior pharynx	Low-dose SC L-hyoscyamine every 4–6 hours
Cheyne–Stokes respiration	Slowed circulation	No treatment; explain sign to family

* Major bleeds are rare.

Table 49-5
Aggressive Pain Management in Hospice or Home Care*

Always start with the simplest, effective analgesics and narcotics.

Increase pain-controlling drugs as necessary to bring pain under control.

Calculate initial doses by standard methods (see Chap. 44) but increase doses according to need because addiction is not an issue.

Oral medication is preferred, although rectal, sublingual, intramuscular, or intravenous administration and subcutaneous pumps offer alternative routes.

Morphine is most frequently the drug of choice.

Persist in determining best combination of pain-controlling drugs for each patient.

* Also see Chapter 44.

These circumstances also raise many fears in parents about their own stability, and their ability to ever love again or to procreate. At a time when the marital relationship needs to be strong and sustaining, it is buffeted by self-doubts, recriminations, and even jealousy. Without strong support systems, parents may find themselves in serious difficulty, with the ultimate loss of the child precipitating a divorce. Efforts by counselors and staff must focus on strengthening family ties and demonstrating to the parents their responsibility to support one another and to provide sustenance for other family members.

During the terminal stage, the parents need to busy themselves in all aspects of the care of the child as part of the bonding between the child and parents. The primary concern of the parents in the terminal stage should be to make each day count.

Siblings

Brothers and sisters need not be excluded from the death bed; if they are not present, the event should be described to them with repeated reassurance that the child was well cared for and did not suffer. The siblings should also be encouraged to participate in the funeral events. The reality and finality of the funeral will help bring closure to this critical life experience.

Health Care Professionals

Caring for the dying child and the family should be perceived as a professional challenge. Providing appropriate comfort care to the child and adequate supportive care to the family members is demanding and requires skill, finesse, and tact. In turn, the providers must identify their own support systems and outlets. Whereas the health professionals have many roles to play daily, the family and child have no alternatives and depend heavily on their interaction with physician and nurse for nurturance, and are grateful for the professional involvement.

POST-TERMINAL PHASE

No degree of education or anticipation adequately prepares one for the reality of death until all bodily functions cease permanently. The anguish and pain of grief on seeing a beloved child dead cannot be allayed and must be allowed to run its course. Most family members want to remain with the child, to hold, to touch, to cry, and to say goodbye, and this wish should be honored. At times there may be an overwhelming sense of relief that the child is no longer suffering.

Value of the Postmortem

Despite the tendency to avoid the uncomfortable task of requesting a postmortem, this subject should be broached in quiet, thoughtful conversation with the parents before the last days of the child's life. After death, the final formality that needs to be completed is obtaining the signatures for the autopsy and signing the death certificate.

The parents should be well informed that the postmortem is not only of value to the caregivers to testify to the accuracy of their clinical judgments and to the scientists working to learn more about specific diseases and the effects of therapy, but also to the family members, who can gain peace of mind in knowing the correct diagnosis and the impact of the treatment, and in having the reassurance that nothing more could have been done that would have substantially prolonged the life of their child. The postmortem stands as moot evidence of the finality of death.

The postmortem also provides the medical and nursing staff with a valuable opportunity to ask to meet with the parents several weeks after the child's death, when the immediacy of the grief is subsiding, to review with them the cardinal events of the illness and death and the details of the postmortem findings. The family always suffers from many self-doubts about their decisions and their actions. The physician and nurse have a duty not only to provide factual information, but to sincerely praise the family, attesting to how well they handled themselves and their child, and to reiterate, when appropriate, that the child died knowing he was surrounded by the love of his family. Almost all families are in need of this approval and affirmation from both the medical and nursing staff on whom they were so dependent throughout the illness.

Bereavement

No matter how prepared family members believe themselves to be, the actual death of the child initiates an extended period of grieving that is both intense and slow to resolve. Shock and numbness interfere with the ability to make decisions or function effectively in routine activities. Gradually, this phase will be replaced by guilt and anger, restlessness, reality testing, depression, and, ultimately, an acceptance of the reality of the child's death. Dates of special significance for the family bring back memories and the pain and loss. Over time, enriching memories soften the pain. Life becomes more meaningful for many families.

The need for supportive family, friends, and professional associates cannot be underestimated. The most frequently denied need of those who mourn is to be allowed to talk and reminisce about the child. It is impossible to put such a loss out of mind. The goal of mourning, as described by Cantor, is "not forgetfulness, but enriched remembrance."[27] The content of the reminiscing and the questions raised rarely need a response but rather empathetic listening to assist the bereaved parent in the necessary process of exorcising the pain of loss. Without verbal release, the memories provoke guilt, anger, and other nonhealing reactions that delay recovery from grief. Following the death of the child, the siblings should be helped to talk freely of the event and the loss, and to learn that their parents are experiencing the same feelings. The reassurance by parents that life will go on and that the parents believe that they and the children can all live a long life will support them as they pass through the bereavement, develop healthy attitudes toward death, and are finally at peace with their loss.

In the follow-up study on 54 of the original 58 families in Martinson's home care project for children with terminal cancer, 84% of parents reported a return to a normal lifestyle by 24 months after the death, with 86% describing their adjustment to the death as good.[16] The many and rapid changes in care of the dying child over the past 5 years preclude comparison of these results to previous studies, but together with the research by Lauer and colleagues[15] measuring parental recovery from guilt, they provide an important argument for continued assistance to the family to reduce the length of their bereavement and hasten their return to normal function and enjoyment.

Research and Evaluation

The purpose of careful evaluation of existing programs and methods of care provided for terminally ill children is to improve the quality of the last days of the child's life and determine ways in which the grief of the family members can be assuaged and the mourning brought to closure. The multifactorial nature of the needs of the dying child will require collaborative, multidisciplinary research on all aspects of the care rendered.

Little has been done to research hospital care beyond the disease orientation, and home and hospice care have been founded largely on clinical experience and testimonials. Nursing research, which emphasizes improved care of the patient, has been taking the leadership role in promoting this necessary effort. The research must address those issues pertinent to the dying patient, the family, and the caregivers, moving beyond the argument of where terminal care should be given to identifying the most effective services leading to a more tranquil death, regardless of location. Scientific rigor must be as critical in determining the appropriate care and support of dying patients as it is in the bench analysis of their diseases.

CONCLUSION

The dying child deserves optimal, competent care and infinite compassion. Not only must the signs and symptoms of impending death be ameliorated, but the personal suffering of the child and that of the family, as they see the child's integrity threatened, must be assuaged. As Cassel has stated, "the relief of suffering is a proper goal of medicine."[27] Only with the collaboration and commitment of health professionals will the best interests of the patient and his family be served.

The untimely and tragic death of a child may not always be prevented, but with careful attention to process and symptom control, a quiet and peaceful death can ensue, providing a bearable memory for the bereaved family.

Special appreciation to Mary Hunter for her perceptive assistance.

REFERENCES

1. Mulhern RK, Lauer ME, Hoffman RG: Death of a child at home or hospital: Subsequent psychological adjustment of the family. Pediatrics 71:743–747, 1983
2. Kohler JA, Radford M: Terminal care for children dying of cancer: Quantity and quality of life. Br Med J 291:115–116, 1985
3. Lauer ME, Mulhern RK, Hoffman RG, Camitta BM: Utilization of hospice/home care in pediatric oncology. Cancer Nurs 9:102–107, 1986
4. Bluebond-Langner M: The Private Worlds of Dying Children. Princeton, NJ, Princeton University Press, 1978
5. Spinetta JJ, Rigler D, Karen M: Personal space as a measure of a dying child's sense of isolation. J Consult Clin Psychol 42:751–757, 1974
6. Wass H, Corr CA: Childhood and death. Issues Compr Pediatr Nurs 8:25–45, 1985
7. Moldow DG, Martinson IM: Home Care: A Manual for Parents. Minneapolis, University of Minnesota, 1979
8. Gronseth EC, Martinson IM, Kersey JH, Nesbit ME: Support system of health professionals as observed in the project of home care for the child with cancer. Death Educ 5:37–50, 1981
9. Stollerman GH: Editorial: Lovable decisions: Re-humanizing dying. J Am Geriatr Soc 34:172, 1986
10. Martinson IM, Nesbit ME, Kersey JH: Physicians role in home care for children with cancer. Death Studies 9:283–293, 1985
11. Joint Commission on Accreditation of Hospitals: Hospice Standards Manual. Chicago, JCAH, 1986
12. Martinson IM, Armstrong GD, Geis DP: Home care for children dying of cancer. Pediatrics 62:106–113, 1978
13. Lauer ME, Mulhern RK: Parental self-selection versus psychosocial predictors of capability in home care referral: A case study. Am J Hospice Care, Spring: 35–38, 1984
14. Lauer ME, Camitta BM: Home care for dying children: A nursing model. J Pediatr 97:1032–1035, 1980
15. Lauer ME, Mulhern RK, Wallskog JM et al: A comparison study of parental adaptation following a child's death at home or hospital. Pediatrics 71:743–747, 1983
16. Corr CA, Corr DM (eds): Hospice Approaches to Pediatric Care. New York, Springer Publishing, 1985
17. McCann BA: Pediatric hospice care. Report of the CHI National Survey, Pediatric Hospice Conference Report, 1985
18. Saunders CM: Care of the Dying. London, Macmillan, 1960
19. Saunders CM: The Management of Terminal Illness. London, Hospital Medicine Publications, 1967
20. Joint Commission on Accreditation of Hospitals: Standards of Care. Chicago, JCAH, 1984
21. Corless IB: Implications of the new hospice legislations and the accompanying regulations. Nurs Clin North Am 20:281–298, 1985
22. Corr CA, Corr DM: Pediatric hospice care. Pediatrics 76:774–780, 1985
23. Martinson IM, Armstrong GD, Geis DP: Home care for children dying of cancer. Pediatrics 62:106–113, 1978
24. Saint Mary's Hospital for Children: Hospice for children. Interior Design February: 192–195, 1986
25. Benoliel JQ: Loss and terminal illness. Nurs Clin North Am 20:439–448, 1985
26. Cantor RC: And a Time to Live: Toward Emotional Well Being During the Crisis of Cancer. New York, Harper & Row, 1978
27. Cassell EJ: The relief of suffering. Arch Intern Med 143:522–523, 1983

Rehabilitation of Long-Term Survivors

part

six

fifty

Late Effects of Childhood Cancer and Its Treatment

Julie Blatt and W. Archie Bleyer

Of the approximately 6600 children under 15 years of age who are found to have cancer in the United States each year, some 60%, or nearly 4000, can expect to be cured of their disease.[1] This dramatic progress, which has been achieved in less than two decades, has provided us with the paradoxical luxury of being able to evaluate the quality of survival—the medical, psychosocial, intellectual, and financial cost of cure. In some systematic studies of the survivors of childhood cancer, disabilities that significantly alter the quality of life have been detected in as many as 40%.[2,3]

Several generalizations can be made about the types of late effects that might be anticipated on the basis of the specific therapy to which a patient was exposed and the age at the time of that exposure. For example, with radiotherapy, adverse effects are usually not apparent acutely and are more likely to surface after a latent period (also see Chap. 11). On the other hand, chemotherapy is most likely to result in acute toxicities, which are usually transient but occasionally persist (also see Chap. 9). Because most chemotherapeutic agents are cell-cycle dependent, their acute toxicities can be related to the proliferation kinetics of individual cell populations. Most susceptible are those tissues or organs with high cell turnover rates, such as the bone marrow, orointestinal mucosa, testes, epidermis, and liver. Least susceptible are those cells that replicate slowly or not at all: neurons, muscle cells, connective tissue, and bone are examples. There are exceptions to this rule: vinca alkaloids, methotrexate and high-dose cytosine arabinoside may cause neural damage, methotrexate may injure bone, and anthracyclines may harm the heart. Moreover, injury that does occur to tissues with low repair potential often results in a longer-lasting, even permanent, deficit. Thus, although children appear to tolerate the acute toxicities of therapy better than do adults, the growing child may be more vulnerable to the delayed adverse sequelae of cancer therapy, such as effects on growth, fertility, and neuropsychologic function.

This chapter reviews many of the late effects seen in survivors of cancer and how they relate to individual therapeutic modalities (surgery, radiation, or single- and multiple-agent chemotherapy) as well as combined-modality regimens, including those used for bone marrow transplantation (Table 50-1). The psychosocial and financial aspects are reviewed in Chapters 41 through 43. An attempt will be made to emphasize documented differences in susceptibility between pediatric and adult patients, to indicate where recognition of late effects already has provided a rationale for modifying therapy, and to summarize current approaches to the long-term follow-up of pediatric oncology patients (Tables 50-2 and 50-3).

GROWTH

Decreased linear growth is a common problem during therapy in children with cancer. Although catch-up may occur, such that the premorbid growth status is regained, in some instances, short stature is permanent or even progressive. For example, severe growth retardation, defined as a standing height below the fifth

Table 50-1
Late Effects of Anticancer Therapy

Treatment	Late Effects of Anticancer Therapy*
Chemotherapy	
Agent(s)	
Alkylators	[Avascular necrosis (cyclophosphamide)]†, azoospermia, amenorrhea (cyclophosphamide, chlorambucil, nitrosoureas, phenylalanine mustard), [cardiomyopathy (cyclophosphamide, DTIC)], [pulmonary fibrosis (BCNU, cyclophosphamide, melphalan, busulfan)], nephritis (nitrosoureas), hemorrhagic cystitis (cyclophosphamide, ifosphamide), second malignancies (cyclophosphamide, mechlorethamine, nitrosoureas)
Antibiotics	Skin/tendon contractures (actinomycin), [cardiomyopathy (actinomycin, mitomycin, bleomycin)], pulmonary fibrosis (bleomycin), [nephritis (actinomycin)], [thrombotic thrombocytopenic purpura (TTP) (mitomycin, bleomycin)]
Anthracyclines	Skin/tendon contractures (Adriamycin, daunomycin), cardiomyopathy/pericarditis (Adriamycin, daunomycin)
Antimetabolites	[Avascular necrosis (methotrexate)], [amputation stump changes (methotrexate)], learning disabilities (methotrexate), [cardiomyopathy (methotrexate)], [pulmonary fibrosis (methotrexate)], hepatitis/fibrosis (methotrexate, actinomycin), nephritis (methotrexate, azacytidine)
Vinca alkaloids	Skin/tendon contractures, neuropathies, [cardiomyopathy (vincristine)], [pulmonary fibrosis (vinblastine)], [TTP]
Miscellaneous	
Steroids	[Obesity], [avascular necrosis], [osteoporosis], [cataracts]
Procarbazine	Azospermia, amenorrhea
Cisplatin	Hearing loss, [gynecomastia], nephritis, [TTP]
MOPP	Azoospermia, amenorrhea, gynecomastia
	Leydig cell dysfunction, [reduced humoral immunity], second malignancies
ABVD	Azoospermia
Radiation	
Area Irradiated	
Cranium/brain	Short stature/short trunk, [obesity], learning disabilities, leukoencephalopathy, cranial neuropathies, alopecia, [cataracts], [hypothyroidism], second malignancies (brain, thyroid)
Head and neck	[Nasolacrimal duct obstruction], [chronic conjunctivitis], [chronic otitis media], alopecia, cataracts, dental abnormalities, voice changes, facial deformities, neuropathies, esophagitis, second malignancies (thyroid, soft-tissue sarcomas, bone tumors)
Mediastinum	Cardiomyopathy, vasoocclusive disease, hypothyroidism, second malignancies (thyroid, ANLL), pneumonitis/fibrosis, pneumonitis, esophagitis, [reduced cell-mediated immunity]
Lungs	Pneumonitis/fibrosis
Spine	Short stature/short trunk, scoliosis, hypo/hyperthyroidism, second malignancies (thyroid), delayed puberty
Abdomen	Soft tissue or bony atrophy/hypoplasia, fibrosis, enteritis, cirrhosis/hepatitis, [hepatic veno-occlusive disease], splenic atrophy
Kidneys	[Vaso-occlusive disease], nephritis (including hypertension), urinary tract infections
Pelvis/gonads	Azoospermia/amenorrhea, Leydig cell/ovarian endocrine dysfunction, [vaso-occlusive disease], hemorrhagic cystitis
Bones	Atrophy/hypoplasia, avascular necrosis, osteoporosis, edema, second malignancies (bone, thyroid, soft-tissue sarcomas), osteochondromas
Total nodal	Reduced cell-mediated immunity, [bone marrow dysfunction]
Surgery	
Procedure	
Thoracotomy	Scoliosis
Laparotomy	Postsplenectomy sepsis, malabsorption (bowel surgery), [hyperammonemic encephalopathy (ureteral diversion)], [hyperchloremic metabolic acidosis (ureteral diversion)], [benign/malignant colonic tumors (ureterosigmoidostomy)]
Amputation	See Chapter 47
Enucleation	Prosthesis complications/blindness (see Chap. 25)
Lymph node dissection	Impotence, retrograde ejaculation, [hydroceles]

* Listed in order of discussion in chapter.

† Square brackets indicate infrequent complications or complications not clearly associated with these agents.

Table 50-2
Information to Obtain During Follow-Up Clinic Visits by Survivors of Childhood Cancer

History of any intercurrent illnesses
Review of systems
Development of any benign tumors or other cancers
Medications: prophylactic antibiotics
Educational status
   Grade completed; special education classes?
   Grade point average; results of IQ tests
   Areas of weakness
Employment status
Insurance coverage
   Individual policy, or coverage through parents?
   Difficulties getting insured
Marital history
Menses, libido, sexual activity
Pregnancy outcome (patient or spouse)

percentile, has been observed in as many as 30% to 35% of survivors of childhood brain tumors[4–9] and in 10% to 15% of patients treated withsome antileukemia regimens.[10,11] Although growth in patients with tumors involving the head and neck, other than the brain, have not been studied exhaustively, there are reports of severe growth retardation in these patients as well.[2,12–17]

Comparison of the growth curves of children with acute lymphocytic leukemia (ALL) treated with different forms of central nervous system prophylaxis has identified whole-brain radiation as the principal cause of short stature.[10,17,18] The effects of cranial radiation appear to be age related, and the consensus is that children younger than 5 years at the time of therapy are particularly susceptible to its growth-inhibiting properties.[19] The effects of cranial radiation also are dose related. After 3000 cGy or more to the hypothalamus or pituitary gland using traditional fractionation schedules, severe growth retardation is seen in more than 50% of brain tumor patients[6–9] (Fig. 50-1). In contrast, chronic growth retardation after 1800 or 2400 cGy, as used in children with ALL, has been less frequent, is generally milder, and has not always been a problem.[20–22]

On the other hand, although few children with ALL fall below the fifth percentile for height, there are large numbers of children who have remained above the fifth percentile but who nevertheless have experienced significant decreases in height percentiles from the time of diagnosis. In two large follow-up series of patients whose only radiation had been 2400 cGy to the cranium, an excess in the proportion of patients in the lower percentiles was noted compared with that expected in a normal population.[11,19] Similar changes in the distribution of height percentiles have been observed after 1800 cGy of cranial radiation, but it is not clear whether the reduction in ultimate stature is less than that seen with the lower dose.[11,18,23]

The precise mechanism by which cranial radiation induces short stature is not clear. Doses as low as 2400 cGy have caused growth hormone deficiency, as indicated by uniform,[24,25] although sometimes transient,[26] blunting of spontaneous growth hormone pulses. However, other biochemical evidence of growth hormone deficiency, including plasma somatomedin C levels and growth hormone responses to a variety of provocative stimuli, have been variable.[9,20,27–31] The pres-

ence or absence of such abnormalities has not correlated fully with the degree of growth failure.

Chemotherapy also may contribute to attenuation of linear growth, but when it is given without radiation, the retardation is usually temporary. When the chemotherapy is discontinued, growth is accelerated, and the patient catches up with his or her peers. Prednisone and methotrexate, when given in a high enough dose or for a long enough time, appear to mediate this effect by their direct effect on bone growth (see Musculoskeletal and Related Tissues).

Direct inhibition of vertebral growth by spinal irradiation often contributes to the short stature. This change is seen most commonly in patients with brain tumors whose entire spinal columns have received doses in excess of 3500 cGy.[32] Moreover, among children with ALL who, in addition to 1800 to 2400 cGy of craniospinal radiation, receive abdominal radiation (1200 cGy), almost 30% have standing heights less than the fifth percentile.[11] This result may be due to irradiation of the gonads, to scatter radiation to the femoral heads, or both.[11,33] Where lower doses (1000–2500 cGy) have been given to ports including part or all of the spine, patients, although not necessarily short, have reduced sitting heights (measured from crown to rump).[9,32,34–36] This is the case for as many as 40% of long-term survivors of Wilms' tumor and Hodgkin's disease and may be more common with the higher doses used for medulloblastoma and soft-tissue sarcoma. This problem has been seen particularly in children who are either less than 6 years old or undergoing their adolescent growth spurt at the time of radiation.

Experience with the chronic effects on growth of total-body irradiation, as in preparation for bone marrow transplantation, is more limited. However, after 1000 cGy given as a single fraction, chronic, severe decreases in growth rates appear in most children.[37,38] The pathogenesis of short stature in these children includes factors other than radiation, notably graft-versus-host (GVH) disease and its therapy.

In some studies, changes in body weight in long-term survivors of childhood cancer are more prominent than changes in height. Chronic weight loss may result from intestinal malabsorption (see Gastrointestinal Function). At the other extreme, obesity has been reported in small groups of children with ALL.[3,23,31,39] This problem has its onset within the first year after discontinuation of chemotherapy and may either progress or stabilize. In one report, an association between obesity and learning disabilities after radiation therapy was noted.[3] The contribution of chemotherapy, particularly adrenocorticosteroids, to the development of obesity is unclear.

Monitoring long-term survivors for growth problems relies on the use of standardized curves familiar to the pediatrician. Because single values for heights and weights are unreliable for children, we recommend frequent serial measurements in order to establish each child's pattern of growth. Preferably, both sitting and standing heights should be obtained, if possible with a stadiometer available in most endocrinology offices. Measurements should be made prior to therapy, every 1 to 3 months during therapy and for the first year thereafter, and then once or twice a year until linear growth is complete.

Because of the above-noted concerns about disproportionate weight gains after the termination of antileukemia therapy, particular attention should be paid to weight during that time, especially during the first year. For those individuals whose growth is abnormal, the additional workup shown in Table 50-3, usually performed with the help of appropriate consultants, may be undertaken. It is important to recognize, however, that even in children in whom growth hormone deficiency has been documented before epiphyseal fusion, clinical

Table 50-3
Suggested Evaluation for Suspected Late Effects

Late Effect*	Screening Test	Additional Studies/Recommendations
Short stature	Growth curve	Basal or pulsatile growth hormone levels
	Sitting height	Provocative growth hormone studies
	Parental heights	Thyroid function tests†
	Bone age	Endocrinologist
Obesity or weight loss	Growth curve	[CT of hypothalamus]‡
	Diet history	Thyroid function tests
		Nutritionist, endocrinologist
Scoliosis	Spine radiography	Evaluate again during adolescent growth spurt
		Orthopedist
Bone asymmetries (hypoplasia, atrophy)	Bone radiography	Orthopedist
		Plastic surgeon
Avascular necrosis/osteoporosis	History of pain, fractures	Bone scan
	Bone radiography	[serum estradiol level; Ca, P]
		Orthopedist
		Physical therapist
Soft tissue hypoplasia, contractures, edema	Physical exam	Plastic surgeon
Dental abnormalities	Physical exam	Dentist, oral surgeon
Learning disabilities	Psychiatric testing	CT scan of head
		Special education classes
Leukoencephalopathy	CT scan	[CSF basic myelin protein]
	(See learning disabilities)	Neurologist
Neuropathy	Physical exam	Nerve conduction studies
		Neurologist
Hearing loss	Audiogram	ENT
		Audiologist
Infertility	History (primary vs. secondary dysfunction)	Endocrinologist
		Obstetrician/gynecologist
	Gonadal function testing†	Sex counseling
		[Chromosomes]
Thyroid dysfunction	Thyroid function testing	Antithyroid antibodies
		Thyroid scan
		Endocrinologist
Cardiomyopathy/pericarditis	ECG	Endomyocardial biopsy
	Echocardiogram	Cardiologist
	Radionuclide angiography	
Vaso-occlusive disease	Angiography	Vascular surgeon
	Doppler pulses	
Pneumonitis/pulmonary fibrosis	Chest radiography	Lung biopsy
	Pulmonary function tests	Pulmonologist
Chronic enteritis	Growth curves	Serum folate, carotene
	Nutritional assessment	Small-bowel studies
		Barium enema
		Gastroenterologist
Hepatitis/cirrhosis	Liver function tests	Liver biopsy
		Liver scan
		Gastroenterologist
Nephritis	Urinalysis	24-hour creatinine clearance or GFR scan
	BUN, creatinine	Intravenous urogram or sonogram
		Nephrologist
Hemorrhagic cystitis	Urinalysis	Cystoscopy
		Urologist
TTP	CBC/platelets	
	Peripheral blood smear	
Sepsis	Compliance with prophylactic antibiotics	
Second malignancy	Studies on an individual basis	Oncologist

* Listed in order of discussion in chapter.

† Thyroid function tests = T_4, thyrotropin, free T_4; gonadal function tests-Tanner staging for males older than 14 years at the time of evaluation or females not yet menstruating by age 12 years or if menses become irregular; FSH, LH, and testosterone (semen analysis) or estradiol, as appropriate.

‡ Square brackets indicate tests or intervention that may be useful; usually done in conjunction with consultants as indicated.

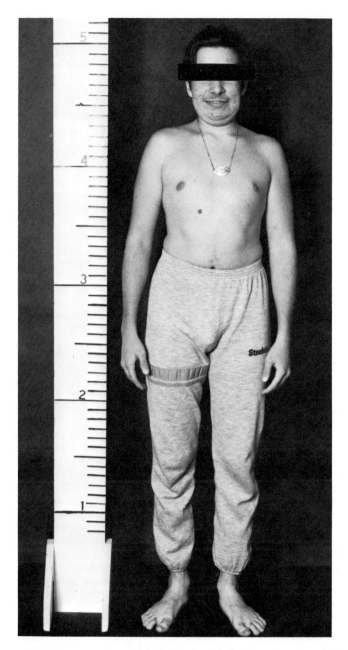

FIGURE 50-1. A 17½ year-old boy with medulloblastoma was treated with 5400 rad to the posterior fossa and 3600 rad to the rest of the neuraxis. The patient's height before treatment was at the 25th percentile; 10 years after radiation, he is well below the 5th percentile; sitting height also is less than the 5th percentile. Parents and siblings are all at least in the 25th percentile.

responses to growth hormone have sometimes been suboptimal.[40]

Current approaches to cancer therapy in children include attempts to spare adverse effects on growth. Leukemia protocols are attempting to use high-dose methotrexate, cytosine arabinoside, or both or intrathecal chemotherapy alone in lieu of radiation for central nervous system prophylaxis (see Chap. 16). Hyperfractionation schedules for radiation therapy and chemotherapy-only regimens are being implemented for treatment of brain tumors and as conditioning regimens in

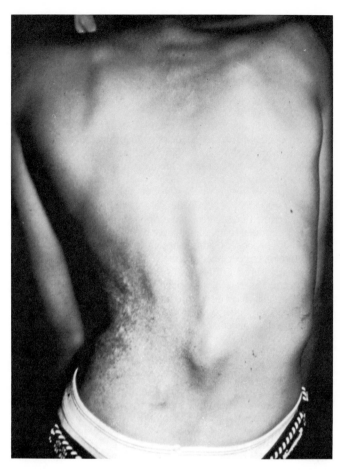

FIGURE 50-2. Kyphoscoliosis in a 15-year-old patient treated 14 years previously with 3000-rad abdominal radiation for a left-sided Wilms' tumor.

bone marrow transplantation. Whether these changes will permit long-term survivors to have normal growth remains to be seen.

MUSCULOSKELETAL AND RELATED TISSUES

Even excluding short stature and second tumors, functional and cosmetic disabilities involving bone, teeth, and muscle and other soft tissues are common, having been reported in 11% to 38% of survivors of a variety of pediatric cancers, notably solid tumors.[2,3] The majority of clinically significant problems involve bony abnormalities: scoliosis, atrophy or hypoplasia, avascular necrosis, and osteoporosis.

Scoliosis is a delayed consequence of radiation to segments of the spinal column. As such, it is seen almost exclusively in patients with solid tumors. Its incidence and severity are inversely related to technologic advances and therefore presumably will decrease in the future. Even with current megavoltage equipment and even when the entire width of each vertebra is included in the field, scoliosis has been reported in about 50% of Wilms' tumor patients given 1800 to 3500 cGy.[35,41] The concavity of the deformity, which is invariably on the side of irradiation (Fig. 50-2), worsens markedly during the adolescent growth spurt, irrespective of the age of the patient at radiation. Nonetheless, in contrast to what had been observed after orthovoltage therapy, today's cases of scoliosis are usually not severe enough to require orthopedic intervention.

In addition to causing scoliosis by direct effects on vertebral growth, abdominal radiation for Wilms' tumor may result in hypoplasia of the ilium and atrophy of muscle, soft tissue, and skin within the field. These fibrosed tissues have been said to "act as a bow string across the vertebrae,"[35] increasing the degree of curvature. With better staging systems, the number of children requiring vertebral or paravertebral radiotherapy for Wilms' tumor or rhabdomyosarcoma has decreased. In addition, symmetric radiation of the entire spine, sparing large volumes of the adjacent soft tissue, as in the treatment of medulloblastoma[32] or as in total-nodal radiation for Hodgkin's disease,[34] appears to carry little risk of scoliosis. Other factors that may contribute to the development of scoliosis include vertebral changes from metastatic tumor, laminectomy, or osteoporosis, processes which are more common in adult patients and in large part account for the development of post-cancer scoliosis in adults. Kyphosis occurs less frequently and rarely in the absence of scoliosis.

Hypoplasia has been reported to follow radiation to most other bones, including the long bones of children with soft-tissue sarcomas of an extremity,[33,42] probably because most patients have already achieved their maximum growth at the time of diagnosis. Shortening of the long bones does not appear to be a significant problem in Ewing's sarcoma, where the entire bone may receive as much as 7000 cGy.

Avascular necrosis of bone and osteoporosis are radiographic diagnoses and may be asymptomatic until the involved bone is subject to fracture or infection. Clinically significant avascular necrosis presenting as pain has been most extensively described in adults with head and neck tumors, particularly those directly involving bone, in whom the incidence has ranged from 5% to 25%,[34,36] and in adults and adolescents with Hodgkin's disease and non-Hodgkin's lymphoma, in whom the incidence has been approximately 3%.[43,44] In the latter group, avascular necrosis most commonly involves the femoral heads, where it may be accompanied by slipped capital femoral epiphysis, but has been described in virtually all locations and may be multifocal. Although necrosis may develop during therapy, the latency period has been as long at 13 years after treatment,[45] which may account for the relatively few reports in children.[46,47] Most avascular necrosis has been attributable to the direct effects of radiation therapy or systemic effects of corticosteroids, and although these appear to show dose dependence, necrosis has been reported after cumulative doses of prednisone as low as 500 mg.[44] In addition to radiation therapy and steroids, avascular necrosis in cancer patients has been anecdotally associated with single-agent cyclophosphamide[43] or methotrexate[48] as well as cyclophosphamide in combination with methotrexate and 5-fluorouracil.[49]

Like avascular necrosis, osteoporosis has been related to steroids and to radiation therapy, the latter in doses used in children with soft-tissue sarcomas or Ewing's sarcoma.[42] Although the link to methotrexate has been more compelling than for avascular necrosis, this appears to be a problem primarily during therapy that resolves once methotrexate has been discontinued:[50] of 110 patients with ALL who survived more than 5 years and received 3 to 5 years of weekly methotrexate, monthly 5-day pulses of prednisone, daily 6-mercaptopurine, and monthly injections of vincristine, only one had residual osteoporosis.[2]

Other bone changes common after radiation are asymptomatic roentgenographic findings including growth-arrest lines, lines of increased density parallel to end plates, and epiphyseal irregularities.[51] In general, these are seen after 2000 cGy or more given in 150- to 200-cGy fractions. Like scoliosis, they are seen primarily in patients who were still growing at the time of therapy and therefore have been reported most commonly in survivors of Wilms' tumor, Hodgkin's disease, neuroblastoma, and medulloblastoma.[34,35,51]

The contribution of irradiation of soft tissue to the development of scoliosis has been noted. In addition, radiation may produce disfiguring soft-tissue hypoplasia and pigmentary changes even without functionally significant abnormalities of neighboring bone (Fig. 50-3). Other connective tissue abnormalities seen in long-term survivors include scarring and contractures due to extravasation of drugs such as vincristine, dactinomycin, and athracyclines; edema resulting from radiation- or tumor-related lymphatic obstruction; nasolacrimal duct obstruction related to radiation fibrosis; chronic conjunctivitis, also caused by radiation;[42] various degrees of alopecia; the sclerodermatous skin manifestations of GVH disease; one or more components of the sicca syndrome (dry eye, dry mouth), also secondary to GVH disease or to radiation therapy involving the lacrimal or salivary glands; and cataracts (see Neurologic Function). The bony and soft-tissue complications resulting from amputation or endoprostheses are discussed elsewhere (see Chaps. 32 and 47).

Dental and maxillofacial abnormalities, although a composite of radiation effects on bone and soft tissue, bear separate mention. One of the few studies of this complication in childhood cancer survivors reported delayed or arrested tooth development in 6 of 14 long-term survivors of childhood ALL treated with 1800 to 3000 cGy and 13 of 14 with Hodgkin's disease treated in the neck or whole mantle with 2000 to 4900 cGy from megavoltage equipment.[52] Severe structural tooth abnormalities including caries, sometimes associated with nasal voice changes, were noted after 4500 to 6500 cGy to ports involving the nasopharynx in all of nine patients treated for rhabdomyosarcoma. Chronic otitis media, although not a feature in this series, has been reported in several similarly treated patients.[13,42] Slight facial deformities were seen in a small number of patients in the series who received a median of 3500 cGy to a variety of ports. The severity of all these defects appeared to vary inversely with age at the time of radiation.

Detection and diagnosis of musculoskeletal and connective tissue toxicities is largely a matter of suspecting them in vulnerable hosts and of a careful history and physical examination. Although soft-tissue or bony asymmetries may be obvious, mild pain or a history of fractures may be the only indication of avascular necrosis or osteoporosis. Dental and connective tissue problems will not be apparent unless they are looked for. Because many of these problems first appear many years after radiation or may progress over time, reevaluation should optimally be done yearly or every other year for life. Particularly when a patient is at high risk for the development of scoliosis, follow-up visits might be scheduled every 6 months during the patient's adolescent growth spurt. The need for diagnostic radiographs and appropriate referral in the case of clinically apparent disease is obvious (Table 50-3). The relative risk:benefit of "routine" radiographs of bones encompassed by radiation ports is less clear. However, some clinicians have advocated such studies every few years in patients who are at least 5 years from diagnosis in order to facilitate conservative medical, dental, or physical therapeutic intervention. Strategies for avoiding these toxicities have focused on refining radiation techniques and on limiting radiation dosages by intensifying chemotherapeutic regimens.

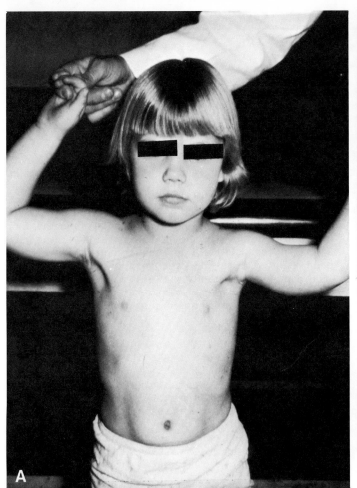

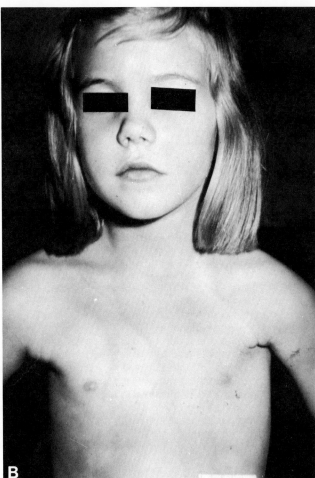

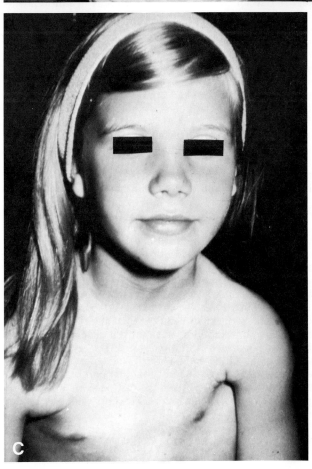

FIGURE 50-3. Progressive pectoral muscle hypoplasia after radiation to a posterior mediastinal neuroblastoma. The child was 10 months old at the time of diagnosis. **A, B,** and **C** were taken, respectively, at 2, 4, and 6 years after radiation. Hypoplasia of the ipsilateral breast can be anticipated.

NEUROLOGIC FUNCTION

Among survivors of all types of pediatric cancer, the incidence of significant neuropsychologic abnormalities has been said to be low.[53,54] However, among children with brain tumors or acute leukemia, in whom neurologic sequelae have been studied most extensively, disabilities necessitating special education or institutionalization have been reported in as many as 8% to 50%[5,55–58] and 8% to 30%,[3,59,60] respectively. Moreover, because leukemia and brain tumors constitute 60% of all childhood cancer, neuropsychologic dysfunction is a significant problem overall for childhood cancer survivors (see Chaps. 16 and 24). Patients with other tumors who have required specific central nervous system treatment appear to be at similar risk. Additional less serious disabilities, not including hypothalamic–pituitary dysfunction (see Gonadal Function, Thyroid) or psychosocial problems (see Chaps. 41 and 42), compatible with most day-to-day activities have been reported in even larger numbers.

Learning difficulties have been of serious concern. These have been associated with cranial radiation and to some degree are dose related. In one report of 36 children with a variety of intracranial tumors who had survived 5 years after treatment, 45% had IQs below 90 and 17% had IQs below 70.[5] These results are consistent with qualitative assessments of intelligence in children with brain tumors treated with high-dose radiation and are clearly more severe than what has been seen in patients treated with neurosurgery alone.[4,32,58,61,62]

Among children with ALL treated with 2400 cGy for central nervous system prophylaxis, retrospective, prospective, controlled, and uncontrolled studies all have reported mean IQs in the 85 to 99 range, significantly lower than those of population normals, healthy siblings, or matched patients with solid tumors who received no central nervous system therapy.[63–70] One study in which a subset of 18 children was prospectively tested before and after such therapy documented drops of 10 or more IQ points in 11.[66] Age below 8 years or IQ below 110 at diagnosis has been associated with increased morbidity.[4,64–68,70] The latter observation has additional significance in that the average IQ of children in the United States prior to therapy for ALL is 110, and it is this level, not 100, that should be considered the baseline mean. Although there is little experience with the long-term effects of 1800 cGy on learning capabilities, in a single study,[71] results appear to be not dissimilar to what has been observed after 2400 cGy.

The deficits seen in children with ALL after preventive central nervous system therapy probably are not only an effect of radiation therapy but also reflect an adverse interaction between cranial irradiation and the accompanying intrathecal methotrexate.[72] Methotrexate by itself has been associated with learning disabilities. A recent comparison between patients randomized to receive either 1800 cGy of cranial irradiation or intrathecal methotrexate during maintenance suggested that full- and performance-scale IQ and visual–motor integration are lower in the irradiated group, whereas attention, concentration, and short-term memory are poorer in the group given intrathecal methotrexate.[71] Such problems also have been seen after long-term low doses of intravenous methotrexate without cranial irradiation. Nonetheless, cranial irradiation is probably the most important factor contributing to learning problems. In both randomized and nonrandomized studies, children with ALL treated with cranial radiation in addition to intrathecal methotrexate have had lower IQs than children whose therapy consisted of intrathecal methotrexate alone, intrathecal methotrexate in combination with other agents, or intravenous methotrexate (500 mg/m^2 every three weeks for 3 doses dur-

ing consolidation). Other iatrogenic factors contributing to the development of learning disabilities may be cerebral thrombosis and hemorrhage from L-asparaginase therapy.[73]

This chronic neurotoxicity may be part of a spectrum, at one extreme of which is a progressive necrotizing leukoencephalopathy. This syndrome is characterized clinically by dementia, dysarthria, dysphagia, ataxia, spasticity, seizures, and coma.[74,75] Blindness also has been described, apparently due to involvement of the optic chiasm.[76] Histopathologic hallmarks of leukoencephalopathy are reactive astrocytosis, gliosis, and demyelinization. As is the case with learning disabilities, the more severe manifestations have been described most frequently in patients treated with a combination of intrathecal or intraventricular and systemic methotrexate as well as at least 2400 cGy of cranial irradiation. Leukoencephalopathy also has been reported in several patients following bone marrow transplantation in patients whose preparative regimens included 1000 cGy total-body irradiation.[77,78] Nearly all the cases reported have been in children, suggesting that the maturing brain is more susceptible.

At the other end of the spectrum are the EEG[60,79] and computed tomography (CT) brain scan abnormalities reported in asymptomatic children with ALL. The latter changes, which also have been seen in rhabdomyosarcoma of the head and neck,[80] include intracerebral calcification, dilatation of the ventricular and subarachnoid space, and a decreased parenchymal attentuation coefficient (white matter hypodensity). These changes usually are seen in patients with clinically evident necrotizing leukoencephalopathy after cranial radiation and methotrexate[59,81] but also have been detected in as many as 53% of functionally normal children[82] even after cranial radiation alone or cranial radiation and intrathecal cytosine arabinoside.[80] In one series, changes were seen only in children who had been less than 8 years of age at diagnosis.[83] In a comparative study of CT scans of patients given one of three methods of central nervous system prophylaxis, although similar minor abnormalities were seen after intrathecal methotrexate alone, intrathecal methotrexate plus intermediate-dose (500 mg/m^2) methotrexate, and intrathecal methotrexate plus 2400 cGy of cranial radiation, significant CT abnormalities were found only in the last group.[81] How neuropsychologic deficits correlate with CT changes is not clear. However, in a recent study, patients with intracerebral calcification (particularly of the basal ganglia) or cortical atrophy demonstrated subtle impairment of attention and memory.[84] These data suggest that CT scan abnormalities presage clinical deficits, a speculation that is especially worrisome in light of the finding that calcifications may first appear more than 7 years after central nervous system prophylaxis.[83]

CT scans of the spinal cord have not been done systematically. Although autopsy findings have shown that the pathologic changes of leukoencephalopathy also can affect the cord (subacute necrotizing leukomyelopathy), this does not seem to be a symptomatic problem in long-term survivors of cancer. However, in patients with solid tumors treated with high doses of radiation (usually greater than 5000 cGy), particularly to the head and neck or brachial plexus, cranial and peripheral neuropathies have developed over months or years as a result of axon necrosis or fibrosis.[85,86] Blindness secondary to radiation-induced necrosis of the optic nerve has been described even at doses as low as 1000 cGy.[87] Sensorimotor neuropathies arising during therapy with vinca alkaloids can persist, although for the most part these are reversible and therefore not seen as late effects of therapy.[88]

Additional neurologic residua include hearing loss from therapy with cisplatin or aminoglycosides or from the chronic otitis media of histiocytosis X (Langerhans' cell histiocytosis) and head and neck rhabdomyosarcoma,[14,42] and blindness from enucleation or radiation-induced cataract formation in patients with retinoblastoma or soft-tissue sarcomas involving the orbit. Less-extensive visual impairment may result from steroid- or radiation-induced posterior capsular cataracts in patients with ALL after cranial irradiation or in patients receiving bone marrow transplants.[37] Other neurologic or neuroendocrine abnormalities may persist in disease-free survivors of childhood cancer and presumably are related to the underlying disease rather than to therapy. These include the ataxia–opsoclonus–myoclonus syndrome seen occasionally in children with neuroblastoma and diabetes insipidus in patients with histiocytosis X.

As suggested in this section, a large number of patients being followed by the pediatric oncologist are at risk for late central nervous system toxicity and therefore need to be monitored carefully. Evaluation of learning disabilities usually is pursued by the school system when a child gets poor grades (see Chap. 51). However, because lesser abnormalities may go undetected and still interfere with optimal learning, we recommend that neuropsychologic screening be done routinely, at least in children who have received cranial radiation, and especially those who were younger than 8 years at the time of diagnosis. An age-standardized battery of tests should be used to measure intellectual ability, visual perception, visual–motor and motor skills, language, memory and learning, academic achievement, and behavior and social functioning. Somewhat arbitrarily, these might first be done 2 years after the completion of all therapy unless clinical difficulties dictate earlier evaluation. Because it is clear from the aforementioned discussion of CT-scan abnormalities that central nervous system toxicity is not static, we believe it is appropriate to repeat neuropsychologic tests every 2 to 3 years until early adulthood. Ideally, results can then be used to individualize remedial instruction. Some oncologists would make the same recommendations with respect to serial CT scans. However, the expense and uncertain meaning of many of the CT abnormalities lead us to recommend that these scans be reserved for children in whom deficits are detected on psychometric testing or in whom there is other evidence of leukoencephalopathy. Although a variety of cerebrospinal fluid proteins, including myelin basic protein, have been proposed as predictors of central nervous system damage, their use is controversial and is not recommended on a routine basis.

Care should be taken to explain to the parent and child that some of their school problems may in fact be related to treatment. Because the vast majority of cancer-related neuropsychologic sequelae result from nonorganic problems and from the attitudes and behaviors of others, a more global approach may need to be taken. This is discussed in Chapters 41 and 42.

The magnitude of neurologic sequelae has emphasized the need to develop alternative approaches to therapy and prevention of central nervous system malignancy. Refinements in radiation techniques, the elimination of radiation altogether in selected lower-risk patients, and its replacement by chemotherapy have been commented on in an earlier section.

GONADAL FUNCTION

Males

Both germ-cell depletion and abnormalities of gonadal endocrine function have been seen in male survivors of cancer.

Most commonly, these have been thought to result from therapy—radiation, surgery, or chemotherapy—with the specific late effects differing as a function of age at diagnosis.

The effects of testicular irradiation on germ cell numbers have been well studied. Reduced sperm production occurs in a dose-dependent manner with fractionated exposures of 10 to 600 cGy.[89–91] In patients with seminoma treated with para-aortic and ipsilateral pelvic radiation after unilateral orchiectomy, incidental doses of 32 to 178 cGy to the remaining testicle have been associated with azoospermia resolving over 6 months to 2 years.[89] Among men with Hodgkin's disease treated with "inverted-Y" radiation, who, despite lead shielding of the scrotum, were estimated to have received a cumulative dose of 140 to 300 cGy to both testes, 100% became azoospermic without recovery after 2 to 40 months of follow-up.[92] Although detailed dosimetry was not reported regarding scatter to the testes from ports encompassing soft-tissue sarcomas of the thigh or abdomen, radiation has been shown to contribute to the 100% incidence of azoospermia in that setting.[93] At doses of 400 to 600 cGy, azoospermia may persist 3 to 5 years, and above 600 cGy, germinal loss with resulting increases in follicle-stimulating hormone (FSH) and decreases in testicular volume usually appears to be irreversible.[90,91] In Seattle, the Bone Marrow Transplantation Group has monitored gonadal function in a large group of male patients who were past puberty at the time of total-body irradiation (1000 cGy single fraction). Azoospermia was universal, and only 2 of 41 patients had recovery 6 years after grafting.[37]

Prepubertal testicular germ cells also appear to be radiosensitive, although tubular damage may be difficult to assess until the patient has gone through puberty. In a follow-up of 10 young men, 17 to 36 years, who had received an estimated 268 to 983 cGy scattered from radiation to a Wilms' tumor during childhood, oligospermia or azoospermia was found in eight.[94] A similar group of eight patients who were still prepubertal at the time of evaluation did not yet show intermittent elevations of FSH, although presumably they, too, had depleted germinal epithelium. Data on gonadal function in boys treated with radiation alone for Hodgkin's disease prior to puberty are limited but are consistent with data from older patients.[95]

Recently, it has become apparent that radiation therapy also is toxic to Leydig cells, with resulting inadequate production of testosterone. Boys treated prepubertally with 2400 cGy for testicular leukemia, in addition to suffering germ-cell depletion, are at high risk for delayed sexual maturation associated with decreased testosterone levels, despite increased luteinizing hormone (LH) levels.[96–99] Similarly, of 16 boys with hematologic malignancy treated prepubertally with total-body irradiation, 11 had delayed onset of puberty.[37] Cranial or craniospinal radiation *per se,* as in children with ALL[100] or primary brain tumors other than those involving the hypothalamic or pituitary glands,[8,101] does not seem to damage testicular function, although precocious onset of puberty has been reported.[102]

Chemotherapy also can interfere with testicular function. In particular, a variety of alkylating agents and the methylhydrazine procarbazine decrease spermatogenesis in long-term survivors. Although much of the data comes from patients with nephritis, studies of adults with non-Hodgkin's lymphoma and soft-tissue sarcomas have confirmed that the effects of cyclophosphamide and chlorambucil are dose dependent but reversible in up to 70% of patients after therapy-free intervals of several years.[93,103–106] Similarly, among pubertal or adult males treated for Hodgkin's disease with five or six cycles of mechlorethamine, vincristine, prednisone, and procarbazine (MOPP) and evaluated 1 to 2 years after completion of therapy, azoospermia is found in 80% to 100%.[106-109] However, this is reversible in only about 20% of cases even 7 years after therapy, a percentage that may increase with fewer MOPP cycles and decrease with pelvic irradiation.[110] After Adriamycin, bleomycin, vinblastine, and dacarbazine (ABVD), the incidence of azoospermia appears to be lower (36%) and the incidence of recovery higher (100%) than after MOPP.[111]

Although evaluation of testicular histology and hormonal status in boys shortly after treatment for ALL with cyclophosphamide, cytosine arabinoside, or both has suggested that germ-cell depletion occurs as an acute toxicity in all age groups,[112] long-term follow-up of patients who received single-agent cyclophosphamide for nephritis or as the pretransplant preparative regimen for aplastic anemia[113] suggests that prepubertal testes are relatively resistant to chronic toxicity. Nonetheless, mild increases of FSH and small testes have been observed several years after prepubertal treatment of boys with nitrosoureas for brain tumors[101] or with MOPP for Hodgkin's disease.[95]

To an even greater extent than its effect on spermatogenesis, the effects of MOPP on Leydig cell function appear to be age related, with normal pubertal progression after therapy prior to puberty, gynecomastia with low testosterone and increased LH in patients treated during adolescence, and compensated Leydig-cell failure (increased LH with low normal testosterone levels or exaggerated FSH and LH responses to luteinizing hormone–releasing hormone) without gynecomastia in adults.[106-108] It is worth noting that compensated Leydig-cell failure has been found at the time of diagnosis in almost half of men with Hodgkin's disease.[114] Decline in libido without impotence may be a common problem and does not correlate with testosterone levels.[109] The reversibility of these abnormalities has not been addressed in the literature. It should be noted that although increased[109] and normal[10,107] levels of prolactin have been described in males years after MOPP or other regimens, the relationship of these findings to serum testosterone levels or the presence of gynecomastia is not clear. Although in children with a history of histiocytosis, hyperprolactinemia caused by hypothalamic involvement by tumor has been associated with galactorrhea,[15] this has not been the case in Hodgkin's disease.

Compensated Leydig-cell failure sometimes associated with gynecomastia also has been described after cisplatin-based therapy in adults.[115] Other combination chemotherapy regimens, including prednisone, vincristine, methotrexate, and 6-mercaptopurine (POMP), as used in adolescent boys with ALL[100] and high-dose methotrexate/vincristine in men with osteosarcoma,[116] appear to cause no or only transient gonadal toxicity. Despite their prominent effects on germ cell epithelium, alkylating agents or antimetabolites have not been reported to produce Leydig cell failure. Whether the even higher doses of methotrexate included in current protocols for high-risk ALL will be as benign remains to be seen.

The effects of surgery on the gonads in males include impotence or retrograde ejaculation following bilateral retroperitoneal lymph node dissection[117] or partial or complete pelvic exenteration. In patients with primary central nervous system tumors involving the hypothalamus or pituitary, surgical resection may be a cause of secondary hypogonadism.[118] Hydroceles have been seen in long-term survivors of Hodgkin's disease[119] and Wilms' tumor (unpublished observation) after retroperitoneal surgery or radiation therapy.

The gonadal toxicities listed in this section, although not life threatening, are of serious concern to patients and their families, particularly in the case of young men who have not already had children at the time of diagnosis. It is this concern

that has popularized pretreatment sperm banking. Cryopreserved semen can in some cases produce normal children.[120] The value of this precaution has been questioned, however, because many men with Hodgkin's disease, primary testicular cancer, and diverse metastatic cancers have lower-than-expected sperm counts and decreased sperm motility at the time of diagnosis.[121-124] These findings correlate with malnutrition,[122] but in men with Hodgkin's disease do not correlate with stage or the presence of B symptoms.[114,124] Whether semen from such patients is adequate for artificial insemination or will tolerate cryopreservation is unclear. Another caveat is the possibility of infertility prior to therapy in males with dysgenetic gonads (e.g., Klinefelter's syndrome) who may be predisposed to gonadal or extragonadal malignancies.[125] Even when semen samples appear adequate, the expense of sperm banking (which frequently is not covered by insurance), the variable quality control among sperm banks, and concern regarding viability and integrity of sperm stored for very long periods makes this a controversial technique. It is one that we mention to our adolescent male patients but do not encourage on a routine basis.

Patients should be routinely screened for problems of gonadal function. This screen should include an age-appropriate history with specific attention to problems with libido, impotence, or fertility and examination for gynecomastia, Tanner staging of body hair, and penile and testicular size. Hormonal evaluation, including at least a single measurement of serum LH, and testosterone levels, should be done in pubertal individuals and in boys whose puberty appears to be delayed. Semen analysis may be helpful. Where abnormalities in gonadal function are detected, close cooperation with an endocrinologist is essential in planning hormonal replacement therapy or in monitoring patients for spontaneous recovery. Where no abnormalities are noted on history and physical examination, but where sexual maturity has not been completed, it is recommended that these studies be repeated every 1 to 2 years.

The value of trying to prevent gonadal dysfunction is obvious. The use of chemotherapeutic regimens such as ABVD (see Chap. 21) that it is hoped will be less toxic but as effective, as well as refinement of radiation techniques, has been mentioned. Extensive surgical procedures have to a large extent been made obsolete by intensive multimodal approaches.

Females

Evaluation of the effects of radiation or chemotherapy on hormonal and reproductive function is more difficult in female survivors of cancer than it is in males. Whereas in the latter orchidometry and semen analysis provide easy measures of germinal reserve, in the former, there are no such easy tests.

Despite these limitations, the effects of radiation on the ovary, as on the testis, have been determined to be both age and dose dependent. Irreversible ovarian failure (primary or secondary amenorrhea, increased LH and FSH levels with or without symptoms of menopause and loss of libido) is an almost universal result of 400 to 700 cGy conventionally fractionated and delivered to both ovaries (as in whole-abdominal radiation for non-Hodgkin's lymphoma) in women older than 40 years.[126] Despite higher doses (1200–5000 cGy), amenorrhea eventually occurred in only 68% of patients treated at a mean age of 6.9 years.[127] In one series, 23% of prepubertal and adolescent girls in whom at least one ovary was at the edge of the radiation field (and therefore had received a dose of only 90–1000 cGy) were found to have ovarian failure.[127] When secondary amenorrhea results from such doses, which are similar to those administered to the ovaries after midline oophoropexy and lead shielding with pelvic radiation in Hodgkin's disease, it appears to be reversible within several months to 4 years in 50% to 60% of patients.[128,129]

Total-body irradiation (1000-cGy single fraction) has been associated with primary amenorrhea and absent secondary sexual characteristics in all 15 patients treated as young girls and followed for as long as 10 years.[38] The effect of craniospinal radiation is less clear. In one report, girls with medulloblastoma treated with craniospinal radiation alone (3000 cGy to the spine) did not experience gonadal toxicity.[101] In contrast, among girls with ALL and a similar age distribution, those receiving craniospinal (1800–2400 cGy) or craniospinal plus abdominal (1200 cGy) radiation experienced incidences of increased FSH and LH in 49% and 93%, respectively, and a large proportion of these children had delayed menses.[130]

Ovarian failure also has been associated with chemotherapy. Although the morbidity is less than in males, single alkylating agents (cyclophosphamide, busulfan, L-phenylalanine mustard)[131–134] and MOPP are the best-described culprits. As with radiation therapy, toxicity is dose and probably age dependent. Women older than 40 may develop amenorrhea with only one to four cycles of MOPP, compared with three to twelve cycles in the 30% of women less than 35 years of age who become amenorrheic.[135] Girls treated prior to puberty with single alkylating agents or MOPP may be capable of normal puberty[108,134] or alternatively, may have pathologic or clinical evidence of ovarian failure.[101,136–138] As with males, treatment of girls with POMP[134] or of women with vincristine/methotrexate[116] has not been associated with gonadal dysfunction.

The diagnostic evaluation of ovarian dysfunction rests on history (primary or secondary amenorrhea, menstrual irregularity, and pregnancies or difficulties becoming pregnant), Tanner staging of breast and genital development, and serum gonadotropin and estradiol levels. These studies might be repeated at intervals similar to those suggested for males. However, because young women may be destined for early menopause, they should have long-term follow-up.

In addition to the above-noted approaches to prevention of gonadal failure, some investigators have begun to examine the use of oral contraceptives to suppress ovarian function and thereby make the ovaries resistant to the effects of chemotherapy.[139]

Pregnancy Outcome

For patients who are fertile after anticancer therapy, there remain concerns about the ability to have normal pregnancies and normal children. The potential teratogenicity or mutagenicity of modern anticancer therapy is difficult to demonstrate in humans for a number of reasons. Few patients have children during or after treatment, and many who conceive elect to have an abortion. Moreover, abortuses and live-born infants have not been scrutinized for defects in morphogenesis, growth, and development. Differences in radiotherapeutic or chemotherapeutic drug combinations and dosages make correlations difficult. Finally, the recent introduction of new agents has thwarted the accumulation of sufficiently similar cases from which to draw definitive conclusions.

Nonetheless, there are enough case reports to suggest a real risk of congenital or developmental abnormalities in the offspring or spontaneous abortuses of patients who have been given intrapartum chemotherapy. The risk appears to vary with the therapeutic regimen and, especially, with the timing of the

pregnancy with respect to drug exposure. On the basis of available information, it is probably reasonable to say that pregnancy outcome is most threatened by chemotherapy given during the first trimester. Chemotherapy appears less commonly, if ever, to have caused serious abnormalities when used later in pregnancy. A detailed summary of the teratogenic effects of anticancer agents administered during pregnancy has been reported elsewhere.[140]

Whether chemotherapy completed before pregnancy is a risk to subsequent offspring is a problem more relevant to the long-term survivor of childhood anticancer therapy. In a preliminary communication, 7.5% of 75 pregnancies that occurred after chemotherapy for Hodgkin's disease resulted in significant malformations.[141] An additional 15% resulted in fetal wastage and another 15% in premature or low-birth-weight babies. These numbers exceed what would be expected in the general population.[141] Unfortunately, this report did not detail the therapeutic regimens, making it difficult to guess at the reasons for these problems. Another report, although not commenting on the occurrence of congenital anomalies, suggested that among children born to young adults of both sexes who had previously been treated for non-Hodgkin's lymphoma, there may be an unusually low son-to-daughter ratio,[142] again suggesting a deleterious effect of chemotherapy on germ cells.

On the other hand, numerous other series[143–145] and case reports have suggested that intensive chemotherapy completed before pregnancy is compatible with normal offspring. Although in several of the series, both major and minor anomalies were observed, these did not appear to occur in excess of what is seen in the population at large. One relatively large series in which the children were examined at 0 to 12 years of age (median 2½ years) did not detect any significant malformations, problems with school performance, or excess of minor abnormalities after a variety of intensive combinations commonly used in the treatment of leukemia, Hodgkin's disease, and sarcomas.[143]

Although chemotherapy has received most of the attention, radiation involving the ovaries also may contribute to compromised pregnancy outcome. Compared with women with Hodgkin's disease treated with chemotherapy alone, women who have received both chemotherapy and radiation therapy have a significantly higher incidence of abnormal offspring.[146] The effects of radiation alone were not studied. However, a recent report documents a greatly increased risk of perinatal death and prematurity in the offspring of female long-term survivors of Wilms' tumor whose therapy included abdominal radiation.[147] The teratogenic influence of chemotherapy or radiation therapy in men has not been addressed, even to the extent it has been in women. However, wives of men with Hodgkin's disease treated with both chemotherapy and radiation therapy, but not those treated with chemotherapy alone, have an increased incidence of spontaneous abortions.[146]

The possibility of mutagenic (as opposed to teratogenic) effects of anticancer therapy also has been raised. One cytogenetic study showed nonclonal chromosomal abnormalities in peripheral blood lymphocytes of six of nine long-term survivors of childhood ALL a median of 7 years after therapy, suggesting that genetic damage can be sustained, at least by somatic cells.[148] However, neither a study of 2308 offspring of long-term survivors who had been treated during childhood or adolescence with chemotherapy with or without radiation therapy[149] nor the above-mentioned study of children of Wilms' tumor patients treated with radiation therapy and chemotherapy[145] found an excess of cancer. One subset of patients—those whose own cancers are due to a genetic predisposition

—may have children with the same predisposition to malignancy. The genetics of embryonal tumors such as retinoblastoma or Wilms' tumor and the risks of malignancy for patients with inherited nonmalignant conditions such as von Recklinghausen's disease have been discussed elsewhere.[150]

We encourage patients who are interested in having children after the completion of therapy, although we advise them to wait 1 year or more in order to be more certain that they are disease free. Difficulties in becoming pregnant can be evaluated as described in the prior section. Because relatively little is known about the problems of children born to survivors of childhood cancer, long-term general follow-up should be emphasized. The importance of optimizing the accrual and dispersal of information about pregnancy outcome in patients with a history of cancer cannot be overemphasized. A central registry is being developed at the National Cancer Institute.

THYROID

Hypothyroidism is the most common nonmalignant late effect involving this gland and almost always is due to radiation to the neck for nonthyroid malignancy. Between 1.5 and 6 years after radiation doses of 1500 to 7000 cGy, laboratory evidence of primary hypothyroidism (increased serum thyrotropin with normal or low T_4 levels) has been demonstrated in 40% to 90% of patients with Hodgkin's disease, non-Hodgkin's lymphoma, and primary intracranial or head and neck tumors[9,13,151–159] and in 25% of children after bone marrow transplants for hematologic malignancy.[38] In some instances, this has been reversible after as long as 3 years even without replacement therapy.[156] Thyroid cancers (see Second Malignancies), thyroid nodularity, exophthalmos, and symptoms of hypothyroidism including myxedema coma have been reported in some of these patients.

However, much lower doses of radiation also appear to carry a risk of primary hypothyroidism. In a recent study by the Children's Cancer Study Group (CCSG), thyroid function was evaluated in 175 children with ALL who were off therapy and at least 7 years from diagnosis.[160] All had received 2400 cGy to the cranium. On the basis of dosimetric measurements, it has been estimated that cranial radiation can deliver up to 7.5% of the total dose to the thyroid;[161] thus, these patients' thyroids would have received as much as 180 cGy. Five of the 175 patients (3%) had low serum T_4 and increased thyrotropin levels, and 11 others (6%) had normal T_4 levels at the expense of increases in thyrotropin, figures that appear to be in excess of what is seen in the general population. The relative incidence and natural history of thyroid dysfunction in patients treated with or without cranial radiation remain to be studied. Secondary hypothyroidism with low thyrotropin and T_4 levels, although reported,[9,13] appears to be uncommon after radiation to the head or neck.

Whether chemotherapy contributes to the development of hypothyroidism is less clear. Evaluation of patients with Hodgkin's disease treated with MOPP without radiation has not detected a significant incidence of thyroid dysfunction.[153,156] L-asparaginase (a drug common to all the patients tested as part of the above-noted ALL study) inhibits synthesis of thyroid-binding globulin, although T_4 levels apparently are not affected.[162,163]

Other factors that may contribute to the development of hypothyroidism in survivors of cancer include hemithyroidectomy, use of iodide-containing contrast material as in lymphangiography, and—arguably—age at the time of irradiation. Although several studies have not detected an age factor,[153,156,158] in one series, 48% of patients with Hodgkin's disease less than

20 years old had elevated thyrotropin levels compared with only 33% of older patients, a difference that was believed to be significant.[154] In another follow-up of 32 children with Hodgkin's disease,[152] although only 22 (69%) had increased thyrotropin levels (an incidence similar to that described in many adult series), with more sensitive clinical techniques, 91% appeared to have some degree of abnormality. This high percentage seems particularly striking because patients were treated with only 2500 to 3000 cGy to the neck.

Hyperthyroidism has been described after radiation for Hodgkin's disease,[153,164] other nonthyroid neoplasms of the neck,[165] and in preparation for bone marrow transplantation,[38] although the incidence is low and the mechanism unclear.

Patients who have received 1000 cGy or more to the neck should be routinely screened for thyroid abnormalities by physical examination and by measuring serum thyrotropin, T_4, and free T_4 levels on a yearly basis for at least 6 years from the conclusion of therapy. Patients with ALL who have had cranial irradiation should probably be screened also, although at what time is less clear. Certainly, regular examinations for exophthalamus, thyroid nodules, or bruits can conveniently be done at the time of yearly follow-up. Evaluation and treatment by an endocrinologist is recommended if any abnormalities are detected. Careful shielding of the thyroid during irradiation, elimination of radiation or the use of lower doses (as is now being advocated in some centers for patients with Hodgkin's disease) and avoidance of the concurrent use of radiation and iodide-containing contrast materials should help decrease the incidence of thyroid abnormalities.

CARDIOVASCULAR FUNCTION

Chronic cardiotoxicity most commonly takes the form of cardiomyopathy, pericarditis, or both. The anthracyclines doxorubicin and daunomycin are well-known causes of cardiomyopathy, and the natural history of anthracycline-induced cardiotoxicity has been carefully defined. Chronic cardiomyopathy appears to be unrelated to the transient ECG changes frequently are seen during therapy. Although an acute-onset myocarditis–pericarditis syndrome is thought to predict chronic cardiomyopathy,[166] prospective evaluation of patients during therapy has demonstrated that even full-blown congestive heart failure with or without arrhythmias can occur at any time without warning.[167,168] Onset has been reported even years after completion of therapy. The incidence of cardiomyopathy is related to the cumulative dose of anthracyclines and among patients given more than 600 mg/m² exceeds 30%.[169,170] With a total dose of 500 to 600 mg/m² the incidence is 11%, falling to less than 1% with total doses below 500 mg/m². Because overt anthracycline cardiomyopathy has been rapidly fatal in as many as 80% of cases[170] and is reversible in others, the incidence presumably is a good deal lower in patients who have been off therapy for many years. The incidence in long-term survivors of subclinical postanthracycline myocardial damage is not known.

Other factors that are thought to enhance the myocardial toxicity of anthracyclines are mediastinal radiation,[167,171,172]; underlying cardiac abnormalities, including involvement by tumor[168,169]; uncontrolled hypertension[168,169]; exposure to other chemotherapeutic agents, particularly cyclophosphamide,[169] dactinomycin,[173] mitomycin,[173] DTIC,[174] vincristine, bleomycin, and methotrexate[175]; and younger age. Above cumulative doses of 550 mg/m², both daunomycin and doxorubicin are more likely to induce congestive heart failure in children than in adults less than 40 years of age.[167,176,177] In a study of 5613 patients given daunomycin, the dose–response curve for congestive heart failure was steeper in the 2861 children than in the 2752 adults.[177] As with daunomycin, the cumulative threshold dose of doxorubicin below which congestive heart failure rarely occurs is the same for children and adults. Above the threshold dose, however, patients younger than 15 years are more likely to develop cardiomyopathy than older patients. The schedule of anthracycline administration also is important, with lesser toxicity from continuous infusions or weekly doxorubicin compared with every-3-week boluses.[170,178,179]

Chronic toxicity caused by radiation alone usually involves pericardial effusions or constrictive pericarditis, sometimes in association with pancarditis. Although 4000 cGy of total-heart irradiation appears to be the usual threshold, pericarditis has been reported after as little as 1500 cGy, even in the absence of radiomimetic chemotherapy.[180,181] In one series of adults with Hodgkin's disease, 62% had dyspnea on exertion when evaluated a mean of 8 years after 4000 cGy mantle irradiation administered via anterior ports.[182] Cardiac evaluations in these and other similarly treated patients[171,183] suggest an incidence of overt or subclinical constrictive pericarditis of about 50% in long-term survivors and a similar incidence of biventricular dysfunction due both to constriction and to myocardial disease. More recent studies of patients in whom combined anterior and posterior ports were used found asymptomatic pericardial effusions in 5% to 30% shortly after therapy, with half of these resolving over 1 year.[180,184] Symptomatic pericarditis, which usually develops 10 to 30 months after radiation, is found in 2% to 10%.[180,181,185] In such patients, including children, who have been off therapy for a number of years, subclinical pericardial and myocardial damage as well as valvular thickening without stenosis or insufficiency may be common.[186,187] It is worth noting, however, that symptomatic pericarditis may first appear as late as 45 years after therapy.[188,189]

Vaso-occlusive disease involving the carotid, coronary, iliofemoral, vertebral, renal, and mesenteric arteries also has been reported after local radiation therapy.[190–196] Carotid disease, which has occurred from several months to 39 years after as little as 1400 cGy, has been reported in 0.25% of Hodgkin's disease survivors treated with radiation to the neck. However, that radiation is the immediate cause is not entirely clear. In one cohort analysis of 4258 person-years at risk, the relative mortality rate from coronary artery disease was not significantly higher in Hodgkin's disease patients who had received mediastinal radiation than in the population at large.[194] Vaso-occlusive disease has not been reported to date in patients who received radiation as children.

Diagnosis of cardiovascular disease requires, first, a high level of suspicion in patients treated with anthracyclines or radiation. Because of the known long latency of cardiotoxicity in some cases, and because of the as-yet poorly defined late natural history of cardiovascular problems in patients treated as children, we recommend a yearly standard history and physical examination for life in patients at high risk. In addition, because subclinical myocardial damage evidenced by a decreased left ventricular ejection fraction may be predictive of congestive heart failure,[166,171,197] gated radionuclide angiography or echocardiography every 2 to 5 years is recommended for patients treated with 500 mg/m[2] or more of the antracyclines or with lower doses together with mediastinal radiation. An ECG also is recommended to look for carditis. For individuals in whom there is any evidence of carditis, more frequent evaluations may be useful to establish the pattern of progression. Although some investigators have used endomyocardial biopsy as a sensitive indicator of myocardial disease, such an invasive procedure probably should not be used routinely. We

know of no evidence that prophylactic digitalis use is helpful in patients with worsening but still asymptomatic cardiac function secondary to anthracyclines or radiation therapy. Nonetheless, close interaction with cardiology specialists is important should asymptomatic disease be detected. In the case of severe anthracycline-induced cardiomyopathy refractory to medical management, cardiac transplantation might be an option for some long-term survivors.

Prevention of cardiotoxicity is a primary focus of investigation. A number of analogues of doxorubicin and daunomycin, which it is hoped will have equal antitumor activity with less cardiotoxicity, continue to undergo phase I and phase II clinical testing. The use of less toxic infusion schedules (see above) and the use of agents that may rescue the heart from anthracycline toxicity also are being explored (see Chap. 9). More conservative use of radiation therapy (smaller doses and reduced port sizes), may decrease the incidence of carditis.

PULMONARY FUNCTION

Both the airways and the pulmonary interstitium are sites of significant late toxicity of anticancer therapy. In adults, where these problems have been looked for and studied most extensively, pulmonary fibrosis—with loss of lung volume, lung compliance and diffusing capacity of carbon monoxide (DLCO)—and pneumonitis are most commonly a result of pulmonary radiation. These problems thus are most often seen in patients with thoracic malignancies, notably Hodgkin's disease and carcinoma of the lung. In such individuals, asymptomatic radiographic findings or restrictive findings on pulmonary function testing consistent with fibrosis or pneumonitis have been reported in 50% to 100%.[198,199] These changes have been detected months to years after radiation therapy, most often in patients who suffered radiation pneumonitis as an acute toxicity.[200] However, clinically apparent pneumonitis with cough, fever, or dyspnea has been found in only 5% to 15% of patients and generally does not develop except when more than 3000 cGy in standard fractions has been delivered to more than 50% of the lung.[200–202]

On the basis of a relatively few pediatric series, it appears that the mechanism for respiratory damage in young children is different from that in the adult or adolescent. In one study of 12 survivors of Wilms' tumor 7 to 14 years after treatment with bilateral pulmonary radiation for metastatic disease,[203] several patients had dyspnea on exertion and radiographic evidence of interstitial and pleural thickening. Mean total lung volumes and DLCO were reduced to approximately 60% of predicted values in the face of normal "static elastic properties" of the lung after median total doses of approximately 2000 cGy. In contrast to older children and adults, in whom, as noted above, radiation for thoracic malignancy results in pulmonary fibrosis with loss of lung volume alone, these data were felt to be consistent with a proportionate interference with the growth of both the lung and the chest wall. Restrictive lung changes after lower doses of whole-lung radiation (1100–1400 cGy) have been reported in several other studies of children with a variety of malignancies.[204–206] There is some suggestion that children younger than 3 years at the time of therapy experience more chronic toxicity.[206]

Obstructive changes also have been reported after conventional therapy.[204] Obstructive lung disease was the chief problem in a large prospective series of patients with hematologic malignancy or aplastic anemia undergoing bone marrow transplantation. After 1000 cGy total-body irradiation in a single fraction, 8% of patients had an FEV$_1$/vital capacity (VC) (a measure of obstructive lung disease) below 50% of normal at 3 years, and 29% had an FEV_1/VC below 70% by that time. Unlike the transient acute restrictive changes observed in the same population, obstructive changes were not associated with a history of interstitial pneumonia, nor were they associated with chronic GVH disease.[207]

In addition to radiation therapy, a growing list of chemotherapeutic agents appears to be responsible for pulmonary disease in long-term survivors. Bleomycin toxicity is the prototype for chemotherapy-related lung injury. Although this problem has been reported in children,[208] clinically apparent bleomycin pneumonopathy is most frequent in adults, particularly those older than 70 years.[209–211] The chronic lung toxicity appears to result from persistence or progression of abnormalities developing within 3 months of therapy. Like the acute toxicity, it is dose dependent above a threshold cumulative dose of 400 units and exacerbated by concurrent or prior radiation therapy[209,212,213] or cyclophosphamide[209,214,215] or subsequent oxygen therapy.[216] At doses above 400 units, 10% of patients experience fibrosis, and 35% to 55% suffer severe symptoms in the face of combinations of the above-noted factors.[213,217] At lower doses, fibrosis occurs sporadically in 5% of patients, with a 1% to 2% mortality rate. In some series, bleomycin toxicity could be anticipated on the basis of DLCO abnormalities.[218]

Alkylating agents also are thought to cause chronic lung injury. As with bleomycin, BCNU pulmonary toxicity is dose related. Although toxicity has been seen with as little as 800 mg/m²,[219] doses greater than 1500 mg/m² result in a 50% incidence of symptoms.[220] Other contributing factors include the number of courses over which the drug has been given and a history of underlying lung disease including asthma.[220] In two children, cyclophosphamide is thought to have caused delayed onset of pulmonary fibrosis with severe restrictive lung disease in association with marked reductions in the anteroposterior diameter of the chest.[221] This was postulated to result from failure of lung growth during a period of rapid body growth. Melphalan[222] and busulfan[223] also have caused pulmonary fibrosis.

Other drugs that have been associated with chronic pneumonitis and fibrosis are vinblastine[224] and methotrexate. Methotrexate toxicity, which probably occurs with an incidence below 1%, has generally been associated with low-dose oral administration over more than 3 years.[225] Intravenous and, rarely, intrathecal[226] administration also may be responsible. The problem has been seen after cumulative methotrexate dosages of as little as 40 mg to more than 4500 mg and has first been noted at the beginning of maintenance methotrexate for treatment of ALL or after 18 years of low-dose therapy, as used in the management of psoriasis.[225]

Other factors contributing to chronic pulmonary toxicity include spinal radiation with possible scatter to the lung, superimposed infection, underlying pneumonopathy (e.g., asthma), cigarette or respirator toxicity, and the effects of chronic pulmonary involvement by tumor or reaction to tumor. For example, a subset of patients with histiocytosis X (Langerhans cell histiocytosis) develops histiocytic pulmonary infiltrates or honeycombing with severe chronic restrictive lung disease unrelated to therapy or the presence of active tumor (also see Chap. 23).[227]

Symptoms of pulmonary dysfunction such as chronic cough (with or without fever) or dyspnea should be looked for on yearly follow-up, particularly in patients treated with thoracic radiation or bleomycin, in patients who experienced acute pulmonary toxicity during therapy, and in patients with structural abnormalities of the thorax. It is important to em-

phasize to all patients the risks of smoking. Whether or how often to recommend pulmonary function tests or chest radiographs in the long-term survivor in the absence of symptoms is not clear. Pulmonary function tests (including DLCO) should be performed in patients with symptoms or in those who will require general anesthesia for any reason. Because knowledge of baseline radiographs may be useful in managing intercurrent disease, it is recommended that chest radiographs be done, even in the absence of symptoms, every 2 to 5 years. Pulmonary function tests and possibly lung biopsy may be indicated if the chest radiograph suggests fibrosis.

The best approach to chronic pulmonary toxicity of anticancer therapy is a preventive one, with careful monitoring of pulmonary function tests and chest radiographs before and during bleomycin or radiation therapy; respecting cumulative dosage restrictions on bleomycin administration; and limiting radiation dosage and port sizes.

GASTROINTESTINAL FUNCTION

Fibrosis and enteritis are the most common pathologic abnormalities of the gastrointestinal tract in long-term survivors of cancer. These can arise as late complications of radiation to any site from the esophagus to the rectum[228–233] and have been associated with adhesions or stricture formation, sometimes with obstruction, with ulcers, and with malabsorption syndromes.[228,232] Their frequency depends on the radiation dosage delivered by external beam or by internal implants (as in patients with cervical or uterine carcinoma). The stomach and small intestine appear to be more radiation sensitive than the colon or rectum. Overall, there is a 5% incidence of fibrosis after 4000 to 5000 cGy and an incidence as high as 36% after 6000 cGy or more. Most complications of intestinal fibrosis arise within 5 years, but there have been reports of strictures developing as long as 20 years after therapy.[228,233] Once they occur, radiation-induced gastrointestinal strictures may be progressive or recurrent. The incidence of clinically significant problems is enhanced by radiomimetic chemotherapy[229] or abdominal surgery.[228,233] These modalities by themselves can cause a similar array of problems.

Fibrosis also is widely mentioned with respect to the liver. Unfortunately, although much information is available about the acute hepatotoxicities of anticancer therapy, there are few data concerning the incidence either of fibrosis–cirrhosis or hepatitis in long-term survivors. The Late Effects Study Group identified "liver disease" in only one of 110 patients with childhood ALL and in one of 15 with Wilms' tumor.[2] However, the true incidence of subclinical hepatic pathology undoubtedly is higher because the presence of cirrhosis is seldom reflected by abnormal liver function tests or hepatomegaly,[234] because hypertransaminasemia may be asymptomatic, and because liver biopsies or liver scans are not routinely done after therapy.

Radiation given in now-obsolete doses is one cause of chronic hepatic fibrosis, notably in patients treated for Wilms' tumor or abdominal neuroblastoma. The degree of damage increases with the volume irradiated, prior partial hepatectomy, concomitant use of dactinomycin, the presence of large intra-abdominal masses compressing the liver or hepatic venous system, and, possibly, younger age.[235–237] There also has been a statistically insignificant trend toward increasing damage (both clinically appreciable and asymptomatic) with increasing dosage between 1200 and 5800 cGy.[235] It is of note that in one series of 99 patient evaluated within 6 months of radiation and again an average of 47 months after radiation, 36 who were thought to be normal during the acute phase by physical examination (liver function testing and liver scans with or without biopsy) developed abnormalities.[235]

Methotrexate also has been implicated as a cause of chronic hepatopathy. In several early prospective studies of patients given the drug for ALL or psoriasis, the incidence of biopsy-proven hepatic fibrosis was as high as 80% after 2½ to 5 years of low-dose daily oral methotrexate.[238,239] With intermediate doses of intravenous methotrexate, the incidence of fibrosis has been below 5%.[240] In general, and apparently in contrast to what is seen after radiation therapy, methotrexate-related hepatic fibrosis stabilizes or resolves after discontinuation of the drug.[234] The contribution of other acute hepatotoxins (for example, 6-mercaptopurine) to chronic liver disease has not been evaluated.

Other late effects involving the gastrointestinal tract are postsurgical blind loop syndromes and transfusion-related hepatitis. Radiation- or chemotherapy-related veno-occlusive disease, usually fatal but sometimes transient, has persisted in a few cases.[241] Secondary malignancies will be discussed in another section.

Because significant hepatitis or cirrhosis with their attendant risks of liver failure or hepatic tumors may be impossible to detect without liver biopsy, it is difficult to suggest foolproof guidelines for long-term follow-up. We monitor patients during physical examination for hepatomegaly, icterus, and malabsorption. For those patients who had acute hepatotoxicity during therapy and for patients treated with hepatectomy, methotrexate, or hepatic radiation (or right-sided abdominal radiation as used in some Wilms' tumor patients), we consider a chemistry screen including transaminase and bilirubin levels every 2 to 5 years to be cost effective. If persistent, abnormalities are further evaluated in collaboration with a gastroenterologist. Given the trend toward lower doses of hepatic radiation, shorter courses of oral methotrexate, and the relatively infrequent development of end-stage liver disease with current anticancer regimens, we do not advocate routine liver scans or biopsies.

A number of newer approaches to the treatment of gastrointestinal malignancy, including both administration of radiolabeled monoclonal antibodies for the therapy of hepatomas and intrahepatic arterial chemotherapy, have not yet been examined with respect to possible delayed effects. Chronic gastrointestinal manifestations of GVH disease or total-body irradiation also remain to be documented.

URINARY TRACT

Both the upper and lower urinary tracts are sites of late effects of anticancer therapy. The clinical presentation of chronic nephritis in this setting is the same as that in other settings and may include fatigue, anemia, nocturia, hyposthenuria, edema, abnormal urinary sediment, salt wasting, hyperuricemia with or without gout, hypertension, and progressive renal failure. Intermittent or persistent proteinuria[242] or renovascular hypertension[243] may be isolated findings or may evolve into chronic renal failure.

Radiation in doses exceeding 2300 cGy given over 4 to 5 weeks is a well-defined cause of chronic nephritis most commonly reported in patients with soft-tissue sarcomas of the abdomen and pelvis; primary tumors of the kidney, adrenal or gastrointestinal tract; or abdominal lymphomas. It may have its onset months to as long as 13 years after therapy and may occur *de novo* or following acute nephrotoxicity.[242,244,245] Although direct radiation nephrotoxicity is the usual cause, a recent report suggests that radiation may cause retroperitoneal fibrosis with ureteral obstruction.[244]

Chemotherapy—dactinomycin,[246] anthracyclines,[247] azacytidine,[247] methotrexate,[248] the nitrosoureas,[249] and cisplatin[250,251]—either enhance the effects of radiation (earlier onset, lower threshold dose) or themselves cause renal failure. Renal failure secondary to chemotherapy generally represents persistence of an acute toxicity and does not develop in patients who had no problems during or shortly after therapy. Cisplatin renal toxicity, which occurs in 50% to 75% of patients, appears to depend on the duration of treatment and the dose: it has not as a rule been seen at total doses below 50 mg/m² per course. Reversibility has been reported in some series, although in several studies in which cisplatin was given as 20 mg/m² per day for 5 days every 3 weeks, a decrease in creatinine clearance of as much as 40% persisted at least 2 to 4 years.[252,253] These decreases may or may not be accompanied by parallel increases in serum creatinine levels. Long-term tubular defects (for example, hypomagnesemia) do not appear to be a problem.[252] Factors that may encourage kidney failure include nephrotoxic antimicrobial agents,[245] such as aminoglycosides, vancomycin, or amphotericin; inadequate alkalinization of the urine prior to methotrexate administration; ectopic kidneys, which may sustain inadvertent radiation damage; retroperitoneal radiation fibrosis with hydronephrosis; secondary urinary tract infections; and renovascular stenosis. Nephrectomy, notably in children with Wilms' tumor, while not itself a problem, may amplify any subsequent injury to the remaining kidney.

Cystitis, the development of which has been epidemiologically linked to a variety of viruses,[254] also is seen following radiation. Doses to the bladder below 4000 cGy have resulted in a 5% incidence of hemorrhagic cystitis, a figure that is increased with distal urinary tract obstruction, infection, or the concurrent use of radiomimetic agents. Cyclophosphamide by itself has been associated with an incidence of hemorrhagic cystitis of about 10%, with occasional cases occurring several decades after therapy.[255,256] With ifosfamide, a cyclophosphamide analogue, the incidence has been as high as 45%.[257] Presumably, these figures have been reduced by the use of prophylactic measures such as vigorous hydration and diuresis, mesna, and less use of long-term oral cyclophosphamide. (see Chap. 9).

Thrombotic thrombocytopenic purpura, a poorly understood multisystem disease in which the kidneys are a primary target, has preceded institution of chemotherapy in adults with carcinomas.[258] Recently, the condition was described after use of mithramycin[259] or the combination of cisplatin, bleomycin, and vinca alkaloids.[260] Although an acute toxicity, usually occurring within 6 months of chemotherapy, it can lead to chronic renal failure and therefore is a potential problem in long-term survivors.

Other systemic late effects related to the urinary tract include hyperammonemic encephalopathy[261] and hyperchloremic metabolic acidosis,[262] both of which have been described as rare complications of ureteral diversion.

Monitoring long-term survivors at risk for urologic toxicity on the basis of their having received any of the above therapies is straightforward. It should include questioning the patient for the signs and symptoms of chronic renal failure listed in this section, as well as for symptoms of hypertension or urinary tract infections; measurement of blood pressure, serum urea nitrogen, and creatinine levels; and urinalysis. Measurement of creatinine clearance or glomerular filtration, which are more sensitive than simple urea nitrogen and creatinine measurements, can be implemented if the level of suspicion is particularly high. Because urologic toxicity is not likely to develop in the absence of acute toxicity after chemotherapy alone, we feel it is reasonable, under this circumstance, for a patient to undergo this type of evaluation on a single occasion within several months of completion of therapy. For patients also treated with radiation, evaluation yearly or every other year may be indicated.

Prevention of hemorrhagic cystitis has been mentioned earlier. Hydration and diuresis with hypertonic saline or mannitol as well as slower infusions may all reduce cisplatin-induced renal toxicity. Management of patients who have hemorrhagic cystitis is usually supportive with simple hydration for mild cystitis. For more severe disease, cystoscopy with fulguration of bleeding points, intravesical infusions of formalin, or ureteral diversion may be necessary.

HEMATOLOGIC AND IMMUNOLOGIC FUNCTION

The long-term hematologic sequelae of anticancer therapy include compromised immune function and decreased bone-marrow reserve. One of the best-defined alterations in immune function is the impaired humoral immunity that follows splenectomy. Splenectomy has been associated with overall decreases in serum levels of IgM and IgA[263] as well as with reductions in specific opsonins. In a literature review of 403 children with Hodgkin's disease who had undergone splenectomy as part of a staging laparotomy, 32, or 7.9%, developed fulminant infections, generally with encapsulated organisms;[264] 16 of these died. Patients were as long as 3 years from diagnosis at the time of their infection, confirming already-abundant evidence that the risk of sepsis persists. Splenic atrophy with similar consequences has been reported following splenic irradiation (approximately 4000 cGy) of Hodgkin's disease and non-Hodgkin's lymphoma.[265] More recent experience suggests that pneumococcal vaccination and the use of prophylactic penicillin for indefinite periods diminishes that risk in survivors of Hodgkin's disease.[266]

Decreases in serum levels of IgM and specific anti-*H. influenzae* capsular antigen also have been seen in patients with Hodgkin's disease as late as 7 years after therapy with MOPP.[267] This effect may be potentiated by total-nodal irradiation, although in the absence of a splenic port, total-nodal irradiation does not chronically impair antibody production.

Impairment of cell-mediated immunity, as indicated by decreased numbers of peripheral T cells[268] and severely decreased *in vitro* protein synthesis in response to phytohemagglutinin, also has followed total-nodal irradiation in patients with Hodgkin's disease. This may present as late as 8 years after therapy.[269] This defect, which is greater in patients with more advanced disease, may in part reflect pretreatment abnormalities[269] rather than result entirely from therapy. Total-body irradiation (1000 cGy) also impairs cell-mediated immunity, and incomplete T-cell reconstitution has been reported as long as 4 years after marrow transplantation (1000 cGy). Quantitative and functional abnormalities, including decreases in OKT4 and increases in OKT8 cells with inversion of OKT4/OKT8 ratios and depression of *in vitro* responsiveness to mitogens, may be more pronounced after allogeneic than autologous transplantation.[270]

When irradiation has involved smaller nodal or marrow fields, long-term effects on the immune system have been variable. In patients with gynecologic malignancy, no significant abnormalities either of humoral or cellular immunity have been noted several years from diagnosis.[271] On the other hand, 4 to 15 years after radiation for localized laryngopharyngeal malignancy, depressed numbers of peripheral T cells and phy-

tohemagglutinin reactivity have been noted.[272] Similar results have been reported after radiation for carcinoma of the breast.[273]

In addition to its effect on lymphocytes, irradiation may compromise other bone marrow lineages in long-term survivors. Long-term marrow suppression after 3000 cGy or more has been demonstrated by hypoplastic or aplastic aspirates and diminished uptake of radioisotopes with an affinity for active marrow,[274–277] by decreased granulocyte increments in response to endotoxins,[278] and, less commonly, by peripheral cytopenia. The degree of marrow damage and therefore the clinical consequences depend on the dosage used and the volume irradiated: with 4000 cGy of total-nodal irradiation, peripheral granulocyte counts and bone marrow reserve can be impaired as long as 7 years after therapy.[199,278] After 4000 to 5000 cGy in 4 to 6 weeks, complete recovery of marrow function may take more than 2 years.[276] After 850 to 1000 cGy of single-dose total-body irradiation and marrow transplantation for a variety of hematologic abnormalities, about 25% of patients have had platelet counts below 100,000 per mm[3] even after 4 months.[279] Thrombopenia in this setting appears to correlate with the presence of GVH disease. Whether this will be a problem for long-term survivors is not clear. Concomitant chemotherapy may increase the degree of radiation-induced marrow damage.[36,276]

The chronic effects of chemotherapy on bone marrow function have not been exhaustively evaluated despite the well-documented short-term effects. However, it is clear that chemotherapy instituted as long as 3 years after radiation in patients with Hodgkin's disease[280] or methotrexate given as much as 18 months after craniospinal radiation in patients with ALL[281] may result in long-term excessive myelosuppression. Biologic response modifiers, whose therapeutic efficacy presumably relies on altering host immune function, cause acute immunohematologic changes. Their long-term effects are seldom an issue, as patients are usually near death at the time of therapy. Anemia secondary to chemotherapy-related chronic renal failure or hypothyroidism is in general only a theoretical possibility.

Monitoring long-term survivors for immunohematologic dysfunction is most conveniently done by a detailed history and physical examination for signs and symptoms of recurrent infection, anemia, or bleeding diathesis. Peripheral cytopenia is useful, but, as indicated above, an abnormal complete blood count is not a sensitive marker of compromised bone-marrow reserve. The approach to prevention or prophylactic management of immune compromise has been most aggressively pursued in patients with Hodgkin's disease, in whom lifelong use of prophylactic antibiotics and single or serial injections of pneumococcal vaccine have already changed the natural history of postsplenectomy sepsis (see Chap. 39). In patients younger than 6 years at the time of splenectomy, the current recommendations are that *H. influenzae* vaccination be given as well. A trend in some institutions away from staging laparotomy, the use of partial rather than total splenectomy, and reduced reliance on larger doses of extensive radiation should eliminate some of these problems. How newer regimens of more intensive but shorter courses of chemotherapy will affect immune and marrow function is as yet unclear.

SECOND MALIGNANT NEOPLASMS

Individuals with a history of childhood cancer have been estimated to have 10 to 20 times the lifetime risk of a second cancer compared with age-matched controls.[282] Although the lifetime incidence of second malignancies has not yet been defined, within the first 20 years after the initial diagnosis, it is on the order of 3% to 12%.[282-284] However, these figures, as well as the types of second malignancy, differ considerably according to the original diagnosis, patient age, specifics of therapy, and presence of genetic conditions. Patients with Hodgkin's disease, multiple myeloma, ovarian cancer, retinoblastoma, or the genetic form of Wilms' tumor; patients treated with kilovoltage radiotherapy or alkylating agents; and patients with von Recklinghausen's neurofibromatosis xeroderma pigmentosum, Klinefelter's disease, or immunodeficiency syndromes are among those at particularly high risk.

Hodgkin's disease appears to be the most common tumor to precede both hematologic and a range of nonhematologic secondary malignancies (see also Chap. 21). Acute nonlymphocytic leukemia has been reported in approximately 3% to 7% of patients given total-lymphoid irradiation in combination with mechlorethamine or cyclophosphamide, and vincristine or vinblastine, and prednisone and procarbazine (*i.e.,* MOPP, COPP, MVPP) 3 months to 21 years (median 5.5 years) after the initial diagnosis.[285-293] The relative causative role of these two modalities is unclear. Data from some[286,288,289] but not all[290,291] series suggest that after radiation alone, the risk of secondary acute nonlymphocytic leukemia is slight and that MOPP alone carries the same risk as MOPP plus radiation. The alkylating agents mechlorethamine and cyclophosphamide have been singled out as the likely leukemogens.[292] In contrast, among patients treated with total-lymphoid irradiation and ABVD, acute nonlymphocytic leukemia has been infrequent.[293,294] To date, both ALL and chronic myelogenous leukemia have been reported in patients with Hodgkin's disease,[295] but the incidence does not appear to exceed that expected on the basis of chance. The occurrence of non-Hodgkin's lymphoma, with a 1% incidence at 12 years,[296] also may reflect random association rather than carcinogenicity of the therapy.

Nonhematologic tumors after Hodgkin's disease are more convincingly associated with radiation therapy, with two-thirds occurring within radiation ports.[285] These tumors, principally bone and soft-tissue sarcomas and skin and thyroid carcinomas, appear after a median latency of 9.5 to 12 years with an actuarial incidence of 5.8% at 12 years. Unlike the risk of secondary leukemias, which seems to plateau by 10 years, the risk of nonhematologic malignancy may increase over time.[286,287]

After nonhematologic primaries, radiation therapy also appears to be the therapeutic modality most often associated with secondary solid tumors. As reported by the Late Effects Study Group,[2] as well as by the Intergroup Rhabdomyosarcoma Study I-III,[297] osteosarcoma and chondroblastic sarcoma, soft-tissue sarcomas, and thyroid carcinoma account for most radiation-related second malignancies. Carcinomas of the skin and breast also are seen more often after radiation therapy. Malignant tumors following nonhematologic primary tumors appear to be associated with radiation therapy in a dose-dependent manner,[298] although the incidence may be less after megavoltage than orthovoltage therapy.[299] Benign tumors, notably osteochondromas, also occur in irradiated fields and have been most carefully looked for in survivors of Wilms' tumor.[35,41] Their malignant potential has not been defined.

As is the case after Hodgkin's disease, secondary hematopoietic malignancies after nonlymphoid primaries are more likely to be related to exposure to chemotherapy. In survivors of ovarian,[300] lung,[301] gastrointestinal,[302] and germ cell[303] malignancies or of multiple myeloma[304] who were treated with alkylating agents, the incidence of acute nonlymphocytic leukemia has been 5% to 20%. Carcinogenicity of other chemotherapy is not strongly suggested by available data. Indeed,

dactinomycin, despite its potentiation of radiation with respect to other toxicities, appears to diminish the risk of radiation-associated second malignancies.[305]

In the large number of long-term survivors of ALL, the incidence of second malignancies appears to be relatively low, on the order of 62 per 100,000 patients per year compared with 280 per 100,000 for Hodgkin's disease.[282] In the Late Effects Study Group's compilation, the most common malignancies were other leukemias and non-Hodgkin's lymphoma. A 2.3% incidence of brain tumors within 10 years of diagnosis also has been reported.[306] Among 468 long-term survivors, four gliomas, four astrocytomas, and one ependymoma occurred after therapy that included 2400 cGy of cranial radiation for central nervous system prophylaxis.[306] The etiology of these second malignancies is unclear. It has been suggested that the development of central nervous system and hematologic malignancies in the same patient may not be a function of therapy but rather may reflect a genetic connection between these two cancer types similar to that between retinoblastoma and osteosarcoma (see Chaps. 25 and 32).[284,307] In other settings, a clear relation between lower doses of radiation (less than several hundred cGy) and the development of carcinomas of the salivary and thyroid glands has been demonstrated.[308] After therapy for ALL with cranial radiation, where the estimated dose delivered to the thyroid may be as much as 7.5% of the total,[161] there have been a small number of cases of thyroid cancer and a similar number of adenomas.[309-313]

Surgery plays a much more limited role in the development of second malignancies. However, the occurrence of benign and malignant colonic tumors at the anastomosis site of ureterosigmoidostomies at 500 times the expected rate deserves mention.[314] Although surgical debulking of Wilms' tumor and soft-tissue sarcomas has been supplanted by preoperative chemotherapy, there are still many adults and some survivors of pediatric cancers with long-established ureterosigmoidostomies who are at risk for colonic neoplasia. The average latency until the discovery of these cancers has been 26 years. A recent observation is the association between splenectomy and the development of secondary acute myeloid leukemia in patients who have been treated with MOPP for Hodgkin's disease.[315]

In assessing these statistics, it is worth remembering, as has been pointed out by others,[285] that the mean latency for solid tumors after radiation therapy is more than 15 years and that it is still too early to expect the common adult cancers to appear in survivors of childhood cancer, even if their incidence ultimately will be increased. Moreover, for newer therapeutic approaches—including total-body irradiation and intensive chemotherapy as used in bone marrow transplantation and monoclonal antibody-directed radiation—insufficient time has elapsed to determine the carcinogenic potential. We therefore stress to our patients their need for lifelong surveillance for secondary malignancies. The signs and symptoms of these tumors are the same as for malignancies occurring *de novo* and will not be detailed here. We do obtain yearly complete blood counts, but not bone marrow aspirates, in patients at risk for secondary hematologic malignancy. The relative merits of routine radiographic evaluation of bones or soft tissues encompassed by radiation therapy ports have been discussed in an earlier section.

SURVEILLANCE

Recognition of what delayed consequences can emerge after cancer therapy is one aspect of the study of late effects. Another, more practical, aspect is the actual tracking of patients in order to monitor their status, offer counseling, and treat problems as they arise. This is usually done through each institution's tumor registry in the form of an annual letter or phone contact. However, to avoid the pitfalls of long-distance interactions, many centers have organized follow-up clinics where patients can be interviewed and examined in some detail. A typical interim history designed to focus on significant medical problems and problems of psychosocial readjustment, school and job performance, and insurance is summarized in Table 50-2. Table 50-1 summarizes the late effects that should be looked for in patients who have received particular forms of chemotherapy, radiation, or surgery. A complete physical examination looking for these late effects is routine. As noted in the pertinent chapter sections, because of the delayed onset or potentially progressive nature of some of these problems, such evaluations will often bear repetition yearly or every other year. Recommendations for laboratory tests are individualized according to what problems the physician should anticipate based on the patient's disease and, especially, on therapeutic history. These have been discussed and are summarized in Table 50-3.

REFERENCES

1. Young JL, Ries LG, Silverberg E, Horm JW, Miller RW: Cancer incidence, survival, and mortality for children younger than 15 years. Cancer 58:598–602, 1986
2. Meadows AT, Krejmas NL, Belasco JB: The medical cost of cure: sequelae in survivors of childhood cancer. In Van Eys J, Sullivan MP (eds): Status of the Curability of Childhood Cancers, pp 263–276. New York, Raven Press, 1980
3. Meadows AT, Hobbie W, Jarrett P et al: Disabilities in long-term survivors of childhood cancer: Results of a systematic follow-up program (abstract). Proc Am Soc Clin Oncol 5:211, 1986
4. Bamford FN, Morris-Jones P, Pearson D et al: Residual disabilities in children treated for intracranial space occupying lesions. Cancer 37:1149–1151, 1976
5. Danoff BF, Cowchock FS, Marquette C, Mulgrew L, Kramer S: Assessment of the long-term effects of primary radiation therapy for brain tumors in children. Cancer 49:1580–1586, 1982
6. Onoyama Y, Mitsuyuki A, Takahashi M, Yabumoto E, Sakamoto T: Radiation therapy of brain tumors in children. Radiology 115:687–693, 1977
7. Shalet SM, Beardwell CG, Morris-Jones PH et al: Growth hormone deficiency in children with brain tumors. Cancer 37:1144–1148, 1976
8. Shalet SM, Beardwell CG, Pearson D, Morris-Jones PH, MacFarlane IA: Endocrine morbidity in adults treated with cerebral irradiation for brain tumors during childhood. Acta Endocrinol 84:673–680, 1977
9. Oberfield SE, Allen JC, Pollack J, New MI, Levine LS: Long-term endocrine sequelae after treatment of medulloblastoma: Prospective study of growth and thyroid function. J Pediatr 108:219–223, 1986
10. Oliff A, Bode U, Bercu BB et al: Hypothalamic–pituitary dysfunction following CNS prophylaxis in acute lymphocytic leukemia: Correlation with CT scan abnormalities. Med Pediatr Oncol 7:141–151, 1979
11. Robison LL, Nesbit ME, Sather HN et al: Height of children successfully treated for acute lymphoblastic leukemia: A report from the late effects study committee of children's cancer study group. Med Pediatr Oncol 13:14–21, 1985
12. Bajorunas DR, Chavimi F, Jereb B, Sonenberg M: Endocrine sequelae of antineoplastic therapy in childhood and head and neck malignancies. J Clin Endocrinol Metab 50:329–335, 1980
13. Richards GE, Wara WM, Grumbach MM et al: Delayed onset of hypopituitarism: Sequelae of therapeutic irradiation of central nervous system, eye, and middle ear tumors. J Pediatr 89:553–559, 1976
14. Komp D, El-Mahdi A, Starling K et al: Quality of survival in histiocytosis X (abstract). Pediatr Res 10:455, 1976
15. Braunstein GD, Kohler PO: Endocrine manifestations of histiocytosis. Am J Pediatr Hematol Oncol 3:68–75, 1981
16. Samaan NA, Vieto R, Schultz PN: Hypothalamic, pituitary and thyroid dysfunction after radiotherapy to the head and neck. Int J Radiat Oncol Biol Phys 8:1857–1867, 1982
17. Perry-Keene DA, Connelly JF, Young RA, Wettenhall HNB, Martin FIR: Hypothalamic hypopituitarism following external radiotherapy for tumors distant from the adenohypophysis. Clin Endocrinol 5:373–380, 1976
18. Wells RJ, Foster MB, D'Ercole AJ, McMillan CW: The impact of cranial irradiation on the growth of children with acute lymphocytic leukemia. Am J Dis Child 137:37–39, 1983
19. Berry DH, Elders MJ, Crist W et al: Growth in children with acute lymphocytic leukemia: A Pediatric Oncology Group study. Med Pediatr Oncol 11:39–45, 1983
20. Shalet SM, Price DA, Beardwell CG, Morris-Jones PH, Pearson D: Normal growth despite abnormalities of growth hormone secretion in children treated for acute leukemia. J Pediatr 94:719–722, 1979
21. Verzosa MS, Aur RJA, Simone JV, Hustu HO, Pinkel DP: Five years after central nervous system irradiation of children with leukemia. Int J Radiat Oncol Biol Phys 1:209–215, 1976
22. Hakimi N, Mohammad A, Mayer JW: Growth and growth hormone of children with acute lymphocytic leukemia following central nervous system prophylaxis with and without cranial radiation. Am J Pediatr Hematol Oncol 2:311–316, 1980
23. Starceski PJ, Lee PA, Blatt J, Finegold D, Brown D: Comparable effects of 1800 and 2400 rad cranial irradiation on height and weight in children treated for acute lymphocytic leukemia. Am J Dis Child 141:550–552, 1987
24. Blatt J, Bercu BB, Gillin JC, Mendelson WB, Poplack DG: Reduced pulsatile growth hormone secretion in children after therapy for acute lymphoblastic leukemia. J Pediatr 104:182–186, 1984
25. Romshe CA, Zipf WB, Miser A et al: Evaluation of growth hormone release and human growth hormone treatment in children with cranial irradiation-associated short stature. J Pediatr 104:177–181, 1984
26. Dacou-Voutetakis C, Xypolyta A, Haidas St Constantinidis M, Papavasiliou C, Zannos-Mariolea L: Irradiation of the head: Immediate effect on growth hormone secretion in children. J Clin Endocrinol Metab 44:791–794, 1977
27. Shalet SM, Beardwell CG, Morris-Jones PH, Pearson D: Growth hormone deficiency after treatment of acute leukaemia in children. Arch Dis Child 51:489–493, 1976
28. Swift PGF, Kearney PJ, Dalton RG et al: Growth and hormonal status of children treated for acute lymphoblastic leukaemia. Arch Dis Child 53:890–894, 1978
29. Griffin NK, Wadsworth J: Effect of treatment of malignant disease on growth in children. Arch Dis Child 55:600–603, 1980
30. Dickinson WP, Berry H, Dickinson L et al: Differential effects of cranial radiation on growth hormone response to arginine and insulin infusion. J Pediatr 92:754–757, 1978
31. Moëll C, Westgren U, Aronson S, Wiebe T, Landberg T: Height, weight, and growth hormone secretion in children treated for acute leukemia. Eur J Pediatr Hematol Oncol 1:167–172, 1984
32. Bloom HJ, Wallace EN, Henk JM: The treatment and prognosis of medulloblastoma in children: A study of 82 verified cases. Am J Roentgenol 105:43–62, 1969
33. Dawson WB: Growth impairment following radiotherapy in childhood. Clin Radiol 19:241–256, 1968
34. Probert JC, Parker BR: The effects of radiation therapy on bone growth. Radiology 114:155–162, 1975
35. Thomas PRM, Griffith KD, Fineberg BB, Perez CA, Land VJ: Late effects of treatment for Wilms' tumor. Int J Radiat Oncol Biol Phys 9:651–657, 1983
36. Parker RG, Berry HC: Late effects of therapeutic irradiation on the skeleton and bone marrow. Cancer 37:1162–1171, 1976
37. Deeg HJ, Storb R, Thomas ED: Bone marrow transplantation: A review of delayed complications. Br J Haematol 57:185–208, 1984
38. Mahoney P, Amos D, Buckner CD et al: Growth and development following marrow transplantation for leukemia. Blood 68:1129–1135, 1986
39. Sainsbury CPQ, Newcombe RG, Hughes IA: Weight gain and height velocity during prolonged first remission for acute lymphoblastic leukemia. Arch Dis Child 60:832–836, 1985
40. Winter RJ, Green OC: Irradiation-induced growth hormone deficiency: Blunted growth response and accelerated skeletal maturation to growth hormone therapy. J Pediatr 106:609–612, 1985
41. Heaston DK, Libshitz HI, Chan RC: Skeletal effects of megavoltage irradiation in survivors of Wilms' tumor. AJR 113:389–395, 1979
42. Tefft M, Lattin PB, Jereb B et al: Acute and late effects on normal tissue following combined chemo- and radiotherapy for childhood rhabdomyosarcoma and Ewing's sarcoma. Cancer 37:1201–1213, 1976
43. Ihde DC, DeVita VT: Osteonecrosis of the femoral head in patients with

lymphoma treated with intermittent combination chemotherapy (including corticosteroids). Cancer 36:1585–1588, 1975

44. Timothy AR, Tucker AK: Osteonecrosis in Hodgkin's disease. Br J Radiol 51:328–332, 1978
45. Libshitz HI, Edeiken BS: Radiotherapy changes of the pediatric hip. AJR 137:585–588, 1981
46. Felix C, Blatt J, Goodman MA, Medina J: Avascular necrosis of bone following combination chemotherapy for acute lymphocytic leukemia. Med Pediatr Oncol 13:269–272, 1985
47. Prindull G, Weigel W, Jentsh E, Enderle A, Willert HG: Aseptic osteonecrosis in children treated for acute lymphoblastic leukemia and aplastic anemia. Eur J Pediatr 139:48–51, 1982
48. Sty JR, Babbitt DP, Boedecker RA: Bone scintigraphy: Methotrexate associated bone necrosis. Wis Med J 78:32–33, 1979
49. Obrist R, Hartmann D, Obrecht JP: Osteonecrosis after chemotherapy. Lancet 1:1316, 1978
50. Nesbit M, Krivit W, Heyn R, Sharp H: Acute and chronic effects of methotrexate on hepatic, biliary, and skeletal systems. Cancer 37:1048–1054, 1976
51. Riseborough EJ, Grabias SL, Burton RI, Jaffe N: Skeletal alterations following irradiation for Wilms' tumor. J Bone Joint Surg [Am] 58:526–536, 1976
52. Jaffe N, Toth BB, Hoar RE et al: Dental and maxillofacial abnormalities in long term survivors of childhood cancer: Effects of treatment with chemotherapy and radiation to the head and neck. Pediatrics 73:816–823, 1984
53. Holmes GE, Holmes FF: After 10 years, what are the handicaps and lifestyles of children treated for cancer? Clin Paediatr 14:819–823, 1975
54. Li FP, Stone R: Survivors of cancer in childhood. Ann Intern Med 84:551–553, 1976
55. Kun LE, Mulhern RK, Crisco JJ: Quality of life in children treated for brain tumors: Intellectual, emotional, and academic function. J Neurosurg 58:1–6, 1986
56. Li FP, Winston KR, Gimbrere K: Follow-up of children with brain tumors. Cancer 54:135–138, 1984
57. Duffner PK, Cohen ME, Thomas PM: Late effects of treatment on the intelligence of children with posterior fossa tumors. Cancer 51:233–237, 1983
58. Deutsch M: Radiotherapy for 10 primary brain tumors in very young children. Cancer 50:2785–2789, 1982
59. McIntosh S, Klatskin EH, O'Brien RT et al: Chronic neurologic disturbance in childhood leukemia. Cancer 37:853–857, 1976
60. Meadows AT, Evans AE: Effects of chemotherapy on the central nervous system. Cancer 37:1079–1085, 1976
61. Raimondi AJ, Tomita T: The disadvantages of prophylactic whole CNS post-operative radiation therapy for medulloblastoma. In Paolitti P, Walker MD, Butti G, Knerick R (eds): Multidisciplinary Aspects of Brain Tumor Therapy, pp 209–218. New York, Elsevier/North Holland, 1979
62. Hirsch JF, Pierre-Kahn A, Benveniste L, George B: Les medulloblastomes de l'enfant: Survie et résultats fonctionnels. Neurochirurgie 24:391–397, 1978
63. Tamaroff M, Miller DR, Murphy ML et al: Immediate and long-term post-therapy neuropsychologic performance in children with acute lymphoblastic leukemia treated without central nervous system radiation. J Pediatr 101:524–529, 1982
64. Moss HA, Nannis ED, Poplack DG: The effects of prophylactic treatment of the central nervous system on the intellectual functioning of children with acute lymphocytic leukemia. Am J Med 71:47–52, 1981
65. Goff JR, Anderson HR Jr, Cooper PF: Distractibility and memory deficits in long-term survivors of acute lymphoblastic leukemia. J Dev Behav Pediatr 1:158–163, 1980
66. Meadows AT, Gordon J, Massari DJ et al: Declines in IQ scores and cognitive dysfunctions in children with acute lymphocytic leukaemia treated with cranial irradiation. Lancet 2:1015–1018, 1981
67. Copeland DR, Fletcher JM, Pfefferbaum-Levine B et al: Neuropsychological sequelae of childhood cancer in long-term survivors. Pediatrics 75:745–753, 1985
68. Rowland JH, Glidewell OJ, Sibley RF et al: Effects of different forms of central nervous system prophylaxis on neuropsychologic function in childhood leukemia. J Clin Oncol 2:1327–1335, 1984
69. Robison LL, Nesbit ME Jr, Sather HN et al: Factors associated with IQ scores in long-term survivors of childhood acute lymphoblastic leukemia. Am J Pediatr Hematol Oncol 6:115–121, 1984
70. Eiser C, Lansdown R: Retrospective study of intellectual development in children treated for lymphoblastic leukemia. Arch Dis Child 52:525–529, 1977
71. Tamaroff M, Salwen R, Miller DR, Murphy ML, Nir Y: Comparison of neuropsychologic performance in children treated for acute lymphoblastic leukemia with 1800 rads cranial radiation plus intrathecal methotrexate or intrathecal methotrexate alone (abstract). Proc Am Soc Clin Oncol 3:198, 1984
72. Bleyer WA, Griffin TW: White matter necrosis, mineralizing microangiopathy, and intellectual abilities in survivors of childhood leukemia; associations with central nervous system irradiation and methotrexate therapy. In Gilbert HA, Kagan AR (eds): Radiation Damage to the Nervous System, pp 115–174. New York, Raven Press, 1980
73. Priest JR, Ramsay NKC, Latchaw RR et al: Thrombotic and hemorrhagic strokes complicating early therapy for childhood acute lymphoblastic leukemia. Cancer 46:1548–1554, 1980
74. Pizzo P, Poplack DG, Bleyer WA: Neurotoxicities of current leukemia therapy. Am J Pediatr Hematol Oncol 1:127–138, 1979
75. Price RA, Jamieson PA: The central nervous system in childhood leukemia II: Leukoencephalopathy. Cancer 35:306–318, 1975
76. Kay HEM, Knapton PJ, O'Sullivan JP et al: Encephalopathy in acute leukemia associated with methotrexate therapy. Arch Dis Child 47:344–354, 1972
77. Atkinson K, Clink H, Lawler S et al: Encephalopathy following bone marrow transplantation. Eur J Cancer 13:623–625, 1977
78. Johnson FL, Thomas ED, Clark BS et al: A comparison of marrow transplantation to chemotherapy for children with acute lymphoblastic leukemia in second or subsequent remission. N Engl J Med 305:846–851, 1981
79. Obetz SW, Ivnik RJ, Smithson WA et al: Neuropsychologic follow-up study of children with acute lymphocytic leukemia: A preliminary report. Am J Pediatr Hematol Oncol 1:207–213, 1979
80. Fusner JE, Poplack DG, Pizzo PA, DiChiro G: Leukoencephalopathy following chemotherapy for rhabdomyosarcoma: Reversibility of cerebral changes demonstrated by computed tomography. J Pediatr 91:77–79, 1977
81. Brecher ML, Berger P, Freeman AI et al: Computerized tomography scan findings in children with acute lymphocytic leukemia treated with three different methods of central nervous system prophylaxis. Cancer 56:2430–2433, 1985
82. Peylan-Ramu N, Poplack DG, Pizzo PA, Adornato BT, DiChiro G: Abnormal CT scans of the brain in asymptomatic children with acute lymphocytic leukemia after prophylactic treatment of the central nervous system with radiation and intrathecal chemotherapy. N Engl J Med 298:815–819, 1978
83. Riccardi R, Brouwers P, DiChiro G, Poplack DG: Abnormal computed tomography brain scans in children with acute lymphoblastic leukemia: Serial long-term follow-up. J Clin Oncol 3:12–18, 1985
84. Brouwers P, Riccardi R, Poplack DG et al: Attentional deficits in long-term survivors of childhood acute lymphoblastic leukemia. J Clin Neuropsychol 6:325–336, 1984
85. Cheng VST, Schultz MS: Unilateral hypoglossal nerve atrophy as a late complication of radiation therapy of head and neck carcinoma: A report of four cases and a review of the literature on peripheral and cranial nerve damage after radiation therapy. Cancer 35:1537–1544, 1975
86. Berger PS, Batanini JP: Radiation-induced cranial nerve palsy. Cancer 40:152–155, 1977
87. Margileth DA, Poplack DG, Pizzo, PA, Leventhal BD: Blindness during remission in two patients with acute lymphoblastic leukemia. Cancer 39:58–61, 1977
88. Casey EG, Jellife AM, LeQuesne PM, Millett YL: Vincristine neuropathy: Clinical and electrophysiological observations. Brain 96:69–86, 1973
89. Hahn EW, Feingold BS, Simpson L, Batata M: Recovery from aspermia induced by low dose radiation in seminoma patients. Cancer 50:337–340, 1982
90. Clifton DK, Bremner WJ: The effect of testicular x-irradiation on spermatogenesis in man. J Androl 4:387–392, 1983
91. Rowley MM, Leach DR, Warner GA, Heller CG: Effect of graded doses of ionizing radiation on the human testes. Radiat Res 59:665–678, 1974
92. Speiser B, Rubin P, Casarett G: Aspermia following lower truncal irradiation in Hodgkin's disease. Cancer 32:692–698, 1973
93. Shamberger RC, Sherins RJ, Rosenberg SA: The effects of postoperative adjuvant chemotherapy and radiotherapy on testicular function in men undergoing treatment for soft tissue sarcoma. Cancer 47:2368–2374, 1981
94. Shalet SM, Beardwell CG, Jacobs HS, Pearson D: Testicular function following irradiation of the human prepubertal testes. Clin Endocrinol 9:483–490, 1978
95. Green DM, Brecher ML, Lindsay AN et al: Gonadal function in pediatric patients following treatment of Hodgkin's disease. Pediatr Oncol 9:235–244, 1981

96. Blatt J, Sherins RJ, Niebrugge D, Bleyer WA, Poplack DG: Leydig cell function in boys following treatment for testicular relapse of acute lymphoblastic leukemia. J Clin Oncol 3:1227–1231, 1985

97. Brauner R, Czernichow P, Cramer P, Schaison G, Rappaport R: Leydig-cell function in children after direct testicular irradiation for acute lymphoblastic leukemia. N Engl J Med 309:25–28, 1983

98. Leiper AD, Grant DB, Chessells JM: The effect of testicular irradiation on Leydig cell function in prepubertal boys with acute lymphoblastic leukemia. Arch Dis Child 58:906–910, 1983

99. Shalet SM, Horner A, Ahmed SR, Morris–Jones PH: Leydig cell damage after testicular irradiation for lymphoblastic leukaemia. Med Pediatr Oncol 13:65–68, 1985

100. Blatt J, Poplack DG, Sherins RJ: Testicular function in boys after chemotherapy for acute lymphoblastic leukemia. N Engl J Med 304:1121–1124, 1981

101. Ahmed SR, Shalet SM, Campbell RHA, Deakin DP: Primary gonadal damage following treatment of brain tumors in childhood. J Pediatr 103:562–565, 1983

102. Brauner R, Czernichow P, Rappaport R: Precocious puberty after hypothalamic and pituitary irradiation in young children. N Engl J Med 311:920, 1984

103. Schilsky RL, Sherins RJ: Gonadal dysfunction. In DeVita VT Jr, Hillman S, Rosenberg SA (eds): Cancer: Principles and Practice of Oncology. Philadelphia, JB Lippincott, 1982 pp 1713–1719

104. Richter P, Calamera JC, Morgenfeld MC et al: Effect of chlorambucil on spermatogenesis in the human with malignant lymphoma. Cancer 25:1026–1030, 1970

105. Cheviakoff S, Calamera JC, Morgenfeld M, Mancini RE: Recovery of spermatogenesis in patients with lymphoma after treatment with chlorambucil. J Reprod Fertil 33:155–157, 1973

106. Sherins RJ, DeVita VT: Effect of drug treatment for lymphoma on male reproductive capacity. Ann Intern Med 79:216–220, 1973

107. Sherins RJ, Olweny CLM, Ziegler JL: Gynecomastia and gonadal dysfunction in adolescent boys treated with combination chemotherapy for Hodgkin's disease. N Engl J Med 299:12–16, 1978

108. Whitehead E, Shalet SM, Morris–Jones PH, Beardwell CG, Deakin DP: Gonadal function after combination chemotherapy for Hodgkin's disease in childhood. Arch Dis Child 57:287–291, 1982

109. Chapman RM, Rees LH, Sutcliffe SB, Edwards CRW, Malpas JS: Cyclical combination chemotherapy and gonadal function. Lancet 1:285–289, 1979

110. da Cunha MF, Meistrich ML, Fuller LM et al: Recovery of spermatogenesis after treatment for Hodgkin's disease with limiting dose of MOPP chemotherapy. J Clin Oncol 2:571–577, 1984

111. Santoro A, Viviani S, Pagnoni AM et al: Long-term therapeutic and toxicologic results of MOPP–radiation–MOPP versus ABVD–radiation–ABVD in PS2B-3 (A, B) Hodgkin's disease (abstract). Proc Am Soc Clin Oncol 4:199, 1985

112. Lendon M, Palmer MK, Hann IM, Shalet SM, Morris–Jones PH: Testicular histology after combination chemotherapy in childhood for acute lymphoblastic leukaemia. Lancet 2:439–441, 1978

113. Sanders JE, Buckner CD, Leonard JM et al: Late effects on gonadal function of cyclophosphamide, total body irradiation, and marrow transplantation. Transplantation 36:252–255, 1983

114. Chapman RM, Sutcliffe SB, Malpas JS: Male gonadal dysfunction in Hodgkin's disease: A prospective study. JAMA 245:1323–1328, 1981

115. Trump DL, Anderson SA: Painful gynecomastia following cytotoxic therapy for testicular cancer: A potentially favorable prognostic sign. J Clin Oncol 1:416–420, 1983

116. Shamberger RC, Rosenberg SA, Seipp CA, Sherins RJ: Effects of high-dose methotrexate and vincristine on ovarian and testicular function in patients undergoing postoperative adjuvant treatment for osteosarcoma. Cancer Treat Rep 65:739–746, 1981

117. Lawrence W, Hays DM, Moon TE: Lymphatic metastasis in childhood rhabdomyosarcoma. Cancer 39:556–559, 1977

118. Thomsett MJ, Conte FA, Kaplan SL, Gumbuark MM: Endocrine and neurologic outcome in childhood craniopharyngioma: Review of effect of treatment on 42 patients. J Pediatr 97:728–735, 1980

119. Duffey P, Campbell EW, Wiernik PH: Hydrocele following treatment for Hodgkin's disease. Cancer 50:305–307, 1982

120. Scammell GE, White N, Stedionska J et al: Cryopreservation of semen in men with testicular tumors or Hodgkin's disease: Results of artificial insemination of their partners. Lancet 1:31–32, 1985

121. Bracken RB, Smith KD: Is semen cryopreservation helpful in testicular cancer? Urology 15:581–585, 1980

122. Chlebowski RT, Heber D: Hypogonadism in male patients with metastatic cancer prior to chemotherapy. Cancer Res 42:2495–2498, 1982

123. Thachil JV, Jewett MAS, Rider WD: The effects of cancer and cancer therapy on male fertility. J Urol 126:141–145, 1981

124. Vigersky RA, Chapman RM, Berenberg J, Glass AR: Testicular dysfunction in untreated Hodgkin's disease. Am J Med 73:482–486, 1982

125. Nichols CR, Hoffman R, Einhorn LH et al: Hematologic malignancies associated with primary mediastinal germ cell tumors. Ann Intern Med 102:603–609, 1985

126. Lushbaugh CC, Casarett GW: The effects of gonadal irradiation in clinical radiation therapy: A review. Cancer 37:1111–1120, 1976

127. Stillman RJ, Schinfeld JS, Schiff I et al: Ovarian failure in long-term survivors of childhood malignancy. Am J Obstet Gynecol 139:62–66, 1981

128. Horning SJ, Hoppe RT, Kaplan HS, Rosenberg SA: Female reproductive potential after treatment for Hodgkin's disease. N Engl J Med 304:1377–1382, 1981

129. Thomas PRM, Winstanly D, Peckham MJ et al: Reproductive and endocrine function in patients with Hodgkin's disease: Effects of oophoropexy and irradiation. Br J Cancer 33:226–231, 1976

130. Hamre MR, Robison LL, Nesbit ME et al: Gonadal function in survivors of childhood acute lymphoblastic leukemia: A report from the Late Effects Study Committee of Children's Cancer Study Group (abstract). Proc Am Soc Clin Oncol 4:166, 1985

131. Rose DP, Davis TE: Ovarian function in patients receiving adjuvant chemotherapy for breast cancer. Lancet 1:1174–1176, 1977

132. Koyama H, Wada T, Nishizawa Y et al: Cyclophosphamide-induced ovarian failure and its therapeutic significance in patients with breast cancer. Cancer 39:1403–1409, 1977

133. Fisher B, Sherman B, Rockette H et al: L-phenylalanine mustard in the management of premenopausal patients with primary breast cancer. Cancer 44:847–857, 1979

134. Siris ES, Leventhal BG, Vaitukaitis JL: Effects of childhood leukemia and chemotherapy on puberty and reproductive function in girls. N Engl J Med 294:1143–1146, 1976

135. Chapman RM, Sutcliffe SB, Malpas JS: Cytotoxic-induced ovarian failure in women with Hodgkin's disease. JAMA 242:1877–1884, 1979

136. Himelstein–Braw R, Peters H, Faber M: Influence of irradiation and chemotherapy on the ovaries of children with abdominal tumours. Br J Cancer 36:269–275, 1977

137. Morris Jones PH, Beardwell CG, Deakin DP: Gonadal function after combination chemotherapy for Hodgkin's disease in childhood. Arch Dis Child 47:287–291, 1982

138. Nicosia SV, Matus–Ridley M, Meadows AT: Gonadal effects of cancer therapy in girls. Cancer 55:2364–2372, 1985

139. Chapman RM, Sutcliffe SB: Protection of ovarian function by oral contraceptives in woman receiving chemotherapy for Hodgkin's disease. Blood 58:849–851, 1981

140. Briggs GG, Freeman RK, Yaffe SJ: In Drugs in Pregnancy and Lactation, 2nd ed, p 537. Baltimore, Williams & Wilkins, 1986

141. McKeen EA, Mulvihill JJ, Rosner F, Zarrabi MH: Pregnancy outcome in Hodgkin's disease. Lancet 2:590, 1979

142. Olsson H, Brandt L: Sex ratio in offspring of patients with non-Hodgkin's lymphoma. N Engl J Med 306:367–368, 1982

143. Blatt J, Mulvihill JJ, Ziegler JL, Young RC, Poplack DG: Pregnancy outcome following cancer chemotherapy. Am J Med 69:828–832, 1980

144. Li FP, Fine W, Jaffe N, Holmes GE, Holmes FF: Offspring of patients treated for cancer in childhood. JNCI 62:1193–1197, 1979

145. Li FP, Jaffe N: Progeny of childhood cancer survivors. Lancet 2:704–714, 1974

146. Holmes GE, Holmes FF: Pregnancy outcome of patients treated for Hodgkin's disease. Cancer 41:1317–1322, 1978

147. Li FP, Gimbrere K, Gelber RD et al: Adverse pregnancy outcome after radiation therapy for childhood Wilms' tumor (abstract). Proc Am Soc Clin Oncol 5:202, 1986

148. Rubin CM, Robison LL, Nesbit ME, Arthur DC: Cytogenetic studies of long-term survivors of childhood acute lymphoblastic leukemia: A follow-up report. Med Pediatr Oncol 14:295–299, 1986

149. Mulvihill JJ, Myers MH, Connelly RR et al: Cancer in offspring of long-term survivors of childhood and adolescent cancer (abstract). Proc Am Soc Clin Oncol 5:216, 1986

150. Meadows AT: Second malignant neoplasms. Clin Oncol 4:247–257, 1985

151. Kaplan MM, Garnick MB, Gelber R et al: Risk factors for thyroid abnormalities after neck irradiation for childhood cancer. Am J Med 74:272–280, 1983

152. Shalet SM, Rosenstock JD, Beardwell CG, Pearson D, Morris–Jones PH: Thyroid dysfunction following external irradiation to the neck for Hodgkin's disease in childhood. Clin Radiol 28:511–515, 1977

153. Schimpff SC, Diggs CH, Wiswell JG, Salvatore PC, Wiernik PH: Radiation-related thyroid dysfunction: Implications for the treatment of Hodgkin's disease. Ann Intern Med 92:91–98, 1980

154. Glatstein E, McHardy–Young S, Brast N, Eltringham JR, Kriss JP: Alterations in serum thyrotropin (TSH) and thyroid function following radiotherapy in patients with malignant lymphoma. J Clin Endocrinol Metab 32:833–841, 1971

155. Fuks Z, Glatstein E, Marsa GW, Gabshaw MA, Kaplan HS: Long-term effects of external radiation on the pituitary and thyroid glands. Cancer 35:1152–1161, 1976

156. Devney RB, Sklar CA, Nesbit ME Jr et al: Serial thyroid function measurements in children with Hodgkin's disease. J Pediatr 105:223–227, 1984

157. Poussin–Rosillo H, Nisce LZ, Lee BJ: Complications of total nodal irradiation of Hodgkin's disease stages III and IV. Cancer 42:437–441, 1978

158. Rosenthal MB, Goldfine ID: Primary and secondary hypothyroidism in nasopharyngeal carcinoma. JAMA 236:1591–1593, 1976

159. Murken RE, Duvall AJV: Hypothyroidism following combined therapy in carcinoma of the laryngopharynx. Laryngoscope 82:1306–1314, 1972

160. Robison LL, Nesbit ME, Sather HN et al: Evaluation of a cohort of long-term survivors of childhood acute lymphoblastic leukemia (ALL) treated on Children's Cancer Study Group (CCSG) protocols. Presented at the Late Effects Conference, Houston, Texas, April 11–12, 1985

161. Rogers PC, Fryer CJ, Hussein S: Radiation dose to the thyroid in the treatment of acute lymphoblastic leukemia (ALL). Med Pediatr Oncol 10:385–388, 1982

162. Garnick MB, Larsen PR: Acute deficiency of thyroxine-binding globulin during L-asparaginase therapy. N Engl J Med 101:252, 1979

163. Heidemann PH, Stubbe P, Beck W: Transient secondary hypothyroidism and thyroxine binding globulin deficiency in leukemic children during polychemotherapy: An effect of L-asparaginase. Eur J Pediatr 136:291–295, 1981

164. Jackson R, Rosenberg C, Kleinmann R, Vagenalsis AG, Braverman LE: Ophthalmopathy following neck irradiation for Hodgkin's disease. Cancer Treat Rep 63:1393–1395, 1979

165. Wasnich RD, Grumet CF, Payne RO, Kriss JP: Grave's ophthalmopathy following external neck irradiation for nonthyroidal neoplastic disease. J Clin Endocrinol Metab 37:703–713, 1973

166. Bristow MR, Mason JW, Billingham ME, Daniels JR: Doxorubicin cardiomyopathy: Evaluation by phonocardiograph, endomyocardial biopsy, and cardiac catheterization. Ann Intern Med 88:168–175, 1978

167. Prout MN, Richards MJS, Chung KJ, Joo P, Davis HL: Adriamycin cardiotoxicity in children. Cancer 39:62–65, 1977

168. Von Hoff DD, Layard MW, Basa P et al: Risk factors for Adriamycin-induced congestive heart failure. Ann Intern Med 91:710–717, 1979

169. Minow RA, Benjamin RS, Gottlieb JA: Adriamycin (NSC-123127) cardiomyopathy: An overview with determination of risk factors. Cancer Chemother Rep 6:195–201, 1975

170. Cortes EP, Lutman G, Wanka J et al: Adriamycin (NSC 123127) cardiotoxicity: A clinicopathologic correlation. Cancer Chemother Rep 6:215–225, 1975

171. Billingham ME, Mason JW, Bristow MR, Daniels JR: Anthracycline cardiomyopathy monitored by morphologic changes. Cancer Treat Rep 62:865–872, 1978

172. Gilladoga AC, Manuel C, Tan CTC et al: The cardiotoxicity of Adriamycin and daunomycin in children. Cancer 37:1070–1078, 1976

173. Kushner JR, Hansen VL, Hammar SP: Cardiomyopathy after widely separated courses of Adriamycin exacerbated by actinomycin D and mithramycin. Cancer 36:1577–1584, 1975

174. Smith PJ, Eckert H, Waters KD, Matthews RN: High incidence of cardiomyopathy in children treated with Adriamycin and DTIC in combination chemotherapy. Cancer Treat Rep 61:1736–1738, 1977

175. Von Hoff DD, Rozencweig M, Piccart M: The cardiotoxicity of anticancer agents. Semin Oncol 9:23–33, 1982

176. Pratt CB, Ransom JL, Evans WE: Age-related Adriamycin cardiotoxicity in children. Cancer Treat Rep 62:1381–1384, 1978

177. Von Hoff DD, Rozencweig M, Layard M, Slavik M, Muggio FM: Daunomycin induced cardiotoxicity in children and adults. Am J Med 62:200–208, 1977

178. Weiss AJ, Manthel RW: Experience with the use of Adriamycin in combination with other anticancer agents using a weekly schedule with particular reference to lack of cardiac toxicity. Cancer 40:2046–2052, 1977

179. Legha SS, Benjamin RS, Mackay B et al: Reduction of doxorubicin cardiotoxicity by prolonged continuous intravenous infusion. Ann Intern Med 96:133–139, 1982

180. Martin RG, Rukdeschel JC, Chang P et al: Radiation-related pericarditis. Am J Cardiol 35:216–220, 1975

181. Marks RD Jr, Agarwal SK, Constable WC: Radiation induced pericarditis in Hodgkin's disease. Acta Radiol Ther Phys Biol 12:305–312, 1973

182. Applefeld MM, Wiernik PH: Cardiac disease after radiation therapy for Hodgkin's disease: Analysis of 48 patients. Am J Cardiol 51:1679–1681, 1983

183. Gottdiener JS, Katin MJ, Borer JS, Bacharach SL, Green MV: Late cardiac effects of therapeutic mediastinal irradiation assessment by echocardiography and radionuclide angiography. N Engl J Med 308:569–572, 1983

184. Ruckdeschel JC, Chang P, Martin RG et al: Radiation related pericardial effusions in patients with Hodgkin's disease. Medicine 54:245–259, 1975

185. Mill WB, Baglan RJ, Kurichetz P et al: Symptomatic radiation induced pericarditis in Hodgkin's disease. Int J Radiat Oncol Biol Phys 10:2061–2065, 1984

186. Kadota RP, Burgert EO, Driscoll DJ, Evans RG, Gilchrist GS: Cardiopulmonary function in long-term survivors of childhood Hodgkin's lymphoma: A pilot study. Proc Am Soc Clin Oncol 5:198, 1986

187. Perrault DJ, Levy M, Herman JD et al: Echocardiographic abnormalities following cardiac radiation. J Clin Oncol 3:546–551, 1985

188. Scott DL, Thomas RD: Late onset constrictive pericarditis after thoracic radiotherapy. Br Med J 1:341–342, 1978

189. Haas JM: Symptomatic constrictive pericarditis developing 45 years after radiation therapy to the mediastinum: A review of radiation pericarditis. Am Heart J 77:89–95, 1969

190. Silverberg GD, Britt RH, Goffinet DR: Radiation-induced carotid artery disease. Cancer 41:130–137, 1975

191. McReynolds RA, Gold GL, Roberts UC: Coronary heart disease after irradiation for Hodgkin's disease. Ann Intern Med 60:39–45, 1976

192. Miller DD, Waters DP, Dangoisse V, David P: Symptomatic coronary artery spasm following radiotherapy for Hodgkin's disease. Chest 83:284, 1984

193. Yahalom J, Hasin Y, Fuks Z: Acute myocardial infarction with normal coronary arteriogram after mantle field radiation therapy for Hodgkin's disease. Cancer 52:637–641, 1983

194. Boivin JF, Hutchison GB: Coronary heart disease mortality after irradiation for Hodgkin's disease. Cancer 49:2470–2475, 1982

195. Saulov ED, Nahhas WA, Mag AG: Iliac and femoral arteriosclerosis following pelvic irradiation for carcinoma of the ovary. Obstet Gynecol 34:345–351, 1969

196. Nylander G, Pettersson F, Swedenborg J: Localized arterial occlusions in patients treated with pelvic field radiation for cancer. Cancer 41:2158–2161, 1978

197. Burns BJ, Bar-Shlomo B, Druck MN et al: Detection of radiation cardiomyopathy by gated radionuclide angiography. Am J Med 74:297–302, 1983

198. Gross NJ: Pulmonary effects of radiation therapy. Ann Intern Med 86:81–92, 1977

199. Slanina J, Mussoff K, Rhaner T, Stiasny R: Long-term side effects of irradiated patients with Hodgkin's disease. Int J Radiat Oncol Biol Phys 2:1–19, 1977

200. Wara WM, Phillips TL, Margolis LW, Smith V: Radiation pneumonitis: A new approach to the derivation of time–dose factors. Cancer 32:547–552, 1973

201. White DDC: The histopathologic basis for functional decrements in late radiation injury in diverse organs. Cancer 37:1126–1143, 1976

202. Libshitz HI, Southard ME: Complications of radiation therapy. Semin Roentgenol 9:41–49, 1974

203. Wohl ME, Griscom NT, Traggis DG, Jaffe N: Effects of therapeutic irradiation delivered in early childhood upon subsequent lung function. Pediatrics 55:507–514, 1975

204. Littman P, Meadows AT, Polgar G, Borns PF, Rubin E: Pulmonary function in survivors of Wilms' tumor: Patterns of impairment. Cancer 37:2773–2776, 1976

205. Benoist MR, Lemerle J, Jean R et al: Effects on pulmonary function of whole lung irradiation for Wilms' tumour in children. Thorax 37:175–180, 1982

206. Miller RW, Fusner JE, Fink RJ et al: Pulmonary function abnormalities in long-term survivors of childhood cancer. Med Pediatr Oncol 14:202–207, 1986

207. Springmeyer SC, Flournay N, Sullivan KM, Storb R, Thomas ED: Pulmonary function changes in long-term survivors of allogeneic marrow transplantation. In Gale RP (ed): Recent Advances in Bone Marrow Transplantation, pp 343–353. New York, Alan R Liss, 1983

208. Eigen H, Wyszomierski D: Bleomycin lung injury in children: Pathophysiology and guidelines for management. Am J Pediatr Hematol Oncol 7:71–78, 1985

209. Ginsberg SJ, Comis RL: The pulmonary toxicity of antineoplastic agents. Semin Oncol 9:34–51, 1982

210. Yagoda A, Mukherji B, Young C et al: Bleomycin, an antitumor antibiotic: Clinical experience in 274 patients. Ann Intern Med 77:861–870, 1972

211. Comis RL: Bleomycin pulmonary toxicity. In Carter SK, Crooke ST, Umezawa H (eds): Bleomycin: Current Status and New Developments, pp 279–291. New York, Academic Press, 1978

212. Einhorn L, Krause M, Hornback N, Furnas B: Enhanced pulmonary toxicity with bleomycin and radiotherapy in oat cell lung cancer. Cancer 37:2414–2416, 1976

213. Samuels ML, Johnson DE, Holoye PY, Lanzotti VJ: Large-dose bleomycin therapy and pulmonary toxicity: A possible role of prior radiotherapy. JAMA 235:1117–1120, 1976

214. Coltman CA, Luce JK, McKelvey EM, Jones SE, Moon TE: Chemotherapy of non-Hodgkin's lymphoma: 10 years experience in the Southwest Oncology Group. Cancer Treat Rep 61:1067–1078, 1977

215. Bauer KA, Skarin AT, Balikian JP et al: Pulmonary complications associated with combination chemotherapy programs containing bleomycin. Am J Med 74:557–563, 1983

216. Goldiner PL, Schweizer O: The hazards of anaesthesia and surgery in bleomycin-treated patients. Semin Oncol 6:121–124, 1979

217. Germon PA, Brady LW: Physiologic changes before and after radiation treatment for carcinoma of the lung. JAMA 206:809–814, 1968

218. Lucraft HH, Wilkinson PM, Stretton TB, Read G: Role of pulmonary function tests in the prevention of bleomycin pulmonary toxicity during chemotherapy for metastatic testicular teratoma. Eur J Cancer Clin Oncol 18:133–139, 1982

219. Bailey CC, Marsden HB, Morris–Jones PH: Fatal pulmonary fibrosis following 1,3-bis(2-chlorethyl)-1-nitrosourea (BCNU) therapy. Cancer 42:74–76, 1978

220. Aronin PA, Mahaley MS Jr, Rudnick SA et al: Prediction of BCNU pulmonary toxicity in patients with malignant gliomas: An assessment of risk factors. N Engl J Med 303:183–188, 1980

221. Alvarado CS, Boat TF, Newman AJ: Late-onset pulmonary fibrosis and chest deformity in two children treated with cyclophosphamide. J Pediatr 92:443–446, 1978

222. Codling BW, Chakera TM: Pulmonary fibrosis following therapy with melphalan for multiple myeloma. J Clin Pathol 25:668–676, 1972

223. Oliner H, Fords R, Rubio F, Dameschek W: Interstitial pulmonary fibrosis following busulfan therapy. Am J Med 31:134–139, 1961

224. Konits PH, Aisner J, Sutherland JC, Wiernik PH: Possible pulmonary toxicity secondary to vinblastine. Cancer 50:2771–2774, 1982

225. Kamen BA: Pulmonary toxicity from methotrexate. Methotrexate Update 4:23–26, 1986

226. Gutin PH, Green MR, Bleyer WA et al: Methotrexate pneumonitis induced by intrathecal methotrexate therapy: A case report with pharmacokinetic data. Cancer 38:1529–1534, 1976

227. Komp DM: Long-term sequelae of histiocytosis X. Am J Pediatr Hematol Oncol 3:165–168, 1981

228. Roswit B: Complications of radiation therapy: The alimentary tract. Semin Roentgenol 9:115–131, 1974

229. Donaldson SS, Jundi S, Ricour C et al: Radiation enteritis in children: A retrospective review, clinco-pathologic correlation, and dietary management. Cancer 35:1167–1178, 1975

230. Requarth W, Roberts S: Intestinal injuries following irradiation of pelvic viscera for malignancy. Arch Surg 73:682–687, 1956

231. Ehinger DS, Slavin RE: Chronic radiation enteritits complicating non-Hodgkin's lymphoma. South Med J 70:960–961, 1977

232. Wellwood JM, Jackson BT: The intestinal complications of radiotherapy. Br J Surg 60:814–818, 1973

233. Localio SA, Stone A, Friedman M: Surgical aspects of radiation enteritis. Surg Gynecol Obstet 129:302–307, 1969

234. Dahl MGC, Gregory MM, Schever PJ: Liver damage due to methotrexate in patients with psoriasis. Br Med J 1:625–630, 1971

235. Tefft M, Mitus A, Das L et al: Irradiation of the liver in children: Review of experience in the acute and chronic phases and in the intact normal and partially resected. Am J Roentgen 108:365–385, 1970

236. D'Angio GJ, Farber S, Maddock CL: Potentiation of x-ray effects by actinomycin D. Radiology 73:175–177, 1959

237. Philips TL: Chemical modifications of radiation effect. Cancer 39:987–999, 1977

238. Hutter RVP, Shipkey FH, Tan CTC, Muraty ML, Chowdhury M: Hepatic fibrosis in children with acute leukemia: A complication of therapy. Cancer 13:288–307, 1960

239. Sharp H, Nesbit M, White J, Krivit W: Methotrexate liver toxicity. J Pediatr 74:818, 1969

240. McIntosh S, Davidson DL, O'Brien RT, Pearson HA: Methotrexate hepatotoxicity in children with leukemia. J Pediatr 90:1019–1021, 1977

241. Johnson FL, Balis FM: Hepatopathy following radiation and chemotherapy for Wilms' tumor. Am J Pediatr Hematol Oncol 4:217–221, 1983

242. Van Slyck EJ, Bermudez GO: Radiation nephritis. Yale J Biol Med 41:243–256, 1968

243. Shapiro AP, Cavallo T, Cooper W et al: Hypertension in radiation nephritis. Arch Intern Med 137:848–851, 1977

244. Chao N, Levine J, Horning SJ: Retroperitoneal fibrosis following treatment for Hodgkin's disease. J Clin Oncol 5:231–232, 1987

245. Maher JF: Toxic and irradiation nephropathies. In Earley LE, Gottschalk CW (eds): Strauss and Welt's Diseases of the Kidney, 3rd Ed, pp 1431–1472. Boston, Little, Brown, 1979

246. Arneil GC, Emmanuel TC, Flatman GE et al: Nephritis in two children after irradiation and chemotherapy for nephroblastoma. Lancet 1:960–963, 1974

247. Garnick MB, Mayer RJ: Acute renal failure associated with neoplastic disease and its treatment. Semin Oncol 5:155–165, 1978

248. Condit PT, Chanes RE, Joel W: Renal toxicity of methotrexate. Cancer 23:126–131, 1969

249. Schein PS, O'Connell MH, Blom J et al: Clinical antitumor activity and toxicity of streptozotocin (NSC 85998). Cancer 34:993–1,000, 1974

250. Comis RL: Cisplatin nephrotoxicity: The effect of dose, schedule, and hydration schedule. In Prestayko AW, Crooke ST, Carter SK (eds): Cisplatin: Current Status and New Developments, pp 485–494. New York, Academic Press, 1980

251. Blachley JD, Hill JB: Renal and electrolyte disturbances associated with cisplatin. Ann Intern Med 95:628–632, 1981

252. Fjelborg P, Sorensen J, Helkjaer PE: The long-term effect of cisplatin on renal function. Cancer 58:2214–2217, 1986

253. Dentino M, Luft FC, Yum MN, Williams SD, Einhorn LH: Long term effect of cis-diamminedichloride platinum (CDDP) on renal function and structure in man. Cancer 41:1274–1281, 1978

254. Arthur RR, Shah KV, Baust SJ, Santos GW, Saral R: Association of BK viruia with hemorrhagic cystitis in recipients of bone marrow transplants. N Engl J Med 315:230–234, 1986

255. Lawrence HJ, Simone J, Aur RJA: Cyclophosphamide-induced hemorrhagic cystitis in children with leukemia. Cancer 36:1572–1576, 1975

256. Johnson WW, Meadows DC: Urinary-bladder fibrosis and telangiectasia associated with long-term cyclophosphamide therapy. N Engl J Med 284:290–294, 1971

257. Klein HO, Wickramanayake P Dias, Coerper C et al: High dose ifosfamide and mesna as continuous infusion over 5 days—a phase I/II trial. Cancer Treat Rev 10A:167–173, 1983

258. Laffay DL, Tubbs RR, Valenzuela MD, Hall PM, McCormack LJ: Chronic glomerular microangiopathy and metastatic carcinoma. Hum Pathol 10:433–438, 1979

259. Jackson AM, Rose BD, Graff LG et al: Thrombotic microangiopathy and renal failure associated with antineoplastic chemotherapy. Ann Intern Med 101:41–44, 1984

260. Harrell RM, Sibley R, Vogelzang NJ: Renal vascular lesions after chemotherapy with vinblastine, bleomycin, and cisplatin. Am J Med 73:429–433, 1982

261. Kaufman JJ: Ammonogenic coma following ureterosigmoidostomy. J Urol 131:743–745, 1984

262. Zincke H, Segura SW: Ureterosigmoidostomy: Critical review of 173 cases. J Urol 113:324–327, 1975

263. Hancock BW, Bruce L, Ward AM, Richmond J: Changes in immune status in patients undergoing splenectomy for the staging of Hodgkin's disease. Br Med J 1:313–315, 1976

264. Lanzkowsky P, Shende A, Karayalcin G, Aral I: Staging laparotomy and splenectomy: Treatment and complications of Hodgkin's disease in children. Am J Hematol 1:393–404, 1976

265. Dailey MO, Coleman CN, Kaplan HS: Radiation-induced splenic atrophy in patients with Hodgkin's disease and non-Hodgkin's lymphomas. N Engl J Med 302:215–217, 1980

266. Hays DM, Ternberg JL, Chen TT et al: Complications related to 234 staging laparotomies performed in the Intergroup Hodgkin's Disease in Childhood Study. Surgery 96:471–478, 1984

267. Weitzman SA, Aisenberg AC, Siber GR, Smith DH: Impaired humoral immunity in treated Hodgkin's disease. N Engl J Med 297:245–248, 1977

268. Fuks Z, Strober S, Bobrove AM et al: Long-term effects of radiation on T and

B lymphocytes in peripheral blood of patients with Hodgkin's disease. J Clin Invest 58:803–814, 1976

269. Levy R, Kaplan HS: Impaired lymphocyte function in untreated Hodgkin's disease. N Engl J Med 290:181–186, 1974

270. Ueda M, Harada M, Shiobara S et al: T lymphocyte reconstitution in long-term survivors after allogeneic and autologous marrow transplantation. Transplantation 37:552–556, 1984

271. Halili M, Bosworth J, Romney S, Moukhtar M, Ghossein NA: The long-term effect of radiotherapy on the immune status of patients cured of a gynecologic malignancy. Cancer 37:3875–3878, 1976

272. Tarpley JL, Potvin C, Chretien PB: Prolonged depression of cellular immunity in cured laryngopharyngeal cancer patients treated with radiation therapy. Cancer 35:638–644, 1975

273. Stjernsward J, Jondal M, Vanky F, Wigzell H, Sealy R: Lymphopenia and change in distribution of human B and T lymphocytes in peripheral blood induced by irradiation for mammary carcinoma. Lancet 1:1352–1356, 1972

274. Sykes MP, Sauel H, Chu FC et al: Long-term effects of therapeutic irradiation upon bone marrow. Cancer 17:1144–1148, 1964

275. Goswitz FA, Andrews GA, Kniseley RM: Effects of local irradiation Co⁶⁰ teletherapy on the peripheral blood and bone marrow. Blood 21:605–619, 1963

276. Rubin P, Landman S, Mayer E, Keller B, Ciccio S: Bone marrow regeneration after extended field irradiation in Hodgkin's disease. Cancer 32:699–711, 1973

277. Kjellgren O, Jonsson L: Bone marrow depression in the pelvis after megavoltage irradiation for ovarian cancer. Am J Obstet Gynecol 105:849–855, 1969

278. Vogel JM, Kimball HR, Foley HT, Wolff SM, Perry S: Effect of extensive radiotherapy on the marrow granulocyte reserves of patients with Hodgkin's disease. Cancer 21:798–804, 1968

279. First LR, Smith BR, Lipton J et al: Isolated thrombocytopenia after allogeneic bone marrow transplantation: Existence of transient or chronic thrombocytopenia syndromes. Blood 65:368–374, 1985

280. Curran RE, Johnson RB: Tolerance to chemotherapy after prior irradiation for Hodgkin's disease. Ann Intern Med 72:505–509, 1970

281. McLennan ICM, Ray HEM, Festenstein M, Smith PG: Analysis of treatments in childhood leukemia I: Predisposition to methotrexate-induced neutropenia after craniospinal irradiation. Br Med J 1:563–566, 1975

282. Mike V, Meadows AT, D'Angio GJ: Incidence of second malignant neoplasms in children: Results of an international study. Lancet 2:1326–1331, 1982

283. Li FP: Second malignant tumors after cancer in childhood. Cancer 40:1899–1902, 1977

284. Meadows AT, D'Angio GJ, Mike V et al: Patterns of second malignant neoplasms in children. Cancer 40:1903–1911, 1977

285. Meadows AT, Baum E, Fossati–Bellani F et al: Second malignant neoplasms in children: An update from the Late Effects Study Group. J Clin Oncol 3:532–538, 1985

286. Coleman CN, Williams CJ, Flint A et al: Hematologic neoplasia in patients treated for Hodgkin's disease. N Engl J Med 297:1249–1252, 1977

287. Meadows AT, Silber J: Delayed consequences of therapy for childhood cancer. CA 35:271–284, 1985

288. Coltman CA, Dixon DO: Second malignancies complicating Hodgkin's disease: A Southwest Oncology Group 10-year follow-up. Cancer Treat Rep 66:1023–1033, 1982

289. Baccarani M, Bosi A, Papa G: Second malignancy in patients treated for Hodgkin's disease. Cancer 46:1735–1740, 1980

290. Arseneau JC, Sponzo RW, Levin DL et al: Nonlymphomatous malignant tumors complicating Hodgkin's disease. N Engl J Med 287:1119–1148, 1972

291. Nelson DF, Coopers S, Weston MG, Rubin P: Second malignant neoplasms in patients treated for Hodgkin's disease with radiotherapy or radiotherapy and chemotherapy. Cancer 48:2386–2393, 1981

292. Coleman CN: Secondary malignancies after treatment of Hodgkin's disease: An evolving picture. J Clin Oncol 4:821–824, 1986

293. Valagussa P, Santoro A, Fossati–Bellani F, Banfi A, Bonadonna F: Second acute leukemia and other malignancies following treatment for Hodgkin's disease. J Clin Oncol 4:830–837, 1986

294. Amadori S, Papa G, Anselmo AP, Mondelli F: Acute promyelocytic leukemia following ABVD and radiotherapy for Hodgkin's disease. Cancer Treat Rep 67:603, 1983

295. Rosner F, Grunwald H: Hodgkin's disease and acute leukemia: A report of eight cases and review of the literature. Am J Med 58:339–353, 1975

296. Krikorian JG, Burke JS, Rosenberg SA et al: Occurrence of non-Hodgkin's lymphoma after therapy for Hodgkin's disease: A study of 21 patients. N Engl J Med 300:452–458, 1979

297. Heyn R, Newton WA, Ragab A et al: Second malignant neoplasms in patients treated on the intergroup rhabdomyosarcoma study I–II (abstract). Proc Assoc Soc Clin Oncol 5:215, 1986

298. Tucker MA, Meadows AT, Boice JD et al: Bone cancer linked to radiotherapy and chemotherapy in children (abstract). Proc Am Soc Clin Oncol 4:239, 1985

299. Hazelow RE, Nesbit M, Dehner LP: Second neoplasms following megavoltage radiation in a pediatric population. Cancer 42:1185–1191, 1978

300. Greene MH, Boice JD, Greer BE, Blessing JA, Dembo AJ: Acute nonlymphocytic leukemia after therapy with alkylating agents for ovarian cancer: A study of five randomized clinical trials. N Engl J Med 307:1416–1421, 1982

301. Rose VL, Kepper MD, Eichner ER, Pitha JV, Murray JL: Acute leukemia after successful chemotherapy for oat cell carcinoma. Am J Clin Pathol 79:122–124, 1983

302. Boice JD, Greene MH, Keehn RJ, Higgins GA, Fraumeni JF: Late effects of low-dose adjuvant chemotherapy in colorectal cancer. J NCI 64:501–511, 1980

303. Redman JR, Vugrin D, Arlin ZA et al: Leukemia following treatment of germ cell tumors in men. J Clin Oncol 2:1080–1086, 1984

304. Wahlin A, Roos G, Rudolphi O, Holm J: Melphalan-related leukemia in multiple myeloma. Acta Med Scand 21:203–208, 1982

305. D'Angio GJ, Meadows A, Mike V et al: Decreased risk of radiation-associated second malignant neoplasms in actinomycin D-treated patients. Cancer 37:1177–1185, 1976

306. Albo V, Miller D, Leiken S, Sather H, Hammond D: Nine brain tumors as a late effect in children "cured" of acute lymphoblastic leukemia from a single protocol study (abstract). Proc Am Soc Clin Oncol 4:172, 1985

307. Farwell J, Flannery JT: Cancer in relatives of children with central nervous system neoplasms. N Engl J Med 311:749–753, 1984

308. Modan B, Baidatz D, Mart H, Steinitz R, Levin SG: Radiation-induced head and neck tumours. Lancet 1:277–279, 1974

309. Tang T, Holcenberg J, Duck S et al: Thyroid carcinoma following treatment for acute lymphoblastic leukemia. Cancer 46:1572–1576, 1980

310. Caulet T, Hibon E, Roth A et al: Sarcome de Kaposi viscéral associé à un carcinome médullaire thyroïdien chez une enfant en très longue rémission de leucémie lymphoblastique. Nouv Presse Med 6:2673–2676, 1977

311. Hosoya R, Eiraku K, Saiki S, Nishimura K: Thyroid carcinoma and acute lymphoblastic leukemia in childhood. Cancer 51:1931–1933, 1983

312. Nesbit M, Robison L, Sather H et al: Evaluation of long-term survivors of childhood acute lymphoblastic leukemia (abstract). Proc Am Assoc Cancer Res 419:107, 1982

313. Ribeiro–Ayeh J: Shilddrusenkarzinom nach Behandlung einer akuten lymphatischen Leukämie. Klin Pädiatr 191:148–151, 1979

314. Lasser A, Acosta AE: Colonic neoplasms complicating ureterosigmoidostomy. Cancer 35:1218–1222, 1975

315. Van Leeuwen FE, Somers R, Hart AAM: Splenectomy in Hodgkin's diesase and second leukaemias. Lancet 2:210–211, 1987

fifty-one

Educational Issues for Children with Cancer

Patricia Deasy-Spinetta and John J. Spinetta

Significant advances in diagnosis, treatment, and patient management have enabled more children to be cured of cancer today than at any other time in history. It is estimated that by 1990, one of every 1000 young adults reaching the age of 20 will be a survivor of childhood cancer.[1] As children live longer with their disease, physicians and parents face the added responsibility of promoting sound academic and social development as the child goes through the treatment process. It is not enough for children simply to survive a life-threatening illness. They must survive as fully functioning, productive members of society. Consequently, the school is now a partner, along with the hospital and the home, in providing the child's total care and cure.

The purpose of this chapter is to discuss the education of the young person with cancer. We offer basic principles of school intervention, review Public Law (PL) 94-142 and its implementation on behalf of the student with cancer, discuss specific school issues impacting on the education of the young person with a malignancy, and offer strategies for intervention on the children's behalf.

PRINCIPLES OF SCHOOL INTERVENTION

No single intervention strategy can be universally applied to all young people with cancer because these children attend school in a variety of settings and have a range of grade and developmental levels, with a wide spectrum of medical involvement. This section offers basic principles of school intervention geared to maximize cooperation and communication among parents, hospital staff, and school personnel. Applications of these principles can then be modified to correspond to the individual and unique characteristics of the young person with cancer, the family, the treatment center, and the school district involved.

Four basic principles underlie school intervention efforts for children with cancer. First, school intervention is an ongoing process. To be fully effective, it must take a proactive, preventive approach and be an integral part of the treatment process and long-term follow-up. Second, children and adolescents should reenter school in the regular classroom as soon after diagnosis as medically possible. Third, care must be taken in choosing the words to discuss children with cancer, because words are keys to attitudes. Accordingly, while in school the child is a *student,* not a patient. The teacher's role is to educate and not to medicate. Finally, because the home, hospital, and school are partners in the total care of the child, each with a unique role and responsibility, it is necessary to define individual roles and to communicate accordingly.

Long-Term Intervention

Long-term school intervention is an ongoing process. There is a growing awareness among parents and health care professionals of intervention strategies to help the newly diagnosed patient.[2,3] However, the educational needs of the young person with cancer encompass far more than reentry issues. School intervention is a dynamic, ongoing process. Communication among the home, school, and hospital is necessary during the entire course of treatment. Progressive medical success in the treatment of pediatric cancer has brought about a shift in the definition of what constitutes care and the amount and types of services required to ensure optimal care. Through the 1960s, care had a single dimension: medical. Beginning in the 1970s, physicians became aware of the need for psychological intervention to help the patient and family cope with both the treatment and its psychological sequelae. Pediatric oncology social workers, psychologists, play therapists, and other psychology-related professionals were added to the team. Care then took on a two-dimensional approach: medical and psychological.

Today, more children are cured of cancer than at any other time in history. To survive childhood cancer in the 1980s and 1990s means surviving not only medically and psychologically but also educationally and socially. The child must be prepared to eventually become a fully functioning, productive member of society. This is the third dimension, a dimension critical to the child's total cure and one that, along with the medical and the psychological, must be present from diagnosis as part and parcel of the child's total treatment. To be fully effective, long-term intervention must take a proactive, preventive approach rather than a reactive crisis approach. Such intervention must begin at the point of diagnosis for all children, preschool through secondary school age.[4]

School intervention needs to be part of the total treatment program, managed by a skilled professional with a background in education, rather than a service that may or may not be provided, depending on the interest or skill of staff at the medical facility. A school liaison, whose role is to be both an advocate with the parent for the child and a bridge between the medical and educational establishment, is a necessary part of the pediatric hematology/oncology team. That nurses, social workers, physicians, and other health care professionals require specialized preparation to provide care for the young person with cancer is well recognized. An effective school advocate also requires specialized training and preparation. He or she must have a thorough understanding of the educational system and curriculum, as well as special education programs. This person must have the ability to identify resources in the school, both individuals and programs, to benefit the child; to work with teachers and curriculum developers; and to write child-specific educational plans. The school liaison must also understand Public Law 94-142 and the individualized education plan (IEP) process in order to work with parents to ensure that the young person with cancer has the best possible program in the least restrictive environment. The school liaison must assist teachers if and when the child reaches the terminal phase. For children cured of cancer, the liaison must work as a long-term advocate who can help those living with any residual effects of therapy, which impact daily on school life. This responsibility requires specialized training and cannot be undertaken haphazardly.

Early School Reentry

School reentry should take place as soon as medically possible after initial diagnosis. Within the first weeks after diagnosis, parents and children look for new ways of coping with the crisis.[5] If return to school becomes part of the information initially offered by the primary physician, it is then incorporated into the coping repertoire of the family. The question of return to school becomes one of "when" rather than "if." School participation, although complicated by the diagnosis, becomes an expected part of the child's life. The commitment to return to school, supported by the entire health care team, not only means a commitment to the child's academic future but, more fundamentally, symbolizes the team's belief that this child will indeed have a future. The sooner the child returns to the regular school program, the sooner he or she will regain the equilibrium and sense of self that are often lost during the emotional trauma of diagnosis.

Semantics of Intervention

The words we use are the key to our attitudes.[6] Attitudes of the medical staff, teachers, friends, and the individual child may determine success in achieving and maintaining school functioning. Physicians can help prevent problems for the children they treat by communicating more effectively through careful use of words.

While in school, the child is a student and not a patient. It is acceptable and usual for a child with cancer to be referred to as a patient by health care providers. However, when this word is used to describe the child in school or to school personnel, it has another connotation. Schools are geared to educate children. This is their purpose; this is the area in which they function as contributors to the total care of the young person with cancer. By stressing "student" rather than "patient" in letters and other communications with the school, physicians and nurses place the emphasis on function—what the child can and is expected to do—rather than dysfunction—what the child cannot do.

Further, if the child is seen as a student, teachers are better prepared and more comfortable in their role as educators. If the child is referred to as a patient, teachers see themselves as unprepared, untrained quasi-paramedics and find themselves always waiting for a medical emergency.[7] The child, too, picks up the nuances of meaning. As a student, he or she has a responsibility to study and complete assignments just like classmates. As a student, the child with cancer also has the opportunity to socialize and master the developmental tasks of childhood and adolescence that center on school-related activities. If the school continues to be a center of the child's life, it can also be a place free of the concerns and worry of the illness. However, if the child is seen by teachers and classmates as a patient with a life-threatening illness, he or she will sense this at a nonverbal level, and school will be a very uncomfortable, unpleasant environment. The child will then manufacture many legitimate reasons for not attending on a regular basis. Thus, the words used are more than an exercise in semantics. They set the tone for the way people feel and act toward the young person with cancer.

Role Definition

An additional basic principle of school intervention involves role clarification and definition between and among the institutions responsible for the long-term care of the child: the home, the school, and the hospital.

The Home

Parents are ultimately responsible for their child's care in the hospital. They are also the primary long-term advocates for the child in school. Parents set the tone for effective communication with the school.[8] If they are confident in their parenting role and knowledgeable about the child's medical status and treatment plan, and if they communicate accurately and regularly with school personnel, a long-term relationship of trust develops between the home and the school. Once this mutual trust is established, then adjustments necessitated by changes in the child's medical or educational status can be facilitated. If the parents do not communicate and if principals and teachers must depend on hearsay for information, then trust never develops and problems ensue. Parents need support and information at the point of diagnosis to assume this long-term responsibility.

The school liaison, who is knowledgeable about the issues surrounding school reentry, is in a good position to work with parents to facilitate the child's initial return to school after diagnosis. Most parents, regardless of the age of the child, share common concerns: how and what to tell teachers, how to protect their child from teasing by classmates, how to inform school personnel about communicable diseases, and how to deal with a child's initial reluctance. These issues must be addressed in such a way that the parents are educated to handle their new responsibilities and can become effective advocates for their child as the child continues through treatment.

Understandably, some parents are initially reluctant to allow their children to return to school. Ethnic mores may lead some parents to regard the child's return to school as a contradiction of their cultural expectations of caring for a sick child. This reluctance needs to be understood and respected. When parents are themselves overwhelmed by the seriousness of the task they face, the tendency is to protect the child. This protection often leads to keeping the child from participating in the types of activities that, by virtue of the challenges they entail, provide opportunity for growth.[9] These parents need help working through these feelings from the very beginning, so that they can give their children the opportunity to return to school and participate as fully as possible in activities that promote normal growth and development.

Social workers, in their frequent contacts with parents, are in a good position to help parents deal with reluctance to allow the child to return to school. Clinical experience has demonstrated that when other parents—who themselves were initially reluctant to allow their child to go to school—talk with the family of the newly diagnosed child, they are effective in alleviating many fears and apprehensions. Some parents continue to be apprehensive, regardless of the intervention used. It is only when their child actually goes to school and is successful and happy about returning to normal life activities that parental fears abate.

The School

The school is primarily responsible for the education of the child. Although there are legitimate medical issues that must be addressed, the essence of the school's responsibility centers on the delivery of optimal educational services to a student who is undergoing or has undergone treatment for a medical condition. Information transmitted by the physician and parents should be focused on issues for which the school is accountable.

There are those who operate on the premise that before a student returns to school, the teachers, school nurses, and other staff need intensive in-service education on the medical aspects of cancer. That emphasis, although comfortable for the medical practitioners, tends to blind educators to the student's educational needs. Instead of evaluating the student's previous academic record, assessing strengths and weaknesses, initiat-

ing peer group awareness and support, evaluating the impact of absences, and developing an individual educational plan, the focus is shifted to an approach ("You poor child—let me help take care of you—look what you are going through") that is paternalistic and ineffective.

Although there are legitimate medical issues that must be transmitted to school officials, the medical information shared is often excessive, much too general to be informative regarding the child in question, and educationally irrelevant. Given the primary responsibility of the school for the education of the child, what kind of educationally relevant medical information should the health care team share?

The Hospital

Information transmitted to the school must be child specific and education related. Physicians need to evaluate treatment protocols in terms of how the administration of chemotherapy on an outpatient or inpatient basis will affect school attendance. Some protocols require frequent hospitalizations. This has a direct educational implication, in that frequent absences can be anticipated and planned for during the planned duration of the treatment. Chemotherapies must also be evaluated in terms of known side-effects that may impact on school performance or social interaction. Some chemotherapies affect fine and gross motor control; others cause hair loss, fatigue, increased activity, or irritability. Some treatments cause residual long-term neuropsychological effects, as discussed in detail in Chapter 50. These side-effects are real. Teachers made aware of treatment side-effects in this manner can make creative and appropriate adjustments on behalf of the student. Further, when information is presented in this manner, school site personnel become cognizant of the need to involve others —school nurses, curriculum planners, school psychologists, resource specialists, reading specialists, adaptive physical education teachers, and speech and language therapists—to help them develop appropriate child-specific educational programs that will meet the short- and long-term academic, social, and developmental needs of the student. Table 51-1 offers a list of issues to be evaluated by physicians when they communicate with schools. Issues for an individual child change as that child progresses through treatment. Issues that may be paramount for a newly diagnosed child will change as the child progresses through treatment and becomes a long-term survivor.

In brief, modern medical advances and quality medical care make it possible for children to live with cancer. Accordingly, the home, the hospital, and the school must work as a team. Although each has a distinct contribution to make to the child, it is important for each to have an understanding of the role and purpose of the other, as all work together to maximize the child's or adolescent's potential to continue normal growth and development as he or she enters the treatment process. Any weak link can jeopardize the efforts of the others.

PUBLIC LAW 94-142 AND THE STUDENT WITH CANCER

Public Law 94-142, the Education for All Handicapped Children Act, was signed into law by President Ford on November 29, 1975. It is the culmination of a movement to provide equal educational opportunity for all handicapped children. Its roots lie in federal legislation dating back to the 1950s. Although it is relatively new, PL 94-142 has become landmark legislation whose impact on public school systems is likely to equal that of the Elementary and Secondary Education Act of 1965 and the Supreme Court decision in *Brown v. Board of Education* in 1954. Many of the major provisions of PL 94-142 were in fact

Table 51-1
Checklist for Physicians and Nurses in Communicating with Educators

A. Factors Affecting Attendance
1. Frequency of outpatient visits
2. Frequency and duration of inpatient treatment

B. Factors Affecting Peer and Social Interaction
1. Possible changes in physical appearance due to surgery or chemotherapy
   a. Amputation
   b. Weight gain/weight loss
   c. Hair loss
2. Chemotherapy-induced mood changes
3. Suppressed appetite
4. Increased frequency of urination

C. Factors Affecting Education
1. Possible neuropsychological side-effects of treatment
2. Changes in fine or gross motor coordination
3. Possible vision or hearing impairments
4. Limitations on physical activity
5. Possible fatigue

D. Factors Affecting Medical Compliance
1. Medication to be administered at school (name, dosage, frequency)
2. Specific information on communicable diseases
3. Methods for reporting communicable diseases
4. Name and telephone number of hospital contact person in case of questions or emergency

required in earlier federal laws, so it is the descendent of a long line of legislation aimed at the education of handicapped children.

Public Law 94-142 is unique in several aspects. It addresses actual instruction at the classroom level more explicitly than does any other federal statute. It is the mandate for the development of an IEP for each handicapped child. The aspect most open to controversy and challenge is PL 94-142's spelling out nine components of that program. It is, moreover, the first federal law to require preservice education (*i.e.,* in a teacher training institution), for both regular and special educators concerning handicapped children. It is noteworthy that the act is codified as both education and civil rights legislation.[10]

Public Law 94-142 requires every state to provide a free and appropriate education in the least restrictive environment for all handicapped individuals between the ages of 3 and 21. Therefore, school districts in all 50 states are mandated through PL 94-142 to provide an appropriate education for students with cancer, ages 3 through 21, whose medical problems adversely affect their educational performance. This section gives an overview of the legal, organizational, and practical aspects of the law; discusses in detail the IEP mandated by the law; and offers suggestions for the development of an appropriate IEP for the student with cancer.[11] It should be noted that because of significant medical advances in pediatrics in general in the last decade, children with other chronic and life-threatening illnesses who were unable to attend school previously are now attending in the regular classroom. There are no clear-cut, ready answers to the multifaceted educational issues posed by these students. The IEP process mandated by PL 94-142 is the vehicle through which educators and parents work together to plan the education of these children. Young people with cancer are another new population needing service, and they can benefit from being involved in a process that not only protects their rights but also is familiar and comfortable to the educational community.

There are school districts that resist implementing PL 94-142 and developing IEPs for children with cancer. In some districts, the reasons for this are budgetary. However, most resistance comes from ignorance. The school forms a part of the larger community in which children must live out their struggle with their disease. Many in the larger community still view cancer as a death sentence. They may be willing to give money to help a dying child fulfill his or her last wish, but have yet to come to terms with the child who does not die and who must be educated toward a future. The educational community must be trained to move from a focus on death to a focus on life, with all the implications for an appropriate education for the child with a serious medical problem.[9] The IEP process discussed below will not only provide a vehicle to obtain appropriate services for a specific child but, through the efforts of parents and hospital personnel involved, will provide information to the larger educational community that will impact not only on the child in question but on future children with cancer who will need services from the school district.

Definition

Public Law 94-142 includes children with cancer as "other health impaired" (OHI), and defines that term as follows:

> "Other Health Impaired" means limited strength, vitality, or alertness due to chronic or acute health problems such as heart condition, tuberculosis, rheumatic fever, nephritis, asthma, sickle cell anemia, hemophilia, epilepsy, lead poisoning, leukemia, or diabetes, which adversely affects a child's educational performance. (#121 a.5 [b] [7])

Each state, in its administrative codes, has its own interpretation of this statute. Some students with cancer can and should attend school without any program modification. Special education is appropriate only when it is necessary to bridge the gap between the child's ability to function in the general school program and any deficits in doing so that result from the handicap.[10] In addition, PL 94-142 requires that the focus of special intervention is not the handicap, but the educational needs that result from the handicap. Every child with cancer is not affected the same way, medically or educationally. Therefore, interventions must be highly individualized.

School District Responsibility

Under PL 94-142, school districts have the following responsibility to all students with handicaps in implementing the law:

1. Assess any handicapped child who is referred to determine how the handicap affects the child's ability to function within the educational system.
2. Construct an IEP for each child whose handicap prevents him or her from progressing normally through the regular educational system. The plan must address the following questions:
   a. What long-term goals and short-term objectives are to be met by the child during the term of the IEP?
   b. What types of specialized services are needed to permit the child to function within the setting in which he or she is placed?
   c. What type of assistance, if any, is needed for a child who speaks no English or only limited English?

d. What type of modifications, if any, are needed for the child to meet the graduation and competency standards of the school district?

e. What type of vocational education is most appropriate to the child's needs?

f. What type of physical education is most appropriate to the child's needs?

g. In what setting can the child be served most appropriately: [1] in regular classes with designated services, [2] in the resource room for part of the day, or [3] in a special class all or most of the day?

h. What is the child's current level of functioning (academic, social, behavioral, physical) as compared with others in the same age group?

3. Provide for review of the IEP at least once a year.

4. Ensure that the rights of the parent and child to due processes—including provisions for parental consent before the IEP is implemented—are upheld throughout the entire process.

5. Provide the services listed in the IEP without cost to the parent or child.

Students with special needs who attend parochial or private schools also have the right to receive some special education and related services from the public school system. How services are provided differs greatly from state to state and from district to district. Parents are ultimately responsible for establishing communication between private schools and local school districts to implement services.

School District Jurisdiction

The school district of residence is responsible for providing services to the child. However, states differ on whose responsibility it is to provide service when a child is hospitalized. AB1689, passed by the California legislature and approved by the Governor in May 1986, clarified the issue in California and could provide model legislation for other states. The law provides that a pupil with a temporary disability, who is in a hospital that is located outside the school district in which the pupil's parent or guardian resides, shall have complied with the residency requirements for school attendance in the school district in which the hospital is located. The law further requires the district in which the hospital is located to provide the pupil with individualized instruction while he or she is in the hospital, within 5 working days of notification. It is the parent's responsibility to notify the school district of the pupil's presence in a qualifying hospital. The law also states in Section 48206.4(2) that the school district in which the hospital is located may enter into an agreement with the school district in which the pupil previously attended regular day classes or an alternative educational program to have that school district provide the pupil with individualized instruction. This allows both flexibility and continuity of the program.

Development of the Individualized Education Plan

Referral

Children and adolescents newly diagnosed with cancer should be referred to the school district for an assessment and evaluation of their eligibility for services under PL 94-142. In most cases, pupils are referred to their home school district; however, in some circumstances, the school district in which the hospital is located develops the IEP, and the parents present the completed document to the home school when the student returns. In addition to newly diagnosed patients, the following should also be referred: children diagnosed in preschool years who are entering kindergarten or first grade and are still undergoing treatment, and children who may have completed treatment but are at high risk for learning problems because of central nervous system involvement (specifically, children who had brain tumors and those with leukemia who had cranial irradiation at a young age, *e.g.,* before the age of 6).

Assessment and Plan Preparation

The assessment by the school district should include academic and psychological testing—done within the context of that district's policies—as well as a complete review of the child's developmental, health, and medical status. These tests will ensure that possible learning disabilities are considered when the IEP is developed. They will also provide a baseline for determining whether progression of the disease or its treatment is likely to cause learning problems in the future.

When the hospital is involved in neuropsychological testing of children, the process of assessment will be less stressful for the child if the results can be shared with the school district.

The school professional who oversees the assessment will also need the assistance of the hospital or clinic team in collecting data that will be important to the IEP team. The IEP team needs to know the following:

1. The type of cancer and treatment.

2. The possible medical side effects and complications of treatment that could affect school functioning.

3. The possible side-effects of surgery, radiation, or chemotherapy that might affect the student's ability to learn.[12–16]

4. The educational and social implications of the disease and treatment (*e.g.,* the likelihood of fatigue; absences; change in physical appearance caused by weight fluctuations, hair loss, or amputations; problems with fine and gross motor control).

5. Problems related to exposure to infectious diseases, especially chicken pox, and clinic guidelines for reporting exposures to the parent or designated clinic staff member.

6. The name of the pediatric hematology/oncology team member who is designated to serve as a contact with the school.

Finally, it is important for the school personnel to be assured that the child's medical condition is monitored closely by the physician, that the parents are knowledgeable about and responsible for the child's care, and that the child will be kept out of school if the physician judges that the child is physically unable to be there. School personnel require these assurances to be able to focus on the educational needs of the child rather than expending energy anticipating a medical emergency.

When the individual educational assessment has been completed, the case manager calls an IEP meeting within 50 school days after the referral is received. The parents should be encouraged to attend and to bring a professional from the hospital or clinic. The IEP team reviews the assessment, receives input from other people attending the meeting, and constructs a plan that will provide the student with the class placement and services most appropriate to his or her needs. The IEP should be written to encompass possible changes in the child's medical status and needs during the term it covers (usually one year), so that additional meetings to alter placement or services will be unnecessary. This will cause team members to look ahead rather than concentrating only on the child's immediate status.

Implementation of the IEP

At the IEP meeting, a special education teacher will be assigned to see that all phases of the plan are implemented. This professional—who may be the special class teacher, the resource specialist teacher, or a designated instructional services person—is the liaison with the hospital or clinic team and coordinates the activities of all other persons and services set forth in the IEP. Typical types of services provided in IEPs for children with cancer include the following:

1. Liaison with regular class teachers regarding the effects of the disease or its treatment on classroom behavior and performance.
2. Assistance of the school nurse or other health office personnel in administering drugs, dealing with illness at school, notifying other school staff of the physicians' recommendations, coordinating plans to monitor and report chicken pox outbreaks, and so forth.
3. Special tutoring for subjects in which the child has fallen behind because of frequent treatment- or illness-related absences.
4. Instruction at home or in the hospital when the child must be out of school for more than a few days.
5. Special class placement for the child who has a diagnosed disability.
6. Counseling related to problems involving school adjustment or peer relationships.
7. Adjustment of the class schedule.
8. Development of independent study programs.
9. Specialized physical education.
10. Special arrangements for taking make-up tests.
11. Waiver of automatic absence penalties.
12. Special equipment, if needed.
13. Transportation to and from school, if necessary.

If the placement and services appear to be incomplete or inappropriate, any member of the IEP team may call an additional meeting to modify the plan. A copy of the IEP is given to the parents, who are urged to permit a copy to be placed in the child's medical file.

If the family moves to another school district or state, the parents should present the IEP on registering the child at the new school to expedite service. The student may be reevaluated by the new district, depending on the educational and administrative code of the state and the guidelines of the school district.

SPECIFIC SCHOOL ISSUES AND STRATEGIES FOR IMPLEMENTATION

School History

School-age children diagnosed with a malignancy bring to the cancer experience a history of school functioning. Established patterns of school performance do not change when a student is diagnosed. In fact, the pattern tends to become more pronounced.[2,3] It is therefore imperative to identify the student's previous history of school functioning before initiating school reentry. This can be done, with the parents' permission, by a review of the cumulative record and a brief telephone conversation with the school principal or counselor. If the child or adolescent has a previous history of behavior, attendance,

learning, or emotional problems, this information is critical to reentry and long-term planning strategies. If the parents have a history of being uncooperative and critical of school personnel and are unrealistic about their child's performance and ability, this also needs to be ascertained. The child's functioning and parents' attitudes before diagnosis need to be known, not only for reentry planning but also so that retrospective review does not attribute these behaviors to the disease process or to the emotional effects of the disease on the child or parent.

Patient Involvement

Since the child or adolescent is the one who lives and develops with the disease and who, in the long run, must become his or her own advocate, the child must be fully involved, in an age-appropriate manner, in decisions regarding the return to school and in ongoing school issues. The child needs to be prepared to answer classmates' questions, and adolescents especially need to have a voice in how information is given to teachers and peers. Issues of changes in physical appearance and peer acceptance are paramount concerns of the young person. These problems cannot be avoided and must be addressed directly and consistently, but not elevated to such a level as to become a major emotional deterrent to school reentry.

For example, a child we will call Andrew entered kindergarten while undergoing treatment for acute lymphocytic leukemia. He was always reluctant to return to school after an absence for treatment with chemotherapy. Andrew's teacher decided on a way to help him discuss his medical situation with peers in a manner that was age appropriate. Each child in the class was assigned a week to prepare a bulletin board on the theme "this is your life." When it was Andrew's week, he brought a camera to the clinic and photographed his "clinic family." In this way, he was able to share in his own turn with his classmates what he was experiencing at the clinic, without having to stand out as different from the other children.

Joan was a high school track star before she underwent a limb salvage procedure for osteogenic sarcoma. An honor student, she very much wanted to return to school. However, she did not want the entire student body to know of her problem. Joan was encouraged to bring her best friend, Carole, with her to clinic and to the adolescent group meetings. For the next two years, Carole acted as a buffer for Joan at the high school. Students who were curious about Joan's limp asked Carole what was going on, and Carole was well prepared to answer. Carole determined which questioners were merely curious and which really were interested and supportive. In this way, she removed from Joan the burden of being asked all sorts of questions by people who were merely prying. Carole's friendship and support—and her education from direct experience at the clinic and at the adolescent groups—made Joan's return to school a happy experience.

Stanley, a budding fifth-grade scientist, chose to have his mother and the school nurse provide a presentation to his class. Halfway through the presentation, he announced that he had more accurate information about his diagnosis and treatment than the nurse and his mother did, and he took over the rest of the presentation himself. By having his mother and the school nurse begin the presentation, he was given the opportunity to involve himself more directly—with the nurse and his mother still in the room in case he needed them.

All three students described above, representing three different developmental levels and stages in school, were initially afraid to return to school. Although their fears were acknowledged, the fact that they would return to school never became an issue. Rather, the school liaison, with help from the physicians, nurses, and social workers who shared the same goals, helped the students to work through their fears and develop strategies to help them gain control of the situation.

How teachers are prepared to work with a young person with cancer varies, depending on circumstances, staff, and distances. Faculty in-service programs, telephone contacts, and individual classroom visits are all acceptable possibilities. Regardless of method, however, the basic objectives are the same.

1. To provide accurate, up-to-date medical information to replace archaic ideas, antiquated attitudes, misconceptions, and myths about the disease.
2. To provide general information on children's developmental understanding of illness and treatment so that teachers focus on the child's perception of what he or she is experiencing at a particular developmental level, rather than imposing adult fears and concerns on the child.
3. To provide an avenue for school personnel to discuss their own feelings and experiences with cancer. The presence of a child with a serious, possibly life-threatening disease triggers strong feelings and emotions in the adults who come in contact with that child. Often these adults must reevaluate their own attitudes toward death or the purpose of life. Some may have to come to terms once again with the pain of the loss of a loved one to cancer, or the accidental death of their own child. One can never know or anticipate the personal experiences of a school faculty when reintegrating a newly diagnosed child. Nor can one resolve these issues. However, by discussing them openly, especially at a faculty meeting, they then become acceptable issues to be further explored informally by the faculty members.
4. To provide the young person's classroom teacher with the specific information and support necessary to prepare the child's class and to accept and understand the social, physical, academic, and emotional consequences of the diagnosis and treatment.
5. To identify long-term educational implications of the disease and treatment on the young person's academic and social performance in school.
6. To develop an individualized educational plan, as discussed in detail above.

Curriculum Modification

The development of well-designed and well-researched treatment protocols is responsible for many of the advances in pediatric cancer. It is important to ascertain the educational implications of treatment protocols so that educators can make long-term curriculum modifications. For example, if a child's protocol requires treatment for 3 years, then the educational plan should be viewed from the same 3-year perspective. To do this, the classroom teacher needs systematic assistance and direction from a district curriculum planner. A long-term plan must be developed so that at the end of treatment the child is not lagging academically. How this curriculum is mastered must be open to great flexibility and ingenuity and will depend on the child's age, ability, and medical involvement.

Plans must be developed that allow the child to fully participate in classroom activities when possible and to pursue individual interests with individualized instruction when he or she cannot participate or is hospitalized. Models for such individualized instruction are available in both gifted and special education programs. For example, the teacher and the child together may explore the child's interests to determine what

specific projects the child would like to investigate. The child's natural motivation can be used to develop his or her interests, enhance a sense of self-worth and self-direction, and introduce basic skills while the student continues in pursuit of his or her own interests.[17] A fourth grader, for example, may be fascinated by aviation. Together, the child and his or her teacher may structure a project on the history of commercial aviation that would involve basic reading, math, language, spelling, vocabulary, art, and writing skills. The child might be encouraged to visit an aviation museum and, if treated for cancer in a major medical center that is a great distance from home, to log his or her mileage, estimate airline fuel consumption, and record ticket cost. This type of assignment provides continuity in the child's education, whether in school or in the hospital, allows him or her to pursue individual interests in a responsible manner, and, at the same time, ensures that the core curriculum is mastered.

Educational technology is another boon to the child with cancer. Computer programs and audiotapes provide the child with many options when integrated into the curriculum. These can be used to supplement classroom instruction or to substitute for it if the child is at home or in the hospital.

School districts and individual schools within districts differ widely in their use of educational technology. Most large or county-wide school districts have professionals responsible for developing computer programs to supplement the basic curriculum. The school liaison should contact the child's school district to identify programs available within the district and to learn how to work with the educational technicians and teachers in the district to adapt available materials to meet the child's individual needs.

Such programs are not easily developed and require work and input from parents, students, teachers, curriculum planners, and other involved school personnel. However, educators, along with the home and hospital, are involved in the total care of the child, and this is the type of program that challenges their expertise and fully involves them in the care of the young person with cancer.

Issues Specific to Neurologically Impaired Students

Research into the late effects of treatment has confirmed the occurrence of long-term neuropsychological sequelae that impact on educational performance, especially among children diagnosed with leukemia as preschoolers who received cranial irradiation as part of their treatment.[12–16]

A subset of these children are severely damaged by the disease and its sequelae. Because of the severity and visibility of the damage, these children are usually easily identified by school personnel, and remedial services in classes for the severely learning handicapped, communicatively handicapped, or vision impaired, for example, are made available. Other children have hidden handicaps. Many have survived their illness without highly visible indicators of residual effects of treatment. There is very little in the literature on methods of remediation to assist these children. Identification of their educational needs is further hampered by the fact that while the pediatric hematology/oncology community is aware of the neuropsychological effects of cranial irradiation, the educational community is not. As a result, without information from the hospital, a well-intentioned school psychologist or educator may attribute the long-term survivor's academic problems to anxiety.

Most of these children are characterized by teachers as hard-working students with well-developed verbal skills. However, difficulties with tasks requiring long- and short-term memory, speed of processing, and acquisition of new information impact significantly on overall achievement.[3] Despite parental support and tutoring, these students, if left unassisted, find themselves lagging farther and farther behind classmates as they progress in school. Academic frustrations offset feelings of self-worth and impinge on all areas of the student's academic, personal, and social life. If these students do not get the remedial help they need, either because educators do not identify the problem and offer appropriate services as mandated under PL 94-142 or because their parents deny the problem, a crisis of major proportions can be anticipated by the time they enter junior high school.

On the other hand, if the problem is recognized and remedial services are made available to the student, then the frustration and anger these children often experience can be dissipated and they can be taught to use their skills to compensate for their deficits.

The student must become his or her own advocate. This is especially true of long-term survivors with hidden handicaps who experience daily the sequelae of cranial irradiation. As these children progress from elementary through junior high to high school and college, they need the concerted efforts of the home, school, and hospital to help them develop the coping skills that will assist them not only with academic tasks but also with the issues of living.

Issues Specific to Adolescents

Adolescents have unique needs not only in the psychosocial management of their illness but in educational issues specific to age and stage in school. The adolescent has the most to lose if educational intervention is undertaken haphazardly.

Upon graduation, most adolescents have one of two goals: employment or college. Most jobs today require a high school diploma or a comparable technical certificate. All colleges have entrance requirements. If the adolescent with cancer is to achieve either goal, systematic intervention is required. Just as the child in elementary school must master the basic skills of one grade to be prepared for the next, the adolescent must also meet certain requirements for graduation and college entrance.

The adolescent's current medical treatment or the neurologic sequelae of past treatment must also be carefully scrutinized to identify possible impacts on educational performance. The academic counselor is the key to coordinating the adolescent's schedule, ensuring that attendance requirements are waived if necessary, and seeing that all requirements for graduation or college entrance are met. The student may have five or six different teachers and classes, and all teachers must be informed each semester, either individually or in a group, of the educational implications of the student's medical status or history. Individual class assignments and requirements need to be negotiated at the beginning of each semester, and alternative independent study plans developed for use during a long-term hospitalization or home stay. This proactive approach is essential if the adolescent is to complete treatment not only medically cured but also prepared to enter the job market or go to college. The adolescent with cancer also needs to be involved in vocational counseling, job placement, or vocational rehabilitation when appropriate (see also Chap. 52). Those seeking to help these adolescents pursue vocational and educational goals will find ready support through well-trained school counselors who—although not versed specifically in issues related to childhood cancer—have expertise in dealing with adolescents with learning or physical disabilities.

Although the above approach to intervention has proved effective, it is difficult to convince some newly diagnosed adolescents or long-term survivors to risk such an approach. Many adolescents initially do not want teachers or peers to know of their illness; their desire not to stand out from the crowd interferes with their need to protect their own best interests. Advocates for these adolescents must take into account a young person's developmental needs but must not let those needs jeopardize his or her future. In the long run, such planning on the part of the young person, parents, guidance counselor, and faculty promotes rather than hinders independence and feelings of self-worth and accomplishment.

Issues Specific to Terminally Ill Children

Despite the successes, some children still die from cancer. Many of these children continue to attend school to the very end. If effective communication has been established among the home, school, and hospital before this stage, then, despite the pain involved, teachers and parents are able to make the necessary adjustments for school to be a life-sustaining experience for the child. In addition, if an IEP is in effect, alternative educational options for home tutors, modified (*i.e.,* shortened) day, and individual instruction will have been identified and can be easily implemented.

At the terminal stage, the siblings are often the ones who become the center of need in the school. If the whole faculty is involved in intervention efforts, then teachers of siblings can be extremely supportive at a time when the parents' energy is of necessity focused on the dying child. This sibling support continues after the child dies.[3]

Teachers also need assistance at this point. Not only have they invested personally in educating the child through difficult circumstances, but they have the added responsibility of supporting the other children in the class.

The time to establish the groundwork for this type of support is at the beginning, when the child first enters the school or is newly diagnosed. The terminal phase is too late to plan and initiate effective intervention.

CONCLUSION

Quality communication with the educational community is essential to ensure the success of the young person with cancer in school. Communication with teachers is a vital element in the total care of these children and cannot be accomplished haphazardly.

School Advocate

A school liaison, whose role is to be both an advocate with the parent for the child and a bridge between the medical and educational establishment, is a necessary part of the pediatric hematology/oncology team. An effective school advocate requires specialized training and preparation. He or she must have a thorough understanding of the educational system and curriculum, as well as special educational programs. This person must have the ability to identify resources in the school, both individuals and programs, to benefit the child; work with teachers and curriculum developers; and write child-specific educational plans; and must understand PL 94-142 and the IEP process in order to work with parents to ensure that the young person with cancer has the best possible program in the least restrictive environment.

Now that the care of the child with cancer has taken on a third dimension—educational and social—it is critical that a specific person be identified as a school liaison, a person whose background is educational rather than medical. How this position is funded and to what extent is up to the medical facility; that it *is* funded is critical to the success of the total program.

Long-Term Objectives

The overall approach to the education of the young person with cancer must be based on four long-term objectives:

1. To prepare the parent to work effectively with the school, not only at the point of diagnosis but also during and after the years of treatment.
2. To prepare the educational community to recognize and accept their responsibility to contribute to the total care of the child, and to identify long-term educational strategies to accomplish this.
3. To prepare the medical community to establish quality and appropriate communication with the school and provide child-specific information on the educational implications of the disease and its treatment, not only at the point of diagnosis but also as the need arises.
4. To provide for the student an area in life where he or she is free of medical concerns and can focus energy on school life.

REFERENCES

1. Meadows AT, Kremas NL, Belasco JB: The medical cost of cure: Sequelae in survivors of childhood cancer. In van Eyes J, Sullivan MP (eds): The Status of the Curability of Childhood Cancers. New York, Raven Press, 1980
2. Katz E: School and Social Reintegration of Children with Cancer: School Reintegration Project: Final Report. Oakland, CA, American Cancer Society, California Division, 1985
3. Deasy-Spinetta P: School Intervention Program for Children with Cancer: Final Report. ACS, CD 542-5-E. Oakland, CA, American Cancer Society, California Division, 1985
4. Deasy-Spinetta P, Spinetta JJ: Remedial and school experiences of child survivors. Cancer (in press)
5. Kaplan DM: Interventions for acute stress experiences. In Spinetta JJ, Deasy-Spinetta P (eds): Living with Childhood Cancer. St Louis, CV Mosby, 1981
6. Mellette SJ: The Semantics of Disability. Proceedings: Workshop on Employment Insurance and the Cancer Patient. American Cancer Society, New Orleans, December 16–17, 1986
7. Deasy-Spinetta P: School intervention: An ongoing process. Candlelighters Progress Reports 4:9–10, 1984
8. Chesler MA, Barbarin OA: Childhood Cancer and the Family: Meeting the Challenge of Stress and Support. New York, Brunner/Mazel, 1987
9. Spinetta JJ, Deasy-Spinetta P: The patient's socialization in the community and school during therapy. Cancer 58:512–515, 1986
10. Shrybman JA: Due Process in Special Education. Rockville, MD, Aspen, 1982
11. Deasy-Spinetta P, Tarr D: Public Law 94-142 and the student with cancer. J Psychosoc Oncol 3(2):1985
12. Goff J, Anderson A, Cooper M: Distractibility and memory deficits in long-term survivors of acute lymphoblastic leukemia. J Dev Behav Pediatr 1:158–163, 1980
13. Lansky SB, Cairns NU, Lansky LL, Cairns GF, Stephenson L, Garin G: Central nervous system prophylaxis. Am J Pediatr Hematol Oncol 6:183–190, 1984
14. Meadows AT, Masari DJ, Ferguson J: Declines in IQ scores and cognitive dysfunctions in children with acute lymphocytic leukemia treated with cranial radiation. Lancet 2:1015–1018, 1981
15. Pfefferbaum-Levine B, Copeland DR, Fletcher JM, Reid HL, Jaffe N, McKinnon WR: Neuropsychologic assessment of long-term survivors of childhood leukemia. Am J Pediatr Hematol Oncol 6:123–128, 1984
16. Robinson LL, Nesbit ME, Sather HN, Meadows AT, Ortega JA, Hammond GD: Factors associated with IQ scores in long-term survivors of childhood acute lymphoblastic leukemia. Am J Pediatr Hematol Oncol 6:115–120, 1984
17. Stallings C: California Model Program: Learning Through Methods of Inquiry: An Individualized Instructional Model. San Diego City Schools, 1979

fifty-two

Occupation and Employment Issues in Pediatric Oncology

Sherry L. Phillips

With the steady increase in survival rates for children with cancer, those who provide their medical treatment face new challenges. In the past, it was acceptable to treat the malignancy and to be satisfied that the child survived. Now, the goal of treatment is to achieve a totally cured child, defined as one who is mentally as well as physically healthy and can function in society. Thus, our responsibilities extend beyond simply rendering our patients free of disease.

We must ensure that patients are able to grow and develop and realize their greatest potential. Thus, a major treatment goal for the child with cancer is that he or she reach adulthood with the ability to obtain employment and achieve competence in adult roles. Concern about having the opportunity to meet this goal becomes a central issue for patients and their families after the child survives the acute phase of the illness.

A review of the literature yields mixed conclusions about the fate of childhood cancer survivors. Initial studies showed that children who had survived cancer made good adjustments and were leading fully active lives,[1,2] but subsequent studies have failed to substantiate these conclusions.[3-8]

In a survey of the vocational status of adults treated for cancer as children at the National Cancer Institute (NCI), 95% of those who responded were employed (70%), in college (17%), or were homemakers (8%).[5] These occupational statuses were similar to those of an age- and sex-matched sample of the U.S. population in the areas of work and homemaker, although a greater percentage of the study patients were students. A comparison of salaries also indicated a similarity between the two samples.[5] Thus, at first glance, these survivors of childhood cancer appeared to be functioning on a par with the U.S. population with regard to employment and earnings. However, closer scrutiny of the data suggested that some of the respondents come from families of higher socioeconomic status, and did not appear to be reaching their expected, preillness potential. Comparisons of the occupational status of 25 age- and sex-matched sibling–patient pairs confirmed this suspicion. More than half of the patients had lower level jobs than their siblings.[5]

Job discrimination on the basis of a cancer health history is difficult to quantify. However, discrimination encountered by childhood cancer survivors when applying for jobs, the military, and health and life insurance has been documented.[3-8] Incidences of being denied access to a job were reported by 55% of the respondents in the NCI survey noted above. Of these, 46% reported that they were denied a job because they needed more training or experience, whereas 44% related their denial of a job to their cancer history.[5]

A survey by the American Cancer Society, California Division, reported that half of all respondents who were working or looking for work reported unfair work experiences. One third of the respondents described one or more incidences of discrimination.[3]

In the NCI study sample, 77% reported having health insurance, compared to an estimated rate for Americans of 90%.[5] Another study revealed that compared to their same-sex siblings, childhood cancer survivors had significantly more difficulty in securing life and health insurance. Although most survivors had health insurance coverage, they were less likely than siblings to be covered by life insurance.[7]

A review of these studies suggests that children who survive cancer may experience disproportionate difficulty achieving success in the workplace but are able to obtain employment and insurance, although they may not be reaching their full potential.

Because most children with cancer are now surviving beyond the acute phase of the disease and are reaching adulthood, it is important to learn about the challenges that face these children. We need to learn why survivors do not achieve their greatest potential in the workplace. Is this simply a result of discrimination, or are these people insufficiently prepared for competing in the world of work? Prospective longitudinal studies are needed to accurately assess the situation.

IMPORTANCE OF WORK

When asked for a definition of mental health, Sigmund Freud cited two characteristics—the abilities to work and to love. Subsequent observers have suggested that the opportunity to work is central to a healthy psychological identity and sense of self-worth.[9] Young people in our society generally grow up with the expectation that they will become wage earners. Parents are expected to instill in their children the notion that they will make a vocational choice that in later years will enable them to support themselves and their families.

Education is often viewed as an entryway into the adult world of work rather than an opportunity to broaden knowledge. Employment generally symbolizes maturity, independence, and other qualities that result in fulfillment of adult roles. Therefore, work is an irreplaceable element in establishing the sense of worth that is a vital component of the individual's psychosocial and economic functioning.[3]

Occupational choice has been viewed as a developmental process that begins in childhood and extends throughout life.[10,11] Young people face many crossroads at which their lives can take decisive turns that narrow the range of alternatives, ultimately influencing their choice of occupation.[12] The road travelled by children with cancer need not be one filled with obstacles; it should be one of opportunity that permits them to pursue their goals and aspirations, unhindered by their disease experience.

DEVELOPMENT AND WORK

Treatment of the child with cancer must be directed toward enhancing normal development. Individuals working with children require a basic understanding of normal childhood development and should realize that each child with cancer is at risk for developmental delays. For example, cognitive and behavioral problems have become evident in some patients with acute lymphoblastic leukemia who have received central nervous system (CNS) preventive therapy (see Chaps. 16 and 24).[13–15] One study discovered that survivors of childhood cancer are at substantially greater risk of developing psychological problems than are survivors of other chronic but not life-threatening childhood illnesses.[4]

All healthy children begin life with an intrinsic drive to explore and master their environment. As they grow and develop, children acquire new inner resources, such as control over their bodily functions, ability to think and solve problems, and physical strength and coordination. They use these resources to explore their world, and eventually encounter societal expectations and demands. Havighurst[16] introduced the idea of "developmental tasks" to signify a progression of necessary learning experiences that a person encounters in successive life stages. Each task must be mastered in sequence for normal development to occur. Personal values and aspirations that become part of one's personality emerge out of interactions between one's organic being and the environmental forces exerted upon that being.

The expectations and demands placed on children by family, health care providers, and teachers are an integral part of normal development for the childhood cancer patient. These outside forces help spur the child to reach high levels of achievement that ultimately lead to developing competent occupational behavior. All children need to be viewed as capable, and they should feel that they deserve to achieve success. This is especially true for children with cancer, who are subjected to numerous stresses that they may misinterpret as an indication that they are bad and do not deserve success.

Abnormal development in the child with cancer can manifest itself physically, cognitively, and emotionally. These developmental deficits can stem directly from the disease and its treatment and indirectly from personal and societal responses.

Often, treatment for childhood malignancy requires radical treatments that are necessary to prolong the patients' lives yet may render them physically disabled. The most common example is amputation of a limb to treat an osteogenic sarcoma. More subtle or delayed effects include the neuropsychological sequelae of cranial irradiation.[13–15,17] It is essential that these children be identified early so that appropriate educational and vocational planning can be implemented.

The adverse effects of cancer and therapy can be both physiologic and psychological. Anxiety about the disease and treatment, adjustment problems at home or school, and feeling somehow responsible for the cancer can seriously scar the child if these issues are not recognized and resolved. One should assume that there will always be some psychological fallout from the diagnosis of cancer.

The Child

Occupational behavior in young children is expressed through play. This begins the developmental process, laying the foundation for occupational roles in adult life. Play is the major vehicle through which the child first explores and learns to master the environment. Young children must have opportunities for play. Occupational and recreational therapists are the ideal professionals to facilitate this (see also Chap. 46). Often, they will be able to identify functional and emotional problems as they are first manifested during play activities.

As the child reaches school age, play as the primary form of occupational activity is supplemented with school. School-age children with cancer must be expected to go to school and participate as fully as possible. Most hospitals have classrooms or visiting teachers, so there is little excuse for a child not to participate in school on some level while undergoing cancer therapy. Teachers should be sensitive to the stresses faced by children with cancer so that realistic expectations can be established.

School is the appropriate arena in which to explore interests, talents, and strengths (see also Chap. 51). Interest in arts and crafts develops during the early school years. Through crafts, the child learns mastery over materials and self, develops problem-solving skills, and acquires work habits and attitudes regarding persistence and pride in doing a good job.[18]

School work provides the child the experience of organizing time and energy to accomplish a task.

The Adolescent

The adolescent poses unique challenges to the family and health care provider because adolescence is a time of confusion and of development of self-identity. The experiences of cancer and its treatment often force the adolescent to be dependent at a time when the goal of independence is paramount.

The development of abstract reasoning occurs in adolescence. Adolescents become better able to think beyond the present and conceptualize the future. It is not too soon for the patient to begin thinking about his or her interests, dreams, and future goals, and perceived obstacles to attaining these goals. A good place to start is by identifying the patient's strengths and by helping him or her acquire the experiences that will capitalize on those strengths. Often, compromised physical strength and stamina require the therapist to assist an adolescent in identifying other areas of ability and to recommend activities that will maximize ability and minimize disability.

The Young Adult

The young adult with cancer is faced with a myriad of feelings of inadequacy and insecurity. Often, this is the time of life when one begins college, marries, or obtains a job. Having cancer may delay these stages. Accordingly, the patient with cancer often substitutes other experiences, such as volunteer jobs or "work therapy." For example, a volunteer job designed by the occupational therapist or vocational counselor may enable the patient to explore interests, restore self-confidence, or learn new skills. In the setting of a volunteer job, perhaps in the hospital, expectations can be easily adjusted to accommodate the patient's condition and treatment schedule.

Recently diagnosed young adults may need to change their plans for work to incorporate physical constraints. An occupational therapist or vocational counselor can help the patient identify strengths and weaknesses, as well as interests, values, and goals. Vocational rehabilitation is best accomplished within the framework of an interdisciplinary treatment team.

VOCATIONAL REHABILITATION

Competent work behavior does not automatically begin at the societally defined work age, nor does it begin when the disease has stabilized.[10] Rehabilitation of the child, adolescent, or young adult with cancer should begin soon after diagnosis. The quality of life and potential of the child are maximized when a future orientation is projected.[19] The key to successfully addressing the vocational needs of the childhood cancer patient is anticipating the problems before they manifest themselves. School-age children, for example, should be enrolled in a school program.

Interdisciplinary team meetings are the appropriate forum for sharing information about the patient. These team meetings are essential for quality treatment of children who have been identified as suffering late effects of treatment. Individual members of the team, with different relationships to the patient, often have different insights that become useful when shared. At least one of the members of the treatment team will need to facilitate interactions with the patient's community. This may involve talking with the local school authority or making the appropriate referral to the state's Division of Vocational Rehabilitation. This health professional acts as an advocate for patients and helps them through the bureaucratic maze.

The Vocational Rehabilitation Specialist

The vocational rehabilitation specialist can be either an occupational therapist (OT) or vocational rehabilitation counselor. Either can be consulted when vocational rehabilitation is warranted; however, the OT has generally been consulted early in the patient's treatment and can subsequently determine the need to refer the patient to a vocational rehabilitation counselor.

Screening and Evaluation

Pediatric oncology patients should be evaluated by an occupational therapist to identify potential areas of dysfunction. A history of performance related to age-appropriate tasks and roles helps to guide further evaluation of the patient's functional capacities, performance skills, and future vocational goals.[20] The evaluation may employ record reviews, standardized tests, specific observations, and interviews.[20] In addition, it is important to determine whether the patient expects to encounter success when pursuing activities. Do the activities the patient has chosen support his or her identified roles? Does the social environment support successful occupational behavior?

Treatment

Following the evaluation, a treatment plan can be implemented. The treatment process involves the use of selected activities, assistive devices, and educational techniques to restore the patient to the highest level of independent function. Activity is directed toward improving muscle strength, range of motion, coordination, endurance, and sensory function. Activities are also used to improve working capacity, cognitive function, social relatedness, personal habits, time management, and role function.[20]

Patients are advised to engage in tasks specifically designed to foster competence. Competence is derived from the actual experience of succeeding in a socially important task. Low self-esteem can result from engaging in tasks that result in failure or have little social importance.

Once the restorative phase of treatment has been completed, the therapist determines whether there is residual disability that will interfere with the patient's ability to return to his or her preillness existence. When residual disability exists, the therapist will initiate a prevocational evaluation.

Prevocational Evaluation and Training

The occupational therapist initiates the prevocational evaluation by identifying the patient's vocational interests and goals. This is accomplished through a series of interviews, history taking, and standardized tests. The goal of this evaluation is to assess and predict work behavior and vocational potential.[20] Those patients who have disabilities that may interfere with returning to their preillness existence should be identified and given direct treatment. In many instances, the patient should be referred to the local Division of Vocational Rehabilitation office for evaluation and treatment.

Vocational rehabilitation services are available to U.S. residents through PL 93-112. For a person to be eligible for federally funded vocational rehabilitation, the following conditions must be met: [1] the person possesses a mental or physical disability; [2] the disability constitutes a substantial handicap to employment; and [3] there is reasonable expectation that the patient's employability will benefit from provision of rehabilitation services.[21]

Successful job training and placement is dependent on a thorough evaluation of the patient's interests, values, and goals. However, it must be remembered that vocational rehabilitation is more than job training. It requires enlisting a skilled professional who can conduct a comprehensive evaluation of the patient and later recommend the appropriate job training that considers skills, handicaps, and personal needs. It is a dynamic process that makes allowances for changes in physical condition and environmental constraints.

REFERENCES

1. Holmes HA, Holmes FF: After ten years, what are the handicaps and lifestyles of children treated for cancer? Clin Pediatr 14:819–823, 1975
2. Li FP, Stone R: Survivors of cancer in childhood. Ann Intern Med 84:551–553, 1976
3. Feldman FL: Work and Cancer Health Histories: Work Expectations and Experiences of Youth (Ages 13–23) with Cancer Histories. Oakland, CA, American Cancer Society, California Division, 1980
4. Koocher GP, O'Malley JE: The Damocles Syndrome: Psycholosocial Consequences of Surviving Childhood Cancer. New York, McGraw-Hill, 1981
5. Phillips SL: Vocational Experiences of Childhood Cancer Survivors. Unpublished Master's thesis, Seattle University, Seattle, WA, 1985
6. Teta MJ, Del Po MC, Kasl SV, Meigs JW, Myers MH, Mulvihill JJ: Psychosocial consequences of childhood and adolescent cancer survival. J Chronic Dis 39:751–759, 1986
7. Holmes GE, Baker A, Hassanein RS, Bovee EC, Mulvihill JJ, Myers MH, Holmes FF: The availability of insurance to long-time survivors of childhood cancer. Cancer 57:190–193, 1986
8. Monaco G: Advocacy and legal issues. In Pizzo PA, Poplack DG (eds): Principles and Practice of Pediatric Oncology, chap 53. Philadelphia, JB Lippincott, 1989
9. Cunnick WR: Advances in the employability of the cancer patient. Proceedings of the American Cancer Society Second National Conference on Human Values and Cancer, p 188, 1977
10. Super DE: The Psychology of Careers—An Introduction to Vocational Development. New York, Harper & Brothers, 1957
11. Ginzberg E, Ginsburg S, Axelrod S, Herma J: Occupational Choice: An Approach to General Theory. New York, Columbia University Press, 1951
12. Smelser N, Smelser W: Personality and Social Systems. New York, John Wiley & Sons, 1963
13. Brouwers P, Riccardi R, Poplack D, Fedio P: Attentional deficits in long-term survivors of childhood acute lymphoblastic leukemia (ALL). J Clin Neuropsychol 6:325–336, 1984
14. Meadows AT, Massari DJ, Fergusson J, Gordon J, Littman P, Moss K: Declines in IQ scores and cognitive dysfunctions in children with acute lymphocytic leukemia treated with cranial irradiation. Lancet 2:1015–1018, 1981
15. Moss HA, Nannis ED, Poplack DG: The effects of prophylactic treatment of the central nervous system on the intellectual functioning of children with acute lymphocytic leukemia. Am J Med 71:47–52, 1981
16. Havighurst RJ: Human Development and Education. New York, Longmans Green, 1953
17. Blatt J, Bleyer WA: Late effects of childhood cancer and its treatment. In Pizzo PA, Poplack DG (eds): Principles and Practice of Pediatric Oncology, chap 50. Philadelphia, JB Lippincott, 1989
18. Pezzutti L: An exploration of adolescent feminine and occupational behavior development. Am J Occup Ther 33(2):84–91, 1979
19. van Eys J: The truly cured child. In Spinetta J, Deasy-Spinetta P (eds): Living With Childhood Cancer, pp 30–40. St Louis, CV Mosby, 1981
20. American Occupational Therapy Association: The role of occupational therapy in the vocational rehabilitation process. Am J Occup Ther 34:881–883, 1980
21. Moriarty JP: Issues in the evaluation of vocational rehabilitation. Professional Psychol 8(4):641–649, 1977

fifty-three

Advocacy and Legal Issues in Pediatric Oncology

Grace Powers Monaco

As defined by *Webster's Ninth New Collegiate Dictionary* (1987), an advocate is "one that pleads the cause of another." In childhood cancer, advocates may be individual members of a family or health care team pleading or acting on behalf of a particular child, or groups of parents or professionals or parent/professional partnerships advocating on behalf of all children with cancer or of specific groups of affected children (*e.g.,* those at a particular treatment center, those needing a particular therapy, or those who are cured survivors). Advocacy can take the form of a parent seeking information on how to support a child through the illness, group efforts toward changing policy or procedures in the treatment of children, individual court cases brought to protect a child's right to adequate treatment, or lobbying for legislation to ensure medical care for children with cancer.

PERSONAL ADVOCACY

The family of a child with cancer continues its nuturing role with a new dimension, assuming the position of questioner, information evaluator, and ultimately decision maker of what medical path to choose. Parents advocate for their family's psychosocial needs, their ill child's psychosocial and medical needs, and their own needs to be informed partners in their child's care—both that given by the medical team at the treatment center and the medical care regimen carried out by the family at home.

The decision making faced by parents of children with a life-threatening illness is continual and not usually clear-cut. It does not always involve choices as final as "pulling the plug" or accepting or declining treatment.[1] There may be decisions about whether to seek a second opinion or a different treatment center; whether or not to accept a protocol that involves a randomization; whether and what to tell the child, his or her siblings, families, neighbors, and schools; and whether to accept the offer of a well-meaning proponent of quackery to give a child injections secretly. Many of these major decisions may have to be made within the first period after diagnosis, a time of shock when parents are suddenly confronted with the unthinkable in this day and age—the possible death of their child (see also Chaps. 41, 42, and 46).[1]

Later in treatment, there may be other agonizing decisions: what to do about a child who does not seem able to tolerate the protocol's prescribed amount of radiation; whether to allow another drug trial; whether to allow completion of a trial that does not seem to be working; and whether or when to stop treatment (see also Chap. 15). The decision between living at all and living a quality life may seem obvious. For parents confronted with the weakened, exhausted shade of their formerly robust child, it may be neither obvious nor clear.[1]

The issue of parental competence and the responsibility of the practitioner to foster and accept it is critical in the area of decision making. The parents' role as advocate requires belief in their competence as parents and the establishment of credibility with the medical staff. How do parents do that? Margaret Saphier, a pediatric nurse practitioner and parent, emphasizes that parents are the experts on their children and are an important part of the surveillance checks and balances that ensure the best medical and psychosocial care.[2] Parents may need reassurance of their competence and may receive such reassurance through a variety of sources, including other parents and family, the medical care team, and parent advocate and peer support groups.

The family is the recognized principal caregiver and major advocate in the "family disease" of childhood cancer (see Chap. 42).[3-8] Studies link childhood cancer patients' favorable adjustment to treatment and rehabilitation with the positive social supports, communication, education, and understanding provided by their parents and family unit.[3-6]

Families cannot effectively advocate for their children and provide the positive supports they need without access to information on the obstacles and opportunities challenging them and their children, as well as empowerment to act as their advocates. Allies in informing, supporting, and empowering the family to advocate effectively for their children include the medical, psychosocial, and educational teams, as well as experiential parent peer support groups that both reinforce parental competence and control and open the avenues for advocacy.

The medical care team's role as allied advocates focuses on presentation of the best medical options to the family, surveillance of the delivery of care, provision of professional psychosocial support, and aid in tapping community resources as needed.[8] In its best form, the medical care team serves as ombudsman for the child both during and after treatment, as, for example, in outreach programs for schoolteachers, nurses, and students designed to enhance the opportunities for their patients to receive the best in education;[9] in formulating arguments to support insurance reimbursement for necessary treatment;[10,11] or in documenting cure, as is necessary for admission on waivers to the armed forces.[12]

Medical care teams and parent groups participate in preparing parents to be the best possible advocates for their child through their development of "how to" manuals for home use.[1] One example is Memorial Sloan-Kettering Cancer Center's chemotherapy and patient care manual for families of pediatric patients, which covers side-effects of treatment; home care management, including how to deal with diarrhea, bruising, nutrition, and fluids; and clinical events that require physician contact. Such specialized materials address the fact that families rarely have the opportunity to process the overload of information received while they are in the hospital setting but can process, understand, and act on information materials they take home and read later.[13]

Advocacy for family and child is assisted at a growing number of centers by a "parent consultant." This member of the medical care team is a parent who has or has had a child with cancer. One of the best known of these programs and the national model is located at Rhode Island Hospital. The parent consultants are fully participating members of the pediatric oncology staff, under the supervision of the physician head of the team, with primary responsibilities as liaison between family, staff, and center and as family advocates ensuring that the health care system is responsive to their needs.[14-16] The job description is as follows:

The Parent Consultant is a professional member of the Core Team with primary responsibilities as liaison and advocate for families and the child with cancer. This encompasses the entire treatment cycle including inpatient, outpatient, home care, and the bereavement process. Secondary functions include counseling and teaching for fam-

ilies, pediatric oncology staff, general hospital staff, and the broader community, as well as acting as a professional parent consultant and hospital representative to community groups, professional organizations, educational institutions, and federal agencies.

The following skills are considered necessary to perform the functions of parent consultant:[17]

Because the care system is constantly changing, this job involves an ongoing process of observation of the functioning of various hospital services and suggesting improvement. Analyzing the system involves interviewing staff and parents for data and identifying obstacles to change, both mechanical and attitudinal, as well as devising programs that lead to solutions. Some examples are: shortening waiting time in clinic; prioritizing delivery of services; expediting parking, billing, blood services; providing more effective patient/family education.

In acting as an advocate for staff, family members and patients, the advocates seek out solutions to routine and special problems employing tact and timing as well as careful thought in the performance of daily responsibilities.

The parent consultant at Children's Hospital in San Diego is supervised by a social worker and meets with families, represents the care team at parent group meetings, encourages participation in support group programs, and responds to parents' requests for reading material in consultation with staff.

Another ally in advocacy, particularly in empowering the family to act forcefully at the home, hospital, school, community, and governmental levels on behalf of their child, is the parent peer support group. The significance of such groups in the socialization, empowerment, and support of the family faced with a child or adolescent with cancer was studied extensively and discussed in *Childhood Cancer and the Family: Meeting the Challenge of Stress and Support.*[18] The studies of Chesler and colleagues, which support the value of experiential parent peer support in childhood cancer, focused on a sample of several different models of such support groups in the informal communication, education, information, and organizational support network of the Candlelighters Childhood Cancer Foundation.[19] They studied 49 self-help groups. Some of these groups were small (fewer than 10 members) and others were large (over 100 active members); some were informal in structure, while others were formal and structured, with bylaws, educational programs, self-help sharing sessions, social events, and assistance programs. Some were parent-led, some were led by professionals, and others were coordinated by parent/professional partnerships. Those authors found that the empowerment skills learned through experiential peer support groups assist families in serving as advocates for and promoting the wellness of their child with cancer as well as in supporting the integrity and harmony of the family structure.[20] An example of such a group is the Candlelighters Childhood Cancer Foundation network.[21,22] Candlelighters started in 1970 to fill the void in information published for parents, to provide access to parents for friendship and sharing, to promote the development of peer support groups, and to advocate in the legislative arena for programs and resources needed by families. As an advocate for parent peer support groups, the Candlelighters network provides information that plays an important role in the empowerment of the family focused on the challenges and opportunities presented by a child with cancer.[18-20,23-25] In its international network of over 200 groups, it fosters a continuum of sharing through newsletters for parents, youths with cancer, and the care team; support group and educational meetings; and publications such as a parent group organization handbook,[26] visitor training program manual,[26a] and annotated bibliography and resource guide[27] (available from the Foundation's offices at 1901 Pennsylvania Ave., NW, Suite 1001, Washington, DC 20006).

GROUP ADVOCACY

The issues addressed by group-supported advocacy are constantly changing. In the early 1970s, the needs of families were for informational material to use in making decisions, for respect as a partner in the care process, for acceptance of the value of peer support groups, and for support for additional social service personnel and home care programs. In the mid 1970s, as children were being seen as potential survivors, the needs were to reduce risks to survivors and other family members from environmental cancer causes, to increase access to information on good nutrition, to find ways to remediate educational deficits, and to provide housing for families away from home for treatment.[28] In the 1980s, the discriminatory effects of a cancer history on work and insurance opportunities have become evident,[29] and support groups have begun to focus on federal and state initiatives to provide insurance and job access for childhood cancer survivors.[30]

Table 53-1 delineates some activities undertaken by support groups, often with the assistance of treatment team members, to respond to problems affecting children and families.

Increasingly, group advocacy efforts are addressed to finding financial resources for treatment perceived by medical staff and parents as necessary to preserve a child's life or obtain a long-term remission. In the United States, medical care for impoverished families is provided by the Medicaid program. For the rest of the young population, care is funded through private insurance programs that pay for treatment deemed "reasonable" or "necessary" but usually exclude reimbursement for "investigational" or "experimental" treatment.

Bone marrow transplantation is an example of an exclusion that has been a particular problem. Costs can range from $75,000 to $250,000. Facilities will not perform transplantation without payment, so that without insurance the procedure usually is not possible. In the 1979 case of a child needing a bone marrow transplant (*Clifton Guilot, et al, v. Dr. William Cherry*), the New Orleans Candlelighters group lobbied and went to court and won. But payment from the state came too late; the child relapsed, lost his opportunity for cure, and died.

Insurers now regularly pay for matched transplants in leukemias and neuroblastoma and are beginning to consider payment for other pediatric cancers, such as Ewing's sarcoma.[51] However, the treatment field evolves more quickly than insurance policy, and parents need medical care teams to educate insurers on which treatments have emerged from investigational status to standard or preferred therapy. If the *Guilot* case occurred today, the insurer could be liable to the family for damages under the rationale articulated in the Wickline case.[52] Under that ruling, if treatment is withheld or delayed for financial reasons, the insurer, and potentially the health care provider, could be liable for injuries suffered by a patient or, if death occurs, the family.

The coverage issue for drugs usually considered experimental is complicated by the Food and Drug Administration's (FDA) new category of "treatment IND" (investigational new drug).[53] Under this category, physicians could use a drug during the investigational new drug (IND) application phase for study in the treatment of private patients who have serious or immediately life-threatening illness and no alternatives or are unmanageable by existing alternatives. The patients would have to pay for these drugs, which could be released as early as Phase II. Because the FDA proposal indicates that release of the drug is intended "to provide the best available therapy to an individual patient," it can be expected that insurers will be pressured to pay for more and more investigational treatment. If this proved too expensive, it could lead to specific exclusions in the payment of benefits, beginning with the more expensive therapies such as transplantation.

This new initiative raises serious advocacy issues. Usually, not enough is known about the long-term toxicities of a drug after Phase I trials to recommend its widespread use outside the tightly controlled investigative setting. Is there danger for a child if private physicians have access to new drugs as early as Phase II for their patients? And what about the reporting of adverse effects that helps to fine tune future use? Compared to the physician performing institution-centered research, a local physician may be less likely to insist on an autopsy to discover if a child's death was related to, caused by, or hastened by the effects of an experimental drug that may have been released improvidently.

LEGAL ISSUES

Informed Consent and Refusal

Fifteen years ago, a parent's choice of cancer treatment usually did not determine a child's chance for survival because the opportunity for cure was not a consistent reality. Today, with a cure rate of over 65%, wrong choices can deprive a child of a chance for survival or deprive parents of their child. The far-reaching impact of a family proxy's wrong decision and the consumer movement's emphasis on individuals being aware, involved, and in charge of their own personal health[54] has created new problems and tensions between the emerging rights of children to exercise self-determination and the traditionally held rights of parents and states to act with the medical care team to determine what is in the child's best interest (see also Chap. 15).[55]

This tension is evident in the court's treatment of parental versus children's rights in the headline-grabbing cases of Chad Green* and Joey Hofbauer, involving laetrile, metabolic therapy and unproven methods,[56,57] and the court-enforced decree ordering chemotherapy for 12-year-old Pamela Hamilton, whose father, a minister, refused cancer chemotherapy on religious grounds.[58] Fortunately, the vast majority of families with a child with cancer are involved with making choices among sound, proven medical alternatives offered in cooperative trial programs and with confronting the daily decisional and compliance problems associated with effective therapy, rather than seeking questionable remedies.

Parents and Caregivers

In the usual circumstances, parents stand in the shoes of their child to exercise rights to self-determination, privacy, informed consent, and bodily function.[56] This is the "private realm of family life which the State cannot enter."[59–61] When the parental role is overridden, courts substitute their judg-

---

* The Chad Green case raises some interesting questions in the informed consent area. The transcript in that case contains statements by the doctors testifying for the Greens that laetrile is not recognized to be effective against leukemias (see trial transcript). This accords with statements made in laetrile labeling prior to 1962.

Table 53-1
Advocacy by Parent Support Groups

Problem	Solutions
Lack of financial resources may deprive a child of a needed medical procedure, such as bone marrow transplantation.	Parent group gathers facts to support need, lobbies legislature for mandated benefits, and files suits to change the law or compel payment.[10,11]
A chemical dump is linked to excess childhood cancers and deaths.	Parents and support groups spend years gathering data, reporting violations, and winning cooperation and cleanup through court action.[31]
Childhood cancer survivors are denied entry into the armed services.	Candlelighters Childhood Cancer Foundation provides consultation, support, and encouragement in attempts to gain admission to the armed services under the new Department of Defense directive pertaining to survivors of childhood cancer, which provides that "Individuals who have a history of childhood cancer and who have not received any surgical or medical cancer therapy for five years and are free of cancer will be considered, on a case by case basis, fit for acceptance into the Armed Forces." [12]
Parents seek information about alleged nutritional cures and answers to their observations that on some diets their children experience fewer drug side-effects.	Candlelighters encourages research on diet and nutrition at NCI and testifies on lack of centralized reporting on progress and need for additional research, resulting in Congressional mandate for Diet, Nutrition and Cancer Program within NCI.[32]
Parents observe that their children are often discriminated against at school, not permitted to take physical education, treated as retarded rather than physically ill, and sometimes need special education.	Parent groups initiate programs to educate teachers about their chidren's cancer and their potential; encourage hospital intervention as ombudsman; seek answers to effects of treatment on learning; and set up tutorial programs.[33,34]
Parents express concern that they do not always get to meet other parents at hospitals; professionals observe that parents are sometimes reluctant to talk about their real problems with medical staff.	Parent groups and hospital care teams initiate parent ombudsman programs.[14-16]
Families burdened with expenses of illness cannot pay for health insurance, mortgage, food, clothes, lodging away from home, protheses, transportation to treatment center.	Groups raise funds to pay direct and indirect costs associated with illness, set up McDonald Houses, and provide financial counseling.[4,35,36]
Family resources are depleted by the time survivors or siblings reach college age.	Groups support scholarship programs.[36-38]
Lack of consistent funding threatens pediatric cancer research and clinical trials programs.	Groups lobby on federal and state levels for increased funding.[39]
Funding cutbacks reduce personnel and care for children.	Groups support and fund additional personnel for hospitals and clinics.[40]
Children in treatment lack recreational opportunities; families need places to go away together, with medical support available if needed.	Groups develop camps and respite care programs.[4,41]
Families find civil service barriers to employment of cured cancer survivors.	Candlelighters Childhood Cancer Foundation provides resources to individual surviving patients; Long Island Candlelighters lobby New York legislature to change prohibitive regulations.[42]
Parents are fired, demoted, or leave work to spend time with their child with cancer.	Parent groups support fair medical and parental leave legislation and policies.[43]
Parents are concerned with prevention and early detection of cancers that appear to have a genetic basis.	Groups support research in genetic predispositions to childhood cancers and efforts to ensure access to medical and psychosocial surveillance for affected families.[44]
Parents are forced to accept reclassification as consultants or part-time employees because employer does not wish to bear insurance responsibility for a child with cancer.	Parent groups support legislation such as pooled insurance to ease the barriers to employment.[45,46]
Parents observe that their cured children cannot obtain health insurance.	Parent groups organize group advocacy for creation of legislation and enforcement policies to eliminate discrimination against cancer survivors in health insurance and employment.[47]
Families and medical care team are concerned about physical, emotional, and psychosocial late effects on childhood cancer survivors.	Groups, parents, and medical teams advocate for medical and psychosocial surveillance programs to maximize survivors' chances in overcoming secondary neoplasms and for programs of detection and remediation of residual physical, emotional, and learning deficits.[36,48,49]
Families and medical care teams become concerned about the care of children who develop transfusion-related acquired immune deficiency syndrome.	Parents work to create a support and advocacy system to meet those special needs.[50]

ment for what the child would decide, if competent to do so, and justify their intervention under *parens patria* and "best interest of the child" principles[62] or "neglect."[63-66]

Parents may be free to become martyrs themselves, but it does not follow that they are free in identical circumstances to make martyrs of their minor children.[59] Parental prerogatives have been limited where the absence of parents' consent to medical care would cause the child serious injury, and courts are beginning to take a more protective role.[63,65,67]

The question is more difficult when life does not hang in the balance or when treatment is only minimally life-prolonging.[68] Usually, if the treatment would only prolong life rather than providing the opportunity for cure, or when gains are offset by the devastating effects of treatment, the court will not order treatment. For example, to a family or child, amputation of a limb may be an appropriate trade-off for a cure, but necrotizing leukoencephalopathy (see Chaps. 15 and 50) may not be.[69]

In one case, a family was taken to court by the treatment facility when they declined to allow their child to complete a course of chemotherapy and opted instead for a "nutritional therapy" program. The court declined to intervene to order the child to continue chemotherapy even though the earlier course of chemotherapy had put her into remission and even though her physicians testified that her remission would be short-lived.[70] This case demonstrates the need to educate the legal system on the illusion of health that is quickly stolen if curative therapy is not completed. Rules[70] should govern physicians' decisions to intervene in opposition to parental decisions: Will the intervention alter the end result for the child? Will it improve the child's comfort and quality of life?[70]

The Minor

The traditional role of the minor in medical treatment was "enforced passivity," in which a physician could not treat a child without parental or guardian consent. This legal view of children as chattel has undergone considerable erosion. It is a given in the structure of pediatric cancer care that the child be involved in the consent process to the fullest extent possible, consistent with age and understanding.[71,72] Children age 6 and older are usually able to understand and assent, and children 14 years or older are expected to be able to consent independently,[73,74] even though their consent, if they are under their parents' care, cannot be legally enforced.[74]

Emancipated and Mature Minors

Although most children are the responsibility of their parents until age 18,[75] in some jurisdictions a legally emancipated minor can consent to medical care. A minor may be deemed emancipated if he or she is married, in the armed services, or self-supporting and living apart from parents; or if the parents have failed to meet their legal responsibilities or a judicial decree has been issued.[68] The mature minor's decision to receive treatment may permit the omission of parental consent if the minor is 15 years old or older and able to understand procedures and risks, the medical procedure is for the patient's benefit, and the treatment is considered necessary when measured against conservative medical opinion or there are good reasons (*e.g.,* absence) why parental consent cannot be obtained.[76] However, when serious surgery, as for the treatment of a brain tumor, is involved, it is considered unthinkable that parental consent would be omitted when dealing with a mature, as opposed to an emancipated, minor.[69,76] As an intervention increases in potential risks or benefits, the level of ability required to make a competent judgment to choose or refuse the procedure should also increase.[69,76,77]

Medical Care Team's Role

The medical care community has an option—court intervention—when irrational decisions by parent, guardian, minor, or physician imperil life.[56,57,70] In the usual model for dealing with adult patients, the caregiver must determine if refusal of treatment is related to psychological distortion, interpersonal dysfunction, medical systems dysfunction, depression, or organic mental disorder; resolution of dysfunction may resolve the refusal.[78,79] If none of these factors precipitated refusal, and if there is truly informed refusal based on a value system entitled to respect and in keeping with the risks and benefits of treatment alternatives, refusal would be respected in adults and should therefore be respected in emancipated minors.[69,78,79] This same system should be employed to examine parents' motives for refusing treatment for their child. For example, in a case of irreversible disease, parental refusal of life-prolonging treatment and substitution of "laying on of hands" or prayer may be preferable to court action wresting a child from the comfort of his or her family.

Courts and families need to be aware that cooperation with the medical regimen does make a difference in survival and length of remission in childhood cancers.[80] When considering informed consent, refusal, and rehabilitation issues, the medical care team should be aware of findings that those cooperating and choosing curative paths had positive self-images and supportive family relationships,[80] belief in control of personal health,[81] and the opportunity to participate in informal patient support groups.[82]

The more supportive and open the relationship between medical caretakers and parents, the less likely it is that the needs of the child will be concealed or overlooked, and the greater the opportunity to mediate a settlement of medical care differences without recourse to the courts.[83] Full and open disclosure and communication may provoke anxiety but is the only course that balances and protects the rights of all participants in cure.[84,85]

Faith Healing

The balance of parental and medical caretakers' rights and obligations is most apparent in the area of faith healing. Faith healing is the belief that prayer and faith alone can cure disease and that medical means are superfluous. This is to be distinguished from deep religious faith and belief that the laying on of hands and praying for divine intervention can achieve a cure *along* with medical help, as a God-given tool for mankind. Faith healing poses a danger only if it deprives a child of recourse to potentially beneficial care. Forty-four states have statutes that protect parents from prosecution for child abuse because their child is receiving spiritual healing instead of medical care.[86] However, these protections do not diminish the court's obligation to compel medical treatment when needed to prevent the endangerment of the child's life,[87] even in some cases when the situation is not life-threatening. For example, chemotherapy treatment was mandated by a court for a 12-year-old girl with Ewing's sarcoma on the rationale that the state as *parens patriae* has a special duty to protect minors and make decisions on their behalf where life-threatening issues are involved, even though the child and her family insisted that the only help they wanted was through their religion.[58]

Innovative Treatments

Families cannot be truly informed advocates without full information on the risks and benefits of innovative research therapy. Information required[88] will vary with the therapy. For ethical and·legal protection, it is imperative that treatment facilities have a process to test patient and family satisfaction with the consent process as a check on whether they are doing their job of communicating information effectively.[88-91] The three most frequently cited reasons for parental acceptance of innovative or research treatment are the belief that it will effect cure, belief that the child's illness will worsen otherwise, and desire to be part of a research effort.[88,89,92,93]

When randomized trials are involved, for example, are both alternatives really equal? To parents, randomized trials can sound like Russian roulette: "Why should we go with an unknown?" "How can we advocate for our child if we don't have a choice?" These are hard questions, but not impossible to answer if families understand that randomization only pits two options of equal value or equal ambiguity against each other[92] and that their physician would not suggest randomization if one treatment was proven to be of more benefit than the other (see also Chaps. 13 and 15).[84,85,92]

Treatments of Last Resort

What of the family that has exhausted therapy of proven curative potential and still seeks treatment? It is at this stage of the discussion of treatments that the family is most vulnerable.[92-95] Holland and others suggest that Phase I and II studies are viewed as the *expected* continuation of the therapeutic process and "a nondecision."[93] As suggested by the Holland study, informed consent is more a process to test the capacity to trust the physician and his or her medical judgment in the last-resort cases than to make an independent medical decision,[96] and the legal and ethical implications of such shared responsibility reinforce the need for physicians' continued assessment of "their role as influencers of the decisions-making process."[96] Thus, caregivers must be prepared to be the primary advocates,[93-95] ensuring that families have received the same information on the ambiguity of early-phase clinical trial potential, its impact on quality of life, and its risks and benefits that they would insist on if they were the patient.[92-95]

Donors

Bone marrow transplants are becoming an increasing treatment of choice in childhood cancers. Special consents must be obtained from the related or unrelated donors[92,97-99] and protection of the donor from coercion must be provided, particularly for minors,[92,97] because there may be a conflict of interest for the parents as both advocate for the transplant and consentor for the related minor donor (see also Chap. 48).[92,97-99]

Questionable Therapies

There are few reported cases involving the seduction of families of children with cancer to unproven, questionable therapies. For the most part, parent inquiry into such therapies occurs either when children are in end-stage disease[101-104] or when parents seeking to enhance their child's overall health add alleged nutritional therapies to the proven therapies.[70,101,105] Those advocating questionable therapies prey on the natural desire of parents to protect their children from needless suffering, advising avoidance of surgery and treatment side-effects by use of their "nontoxic" therapies.[100,104-108] Questionable publications contain glowing reports of success in treating childhood cancers with laetrile and metabolic therapy.[107] The Chad Green case provides an excellent discussion of the results when the potential for cure is threatened by parental recourse to a questionable therapy. In this case, which evaluated the use of laetrile in place of chemotherapy for leuke-

mia,[56] the judge invoked the doctrine of substituted judgment and decided that, balancing the factors for and against treatment, a rational competent person would undergo chemotherapy. The decision focused on the medical consequences to the child if he was left untreated.

The Massachusetts Supreme Court affirmed this decision and held that the record supported the lower court's four tenets:

(1) That acute lymphocytic leukemia in children is fatal if untreated; (2) that chemotherapy is the only available medical treatment offering a hope for cure; (3) that the risks of the treatment are minimal when compared to the consequences of allowing the disease to go untreated; and (4) that the parents are unwilling to continue the child's chemotherapy, regardless of the consequences. We conclude that these findings were supported by the evidence and were sufficient to meet the requirements of the care and protection statute.

Judge Volterra found the Greens sincere but their medical policy untenable because their fear of chemotherapy was unsubstantiated and they failed to propose a reasonable alternate treatment. He found the parents' conduct indicated an unwillingness to provide necessary and proper care and ordered the child placed in legal custody of the Massachusetts Department of Public Welfare to undergo chemotherapy. Physical custody of the child remained with the parents.

In contrast, in *in re Hofbauer,*[109] the New York Appellate Court affirmed a lower court ruling that parents could decide to have their child, who had Hodgkin's disease, undergo alleged metabolic therapy that consisted of laetrile, enzymes, and vitamins. This court did not rule on the merits of a proven therapy versus laetrile, which was the issue in the Chad Green case, but rather on whether the parents supplied the child with adequate medical treatment. Using a child abuse criterion, the judge found that the parent has the primary right to select medical care and that the state had failed to prove that the choice of laetrile therapy instead of proven therapy constituted parental neglect. A factor in the court decision was that a local doctor was giving the questionable treatment and had promised to bring the child for appropriate proven therapy if his condition deteriorated. This, however, did not happen; the child went from metabolic to immunoaugmentive therapy and finally died of a truly curable cancer. In contrast, the ruling in the Chad Green case distinguished the Hofbauer ruling by stating that, unlike Chad Green, the Hofbauer child's condition was stable, his parents had expressed an intent to resort to chemotherapy should it deteriorate, and a course of parental conduct that was demonstrably threatening the child's well-being was not established.

In the *Green* case, the appropriateness of laetrile therapy was the substantive medical question. In *Hofbauer,* the issue of the medical treatment was secondary to parental neglect; that is, the issue was not the merits of individual treatments or selection of the right or best therapy, but whether the parents had made an unreasonable choice among medical alternatives. Because the laetrile therapy was recommended by a doctor licensed to practice in the state, it was the court's view that the parents could not be charged with neglect. These cases demonstrate the need for medical advocates to be fully prepared to disprove or debunk questionable therapies when they go into court to attempt to enforce potentially curative care. Their word alone will not suffice. They must be in a position to prove that delay or interruption of therapy will derail a potentially curative path for the child.

The legal framework for actions against physicians, manufacturers, and distributors by families who have been prosyletized to accept questionable therapies implies a great potential for successful judicial recourse in informed consent and consumer fraud actions, and also has potential in the area of malpractice. The crux is whether a patient is properly informed as to the risks and benefits of a particular treatment. The lack of candor in messages directed at parents of children with cancer as to the effectiveness of questionable therapies makes a binding informed consent impossible.[101,102,110] There have been few malpractice cases involving questionable therapies; those that have been argued primarily involved consumer fraud, not malpractice.[102,103] The reluctance of families to sue often stems from their reluctance to relive a painful experience or a need to avoid the horrifying concept that a road they chose because of pressure and bad information may have contributed to their child's death.

Some of the "new approaches" of which medical caretakers should be aware in the area of questionable therapies include "gentle" chemotherapy (chemotherapy given in homeopathic dosages)[103] coupled with imagery, nutritional, metabolic, or immune therapies; and chelation, allergy, or detoxification treatments to eliminate toxicities from mercury fillings, pollutants, and "immune dysregulation" that purportedly "caused" or exacerbates the cancer.[106]

Because nutritional therapies are the adjuncts to therapy that families of pediatric cancer patients most often have recourse to, and since parents rarely disclose their use, caregivers should be aware of how these therapies are depicted by their purveyors. Most often, these purveyors inform families that doctors are not nutrition experts, and advise them that if their doctor has not heard of some special diet that supports their therapy, it proves that the physician is not knowledgeable and that talking to him or her is a waste of time. Suggestion: bring in a registered dietitian whenever a family wants nutritional advice and help to tailor a program that convinces the family you are providing the most sensible nutritional support. Point out the dangers of multi-vitamin A therapy and the possibility that some high-dose vitamin regimens might interfere with chemotherapy and laboratory tests. If you have this discussion early in treatment, you may lose your "silent" nutritional partner and the potential dangers that person may pose to curative care.

PUBLIC ADVOCACY

Children with cancer are a minority group; they do not have the overwhelming numbers that make for successful lobbying for appropriations or policies needed for their survival and sustenance. Their families are young, struggling, and usually without the financial support to buy publicity or fund social services and research. More and more children are being cured, but this means fewer "terminal" sob stories that attract press coverage and rally the greater public to expend necessary resources to attack the childhood cancers that are resistant to cure. Families of children with cancer want to be normal and do not willingly seek publicity to push their agenda.

Effective advocacy therefore must involve the professionals who serve our children, along with our challenged families. Childhood cancer needs to be adopted as a social cause as well as a medical cause by those who treat children and by their professional societies, which have the necessary clout to remove barriers both to cure and to full, productive lives following cure.

REFERENCES

1. Nathanson MN: Family roles in medical decisions. Candlelighters Childhood Cancer Foundation Quarterly Newsletter 6(1):1,3, 1982
2. Saphier MK: When being challenged, know your role as a parent. Candlelighters Childhood Cancer Foundation Progress Reports 4:4–13, 1984
3. Blotcky AD: Helping adolescents with cancer cope with their disease. Semin Oncol Nurs 2(2):117–122, 1986
4. Koocher GP: Psychosocial issues during the acute treatment of pediatric cancer. Cancer 58:468–472, 1986
5. Adams-Greely M: Psychological staging of pediatric cancer patients and their families. Cancer 58(2, Suppl):449–453, 1986
6. Pizzo P: Parent to Parent: Working Together for Ourselves and Our Children. Boston, Beacon Press, 1983
7. Tebbi CK, Stern M, Boyle M, Mittin CJ, Mindell E: The role of social support systems in adolescent cancer amputees. Cancer 56:965–971, 1985
8. Monaco GP: Resources available to the family of the child with cancer. Cancer 58(2, Suppl):516–521, 1986
9. Candlelighters Childhood Cancer Foundation Quarterly Newsletter 8:3, Summer 1984
10. Petrovich v. California Western States Life Insurance, Case No. 3100 85, Superior Court of California, County of Sacramento; Ruling of May 17, 1984 [The procedure was not experimental because life and death were in the balance: "This was . . . a treatment medically approved . . . to treat and possibly to save the life of the patient, consistent with the opinion of the most eminent oncologists."]
11. Clifton Guilot, et al v. Dr. William Cherry, Director DHHR, Louisiana, Civil Action No. 79-4371, United States District Court, Eastern District of Louisiana [State medical aid programs should include bone marrow transplantation as medically necessary.]
12. Department of Defense Directive, Physical Standards for Enlistment, Appointment, and Induction Number 6130.3, 1–45, March 1986
13. Redd E: Families of pediatric patients get help from treatment guides. Oncol Times 3:32, March 1986
14. Richards HG, Benson J, Pitel AU, Pitel PA, Forman EN: The parent consultant role in pediatric oncology. Candlelighters Childhood Cancer Foundation Progress Reports 6(2/3):5–8, 1986
15. Wild E: Alternative methods of communication. Proceedings of the American Cancer Society Third National Conference on Human Values and Cancer, Washington, DC, April 23–25, 1981
16. Lansky SB, Lowman JT, Gyulay JE, Briscoe K: A team approach to coping with cancer. In Cullen JW, Fox BH, Isom RN (eds): Cancer: The Behavioral Dimensions, pp 295–308. New York, Raven Press, 1976
17. Wild E: Alternative methods of communication. In Proceedings of the American Cancer Society Third National Conference on Human Values and Cancer, p 42, April 23–25, 1981, Washington, DC. New York, American Cancer Society, 1981
18. Chesler M, Barbarin O: Childhood Cancer and the Family. New York, Brunner/Mazel, in press
19. Chesler M, Yoak M: Self-help groups for parents of children with cancer. In Roback HB (ed): Helping Patients and Their Families Cope with Medical Problems. San Francisco, Jossey-Bass, 1984
20. Yoak M, Chesney B, Schwartz N: Active roles in self-help groups for parents of children with cancer. Child Health Care 14(1):38–45, 1985
21. Toseland RW, Hacker L: Social workers' use of self-help groups as a resource for clients. Social Work 30:232–237, 1985
22. Toseland RW, Hacker L: Self-help groups and professional involvement. Social Work 27:341–347, 1982
23. Chesler M, Barbarin O: Difficulties of providing help in crisis: Relationships between parents of children with cancer and their friends. Social Issues 40(4):113–134, 1984
24. Nathanson MN, Monaco GP: Meeting the educational and psychosocial needs produced by a diagnosis of pediatric/adolescent cancer. Health Educ 10(Suppl):67–75, Spring 1984
25. Monaco GP, Nathanson MN: Candlelighters parent groups as a preventive mental health factor in the loss and grieving process. Proceedings of the Foundation Thanatology Symposium, Children and Death: Perspectives from Birth Through Adolescence, 1983 (in press)
26. Nathanson MN: Organizing and Maintaining Support Groups for Parents of Children with Chronic Illness and Handicapping Conditions. Washington, DC, Association for Care of Children's Health, 1986
26a. Bogue E-L, Chesney BK: Making contact: A parent-to-parent visitation manual. Washington, DC, Candlelighters Childhood Cancer Foundation, 1987
27. Candlelighters Childhood Cancer Foundation: Annotated Bibliography and Resource Guide. Washington, DC, Candlelighters Childhood Cancer Foundation, 1987
28. Candlelighters lobby for cancer research. Voluntary Action News 5, September/October 1974
29. Teta MJ et al: Psychosocial consequences of childhood cancer and adolescent cancer survival. Chronic Dis 39:751–759, 1986
30. Monaco GP: Socioeconomic considerations in childhood cancer survival:

Society's obligation. The University of Texas M. D. Anderson Hospital and Tumor Institute Tenth Annual Mental Health Conference, Childhood Cancer Survivors: Living Beyond Cure, April 11–12, 1985

31. Cutter JJ, et al: Childhood leukemia in Woburn, Massachusetts. Public Health Rep 101(2):201–205, 1986

32. US House of Representatives, 93rd Congress, 2nd Session, Report No. 93-954, National Cancer Amendments of 1974, Report to accompany HR 13053, p 12

33. Connecticut Candlelighters: The changing scene of childhood cancer workshop. Candlelighters Foundation Organization and Information Handbook, revised edition, 1980

34. Deasy-Spinetta P: School intervention and ongoing process; Meadows A: Learning problems associated with therapy for acute lymphocytic leukemia (ALL); Gustafson M: School experiences for children with cancer. Candlelighters Foundation Progress Reports 6(3):9–12, 1984

35. Williams L: Easing medical bills: Childhood cancer assistance program funds help families in need. New Berlin Citizen (WI), December 8, 1983

36. Pommer B: A battle lost, a dream born. Candlelighters Childhood Cancer Foundation Quarterly Newsletter 7(4):7, 1983

37. COPE (Cincinnati Oncology Parents Endeavor) scholarship program guidelines. Candlelighters Foundation Quarterly Newsletter 5(1):3, 1981

38. Steven J: Sackler scholarship. Candlelighters Childhood Cancer Foundation Quarterly Newsletter 11(1):6, 1987

39. Statement of the Candlelighters before the Subcommittee on Labor, Health, Education and Welfare of the Committee on Appropriations, United States Senate, 1970–1986: Statement of the Candlelighters before the Subcommittee on Labor-HEW, of the House Committee on Appropriations, 1970–1986. Group News: Missouri. Candlelighters Foundation Quarterly Newsletter 5(3):10, 1981

40. Group News: Missouri. Candlelighters Foundation Quarterly Newsletter 5(3):10, 1981

41. Camps for children with cancer and their siblings. Candlelighters Childhood Cancer Foundation Quarterly Newsletter 7(2):1,4, 1983

42. Zeldis N: Beating cancer discrimination. New York Times, July 27, 1986

43. Schroeder P: US House of Representatives, 99th Congress, 2nd Session, HR 2020, 1985 ["To require that employees be allowed parental leave in cases involving birth, adoption or serious illness of a child and temporary disability leave in cases involving inability to work. . . ."]

44. Etaganti RSK, German J (eds): Genetics in Clinical Oncology, pp 35–54; 237–238. New York, Oxford University Press, 1985

45. Klagstad N: Coping with insurance. Candlelighters Childhood Cancer Foundation Quarterly Newsletter 7(4):7, 1983

46. Cystic Fibrosis Foundation: Pooled risk insurance: New bills in congress. Commitment, Spring/Summer 1986

47. Biaggi M: US House of Representatives, 99th Congress, 1st Session, HR 1294, 1985 [To amend Title VII of the Civil Rights Act of 1964 to prohibit employment discrimination on the basis of a cancer history]

48. Dobkin PL, Morrow GR: Long-term side effects in patients who have been treated successfully for cancer. J Psychosoc Oncol 34(4):23–51, 1986

49. D'Angio GJ: The child cured of cancer: A problem for the internist. In Perry MC, Yarbro JW (eds): Toxicity of Chemotherapy, pp 507–519. New York, Grune & Stratton, 1984

50. Board of Education of the City of Plainfield v. Cooperman, 507 A 2d 253 (N.J. Super. 1986)

51. Hartmann O, et al: Treatment of advanced neuroblastoma with high-dose melphalan and autologous bone marrow transplantation. Cancer Chemother Pharmacol 16:165–169, 1986

52. Wickline v. State of California, 228 Cal. Rptr. 661,671 (Cal. App. 2 Dist, 1986)

53. Investigational new drug, antibiotic and biological drug product regulations: Treatment used and sale. Fed Register 521(53):8850–8857, March 19, 1987

54. Applebaum PS: The rising tide of patients rights' advocacy. Hosp Community Psychiatry 37:9–10, 1986

55. Truman JT, Brant J: Ethical and legal issues in the treatment of children with cancer. Am J Pediatr Hematol Oncol 6(3):313–317, 1984

56. Custody of a Minor (Chad Green), 379 N.E. 2d 1053 (Massachusetts 1978), on review aff'd 393 N.E. 2d 836 (1979)

57. Hofbauer: May parents choose unorthodox medical care for their child? Albany Law Review 44:818, 1980

58. In re Hamilton; 657 S.W. 2d 425 (Tenn. App. 1983)

59. Prince v. Massachusetts, 321 U.S. 158, 168 (1944)

60. Brown A, Truitt B: The rights of minors to medical treatment. De Paul Law Review 28:289, 1979

61. Judicial limitations on parental autonomy in the medical treatment of minors. Nebraska Law Review 59:1093, 1980

62. The minor's right to consent to medical treatment; A corollary of the constitutional right to privacy. Southern California Law Review 48:1417, 1434–1443, 1979

63. People ex rel. Wallace v. Labrenz, 411 lll, 618,104 N.E. 2d 769,773 (1952). [Parents' refusal to permit emergency transfusion warranted finding of child neglect.]

64. Morrison v. State, 252 S.W. 2d 97,102 (K.C. App. 1952). [Parents refusal to permit emergency transfusion violated natural law duty of parents to provide for children.]

65. State v. Perricone, 37 N.J. 462, 181 A. 2d 751, 759. [Parents' refusal to permit emergency transfusion warranted finding of neglect.]

66. In re Santos v. Goldstein, 16 A.D. 755, 277 N.Y.S. 2d 750, 751 (1962)

67. In re Clark, 900 Ind. L. Abs. 21, 185 N.E. 2d 128 (1962). [Emergency blood infusion.]

68. Baron CH: Medicine and human rights; Emergency substantive standards and procedural protections for medical decision making with the American family. Family Law Q 17(1):4–6, 1983

69. Holder AR: Legal Issues in Pediatrics and Adolescent Medicine, 2nd ed, pp 119–141. New Haven, Yale University Press, 1985

70. In the Interest of M.H., A Minor, Docket No. 22B, Court of Common Pleas of Somerset Co. PA (November 17, 1983), Slip opinion at 30

71. Van Eys J, Vietti TJ: Pediatric cooperative trial groups in the 80's; Challenges and opportunities. Cancer Bull 34:117–120, 1982

72. Bartholome WG: The ethical rights of the child patient. Front Radiat Ther Oncol 16:156–166, 1982

73. Cogliano-Shulta NA: Pediatric Phase I clinical trials: Ethical issues and nursing considerations. Oncol Nurs Forum 13(2):29–32, 1986

74. Rae WA, Fournier EJ: Ethical issues in pediatric research: Preserving psychosocial care in scientific inquiry. Child Health Care 14:242–248, 1986

75. Kjonstad A: Informed consent in medical research. Med Law 5:11–15, 1986

76. Holder AR: Legal issues in pediatrics and adolescent medicine, 2nd ed, pp 134–135. New Haven, Yale University Press, 1985

77. President's Commission: Making Health Care Decisions, vol 1, p 60. Washington, DC, US Government Printing Office, 1982

78. Goldberg RJ: Systemic understanding of cancer patients who refuse treatment. Psychother Psychosom 39:180–189, 1983

79. Culver CM, Gert B: Philosophy in Medicine: Conceptual and Ethical Issues in Medicine and Psychiatry. New York, Oxford University Press, 1982

80. Smith SD, Rosen D, Truesworthy RC et al: A reliable method for evaluating drug compliance in children with cancer. Cancer 43:169–173, 1979

81. Jameson RN, Lewis S, Burgich T: Cooperation with treatment in adolescent cancer patients. J Adolesc Health Care 7:162–167, 1986

82. Waller DA, Altshuler KZ: Perspectives on patient noncompliance. Hosp Community Psychiatry 37:490–496, 1986

83. Note: Faith healing exemptions to child protection laws: Keeping the faith versus medical care for children. J Legislation 12:243–263, 1985

84. Simes RJ et al: Randomized comparison of procedures for obtaining informed consent in clinical trials of treatment for cancer. Br Med J 293:1065, 1986

85. Miller DR, Haupt EA: Clinical Cancer Research: Patient, Parent and Physician Interactions 5:43–65, 1984

86. Report H: Religious exemptions in child abuse legislation. American Medical Association, Report of the Board of Trustees, Reference Committee B, 1986

87. Child Health Care Is a Legal Duty. Sioux City, IA, CHILD, Inc, 1987

88. Monaco GP: Informed consent: Does the consent process reflect the realities of current treatment, procedures and side effects? Am J Pediatr Hematol Oncol 5:401–407, 1983

89. Annas GJ: The care of private patients in teaching hospitals: Legal complications. Bull NY Acad Med 56:403–411, 1980

90. Morrow G, Gottnick J, Schmale A: A simple technique for increasing cancer patients' knowledge of informed consent to treatment. Cancer 42:793–799, 1978

91. Eth S, Eth C, Edgar H: Case studies: Can a research subject be too eager to consent? Hastings Center Rep 11:20–21, 1981

92. Bone Marrow Transplantation in Childhood Cancer. Candlelighters Childhood Cancer Foundation Progress Reports, Special Issue 5, 1985

93. Lesko LM et al: Parental and physician perception of informed consent for pediatric allogeneic bone marrow transplantation. Proc Am Soc Oncology 5:240, 1986

94. Leikin S et al: Beyond pro forma consent for childhood cancer research. J Clin Oncol 3:420–428, 1985

95. Light SE, Holland JC, Tan C: Attitude of parents toward phase chemotherapy for their child. Proc Am Soc Clin Oncol 3:73, 1984

96. Patenaude AF et al: The physician's influence on informed consent for bone marrow transplantation. Theor Med 7:165–179, 1986

97. Brant J: Legal issues involving BMT to minors. Am J Pediatr Hematol Oncol 6:89–91, 1984

98. Briggs NC et al: On willingness to be a bone marrow donor. Transfusion 26:324–330, 1986

99. Mallory SD et al: Family coercion and valid consent. Theor Med 7:123–126, 1986

100. Cassileth BR et al: Contemporary unorthodox treatments in cancer medicine. Ann Intern Med 101:105–112, 1984

101. Peters v. Dr. Harold Manner et al, Docket No. 83L 22441, Circuit Court of Cook County, Illinois County Department, Law Division. [Vitamin A toxicity, metabolic therapy, consumer fraud.]

102. Zabodyn v. Dr. Stanislaw R. Burzynski, Docket No. 83-29081, District Court, Harris County, Texas 269th Judicial District. [Settled; antineoplastic treatment, consumer fraud.]

103. RA et al v. Prudential Insurance Company of America, Docket No. L 8093-79, Superior Court of New Jersey, Law Division (August 6, 1982)

104. Holland JC: Why patients seek unproven cancer remedies: A psychological perspective. CA 32(1):10–14, 1982

105. Monaco GP: The impact of the laetrile phenomenon on the legal profession: Technology by experiment or technology by oath helpers. Jurimetrics J Law Sci Technol 21(2/3): Winter 1980, Spring 1981

106. Monaco GP: The primary care physician: The first line of defense in the battle against health fraud. Med Times, May 1986

107. Chemotherapy and radiation damage and side effects. Cancer Control J 5:3–6, 1978

108. Herbert V: Unproven (questionable) dietary and nutritional methods on cancer prevention and treatment. Cancer 58:1930–1941, 1986

109. *In re* Hofbauer, 65 A.D. 2d 108, 411 N.Y.S. 2d 416 (1978) affirmed, 47 N.Y.S. 2d 648, 393 N.E. 2d 1009, 419 N.Y.S. 2d 936 (1979)

110. Floyd, Lewis v. American International Hospital, Docket No. 80-1020799A, Circuit Court of Cook County, Illinois County Department, Law Division. [Metabolic therapy for cancer; malpractice.]

Future Perspectives

part seven

fifty-four

Strategies for Applying the Principles of Pediatric Oncology to the Developing World

Ian T. Magrath,
Nazli Gad-el-Mawla,
Hai Peng Lin,
Christopher Williams,
V. Shanta, Saresh Advani,
Beatriz de Camargo,
Sergio Petrilli,
Blanca Diez,
and Luis Becu

Pediatric neoplasms account for a small proportion of all cancers, but their importance to the understanding of neoplasia and to the evolution of cancer therapy far outweighs their relative contribution to cancer deaths. Moreover, the sociologic impact of these diseases is also much greater than might be anticipated from incidence figures—childhood cancer usually disrupts family life to a much greater degree than does cancer in the elderly, can result in the loss of many more productive years of life, and arouses more poignant sympathy for its victims. Fortunately, more than half of all children with cancer can now be expected to achieve long-term survival if treated according to current optimal therapeutic standards.[1] However, on a global level this progress has not yet had a major impact on mortality rates in childhood malignancy because only a small fraction of children with cancer throughout the world have access to state-of-the-art treatment.

The 129 less developed countries account for some 76% of the world's population and 84% of all children younger than 15 years of age. If the incidence of childhood cancer throughout the world were similar to that for white children in the United States (about 130 per million children per year), there would be some 178,165 new cases of cancer in children in the less developed countries each year, as compared to 33,878 in the more developed countries—a difference of more than fivefold, and one which is steadily increasing. Thus, even without any further therapeutic developments, the worldwide mortality from pediatric cancer could be greatly reduced simply by raising the standards of treatment received by children in the less developed countries to the level of the more developed nations. Although such estimates are of necessity crude, they serve to illustrate the size of the problem.

Contrasts Between Less and More Developed Nations

In this chapter, we consider the problems that beset the oncologist treating childhood cancer in the less developed countries. Although common themes recur, it must be realized that these countries represent a broad spectrum with regard to general levels of development and standards of medical care. In some countries, issues of food and water supply and sanitation eclipse all other health issues. Where such basic problems have largely been surmounted, more resources can be devoted to dealing with other health problems such as cancer, and cancer assumes a much greater significance as a cause of morbidity and mortality. Even within individual countries, there are enormous differences in the incomes and lifestyles of different segments of the population. In some parts of Africa and the South American jungles, for example, some people still live as hunter-gatherers or herdsmen, with limited or no access to modern medicine and very little comprehension of 20th century community life. Yet the same nations often possess large cities and abundant industry.

Although economic disparity is the most obvious difference in overall living

LESS DEVELOPED REGIONS
POPULATION BY AGE (MALES AND FEMALES)

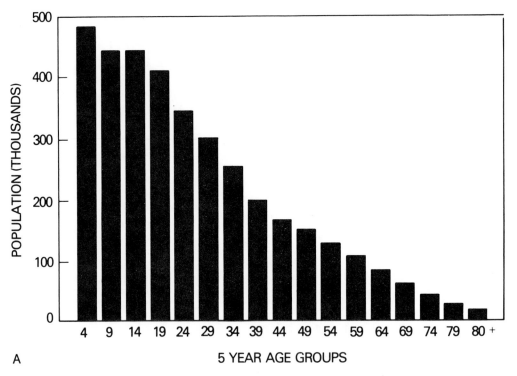

A

MORE DEVELOPED REGIONS
POPULATION BY AGE (MALES AND FEMALES)

FIGURE 54-1. Histograms showing the proportions of the population in different age groups in less developed regions (**A**) and more developed regions (**B**). Figures are 1985 estimates projected in 1982 and were obtained from Reference 7. More developed regions include Europe, North America, the USSR, Japan, Australia, and New Zealand. All other countries are included in the less developed regions. Data are arranged in 5-year age groups, indicated on the histograms by the highest year in the 5-year group (*e.g.,* 0–4 yrs is depicted as 4). All individuals older than 85 years of age are included as a single group.

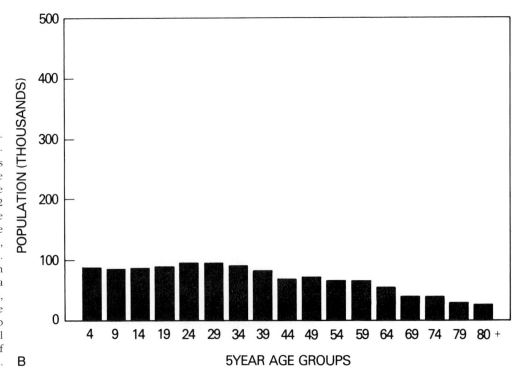

B

standards between the more and less developed nations, simply infusing money—although an essential component of efforts to redress inequalities—would not produce immediate resolution of these differences. Improvement of health care in the less developed nations, particularly in the context of diseases that require relatively prolonged and complex treatment, will require major efforts, sustained over many years, which take into consideration the vast differences in values, education, and beliefs between populations of less and more developed countries. In the specific context of childhood neoplasms, there may also be biological, and consequently clinical, differences leading to differences in the response to treatment. Further, toxicities of chemotherapeutic agents may differ significantly in populations where chronic malnourishment and infections are the rule, and where standards of hygiene often differ markedly from those of the more developed nations. Consequently, it is essential to develop approaches to diagnosis and treatment relevant to the circumstances that exist in specific less developed countries.

Research Opportunities

Despite the often overwhelming logistic and financial problems in many developing countries, there are also numerous important research opportunities that are likely to benefit pediatric oncology in general. For example, the less developed countries provide a much better paradigm for exploring the influence of environmental factors on the incidence of neoplasms because of the extreme contrasts in lifestyles that exist within a given country. In the more developed countries, standards of hygiene, exposure to infectious agents, access to and standards of health care, and the overall standard of living differ much less between the richest and poorest segments of the populations. Moreover, as living standards of the most un-

derprivileged communities of the less developed countries improve, there will be opportunities to examine the consequent alterations in the spectrum of neoplasms. A precedent for such alterations exists in the observed changes in the pattern of lymphoid neoplasms seen in the Gaza Strip during a period of rapid socioeconomic development.[2] It is probable that some tumors occur much more frequently, or even exclusively, in the less developed countries. Such tumors are far from being irrelevant to the rest of the world, and may provide important insights into oncogenesis and valuable information relevant to all aspects of oncology. A good example is endemic Burkitt's lymphoma (see Chap. 20). Also, clinical trials can sometimes be completed more rapidly than in the more developed nations, because single centers often see very large numbers of patients. This is a consequence both of the limited number of specialized centers and of the increased proportion of children in the populations of these countries.

It is clear that devoting greater resources to the study of pediatric neoplasms in the less developed nations will provide benefits that transcend the immediate social and humanitarian implications. Accordingly, there is much to be gained from the establishment of effective collaborative efforts between the less and more developed countries. However, to accomplish this, a greater awareness of the opportunities for scientific re-

FIGURE 54-2. Percentages of world births in different world regions. Estimates are based on live birth-rates between 1980 and 1985 and latest available population estimates during this period and were obtained from data in Reference 3. The more developed region is defined as in Figure 54-1.

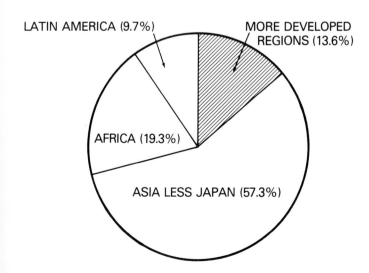

WORLD BIRTHS 1980—85
PERCENT BY REGION

LATIN AMERICA (9.7%)

MORE DEVELOPED REGIONS (13.6%)

AFRICA (19.3%)

ASIA LESS JAPAN (57.3%)

Table 54-1
Population Estimates by Age Groups (1985)

	Total Population (millions)	*Percentage by Age Group*		
		<15 Years	*15–64 Years*	*65+ Years*
World	4,842	34	61	6
Macro Regions				
Africa	553	45	52	3
Asia (all)	2,824	35	61	4
Latin America	406	38	58	4
North America*	263	22	67	11
Europe	492	21	67	12
USSR†	278	25	66	9
Oceania‡	24.8	28	63	8
Less developed regions§	3,668.8	37	59	4
More developed regions	1,172	22	67	11
Selected Regions				
West Africa	168	45	52	3
East Africa	161	47	50	3
North Africa	125	43	53	4
Japan	120	21	69	10
China	1,063	31	64	5
South Asia	1,572	39	57	3
West Europe	154	18	69	13
East Europe	113	24	66	11
Australia/N.Z.	19	24	66	10
Other Oceania	5.8	43	54	3

(From the Demographic Year Book, United Nations, 1984)

* Including Hawaii.

† Not included with Europe or Asia.

‡ Excluding Hawaii.

§ Here taken as Africa; Asia minus Japan; Latin America; and Oceania minus Australia and New Zealand. Newly industrialized nations (Taiwan, Hong Kong, Singapore, and South Korea) are included with the less developed nations.

search and of the problems encountered in the developing countries must first be instilled into the academic medical community of the more developed nations.

DEMOGRAPHIC CONSIDERATIONS

Population Structure, Births, and Deaths

Several characteristics relevant to pediatric neoplasms distinguish the population structures of the less developed from the more developed countries.[3-7] The less developed countries have a relatively high proportion of children in their populations because of their higher birthrates and shorter life expectancies (Figs. 54-1 and 54-2; Tables 54-1 and 54-2). In the 20 countries that have the lowest age structure (all less developed nations), between 46% and 52% of the population was younger than 15 years in 1984—more than twice the percentage in the 20 countries (all more developed) with the highest age structure (16%–23%).[7] The less developed nations, with an overall crude birthrate of 31.2 per 1000 between 1980 and 1985 (compared to 15.5 per 1000 for the more developed nations), account for more than 86% of all births in the world, and have almost 10 times the average annual increment in population of the more developed countries—70.4 million compared to 7.4 million between 1980 and 1985. Estimated life expectancy at birth (1980–1985) in the less developed regions is 56.6 years as compared to 73 years in the more developed regions.[7] Although the perinatal mortality rate is considerably higher in the less developed countries—91 per 1000 births, compared to 17 per 1000 births between 1980 and 1985 in the more developed countries—this has a relatively small impact on the rate of increase of the population, although it could conceivably influence the pattern of disease in childhood.

These figures strongly suggest that pediatric neoplasms are likely to account for a much higher proportion of cancer deaths in the less developed nations. This is, in fact, the case as is demonstrated in Table 54-3, which lists childhood deaths from cancer as a percentage of all cancer deaths in selected

countries. In the less developed countries, the proportion of cancer deaths due to childhood neoplasms is quite variable—between 0.77% and 10.06%. In contrast, in the more developed countries, 0.26% to 1.19% of all cancer deaths occur in children. It is probable that the magnitude of the difference is much greater than is suggested in Table 54-3 because most of the less developed countries included are in Latin America. In the least developed nations, for which recent data are not available, childhood cancer deaths probably account for an even greater proportion of all cancer deaths, so that the overall difference between more and less developed countries is probably greater than 10-fold. It should be borne in mind that these figures are for cancer deaths, not incidence, for which relatively little information is available in most of the less developed countries. Interestingly, there are not clear-cut differences in mortality rates for childhood neoplasms between the more and less developed countries (Table 54-4). Available figures, however, are probably inaccurate because of incomplete and incorrect reporting of the causes of death, a problem that increases with decreasing levels of development of a country.

Although childhood cancer in the less developed countries is relatively more important as a fraction of cancer deaths in all age groups, it usually accounts for a much lower proportion of all deaths in childhood because of the very high perinatal mortality rates and the high frequency of deaths from infectious and parasitic diseases (Fig. 54-3 and Table 54-5). Because deaths from infection decrease markedly after the age of 1, cancer as a cause of death in childhood becomes relatively more important. From age 5 years on, death rates from cancer become similar to those from infection in the most advanced of the less developed nations, and in these countries assume a similar degree of importance as a cause of all deaths in children age 5 years or older (Table 54-5). Because the highest mortality rates in children, particularly in the less developed countries, are in the very young, one crude measure of the level of development of a country is the percentage of infants who fail to survive to the age of 5 years. In equatorial African countries and many Asian countries, this figure was between 15% and 25% in 1980 to 1985.[3] In only a few African or Asian

Table 54-2
Birth and Death Rates, Life Expectancy, and Rate of Increase in Population

	Population*		Rate of Increase†	Birth Rate‡	Death Rate§	Life Expectancy‖
Region	*1950*	*1984*				
World	2,504	4,763	1.7	27	11	58.9
Africa	222	537	3.0	46	17	49.7
Asia	1,366	2,731	1.7	27	10	57.9
South Asia	695	1,539	2.2	35	13	51.8
East Asia	671	1,239	1.1	18	7	68.0
North America	166	261	0.9	16	9	74.1
Latin America	165	397	2.3	32	8	64.1
Europe	392	490	0.4	14	11	73.2
USSR	180	276	1.0	19	9	70.9
Oceania	12.6	24.5	1.5	21	8	67.6

(From the Demographic Yearbook, United Nations, 1984)

* Midyear estimates, in millions.

† Annual rate of population increase (percentage), 1980–1985.

‡ Per thousand, 1980–1985.

§ Per thousand, 1980–1985.

‖ At birth, both sexes. Estimate for 1980–1985 as assessed in 1982. Medium variant. (From World Population Prospects, United Nations, Population Studies no. 86, 1985).

countries (China, Mongolia, Thailand, Malaysia, and the newly industrialized nations) do fewer than 10% of infants fail to reach age 5, and in the poorest of nations, more than 25% of children may die in the first 5 years of life. In the more developed countries and in some South American countries (*e.g.,* Argentina and Chile), fewer than 5% of children die before 5 years, whereas in most other Latin American countries, between 5% and 10% of children die in their first 5 years of life.[3] The high mortality in young children, quite unrelated to cancer, must be taken into account when allocating health care resources, particularly since the cost of treating childhood cancer is very high, whereas many of the most important causes of death in children, such as diarrhea and enteritis, can be dealt with at very little expense. Such acute diseases require short durations of treatment, and expensive diagnostic and treatment facilities are not necessary.

The very high birthrates in the less developed countries represent a major obstacle to socioeconomic improvement. The countries with the most severe economic difficulties and most immature social (including health care) and political structures are unfortunately also the countries with the most rapid rates of increase in population, despite the fact that in such countries more than one quarter of all children fail to reach the age of 5. Whereas the population of Western Europe increased from 122 million in 1950 to 154 million in 1985 (26%), the population of Africa increased from 222 to 553 million (149%) and that of Southeast Asia from 181 to 401 million (122%) in the same period (see Table 54-2). The impact of such dramatic population increases in economically deprived areas is not difficult to envision.

Urban/Rural Distribution of Population

Apart from differences in the age structure of the population, there are many other demographic differences between the less and more developed countries. Living conditions, and thus the overall environment, differ markedly. There is little doubt that the environment (including dietary habits, tobacco consumption, exposure to certain viral infections) has a major influence on the patterns of malignant disease in general, although little information is available with regard to pediatric tumors. Crude, overall statistics may provide few insights regarding etiology, but they do provide a measure of the extent of the environmental differences. One gross but readily measurable difference in environment is whether an individual lives in a rural or urban setting. Although the precise definitions of these terms are not universally agreed upon, in the less developed countries as a whole (notwithstanding marked variation between individual countries), a much larger proportion of people live in rural areas and work on the land. The percentage of the population living in urban areas ranges from 4.6% (Rwanda) to 52% (Algeria) in Africa, 6.4% (Nepal) to 80.9% (United Arab Emirates) in Asia, and 28.0% (Haiti) to 84.3%

Table 54-3
Proportion of Annual Cancer Deaths Occurring in Children Younger Than 15 Years

	Absolute Number of Deaths from Cancer				Percentage <15 Years
	All Ages	<1 Year	1–4 Years	5–14 Years	
Less Developed Countries					
Jordan (79)*	308	4	10	17	10.06
Kuwait (85)	509	1	12	22	6.88
Egypt (80)	7,808	80	84	261	5.44
Mexico (82)	29,415	108	373	864	4.57
Sri Lanka (80)	4,120	51	67	82	4.85
Thailand (79)	9,672	24	113	258	4.08
Venezuela (83)	8,901	26	106	188	3.60
Costa Rica (83)	1,853	5	20	26	2.75
Argentina (81)	42,700	47	218	384	1.52
Uruguay (84)	6,372	1	14	34	0.77
Newly Industrialized Countries					
Singapore (85)	2,893	6	12	20	1.31
Hong Kong (85)	7,535	5	12	42	0.78
More Developed Countries					
Bulgaria (84)	14,388	6	62	103	1.19
Ireland (83)	6,471	2	16	26	0.68
Japan (85)	187,714	55	240	728	0.54
Australia (84)	25,820	8	53	126	0.72
France (84)	130,933	44	166	350	0.43
United States (83)	442,986	132	654	1,318	0.47
England/Wales (84)	138,326	22	140	264	0.31
Netherlands (84)	32,815	6	32	89	0.39
Hungary (84)	28,523	10	34	87	0.46
Austria (85)	18,837	5	16	28	0.26

(World Health Organization Statistics, 1981, 1985, and 1986)

* Numbers in parentheses indicate the year these data were collected (latest available).

Table 54-4

Mortality Rate per 100,000 Population (or Live Births for Infants) for Infectious Diseases and Cancer

	Infectious and Parasitic Diseases			Cancer		
	<1 Year	1-4 Years	5-14 Years	<1 Year	1-4 Years	5-14 Years
Less Developed Countries						
Jordan (79)*	243.4	34.8	3.8	4.4	3.2	2.4
Kuwait (85)	121.7	6.1	2.1	1.8	6.1	5.7
Egypt (80)	298.0	11.2	6.5	5.1	1.7	2.4
Mexico (82)	872.0	87.4	9.6	4.5	4.0	4.2
Sri Lanka (80)	356.1	65.6	16.6	12.2	4.4	2.2
Thailand (79)	238.7	52.7	21.3	2.2	2.0	2.1
Venezuela (83)	712.7	56.3	5.7	5.1	5.4	4.6
Costa Rica (83)	201.0	21.8	2.5	6.9	8.9	4.7
Argentina (81)	358.2	40.3	4.0	6.9	12.0	9.3
Uruguay (84)	374.7	10.6	1.3	1.9	6.5	6.4
Newly Industrialized Countries						
Singapore (85)	44.7	3.0	0.5	14.1	7.3	4.8
Hong Kong (85)	11.8	1.5	0.5	6.5	3.5	1.9
More Developed Countries						
Bulgaria (84)	65.4	6.8	1.6	4.9	12.4	7.7
Ireland (83)	22.5	7.0	0.4	3.0	5.6	3.7
Japan (85)	13.2	1.9	0.4	3.8	4.0	3.9
Australia (84)	12.0	0.8	0.4	3.4	5.6	4.9
France (84)	13.9	2.1	0.7	5.8	5.4	4.6
United States (83)	20.4	2.0	0.6	3.7	4.7	3.8
England/Wales (84)	14.4	1.9	0.5	3.5	5.6	4.1
Netherlands (84)	9.7	0.9	0.5	3.4	4.5	4.4
Hungary (84)	19.1	1.1	0.2	8.0	6.1	5.3
Austria (84)	17.9	1.9	0.7	3.4	7.4	4.0

(World Health Organization Statistics, 1981, 1985, and 1986)

* Numbers in parentheses indicate the years in which these data were collected (latest available).

(Uruguay) in South and Central America. In the more developed countries, this percentage ranges from 29.7% (Portugal) to 94.6% (Belgium). A mean of approximately 30% of the people in less developed countries live in an urban setting, compared to approximately 75% of the population in the more developed countries.[3,4]

Of course, it would be incorrect to assume that rural (or urban) environments in the less and more developed countries are in any way equivalent. In the latter, there may be rather minor differences in standards of hygiene, health care, exposure to infectious diseases, income, and education between urban and rural environments, whereas in the former, rural and urban communities usually differ markedly with respect to these criteria. In general, there is more poverty and illiteracy in rural communities in less developed regions, but hygiene is not necessarily worse than in urban communities, although exposure to certain infections and infestations (malaria, nematodes, and viruses harbored in animals and vectored by insects) may be greater. Hygiene in general, however, is poor in the less developed countries. For example, according to World Health Organization statistics,[3] only 17% of the population in the 36 least developed countries has adequate sanitary facilities, compared to 77% in the more developed countries; similarly, in these same 36 countries only 36% of the population has access to a safe water supply within 15 minutes of the home, compared to 96% in more developed regions.[3] Comparable figures for rural areas of these 36 nations are even lower

—less than 5% have adequate sanitary facilities and less than 10% a safe water supply.

Educational Standards

The educational standards of a country have a significant impact on the practice of pediatric oncology. For example, educational attainment influences income, which in turn alters lifestyle, patterns of disease, and the ability to meet the costs of illness. In the poorest of countries, it is not unusual for more than 80% of the population above the age of 25 years to have had less than a year of schooling. In such communities, hygiene is usually poor and the pattern of infectious disease (particularly relevant to the neutropenic patient) is quite different from that of communities that have reached a higher level of sophistication. Educational deficits also have consequences that are not directly dependent on economic considerations. Among the most relevant of these are the readiness of families to seek medical attention and their ability to comprehend the necessity of the prolonged therapies usually required for pediatric malignancies. In many parts of the world (*e.g.,* some African countries), modern medical care may never be sought (another reason for inaccurate statistics). Alternatively, medical advice may be sought only when the disease is at an advanced stage. This delay may be influenced by local forms of traditional or tribal medicine, or by the belief that cancer is

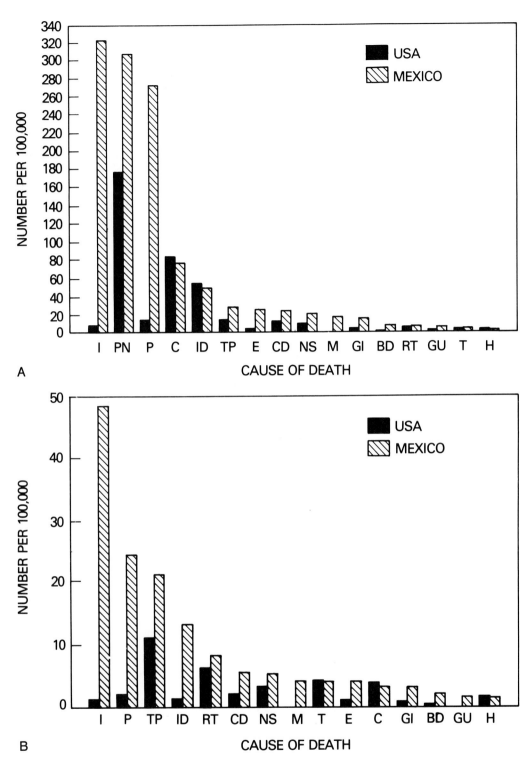

FIGURE 54-3. Comparison of the mortality rates from different causes in children in representative less (Mexico) and more developed (USA) countries. **A.** Deaths from birth to the 15th birthday. **B.** Deaths from the 1st to the 15th birthday. The histograms are arranged in descending order of frequency of each cause for Mexican children. The causes of death shown are the first 16 of a total of 21 categories in order of frequency for both countries in these age groups. The indicated causes on the X-axis follow the classification in the *Manual of the International Statistical Classification of Diseases, Injuries and Causes of Death,* Ninth revision (ICD-9), and are indicated on the histograms as follows: I, Infectious and parasitic diseases (01–07); PN, obstetric trauma and other perinatal afflictions; P, pulmonary and respiratory diseases; C, congenital anomalies; ID, ill-defined conditions; TP, accidents and adverse effects, poisoning; E, endocrine diseases; CD, circulatory disorders; NS, diseases of the nervous system; M, protein–calorie malnutrition, GI, gastrointestinal diseases; BD, anemia and other blood disorders; RT, road traffic accidents; GU, diseases of the genitourinary system; T, malignant tumors; H, homicide. (Data were obtained from World Health Statistics Annual 1986. Geneva, World Health Organization, 1986)

incurable. Even when medical attention is obtained, the administration of optimal therapy may be hindered by a family's lack of understanding of the need to return at intervals for additional treatment, coupled with the urgent necessity to return home in order to obtain a livelihood or to fend for other family members. Religious mores, customs, or simply ignorance may influence the readiness with which important tests will be permitted, or blood donated. The inability of the family to understand the need for careful surveillance for fever in a potentially neutropenic patient, or to undertake the care of an

indwelling venous catheter, may require modification of treatment plans.

Although not necessarily correlated with all of these issues, the degree of illiteracy (defined simply as an inability to read and write) provides a reasonable measure of a country's overall level of education. The illiteracy rate varies greatly among countries and among different communities or ethnic groups in a single country. In the more developed countries, illiteracy rates for people older than 25 years are nearly always below 1%, whereas rates are considerably higher in the less

Table 54-5
*Proportion of Annual Deaths Caused by Cancer in Children Younger Than 15 Years**

	<1 Year			1-4 Years			5-14 Years		
	Total	*Cancer*	*%*	*Total*	*Cancer*	*%*	*Total*	*Cancer*	*%*
Less Developed Countries									
Jordan	1,203	4	0.3	713	10	1.4	468	17	3.6
Kuwait	1,016	1	0.1	162	12	7.4	197	22	11.2
Egypt	119,290	80	0.1	52,437	84	0.2	15,954	261	1.6
Mexico	78,492	108	0.1	21,786	373	1.7	13,472	864	6.4
Sri Lanka	14,391	51	0.4	4,256	67	1.6	3,082	82	2.7
Thailand	15,224	24	0.2	16,469	113	0.7	15,075	258	1.7
Venezuela	14,106	26	0.2	3,438	106	3.1	2,052	188	9.2
Costa Rica	1,306	5	0.4	264	20	7.6	181	26	14.4
Argentina	22,881	47	0.2	4,023	218	5.4	2,664	384	14.4
Uruguay	1,593	1	0.1	212	14	6.6	184	34	18.5
Newly Industrialized Countries									
Singapore	394	6	1.5	65	12	18.5	100	20	20.0
Hong Kong	580	5	0.9	134	12	9.0	180	42	23.3
More Developed Countries									
Bulgaria	1,968	6	0.3	548	62	11.3	582	103	17.7
Ireland	677	2	0.3	161	16	9.9	153	26	17.0
Japan	7,899	55	0.7	2,935	240	8.2	3,440	728	21.2
Australia	2,163	8	0.4	456	53	11.6	578	126	21.8
France	6,297	44	0.7	1,477	166	11.2	1,939	350	18.1
United States	40,627	132	0.3	7,801	654	8.4	9,143	1,318	14.4
England/Wales	6,037	22	0.4	1,064	140	13.2	1,411	264	18.7
Netherlands	1,459	6	0.4	311	32	10.3	448	89	19.9
Hungary	2,558	10	0.4	286	34	11.9	420	87	20.7
Austria	1,018	3	0.3	201	27	13.4	242	38	15.7

(World Health Organization Statistics, 1985 and 1986)

* Numbers of total deaths and deaths from cancer, and percentage of deaths caused by cancer, in different age groups. Years as in Tables 54-1 and 54-2.

developed regions, frequently exceeding 90% in African and Asian countries. The illiteracy rate is higher in females, and also much higher in rural than urban areas, factors that may impinge on the pattern of disease in infants. More detailed information on educational achievements is obtainable from UNESCO.[7]

Socioeconomic Considerations

Socioeconomic considerations are important to the practice of pediatric oncology in the developing countries for a variety of reasons and at a variety of levels. Of course, poverty is the root cause of poor living conditions, including not only dietary and sanitary inadequacies but also the low standards of education. But economic considerations at both national and personal levels are important to pediatric oncology for other reasons. The proportion of the national budget devoted to education and health care has an impact on the number of doctors trained (and hence the extent to which specialization in pediatric oncology is feasible) and the number of cancer units or facilities that can deliver appropriate care for children with cancer. The per capita income influences the ability of the average family to meet the cost of travel to a specialized center (likely to be a considerable distance away) or to pay for expensive drugs that may not be provided by the hospital or the government. Further, the family may lose its means of livelihood when adult members are away from home. Frequently, many family members accompany the patient to treatment centers. Moreover, families are usually large, so that the problem of caring for the other siblings arises. Babies are almost invariably breast fed and must accompany the mother.

The dramatic economic differences between the less and more developed countries are illustrated by the average annual per capita income, which can be as low as $120 (*e.g.,* in Bangladesh) and is frequently only a few hundred dollars in African and Asian nations.[5] In India, the average income is $260 and in Pakistan it is $363. In South American countries, and some of the North African countries, the average income is usually between $1500 and $2500, whereas in the more developed countries it is usually in excess of $5000 (France, $10,552; the United States, $12,700; and Switzerland, $16,400). It should be borne in mind that since these are average figures, a large proportion of the population earns considerably less than these amounts; however, the cost of living is also less in the less developed countries (in some cases, 10 times less).

HEALTH CARE RESOURCES

General Considerations

In evaluating discrepancies between the health services and resources of the more and less developed countries, no single statistic can provide an accurate index. All statistics should, in any event, be considered only as estimates because of inaccuracies in data collection, the unavailability of different statistics in the same year, and the large variations in definitions (*e.g.,* the term "hospital"). It should also be realized that in all countries, and particularly the less developed countries, the distribution of health care is uneven. There are frequently large discrepancies in doctor/patient ratios between rural and urban districts, and advanced or specialized medical assistance may be available in relatively few regions (usually the major cities). This problem is compounded by the generally poor communications and transportation systems. When transportation is available, the cost may be disproportionately high in relation to income, a factor that weighs heavily against early medical intervention and patient compliance. If a patient does arrive at a specialized facility and is extremely ill (possibly as a consequence of delay in seeking medical attention), he or she may be refused admission because of the low chance of survival. The scant resources that exist cannot be wasted, and are therefore reserved for patients who have a reasonable chance of responding to therapy.

A useful comparative index of health care resources is the doctor/patient ratio, or the "medical index." In the more developed countries, there is approximately 1 doctor for every 500 people. In the less developed countries, although there are notable exceptions (*e.g.,* Egypt), the ratio is usually 1 to several thousand, and may be as low as 1 to 30,000 (Table 54-6). Another index shown in Table 54-6 is the number of hospital beds relative to the population. These figures provide, however, only the crudest illustration of differences in health care resources. Public health measures and improved social circumstances have markedly reduced the incidence of infectious diseases in the more developed countries (see Table

54-4). But in some countries, fewer than 10% of children receive three diphtheria–pertussis–tetanus immunizations (*e.g.,* Chad, Angola, Burma, Bangladesh, and Indonesia).[3] Thus, the overall incidence of serious ill health, at least in children, is significantly greater in such countries, so that the smaller medically trained work force is stretched even further. In such circumstances, specialization in rare diseases is more difficult to justify. Thus, ironically, even if a cancer patient does seek medical aid early in the course of the disease, considerable delay in diagnosis may occur while the patient receives standard therapeutic manipulations, or because the doctor holds antiquated views regarding cancer. Malignant diseases are also less readily apparent in the setting of rampant infectious disease and parasitic infestation. The rare case of acute lymphoblastic leukemia, for example, will not be clinically obvious in a setting where anemia is almost invariably present as a consequence of hookworm infestation, lymphadenopathy is usually tuberculous, and splenomegaly is frequently due to malaria.

Where trained staff and equipment are scarce and patient numbers are very large, it is often more practical, and indeed preferable, to administer therapy for the likeliest cause of the malaise. Failure to emphasize empirical therapy, with a minimum of time- and money-consuming diagnostic tests in order to provide treatment for the greatest number of patients, could lead to even greater loss of life than the inappropriate treatment of some patients with less common diseases (see Chap. 39). Moreover, the use of "standard" therapies, such as the administration of chloroquine and penicillin for febrile patients in Africa, permits far wider use of ancillary medical personnel. This is why most developing countries have instituted local health care "dispensaries" where treatment for the commonest illnesses can be administered by minimally trained personnel; only patients who do not respond to initial therapy or who are clearly suffering from an unusual condition (*e.g.,* a visible tumor) are referred to a larger hospital for more expert attention.

Pediatric Oncology

Both diagnostic and therapeutic facilities for pediatric oncology are very rare in less developed countries. Even in the most advanced centers in some countries, the availability of instruments such as computed tomographic (CT) scanners, gamma cameras, and ultrasonic scanners is very limited. Because of the expense of chemotherapeutic agents, treatment is frequently based on the availability of drugs rather than the optimal drug combination, and treatment regimens are generally pursued with timidity because of the poor quality of supportive care. Infectious complications are usually inadequately treated because of the unavailability of the more expensive broad-spectrum antibiotics that play such an important role in the management of the febrile neutropenic patient, and the lack of adequate blood banking facilities (particularly for the production of blood components such as platelet concentrates), coupled with the relative inefficiency or even absence of organized blood collection schemes, results in inadequate support of the thrombocytopenic patient. In addition, laboratory monitoring (*e.g.,* blood counts; coagulation studies; electrolyte, renal, and liver function tests; and even blood cultures) is sporadic at best because of financial constraints. On the whole, primary care for the patient with cancer is still provided predominantly by surgeons and radiotherapists in the less developed countries, and because there are relatively few medical oncologists and even fewer pediatric oncologists, chemotherapy and appropriate supportive care are rarely administered optimally, even when the necessary diagnostic tools and drugs are available.

Table 54-6
Measures of Health Care

Country	People per Hospital Bed	People per Physician
Africa		
Benin	771	18,774
Tanzania	924	32,938
Egypt	539	629
Tunisia	530	5,760
Asia		
Pakistan	1,748	3,000
Nepal	6,225	38,333
Iran	706	4,359
Iraq	649	2,957
Latin America		
Mexico	928	1,157
Haiti	1,533	15,663
Honduras	770	3,095
United States	171	500
USSR	789	250
Europe		
West Germany	90	420
France	87	503
Poland	152	544

(Paxton J [ed]: The Statesman's Year-Book, 1985–86. New York, St. Martins Press 1986)

A particularly important aspect of primary patient care is the quality of nursing. The nursing care of the patient with cancer requires special training and skills, that are largely unavailable in the less developed countries. In general, nursing staff have a much smaller role in the care of the patient in these countries, and skills such as the management of intravenous infusions—an essential component of optimal chemotherapy —tend to be rudimentary. In many circumstances, family members carry out a high proportion of what would be considered nursing care in the more developed countries. Similarly, teams of ancillary staff, including social workers, teachers, religious advisors, occupational therapists, and sometimes psychologists and psychiatrists, who play such an important role in assisting patients and their families through the major upheavals of serious illness in the more developed countries, are in most cases totally absent.

It is clear that the problems of health care in general, and of pediatric oncology in particular, in the less developed countries encompass the availability of educational opportunities for potential health care professionals; the structure of the medical, nursing, and ancillary professions; the paucity of adequate physical resources; and the need for efficient health programs that emphasize prevention (*e.g.,* vaccination and other public health measures) but include the organization at a regional level of diagnostic and therapeutic facilities. Of course, intimately related to any improvement in health care are efforts to improve the educational and economic standards of the general population.

INCIDENCE AND REGIONAL VARIATIONS OF PEDIATRIC MALIGNANCIES

Most cancers are a consequence of the interaction of environmental factors with the genetic make-up of the individual at risk. The relative importance of nature versus nurture varies considerably with tumor type. Some neoplasms, such as familial retinoblastoma and familial Wilms' tumor, appear to arise almost exclusively as a consequence of inherited genetic factors. The genesis of other tumors, particularly those arising from tissues that interact directly with environmental elements (*e.g.,* the immune system, bowel, and lung) is likely to be influenced considerably by environmental factors. Whether or not a specific individual develops cancer may also involve a significant element of chance. This is because only a limited number of somatic genetic changes are consistent with the particular pattern of cellular behavior that is characteristic of a specific cancer, and whether or not the required genetic changes develop in an individual cell is, to a degree, a random event (see Chaps. 2 and 3). Thus, nearly all factors that influence the development of cancer do so by altering the relative risk. (An exception is cancer in animals caused directly by the acute transforming retroviruses; whether an analogous situation exists in man is not known.) Although genetic factors may have a role, it seems probable that the vastly different lifestyles and environments of the populations of the less and more developed countries are the predominant reason for the often dramatic differences in the spectra of neoplasms. Examples include the very high incidence of squamous bladder cancer consequent upon endemic bilharzia in Egypt, and hepatoma secondary to hepatitis in Africa. Some information exists regarding genetic factors that predispose to pediatric cancers such as retinoblastoma, Wilms' tumor, and hematopoietic neoplasms in a small number of genetic disorders such as Down's, Fanconi's, and Bloom's syndromes and ataxia telangiectasia, but little is known of the environmental factors (apart from

ionizing radiation) that may predispose to cancer. However, several observations, particularly regarding geographic differences in incidence (Table 54-7), suggest that environmental factors may heavily influence the spectrum of pediatric neoplasms in any given location. Although the nature of the relevant factors is currently a matter for speculation, there are a number of candidate factors, which are likely to be of varying importance in different tumors. These include general nutritional status and specific components of diet; infectious agents, including DNA viruses, retroviruses, protozoans, and a variety of parasites; local minerals and chemicals, possibly including naturally occurring radioisotopes; and a variety of local or regional cultural practices and habits (exemplified in adults by tobacco consumption and the chewing of betel nut leaf mixed with lime).

Chemical exposure is less likely to play a role in childhood cancer because of the long latent period required for tumorigenesis. As a corollary, childhood cancers are less likely to arise in cells that have preexisting resistance to environmental chemicals, a phenomenon that could be a component of intrinsic resistance to chemotherapy in some adult tumors, particularly colorectal and renal cancers.[8] These considerations may be relevant to the general chemosensitivity of pediatric cancers and also favor a relatively more frequent role (compared to adult cancers) for infectious agents in their etiology. It must also be recognized that in cancers occurring in the first few years of life, predisposing factors, including components of diet, infection, and ionizing radiation may operate *in utero.*

Although there may be wide variations in the incidence of a given neoplasm in different parts of the world, these differences do not necessarily correlate with a country's developmental status. In different parts of the world, populations of similar socioeconomic status are likely to have a quite different exposure to a variety of environmental factors. This, coupled with the broad range of levels of development among the less

Table 54-7

*Incidence of Pediatric Neoplasms in Selected Countries**

Type of Cancer	United States†	India	Malaysia	Brazil
Overall	13.0	7.2	7.0	12.1
ALL	2.9	1.0	1.5	3.1
AML	0.5	0.3	0.7	
Hodgkin's	0.7	0.5	0.2	0.8
NHL	0.9	0.4	0.2	0.6
All hematopoietic	5.0	2.5	3.5	
Brain and CNS	2.5	1.0‡	1.0	2.0
Neuroblastoma	0.9		0.2	
Soft tissue sarcomas	0.8	0.2	0.3	0.6
Wilms' tumor	0.8	0.3	0.5	1.5
Osteosarcoma	0.3	0.5§		1.0
Ewing's sarcoma	0.3		0.2	
Retinoblastoma	0.3	0.5	0.5	0.5

* Average annual incidence per 100,000. All data are for children younger than 15 years, except Malaysia (<13 years). U.S. figures are from the SEER program, 1973–1982. Other sources are as follows: Bombay Cancer Registry, 1973–1975; Malaysian Childhood Cancer Incidence Study, 1986; and Sao Paulo Cancer Registry, 1973–1975.

† Incidence for whites only (both sexes).

‡ Includes all CNS and sympathetic nervous system tumors.

§ Includes all bone tumors.

developed nations, makes a simple division into more and less developed countries inadequate for comparative purposes and reinforces the need for accurate, population-based tumor registries in all countries.

Another problem that must be faced in comparing tumor incidences geographically is the limitations of diagnoses based purely on morphology. This reflects not only the marked variability in technical expertise but also the inherent limitations of this approach. For an increasing number of tumors, an array of diagnostic techniques can be applied, including monoclonal antibodies, biochemical examination of tumor markers, electron microscopy, cytogenetics, and molecular biology. In general, such diagnostic modalities are unavailable, or available to a very limited extent, in the less developed countries, and it could be argued that their application is of limited relevance to the predominant consideration of providing adequate treatment to children with cancer. Yet precise diagnosis can be critically important to the application of appropriate therapy and to the definition of patient subgroups with differing prognoses—a prerequisite to the development of appropriate therapy. If optimal strategies are to be developed for pediatric cancer in the less developed countries, it will be essential to study the biology of the tumors so that similarities to and differences from tumors in the more developed countries can be discerned and subtypes of possible therapeutic significance can be identified within a morphologically homogeneous group. Which additional diagnostic modalities should be used and to what extent is an issue that can only be decided in the context of the local situation. Immunohistochemistry and cytogenetics, for example, are likely to become of increasing importance to precise diagnosis and require relatively minor additional resources. It seems appropriate that at least the major centers in less developed countries move toward developing the necessary expertise in these areas. This is a particularly fertile area for collaboration with centers in more developed countries.

The importance of the above points is best illustrated by a brief consideration of some of the known differences in the spectra of pediatric neoplasms in different populations. In this regard, it should be recognized that in the least developed countries, few reliable incidence figures are available because of the lack of population-based registries. Even the few existing registries (Table 54-8) suffer from the tendency to categorize tumor data on an organ or system basis rather than by histology, and also from inherent inaccuracies of unknown magnitude that result from inadequate demographic statistics and incomplete registration. However, there are some observations that have been made repeatedly, and that come from sources sufficiently reliable that their validity is not in question.

Acute Lymphoblastic Leukemia

Acute lymphoblastic leukemia (ALL) appears to be the commonest childhood leukemia throughout the world, but there seem to be highly significant differences in its incidence, with the lowest rates occurring in equatorial Africa and the highest rates in the more developed countries (see Chaps. 1, 2, and 16). Although population-based data still frequently fail to distinguish between different types of acute leukemia, there does appear to be an overall correlation between affluence and the incidence of leukemias in children, which is almost certainly due to differences in the incidence of ALL (see Table 54-8).[2,9] In the United States, there is a significantly lower incidence of ALL in blacks and Puerto Ricans than in whites (Table 54-9), while South African blacks also have a markedly lower incidence of ALL than South African whites.[10]

There is little possibility of comprehending these differences when ALL is considered as a single disease—and even less when all leukemias are lumped together. Immunophenotyping and, more recently, cytogenetic examination have shown that ALL consists of several diseases (see Chaps. 3, 4, and 16). There are differences in the prognosis of these subtypes (depending on the treatment regimen employed) and, because it is highly likely that the relative proportions of these subgroups differ geographically, and even that previously unrecognized subgroups may be discovered, the development of optimal treatment regimens requires the characterization of ALL at both clinical and biological levels in different populations. It is possible that the generally more advanced stage of ALL in the developing countries depends less on late presentation to medical aid (although this is an important consideration) than on differences in the biology of the disease. The

---

Table 54-8

*International Variations in Incidence of Childhood Leukemia, Non-Hodgkin's Lymphoma, and Hodgkin's Disease; Observed (OBS) and Expected (EXP) Numbers of Cases**

Registry	Hodgkin's Disease			Non-Hodgkin's Lymphoma			Leukemia		
	OBS	EXP	OBS/EXP	OBS	EXP	OBS/EXP	OBS	EXP	OBS/EXP
Bombay	83	82.6	1.01	109	144.3	0.76†	406	703.4	0.58†
Kingston	19	15.1	1.26	22	28.2	0.78	89	145.0	0.61†
Ibadan	13	7.1	1.83‡	171	13.0	13.20†	25	65.7	0.38†
Cuba	169	134.6	1.26§	435	236.7	1.84†	1018	1157.0	0.88†
São Paulo	33	16.5	2.00†	69	28.6	2.41†	131	140.6	0.93

* Expected numbers are based on age-specific rates for all 42 registries reporting to the International Agency for Research in Cancer for the compilation of *Cancer Incidence in Five Continents* (first four volumes). Childhood leukemia is not subdivided and includes both lymphoblastic and myeloid as well as rare chronic leukemias (after Breslow and Langholz[9]).

† *p* < 0.001.

‡ *p* < 0.05.

§ *p* < 0.01.

Table 54-9

Ethnic Variations in the Observed and Expected Numbers of Cases of Various Childhood Neoplasms Within the United States*

Neoplasm	Black			New Mexico Hispanic			Puerto Rican		
	OBS	EXP	OBS/EXP	OBS	EXP	OBS/EXP	OBS	EXP	OBS/EXP
ALL	43	87	0.49†	22	26	0.84	139	184	0.76‡
ANLL	18	16	1.11	6	5	1.2	21	34	0.61
Brain tumors									
Gliomas	38	45	0.85	4	14	0.28§	46	94	0.49†
Medulloblastoma	20	15	1.34	2	5	0.42	8	32	0.25†
Neuroblastoma	21	28	0.75	5	8	0.64	28	58	0.48†

(Data derived from SEER, 1973–1977, after Breslow and Langholz[9])

* Expected incidence is based on age-specific rates for U.S. whites.

† $p < 0.0001$.

‡ $p < 0.01$.

§ $p < 0.001$.

duration of symptoms may, in fact, be shorter in patients with particularly aggressive forms of ALL.

A good marker of phenotypic differences in ALL is the presence of a sharp early age peak (2–5 years) in the incidence of the disease.[11] The vast majority of patients at this age have "common ALL," characterized by the presence of the common ALL antigen in blast cells with a B-cell precursor phenotype. T-cell leukemia has a much broader incidence peak, distributed throughout the first two decades of life. This early age peak was first detected in the United Kingdom in the 1920s and subsequently appeared in the United States, first in whites and then in blacks, and in Japan.[12] It still appears to be absent in the least developed countries, although a somewhat broader early age peak has appeared in recent years in some of the more economically advanced developing countries (*e.g.*, China, Malaysia, and some South American countries).[13–15] This suggests strongly that the frequency of common ALL is likely to be much lower in the less developed countries, with a corresponding increase in T-cell ALL—a phenotype with a worse prognosis in most ALL clinical trials. Recently, phenotyping studies from several countries have confirmed the hypothesis of varying incidences of immunophenotypes in ALL.[9] For example, T-cell ALL comprises a third to a half of childhood ALL cases in series from centers in Egypt and India, with the distribution of phenotypic subgroups being similar in children and adults.[16–18] Because the early age peak is present in patients with high white counts,[19] the lack of an early age peak cannot be explained on the basis of delayed diagnosis.

The development of an early age peak in the industrialized countries coincided with an increase in the incidence of ALL, so the lower incidence of ALL in the less developed countries is probably due primarily to a deficit of common ALL. As economic progress is made, the incidence of common ALL is likely to increase. With many treatment regimens, this subtype of ALL has a better prognosis than others, a factor that must be taken into account when comparing treatment results from different parts of the world.

Acute Nonlymphocytic Leukemia

The incidence of acute nonlymphocytic (myeloid) leukemia (ANLL) does not seem to correlate with the economic level of a population. There is no difference in incidence, for example,

between whites and blacks in South Africa or the United States.[1,10] However, clinical features do differ. There is, for example, a higher frequency of gingival hypertrophy, hepatosplenomegaly, necrotic or infected oropharyngeal lesions, and chloromas in black than white South African children with ANLL.[10] In one series, 24% of black children but no white children had orbital chloromas.[10] A high frequency of orbital chloroma in ANLL has also been reported in equatorial Africa; in Egypt, where 24% of patients with ANLL have orbital chloromas (Nazli Gad el Mawla, personal communication); and in Turkey, where the frequency may be even higher (20 of 56 patients in one series).[20] It is likely that the increased frequency of chloromas in less developed countries reflects differences in the leukemic cell type.

Hodgkin's Disease

Geographic variations in the incidence, sex ratio, and relative proportions of different histologic subtypes of Hodgkin's disease in children have been recognized for some years. In the less developed countries, there is usually a relatively high incidence in childhood (the predominant incidence peak is often in the 0-15 year age group), a marked male preponderance, and a higher proportion of mixed cellular or lymphocyte-depleted histologic types.[21] Nodular sclerosis, the predominant histologic type in the United States and Western Europe, is generally much less common in the developing countries (Table 54-10), although there are exceptions to this.[15] The pattern of Hodgkin's disease appears to correlate with socioeconomic conditions, although whether this disease is a single entity or several related diseases with different etiologies is not known.

Non-Hodgkin's Lymphoma

Marked variations in the incidence of different histologic types of non-Hodgkin's lymphoma (NHL) have been observed in different parts of the world. Although incidence figures are available from only a few population-based registries in the less developed countries, significant geographic differences in the overall incidence of NHL have also been documented (see

Table 54-10
Geographic Comparison of Histologic Subtypes of Hodgkin's Disease

Histology	Egypt	East Africa	India	Argentina	United States
Lymphoid predominance	13.6	19.5	23	21	13
Nodular sclerosis	13.6	10.5	9	21	43
Mixed cell	60.7	32	54	47	32
Lymphocyte depleted	3.7	38	14	11	12
Unclassified	8.4				

Table 54-8). In children, this appears to be primarily due to large differences in the incidence of Burkitt's lymphoma. Although Burkitt's lymphoma (defined histologically) occurs throughout the world, its incidence is some 25- to 50-fold higher in equatorial Africa than in the more developed countries, and its clinical and biological features differ significantly in these two settings (see Chap. 20). There is little accurate information regarding NHL from other less developed countries, although it appears that the North African and Middle Eastern countries have a rather high incidence of Burkitt's lymphoma, intermediate between that of equatorial Africa and the more developed countries.

Brain Tumors

Second to ALL, brain tumors are the commonest group of pediatric neoplasms in the United States and Europe. This is not the case in many of the less developed countries (*e.g.,* India, Africa), where brain tumors, like ALL, are much less common.[9] However, it is not clear that these differences are a consequence of socioeconomic factors; Singapore has a lower incidence than Shanghai, and even within countries such as Japan and the United States, there is marked regional variation.[9] Little information is available with regard to the histologic spectrum in the less developed countries, so it is not clear whether these differences extend to all histologic types or represent variations in the frequency of a particular variety of brain tumor. In Puerto Rico, however, there is a significantly lower incidence of both glial neoplasms and medulloblastoma compared to that in whites in the United States (see Table 54-9).

Retinoblastoma

In some parts of the world, notably some regions in India (*e.g.,* Chandigahr) and Pakistan (Karachi), retinoblastoma is the commonest childhood tumor.[22,23] In Brazil, retinoblastoma appears to be the second commonest childhood neoplasm, at least in Sao Paulo,[24] and it is noticeably more frequent in Malays and Indians than in Chinese in Malaysia.[25] In equatorial African countries, retinoblastoma is at least three times as common as neuroblastoma, the reverse of the situation in more developed countries.[26] There does not seem to be an increase in the familial form of the tumor in these areas, so the basis for these findings is not simply an increased inheritance of a defective retinoblastoma gene (see Chaps. 3 and 25). Nor is there an obvious correlation with the level of socioeconomic development. At least some osteosarcomas carry the same genetic lesion as retinoblastoma, so it would be worthwhile to corre-

late the incidence of these two tumors in various geographic regions. However, inadequate data exist currently to do this.

Neuroblastoma

There is a substantial variability in the incidence of neuroblastoma throughout the world, and this tumor appears to be more common in the more developed than the less developed countries. For example, neuroblastoma appears to be only one tenth as common in central Africa as in the United States, and India and Pakistan also appear to have a low incidence.[22,27] There is at least a relative paucity in Egypt.[28] A significantly lower incidence of neuroblastoma is seen in Puerto Rico compared to whites in the United States (see Table 54-9). Unfortunately, the major population-based registries often include neuroblastoma with brain tumors, as neoplasms of the nervous system, so that accurate incidence data are not readily obtainable.

Wilms' Tumor

Although Wilms' tumor was for some time believed to be of similar incidence throughout the world, it has recently become clear that this is not the case. Japan, for example, has an incidence of only about 60% of that in the United States and Europe, and incidence rates are also low in Singapore and India. In Scandinavia, Nigeria, and Brazil the incidence appears to be higher than in the United States.[9] Thus, there is no clear relationship to socioeconomic status, and factors that influence the incidence of the nonfamilial form of Wilms' tumor are not known.

THE STATUS OF PEDIATRIC ONCOLOGY IN REPRESENTATIVE REGIONS

The current status of pediatric oncology in the less developed countries is best illustrated by some specific examples, selected from regions of the world with different levels of development.

Africa

Sub-Saharan Africa

The African continent includes the least developed countries in the world. Gross national product per capita is generally about U.S. $200 to $500. Moreover, political turmoil and repeated famines, droughts, and consequent epidemics of infectious diseases in many sub-Saharan African countries make it difficult or impossible to create an ordered approach to health care in general, and the problem of pediatric malignancies shrinks to insignificance on a national scale. This part of the world epitomizes the health problems faced by the less developed countries. There is a paucity of doctors relative to the population and a lack of drugs, equipment, hospital facilities, trained ancillary personnel, and interdisciplinary organization. There are very few trained pediatric oncologists by any standards. Radiation therapy is available in only a limited number of countries, and advanced diagnostic facilities are scarce. The available range of cytotoxic drugs and antibiotics is extremely limited in the majority of countries, and there are no cooperative pediatric oncology groups. Training in oncology is limited by the small number of experienced pediatric or adult oncologists. Thus, the quality of pediatric oncology is extremely variable, and the field depends largely for its existence on the presence of a small number of interested pediatricians and pediatric surgeons, or physicians of other specialties who have developed an interest in a particular tumor or group of tumors. Some African cancer societies do exist, however. For example AORTIC—the African Organization for Research and Teaching in Cancer—was founded a few years ago with the objective of improving scientific interchange and teaching in the general area of cancer.

Nigeria provides an example of the problems faced in a country at the upper end of the economic spectrum in sub-Saharan Africa. In this country of some 100 million people, with 47% of the population younger than 15 years, there was until quite recently only a single pediatric hospital (of about 50 beds), and pediatrics was not considered a separate specialty. Most Nigerians (90%) live in rural regions, whereas most of the country's several thousand doctors practice in urban communities, so that the majority of Nigerians never encounter a trained physician. In 1985 there were five formally trained oncologists in the country, one medical oncologist, and five radiotherapists, but no pediatric oncologist. Radiotherapy is available only at the teaching hospital at Lagos, although another unit is about to be commissioned in Ibadan. The existing unit is severely hampered by frequent and often prolonged power failures and breakdowns, with long delays before repairs can be accomplished. Thus, the vast majority of Nigerian patients, including children with radioresponsive tumors, have no access to radiotherapy. Chemotherapy is usually given by surgeons, who provide primary care for the majority of cancer patients in the country. Cancer chemotherapy drugs are in short supply and often used poorly, with the object of avoiding toxicity. Nigerian families can rarely comprehend the need for prolonged chemotherapy or specialized care of any form, and doctors often see only terminally ill patients. For the few who come to medical attention earlier in the disease course, follow-up is fraught with difficulties. In Ibadan, for example, over 50% of the population live in areas without street names, and people may not be known by the names registered in the hospital. Rural dwellers can rarely afford the cost of travel to the city hospital.

The commonest childhood neoplasm in Nigeria is Burkitt's lymphoma, followed by retinoblastoma and then other lymphomas. Leukemia is sixth in frequency after sarcomas and Wilms' tumor.[29] Naturally, pediatric oncologic research has focused on Burkitt's lymphoma, but the conduct of a clinical trial in this setting is fraught with difficulty. In a recent trial conducted in the Department of Medical Oncology in Ibadan, patients were preselected and kept in hospital for the duration of treatment.[30] Even so, there was a high rate of protocol devia-

tions and many patients were lost to follow-up. A particular problem has been the variability in the hospital budget, resulting in an erratic supply of antibiotics and intravenous fluids. Supplies such as intravenous infusion sets, needles, and syringes are not always available, and funds must be found for patient travel and tracing. Yet, despite these difficulties, research opportunities abound, and progress can be made. The introduction of combination therapy for the treatment of Burkitt's lymphoma, for example, more than doubled the complete response and survival rates.[31]

North Africa

The countries of North Africa have enjoyed a more active scientific exchange with the adjacent European countries, and are also more prosperous than the sub-Saharan countries of Africa. A number of major cancer centers exist in countries such as Algeria, Tunisia, and Egypt. These usually offer reasonably good diagnostic facilities, usually including CT scanners, excellent surgical capabilities, radiotherapy (although usually with cobalt machines rather than linear accelerators), and medical oncologists, sometimes including pediatric oncology specialists. Some of these centers (e.g., the National Cancer Institute in Cairo), provide the major base for training oncologists as well as treating a very high proportion of all patients with cancer in the country. In general, the cancer centers tend to function individually and rarely develop cooperative treatment programs with other centers in the same country or in other North African countries, although significant collaboration is undertaken with investigators in Europe and, to a lesser extent, the United States. Most of the major North African centers have the capability and patient populations to carry out meaningful clinical trials. Limiting factors tend to be predominantly financial.

Pediatric oncology in North Africa is well exemplified by the situation in Egypt. In this country of about 46 million inhabitants and a gross national product per capita of U.S. $650 in 1981, pediatric oncology is concentrated in Cairo (the population of greater Cairo is 8.54 million). The primary facility for pediatric oncology is the Pediatric Unit of the Medical Oncology Department of the National Cancer Institute (Cairo NCI). Smaller numbers of cases are treated in other units associated with universities in Cairo and Alexandria. General pediatric units exist in most of the general hospitals in the capital cities of the governorates, but almost all pediatric cancer patients are referred to Cairo. There are about 15 specialists in pediatric oncology in Egypt, many of whom have had additional training in the United States or Europe. Pediatric surgery is carried out at the Cairo NCI or at the School of Medicine, Cairo University, and telecobalt radiotherapy is also available at both these facilities. A CT scanner is available, although the demand is far greater than can be met by the single instrument. Some of the newer diagnostic modalities, including phenotyping of hematopoietic neoplasms, are available in these major centers. Although there are separate facilities for patients with pediatric cancer, there are no critical care units. Blood products are in very short supply because the people are reluctant to donate blood and facilities for processing blood components are limited. All chemotherapy drugs can be obtained, but the more expensive cytotoxic drugs and antibiotics are rarely at hand. In some circumstances, drugs are provided by pharmaceutical companies as part of approved clinical trials.

Some 300 new pediatric cancer patients are seen each year at the Cairo NCI, of whom 70% have leukemia or lymphoma. Patients with leukemia have been treated with moderately intensive therapy but, in AML particularly, there is a very high incidence of early death—28%—most of these (80%) being due to infection. The mean survival of patients with AML is less than 2 months. In ALL, like other pediatric neoplasms where chemotherapy is a critical component of treatment, the dilemma faced in Egypt is similar to that in other less developed countries. That is, whereas relatively nonaggressive treatment produces poor disease-free survival rates, more aggressive treatment results in increased infection rates. The lack of adequate support for the neutropenic patient (including antibiotics and blood products) is a major obstacle to the delivery of modern intensive antileukemic therapy. Bone marrow transplantation has not yet been done in Egypt.

Follow-up of patients in Egypt is difficult since families are usually large and there are few or no social supports. Thus, most parents find it increasingly difficult to continue making often long and expensive journeys to the major pediatric cancer facilities, even though the treatment is free.

Asia

India

The level of development in pediatric oncology in India is, at its best, similar to that in North Africa. In this country of over 750 million people and a gross national product per capita of U.S. $260 (1981), there are only a few major cancer centers, the largest being in Bombay (the Tata Memorial), New Delhi (in the All India Institute of Medical Science), Madras (the Cancer Institute at Adyar), Bangalore (the Kidwai Memorial Cancer Institute), and Chandigarh (the Post Graduate Medical Institute). Pediatric oncology in these centers is usually practiced by members of the medical oncology department who focus on childhood cancer. The pediatric ward is, however, usually separate from the adult oncology wards. Pediatric oncology is also practiced in some pediatric hospitals (where patients may be housed on a general ward that includes patients with infectious diseases), and a small number of hospitals in various cities have established pediatric surgery units. Most of the major centers have access to good diagnostic equipment, including CT scanning. In the above mentioned centers, additional diagnostic studies, such as immunologic characterization and cytogenetics, can also be performed, although to date there is limited experience in this area. Good radiotherapy facilities, including linear accelerators, are available in all the major centers, and, as in Egypt, although all chemotherapeutic drugs can be obtained most of the time, the more expensive cytotoxic drugs and antibiotics are rarely available. Thus, patients are often treated with whatever drugs are available rather than the most appropriate drugs. There are no critical care units, but facilities and expertise for bone marrow transplantation do exist in Bombay, and are planned for the future in Madras.

Among the most pressing problems are the limited number of specialists in pediatric oncology and the financial difficulties that frequently lead to gross inadequacies in the supply of chemotherapeutic agents and broad-spectrum antibiotics. This combination of circumstances leads to a limited ability to treat many patients and, with some exceptions, to overall poor results, even in the major centers. Quite high proportions of patients are turned away without treatment because resources must be conserved for those more likely to survive treatment. The principles of supportive care are rarely adhered to outside the major centers.

Pediatric surgery has developed significantly in recent years, and the major centers have linear accelerators, so that the highest priority is improvement in the ability to administer and support patients through intensive drug programs.

Southeast Asia

Although there is considerable variability in the level of development in Southeast Asia, economic growth in this region is extremely rapid, and health care facilities are therefore improving rapidly. In some parts of the region (*i.e.,* the "newly industrialized nations"—Singapore, Hong Kong, Taiwan, and South Korea), the best facilities differ little from those available in Europe and the United States. Malaysia will be taken as an example of the state of pediatric oncology in this region.

Pediatric oncology has existed in Malaysia, a country of some 15 million inhabitants and a gross national product per capita of U.S. $1840, for about 10 years. All three of the main treatment centers, which are associated with the University and the General Hospital, are situated in Kuala Lumpur, and the majority of childhood cancers are managed in the pediatric departments of these centers. Some cases of solid tumors, including retinoblastoma, Wilms' tumor, and bone and soft tissue sarcomas, are managed by local surgeons. Most diagnostic facilities, including CT scanning, are available, as are good support facilities, including blood banking and critical care facilities. The demand for these specialized services, however, is greater than their capacity, and blood banking is hindered by culturally based reluctance to donate blood. Most chemotherapeutic drugs are available, but the most expensive ones and the newer antibiotics are not supplied by the hospital and must be purchased (if possible) by the patient.

There are only three pediatric oncologists in the country (all in Kuala Lumpur) and there is no formal training in this discipline, although interested postgraduates supplement on-the-job training by short periods overseas.

About 100 new cases of childhood cancer are seen each year at the University Hospital. Results on the whole are superior to those obtained in the less developed countries discussed so far, and, although numbers are small, survival rates are similar to those obtained in the United States and Europe. Most patients in the main centers are treated on formal protocols. Bone marrow transplantation is likely to be performed in the near future in Kuala Lumpur.

Follow-up of patients in Malaysia varies with locality, but in general is very good. Those referred from outlying regions are followed up predominantly in local hospitals but are seen at the University Hospital several times a year, and the considerable financial difficulties relating to travel appear to be somehow overcome in the majority of cases.

Latin America

Latin America, like Southeast Asia, falls into the category of a more advanced region of the less developed world. This means that, although there is considerable variation, major cancer centers are able to deliver good care, and treatment in the better centers is not markedly inferior to that in the United States and Europe. Two countries will be discussed as representative of the region.

Argentina

Argentina is a country of approximately 30 million inhabitants and a gross national product per capita of U.S. $1550. The major Children's Hospital, in Buenos Aires, provides specialized consultations in pediatric oncology, but there is less centralization in Argentina than in some of the other countries discussed here. Diagnostic facilities are good, with the availability of CT scanning and specialized testing such as immunologic phenotyping. All cytotoxic drugs and antibiotics are available, and supportive care facilities are relatively good. There is a critical care unit in the Children's Hospital in Buenos Aires.

There are approximately 20 pediatric oncologists in Argentina, but these physicians typically function in an advisory capacity, and separate pediatric oncology units do not exist. Approximately 25% of the general pediatric beds in the Children's Hospital in Buenos Aires are occupied by children with cancer.

All patients in the major centers are treated according to standard protocols, and cooperative groups exist, such as GATLA, the Argentinean group for the treatment of acute leukemia, which is a member of GLATHEM, the Latin American group for the treatment of hematopoietic malignancies. The latter includes member institutions in Argentina, Costa Rica, Cuba, Chile, and Uruguay. By 1985, 3180 patients had been accrued on GLATHEM protocols for the treatment of acute leukemia in adults and children. The results of these protocols are approaching those seen in the more developed countries.

Brazil

Brazil (population = approximately 140 million; gross national product per capita = $2050) is a country of marked regional contrasts, with most of the economic resources concentrated in the south. Cancer is the fifth or sixth cause of mortality in children. The contrast in medical resources is reflected in the doctor to patient ratio, which ranges from 1 to 610 in Rio de Janeiro to 1 to 7000 in the northeastern states. There are few oncology centers in Brazil, although in São Paulo there is a major cancer center with a pediatric oncology department that includes six pediatric oncologists and sees over 400 new cases per year, a pediatric oncology department in the university hospital, and a separate pediatric oncology hospital. The major centers in São Paulo provide training programs in pediatric oncology and in general are well provided with drugs and equipment. There is also a pediatric oncology center in Salvador, which sees some 300 patients per year but has greater problems regarding drug supply and patient compliance.

In the cancer center in São Paulo, the commonest pediatric tumors in the period 1953 to 1983 were non-Hodgkin's lymphomas (18% of all patients) and retinoblastoma, (17%). Leukemias accounted for 12% of patients. Although it is hazardous to use hospital-based statistics to provide a picture of even the relative frequency of various tumors, it is difficult to avoid the conclusion that in São Paulo, as in some regions on the Indian subcontinent, there is an excess of retinoblastoma. There has been marked improvement in the survival of patients with pediatric neoplasms and, overall, the results in the major centers are not dissimilar from those obtained in the more developed countries.

Brazil has a pediatric oncology society, founded in 1981, which currently has 160 members. An important function of this society is to develop treatment protocols relevant to the situation in Brazil. In 1986, a Brazilian cooperative group for the treatment of Wilms' tumor was established, and more recently, groups have been formed for non-Hodgkin's lymphoma and leukemias. There seems to be little doubt that the development of more interest in pediatric oncology, the standardization of protocols, and the greater efforts to educate the people and the medical profession are the major reasons for these improvements. A very important factor in improving the ability of patients to tolerate chemotherapy has been the introduction of standard protocols for the management of the febrile neutropenic patient in at least one of the major centers. Standard treatment has been amikacin, cefoxitin, and carbenicillin, and more than 80% of patients with documented infections are now surviving—a considerable improvement from previous years.

STRATEGIES FOR IMPROVING THE RESULTS OF TREATMENT

General Considerations

The practice of pediatric oncology in the less developed countries is hindered by problems that transcend the purely medical and are intimately bound up with the spectrum of socioeconomic hardships faced by such countries. Even the most conscientious and philanthropic of governments in a poorly developed nation, when faced with the difficult problem of how best to use meager resources, is unlikely to give pediatric oncology a high priority because of the rarity of pediatric cancers and the extremely high cost of their treatment. In contrast, an enormous impact can be made on major causes of infant mortality such as infantile diarrhea, where thousands of lives can be saved by simple and inexpensive rehydration solutions such as glucose/saline or boiled rice water. Clearly, in such a situation, it would be inappropriate to divert educational programs and precious funds from the common infectious diseases to pediatric cancer. Yet lives *are* lost from pediatric cancer in these countries—lives that might be saved with more adequate facilities and availability of appropriate drugs. Moreover, as economic development occurs, pediatric cancer will loom larger and larger as a cause of death in children until, as in the United States, it is exceeded only by accidental death. This issue is sociopolitical rather than medical and thus perhaps not an appropriate topic for discussion here.

There is, however, a potential answer to this problem. Since childhood cancer is an extremely important health issue in the more developed countries, and since there is much to be gained from studies conducted in the less developed countries, this would seem to be a valuable area for international collaboration between the more and less developed countries, with a substantial proportion of the financial expenditure coming from the richer partner. Diversion of skilled personnel from other tasks related to public health should not pose an ethical dilemma, because the management of major causes of infant death such as diarrhea and enteritis often does not require sophisticated skills or complex equipment. Medical assistants, suitably directed, should be well able to deal with these common health problems. A major challenge is to develop a coordinated approach to the study of the epidemiology, biology, clinical features, and management of pediatric neoplasms in selected countries or regions representing the least developed areas of the world. Although at first glance it may seem inappropriate to use scarce resources for research, the added costs of good characterization of tumors and of accurate record keeping of toxicity and treatment results are not large, and such information is essential if regional and national treatment strategies are to be efficiently directed toward the local patient population. Moreover, oncology represents an area of medicine where good clinical practice and research go hand in glove. There is no room for arbitrary decisions or inadequate documentation of results achieved. Moreover, although patients are the unfortunate victims of their diseases, they also represent the major resource for research efforts designed to improve the results of therapy. One might ask whether it is appropriate to overlook such a rich resource in a group of diseases that are so rare but can be so devastating—particularly when benefit will accrue not only to the present victims but to children who will develop cancer in the future.

Some countries in Southeast Asia and Latin America have developed to the point where advanced treatment protocols can be conducted in the major centers, but economic problems remain, biological and epidemiologic questions are little studied, and there is often a lack of communication between the outlying hospitals and the major centers. Supportive care and the overall results of therapy are usually, but not invariably, inferior to those achieved in the United States and Europe. Further, some of the more remote regions have a high illiteracy rate and inadequate numbers of medical personnel, and are sorely in need of educational programs—both for the people and for primary health care personnel (who are not always physicians and nurses). Even in Latin America, therefore, it is necessary for each country to develop its own plan, and to do so in the light of the important questions that need to be asked if pediatric oncology is to develop optimally. Of the several benefits that could accrue from collaboration between the more and less developed countries, not the least is the opportunity to rethink the essentials of pediatric oncology and to design clinical trials that pay attention to simplicity, economy, and safety as well as to efficiency. Moreover, the opportunity to gain information about the relevance of the environment to pediatric neoplasia is one that should not be missed, for without knowledge of cause, even in the most simplistic terms, prevention cannot be entertained. Nor can we hope to develop new and more specific approaches to treatment.

Specific Measures

In considering strategies for improving the treatment of pediatric cancer in the less developed countries, it is clear that this is a multifaceted problem, and that the component parts of an optimal overall approach exist to varying degrees in different parts of the world. Even in the United States and Europe, where coordination of effort is at its highest level, not all children are cared for with the same high standards of practice that pertain in the major centers. Thus, even though some countries, or regions of countries, in the developing world have already established the kinds of approaches outlined below, it remains worthwhile to consider the absolute essentials for the development of a pediatric oncology program that is acceptable by the criteria of the more developed countries.

The complicated therapies currently necessary for most childhood cancers demand not only care by specialists, but also a team approach. Further, because of the rarity of these diseases, experience in their management can only be gained in centers or units dedicated to pediatric oncology. Thus, the approach to pediatric oncology must begin with the establishment of special pediatric oncology units staffed by physicians and nurses experienced in the management of childhood cancer. In the poorest countries, even a single unit would provide a foundation on which to build a national pediatric oncology program focused on the particular problems of the country. The center should not only provide a focus for the treatment of children with cancer but also coordinate research efforts in pediatric oncology, provide a registry (preferably population based) for childhood cancer (an essential component of any meaningful epidemiologic studies), and establish educational programs at both professional and public levels. The association of the unit or center will differ depending on circumstances. It may be a part of a comprehensive cancer center, which in turn may be independent or may be a part of a university, a medical school, or a children's hospital. Ideally, there should be readily available expertise in pediatric surgery and anesthesiology, as well as access to good radiotherapy facilities with at least one individual familiar with pediatric oncology patients. Figure 54-4 summarizes these concepts.

The Pediatric Oncology Unit

The establishment of specialized, physically separate pediatric oncology units has many potential advantages:

1. Potentially immunocompromised cancer patients are not in close proximity to children suffering from the common infectious diseases.
2. The unit provides a focus for the development of a cadre of doctors, nurses, and ancillary staff (including social workers, teachers, and religious advisors) familiar with the problems encountered in treating childhood cancer and able to devote the necessary time and effort required by those problems.
3. Better opportunities exist for the training of health care professionals in their respective disciplines within the general field of pediatric oncology. Trained personnel may then establish similar units in other parts of the country (or world).
4. Programs can be more readily established for education, and for support of all kinds, for families with children suffering from cancer. This includes the support that families obtain from discussing common problems with each other (whether informally or in supervised meetings) and the provision of social assistance, including lodging during prolonged inpatient or outpatient treatment periods.

The pediatric unit does not have to be technically sophisticated, with piped oxygen or wall suction, but it should be kept scrupulously clean and there must be facilities for washing hands between patient examinations. Ideally, there should be several separate areas so that patients requiring different levels of care can be segregated. At least one area should be reserved for isolation purposes. Isolation facilities are likely to be used even more than in the more developed countries because, depending on the local spectrum of infectious diseases, they may at different times house patients suffering from diarrheal illnesses, typhoid fever, open tuberculosis, measles, chicken pox, and herpes zoster. The size of the isolation unit should be based on its anticipated use and its location planned to take into account traffic patterns of personnel, storage areas, and, where relevant, usual airflow patterns.

Another valuable component of the pediatric oncology unit is a facility where chemotherapy or blood product transfusions can be given on an outpatient basis. This may be less valuable in some parts of the world because many patients must travel long distances to reach the treatment center, and outpatient therapy according to the western model is not always practical.

Laminar air-flow units would seem, in general, to be an unwarranted luxury in the less developed countries. In this environment, the possible benefits of such facilities are far outweighed by their cost.

Training Programs for Professionals

If care is to reach appropriately high standards, training programs for health care professionals of all categories must be established. These are appropriately centered around the pediatric oncology unit. The exchange of personnel between the more and less developed countries can help considerably in this effort. However, there are several potential problems. Because opportunities are greater in the more developed countries, young trainees are often reluctant to return to their countries of origin. Moreover, the training programs are not adapted to the requirements in the trainee's country. Very often, even if the trainee does return to his or her own country, the lack of similar facilities may significantly hinder the application of principles learned during training. An alternative approach is to establish visiting programs for senior staff from the more developed countries. However, the visiting professor is un-

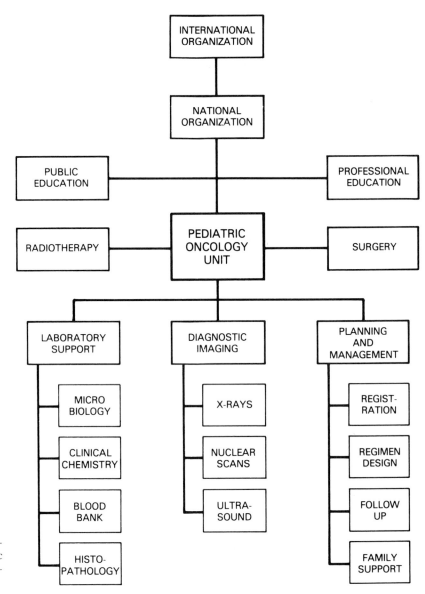

FIGURE 54-4. Diagrammatic depiction of the development of a pediatric oncology program. The pediatric oncology units form nodes on a network linked at national and international levels.

likely to be familiar with the problems encountered in the less developed countries, so that the teaching may be of limited practical value. Perhaps the most valuable exchange programs are those involving scientific collaborations or clinical trials— longer term relationships from which all participants stand to gain.

Necessary Ancillary Services

Clearly, no pediatric oncology unit can function without access to good diagnostic facilities and laboratory support in microbiology, hematology, clinical chemistry, and blood banking. Considerable thought should be given to the priorities regarding diagnosis and staging of patients (*i.e.,* determination of the extent of disease). Histology is still the backbone of diagnosis, although there is considerable variation in the technical standards achieved and the experience of histopathologists in evaluating pediatric neoplasms. There are circumstances when cytologic diagnosis may be adequate, particularly when supplemented by immunocytochemical studies. Electron mi-

croscopy, however, cannot be accorded a high priority because of its expense and the unusual expertise required, even though it can provide valuable information not obtainable by histologic examination in some cases.

Imaging studies, which play such an important role in the management of pediatric neoplasms in the more developed countries, should be carefully weighed in the list of priorities (see also Chap. 7). Standard radiographs are almost always available, but CT scanning and radionuclide imaging must take second place to drug availability and supportive care. Ultrasound examination may provide a less expensive alternative to CT scanning if the necessary expertise is available. It is possible to treat patients effectively using only clinical examination and chest radiographs, supplemented by an intravenous pyelogram, cavagram, and skeletal films, where necessary, for determining the extent of tumor. This range of radiologic capabilities can be provided by the simplest of equipment. It is not possible, however, to treat patients effectively without radiotherapy facilities, cytotoxic drugs, and the availability of good supportive care, including blood products and broad-spectrum antibiotics.

Specific Therapy

The requirements for specific therapy should also be carefully considered. For many pediatric tumors, radiation therapy is still an important or essential component of therapy (see Chap. 11). There are few countries that totally lack radiotherapy facilities, but often the existing facilities are so overloaded that delays are incurred in instituting therapy, and the machines are sometimes run through the night to deal with the heavy load. Because megavoltage units are expensive, it is imperative to carefully determine the role of radiation therapy in each pediatric neoplasm. The reluctance that still persists in the industrialized nations to relinquish radiotherapy—even in situations where chemotherapy has become the primary modality and radiation may add only toxicity—cannot be indulged in the less developed countries. If necessary, clinical trials must be undertaken to determine the role of radiation therapy in diseases traditionally treated with this modality, where chemotherapy has been shown to be highly effective. For example, there is probably only a very limited role for radiation therapy in non-Hodgkin's lymphoma treated with chemotherapy, and even Hodgkin's disease can be treated quite adequately with chemotherapy alone. In general, the radiotherapy facility will be used primarily for adult cancers, so that considerations of cost are not likely to involve the pediatric oncologist exclusively. Even in the context of a pediatric hospital, it is usually possible for children to receive radiation therapy in another hospital, and this is much less expensive than providing a separate radiotherapy suite.

Ideally, standardized clinical protocols should be developed in designated pediatric oncology units (see Chap. 13). In general, the quality of care received by patients is higher and the outcome of therapy better when standardized treatment protocols are adhered to. Further, information collected systematically from such studies, including the redefinition of prognostic groups in the setting of the less developed countries, should provide a foundation for future treatment protocols tailored to the region. Such standardized treatment protocols are more likely to be supported financially by pharmaceutical companies or granting bodies, which increases the likelihood of drugs being available to a greater number of patients. Finally, as noted, clinical trials provide a mutually beneficial medium for collaboration between the more and less developed countries. The institution of good clinical trials, preferably involving collaboration between the more and less developed countries, could provide the seed for developing improved care for patients in the less affluent parts of the world.

The nature of the chemotherapy protocols requires some discussion. The goal must be to provide therapy that produces results equivalent to those in the more developed countries, where some 57% of all children with cancer are alive at 5 years.[1] However, it is not necessarily appropriate to simply transpose regimens from the more developed countries, although they should represent the basis for developing more locally appropriate protocols. Intensive regimens require excellent supportive care that must be developed *pari passu* with chemotherapy regimens. The toxicities of drugs may differ in the less developed countries as a consequence of patients' poor nutritional status and exposure to a different spectrum of infectious diseases, including latent infections—to say nothing of possible genetic factors (see also Chaps. 9 and 39). Information relevant to differences in drug toxicities must be obtained. In addition, certain drug regimens that entail a potentially high risk if incorrectly administered should be avoided unless their use is considered to be absolutely necessary. High-dose methotrexate falls into this category because its safe

administration requires very careful monitoring, including the ability to measure methotrexate levels. Drug regimens that are very complicated should also be viewed with skepticism unless it has been clearly shown that they have a significant advantage over simpler regimens. Complicated regimens are more expensive, require more nursing and medical input, and are generally less likely to meet with full compliance by patient or doctor. The duration of therapy should be carefully considered because the strain of prolonged therapy on the patient's family is even greater in the less developed countries, for reasons discussed above. Moreover, when drugs are in such short supply, abbreviated therapy may permit the treatment of a greater number of patients and limit the need to select better risk patients or patients more able to comply with the requirements of the treatment protocol.

The advisability of developing bone marrow transplantation (BMT) programs in the less developed countries is an issue that frequently surfaces. This would not seem to be a high priority at the present time because BMT is extremely expensive, requires excellent supportive care, and is applicable to only a minority of patients, many of whom will have relapsed from primary therapy. However, some patients may travel to other countries for such procedures, at great personal or governmental expense. Such funds might be more efficiently used locally. In addition, the attention received by a BMT program may inspire voluntary or charitable contributions. Establishing a transplantation program, however, requires an efficient network of support services, as well as highly trained staff. Clearly, this issue is one that cannot be generalized and requires careful consideration at the national level. The establishment of a small number of regional centers (possibly serving more than one country), based in centers that have all the requirements for an efficient general program, may not be unreasonable in certain circumstances. However, BMT ought not to represent an end in itself, or be introduced at the expense of developing more important basic necessities.

Supportive Care

Because the treatment of almost all pediatric neoplasms involves cytotoxic chemotherapy, the need for supportive care during periods of myelosuppression must be given a high priority. There is no justification for the reduction of drug doses specifically to avoid significant myelosuppression—an approach that is almost certainly doomed to failure in terms of ultimate patient survival. The only alternative at present is the improvement of supportive care to a level such that the majority of patients will survive episodes of myelosuppression. This may necessitate accepting higher rates of treatment-related deaths at first, but as competence improves, mortality rates are likely to lessen considerably. Even with suboptimal supportive care, overall survival may well be better for patients treated with an appropriately intensive regimen than for those treated halfheartedly with regimens designed to minimize potentially life-threatening myelosuppression.

THE FEBRILE NEUTROPENIC PATIENT. Paramount in the provision of supportive care is strict adherence to the rule that febrile neutropenic patients are treated as medical emergencies requiring the immediate institution of broad-spectrum antibiotics (see Chap. 39). It is important that each pediatric unit establish the pattern of infection among its own patients because patterns are likely to differ considerably in various parts of the world. This requires developing a standard protocol for the routine workup of febrile neutropenic patients that includes blood, throat, urine, and stool cultures, chest radiographs, and a series of additional studies that should be based on the likeliest local causes of fever. In the majority of the less developed countries, tuberculosis is still rampant, and typhoid fever and shigellosis may be common infectious problems. Protozoal infections such as malaria, schistosomiasis, and trypanosomiasis may need to be considered, and in some parts of the world (*e.g.,* South America), fungal infection may be of much greater importance than in the United States and Europe. The possibility of massive nematode infestation and visceral migration should be borne in mind, particularly in the presence of polymicrobial sepsis, and viral infections may also assume a significantly greater degree of importance. Measles tends to be a much more serious and more common infection, particularly in countries where few people are vaccinated, while viral infections of the gastrointestinal tract, as well as arbovirus infections, should be considered in endemic areas. Not all of these infections are necessarily more common in the immunocompromised host, but their high incidence requires due attention.

Regardless of possible differences in microbiological flora, it is crucial to provide adequate (*i.e.,* broad spectrum) antibiotic coverage for bacterial infections which, throughout the world, are the most important pathogens in the febrile neutropenic patient. A number of antibiotics or antibiotic combinations may be considered. Until systematic studies become available of the microbiology of the immunocompromised host in different regions, including the sensitivity of bacterial pathogens to antibiotics, combinations of an aminoglycoside and a second-generation cephalosporin or an extended-spectrum penicillin, or all three classes of antibiotic, would seem the most reasonable choices. In holoendemic malarial regions, it may be appropriate to add antimalarials, although rapid diagnosis with thick and thin blood films may obviate their routine use. Acyclovir is a useful drug for varicella/zoster infections but has a lower priority than broad-spectrum antibiotics, if choices must be made, because of the relative rarity of these infections compared to bacterial infections in the immunocompromised host. Amphotericin is another important agent for use in patients with documented fungal infections and in the neutropenic patient whose fever persists in spite of broad-spectrum antibiotic coverage, and its earlier introduction (or the use of other antifungals) during the period of neutropenia could be particularly important in some regions.

The need for a critical care unit requires careful consideration. Although the lives of a small number of patients might be saved by the special facilities available in a critical care unit (*e.g.,* a proportion of those with sepsis), such units cannot be considered essential because of the relative infrequency of the need for critical care medicine (assuming that the chemotherapy regimens used do not have an extremely high degree of toxicity). Further, the cost of establishing and maintaining such a unit can only be justified after attention has been given to the essential components of supportive care. Many patients will die if broad-spectrum antibiotics are not given for febrile neutropenic episodes, but only a very few will die for lack of a critical care unit.

BLOOD PRODUCT SUPPORT. Packed red cell and platelet transfusions have become an essential adjunct to modern intensive chemotherapy protocols and must be made available where such regimens are used (see Chap. 38). This raises a number of problems, one of the most important being the frequent reluctance of people in some countries to donate blood, and the consequent lack of blood products. This can often be overcome by instituting a program whereby blood is primarily donated by relatives. The sophistication required for the collection of whole blood is minimal, but the need for platelet transfusions often provides a significant obstacle. It is necessary to scrupulously examine the criteria for determining the need for platelet transfusions to ensure that precious resources are used most efficiently. The possibility of vitamin K deficiency or liver disease adding to bleeding problems must also be kept in mind. Where cell separators are not available, platelet-rich plasma provides an acceptable substitute.

PSYCHOLOGICAL SUPPORT. Psychological support, an increasingly important component in the overall management of the cancer patient and his or her family in the more developed countries, is a particularly difficult area in the developing countries. Because of the major problems in providing adequate medical care, psychological aspects must take second place. However, education of patients is crucially important to obtaining cooperation during therapy, and there is much to recommend the addition of ancillary personnel who take a major role in this area (see Chaps. 41 and 42). Such a team, with a knowledge of local mores and traditional fears, could do much to allay anxiety and improve patient compliance. The availability of videorecording equipment also raises the possibility that patient education could be carried out, at least in part, by means of educational films. This approach has the advantages of saving time, ensuring completeness, and providing whatever incentives may be deemed helpful, such as the depiction of successfully treated patients. Written materials are generally unlikely to be of value because of the high illiteracy rates (although they could be made available to those who could benefit). By the same token, written documentation of informed consent for a clinical study must be carefully considered in the context of the educational level of the parents and the rules pertaining to clinical research in the particular country. Although explanations of the nature of the disease and its treatment are always desirable, different approaches to the process of informed consent may be necessary. Clearly, educational programs must be tailored to specific regions because of the enormous geographic differences in language, customs, and beliefs.

Patient Follow-Up

In the less developed countries, follow-up may be a major problem that can hinder the delivery of adequate care and the collection of accurate data on the immediate and long-term beneficial and toxic results of therapy. Schemes must be developed to provide expenses for traveling to the treatment center. In many parts of the world, such as India, federal or regional governments subsidize travel for cancer patients. This must be supplemented by adequate systems for ensuring that defaulting patients are immediately contacted (often a major undertaking, particularly in rural regions where the concept of "address" is much vaguer than in the more developed countries) and, wherever possible, by a system to provide families in need with a means of livelihood during periods when the child is hospitalized. The need for, and approach to, such efforts will naturally vary from country to country. Very often the income necessary to sustain the family at their usual level is quite small. In some cases, work can be found at the treatment center that is sufficient to provide a small income. Alternatively, research funds can often be used for subsistence and travel allowances. Since the relative costs of both travel and subsistence are usually extremely low in the less developed countries, this component of the cost of clinical trials is often minor compared to, for example, the cost of drugs.

Assistance for travel and subsistence cannot be separated from the importance of impressing on families the need to return to the cancer unit for further therapy or follow-up. Simply providing money is often the wrong approach, because cash may well be used for other purposes. Giving families passes or vouchers for buses and trains is often preferable, although subsistence allowances may need to be given as cash. The family's realization that they will receive support for future visits may well provide an additional incentive to return.

Good follow-up is so vitally important to the ability to obtain accurate data, and hence to the conduct of good clinical research, that it is often worth assigning a specific person (or team, depending on the size of the unit) to the task of detecting defaulters.

Organization at a National Level

It is clear that the most efficient approach to childhood cancer in the less developed countries entails a regional or, preferably, a national plan whereby resources are used optimally and organized approaches are developed for training appropriate professionals, identifying regional sites for pediatric oncology units, and providing appropriate diagnostic facilities and treatment protocols tailored to the specific needs of the country in question. National bodies are also in a good position to institute or encourage the institution of degrees or diplomas relevant to training schemes, to establish collaboration (including exchange of personnel and financial support) with the more developed countries, and to institute subsidized transportation to and from the hospital. Another important role for national and regional bodies is the development of educational programs directed toward increasing the average person's understanding of cancer. A variety of approaches can be envisioned. Films can be shown on national television (even the poorest of villages may own a communal television), visits of health professionals to local communities can be arranged, and information disseminated through regional health authorities. Even schemes to support families who lose their income when uprooted to a regional cancer center may be more readily instituted when introduced with the authority of a national body.

National bodies should also organize conferences and committees to deal with problems of particular importance to pediatric oncology in their own countries. Among the many issues to be grappled with, particularly in the poorest of countries, is the possibility of establishing small industries that can provide many of the goods required for the development of the more complex medical practice required in pediatric oncology. Such industries can be readily justified because they will be relevant to a much broader area of medical practice than simply pediatric oncology. Appropriate items for consideration include disposable plastic ware such as syringes and intravenous infusion sets, intravenous solutions, and even some of the more easily manufactured chemotherapeutic agents and antibiotics. In the smaller countries, and even some of the larger ones, most of these items are currently imported from abroad at great expense.

The precise nature of the most appropriate national body will vary from country to country, and also according to the nature of the task that must be performed. In some circumstances, a government agency will be the most useful, or even the only, body likely to succeed. In other situations, a professional organization or branch thereof, such as an oncology society, may take the lead role or propose solutions to the government.

The Role of International Organizations

International organizations of all types could have a major impact on the development of pediatric oncology throughout the world. Among the more important of these are the interna-

tional health and cancer organizations, but international financial bodies that are often involved in shaping the development of a country could also have an important role.

International cancer organizations might be expected to provide the lead role by convening committees with broad international representation to assist in determining priorities and to provide guidelines for evolving national policy. Detailed guidance could also be provided at the level of the pediatric cancer unit itself regarding the determination of the basic components of such a unit and its supporting facilities, the development of curricula for training programs at all levels, and the promotion of international scientific exchanges (e.g., conferences or the establishment of individual scholarships and grants). The Committee on International Collaborative Activities of the International Union Against Cancer (UICC) has already given a great deal of thought to establishing guidelines for the development of comprehensive cancer centers, aimed at providing comprehensive management, clinical and basic research, and educational programs for professionals and for patients' families. Although not specifically directed toward pediatric oncology, the UICC's published guidelines contain much useful information.[32] International granting bodies could help by establishing funds to be used specifically for encouraging scientific work in pediatric oncology in the less developed countries and for supporting the travel of trainees or experts to and from such countries. International bodies such as the UICC have an important role in encouraging international collaborative studies and fostering the exchange of clinical information (e.g., through the International Cancer Patient Data Exchange System). Pharmaceutical companies can (and often do) provide valuable support for clinical trials, for example, by providing drugs and assisting with protocol design and monitoring and by contributing funding for conferences in which participants discuss the results of such studies. A more specific role could be played by employing local representatives of the drug company and increasing the manufacture of chemotherapeutic agents in the less developed countries themselves. The development of new agents particularly suitable for the less developed regions of the world is another possible contribution that could be made by the pharmaceutical industry.

It is clear that, despite the sometimes extremely limited resources of the poorest of the world's countries, there are numerous mechanisms whereby improvements in the practice of pediatric oncology can be accomplished. Many of the approaches mentioned already exist to some extent, but obviously at a grossly inadequate level. Although it is true that pediatric oncology is not the primary health-related issue in the less developed countries, as long as it can be developed without draining resources from projects of more immediate import, there is much to be gained not only by the victims of these diseases but by researchers in all parts of the world. Further, as anticipated improvements in socioeconomic standards take place, mechanisms will already exist whereby the increasing importance of malignancies as a cause of death in children can be dealt with effectively. It is worth remembering that major improvements in health care in the more developed countries have occurred only in the course of this century. In the early 1900s, the infant mortality rates for New York (140 per 1000) and Birmingham, United Kingdom (200/1000), were as high or higher than those in any of the less developed countries today.[33] The major socioeconomic changes needed to bring about improved sanitation and nutrition and, with these, improved health in the less developed countries may not be as far off as they now seem. Dramatic changes are likely to take place in at least some countries in the lifetime of its present children. The children of a country represent its future, and all possible measures should be taken to ensure that the future is bright.

REFERENCES

1. Young JL, Ries LG, Silverberg E, Horm JW, Miller RW: Cancer incidence, survival and mortality for children younger than age 15 years. Cancer 58:598–602, 1986
2. Ramot B, Magrath IT: Hypothesis: The environment is a major determinant of the immunological sub-type of lymphoma and acute lymphoblastic leukaemia in children. Br J Haematol 52:183–189, 1982
3. World Health Statistics Annual 1986. Geneva, Switzerland, World Health Organization, 1986
4. Demographic Yearbook 1984. New York, United Nations, 1984
5. The 1986 Information Almanac. Boston, Houghton Mifflin, 1986
6. Paxton J (ed): The Stateman's Yearbook 1985–86. New York, St Martin's Press, 1986
7. World Population Prospects. Estimates and Projections as Assessed in 1982. New York, United Nations, 1985
8. Ivy PS, Ozols RY, Cowan KN: Drug resistance in cancer. In Magrath IT (ed): New Directions in Cancer Research. Heidelberg, Springer (in press)
9. Breslow NE, Landholz B: Childhood cancer incidence: Geographical and temporal variations. Int J Cancer 32:703–716, 1983
10. Macdougall LG, Jankowitz P, Cohn R, Berstein R: Acute childhood leukemia in Johannesburg. Am J Pediatr Hematol Oncol 8:43–51, 1986
11. Greaves MF: Subtypes of acute lymphoblastic leukemia: Implications for the pathogenesis and epidemiology of leukemia. In Magrath IT, O'Conor GT, Ramot B (eds): The Pathogenesis of Leukemias and Lymphomas: Role of the Environment, pp 129–139. New York, Raven Press, 1984
12. Court-Brown WM, Doll R: Leukaemia in childhood and young adult life. Trends in mortality in relation to aetiology. Br Med J 26:981, 1961
13. Li FP, Jin F, Tu CT, Gao YT: Incidence of childhood leukemia in Shanghai. Int J Cancer 25:701–703, 1980
14. Bosco J, Cherian R, Lin HP, Pang T: A survey of lymphoid malignancies at University Hospital, Kuala Lumpur, Malaysia. In Magrath IT, O'Conor GT, Ramot B (eds): The Pathogenesis of Leukemias and Lymphomas: Role of the Environment, pp 61–65. New York, Raven Press, 1984
15. Misad O, Solidaro A, Quiroz L, Olivares L: An overview of lymphoreticular malignancies in Peru. In Magrath IT, O'Conor GT, Ramot B (eds): The Pathogenesis of Leukemias and Lymphomas: Role of the Environment, pp 85–97. New York, Raven Press, 1984
16. Kamat DM, Gopal R, Advani SH, Nair CN, et al: Pattern of subtypes of acute lymphoblastic leukemia in India. Leuk Res 9:927–934, 1985
17. Greaves MF, Pegram SM, Chan LC: Collaborative group study of the epidemiology of acute lymphoblastic leukemia subtypes. Background and first report. Leuk Res 9:715–733, 1985
18. Bhargava M (New Delhi), Kamel A (Cairo): Personal communication
19. Magrath IT: Selected epidemiological data pertinent to topics discussed in this volume. In Magrath IT, O'Conor GT, Ramot B (eds): The Pathogenesis of Leukemias and Lymphomas: Role of the Environment, pp 379–386. New York, Raven Press, 1984
20. Cavdar AO, Arcossy A, Babacan E, Golzdasogh S, Topuz U, Fraumeni JF: Ocular granulocytic sarcoma (chloroma) with acute myelomonocytic leukemia in Turkish children. Cancer 41:1606–1609, 1978
21. Correa P, O'Conor GT: Epidemiological patterns of Hodgkin's disease. Int J Cancer 8:192–201, 1971
22. McKeen EA, Khan AB, Kaid S: Childhood cancer in Pakistan. Proc Am Assoc Cancer Res 21:47, 1980
23. Gupta BD, Grover RK: Hospital cancer registry at Post-Graduate Institute of Medical Education and Research, Chandigahr: Annual report. In Annual Report, National Cancer Registry of the Indian Council of Medical Research, pp 121–140. New Delhi, ICMR, 1982
24. Camargo B, Petrilli S: Personal communication
25. Lin H-P: Personal communication
26. Nkrumah FK: Pediatric oncology in the developing world: An African perspective. Ann Trop Paediatr 7:155–158, 1987
27. Grover S, Hardas UD: Childhood malignancies in Central India. J Natl Cancer Inst 99:953–958, 1972
28. Gad-el-Mawla N: Personal communication
29. Williams CKO: Epidemiology of childhood leukemias and lymphomas with special reference to Ibadan. Niger J Pediatr 12:1–9, 1985
30. Williams CKO, Akingbehin NH, Seriki O, Folami OA: Efficacy of high-dose cytosine arabinoside (ara-C) containing regimen in the control of advanced Burkitt's lymphoma—A preliminary assessment. Proc Am Soc Clin Oncol 4:197, 1985
31. Johnson AOK, Williams CKO: A reappraisal of the management of common childhood abdominal malignancies in Ibadan. Niger J Pediatr 11:29–39, 1984
32. Committee on International Collaborative Activities (CICA): Guidelines for developing a comprehensive cancer center. In UICC Technical Reports, vol 53. Geneva, Switzerland, UICC, 1980
33. Davis R, Butler N, Goldstein H: From Birth to Seven. London, Longman, 1973

fifty-five

Preventive Pediatric Oncology: The Childhood Origins of Adult Cancer

Frederick P. Li and John J. Mulvihill

Approximately 900,000 new cases of cancer are diagnosed annually in the United States. Of these, 1% (6500) occur in children under 15 years of age.[1] The remainder develop in adults, and most are carcinomas in persons over 50 years of age (Table 55-1).[2] The number of cancers nationwide is rising, primarily because of the aging and growth of the population.[3] Cancer prevention, early detection, and improved therapy are important approaches to cancer control.

Most human cancers are diagnosed decades after initial exposure to the causal agent.[4] For asbestos-associated mesothelioma, for example, the latency period is usually 30 years or longer. For radiation, as revealed by follow-up studies of atomic bomb survivors, the briefest interval was 2 to 3 years for acute leukemia, whereas an excess of radiogenic breast cancer is still being seen in those exposed as children. Therefore, cancers that appear later in life might be due to influences present during childhood. These factors may involve environmental exposure associated with personal habits, diet, ambient pollutants, medicinal agents, and viruses.[4-6] In addition, genetic factors, particularly cancer genes, can radically elevate the risk of specific cancers (see Chap. 2).[7] This chapter reviews the available data on childhood influences that increase the risk of cancer in adult life and explores interventions to reduce cancer morbidity and mortality in later life.

ENVIRONMENTAL CARCINOGENS

Data suggest that up to 80% of cancers in adults are due in large part to environmental factors.[8] This figure is derived from findings that cancer incidence rates differ substantially among the populations of the world and change over time and with migration. The findings suggest that elimination of environmental carcinogens may be sufficient to prevent many cancers, and much effort has, therefore, been expended to investigate and identify human carcinogens.

Human carcinogens include physical, chemical, and biological agents that can induce neoplasms in a single organ site or multiple sites (Table 55-2).[4,6,9] Ultraviolet and ionizing radiation produce cancer through their physical properties. Among the many chemicals that have been evaluated for carcinogenic effects, approximately 20 have been shown to be carcinogenic in humans.[9] Other chemicals can induce cancer in laboratory animals, but data for humans are insufficient or inconsistent. Viruses have been known for decades to be carcinogenic in experimental systems, but only recently have studies provided compelling evidence of viral oncogenesis in humans.[10-12]

Personal Habits

Tobacco Use

Tobacco is by far the most important cause of carcinoma of the lung.[13] In the United States, lung cancer has been the leading cause of cancer death among males for nearly three decades and is replacing breast cancer as the leading cause of cancer mortality among women. Cigarette smoking accounts for more cancer deaths nationally than all other known carcinogens combined. An estimated 100,000 men and more than 40,000 women died of lung cancer in 1987. More than 125,000 deaths each year in the United States, or 25% of all cancer deaths, are attributable to tobacco consumption.

Cigarette smoking is associated with all the major histologic types of primary lung cancer and accounts for the large majority of squamous and oat cell carcinomas of the lung. Smoking also causes cancers of the oral cavity, larynx, esophagus, bladder, and perhaps other sites. Data on the causal role of smoking in human cancers, as summarized in the reports of the Surgeon General of the United States, are convincing and consistent.[14] Studies show that the risk of lung cancer increases with dose, as measured by the number of cigarettes consumed per day; the total duration of smoking; and the amount of inhaled tobacco smoke.

One of the single most effective strategies to cancer prevention in adults will be the cessation of smoking and tobacco use. Because a decade elapses before the maximum benefit of cessation is attained, smokers should stop as soon as possible. More importantly, adolescents and young adults should be strongly encouraged not to start smoking.

Of note, the per capita tobacco consumption has been declining for a number of years in the United States.[15] The decline has been substantial among adult males, leading to predictions that lung cancer rates in men will decrease. This trend can be attributed to success in public education, legislation requiring warning labels on cigarette packages, prohibition of certain forms of advertising, and establishment of nonsmoking areas in public places. However, cigarette smoking remains a common habit among certain segments of the population, notably nonwhites and teenage girls.[14] Because cigarette smoking often begins in adolescence and cessation is difficult once the habit is initiated, efforts should be focused on discouraging teenagers from starting to smoke.

Several strategies based on studies of smoking behavior have been developed to limit smoking among adolescents and young adults.[16] Self-help, counseling, hypnosis, and other interventions have been applied to individual smokers. Some school programs emphasize education of students regarding the deleterious effects of smoking, and others use psychosocial approaches to help adolescents resist peer pressures to smoke. Both methods seem to have some benefit, particularly when directed at children who have not started smoking. Cigarette smoking is often a family habit, and cessation programs should also be targeted at the family unit as well as the larger community. For people who cannot be motivated to protect their own health, knowledge of the harmful effects of passive smoking on their friends and family members may provide the incentive to quit.[17]

Table 55-1
Most Common Forms of Cancer Among Children and Adults in the United States*

Adults (ages 15 and older)		Children (ages 0–14)	
Cancer Site	Annual Incidence	Cancer Site	Annual Incidence
Lung	149,000	Leukemias	2000
Colon and rectum	140,000	Brain tumors	1200
Breast	123,900	Lymphomas	800
Prostate	90,000	Neuroblastoma	400
Bladder	40,500	Soft tissue sarcoma	400
Other	386,600	Other	1700
All cancers	930,000	All cancers	6500

* Based on data of the Statistics, Epidemiology and End Results Program of the National Cancer Institute.

Table 55-2
Environmental Exposures in Childhood and Adolescence Associated with Cancer Development in Later Life

Type	Carcinogenic Agent	Associated Cancers
Personal habits	Tobacco	Lung, oral cavity, larynx, esophagus, bladder
	Alcohol	Oral cavity, larynx, esophagus, liver
	Diet	Gastrointestinal tract
	Sunlight	Skin, ocular melanoma
Medicinal	Alkylating agents	Acute nonlymphocytic leukemia, bladder (cyclophosphamide)
	Androgens	Liver
	Immunosuppressives (azathioprine, cyclosporine)	Non-Hodgkin's lymphoma
	Prenatal diethylstilbestrol	Vaginal adenocarcinoma
	Ionizing radiation	Diverse cancers
	Phenacetin	Bladder, renal pelvis
Pollutants and occupational (parental) exposures	Asbestos	Lung, mesothelioma
	Arsenic	Skin
	Benzene	Acute myelocytic leukemia
	Polycyclic hydrocarbons	Lung, scrotum
Infection	Hepatitis B virus	Liver
	HIV	Kaposi's sarcoma, lymphoma
	HTLV-I	Adult T-cell leukemia/lymphoma
	Papilloma virus	Cervix

Nearly all clinicians, including pediatricians, have experienced the difficulty of convincing patients to cease smoking.[13] At times, the effort seems futile. Nevertheless, the value of education regarding the hazards of smoking has been demonstrated by the decline in tobacco use among health care providers, including physicians, dentists, and pharmacists.[18] Pediatricians can help to prevent children and adolescents from starting to smoke by acting as role models and providing support for the antismoking efforts of schoolteachers, family members, and other health providers.

In recent years, the use of smokeless tobacco has increased, particularly among adolescent and adult males.[19] This trend has resulted in part from extensive advertising campaigns by tobacco producers and pressures against smoking in some public places. Oral cancers have been reported with increasing frequency among users of smokeless tobacco, and interventions against smoking should also include attention to other forms of tobacco consumption (see also Chap. 35).

Alcohol

Excessive alcohol consumption is another addictive habit that often starts in adolescence.[16] Alcohol abuse is due partly to the same social, psychological, and peer influences that promote cigarette smoking. Alcoholism is associated with cancers of the mouth, larynx, esophagus, liver, and perhaps other sites.[20,21] The risk of these cancers is particularly high in drinkers who also smoke, suggesting that alcohol is a cocarcinogen with tobacco. In addition, suicide, homicide, and injuries, and death from automobile and industrial accidents occur with high frequency among alcoholics. Prevention of addiction to drugs and alcohol has begun to receive much needed attention by schools and social and legal agencies.

Sunlight

Lifelong exposure to sunlight increases the risk of several forms of skin cancer in exposed surfaces.[4,22,23] The risk of cancer is higher among fair-skinned individuals of Celtic origin, and in susceptible groups such as persons with xeroderma pigmentosum and dysplastic nevus syndrome.[24] In recent years, the increased popularity of sunbathing and outdoor activities, particularly among adolescents and young adults, has heightened the exposure to ultraviolet radiation (see Chap. 35). Education regarding the protective effects of topical sunscreens appears to be the most effective and acceptable method of reducing exposure to sunlight among sensitive individuals.

Diet

Available epidemiologic data implicate diet in the etiology of cancers of the digestive tract and other sites.[5] However, precise dietary causes of cancers in humans remain uncertain, despite a long list of suspects.[25] These include the basic ingredients of foods (fat, caloric, and fiber content), food additives (dyes), flavoring agents (saccharin), contaminants (aflatoxin), and cooking methods (charcoal broiling) (see also Chap. 40). Studies also suggest that there may also be protective dietary factors, such as calcium, selenium, and vitamins A, C, D, and E. Controversy remains regarding the appropriate recommendations regarding dietary modification as an approach to cancer prevention. Some observers have advocated major public education to modify the diet of the U.S. population.[26] The objective is to encourage consumption of a balanced diet adequate in protein and other needed nutrients, with energy content sufficient to maintain a stable and normal body weight. These measures include reducing caloric and alcohol intake, decreasing fats to less than 30% of total calories, and increasing consumption of fresh fruits and vegetables.[26] While research continues, these recommendations seem prudent. Even if benefits in terms of cancer prevention were small, these measures would probably provide protection against cardiovascular diseases, still the leading cause of death in adults nationally. To date, a few trials of diet modification and supplementation have been instituted, but definitive results are not yet available. Nutritional education in schools can be presented in conjunction with programs directed against tobacco and alcohol use. In addition, fads in diet such as high-dose vitamin supplements should be discouraged until their consequences are determined.

Ionizing Radiation

Ionizing radiation is probably the most thoroughly studied human carcinogen.[6] Cancers induced by this agent include leukemias, carcinomas, and sarcomas. The leukemias start to appear within several years after radiation exposure and the solid tumors develop after a lapse of a decade or more. The excess risk of cancer persists for many years, perhaps a lifetime (see also Chaps. 1 and 2). Radiation-induced cancers have been reported in persons exposed during childhood to the detonation of nuclear weapons and to treatments for neoplasia and benign conditions such as thymic and tonsillar enlargement and tinea capitis. At the time of their use, such procedures were accepted clinical practice, but they proved to have devastating risks later in life. Pediatricians must be ever vigilant to the lifelong consequences of seemingly rational new practices. After high-dose orthovoltage radiotherapy for childhood cancers, the risk of a second neoplasm is as high as 0.5% per year, or 15% over the 30 years after treatment (see Chaps. 11 and 50).

The recognition of the carcinogenic effects of ionizing radiation has led to efforts to reduce exposure in childhood. Unnecessary exposures have been eliminated, and radiography and radiotherapy equipment have been modernized to reduce absorbed dose. It is theoretically plausible that every single exposure to ionizing radiation may contribute to the eventual initiation of cancer, so pediatricians should be scrupulous in ordering radiography for only the best medical reasons.

Medicinal Agents

Among the hundreds of drugs administered to children today, it is remarkable that only a handful have been shown to cause cancer (see Table 55-2).

Patients who survive a childhood cancer have been reported to develop acute nonlymphocytic leukemia after receiving alkylating agents, such as cyclophosphamide, melphalan, chlorambucil, nitrogen mustard, and the nitrosoureas (see also Chaps. 9 and 50).[27] The leukemia risk, which appears to increase with drug dose, is a few percent within the first decade after exposure. The risk of other cancers has not been established for most alkylating agents. To date, no carcinogenic effect has been detected in patients exposed to the antimetabolites, vinca alkyloids, and anthracyclines. Knowledge of the leukemogenic and other toxic effects of alkylating agents has led to studies to find alternative therapies. For Hodgkin's disease, investigators have examined the use of the ABVD combination as a substitute for MOPP chemotherapy (see Chap. 21).[28]

Cancer in later life can result from carcinogenic exposures during fetal development. The first transplacental carcinogen identified in humans was diethylstilbestrol.[29] Maternal ingestion of this drug during pregnancy increases the risk in daughters of vaginal adenocarcinoma, a rare neoplasm in the general population (see Chaps. 1, 2, and 35). A few hundred cases of this association have been reported, and the risk of developing the cancer is approximately 1 per 1000 women exposed *in utero* to this drug.[30] Transplacental effects have also been reported with cigarette smoking and use of hydantoin and other drugs.

Several other drug therapies in childhood have been linked to the development of cancers in later life. These include non-Hodgkin's lymphomas in organ transplant recipients after immunosupressive treatments with azothioprine and cyclosporine; primary liver cancer in patients treated with androgens for bone marrow failure; and renal pelvis and bladder carcinoma after prolonged phenacetin therapy for chronic pain.[4,31,32]

Viruses

Hepatitis B Virus

Evidence shows that the hepatitis B virus is a likely cause of primary liver cancer (see also Chap. 26).[10] This neoplasm is rare in the United States but is a leading cause of cancer death in many areas of Asia and Africa. Geographically, the patterns of hepatitis B infection and liver cancer overlap. The risk of liver cancer rates is increased nearly 200-fold among patients with chronic hepatitis B infection, a condition often acquired in infancy.[33] An etiologic role of the virus has been supported by laboratory investigations showing viral DNA integration into the host cell genome and presence of the agent in liver cancer cells, and by animal models of liver cancer after infection by hepatitis B-like viruses. In recent years, the development of vaccines has led to effective prevention of hepatitis B infection, and studies to examine possible prevention of primary liver cancer are in progress.

Human T Lymphoma-Leukemia Viruses (HTLV)

Recent identification of the HTLV viruses has strengthened the evidence for an oncogenic role of viruses in humans.[12] The HTLV-I virus is associated with an aggressive form of T-cell lymphoma in young adults (see also Chaps. 20 and 22). The disease shows an unusual geographic distribution, with high rate areas in Japan and the Caribbean. Infection with this virus in childhood can lead to the development of the hematologic neoplasm years later. An apparently related agent is the human immunodeficiency virus (HIV, or HTLV-III), the causal agent in acquired immunodeficiency syndrome (AIDS) (see Chap. 36).[34] The disease is now widespread and in the United States alone has caused more than 15,000 deaths.[33] Serologic studies of the prevalence of infection in the general population indicate that this number will rise sharply. The disease is transmitted by intimate contact and in the United States is prevalent in homosexual males. Infection in infancy can be acquired from an affected mother. Blood transfusion is another route of infection, particularly among transfusion-dependent hemophiliacs. Blood products are now routinely screened for evidence of HIV contamination. Avoidance of intimate contact with infected persons is effective in preventing AIDS-associated diseases, including Kaposi's sarcoma and lymphomas.

Other Viruses

Despite extensive use of the Papanicolaou smear to detect early disease, cervical carcinoma remains a persistent problem in certain segments of the population.[16] Epidemiologic data indicate that the cervical cancer risk increases with early age at first coitus, multiple sexual partners, history of venereal diseases, and work as a prostitute. Findings suggest that carcinoma of the cervix is a sexually transmitted neoplasm that can be acquired initially in adolescence. The transmissible agent has long been suspected to be a virus, and recent attention has focused on the papilloma virus, type 6 (see Chaps. 1 and 35).[11] Members of the herpes simplex virus family have been implicated in the development of cervical and oral cancers, although the evidence is more tenuous.

Some virus-induced cancers are preventable by appropriate intervention in childhood. Screening of pregnant women to detect chronic hepatitis carriers, and vaccination of their newborns, may prevent liver cancer in later life. Counseling of adolescents regarding sexual activity can reduce the risk of cervical cancer and HIV-associated cancer. Appropriate intervention includes taking a confidential sexual history from adolescent patients, discussing the hazards of sexually transmitted diseases, instructing sexually active patients in the proper use of barrier contraceptives, and introducing early cervical cancer screening in susceptible patients.[16]

Ambient Exposures

Asbestos

Asbestos is an important cause of lung cancer and is the predominant cause of peritoneal and pleural mesotheliomas.[35] Asbestos, a valuable insulating fiber, has been mined in large quantities over the last century. The material is virtually indestructible, and heavy exposure has produced mesothelioma and lung cancers among asbestos miners, shipyard workers, pipefitters, and plumbers. Each year in the United States, asbestos is estimated to cause several thousand cancers.[36] An interaction has been found between asbestos and cigarette smoking, and the risk of lung cancer is markedly increased in persons with both exposures. The carcinogenic effect of asbestos appears to be due to the long, needle-like physical configuration of the fiber. Mesothelioma after asbestos exposure has a latent period of several decades, and has been reported after a relatively minimal exposure. Mesothelioma in young adults has occurred after childhood residence near asbestos mines and exposure to asbestos fibers carried home on workers' clothing. Currently, concern is focused on the effects of contamination of nearly 10% of U.S. schools by asbestos installed as a fire retardant in ceiling material.[37] To date, no cancers have been shown to arise from attendance at these schools, but the time elapsed is still short.

Waste products of industry are discarded into the environment, either by accident or intentionally. The refuse may contain carcinogens such as aromatic amines, metals, radioisotopes, and solvents that have been shown to cause cancer in workers. Increasing numbers of contaminated dump sites have been identified throughout the United States. Residents of these areas have become alarmed about possible carcinogenic hazards, particularly in children. In Woburn, Massachusetts, an excess of leukemias has been associated with chemical contamination of the soil and water, although a causal relationship remains uncertain.[38] Extensive studies of other dump sites, such as Love Canal in New York State, have not yet shown any excess cancers in the local population.[39] Monitoring for early evidence of harmful effects is continuing at many of these sites (see also Chaps. 1 and 2).

HEREDITARY CANCERS

Efforts in cancer prevention have focused on the elimination of environmental carcinogens.[8] Primary and secondary prevention of hereditary cancers has received little attention because of the perception that effective intervention is not possible. However, data show that prevention of hereditary cancers can be achieved through genetic counseling, periodic surveillance, and early intervention in affected kindreds.[40]

A hereditary component has been identified in virtually all forms of human cancers, including cancers of the colon, breast, and other common sites.[41] Members of families with a hereditary cancer are often affected in childhood or early adulthood. The occurrence of hereditary cancer within a family is typically limited to one or a few organs, which helps simplify early detection efforts. However, multiple foci of tumor may develop in the target organ(s), and successful treatment of one tumor may be followed by the appearance of additional primary lesions.

Cancers in some families are inherited as single gene (Mendelian) traits. An offspring of the carrier of a dominant gene, such as the retinoblastoma gene, has a 50% probability of inheriting the defect, and risk of developing cancer is determined by gene penetrance.[42] *In utero* diagnosis of carriers of the retinoblastoma gene is now possible in some families, and these techniques can be extended in the future to detection of carriers of other cancer genes (see Chap. 25).[43] Even without an applicable laboratory test, patients in cancer families should be counseled regarding possible transmission of the susceptibility to cancer. The benefits of genetic counseling may accrue over the same period of time required to achieve maximal benefit from smoking cessation (*i.e.*, longer than a decade).[14]

Hereditary cancers can be recognized early in some patients, and this can lead to appropriate measures for early intervention. Precursor moles identify affected members of families with dominantly transmitted dysplastic nevus syndrome who should be watched for treatable localized malignant melanoma.[23] Dominantly inherited polyposis coli antedates the development of adenocarcinoma of the colon and can be diagnosed through the family history and a colon examination; prophylactic colectomy before the development of unresectable colon carcinoma is the treatment of choice (see Chap. 35).[44] Identification of cancer gene carriers through a detailed family history also provides opportunities to employ laboratory markers of early cancer, such as elevated calcitonin levels in patients with familial medullary thyroid carcinoma.[45] When inherited predisposition to cancer is recognized, attention should be given to the avoidance of environmental factors that may enhance oncogenesis. For example, avoidance of sunlight in patients with xeroderma pigmentosum and albinism can substantially delay the development of skin cancer.[46]

Survivors of childhood cancers are at increased risk of developing second primary cancers.[47] Patients with hereditary retinoblastoma develop an excess of osteosarcoma, pinealoma, and other cancers (see Chaps. 25 and 50).[48] Children with other forms of cancer may also have an underlying genetic disorder, such as von Recklinghausen's neurofibromatosis, which may not be discernible until the later development of additional cancers.[49] Recently, studies of survivors of hepatoblastoma suggest that this neoplasm is a rare feature of the polyposis coli gene.[50] Among survivors of hepatoblastoma due to the polyposis coli gene, the risk of colonic neoplasms in later life approaches 100%. Early intervention to detect polyposis coli in these patients can reduce their risk of dying from colon cancer.

REFERENCES

1. Young JL Jr, Ries LG, Silverberg E et al: Cancer incidence, survival, and mortality for children younger than age 15 years. Cancer 58:598–602, 1986
2. Young JL Jr, Percy CL, Asire AJ (eds): Surveillance, Epidemiology, and End Results: Incidence and Mortality Data, 1973–1977. Natl Cancer Inst Monogr 57:66–67, 1981
3. Bailar JC III, Smith EL: Progress against cancer? N Engl J Med 314:1226–1232, 1986
4. Schottenfeld D, Fraumeni JF Jr: Cancer Epidemiology and Prevention. Philadelphia, WB Saunders, 1982
5. Willet WC, MacMahon B: Diet and cancer—an overview. N Engl J Med 310:633–638, 697–703, 1984
6. Boice JD Jr, Fraumeni JF Jr (eds): Radiation Carcinogenesis: Epidemiology and Biological Significance. New York, Raven Press, 1984
7. Mulvihill JJ, Miller RW, Fraumeni JF Jr (eds): Genetics of Human Cancer. New York, Raven Press, 1977
8. Doll R, Peto R: The causes of cancer: Quantitative estimates of avoidable risks of cancer in the United States today. J Natl Cancer Inst 66:1192–1308, 1981
9. IARC Working Group: An evaluation of chemicals and industrial processes associated with cancer in humans based on human and animal data. Cancer Res 40:1–12, 1980
10. Blumberg BS, London WT: Hepatitis B virus and the prevention of primary cancer of the liver. J Natl Cancer Inst 74:267–274, 1985
11. Macnab JCM, Walkinshaw SA, Cordiner JW et al: Human papillomavirus in clinically and histologically normal tissue of patients with genital cancer. N Engl J Med 315:1052–1058, 1986
12. Wong-Staal F, Gallo RC: Human T-lymphotrophic retroviruses. Nature 317:395–403, 1985
13. Fielding JE: Smoking: Health effects and control. N Engl J Med 313:491–498, 555–561, 1985
14. Smoking and Health: A Report of the Surgeon General. US Department of Health, Education, and Welfare, DHEW Publication No. (PHS) 79-50066. Washington, DC, US Government Printing Office, 1979
15. Iglehart JK: The campaign against smoking gains momentum. N Engl J Med 314:1059–1064, 1986
16. Marino LB, Levy SM: Primary and secondary prevention of cancer in children and adolescents: Current status and issues. Pediatr Clin North Am 33:975–993, 1986
17. White JR, Froeb HF: Small-airways dysfunction in nonsmokers chronically exposed to tobacco smoke. N Engl J Med 302:720–723, 1980
18. Enstrom JE: Trends in mortality among California physicians after giving up smoking: 1950–1979. Br Med J 286:1101–1105, 1983
19. Connolly GN, Winn DM, Hecht SS et al: The reemergence of smokeless tobacco. N Engl J Med 314:1020–1027, 1986
20. Rothman KJ: Alcohol. In Fraumeni JF Jr (ed): Persons at High Risk of Cancer: An Approach to Cancer Etiology and Control, pp 139–150. New York, Academic Press, 1975
21. Decker J, Goldstein JC: Risk factors in head and neck cancer. N Engl J Med 306:1151–1155, 1982
22. Kripke ML, Sass ER (eds): International Conference on Ultraviolet Carcinogenesis. DHEW Publication No. (NIH) 78-1532. Washington, DC, US Government Printing Office, 1977
23. Tucker MA, Shields JA, Hartge P et al: Sunlight exposure as risk factor for intraocular malignant melanoma. N Engl J Med 313:789–792, 1985
24. Greene MH, Clark WH Jr, Tucker MA et al: Acquired precursors of cutaneous malignant melanoma: The familial dysplastic nevus syndrome. N Engl J Med 312:91–97, 1985
25. Pariza MW: A perspective on diet, nutrition, and cancer. JAMA 251:1455–1458, 1984
26. Greenwald P: Manipulation of nutrients to prevent cancer. Hosp Pract 19:119–134, 1984
27. Pedersen-Bjergaard J, Larsen SO: Incidence of acute nonlymphocytic leukemia, preleukemia, and acute myeloproliferative syndrome up to 10 years after treatment of Hodgkin's disease. N Engl J Med 307:965, 1982

28. Santoro A, Bonadonna G, Bonfante V et al: Alternating drug combinations in the treatment of advanced Hodgkin's disease. N Engl J Med 306:770–775, 1982

29. Herbst AL, Ulfelder H, Poskanzer DC: Adenocarcinoma of the vagina: Association of maternal stilbestrol therapy with tumor appearance in young women. N Engl J Med 284:878–881, 1971

30. Lanier AP, Noller KL, Decker DG et al: Cancer and stilbestrol: A follow up of 1719 persons exposed to estrogens in utero and born 1943–1959. Mayo Clin Proc 48:793–799, 1973

31. Hoover R, Fraumeni JF JR: Risk of cancer in renal-transplant recipients. Lancet 2:55–57, 1973

32. Piper JM, Tonascia J, Matanoski GM: Heavy phenacetin use and bladder cancer in women aged 20 to 49 years. N Engl J Med 313:292–295, 1985

33. Beasley RP, Lin C, Hwang L et al: Hepatocellular carcinoma and hepatitus B virus: A prospective study of 22,707 men in Taiwan. Lancet 11:1129–1132, 1981

34. Quinn TC, Mann JM, Curran JW et al: AIDS in Africa: An epidemiologic paradigm. Science 234:955–963, 1986

35. Selikoff IJ, Hammond EC, Churg J: Asbestos exposure, smoking, and neoplasia. JAMA 204:106, 1968

36. Walker AM, Loughlin JE, Friedlander ER et al: Projections of asbestos-related disease 1980-2009. J Occup Med 25:409–425, 1983

37. Spooner CM: Asbestos in schools: A public health problem. N Engl J Med 301:782–784, 1979

38. Lagakos SW, Wessen BJ, Zelen M: An analysis of contaminated well water and health effects in Woburn, Massachusetts. J Am Stat Assoc 395:583–614, 1986

39. Janerich DT, Burnett WS, Feck G et al: Cancer incidence in the Love Canal area. Science 212:1404–1407, 1981

40. Li FP: Genetic and familial cancer: Opportunities for prevention and early detection. Cancer Detect Prev 9:41–45, 1986

41. Knudson AG Jr, Strong LC, Anderson DE: Heredity and cancer in man. Prog Med Genet 9:113–158, 1973

42. Cavenee WK, Dryja TP, Phillips RA et al: Expression of recessive alleles by chromosomal mechanisms in retinoblastoma. Nature 305:779–784, 1983

43. Cavenee WK, Murphree AL, Shull MM et al: Prediction of familial predisposition to retinoblastoma. N Engl J Med 314:1201–1207, 1986

44. Erbe RW: Inherited gastrointestinal-polyposis syndromes. N Engl J Med 294:1101–1104, 1976

45. Graze K, Spiler IJ, Tashjian AH et al: Natural history of familial medullary thyroid carcinoma: Effect of a program for early diagnosis. N Engl J Med 299:980–985, 1978

46. Robbins JH, Kraemer KH, Lutzner MA et al: Xeroderma pigmentosum: An inherited disease with sun sensitivity, multiple cutaneous neoplasms, and abnormal DNA repair. Ann Intern Med 80:221–248, 1974

47. Tucker MA, Meadows AT, Boice JD Jr et al: Cancer risk following treatment of childhood cancer. In Boice JD, Fraumeni JF Jr (eds): Radiation Carcinogenesis: Epidemiology and Biological Significance, pp 211–224. New York, Raven Press, 1984

48. Hansen MF, Koufos A, Gallie BL et al: Osteosarcoma and retinoblastoma: A shared chromosomal mechanism revealing recessive predisposition. Genetics 82:6216–6220, 1985

49. Sorensen SA, Mulvihill JJ, Nielsen A: Long-term follow-up of von Recklinghausen neurofibromatosis. N Engl J Med 314:1010–1015, 1986

50. Kingston JE, Herbert A, Draper GJ et al: Association between hepatoblastoma and polyposis coli. Arch Dis Child 58:959–962, 1983

Index

Numbers followed by an *f* indicate a figure; *t* following a page number indicates tabular material.

ISBN 0-397-50821-2

90000

9 780397 508211

PRODUCT IDENTIFICATION &
PROCESSING SYSTEMS, INC
436 EAST 87TH STREET
NEW YORK, NY 10128-6502
(212) 996-6000

P
I
P
S

0993/ND MAG 0.92 BWR .0020in
PS 9792A PIZZO

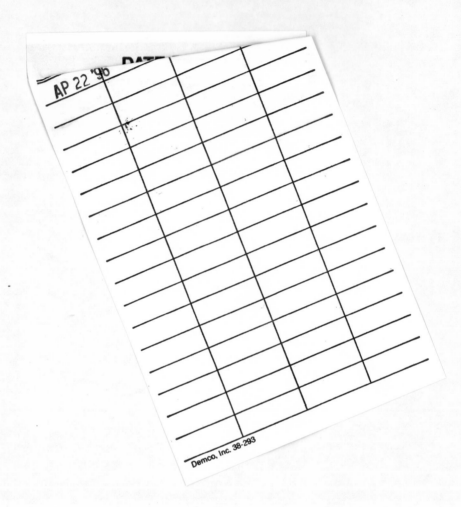

DATE

Demco, Inc. 38-293